D0927000

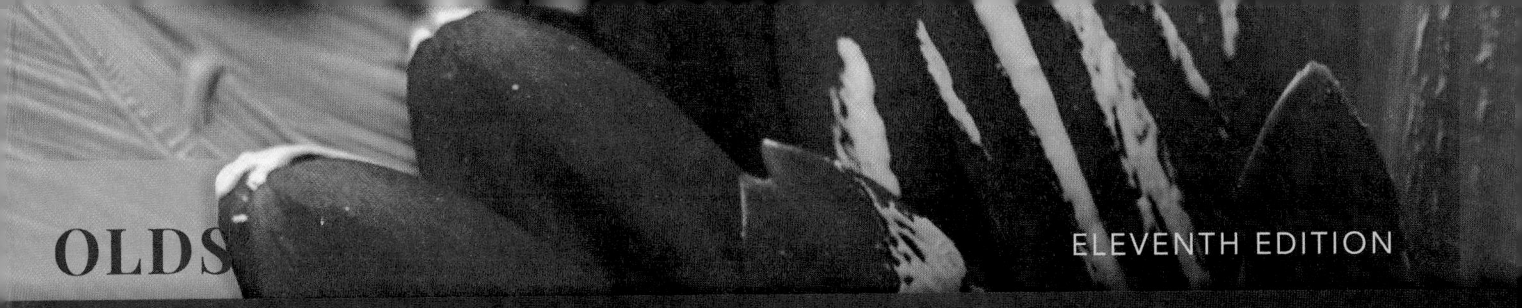

OLDS'

ELEVENTH EDITION

Maternal-Newborn Nursing & Women's Health ACROSS THE LIFESPAN

Michele R. Davidson, PhD, CNM, PMHNP, CFN, SANE, FNE, RN
Professor of Nursing
Sentara College of Health Sciences
Chesapeake, Virginia
Leta Psychiatry
Virginia Beach, Virginia

Marcia L. London, RN, MSN, APRN, CNS, NNP-BC-E
Senior Clinical Instructor and Director of Neonatal Nurse Practitioner Program (Ret.)
Beth-El College of Nursing and Health Sciences
University of Colorado
Colorado Springs, Colorado

Patricia A. Wieland Ladewig, PhD, RN
Provost Emerita
Regis University
Denver, Colorado

Pearson

Senior Vice President, Portfolio Management: Adam Jaworski
Director, Portfolio Management: Katrin Beacom
Portfolio Manager: Hilarie Surrena
Development Editor: Lynda Hatch
Portfolio Management Assistant: Erin Sullivan
Vice President, Content Production and Digital Studio: Paul DeLuca
Managing Producer, Health Science: Melissa Bashe
Content Producer: Faye Gemmellaro
Editorial Project Manager: Dan Knott, Pearson CSC
Operations Specialist: Maura Zaldivar-Garcia
Creative Digital Lead: Mary Siener
Director, Digital Production: Amy Peltier
Digital Studio Producer, REVEL and e-text 2.0: Jeff Henn
Digital Content Team Lead: Brian Prybella
Digital Content Project Lead: William Johnson
Vice President, Product Marketing: Brad Parkins
Executive Product Marketing Manager: Christopher Barry
Sr. Field Marketing Manager: Brittany Hammond
Full-Service Vendor: Pearson CSC
Full-Service Project Management: Pearson CSC, Monica Moosang
Composition: Pearson CSC
Inventory Manager: Vatche Demirdjian
Manager, Rights & Permissions: Gina Cheselka
Interior Design: Pearson CSC
Cover Design: Studio Montage
Cover Art: Nik Merkulov/Shutterstock
Printer/Binder: LSC Communications, Inc.
Cover Printer: LSC Communications, Inc.

Copyright © 2020, 2016, 2012 by Pearson Education, Inc. 221 River Street, Hoboken, NJ 07030. All Rights Reserved. Printed in the United States of America. This publication is protected by copyright, and permission should be obtained from the publisher prior to any prohibited reproduction, storage in a retrieval system, or transmission in any form or by any means, electronic, mechanical, photocopying, recording, or otherwise. For information regarding permissions, request forms and the appropriate contacts within the Pearson Education Global Rights & Permissions department, please visit https://www.pearsoned.com/permissions/.

Many of the designations by manufacturers and sellers to distinguish their products are claimed as trademarks. Where those designations appear in this book, and the publisher was aware of a trademark claim, the designations have been printed in initial caps or all caps.

Notice: Care has been taken to confirm the accuracy of information presented in this book. The authors, editors, and the publisher, however, cannot accept any responsibility for errors or omissions or for consequences from application of the information in this book and make no warranty, express or implied, with respect to its contents.

The authors and publisher have exerted every effort to ensure that drug selections and dosages set forth in this text are in accord with current recommendations and practice at time of publication. However, in view of ongoing research, changes in government regulations, and the constant flow of information relating to drug therapy and reactions, the reader is urged to check the package inserts of all drugs for any change in indications or dosage and for added warning and precautions. This is particularly important when the recommended agent is a new and/or infrequently employed drug.

A note about nursing diagnoses: Nursing diagnoses in this text are taken from T. Heather Herdman / Shigemi Kamitsuru (Eds.), NANDA International, Inc. *Nursing Diagnoses: Definitions and Classification 2018–2020*, Eleventh Edition © 2017 NANDA International, ISBN 978-1-62623-929-6. Used by arrangement with the Thieme Group, Stuttgart/New York.

Library of Congress Cataloging-in-Publication Data
Names: Davidson, Michele R., author. | London, Marcia L., author. | Ladewig, Patricia W., author.
Title: Olds' maternal-newborn nursing & women's health across the lifespan / Michele R. Davidson, Marcia L. London, Patricia A. Wieland Ladewig.
Other titles: Olds' maternal-newborn nursing and women's health across the lifespan | Maternal-newborn nursing & women's health across the lifespan
Description: Eleventh edition. | Boston : Pearson, [2020] | Includes bibliographical references and index.
Identifiers: LCCN 2018047082 | ISBN 9780135206881 (student edition) | ISBN 013520688X (student edition)
Subjects: | MESH: Maternal-Child Nursing—methods | Women's Health | Neonatal Nursing—methods | Pregnancy Complications—nursing | Nursing Assessment—methods | Prenatal Care—methods
Classification: LCC RG951 | NLM WY 157.3 | DDC 618.2/0231—dc23

1 18

Pearson

ISBN 10: 0-13-520688-X
ISBN 13: 978-0-13-520688-1

Sally B. Olds was the quintessential nurse and teacher—

She saw possibilities where others saw problems, abilities where others saw limitations.

She cared passionately about childbearing families and had a clear vision of what excellent nursing means.

She stressed the importance of clinical skill and acumen but never lost sight of the human side of caregiving.

She was committed to students, to helping them to learn and grow, to develop their own sense of the difference a nurse can make.

She was the best of the best of nursing.

And so, with the deepest affection and respect we dedicate this book to Sally, who was our dear friend and colleague, who left this world too soon.

We thank her for the inspiration she provided, the warmth she brought, and the expertise she shared.

And, as always, to our beloved families

To Nathan Davidson, Hayden, Chloe, Caroline, and Grant

To David London, Craig, Jennifer, Hannah, and Matthew

To Tim Ladewig, Ryan, Amanda, Reed, and Addison; Erik, Kedri, Emma, and Camden

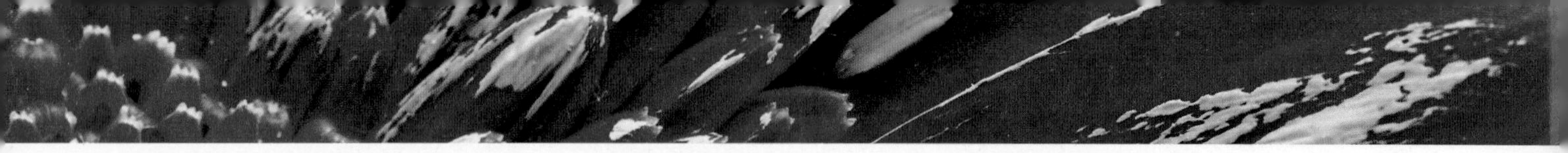

About the Authors

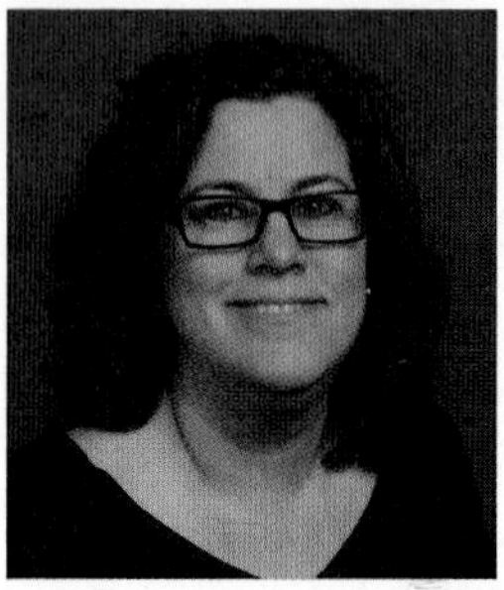

Michele R. Davidson

Michele R. Davidson completed her ADN degree from Marymount University and worked in multiple women's health specialty areas including postpartum, newborn nursery, high-risk nursery, labor and delivery, reproductive endocrinology, gynecology medical-surgical, and oncology units as a registered nurse while obtaining a BSN from George Mason University. She earned her MSN and a nurse-midwifery certificate at Case Western Reserve University and continued to work as a full-scope nurse-midwife for 16 years. Dr. Davidson has delivered over 1,000 babies during her career as a nurse-midwife. She completed her PhD in nursing administration and healthcare policy at George Mason University (GMU) and began teaching at GMU in 1999 while continuing in her role as a nurse-midwife. In 2018, Dr. Davidson earned an additional degree as a psychiatric mental health nurse practitioner (PMHNP). She has an ongoing interest in women's mental health and focuses her research on perinatal and postpartum mood and anxiety disorders. Dr. Davidson also has an interest in the care of individuals with disabilities; she has served as a member of the Loudoun County Disability Advisory Committee and is a disability advocate in her community. She was a member of the American College of Nurse-Midwives Certification Council, the body that writes the national certification examination for certified nurse-midwives. Dr. Davidson was recently appointed to the Virginia State Maternal Mortality Review Board and has served on several federal task forces for the prevention of maternal mortality. She is a member of numerous editorial and advisory boards and has a passion for writing. In 2003, Dr. Davidson founded the Smith Island Foundation, a nonprofit organization in which she served as executive director for 8 years and later held an appointment as the vice-president of Smith Island United, a community advocacy group. Dr. Davidson has also completed certifications in lactation consulting, forensic nursing, and as a surgical first assistant. In 2012, her book, *A Nurse's Guide to Women's Mental Health*, won an American Journal of Nursing Book Award. In her free time, she enjoys spending time with her mother, writing, gardening, internet surfing, and spending time on Smith Island with her nurse-practitioner husband, Nathan, and their four children, Hayden, Chloe, Caroline, and Grant. Dr. Davidson and her family love the Eastern Shore of Maryland and Virginia and continue to be part-time residents of Smith Island.

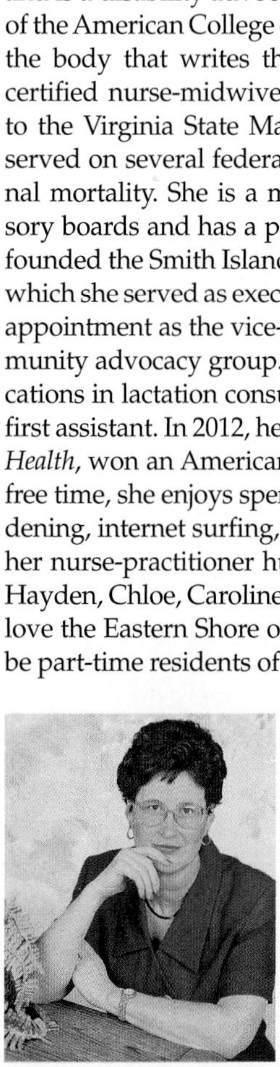

Marcia L. London

Marcia L. London received her BSN and School Nurse Certificate from Plattsburgh State University in Plattsburgh, New York, and her MSN in pediatrics as a clinical nurse specialist from the University of Pittsburgh in Pennsylvania. She worked as a pediatric nurse and began her teaching career at the Pittsburgh Children's Hospital Affiliate Program. Mrs. London began teaching at Beth-El School of Nursing and Health Science in 1974 (now part of the University of Colorado, Colorado Springs) after opening the first intensive care nursery at Memorial Hospital of Colorado Springs. She has served in many faculty positions at Beth-El, including assistant director of the School of Nursing. Mrs. London obtained her postmaster's Neonatal Nurse Practitioner certificate in 1983 and subsequently developed the Neonatal Nurse Practitioner (NNP) certificate and the master's NNP program at Beth-El. She is active nationally in neonatal nursing and was involved in the development of National Neonatal Nurse Practitioner educational program guidelines. Mrs. London pursued her interest in college student learning by taking doctoral classes in higher education administration and adult learning at the University of Denver in Colorado. She feels fortunate to be involved in the education of her future colleagues and teaches undergraduate education. Mrs. London and her husband, David, enjoy reading, travel, and hockey games. They have two sons. Craig, who lives in Florida with his wife Jennifer and daughter Hannah, works with Internet companies. Matthew works in computer teleresearch. Both are more than willing to give Mom helpful hints about computers.

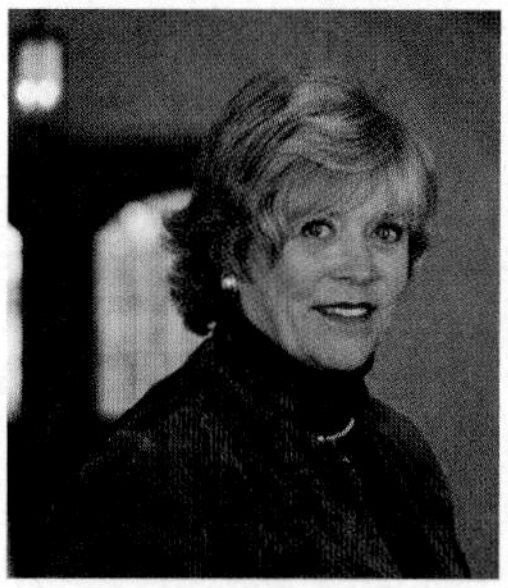

Patricia A. Wieland Ladewig

Patricia A. Wieland Ladewig received her BS from the College of Saint Teresa in Winona, Minnesota; her MSN from Catholic University of America in Washington, DC; and her PhD in higher education administration from the University of Denver in Colorado. She served as an Air Force nurse and discovered her passion for teaching as a faculty member at Florida State University. Over the years, she has taught at several schools of nursing. In addition, she became a women's health nurse practitioner and maintained a part-time clinical practice for many years. In 1988, Dr. Ladewig became the first director of the nursing program at Regis College in Denver. In 1991, when the college became Regis University, she became academic dean of the Rueckert-Hartman College for Health Professions. Under her guidance, the School of Nursing added a graduate program. In addition, the college added a School of Physical Therapy and a School of Pharmacy. In 2009 Dr. Ladewig became Vice President for Academic Affairs, and in 2012 she became Provost at Regis University. She retired in 2016. She remains active professionally, serving on the Community Health Values Committee of Centura Health. She and her husband, Tim, enjoy traveling, skiing, and baseball games. However, their greatest pleasure comes from their family: son Ryan, his wife Amanda, and grandchildren Reed and Addison Grace; and son Erik, his wife Kedri, and grandchildren Emma and Camden.

Thank You

Contributors

We are grateful to the contributors to the 11th edition of *Olds' Maternal-Newborn Nursing & Women's Health Across the Lifespan*.

Jessica Anderson, DNP, CNM, WHNP-BC, FACNM
University of Colorado
Denver, Colorado
Chapter 12: Antepartum Nursing Assessment

Wendelyn M. Barrett, MSN, NNP, APRN
Children's Hospital Colorado
Aurora, Colorado
Chapter 31: The Newborn at Risk: Birth-Related Stressors

Nancy Benner RNC, BSN
St. George, Utah
Chapter 28: The Normal Newborn: Needs and Care

Jenny Clapp RN-OB, MSN
University of North Carolina
Greensboro, North Carolina
Chapter 32: Postpartum Adaptation and Nursing Assessment

Robin Webb Corbett, PhD, FNP-C, RNC
East Carolina University
Greenville, North Carolina
Chapter 5: Commonly Occurring Infections
Chapter 6: Women's Health Problems

Nathan S. Davidson, II, CFNP, MSN, RN
George Mason University
Fairfax, Virginia
Concept Map features

Katherine Heatherington Endres, RNC
Inova Alexandria Hospital
Alexandria, Virginia
Chapter 22: Pharmacologic Pain Management

Cori Feist, MS, CGC
Oregon Health & Science University
Portland, Oregon
Chapter 10: Reproductive Genetics

Victoria A. Flanagan RN, MS
Geisel School of Medicine at Dartmouth
Dartmouth University
Lebanon, New Hampshire
Chapter 17: Pregnancy at Risk: Pregestational Problems

Jennifer G. Hensley, EdD, CNM, WHNP, RN, LCCE
The University of Texas at Austin
Austin, Texas
Chapter 4: Family Planning
Chapter 18: Pregnancy at Risk: Gestational Onset

Sharon Holley, DNP, CNM, FACNM
Baystate Medical Center
Springfield, Massachusetts
Chapter 20: Intrapartum Nursing Assessment

Janet L. Houser, PhD, RN
Regis University
Denver, Colorado
Evidence-Based Practice features

Jessica Howard, CNM, MSN, MSW
University of Colorado
Denver, Colorado
Chapter 8: Violence Against Women

Vanessa Howell RN, MSN
Beth-El College of Nursing and Health Sciences
Colorado Springs, Colorado
Chapter 27: Nursing Assessment of the Newborn

Laura R. Muñoz, PhD, RNC, NNP
University of the Incarnate Word
San Antonio, Texas
Chapter 25: Birth-Related Procedures

Julie W. Nadeau, EdD, MSN, RN, CNE
University of the Incarnate Word
San Antonio, Texas
Chapter 33: The Postpartum Family: Needs and Care
Chapter 34: Home Care of the Postpartum Family

Deborah Pollard, PhD, RNC-OB, C-EFM, CNE, IBCLC, RLC
Beth-El College of Nursing and Health Sciences
Colorado Springs, Colorado
Chapter 29: Newborn Nutrition

Mary Claire Wahl, MSN, CNM, RN
Beth-El College of Nursing and Health Sciences
Colorado Springs, Colorado
Chapter 35: The Postpartum Family at Risk

Reviewers

We are grateful to all the nurses, both clinicians and educators, who reviewed the manuscript of this textbook. Their insights, suggestions, and eye for detail helped us prepare a more relevant and useful textbook, one that will prepare caring and competent nurses in the field of maternal-newborn and women's health nursing.

Rachel Choudhury, PHD(C), MSN, MS, RN, CNE
Brandman University
Irvine, California

Marcia Clevesy, MSN, APRN
University of Nevada
Las Vegas, Nevada

Holly Diesel, PHD, RN
Barnes Jewish College
St. Louis, Missouri

Susan Dougherty, RNC, WHNP, DNP
Augusta University
Augusta, Georgia

Barbara Gross, MSN, RN
University of Central Florida
Orlando, Florida

Susan Groth, PhD, WHNP-BC, FAANP
University of Rochester
Rochester, New York

Dr. Carole McKenzie, CNM, RN
Texas A&M University
Commerce, Texas

Diane E. Mosqueda, DNP, RN, FNP-c, CNE
University of Texas
Galveston, Texas

Patricia Novak, MSN
Gateway Community College
New Haven, Connecticut

Erin F. Sullivan, MSN, RN, CCRN
Texas Woman's University
Dallas, Texas

Patricia D. Suplee PhD, RNC-OB
Rutgers University
Camden, New Jersey

Jennifer Swendsen, MSN
University of Texas of the Permian Basin
Odessa, Texas

Jennifer L. Talleff, MSN, RN, FNP-BC
Texas Woman's University
Dallas, Texas

Amber Welborn, RN, MSN
University of North Carolina
Greensboro, North Carolina

Acknowledgments

Our goal with every revision is to incorporate the latest research and information from the literature of nursing and related fields to make our text as relevant and useful as possible. This would not be possible without the support and encouragement of our colleagues in nursing. The comments and suggestions we have received from nurse educators and practitioners around the country have helped us keep this text accurate and up to date. Whenever a nurse takes the time to write or to speak to one of us at a professional gathering, we recognize again the intense commitment of nurses to excellence in practice. And so we thank our colleagues.

We are grateful, too, to our students—past, present, and future. They stimulate us with their interest; they reinvigorate us with their enthusiasm; they challenge us with their questions to make each edition of this text clear and understandable. We learn so much from them.

In publishing, as in healthcare, quality assurance is an essential part of the process. That is the dimension our reviewers have added. Some reviewers assist us by validating the accuracy of the content, some by their attention to detail, and some by challenging us to examine our ways of thinking and to develop a new awareness about a given topic. Thus, we extend our sincere thanks to all those who reviewed the manuscript for this book. Their names and affiliations are listed on the preceding pages.

We are also grateful to the contributors to the 11th edition of *Olds' Maternal-Newborn Nursing & Women's Health Across the Lifespan*. Their knowledge of clinical practice and current literature in their areas of expertise helps make the chapters relevant and accurate. They, too, are listed on the preceding pages.

We cannot say enough good things about our development editor, Lynda Hatch. She is a godsend. Her wonderful eye for detail, her truly supportive approach, and her calmness under pressure help us stay focused and on track (mostly!). Thank you, Lynda! We would be lost without you! Without your support in these crucial areas, our work would not be as visually appealing and accurate as it is.

During these times of change in the healthcare environment, we are sustained by our passion for nursing and our vision of what childbirth means. Time and again, we have seen the difference a skilled nurse can make in the lives of people in need. We, like you, are committed to helping all nurses recognize and take pride in that fact. Thank you for your letters, your comments, and your suggestions. We are renewed by your support.

Michele R. Davidson
Marcia L. London
Patricia W. Ladewig

Preface

Nurses play a central role in all aspects of the childbearing experience, from the earliest days of pregnancy, through the moments of birth, and during the early days of parenthood. Most often, pregnancy and childbirth are times of great joy, a celebration of life, and a promise of the future. But they may also be times of deepest sorrow as families deal with illness, complications, and loss. Often the quality of the nursing care that a family receives profoundly influences their perceptions of the entire experience—for better or for worse. However, the changes occurring in the healthcare delivery system are altering the way we practice nursing and have staggering implications for nurses everywhere.

Now, more than ever, nurses must be flexible, creative, and open to change. They must be able to think critically and problem-solve effectively. They must be able to meet the teaching needs of their patients so that their patients can, in turn, better meet their own healthcare needs. They must be open to an increasingly multicultural population. They must understand and use the healthcare technology available in their chosen area of practice. Most crucially, they must never lose sight of the importance of excellent nursing care to promote patient safety and in improving the quality of people's lives.

Important Themes in This Edition

The underlying philosophy of *Olds' Maternal-Newborn Nursing & Women's Health Across the Lifespan* remains unchanged. We believe that pregnancy and birth are normal life processes and that family members are partners in care. We believe that women's healthcare is an important aspect of nursing. We remain committed to providing a text that is accurate and readable—a text that helps students develop the skills and abilities they need now and in the future in an ever-changing healthcare environment.

Partnering with Families Through Health Promotion Education

Developing a partnership with women and their families is a pivotal aspect of maternal-newborn nursing, and one key element of that partnership is patient and family health promotion teaching. It is a crucial responsibility of the maternal-newborn nurse to find opportunities to educate patients and their families, and we continue to emphasize and highlight this in the 11th edition. Again, the focus is on the teaching that nurses do at all stages of pregnancy and the childbearing process, including the important postpartum teaching that is done before and immediately after families are discharged.

In this textbook, we also subscribe to the paradigm that women and childbearing families need health promotion and health maintenance interventions, no matter where they seek healthcare or what health conditions they may be experiencing. Nurses integrate health promotion and health maintenance into the care for women and childbearing families in a variety of birthing and community settings where they go to obtain health supervision care. This textbook integrates health promotion and health maintenance content throughout, most visibly in Part II, *Women's Health Across the Lifespan*, and Chapter 34, *Home Care of the Postpartum Family*.

Because we believe that nursing excellence must include partnering with women and their families for all outcomes, we have included Chapter 36, *Grief and Loss in the Childbearing Family*. It is designed to assist nurses to support families as they deal with the painful losses—maternal, fetal, and neonatal—that sometimes turn expected moments of great joy into times of deep sorrow. We know that it often takes time for nurses to find authentic ways to support grieving families. Our aim in having this chapter is to help you understand the dynamics of loss and to offer concrete guidance about effective nursing approaches.

Women's Healthcare

This edition continues to provide expanded coverage of women's healthcare with updated information on contraception, commonly occurring infections, health maintenance recommendations, menopause, and a variety of gynecologic conditions such as polycystic ovarian syndrome and pelvic relaxation. Special attention is given to violence against women, which is the focus of a separate chapter. Other pressing societal issues are also covered in a separate chapter, as well as throughout the women's health unit. Moreover, because of the text's focus on community-based care, gynecologic cancers are covered briefly.

Nursing Excellence in Maternal-Newborn and Women's Health

Truly effective nurses have both a solid understanding of underlying nursing theory and excellent clinical skills. Perhaps equally important, they have a deep appreciation of the essential need to partner with childbearing women and their families to ensure optimum outcomes for all. But how do we help students develop this level of expertise? We believe that nursing excellence as it relates to women's health and to childbearing families starts here, in the pages of this text. This book provides essential theoretical content within a contemporary, holistic, family-centered context. Our goal is to lay a foundation that you can build on with each clinical experience you have.

Evidence-Based Practice

Nursing professionals are increasingly aware of the importance of using evidence-based approaches as the foundation for planning and providing effective care and to foster patient safety and quality improvement. The approach of evidence-based practice draws on information from a variety of sources, including nursing research. To help nurses become more comfortable integrating new knowledge into their nursing practice, a brief discussion of evidence-based practice is included in Chapter 1, *Contemporary Maternal-Newborn Nursing*.

A feature titled **Evidence-Based Practice** further enhances the approach of using research to determine nursing actions. It describes a particular problem or clinical question and investigates the research evidence from a variety of sources—including systematic reviews of research literature, recent research findings, and national organization policy—that have direct application to nursing practice. The feature asks the student to use clinical reasoning and clinical judgment to determine what additional information is needed and what the evidence shows to be best practice at this time and invites the student to apply critical thinking skills to further identify nursing approaches to meet women's health and maternal-newborn nursing care issues.

Healthy People 2020

At the national level, the government has developed a set of ambitious, measurable goals designed to improve the health of Americans by 2020. Many of these goals, which are arranged by categories, have direct relevance to maternal, newborn, and women's healthcare nurses. To help you become aware of these goals, we have incorporated them at the beginning of each chapter. We hope you will take time to visit the *Healthy People 2020* website and become more knowledgeable about the effort.

Commitment to Diversity

As nurses and as educators, we recognize the importance of honoring diversity and of providing culturally competent care. Thus, we continually strive to make our text ever more inclusive. Chapter 1, *Contemporary Maternal-Newborn Nursing*, briefly introduces cultural issues relevant to maternity and newborn nursing care. Chapter 2, *Families, Cultures, and Complementary Therapies*, provides the theoretical basis for the consideration of cultural factors that influence a family's expectations of their healthcare providers and their experience with the healthcare system. We elaborate upon this information throughout the text in a boxed feature titled **Developing Cultural Competence**. In addition, we have worked hard to ensure that our photos, illustrations, charts, and case scenarios are inclusive in their appearance and in the information they provide. As our society becomes more global in nature, nurses need to cultivate their awareness of these issues because they ultimately do affect how we deliver healthcare in this country.

Women with Special Needs

Women who seek healthcare represent a range of ages, backgrounds, and requirements for effective care. In many cases, women have individualized needs that nurses may not encounter routinely. We are especially proud of a feature titled **Women with Special Needs**, which is designed to help you consider ways in which care must be modified to address the needs of all women regardless of their circumstances.

Case Study

As educators we recognize how crucial it is to help students apply the theory they learn to specific patients—patients with unique needs and concerns. To accomplish this goal, we have developed a new clinical feature for this edition called **Case Study**. In this feature we follow four women through their pregnancies, birth experiences, and postpartum issues. Each Case Study is designed to enable students to consider specific issues that might have implications for patient care. The women are:

- Melissa Bond-James, a 40-year-old Caucasian American who has experienced preterm labor during her pregnancy. She is a lesbian, whose wife, Nancy James, is supportive and extremely excited about the pregnancy.
- Benita Cartier is a 26-year-old, married, African American woman who is being treated for chronic hypertension. Her husband is an airline pilot and they have a toddler daughter.
- Azia Askari is a 32-year-old married woman who immigrated to the United States from Iran in 2014. She has two children and is experiencing an uneventful pregnancy. She is dealing with some cultural issues related to her life in the United States.
- Angelina Newman is a 16-year-old, single Caucasian American young woman who is a sophomore in high school. She has a sexually transmitted infection and possible labor/birth complication.

Nursing Professionalism

Professionalism requires that the astute professional nurse demonstrate professional standards of moral, ethical, and legal conduct and model the values of the nursing profession as he or she cares for women and childbearing families. This requires a commitment to *quality improvement* in all areas of care. With these expectations, the feature called **Professionalism in Practice** focuses on topics such as legal considerations, contemporary nursing practice issues, professional accountability, patient advocacy, and home and community care considerations.

Two features strengthen this emphasis on professionalism:

- **Ethics in Action!** challenges you with thought-provoking questions about many of the ethical dilemmas nurses may face in providing care.
- **Safety Alert!** calls your attention to issues that represent a situation that requires careful attention to avoid putting a patient at risk. Not surprisingly, many of these alerts—but not all—relate to the administration of medications.

Patient Teaching

Patient teaching remains a critical element of effective *patient-centered care*, one that we emphasize in this text. Nurses teach their patients during the care of women, through all stages of pregnancy, during the childbearing process, and while providing care for specific conditions. Throughout the book, we include **Teaching Highlights** features that present a special healthcare issue or problem and the related key teaching points for care by the patient and family.

Pearson Nursing's MAP App includes a section on **Patient/Family Teaching**, which supplies useful information and strategies for educating parents and families in a variety of situations and settings.

Complementary Health Approaches

Nurses and other healthcare professionals recognize that today, more than ever, complementary health approaches have become a credible component of holistic care. To help nurses become more familiar with these therapies, Chapter 2, *Families, Cultures, and Complementary Therapies*, provides basic information on some of the more commonly used therapies. Then throughout the text, we expand on the topic by providing a special boxed feature, **Complementary Health Approaches**, which discusses therapies your patients might be using or therapies you might suggest, keeping patient safety upmost in our thoughts. In all cases, research is cited for safe practice of these therapies.

Community-Based Nursing Care

By its very nature, maternal-newborn nursing is community-based nursing. Only a brief portion of the entire pregnancy and birth is spent in a birthing center or hospital. Moreover, because of changes in practice, even women with high-risk pregnancies are receiving more care in their homes and in the community and spending less time in hospital settings. Similarly, most aspects of women's healthcare are addressed in ambulatory settings.

The provision of nursing care in community-based settings is a driving force in healthcare today and, consequently, is a dominant theme throughout this edition. Four chapters provide a theoretical perspective and important tools in caring for childbearing families in the community setting: Chapter 12, *Antepartum Nursing Assessment*; Chapter 13, *The Expectant Family: Needs and Care*; Chapter 33, *The Postpartum Family: Needs and Care*; and Chapter 34, *Home Care of the Postpartum Family*. We have addressed this topic in a variety of ways. **Community-Based Nursing Care** is a heading used throughout the Nursing Management sections to assist you in identifying specific aspects of this content. Because we consider **Home Care** to be one form of community-based care, it is often a separate heading under Community-Based Nursing Care.

Other New or Expanded Concepts in This Edition

Nursing is a dynamic profession that requires specific information that reflects current practice. As such, we have expanded or added several important areas of content in the 11th edition.

- **NEW! Reproductive Genetics** This chapter was added to the 11th edition to reflect an emerging understanding of genome science, its impact on health and illness in childbearing families, and the expanding role that nurses play in applying genetics in clinical practice.
- **NEW! Genetic Facts** This feature provides information on the genetic implications of topics being addressed in the chapter.
- **NEW! Case Study** This feature shows students how to apply theory to clinical practice as they follow the experiences of four pregnant women with various issues and concerns.
- **NEW!** A two-page, 16-photograph *Birth Sequence* in Chapter 19 provides a moment-by-moment visual presentation of the birth of a baby.
- **Concept maps** provide an algorithm or flow chart to assist nurses in planning and providing care. The map provides a visual description of data to be analyzed in making decisions about care.
- **Key Facts to Remember** is a feature that summarizes major elements related to a specific topic. We believe you will find this feature to be especially helpful.
- **Nutrition** during pregnancy and infancy is important to promote growth, development, and health. A growing national focus on healthy nutrition patterns underscores the importance of this information. Chapter 14, *Maternal Nutrition*, and Chapter 29, *Newborn Nutrition*, address ensuring appropriate nutrition for pregnant women and newborns.
- **Pain management** is a priority in healthcare settings. All of the chapters in Part V, *Labor and Birth*, address pain assessment and management, and it is the primary focus in Chapter 22, *Pharmacologic Pain Management*. We discuss applicable pain assessment and management when appropriate in other chapters in Part VI, *The Newborn*, and Part VII, *Postpartum*.
- **Women with intellectual disabilities** information and specific care has been added to Chapter 7, *Social Issues*. Such women are more commonly choosing to

live independently and even become mothers. Therefore, we have also added coverage addressing the care of mothers with intellectual disabilities in Chapter 33, *The Postpartum Family: Needs and Care.*

Organization: A Nursing Management Framework

Nurses today must be able to think critically and to solve problems effectively. For these reasons, we begin with an introductory unit to set the stage by providing information about maternal-newborn nursing and important related concepts. Subsequent units progress in a way that closely reflects the steps of the nursing process. We clearly delineate the nurse's role within this framework. Thus, the units related to pregnancy, labor and birth, the newborn period, and postpartum care begin with a discussion of basic theory followed by chapters on nursing assessment and nursing care for essentially healthy women or infants. Within the nursing care chapters and content areas, we use the heading **Nursing Management** and the subheadings **Nursing Assessment and Diagnosis**, **Planning and Implementation**, and **Evaluation**.

Complications of a specific period appear in the last chapter or chapters of each unit. The chapters also use the nursing process as an organizational framework. We believe that students can more clearly grasp the complicated content of the high-risk conditions once they have a good understanding of the normal processes of pregnancy, birth, and postpartum and newborn care. However, to avoid overemphasizing the prevalence of complications in such a wonderfully normal process as pregnancy and birth, we avoid including an entire unit that focuses only on complications.

●○● NURSING MANAGEMENT

The *Nursing Management* sections delineate the important care management role of the nurse within the organizing framework of the nursing process to help you understand what nursing actions are needed. Numerous special features reinforce the nursing management role.

Nursing Care Plan

Nursing Care Plans address nursing care for patients who have complications, such as a woman with preeclampsia. We designed this feature to help you approach care from the nursing process perspective. These care plans use a nursing diagnosis approach in planning and providing care when pregnancy-related and newborn complications arise.

Assessment Guide

Assessment Guides help you organize your questions and steps during a physical assessment and provide normal findings, alterations, and possible causes, as well as guidelines for nursing interventions.

Resources for Student Success

- **Online Resources** are available for download at *www.pearsonhighered.com/nursingresources*, including:
  - NCLEX-RN®-Style Review Questions
  - Case Studies
  - Care Plans
  - Thinking Critically exercises, and more!
- **NEW! Pearson Nursing's MAP App** provides a collection of handy tools and additional content for students to use while studying maternity or pediatrics or for quick reference in the clinical setting. The maternity content includes a section on **Patient/Family Teaching**, which supplies useful information, tips, and strategies for educating parents and families in a variety of situations and settings. The colorful **Maternal-Fetal Growth and Development Timeline** depicts maternal/fetal development month by month and provides specific teaching guidelines for each stage of pregnancy. We are excited to offer students the opportunity to have all of this valuable information in one convenient place for on-the-go reference.

Resources for Faculty Success

Pearson is pleased to offer a complete suite of resources to support teaching and learning, including:

- **TestGen Test Bank**
- **Lecture Note PowerPoints**
- **Classroom Response System PowerPoints**

Features That Help You Use This Text Successfully

Instructors and students alike value the in-text learning aids that we include in our textbooks. The following guide will help you use the features and resources from *Olds' Maternal-Newborn Nursing & Women's Health Across the Lifespan*, 11th edition, to be successful in the classroom, in the clinical setting, on the NCLEX-RN® examination, and in nursing practice.

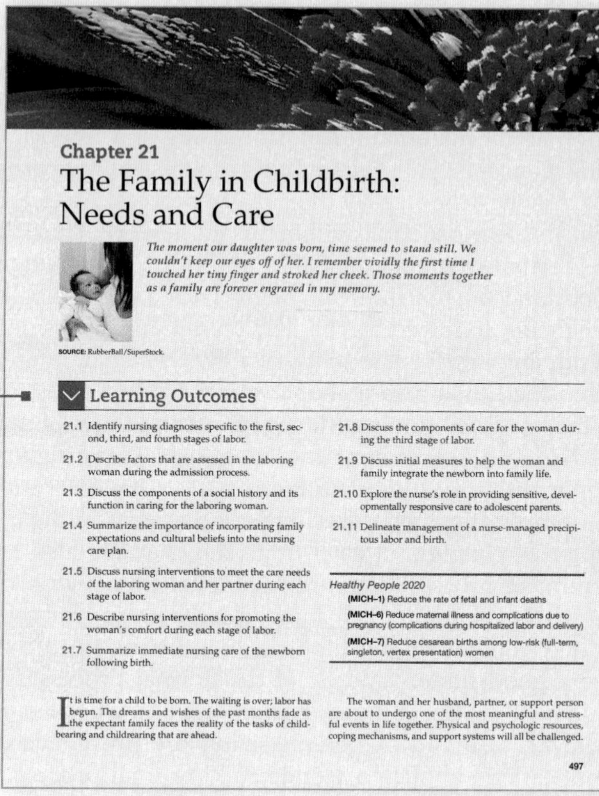

Chapter 21

The Family in Childbirth: Needs and Care

The moment our daughter was born, time seemed to stand still. We couldn't keep our eyes off of her. I remember vividly the first time I touched her tiny finger and stroked her cheek. Those moments together as a family are forever engraved in my memory.

SOURCE: RubberBall/SuperStock.

Learning Outcomes

21.1 Identify nursing diagnoses specific to the first, second, third, and fourth stages of labor.

21.2 Describe factors that are assessed in the laboring woman during the admission process.

21.3 Discuss the components of a social history and its function in caring for the laboring woman.

21.4 Summarize the importance of incorporating family expectations and cultural beliefs into the nursing care plan.

21.5 Discuss nursing interventions to meet the care needs of the laboring woman and her partner during each stage of labor.

21.6 Describe nursing interventions for promoting the woman's comfort during each stage of labor.

21.7 Summarize immediate nursing care of the newborn following birth.

21.8 Discuss the components of care for the woman during the third stage of labor.

21.9 Discuss initial measures to help the woman and family integrate the newborn into family life.

21.10 Explore the nurse's role in providing sensitive, developmentally responsive care to adolescent parents.

21.11 Delineate management of a nurse-managed precipitous labor and birth.

Healthy People 2020

(MICH-1) Reduce the rate of fetal and infant deaths

(MICH-6) Reduce maternal illness and complications due to pregnancy (complications during hospitalized labor and delivery)

(MICH-7) Reduce cesarean births among low-risk (full-term, singleton, vertex presentation) women

It is time for a child to be born. The waiting is over; labor has begun. The dreams and wishes of the past months fade as the expectant family faces the reality of the tasks of childbearing and childrearing that are ahead.

The woman and her husband, partner, or support person are about to undergo one of the most meaningful and stressful events in life together. Physical and psychologic resources, coping mechanisms, and support systems will all be challenged.

497

Each chapter begins with a **personal vignette** and photo that sets the tone for the chapter.

Learning Outcomes introduce you to the topics covered in each chapter.

Healthy People 2020 features at the beginning of each chapter assist you in becoming aware of the *Healthy People 2020* goals that have direct relevance to maternal, newborn, and women's healthcare nurses.

The following features are found throughout the text:

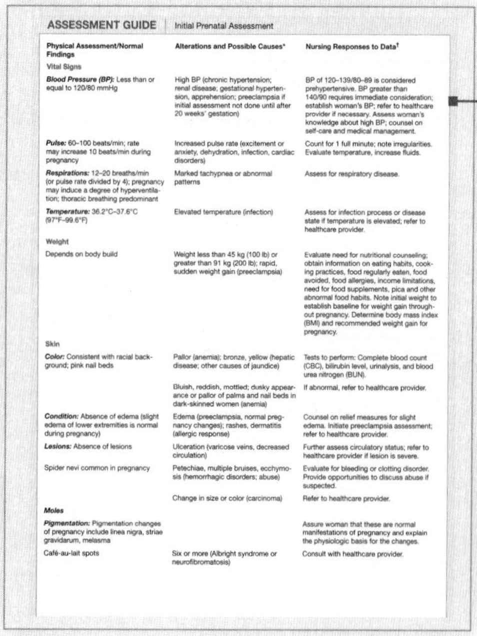

ASSESSMENT GUIDE | Initial Prenatal Assessment

Physical Assessment/Normal Findings	Alterations and Possible Causes*	Nursing Responses to Data†
Vital Signs		
Blood Pressure (BP): Less than or equal to 120/80 mmHg	High BP (chronic hypertension; renal disease; gestational hypertension, apprehension; preeclampsia if initial assessment not done until after 20 weeks' gestation)	BP of 120–139/80–89 is considered prehypertensive. BP greater than 140/90 requires immediate consideration; establish woman's BP; refer to healthcare provider if necessary. Assess woman's knowledge about high BP; counsel on self-care and medical management.
Pulse: 60–100 beats/min; rate may increase 10 beats/min during pregnancy	Increased pulse rate (excitement or anxiety, dehydration, infection, cardiac disorders)	Count for 1 full minute; note irregularities. Evaluate temperature, increase fluids.
Respirations: 12–20 breaths/min (or pulse rate divided by 4); pregnancy may induce a degree of hyperventilation; thoracic breathing predominant	Marked tachypnea or abnormal patterns	Assess for respiratory disease.
Temperature: 36.2°C–37.6°C (97°F–99.6°F)	Elevated temperature (infection)	Assess for infection process or disease state if temperature is elevated; refer to healthcare provider.
Weight		
Depends on body build	Weight less than 45 kg (100 lb) or greater than 91 kg (200 lb); rapid, sudden weight gain (preeclampsia)	Evaluate need for nutritional counseling; obtain information on eating habits, cooking practices, food regularly eaten, food avoided, food allergies, income limitations, need for food supplements, pica and other abnormal food habits. Note initial weight to establish baseline for weight gain throughout pregnancy. Determine body mass index (BMI) and recommended weight gain for pregnancy.
Skin		
Color: Consistent with racial background; pink nail beds	Pallor (anemia); bronze, yellow (hepatic disease; other causes of jaundice)	Tests to perform: Complete blood count (CBC), bilirubin level, urinalysis, and blood urea nitrogen (BUN).
	Bluish, reddish, mottled; dusky appearance or pallor of palms and nail beds in dark-skinned women (anemia)	If abnormal, refer to healthcare provider.
Condition: Absence of edema (slight edema of lower extremities is normal during pregnancy)	Edema (preeclampsia, normal pregnancy changes); rashes, dermatitis (allergic response)	Counsel on relief measures for slight edema. Initiate preeclampsia assessment; refer to healthcare provider.
Lesions: Absence of lesions	Ulceration (varicose veins, decreased circulation)	Further assess circulatory status; refer to healthcare provider if lesion is severe.
Spider nevi common in pregnancy	Petechiae, multiple bruises, ecchymosis (hemorrhagic disorders; abuse)	Evaluate for bleeding or clotting disorder. Provide opportunities to discuss abuse if suspected.
	Change in size or color (carcinoma)	Refer to healthcare provider.
Moles		
Pigmentation: Pigmentation changes of pregnancy include linea nigra, striae gravidarum, melasma		Assure woman that these are normal manifestations of pregnancy and explain the physiologic basis for the changes.
Café-au-lait spots	Six or more (Albright syndrome or neurofibromatosis)	Consult with healthcare provider.

Assessment Guides assist you with diagnoses by incorporating physical assessment and normal findings, alterations and possible causes, and guidelines for nursing interventions.

CASE STUDY: Azia Askari

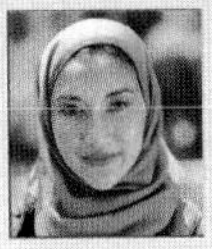

Azia presents to the local hospital with reports of beginning contractions yesterday after walking with her daughters outdoors to a nearby playground. Her sister-in-law has brought her to the hospital and is translating for the nurse. The hospital has an interpreter who speaks Farsi who is en route to the hospital to translate. Her sister-in-law reports that the contractions have increased in frequency, duration, and strength and they are now occurring every 3 to 5 minutes, lasting 45 to 60 seconds, and they are getting stronger. She stresses that the family has a firm preference for female-only care providers based on their cultural beliefs and Muslim religion.

Question to Ponder

What steps would you take to support Azia's cultural beliefs in this situation?

Case Study This feature shows students how to apply theory to clinical practice as they follow the experiences of four pregnant women with various issues and concerns.

Clinical Skill boxes offer step-by-step techniques that show you the tasks expected of a nurse in clinical situations, preparing you for your clinical experiences. Included in each box are the preparation steps with rationales, equipment and supplies needed, and steps for the procedure itself, with rationales for the nurse's actions.

CLINICAL SKILL 21–1

Performing Nasal Pharyngeal Suctioning

NURSING ACTION

Preparation

- Suction equipment is always available in the birthing area to clear secretions from the newborn's nose or oropharnyx if respirations are depressed or if amniotic fluid was meconium stained.
- Tighten the lid on the DeLee mucus trap or other suction device collection bottle.

Rationale: *This avoids spillage of secretions and prevents air from leaking out of the lid.*

- Connect one end of the DeLee tubing to low suction.

Equipment and Supplies

DeLee mucus trap or other suction device

Procedure: Clean Gloves

1. Don gloves.
2. Without applying suction, insert the free end of the DeLee tubing 3 to 5 inches into the newborn's nose or mouth (Figure 21–7).

Rationale: *Applying suction while passing the tube would interfere with smooth passage of the tube.*

3. Place your thumb over the suction control and begin to apply suction. Continue to suction as you slowly remove the tube, rotating it slightly.

Rationale: *Suctioning during withdrawal removes fluid and avoids redepositing secretions in the newborn's nasopharnyx.*

4. Continue to reinsert the tube and provide suction for as long as fluid is aspirated.

Note: Excessive suctioning can cause vagal stimulation, which decreases the heart rate.

5. If it is necessary to pass the tube into the newborn's stomach to remove meconium secretions that the newborn swallowed before birth, insert the tube through the newborn's mouth into the stomach. Apply suction and continue to suction as you withdraw the tube.

Rationale: *Because the newborn's nares are small and delicate, it is easier and faster to pass the suction tube through the mouth.*

6. Document the completion of the procedure and the amount and type of secretions.

Rationale: *This documentation provides a record of the intervention and the status of the neonate at birth.*

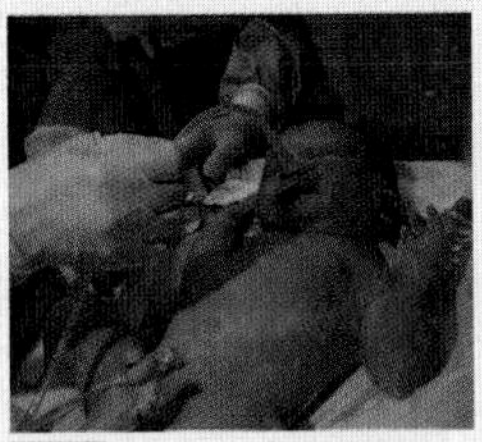

Figure 21–7 DeLee mucus trap being used to suction a newborn's mouth to remove excess secretions. One end of the suction tubing is connected to low suction, and the other end of the tubing is inserted 3 to 5 inches into the newborn's nose or mouth. Suction is applied as the tubing is pulled out. The process is repeated for as long as fluid is aspirated.

SOURCE: Wilson Garcia.

Clinical Tip

Screening for aneuploidy should be presented as an informed choice. The decision to proceed with screening is a personal choice and stems from one's values, beliefs, and interests. The nurse should be knowledgeable about the options available for screening and next steps if an abnormal result occurs.

Clinical Tip features offer hands-on suggestions for specific procedures and interventions. The authors' wealth of clinical knowledge—reflecting many decades of experience—are reflected in these pearls of wisdom.

Complementary Health Approaches have become a credible component of holistic care. We have featured this content to help you to become more familiar with it and to inform you about therapies your patients might be using or those you might safely suggest. In all cases, research is cited for safe practice of these methods.

Complementary Health Approaches

Treatment of Endometriosis

Complementary therapies that may play a role in the treatment of endometriosis include (Oyelowo & Johnson, 2018):

- Acupuncture to help with pain control
- Vag Packs (suppositories with vitamins, minerals, and herbs)
- Yoga for relaxation and stress reduction
- Massage
- Traditional Chinese herbal medicine for symptomatic relief
- Spiritual therapies such as prayer, religious rituals, meditation, and support groups.

Concept Maps provide a visual description of data to be analyzed as nurses plan and provide care.

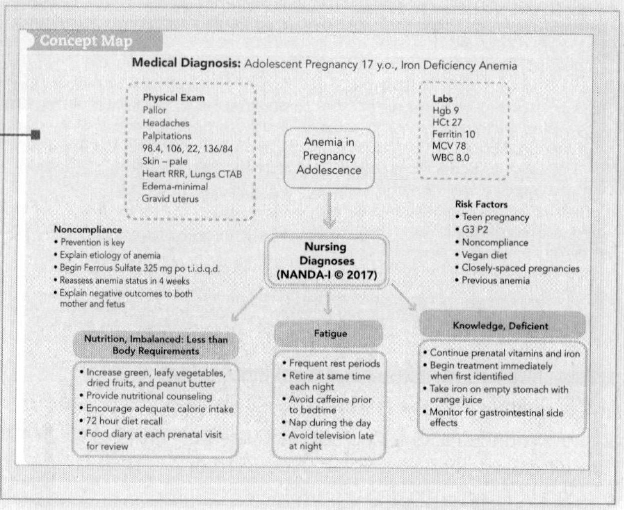

Developing Cultural Competence Home Births in Amish Communities

Approximately 40 to 80% of Amish women give birth at home or in an Amish-run birthing center. The factors for these choices are often driven by costs (the Amish have no commercial health insurance), geographic distance, and preference to be cared for in the home setting. Amish women in the United States, many of whom have eight or more children, are cared for by CNMs, lay midwives, and, in rare cases, physicians who attend home births. Because the Amish do not utilize electricity, caregivers must bring specialized equipment for the birth. At most Amish births, the husband is the only family member in attendance. Many Amish families decline medical interventions, such as vitamin K injections, eye ointment, hepatitis B vaccines, or circumcision. Once an Amish woman gives birth, a young single Amish girl is typically employed as a maid in the home for 4 to 6 weeks to perform household chores for the family (Wente, 2015).

Note: It is unwise to attribute specific attitudes or beliefs to all members of a cultural group. The information in the Developing Cultural Competence boxes offers possible insights into caring for women from different cultural groups.

Developing Cultural Competence boxes foster your awareness of cultural factors that influence a family's expectations of and responses to their healthcare provider and their experiences with the healthcare system.

Drug Guide boxes for selected medications commonly used in maternal-newborn nursing guide you in correctly administering the medications and evaluating your actions.

Drug Guide
Carboprost Tromethamine (Hemabate)

PREGNANCY RISK CATEGORY: D

OVERVIEW OF ACTION

Carboprost tromethamine (Hemabate) is used to reduce blood loss secondary to uterine atony. It stimulates myometrial contractions to control postpartum hemorrhaging that is unresponsive to usual techniques. Carboprost tromethamine can also be used to induce labor in women desiring an elective termination of a pregnancy. The drug is also used to induce labor in cases of intrauterine fetal death and hydatidiform mole (Wilson et al., 2017).

ROUTE, DOSAGE, FREQUENCY

In cases of immediate postpartum hemorrhage, when other measures have failed, the usual intramuscular dose is 250 mcg (1 mL), which can be repeated every 1.5 to 3.5 hours if uterine atony persists. In severe bleeding, an initial dose of 400 mcg may be considered. The dosage can be increased to 500 mcg (2 mL) if uterine contractility is inadequate after several doses of 250 mcg. The total dosage should not exceed 12 mg. The maximum duration of use is 48 hours (Wilson et al., 2017).

CONTRAINDICATIONS

The drug is contraindicated in women with active cardiac, pulmonary, hepatic, or renal disease. It should not be administered during pregnancy or in women with acute pelvic inflammatory disease (Wilson et al., 2017).

SIDE EFFECTS

The most common side effects are nausea and vomiting and diarrhea. Fever, chills, and flushing can occur. Headache and muscle, joint, abdominal, or eye pain can also occur (Wilson et al., 2017).

NURSING CONSIDERATIONS

1. Pretreatment or concurrent administration of antiemetic and antidiarrheal drugs may be given to decrease nausea and vomiting and diarrhea.
2. The injection should be given in a large muscle with a tuberculin syringe. Aspiration should be performed to avoid injection into a blood vessel, which can result in bronchospasm, tetanic contractions, and shock.
3. After administration, monitor uterine status and bleeding carefully.
4. Report excess bleeding to the physician/CNM.
5. Check vital signs routinely, observing for an increase in temperature, elevated pulse, and decreased blood pressure.
6. Breastfeeding should be delayed for 24 hours after administration (Wilson et al., 2017).

Ethics In Action!

A patient in your practice has finally disclosed to you after repeated IPV screenings that her husband is physically abusive to her. You practice in a state where you are covered by the IPV mandatory reporting law, but your patient has asked you to not report as she is scared for her life. How do you respond to this situation?

Ethics in Action! features challenge you with thought-provoking questions that reflect myriad ethical dilemmas that nurses providing care may face.

Evidence-Based Practice boxes relate research evidence to women's health and maternal-newborn nursing. Each feature asks you to use critical thinking skills to analyze the data to best meet women's health and maternal-newborn nursing care needs and to help you understand the use of reliable information to plan and provide effective nursing care.

EVIDENCE-BASED PRACTICE | Ectopic Pregnancy

Clinical Question

What is best practice in diagnosing and treating an ectopic pregnancy?

The Evidence

An ectopic pregnancy is one that occurs outside the uterine cavity. The most common site for an ectopic pregnancy is in the fallopian tube. If these pregnancies progress to the point of rupture, they account for significant morbidity and even maternal death. Suspicion of an ectopic pregnancy, then, is considered a medical emergency. If detected early, ectopic pregnancy can be effectively treated with surgical or pharmacological intervention. More than half of women who receive a diagnosis of ectopic pregnancy do not have any known risk factors. Those at highest risk are those with a previous ectopic pregnancy, damaged fallopian tubes, ascending pelvic infection, or prior pelvic or fallopian tube surgery. Contrary to a widely held belief, women who use an IUD for contraception are at a *lower risk* of ectopic pregnancy because of the effectiveness of this contraceptive method. However, if a woman with an IUD in place becomes pregnant, more than half will have an ectopic pregnancy. No other contraceptive methods have been associated with extrauterine pregnancy (ACOG, 2018c).

The American College of Obstetricians and Gynecologists (2018c) reviewed the evidence related to the diagnosis and treatment of ectopic pregnancy and updated their existing practice guidelines. This type of guideline, created by a professional medical organization evaluating and integrating evidence from randomized trials, systematic reviews, and the opinions of clinical experts, is the strongest evidence for practice.

Every sexually active reproductive-age woman who presents with abdominal pain and bleeding should be screened for pregnancy, regardless of whether she believes she is pregnant. Rupture of an ectopic pregnancy can occur very early in a pregnancy, even before the woman suspects she is pregnant. If a woman is pregnant and presents with an acute abdomen, including severe pain of unknown origin, the minimum diagnostic evaluation is a transvaginal ultrasound evaluation and confirmation of pregnancy through serum hCG-level measurement. However, serum hCG alone cannot be used to diagnose an ectopic pregnancy. The absence of a possible gestational sac on ultrasound examination in the presence of a positive hCG measurement strongly suggests a nonviable gestation. In 50 to 70% of these cases, these findings are consistent with ectopic pregnancy (ACOG, 2018c).

Treatment of a confirmed ectopic pregnancy that has not ruptured may be via laparoscopic surgery or intramuscular administration of methotrexate. Both treatments are safe and effective. The decision for surgical or medical management is guided by clinician assessment as well as patient-informed choice. Surgical management is required if the patient is experiencing hemodynamic instability, symptoms of a ruptured ectopic mass, or signs of intraperitoneal bleeding (ACOG, 2018c).

Best Practice

Women who present with acute abdominal pain and bleeding should be screened for pregnancy. If hCG levels are elevated, then a transvaginal ultrasound is indicated to determine if an ectopic pregnancy exists. An ectopic pregnancy constitutes a medical emergency, as rupture of the fallopian tubes is associated with significant morbidity and mortality. Best practice in treatment of ectopic pregnancy includes laparoscopic surgery or administration of methotrexate. Women suffering from ectopic pregnancy can be counseled that both treatments are safe and effective (ACOG, 2018c).

Clinical Reasoning

What elements of a nursing history could raise suspicion about the potential for an ectopic pregnancy? What questions should be asked of every woman who presents with acute abdominal pain?

Genetic Facts **Exposure to Toxins**

Environmental factors can impact future generations when people are exposed to toxins. Epigenetic changes in gene expression can occur when a woman is exposed to various environmental toxins. Depending on the agent and exposure, the cell nucleus can be altered at the molecular level and can impact if a gene is expressed or silenced (Stahl, 2017).

Genetic Facts provides information on the genetic implications of various topics being addressed in the chapter.

Health Promotion boxes emphasize the patient teaching that often involves empowering patients in their own health promotion.

Health Promotion **Reducing Discomforts of Menopause**

A variety of therapeutic modalities have been proposed as treatment or prevention measures for the discomforts and ailments of the perimenopausal, menopausal, and postmenopausal years. These include nutrition supplements, such as a diet rich in calcium and vitamins E, D, and B complex. Mind–body practices, such as yoga, t'ai chi, and meditation, are also helpful in reducing symptoms.

Key Facts to Remember summarize the elements of particular importance related to a specific topic.

Key Facts To Remember

Recommendations for Parents to Help Their Teens Avoid Pregnancy

- Parents should be clear about their own sexual attitudes and values in order to communicate clearly with children.
- Parents need to talk with their children about sex early and often and be specific in the discussions.
- Parents should supervise and monitor their children and teens with well-established rules, expectations, curfews, and standards of behavior.
- Parents should know their children's friends and their families.
- Parents need to clearly discourage early dating as well as frequent and steady dating.
- Parents should take a strong stand against allowing a daughter to date a much older boy; similarly, they should not allow a son to develop an intense relationship with a much younger girl.
- Parents need to help children set goals for their future and have options that are more attractive than early pregnancy and childrearing.
- Parents should show their children that they value education and take school performance seriously.
- Parents need to monitor what their children are reading, listening to, and watching.
- It is especially important for parents to build a strong, loving relationship with their children from an early age by showing affection clearly and regularly, spending time with them doing age-appropriate activities, building children's self-esteem, and having meals together as a family often.

NURSING CARE PLAN: The Woman with HIV Infection

1. Nursing Diagnosis: ***Infection, Risk for*****, related to inadequate defenses (leukopenia, suppressed inflammatory response) secondary to HIV-positive status (NANDA-I © 2017)**

Goal: Patient will remain free of opportunistic infection during the course of pregnancy.

INTERVENTION	RATIONALE
• Obtain a complete health history and physical examination during first prenatal visit.	• A complete health history will help determine risk factors for the development of opportunistic infections, and a physical examination will assist in identifying any underlying problem symptoms or illnesses that may compromise the pregnancy or complicate the treatment of HIV.
• Educate the woman as to the signs and symptoms of infection.	• Early recognition of signs and symptoms of infection will allow for immediate treatment, which may decrease the severity of the infection. Signs and symptoms of infection include fever, weight loss, fatigue, persistent candidiasis, diarrhea, cough, and skin lesions (Kaposi sarcoma and hairy leukoplakia in the mouth).
• Obtain nutritional history and monitor weight gain at each prenatal visit.	• The HIV-infected woman needs to maintain optimal nutritional intake. A compromised nutritional status may affect maternal and fetal well-being. Depleted reserves of protein and iron may decrease the patient's ability to fight infection, thereby making her more susceptible to opportunistic infections.
• **Collaborative:** Monitor the absolute $CD4^+$ T lymphocyte count, erythrocyte sedimentation rate (ESR), complete blood count (CBC) with differential, and hemoglobin and hematocrit (H & H) as indicated.	• Laboratory results provide information about the woman's immune system and the potential for disease progression. Opportunistic infections are more likely to occur when the $CD4^+$ T lymphocyte count drops below a level of 200/mm^3. ESR can rise above 20 mm/hr with anemia and with acute and chronic inflammation. CBC with differential and platelet count helps identify anemia, thrombocytopenia, and leukopenia. H & H can also identify anemia.

EXPECTED OUTCOME: Patient will remain free of opportunistic infection as evidenced by $CD4^+$ T lymphocyte count within normal limits; no complaints of chills, fever, or sore throat; normal weight gain throughout pregnancy.

2. Nursing Diagnosis: ***Health Maintenance, Ineffective*****, related to a lack of information about HIV/AIDS and its long-term implications for the woman, her unborn child, and her family (NANDA-I © 2017)**

Goal: The patient and her family will verbalize the importance of following her medication regimen and of regular prenatal care.

INTERVENTION	RATIONALE
• Assess the patient's and family's level of understanding of HIV infection, its modes of transmission, and the long-term implications.	• Knowledge of the woman's (and her family's) level of understanding about her HIV infection forms a starting point for further health teaching.
• Explain the risks of mother-to-child transmission of HIV infection.	• In untreated women the risk of transmission is 25%. That risk can be reduced to 1% or less with the use of antiretroviral therapy throughout pregnancy, labor, and birth; the use of cesarean birth when indicated; and formula-feeding rather than breastfeeding.
• Describe ART. Include the regimen prescribed, its purposes, and the procedures for taking it.	• ART approaches vary based on the health status of the individual woman and whether she is currently on ART. Generally it includes IV ZDV during labor through birth and therapy for the baby for 6 weeks following birth.
• Discuss signs the woman should be alert for, including fever, fatigue, weight loss, cough, skin lesions, and behavior changes.	• These symptoms may indicate that the woman is developing symptomatic loss, persistent candidiasis, diarrhea, and HIV infection.

EXPECTED OUTCOME: Woman will actively seek information about her condition, her treatment regimen, and her pregnancy and will cooperate with her caregivers.

Nursing Care Plans address nursing care for women who have complications such as preeclampsia or diabetes mellitus, as well as for high-risk newborns. We designed this information to enhance your preparation for the clinical setting.

Professionalism in Practice helps you to identify how to remain professional in nursing practice and focus on topics such as legal and ethical considerations, contemporary nursing practice issues, professional accountability, patient advocacy, and home and community care considerations.

Professionalism in Practice Using Contraception Resources During Patient Teaching

In your role as teacher, it is important to have resources on hand for women seeking a method of contraception. Having IUC models or a female condom plus informational handouts for the various methods of contraception is invaluable. Describing correct use of the method along with important tips, its side effects, and the warning signs for serious adverse reactions is essential. Women can refer to the informational sheets at home. Be sure to include the office or clinic phone number, and always remember to mention emergency contraception (EC).

SAFETY ALERT!
Lack of fetal movement can be an indication of chronic placental insufficiency or even fetal death; thus, the woman should be advised how to handle nonreassuring findings. The woman should call her healthcare provider, and if advised she should come in for testing. The need to retain a sense of calm is imperative for the mother who is transporting herself to the medical setting for these tests.

Safety Alert! features bring forward critical information for safe and effective nursing practice.

Teaching Highlights help you to plan and organize your patient teaching. The teaching that nurses do at all stages of pregnancy and childbearing and throughout the life of a woman is one of the most important aspects of their work.

TEACHING HIGHLIGHTS | What to Tell the Pregnant Woman About Assessing Fetal Activity

- Explain that fetal movements are first felt around 18 weeks of gestation, but some women may not feel fetal movement until 25 weeks. This is called *quickening*. From that time, the fetal movements get stronger and easier to detect. A slowing or stopping of fetal movement may be an indication that the fetus needs some attention and evaluation. The mother's perception of decreased fetal movement is sufficient in most cases. Formal tracking of fetal movement does not lead to improved outcomes in low-risk pregnancies but may have value in high-risk situations.
- Describe the procedures and demonstrate how to assess fetal movement. Sit beside the woman and show her how to place her hand on the fundus to feel fetal movement. Advise the woman to keep a daily record of fetal movements beginning at about 28 weeks of gestation.
- Explain the procedure for the Cardiff Count-to-Ten method:
  1. Beginning at the same time each day, have the woman place an X on the Cardiff card (Figure 16–11) for each fetal movement she perceives during normal everyday activity until she has recorded 10 of them.
  2. Movement varies considerably, but the woman should feel fetal movement at least 10 times in 12 hours, and many women will feel 10 fetal movements in much less time, possibly 2 hours or less.
- Explain the procedure for the DFMR method:
  1. The woman should begin counting at about the same time each day, after taking food.
  2. She should lie quietly in a side-lying position.
  3. The woman should feel at least three fetal movements within 1 hour.
- Instruct the woman to contact her care provider in the following situations:
  1. Using the Cardiff method: If there are fewer than 10 movements in 12 hours.
  2. Using the DFMR method: If there are fewer than three movements in 1 hour.
  3. Both methods: If overall the fetus's movements are slowing, and it takes much longer each day to note the minimum number of movements in the specified time period, and if there are no movements in the morning.
- Whichever method she is using, encourage the woman to complete her fetal movement record daily and to bring it with her during each prenatal visit. Assure her that the record will be discussed at each prenatal visit and that questions may be addressed at that time if desired.
- Provide the woman with a name and phone number in case she has further questions.

Women with Special Needs **Women with Paralysis**
Women with paralysis often warrant intermittent fetal surveillance since they are unable to feel fetal movement or premature contractions. These women are at risk for unattended birth since they cannot perceive their contractions. Their partner or care provider should be trained to palpate contractions and observe for fetal movement on a regular basis.

Women with Special Needs features serve as alerts that women with individualized needs may require modified plans of care.

Focus Your Study ends each chapter with an outline of the main points of the chapter so that you can review chapter content in an easy, quick-view format.

Focus Your Study

- Nurses often play a key role not only in teaching families about various testing procedures, but also in providing clarity and emotional support to the woman and her family undergoing antenatal testing.
- Ultrasound offers a valuable means of assessing intrauterine fetal growth because the growth can be followed over a period of time. It is noninvasive and painless, allows the practitioner to study the gestation serially, is nonradiating to both the woman and her fetus, and to date has shown no known harmful effects.
- Using ultrasound, the gestational sac may be detected as early as 5 or 6 weeks after the last menstrual period. Measurement of the crown–rump length in early pregnancy is most useful for accurate dating of a pregnancy. The most important and frequently used ultrasound measurements in the second trimester are biparietal diameter, head circumference, abdominal circumference, and femur length.
- Maternal assessment of fetal activity is very useful as a screening procedure in evaluation of fetal status.
- A nonstress test (NST) measures fetal heart rate (FHR) during fetal activity; FHR normally increases in response to fetal activity. The desired result is a reactive test.
- A contraction stress test (CST) provides a method for observing the response of the FHR to the stress of uterine contractions. The desired result is a negative test.
- A fetal biophysical profile (BPP) includes five fetal variables (breathing movement, body movement, tone, amniotic fluid volume, and FHR reactivity). It assesses the fetus at risk for intrauterine compromise.
- Aneuploidy screening includes first-trimester single test screening (nuchal translucency and PAPP-A and beta hCG); stepwise sequential, integrated, or contingent screening; cell-free DNA testing; or quadruple screening of AFP, hCG, diameric inhibin-A, and estriol.
- Amniocentesis can be used to obtain amniotic fluid for testing. A variety of tests is available to evaluate the presence of disease, genetic conditions, and fetal maturity.
- Chorionic villus sampling (CVS) is a procedure that obtains fetal karyotype in the first trimester. It is used to diagnose hemoglobinopathies (e.g., sickle cell disease and alpha and some beta thalassemias), phenylketonuria, alpha antitrypsin deficiency, Down syndrome, Duchenne muscular dystrophy, and factor IX deficiency.
- The lecithin/sphingomyelin (L/S) ratio of the amniotic fluid can be used to assess fetal lung maturity. The presence of phosphatidylglycerol (PG) may also provide information about fetal lung maturity.
- Lamellar body counts (LBCs) testing can be used as a predictive indicator for predicting respiratory distress syndrome (RDS) in preterm newborns. Optical density at 650 nm is an indirect measure of LBCs.

Contents

Introduction to Maternal-Newborn Nursing

Part I

Chapter 1

Contemporary Maternal-Newborn Nursing

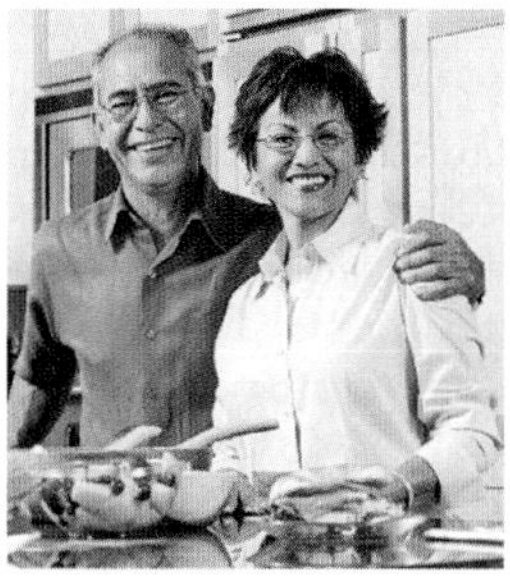

SOURCE: Corbis/SuperStock.

Our daughter just told us that she is 3 months pregnant with our first grandchild. As a labor and delivery nurse for 30 years, I've helped with hundreds of births, but it still seems magical to me, especially now. I'm excited for her and a little worried because I know all the risks as well as the joys. She is so happy; when I am with her, I just want to laugh out loud. I already know I love being a grandmother!

Learning Outcomes

1.1 Discuss the impact of the self-care movement on contemporary childbirth.

1.2 Compare the nursing roles available to the maternal-newborn nurse.

1.3 Describe the use of community-based nursing care in meeting the needs of childbearing families.

1.4 Identify specific factors that contribute to a family's value system.

1.5 Delineate significant legal and ethical issues that influence the practice of nursing for childbearing families.

1.6 Evaluate the potential impact of some of the special situations in contemporary maternity care.

1.7 Contrast descriptive and inferential statistics.

1.8 Identify the impact of evidence-based practice in improving the quality of nursing care for childbearing families.

Healthy People 2020

(MICH-10) Increase the proportion of pregnant women who receive early and adequate prenatal care

(MICH-1) Reduce the rate of fetal and infant deaths

(MICH-7) Reduce cesarean births among low-risk (full-term, singleton, and vertex presentation) women

(MICH-5) Reduce the rate of maternal mortality

The practice of most nurses is filled with special moments, shared experiences, times in which they know they have practiced the essence of nursing and, in doing so, have touched a life. What is the essence of nursing? Simply stated, nurses care for people, care about people, and use their expertise to help people help themselves.

"I like working with students. I enjoy the enthusiasm they bring, the questions they ask, the ways they cause me to examine my practice. I love being a nurse. I am passionate about the importance of what I do, and I feel the need to seize every chance to influence those who will be practicing beside me someday. Last week was a perfect example. I had a nursing student working with me in one of our birthing rooms. It was her first day caring for a laboring woman, and she was scared and excited at the same time. We were taking care of a healthy woman who had two boys at home and really wanted a girl."

"As labor progressed, the student and I worked closely together monitoring contractions, teaching the woman and her partner, doing what we could to ease her discomfort. Sometimes the student would ask how I knew when to do something—a vaginal exam, for example—and I'd have to think beyond 'I just do' to give her some clues. At the birth, the student stayed close to the mother, coaching and helping with breathing. The student was excited but felt she had an important role to play, and she handled it beautifully. At the moment of birth, the student and the dad were leaning forward watching as the baby just slipped into the world. There wasn't a sound until the student said in a voice filled with awe, 'Oh, it's a girl!' Then we all laughed and hugged each other. What a day—using my expertise to help others and helping a future nurse recognize the importance of what we do! ”

All nurses who provide care and support to childbearing women and their families can make a difference. Expert nurses, like the nurse in the preceding quotation, have a clear vision of what is possible in a given situation. This holistic perspective that expert nurses develop is based on a wealth of knowledge bred of experience and enables them to act "intuitively" to provide effective care. In reality, nurses' intuition reflects their internalization of information. When faced with a clinical situation, expert nurses draw almost subconsciously on their stored knowledge and judgment. New nurses need time to develop this level of skill and can benefit greatly from mentoring and coaching by their more seasoned colleagues.

This intuitive perception is integral to the "art of nursing," especially in areas such as maternal-newborn nursing, where change occurs quickly and families look to the nurse for help and guidance. Labor nurses become attuned to a woman's progress or lack of progress; nursery nurses detect subtle changes in the newborns under their care; antepartum and postpartum nurses become adept at assessing and teaching. Similarly, nurses who are cross-trained as labor, delivery, recovery, and postpartum (LDRP) nurses become skilled at caring for childbearing families during all phases of childbirth. Thus, skilled nursing practice depends on a solid base of knowledge and clinical expertise delivered in a caring, holistic manner.

“My first pregnancy ended in spontaneous abortion at 8 weeks, so this time I decided not to tell anyone I was pregnant until I was 3 months along. We had just told both families the news the preceding day when it happened again. We rushed to the hospital and, a short time later, I passed a small fetus into the Johnny cap. My poor baby—so tiny, maybe 3 or 4 inches long. My husband sat with his arm around me as I cried while the nurse took our baby out. A few minutes later, she came back and said, 'I saw on your record that you are Catholic. Would you like me to baptize your baby?' I said, 'Oh, yes, please,' and she left. Even in my grief, I recognized the meaningfulness of her act. She showed me so very clearly that I was an individual in need of individualized care. I vowed that I would practice nursing in the same holistic way. ”

Many nurses who work with childbearing families are sensitive, intuitive, knowledgeable, critical thinkers. They are technically skilled, empowered professionals who can collaborate effectively with others and advocate for those individuals and families who need their support. Such nurses do make a difference in the quality of care that childbearing families receive.

Contemporary Childbirth

The scope of practice of maternal and newborn nurses has changed dramatically in the past 30 years. Today's maternal-newborn nurses have far broader responsibilities and focus more on the specific goals of the individual childbearing woman and her family (Figure 1–1).

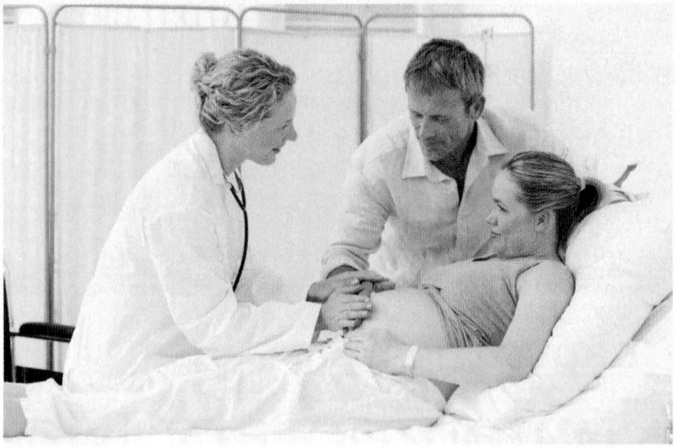

Figure 1–1 Individualized education for childbearing couples is one of the prime responsibilities of the maternal-newborn nurse.

SOURCE: Wavebreak Media Ltd/123 RF

Family-centered care, characterized by an emphasis on the family and family involvement throughout the pregnancy, birth, and postpartum period, is accepted and encouraged. Fathers are active participants in the childbirth experience. Families and friends are also often included. Siblings are encouraged to visit and meet their newest family member and may even attend the birth.

As new definitions of *family* evolve, as discussed in Chapter 2, family-centered care changes and evolves as well. For example, the family of the single mother may include her mother, sister, another relative, a close friend, her partner, or the father of the child. Many cultures also recognize the importance of extended families, where several family members often provide care and support.

In addition to the emphasis on the family, contemporary childbirth is also characterized by an increasing number of choices about many aspects of the childbirth experience, including the place of birth (hospital, free-standing birthing center, or home birth); the primary caregiver (physician, certified nurse-midwife, or certified midwife); the use of a *doula* to provide labor support (see Chapter 21 for more information on doulas); and birth-related experiences (methods of childbirth preparation, use of analgesia and anesthesia, and position for labor and birth, for example).

It seems likely that home follow-up nursing care will continue to gain acceptance because it is a cost-effective approach with favorable long-term family outcomes. In addition, families can access a variety of community resources, from local programs focusing on specific topics such as parenting or postpartum exercise to the widely recognized support provided by national organizations such as La Leche League.

For families with access to the internet, a wealth of information and advice is available. For example, the U.S. Department of Health and Human Services' Office on Women's Health offers a wide variety of educational resources designed to help promote women's health and well-being. Web links to a variety of other organizations and consumer publications also exist.

Interest in complementary and alternative medicine (CAM) practices is growing nationwide and is having an impact on the care of childbearing families. In response to this trend, the National Institutes of Health has established the National Center for Complementary and Integrative Health (NCCIH), which is a valuable resource for both families and healthcare professionals. Nurses caring for childbearing families need to recognize that a significant percentage of Americans are using some form of unconventional or alternative practice, although they may not share this information with their healthcare provider. It is important for nurses to communicate a willingness to work with the women and their families to recognize and respect these alternative approaches. Complementary health approaches are discussed in Chapter 2.

Many women elect to have their pregnancy and birth managed by a certified nurse-midwife (CNM), a registered nurse who is also prepared as a midwife. Midwives who are not registered nurses but who complete a direct-entry midwifery education program that meets the standards established by the American College of Nurse-Midwives (ACNM) may take a certification exam to become a *certified midwife (CM)*. The CM credential is not recognized in all states. In 2014, CNMs and CMs attended 8.3% of all births in the United States and 12.1% of all vaginal births (American College of Nurse-Midwives [ACNM], 2016). Education and certification standards are the same for CNMs and CMs. As of 2010, a graduate degree is required for either credential (ACNM, 2016). Most states mandate that private insurers provide reimbursement for midwifery services; Medicaid reimbursement for these services is mandatory in all states (ACNM, 2016).

The North American Registry of Midwives (NARM) is also a certification agency. NARM midwifery certification is a competency-based model. Midwives certified through NARM may become midwives through a formal educational program at a college, university, or midwifery school or through apprenticeship or self-study. They are eligible to use the credential *certified professional midwife (CPM)* (NARM, 2014).

Traditional midwives, sometimes called *lay midwives*, are midwives who do not become certified or licensed, often for religious or personal reasons. They typically serve a specific community and are a reflection of historical approaches to midwifery (Midwives Alliance of North America [MANA], 2016).

The place of birth is an important decision. Birthing centers and special homelike labor, delivery, recovery, postpartum (LDRP) rooms in hospitals have become increasingly popular. Some women choose to give birth at home, although healthcare professionals do not generally recommend this approach. Most professionals are concerned that, in the event of an unanticipated complication that threatens the well-being of the mother or her baby, delay in obtaining emergency assistance might result. Some CNMs do attend home births; however, the majority of home births are attended by CMs, CPMs, or traditional midwives. In 2015, 1.5% of births occurred outside of a hospital. Of these, 63.1% were home births, while the remainder occurred in a freestanding birthing center; this is the highest number of home births reported since this information began to be collected in 1989 (Martin, Hamilton, Osterman, et al., 2017).

The Self-Care Movement

The *self-care* movement began to emerge in the late 1960s as consumers sought to understand technology and take an interest in their own health and basic self-care skills. More and more people have begun to exercise, control their diet, and monitor their psychologic and physiologic status. Thus, they assume many primary care functions. Furthermore, today's healthcare consumers are requiring greater information and accountability from their healthcare providers. These consumers recognize that knowledge, indeed, is power.

Practicing self-care—assuming responsibility for one's own health—often requires patients to be assertive and to take an active role in seeking necessary information. Healthcare providers can help foster self-care by focusing on *health promotion education* during every patient encounter. This may be as simple as discussing actions that foster a healthy lifestyle, such as exercising regularly or wearing a helmet when biking, skiing, or snowboarding, or it may be more involved for a person with a chronic health condition. Health promotion education can be especially effective when it is related to a specific health concern. For example, discussion about the importance of a healthy diet, weight control, and regular exercise may be particularly impactful for a woman who learns she has high cholesterol or who is diagnosed with gestational diabetes mellitus. Nurses can foster self-care by providing information readily and by acknowledging people's right to ask questions and become actively involved in their own care.

Gradually, as more and more people have come to recognize that promoting health can help decrease healthcare costs, health promotion education activities have increased significantly. Literature and handouts are available in offices, pharmacies, stores, and other public places. Television, radio, newspapers, and magazines regularly address health-related topics. Community organizations have become more active in promoting health through events, such as bicycle safety camps for youngsters and by providing car seats to low-income families so that newborns are protected from the moment they leave their places of birth.

Maternal-newborn care offers a special opportunity to promote health-related activities and to foster active participation in healthcare because it is essentially health focused; in most cases, patients are well when they enter the system. The consumer movement, which has already influenced childbirth, encourages people to speak up about their preferences in dealing with healthcare providers.

We believe that health promotion education and its natural outcome, self-care, will be vital parts of healthcare for years to come. Obviously, self-care is not always realistic or appropriate, especially in acute emergencies, but in many situations it is appropriate. With this in mind, throughout this book we have attempted to suggest ways in which nurses might offer health promotion education that would enable the childbearing family to meet its own healthcare needs. We see this as one of nursing's most important functions and one that nurses are especially well qualified to perform. The nursing profession has been at the forefront in recognizing that people who are able to do so should take an active role in their own healthcare, and we agree.

The Healthcare Environment

Healthcare issues are at the top of policy and legislative agendas. Cost, access, and quality of healthcare have become the "bywords" of the times. In 2016, healthcare expenditures in the United States were $2.7 trillion. The healthcare share of the gross domestic product was 17.8% (National Center for Health Statistics [NCHS], 2016).

Almost all adults over age 65 are covered by Medicare, so the vast majority of the uninsured are under age 65. In 2013, the percentage of uninsured individuals was 20.4%; that decreased to 12.4% during the first 6 months of 2016 (NCHS, 2017) (Figure 1–2). The percentage of uninsured people is changing, however, as the Federal government makes changes to healthcare coverage.

For women who become pregnant, early prenatal care is one of the most important approaches available to reduce adverse pregnancy outcomes. In 2016, 77.1% of pregnant women in the United States began prenatal care in the first trimester, 16.7% began prenatal care in the second trimester, and 6.2% began prenatal care in the third trimester or received no prenatal care (Martin, Hamilton, Osterman, et al., 2018).

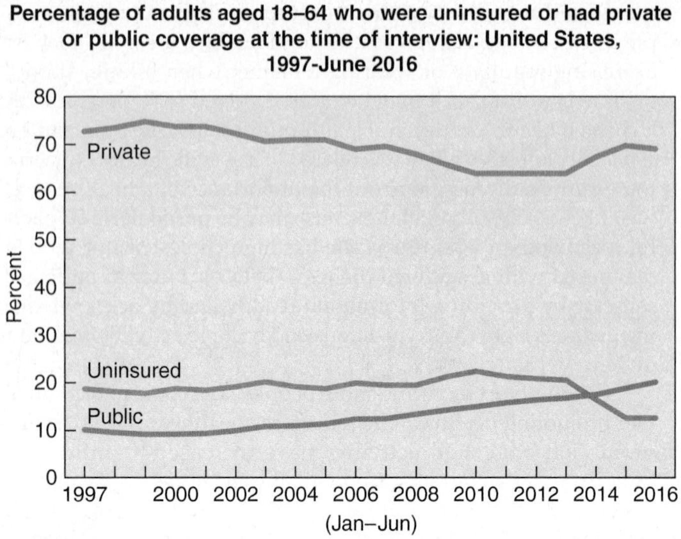

Figure 1–2 **Graph showing percentage of U.S. adults 18–64 years of age who either were uninsured, had public insurance coverage, or had private insurance coverage from 1997 through the first 6 months of June 2016.**

SOURCE: Centers for Disease Control and Prevention/National Center for Health Statistics (CDC/NCHS). (2017). *NCHS Fact Sheet*. Data from the National Health Interview Survey 1997–2016.

Changes in the healthcare environment are influencing women's health and maternal-newborn nursing. Several factors contribute to this, including:

- Demographic changes
- Recognition of the need to improve access to care
- Availability of healthcare
- Public demand for more effective healthcare options
- New research findings
- Women's preferences for healthcare.

Changes are also predicted to occur in clinical procedures, provider roles, care settings, and financing of care. As access to healthcare and the need to control costs increase, so will the need for, and use of, nurses in many roles—especially in advanced practice.

Changing the current system requires a new way of thinking and providing services. Primary healthcare services should be the base on which all other secondary and tertiary services are built. Today in the United States, the opposite is still the case. The system emphasizes high-technology care rather than prevention. However, morbidity and mortality from disease are reduced significantly when people use preventive health services.

Providing all segments of the population with access to primary healthcare should be the chief criterion for meaningful reform of the U.S. healthcare system. This includes a focus on health promotion, prevention, and individual responsibility for one's own health. In this model, secondary healthcare services would use a smaller proportion of the healthcare dollar.

Culturally Competent Care

Culture develops from socially learned beliefs, lifestyles, values, and integrated patterns of behavior that are characteristic of the family, cultural group, and community. The U.S. population has a varied mix of cultural groups with ever-increasing diversity. Estimates suggest that by 2020, fewer than half of all children in the United States will be non-Hispanic White, down from 52% in 2015. By 2050, this number decreases to 39% (Federal Interagency Forum on Child and Family Statistics, 2016). Thus, it is vitally important that nurses who care for women and for childbearing families recognize the importance of a family's cultural values and beliefs, which may be different from those of the nurse (Figure 1–3).

Specific elements that contribute to a family's value system include:

- Religion and social beliefs
- Presence and influence of the extended family as well as socialization within the ethnic group
- Communication patterns
- Beliefs and understanding about the concepts of health and illness
- Permissible physical contact with strangers
- Education.

Specific differences in beliefs between families and healthcare providers are common in the following areas:

- Help-seeking behaviors
- Pregnancy and childbirth practices
- Causes of diseases or illnesses
- Death and dying
- Caretaking and caregiving
- Childrearing practices.

These elements in differing degrees influence the cultural beliefs and values of an ethnic group, making the group unique. Misunderstandings may occur when the healthcare professional and the family come from different cultural groups. In addition, past experiences with care may have made the family angry or suspicious of providers.

When the family's cultural values are incorporated into the care plan, the family is more likely to accept and comply with the needed care, especially in the home care setting. It is important for nurses to avoid imposing personal cultural values on the women and families in their care. By learning about the values of the different ethnic groups in the community—their religious beliefs that have an impact on healthcare practices, their beliefs about common illnesses, and their specific healing practices—nurses can develop an individualized nursing care plan for each childbearing woman and her family. See *Developing Cultural Competence: Values Conflicts*.

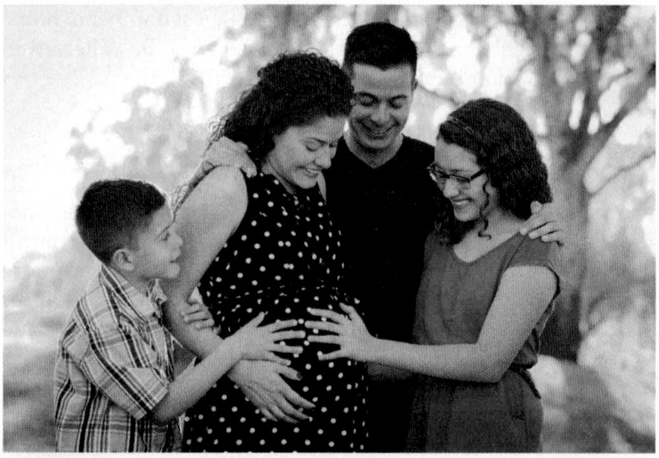

Figure 1–3 **Nurses who care for childbearing families must recognize the importance of each family's cultural values and beliefs.**

SOURCE: Andy Dean/Fotolia.

Developing Cultural Competence
Values Conflicts

Conflicts with a childbearing woman and her family can occur when traditional rituals and practices of the family's elders do not conform to current healthcare practices (Spector, 2017). Nurses need to be sensitive to the potential implications for the woman's health and that of her newborn, especially after they are discharged home. When cultural values are not part of the nursing care plan, a woman and her family may be forced to decide whether the family's beliefs should take priority over the healthcare professional's guidance. Nurses need to be able to recognize, respect, and respond to ethnic diversity in a way that leads to an outcome that is satisfactory to both the patient and the healthcare provider.

Because of the importance of culturally competent care, this topic is discussed in more depth in Chapter 2 and throughout the book as well.

Professional Options in Maternal-Newborn Nursing Practice

“As a man, I don't always find it easy to be a labor and delivery nurse. I have three children of my own and attended all their births. It meant a lot to me to be there, and I like helping others to have good childbirth experiences, too. I don't fit some people's image of a nurse, so they refer to me as a 'male nurse' as opposed to a real nurse, and they ask why I didn't go into medicine instead. Why can't they understand that I'm a nurse because it's what I really want to be? And I'm darned good at it, too. More men are choosing nursing now, and I think that will help. I hope to see the day when we don't have 'female doctors' and 'male nurses,' but doctors and nurses, period!”

Maternal-newborn nurses are found in the maternity departments of acute care facilities, in physicians' offices, in clinics, in college health services, in school-based programs dealing with sex education or adolescent pregnancies, in community health services, and in any other setting in which a patient has a need for maternity care. The depth of nursing involvement in various settings is determined by the qualifications and the role or function of the nurse employed. Many different titles have evolved to describe the professional requirements of the nurse in various maternity care roles. These titles include:

- A **professional nurse** is a graduate of an accredited basic program in nursing who has successfully completed the nursing examination (NCLEX-RN) and is currently licensed as a registered nurse (RN). Professional nurses are typically educated as generalists.
- A **certified registered nurse (RNC)** has shown expertise in a particular field of nursing such as labor and birth by passing a national certification examination.
- A **nurse practitioner (NP)** is a professional nurse who has received specialized education in either a *Doctor of Nursing Practice (DNP)* or a master's degree program and can function in an expanded role. The area of specialization determines the NP's title, so there are family nurse practitioners, neonatal nurse practitioners, pediatric nurse practitioners, women's health nurse practitioners, and so forth. Nurse practitioners often provide ambulatory care services to the expectant family (women's health nurse practitioner, family nurse practitioner); some NPs also function in acute care settings (neonatal nurse practitioner, perinatal nurse practitioner). NPs focus on physical and psychosocial assessment, including health history, physical examination, and certain diagnostic tests and procedures. The nurse practitioner makes clinical judgments and begins appropriate treatments, seeking physician consultation when necessary.
- A **clinical nurse specialist (CNS)** is a professional nurse with a master's degree who has additional specialized knowledge and competence in a specific clinical area. CNSs assume a leadership role within their specialty and work to improve patient care both directly and indirectly.
- A **certified nurse-midwife (CNM)** is educated in the two disciplines of nursing and midwifery and is certified by the American College of Nurse-Midwives (ACNM). The certified nurse-midwife is prepared to manage independently the care of women at low risk for complications during pregnancy and birth and the care of normal newborns (Figure 1–4).

The term *advanced practice nurse* is used to describe nurses who, by education and practice, function in an expanded nursing role. The term, often used in a legal sense in state nurse practice acts, most frequently applies to NPs, CNSs, certified registered nurse anesthetists (CRNAs), and CNMs. As NPs assume a more prominent role in providing care, the distinctions between the roles of the nurse practitioner and the clinical nurse specialist are beginning to blur, and these roles may ultimately merge.

The **nurse researcher** has an advanced doctoral degree, typically a Doctor of Philosophy (PhD), and assumes a leadership role in generating new research. Nurse researchers are typically found in university settings, although more and more hospitals are employing them to conduct research relevant to patient care, administrative issues, and the like. Nurses who have earned a DNP often participate in nursing research; they also play a key role in advancing evidence-based practices that improve patient outcomes and the quality of patient care.

Interprofessional Cooperation and Collaborative Practice

Managed care has led to a rethinking of care delivery and an increased recognition of the importance of interprofessional care

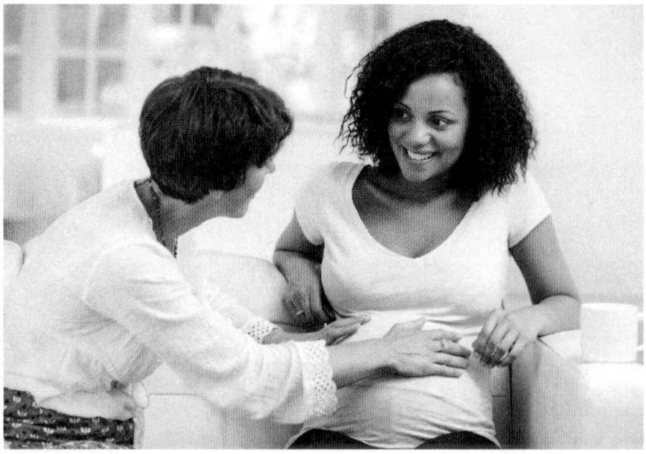

Figure 1–4 A certified nurse-midwife confers with her patient.

SOURCE: Monkey Business Images/Shutterstock.

and collaborative practice. Most groups that accredit programs in the health professions have developed specific standards that address the importance of this acknowledgment of the complementary roles of the various health professions.

Collaborative practice is a comprehensive model of healthcare that uses a multidisciplinary team of health professionals to provide cost-effective, high-quality care. In maternal-newborn settings, the team generally includes CNMs and NPs in practice with physicians (often obstetricians or family practice physicians) and may include other health professionals, such as lactation consultants, social workers, or CNSs (Figure 1–5).

In a successful team, each individual has autonomy but functions within a clearly defined scope of practice. In such a collaborative approach, no single profession "owns the patient." Rather, the team seeks to empower patients and families and include them as partners in their care and in decision making.

Community-Based Nursing Care

Primary care is the focus of much attention as healthcare professionals search for a new, more effective direction for healthcare. Primary care includes a focus on health promotion, illness prevention, and individual responsibility for one's own health. These services are best provided in community-based settings. Community-based health services providing primary care and some secondary care will be available in schools, workplaces, homes, churches, clinics, transitional care programs, and other ambulatory settings.

The growth and diversity of healthcare plans offer both opportunities and challenges for women's and children's healthcare. Opportunities for improved delivery of screening and preventive services exist in community-based models of coordinated and comprehensive well-woman and well-child care. A challenge that healthcare plans face is how to relate to essential community providers of care, such as family-planning clinics, women's health centers, and child health centers, that offer a unique service or serve groups of women and children with special needs (adolescents, women and children with disabilities, and ethnic or racial minorities).

Community-based care is also part of a trend initiated by consumers, who are asking for a "seamless" system of family-centered, comprehensive, coordinated healthcare, health education, and social services. This type of system requires coordination as patients move from primary care services to acute care facilities and then back into the community. Nurses can assume this care-management role and perform an important service for individuals and families.

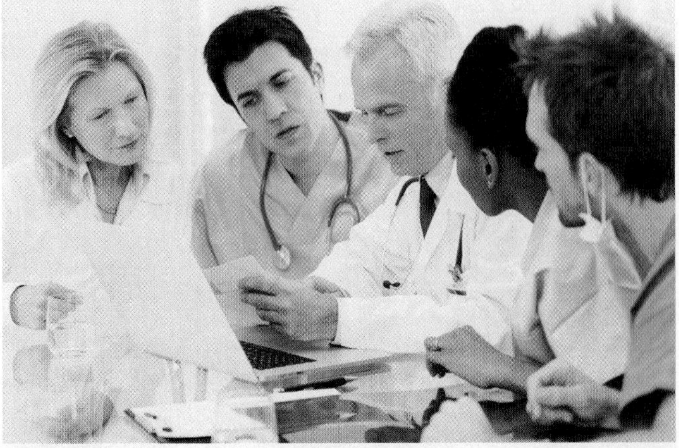

Figure 1–5 A collaborative relationship between nurses and physicians contributes to excellent patient care.

SOURCE: Rido/Fotolia.

Community-based care is especially important in maternal-child nursing because the vast majority of healthcare provided to childbearing women and their families takes place outside of hospitals in clinics, offices, community-based organizations, and private homes. In addition, maternal-child nurses offer specialized services such as childbirth preparation classes and postpartum exercise classes that typically take place outside of hospitals. In essence, we are expert at providing community-based nursing care.

HOME CARE

The provision of healthcare in the home is emerging as an especially important dimension of community-based nursing care. The shortened length of hospital stays has resulted in the discharge of individuals who still require support, assistance, and teaching. Home care can help fill this gap. Conversely, home care also enables individuals with conditions that formerly would have required hospitalization to remain at home.

Nurses are the major providers of home care services. Home care nurses perform direct nursing care and also supervise unlicensed assistive personnel who provide less skilled levels of service. In a home setting, nurses can use their skills in assessment, therapeutics, communication, teaching, problem solving, and organization to meet the needs of childbearing families. They also play a major role in coordinating services from other providers, such as physical therapists or lactation consultants.

Postpartum and newborn home visits are becoming a recognized way of ensuring that childbearing families make a satisfactory transition from the hospital or birthing center to the home. We see this trend as positive and hope that this method of meeting the needs of childbearing families becomes standard practice. Chapter 34 discusses postpartum home care in detail and provides guidance about making a home visit. In addition, throughout the text we have provided information on how home care can meet the needs of women with health problems, such as diabetes or preterm labor, which put them at risk during pregnancy. We believe that home care offers nurses the opportunity to function in an autonomous role and make a significant difference for individuals and families.

Healthy People 2020 Goals

For over 30 years, the *Healthy People* initiative has been providing science-based, national agendas for improving the health of all Americans. This effort is based on the recognition that it is possible to motivate action by setting national objectives and monitoring progress. Analysis indicates that this approach has led to significant progress in many areas.

Healthy People 2020 is grouped by topic area and objectives. Maternal-newborn, pediatric, and women's health nurses focus directly on many of the topics, including:

- Maternal, infant, and child health
- Adolescent health (new)
- Family planning
- Injury and violence prevention
- Lesbian, gay, bisexual, and transgender health (new)
- Sexually transmitted infections
- Genomics.

Because of the role women play in maintaining their family's health, many other topics may also be of importance to them, such as immunization and infectious diseases, diabetes, and nutrition and weight status. Nurses of all disciplines will find it helpful to become familiar with the *2020* topics and objectives, which may be found at the *Healthy People* website (U.S. Department of Health and Human Services, 2017). To increase your familiarity with the objectives, we have created a boxed feature at the beginning of each chapter that identifies *Healthy People 2020* objectives that are relevant for the topic presented in the text.

Legal and Ethical Considerations

Professional nursing practice requires full understanding of practice standards; institutional or agency policies; and local, state, and federal laws. Professional practice also requires an understanding of the ethical implications of those standards, policies, and laws that impact care, care providers, and care recipients. Ethical dilemmas are common in maternal-newborn nursing, and often they are especially challenging. To help you begin identifying ethical dilemmas and to prepare you for professional practice, we have added a new boxed feature called *Ethics in Action!* It asks you to consider how you would respond to ethical issues you might encounter in practice.

Scope of Practice

State nurse practice acts protect the public by broadly defining the legal *scope of practice* within which every nurse must function and by excluding untrained or unlicensed individuals from practicing nursing. Although some state practice acts continue to limit nursing practice to the traditional responsibilities of providing patient care related to health maintenance and disease prevention, most state practice acts cover expanded practice roles that include collaboration with other professionals in planning and providing care, diagnostic and prescriptive privileges, and the delegation of patient care tasks to other specified licensed and unlicensed personnel. A nurse must function within his or her scope of practice or risk being accused of practicing medicine without a license.

Correctly interpreting and understanding state practice acts enables the nurse to provide safe care within the limits of nursing practice. State boards of nursing may provide official interpretation of practice acts when the limits are not clear. On occasion, hospital policy may conflict with a state's nurse practice act. It is important to recognize that hospital or agency policy may restrict the scope of practice specified in a state practice act, but such policy cannot legally expand the scope of practice beyond the limits stated in the practice act.

Standards of Nursing Care

Standards of care establish minimum criteria for competent, proficient delivery of nursing care. Such standards are designed to protect the public and are used to judge the quality of care provided. Legal interpretation of actions within standards of care is based on what a reasonably prudent nurse with similar education and experience would do in similar circumstances.

The American Nurses Association (ANA) has published standards of professional practice for maternal-child health. Organizations such as the Association of Women's Health, Obstetric and Neonatal Nurses (AWHONN), the National Association of Neonatal Nurses (NANN), and the Association of periOperative Registered Nurses (AORN) have developed standards for specialty practice. Agency policies, procedures, and protocols also provide appropriate guidelines for care standards. For example, **clinical practice guidelines** are comprehensive interdisciplinary care plans for a specific condition that describe the sequence and timing of interventions that should result in expected patient outcomes. Clinical practice guidelines are adopted within a healthcare setting to reduce variation in care management, to limit costs of care, and to evaluate the effectiveness of care.

While standards of care do not carry the force of law, they have important legal significance. Any nurse who fails to meet appropriate standards of care invites allegations of negligence or malpractice. Practicing within the guidelines established by an agency or following local or national standards decreases the potential for litigation.

Ethics in Action!

What would you do if you knew that a colleague administered an antibiotic late but recorded it on the electronic health record (EHR) (sometimes called electronic medical record [EMR]) as being administered on time?

Patients' Rights

Patients' rights encompass such topics as patient safety, informed consent, privacy, and confidentiality.

PATIENT SAFETY

The Joint Commission, a nongovernmental agency that audits the operation of hospitals and healthcare facilities, has identified patient safety as an important responsibility of healthcare providers and provides an annual list of specific patient safety goals. These goals and recommendations can be found on The Joint Commission website.

Safety is a major focus of nursing education programs. The Quality and Safety Education for Nurses (QSEN) project, established in 2005, is designed to address " . . . the challenge of preparing future nurses with the knowledge, skills, and attitudes (KSAs) necessary to continuously improve the quality and safety of the healthcare systems within which they work" (2014, p. 1). The project focuses on competencies in six areas:

1. Patient-centered care
2. Teamwork and collaboration
3. Evidence-based practice
4. Quality improvement
5. Safety
6. Informatics.

To support the efforts of The Joint Commission and to draw special attention to the importance of the QSEN project's emphasis on safety, key issues related to safety are noted throughout this text in a feature titled **SAFETY ALERT!**

INFORMED CONSENT

Informed consent is a legal concept designed to allow patients to make intelligent decisions regarding their own healthcare. Informed consent means that a patient, or a legally designated decision maker, has granted permission for a specific treatment or procedure based on full information about that specific treatment or procedure as it relates to that patient under the specific circumstances of the permission. Although this policy is usually enforced for such major procedures as surgery or regional anesthesia, it pertains to any nursing, medical, or surgical intervention. To touch a person without consent (except in an emergency) constitutes battery.

Several elements must be addressed to ensure that the patient has given informed consent. The information must be clearly and concisely presented in a manner understandable to the patient and must include risks and benefits, the probability of success, and significant treatment alternatives. The patient also needs to be told the consequences of receiving no treatment or procedure. Finally, the patient must be told of the right to refuse a specific treatment or procedure. Each patient should be told that refusing the specified treatment or procedure does not result in the withdrawal of all support or care.

The individual who is ultimately responsible for the treatment or procedure should provide the information necessary to obtain informed consent. In most instances, this is a physician. In such cases, the nurse's role may be to witness the patient's signature giving consent. A nurse who knows the patient and the procedure may certainly help the physician obtain the patient's consent by clarifying the information the physician provides. It is also part of the nurse's role to determine that the patient understands the information before making a decision. Anxiety, fear, pain, and medications that alter consciousness may influence an individual's ability to give informed consent. An oral consent is legal, but written consent is easier to defend in a court of law.

Society grants parents the authority and responsibility to give consent for their minor children. Parents are presumed to possess what a child lacks in maturity, experience, and capacity for judgment in life's difficult decisions. Although the age of majority is 18 years in most states, variations in certain states require that nurses be aware of the law in the state where they practice. Children under 18 or 21 years of age, depending on state law, can legally give informed consent in the following circumstances:

- When they are minor parents of the newborn, infant, or child patient
- When they are *emancipated minors* (self-supporting adolescents under 18 years of age, not living at home, married, or on active duty in the military)

In some states, *mature minors* (14- and 15-year-old adolescents who are able to understand treatment risks) can give independent consent for treatment or refuse treatment for some limited conditions, such as testing and treatment for sexually transmitted infections, family planning, drug and alcohol abuse, blood donation, and mental healthcare. Special problems can occur in maternity nursing when a minor gives birth. It is possible, depending on state law, that a minor might be able to consent to treatment for her baby but not allowed to consent to treatment for herself. In most states, however, a pregnant teenager is considered an emancipated minor and may, therefore, give consent for herself as well.

Refusal of a treatment, medication, or procedure after appropriate information also requires that the patient sign a form to release the physician and agency from liability. For example, a person who is a Jehovah's Witness may refuse a transfusion of blood or Rh immune globulin.

Nurses are responsible for educating patients about any nursing care provided. Before each nursing intervention, the maternal-child nurse lets the individual and/or family know what to expect, thus ensuring cooperation and obtaining consent. Afterward, the nurse documents the teaching and the learning outcomes in the person's record. The importance of clear, concise, and complete nursing records cannot be overemphasized. These records are evidence that the nurse obtained consent, performed prescribed treatments, reported important observations to the appropriate staff, and adhered to acceptable standards of care.

RIGHT TO PRIVACY

The *right to privacy* is the right of a person to keep his or her person and property free from public scrutiny. Maternity nurses need to remember that this includes avoiding unnecessary exposure of the childbearing woman's body. In the context of healthcare, the right to privacy dictates that only those responsible for a person's care should examine the person or discuss his or her case.

Most states have recognized the right to privacy through statutory or common law, and some states have written that right into their constitution. The ANA, the National League for Nursing (NLN), and The Joint Commission have adopted professional standards protecting patients' privacy. Healthcare agencies should also have written policies dealing with patient privacy. The Health Insurance Portability and Accountability Act (HIPAA) of 1996 also has a provision to guarantee the security and privacy of health information.

Laws, standards, and policies about privacy specify that information about an individual's treatment, condition, and prognosis can be shared only by the health professionals responsible for his or her care. Authorization for the release of any patient information should be obtained from competent individuals or their surrogate decision makers. Although it may be legal to reveal vital statistics such as name, age, occupation, and prognosis, such information is often withheld because of ethical considerations. The patient should be consulted regarding what information may be released and to whom.

CONFIDENTIALITY

Given the highly personal and intimate information requested of patients, the need for maintaining confidentiality is crucial for the development of trust in the relationship between the individual and the provider. Privileged communications exist between patient and physician, patient and attorney, husband and wife, and clergy and those who seek their counsel. In some states, laws of privilege also protect nurses. Nurses should become well informed about privileged communication laws in their state.

The Federal Patient Self-Determination Act requires all healthcare institutions that are reimbursed by Medicare or Medicaid to provide all hospitalized individuals with written information about their rights, which include expressing a preference for treatment options and making *advance directives* (writing a living will or authorizing a durable power of attorney for healthcare decisions on the individual's behalf). This often comes as a surprise to young women and couples of childbearing age who may have no experience with hospitals. However, with an advance directive in place, a childbearing woman can be certain that, even if she becomes incompetent, she can retain her autonomy about healthcare decisions. See *Professionalism in Practice: Confidentiality and the Pregnant Adolescent.*

Professionalism in Practice **Confidentiality and the Pregnant Adolescent**

Breaching confidentiality is a potential problem for pregnant adolescents, who are just learning whom they can trust in the healthcare system. Make sure you openly discuss the limits of confidentiality for such things as mandatory reporting requirements with the patient and family. Inadvertent disclosure of personal information may lead to psychologic, social, or physical harm for some patients.

Special Ethical Situations in Maternity Care

While ethical dilemmas confront nurses in all areas of practice, those related to pregnancy, birth, and the newborn can be especially complex and difficult to resolve.

Maternal–Fetal Conflict

Until fairly recently, the fetus was viewed legally as a nonperson. Mother and fetus were viewed as one complex patient—the pregnant woman—of which the fetus was an essential part. However, advances in technology have permitted the physician to treat the fetus and monitor fetal development. The fetus is increasingly viewed as a patient separate from the mother, although treatment of the fetus necessarily involves the mother. This type of approach, by nature adversarial, tends to emphasize the divergent interests of the mother and her fetus rather than focus on their shared interests. This focus on the fetus intensified in 2002 when President George W. Bush announced that "unborn children" would qualify for government healthcare benefits. The move was designed to promote prenatal care, but it represented the first time that any U.S. federal policy had defined childhood as starting at conception.

Most women are strongly motivated to protect the health and well-being of their fetuses. In some instances, however, women have refused interventions on behalf of the fetus, and forced interventions have occurred. These include forced cesarean birth, coercion of mothers who practice high-risk behaviors such as substance abuse to enter treatment, and, perhaps most controversial, mandating experimental in utero therapy or surgery in an attempt to correct a specific birth defect. These interventions infringe on the autonomy of the mother. They may also be detrimental to the baby if, as a result, maternal bonding is hindered, the mother is afraid to seek prenatal care, or the mother is herself harmed by the actions taken. Attempts have also been made to criminalize the behavior of women who fail to follow a physician's advice or who engage in behaviors that are considered harmful to the fetus. These forced interventions raise two thorny questions: (1) What practices should be monitored? and (2) Who will determine when the behaviors pose such a risk to the fetus that the courts should intervene?

The American College of Obstetricians and Gynecologists (ACOG) Committee on Ethics (2016b) has affirmed the fundamental right of pregnant women to make informed, uncoerced decisions about medical interventions and has taken a direct stand against coercive and punitive approaches to the maternal–fetal relationship.

Cases of maternal–fetal conflict involve two patients, both of whom deserve respect and treatment. Such cases are best resolved by using internal hospital mechanisms including counseling, the intervention of specialists, and consultation with an institutional ethics committee. Court intervention should be considered a last resort, appropriate only in extraordinary circumstances.

Abortion

Since the 1973 *Roe v. Wade* Supreme Court decision, abortion has been legal in the United States. It can be performed until the *period of viability*, that is, the point at which the fetus can survive independently of the mother. After viability, abortion is permissible only when the life or health of the mother is threatened. Before viability, the mother's rights are paramount; after viability, the rights of the fetus take precedence.

Personal beliefs, cultural norms, life experiences, and religious convictions shape people's attitudes about abortion. Ethicists have thoughtfully and thoroughly argued positions supporting both sides of the question. Nevertheless, few issues spark the intensity of responses seen when the issue of abortion is raised.

At present, decisions about abortion are made by a woman and her physician. Nurses (and other caregivers) have the right to refuse to assist with the procedure if abortion is contrary to their moral and ethical beliefs. However, if a nurse works in an institution where abortions may be performed, the nurse can be dismissed for refusing. To avoid being placed in a situation contrary to their values and beliefs, nurses should determine the philosophy and practices of an institution before going to work there. A nurse who refuses to participate in an abortion because of moral or ethical beliefs does have a responsibility to ensure that someone with similar qualifications is able to provide appropriate care for the patient. Patients may never be abandoned, regardless of the nurse's beliefs.

Fetal Research

Research with fetal tissue has been responsible for remarkable advances in the care and treatment of fetuses with health problems and advances in the treatment of progressive, debilitating adult diseases, such as Parkinson disease, Alzheimer disease, and DiGeorge syndrome. Therapeutic research with living fetuses has been instrumental in the treatment of newborns who are Rh sensitized, the evaluation of lung maturity using the lecithin/sphingomyelin ratio, and the treatment of pulmonary immaturity in the newborn. Because it is aimed at treating a fetal condition, therapeutic fetal research raises fewer ethical questions than does nontherapeutic fetal research. To be approved, nontherapeutic research requires that the risk to the fetus be minimal, that the knowledge to be gained be important, and that the information be unobtainable by any other means. Control over research standards and attention to state and federal regulations remain foci of debate regarding fetal research.

Intrauterine fetal surgery, which is generally considered experimental, is a therapy for anatomic lesions that can be corrected surgically and are incompatible with life if not treated. Examples include surgery for myelomeningocele and some congenital cardiac defects.

Intrauterine fetal surgery involves opening the uterus during the second trimester (before viability), treating the fetal lesion, and replacing the fetus in the uterus. The risks to the fetus are substantial, and the mother is committed to cesarean births for this and subsequent pregnancies because the upper, active segment of the uterus is incised during the surgery. The parents must be informed of the experimental nature of the treatment, the risks of the surgery, the commitment to cesarean birth, and alternatives to the treatment.

As with other aspects of maternity care, caregivers must respect the pregnant woman's autonomy. The procedure does involve health risks to the woman, and she retains the right to refuse any surgical procedure. Healthcare providers must be careful that their zeal for new technology does not lead them to focus unilaterally on the fetus at the expense of the mother.

Reproductive Assistance

The number and sophistication of reproductive assistance techniques continue to grow. Infertile couples now have available a wide range of reproductive options, from intrauterine insemination to in vitro fertilization and beyond. The ethical dimensions of such techniques are discussed here. The techniques themselves are identified and described in detail in Chapter 6.

Intrauterine insemination (IUI) is accomplished by depositing sperm obtained from her husband or partner into a woman. The term *donor insemination (DI)* is used when the sperm is obtained from a donor rather than the woman's husband or partner. Some women who are single are choosing IUI or DI as a childbearing option. No states prohibit intrauterine insemination using a husband's sperm because there is no question of the child's legitimacy. Legal problems may occur with DI, however. Because the child is the biologic child of the mother, legal concerns center on the donor. A donor must sign a form waiving all parental rights. The donor must also furnish accurate health information, particularly regarding genetic traits or diseases. Donor sperm must be tested for HIV. Husbands/partners are often requested to sign a form to agree to the insemination and to assume parental responsibility for the child. Some men legally adopt the child so there is no question of parental rights and responsibilities. Several states have enacted legislation regarding paternity of the child conceived by insemination with donor sperm.

Assisted reproductive technology (ART) is the term used to describe highly technologic approaches used to produce pregnancy. *In vitro fertilization–embryo transfer (IVF–ET)*, a therapy offered to select infertile couples, is perhaps the best-known ART technique.

Multifetal pregnancy may occur with ART because the use of ovulation-inducing medications typically triggers the release of multiple eggs, which, when fertilized, produce multiple embryos, which are then implanted. Multifetal pregnancy increases the risk of miscarriage, preterm birth, and neonatal morbidity and mortality. It also increases the mother's risk of complications, including cesarean birth. To help prevent a high-order multifetal pregnancy (presence of three or more fetuses), the American Society for Reproductive Medicine (ASRM) and the Society for Assisted Reproductive Technology (SART) have jointly issued guidelines to limit the number of embryos transferred. Specifically, women under age 35 and ages 35 to 37 should be strongly encouraged to have a single embryo transferred. The number recommended for transfer increases for women ages 38 to 40 and for women age 41 and older. These guidelines are designed to decrease risk while allowing for individualized care (ASRM & SART, 2017).

This practice raises ethical considerations about the handling of unused embryos. However, when a multifetal pregnancy does occur, the physician may suggest that the woman consider fetal reduction, in which some of the embryos are aborted in the first trimester or early in the second trimester to give the remaining ones a better chance for survival. Clearly, this procedure raises ethical concerns about the sacrifice of some so that the remainder can survive.

Prevention should be the first approach to the problem of multifetal pregnancy. It begins with careful counseling about the risks of multiple gestation and the ethical issues that relate to fetal reduction. Ultimately, the ethical principle of autonomy indicates that it is the woman who needs to assess the issues involved and decide whether to opt for fetal reduction. No physician who is morally opposed to fetal reduction should be expected to perform the procedure; the patient should be referred to a physician who has the necessary expertise. However, physicians should be aware of the ethical and medical issues involved and be prepared to respond to families in a professional and ethical manner (ACOG, 2016a).

Surrogate childbearing is another approach to addressing the issue of infertility. Surrogate childbearing occurs when a woman agrees to become pregnant for another woman or for a couple, who are usually childless. Depending on the infertile woman's or couple's needs, the surrogate may be inseminated with the male partner's sperm or a donor's sperm, or she may receive a gamete transfer depending on the infertile couple's needs. If fertilization occurs, the woman carries the fetus to term and then releases the newborn to the couple after birth.

These methods of resolving infertility raise many ethical questions, including the problem of religious objections to artificial conception, the question of who will assume financial and moral responsibility for a child born with a congenital defect, the issue of candidate selection, and the threat of genetic engineering. Other ethical questions include:

- What should be done with surplus fertilized oocytes?
- To whom do frozen embryos belong—parents together or separately? The hospital or infertility clinic?
- Who is liable if a woman or her offspring contracts HIV disease from donated sperm?
- Should children be told the method of their conception?

“Our son was born after artificial insemination. Nick, my husband, was sterile because of radiation therapy, so his cousin was the donor for us. I thought that might be awkward but the whole family was so excited that there was a way to help us after Nick's battle with cancer that it has been OK. Every time we look at Vincent Joseph (he is named for his grandfathers) and see him smile, we know that we would do it again in an instant.”

Embryonic Stem Cell Research

Human stem cells can be found in embryonic tissue and in the primordial germ cells of a fetus. Research has demonstrated that in tissue cultures these cells can be made to differentiate into other types of cells such as blood, nerve, or heart cells, which might then be used to treat problems, such as diabetes, Parkinson and Alzheimer diseases, spinal cord injury, or metabolic disorders. The availability of specialized tissue or even organs grown from stem cells might also decrease society's dependence on donated organs for organ transplants.

Positions about embryonic stem cell research vary dramatically, from the view that any use of human embryos for research is wrong to the view that any form of embryonic stem cell research is acceptable, with a variety of other positions that fall somewhere in between these extremes. Other questions also arise: What sources of embryonic tissue are acceptable for research? Is it ever ethical to clone embryos solely for stem cell research? Is there justification for using embryos remaining after fertility treatments?

The question of how an embryo should be viewed—with the status in some way of a person or in some sense of property (and, if property, whose?)—is a key question in the debate. Ethicists recognize that it is not necessary to advocate full moral status or personhood for an embryo to have significant moral qualms about the instrumental use of a human embryo in the "interests" of society. The issue of consent, which links directly to an embryo's status, also merits consideration. In truth, the ethical questions and dilemmas associated with embryonic stem cell research are staggeringly complex and require careful analysis and thoughtful dialogue.

Implications for Nursing Practice

The complex ethical issues facing maternal-newborn nurses have many social, cultural, legal, and professional ramifications. Nurses, like all healthcare professionals, need to learn to anticipate ethical dilemmas, clarify their own positions and values related to the issues, understand the legal implications of the issues, and develop appropriate strategies for ethical decision making. To accomplish these tasks, they may read about bioethical issues, participate in discussion groups, or attend courses and workshops on ethical topics pertinent to their areas of practice. Most nurses develop solid skills in logical thinking and critical analysis. These skills, coupled with theoretical knowledge about ethical decision making, can serve nurses well in dealing with the many ethical dilemmas found in healthcare.

Evidence-Based Practice in Maternal-Child Nursing

Evidence-based practice—that is, nursing care in which all interventions are supported by current, valid research or other forms of evidence, such as committee opinions or task force recommendations, is emerging as a major force in healthcare. It provides a useful approach to problem solving/decision making and to self-directed, patient-centered, lifelong learning. Evidence-based practice builds on the actions necessary to transform research findings into clinical practice by also considering other forms of evidence that can be useful in making clinical practice decisions. These other forms of evidence may include, for example, statistical data, quality improvement measurements, risk management measures, and information from support services such as infection control.

As clinicians, nurses need to meet three basic competencies related to evidence-based practice:

1. To recognize which clinical practices are supported by sound evidence, which practices have conflicting findings as to their effect on patient outcomes, and which practices have no evidence to support their use
2. To use data in their clinical work to evaluate outcomes of care
3. To appraise and integrate scientific bases into practice.

Some agencies and clinical units where nurses practice still operate in the old style, which sometimes generates conflict for nurses who recognize the need for more responsible clinical practice. More often, however, market pressures are forcing nurses and other healthcare providers to evaluate routines to improve efficiencies and provide better outcomes for patients.

Nurses need to know what data are being tracked in their workplaces and how care practices and outcomes are improved as a result of quality improvement initiatives. However, there is more to evidence-based practice than simply knowing what is being tracked and how the results are being used. Competent, effective nurses learn to question the very basis of their clinical work.

Throughout this text we have provided snapshots of evidence-based practice related to childbearing women, children, and families in the *Evidence-Based Practice* features. We believe that these snapshots will help you understand the concept more clearly. We also expect that these examples will challenge you to question the usefulness of some of the routine care you observe in clinical practice. That is the impact of evidence-based practice—it moves clinicians beyond practices of habit and opinion to practices based on reliable, valid, current science.

Nursing Research

Research is vital to expanding the science of nursing, fostering evidence-based practice, and improving patient care. Research also plays an important role in advancing the profession of nursing. For example, nursing research can help determine the psychosocial and physical risks and benefits of both nursing and medical interventions.

The gap between research and practice is being narrowed by the publication of research findings in popular nursing journals, the establishment of departments of nursing research in hospitals, and collaborative research efforts by nurse researchers and clinical practitioners. Interdisciplinary research between nurses and other healthcare professionals is also becoming more common. This ever-increasing recognition of the value of nursing research is important because well-done research supports the goals of evidence-based practice.

Nursing Care Plans and Concept Maps

Nursing care plans, which use the nursing process as an organizing framework, are invaluable in planning and organizing care. Care plans are especially valuable for nursing students and novice nurses. To help organize care, this text provides several examples of nursing care plans.

Concept maps are becoming increasingly popular in planning nursing care. They provide a visual depiction of nursing management. For your reference, we have included several examples throughout the text.

Statistical Data and Maternal-Newborn Care

Nurses are increasingly recognizing the value and usefulness of statistics. Health-related statistics provide an objective basis for projecting patient needs, planning use of resources, and determining the effectiveness of specific treatments.

There are two major types of statistics: Descriptive and inferential. *Descriptive statistics* describe or summarize a set of data. They report the facts—what is—in a concise and easily retrievable way. An example of a descriptive statistic is the birth rate in the United States. Although no conclusion may be drawn from these statistics about why some phenomenon has occurred, they can identify certain trends and high-risk "target groups" and generate possible research questions.

Inferential statistics allow the investigator to draw conclusions or inferences about what is happening between two or more variables in a population and to suggest or refute causal relationships between them. For example, descriptive statistics reveal that the overall infant mortality rate in the United States has declined over the past decade (Mathews, Ely, & Driscoll, 2018). Exactly why that trend has occurred cannot be answered by simply looking at these data, however. More data and inferential statistics using smaller samples of the population of pregnant women are needed to determine whether this finding is because of earlier prenatal care, improved maternal nutrition, use of electronic fetal monitoring during labor, and/or any number of factors potentially associated with maternal-fetal survival.

Descriptive statistics are the starting point for the formation of research questions. Inferential statistics answer specific questions and generate theories to explain relationships between variables. Theory applied in nursing practice can help change the specific variables that may cause or contribute to certain health problems.

TABLE 1–1 Births and Birth Rates by Race, 2016

RACE OF MOTHER	BIRTHS	BIRTH RATE
All races	3,945,875	12.2
White	2,056,332	10.5
Black	558,622	14.0
Native American or Alaska Native	31,452	13.3
Asian	254,471	14.6
Native Hawaiian or Other Pacific Islander	9,342	16.8

SOURCE: Martin, J. A., Hamilton, B. E., Osterman, M. J. K., Driscoll, A. K., & Drake, P. (2018). Births: Final data for 2016. *National Vital Statistics Reports, 67*(1), 1–55.

This section discusses descriptive statistics that are particularly important to maternal-newborn healthcare. Inferences that may be drawn from these descriptive statistics are addressed as possible research questions that may help identify relevant variables.

BIRTH RATE

Birth rate refers to the number of live births per 1000 people in a given population. In 2016, the U.S. birth rate was 12.2 per 1000. The birth rate fell for women 15 through 29 years of age, increased for women 30 to 49 years of age, and remained unchanged for girls 10 to 14 years of age. The actual number of live births declined in 2016 by 1% to 3,945,875 (Martin et al., 2018). Table 1–1 provides information about the number of births and the birth rate by race in 2016.

In 2016, childbearing by unmarried women was 42.4 births per 1000 unmarried women, a drop of 18% from the high rate of 51.8 in 2007 and 2008. Statistics also indicate that the caesarean birth rate in 2016 was 31.9%, the lowest rate since 2007 (Martin et al., 2018).

Birth rates also vary dramatically from country to country. Table 1–2 identifies the birth rates for selected countries. Factors affecting birth rates may be identified by considering the following research questions:

- Is there an association between birth rates and changing societal values?
- Do the differences in birth rates between various age groups reflect education? Changed attitudes toward motherhood?
- Do the differences in birth rates among various countries reflect cultural differences? Do they represent availability of contraceptive information? Are there other factors at work?

TABLE 1–2 Live Birth Rates and Infant Mortality Rates for Selected Countries

COUNTRY	BIRTH RATE*	INFANT MORTALITY RATE
Afghanistan	37.9	110.6
Argentina	16.7	9.8
Australia	12.1	4.3
Cambodia	23.0	47.4
Canada	10.3	4.5
China	12.3	12.0
Egypt	29.6	19.0
Germany	8.6	3.4
Ghana	30.5	35.2
India	19.0	39.1
Iraq	30.4	37.5
Japan	7.7	2.0
Mexico	18.3	11.6
Russia	11.0	6.8
United Kingdom	12.1	4.3
United States	12.5	5.8

*Based on 2017 estimates.

SOURCE: Data from *The World Fact Book.* (2018). Washington, DC: Central Intelligence Agency. Retrieved from https://www.cia.gov/library/publications/the-world-factbook/.

INFANT MORTALITY

The **infant mortality rate** is the number of deaths of infants under 1 year of age per 1000 live births in a given population. *Neonatal mortality* is the number of deaths of newborns less than 28 days of age per 1000 live births. *Postneonatal mortality* refers to the number of deaths of infants between 28 days and 1 year of age. *Perinatal mortality* includes both neonatal deaths and fetal deaths per 1000 live births. (*Fetal death* is death in utero at 20 weeks' or more gestation.)

In 2015, the infant mortality rate in the United States was 5.90 per 1000 live births (Mathews et al., 2018). (*Note:* The federal definition of "infant" includes both neonates and infants.) The neonatal mortality rate was 3.93 while the postneonatal mortality rate was 1.96 (Murphy, Xu, Kochanek, et al., 2017). This rate varied widely by the race of the mother, from 4.82 for non-Hispanic White infants to 5.20 for Hispanic infants to 11.73 for non-Hispanic Black infants (Murphy et al., 2017). It also varied by the state in which the infant was born, ranging from a low of 4.28 per 1000 live births in Massachusetts to 9.08 in Mississippi (Mathews et al., 2018). Infant mortality rates are higher among infants born in multiple births, infants born prematurely, and those born to unmarried mothers. Figure 1–6 shows the changes in infant, neonatal, and postneonatal mortality since 1960. Table 1–3 identifies the five leading causes of deaths of infants in the United States and their respective rates.

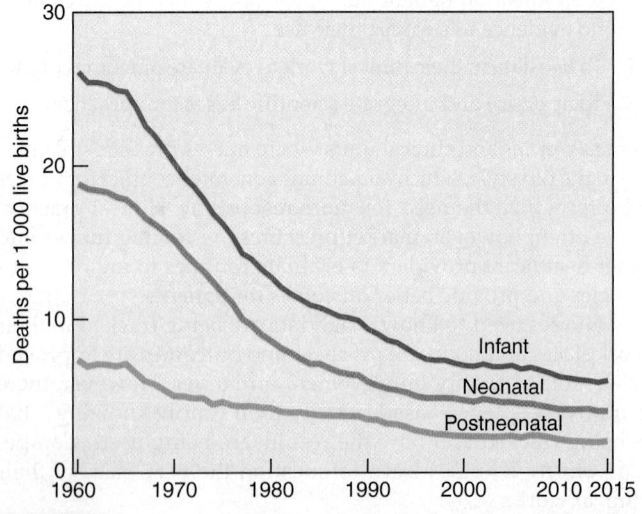

Figure 1–6 Infant, neonatal, and postneonatal mortality rates in the United States from 1960 to 2015. In 2015, the infant mortality rate was 5.90, the neonatal mortality rate was 3.93, and the postneonatal mortality rate was 1.96 per 1000 live births.

Note: Rates are infant (under 1 year), neonatal (under 28 days), and postneonatal (28 days to 11 months) deaths per 1000 live births in the specified group.

SOURCE: CDC/NCHS, National Vital Statistics Report: 2015.

TABLE 1–3 2015 U.S. Infant Mortality Rates for the Five Leading Causes of Newborn/Infant Deaths

CAUSE	RATE PER 100,000 LIVE BIRTHS
Congenital malformations, chromosomal abnormalities	121.3
Short gestation, low birth weight	102.7
Sudden Infant Death Syndrome (SIDS)	39.4
Maternal complications of pregnancy	38.3
Accidents (Unintentional injuries)	32.4

SOURCE: Data from Murphy, S. L., Xu, J., Kochanek, K. D., Curtin, S. C., & Arias, E. (2017). Deaths: Final data for 2015. *National Vital Statistics Reports, 66*(7), 1–75.

The U.S. infant mortality rate continues to be an area of concern because the United States ranks significantly higher than many industrialized nations. Much of this high rate has been attributed to the high percentage of preterm births in the United States. Healthcare professionals, policymakers, and the public continue to stress the need for better prenatal care, coordination of health services, and provision of comprehensive maternal-child services in the United States.

Table 1–2 identifies infant mortality rates for selected countries. As the data indicate, the range is dramatic among the countries listed. Unfortunately, information about birth rates and mortality rates is limited for some countries because of a lack of organized reporting mechanisms.

The information prompts questions about access to healthcare during pregnancy and following birth, standards of living, nutrition, sociocultural factors, and more. Additional factors affecting the infant mortality rate may be identified by considering the following research questions:

- Does infant mortality correlate with a specific maternal age?
- What are the leading causes of infant mortality in each country?
- Is there a difference in mortality rates among racial groups? If so, is it associated with the availability of prenatal care? With the educational level of the mother or father?

MATERNAL MORTALITY AND PREGNANCY-RELATED DEATHS

The **maternal mortality rate** is the number of deaths from any cause related to or aggravated by pregnancy or its management during the pregnancy cycle (including the 42-day postpartum period) per 100,000 live births. It does not include accidental or unrelated causes. Since 1986, the Centers for Disease Control and Prevention (CDC) has tracked pregnancy-related deaths. **Pregnancy-related death** is defined as the death of a woman while pregnant or within 1 year of the termination of pregnancy (regardless of the length of the pregnancy or the site of implantation) from any cause aggravated by pregnancy or related to it (NCHS, 2016). The pregnancy-related mortality rate in the United States in 2015 was 17.3 deaths per 100,000 live births (Centers for Disease Control and Prevention [CDC], 2017). Black women have 43.5 maternal deaths per 100,000 live births, White women have 12.7 deaths, and women of other races have 14.4 deaths (CDC, 2017) (Figure 1–7).

In general, worldwide, maternal mortality rates fell by nearly 44% over the past 25 years, from an approximate rate of 385 per 100,000 live births in 1990 to an approximate rate of 216 in 2015. Nevertheless, in 2015 an estimated 303,000 women died during and following pregnancy and childbirth (World Health Organization [WHO], 2015). Developing regions accounted for the vast majority (99%) of maternal deaths, especially sub-Saharan Africa, which accounted for 66% of deaths, followed by southern Asia. Among countries, Nigeria and India account for over one-third of worldwide maternal deaths (WHO, 2015).

Factors influencing the overall decrease in maternal mortality worldwide include the increased use of hospitals and specialized healthcare personnel by antepartum, intrapartum, and postpartum maternity patients; the establishment of care centers for high-risk mothers and neonates; the prevention and control of

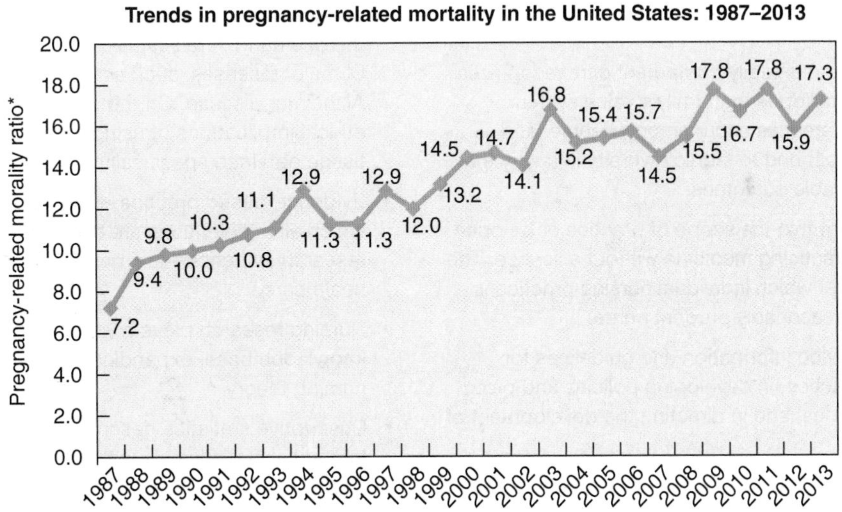

Figure 1–7 **Trends in Pregnancy-Related Mortality in the United States, 1987–2013.**

**Note:* Number of pregnancy-related deaths per 100,000 live births per year.

SOURCE: National Center for Health Statistics (NCHS). (2017). *Pregnancy Mortality Surveillance System.*

infection with antibiotics and improved techniques; the availability of blood and blood products for transfusions; and the lowered rates of anesthesia-related deaths.

Additional factors to consider may be identified by asking the following research questions:

- Is there a correlation between maternal mortality and age?
- Is there a correlation with availability of healthcare? Socioeconomic status?

IMPLICATIONS FOR NURSING PRACTICE

Nurses can use statistics in a number of ways. For example, statistical data may be used to do the following:

- Determine populations at risk.
- Assess the relationship between specific factors.
- Help establish databases for specific patient populations.
- Determine the levels of care needed by particular patient populations.
- Evaluate the success of specific nursing interventions.
- Determine priorities in caseloads.
- Estimate staffing and equipment needs of hospital units and clinics.

Statistical information is available through many sources, including professional literature; state and city health departments; vital statistics sections of private, county, state, and federal agencies; special programs or agencies (family-planning and similar agencies); and demographic profiles of specific geographic areas. Most of these sources are accessible via the internet. Nurses who use this information will be better prepared to promote the health needs of maternal-newborn patients and their families.

Focus Your Study

- Many nurses working with childbearing families are expert practitioners who are able to serve as role models for nurses who have not yet attained the same level of competence.
- Contemporary childbirth is family centered, offers choices about birth, and recognizes the needs of siblings and other family members.
- The self-care movement, which emerged in the late 1960s, emphasizes personal health goals, a holistic approach, and preventive care.
- The U.S. healthcare system is facing a variety of challenges including the high cost of healthcare and the need for cost containment while retaining quality; the large numbers of uninsured and underinsured people; high infant mortality rates as compared with other industrialized nations; and a high incidence of poverty, especially among children and women-headed households.
- The nurse who provides culturally competent care recognizes the importance of the childbearing family's value system, acknowledges that differences occur among people, and seeks to respect and respond to ethnic diversity in a way that leads to mutually desirable outcomes.
- A nurse must practice within the scope of practice or be open to the accusation of practicing medicine without a license. The standard of care against which individual nursing practice is compared is that of a reasonably prudent nurse.
- Nursing standards provide information and guidelines for nurses in their own practice, in developing policies and protocols in healthcare settings, and in directing the development of quality nursing care.
- Informed consent—based on knowledge of a procedure and its benefits, risks, and alternatives—must be secured before providing treatment.
- State constitutions, statutes, and common law protect the right to privacy.
- Maternal–fetal conflict may arise when the fetus is viewed as a person of equal rights to those of the mother and external agents attempt to force the mother to accept a therapy she wishes to refuse or similarly attempt to restrict a mother's actions to support the well-being of the fetus.
- Abortion can be performed until the age of viability. Caregivers have the right to refuse to perform an abortion or assist with the procedure.
- A variety of procedures are available to help infertile couples achieve a pregnancy. However, some of these procedures provoke serious ethical dilemmas.
- Embryonic stem cell research using human stem cells obtained from a human embryo is marked by controversy. On the one hand, it raises the possibility of treatment for a variety of major diseases, such as diabetes, Parkinson disease, and Alzheimer disease. On the other hand, ethicists question the ethical implications of using embryonic tissue—especially tissue obtained specifically for stem cell research.
- Evidence-based practice—that is, nursing care in which all interventions are supported by current, valid research evidence—is emerging as a positive force in healthcare.
- Nursing research plays a vital role in adding to the nursing knowledge base, expanding clinical practice, and expanding nursing theory.
- Descriptive statistics describe or summarize a set of data. Inferential statistics allow the investigator to draw conclusions about what is happening between two or more variables in a population.

References

American College of Nurse-Midwives (ACNM). (2016). *Essential facts about midwives.* Retrieved from http://www.midwife.org/Essential-Facts-about-Midwives

American College of Obstetricians and Gynecologists (ACOG). (2016a). *Multifetal pregnancy reduction* (ACOG Committee Opinion No. 553). Washington, DC: Author.

American College of Obstetricians and Gynecologists (ACOG). (2016b). *Refusal of medically recommended treatment during pregnancy* (ACOG Committee Opinion No. 664). Washington, DC: Author.

American Society for Reproductive Medicine & the Society for Assisted Reproductive Technology (ASRM & SART). (2017). Guidance on the limits to the number of embryos to transfer: A committee opinion. *Fertility and Sterility, 107*(4), 901–903.

Centers for Disease Control and Prevention (CDC). (2017). *Pregnancy mortality surveillance system.* Retrieved from https://www.cdc.gov/reproductivehealth/maternalinfanthealth/pmss.html

Federal Interagency Forum on Child and Family Statistics. (2016). *America's children: Key national indicators of well-being, 2016.* Retrieved from https://www.childstats.gov/pdf/ac2016/ac_16.pdf

Martin, J. A., Hamilton, B. E., Osterman, M. J. K., Driscoll, A. K., & Mathews, T. J. (2017). Births: Final data for 2015. *National Vital Statistics Reports, 66*(1), 1–69.

Martin, J. A., Hamilton, B. E., Osterman, M. J. K., Driscoll, A. K., & Drake, P. (2018). Births: Final data for 2016. *National Vital Statistics Reports, 67*(1), 1–55.

Mathews, T. J., Ely, D. M., & Driscoll, A. K. (2018). State variations in infant mortality by race and Hispanic origin of mother, 2013–2015. *NCHS Data Brief No. 295.* Hyattsville, MD: National Center for Health Statistics.

Midwives Alliance of North America (MANA). (2016). *Become a midwife.* Retrieved from https://mana.org/resources/become-a-midwife

Murphy, S. L., Xu, J., Kochanek, K. D., Curtin, S. C., & Arias, E. (2017). Deaths: Final data for 2015. *National Vital Statistics Reports, 66*(7), 1–75.

National Center for Health Statistics (NCHS). (2016). *Health, United States, 2016. With chartbook on long-term trends in health.* Retrieved from https://www.cdc.gov/nchs/data/hus/hus16.pdf

National Center for Health Statistics (NCHS). (2017). *Health insurance and access to care.* Retrieved from https://www.cdc.gov/nchs/data/factsheets/factsheet_hiac.htm

North American Registry of Midwives (NARM). (2014). *Equivalency applicants: Updates to CPM eligibility requirements.* Retrieved from http://narm.org/req-updates

Quality and Safety Education for Nurses (QSEN). (2014). *About QSEN.* Retrieved from http://qsen.org/about-qsen

Spector, R. E. (2017). *Cultural diversity in health and illness* (8th ed.). Hoboken, NJ: Pearson.

U.S. Department of Health and Human Services. (2017). *Healthy People 2020.* Washington, DC: Author. Retrieved from http://www.healthypeople.gov/2020/about-Healthy-People

World Health Organization (WHO). (2015). *Trends in maternal mortality: 1990–2015.* Retrieved from http://apps.who.int/iris/bitstream/10665/193994/1/WHO_RHR_15.23_eng.pdf?ua=1

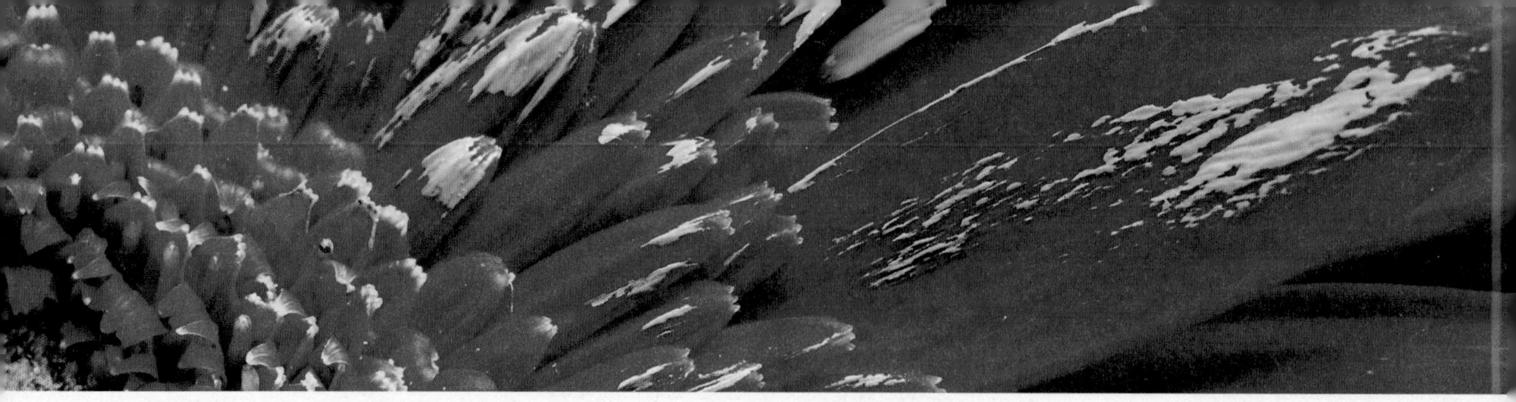

Chapter 2

Families, Cultures, and Complementary Therapies

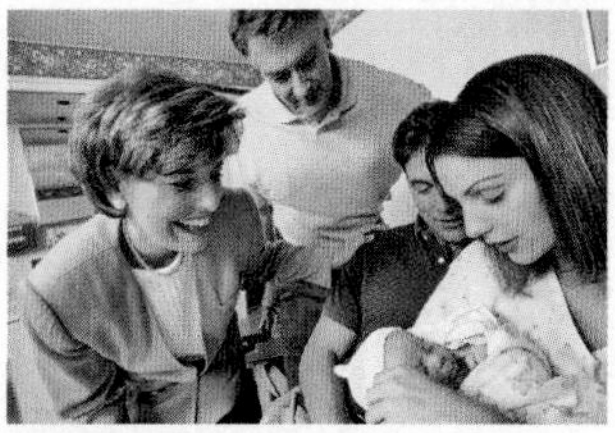

SOURCE: Purestock/Florian Flake/Superstock.

I can't imagine going through pregnancy, birth, or those initial few weeks after my daughter was born without my family. My brother called regularly throughout my pregnancy to check on me. Dad gave me pep talks on eating right and taking care of myself. My husband and my mom were both with me during my labor and my unexpected cesarean birth. After Rosario was born, my husband accompanied our new daughter to the nursery and mom stayed with me, talking and holding my hand. What a difference a family can make.

Learning Outcomes

2.1 Compare the characteristics of different types of families.

2.2 Identify the stages of a family life cycle.

2.3 Identify prevalent cultural norms related to childbearing and childrearing.

2.4 Summarize the importance of cultural competency in providing nursing care.

2.5 Discuss the use of a cultural assessment tool as a means of providing culturally sensitive care.

2.6 Identify key considerations in providing spiritually sensitive care.

2.7 Differentiate between complementary and alternative therapies.

2.8 Summarize the benefits and risks of complementary health approaches.

2.9 Describe complementary therapies appropriate for the nurse to use with childbearing and childrearing families.

Individuals do not live in isolation. Their values, beliefs, behaviors, decisions, attitudes, and biases are shaped by many factors, including their families, cultures, and religious beliefs. Nurses who provide comprehensive, holistic care recognize this reality and seek to learn about and care for the entire family.

This chapter begins with a brief discussion of family types, functioning, and assessment. It then addresses the impact of culture on the family and concludes with a brief examination of some of the complementary health approaches a family might use. Also in this chapter, four individual mothers and their families are introduced in a new feature called *Case Study*: Melissa Bond-James, Benita Cartier, Azia Askari, and Angelina Newman. Throughout the text, you will accompany them as they go through pregnancy, birth, and the postpartum period with various physical, social, emotional, and cultural issues that can occur in real-life pregnancies. Because effective learning involves repetition, application, analysis, and synthesis, these women's experiences appear in various chapters illustrating issues that will allow you to see the true nature and challenges faced by childbearing women and their families, and that will ask you to think critically while applying holistic approaches to caring for them. *Case Study* includes questions for discussion and classroom engagement.

The Family

The U.S. Census Bureau defines **family** as two or more individuals who are joined together by marriage, birth, or adoption and live together in the same household. This definition has remained unchanged since 1930 (U.S. Census Bureau, 2017). Because some contemporary families may not fall within this definition, others define families more broadly by using a definition that characterizes families as individuals who have established bonds of emotional closeness, sharing, and support.

Families are guided by a common set of values or beliefs about the worth and importance of certain ideas and traditions. These values often bind family members together, and these values are greatly influenced by external factors including cultural background, social norms, education, environmental influences, socioeconomic status, and beliefs held by peers, coworkers, political and community leaders, and other individuals outside the family unit. Because of the influence of these external factors, a family's values may change considerably over the years.

Types of Families

Families are diverse in structure, roles, and relationships. Various types of families—those considered both traditional and nontraditional—exist in contemporary American society. This section identifies common types of family structures.

- In the *nuclear family*, children live in a household with both biologic parents and no other relatives or persons. One parent may stay home to rear the children while one parent works, but more commonly, both parents are employed by choice or necessity. Two-income families must address important issues, such as child care arrangements, household chores, and how to ensure quality family time. *Dual-career/dual-earner families* are now considered the norm in modern society. See *Case Study: Introducing Benita Cartier*.
- The *child-free (childless) family* is a growing trend. In some cases, a family is child free by choice; in other cases, a family is child free because of issues related to infertility.
- In an *extended family*, a couple shares household and childrearing responsibilities with parents, siblings, or other relatives. Families may reside together to share housing expenses and child care. However, in many cases, a child may be residing with a grandparent and one parent because of issues associated with unemployment, parental separation, parental death, or parental substance abuse. Grandparents may raise children due to the inability of parents to care for their own children.
- An *extended kin network family* is a specific form of an extended family in which two nuclear families of primary or unmarried kin live in proximity to each other. The family shares a social support network, chores, goods, and services.
- The *single-parent family* is becoming increasingly common. In some cases, the head of the household is widowed, divorced, abandoned, or separated. In other cases, the head of the household, most often the mother, remains unmarried. The mother in a single-parent family may be an adolescent or may have had her child(ren) during her teenage years. Single-parent families often face difficulties because the sole parent may lack social and emotional support, need assistance with childrearing issues, and face financial strain (Figure 2–1). See *Case Study: Introducing Angelina Newman*.

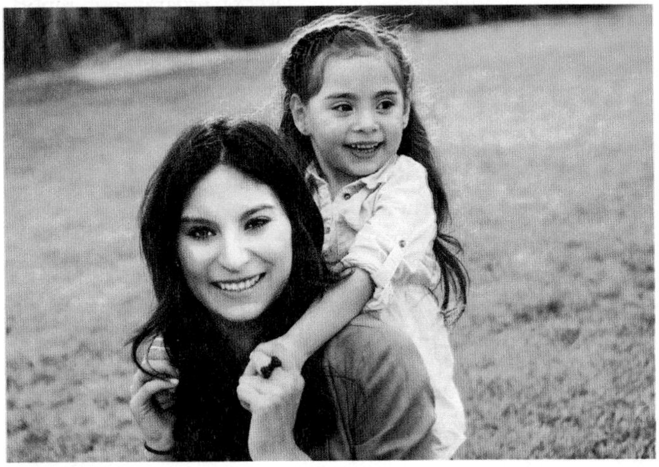

Figure 2–1 Single-parent families account for nearly one-third of all U.S. families. What types of challenges do single-parent families face?

SOURCE: Phase4Photography/Fotolia.

CASE STUDY: Introducing Benita Cartier

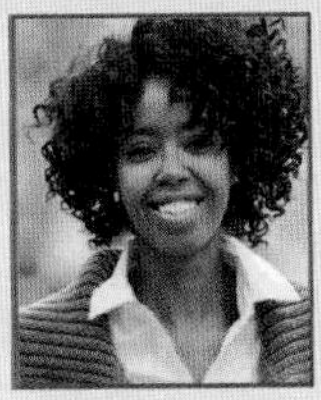

SOURCE: blvdone/Shutterstock

Benita Cartier is a 26-year-old, G2P1 (gravida indicates number of pregnancies, para indicates the number of births), married, African American woman who is being treated for chronic hypertension. In her previous pregnancy with her now 25-month-old daughter, she was treated for chronic hypertension and developed preeclampsia at 31 weeks. Her husband, Gerald, is supportive and helps her at home with their daughter and housework, but he is an airline pilot and is away from home on a regular basis. Because of complications with her previous pregnancy, Benita was seen by the perinatologist at the beginning of her pregnancy and is scheduled for a consult at least every trimester during this pregnancy.

CASE STUDY: Introducing Angelina Newman

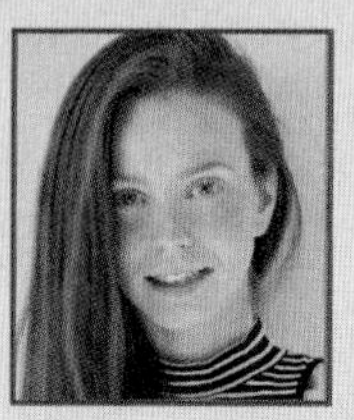
SOURCE: WAYHOME studio/Shutterstock

Angelina Newman is a 16-year-old, G1P0, single, Caucasian American young woman who is a sophomore at a local high school. Angelina is an honor student and was on the junior varsity basketball team last year. She lives at home with her mother, stepfather, and younger brother. When Angelina found out she was pregnant, she immediately told her boyfriend, a 17-year-old junior who also plays high school basketball. While he attempts to be supportive, he is spending less and less time with her. Last week, she was diagnosed with chlamydia. When she told her boyfriend, he accused her of cheating on him, and they are no longer speaking.

- The *single mother by choice family* represents a family composed of an unmarried woman who chooses to conceive or adopt without a life partner (Single Mothers by Choice, 2016). Although these families are statistically included in the single-parent family statistics, they differ significantly in that these women are typically older, college educated, and financially stable and have contemplated pregnancy significantly prior to conceiving (Single Mothers by Choice, 2016). While there is currently little or no tracking on the number of these types of families, one organization reports that women who are single mothers by choice are generally in their 30s and 40s at the time of birth. These women enter motherhood in a variety of ways, including donor insemination (60%), adoption (20%), or known donors or sex partners (20%) (Single Mothers by Choice, 2016). While some of these women may later marry or join with a life partner, they enter motherhood with the expectation that they will independently parent.
- The *blended or reconstituted nuclear family* includes two parents with biologic children from a previous marriage or relationship who marry or cohabitate. This family structure has become increasingly common due to high rates of divorce and remarriage. Potential advantages to the children include better financial support and a new supportive role model. Stresses can include lack of a clear role for the stepparent, lack of acceptance of the stepparent, financial stresses when two families must be supported by stepparents, and communication problems.
- A *binuclear family* is a postdivorce family in which the biologic children are members of two nuclear households, with parenting by both the father and the mother. The children alternate between the two homes, spending varying amounts of time with each parent in a situation called co-parenting, usually involving joint custody. Joint custody is a legal situation in which both parents have equal responsibility and legal rights, regardless of where the children live. The binuclear family is a model for effective communication. It enables both biologic parents to be involved in a child's upbringing and provides additional support and role models in the form of extended family members.
- A *heterosexual cohabitating family* describes a heterosexual couple who may or may not have children and who live together outside of marriage. This may include never-married individuals as well as divorced or widowed persons. While some individuals choose this model for personal reasons, others do so for financial reasons or for companionship.
- *Gay and lesbian families* include those in which two adults of the same sex live together and are married or who live together as domestic partners with or without children. Gay and lesbian families also include gay or lesbian single parents who are rearing children. Children in these families may be from a previous heterosexual union or be born to or adopted by one or both members of the same-sex couple. A biologic child may be born to one of the partners through artificial insemination or through a surrogate mother. See *Case Study: Introducing Melissa Bond-James*.

Clinical Tip

It is important to establish which parent has legal custody, current visitation policies, and other variables (restraining orders, supervised visitation, etc.) when communicating information to parents about their children. Certain legal issues may prohibit the nurse from sharing some information with the noncustodial parent.

CASE STUDY: Introducing Melissa Bond-James

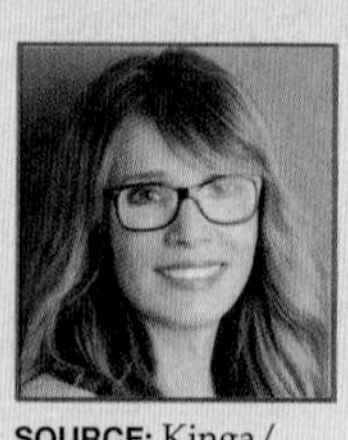
SOURCE: Kinga/Shutterstock

Melissa Bond-James is a 40-year-old, G1P0. She is a married, lesbian Caucasian American woman who has experienced preterm labor during her pregnancy. Melissa conceived via intrauterine insemination after 4 months of attempting pregnancy and began prenatal care at 7 weeks. Her wife, Nancy James, is supportive and is extremely excited about the pregnancy. Melissa is a successful real estate agent and a long-time runner. She has continued exercising throughout her pregnancy and ran a half marathon when she was 13 weeks pregnant.

Family Development Frameworks

Family development theories use a framework to categorize a family's progression over time according to specific, typical stages in family life. These are predictable stages in the life cycle of every family, but they follow no rigid pattern. Duvall's eight stages in the family life cycle of a traditional nuclear family have been used as the foundation for contemporary models of the family life cycle that describe the developmental processes and role expectations for different family types (Duvall & Miller, 1985). Table 2–1 lists Duvall's eight stages to illustrate important developmental transitions that occur at some point in most families.

Other family development models have been developed to address the stages and developmental tasks facing the unattached young adult, the gay and lesbian family, those who divorce, and those who remarry. Textbooks on families and developmental psychology provide further information on this topic.

Family Assessment

The nurse's understanding of a family's structure helps provide insight into the family's support system and needs. A *family assessment* is a collection of data about the family's type and structure, current level of functioning, support system, sociocultural background, environment, and needs.

To obtain an accurate and concise family assessment, the nurse needs to establish a trusting relationship with the woman and the family. Data are best collected in a comfortable, private environment, free from interruptions.

Basic information should include:

- Name, age, sex, and family relationship of all people residing in the household
- Family type, structure, roles, and values
- Cultural associations, including cultural norms and customs related to childbearing, childrearing, and newborn/infant feeding

TABLE 2–1 Eight-Stage Family Life Cycle

STAGES	CHARACTERISTICS
Stage I	Beginning family, newly married couples*
Stage II	Childbearing family (oldest child is an infant through 30 months of age)
Stage III	Families with preschool-age children (oldest child is between 2.5 and 6 years of age)
Stage IV	Families with schoolchildren (oldest child is between 6 and 13 years of age)
Stage V	Families with teenagers (oldest child is between 13 and 20 years of age)
Stage VI	Families launching young adults (all children leave home)
Stage VII	Middle-aged parents (empty nest through retirement)
Stage VIII	Family in retirement and old age (retirement to death of both spouses)

*Keep in mind that this was the norm at the time the model was developed, but today families form through many different types of relationships.

Sources: Data from Duvall, E. M., & Miller, B. C. (1985). *Marriage and family development* (6th ed.). New York, NY: HarperCollins; White, J. M., & Klein, D. M. (2014). *Family theories: An introduction.* Thousand Oaks, CA: Sage; Allen, K. R., & Henderson, A. C. (2016). *Family theories: Family and applications.* Hoboken, NJ: Wiley-Blackwell; Thomilson, B. (2015). *Family assessment handbook: An introductory practice guide to family assessment* (4th ed.). Boston, MA: Cengage Learning.

- Religious affiliations, including specific religious beliefs and practices related to childbearing
- Support network, including extended family, friends, and religious and community associations
- Communication patterns, including language barriers
- Disabilities in any family member, including impact on family and caregiving needs

Other factors can play a role in a holistic family assessment, including information on the health of other family members and the home environment, which is ideally assessed during a home visit, when possible.

Cultural Influences Affecting the Family

When caring for families, it is critical to consider the influence of culture, which may affect how a family responds to health-related issues. In 2015, the National Institute of Health convened a panel to examine, define, and identify interventions that incorporate culture as a component in the research process.

Culture is a multilevel, multidimensional concept that is fluid and changing. It encompasses a large number of complex variables that impact an individual, family, group, or population. Culture consists of dynamic and ecologically based interrelated elements that function together as a living, adapting system. To delineate culture, multiple variables are considered and include biopsychosocial, ecological, geographic, historical, social, and political realities that vary within diverse communities. All of these elements constitute the cultural framework its members use to "see" the world and attribute meaning to their daily lives (Ellwood, 2016).

Transcultural nursing theory, developed in 1961 by Dr. Madeleine Leininger, has its foundation in anthropology and nursing. Transcultural nursing theory is rooted in the caring that embraces the beliefs and practices of individuals or groups of similar or different cultures. Leininger was a pioneer who recognized that individuals' cultural beliefs greatly influenced their perceptions of health and wellness. Culture is characterized by certain key elements, including:

- ***Culture is based on shared values and beliefs.*** Each culture identifies and articulates its shared values and beliefs. Thus, behaviors and roles emerge that are consistent with those specific values and beliefs.
- ***Culture is learned and dynamic.*** A child is born into a culture and starts learning the beliefs and practices of the group from birth. Children who are members of two cultural groups, such as African and immigrant, learn about both groups as they grow and develop. Immigrants may face challenges when integrating the rules of the dominant culture. Children who have family members from two or more cultural groups integrate parts of the worldview from each group. Therefore, although culture is connected with groups, each individual's manifestation of his or her own cultural background will be unique. Culture evolves and adapts as new members are born into or join the group and as the surrounding social and physical environments change. For example, as first-generation immigrants enter a new country, they generally closely follow the cultural patterns of their native lands. As their children grow, the youth maintain some of the family cultural patterns but begin to incorporate some of the new culture (Figure 2–2).

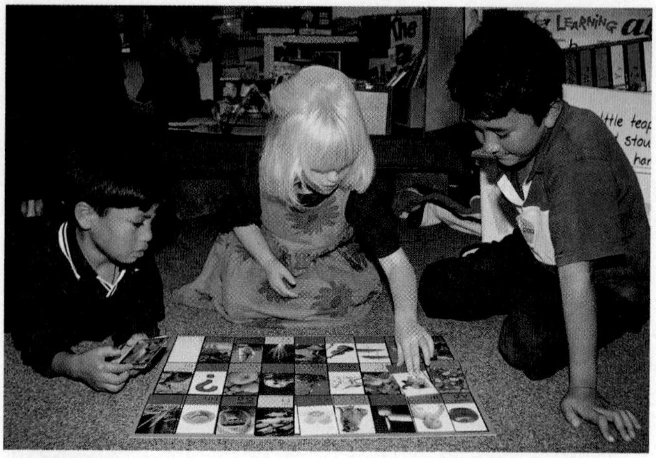

Figure 2–2 **Preschoolers from various cultural backgrounds play together. How can nurses partner with families to assist children to understand and respect cultural differences?**

- ***Culture is integrated into life and uses symbols.*** Culture is integrated through social institutions, such as schools, places of worship, friendships, families, and occupations. This provides a variety of opportunities for learning about one's culture. Symbols are an important way that many cultures communicate with each other and with the outside world. Language, dress, music, tools, and nonverbal gestures are symbols a culture uses to display and transmit the culture. See *Case Study: Introducing Azia Askari.*

Race is a concept that categorizes groups of people who share biologic similarities, such as skin color, bone structure, and genetic traits. Examples of races include White (also called Caucasian or European American), Black (also called African American in the United States), Hispanic, Native (such as Native Americans, Alaskan Native, Hawaiian Native, and First Nation people of Canada), and Asian.

Ethnicity describes a cultural group's identity, which is associated with the group's social and cultural heritage (McFarland & Wehbe-Almah, 2014). Examples of ethnic groups include Hmong, Jewish, Irish, Dutch, Serbs, Koreans, Persians, and so forth. Even the mainstream or majority of groups usually identify with an ethnic group. People sometimes define ethnicity by physical characteristics, such as skin color. However, many people consider themselves to be biracial or multiracial or identify themselves with a specific group not because of skin color but because of a shared ideology or attitudes. More and more, individuals are blends of ethnic and racial backgrounds, and it is often difficult to assign a specific ethnic or racial identity to someone.

While some beliefs and practices are common among certain ethnic groups, it is important to avoid *stereotyping* individuals, that is, assuming that all members of a group have the same characteristics. The term *individuality* describes a person's own unique characteristics, beliefs, and self-perceptions. The nurse should assess the woman and her family to determine her specific cultural beliefs rather than assuming that because she identifies with a specific cultural group or ethnicity that she will automatically practice predetermined customs or hold specific beliefs.

Acculturation refers to the process of modifying one's culture to fit within the new or dominant culture. **Assimilation** is related to acculturation and is described as adopting and incorporating traits of the new culture within one's practice (McFarland & Wehbe-Almah, 2014). Acculturation frequently occurs when people leave their country of origin and immigrate to a new country. Often acculturation is associated with improved health status and health behaviors, especially if the new country is associated with improved socioeconomic status, which leads to better nutrition and access to healthcare. This is frequently true for people who immigrate to the United States from a developing country. On the other hand, health sometimes declines with acculturation. For example, obesity is a problem that is growing rapidly within the United States and particularly among immigrant populations.

Family Roles and Structure

A family's organization and the roles played by individual family members are largely dependent on cultural influences combined with a family's individualized beliefs and past behaviors in earlier generations. The family structure defines acceptable roles and behavior of family members. For example, culture may determine who has authority (head of household) and is the primary decision maker for other members of the family. Additionally, the role of decision maker may change according to specific decisions. In some cultures, decisions regarding the family's healthcare are primarily the responsibility of the female, while other decisions are male dominated. Family dominance patterns may be *patriarchal*, as may be seen in Appalachian cultures; *matriarchal*, as may be seen in African American cultures; or more *egalitarian* (equal), as may be seen in European American cultures. Nurses need to be alert to the roles and functions in families since teaching may need to be directed to those responsible for decision making in order to promote health for all family members.

Culture also defines gender roles, the role of older adults, and the role of the extended family. For example, Native Americans may consult tribal elders (considered part of the extended family) before agreeing to medical care for a pregnant woman or newborn. In some cultures, major decisions for the family include input from grandparents and other extended family members (Figure 2–3). Grandparents may even assume responsibility for

CASE STUDY: Introducing Azia Askari

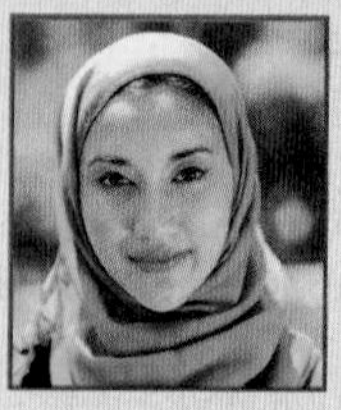

SOURCE: HONGQI ZHANG/123RF

Azia Askari is a 32-year-old, G3P2, married woman who immigrated to the United States from Iran in 2014. Azia speaks some English but is hesitant to do so because she is not confident in her English language skills. She considers herself to be more culturally aligned with her native ancestry and the Muslim religion and beliefs. She wears a hijab and has requested female-only providers in the clinic setting. This has created stress for her on two occasions when male providers were the only clinicians available. On one of these occasions, she was scheduled for a vaginal culture, but the registered nurse advocated for the testing to be delayed until the following week. She has had two normal pregnancies with spontaneous vaginal births in Iran.

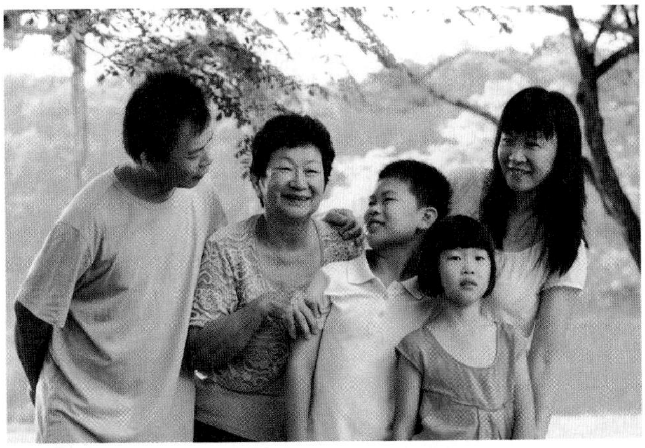

Figure 2–3 **Many cultures value the input of grandparents and other elders in the family or group. In this multigenerational family, the grandmother's guidance is highly valued and significantly influences the family's childrearing practices.**

SOURCE: Wong yu liang/Fotolia.

care of the children in the family. In these cases, nurses must direct teaching for health promotion and demonstration for treatment procedures to the grandparents. See *Developing Cultural Competence: Including Grandparents and Cultural Health Practices in the Teaching Plan*.

Developing Cultural Competence Including Grandparents and Cultural Health Practices in the Teaching Plan

When you care for a family in which the grandparents play a key role in decision making, be sure that they are present when you are teaching something that is important for the family to understand and act on. This might include, for example, signs of illness in the newborn that need immediate follow-up.

If a specific cultural health practice is important to the family and will not cause harm, such as prayer, chanting, or specific foods, respect the family's beliefs and develop a teaching plan that includes those practices. Respecting a family's values improves the likelihood that the newly recommended healthcare actions will be accepted.

Family goals are also determined by cultural values and practices, as are family member roles and childbearing and childrearing practices and beliefs.

Health Beliefs, Approaches, and Practices

The importance of spirituality within healthcare and nursing was identified by early nursing theorists, such as Betty Neuman. She recognized that holistic nursing care incorporated spirituality and that beliefs in God, gods, magic, spirits, or fate had significant impact for many patients. In some cultures or certain religions, a miscarriage or the illness of a pregnant woman may be perceived as a punishment for actions. In other religions, adverse events may be viewed as God's will, not to be questioned. It is wise to ask the woman and her family what they think caused an illness or how they believe they can stay well. People with strong associations with spirituality may gain comfort from prayer, healing rituals, and faith healing.

There are a variety of models and theories that provide evidence of how an individual or family perceives health, illness, and wellness. Some families may believe in a strictly *scientific* or *biomedical health paradigm*, which assumes that physiology explains every aspect of illness and life itself (Andrews & Boyle, 2015). Western medicine is a facet of this paradigm and assumes that all illness results from viruses, bacteria, or bodily damage. Families who hold this view expect a traditional Western medical intervention, such as medication, treatment, or surgery, to treat the specific health problem. Within this belief system, it is very difficult to understand certain health conditions. Families may struggle to "explain" an illness by wondering if the newborn was exposed to something harmful during fetal life or exposed to something in the environment. A physiological reason for the condition is needed in order for the family to understand it. For families with this belief system, health professionals sometimes need to emphasize that certain conditions have no known cause and might suggest treatments other than traditional Western medicine if other approaches may be helpful.

Many nurses in contemporary practice embrace a *holistic health belief* in which biopsychosocial, cultural, and spiritual beliefs guide their practice. They believe these concepts play a primary role in the development and treatment of illness and disease and also heavily influence the foundation for wellness. Many nurse theorists ascribe to holistic models of health and wellness. It is important to remember that cultural, family, and environmental factors are also included within the holistic paradigm. Balance and harmony of the body and nature are important concepts in the holistic health belief. It is believed that illness results when the natural balance or harmony is disturbed. Infections and other illnesses gain entry into the body when it is not in balance. This health belief is most common in North American Native and Asian cultures (Andrews & Boyle, 2015). Increasingly, holistic health practices are being integrated into Western healthcare and combined with other approaches. An example of integration of approaches is use of a medication or radiation for illness in combination with adequate rest and a diet that is designed to increase immune function.

An associated holistic health belief is the hot and cold theory of disease, according to which illnesses and diseases are a result of disruption in the hot and cold balance of the body. Therefore, consuming foods of the opposite variety can cure or prevent specific hot and cold illnesses (Table 2–2). Hot and cold therapies related to healing are practiced in some African American, Asian, Latino, Arab, Muslim, and Caribbean cultures (Andrews & Boyle, 2015).

Healthcare Practitioners

The family seeking care for its members may choose from a variety of healthcare practitioners or a combination of magicoreligious, holistic, or biomedical healthcare providers. The use of *folk healers* varies according to the culture. Though the healer's role and position in the community differ among cultures, generally healers do share commonalities. Healers speak the language of the cultural group, use common methods of communication for the culture, and live in the same community.

Hispanic Americans may seek healing by a *curandero* (male healer) or *curandera* (female healer), a holistic healer who deals with physical, psychologic, and social problems (Golden, 2017). The *curandero/a*'s holistic treatment may include use of herbs,

TABLE 2–2 Hot and Cold Conditions and Foods

HOT CONDITION	COLD FOOD USED TO TREAT HOT CONDITION	COLD CONDITION	HOT FOOD USED TO TREAT COLD CONDITION
Diarrhea	Barley water	Cancer	Beef
Fever	Chicken	Earaches	Cheese
Constipation	Dairy products	Headaches	Eggs
Infection	Raisins	Musculoskeletal conditions	Grains (other than barley)
Kidney problems	Fish	Pneumonia	Liquor
Liver conditions	Cucumber	Menstrual cramps	Pork
Sore throats	Fresh fruits	Malaria	Onions
Stomach ulcers	Fresh vegetables	Arthritis	Spicy foods
	Goat meat	Rhinitis	Chocolate
		Colic	Warm water and honey

Sources: Data from Purnell, L. D. (2014). *Guide to culturally competent healthcare* (3rd ed.). Philadelphia, PA: F. A. Davis; Andrews, M. M., & Boyle, J. S. (2015). *Transcultural concepts in nursing care* (7th ed.). Philadelphia, PA: Wolters Kluwer Health; Lincoln, B., & Dodge, J. (2016). *Reflections from common ground: Cultural awareness in healthcare.* Atlanta, GA: Create Space Independent Publishing Platform.

laying-on of hands, massaging the afflicted area, cleansing the body with herbs, preparing an amulet to be worn, burning a candle with a specific prayer printed on the candle jar, or calling the spirit of a saint to bless the individual. Essential to the *curandero/a* and the family is the faith the family has in his or her abilities. Families may combine *curanderismo* (Hispanic medical system) with a Western approach for some conditions. For example, a baby with seizures may be given medications for the disorder obtained from Western care and may be fed a tea that the healer believes will treat the condition.

Espiritistas is the Spanish word meaning "spiritism." In Latin America and the Caribbean, it is used to describe a healer who communicates with spirits for the physical and emotional development of the patient (Spector, 2017). Hispanic Americans may use this type of healer when the ailment is thought to be caused by witchcraft. However, use of an *espiritistas* is frowned on in some Hispanic cultures. A *sobador*, an individual who uses massage and manipulation to treat patients with joint and muscle problems, is another type of healer who might be used by Hispanic Americans (Graham, Sandberg, Quandt, et al., 2016).

People of African heritage may combine Western and traditional beliefs about illness. Some believe in spirits as causes of illness and may use powders, oils, and ceremonies to maintain health.

Native Americans may seek healing from a *shaman*, an individual with "access to, and influence in, the world of good and evil spirits," who often enters a trancelike state during a ritualistic healing practice. Shaman healers are most commonly used in northern Asia and North America (Oxford Dictionaries, 2016). Native Americans generally believe in the balance of nature and a state of harmony and may seek advice to identify potential causes of disruptions in body harmony. The healer will then prescribe the required treatment for restoration of balance and harmony. Teas, other herbal products, sweats, smudges, meditation, and other approaches are common. Returning to one's family, home, and roots may produce a sense of balance.

Impact of Religion and Spirituality

The terms *religion* and *spirituality* mean different things to different people. Many people view religion, which is sometimes termed *faith-based belief*, as an organized system that shares a common set of beliefs and practices about the significance, cause, and purpose of life and the universe. Religion is usually centered on the belief in or worshipping of a supernatural being or Supreme Being (such as God or Allah). **Spirituality** refers to the individual's experience and own interpretation of his or her relationship with a Supreme Being. Prayer, one of the most common expressions of religious faith, is a frequently used therapy in which many families engage (Krause, Pargament, Hill, et al., 2016).

A family's religious beliefs, affiliation, and practices can deeply influence their experiences and attitudes toward healthcare, childbearing, and childrearing. Members of certain religious groups, such as Christian Scientists, may attempt to avoid all medical interventions, whereas others, such as Jehovah's Witnesses, may refuse specific interventions, such as blood transfusions. Roman Catholics may refuse contraception. In most cases, families gain comfort from acknowledgment of and respect for their religious beliefs and practices in the healthcare setting. However, the *agnostic* (one who has doubts about the existence of a transcendent being) or the *atheist* (one who believes that there is no higher power) may be offended if healthcare providers assume that references to God or to a higher power will be comforting.

A religious or spiritual history is often completed when a woman is admitted to a clinic or labor setting. The assessment can include questions about current spiritual beliefs and practices and preferences for religious rituals. Whenever possible the nurse should attempt to accommodate religious rituals and practices requested by the family.

Considering the diversity of religious beliefs, it is not unusual for nurses to encounter childbearing families whose beliefs conflict with their own. This is not problematic as long as the nurse does not attempt to influence the family's decision making. For example, a nurse who does not believe in baptism should avoid revealing this to a Catholic mother seeking baptism for her stillborn baby. Nurses should also examine their religious beliefs related to genetic screening procedures, use of assisted reproductive technology to achieve pregnancy, abortion, use of technology to support life in a severely compromised newborn or a terminally ill baby, and even less dramatic issues, such as methods of contraception, circumcision, and newborn/infant feeding.

Although adherence to a religious tradition is predominant in the United States, it should not be assumed that all individuals believe in or practice organized religion. It is estimated that

20% of Americans do not identify with any religious group nor consider themselves followers of any specific religion; an additional 7% classify themselves as agnostic or atheist (Pew Research Center, 2016). The nurse should always ask the family if they follow a faith tradition and if they would like a leader from that faith to visit when in the hospital. Adolescents may follow different faith traditions than their parents and should be asked the question individually.

Some religions may be unaccepting of homosexual or transgendered persons. In some cultures, homosexual practices may be considered a sin or may be viewed negatively, whereas in other cultures they are accepted as one of many different ways of being human. Sensitivity to lesbian women who might not be "out" to their families is important in establishing trust with the nurse.

Collaboration between the healthcare team and family is essential to providing care congruent with the family's expectations. Although spirituality is important for many families, it is often overlooked as a healing strategy. Illness and injury may cause the family to turn to spiritual guidance as a method of understanding and coping. Assessment of the family's spiritual needs is an important aspect of nursing care (Denham & Eggenberger, 2015). The nurse must respect the family's view and avoid being judgmental about their beliefs. Partnering with the family to incorporate its traditional practices and beliefs with prescribed therapies will help to ensure the delivery of safe and effective care.

Ethics in Action!

You find yourself in a clinical situation that is in direct violation of your own moral or religious beliefs, and there is no other staff member available to care for the family. What are your obligations in providing nursing care to the family?

Childbearing Practices

Children are generally valued all over the world, not only for the joy they bring, but also because they ensure continuation of the family and cultural values. The valuing of children may manifest itself in different ways. Families in the United States and many Western countries commonly have only one or two children out of a desire to provide them with the best home and education they can afford and to spend as much free time with them as possible. In contrast, in many cultures throughout the world, it is common to have as many children as possible. In the western United States, people of the Mormon faith view motherhood as the most important aspect of a woman's life, comparable with the male role of priesthood (Sorenson, 2015). In Mexican American society and among many other Latino groups, having children is evidence of the male's virility and is a sign of *machismo* (manliness), a desired trait.

In some cultures, a woman who gives birth attains a higher status, especially if the child is male. Although known to be prevalent in China, this trend is increasingly becoming common in other parts of the world, including Asia, Southeastern Europe, the Middle East, and some parts of Africa (Hendl & Rothman, 2016). In nature, gender ratios begin with a higher male to female ratio (105:100), but typically equalize by the age of 55. Gender imbalance and gender manipulation (favoring males) can be influenced via advanced technological interventions, ultrasound assessment, and serological testing; female infanticide; and purposeful neglectful care of female babies that leads to death. In 1995, there were six countries with such gender imbalances; however, the number of countries with gender imbalances has increased to 21 in the 21st century (Brink, 2015).

Culture may also influence attitudes and beliefs about contraception. For example, many Muslims from the Middle East may use birth control but do not believe in sterilization because it is a permanent method (Arousell & Carlbom, 2016). Other Muslims might not practice contraception because children are highly valued, and it is believed that the traditional role of women is to bear children. In Chinese society, on the other hand, where government policy limits the number of children a couple can have, contraception is common.

Health values and beliefs are also important in understanding reactions and behavior. Certain behaviors can be expected if a culture views pregnancy as a sickness, whereas other behaviors can be expected if the culture views pregnancy as a natural occurrence. For example, because Native Americans, African Americans, and Mexican Americans generally view pregnancy as a natural and desirable condition, prenatal care may not be a priority. In other cultures, pregnancy may be seen as a time of increased vulnerability. In Orthodox Judaism, for example, it is a man's responsibility to procreate, but it is a woman's right, not her obligation, to do so. This is because, according to Orthodox Jewish law, the health of the mother, both physically and mentally, is of primary concern, and she should never be obliged to do something that threatens her life.

Individuals of many cultures take certain protective precautions based on their beliefs. For example, many Southeast Asian women fear that they will have a complicated labor and birth if they sit in a doorway or on a step. Thus, they tend to avoid areas near doors in waiting rooms and examining rooms. In the Mexican American culture, the belief is common that *mal aire*, or "bad air," may enter the body and cause harm. Preventive measures, such as keeping the windows closed or covering the head, are used. Some Latinos may place a raisin on the cord stump of a newborn to prevent drafts from entering their bodies.

A **taboo** is a behavior or thing that is to be avoided. Many cultures, including those found in the United States, have taboos centered on the unborn baby or newborn that are meant to ensure that the baby will survive. For example, it is common among Muslims to avoid naming the baby until after birth; similarly, many Orthodox Jewish women wait to set up the nursery until after the baby is born.

In developing countries, mortality rates among newborns/infants and young children are extremely high; thus, certain traditions focus on protecting the baby from evil spirits. For example, many Muslim parents will pin an amulet, such as a blue stone or a verse from the Qur'an, to the newborn's clothing as protection. Following birth, it is common for a male family member to whisper prayers in the newborn baby's ear to declare faith and protect the baby (Arousell & Carlbom, 2016).

Culture and Nursing Care

Healthcare providers are often unaware of the cultural characteristics they themselves demonstrate. Without cultural awareness, healthcare professionals tend to project their own cultural responses onto foreign-born patients; patients from different socioeconomic, religious, or educational groups; or patients from different regions of the country. This projection leads healthcare providers to assume that the patients are demonstrating a specific behavior for the same reason that they themselves would. Moreover, healthcare professionals often fail to realize that medicine has its own culture, which has been dominated historically by traditional middle-class values and beliefs.

Ethnocentrism is the conviction that the values and beliefs of one's own cultural group are the best or only acceptable ones. It is characterized by an inability to understand the beliefs and worldview of another culture. To a certain extent, everyone is guilty of ethnocentrism, at least some of the time. Thus, the nurse who values stoicism during labor may be uncomfortable with the more vocal response of some Latin American women. Another nurse may be disconcerted by a Southeast Asian woman who believes that pain is something to be endured rather than alleviated and who is intent on maintaining self-control in labor.

Healthcare providers sometimes believe that if members of other cultures do not share Western values and beliefs, they should adopt them. For example, a nurse who believes strongly in equality of the sexes may find it difficult to remain silent if a woman from a Middle Eastern culture defers to her husband in decision making. It is important to remember that pressure to defy cultural values and beliefs can be stressful and anxiety provoking for these women. See *Developing Cultural Competence: Culture Shock*.

Developing Cultural Competence Culture Shock

The experience that people have in attempting to understand or adapt to a culture that is fundamentally different from their own culture is known as *culture shock*. It may produce feelings of discomfort, powerlessness, anxiety, and disorientation. Immigrants to the United States may experience culture shock when differences or conflicts arise between their own values, beliefs, and customs and the ways of their new surroundings (Spector, 2017). The nurse should assess childbearing women and their families who have recently immigrated for indications of culture shock. Referring the family to counseling or support from representatives of the family's culture, such as a translator or community group, may be helpful (Ono & Aczel, 2016).

To address issues of cultural diversity in the provision of healthcare, emphasis is being placed on developing **cultural competence**—that is, the ability to understand and effectively respond to the needs of individuals and families from different cultural backgrounds. Cultural competence encompasses congruent behaviors, attitudes, and policies that come together, enabling effective interactions in cross-cultural situations. Cultural competence is a unique complex combination of knowledge, attitudes, and skills that evolves and may change over time (Centers for Disease Control and Prevention [CDC], 2017). It involves identifying and integrating a family's health beliefs, practices, and cultural and linguistic needs into patient care (CDC, 2017).

Culturally Influenced Responses

The nurse can begin developing cultural competence by becoming knowledgeable about the cultural differences and practices of various groups. Nurses who are knowledgeable about differences and who take them into account in planning and providing nursing care will be far more effective caregivers than those who do not.

BIOLOGIC DIFFERENCES

Genetic and physical differences occur among cultural groups and can lead to disparity in needs and care. Differences include blood type, body build, skin color, drug metabolism, and susceptibility to certain diseases. Other disparities occur because of fundamental differences between genders, ages, and races. For example, males are more likely to manifest pyloric stenosis and attention-deficit disorder, whereas females more often have congenital hip dysplasia and systemic lupus erythematosus. Age provides another biologic variation, as infants are more likely to manifest the cancer neuroblastoma, whereas adolescents have a higher incidence of Hodgkin disease. Race is also connected with certain disease processes. Sickle cell disease occurs predominantly in African Americans, who also have a higher incidence of hypertension. Native Americans have the highest incidence of diabetes by percentage of population in the United States. However, type 1 diabetes is more common in Caucasian Americans, while type 2 diabetes has a higher incidence in Hispanic Americans and Native Americans. Thalassemia, a type of anemia, and other genetic disorders of the red blood cells are most common in people of Asian, African, and Mediterranean heritage. Lactose intolerance is common in Mexican Americans, African Americans, Native Americans, and Asians (Kuzawa & Gravlee, 2016). See *Genetic Facts: Genetic Variations and Tay-Sachs Disease*.

Genetic Facts Genetic Variations and Tay-Sachs Disease

While an individual's cultural background is imperative to providing competent satisfying nursing care, additional assessments should obtain one's ethnic status because certain genetic variations occur in different ethnic groups. For example, Ashkenazi Jews (90% of the American Jewish population are Ashkenazi) have a higher carrier frequency for Tay-Sachs disease and 16 other genetic diseases. Individuals of Irish, British, French Canadian, or Cajun background also have an increased genetic risk of Tay-Sachs (Genetic Disease Foundation, 2017).

Nurses need to understand other genetic characteristics in order to perform culturally competent nursing assessments and interventions. Differences in skin color and tone may make cyanosis, pallor, and jaundice difficult to recognize and describe. Mongolian spots are darkened skin on the lower back and buttocks of some babies with dark skin tones. Variations in texture of hair require different approaches to hygiene among various racial groups.

COMMUNICATION PATTERNS

Communication is the method by which members of cultural groups share information and preserve their beliefs, values, norms, and practices. To ensure effective care, it is essential for families to be able to communicate with nurses and other healthcare providers. This becomes an issue when the family does not speak the language of the health professionals. In such cases it is best if the healthcare facility provides translators. Children are most likely to speak both the language of the parents and that of the healthcare providers and may appear to be likely interpreters. However, it is recommended that children never be used to interpret in healthcare situations due to the confidentiality needs of both parent and child. Additionally, if children are used as interpreters, it can create an imbalance in power that could adversely affect parental authority. Signs, posted literature, and brochures should also be available in the languages of the families served. Written material must be provided at a level that the family can read and understand.

Language can also affect health literacy skills because a large number of instructions are given in writing, including prescriptions and directions on medication bottles, signs hanging in health facilities, consent forms for procedures and surgery, insurance forms, directions for techniques or procedures, future appointment dates, and health promotion materials. Nurses need to verify what the patient and family can read and whether alternative ways of providing the information are needed. For example, nurses could verbally give the information and provide paper and pencil so that the family can take notes in their own language. Translation services should be available in all healthcare settings. See *Women with Special Needs: Helping Women Who Are Deaf*.

Women with Special Needs Helping Women Who Are Deaf

Women who are deaf may read lips or may need interpreters to ensure that relevant healthcare assessments and patient teaching can be performed. Ask the woman if she would like an interpreter to be present. If she declines, preferring to read lips, ensure that you are in close contact and facing the woman directly. Use a normal rate and volume of speech. Ask the woman if she has any questions and if she is able to adequately understand what you have said and the information that has been provided.

Variations in communication among cultures are reflected in their word meaning, voice inflection and quality, and verbal styles. Culture influences not only the manner in which feelings are expressed, but also which verbal and nonverbal expressions of communication are considered appropriate. An individual's willingness to discuss certain topics or to express or conceal certain thoughts and feelings is also influenced by cultural norms. Some groups may be expected to remain quiet when experiencing pain, while other cultures may loudly and dramatically express pain.

Clinical Tip

Speaking and reading may not occur in the same language. For example, an immigrant may read and speak fluently in his or her primary language and speak but not read the language of the new country. Always ask about both reading and speaking preferences.

Use of first names and surnames varies among cultural groups, so nurses should not make assumptions because the use of a person's first name may be considered disrespectful. Address family members respectfully, usually using terms such as Mr., Mrs., and Ms. If the person has a title, such as doctor, judge, or senator, it should be used. The nurse should ask what the person prefers to be called and record this in the health record for future reference. In some cultures, such as Korean, Cambodian, and Filipino, the first name used is actually the family name. Asking for the "family name" rather than the "last name" may clarify this practice.

Nonverbal Communication. Nonverbal communication refers to body language, such as posture, gestures, facial expressions, eye contact, and touch, as well as the use of silence. The nurse's use of nonverbal communication may hinder or help communication. Gestures and body language may be misunderstood or misinterpreted. Eye contact has different meanings among different cultures. European Americans, for example, value eye contact with communication and interpret this as a sign of sincerity and interest. In other cultures, such as Asian and Native American, sustained eye contact may be considered rude or disrespectful. Some people of African heritage may misinterpret direct eye contact as aggressive behavior (Purnell, 2013).

Silence is considered a sign of respect in some cultures. Among those groups, offering an immediate response to a question may be viewed as being disrespectful because an instant reply could indicate that no thought was given to the matter. Nurses should watch for patterns in various cultures and alter their approach to be more congruent. For example, many nurses commonly nod and say "Yes" or "Oh, I see" when a patient is speaking. This may seem disruptive to some cultures. If the patient or family member is silent and does not use such patterns of agreement, the nurse should alter his or her response to match more closely the acceptable method of communication for the family.

Touch. The appropriateness of touch varies with each culture. For example, an Asian may consider touching an unfamiliar person of the opposite gender to be inappropriate, whereas touch between men and women may be viewed as appropriate by another culture. Adults commonly feel that it is acceptable to touch children of all ages, but this may not be accurate. It is best to look for responses from the family regarding touch and progress accordingly.

Space. An individual's sense of personal space also differs by culture. Space refers to the physical distance and relationships between the individual and other persons and objects in the environment. Certain cultures may have specific spatial preferences, such as personal distance and social distance. Some cultures tend to prefer close contact with less space since they use touch as a form of communication. The nurse should be aware of how close a patient or her family members come to other individuals and try to maintain this space during interactions. Nursing procedures often cause the space barrier to be broken. Nurses need to touch patients to take vital signs, administer injections, change dressings, and the like. This does not mean that close touch is appropriate at all times. It is essential to tell all patients before touching them for procedures so they understand what is happening.

TIME ORIENTATION

Cultures have specific values and meanings regarding time orientation. Cultural groups may place emphasis on the events of the past, events that occur in the present, or those events that will occur in the future.

Cultures that are oriented predominantly to the past may want to begin healthcare encounters with lengthy descriptions of past healthcare treatments, family history of diseases, or individual past experiences with health. There may be little interest in learning methods of adapting to or maintaining a new plan of care.

For cultures that are oriented predominantly to the present, little consideration may be given to either the past or the future. For example, adolescents commonly focus on the present and may not engage in preventive health practices for long-term health. Therefore, short-term goals often provide more incentive to them.

Cultures that are oriented predominantly to the future may not focus on what is important at the present time. For example, the family focusing on the future may focus on the dreams they had for a new baby's education or talents and have trouble setting present goals for treatment of an at-risk baby. One commonly hears that it is a big adjustment to learn to "take it one day at a time."

Time also refers to punctuality regarding schedules and appointments. In the United States, the predominant culture respects being on time and considers time valuable and not to be wasted. Other cultures may not emphasize a concern for time. This may be manifested by a family's inability to follow timed medication schedules or treatments or to show up as scheduled for an appointment. In these cases it is not intended as a sign of disrespect.

NUTRITION

Nutritional practices begin even before birth, as many cultural groups have beliefs that determine foods that are healthy to eat or that should be avoided during pregnancy. Nutritional habits and patterns vary among cultures and are related to both religious practices and health beliefs. Certain cultures and religions have restrictions on or proscriptions about specific foods and preparation methods. Ritualistic behaviors involving eating and drinking—for example, on special occasions and holidays—are observed by most cultures. Many religions recommend fasts during specific holy seasons, such as Lent for Roman Catholics, Yom Kippur for Jewish people, and Ramadan for Muslims; however, in most cases, small children, pregnant women, older adults, and sick individuals are not required to fast.

While there is ongoing debate on the safety and potential outcomes of fasting in pregnant women, cultural norms, fears of adverse pregnancy outcomes, prepregnancy body mass index (BMI), gestational age, maternal guilt for breaking tradition, and the opinion and attitude of the husband all impact the woman's decision making (van Bilsen et al., 2016). Most practitioners agree that any woman with risk factors, such as a history of preterm birth, preterm labor, diabetes, or any other risk factors, should abstain from prolonged fasting. Ramadan fasting can actually be made up by a woman who chose not to participate during pregnancy once the woman has given birth and recovered beyond the immediate postpartum period. Fasting is also not recommended for breastfeeding women due to dehydration that can decrease the milk supply (van Bilsen et al., 2016).

Some cultures value large size or may associate a healthy baby with being large. Many Western cultures honor being slim in the media but reinforce overeating and large size by positive images of large sports stars, which can result in confusion about health and body image. In the United States, the availability of prepared foods, large portion sizes, and frequent consumption of fast foods and high-calorie foods has led to an obesity epidemic. Although most Americans favor slim body builds, the rising epidemic of obesity has led to adverse health outcomes, both physical and psychologic.

Nutrition may also be essential to a culture's practices for health promotion and care during illness. Health problems associated with specific cultures that may require dietary changes should be identified. Nutrition can be closely related to environmental situations, and families with few resources may not be able to obtain or eat cultural foods due to access or financial issues. Nutrition plays a powerful role in maintaining health, so resources for nutritious and desired foods may be needed.

●○● NURSING MANAGEMENT

For Providing Culturally Competent Care

The focus of nursing care is assessment of cultural influences on the patient's health. To provide culturally competent care, you must consider all facets of the patient's culture, including cultural influences and cultural barriers.

Nursing Assessment

Assessment of the woman or family includes determining the family's cultural healthcare beliefs and practices. Questions may include:

- Who in the family must be consulted before decisions are made about the patient's care?
- Does the patient see primarily in the present or does she have a futuristic time orientation?
- What type of health provider is most appropriate for (or preferred by) the woman or the family?
- Does the family have beliefs or traditions that may affect the plan of care?

Several cultural assessment tools are available to assist in gathering this information. These tools are becoming increasingly common at healthcare agencies as providers act in response to the expectation of culturally competent care. Respecting cultural diversity makes you an asset to the childbearing family as they adjust to their new role. Establishing a trusting relationship enables you to assist the family in meeting educational needs. A sample cultural assessment tool is presented in Table 2–3.

The use of North American Nursing Diagnosis Association (NANDA) nursing diagnoses to describe situations specifically related to culture may in itself be culturally biased because the foci of these diagnoses are based on Western cultural beliefs. Diagnoses such as *Communication: Verbal, Impaired* or *Knowledge, Deficient* should not be used solely because a person does not speak English. Is someone who speaks a different language "impaired" in communication?

Specific nursing diagnoses are dependent on the reason the family seeks contact with healthcare professionals, ranging from a woman's health problems, to pregnancy, to a newborn's health promotion and health maintenance. Examples include:

- ***Health Management: Ineffective***, related to mistrust of healthcare personnel
- ***Fear*** related to separation from support system in stressful situation, such as hospitalization
- ***Spiritual Distress*** related to discrepancy between spiritual beliefs and prescribed treatment
- ***Family Processes, Interrupted***, related to a shift in family roles due to illness

(NANDA-I © 2017)

Nursing Plan and Implementation

The planning and implementation of nursing care for the culturally diverse family depend specifically on the findings of the previous assessments. By partnering with the family, you can establish a safe, effective, and desirable plan of care. Ensure access to an interpreter, if necessary, and evaluate whether the match with a particular interpreter is appropriate for the woman and her family members.

A culturally competent nurse finds effective ways to partner with the woman and family members to assist them in determining how they can incorporate medically prescribed therapies with their own healthcare practices. Ensure that the woman and the family understand the problem or illness, treatment, and health promotion activities. Apply culturally sensitive techniques when dispelling any cultural myths.

TABLE 2–3 Sample Cultural Assessment

1. How do you view healthcare (e.g., accepting, fearful, suspicious)?	2. How do you relate to individuals outside of your cultural group (e.g., openly, fearfully, withdrawn, quiet, talkative, with trust)?
3. How do you express emotions in your culture?	4. How is religion or spirituality expressed in your culture? How does your culture view death, dying, and grief? How does your culture view modesty?
5. What are norms for male–female interactions and relationships? What are your expectations for the nurse–patient relationship?	6. Does your cultural group have any restrictions on medication use, medical procedures, or surgery? How does your culture view sexuality? Is there any fear of the dead or is it preferred that deceased persons not be discussed?
7. What is your native language? What language is spoken at home? What language do you read? What is your preferred language for healthcare discussions? What is your fluency level? Do you prefer an interpreter?	8. How do you prefer to be addressed? Are there any communication factors that are the norm in your culture (e.g., eye contact, avoidance of certain topics, confidentiality, speed of conversation)? What types of nonverbal communication are common in your culture?
9. Do you prefer healthcare providers from the same cultural group? What are your feelings about having healthcare providers from different backgrounds, gender, and age?	10. What things do you feel contribute to health and illness (e.g., moral transgressions, divine wrath, imbalances of hot and cold)? What is your cultural belief about the ideal body shape and size? What things do you believe promote health (e.g., exercise, diet, prayer)?
11. What are your religious beliefs? How strongly do you affiliate with these beliefs? Do you utilize cultural healers?	12. What complementary and alternative medicine practices do you routinely use? How do you perceive healthcare workers and nurses? What expectations do you have for your nurse? How do you perceive the "sick role"? How do people from your culture perceive being ill? What are your cultural views on mental illness?
13. What are traditional foods you eat? Avoid? How is food prepared? Are there certain foods you do not eat? Who purchases and prepares meals? How often are meals consumed? Where do you purchase food? Are you on any special diet? Does your culture or religious beliefs forbid you to eat certain foods?	14. Who is in your social network? Who provides support and caring to your family? What activities of health promotion does your family engage in? Are any self-care activities performed by family members? Is there a key decision maker within the family for healthcare decisions?
15. What is the family's economic status? Who is the primary wage earner? Do you have insurance coverage? How does your income affect your living conditions and ability to provide basic needs?	16. Are there any specific genetic or acquired disorders associated with your cultural group? Are there any socioenvironmental conditions more prominent in your cultural group?
17. What are your cultural beliefs regarding newborns, children, and older adults?	

Sources: Data from Andrews, M. M., & Boyle, J. S. (2015). *Transcultural concepts in nursing care* (7th ed.). Philadelphia, PA: Lippincott Williams & Wilkins; Spector, R. E. (2017). *Cultural diversity in health and illness* (8th ed.). Boston, MA: Pearson.

Collaborate with a multidisciplinary team, including social workers and language specialists, to assist the family in receiving assistance with barriers to care, such as transportation, financial issues, remote access, and others.

Complementary Health Approaches and the Family

Throughout most of the 20th century in the United States, it was rare for European American childbearing families to consult anyone except their obstetrician for advice about their pregnancy, birth, and postpartum period. Though such patients are still encountered today, nurses are more likely to care for families who integrate other types of practitioners and therapies with traditional Western medicine.

Although the terms *complementary*, *integrative*, and *alternative* are often used interchangeably, they have different meanings and applications. A **complementary therapy** may be defined as any procedure or product that is used as an adjunct to conventional medical treatment (National Center for Complementary and Integrative Health [NCCIH], 2016). Although complementary therapies were absent from clinics and hospitals until the past few decades, therapies such as acupuncture, acupressure, and massage therapy are now often used with conventional medical care, and many health insurance plans cover at least a portion of the cost of such therapies.

Integrative health approaches involve using complementary and conventional medical techniques together in a coordinated manner to relieve pain, address side effects of drug therapies and pain in cancer patients, and foster programs to promote healthy behaviors, among other practices.

In contrast, an **alternative therapy** is usually considered a substance or procedure that is used in place of conventional medicine (NCCIH, 2016). It usually has not undergone rigorous scientific testing in this country, although it might have been thoroughly tested in other countries. Alternative therapies are not usually available in conventional clinics and hospitals, and their costs typically are not covered under most health insurance policies. An example of an alternative therapy is the use of herbal medicines instead of biomedicines for the treatment of an individual's health condition. In other words, the person would not receive traditional Western medical care for the condition, such as surgery, radiation, prescribed medications, or other medical interventions.

The dramatic increase in complementary health approaches that began in the final decade of the 20th century was probably the result of a combination of several factors:

- Increased consumer awareness of the limitations of conventional Western medicine
- Increased international travel
- Increased media attention
- Advent of the internet.

In this century, it seems clear that Western healthcare will see an ever-increasing integration between conventional medicine and complementary approaches. Some obvious examples of this new integration in perinatal settings include the acceptance of certain herbal teas for antepartum discomforts; the use of massage, Reiki, or therapeutic touch during the first stage of labor; music during childbirth; and the increased emphasis on skin-to-skin mother-to-baby bonding in the immediate postpartum period. See *Women with Special Needs: Utilizing Complementary Therapies*.

Women with Special Needs **Utilizing Complementary Therapies**

Complementary therapies in combination with traditional Western medicine interventions are used with increasing frequency by women with physical and mental disabilities. Many treatment options are limited for women with disabilities because of lack of insurance or public assistance funding. Alternative therapies may be beneficial for women with certain chronic medical conditions (Nathenson & Nathenson, 2013).

Benefits and Risks

Complementary or alternative health approaches have many benefits. Many complementary or alternative therapies emphasize prevention and wellness and place a higher value on holistic healing than on physical cure.

SAFETY ALERT!

Complementary or alternative health approaches must be assessed for safety, including positive and negative benefits, cost, efficacy, and clinical usefulness. The use of herbs and natural products raises many issues, including standards of products, misleading claims, and safety related to megadoses of some products. This is especially important in pregnant women since any medication or alternative therapy can directly impact the developing fetus.

Determine the family's use of alternative therapies, such as the type of remedies and healthcare practices used. Also determine the side effects, risks, and other implications to the individual receiving this type of therapy. Work with the family to ensure safe practices with the use of complementary and/or alternative modalities.

Types of Complementary Health Approaches

Numerous forms of complementary therapies are available. Only a few of the most commonly used approaches are presented here.

HOMEOPATHY

Homeopathy is a healing approach in which a person is treated with small doses of medicines that would cause illness when given to someone who is healthy. Traditional Western (or allopathic) medicine generally gives medicine or treatments that suppress symptoms. Analgesics for pain or antibiotics for infection are examples of such treatments. In homeopathy, the symptoms are viewed as the body's method of healing, and small doses of medications are given to enhance the symptoms. For example, medications are chosen to promote fever and inflammation since they are thought to be healing forces (Fontaine, 2011; Spector, 2017).

NATUROPATHY

Naturopathy is a form of medicine that utilizes the healing forces of nature and is commonly referred to as natural medicine. It is more precisely defined as a healing system that combines safe and effective traditional means of preventing and treating human disease with the most current advances in modern medicine (American Association of Naturopathic Physicians [AANP], 2017). Many naturopathic physicians are eclectic, employing a variety of therapies in their practice. These might include clinical nutrition, botanical medicine, homeopathy, natural childbirth, traditional Chinese medicine, hydrotherapy, naturopathic manipulative therapy, pharmacology, minor surgery, and counseling for lifestyle modifications (AANP, 2017).

TRADITIONAL CHINESE MEDICINE

Traditional Chinese medicine (TCM) was developed more than 3000 years ago in the Chinese culture and then gradually spread with modifications to other Asian countries. The underlying focus of TCM is prevention, although diagnosis and treatment of disease also play an important role.

TCM seeks to ensure the balance of energy, which is called *chi* or *qi* (pronounced "chee"). Chi is the invisible flow of energy in the body that maintains health and energy and enables the body to carry out its physiologic functions. Chi flows along certain pathways or meridians.

Another important concept in TCM is that of *yin* and *yang*, opposing internal and external forces that, together, represent the whole (Figure 2–4).

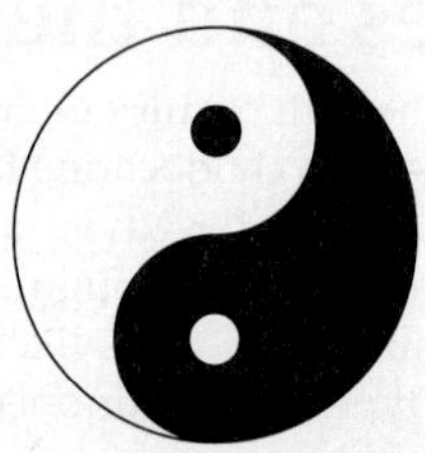

Figure 2-4 **Traditional Chinese symbol of the opposing forces of *yin* and *yang* in perfect balance, representing integration and wholeness.**

TCM includes the following therapeutic techniques:

- *Acupuncture* uses very fine (hairlike) stainless steel needles to stimulate specific acupuncture points, depending on the patient's medical assessment and condition.
- *Acupressure* (Chinese massage) uses pressure from the fingers and thumbs to stimulate pressure points.
- *Herbal therapy* is an important part of TCM, but it is sometimes difficult to locate a skilled herbalist because there are relatively few in the United States and other English-speaking countries.
- *Qi gong* (pronounced "chee-goong") is a self-discipline that involves the use of breathing, meditation, self-massage, and movement. Typically practiced daily, the movements are nontiring and are designed to stimulate the flow of chi (Figure 2–5).
- *T'ai chi* (pronounced "ty chee") is a form of martial art. It originally focused on physical fitness and self-defense, but it is currently used to improve health as well (Spector, 2017).
- *Moxibustion* involves the application of heat from a small piece of burning herb called *moxa (Artemisia vulgaris)*. The moxa stick is typically burned at the lateral side of the little toe. In TCM moxibustion has many uses. For example, studies from China demonstrate good success when moxibustion is used to help turn a fetus that is breech to a vertex presentation (Cuneo, 2017).

"I am so glad that complementary therapies are becoming more accepted. I don't plan to stop going to see my doctor, but now that I am pregnant I like doing things on my own to improve my health. I used acupressure wrist bands early on and felt they really helped my nausea. I'm taking Qi gong classes now, and I feel terrific!"

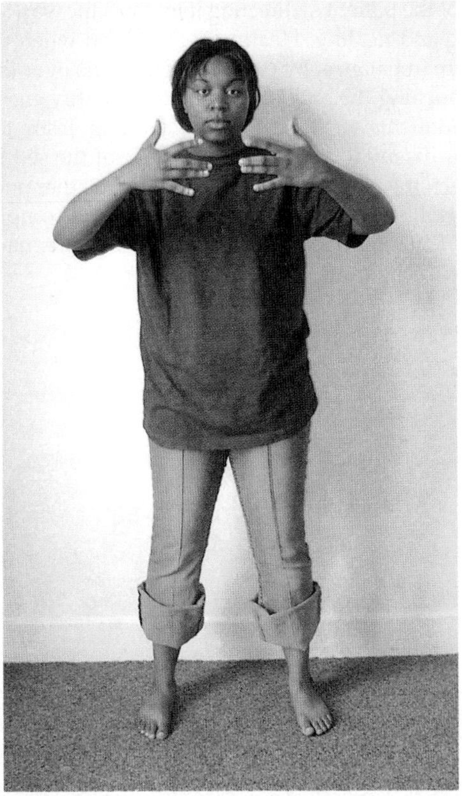

Figure 2–5 **Pregnant woman practices the movements of Qi gong.**

SOURCE: Michele Davidson.

MIND-BASED THERAPIES

- ***Biofeedback*** is a method used to help individuals learn to control their physiologic responses based on the concept that the mind controls the body. An individual is hooked up to a system of highly sensitive instruments that relay information about the body back to that person. Currently, biofeedback has more than 150 applications for disease prevention and the restoration of health. The effectiveness of biofeedback has been proven in countless studies, and it is now considered a conventional therapy more than a complementary one.
- ***Hypnosis***, whether guided by a trained hypnotherapist or induced through self-hypnosis, is a state of great mental and physical relaxation during which a person is very open to suggestions. In this state the individual is able to modify body responses. Pregnant women who receive hypnosis before childbirth have reported shorter, less painful labors and births.
- ***Visualization*** is a complementary therapy in which a person goes into a relaxed state and focuses on or "visualizes" soothing or positive scenes, such as a beach or a mountain glade. Visualization helps reduce stress and encourage relaxation.
- ***Guided imagery*** is a state of intense, focused concentration used to create compelling mental images. It is sometimes considered a form of hypnosis. Guided imagery is useful in imagining a desired effect, such as weight loss, or in mentally rehearsing a new procedure or activity.

CHIROPRACTIC

Chiropractic, the third largest independent health profession in the United States (behind medicine and dentistry), is based on concepts of manipulation to address health problems that are thought to be the result of abnormal nerve transmissions (subluxation) caused by misalignment of the spine. In the United States doctors of chiropractic perform more than 90% of all spinal manipulations (American Chiropractic Association, 2017). Chiropractors also stress the importance of proper nutrition and regular exercise for good health. Chiropractic is widely available, and popular demand has earned it a higher level of insurance coverage than most other alternative therapies.

MASSAGE THERAPY

Massage has been used for centuries as a form of therapy. *Massage therapy* involves manipulation of the soft tissues of the body to reduce stress and tension, increase circulation, diminish pain, and promote a sense of well-being. Different techniques have been developed, including Swedish massage, shiatsu massage, Rolfing, and trigger point massage. Most forms use techniques, such as pressing, kneading, gliding, circular motion, tapping, and vibrational strokes.

Certain massage therapists specialize in massage for women during pregnancy (Figure 2–6). Massage is often helpful as women adapt to the discomforts of their changing bodies. Certified nurse-midwives often use perineal massage prior to labor to stretch the muscles of the perineum around the vaginal opening and thereby prevent tearing of the tissues during childbirth. During labor, massage of the back and buttocks by the nurse, labor coach, or doula can help the woman relax and may help decrease her discomfort.

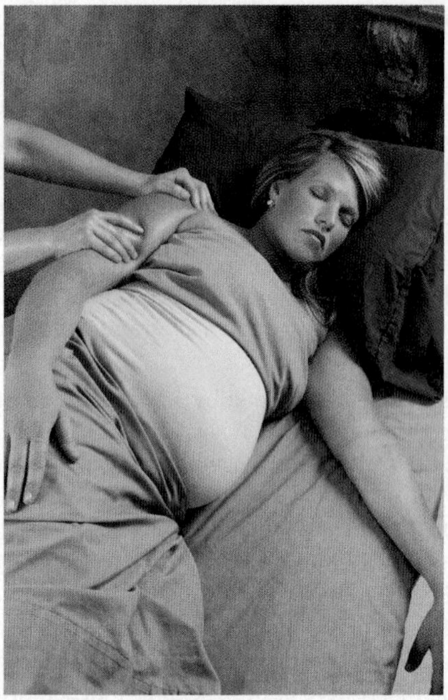

Figure 2–6 **Massage is often useful in helping a pregnant woman cope with the discomforts of pregnancy.**

SOURCE: Alfred Wekelo/Fotolia.

Infant massage is also growing in popularity in the United States, and many parents have learned to massage their infants and young children (Figure 2–7).

> “I got into infant massage when Ryan was born. I loved the time we spent together, and I am convinced it was part of the reason he was such a good baby.”

HERBAL THERAPIES

Herbal therapy or herbal medicine has been used since ancient times to treat illnesses and ailments. Well-known herbal remedies include ginger, rosemary, ginseng, ginkgo, chamomile, oil of evening primrose, echinacea, garlic, lemon balm, and black cohosh.

Herbs are categorized as dietary supplements and are controlled by the Dietary Supplement Health Education Act. They do not require approval by the Food and Drug Administration (FDA) as do prescription and over-the-counter medications; however, the FDA does have the authority to pull a product off the market if it is proven to be dangerous (FDA, 2017). Consequently, most of what is known about herbs comes from Germany, where they have been studied for some time (Fontaine, 2014). See *Developing Cultural Competence: Herbalism.*

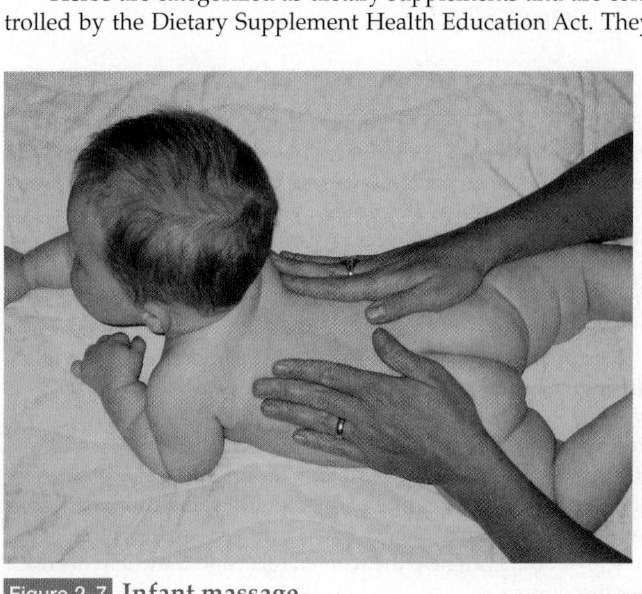

Figure 2–7 **Infant massage.**

SOURCE: Michele Davidson.

SAFETY ALERT!

The use of herbs during pregnancy is an especially important consideration for nurses working with childbearing families. Pregnant and lactating women interested in using herbs are best advised to consult with their healthcare provider before taking any herbs, even as teas. Lists identifying common herbs that women are advised to avoid or use with caution during pregnancy and lactation are available.

Developing Cultural Competence Herbalism

The World Health Organization estimates that 80% of the earth's population depends on plants to treat common ailments. Herbalism is an essential part of traditional Indian, Asian, Native American, and naturopathic medicines. Many homeopathic remedies are also developed from herbs (University of Maryland Medical Center, 2012).

THERAPEUTIC TOUCH

Therapeutic touch (TT) is grounded in the belief that people are a system of energy with a self-healing potential. The therapeutic touch practitioner, often a nurse, can unite his or her energy field with that of the patient's, directing it in a specific way to promote well-being and healing. Healing is promoted when the body's energies are in balance. By passing their hands over the patient, without touching the patient, healers can identify energy imbalances. Proponents of TT believe that a strong desire to help the recipient is essential, as is a conscious use of the self to act as a link between the universal life energy and the other person (Fontaine, 2014). Like many other conventional and complementary therapies, TT should be applied cautiously to pregnant women and newborns by trained providers (Figure 2–8).

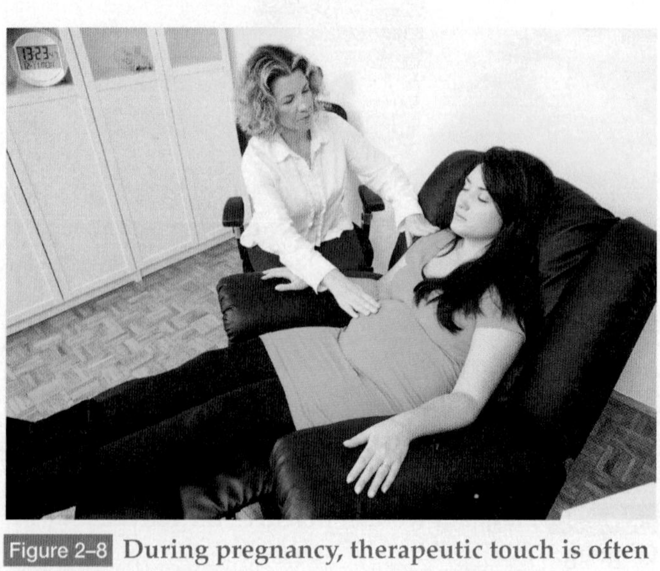

Figure 2–8 **During pregnancy, therapeutic touch is often helpful in easing pain and reducing anxiety.**

SOURCE: Dean Bertoncelj/Shutterstock.

OTHER TYPES OF COMPLEMENTARY HEALTH APPROACHES

This discussion has touched on only some of the most common forms of complementary health therapies. Other examples include *ayurveda* (the traditional medicine of India), meditation, craniosacral therapy, reflexology, hydrotherapy, hatha yoga, regular physical exercise, aromatherapy, color and light therapy, music and sound therapies, magnetic therapy, and Reiki. Readers interested in these therapies are referred to specialty texts.

Nursing Care of the Family Using Complementary Therapies

According to a 2012 National Health Interview Survey conducted by the NCCIH, some form of complementary health approach is used by 33.2% of adults and 11.6% of children in the United States (Fontaine, 2014). When prayer for health reasons and megavitamin therapy are added to the definition, the number increases to 62%. Women use *complementary and alternative medicine (CAM)* more often than men do, as do people with higher educational levels and people who have been hospitalized within the past year. Use of CAM in pregnancy was associated with a desire for a normal birth and a rewarding emotional birth experience (Fontaine, 2014).

The possibility that families may use CAM and not reveal it to healthcare professionals raises some concern. Certain CAM modalities, such as biofeedback, acupuncture, aromatherapy, and massage, are not likely to cause adverse effects. However, the possibility exists that there might be interactions between herbal therapies and other medications prescribed by the healthcare provider (Fontaine, 2014). Complications may also develop from the use of vitamin supplements.

Nurses who create a climate of respect and openness tend to be more effective in gathering information about a family's use of complementary or alternative therapies. The nurse should use a nonjudgmental approach in assessing pregnant women and families for the use of complementary health approaches. Identify the expected outcome of the herbal or dietary supplement. The nurse should ask specifically about the use of herbs and other supplements, as the pregnant woman may not think to include them in her list of medications. The nurse should discuss therapies in depth with the woman because some CAM practices could be harmful in pregnancy and should be avoided.

Nurses should use complementary modalities that are in the scope of their nursing practice and the nursing practice act in their state. Their use should also be supported by evidence-based research. Nurses working with pregnant women might use acupressure wristbands for the treatment of nausea. Other therapies nurses often employ include progressive relaxation, exercise and movement, therapeutic touch, visualization and guided imagery, prayer, meditation, music therapy, massage, storytelling, aromatherapy, and journaling.

Nurses who use complementary modalities should document their use within the context of nursing practice. This is most effective when the modality is identified as an intervention to address a specific nursing diagnosis or identified patient need. Thus, music therapy might be used for a laboring woman to help address the identified nursing diagnosis of *Pain, Acute* (NANDA-I © 2017).

Nurses have a role in conducting and supporting research on complementary health approaches. Because of the variety of complementary therapies in use, research is needed in a host of areas. The results of research on complementary health approaches can be found in professional journals and at the NCCIH website. As the evidence supporting the use of certain interventions grows, nurses and other healthcare providers are incorporating the results as part of their evidence-based practice.Source: Wong yu liang/Fotolia.Source: Kinga/Shutterstock

Focus Your Study

- Family values, roles, and power are important to consider when attempting to provide holistic healthcare to childbearing families.
- Nuclear families consist of a mother, father, and children.
- Dual-career/dual-earner families comprise the majority of contemporary families in the United States.
- Child-free families are a growing trend in American culture.
- Extended family members can play an active role in family life, decision making, and family roles.
- Single-parent families account for almost one-third of all U.S. families, and stepparent and binuclear families are increasingly common.
- The single mother by choice family represents a family composed of an unmarried woman who chooses to conceive or adopt without a life partner.
- A binuclear family is a postdivorce family in which the biologic children are members of two nuclear households, with co-parenting by the parents.
- A heterosexual cohabitating family describes a heterosexual couple who may or may not have children and who live together outside of marriage.
- Gay and lesbian families include those in which two adults of the same sex live together as spouses or domestic partners with or without children and those in which a gay or lesbian single parent rears a child.
- The developmental framework looks at a family over time as it progresses through predictable stages within the life cycle.
- A family assessment provides an in-depth tool to collect pertinent family life information that can assist the nurse in planning care.
- Culture plays a significant part in a family's development, assignment of roles, and observance of traditions, customs, and taboos.
- Cultural norms influence a family's beliefs about the importance of children, pregnancy, health practices, and newborn/infant feeding.

- Providing culturally competent care involves recognizing the importance of the childbearing family's value system, acknowledging that differences occur among people, and respecting and responding to ethnic diversity in a way that leads to mutually desirable outcomes.
- A cultural assessment can assist the nurse in identifying cultural norms and in providing culturally appropriate nursing care. It should focus on factors that will influence the practices of the childbearing family with regard to health needs and may include a religious history.
- Providing spiritually sensitive care involves determining the current spiritual and religious beliefs and practices that will affect the mother and baby, accommodating these practices where possible, and examining one's own spiritual or religious beliefs to be more aware and able to provide nonjudgmental care.
- A complementary therapy is an adjunct to conventional medical treatment, whereas an alternative therapy is used in place of prescribed medical therapy.
- Complementary health approaches have several benefits. Many of them emphasize prevention and wellness, place a higher value on holistic healing than on physical cure, are noninvasive, and have few side effects. In addition, many are more affordable and available than conventional therapies.
- Risks of using complementary therapies include lack of standardization, lack of regulation and research substantiating safety and effectiveness, inadequate training and certification of some healers, and financial and health risks of unproven methods.
- Homeopathy is a healing system that uses like to cure like; that is, homeopathic remedies are minute dilutions of substances that, if ingested in larger amounts, would produce effects *similar* to the symptoms of the disorder being treated.
- Traditional Chinese medicine (TCM) seeks to ensure the balance of energy, called *chi* or *qi*. TCM techniques include acupuncture, acupressure, herbal therapy, Qi gong, t'ai chi, and moxibustion.
- Biofeedback is a method used to help individuals learn to control their physiologic responses based on the concept that the mind controls the body.
- Hypnosis, whether guided by a trained hypnotherapist or induced through self-hypnosis, is a state of great mental and physical relaxation during which a person is very open to suggestions.
- Guided imagery is a state of intense, focused concentration used to create compelling mental images.
- Chiropractic, a profession practiced by licensed chiropractors, is based on concepts of manipulation, especially spinal manipulation.
- Massage therapy involves manipulation of the soft tissues of the body to reduce stress and tension, increase circulation, diminish pain, and promote a sense of well-being.
- Herbal therapy has been used since ancient times; well-known herbal remedies include ginger, rosemary, ginseng, ginkgo, chamomile, oil of evening primrose, echinacea, garlic, lemon balm, and black cohosh.
- Therapeutic touch is based on the belief that people are a system of energy with a self-healing potential. The therapeutic touch practitioner, often a nurse, can unite his or her energy field with that of the patient's, directing it in a specific way to promote well-being and healing.
- Many nurses are open to and supportive of complementary and alternative therapies. Nurses who incorporate such therapies into their practice must be certain that they are practicing within the framework of their nurse practice act and with the informed consent of their patients.

In order to make safe and effective judgments using NANDA-I © 2017 nursing diagnoses, it is essential that nurses refer to the definitions and defining characteristics of the diagnoses used in this text, which can be found in Appendix C.

References

American Association of Naturopathic Physicians (AANP). (2017). *Definition of naturopathic medicine.* Retrieved from http://naturopathic.org/content.asp?contentid=59

American Chiropractic Association. (2017). *Spinal manipulation.* Retrieved from https://www.acatoday.org/Patients/Why-Choose-Chiropractic/What-is-Chiropractic

Andrews, M. M., & Boyle, J. S. (2015). *Transcultural concepts in nursing care* (7th ed.). Philadelphia, PA: Lippincott Williams & Wilkins.

Arousell, J., & Carlbom, A. (2016). Culture and religious beliefs in relation to reproductive health. *Best Practice and Research: Clinical Obstetrics and Gynaecology, 32,* 77–87.

Brink, S. (2015). Selecting boys over girls is a trend in more and more countries. National Public Radio (NPR). Retrieved from http://www.npr.org/sections/goatsandsoda/2015/08/26/434616512/selecting-boys-over-girls-is-a-trend-in-more-and-more-countries

Centers for Disease Control and Prevention. (CDC). (2017). *Cultural competence.* Retrieved from https://npin.cdc.gov/pages/cultural-competence

Cuneo, J. (2017). Women's health: Pregnancy and conception. *Primary Care: Clinics in Office Practice, 44*(2), 369–376.

Denham, S.A., & Eggenberger, S. (2015). *Family-focused nursing care.* Philadelphia: F.A. Davis.

Duvall, E. M., & Miller, B. L. (1985). *Marriage and family development* (6th ed.). New York, NY: HarperCollins.

Ellwood, W. (2016). *The cultural framework for health. Culture: Oft-missed key explanatory variable in health research.* Bethesda, MD: National Institutes of Health.

Fontaine, K. L. (2014). *Complementary and alternative therapies for nursing practice* (4th ed.). Upper Saddle River, NJ: Pearson.

Food and Drug Administration (FDA). (2017). *Dietary supplements.* Retrieved from http://www.fda.gov/Food/DietarySupplements/

Genetic Disease Foundation. (2017). *Genetic testing and pregnancy.* Retrieved from http://www.knowyourgenes.org/planning-carrier-screening.shtml

Golden, J. (2017). "Doctor's don't do so much good": Traditional practices, biomedicine, and infant care in the 20th-century United States. *Nursing History Review, 25,* 86. Retrieved from http://dx.doi.org/10.1891/1062-8061.25.86

Graham, A., Sandberg, J. C., Quandt, S. A., Mora, D. C., & Arcury, T. A. (2016). Manual therapy practices of sobadores in North Carolina. *Journal of Alternative and Complementary Medicine, 22*(10), 841–846. DOI:10.1089/acm.2015.0323

Hendl, T., & Rothman, B. K. (2016). Sex selection. In N. A. Naples, R. C. Hoogland, M. Wickramasinghe, & W. C. A. Wong (Eds.), *The Wiley Blackwell encyclopedia of gender and sexuality studies.* Hoboken, NJ: Wiley.

Krause, N., Pargament, K. I., Hill, P. C., & Ironson, G. (2016). Humility, stressful life events, and psychological well-being: Findings from the landmark spirituality and health survey. *The Journal of Positive Psychology, 11*(5), 1–12.

Kuzawa, C. W., & Gravlee, C. C. (2016). Beyond genetic race: Biocultural insights into the causes of racial health disparities. In M. K. Zuckerman & D. L. Martin (Eds.), *New directions in biocultural anthropology.* Hoboken, NJ: Wiley.

McFarland, M. R., & Wehbe-Almah, H. B. (2014). *Leininger's culture care diversity and universality.* Boston, MA: Jones & Bartlett.

Nathenson, S. L., & Nathenson, P. (2013). Integrative wellness in rehabilitation: Social and behavioral aspects of healthcare and clinical applications. *Rehabilitation Nursing, 38*(6), 276–283. DOI:10.1002/rnj.80

National Center for Complementary and Integrative Health (NCCIH). (2016). *Complementary, alternative, or integrative health: What's in a name?* Retrieved from https://nccih.nih.gov/health/integrative-health

Ono, K., & Aczel, A. D. (2016). *My search for Ramanujan: How I learned to count.* New York, NY: Springer.

Oxford Dictionaries. (2016). *Shaman.* Retrieved from https://en.oxforddictionaries.com/definition/shaman

Pew Research Center. (2016). *Religious landscape study.* Retrieved from http://www.pewforum.org/religious-landscape-study

Purnell, L. D. (2013). *Transcultural healthcare: A culturally competent approach* (4th ed.). Philadelphia, PA: F. A. Davis.

Single Mothers by Choice. (2016). *About single mothers by choice.* Retrieved from http://www.singlemothersbychoice.org

Sorenson, E. (2015). *An analysis of hegemony in LDS discourse on motherhood.* Doctoral dissertation, Utah State University. Retrieved from http://digitalcommons.usu.edu/cgi/viewcontent.cgi?article=1729&context=gradreports

Spector, R. E. (2017). *Cultural diversity in health and illness* (9th ed.). Hoboken, NJ: Pearson.

University of Maryland Medical Center. (2012). *Herbal medicine.* Retrieved from https://www.umms.org/ummc/patients-visitors/health-library/medical-encyclopedia/carepoints/a-guide-to-herbal-remedies

U.S. Census Bureau. (2017). *Definition: Household and family.* Retrieved from https://ask.census.gov

van Bilsen, L. A., Savitri, A. I., Amelia, D., Baharuddin, M., Grobbee, D. E., & Uiterwaal, C. S. (2016). Predictors of Ramadan fasting during pregnancy. *Journal of Epidemiology and Global Health, 6*(4), 267–275.

Women's Health Across the Lifespan

Part II

Chapter 3

Health Promotion

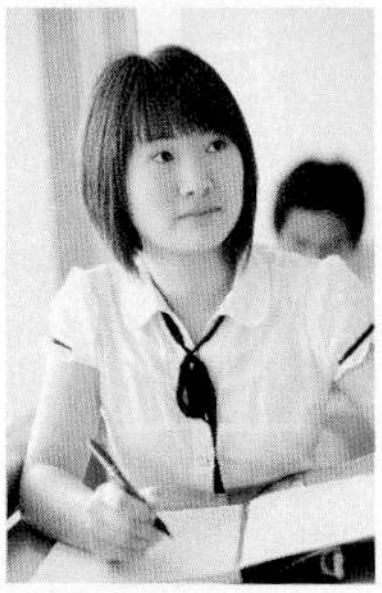

SOURCE: Glow Asia/SuperStock.

This is a great time to be a woman. I feel like I can accomplish just about whatever I put my mind to. There are more opportunities for women now in education, sports, and involvement in the community. I intend to take good care of this body and mind and strive for something great.

Learning Outcomes

3.1 Discuss the key points a nurse should consider when taking a sexual history.

3.2 Summarize information that women may need in order to implement appropriate self-care measures for dealing with menstruation.

3.3 Identify causes of amenorrhea.

3.4 Contrast the signs, symptoms, and nursing management of women with dysmenorrhea and those with premenstrual syndrome.

3.5 Delineate the physical and psychologic aspects of menopause.

3.6 Explain the relationship between menopause and osteoporosis.

3.7 Identify medical and complementary therapies to alleviate the discomforts of menopause.

Healthy People 2020

(AOCBC-10) Reduce the proportion of adults with osteoporosis

(AOCBC-11) Reduce hip fractures among older adults

(DIA-1) (Developmental) Increase the proportion of persons with diagnosed Alzheimer disease and other dementias, or their caregivers, who are aware of the diagnosis

(DIA-2) (Developmental) Reduce the proportion of preventable hospitalizations in persons with diagnosed Alzheimer disease and other dementias

A woman's healthcare needs change throughout her lifetime. As a young girl, she requires health teaching about menstruation, sexuality, and personal responsibility. As a teen she needs information about reproductive choices and safe sexual activity. During this time, she should also be introduced to the importance of healthcare practices, such as regular Pap smears. The mature woman may need to be reminded of these self-care issues and prepare for physical changes that accompany childbirth and aging. By educating women about their bodies, their healthcare choices, and their rights and responsibilities, nurses can help women be knowledgeable consumers who assume responsibility for the healthcare they receive.

Community-Based Nursing Care

Women's health refers to a holistic view of women and their health-related needs within the context of their everyday lives. It is based on the awareness that a woman's physical, mental, and social statuses are interdependent and determine her state of health or illness. The woman's perception of her situation and her assessment of her needs, her values, and her beliefs are valid, important factors to be incorporated into any healthcare intervention.

Clinical Tip

When making decisions about effective methods for communicating with a family about healthcare issues, remember that a woman's views frequently influence the healthcare of her entire family because women typically coordinate the family's healthcare needs.

Nurses can provide health teaching and information about self-care practices in schools, during routine examinations in a clinic or office, at senior centers, at meetings of volunteer organizations, through classes offered by the local health department or community college, or in the home. Nurses can also help women with various forms of disability to address their unique healthcare needs and optimize their state of wellness. This community-based focus is the key to providing effective nursing care to women of all ages.

In reality, the vast majority of women's healthcare is provided outside of acute care settings. Nurses oriented to community-based care are especially effective in recognizing the autonomy of each individual and in dealing with patients holistically. This approach is important in addressing not only physical problems but also major health issues, such as violence against women, which may go undetected unless care providers ask women specifically about violence and are alert for signs of it. See *Developing Cultural Competence: Understanding Cultural Differences*.

Developing Cultural Competence Understanding Cultural Differences

The U.S. population is made up of many ethnic and cultural groups. The U.S. Census Bureau (2016) reports that the immigrant population in the United States has reached about 40.1 million people, or almost 13% of the total population. As a nurse you will be caring for women and families from diverse cultures. It is important to avoid ethnocentrism and to approach the childbearing woman with openness to learning about her traditions and cultural preferences. Understanding subtle differences in various cultures will help you initiate conversation and ask questions that will allow the woman to offer information about her preferences.

The Nurse's Role in Addressing Issues of Women's Wellness and Sexuality

Women expect the nurses who care for them to be knowledgeable not only about gynecologic health, but also about a wide variety of health topics. Thus, it is important that nurses expand their knowledge about the issues healthy women and their families may face. These include, for example, a general knowledge of normal growth and development; recommended screening procedures for both women and men and the ages at which these procedures are indicated; signs and symptoms of substance abuse, including alcoholism; health issues that well men face; signs of emotional stress and depression; and community resources. By keeping abreast of issues well families may face, the nurse becomes a more complete resource and is better able to promote overall health.

On occasion women experience concern and even anxiety about some aspect of menstruation, contraception, or sexual activity. Societal standards and pressures can cause girls and adolescents to evaluate and compare with others their experiences with menstruation, sexual attractiveness, and beliefs and values about engaging in sexual activity. Young adults may be more concerned about the reproductive and health implications of sexual intercourse. The desire to achieve or avoid pregnancy and the fear of sexually transmitted infections may cause many women to modify their sexual practices and activities. Although older women share many of these same concerns, they may also experience anxiety about the onset of menopausal changes and wonder how these changes will affect their sexuality. Furthermore, throughout the lifespan women may have concerns, problems, and questions about sex roles, sexual orientation, behaviors, inhibitions, morality, and related areas, such as family planning. Recently divorced or widowed women who have been in long-term marriages may need education about sexual activity and sexually transmitted infections if they are reentering the dating world. Women frequently voice these concerns to the nurse in a clinic or ambulatory setting. Thus, the nurse may need to assume the role of counselor on sexual and reproductive matters.

Nurses who assume this role must develop an awareness of their own feelings, values, and attitudes about sexuality so that they can be more sensitive and objective when they encounter the values and beliefs of others. It is important for nurses to understand the structures and functions of the female and male reproductive systems (see Chapter 9) and to have accurate, up-to-date information about topics related to menstruation, sexuality, sexual practices, cultural differences, menopause, and common gynecologic problems.

Staying up to date on issues of sexuality and women's health requires constant vigilance: Regular journal review, attendance at reputable conferences, library and internet searches, and diligent perusal of women's health literature are essential activities. Continuing education for the practicing nurse and appropriate courses in undergraduate and graduate nursing education programs can also help nurses achieve and maintain the requisite knowledge. These activities enhance nurses' knowledge about these topics and improve their effectiveness in teaching and providing care for their patients.

Taking a Sexual History

Nurses today are often responsible for taking a woman's initial health history, including her gynecologic and sexual history. To be effective in this role, the nurse must have good communication skills and should ideally conduct the interview in a quiet, private place free of distractions.

Clinical Tip

When taking a history, start your interview with less intimate areas, such as medical and surgical history, and then proceed to the sexual history toward the end of the history-taking session. This approach helps the woman develop a comfort level with you before disclosing personal information.

Opening the sexual history discussion with a brief explanation of the purpose of such questions is often helpful. For example, the nurse might say, "As your nurse I'm interested in all aspects of your well-being. Often women have concerns or questions about sexual issues, especially as their life situations change. I will be asking you some questions about your sexual history as part of your general health history." This explanation will help women understand the nature of this part of the history and allow for more open, honest answers.

It may be helpful to use direct eye contact as much as possible unless the nurse knows it is culturally unacceptable to the woman. When possible, the nurse should limit the amount of writing or typing into a computer during this part of the interview. Open-ended questions are often useful in eliciting information. For example, "What, if anything, would you change about your sex life?" will elicit more information than "Are you happy with your sex life now?" The nurse should also clarify terminology to ensure accurate information is being conveyed. Proceeding from easier topics to those that are more difficult will help elicit a natural flow of information. Throughout the interview, the nurse should be alert to the woman's body language and nonverbal cues. It is essential that the nurse listen, react in a nonjudgmental manner, and use teachable moments to educate women about their bodies. It is also important that the nurse not assume that the woman is heterosexual. Some women are open about lesbian relationships or transgender surgery; others are more reserved until they develop a sense of trust in their caregivers.

After completing the sexual history, the nurse assesses the information obtained. If there is a concern that requires further medical tests and assessments, the nurse refers the woman to a nurse practitioner, certified nurse-midwife (CNM), physician, or counselor as necessary. In many instances the nurse alone will be able to develop a nursing diagnosis and then plan and implement an appropriate intervention. For example, if the nurse determines that a woman who is interested in conceiving a child does not have a clear understanding of when she ovulates, the nurse may formulate the nursing diagnosis *Knowledge, Deficient* (NANDA-I © 2017) related to lack of information about the timing of ovulation. The nurse can implement a plan of care to evaluate the woman's knowledge and then provide the necessary education.

The nurse must be realistic in making assessments and planning interventions. It requires insight and skill to recognize when a woman's problem requires interventions that are beyond a nurse's preparation and ability. In such cases, the nurse must make appropriate referrals.

Menstruation

Girls today begin to learn about puberty and menstruation at a young age. Unfortunately, the source of their "education" is sometimes their peers or the media; thus, the information is frequently incomplete, inaccurate, and sensationalized. Nurses who work with young girls and adolescents recognize this and strive to provide accurate health teaching and to correct any misinformation they have been given about *menarche* (the onset of menstruation) and the menstrual cycle.

Cultural, religious, and personal attitudes about menstruation play an integral part in the menstrual experience. Historically, misconceptions surrounding menstruation have led women to feelings of isolation and restricted women to the company of other women during their menstrual cycle because they were considered "unclean." Currently in the Western world, there are few customs associated with menstruation. Sexual intercourse during menstruation is a common practice and is not generally contraindicated. For most couples, the decision is one of personal preference. (The physiology of menstruation is discussed in Chapter 9.)

Counseling the Premenstrual Girl About Menarche

Menarche for well-nourished girls in developed countries generally occurs between 12 and 13 years of age (the median is 12.43 years), with a range between 9 and 15 years of age (American College of Obstetricians and Gynecologists [ACOG], 2015). It tends to occur earlier in girls who are obese, probably because they have gained a minimal required body mass index (BMI). Genetics is the most important factor in determining the age at which menarche starts but geographical location, nutrition, weight, and general health also play a role. Two years prior to menarche, a young girl begins to experience a series of physical changes as her body develops. Maturity level and self-confidence often influence a young girl's comfort in discussing these changes. However, the most critical factor in successful adaptation to menarche is the young girl's level of knowledge and understanding of correct information. The nurse is an excellent source of reliable information about puberty and menarche. Information should be clear and straightforward and offered as it relates to each girl's individual situation and maturation level. The following basic information is helpful for young patients:

- ***Cycle length:*** Cycle length is determined from the first day of one menses to the first day of the next menses. Initially, cycle length may be irregular. It is not unusual for cycles to be unpredictable for the first year. Once established, the cycle is about 28 to 30 days, but the normal length may vary from 21 to 35 days (Joshi & Jamshidl, 2017). Cycle length often varies by a day or two from one cycle to the next, although greater normal variations may also occur.
- ***Amount of flow:*** The average amount of flow is approximately 25 to 60 mL per period. Blood loss greater than 80 mL/cycle is considered abnormal. Usually women characterize the amount of flow in terms of the number of pads or tampons used. Flow is often heavier at first and lighter toward the end of the period.
- ***Length of menses:*** Menses usually lasts from 4 to 6 days, although the length may vary, and may last up to 7 days (Joshi & Jamshidl, 2017).

The nurse should stress that variations in age at menarche, length of cycle, and duration of menses are normal because girls are likely to be concerned if their experiences vary from those of their peers. It is also helpful to acknowledge the negative aspects of menstruation (messiness and embarrassment) while stressing its positive role as a symbol of maturity and womanhood.

Cultural factors may play an important role in menstruation for girls and women of some cultures. See *Developing Cultural Competence: Islamic Women and Menstruation*.

Developing Cultural Competence Islamic Women and Menstruation

Islamic women who are menstruating are not required to fast during the month of Ramadan, but if they elect not to fast, they are expected to make up the missed fasting days before the next Ramadan. Because it may be harder to fast alone, some Muslim women use oral contraceptives to delay their menses (Huda, 2016; Kridli, 2011). Others choose to fast even when menstruating.

Note: It is unwise to attribute specific attitudes or beliefs to all members of a cultural group. The information in the Developing Cultural Competence boxes offers possible insights into caring for women from different cultural groups.

Educational Topics

The nurse's primary role is to provide accurate information and assist in clarifying misconceptions so that girls will develop positive self-images and progress smoothly through this phase of maturation.

PADS AND TAMPONS

Since early times women have made pads from cloth or rags, which required washing but were reusable. Some women made them from gauze or cotton balls. Commercial tampons were introduced in the 1930s.

Today, adhesive-stripped, disposable minipads and maxipads and flushable tampons are readily available. However, the deodorants and increased absorbency that manufacturers have added to both sanitary napkins and tampons may prove harmful. The chemicals used to deodorize and increase absorbency can create irritation of the vulva and inner aspects of the vagina. This irritation may cause an external rash or internal sores from trauma to the tender mucosal lining of the vagina.

Interest is growing in the use of eco-friendly menstrual products, including reusable menstrual pads made of washable cotton, menstrual cups, and menstrual sponges (Figure 3–1). These products are becoming more readily available at pharmacies and major discount stores.

When taking a menstrual history, the nurse should attempt to determine the amount of bleeding each month. The woman can be asked what type of pad or tampon she uses, how frequently she changes it, and how much blood has been absorbed. Women should be advised to change pads frequently, every 3 to 6 hours when awake, regardless of the amount of blood that is absorbed. If a woman reports that she supersaturates a maxipad every 1 to 2 hours for 2 to 3 days, she may be experiencing a gynecologic problem requiring the need for further evaluation. Heavy menstrual flow is a leading cause of anemia in women; thus, an accurate estimation of blood loss is essential to anticipate health concerns.

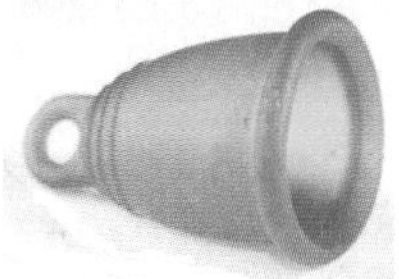

Figure 3–1 A menstrual cup is an eco-friendly way to manage menstrual flow.

SOURCE: Aguadeluna/Fotolia.

Women should be instructed to use tampons with the minimum absorbency needed to control menstrual flow to avoid complications, such as toxic shock syndrome (TSS). Like pads, tampons should be changed every 3 to 6 hours and should not be used for vaginal discharge or abnormal bleeding that occurs outside of menstruation. Because *Staphylococcus aureus*, the causative organism of TSS, is frequently found on the hands, a woman should wash her hands before inserting a fresh tampon and should avoid touching the tip of the tampon when unwrapping it or before insertion. When a tampon is removed, it should first be wrapped in toilet tissue or placed in a disposable bag and then discarded in a trash receptacle or designated container. The woman should be instructed to again wash her hands after removing and discarding the tampon.

Education on the appropriate times to use a tampon is also important and should include instruction to avoid using tampons in the absence of a heavy menstrual flow because tampons absorb moisture, leaving the vaginal walls dry and subject to injury. A woman may want to use tampons only during the day and switch to pads at night to avoid vaginal irritation. If a woman experiences vaginal irritation, itching, or soreness or notices an unusual odor while using tampons, she should stop using them and be evaluated for infection.

The choice of sanitary protection must meet the individual's needs and feel comfortable, whether it be pads or tampons. Cultural factors may play a role in this decision. Young women should be taught to track their periods and to carry feminine hygiene products when their menses is due so that they are prepared for its onset.

Clinical Tip

If you work with teens and preteens, keep samples of menstrual cups and menstrual sponges as well as a variety of pads and tampons on hand so that you can help these young girls become familiar with the options available for dealing with menstruation. You can also put colored water in a small glass and insert a tampon to show a girl how much fluid a tampon absorbs. Girls often think that they lose far more blood with a period than they actually do.

VAGINAL SPRAYS AND DOUCHING

Vaginal sprays are unnecessary and can cause itching, burning, rashes, and other problems. Healthcare providers do not generally recommend that women use them. If a woman chooses to use a spray, she needs to know that these sprays are for external use only, should be used infrequently, and should never be applied to irritated or itching skin.

Douching as a hygiene practice is unnecessary because the vagina has numerous glands that provide a natural cleansing. The vagina has naturally occurring bacteria that aid in maintaining a pH balance to keep fungal and bacterial growth at bay. Douching upsets this vaginal flora, which can make the vagina more susceptible to infection. Douching with one of the perfumed or flavored douches can cause an allergic reaction. Propelling water up the vagina may force bacteria and germs from the vagina into the uterus. It is essential that women avoid douching during menstruation because the cervix is dilated to permit the downward flow of menstrual fluids from the uterine lining. Douching is also contraindicated during pregnancy.

CLEANSING THE PERINEUM

The secretions that continually bathe the vagina are completely odor free while they are in the vagina; only when they combine with perspiration and become exposed to the air does odor develop. Keeping one's skin clean and free of bacteria with plain soap and water is the most effective method of controlling odor. Bathing is as important during menses as at any other time. A long leisurely soak in a warm tub may also help to relieve cramps.

A woman can ensure herself of adequate ventilation by wearing cotton panties and clothes loose enough to allow air to circulate. After using the toilet, a woman should always wipe herself from front to back and, if necessary, follow up with a moistened paper towel or toilet paper.

If an unusual odor persists despite these efforts, a visit to one's healthcare provider is indicated. Certain conditions, such as vaginitis, produce a foul-smelling discharge that women often describe as having a "fishy" odor.

Associated Menstrual Conditions

A variety of menstrual irregularities have been identified. *Abnormal uterine bleeding (AUB)* refers to any uterine bleeding that is abnormal in duration, frequency, volume, or regularity (ACOG, 2014). Amenorrhea and dysmenorrhea are discussed in this chapter. AUB is discussed in more detail in Chapter 6.

Table 3–1 identifies the current terminology that is used to identify types of menstrual conditions considered to be AUB.

AMENORRHEA

Amenorrhea, the absence of menses, is classified as primary or secondary. Primary amenorrhea is said to occur if menstruation has not been established by 16 years of age or within 4 years of breast development. Secondary amenorrhea is said to occur when an established menses (of longer than 3 months) ceases. Secondary amenorrhea is caused most frequently by pregnancy. Typically, the causes of amenorrhea are categorized into one of four groups:

1. ***Hypothalamic dysfunction:*** Several types of hypothalamic disorders can occur. Some are very rare disorders and may be related to a failure of the central structures of the hypothalamus to develop properly. Other disorders may be caused by a tumor. More common forms of hypothalamic dysfunction are triggered by systemic stress related to marked weight loss (anorexia, bulimia, fad dieting), excessive exercise (associated with long-distance runners, dancers, and other athletes with a low body fat ratio), or severe or prolonged stress. See *Evidence-Based Practice: Amenorrhea in Female Athletes.*
2. ***Pituitary dysfunction:*** Pituitary disease and pituitary tumors, such as a pituitary adenoma, can cause changes in the many hormones, including prolactin, that the pituitary manufactures. A variety of medications, including several used to treat anxiety and other psychiatric disorders, can induce a mild increase in prolactin levels, resulting in amenorrhea. Amenorrhea may also be related to low prolactin levels resulting from pituitary failure. Sheehan syndrome, head trauma, and cancer are also serious causes of hypopituitarism.
3. ***Chronic anovulation or ovarian failure:*** Some forms of ovarian failure are caused by genetic disorders often related to the sex chromosomes and are not treatable. Turner syndrome (see Chapter 10) is one of the most common genetic disorders. Causes of chronic anovulation include polycystic ovarian syndrome or thyroid or adrenal disorders. Ovarian failure is related to exposure to radiation, chemotherapy, viral infection, and surgical removal of the ovary.
4. ***Anatomic abnormalities:*** This category includes a variety of structural disorders, such as congenital absence of the uterus, ovaries, or vagina; congenital obstruction; and imperforate hymen.

Diagnosis begins with a thorough history and careful physical examination. For women who have had at least one menstrual period, this evaluation begins with a pregnancy test. For a woman who has never menstruated, the pelvic examination is a crucial assessment tool in determining that she has a normal vagina, uterus, and ovaries. Regardless of type of amenorrhea, based on initial findings, further, more specific tests are indicated. To evaluate pituitary function, a serum prolactin level is often obtained as a screening test. If serum prolactin levels are elevated, magnetic resonance imaging (MRI) will be ordered to rule out a pituitary tumor. Other pituitary hormones can be evaluated, if necessary. Similarly, elevated serum follicle-stimulating hormone (FSH) levels indicate ovarian failure. A thyroid-stimulating hormone (TSH) level is assessed to rule out thyroid disease. A condition known as polycystic ovarian syndrome (PCOS) should be ruled out based on several diagnostic parameters as well (see Chapter 6).

Treatment is dictated by the causative factors. Some conditions, such as imperforate hymen, are easily corrected. Other causes are not treatable. The nurse can explain that once the underlying condition has been corrected, menses will resume.

TABLE 3–1 Abnormal Uterine Bleeding: Terminology and Definitions

CURRENT TERMINOLOGY	FORMER TERMINOLOGY	DEFINITION
Amenorrhea	Same	No periods for at least 3 months (See discussion on amenorrhea)
Intermenstrual bleeding (IMB)	Metrorrhagia	Bleeding or spotting between regular periods
Heavy menstrual bleeding (HMB)	Menorrhagia or hypermenorrhea	Excessive menstrual bleeding that occurs at regular intervals; prolonged duration (greater than 7 days) or excessive amount of bleeding (greater than or equal to 80 mL/cycle); woman's perception of heavy bleeding
Polymenorrhea	Same	Regular, frequent menses (cycles less than 21 days)
Oligomenorrhea	Same	Bleeding that occurs less often than every 35 days

SOURCES: Adapted from American College of Nurse-Midwives (ACNM). (2016). *Abnormal uterine bleeding.* Clinical Bulletin No. 15. Washington, DC: Author; American College of Obstetricians and Gynecologists (ACOG). (2014). *Guidelines for women's health care: A resource manual* (4th ed.). Washington, DC: Author.

EVIDENCE-BASED PRACTICE | Amenorrhea in Female Athletes

Clinical Question

What is the incidence of amenorrhea in female athletes? What is the attitude of athletes toward amenorrhea, particularly elite athletes?

The Evidence

Hormonal changes brought about by extreme exercise and related low energy may result in menstrual dysfunction in female athletes, even those with normal eating patterns. Two studies focused on amenorrhea in female athletes. One study included 245 female athletes in National Collegiate Athletics Association (NCAA) Division 1 sports and focused on both the prevalence of menstrual irregularities and the attitudes of athletes toward amenorrhea. A second, year-long study conducted in Sweden focused on 149 elite athletes—those ranked in the top 10 nationally for their sport. These are descriptive studies, but taken together form a strong level of evidence.

In the general population, the prevalence of amenorrhea is approximately 1%. In contrast, 18% of the NCAA Division I athletes reported amenorrhea and 36% reported fewer than 10 cycles in a year (oligomenorrhea). Twenty-five percent of the elite athletes reported a history of amenorrhea (Rost, Jacobsson, Dahlstrom, et al., 2014). Runners with lower BMI had a higher prevalence of amenorrhea, as did women who participated in sports with high demands on aerobic performance, such as long-distance running.

Missed or irregular menses are often the first sign of a health disturbance, yet some athletes interpret missed menses as a sign of fitness. Fifty-seven percent of the NCAA athletes believed missing menses was normal, 58% believed it was not harmful, and 67% believed it is common among all women (Myrisk, Reinn, & Harkins, 2014). This normalization of amenorrhea is problematic from a clinical standpoint in that amenorrhea is one element of the "female athlete triad" that includes menstrual dysfunction, eating disorders, and osteoporosis. The long-term consequences of menstrual irregularities can include loss of bone mineral density and a three-fold greater risk of musculoskeletal injury.

Best Practice

Coaches, athletic trainers, and athletes need education regarding the serious consequences of menstrual dysfunction and the "female athlete triad" in general. The most common reported cause of amenorrhea among athletes is energy deficiency brought on by consuming too few calories relative to energy expenditure. Adequate nutrition for female athletes is essential to avoid the long-term consequences of menstrual dysfunction.

Clinical Reasoning

How can the nurse affect the attitudes of athletes about normal menstrual function and the importance of adequate nutrition? How can coaches and athletic trainers be motivated to attend to menstrual dysfunction as a signal of a health disturbance?

DYSMENORRHEA

Dysmenorrhea, or painful menstruation, occurs at, or a day before, the onset of menstruation and disappears by the end of menses. Dysmenorrhea is classified as primary or secondary.

Primary dysmenorrhea is defined as cramps without underlying disease. Prostaglandins F_2 and $F_{2\alpha}$, which are produced by the uterus in higher concentrations during menses, are the primary cause. They increase uterine contractility and decrease uterine artery blood flow, causing ischemia. The end result is the painful sensation of cramps. Dysmenorrhea typically disappears after a first pregnancy and may not occur if cycles are anovulatory.

Treatment of primary dysmenorrhea includes combined oral contraceptives (COCs), which inhibit ovulation, and nonsteroidal anti-inflammatory drugs (NSAIDs) (such as ibuprofen, aspirin, and naproxen), which act as prostaglandin inhibitors. See *Health Promotion: Self-Care Measures for Dysmenorrhea.*

Health Promotion Self-Care Measures for Dysmenorrhea

- Regular exercise (Figure 3–2), rest, application of heat, and good nutrition
- Avoidance of salt to decrease discomfort from fluid retention
- Vitamin B_6, which may help relieve the premenstrual bloating and irritability some women experience
- Vitamin E, a mild prostaglandin inhibitor, may ease cramping.

Secondary dysmenorrhea is associated with pathology of the reproductive tract and usually appears after menstruation has been established. Conditions that most frequently cause secondary dysmenorrhea include endometriosis, residual pelvic inflammatory disease (PID), cervical stenosis, uterine fibroids, ovarian cysts, benign or malignant tumors of the pelvis or abdomen, and the presence of an intrauterine contraceptive device (IUCD). Because primary and secondary dysmenorrhea may coexist, accurate differential diagnosis is essential for appropriate treatment.

For women with severe dysmenorrhea, use of continuous oral contraceptive therapy, which does not allow ovulation or menstruation to occur, may be of benefit. Hysterectomy may be the treatment of choice if there are anatomic disorders and childbearing is not desired. Presacral neurectomy may control severe dysmenorrhea caused by endometriosis.

PREMENSTRUAL SYNDROME

Premenstrual syndrome (PMS) refers to a symptom complex characterized by behavioral and physical changes that occur during the luteal phase of the menstrual cycle, anywhere from several days to 2 weeks before the onset of menstrual flow. The symptoms are relieved once menses has started. While 20 to 40% of women who experience symptoms view them as difficult, severe PMS, resulting in emotional distress that impairs work, relationships, and activity levels, occur in only 3 to 5% of menstruating women (ACOG, 2014). The majority of women seeking help with these symptoms are in their mid-20s to late 30s. A diagnosis of PMS occurs when a woman experiences one to three troublesome symptoms.

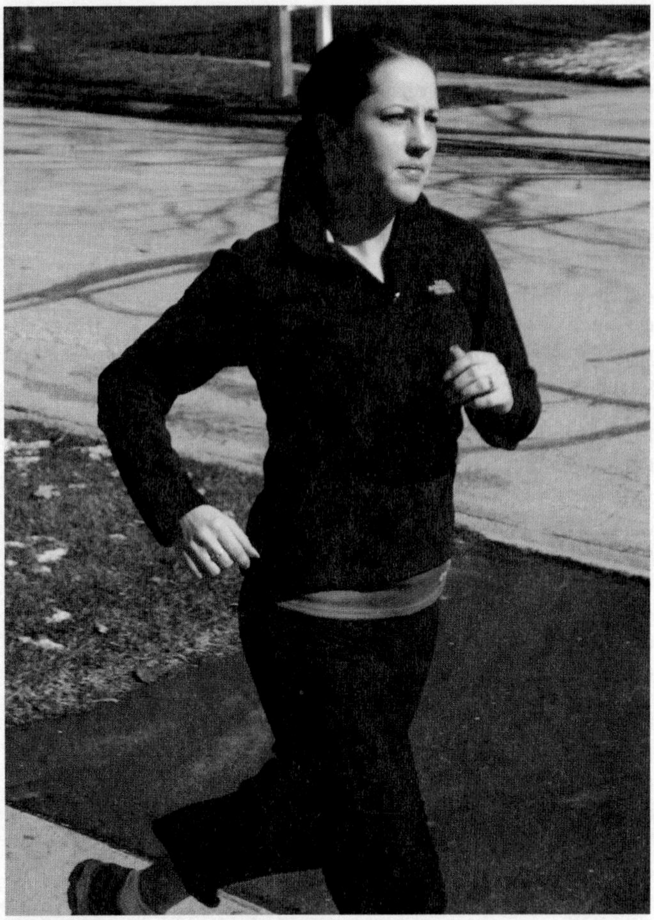

Figure 3–2 **Regular exercise is an important part of therapy for dysmenorrhea.**

Premenstrual dysphoric disorder (PMDD), a more serious form of PMS, is characterized primarily by emotional symptoms as identified in the fifth edition of the *Diagnostic and Statistical Manual of Mental Disorders (DSM-5)* (Ryu & Kim, 2015). It affects 1.3 to 8% of women of childbearing age (Janda, Kues, Andersson et al., 2017). Evidence suggests that a history of severe exposure to stress has been associated with PMDD (Hantsoo & Epperson, 2015). These symptoms are relieved by menstruation and occur in most menstrual cycles. Experts compare the difference between PMS and PMDD to the difference between a mild tension headache and a migraine.

Premenstrual syndrome symptoms include, but are not limited to:

- *Psychologic:* irritability, lethargy, depression, low morale, anxiety, sleep disorders, crying spells, hostility, decreased concentration, social withdrawal
- *Neurologic:* headache, classic migraine
- *Respiratory:* rhinitis, hoarseness
- *Gastrointestinal:* abdominal bloating, weight gain, nausea and vomiting, constipation, increased appetite or food cravings
- *Urinary:* retention and oliguria
- *Dermatologic:* acne
- *Mammary:* swelling and tenderness
- *Musculoskeletal:* joint or muscle pain, swelling of the extremities

The exact cause of PMS is unknown, although a variety of theories have been put forth to explain it. Evidence suggests that progesterone and estradiol levels are involved, although no consistent differences in these levels have been identified. Newer theories suggest that some women have an abnormal sensitivity to the normal changes of these hormones during the menstrual cycle (Ryu & Kim, 2015). Central nervous system–mediated interactions between neurohormones and sex steroids may also account for the occurrence of PMS. Certain risk factors, such as stress, genetics, obesity, or a history of depression or other psychiatric disorders, may predispose women to these disorders.

Diagnosis is generally made after having the woman keep a menstrual calendar for 3 months on which she carefully records daily symptoms, rating them on a scale of 0 to 4, with 0 used for no symptoms and 4 used for severe, debilitating symptoms. The information provided by the diary should be very helpful. Women with PMDD may benefit from selective serotonin reuptake inhibitors (SSRIs), such as fluoxetine hydrochloride (Prozac), sertraline hydrochloride (Zoloft), and paroxetine CR (Paxil CR), taken during the entire cycle or intermittently (half the cycle).

NURSING MANAGEMENT

For the Woman with PMS

Help the woman with PMS identify specific symptoms and develop healthy new behaviors. After assessment, you may advise the woman to restrict her intake of foods containing methylxanthines, such as chocolate, cola, and coffee. It is advisable for the woman to restrict her intake of alcohol, nicotine, red meat, animal fats, and foods containing salt and sugar. Concurrently, she should increase her intake of complex carbohydrates (such as whole grains, brown rice, oatmeal), protein, fruits, vegetables, and vegetable oils and increase the frequency of meals.

Supplementation with 50 to 100 mg daily of vitamin B_6 may help women with some symptoms. A calcium supplement of 1200 mg per day is occasionally effective in reducing physical and psychologic symptoms of PMS. A magnesium supplement of 400 mg daily may help reduce fluid retention and bloating. Vitamin E taken in 400 international units daily may reduce cramping

Complementary Health Approaches

Herbal Remedies for PMS

Herbal remedies for PMS may include (Schuiling & Likis, 2017):

- Black cohosh
- Ginger
- Red raspberry leaf
- Evening primrose oil.

Natural progesterone creams derived from wild yams or soybeans may provide relief to some women; however, no scientific studies have shown this to be true (Schuiling & Likis, 2017).

Note: Underlying health conditions may contraindicate the use of herbal or vitamin supplements, however, and must be considered when recommending them.

and breast tenderness. See *Complementary Health Approaches: Herbal Remedies for PMS*.

A program of aerobic exercise, such as fast walking, jogging, or aerobic dancing, is generally beneficial. In fact, women who exercise regularly tend to have fewer, less severe symptoms.

An empathic relationship with a healthcare professional to whom the woman feels free to voice concerns is highly beneficial. Encourage the woman to keep a journal to help identify life events associated with PMS. Stress reduction education, self-care groups, and self-help literature can also help women gain control over their bodies.

Health Promotion Education

Healthcare providers are becoming increasingly aware of the value of health maintenance and disease prevention, as are many consumers of healthcare services. Women can be advised to make lifestyle choices that promote health and well-being, including:

- Eat a nutritious, balanced diet.
- Maintain normal weight for height (no fad dieting).
- Perform regular aerobic exercise and weight training several times a week.
- Get adequate sleep.
- Avoid smoking and/or stop smoking.
- Consume alcohol in moderation.
- Manage stress effectively.
- Develop enjoyable hobbies and leisure activities.
- Develop an inner life in some form through religion, spirituality, personal reflection, yoga, and so forth.
- Foster bonds of support and affection with family and friends.
- Obtain regular health screenings and assessments.
- Ensure that immunizations are up to date.

Health screening recommendations vary by age, as do recommendations for vaccines. Table 3–2 identifies general screening tests recommended for low-risk women based on their ages. Nurses can share this information with well women so that they can be aware of indicated screening procedures.

TABLE 3–2 Recommended Screening Tests for Low-Risk Women

SCREENING TEST	AGES 18–39	AGES 40–49	AGES 50–64	AGES 65 AND OLDER
Blood pressure	Get tested at least every 3–5 years if you have normal blood pressure (lower than 120/80). Get tested once a year if you have blood pressure between 120/80 and 139/89. Discuss treatment with your doctor or nurse if you have blood pressure 140/90 or higher.	Get tested at least every 2 years if you have normal blood pressure (lower than 120/80). Get tested once a year if you have blood pressure between 120/80 and 139/89. Discuss treatment with your doctor or nurse if you have blood pressure 140/90 or higher.	Get tested at least every 2 years if you have normal blood pressure (lower than 120/80). Get tested once a year if you have blood pressure between 120/80 and 139/89. Discuss treatment with your doctor or nurse if you have blood pressure 140/90 or higher.	Get tested at least every 2 years if you have normal blood pressure (lower than 120/80). Get tested once a year if you have blood pressure between 120/80 and 139/89. Discuss treatment with your doctor or nurse if you have blood pressure 140/90 or higher.
Bone mineral density		Discuss with your doctor or nurse.	Discuss with your doctor or nurse if you are at risk of osteoporosis. Women over 50 with fractures should have a bone density test (DEXA scan).	Get this test at least once at age 65 or older. Talk to your doctor or nurse about repeat testing based on results and screening test used.
Breast cancer (mammogram)		Discuss with your doctor or nurse. Women ages 40–49 may have a mammogram every 1–2 years.	Starting at age 50, get screened every 2 years.	Get screened every 2 years through age 74. Age 75 and older, ask your doctor or nurse if you need to be screened. Decision is a shared one based on your health status and longevity. ACOG supports discontinuing routine screening over age 75.
Cervical cancer (Pap test)	Get a pelvic exam and Pap test every 3 years if you are 21 or older and have a cervix. If you are 30 or older, you can get a Pap test and HPV test together every 5 years.	Get a Pap test and HPV test together every 5 years if you have a cervix.	Get a Pap test and HPV test together every 5 years if you have a cervix.	Ask your doctor or nurse if you need to get a Pap test.

(continued)

TABLE 3–2 Recommended Screening Tests for Low-Risk Women *(continued)*

SCREENING TEST	AGES 18–39	AGES 40–49	AGES 50–64	AGES 65 AND OLDER
Chlamydia	Get tested for chlamydia yearly through age 24 if you are sexually active or pregnant. Age 25 and older, get tested for chlamydia if you are at increased risk, pregnant or not pregnant.	Get tested for chlamydia if you are sexually active and at increased risk, pregnant or not pregnant.	Get tested for chlamydia if you are sexually active and at increased risk.	Get tested for chlamydia if you are sexually active and at increased risk.
Dental exam	See dentist once or twice each year for examination and cleaning.	See dentist once or twice each year for examination and cleaning.	See dentist once or twice each year for examination and cleaning.	See dentist once or twice each year for examination and cleaning.
Lung cancer screening			Lung cancer screening with low-dose computed tomography recommended in adults ages 55–80 who have a 30-pack/year smoking history AND currently smoke or have quit in past 15 years.	Lung cancer screening with low-dose computed tomography recommended in adults ages 55–80 who have a 30-pack/year smoking history AND currently smoke or have quit in past 15 years.
Colorectal cancer (using fecal occult blood testing, sigmoidoscopy, or colonoscopy)			Starting at age 50, get screened for colorectal cancer. Talk to your doctor or nurse about which screening test is best for you and how often you need it.	Get screened for colorectal cancer through age 75. Talk to your doctor or nurse about which screening test is best for you and how often you need it.
Diabetes screening	Get screened for diabetes if your blood pressure is higher than 135/80, your body mass index (BMI) is greater than 25, and you have other risk factors for diabetes.	Get screened for diabetes if your blood pressure is higher than 135/80 or if you take medicine for high blood pressure.	Get screened for diabetes if your blood pressure is higher than 135/80 or if you take medicine for high blood pressure.	Get screened for diabetes if your blood pressure is higher than 135/80 or if you take medicine for high blood pressure.
HIV	Get tested for HIV at least once. Discuss your risk with your doctor or nurse because you may need more frequent tests. All pregnant women need to be tested for HIV.	Get tested for HIV at least once. Discuss your risk with your doctor or nurse because you may need more frequent tests. All pregnant women need to be tested for HIV.	Get tested for HIV at least once. Discuss your risk with your doctor or nurse because you may need more frequent tests.	Get tested for HIV at least once if you are age 65 and have never been tested. Get tested if you are at increased risk for HIV. Discuss your risk with your doctor or nurse.

SOURCES: Data from ACOG. (2017). Well-woman recommendations. Washington, DC: Author; MedlinePlus. (2018). Health screenings for women ages 18 to 39. Retrieved from https://medlineplus.gov/ency/article/007462.htm; MedlinePlus. (2018). Health screenings for women ages 40 to 64. Retrieved from https://medlineplus.gov/ency/article/007467.htm; Office of Women's Health. (2018). Steps for better health by age. Retrieved from https://www.womenshealth.gov/nwhw/by-age/

Body Piercing and Tattoos

Body piercing, tattooing, and scarification, often called *body art*, are rapidly becoming commonplace in today's culture among people of all ages (Figure 3–3).

Tattooing is the application of minute amounts of pigments into the skin with indelible inks. Body piercing sites include earlobes and ear cartilage, lips, nose, tongue, eyebrow, nipples, navel, penis, scrotum, clitoris, perineum, and labia for the purpose of displaying some form of adornment or jewelry. *Scarification* involves the creation of a permanent scar by cutting into the skin and allowing the lesion to heal. Depending on the incisions made, this may result in a simple design or an intricate pattern. Estimates suggest that up to 38% of Americans have some form of body art (Perper, Aldahan, Tsatalis, et al., 2017).

Each of these forms of body art carries with it an element of health risk. For tattooing and body piercing, risks include infections, such as HIV and hepatitis B and C, because of the use of inadequately sterilized equipment, as well as allergic reactions, local swelling and burns, granulomas, and keloid formation (more common in people of African descent). Oral piercing has been associated with tooth and gum damage. Among pregnant or breastfeeding women, nipple piercing has been associated

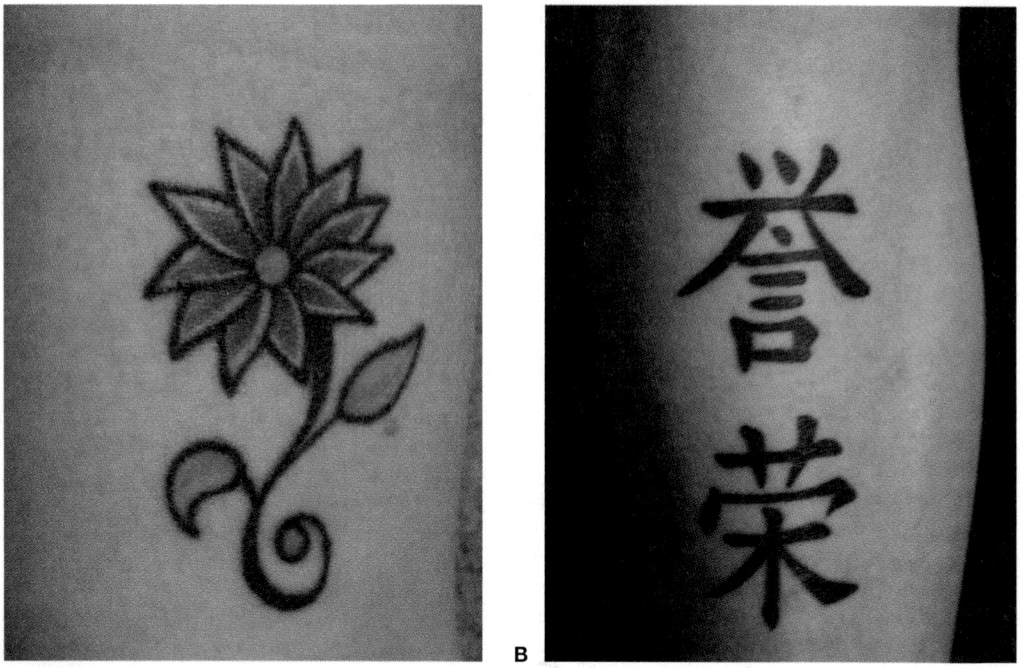

A B

Figure 3–3 **Tattoos vary greatly in size, complexity, and meaning to the individual. A. This tattoo, on the ankle of a young woman, is purely decorative. B. This tattoo, on the shin of a young man, is the Chinese symbol for honor. He chose it to express a personal commitment to live a life of integrity.**

SOURCE: A.–B. Michele Davidson.

with mastitis, damaged milk ducts, leaking milk from piercing holes, and difficulty with breastfeeding (Roche-Paull, 2015). See *Case Study: Angelina Newman*.

Educating patients about the risks associated with these practices should include information about infection, permanent scarring, keloid formation, and care afterward. It is important for the nurse to avoid passing judgment or making generalizations about individuals who have these types of body alterations.

Menopause

Menopause, defined as the absence of menstruation for 1 full year, is a time of transition for a woman, marking the end of her reproductive abilities. Although it usually occurs between 45 and 58 years of age, the average age of menopause in the United States is 51 years (National Institute on Aging, 2016). Not all of the physiologic mechanisms initiating menopause are precisely understood; however, it is known that the onset occurs when estrogen levels drop because of cessation of ovarian function. In addition, most researchers agree that the age of onset is influenced by such factors as the woman's overall health, weight, nutrition, lifestyle, culture, and genetic factors. See *Genetic Facts: Family History*.

Genetic Facts Family History

Knowledge of family history is an essential element in identifying risk factors for many of the changes and conditions associated with aging, including age at onset of menopause, osteoporosis, cardiovascular disease, certain cancers, and Alzheimer disease. Thus, it is important that women be familiar with their family history and that they share relevant information with their children.

CASE STUDY: Angelina Newman

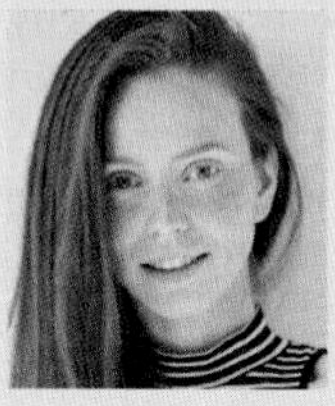

SOURCE: WAYHOME studio/Shutterstock.

Angelina mentions at her 14-week prenatal visit that she is interested in getting a tattoo of a baby on her abdomen as a remembrance of her pregnancy. Her boyfriend has already gotten a small baby tattooed on his abdomen and has a tattoo artist in mind for her. Angelina's mother is concerned there would be hazards that could occur during pregnancy and states that Angelina needs to get clearance from her nurse-midwife before she will allow her to get this tattoo.

Question to Ponder

What are the potential risks associated with getting a tattoo during pregnancy?

Climacteric, or *change of life* (often used synonymously with *menopause*), refers to the host of psychologic and physical alterations that occur around the time of menopause. These aspects are discussed separately.

Perimenopause

Perimenopause refers to the period of time before menopause during which the woman moves from normal ovulatory cycles to cessation of menses. Women in perimenopause will generally begin having menstrual irregularities and changes in estrogen and FSH. On average, perimenopause lasts 5 years but women may have symptoms for up to 8 years before the final menstrual period (McNamara, Batur, & DeSapri, 2015).

Symptoms of perimenopause vary significantly in women. It is estimated that more than 80% of women in perimenopause report some degree of vasomotor symptoms (hot flashes). It is important that women in this age group be screened thoroughly to rule out other causes of vasomotor symptoms. Mood and cognitive changes are also a common complaint, with women expressing concern over emotional instability and a decrease in memory. These may, in fact, be the more concerning symptoms women express to their healthcare providers. Changes in sexuality are common and may include decreased libido, vaginal lubrication, and comfort with sexual intercourse.

Contraception remains a major concern for many perimenopausal women. In fact, women over age 40 have the second highest abortion rate because of unintended pregnancy (Zieman, Hatcher, & Allen, 2015). As women age, fertility decreases and the risk of spontaneous abortion increases. In women who delay pregnancy until after age 40, risks for pregnancy complications are approximately twofold to sixfold higher. These complications include hypertensive disorders, diabetes, placenta previa, and placental abruption. These complications in turn increase the rate of preterm birth, intrauterine growth restriction, and serious neonatal complications.

In the United States, 50% of women over age 40 have been sterilized, and sterilization remains a reliable option for women (Zieman et al., 2015). However, combined hormonal contraceptives (the pill, patches, and vaginal rings) continue to be popular forms of contraception during this time in a woman's reproductive life. Combined hormonal contraceptives prevent pregnancy and provide noncontraceptive benefits. Healthy nonsmokers benefit from effective contraception; regulation of menses; treatment of anovulatory bleeding; relief of symptoms of estrogen deficiency and variability, such as hot flashes, sleep disturbances, menorrhagia, and vaginal dryness; and a decreased risk of endometrial and ovarian cancer. They may also experience less acne and *hirsutism* (abnormal hair growth, often on the face and neck) and decreased osteopenia. Thus, combined hormonal contraceptives are considered by many to be an optimal approach to this transition, even when contraception is not a concern. Other contraceptive options for perimenopausal women include sterilization; contraceptive intrauterine devices (IUDs); progestin-only methods of contraception; and barrier methods of contraception, such as male and female condoms, diaphragm, cervical cap, and spermicides. (See Chapter 4 for a discussion of these methods.)

Women describing problems that suggest perimenopause should be referred to their care providers. If oral contraceptives are not an option, other alternatives are available. Exercise, calcium and vitamin D, and other supplements or medications may be effective.

Psychologic Aspects of Menopause

A woman's psychologic adaptation to menopause and the climacteric is multifactorial. It is often further complicated because women of this age may be dealing with other life circumstances, such as adjustment to an "empty nest" or caring for aging parents. Numerous personal factors influence a woman's ability to transition and cope with these changes, such as self-concept, physical health, marital stability, relationships with others, and cultural values. Some women express disappointment in approaching this time of their lives, whereas others may see it as a positive transition that offers freedom from menses or concern about contraception. Women who are dealing with aging, ill parents may have increased stressors that affect their emotional health and ability to deal with their symptoms. Often night sweats and insomnia affect a woman's capability to cope because of increased fatigue.

As a nurse, understanding the basic physiology of menopause offers an opportunity to provide education, supportive resources, and encouragement to women at this time in their lives. Suggesting exercises and teaching proper nutrition are critical for overall health and may help these women improve the emotional aspects associated with menopause. It is important to help women understand the changes that come with menopause and deal with their feelings during this period. Moreover, caregivers need to be alert for signs that distinguish between the mood swings that are related to hormonal changes and true clinical depression.

Today, the average woman in the United States will live one-third of her life after menopause. The changing perceptions of menopause and beyond are enabling menopausal women to cope more effectively and to view menopause as a time of personal growth.

> "My personal response to menopause has surprised me a little. Suddenly, 52 doesn't really seem old. I look at pictures of my mother in her early 50s, and she seems so much older. I imagine each generation looks back and thinks the same thing. I do wish I had known at 22 what I know now, but I still see myself as learning and growing. I know I have a lot to offer and a lot of choices in how to accomplish that. One thing I'm committed to is trying to live each day as well as I can, to stay positive, and to keep looking forward."

Physical Aspects of Menopause

CHANGES IN THE REPRODUCTIVE SYSTEM

The physical characteristics of menopause are linked to the shift from a cyclic to a noncyclic hormonal pattern. Beginning 2 to 8 years before menopause, women experience episodes of anovulation, reduced fertility, decreased or increased menstrual flow, menstrual cycle irregularities, and then, ultimately, amenorrhea. Generally, ovulation ceases 1 to 2 years before menopause, but individual variations exist. FSH levels rise, and ovarian follicles cease to produce estrogen. As estrogen levels decline, physiologic changes occur within the reproductive organs. The uterine lining, or endometrium, thins and the uterine muscle layer, or myometrium, atrophies. The fallopian tubes and ovaries atrophy. The vaginal mucosa loses its elasticity and becomes thinner and smoother. The loss of cervical gland function leads to dryness of the mucous membranes of the vagina, which can lead to burning and itching. The vaginal pH level increases as the number of Döderlein's bacilli decreases. This change in the vaginal ecology can lead to a condition known as atrophic vaginitis and increases the woman's risk of vaginal infections.

Pubic hair thins, turns gray or white, and may ultimately disappear. The labia shrink and lose their heightened pigmentation. Menopausal women may experience a general loss of pelvic tone and support, which can lead to prolapse of reproductive and urinary tract organs and subsequent urinary incontinence. Kegel exercises (see Chapter 13) and regular sexual activity help prevent this change. Breasts lose their density and are replaced by fat, which makes them more pendulous and less firm.

Sexual functioning declines with age. Contributing factors to the decline in both interest and occurrence of sexual activity are widespread. Pain during intercourse due to lack of lubrication and thinning vaginal walls is a common cause. Other factors may include a lack of partners, stress in current relationships, psychosocial factors, and a decline in general health. Completing a good sexual history will help the nurse to assess the woman's sexual health and allow the woman to ask questions and express concerns or frustrations.

VASOMOTOR CHANGES

Many women who are perimenopausal or menopausal experience a vasomotor disturbance commonly known as a *hot flash.* Hot flashes are typically described as a feeling of heat rising from the chest and spreading to the neck and face. Hot flashes at night are often accompanied by sleep disturbances triggered by profuse sweating (*night sweats*) in which a woman awakens with drenched night clothes and bedding. These episodes may occur as often as 20 to 30 times a day and generally last 3 to 5 minutes or less. Some women also experience dizzy spells, palpitations, and weakness. Many women find their own most effective ways to deal with the hot flashes. Some report that dressing in layers, using a fan, avoiding alcoholic beverages, or drinking a cool liquid helps relieve distress. Still others seek relief through hormone therapy or complementary therapies, such as herbs or acupuncture.

CHANGES IN THE MUSCULOSKELETAL SYSTEM AND SKIN

Osteoporosis, a decrease in bone strength related to diminished bone density and bone quality, is a major health concern for women, particularly after menopause. Women who experience menopause at a younger age and those with less bone mass when entering menopause predicatively will have the most severe bone loss. This change is associated with lowered estrogen levels; however, the greatest influencing factor is a family history of osteoporosis. Osteoporosis puts an individual at increased risk for fractures of the hip, forearm, and vertebrae. Risk factors associated with osteoporosis are identified in Table 3–3.

As skin ages, collagen and elastin, which are what maintain firmness of the skin, weaken. The skin appears looser and thinner and wrinkles more easily. Past sun exposure and tobacco use influence the amount of skin changes that occur. As women age, the skin becomes drier and may need increased moisturizing. Nurses, as a part of general counseling, can remind women to wear sunscreen with a sun protection factor (SPF) of at least 30 to provide an ultraviolet B (UVB) filter and prevent damage. Evidence suggests that estrogen regulates weight and fat metabolism in women, and during menopause a change in fat distribution occurs. In postmenopausal women compared to premenopausal women, total body fat increases. More specifically, the increase in fat accumulation occurs in the trunk region. Nurses should be especially concerned about central body obesity, which is a predictor of the development of chronic illness. This is done by calculating a waist-to-hip ratio, or dividing the woman's waist measurement by the hip measurement. Women should maintain a waist-to-hip ratio of less than 0.80 to decrease their risk for chronic disease.

TABLE 3–3 Risk Factors for Osteoporosis

- Personal history of fracture after age 50
- Current low bone mass
- History of fracture in a first-degree relative
- Being female
- Being thin (weight less than 127 lb and/or having a small frame)
- Advanced age
- Family history of osteoporosis, especially a maternal hip fracture
- Use of certain medications (e.g., corticosteroids, chemotherapy, barbiturates, anticonvulsants)
- Abnormal absence of menses; early onset of menopause
- Anorexia nervosa
- Low lifetime intake of calcium
- Vitamin D deficiency
- Current cigarette smoking, excessive alcohol use
- Inactive lifestyle
- Being Caucasian or Asian

CHANGES IN THE CARDIOVASCULAR SYSTEM

An important long-range physical change of menopause is a shift in lipid and lipoprotein levels. The presence of normal estrogen levels before menopause contributes to higher levels of high-density lipoprotein cholesterol (HDL-C), or the "good" cholesterol, and lower levels of low-density lipoprotein cholesterol (LDL-C), or "bad" cholesterol. Low levels of HDL-C are a major predictor of coronary heart disease (CHD) in women. As estrogen levels fall during menopause, this protective mechanism ceases, which potentially places a woman at increased risk for coronary heart disease, hypertension, and stroke. During menopause women should be encouraged to have their cholesterol monitored on an annual basis if normal and every 3 to 6 months if abnormal.

Cardiovascular disease (CVD) is the number one killer of women in the United States. Risk factors for CHD are identified in Table 3–4.

Metabolic syndrome is a major predisposing factor for CHD and is defined through a collection of risk factors. It occurs when an individual has three or more of the following findings (American Heart Association, 2016):

- Waist measurement greater than 35 inches in women (40 inches in men)
- Triglycerides of 150 mg/dL or greater
- HDL cholesterol less than 50 in women (less than 40 in men)
- Blood pressure of 130/85 or higher
- Fasting glucose levels of 100 mg/dL or higher.

TABLE 3–4 Risk Factors for Coronary Heart Disease in Women

- Family history of heart disease
- Advancing age—over 55 or postmenopausal
- Overweight and obesity
- Cigarette smoking and/or tobacco use
- Sedentary lifestyle
- Hypertension
- Diabetes
- Elevated cholesterol
- Race (highest incidence in African American women)

CHANGES IN COGNITIVE FUNCTION

Memory and cognitive function change with advancing age. It has been suggested that the brain benefits from circulating estrogen and that declining estrogen levels might contribute to loss of this function as well as to the development of dementia. This change is also influenced by lifestyle, genetics, and socioeconomic status. In the United States, Alzheimer disease (AD) is the most common form of dementia, estimated to affect 5.4 million Americans. Projections indicate that by the year 2025, 7.1 million Americans over the age of 65 will have AD (Alzheimer's Association, 2016b). This projected increase represents a major health concern for the country.

The cause of Alzheimer disease is unknown, although it is believed that risk factors other than advancing age may play a role. These risk factors include specific genotypes, family history, obesity, diabetes, elevated cholesterol, hypertension, and inflammation. At present there are no therapies that slow the progression of the disease; only symptomatic therapies are available. Cholinesterase inhibitors and *N*-methyl-D-aspartate antagonists are the only medications approved by the Food and Drug Administration (FDA) for treating cognitive dysfunction.

The following lifestyle practices may help prevent AD and other dementias (Alzheimer's Association, 2016a):

- Exercise regularly—at least 30 minutes 5 days per week.
- Quit smoking.
- Maintain a healthy blood pressure.
- Maintain a normal weight.
- Eat a healthy diet. Research indicates that the Mediterranean diet and the DASH (Dietary Approaches to Stop Hypertension) diet are beneficial.
- Remain mentally active through activities that keep the brain stimulated, such as reading, writing, playing games, or learning something new, such as a foreign language or how to play a musical instrument.
- Get enough sleep.
- Stay socially engaged through volunteering and sharing activities with family and friends (see Figure 3–4).
- Prevent diabetes. For people who are diabetic, maintain excellent blood glucose control.
- Deal with symptoms of depression, anxiety, or other mental health concerns (medications may be indicated).

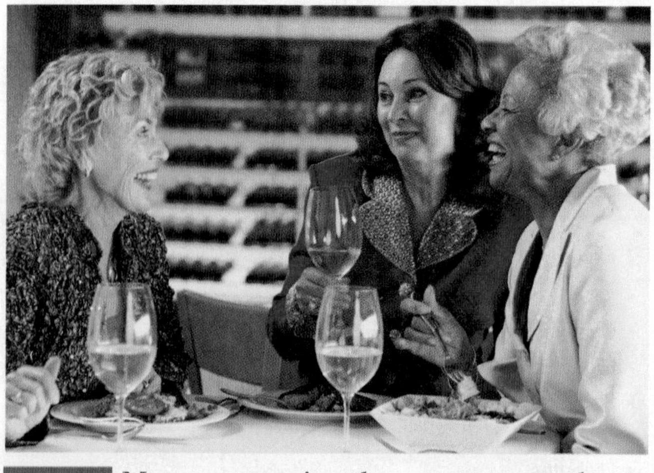

Figure 3–4 Many women view the postmenopausal years as a time of personal growth and enjoyment.

SOURCE: Monkey Business/Fotolia.

Premature Menopause

Premature ovarian insufficiency (POI), resulting in premature menopause, is a devastating event and is not well understood. It occurs in about 0.1% of women by the age of 30 and 1% of women by the age of 40 (Fenton, 2015). It is defined as 4 to 6 months of no menses in women under the age of 40 years who have elevated FSH and low estradiol levels. POI is different from menopause in that women with POI retain intermittent ovarian function, and, although difficult, pregnancy may occur. Women with POI who desire pregnancy may experience emotional trauma and require extra sensitivity from caregivers. Concern for the patient's long-term health should be a consideration.

Women should be encouraged to engage in weight-bearing exercises for 30 minutes at least 3 days per week to strengthen muscle and maintain bone mass. Adequate intakes of calcium and vitamin D are also important. Estrogen, progesterone, and possibly testosterone hormone therapy is recommended for women who experience premature ovarian insufficiency at least until they reach the average age of natural menopause (Baber, Panay, Fenton, & the IMS Writing Group, 2016). Other forms of premature menopause occur with anorexia, chemotherapy or radiation treatments, and oophorectomy (surgical removal of the ovaries).

See *Health Promotion: Reducing Discomforts of Menopause* and *Complementary Health Approaches: Relieving Menopausal Symptoms* for discussions of complementary health approaches a woman might employ during the menopausal years.

Health Promotion Reducing Discomforts of Menopause

A variety of therapeutic modalities have been proposed as treatment or prevention measures for the discomforts and ailments of the perimenopausal, menopausal, and post-menopausal years. These include nutrition supplements, such as a diet rich in calcium and vitamins E, D, and B complex. Mind–body practices, such as yoga, t'ai chi, and meditation, are also helpful in reducing symptoms.

Medical Therapy

MENOPAUSAL HORMONE THERAPY

Menopausal hormone therapy (MHT), formerly called *hormone replacement therapy (HRT)*, refers to the administration of specific hormones to alleviate symptoms associated with the changes of menopause. Estrogen therapy (ET) and combined estrogen-progestogen therapy (EPT) are the individual types currently in use. Hormone therapy containing estrogen only is given to women who have undergone a *hysterectomy* (surgical removal of the uterus), whereas hormone therapy containing estrogen and progestogen (which encompasses both progesterone and progestin) is used for women with an intact uterus. Estrogen alone, in a woman with a uterus (unopposed estrogen), increases the risk of endometrial (the lining of the uterus) cancer by eightfold and, therefore, is never given without progesterone in these women.

MHT can be prescribed in a number of ways, including orally; transdermally (patch); topically as a gel, lotion, mist, or cream; and through a vaginal ring. It is given in a continuous manner, as daily administration of both estrogen and progestogen, or as a cyclic or sequential therapy, with estrogen use daily and a progestogen added on a set sequence. Combination estrogen-progestogen preparations are also available.

Complementary Health Approaches

Relieving Menopausal Symptoms

Very little scientific research has been done on complementary alternative therapy for the treatment of menopause. The following complementary therapies have been used to help relieve menopausal symptoms, but results are mixed (National Center for Complementary and Integrative Health, 2016):

- Black cohosh has received attention for its possible effectiveness, but preliminary research suggests that it is no more effective than a placebo in relieving symptoms. In rare cases it has been associated with liver inflammation.
- Phytoestrogens (isoflavones found in red clover, soy, and other plants) are sometimes used to reduce hot flashes, but research has found inconsistent relief of symptoms and further study is warranted to demonstrate their effectiveness. Women who have had or who are at risk for hormone-dependent cancers, cardiovascular events, or thromboembolic disease should not use phytoestrogens.
- DHEA, a dietary supplement, has been evaluated for possible benefit in dealing with hot flashes and decreased sexual arousal. Evidence to date shows no benefit.
- Mind and body practices
  - Hypnotherapy and mindfulness meditation—these approaches may help improve some menopausal symptoms, including hot flashes, but evidence as to effectiveness is limited
  - Acupuncture—there is insufficient evidence to determine its effectiveness
  - Yoga—there is insufficient evidence to determine whether it has a beneficial effect

Postmenopausal women experiencing decreased libido may experience improved sexual desire, responsiveness, and frequency when testosterone is added to their MHT. Options for providing testosterone in doses low enough for women are still limited and are not approved by the FDA. Estratest, a combined estrogen-androgen pill, is used by some women. Custom-compounded testosterone preparations are available by prescription. Procter & Gamble has developed a low-dose testosterone transdermal patch for women called Intrinsa that is available by prescription in Europe. Another testosterone product, a gel called LibiGel, is currently undergoing testing.

For over a decade, the use of MHT had decreased significantly because of a large study that suggested that the risks of MHT outweighed the benefits, particularly the increased risk of breast cancer, thromboembolic disease, and stroke. In light of findings from more recent clinical trials, that study has been called into question. The International Menopause Society (IMS) has developed the following recommendations about the clinical management of menopausal hormone therapy (Baber et al., 2016):

- MHT remains the most effective therapy for moderate to severe menopausal vasomotor symptoms (hot flashes and night sweats) and urogenital atrophy.
- Consideration of the use of MHT should be part of an overall healthcare strategy that also addresses diet and exercise, smoking cessation, and safe levels of alcohol consumption.
- MHT should be tailored to each individual based on symptoms, family history, personal risk factors (age, time since onset of menopause, risk of venous ischemic heart disease, thromboembolism, and breast cancer), and the woman's preferences and expectations.
- "There are no reasons to place mandatory limitations on the duration of MHT" (Baber et al., 2016, p. 111).
- Intravaginal estrogen is generally recommended to treat vaginal dryness, pruritis, and dyspareunia.
- MHT is effective for the prevention of fractures related to osteoporosis in women who are at risk before age 60 or within 10 years of menopause and can be considered a first-line therapy for them. Individual calculation of risk–benefit ratios and consideration of other available drug treatments should be done before initiating HRT in women ages 60–70, and then at the lowest possible dose. HRT should not be started in women over age 70.
- The risk of venous thromboembolism and stroke does increase with MHT, but the absolute risk is rare in women younger than age 60.
- The risk of breast cancer is complex. It is related to duration of use and is primarily associated with the addition of a progestogen to the estrogen therapy. The risk decreases after therapy is stopped. However, MHT should not be used in breast cancer survivors.
- Estrogen-alone MHT may decrease coronary heart disease in women younger than age 60 and within 10 years of menopause. Findings are mixed about the effects of daily continuous estrogen plus progestogen MHT in this population but other combined therapy approaches appear to be cardioprotective.

A great deal of attention has been given to "bioidentical" hormones lately because of current views, which are not supported by medical literature, that these "more natural" hormones are safer and more effective. A *bioidentical hormone* refers to a hormone that is structurally identical to those found in the body, more specifically, those produced by the ovaries. These hormones are compounded by a specialty pharmacy and are not approved by the FDA, nor have they been proven to have a better safety profile, and their use is not recommended (de Villiers et al., 2013).

PREVENTION AND TREATMENT OF OSTEOPOROSIS

Estimates indicate that 54 million adults in the United States are affected by osteoporosis and low bone mass. Annually, 2 million fractures occur as the result of osteoporosis but fewer than one-fourth of older men and women who break a bone are tested or treated for it (National Osteoporosis Foundation [NOF], 2016).

These numbers are especially worrisome because osteoporosis is a largely preventable disease and a source of significant risk for fracture and subsequent health decline. *Healthy People 2020* addresses the issue of osteoporosis in general and hip fracture in particular.

Bone mineral density (BMD) testing is useful in identifying individuals who are at risk for osteoporosis. NOF (2016) recommends BMD testing of all women ages 65 and older and all men ages 70 and older. The diagnosis and treatment of osteoporosis should be based on a comprehensive approach using history, physical examination, BMD testing, and the WHO 10-year estimated fracture probability assessment developed by the WHO Working Group on Osteoporosis (Cosman et al., 2014). The online tool *FRAX* is designed to assess hip fracture probability based on several individual patient and clinical factors. The FRAX tool serves to project fracture risk through statistical models and integrate individual clinical risk factors (Cosman et al., 2014). BMD testing may also be indicated for premenopausal or postmenopausal women with risk factors, certain medical conditions, such as eating disorders, thyroid disorders, leukemia, rheumatoid arthritis, and multiple sclerosis, and for those women on certain medications, such as corticosteroids or anticonvulsants.

The woman's height should be measured at each visit because a loss of height is often an early sign that vertebrae are being compressed because of reduced bone mass. A variety of conditions—including malabsorption syndrome, cancer, cirrhosis of the liver, chronic use of cortisone, and rheumatoid arthritis—can cause secondary arthritis, which resembles osteoporosis. If these secondary causes are ruled out, treatment for osteoporosis is instituted.

Prevention of osteoporosis is the primary goal. It should include (Cosman et al., 2014):

- Adequate intake of calcium and vitamin D
- Regular weight-bearing, muscle-strengthening exercises
- Smoking cessation
- Moderate intake of alcohol
- Fall prevention strategies.

Postmenopausal women should have a daily intake of 1200 mg of calcium, increasing to 1500 mg if they are not on hormone therapy. Most women require supplements to achieve this level. Calcium supplementation is most effective when single doses do not exceed 500 mg and when taken with a meal.

Vitamin D is a fat-soluble vitamin that has its greatest effect on maintaining adequate levels of serum calcium. It is primarily metabolized by the body through sunlight or dietary intake. The use of sunscreen can result in decreased production of vitamin D in the skin. Low bone density and certain autoimmune diseases are associated with vitamin D deficiency. It is recommended that adults take a vitamin D supplement of 1000 to 2000 international units per day to reduce the incidence of low bone density.

The effectiveness of estrogen in preventing osteoporosis is well documented. Women with no contraindications to estrogen who are showing evidence of bone loss are good candidates for MHT. For women who are unable or unwilling to take estrogen, other medications available to treat or help prevent osteoporosis include:

- *Bisphosphonates* are calcium regulators that act by inhibiting bone resorption and increasing bone mass. Alendronate (Fosamax®) and risedronate (Actonel®) are commonly prescribed. Zoledronic acid (Zometa®) is administered by IV once a year and seems to achieve the same results in treating osteoporosis as other bisphosphonates taken daily or weekly without the troublesome gastrointestinal side effects.
- *Selective estrogen receptor modulators (SERMs)* such as raloxifene (Evista®) preserve the beneficial effects of estrogen, including its protection against osteoporosis, but do not stimulate uterine or breast tissue.
- *Salmon calcitonin* (Miacalcin® or Fortical®) is a calcium regulator that may inhibit bone loss. Administered daily as a nasal spray, its value is less clear than that of the other medications listed.
- *Parathyroid hormone* (teriparatide, brand name Forteo®), taken daily as a subcutaneous injection, activates bone formation, which results in substantial increases in bone density. It is indicated for women who develop fractures while on other medications or who have a severe case of osteoporosis. It should not be taken for more than 18 months (Baber et al., 2016).
- *Receptor activator of nuclear factor kappa-B ligand (RANKL) inhibitor* (denosumab, brand name Prolia®) decreases bone resorption and increases bone mass and strength. It is administered subcutaneously every 6 months.

PREVENTION OF CORONARY HEART DISEASE

Cardiovascular disease (CVD) remains the leading cause of death in women in the United States, accounting for one in three women's deaths. Moreover, fewer women than men survive an initial heart attack (American Heart Association, 2017). The good news is that CVD is largely preventable. Prevention begins with lifestyle choices and with lifestyle modifications as necessary. This includes maintaining ideal body weight, exercising regularly, eating a nutritious diet, avoiding smoking, managing stress effectively, obtaining regular healthcare screenings as indicated, and developing a strong social support system.

It is critical that women be familiar with the signs of myocardial infarction (heart attack) that are commonly seen in women. These include pain in the neck, back, or epigastric region; loss of appetite; shortness of breath; nausea or vomiting; and weakness in the shoulder, arms, and chest. Research indicates that women are more likely than men to delay seeking treatment. Thus, it is important for nurses to stress the need to seek immediate treatment if symptoms develop. See *Developing Cultural Competence: Filipina Women and Aging*.

Developing Cultural Competence Filipina Women and Aging

In the Philippines, menopause is viewed as a positive and liberating event. As women age, they are more respected and admired for their years of gained experiences. Older women gain status and importance as they age and are widely embraced by the younger generations within their family.

Source: Comments from a Filipina nursing student.

Weight-bearing exercise, including such activities as walking, jogging, tennis, and running, is a means of increasing bone mass and potentiating the effect of estrogen on bone mass. Exercise also improves cholesterol profiles and contributes to overall health (Figure 3–5). Pelvic floor, or Kegel, exercises can help

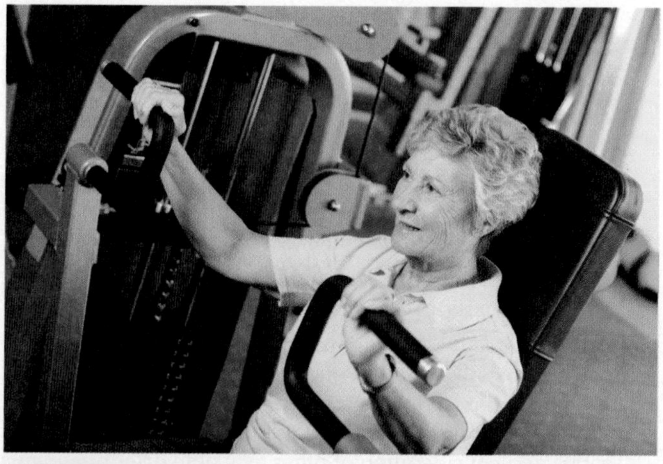

Figure 3–5 Regular exercise is important, especially for postmenopausal women.

SOURCE: Jamstockfoto/Fotolia.

maintain vaginal muscle tone and increase blood circulation to the perineal area. Vaginal lubricants and adequate foreplay can be helpful in maintaining a satisfactory sexual experience. Stress management and relaxation techniques, such as biofeedback, meditation, yoga, visualization, and massage, may provide a sense of well-being.

NURSING MANAGEMENT

For the Woman Experiencing Menopause

Some menopausal women may need counseling to adjust successfully to this developmental phase of life. Others have no difficulty with this life transition. Reaction to menopause is determined to a large extent by the kind of life the woman has lived, by the security she has in her feminine identity, by her feelings of self-worth and self-esteem, and by her relationships with others.

Nurses and other healthcare professionals may be able to help the menopausal woman achieve high-level functioning at this time in her life. Of paramount importance is your ability to understand and provide support for the woman's views and feelings. Whether the woman expresses relief and delight or tearfulness and fear, use an empathetic approach in counseling, health teaching, or providing physical care. See *Women with Special Needs: Assisting the Older Woman with a Physical Disability.*

Women with Special Needs Assisting the Older Woman with a Physical Disability

More than 50% of women over the age of 65 have a physical disability. The most common disabilities in this age group are related to arthritis or rheumatism. Older women with physical disabilities may need assistance getting onto the examination table for a gynecologic examination. The nurse should assist the woman into a semi-Fowler position and move both legs simultaneously to stirrups to prevent muscle strain or injury.

Women may discuss areas of deep concern, including a history of sexual abuse, current distress, or life problems. Have appropriate referrals to domestic violence hotlines and to professional therapists who work with women. Women may also be dealing simultaneously with chronically ill parents, divorce or the death of a spouse, troubled or handicapped children, children leaving home, job stressors, and/or generalized fear and anxiety. Refer your patients to support groups and counselors who are specific to each woman's need. Although this may be a challenge, it is your responsibility in caring for women to be prepared to meet their needs.

Explore the question of the woman's comfort during sexual intercourse. In counseling, you may say, "After menopause, many women notice that their vaginas seem drier, and sex of any kind can be uncomfortable. Have you noticed any changes?" This gives the woman information and may open discussion. Go on to explain that the woman can address dryness and shrinking of the vagina by using a water-soluble lubricant to help provide relief. Use of estrogen, orally or in vaginal creams, may also be indicated. Increased frequency of sexual activity will maintain some elasticity in the vagina. When assessing the menopausal woman, address the question of sexual activity openly but tactfully because the woman may have been socialized to be reticent in discussing sex. Counsel heterosexual women who do not wish to become pregnant to use a method of contraception for 1 year after their last menstrual period. Also advise them to report any bleeding after 1 year of amenorrhea because this may indicate a problem and requires evaluation.

The crucial need of women in the perimenopausal period of life is for adequate information about the changes taking place in their bodies and their lives and support in adjusting to the changes that occur. Supplying that information and providing support as needed present both a challenge and an opportunity for nurses. See *Professionalism in Practice: Personalizing Care During Menopause.*

Professionalism in Practice Personalizing Care During Menopause

Women respond differently to the experience of menopause, so it is important to avoid generalizations. During menopause women are in varying stages of life. In working with menopausal women, being sensitive to their place in life—such as caring for aging parents, empty nest, or change in marital status—will personalize their care and offer appropriate measures to help them through this process.

Focus Your Study

- Nurses should provide girls and women with clear information about menstrual issues, such as the use of pads and tampons (including warnings regarding deodorant and absorbency); vaginal spray and douching practices; and self-care comfort measures during menstruation, such as maintaining good nutrition, exercising, and applying heat and massage.
- Dysmenorrhea usually begins at, or a day before, the onset of menses and disappears by the end. Hormone therapy (e.g., combined oral contraceptives), nonsteroidal anti-inflammatory drugs, or prostaglandin inhibitors can alleviate dysmenorrhea. Self-care measures include improving nutrition, exercising, applying heat, and getting extra rest.
- Premenstrual syndrome occurs most often in women over age 30. The most pronounced symptoms occur 2 to 3 days before onset of menstruation and subside as menstruation starts, with or without treatment. Medical management usually

includes prostaglandin inhibitors and calcium supplementation. Self-care measures include improving nutrition (taking vitamin B complex and E supplements and avoiding methylxanthines, which are found, for example, in chocolate and caffeine), undertaking a program of aerobic exercise, and participating in self-care support groups. In some cases, pharmacologic agents, such as selective serotonin reuptake inhibitors, may be indicated.

- During her adult years, a healthy woman should make healthful lifestyle choices, such as avoiding smoking and exercising regularly. She should also participate in regular health screenings, following a recommended schedule.
- Menopause is a physiologic, maturational change in a woman's life. Physiologic changes include the cessation of menses and a decrease in circulating hormones. Hormonal changes sometimes bring unsettling emotional responses. The more common physiologic symptoms are hot flashes, palpitations, dizziness, and increased perspiration at night. The woman's anatomy also undergoes changes, such as atrophy of the vagina, reduction in size and pigmentation of the labia, and myometrial atrophy. Osteoporosis becomes an increasing concern.
- Osteoporosis is becoming a significant health problem in the United States. Prevention is the preferred approach to addressing the issue. This includes adequate calcium intake and regular weight-bearing exercise. For women who have already developed osteoporosis, medications are available as a treatment option.
- Cardiovascular disease is the number-one killer of women in the United States, accounting for one in three deaths annually. Prevention is the goal of therapy.
- Current management of menopause is focused on minimizing symptoms and managing complications.
- Menopausal hormone therapy (MHT) is recommended for the treatment of vasomotor symptoms in women under age 60 or within 10 years of menopause. The decision to begin MHT should be made jointly by the woman and her caregiver based on a careful analysis of risks and benefits.

In order to make safe and effective judgments using NANDA-I © 2017 nursing diagnoses, it is essential that nurses refer to the definitions and defining characteristics of the diagnoses used in this text, which can be found in Appendix C.

References

Alzheimer's Association. (2016a). *10 ways to love your brain.* Retrieved from http://www.alz.org/brain-health/10_ways-to-love-your-brain.asp

Alzheimer's Association. (2016b). *2016 Alzheimer's disease facts and figures.* Retrieved from http://www.alz.org/documents_custom/2016-facts-and-figures.pdf

American College of Obstetricians and Gynecologists (ACOG). (2014). *Guidelines for women's health care: A resource manual* (4th ed.). Washington, DC: Author.

American College of Obstetricians and Gynecologists (ACOG). (2015). *Menstruation in girls and adolescents: Using the menstrual cycle as a vital sign* (ACOG Committee Opinion No. 651). Washington, DC: Author.

American Heart Association (AHA). (2016). *About metabolic syndrome.* Retrieved from http://www.heart.org/HEARTORG/Conditions/More/MetabolicSyndrome/About-Metabolic-Syndrome_UCM_301920_Article.jsp#.WdPprGhSyUk

American Heart Association (AHA). (2017). *Heart disease statistics at a glance.* Retrieved from https://www.goredforwomen.org/about-heart-disease/facts_about_heart_disease_in_women-sub-category/statistics-at-a-glance

Baber, R. J., Panay, N., Fenton, A., & the IMS Writing Group. (2016). 2016 IMS recommendations on women's midlife health and menopause hormone therapy. *Climacteric, 19*(2), 109–150.

Cosman, F., deBeur, S. J., LeBoff, M. S., Lewiecki, E. M., Tanner, B., Randall, S., & Lindsay, R. (2014). Clinician's guide to prevention and treatment of osteoporosis. *Osteoporosis International, 25*(10), 2359–2381. DOI:10.1007/s00198-014-2794-2

de Villiers, T. J., Gass, M. L. S., Haines, C. J., Hall, J. E., Lobo, R. A., Pierroz, D. D., & Rees, M. (2013). Global consensus statement on menopausal hormone therapy. *Climacteric, 16,* 203–204.

Fenton, A. J. (2015). Premature ovarian insufficiency: Pathogenesis and management. *Journal of Mid-Life Health, 6*(4), 147–153.

Hantsoo, L., & Epperson, N. (2015). Premenstrual dysphoric disorder. *Current Psychiatry Reports, 17,* 86–95. DOI:10.1007/s11920-015-0628-3

Huda. (2016). What does Islam say about delaying menstruation. Retrieved from http://aboutislam.net/counseling/ask-the-scholar/acts-of-worship/pills-delaying-menstruation-ramadan-allowed/

Janda, C., Kues, J. N., Andersson, G., Kleinstäuber, M., & Weise, C. (2017). A symptom diary to assess severe premenstrual syndrome and premenstrual dysphoric disorder. *Women and Health, 57*(7), 837–854.

Joshi, D., & Jamshidl, M. (2017). Abnormal uterine bleeding. In C. T. Johnson, J. L. Hallock, J. L. Bienstock, H. E. Fox, & E. E. Wallach (Eds.), *The Johns Hopkins manual of gynecology and obstetrics* (5th ed.). Philadelphia, PA: Wolters Kluwer.

Kridli, S. (2011). Health beliefs and practices of Muslim women during Ramadan. *MCN, the American Journal of Maternal/Child Nursing, 36*(4), 216–221.

McNamara, M., Batur, P., & DeSapri, K. T. (2015). In the clinic: Perimenopau se. *Annals of Internal Medicine, 162*(3), ITC1–15. DOI:10.7326/AITC201502030

Myrisk, K., Reinn, R., & Harkins, M. (2014). The prevalence of and attitudes toward oligomenorrhea and amenorrhea in Division I female athletes. *International Journal of Athletic Therapy & Training, 19*(6), 41–17.

National Center for Complementary and Integrative Health (NCCIH). (2016). *Menopausal symptoms and complementary health practices: What the science says.* Retrieved from https://nccih.nih.gov/health/providers/digest/menopause-scienceInt

National Institute on Aging. (2016). *Health and aging: Menopause.* Retrieved from https://www.nia.nih.gov/health/topics/menopause

National Osteoporosis Foundation (NOF). (2016). *Medical and scientific leaders in the bone health field gather in Miami for the Interdisciplinary Symposium on Osteoporosis.* Retrieved from https://www.nof.org/news/medical-and-scientific-leaders-in-the-bone-health-field-gather-in-miami-for-the-interdisciplinary-symposium-on-osteoporosis/

Perper, M., Aldahan, A. S., Tsatalis, J. P., & Nouri, K. (2017). Modifications of body surface: Piercings, tattoos, and scarification. *International Journal of Dermatology, 56,* 351–353.

Roche-Paull, R. (2015). Body modifications and breastfeeding: What you need to know. *Journal of Human Lactation, 31*(3), 552–553.

Rost, M., Jacobsson, J., Dahlstrom, O., Hammar, M., & Timpka, T. (2014). Amenorrhea in elite athletics athletes: Prevalence and associations to athletics injury. *British Journal of Sports Medicine, 48*(7), 560–674.

Ryu, A., & Kim, T-H. (2015). Premenstrual syndrome: A mini review. *Maturitas, 82*(4), 436–440.

Schuiling, K. D., & Likis, F. E. (2017). *Women's gynecologic health* (3rd ed.). Burlington, MA: Jones & Bartlett Learning.

U. S. Census Bureau. (2016). *The foreign-born population in the United States, 2010.* Retrieved from https://www.census.gov/topics/population/foreign-born/about.html

Zieman, M., Hatcher, R. A., & Allen, A. Z. (2015). *Managing contraception 2015–2016.* Tiger, GA: Bridging the Gap Foundation.

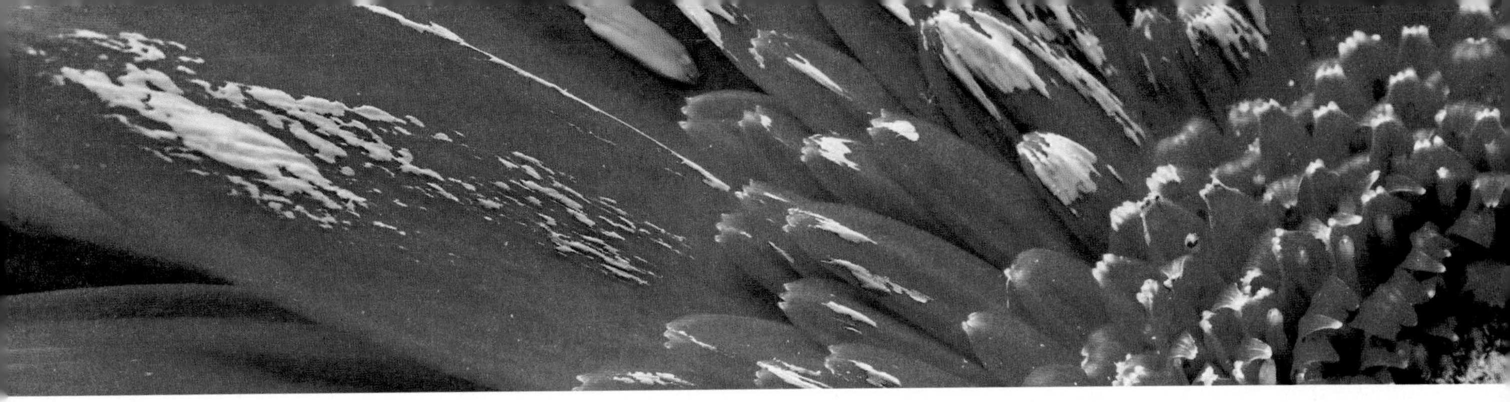

Chapter 4

Family Planning

I was 15 when I fell in love with Trevor, a handsome 17-year-old senior on our high school basketball team. My friends were so envious. We didn't plan on becoming sexually involved. It just happened. I knew I should have used some method of birth control, but I didn't know where to go. I couldn't talk to my mother. She wouldn't understand. Trevor tried condoms, but he didn't like the way they felt. Several months went by and nothing happened. Then one month my period was late. I was SCARED. It really hit me that a pregnancy would be so hard to handle. I was only a sophomore. My best friend took me to see her nurse practitioner. My pregnancy test was negative. The nurse practitioner encouraged me to talk. She taught me about my body and how to protect myself against an unintended pregnancy and sexually transmitted infections. She helped me build my self-esteem. I realize now that I'm not ready to be in a sexual relationship yet, but when I am, I know how to ask for birth control and where to go.

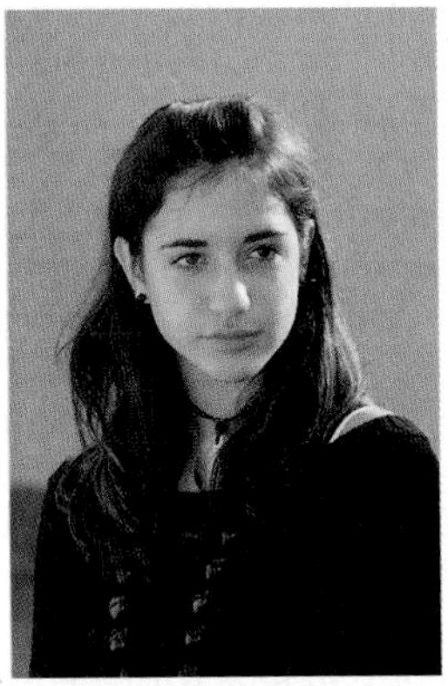

SOURCE: Jules Selmes/Pearson Education Ltd.

Learning Outcomes

4.1 Describe the reasons why women and couples choose to use contraception.

4.2 Discuss types of fertility awareness–based methods (FAB) such as natural family planning (NFP).

4.3 Identify the only spermicide preparation currently available in the United States.

4.4 Compare the barrier methods of contraception with regard to correct use and advantages and disadvantages.

4.5 Summarize the key points that women who use combined hormonal contraceptives (estrogen and a progestin) should know, including the correct procedure for use, common side effects, warning signs, and noncontraceptive benefits of the following: Combined oral contraceptive pills, contraceptive patch (Xulane), and contraceptive vaginal ring (NuvaRing).

4.6 Compare progestin-only hormonal contraceptive methods to combined hormonal estrogen–progestin methods of the following: Medroxyprogesterone acetate injection (Depo-Provera), the norethindrone "mini-pill" (Micronor), and etonogestrel subdermal implant (Nexplanon).

4.7 Delineate the advantages and disadvantages of intrauterine contraception (IUC) as a method of birth control, as well as the differences between the IUCs with hormones and the one with copper.

4.8 Discuss advantages of long-acting reversible contraceptive methods (LARC): IUCs (ParaGard T380A, Mirena, Skyla, Liletta, Kyleena) and the subdermal implant (Nexplanon).

4.9 Identify the appropriate time frame for initiating postcoital emergency contraception (EC).

4.10 Contrast the forms of sterilization (tubal ligation and vasectomy) with regard to risk, effectiveness, advantages, and disadvantages.

4.11 Compare medical and surgical approaches to pregnancy termination.

Healthy People 2020

(FP-1) Increase the proportion of pregnancies that are intended

(FP-2) Reduce the proportion of females experiencing pregnancy despite use of a reversible contraceptive method

Family planning refers to actions an individual or a couple takes to avoid a pregnancy, to plan the timing of a pregnancy, to space future pregnancies, or to gain control over the number of children conceived. A woman who is sexually active and not intending a pregnancy will require contraception for approximately 30 years. Thus, at a given time, a woman may choose one method of contraception and at a later time may elect to use a different method. For example, combined oral contraceptives (COCs) are an excellent method of contraception for women who are healthy, have no medical contraindications, and desire a method that is rapidly reversible. A woman in a stable sexual relationship who desires long-term family planning may choose to use intrauterine contraception (IUC), whereas a woman who has no desire for future children may elect permanent sterilization for herself, or her male partner may choose to undergo a vasectomy (a male sterilization procedure). There are women who are not in need of family planning. These women might not use contraceptive methods for religious reasons (Roman Catholicism, Orthodox Judaism), might not be sexually active, might be attempting to get pregnant or be already pregnant, might be infertile, or might be in the immediate postpartum period. Nurses educate women. To help nurses provide accurate contraceptive information that meets a woman's needs at a particular time in her life, this chapter discusses current contraceptive methods and use, as well as advantages and disadvantages for each.

Women and their partners who do wish to have children face the decision as to the right timing of a pregnancy. A simple question to help a woman decide if she is ready for children is to ask, "Do you want to become pregnant this year?" (American College of Obstetrics and Gynecology [ACOG], 2016a). As a pregnancy can be planned or unintended (failure to use contraception or failure of the contraceptive method), this chapter concludes with a discussion of preconception counseling. Nurses can give women and their partners anticipatory guidance about preconception to ensure that they are in the best possible physical and mental health when, and if, a pregnancy occurs.

Ethics in Action!

Is family planning a basic human right (United Nations Population Fund [UNFPA], 2016)?

Overview of Family Planning

Family planning can reduce poverty and empower women. Women who choose the number of children desired and when to have those children are allowed to complete an education that improves their earning potential and their ability to care for their families. Family planning and contraception also prevents unintended pregnancies and complications associated with pregnancy and birth. "If all women with an unmet need for contraceptives were able to use modern methods, an additional 24 million abortions (14 million of which would be unsafe), 6 million miscarriages, 70,000 maternal deaths and 500,000 infant deaths could be prevented" (UNFPA, 2016). Nurses can help empower women by providing accurate information about family planning.

Demographics

Women of childbearing age are defined as being 15 to 44 years of age. A pregnancy can be considered intended or unintended, with the latter subcategorized into "unintended and mistimed" or "unintended and unwanted" (Schuiling & Likis, 2017). In the United States in 2014, over 20 million sexually active women of reproductive age were at risk for an unintended pregnancy due to unmet contraceptive needs (Frost, Frohwirth, & Zolna, 2016). In part, due to the increased availability and healthcare coverage for long-acting reversible contraception (LARC) under the Affordable Care Act, the rate of unintended pregnancy in the United States declined between 2008 and 2011 from 51 to 45% (Finer & Zolna, 2016). In 2011, of 6.1 million pregnancies, 42% ended in abortion and 58% ended in birth (Guttmacher Institute [GI], 2016d). In 2014, 652,639 pregnancies ended in abortion (Jatlaoui et al., 2017). That same year, publicly funded family planning services helped women avoid 2 million pregnancies that would have resulted in 900,000 births and nearly 700,000 abortions (GI, 2016d). Unintended pregnancies due to unmet contraceptive needs are not only a problem in the United States but across the globe.

Worldwide there are 225 million women of reproductive age living in the poorest countries with unmet modern contraceptive needs (UNFPA, 2016). Every day approximately 830 women die from a preventable pregnancy-related complication (AIDS, hemorrhage, hypertension, infection, and emboli) and 99% of these preventable tragedies occur in developing countries, more than half of which are in sub-Saharan Africa (World Health Organization [WHO], 2016). In 2000, the United Nations endorsed the Millennium Development Goals to reduce extreme poverty by 2015; the fifth goal focused on improving maternal health (WHO, 2015a). Although the maternal mortality rates dropped by 44%, from 385 maternal deaths per 100,000 live births to 216 per 100,000 live births, the rate remains unacceptably high (WHO, 2015b). In 2015 the United Nations developed the Sustainable Development Goals (SDG) of which Goal 3 is to reduce maternal mortality to less than 70 per 100,000 live births (WHO, 2016). Provision of contraceptive services is essential to prevent unintended pregnancies and pregnancy-related complications, as well as to meet SDG Goal 3. If family planning is a human right, women in the United States and across the globe need access to reliable contraception and education about proper use.

Contraception

Contraception is not only about preventing unintended pregnancies, but also about preventing maternal morbidity and mortality due to pregnancy-related complications. Worldwide, women who are able to use contraception and plan the desired number of pregnancies, as well as the interval between those pregnancies, benefit in several ways (UNFPA, 2016):

- They are generally healthier.
  - They enjoy a lower incidence of sexually transmitted infections, including HIV.
  - They have lower rates of induced, often unsafe, abortions.
- They have fewer unwanted pregnancies and births.
- They are better educated.
  - They are more empowered at home, in the community, and are more financially productive.
- Their children are healthier.
- Their children are better educated.

Choosing a Method of Contraception

The decision to use a method of contraception may be made individually by a woman (or, in the case of condoms or vasectomy, by a man) or jointly by a couple. Attitudes about contraceptive methods vary considerably. Since 1982, the two leading contraceptive methods in the United States have been the combined oral contraceptive (COC) pill for women younger than 35 years of age and sterilization for women over the age of 35 years (GI, 2016b). Use of the male **condom** (a thin latex, silicone, polyurethane, or lambskin sheath worn on a man's penis during sexual intercourse as a contraceptive measure) increased from 52 to 93% from 1982 to 2010 because of the effectiveness of condoms in preventing unintended pregnancy and sexually transmitted infections (GI, 2016b).

Any decision by the woman about a contraceptive method should be made voluntarily with full knowledge of its advantages, disadvantages, effectiveness, side effects, contraindications, and adverse and long-term side effects. Many outside factors will influence this choice, including cultural practices, religious beliefs, personality, cost, effectiveness, availability, misinformation, practicality of method, and self-esteem. The possibility of decreased efficacy of hormonal contraceptives in women over 198 pounds, or those who are greater than 130% of their ideal body weight, has not been resolved, a fact that will impact decision making. Different methods of contraception, or perhaps more than one contraceptive method at a time, may be appropriate. In choosing a contraceptive method, consistency of use always outweighs the absolute reliability of the given method. See Table 4–1.

Criteria promulgated by the World Health Organization and the Centers for Disease Control are available to assist the woman and her healthcare provider in determining the best contraceptive method for her (CDC, 2016d, 2016e). The U.S. Medical Eligibility Criteria for Contraceptive Use (MEC) and the U.S. Selected Practice Recommendations for Contraceptive Use (SPR) 2016 are to be used in conjunction with a thorough health history and physical examination to ensure that the contraceptive method is both safe and effective for an individual woman (CDC, 2016b, 2016d, 2016e). See *Women with Special Needs: Contraceptive Counseling*.

TABLE 4–1 Factors to Consider in Choosing a Method of Contraception

- Effectiveness of method in preventing pregnancy
- Safety of the method:
  - Are there inherent risks?
  - Does it offer protection against sexually transmitted infections or other conditions?
- Woman's age and future childbearing plans
- Any contraindications in the woman's health history; see U.S. Medical Eligibility Criteria for Contraceptive Use [MEC] (CDC, 2016d) and U.S. Selected Practice Recommendations for Contraceptive Use [SPR] (CDC, 2016e)
- Religious, cultural, or moral factors influencing choice
- Personal preferences, biases
- Lifestyle:
  - How frequently does the woman have intercourse?
  - Does she have multiple partners?
  - Does she have ready access to medical care in the event of complications?
  - Will unscheduled bleeding (irregular bleeding) preclude coitus with her partner and cause discord in intimacy?
  - Is she comfortable with touching herself?
  - Does she have a fear of needles?
- Is cost a factor?
- Is her partner supportive and willing to cooperate?
- Personal motivation to use method
- Woman's weight in pounds or percent over ideal body weight

Women with Special Needs Contraceptive Counseling

Many healthcare providers assume that women with developmental disabilities are not sexually active and, therefore, do not need contraceptive counseling. Women with developmental disabilities need education on sexual issues including conception and pregnancy prevention. A level of functioning assessment should be performed to determine if the woman is capable of using different types of contraceptives effectively. Contraceptive choices should be discussed and provided as needed.

Fertility Awareness–Based Methods

A woman is fertile once during her menstrual cycle, typically 14 days before the onset of menses, compared with a man, who is fertile every day. **Fertility awareness–based (FAB) methods** include methods that require a woman to monitor her *fertile window* (generally between days 8 and 19 of 26- to 32-day cycles) and abstain from coitus, or use a barrier method, during that time. A woman is most fertile 5 days before ovulation until 1 day post-ovulation. If a woman abstains from coitus until after her fertile window has closed, she is using *natural family planning (NFP)* (Schuiling & Likis, 2017).

NFP is free, safe, and acceptable to many whose religious beliefs prohibit other methods. NFP provides an increased awareness of the menstrual cycle, involves no artificial substances or devices, encourages a couple to communicate about sexual activity and family planning, and, conversely, is useful in helping a couple plan a pregnancy.

To be used effectively, all FAB methods, including NFP, require extensive initial counseling and are best suited for women with regular menstrual cycles. FAB/NFP methods may interfere with sexual spontaneity, require the couple to maintain records for several menstrual cycles (months) before beginning use, may be difficult or impossible for certain groups of women to use, and may not be as reliable in preventing pregnancy as other methods. Women for whom a FAB/NFP method might not be ideal include those with irregular menstrual cycles (such as those with polycystic ovarian syndrome), those who are breastfeeding, or those in perimenopause.

Standard Days Method

The *Standard Days Method (SDM)* is good for women with regular menstrual cycles between 26 and 32 days. Intercourse is avoided, or a barrier method used, during cycle days 8 through 19 (Schuiling & Likis, 2017). CycleBeads® is a color-coded set of beads to be used in conjunction with SDM that represents when to abstain from coitus.

Calendar Rhythm Method

The *calendar rhythm method (CRM)* is based on the assumption that ovulation tends to occur 14 days (plus or minus 2 days) before the start of the next menstrual period. To use this method, the woman must record her menstrual cycle for 6 months to identify the shortest and longest cycles. The first day of menstruation is the first day of the cycle. The fertile phase is calculated from 18 days before the end of the shortest recorded cycle through 11 days from the end of the longest recorded cycle. For example, if a woman's cycle lasts from 24 to 28 days, the fertile phase would be calculated as day 6 through day 17. Once this information is obtained, the woman can identify the fertile and infertile phases of her cycle. For effective use of this method, she must abstain from intercourse during the fertile phase or use a barrier method during that time (Schuiling & Likis, 2017).

Billings Ovulation Method

The *Billings Ovulation Method (BOM)* involves the assessment of cervical mucus changes that occur during the menstrual cycle. The amount and character of cervical mucus changes because of the influences of estrogen and progesterone (see Chapter 9 for a discussion of the female reproductive cycle). During the follicular phase of the cycle (from the end of menses until just before ovulation), cervical mucus is nonmalodorous, thick, white, and sticky. This progesterone-dominant mucus is not friendly to sperm and is known as *hostile mucus*. At the time of ovulation, estrogen-dominant mucus is clearer, waterier, and stretchable (a quality called *spinnbarkeit*) (Figure 4–1A). It has an "egg-white" appearance and is known as *fertile mucus*, which is "friendly" to sperm, as it nourishes and assists passage through the cervix and uterus up into the fallopian tubes. It also shows a characteristic fern leaf pattern when placed on a glass slide and allowed to dry (Figure 4–1B). Following ovulation, during the luteal phase of the cycle (ovulation to menses), cervical mucus is again progesterone-dominant and this thick mucus forms a network that traps sperm, making their passage upward into the female reproductive tract difficult.

Before using this method, the woman abstains from intercourse for at least one entire menstrual cycle, during which time she assesses her cervical mucus daily for amount, feeling of slipperiness or wetness, color, clearness, and spinnbarkeit. Abstinence is essential during this time, not only so that the woman avoids pregnancy, but also because the presence of ejaculate in the vagina in the hours following intercourse could interfere with the woman's assessment of her cervical mucus as the male ejaculate liquefies and can be confused with "fertile" mucus.

When using this method, the woman assumes that the peak day of wetness and clear, stretchable mucus is the day of ovulation. However, she abstains from intercourse from the time she *first* notices the mucus is becoming clearer, more elastic, and slippery until 4 days *after* the peak of mucus (ovulation) is noticed. Because this method evaluates the effects of hormonal changes, women with irregular cycles may still be able to use it. Women who feel uncomfortable checking their mucus should be encouraged to use another method (Schuiling & Likis, 2017).

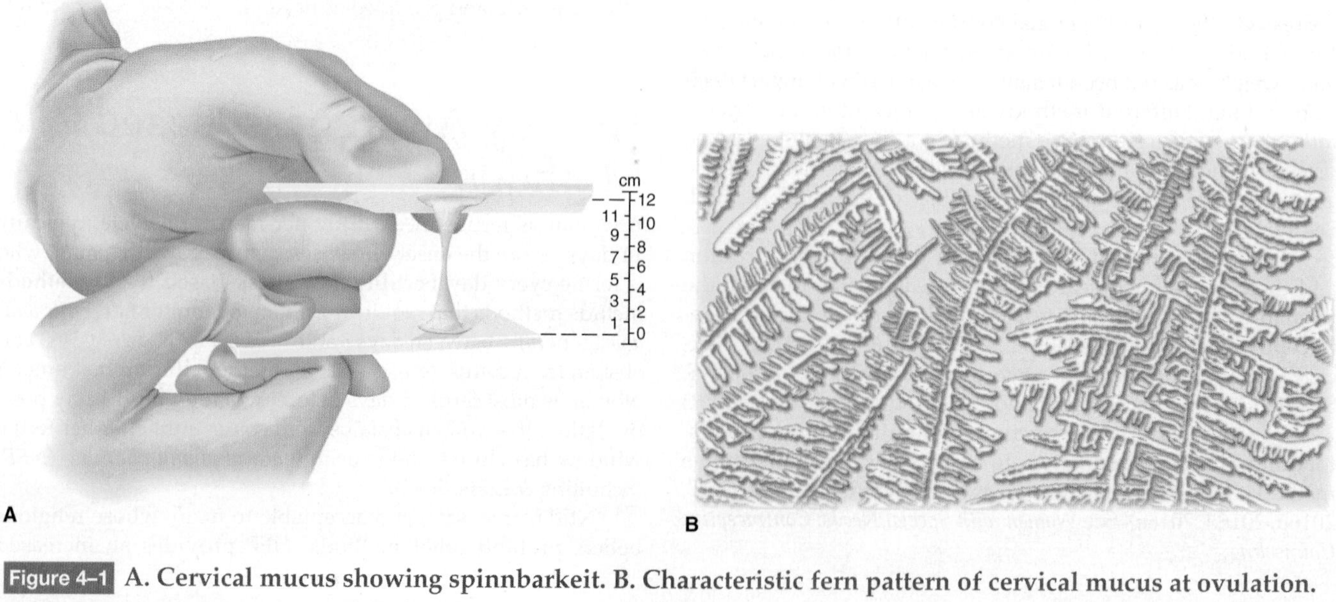

Figure 4–1 A. Cervical mucus showing spinnbarkeit. B. Characteristic fern pattern of cervical mucus at ovulation.

Two-Day Method

The *two-day method* is based on a woman's ability to distinguish the difference between progesterone-mediated and estrogen-mediated cervical mucus that is present at her introitus before she urinates, preferably in the afternoon and evening. If she notices cervical secretions of any type either yesterday or today, she is fertile *today*. If no secretions were noted today or yesterday, she is not fertile *today*—hence the name (Schuiling & Likis, 2017).

Symptothermal Method

The *symptothermal method (STM)* consists of recording various indicators of fertility by the woman and her partner for a number of months. These include cycle length; frequency and timing of coitus; cervical mucus changes; secondary signs of ovulation such as increased libido, abdominal bloating, and *mittelschmerz* (midcycle abdominal pain); and changes in basal body temperature (BBT). In retrospect, using the indicators, the couple learns to recognize signs that indicate ovulation. For couples interested in the symptothermal method, especially for use as NFP, training courses are available through the Couple to Couple League (CCL, 2017).

Basal Body Temperature Method

The *basal body temperature (BBT)* method is incorporated into the symptothermal method and provides an objective record of fertile days. The BBT method is used to detect ovulation by a predictable increase in the basal temperature during the menstrual cycle that follows ovulation. It requires that the woman take her temperature every morning upon awakening (before any activity) and record the findings on a temperature graph. After 3 to 4 months of recording her temperatures, if she has regular cycles, she should be able to predict when ovulation will occur by a retrospective review of temperature charts. This method is based on the fact that the temperature almost always rises and remains elevated after ovulation until the next menses (or during the luteal phase) because of the production of progesterone, a thermogenic (heat-producing) hormone, produced by the corpus luteum cyst. Figure 4–2 shows a sample BBT chart. If a pregnancy is not achieved, the temperature drops prior to menses. If a pregnancy is achieved, the temperature will remain elevated throughout the gestation.

To avoid conception, the woman and her partner abstain from intercourse, or use a barrier method, on the day of the temperature rise and for 3 days following. Because the temperature rise does not occur until after ovulation, if the woman had intercourse just before the rise, she may be at risk of pregnancy.

Other Options

The *lactational amenorrhea method (LAM)* is based on a woman breastfeeding *exclusively* or *almost exclusively* for the first 6 months after childbirth or until her first menses occurs. High levels of prolactin in the woman's body during breastfeeding should prevent ovulation. The woman should breastfeed on demand, and the newborn should suckle both breasts until empty. Breast milk expression by hand or a pump is not a suitable substitute when using LAM. If a formula supplement is used often, a barrier method of contraception should be used. When the woman stops breastfeeding, resumes her menses, or her newborn becomes 6 months old, she should select another method of contraception. This method is most reliable in the United States when used with a barrier method. In developing countries, it is a useful method of pregnancy spacing (Schuiling & Likis, 2017).

Abstinence can be considered a method of contraception and is described as avoidance of penis-in-vagina intercourse. A woman who, by personal choice, has never had sexual intercourse is practicing abstinence. Abstinence may also be culturally dictated before marriage. Abstinence may occur when a woman and her male partner choose to abstain for a period of time. This may occur due to the unavailability of her partner, while she waits for a more reliable method of contraception, or because it is the cultural norm during the postpartum period (Zieman, Hatcher, & Allen, 2015). *Outercourse* is a term used to describe penile–vaginal touch without penetration (Planned Parenthood Federation of America, 2016). Ejaculation on the perineum of a woman who is ovulating during outercourse may result in pregnancy.

Coitus interruptus, or *withdrawal*, is one of the oldest methods of contraception. This method requires that the male withdraw from the female's vagina when he feels that ejaculation is impending. He then ejaculates away from the external genitalia of the woman. Coitus interruptus is forbidden in some religions (Orthodox Judaism, Muslim). Failure of this method tends to occur because of the following:

- This method requires great control on the part of the man, who must withdraw just as he feels the urge for deeper penetration with impending orgasm.
- In some men, the pre-ejaculatory fluid, which a man may release as soon as his penis becomes erect, may contain a

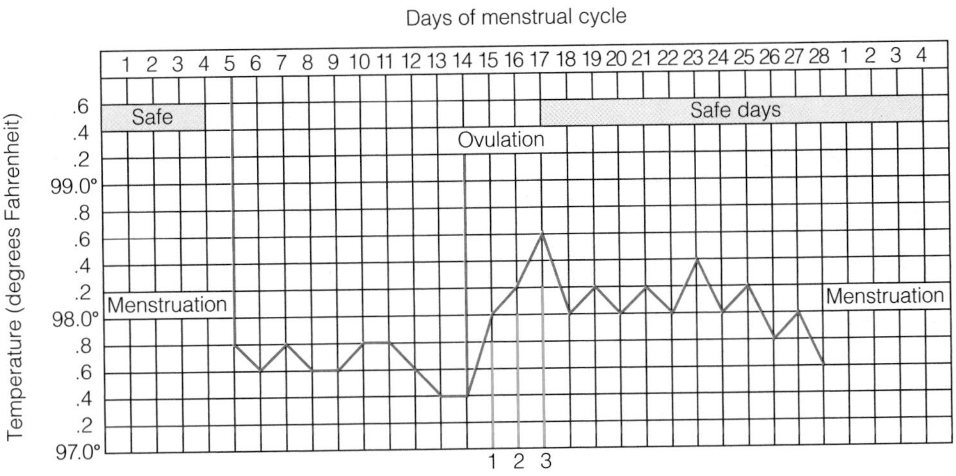

Figure 4–2 **Sample basal body temperature chart.**

small number of sperm. The man may not be aware that he has released pre-ejaculatory fluid. After the first act of coitus, any seminal fluid will contain sperm. If more than one act of intercourse takes place within a short time, the man should urinate first and wipe the tip of his penis to remove any remaining sperm.

Douching after intercourse is an ineffective method of contraception and is *not* recommended. Moreover, it may actually facilitate conception by pushing sperm farther up the birth canal.

Couples who use these methods should be aware of postcoital emergency contraceptive (EC) options. Such options are discussed later in the chapter.

Spermicide

The **spermicide** approved for use in the United States, nonoxynol-9 (N-9), is available as a cream, gel, foam, vaginal film, suppository, or contraceptive sponge. The *contraceptive sponge* (Today® sponge) is both a spermicide and a barrier method, as it contains N-9 and its plastic matrix traps sperm. As a surfactant, spermicides destroy sperm by disrupting the cell membrane.

N-9 is minimally effective when used alone, but its effectiveness increases in conjunction with a barrier method such as the diaphragm, the cervical cap, or male and female condoms. The major advantages of N-9 spermicidal preparations include over-the-counter availability, lack of systemic side effects, and low local toxicity.

The spermicidal preparation is inserted into the vagina before intercourse. A spermicide that effervesces in a moist environment offers more rapid protection, and coitus may take place immediately after it is inserted. A suppository may require up to 15 minutes to dissolve and will not offer protection until it has done so. The nurse needs to instruct the woman to insert any of these spermicidal preparations high in the vagina as close to the cervix as possible. Maintaining a supine position after application, except for use with the cervical sponge, will help keep the preparation in the vagina and close to the cervix after it dissolves. Except for the contraceptive sponge, multiple acts of coitus require repeated doses of the spermicide. In the past, N-9 was thought to offer a modest level of protection against several sexually transmitted infections. However, research suggests that N-9 does not offer protection against the organisms that cause gonorrhea, chlamydia, or HIV/AIDS (Zieman et al., 2015). Moreover, N-9 alone may actually increase a woman's risk of HIV infection because it has a negative effect on the integrity of vaginal cell membranes, making them more susceptible to invasion by organisms such as HIV.

Barrier Methods of Contraception

Barrier methods of contraception block the transport of sperm up the reproductive tract of the woman to the ovum. Included in this category are the male and female condoms, the diaphragm, the cervical cap, and the cervical sponge. Barrier methods are made of latex, silicone, polyurethane, nitrile, plastic, or lambskin, and are often used in conjunction with N-9 to increase contraceptive effectiveness. A trained healthcare provider must examine the woman and fit her for the correct size diaphragm or cervical cap to ensure that the woman's cervix is covered.

Barrier methods require that an individual or couple proactively decide which type to use and then take action to use it prior to every act of coitus. These methods require motivation on the part of the user and cooperation from the partner. A barrier method used with a FAB/NFP method would mean its use is not necessary with every act of coitus, but only during a woman's *fertile window*.

Barrier methods have few side effects, are safe, and offer some level of protection against sexually transmitted infections (STIs), including the human papilloma virus (HPV), which causes cervical dysplasia and cancer. The female condom is the most effective for prevention against STIs.

Barrier methods of contraception are a good choice for women who:

- Have a medical contraindication to using a specific method such as combined oral contraceptives (COCs) or intrauterine contraception (IUCs)
- Are opposed to using contraception that has hormones with or without systemic effects such as hormonal contraceptives, the injection Depo-Provera, the progestin IUCs, or the subdermal implant (Nexplanon)
- Are in the early postpartum period or are lactating
- Need a backup method of contraception for a period of time such as after beginning COCs, after IUC insertion, or after a male partner has just had a vasectomy
- Have intercourse rarely or sporadically
- Are perimenopausal but smoke and thus are not good candidates for COCs.

Women who are allergic to latex should tell their healthcare providers and avoid condoms made of this material. Additionally, they should avoid using oil-based products, such as mineral oil or baby oil, and vaginal medications such as Monistat cream (for a yeast infection) and estrogen creams because these weaken latex. Barrier methods are made of a variety of materials: The diaphragm and cervical cap are made of silicone; the female condom 2 (FC2) is made of nitrile; male condoms are made of latex, silicone, polyurethane, or lambskin; and the Today contraceptive sponge is made of plastic and nonoxynol-9.

Barrier methods can be inserted prior to coitus to increase spontaneity and are more effective when used in conjunction with N-9. Before inserting any female barrier contraceptive, a woman should wash her hands with soap and water to prevent the introduction of microorganisms. After the first act of intercourse, reapplication of N-9 is recommended for each subsequent act. After the last act of intercourse, the diaphragm, cervical sponge, and cervical cap should remain in place for a minimum of 6 to 8 hours to prevent pregnancy. To avoid toxic shock syndrome (TSS), the contraceptive sponge and diaphragm should only be worn for a total of 24 hours, and the cervical cap for 48 hours. Each should be cleaned with mild soap and water after use and should not be shared with other women.

In general, female barrier methods are more effective when used with a male condom, except when using a female condom, as the two condoms can stick to each other, rendering either ineffective. Women who use barrier methods should be alert for symptoms of TSS such as high fever, sore throat, vomiting and/or diarrhea, faintness, weakness, muscle aches, and a rash. Women who use diaphragms should report any symptoms of a urinary tract infection such as dysuria, hematuria, urinary urgency, suprapubic pain, or low-grade fever (Zeimer et al., 2015).

Male Condom

The male condom offers a viable means of contraception when used consistently and properly (Figure 4–3). Acceptance has been increasing for two reasons: (1) A growing number of men are assuming responsibility for regulation of fertility, and (2) condoms provide protection against STIs for both men and women. For women, regardless of age, an STI increases the risk of pelvic inflammatory disease (PID) and may result in infertility. Many women insist that their sexual partners use condoms, and many women carry condoms with them.

The condom is applied to the erect penis, rolled from the tip to the end of the shaft, before vulvar or vaginal contact. Most condoms have a reservoir tip to allow for collection of ejaculate. When using a condom without a reservoir end, a small space must be left at the end to collect the ejaculate, so that the condom does not break at the time of ejaculation. If the condom or vagina is dry, water-soluble lubricants, such as K-Y Jelly or Astroglide, should be used to prevent irritation and possible condom breakage. Oil-based lubricants such as petroleum jelly, baby oil, or hand lotion may weaken the condom and facilitate breakage. Care must be taken in removing the condom after intercourse. For optimal effectiveness, the man should withdraw his penis from the vagina while it is still erect and hold the condom rim to prevent spillage. If, after ejaculation, the penis becomes flaccid while still in the vagina, the man should hold onto the edge of the condom nearest his lower abdomen while withdrawing his penis from the woman's vagina to prevent it from slipping off and to avoid spilling semen.

The effectiveness of male condoms is largely determined by their use. The condom is small, lightweight, disposable, and inexpensive. It has no side effects, as there are polyurethane, silicone, and lambskin condoms for men who are allergic to latex. The male condom requires no medical examination or supervision and offers visual evidence of effectiveness. Condoms are available with ribbed or smooth sides, are tapered or straight-sided, lubricated or unlubricated, and come in a variety of colors, sizes, and flavors, with or without spermicide. Condoms with concurrent use of a vaginal spermicide increase the overall effectiveness in the prevention of pregnancy. Condom use can decrease the transmission of STIs such as gonorrhea, chlamydia, HIV, HPV, syphilis, and herpes simplex I or II.

Slippage, risk of breakage, perineal or vaginal irritation, and dulled sensation are possible disadvantages of male condoms. Condoms should not be stored in hot conditions because heat accelerates their deterioration, making them more susceptible to breaking. Thus, men should avoid placing them in their car glove box or in their wallet in a rear pants pocket.

Ethics in Action!

Does discussion of condom use promote sexual activity in teens?

Female Condom

The *Female Condom 2 (FC2)* (Figure 4–4) is a thin nitrile sheath with a flexible ring at each end. The inner ring, at the closed end of the condom, serves as the means of insertion and fits over the cervix like a diaphragm. The second ring remains outside the vagina and covers a portion of the woman's perineum. It also covers the base of the man's penis during intercourse. A woman needs to be careful not to twist the sheath when she inserts the condom because twisting makes male penetration impossible. The nitrile FC2 replaced the polyurethane condom (Reality Female Condom) due to noisiness during intercourse.

Available over the counter and designed for one-time use, the FC2 may be inserted up to 8 hours before intercourse. The inner sheath is prelubricated but does not contain a spermicide and is not designed to be used with a male condom. Although it also covers only a portion of the vulva, it does not provide

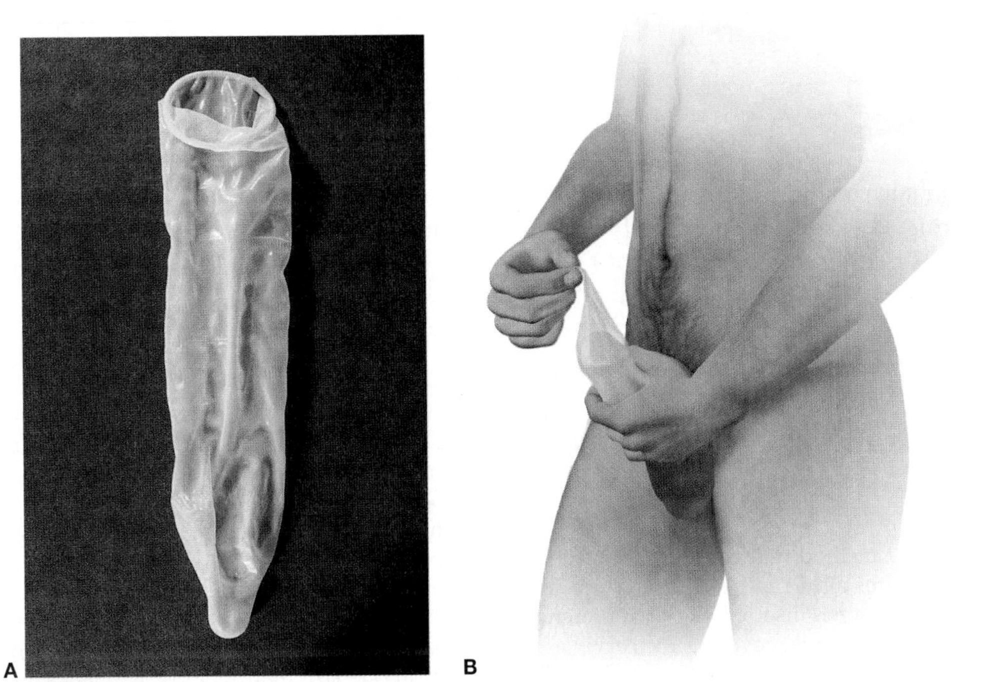

Figure 4–3 A. An unrolled condom with reservoir tip. B. Correct use.

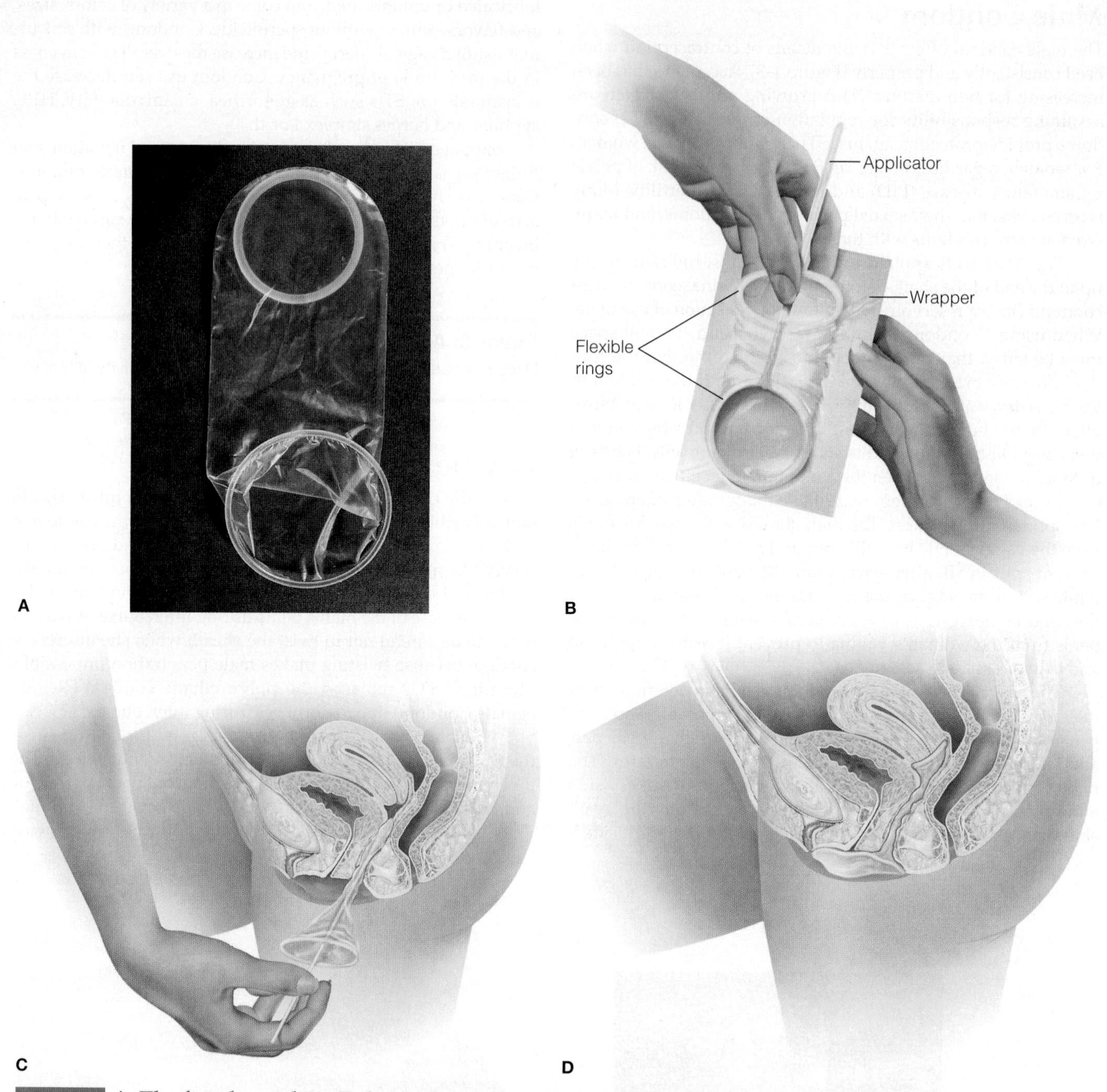

Figure 4–4 **A. The female condom. To insert the condom: B. Remove condom and applicator from wrapper by pulling up on the ring. C. Insert condom slowly by gently pushing the applicator toward the small of the back. D. When properly inserted, the outer ring should rest on the folds of skin around the vaginal opening, and the inner ring (closed end) should fit loosely against the cervix.**

complete protection against STIs, but probably provides better protection than other methods. High cost and the cumbersome feel of the device make acceptability a problem for some couples.

Diaphragm

The **diaphragm** is a barrier method that consists of a steel or nylon round spring that forms a ring and is covered with silicone so that when the diaphragm is inserted, the circumference of the ring lodges high in the vagina, covering the cervix and secured in place behind the symphysis pubis. Use of N-9 spermicidal cream or gel placed inside the diaphragm provides a good level of contraception. The diaphragm potentially reduces the incidence of cervical gonorrhea, chlamydia, and HPV infection, the latter of which can cause cervical neoplasia (Zieman et al., 2015).

The Wide-Seal OmniFlex and Arcing-Style diaphragms manufactured by Cooper Surgical require that a woman be fitted for one of the eight diaphragm sizes and be given instructions by a healthcare provider. The diaphragm should be rechecked for correct size after each childbirth and whenever a woman has gained or lost 10 to 15 pounds or more. The Caya contoured diaphragm comes in one size that fits most women. This is available only by prescription from a healthcare provider, but a fitting is not necessary. The diaphragm must be inserted before intercourse with approximately 1 teaspoonful (or 1.5 inches of spermicide from the tube) of N-9 spermicidal gel placed around its rim and in the cup (Figure 4–5). This N-9 chemical barrier supplements the mechanical barrier of the diaphragm, resulting in disruption of sperm cell membranes and its blockage from ascension to the upper female reproductive tract. The diaphragm is inserted through the vagina and should cover the cervix and anterior portion of the vagina. When the entire diaphragm is inserted and properly in place behind the symphysis, a "popping" sensation may occur. A well-fitting diaphragm should not cause discomfort to the woman or her partner. Correct placement of the diaphragm can be checked by touching the cervix with a fingertip through the cup. The cervix feels like a small rounded structure and has a consistency similar to that of the tip of the nose. It is necessary to leave the diaphragm in place for at least 6 hours after the last act of coitus. If intercourse is desired again within the 6 hours, another type of contraception must be used or additional spermicidal gel placed in the vagina with an applicator, taking care not to disturb the placement of the diaphragm. The diaphragm should not remain in the vagina for more than 24 hours because of the risk of TSS.

Periodically, the diaphragm should be held up to the light or filled with water and inspected for tears or holes. If properly maintained, it can last for several years, so it is a cost-effective method of contraception. The diaphragm should be washed with soap and dried well after each use and then stored in a clean, dry container.

Some couples feel that the use of a diaphragm interferes with the spontaneity of intercourse. However, this perception can be decreased if the woman inserts the diaphragm before intercourse or if insertion of the diaphragm by the male partner becomes part of the intimacy act. Women who object to touching their genitals to insert the diaphragm, check its placement, and remove it may find this method unsatisfactory. Women who are very obese or who have short fingers may find the diaphragm difficult to insert. It may not be recommended for women with a history of urinary tract infections (UTIs) because pressure from the diaphragm on the urethra may interfere with complete bladder emptying and lead to recurrent UTIs. These women should be given information about other methods of contraception. Any woman with a history of TSS should not use the diaphragm, cervical sponge, or cervical cap because these must be left in place

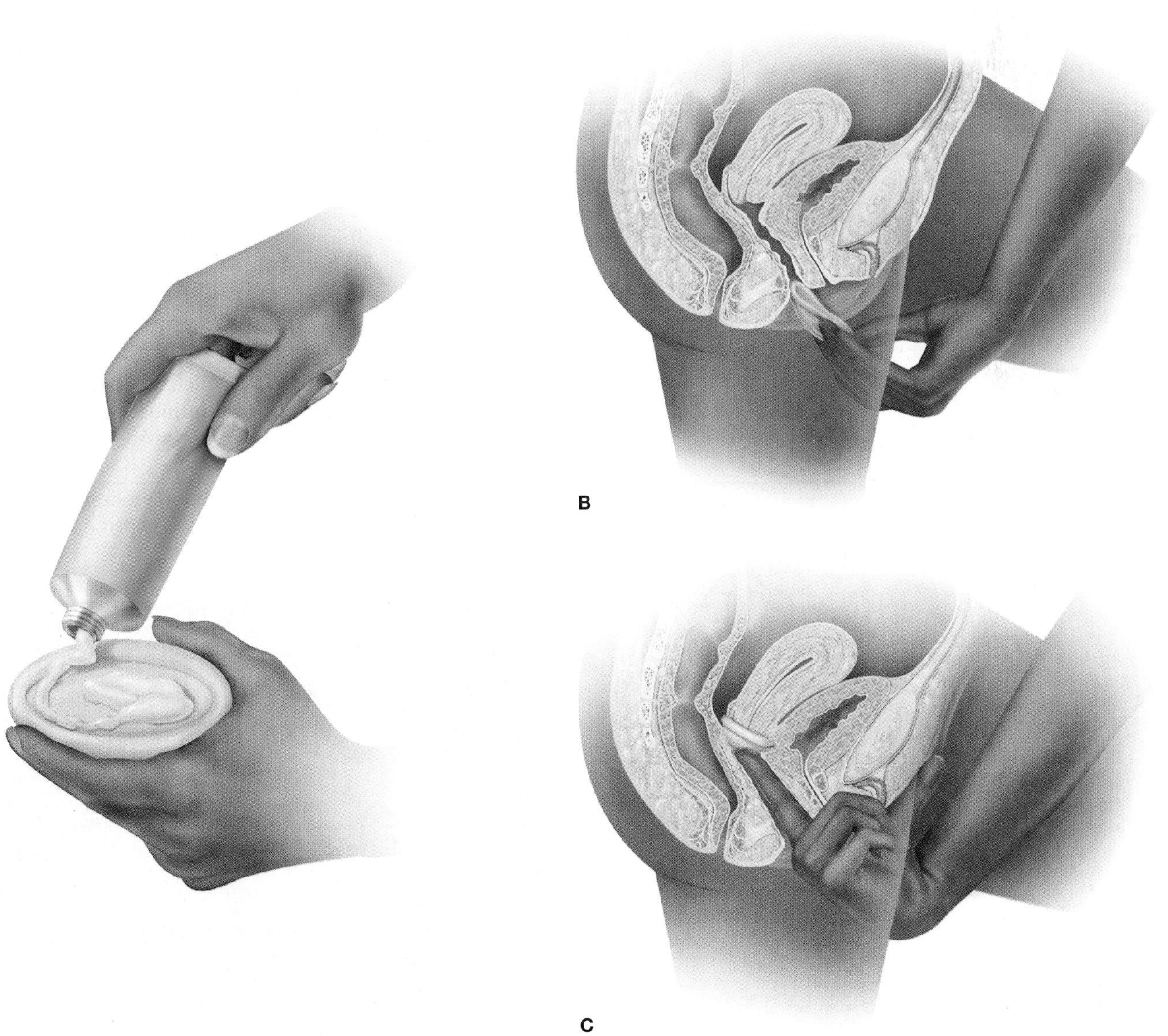

Figure 4–5 Inserting the diaphragm. A. Apply jelly to the rim and center of the diaphragm. B. Insert the diaphragm. C. Push the rim of the diaphragm under the pubic symphysis. Then check placement of the diaphragm. The cervix should be felt through the diaphragm.

for prolonged periods. For the same reason, the diaphragm should not be used during a menstrual period or if a woman has abnormal vaginal discharge.

The Cervical Cap

Advantages, disadvantages, and contraindications for the cervical cap are similar to those associated with the diaphragm. It should be used with N-9 inserted inside the cap. As the cap is smaller than the diaphragm, it does not interfere with emptying of the bladder that can lead to recurrent UTIs. As with the diaphragm, placement of the device requires that it be inserted prior to coitus and left in for 6 to 8 hours afterward. The cervical cap should not remain in the vagina longer than 48 hours due to the risk of TSS.

The *FemCap* cervical cap is reusable, looks like a small sailor's cap, and is made of soft silicone. The dome of the cap fits over the cervix, while the soft brim flares out slightly and conforms to the shape of the vagina. A strap placed over the dome permits easier removal. The cap is available in three sizes according to parity and should be used with a spermicide. In the United States a prescription is required and then the cap can be ordered online or obtained through a pharmacy.

Contraceptive Sponge

The *Today* contraceptive sponge, available without a prescription, is a plastic pillow-shaped, soft, absorbent synthetic sponge containing the spermicide N-9. It is made with a concave or cupped area on one side, which is designed to fit over the cervix. It has a loop to permit easy removal. The sponge acts by releasing the spermicide N-9 gradually over a 24-hour period and by trapping sperm in its matrix, thus making it both a barrier and a spermicidal method of contraception.

The sponge is moistened thoroughly with water before use to activate the spermicide and is then inserted high into the vagina so that the cupped side fits snugly against the cervical os (Figure 4–6). This decreases the chance of the sponge being dislodged during intercourse. It should be left in place for at least 6 hours after intercourse but worn for no more than 24 hours before being removed and discarded.

Advantages of the cervical sponge include professional fitting is not required, it may be used for multiple acts of coitus for up to 24 hours, one size fits all, and it acts as both a barrier method and a spermicidal agent. Problems associated with the sponge include difficulty removing it, local irritation, or allergic reactions. Some women also report that the sponge absorbs vaginal secretions, contributing to vaginal dryness.

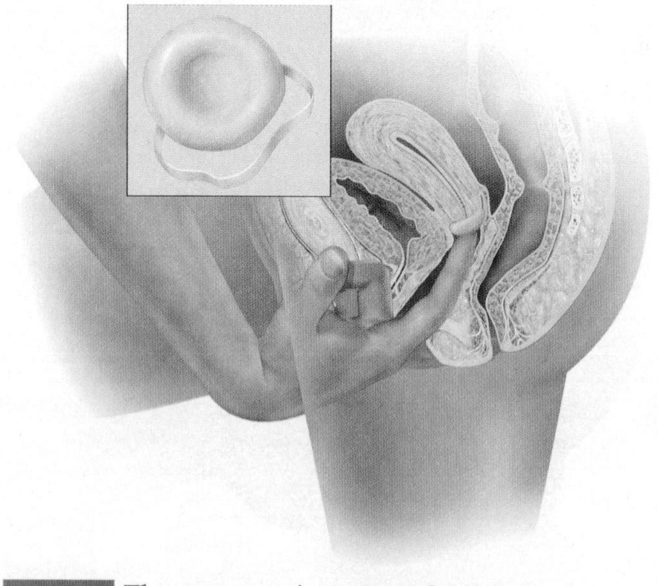

Figure 4–6 The contraceptive sponge is moistened well with water and inserted into the vagina with the concave portion positioned over the cervix.

Long-Acting Reversible Contraception

Long-acting reversible contraceptive methods (LARC) include those that are used for an extended period of time, do not require user compliance, are not associated with the act of coitus, and are reversible upon discontinuation. These cost-effective methods are especially well suited for adolescents and include intrauterine contraception and the subdermal implant. Another term for LARC is the "forgettable method" because the woman does not have to remember to use it prior to coitus.

Intrauterine Contraception

Intrauterine contraception (IUC) refers to the use of an *intrauterine device (IUD)* that is designed to be inserted into the uterus by a qualified healthcare provider and left in place for an extended period, providing continuous contraceptive protection for 3 to 10 years (Figure 4–7). There are five devices used for intrauterine contraception available in the United States.

- The *Copper IUC (ParaGard T 380A)* is a small, radiopaque polyethylene T-shaped device that has copper covering parts of its stem and arms. This IUC is not an option for women allergic to copper but is an excellent choice for women who have medical conditions that preclude use of other contraceptives, hormonal or barrier. It provides effective contraception for 10 years.
- Each of the levonorgestrel-secreting progestin intrauterine contraceptive devices is small and T-shaped, with a reservoir

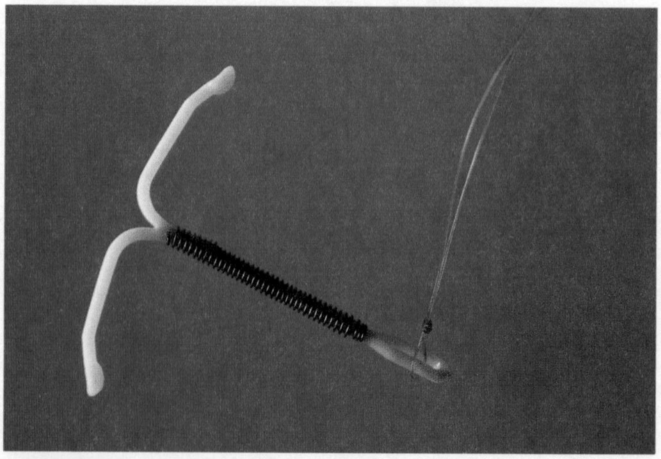

Figure 4–7 An example of IUC.

SOURCE: Boucharlat/AGE Fotostock.

that releases the locally acting progestin over a 24-hour period. There should be little to no systemic effect of the progestin.

- *Mirena* contains a total of 52 mg of levonorgestrel, releasing 20 micrograms per day, and provides 5 years of protection.
- *Skyla* contains a total of 13.5 mg of levonorgestrel and has a 3-year indication. Sklya is smaller than Mirena and may fit into the uterus of a nulliparous woman more easily. Skyla also has a radiopaque silver ring at the top of the "T" so it can easily be identified on ultrasound. If the woman needs an MRI, she must notify the technician.
- *Liletta* contains 52 mg of levonorgestrel and has a 3-year indication.
- *Kyleena* contains 19.5 mg of levonorgestrel and has a 5-year indication.

Mirena, Sklya, Liletta, and Kyleena are progestin-only IUC. Without an estrogen to stabilize the endometrium, unscheduled (irregular) bleeding can occur. Thus, the primary cause of discontinuation of the progestin-only IUC is *unscheduled bleeding*. Women need anticipatory guidance to understand how the progestin-only IUC works and how IUC can affect bleeding patterns and still be a healthy choice. Any type of progesterone-only IUC is an excellent choice for women who are allergic to copper or who have heavy menses and desire decreased bleeding or amenorrhea, as the progestin causes the endometrium to become atrophic, leading to overall less uterine bleeding.

Traditionally, IUC was believed to act by preventing implantation of the fertilized ovum. Thus, it was considered an abortifacient. This belief is not accurate; all IUC is truly contraceptive. The copper IUC is known to have local inflammatory effects on the endometrium and to impair sperm from functioning properly. The levonorgestrel-secreting IUC causes the lining of the uterus (endometrium) to become atrophic and also produces thick cervical mucus that is hostile or unfriendly to sperm. All types of IUC produce a spermicidal intrauterine environment (Schuiling & Likis, 2017).

IUC available today, contrary to common myth, does not increase the risk of ectopic pregnancy or pelvic inflammatory disease (PID). In reality, infections in IUC users are probably related more to the woman's lifestyle than to the presence of the IUC. Advantages of all IUC include a high rate of effectiveness, continuous contraceptive protection, non-coitus-related contraception, and relative inexpensiveness over time. Possible adverse reactions to IUC include discomfort to the wearer

EVIDENCE-BASED PRACTICE | Long-Acting Reversible Contraceptive Methods

Clinical Question

What are the characteristics of women who are acceptable candidates for the long-acting reversible contraceptive methods of intrauterine devices and contraceptive implants? What are the recommendations for optimal initiation and management of these methods?

The Evidence

Long-acting reversible contraceptives (LARC) include intrauterine devices (IUDs) and contraceptive implants. These methods have been demonstrated to be the most effective of the reversible contraceptives. There are many advantages of LARC compared to other reversible contraceptive methods. They do not require any ongoing personal effort to achieve full effectiveness, and the return of fertility is rapid after removal. A practice bulletin produced by the American College of Obstetrics and Gynecology (ACOG; 2017) provides information for patient selection and recommendations for initiation and management of these methods.

The ACOG used a comprehensive systematic review of the MEDLINE database, the Cochrane Library of practice guidelines, and the internal resources and documents of the College to conduct a literature search of articles published over a 17-year period. This type of practice guideline forms the highest level of evidence for practice and is considered the gold standard for nursing practice.

Best Practice

Both LARC methods are safe and effective contraceptive options for nulliparous women and adolescents. Evidence shows that complications associated with IUD insertion are uncommon for all users, including nulliparous women and adolescents. First-attempt success rates for insertion of IUDs surpass 95% and most are performed by advanced practice clinicians. Use of drugs to ease insertion is not recommended. Expulsion rates may be higher for adolescents and multi-parous women; expulsion rates for nulliparous women are low. The risk of infection after IUD insertion is low, and there is no evidence that IUD use is associated with subsequent infertility. While clinicians have traditionally inserted an IUD during menses, there is no evidence that this is superior timing. Indeed, requiring two visits for IUD insertion resulted in a drop to 54% usage. A backup method of contraception should be used for 7 days after insertion of an IUD. Insertion immediately after an induced or spontaneous abortion is safe and effective. Since women who have an abortion are at high risk of repeat unintended pregnancy, prompt initiation of a contraceptive method for women who desire it may reduce repeat unintended pregnancy. An IUD may also safely be inserted in the immediate postbirth period to prevent unintended pregnancy after a live birth. There is no impact on breastfeeding.

Similarly, contraceptive implants are effective for use by all women, including those who are nulliparous and adolescents. Adolescents tended to select the implant method over the IUD when selecting a LARC. Continuation rates for adolescents were highest among these users.

Clinical Reasoning

How does this practice guideline support development of teaching materials for obstetric and gynecological nurses? How should women be counseled regarding long-acting contraception methods following pregnancy, birth, or abortion?

(possible increased cramping), increased bleeding during menses (ParaGard), increased risk of pelvic infection for about 3 weeks following insertion, perforation of the uterus at the time of insertion, unscheduled bleeding, dysmenorrhea, and expulsion of the device.

IUC is an excellent method of contraception for most women. IUC is contraindicated in women who are pregnant and in women who have an active pelvic infection (pelvic inflammatory disease [PID], endometritis, cervicitis, and pelvic tuberculosis). IUC should not be inserted in women with cervical or endometrial cancer or gestational choriocarcinoma. The risk for IUC expulsion is greater in women with anatomic abnormalities of the uterus. IUC is an excellent contraceptive option for women with diabetes; it may also be used in women with a history of breast cancer, cesarean birth, or uterine or cervical surgery (CDC, 2016d; Zeimer et al., 2015).

Women who have had children have a deeper uterine cavity that accepts placement of the IUC more readily. However, women who have not had children can be candidates for insertion of the IUC if the cavity of their uteri are deep enough (6–10 cm). If the woman has multiple sexual partners, she should be cautioned to use a condom in addition to her IUC, primarily for protection against STIs. However, because the levonorgestrel-secreting IUC causes thick cervical mucus, it may have a protective effect against STIs (Schuiling & Likis, 2017).

IUC is inserted into the uterus with its strings protruding through the cervix into the vagina. It may be inserted at any time during the woman's cycle or during the 6-week postpartum check, providing she is not pregnant. After insertion, the clinician instructs the woman to check for the presence of the strings once a week for the first month and then monthly, or after each menses with the ParaGard. She does this by inserting her index finger or middle finger into her vagina to feel the strings; this ensures that the IUC is still in the uterus. She is told that she may have some cramping or bleeding intermittently for 2 to 6 weeks and that irregular bleeding is expected for up to 3 months. Approximately half of women using levonorgestrel-secreting IUC will experience amenorrhea after 6 months of use (Zeimer et al., 2015). Follow-up examination is suggested at 4 to 8 weeks after insertion.

Women with IUC should contact their healthcare providers if they are exposed to an STI or if they develop the following warning signs: Late menses, abnormal spotting or bleeding (different from what she has been experiencing), dyspareunia (pain with intercourse), abdominal pain, abnormal discharge, signs of infection (fever, chills, malaise), missing strings, or lengthening of the strings. If a woman becomes pregnant with IUC in place, the device should be removed as soon as possible to prevent infection and miscarriage (Zeimer et al., 2015).

Nexplanon

Nexplanon, manufactured by Merck & Co., has replaced its predecessor, Implanon. It is a radiopaque, single-capsule implant inserted subdermally in the woman's nondominant upper underarm. It is impregnated with 68 mg of etonogestrel, a progestin, which releases up to 45 mcg the first year, 40 mcg the second year, and 20 mcg the third year. It is good as a contraceptive method for 3 years, and it acts by preventing ovulation. Nexplanon also stimulates the production of thick cervical mucus, which inhibits sperm penetration past the cervix.

Nexplanon provides effective continuous contraception removed from the act of coitus as a LARC or "forgettable" method. Possible side effects include unscheduled bleeding or amenorrhea, an increased incidence of nonproblematic ovarian cysts, weight gain, headaches, fluid retention, acne, hair loss, mood changes, and depression. It was released in the United States in 2012. Nexplanon has not been studied in women who weigh greater than 130% of their ideal body weight. A minor surgical procedure is required to insert and remove the implant (Merck Pharmaceuticals, 2016). Only trained providers should insert Nexplanon, as rods inserted too deeply have been known to migrate to the pulmonary artery (Merck Pharmaceuticals, 2016). See *Case Study: Azia Askari*.

Hormonal Contraception

Hormonal contraceptives are available in a variety of forms such as a pill, an injectable, an implant, a vaginal ring, or a skin patch. They may contain a combination of an estrogen and a progestin or may be progestin-only.

Combination Estrogen–Progestin Approaches

The use of a combination of an estrogen and a progestin is a highly successful, very safe method of contraception that is readily reversible when discontinued. Hormonal contraceptives work by inhibiting the release of an ovum, by creating an atrophic endometrium, and by maintaining thick cervical mucus that slows or prevents sperm transport to the upper female reproductive tract as well as inhibiting the process that allows sperm to penetrate the ovum (capacitation). Most drug trials for combined hormonal contraception limited participants to those weighing less than or equal to 198 pounds. Whether or not weighing more than 198 pounds truly contributes to decreased contraceptive effectiveness has not yet been determined with certainty, although these women should be cautioned.

CASE STUDY: Azia Askari

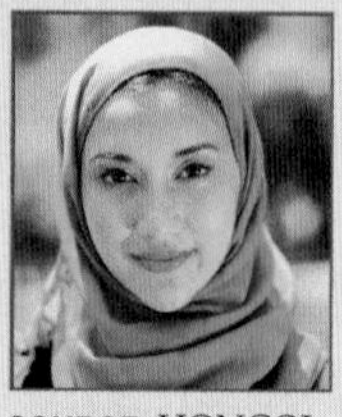

SOURCE: HONGQI ZHANG/123RF

Azia, 29-weeks pregnant, presents to an appointment with her sister-in-law. The nurse asks Azia if she has considered options for postpartum birth control. As the nurse begins to discuss options, the sister-in-law says that permanent sterilization is not a culturally accepted alternative. In addition, Azia prefers not to use hormonal contraceptives.

Question to Ponder

What fertility awareness methods can be taught to Azia that will reduce her risk of pregnancy in the future?

COMBINED ORAL CONTRACEPTIVES

Combined oral contraceptives (COCs)—commonly called *birth control pills* or *"the pill"*—are a combination of a synthetic estrogen and a progestin. COCs are one of the most popular contraceptive options available to women in the United States because they are safe, highly effective, and rapidly reversible (Figure 4–8). Most pill packets include 28 pills, 21 of which are hormones and seven of which are placebos or an iron tablet, although they are also marketed for extended 84-day use. During the week of placebo pills, a hormonally mediated "scheduled" bleed will occur 1 to 4 days after the last pill containing the hormones is taken. For most women, this scheduled bleed will be lighter and of fewer days' duration than a naturally occurring menses. COCs can be initiated using one of these models:

1. ***Day 1 start***. The woman begins taking the pill on the first day of her menstrual cycle. This method prevents ovulation in the first cycle, so no backup method of contraception for 7 days is needed.
2. ***Sunday start***. The woman begins taking the pill on the Sunday after the first day of the menstrual cycle and ends the packet on a Saturday. The Sunday start is common because it tends to prevent "scheduled" bleeding on weekends. However, a backup method of contraception is necessary during the first 7 days of use.
3. ***Quick start***. The woman begins taking the pill in the provider's office if she is reasonably certain she is not pregnant. A backup method is necessary for 7 days. New quick-start COC users are more likely to be using the method 3 months later when compared with the other start models (Zeimer et al., 2015).

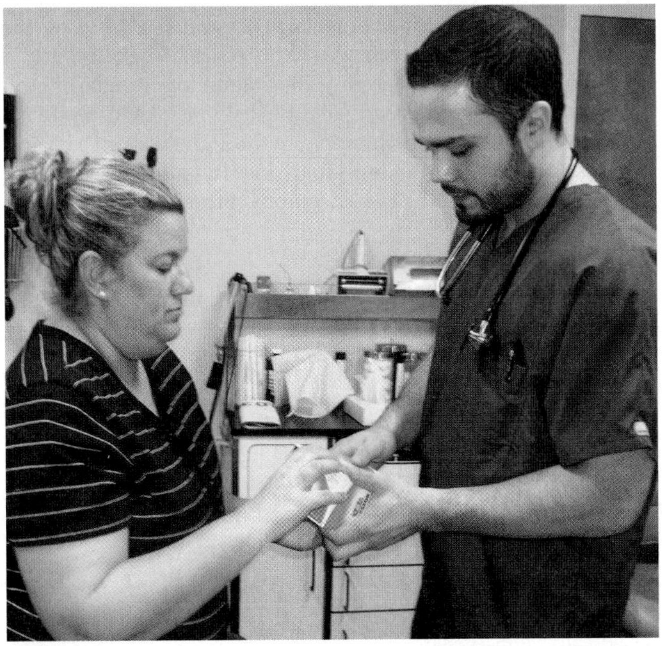

Figure 4–8 The nurse practitioner provides the patient with combined oral contraceptives, discusses their use, and addresses any questions or concerns the patient has about using them.

SOURCE: Nathan Davidson.

Women who desire a scheduled bleed every 4 weeks can be prescribed COC packets with 21 or 28 pills. Women who have 21-day pill packets wait for 7 days after taking the last hormone pill before starting a new 21-day pack of pills. Women who have 28-day pill packets should take the 7 placebo or iron pills so that they never stop taking a pill and thus never forget to start a new pack a week later. Women who use either the 21- or 28-day COC packet will always begin a new pack on the same day. The pill should be taken at approximately the same time each day—usually on arising or before retiring in the evening.

Three COC formulations for extended use are available in the United States. Women taking extended-use COCs have four scheduled bleeds per year (rather than 12). Women who use COCs for menstrual suppression would take an active hormonal pill every day; they should expect complete amenorrhea. Extended-use COCs reduce the nuisance side effects such as bloating, headache, breast tenderness, cramping, and swelling (Schuiling & Likis, 2017). COCs can be used "off label" (i.e., not for contraception) for menstrual suppression due to dysmenorrhea, menorrhagia, or endometriosis, as they inhibit the hypothalamic–pituitary–ovarian axis. Irregular pill taking is one of the major causes of unscheduled bleeding, a side effect that leads many women to discontinue COCs. Although highly effective when taken correctly, improper use of COCs can contribute to an unintended pregnancy.

COCs have been available for more than 50 years. In the United States, the estrogen component ethinyl estradiol (EE) is most commonly used. Initially, COCs contained high levels of estrogen and were linked with an increased risk for myocardial infarction (MI), thromboembolic disorders (blood clots), and stroke. Lowering the estrogen dose in the formulation decreased these risks. Based on this understanding, over the years, the estrogen component in COCs has been decreased from 150 mcg/day to the lowest dose currently available—10 mcg/day (Zeimer et al., 2015). Currently 10 different formulations of progestins are available in the United States. These progestins vary with respect to their biologic activity, including inhibition of ovulation. Synthetic progestins can have androgenic, antiandrogenic, estrogenic, and antiestrogenic effects. These effects are responsible for the varying progestin-related side effects.

COCs are among the most studied medications available. The current generation of COCs are considered safe because they are "low dose," or do not contain more than 35 mcg of estrogen. They would be even safer if smokers over the age of 35 years did not take them. In an effort to reduce complications such as myocardial infarction, stroke, blood clots, and hypertension, regimens have been developed that use very low doses of estrogen (10, 20, or 25 mcg) and progestins that are less androgenic in effect. These very-low-dose pills may result in weaker endometrial control, which leads to more unscheduled bleeding. Unscheduled bleeding is a nuisance and may lead to discontinuation of the COC, but it does not decrease its efficacy as a contraceptive. It is recommended that smokers of all ages who wish to take COCs be prescribed pills with 10 to 20 mcg of estrogen to reduce serious complications.

Side effects are generally identifiable as estrogen related or progestin related. Thus, it is possible to modify some side effects by choosing a different COC preparation. The side effects are identified in Table 4–2.

Whether or not a woman should use a COC can be determined by the U.S. Medical Eligibility Criteria (MEC) for Contraceptive Use (CDC, 2016d). Generally, contraindications to the use of COCs include pregnancy, previous history of thrombophlebitis or thromboembolic disease, acute or chronic liver disease of the

TABLE 4–2 Side Effects Associated with Combined Oral Contraceptives

ESTROGEN EFFECTS	PROGESTIN EFFECTS
Alterations in lipid metabolism	Acne, oily skin
Breast tenderness, engorgement or increased breast size	Breast tenderness; increased breast size
Cerebrovascular accident	Decreased libido
Changes in carbohydrate metabolism	Decreased high-density lipoprotein (HDL) cholesterol levels
Chloasma	Depression
Fluid retention; cyclic weight gain	Fatigue
Headache	Hirsutism
Hepatic adenomas	Increased appetite; weight gain
Hypertension	Increased low-density lipoprotein (LDL) cholesterol levels
Leukorrhea, cervical erosion, ectropion	Oligomenorrhea, amenorrhea
Nausea	Pruritus
Nervousness, irritability	Sebaceous cysts
Telangiectasia	
Thromboembolic complications—thrombophlebitis, pulmonary embolism	

cholestatic type with abnormal liver function tests, presence of estrogen-dependent carcinomas, undiagnosed uterine bleeding, heavy smoking, gallbladder disease, hypertension, diabetes, migraine with visual disturbances, hypercoagulable disorders, and hyperlipidemia. Women who may use COCs with frequent monitoring include women with migraine headaches without visual disturbances, epilepsy, depression, oligomenorrhea, and amenorrhea. Women who choose COCs should be fully advised of the potential side effects and complications. Certain medications can decrease the efficacy of COCs. Generic preparations of COCs are as effective as brand-name COCs (Zeimer et al., 2015). See *Case Study: Benita Cartier*.

COCs have several important noncontraceptive benefits. Many women who use COCs experience relief from uncomfortable menstrual symptoms and premenstrual syndrome; cramps diminish, flow decreases, and the cycle becomes more regular; and mittelschmerz is eliminated. More important, there is a reduction in the incidence of ovarian cancer, endometrial cancer, colorectal cancer, menstrual migraines, and iron deficiency anemia. In addition, COCs can be effective in improving bone mineral density and in treating acne or hirsutism, pelvic pain due to endometriosis, and bleeding due to leiomyomas (ACOG, 2016c). Currently, COCs assist with some of the physiologic changes experienced by women during perimenopause (such as hot flashes) as well as provide contraception. COCs can be used by nonsmoking women until they transition into menopause, at which time hormone therapy may be necessary to control vasomotor symptoms (Zeimer et al., 2015). Because of an increased risk of heart attack, women over age 35 who smoke should not take COCs.

The woman using COCs should contact her healthcare provider if she becomes depressed, develops a breast lump, becomes jaundiced, or experiences any of the following warning signs of the acronym **ACHES**, which could signify a medical complication.

- **A**bdominal or leg pain, severe (deep vein thrombosis)
- **C**hest pain, severe, or shortness of breath (pulmonary embolism or myocardial infarction)
- **H**eadaches, severe, or dizziness (cerebral vascular accident or CVA)
- **E**ye vision loss or blurring (thrombosis of the retinal artery)
- **S**peech problems (CVA)

TRANSDERMAL HORMONAL CONTRACEPTION

Combined hormonal contraception (ethinyl estradiol and norelgestromin) is available as a transdermal *contraceptive skin patch* called Xulane, manufactured by Mylan Pharmaceuticals. Roughly the size of a silver dollar, but square, this patch is applied weekly for 3 weeks on one of four sites: The woman's abdomen, buttocks, upper outer arm, or trunk (excluding the breasts). During the fourth week, no patch is applied and a scheduled bleed typically occurs. The amount of estrogen as ethinyl estradiol absorbed is equivalent to a 35 mcg COC. Systemic absorption of the estrogen component through the skin leads to a higher steady-state serum level than does the pill. This may lead to a small increase in the risk of venous thromboembolism, and

CASE STUDY: Benita Cartier

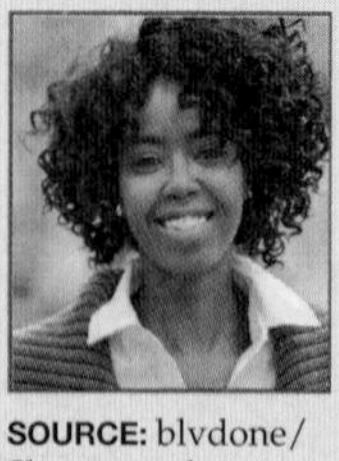

SOURCE: blvdone/ Shutterstock

Benita is currently 13 weeks pregnant and is concerned because she became pregnant while she was taking oral contraceptives. She tells the nurse that her aunt said she should get her tubes tied after this birth because the pill does not work for her. Benita is apprehensive about such a permanent measure of birth control because she may consider having more children in a few years. Benita insists she took her pills on a regular basis without ever missing a day and was very conscientious about taking them every morning. The nurse notes that prior to pregnancy, Benita had chronic urinary tract infections and was placed on Macrobid for a 7-day course. Her primary care provider also advised her to take a Macrobid immediately after intercourse to reduce the risk of infection as a result of sexual activity.

Question to Ponder

Research which medications are known to decrease the efficacy of oral contraceptives. How would you counsel patients on oral contraceptive pills to prevent a medication-related contraceptive failure?

the woman should be cautioned. The patch is highly effective in women who weigh less than 198 pounds; those who weigh more should be cautioned regarding its effectiveness (Mylan Pharmaceuticals, 2016). Users apply their first patch the same as women who start COCs and use a backup method for 7 days if necessary.

The patch is as safe and effective as COCs and has a better rate of user compliance. Generally, women who are candidates for COCs are candidates for the patch unless they weigh more than 198 pounds, have skin disorders that may result in reactions at the site of application, or are at risk of a venous thromboembolus (VT).

VAGINAL CONTRACEPTIVE RING

The NuvaRing (etonogestrel and ethinyl estradiol) vaginal contraceptive ring (manufactured by Merck) is another form of low-dose, sustained-release combined hormonal contraceptive. It is a flexible, soft vaginal ring that is inserted for 3 weeks (Figure 4–9), left in place for 21 days, and then removed for 7 days (Zeimer et al., 2015). Approximately 15 mcg of ethinyl estradiol is absorbed by the vaginal mucosa. This one-size ring fits virtually all women. Women with marked vaginal prolapse should be cautioned to check for expulsion of the ring during early use. As with all combined hormonal methods, the clinician should consult the CDC's Medical Eligibility Criteria for Contraceptive Use (MEC) about its safety for an individual woman (CDC, 2016b). Women who use the NuvaRing should begin its use in the same way as described for the transdermal patch or COCs.

Progestin Contraceptives

PROGESTIN-ONLY PILLS

Another oral contraceptive is the progestin-only pill (norethindrone), also called the *minipill*. It is used primarily by nursing mothers because it does not interfere with breast milk production. It is also used by women who have a medical condition that precludes use of the estrogen component in a combination preparation, such as a history of thrombophlebitis, hypertension, or other estrogen-related side effects. Women who use the minipill must be highly motivated, as the pill must be taken consistently at the same time every day, within a 2-hour window period (Schuiling & Likis, 2017) and is slightly less effective than COCs. Use with a condom will provide added protection against an unintended pregnancy. The major problems with progesterone-only pills are amenorrhea or unscheduled (irregular) bleeding patterns.

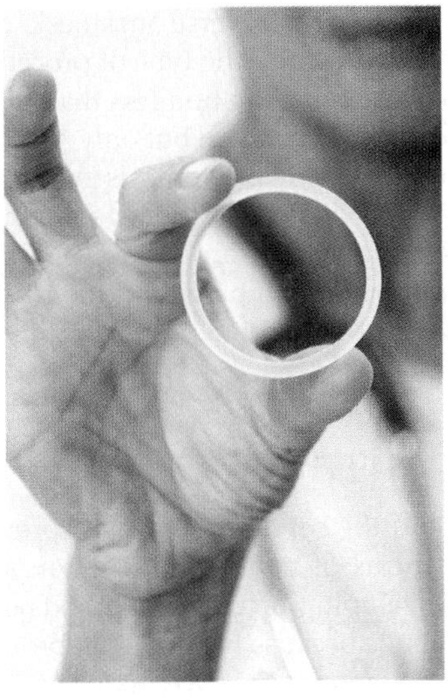

Figure 4–9 The NuvaRing vaginal contraceptive ring.

SOURCE: N. Aubrier/age fotostock/Getty Images.

LONG-ACTING PROGESTIN CONTRACEPTIVES

Long-acting progestin-only contraceptives include Depo-Provera and Nexplanon, the latter of which is also considered a LARC method and was discussed previously. Progestin-only contraceptive methods are recommended for lactating women, women who cannot use estrogen or the copper IUC, women who forget to take COCs on a daily basis, and women who are not bothered by unscheduled bleeding or spotting. Both are safe, reversible forms of contraception.

Depo-Provera or depot-medroxyprogesterone acetate (DMPA), manufactured by Pfizer, is a long-acting, injectable, progestin-only contraceptive. DMPA is manufactured in two doses: DMPA-IM 150 mg for intramuscular use or DMPA-SC 104 mg for subcutaneous use. Both provide highly effective birth control for 3 months after administration with subsequent injections scheduled every 10 to 13 weeks. DMPA-SC may cause less pain than an intramuscular (IM) injection and can be self-administered, increasing compliance by not having to return to the clinic every 3 months.

DMPA, which acts primarily by suppressing ovulation, is safe, convenient, private, and relatively inexpensive. It also separates birth control from the act of coitus. It can be given to nursing mothers because it contains no estrogen. DMPA provides blood levels of progesterone high enough to block the luteinizing hormone (LH) surge, thereby suppressing ovulation. It also thickens the cervical mucus to block sperm penetration. Side effects include unscheduled bleeding, headache, weight gain, breast tenderness, hair loss, and depression. Return of fertility may be delayed for an average of 10 months. Thus, women who seek to become pregnant in the near future may be advised to use an alternative contraceptive that does not delay fertility after discontinuation (Schuiling & Likis, 2017). DMPA is associated with bone demineralization, especially during the first 2 years of use. The rate of calcium loss slows after this time, and bone loss is reversible after discontinuation of DMPA. All women on DMPA should exercise daily and take 1,200 mg of calcium with vitamin D to avoid bone loss.

Postcoital Emergency Contraception

Postcoital **emergency contraception (EC)**, once known as the *morning-after pill*, is indicated when a woman is worried about pregnancy because of unprotected intercourse, sexual assault, or possible contraceptive failure (e.g., broken condom, slipped diaphragm, missed COCs, or too long a time between DMPA injections). Research indicates that oral hormonal EC taken as soon as possible within 72 hours, but up to 5 days, can reduce the risk of pregnancy after a single act of unprotected intercourse by at least 74% (ACOG, 2015a). EC should not be confused with medical abortion, which is discussed elsewhere.

Preparations for EC that inhibit ovulation include (1) high doses of levonorgestrel and ethinyl estradiol (Yuzpe regimen), (2) high doses of levonorgestrel (Plan B; Plan B One-Step), and (3) ulipristal acetate, a progesterone agonist–antagonist (Ella®, manufactured by Watson). Levonorgestrel should only be taken within 72 hours of unprotected intercourse, and the other preparations within 120 hours. Insertion of a ParaGard copper IUD within 5 days of unprotected coitus is effective as abortifacient emergency contraception. The COC preparation with estrogen and a progestin (Yuzpe regimen) confers more side effects, such as nausea, than does the progestin-only levonorgestrel (Plan B) regimen. An antiemetic might be prescribed an hour before the woman takes the COC preparation. The combined regimen remains an option because many women knowledgeable about EC can use their unused COCs within 5 days after consulting with their healthcare provider about appropriate dosing (ACOG, 2015a).

The progestin-only approach uses a high dose of one progestin, levonorgestrel. Plan B® and Plan B One-Step® is an EC method that is more effective than combined hormonal EC; it also has a much lower incidence of associated nausea and vomiting. Plan B comes as two tablets of 0.75 mg levonorgestrel to be taken at once, or as Plan B One-Step, one tablet that contains 1.5 mg of levonorgestrel, the latter which is, as of 2013, available without a prescription and without age restrictions (ACOG, 2015a). Both dosings should be initiated as soon as possible after unprotected coitus, but within 72 hours.

The only contraindication is a diagnosed pregnancy because the pills are ineffective (Zeimer et al., 2015). The woman should have her normal menses 2 weeks after taking EC. If she does not, she should follow up with a pregnancy test. If the pregnancy test is negative, she should be counseled about reliable methods of contraception.

Currently there is considerable debate about the best ways to improve access to EC, as one survey revealed only 64% of emergency department patients knew about it (ACOG, 2015a). It is essential that healthcare providers counsel women about the availability of EC during routine screenings and appointments. This approach ensures that women are familiar with the method before an emergency occurs. It is also helpful to have printed literature on EC available in the waiting areas of clinics and emergency departments.

Operative Sterilization

Operative **sterilization** is an inclusive term that refers to surgical procedures that permanently prevent undesired future fertility and pregnancy. In the man, sterilization is achieved through a procedure called *vasectomy*. In the woman, sterilization is done by *tubal ligation* of the proximal end of the fallopian tubes.

Before sterilization is performed on either partner, a thorough explanation of the procedure is provided. Each person needs to understand that sterilization is not a decision to be taken lightly or entered into at times of psychologic stress, such as during separation or divorce. Even though both male and female procedures are theoretically reversible, the permanency of the procedure should be stressed and understood.

Vasectomy

Male sterilization is achieved through a relatively minor procedure called a **vasectomy**. The scrotal skin is either incised with a scalpel or pierced with dissecting forceps (no-scalpel technique) to locate and surgically severe the vas deferens in both sides of the scrotum by ligation or cautery. It takes about 3 months and 15 to 20 ejaculations to clear the remaining sperm from the vas deferens (Schuiling & Likis, 2017). During that period, the couple is advised to use another contraceptive method until a semen specimen reveals a zero sperm count. At that point, the couple can safely have unprotected sex. Side effects of a vasectomy include regret, pain, infection, hematoma, sperm granulomas, and spontaneous reanastomosis (reconnecting).

Vasectomies can sometimes be reversed up to 90% of the time by using microsurgery techniques. However, pregnancy rates are only 50% following reversal (Zeimer et al., 2015).

“Damien and I married in our mid-twenties. We didn't want children then, so he had a vasectomy when he was 30. As I approached my late thirties I realized I longed for a child. Damien agreed to try a vasectomy reversal and it worked! I had Megan at age 38 and Gina 2 years later. Damien died 4 years ago—pancreatic cancer—and we mourned him deeply. I am 63 now and full of joy because last night Megan gave birth to my first grandchild. Gina will marry in the fall. How different my life would have been if not for Damien's choice.”

Tubal Ligation

Voluntary female sterilization can be accomplished by **tubal ligation**. Three procedures are common in the United States:

- Laparotomy following a cesarean birth or other abdominal surgery
- Minilaparotomy in the postpartum period soon after a vaginal birth
- Laparoscopy done during an “interval period,” when the woman is not pregnant or not postpartum

Tubal ligation can be done at any time the woman is not pregnant. However, the postpartum period is an ideal time to perform a tubal ligation because the uterus is enlarged and the tubes are easy to locate. During these procedures the tubes are ligated, clipped, electrocoagulated, banded, or plugged. This interrupts the patency of the fallopian tube, thus preventing the ovum and the sperm from meeting.

Complications of female sterilization procedures include regret, coagulation burns on the bowel, bowel perforation, pain, infection, hemorrhage, and adverse anesthesia effects. Reversal of a tubal ligation depends on the type of procedure performed. Of women who chose tubal ligation less than age 30 years, 40% requested information on reversal but only 1% did so. The pregnancy rate following tubal reanastomosis (surgical reconnection) is 50%, and dependent on length of time following the initial surgery, the woman's age, type of procedure, amount of scar tissue, length of remaining fallopian tubes and their functionality, and her partner's sperm count (Zeimer et al., 2015).

Male Contraception

The vasectomy and the condom, discussed previously, are currently the only forms of male contraception available in the United States. Developing reversible methods of contraception for men is a challenge because healthy men produce sperm continuously, whereas women produce mature ova cyclically. It is easier to devise a reversible method that interrupts a cyclic process than it is to find ways to interrupt continuous fertility.

Hormonal contraception for men has yet to be developed. Studies using weekly injections of testosterone, a synthetic hormone that significantly inhibits sperm production, had significant side effects such as feminization, an unfavorable lipid profile, loss of libido, and more, which make it largely unacceptable. Future methods will consider how to stop pituitary LH and FSH to block testicular cell function, how to interfere with sperm production, and how to disrupt transport of mature sperm (GI, 2016a; Hatcher et al., 2012).

"I think I'm like a lot of women. During my life I've used a variety of contraceptive methods. I took the pill until I was married and ready to have children, used spermicidal foam without a diaphragm and subsequently had a baby, and later used spermicidal cream and condoms more successfully. I never wanted a tubal, but my husband refuses to consider a vasectomy, so the IUC was a perfect alternative for us. I am 37 and I like using something I don't have to think about every time we want to make love. Maybe someday there will be more contraceptives for men—it seems only fair—but I'm glad that at least I've had some choices."

●○● NURSING MANAGEMENT

For the Woman Choosing a Contraceptive Method

In most cases, you will work with the woman when providing information and guidance about contraceptive methods because most contraceptive methods are female oriented. Because a man can purchase condoms without seeing a healthcare provider, only in the case of vasectomy does a man require counseling and interaction with a nurse. However, men should be encouraged to participate in contraceptive counseling being provided for their female partners. You can play an important role in helping a woman and her partner choose a method of contraception that is acceptable to both. See *Professionalism in Practice: Using Contraception Resources During Patient Teaching*.

In addition to completing a history and assessing for any medical contraindications to specific methods, you should spend time with the woman, learning about her lifestyle, personal attitudes about particular contraceptive methods, religious and cultural beliefs, personal biases, and plans for future childbearing in order to help her select the most effective and acceptable contraceptive method. See *Developing Cultural Competence: Birth Control Attitudes*.

Once the woman chooses a method, the nurse educates about proper use of the method so as to achieve the best effectiveness. *Teaching Highlights: Using a Method of Contraception* provides guidelines for helping women use a method of contraception effectively.

Professionalism in Practice **Using Contraception Resources During Patient Teaching**

In your role as teacher, it is important to have resources on hand for women seeking a method of contraception. Having IUC models or a female condom plus informational handouts for the various methods of contraception is invaluable. Describing correct use of the method along with important tips, its side effects, and the warning signs for serious adverse reactions is essential. Women can refer to the informational sheets at home. Be sure to include the office or clinic phone number, and always remember to mention emergency contraception (EC).

Developing Cultural Competence **Birth Control Attitudes**

Attitudes about birth control may be influenced by cultural factors or ethnicity. Although it is impossible to attribute one attitude to an entire group of people, the following general information may be helpful as a starting point in working with women from a particular cultural group, especially if they are first generation in the United States.

- *Gender inequities* may prohibit some Middle Eastern, Latina, and Eastern Indian women from seeking out or using a contraceptive method unless their husbands agree. After being given appropriate information, the nurse may suggest the couple discuss contraceptive options in private.
- *Attitudes toward bleeding* affect a woman's duties to her family and partner. Vaginal bleeding may be seen as "unclean" by Muslim and Orthodox Jewish women. Any contraceptive method that involves irregular bleeding might not be acceptable (Pinter et al., 2016). On the other hand, among women who feel a monthly period is necessary, any method that ultimately causes amenorrhea would not be acceptable.
- Among Orthodox Jewish couples, contraception is acceptable if it does not work as castration or if it does not "waste" a man's seed. Thus, use of condoms, coitus interruptus, or male sterilization is not acceptable (Pinter et al., 2016).
- The Roman Catholic Church considers all artificial methods of contraception unacceptable. Natural family planning might be an acceptable method for women who closely follow the Church's teaching (Pinter et al., 2016). Among American Catholics, however, attitudes about the proscription regarding birth control may vary, and it is important to determine the woman's beliefs on the subject.
- Large families are valued in many cultures, and contraception may not be desired. Unplanned pregnancies may be welcomed in the Hispanic culture, and unplanned adolescent pregnancies may not necessarily carry a negative stigma for African Americans (Spector, 2017).

Note: It is unwise to attribute specific attitudes or beliefs to all members of a cultural group. The information in the Developing Cultural Competence boxes offers possible insights into caring for women from different cultural groups.

TEACHING HIGHLIGHTS | Using a Method of Contraception

- Discuss factors a woman should consider when choosing a method of contraception (see Table 4–1). Note that different methods may be appropriate at different times in a woman's life.
- Review the woman's reasons for choosing a particular method and confirm the absence of any contraindications to specific methods.
- Give a step-by-step description of the correct procedure for using the method chosen. Provide opportunities for questions.
- If a technique is to be learned, such as charting BBT or inserting a diaphragm, demonstrate and then have the woman do a return demonstration as appropriate. (*Note*: If certain aspects are beyond your level of expertise, such as fitting a diaphragm, review the content about its use and confirm that the woman understands what she is to do.)
- Provide information on what the woman should do if unusual circumstances arise (for example, she misses a pill or forgets to take a morning temperature). These can be presented in a written handout as well.
- Stress warning signs that may require immediate action by the woman and explain why these signs indicate a risk. (These should also be covered in the handout.)
- Arrange to talk with the woman again soon, either by phone or at a return visit, to see if she has any questions or has encountered any problems.

It is a nursing responsibility to review with the woman any possible side effects and warning symptoms related to the chosen method. Also, counsel her about what action to take if she suspects she is pregnant. In many cases, telephone counseling of women who call with questions and concerns about contraception will be helpful. Thus, it is vital to be knowledgeable about this topic and have resources available to find answers to less common questions.

Clinical Interruption of Pregnancy

Abortion is the termination of a pregnancy. Although legalized in the United States in 1973, the moral and legal controversies continue, readily apparent in the medical and nursing professions, as they are in other groups. Despite the controversies, the procedures available for abortion are essential to providing safe obstetrical care and handling of obstetric emergencies such as retained products of conception or removal of gestational trophoblastic disease.

Many women are strongly opposed to abortion for religious, ethical, cultural, or personal reasons. Other women feel that abortion provides a legally available alternative to a pregnancy. A number of physical and psychosocial factors influence a woman's decision to seek an abortion. The presence of a disease or altered health state that jeopardizes the mother's life or serious, life-threatening fetal problems can be indications for abortion. In other instances, the timing or circumstance of the pregnancy creates an inordinate stress on the woman, prompting her to choose an abortion. Some of these situations may involve contraceptive failure, sexual assault, or incest. Poverty, inability to care for the number of children already in the home, and responsibilities for other family members also influence the decision to interrupt an unintended pregnancy.

Usually the decision is best made by the woman or couple involved but may involve family or clergy input. A woman whose life is threatened by the pregnancy may choose to continue the pregnancy, whereas one with no obvious threat may choose to have an abortion. The medical terminology and procedures for termination of pregnancy are the same for an elective abortion as they are for a medically necessary abortion (intrauterine fetal demise, congenital anomalies incompatible with life, missed abortion). The nurse should be sensitive to the needs of the woman and the reason for the abortion.

The legal status of abortion varies greatly worldwide. Whether or not abortion is legal has little to do with whether or not a woman elects to have the procedure. Worldwide, an estimated 56 million abortions took place between 2010 and 2014 (GI, 2016c). Just as in the United States, developed regions that have access to modern contraceptive methods saw a decline in the abortion rate from 46 to 27 per 1000 women of reproductive age while developing countries saw a drop from 39 to 37 per 1000 women (GI, 2016c). Countries with better access to family planning have fewer abortions, and countries where abortion is legal have fewer maternal deaths associated with complications of unsafe and unclean procedures such as infection and hemorrhage. Nonetheless, one in three women by the age of 45 will have had an abortion (ACOG, 2015b).

Prior to abortion, it is essential that an accurate gestational age be determined so the appropriate procedure is performed. The most accurate method is by sonographic determination using biometric measures, such as crown–rump length (CRL) of the fetus. An abortion can be performed medically or surgically in both the first and second trimesters. Which procedure will depend on the volume of uterine contents, the skill of the operator, preference of the woman, and availability of emergency services in the event of a complication.

Medical Interruption of Pregnancy

An elective medical abortion entails taking an oral prescription that will interrupt a pregnancy in the first 70 days (10 weeks) post–last menstrual period (LMP). Available in the United States, medical abortion with mifepristone and misoprostol provides an effective alternative to surgical abortion for many women with unintended pregnancies. Mifepristone is an antiprogesterone that disrupts the pregnancy, and misoprostol is a smooth muscle contractor that expels the products of conception, which leads to complete abortion in approximately 92% of women (ACOG, 2016b). The regimen includes 200 mg of mifepristone administered orally followed in 24 to 48 hours by 800 mcg of misoprostol administered buccally. Between 7 and 14 days after taking the misoprostol, the woman is seen to confirm that the abortion was successful (Food and Drug Administration, 2016). Mifepristone has been associated with bleeding and women on anticoagulants are not candidates for medical abortion. Concomitant intake of folic acid may decrease the efficacy of mifepristone and nonsteroidal anti-inflammatory drugs (NSAIDs) may decrease the efficacy of misoprostol.

Endometritis, an inflammatory condition of the lining of the uterus usually due to infection, is a risk with any abortion, elective or spontaneous. Since 2001, a few deaths have occurred related to the oral mifepristone–vaginal misoprostol regimen and were caused by *Clostridium sordellii* or *perfringens* (Zeimer et al., 2015). Misoprostol inhibits local immunity. Although vaginal mifepristone is still considered safe, the buccal route for misoprostol is almost as effective as the vaginal route and seems safer. The use of routine prophylactic antibiotics is not recommended. A woman who has taken the oral mifepristone–vaginal misoprostol regimen and develops stomach pain, weakness, nausea and vomiting, or diarrhea (with or without fever) within 24 hours should contact her healthcare provider *immediately* to rule out a clostridial infection.

Women who have suffered a *missed abortion* (a pregnancy that is no longer viable) and prefer a medical option to pregnancy termination rather than a surgical one will not require the antiprogesterone agent mifepristone, as the pregnancy has already been interrupted. Misoprostol 400 mcg sublingually or vaginally would be appropriate to help expel the products of conception (Dehbashi, Moosazadeh, & Afshari, 2016).

Surgical Interruption of Pregnancy

Surgical abortion in the first trimester (less than 13 weeks' gestation) is technically easier and safer than abortion in the second trimester. Use of a prophylactic antibiotic such as doxycycline reduces the risk of endometritis. If less than 8 weeks' gestation, a manual vacuum aspiration can be performed, which does not require preparatory dilation of the cervix with osmotic or mechanical dilators. After 8 weeks' gestation, due to pregnancy-related changes, the cervix will require preparatory dilation either mechanically with metal "Pratt" dilators, osmotically with *Laminaria japonica* (sterile seaweed), or medicinally with misoprostol and/or mifepristone. After cervical dilation, either overnight (as with an osmotic dilator) or immediately prior to the procedure, the cervix is anesthetized using 1% lidocaine with epinephrine as a paracervical block. A cannula is placed through the cervix and suction is applied to recover all the products of conception. Mechanical scraping of the uterus with a sharp curette can be an alternative to suction, or these two procedures can be done together to ensure emptying of the uterus. The major risks include perforation of the uterus, laceration of the cervix, systemic reaction to the anesthetic agent, hemorrhage, retained products of conception, and infection (ACOG, 2015b; Zeimer et al, 2015b).

Second-trimester abortion (greater than 13 weeks' gestation up to 24 weeks, or per state law) may be done medically, with induction of labor, or surgically, with dilation and evacuation. Medical termination includes the use of misoprostol, and the woman will need to labor and pass the fetus in the hospital. Surgical termination is done using dilation of the cervix and evacuation of the products of conception with forceps. These procedures may combine suction aspiration and curettage to empty the uterus because any retained products may lead to hemorrhage and infection. If the woman is Rh negative, she should receive Rh immune globulin.

●○● NURSING MANAGEMENT

For the Woman Having an Abortion

The woman deciding to terminate a pregnancy may choose to do so based on an unintended/unwanted pregnancy, sexual assault, lack of finances, her health, or the health of the fetus. The pregnancy needs to be verified early so the proper procedure can be offered. The woman's need for support and/or counseling should also be assessed. If the decision to terminate was difficult for the woman, assist her in finding postprocedure support.

Anticipatory guidance for medical abortion is essential. The woman needs to clearly understand that medical abortion takes time (up to 2 weeks) and that follow-up is essential to be certain all the uterine contents have been expelled. Additionally, the woman needs accurate information about the pain, cramping, bleeding, and passage of tissue that occurs so that she is prepared to deal with the discomfort and the sight of blood and possible uterine contents.

In general, important aspects of nursing care for a woman who chooses to have an abortion include providing information about the methods of abortion and associated risks as well as counseling regarding available alternatives to abortion and their implications (e.g., relinquishment, parenting). Nursing care also includes encouraging the woman to verbalize her feelings; providing support before, during, and after the procedure; monitoring vital signs, intake, and output; providing for physical comfort and privacy throughout the procedure; and teaching the woman self-care, the importance of the postabortion checkup, and use of a reliable contraceptive (including methods that can be started immediately after the procedure).

Preconception Counseling

One of the first questions a couple should ask themselves is whether or not they wish to have children. This involves consideration of each person's goals, expectations of the relationship, and the desire to parent. At times one individual may wish to have a child, whereas the other does not. In such a situation, an open discussion is essential to reach a mutually acceptable decision. In some cases, professional counseling for a couple—be they heterosexual or LGBTQ—may be necessary.

Couples who wish to have children face a decision about the timing of pregnancy. At what point in their lives do they believe it would be best to become parents? Pregnancy comes as a surprise even when the decision about timing is made, but with planning, the couple has some control.

For heterosexual couples who have religious beliefs that do not support contraception or who feel that family planning is unnatural and wrong, planning the timing of pregnancy is unacceptable and irrelevant. These couples should still take steps to ensure that they are in the best possible physical and mental health when, and if, pregnancy occurs.

Ideally, once the decision to become pregnant has been made, the timing as to when should be projected. However, this is not always the case. In 2011, 45% of all pregnancies in the United States were unintended (GI, 2016d), all the more reason to be preconceptually prepared. Couples with unplanned pregnancies may need additional support from the nurse, such as information about community resources that are available for them and their baby. Encouragement and reassurance are especially needed for these families.

Preconception Health Measures

Preconception planning typically begins with a careful health assessment, including a consideration of known or suspected risks.

MODIFIABLE RISK FACTORS

The nurse encourages the woman to address modifiable health risks, including:

- *Smoking.* Pregnancy often provides a strong incentive for women to quit smoking. In fact, research indicates that of women who smoked during the 3 months before becoming pregnant, 55% quit during pregnancy (CDC, 2016c).
- *Alcohol.* Alcohol consumed during pregnancy can result in fetal alcohol syndrome, birth defects, and low birth weight.
- *Social drugs and street drugs.* These substances pose a real threat to the fetus and are associated with a variety of complications including abruptio placentae, intrauterine growth restriction, neonatal abstinence syndrome, and preterm labor.
- *Caffeine.* The effects of caffeine are less clearly understood; however, as a precaution the woman is advised to avoid caffeine or limit her daily intake.
- *Medications.* A woman who uses any prescription or over-the-counter medications needs to discuss the implications of their use with her healthcare provider. It is best to avoid using any medication, if possible.
- *Environmental hazards.* Because of the possible teratogenic effects of environmental hazards in the workplace, the couple contemplating pregnancy needs to determine whether either or both are exposed to any environmental hazards at work or in their community.These risk factors are discussed in detail in Chapter 13.

PHYSICAL EXAMINATION

It is advisable for both partners to have a physical examination to identify any health problems that might affect pregnancy so that they can be corrected, if possible. These might include medical conditions, such as high blood pressure or obesity; problems that pose a threat to fertility, such as certain sexually transmitted infections; or conditions that keep either from achieving optimal health, such as diabetes, anemia, or colitis. If the family history indicates previous genetic disorders or if the couple is planning pregnancy when the woman is over age 35, the healthcare provider may suggest that the couple consider genetic counseling.

In addition to the history and physical exam, the woman may have the following laboratory tests: Urinalysis, complete blood count, blood type and Rh factor, a syphilis test, cervical cancer screening, nucleic acid amplified testing for gonorrhea and chlamydia, and rubella and hepatitis B and/or C screens. Women who are not immune to rubella should be counseled about the possible effects on the fetus should infection occur during pregnancy. If a woman decides to receive the rubella vaccine, the nurse needs to advise her to wait 1 month before conceiving to eliminate any potential risk to a fetus. During this time, she can be counseled to use a condom. Before conception, the woman is also advised to have a dental examination and any necessary dental work completed; dental disease is linked to preterm labor.

Women should also be asked questions regarding their psychologic history and assessed for mental illness. Certain classes of medications may be contraindicated during pregnancy, and drug changes may be needed prior to conception to prevent adverse maternal or fetal effects.

NUTRITION

Before conception, it is advisable for the woman to be at an average weight for her body build and height. The nurse can discuss nutrition and recommend that the woman follow a nutritious diet that contains ample quantities of all the essential nutrients. Some nutritionists advocate emphasizing the following nutrients: Calcium, protein, iron, B-complex vitamins, vitamin C, magnesium, and folic acid. Folic acid supplementation should be initiated before conception because it decreases the incidence of neural tube defects in newborns. (See the discussion in Chapter 14.) The CDC (Centers for Disease Control and Prevention, 2016a) estimates that most of these birth defects could be prevented if all women of childbearing age consume 400 mcg of folic acid daily. Consumption of a balanced diet with the appropriate distribution of the basic food groups as illustrated in the food pyramid is especially important during pregnancy. Excessive intake of lipid-soluble vitamins, especially vitamin A, can cause severe fetal problems and should be avoided.

EXERCISE

A woman is advised to establish a regular exercise plan beginning at least 3 months before she plans to attempt to become pregnant. The exercise should be one she enjoys and will continue. It needs to provide some aerobic conditioning and some general toning. Exercise improves the woman's circulation and general health and tones her muscles. Once an exercise program is well established, the woman is generally encouraged to continue it during pregnancy. Prepregnancy obesity, defined as a body mass index of 30 or above, puts the woman at risk for a variety of complications; therefore, it is advisable to advocate weight reduction for obese women prior to becoming pregnant.

Contraception

A woman who takes COCs is advised to stop and have two or three normal menses before attempting to conceive. This allows the natural hormonal cycle to return and facilitates dating the subsequent pregnancy. A woman using an intrauterine device is advised to have it removed and wait 1 month before attempting to conceive. This allows the endometrium to be restored. Other methods of contraception that women can use during the waiting period include a variety of barrier methods of contraception (condoms, diaphragm, or cervical cap with a spermicide).

Conception

Most preconception recommendations focus on helping the couple attain their best possible health state so that they do not enter pregnancy with unnecessary risks. Conception is a personal and emotional experience, and, even if a couple is prepared, the individuals may feel some ambivalence. This is a normal response, but they may require reassurance that the ambivalence will pass. The prospective parents may get so caught up in preparation and in their efforts to "do things right" that they lose sight of the pleasure they derive from each other and their lives together and cease to value the joy of spontaneity in their relationship. It is often helpful for the nurse to remind an overly zealous couple that moderation is always appropriate and that there is value in "taking time to smell the roses."

Focus Your Study

- The fertility awareness–based (FAB) method of natural family planning (NFP) is a "natural," noninvasive method of contraception often used by people whose religious beliefs prevent them from using artificial methods.
- Other FAB methods can be used in conjunction with a barrier method during the woman's fertile days.
- Situational contraceptives such as coitus interruptus (withdrawal) or abstinence are activities an individual might use in a given situation to avoid pregnancy without benefit of clinical guidance or medical care.
- Barrier contraceptives such as the contraceptive sponge, diaphragm, cervical cap, and condom act by blocking the transport of sperm. These methods are often used in conjunction with a spermicide.
- N-9, the spermicide available in the United States, is far less effective in preventing pregnancy when it is not used with a barrier method.
- The copper IUC (intrauterine contraception) is a mechanical contraceptive. Although its exact method of action is not clearly understood, research suggests it acts by immobilizing sperm or by impeding the progress of sperm from the cervix to the fallopian tubes. In addition, the IUC does have a local inflammatory effect.
- Levonorgestrel-releasing IUC is both hormonal and mechanical. Their action is similar to that of the copper IUC, but they also secrete a progestin, levonorgestrel, that helps the endometrium to become atrophic and the cervical secretions to become thick.
- Combined oral contraceptives (COCs) are combinations of estrogen and a progestin. When taken correctly, they are one of the most effective and reversible method of contraception. They also provide noncontraceptive benefits such as less acne and decreased scheduled bleeding.
- The progestin-only subdermal implant, Nexplanon, is an excellent choice for women desiring long-term contraception who cannot take estrogen.
- Other combined hormonal options (estrogen and progestin) such as the transdermal contraceptive patch (Xulane) and the vaginal ring (NuvaRing) have broadened the range of contraceptive options available.
- The long-acting progestin-only injection, Depo-Provera IM 150 mg or Depo-Provera SC 104 mg, is available for women who cannot take estrogen.
- Permanent sterilization is accomplished by tubal ligation for women and vasectomy for men. Although theoretically reversible, patients are advised that the method should be considered irreversible.
- The termination of pregnancy through abortion can be achieved by either medical or surgical means.
- Preconception counseling can be used to identify risk factors and unhealthy behaviors before a pregnancy occurs. Healthful lifestyle changes can be employed.

References

American College of Obstetricians and Gynecologists (ACOG). (2015a). *Emergency contraception* (ACOG Practice Bulletin No. 152). Washington, DC: Author.

American College of Obstetricians and Gynecologists (ACOG). (2015b). *Second-trimester abortion* (ACOG Practice Bulletin No. 135). Washington, DC: Author.

American College of Obstetricians and Gynecologists (ACOG). (2016a). Committee Opinion No. 654 Summary: Reproductive life planning to reduce unintended pregnancy. *Obstetrics and Gynecology, 2*(127), 415–417.

American College of Obstetricians and Gynecologists (ACOG). (2016b). *Medical management of abortion* (ACOG Practice Bulletin No. 143). Washington, DC: Author.

American College of Obstetricians and Gynecologists (ACOG). (2016c). *Noncontraceptive uses of hormonal contraceptives* (ACOG Practice Bulletin No. 110). Washington, DC: Author.

American College of Obstetricians and Gynecologists (ACOG). (2017). *Long-acting reversible contraception: Implants and intrauterine devices* (ACOG Practice Bulletin No. 186). Washington, DC: Author.

Centers for Disease Control and Prevention (CDC). (2016a). *Folic acid: Recommendations.* Retrieved from http://www.cdc.gov/ncbddd/folicacid/recommendations.html

Centers for Disease Control and Prevention (CDC). (2016b). *Summary chart of U.S. medical eligibility criteria for contraceptive use.* Retrieved from http://www.cdc.gov/reproductivehealth/contraception/pdf/summary-chart-us-medical-eligibility-criteria_508tagged.pdf

Centers for Disease Control and Prevention (CDC). (2016c). *Tobacco use and pregnancy.* Retrieved from https://www.cdc.gov/reproductivehealth/maternalinfanthealth/tobaccousepregnancy/index.htm

Center for Disease Control and Prevention (CDC). (2016d). U.S. medical eligibility criteria for contraceptive use, 2016. *MMWR Recommendations and Reports, 65*(3), 1–108. Retrieved from http://www.cdc.gov/mmwr/volumes/65/rr/pdfs/rr6503.pdf

Center for Disease Control and Prevention (CDC). (2016e). U.S. selected practice recommendations for contraceptive use, 2016. *Morbidity and Mortality Weekly Report, 65*(4), 1–72. Retrieved from http://www.cdc.gov/mmwr/volumes/65/rr/pdfs/rr6504.pdf

Couple to Couple League (CCL). (2017). *Building joyful marriages by teaching Natural Family Planning, couple to couple.* Retrieved from http://ccli.org

Dehbashi, Z., Moosazadeh, M., & Afshari, M. (2016). Comparison between sublingual and vaginal route of misoprostol in management of first trimester miscarriage missing. *Materia Socio Medica, 28*(4), 271–273.

Finer, L. B., & Zolna, M. R. (2016). Declines in unintended pregnancy in the United States, 2008–2011. *New England Journal of Medicine, 374*(9), 843–852. DOI:10.1056/NEJMsa1506575

Food and Drug Administration. (2016). Highlights of prescribing information: Mifeprex. Retrieved from https://www.accessdata.fda.gov/drugsatfda_docs/label/2016/020687s020lbl.pdf

Frost, J. J., Frohwirth, L., & Zolna, M. R. (2016). *Contraceptive needs and services, 2014 update.* Retrieved from https://www.guttmacher.org/report/contraceptive-needs-and-services-2014-update

Guttmacher Institute (GI). (2016a). Abortion in developing regions: What progress since 1990? *News in Context.* Retrieved from https://www.guttmacher.org/article/2016/09/abortion-developing-regions-what-progress-1990

Guttmacher Institute (GI). (2016b). Contraceptive use in the United States. *Fact Sheet.* Retrieved from https://www.guttmacher.org/fact-sheet/contraceptive-use-united-states

Guttmacher Institute (GI). (2016c). Induced abortion in the United States. *Fact Sheet.* Retrieved from https://www.guttmacher.org/sites/default/files/factsheet/fb_induced_abortion_3.pdf

Guttmacher Institute (GI). (2016d). Unintended pregnancy in the United States. *Fact Sheet.* Retrieved from https://www.guttmacher.org/fact-sheet/unintended-pregnancy-united-states

Hatcher, R. A., Trussell, J., Nelson, A., Cates, W., Kawal, D., & Policar, M. S. (2012). *Contraceptive technology* (20th ed.). New York, NY: Ardent Media.

Jatlaoui, T. C., Ewing, A., Shah, J., Mandel, M. G., Krashin, J. W., Suchdev, D. B., Jamieson, D. J., & Pazol, K. (2017). Abortion surveillance—United States, 2014. *MMWR Surveillance Summary, 66*(24), 1–48. DOI:10.15585/mmwr.ss6512a1

Merck Pharmaceuticals. (2016). *Nexplanon prescribing information.* Retrieved from https://www.merck.com/product/usa/pi_circulars/n/nexplanon/nexplanon_pi.pdf

Mylan Pharmaceuticals. (2016). *Xulane prescribing information for U.S. healthcare professionals.* Retrieved from https://www.xulane.com/-/media/xulanecom/files/neets-r12_exhibit-pdf.pdf

Pinter, B., Hakim, M., Seidman, D. S., Kubba, A., Kishen, M., & DiCarlo, C. (2016). Religion and family planning. *European Journal of Contraception and Reproductive Health Care, 21*(6), 486–495.

Planned Parenthood Federation of America. (2016). *Outercourse.* Retrieved from https://www.plannedparenthood.org/learn/birth-control/abstinence-and-outercourse

Schuiling, K. D., & Likis, F. E. (2017). *Women's gynecologic health* (3rd ed.). Burlington, MA: Jones & Bartlett Learning.

Spector, R. E. (2017). *Cultural diversity in health and illness* (9th ed.). Hoboken, NJ: Pearson.

United Nations Population Fund (UNFPA). (2016). *Family planning (Family planning saves lives).* Retrieved from http://www.unfpa.org/family-planning

World Health Organization (WHO). (2015a). *Millennium development goals.* Retrieved from http://www.who.int/en/news-room/fact-sheets/detail/millennium-development-goals-(mdgs)

World Health Organization (WHO). (2015b). *Trends in maternal mortality: 1990–2015.* Retrieved from http://apps.who.int/iris/bitstream/handle/10665/194254/9789241565141_eng.pdf;jsessionid=637A1F288F7BFC7ECA4CF50ED4AB78AF?sequence=1

World Health Organization (WHO). (2016). Maternal mortality [Fact Sheet No. 348]. *Media Centre.* Retrieved from http://www.who.int/mediacentre/factsheets/fs348/en/

Zieman, M., Hatcher, R. A., & Allen, A. Z. (2015). *Managing contraception 2015–2016.* Tiger, GA: Bridging the Gap Foundation.

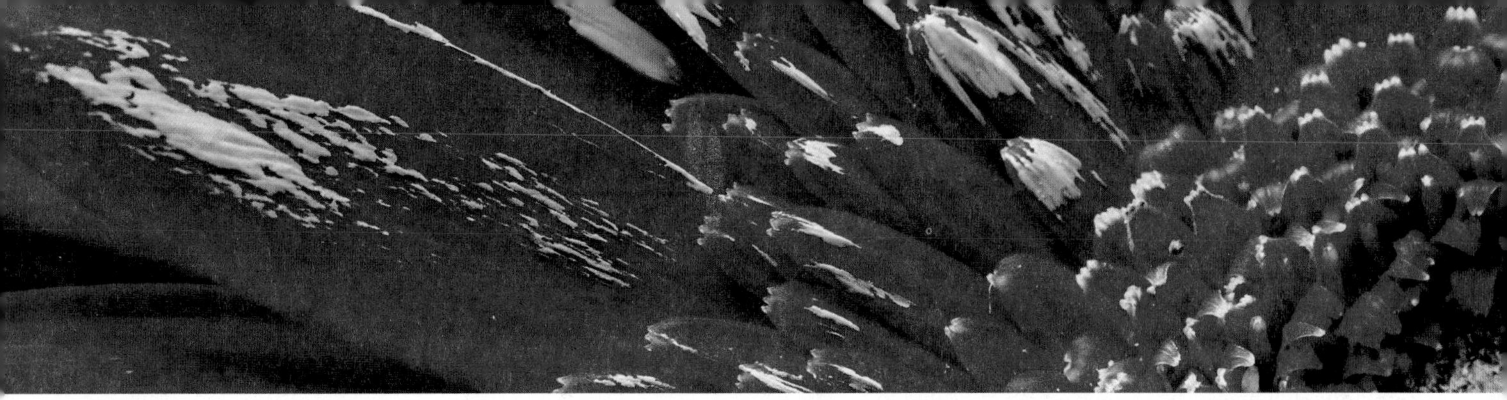

Chapter 5
Commonly Occurring Infections

I just wanted to have a good time when I was young. I only had sex with people I "knew," but eventually I got herpes. When I was 27, I got married, and my husband and I dealt with the herpes pretty effectively. Now I am 52, a widow, and I have started dating. I am seeing a wonderful man who has never had herpes. We are very careful—I don't want him infected because of me. How much simpler life would be if I didn't carry that virus. Too bad that we can't change the past.

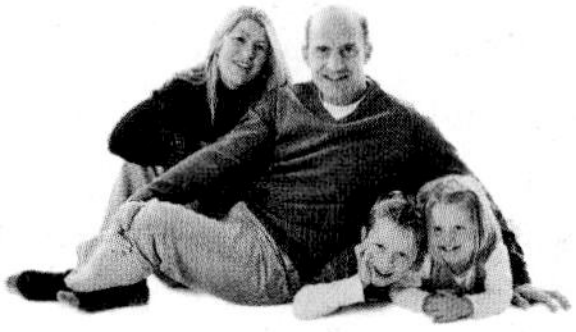

SOURCE: David Morgan/Alamy Stock Photo.

Learning Outcomes

5.1 Compare vulvovaginal candidiasis and bacterial vaginosis.

5.2 Summarize modes of transmission, treatments, and descriptions of the most commonly occurring sexually transmitted infections (STIs).

5.3 Describe the health teaching that a nurse needs to provide to a woman with an STI.

5.4 Relate the implications of pelvic inflammatory disease (PID) for future fertility to its pathologic origin, signs and symptoms, and treatment.

5.5 Contrast cystitis and pyelonephritis.

5.6 Compare the different types of viral hepatitis.

5.7 Summarize the differences between a lower urinary tract infection and an upper urinary tract infection with regard to signs and symptoms, treatment, severity, and nursing care.

Healthy People 2020

(STD-2) Reduce chlamydia rates among females aged 15 to 44 years

(STD-6-1) Reduce gonorrhea rates among females aged 15 to 44 years

Many women seek healthcare because of infections of one sort or another, including those that are sexually transmitted. The nurse caring for a woman with an infection can be most helpful by providing accurate, sensitive, and supportive healthcare and health information. Additionally, the nurse is uniquely able to provide nonjudgmental health promotion, education, and counseling to influence the woman's future health behaviors positively. To meet the woman's needs, the nurse needs to have up-to-date information about a variety of infections, including how they are spread, diagnosed, and treated, and their long-term implications.

This chapter focuses on several types of infections with an emphasis on sexually transmitted infections. It is designed to provide current information to help nurses provide more effective healthcare for women and their families.

Care of the Woman with a Lower Genital Tract Infection (Vaginitis)

Vaginitis is the most common reason why women seek gynecologic care. Symptoms of vaginitis, or *vulvovaginitis*, may include increased vaginal discharge, vulvar irritation and pruritus, external dysuria, dyspareunia (painful sexual intercourse), bleeding with intercourse, or a foul odor. Women with vaginitis may have either infectious abnormal organisms or an abundance or overgrowth of vaginal microorganisms such as *Gardnerella vaginalis*, *Haemophilus*, *Mycoplasma hominis*, *Ureaplasma urealyticum*, and *Mobiluncus*, *Bacteroides*, and *Peptostreptococcus* species. The three most common types of vaginitis are bacterial vaginosis (BV), vulvovaginal candidiasis, and trichomoniasis (Centers for Disease Control and Prevention [CDC], 2015).

Bacterial Vaginosis

Bacterial vaginosis (BV) is the most prevalent form of vaginal infection in the United States and worldwide. BV is more prevalent in sexually active women; however, it is not identified as a sexually transmitted infection because it has also been detected in virginal women. The etiology of BV is related to a change in the normal vaginal flora. Normal hydrogen peroxide–producing lactobacilli are reduced with an overgrowth of vaginal anaerobes and subsequent rise in vaginal pH.

This process is poorly understood, and the causes leading to overgrowth are not clear. Frequent sexual intercourse without condom use (sperm and seminal fluid have pH greater than 7), trauma from douching, having a new sexual partner or multiple partners in the previous 6 months, and an upset in normal vaginal flora are all predisposing or contributing factors. BV can also occur in women who have never had sexual intercourse. An increased rate is also noted in women with same-sex partners (CDC, 2015). The *Gardnerella vaginalis* and *Mycoplasma hominis* organisms have been found in the vast majority of cases, along with an increased concentration of anaerobic bacteria.

The infected woman often notices an excessive amount of thin, watery, white or gray vaginal discharge with a foul odor sometimes described as "fishy." However, the majority of women with BV are asymptomatic. (The characteristic "clue cells" are seen on a wet-mount preparation, and leukocytes are conspicuously absent [Figure 5–1].)The addition of a 10% potassium hydroxide (KOH) solution to the vaginal secretions, called the "whiff" test, releases a strong, fishy, amine-like odor, due to the release of the biologic amines. The vaginal pH is usually greater than 4.5 (normal vaginal pH should be between 3.8 and 4.2). Women with BV have an increased risk of pelvic inflammatory disease (PID), HIV disease, abnormal cervical cytology, postoperative cuff infections after hysterectomy, and postabortion PID. BV infections are associated with negative pregnancy outcomes such as preterm birth, preterm rupture of the membranes, and low birth weight newborns (CDC, 2015; Nasioudis, Linhares, Ledger, et al., 2017).

The nonpregnant woman who is symptomatic is generally treated in one of the following ways:

- Metronidazole (Flagyl): 500 mg orally twice a day for 7 days (see *Drug Guide: Metronidazole*)
- Metronidazole gel (0.75%): One full applicator intravaginally, once daily for 5 days
- Clindamycin cream (2%): One full applicator intravaginally at bedtime for 7 days.

Clindamycin should not be used with latex condoms and diaphragms for 5 days because the cream is oil based and may weaken the barrier method (CDC, 2015). Follow-up visits are not necessary unless symptoms recur. Routine treatment of sex partners is not recommended.

Alternatively, a more expensive treatment is Tinidazole, 2 g orally once daily for 2 days, or Tinidazole, 1 g orally daily for 5 days (CDC, 2015). Prolonged oral or vaginal probiotics following the usual treatment may prevent recurrent BV (Mogha & Prajapati, 2016). Additionally, vitamin B complex may be an effective adjuvant therapy, although dosage and adverse effects are unknown (Sun, Huang, Xu, et al., 2017).

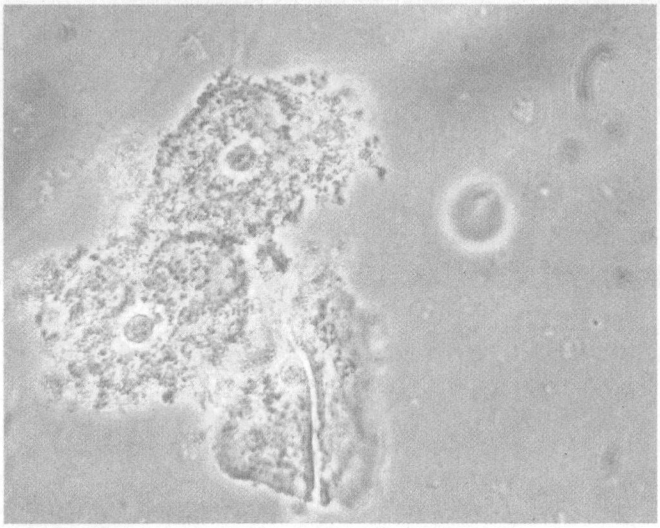

Figure 5–1 The characteristic "clue" cells seen in bacterial vaginosis.

SOURCE: Centers for Disease Control and Prevention.

For many years, metronidazole was regarded as a potential teratogen, particularly in the first trimester, and its use was generally avoided, especially in early pregnancy. However, studies have not demonstrated a consistent relationship between metronidazole use during pregnancy and teratogenic effects on the newborn. Currently, the recommended treatment during pregnancy is the same treatment as for nonpregnant women (CDC, 2015). Nevertheless, some providers still do not treat patients with metronidazole in the first trimester due to the potential for fetal anomalies.

Most providers recommend screening of all pregnant women for BV because it has been associated with preterm labor and birth.

SAFETY ALERT!

Alcohol should be avoided when taking either metronidazole or tinidazole. When combined with alcohol, both metronidazole and tinidazole can produce effects similar to that of alcohol and Antabuse—abdominal pain, flushing, and tremors. The CDC (Centers for Disease Control and Prevention, 2015) recommends abstaining from alcohol for 24 hours after completing metronidazole and 72 hours after completing tinidazole.

Vulvovaginal Candidiasis

Vulvovaginal candidiasis (VVC), also known as *candidiasis*, or *yeast (fungal) infection*, is the second most common cause of vaginitis. It is estimated that in their lifetimes, 75% of women will have at least one episode of VVC (CDC, 2015). *Candida albicans* is responsible for the vast majority of vaginal yeast infections. Non-*albicans* species of *Candida*, such as *C. glabrata*, *C. tropicalis*, and *C. krusei*, can also cause vulvovaginal symptoms and are becoming more prevalent. There is evidence that some of these strains are developing resistance to therapies such as fluconazole. Predisposing factors to yeast infections include glycosuria, use of oral contraceptives, use of antibiotics, pregnancy, diabetes mellitus, and the use of immunosuppressant drugs.

Drug Guide

Metronidazole (Flagyl)

OVERVIEW OF ACTION

Metronidazole is an antimicrobial working in an anaerobic environment. It is an antiprotozoal and antibacterial agent. It possesses direct trichomonacidal and amebicidal activity against *T. vaginalis* and *E. histolytica*. It is used predominantly to treat the following infections in women: *T. vaginalis*, bacterial vaginosis, endometritis, endomyometritis, tubo-ovarian abscess, and postsurgical vaginal cuff infection (*Nursing 2016 Drug Handbook*, 2016).

ROUTE, DOSAGE, AND FREQUENCY

Trichomoniasis—1-day treatment: 2 g orally in a single dose; 7-day treatment: 500 mg orally twice a day for 7 consecutive days (CDC, 2015)

Amebiasis—Adults: 750 mg orally 3 times a day for 5–10 days

Bacterial vaginosis—500 mg orally twice a day for 7 consecutive days or one full applicator of metronidazole gel 0.75% intravaginally once daily for 5 days (CDC, 2015)

CONTRAINDICATIONS

Blood dyscrasias
Breastfeeding women (drug secreted in breast milk)
Impaired kidney or liver function
Active central nervous system (CNS) disease

SIDE EFFECTS

Abdominal cramping
Anorexia
Ataxia
Confusion
Convulsive seizures
Cystitis
Decreased libido
Depression
Diarrhea
Dizziness
Dyspareunia
Dysuria
Epigastric distress
Flattening of the T wave on electrocardiogram (ECG)
Headache
Incontinence
Insomnia
Irritability
Joint pain (fleeting)
Metallic taste in mouth
Nausea and vomiting
Pelvic pressure
Peripheral neuropathy
Polyuria
Proliferation of *Candida* in the vagina and mouth
Reversible leukopenia
Uncoordination
Vertigo
Weakness

NURSING CONSIDERATIONS

- Inform the woman about potential side effects.
- Stress the importance of contraceptive compliance during course of treatment.
- Obtain baseline renal and liver function tests as ordered.
- Teach the woman about the signs, symptoms, and treatment of vulvovaginal candidiasis.
- Counsel the woman to avoid alcoholic beverages while taking the medication.
- Counsel the woman to avoid sexual activity during treatment. If the woman is taking oral contraceptives, a backup nonhormonal contraceptive method is recommended during treatment.
- Take a thorough history to rule out the woman's exposure to this medication within the last 6 weeks.
- Teach the woman to monitor the signs and symptoms of her infection.
- Encourage cooperation with the entire course of treatment.

The woman with VVC often complains of nonmalodorous, thick, white, curdy (cottage cheese–like) vaginal discharge, severe itching, dysuria (external vs. urethral), and dyspareunia. A male sexual partner may experience a rash or excoriation of the skin of the penis, balanitis (inflammation of the glans penis), and possibly pruritus (CDC, 2015). The male can be symptomatic and the female asymptomatic.

On physical examination, the woman's labia may be swollen and excoriated if pruritus has been severe. A speculum examination usually reveals thick, white, tenacious, curdlike patches adhering to the vaginal mucosa. The diagnosis is made by observing mycelia or pseudohyphae upon direct microscopy in a 10% KOH preparation (Figure 5–2). Other diagnostic tests include DNA probe and culture, although cultures are not used for routine diagnosis. The pH of the vagina remains 4 to 4.5 or less (the normal pH of the vagina is about 3.8 to 4.2). This vaginal pH level is in contrast to the pH noted with BV or *Trichomonas*.

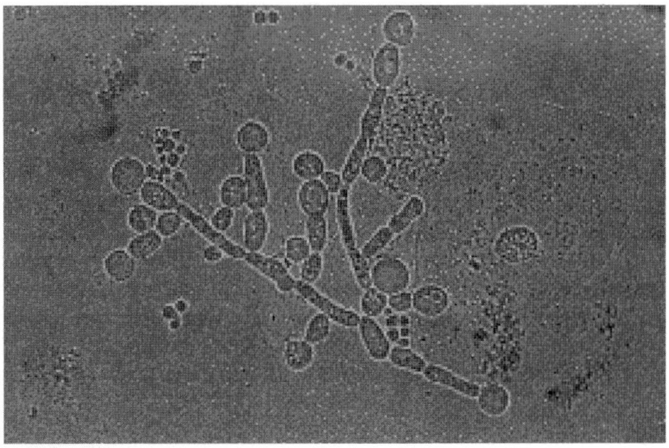

Figure 5–2 Hyphae and spores of *Candida albicans*.

SOURCE: Centers for Disease Control and Prevention.

Medical treatment of VVC includes intravaginal clotrimazole or miconazole cream or suppositories or tioconazole intravaginal ointment, which are available over the counter (OTC). Butoconazole cream, terconazole cream or suppositories, and fluconazole in a single oral dose are available by prescription (CDC, 2016). Single-dose and short-course (3-day) approaches are effective for 80 to 90% of women with uncomplicated VVC. Women who continue to have symptoms after using an OTC preparation and women who have a recurrence of symptoms within 2 months should be evaluated during an office visit because inappropriate use of OTC preparations can lead to a delay in treatment (CDC, 2015).

Treatment of the male partner is generally not indicated, although it may be recommended for partners of women who have recurrent infection. For men who have candidal balanitis, treatment with a topical antifungal medication is indicated (CDC, 2015).

Recurrent VVC, defined as four or more episodes of symptomatic VVC in 1 year, affects less than 5% of women (CDC, 2016). If a woman experiences frequent recurrences of monilial vaginitis, she should be tested for an elevated blood glucose level to determine whether a diabetic or prediabetic condition is present and evaluated for immunosuppression. Women at high risk for sexually transmitted infections should also be tested for HIV infection. In the absence of other risk factors, recurrent VVC treatment should include confirmation of the organism by culture, followed by an intensive regimen of topical agents for 7 to 14 days or oral doses of fluconazole every third day for three doses (days 1, 4, and 7), followed by maintenance antifungal therapy using oral fluconazole 100 mg, 150 mg, or 200 mg weekly for at least 6 months (CDC, 2015). Treatment of the sexual partner is not recommended.

Pregnant women with VVC should be treated only with topical azole preparations applied for 7 days; fluconazole is contraindicated (CDC, 2015). Infection at the time of birth may cause thrush (a *candidal* infection of the mouth) in the newborn.

●○● NURSING MANAGEMENT

For the Woman with Vulvovaginal Candidiasis

Nursing Assessment and Diagnosis

Suspect VVC if the woman complains of intense vulvar itching and a thick, nonodorous white discharge. Women who are HIV positive, are immunosuppressed, are pregnant, or have diabetes mellitus are especially susceptible to this infection; be alert for symptoms in these women. In some areas nurses are trained to do speculum examinations and wet-mount preparations and can confirm the diagnosis themselves. In most cases, however, if you suspect a vaginal infection, report it to the woman's healthcare provider.

Nursing diagnoses that might apply to the woman with VVC include:

- ***Skin Integrity, Risk for Impaired,*** related to scratching secondary to discomfort of the infection
- ***Knowledge, Readiness for Enhanced,*** regarding information about yeast infection related to an expressed desire to know about ways of preventing the development of VVC

(NANDA-I © 2017)

EVIDENCE-BASED PRACTICE | Use of Probiotics for Vulvovaginal Candidiasis

Clinical Questions

Can the ingestion of probiotics enhance antifungal medication effectiveness in women with vulvovaginal candidiasis? Does the use of probiotics reduce long-term recurrence of this condition?

The Evidence

Vulvovaginal candidiasis (VVC) is one of the most commonly occurring infections of the female genitourinary tract. One cause of VVC is an imbalance in the normal vaginal habitat resulting in a decrease of normal lactobacilli and an overgrowth of the *Candida* fungus. Antifungal drugs have been shown to be effective at providing a clinical cure, yet these drugs have side effects, and there is increasing resistance to the drugs resulting in recurrence of the infection. Probiotics are thought to have positive effects on the body's normal microbial habitat, which gives rise to the hypothesis that ingesting probiotics could recover and maintain the normal vaginal microbiota, increasing resistance to reinfection. A team of Cochrane reviewers summarized the evidence from 10 randomized trials that tested pharmacological treatment alone compared with probiotics used as adjuvant therapy to antifungal drugs. These studies, taken together, include more than 1650 subjects. Systematic reviews, particularly those published in the scientifically rigorous *Cochrane Reviews*, form the highest quality of evidence for practice.

Compared with conventional antifungal drugs used alone, the adjuvant therapy of probiotics increased the short term-reduction in symptoms associated with VVC and supported both clinical and mycological cure. At 1 month, relapse rates were reduced for those taking probiotics and antifungal drugs versus those taking antifungal drugs alone (Xie et al., 2017).

However, long-term relapse rates were unaffected by the addition of probiotics. Long-term symptom management, clinical cure, and mycological reduction were not affected by the addition of probiotics to antifungal treatment. The addition of probiotics did not produce any serious or nonserious side effects or adverse events (Xie et al., 2017).

Best Practice

Probiotics as an adjuvant therapy to antifungal medication may enhance symptom reduction and both clinical and mycological cure in women with VVC. No serious or nonserious side effects were associated with the use of probiotics. However, while probiotics may reduce short-term recurrence, this treatment does not inhibit recurrence in the long term. The nurse can advise women to take probiotics in addition to pharmacologic treatment, but will want to counsel them to monitor for longer-term recurrence.

Clinical Reasoning

Why might ingesting probiotics enhance the use of antifungal drugs for VVC? What kinds of women might make the best candidates for adjuvant probiotic therapy?

Nursing Plan and Implementation

Discuss with the woman the factors that contribute to the development of VVC and suggest ways to prevent recurrences, such as wearing cotton underwear and cotton-crotch pantyhose, avoiding tight-fitting clothing, discontinuing oral contraceptives, and avoiding douching and vaginal powders or sprays that can irritate the vulva. Advise women taking antibiotics about the possibility of developing VVC and encourage them to seek treatment early if symptoms develop. Some clinicians recommend that women who are taking antibiotics consume yogurt or probiotics supplements (containing acidophilus and other helpful bacteria) simultaneously to reestablish normal vaginal flora. Women with diabetes mellitus are encouraged to improve glycemic control.

Evaluation

Expected outcomes of nursing care include:

- The woman's symptoms are relieved, and the infection is cured.
- The woman is able to identify self-care measures to prevent further episodes of VVC.

Care of the Woman with a Sexually Transmitted Infection

The occurrence of **sexually transmitted infection (STI)**, or *sexually transmitted disease (STD)*, has increased over the past few decades. In fact, vaginitis and STIs are the most common reasons for outpatient, community-based treatment of women. More than one STI can occur at the same time. All symptomatic women should be tested for other infections. Table 5–1 provides a summary of common vaginal and sexually transmitted infections.

Prevention of Sexually Transmitted Infections

Effective prevention and control of STIs is based on the following concepts (CDC, 2015):

1. Education and counseling for people at risk on ways to practice safer sexual behavior
2. Identification of infected, asymptomatic individuals and of people with symptoms of STI who are not likely to seek diagnostic and treatment services

TABLE 5–1 Summary of Common Vaginal and Sexually Transmitted Infections

			TREATMENT	
DISEASE	ORGANISM	DIAGNOSIS	NONPREGNANT	PREGNANT
Vulvovaginal candidiasis (VVC)	*Candida albicans*	NaCl wet-mount hyphae	Topically applied azole drugs	Topically applied azole drugs
Bacterial vaginosis (BV)	*Gardnerella vaginalis* and *Mycoplasma hominis*	KOH wet-mount clue cells (greater than 20%)	Metronidazole	Metronidazole or clindamycin
Trichomoniasis	*Trichomonas vaginalis*	NaCl wet-mount trichomonads	Metronidazole or tinidazole	Metronidazole
Syphilis	*Treponema pallidum*	Dark-field examination, Venereal Disease Research Laboratories (VDRL), rapid plasma reagin (RPR), or microhemagglutination assay–Treponema pallidum (MHA-TP)	Benzathine Penicillin G	Benzathine Penicillin G
Herpes genitalis	Herpes simplex virus	Herpes culture or titer	Acyclovir, Valacyclovir, Famciclovir	Acyclovir, Valacyclovir
Chlamydia	*Chlamydia trachomatis*	Chlamydia culture	Doxycycline or azithromycin*	Azithromycin or amoxicillin
Gonorrhea	*Neisseria gonorrhoeae*	Gonorrhea culture	Ceftriaxone, plus azithromycin or doxycycline	Ceftriaxone, plus azithromycin
AIDS	HIV	Enzyme-linked immunosorbent assay (ELISA) test and Western blot	Varies	Varies
Condylomata acuminata	Human papilloma virus	Virapap, biopsy, Pap smear, colposcopy	Cryotherapy, trichloroacetic acid (TCA), bichloroacetic acid (BCA), podophyllin, podofilox, excision	Cryotherapy, trichloroacetic acid
Pediculosis pubis	*Pthirus pubis*	Microscopic identification of lice or nits	Permethrin 1% liquid or malathion 0.5% lotion	Permethrin 1% liquid
Scabies	*Sarcoptes scabiei*	Confirmation of symptoms or scraping of furrows	Permethrin 5% cream or crotamiton 10% cream or lotion	Permethrin 5% cream

* Doxycycline is contraindicated during pregnancy.

3. Effective diagnosis and treatment of people with an STI
4. Evaluation, treatment, counseling, and education for individuals who are the sex partners of people with an STI
5. Pre-exposure vaccination of individuals at risk for vaccine-preventable STIs
6. Expedited partner therapy (EPT), whereby partners are treated, as recommended by the CDC.

With EPT, infected individuals deliver medications or prescriptions to their partners to manage and decrease the reinfection rates of STIs. This approach is effective but is not mandated by law in all states.

Individuals are at lowest risk for an STI if they abstain from sexual intercourse (whether vaginal, anal, or oral sex) and if they are in a long-term, monogamous relationship with a partner who is free of infection. Ideally, before entering a new sexual relationship, both partners should be tested for STIs, including HIV infection. If a person decides to have sex without knowing the partner's infection status, a new condom should be used before each act of intercourse (CDC, 2015).

Nurses can play an important role in educating and counseling individuals who have an STI, who are at risk for one, or who are the partners of an infected individual. Information should be tailored to individual needs and specific risk factors. It can include details about actions a person can take to avoid exposure to an STI or to avoid transmitting one. Nurses need to be nonjudgmental and respectful and draw on their counseling skills in sharing information. In addition, nurses may find teaching opportunities by listening attentively to patients to clarify misconceptions about sexual and reproductive health.

Trichomoniasis

Trichomoniasis is a commonly occurring STI caused by *Trichomonas vaginalis*, a microscopic motile protozoan that thrives in an alkaline environment. In young, sexually active women, trichomoniasis is the most common curable nonviral, sexually transmitted infection, affecting approximately 11% of women 40 years of age and younger (CDC, 2015). The single-celled parasite, called a *trichomonad*, is an anaerobe that has the ability to generate hydrogen, which combines with oxygen to create an anaerobic environment. Coinfection with other sexually transmitted infections is common, and HIV has been shown to be transmitted more easily with trichomoniasis present (CDC, 2016). Pregnant women with trichomoniasis may be at increased risk for premature rupture of membranes and preterm birth.

Approximately 70 to 85% of women with trichomoniasis are asymptomatic or have only mild symptoms (CDC, 2015). Symptoms of trichomoniasis include:

- Discharge that is odorous, yellow-green, and frothy
- Vulvar itching
- Dysuria and dyspareunia.

Diagnosis is made based on the following findings:

- Microscopic visualization of mobile trichomonads and increased leukocytes (Figure 5–3)
- Vaginal pH of 5.0 or higher
- Positive whiff test
- Two other tests with greater sensitivity than the wet-mount preparation are also available and are performed on vaginal secretions: The nucleic acid amplification test (NAAT) and the Aptima *T. vaginalis* assay (CDC, 2015).

Recommended treatment for trichomoniasis is metronidazole (Flagyl) administered in a single 2-g dose or tinidazole in a single

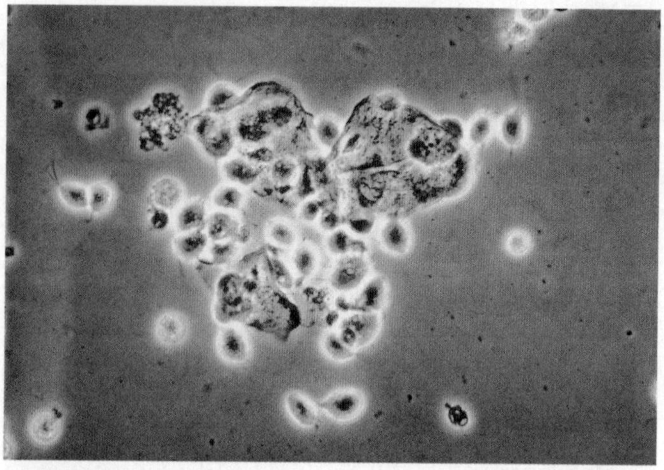

Figure 5–3 Microscopic appearance of *Trichomonas vaginalis*.

SOURCE: Centers for Disease Control and Prevention.

2-g oral dose or, alternatively, metronidazole 500 mg twice daily for 7 days for both male and female sexual partners. Tinidazole has fewer gastrointestinal side effects than metronidazole but is more costly (CDC, 2016). Partners should avoid intercourse until both are cured (therapy is completed and both are symptom free), approximately 7 days. The woman and her partner should be cautioned to avoid alcohol for 24 hours after taking metronidazole and 72 hours after taking tinidazole; the combination has an effect similar to that of alcohol and disulfiram (Antabuse)—abdominal pain, nausea, flushing, or tremors (Wilson, Shannon, & Shields, 2017).

Chlamydial Infection

Chlamydial infection, caused by *Chlamydia trachomatis*, is the most common bacterial STI in the United States (CDC, 2015). It is found most frequently in sexually active adolescents and young adults. Transmission commonly occurs through vaginal sex. The organism is an intracellular bacterium with different immunotypes.

Chlamydia is a major cause of nongonococcal urethritis (NGU) in men. In women it can cause infections similar to those that occur with gonorrhea. However, asymptomatic infection is common in both men and women. Severe sequelae can result from untreated chlamydial infection, including pelvic inflammatory disease (PID), infertility, and ectopic pregnancy. In men, chlamydial infection can result in epididymitis and infertility. In addition, chlamydia infection is associated with an increased risk of acquiring and transmitting HIV infection. The newborn of a woman with untreated chlamydia is at risk of developing ophthalmia neonatorum (a form of conjunctivitis that is contracted by a newborn during passage through the birth canal of an infected mother), which responds to erythromycin ophthalmic ointment prophylaxis at birth. The newborn may also develop chlamydial pneumonia.

Up to half of women are asymptomatic. In females, symptoms of chlamydia include:

- Thin or mucopurulent discharge
- Cervical ectropion
- Friable cervix (bleeds easily)
- Burning and frequency of urination
- Lower abdominal pain.

Of the laboratory tests currently available to diagnose chlamydia, NAAT tests are the most sensitive and several different tests are currently available. Diagnosis is frequently made after treatment of a male partner for NGU or in a symptomatic woman with a negative gonorrhea culture. Routine screening is

CASE STUDY: Angelina Newman

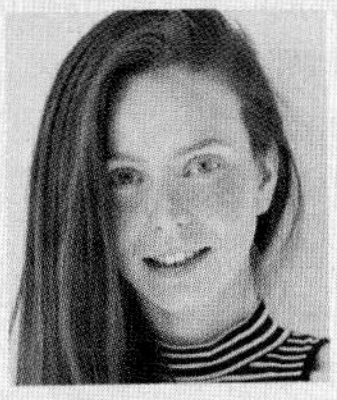

SOURCE: WAYHOME studio/Shutterstock

Angelina recently underwent her first pelvic examination due to pregnancy. Her boyfriend is ambivalent about the pregnancy but attends the follow-up visit after pressure from her. At this visit, Angelina is told she tested positive for chlamydia. The boyfriend is not in the room when she is given the results, but the nurse practitioner has offered to be present as she tells him the test results. Angelina reports she has no symptoms and that her boyfriend is the only sexual partner she has ever had. She tells the NP that she knows her boyfriend had previous sexual relationships prior to them starting a relationship. The boyfriend expresses intense anger when learning that she has tested positive for chlamydia. She informs him that she never slept with anyone else.

Questions to Ponder

What is the necessary next step for treating this couple? What precautions should they use during infection treatment?

recommended in all sexually active women less than 25 years of age (CDC, 2015). See *Case Study: Angelina Newman*.

The recommended treatment is a single dose of azithromycin 1 g orally or doxycycline 100 mg by mouth twice a day for 7 days. Sexual partners should also be treated, and the partners should abstain from intercourse for 7 days. Doxycycline is contraindicated during pregnancy, especially in the second and third trimester. The CDC (2015) recommends that pregnant women be treated with azithromycin 1 gm orally. Alternative treatments include amoxicillin 500 mg orally three times daily for 7 days or erythromycin orally, ranging from 250–800 mg at varied dosing from 7 to 14 days (or erythromycin orally, ranging from 250–800 mg at varied dosing from 7 to 14 days) (CDC, 2015). Because so many people with chlamydia are asymptomatic, screening of the following groups is recommended as a primary method of decreasing the incidence (CDC, 2015):

- Annual screening for sexually active adolescent females and women under age 25
- Annual screening for women over age 25 who are at risk for chlamydia (history of STIs, multiple sexual partners, new sexual partner, inconsistent use of barrier contraceptives)
- Screening of all pregnant women under age 25 and older women at risk for chlamydia at their first prenatal visit and again during the third trimester of pregnancy (*Note:* Many practitioners routinely screen all pregnant women.) Screening using a nucleic amplification test can be done on endocervical and vaginal specimens for women and urine specimens for men. The use of self-obtained vaginal swab specimens is a viable screening option for women who have been given instruction (CDC, 2015).

Gonorrhea

Gonorrhea, an infection caused by the bacterium *Neisseria gonorrhoeae*, is the second most commonly reported STI in the United States, with more than 820,000 cases annually. The highest rates of infection occur in females less than 25 years of age (CDC, 2015). Most men seek treatment for gonorrhea early because of symptoms, but many women with the infection are asymptomatic until complications such as PID occur. Transmission can occur through vaginal, anal, or oral sex.

If a pregnant woman becomes infected after the third month of gestation, the mucous plug in the cervix generally prevents the infection from ascending, and it remains localized in the urethra, cervix, and Bartholin glands until the membranes rupture. Then it can spread upward. A newborn exposed to a gonococcal-infected birth canal is at risk of developing ophthalmia neonatorum. Eye prophylaxis for all newborns is provided to prevent this complication.

Because so many women with gonorrhea are asymptomatic, it is accepted practice to screen for it by doing a cervical culture during the initial prenatal examination. For women at high risk, the culture may be repeated during the last month of pregnancy. Cultures of the urethra, throat, and rectum may also be required for diagnosis, depending on the body orifices used for intercourse.

The most common symptoms of gonorrheal infection, when they occur, include a purulent, greenish-yellow vaginal discharge, dysuria, and urinary frequency. Some women also develop inflammation and swelling of the vulva. The cervix may appear swollen and eroded and may secrete a foul-smelling discharge in which gonococci are present. Symptoms in women may also include cervicitis, acute cystitis, or vaginitis. Bilateral lower abdominal or pelvic pain may occur. The preferred treatment for both nonpregnant and pregnant women consists of antibiotic therapy with a single dose of ceftriaxone 250 mg intramuscularly plus a single 1-gm dose of azithromycin orally. This dual treatment is recommended to minimize secondary antimicrobial resistance and to address the risk of co-infection with chlamydia because gonorrhea and chlamydia often occur together (CDC, 2015).

All sexual partners must be treated or the woman can become reinfected. As with chlamydia, nurses should recommend abstinence for 7 days following treatment.

Retesting is recommended 3 months following treatment because of the risk of reinfection (CDC, 2015). Both sexual partners should be treated if either has a positive test for gonorrhea. Women should also be informed of signs that infection has spread and resulted in PID. A test-of-cure 14 days after treatment is only indicated for individuals with pharyngeal gonorrhea who have been treated with an alternative regimen (CDC, 2015).

Ethics in Action!

How do you respond to a woman who comes in for treatment with her fourth chlamydia/gonorrhea infection in 2 years and states she just wants to have fun?

Herpes Genitalis

The *herpes simplex virus (HSV)* causes herpes infections, which are recurrent, lifelong infections. Two serotypes of HSV cause human infections: HSV-1 and HSV-2. HSV-2 causes most cases of recurrent genital herpes and is spread through vaginal, anal, or oral sex. It can also be spread through skin-to-skin contact with an infected site such as a finger (herpetic whitlow). The clinical symptoms and treatment of both types are the same. At least 50 million people in the United States have been diagnosed with genital HSV-2 infection—**herpes genitalis**. Even so, most people infected with genital herpes have not been diagnosed because they have mild or unrecognized infections but shed the virus intermittently (CDC, 2015).

A primary herpes infection during pregnancy has been associated with an increased risk of spontaneous abortion, low birth weight, and preterm birth. If herpes is present in the genital tract of a woman during childbirth, it can have a devastating effect on the newborn. Women with herpetic lesions when labor begins should give birth by cesarean to prevent neonatal herpes. See Chapter 18 and Table 31–5, Maternally Transmitted Newborn Infections, for more information.

The primary episode (first outbreak) of herpes genitalis is characterized by the development of single or multiple blister-like vesicles, which usually occur in the genital area and sometimes affect the vaginal walls, cervix, urethra, and anus. The vesicles may appear within a few hours to 20 days after exposure and rupture spontaneously to form very painful open, ulcerated lesions. Inflammation and pain secondary to the presence of herpes lesions can cause difficult urination and urinary retention. Enlargement of the inguinal lymph nodes may be present. Flulike symptoms and genital pruritus or tingling also may be noticed. Primary episodes usually last the longest and are the most severe. Lesions heal spontaneously in 2 to 4 weeks.

After the lesions heal, the virus enters a dormant phase, residing in the nerve ganglia of the affected area. Some individuals never have a recurrence, whereas others have regular recurrences. Recurrences are usually less severe than the initial episode and seem to be triggered by emotional stress, menstruation, ovulation, pregnancy, and frequent or vigorous intercourse. Patients with poor health status, a generally run-down physical condition, or who are immunocompromised can experience more frequent recurrences. Diagnosis is made on the basis of the clinical appearance of the lesions, NAAT, viral culture of the lesions, PCR identification, and glycoprotein G-based HSV type-specific assays (CDC, 2015).

No known cure for herpes exists; however, medications are available to partially control the symptoms of herpes and prevent complications from secondary infection. The recommended treatment of the first clinical episode of genital herpes is oral acyclovir, valacyclovir, or famciclovir. These same medications, in somewhat different dosages, are also recommended for recurrent herpes infection and for daily suppressive therapy for people who have frequent recurrences. Therapy should be started during the prodromal period (time before the onset of lesions) for the greatest benefit.

For recurrent infections, suppressive therapy during pregnancy is acyclovir 400 mg orally three times a day or valacyclovir 500 mg orally twice a day starting at 36 gestational weeks. Its use from 36 weeks' gestation to birth may reduce the frequency of cesarean births by decreasing the incidence of recurrences at term but may not prevent neonatal transmission (CDC, 2015).

Keeping the genital area clean and dry, wearing loose clothing, taking sitz baths, and wearing cotton underwear or none at all will promote healing. Primary or recurrent lesions will heal without treatment.

Syphilis

Syphilis is a chronic infection caused by the spirochete *Treponema pallidum*. Syphilis is commonly acquired through vaginal, oral, or anal sex. All patients with syphilis should be screened for HIV because coinfection is common. Men having sex with men (MSM) account for the majority of the cases of primary and secondary syphilis reported.

Syphilis is divided into early and late stages. During the early stage (primary), a chancre appears at the site where the *T. pallidum* organism entered the body. Symptoms include slight fever, loss of weight, and malaise. The chancre persists for about 4 weeks and then disappears. In 6 weeks to 6 months, secondary symptoms appear. Skin eruptions called *condylomata lata*, which resemble wartlike plaques and are highly infectious, may appear on the vulva. Other secondary symptoms are acute arthritis, enlargement of the liver and spleen, nontender enlarged lymph nodes, iritis, and a chronic sore throat with hoarseness. A latent phase with no lesions may be followed by a tertiary stage. Approximately 30% of those patients who are not treated may progress to tertiary syphilis (CDC, 2015).

Syphilis may also be transmitted transplacentally. When infected in utero, the newborn exhibits secondary-stage symptoms of syphilis. Transplacentally transmitted syphilis may cause intrauterine growth restriction, congenital anomalies, preterm birth, and stillbirth. As a result of the disease's impact on the fetus in utero, serologic testing of every pregnant woman is recommended; some state laws require it. Testing is done at the initial prenatal screening and may be repeated in the third trimester. Blood studies in early pregnancy may be negative if the woman has only recently contracted the infection.

Congenital syphilis can cause neonatal death, stillbirth, and congenital anomalies, including deafness, neurologic impairment, and bone and teeth abnormalities (CDC, 2015). See Table 31–5, Maternally Transmitted Newborn Infections.

During the early primary stage, the diagnosis is made by dark-field microscopic examination of the chancre for spirochetes and direct fluorescence antibody testing. Blood tests such as Venereal Disease Research Laboratories (VDRL), rapid plasma reagin (RPR), or the more specific fluorescent treponemal antibody absorption test (FTA-ABS) are commonly done. Nontreponemal test antibody titers (VDRL and RPR) correlate with disease activity and are used to guide treatment, while treponemal tests remain reactive, usually for life (CDC, 2015).

For pregnant and nonpregnant women with syphilis of less than a year's duration (early latent syphilis), the CDC (CDC, 2015) recommends 2.4 million units of benzathine penicillin G intramuscularly in a single dose. If syphilis is of long duration (more than 1 year) or of unknown duration, 2.4 million units of benzathine penicillin G are given intramuscularly once a week for 3 weeks. If a woman is allergic to penicillin and nonpregnant, latent syphilis is treated with doxycycline 100 mg orally twice a day or tetracycline 500 mg orally four times a day for 28 days. Tertiary syphilis is treated with 2.4 million units of benzathine penicillin G IM weekly for 3 weeks. The pregnant woman with syphilis who is allergic to penicillin should be desensitized in a hospital and then treated (CDC, 2015).

Human Papilloma Virus/ Condylomata Acuminata

Condylomata acuminata, also called *genital warts*, is a common STI caused by the human papilloma virus (HPV). Transmission can occur through vaginal, oral, or anal sex.

Because of the evidence of a link between HPV and cervical and anorectal cancers, the condition is receiving increasing attention. Over 100 HPV subtypes have been identified; of these, about 40 types can infect the genital tract (CDC, 2016). Most HPV infections are unrecognized, asymptomatic, or subclinical. HPV types 6 and 11 account for approximately 90% of visible genital warts, but they have a low cancer-causing potential, whereas high-risk types such as 16 and 18 cause 80% of cervical cancers (CDC, 2016). Patients with visible genital warts can be infected concurrently with different HPV types.

A woman often seeks healthcare after noticing single or multiple soft, grayish-pink, cauliflower-like lesions in her genital area (Figure 5–4). These warts are often asymptomatic; however, depending on their location and size, they may cause itching (pruritus) or be friable (bleed easily). The moist, warm environment of the genital area is conducive to the growth of the warts, which may be present on the vulva, perineum, vagina, cervix, urethra, and anus. The incubation period following exposure is 3 weeks to 3 years, with the average being about 3 months.

Because condylomata sometimes resemble other lesions and can become cancerous, all atypical, pigmented, and persistent warts should be biopsied and treatment instituted promptly. Diagnosis is usually made by visual appearance. However, vaginal and cervical warts are more common than warts of the external genitalia. Most of these are flat lesions visible only by colposcopy. Subclinical diagnosis can be made if characteristic changes are present on a Pap smear.

The CDC does not specify a treatment of choice for genital warts but recommends that treatment be determined based on patient preference, available resources, and experience of the healthcare provider (CDC, 2015). No single treatment is best for all types of warts or for all patients. Patient-applied therapies include podofilox solution or gel, imiquimod cream, or sinecatechin 15% ointment.

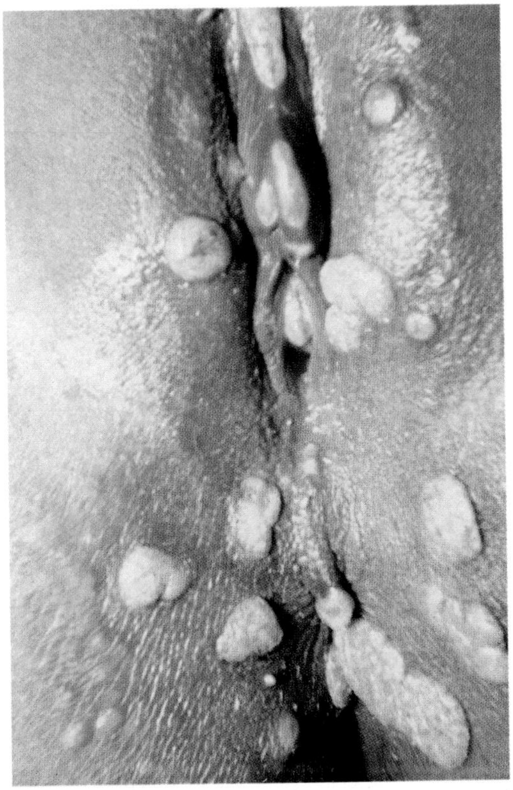

Figure 5–4 Condylomata acuminata on the vulva.

SOURCE: Centers for Disease Control and Prevention.

SAFETY ALERT!

If a patient-applied therapy is prescribed, the patient must understand exactly how to apply the medication and must be able to identify and reach all the warts. These regimens have specific directions for application, frequency, and length of use, which the nurse should review carefully. Both imiquimod and sinecatechin ointment must be washed off after specified time periods.

Provider-administered therapies include cryotherapy with liquid nitrogen or cryoprobe; topical podophyllin; trichloroacetic acid (TCA); bichloroacetic acid (BCA); and surgical removal by tangential scissors excision, shave excision, curettage, or electrosurgery. Alternative therapies include intralesional interferon, podophyllin resin, photodynamic therapy, or topical cidofovir (CDC, 2015).

Warts can proliferate during pregnancy and may obstruct the birth canal. Imiquimod, podophyllin, podofilox, and sinecatechin ointment are not used because their safety during pregnancy has not been determined. TCA, BCA, and surgical removal are safe during pregnancy and may be used secondary to the size of the warts and patient discomfort. Genital and vulvar warts do not warrant cesarean birth.

Three HPV vaccines are now available against herpes simplex virus (HSV) types 16 and 18, which cause 66% of cervical cancers. Gardasil, the first vaccine to receive FDA approval, is a quadrivalent vaccine that provides protection against types 6, 11, 16, and 18. The second vaccine, Cervarix, is a bivalent vaccine that provides protection only against HSV types 16 and 18. Either vaccine is recommended for girls ages 11 to 12 (preferably before they are sexually active) and for 13- to 26-year-old females who did not receive or complete the three-dose vaccine series. A 9-valent vaccine is now available that prevents infection with HPV types 6, 11, 16, 18, 31, 33, 45, 52, and 58. The CDC (2015) recommends that either the quadrivalent or 9-valent vaccine be routinely given to boys ages 11 to 12 to protect against HPV and also help provide indirect protection of women by reducing HPV transmission. All the vaccines are given as a three-dose series of IM injections with the second dose given 1 to 2 months after the initial dose and the third dose given 6 months after the initial dose. Pregnant women should not receive HPV vaccines.

All women, including those who have received the vaccine, should receive regular Pap smears as recommended. Women with diagnosed HPV infections should have more frequent Pap smears to monitor cervical cell changes. Sex partners are probably infected but do not require treatment unless large lesions are present. The use of male or female condoms may reduce the risk of transmitting the virus to an uninfected partner.

“I've finally come to terms with the fact that I carry HPV. I know I will always run the risk of recurrence, but it's just a virus. It doesn't define me as a person.”

Pediculosis Pubis (Pubic or Crab Lice)

Pediculosis pubis is caused by *Pthirus*, a grayish, parasitic “crab” louse that lays eggs that attach to the hair shaft. Transmission is primarily by sexual contact, although shared towels and bed linens of infested persons are also possible sources.

Symptoms include itching, usually in the pubic area. For either pregnant or nonpregnant women, it is treated by applying 1% permethrin cream rinse or pyrethrins with piperonyl butoxide (CDC, 2017b). The treatment is applied to clean hair, saturating the hair and removing it after 10 minutes with warm water. Some providers recommend combing the pubic hair with a fine-toothed comb before rinsing off the medication. Retreatment may be necessary.

Both partners must be treated and tested for other STIs. Bed linens, towels, clothing, and other objects should be machine-washed in hot water and dried in a hot dryer for 20 minutes or dry-cleaned or sealed in an airtight bag for 2 weeks. Sexual contact should be avoided until the woman and her partner(s) have been treated and cured. Treatment may be repeated in 7 days if live lice are noted.

Scabies

Sarcoptes scabiei is a parasitic itch mite. The female mite burrows under the skin to deposit her eggs. Transmission by intimate sexual contact is common in adults, but scabies in children is not generally sexually acquired (CDC, 2015).

Symptoms include itching that worsens at night or when the individual is warm. Noticeable erythematous, papular lesions or furrows may be present. The recommended treatment for scabies is permethrin cream 5% applied to all body areas from the neck down and washed off after 8 to 14 hours or ivermectin 200ug/kg taken orally and repeated in 2 weeks. Treatment is repeated in 7 days if live mites still exist. Other medications include lindane 1% lotion or 30 g of cream that has scabicidal and antipruritic actions. It is applied in a thin layer to all areas of the body from the neck down, with attention to body creases, and rinsed off after 8 hours. Permethrin 5% is used in pregnant women. Clothing and bed linens should be washed and dried in a hot dryer, dry-cleaned, or sealed in a plastic bag for a minimum of 72 hours. Sexual contacts and close household contacts within the previous month need to be examined and treated for scabies as appropriate.

Viral Hepatitis

Hepatitis is an inflammatory process of the liver caused by infection by one of the five distinct viruses: A, B, C, D, and E. Ninety-six percent of deaths from hepatitis are primarily from hepatitis B and C (World Health Organization [WHO], 2017). Currently, immunizations are only available for hepatitis A and B. Table 5–2 compares the five forms of viral hepatitis.

Hepatitis A is characterized by symptoms of jaundice, anorexia, nausea and vomiting, malaise, fever, and gray-colored bowel movements. It is self-limiting and is not a chronic condition. Vaccines are available to prevent hepatitis A and B.

Hepatitis B, C, and D have symptoms similar to those of hepatitis A and can also include arthralgias, arthritis, and skin eruptions or rash. Unlike hepatitis A infection, those of B, C, and D infections are chronic. See Table 17–6 for information about hepatitis B and pregnancy. Hepatitis C is a common bloodborne infection that is transmitted primarily by contact with infected blood. People at high risk for the infection include intravenous (IV) drug users, healthcare workers who receive a needlestick, and people with multiple sexual partners.

Hepatitis D only occurs in people infected with hepatitis B and is uncommon in the United States. Hepatitis E, while uncommon in the United States, is common worldwide, occurring primarily in East and South Asia. Its symptoms are like those of hepatitis A. It is also a self-limiting disease and not a chronic condition.

AIDS

AIDS is a serious, often fatal disorder caused by HIV. A medical-surgical text more fully describes this condition. HIV alters the presentation of STIs and can complicate the treatment of an STI. This is a bidirectional relationship because STIs can facilitate the transmission of HIV (CDC, 2015). Because the diagnosis of HIV/AIDS or the presence of the HIV antibody has implications for a fetus if the woman is pregnant, HIV/AIDS is discussed in greater detail in Chapter 17.

●○● NURSING MANAGEMENT

For the Individual with a Sexually Transmitted Infection

Nursing Assessment and Diagnosis

When working with women, it is important to become adept at taking a thorough history and identifying women at risk for STIs. Risk factors include multiple sexual partners; a partner's involvement with other partners; high-risk sexual behaviors, such as intercourse without barrier contraception or anal intercourse; partners with high-risk behaviors; and young age at onset of sexual activity. Be alert for signs and symptoms of an STI and be familiar with diagnostic procedures if it is suspected.

Although each STI has certain distinctive characteristics, the following complaints suggest the possibility of infection and warrant further investigation:

- Presence of a "sore" or lesion on the vulva
- Increased vaginal discharge or malodorous vaginal discharge
- Burning with urination
- Dyspareunia
- Bleeding after intercourse
- Pelvic pain.

TABLE 5–2 Types of Viral Hepatitis

FORM	PRIMARY ROUTE OF TRANSMISSION	INCUBATION PERIOD	CHRONIC INFECTION?	IMMUNIZATION AVAILABLE?
Hepatitis A	Fecal–oral, contaminated food/water	15–50 days	No	Yes
Hepatitis B	Blood/body fluids	45–108 days	Yes	Yes
Hepatitis C	Blood/blood products	14–180 days	Yes	No
Hepatitis D	Blood/body fluids	45–160 days	Yes	No
Hepatitis E	Fecal–oral	21–56 days	No	Yes (China only)

Developing Cultural Competence STI Rates in the United States

Rates of STIs vary by race/ethnicity. In 2015, for example, the gonorrhea rate in those of African heritage was 424.9 cases per 100,000 population; among Native American/Alaska natives the rate was 192.8 cases per 100,000 population; among Native Hawaiians/other Pacific Islanders the rate was 123.0 cases per 100,000 population; among Hispanics the rate was 80.5 per 100,000 population; among Caucasian Americans the rate was 44.2 cases per 100,000 population; and among Asian Americans the rate was 22.9 cases per 100,000 (CDC, 2016).

In many instances the woman is asymptomatic but may report symptoms in her partner, especially painful urination or urethral discharge. It is often helpful to ask the woman whether her partner is experiencing any symptoms.

Nursing diagnoses that may apply to a woman with an STI include:

- *Family Processes, Interrupted*, related to the effects of a diagnosis of sexually transmitted infection on the couple's relationship
- *Knowledge, Readiness for Enhanced*, related to preventing STIs related to an expressed desire to avoid infection

(NANDA-I © 2017)

While it is important to learn to effectively communicate with all young adults about STIs, it is especially critical with those of minority groups. Efforts to provide effective screening and treatment of STIs need to be expanded, and teaching and prevention strategies that are culturally sensitive need to be developed. These endeavors will contribute to decreasing the long-term consequences of STIs, such as ectopic pregnancy and infertility, and will also help decrease healthcare costs.

Nursing Plan and Implementation

In a supportive, nonjudgmental way, provide the woman who has an STI with information about the infection, methods of transmission, implications for pregnancy or future fertility, and importance of thorough treatment. If treatment of her partner is indicated, the woman must understand that it is necessary to prevent a cycle of reinfection. She should also understand the need to abstain from sexual activity, if necessary, during treatment.

Some STIs, such as trichomoniasis or chlamydia, may cause a woman concern but once diagnosed are rather simply treated. Other STIs can also be fairly simple to treat medically but may carry a stigma and be emotionally devastating for the woman. Stress prevention with all women and encourage them to require partners, especially new partners, to use condoms.

Displaying sensitivity can be especially helpful in encouraging the woman to explore her feelings about the diagnosis. She may experience anger or feel betrayed by a partner; she may feel guilt or see her diagnosis as a form of punishment; or she may feel concern about the long-term implications for future childbearing or ongoing intimate relationships. She may experience a myriad of emotions that she never expected. Opportunities to discuss her feelings in a nonjudgmental environment can be especially helpful. Offer suggestions about support groups, if indicated, and assist the woman in planning for her future with regard to sexual activity.

Health Promotion

The risk of contracting an STI increases with the number of sexual partners. Because of the extended time between infection with HIV and evidence of infection, intercourse with an individual exposes a female or male to all the other sexual partners of that individual for the past 5 or more years. Because of this risk, it is important that women take the following actions:

- Plan ahead, review decision-making skills, and develop strategies to refuse sex (especially important for adolescents who may be less confident about saying "no" to casual sexual encounters) because abstinence is the best method of preventing STIs.
- Limit the number of sexual contacts and practice mutual monogamy.
- Use condoms for every act of vaginal and anal intercourse. Other contraceptives such as the diaphragm, cervical cap, and spermicides also offer limited protection against STIs.
- Plan strategies for negotiating condom use with a partner.
- Reduce high-risk behaviors. Use of recreational drugs and alcohol can increase sexual risk taking.
- Refrain from oral sex if her partner has active sores in the mouth, vagina, or anus or on the penis.
- Seek care as soon as she notices symptoms and make sure her partner gets treatment, if indicated. Absence of symptoms or disappearance of symptoms does not mean that treatment is unnecessary if she suspects an STI. Take all prescribed medications completely.
- The presence of a genital infection can lead to an abnormal Pap smear. Women with certain infections should have regularly scheduled Pap tests according to a schedule recommended by their healthcare provider.

Evaluation

Expected outcomes of nursing care include:

- The infection is identified and cured, if possible. If not, supportive therapy is provided.
- The woman and her partner can describe the infection, its method of transmission, its implications, and the therapy.
- The woman copes successfully with the impact of the diagnosis on her self-concept.

Professionalism in Practice Attitudes About STIs

Many women deal matter-of-factly with an STI diagnosis; other women find it embarrassing and possibly even shameful. The nurse's attitude of straightforward acceptance conveys to the woman that she is still an acceptable person who happens to have an infection and can help the woman deal effectively with her diagnosis and its implications.

Care of the Woman with an Upper Genital Tract Infection (Pelvic Inflammatory Disease)

Pelvic inflammatory disease (PID) occurs most often in women of childbearing age, especially sexually active adolescents (CDC, 2016). Other risk factors include multiple sex partners, a partner who has had more than one sex partner, a history of PID, early onset of sexual activity, recent insertion of an intrauterine device (IUD), and regular douching. Perhaps the greatest problem of PID is postinfection tubal damage, which is closely associated with infertility, ectopic pregnancy, or chronic pelvic infections (CDC, 2017a).

PID is defined as a clinical syndrome resulting from an ascending infection from the vagina and endocervix to the endometrium and fallopian tubes (CDC, 2016). The organisms most frequently identified with PID include *C. trachomatis* and *N. gonorrhoeae*. Other pathogens associated with PID include *G. vaginalis, Haemophilus influenza,* and *Streptococcus agalactiae* (Vanthuyne & Pittrof, 2016). Symptoms of PID include bilateral sharp, cramping pain in the lower quadrants, fever greater than 100.4°F, mucopurulent cervical or vaginal discharge, cervical motion tenderness during intercourse, malaise, and nausea and vomiting. However, it is also possible to be asymptomatic and have normal laboratory values.

Diagnosis is based on examination, cultures for gonorrhea and chlamydia, a complete blood count (CBC) with differential, and a Rapid Plasma Reagin (RPR) or Venereal Disease Research Laboratory (VDRL) test to check for syphilis. The woman may have an elevated C-reactive protein and an elevated sedimentation rate. Physical examination usually reveals direct abdominal tenderness with palpation and, on bimanual examination, adnexal tenderness and cervical and uterine tenderness with movement (chandelier sign). A palpable mass is evaluated with ultrasonography. In confounding cases, laparoscopy can be used to confirm the diagnosis and to enable the examiner to obtain cultures from the fimbriated ends of the fallopian tubes.

Oral outpatient therapy is comparable to inpatient intravenous (IV) therapy in women with PID of mild to moderate severity (CDC, 2015). The decision to hospitalize a woman is based on clinical judgment. The woman should be hospitalized if the diagnosis is uncertain, ectopic pregnancy or appendicitis is suspected, the woman is severely ill (nausea and vomiting, high fever, dehydration), there has been little response to oral therapy after 72 hours, there are complications from pelvic abscesses or pelviperitonitis, the patient is a young adolescent, or the woman is unable to return for follow-up care.

Inpatient treatment includes intravenous (IV) fluids, pain medication, and administration of IV antibiotics, often cefoxitin, cefotetan plus doxycycline, or clindamycin plus gentamicin. Other antibiotic combinations may also be used. In addition, supportive measures are often indicated for severe symptoms. These may include increased oral fluids (up to 2 liters per day), continued bedrest or pelvic rest, acetaminophen for fever, and pain relievers for abdominal pain. Outpatient therapy usually includes ceftriaxone IM plus doxycycline with or without metronidazole. Sexual partners should also be treated if they had sexual contact within the prior 60 days of the patient becoming ill. If the woman has an intrauterine contraceptive (IUC) in place, it does not need to be removed. She should receive recommended treatment and should be followed closely. Healthcare providers need only consider removing the IUC if no improvement occurs after 48 to 72 hours of therapy (CDC, 2015).

NURSING MANAGEMENT

For the Woman with Pelvic Inflammatory Disease

Nursing Assessment and Diagnosis

Be alert to factors in a woman's history that put her at risk for PID. Ask whether the woman has had an IUC inserted within the past 3 weeks because the risk of PID associated with IUC is primarily confined to that period (CDC, 2015). Question the woman about possible symptoms, such as aching pain in the lower abdomen, foul-smelling discharge, malaise, and dyspareunia. The woman who is acutely ill has obvious symptoms, but a low-grade infection is more difficult to detect.

Nursing diagnoses that may apply to a woman with PID include:

- ***Pain, Acute,*** related to peritoneal irritation
- ***Knowledge, Deficient,*** related to a lack of information about the possible effects of PID on fertility

(NANDA-I © 2017)

Nursing Plan and Implementation

You can play a vital role in helping to prevent or detect PID. Spend time with the woman discussing risk factors related to this infection. The woman who uses an IUD for contraception and has multiple sexual partners needs to understand clearly the risk she faces. Discuss signs and symptoms of PID with women at high risk and stress the importance of early detection.

The woman who develops PID needs to understand the importance of completing her antibiotic treatment and of returning for follow-up evaluation. She should also understand that one outcome of the infection may be decreased fertility or infertility.

Evaluation

Expected outcomes of nursing care include:

- The woman describes her condition, her therapy, and the possible long-term implications of PID on her fertility.
- The woman completes her course of therapy and the PID is cured.

Care of the Woman with a Urinary Tract Infection

Urinary tract infection (UTI) is defined as significant bacteriuria in the presence of symptoms. Approximately 50% of women will experience a UTI in their lifetimes (ACOG, 2017). Bacteria usually enter the sterile environment of the urinary tract by way of the urethra. The organisms are capable of migrating against the downward flow of urine. The shortness of the female urethra facilitates the passage of bacteria into the bladder. Other conditions that are associated with bacterial entry are relative incompetence of the urinary sphincter, sexual activity, diabetes mellitus, pregnancy, and urinary catheterization. Wiping from back to front after urination may transfer bacteria from the anorectal area to the urethra.

Voluntarily suppressing the desire to urinate is also a predisposing factor. Retention overdistends the bladder and can lead to an infection. There also seems to be a relationship between recurring UTI and new onset of sexual activity. General poor health or lowered resistance to infection can increase a woman's susceptibility to UTI. The rate of urinary tract infections increases as women age. For postmenopausal women, estrogen deficiency is a risk factor for urinary tract infection. Factors that may inhibit bacterial growth include a low pH (5.5 or less) resulting in more acidic urine and high urea concentration. Urinary tract infections can be classified by location or as complicated or uncomplicated.

Asymptomatic Bacteriuria

Asymptomatic bacteriuria (ASB) refers to bacteria in the urine actively multiplying without accompanying clinical symptoms. This becomes especially significant if the woman is pregnant because it is found in up to 2 to 7% of pregnancies, and as many as 20 to 30% of pregnant women with untreated ASB will develop pyelonephritis (Stewart & Ehsanipoor, 2015). ASB is almost always caused by one organism, *Escherichia coli*. Less commonly causative organisms include *Klebsiella* and *Proteus* and *Pseudomonas* and *Staphylococcus* species. Women with sickle cell trait are twice as likely to develop ASB and should have a urine culture every trimester when pregnant.

A woman who has had a UTI is susceptible to recurrent infection. Although the role of ASB in pregnancy complications remains controversial, the majority of evidence supports the view that bacteriuria does not, as an isolated factor, lead to low birth weight or prematurity. However, an untreated ASB can progress to pyelonephritis in approximately 12.5 to 30% of pregnant women (Blackburn, 2018).

Lower Urinary Tract Infection (Cystitis and Urethritis)

Because UTIs ascend, it is important to recognize and diagnose a lower UTI early to avoid the sequelae associated with upper UTI. **Cystitis**, or *inflammation of the bladder*, usually occurs secondary to an ascending infection. Several factors place a woman at increased risk for cystitis, including sexual intercourse, the use of a diaphragm and a spermicide, pregnancy, and a history of a recent UTI.

E. coli is present in the vast majority of women with UTIs. *Staphylococcus saprophyticus*, *Klebsiella pneumonia*, *Proteus mirabilis*, *Enterobacter* species, and *Pseudomonas* are also causative pathogens (Davis & Rantell, 2017).

When cystitis develops, the classic initial symptoms are often acute and include dysuria, specifically at the end of urination, as well as urgency and frequency. Suprapubic or low back pain may also occur. Cystitis is usually accompanied by a low-grade fever (38.3°C [101°F] or lower), and hematuria is occasionally seen. Urine specimens often contain an abnormal number of leukocytes and bacteria and may contain protein.

The diagnosis can be made with a urine culture. Bacteriuria dipstick screening tests are quick office screening tests; however, they have high false-positive and false-negative rates. Before treatment, the diagnosis should be confirmed by clinical evaluation and urine culture and sensitivity results. The treatment depends on the causative pathogen. A 3-day treatment is indicated using either trimethoprim-sulfamethoxazole (TMP-SMZ) 200 mg twice daily or nitrofurantoin 100 mg twice daily. Other antibiotics that may be used include amoxicillin, cephalexin, and ampicillin (Duff & Birsner, 2017). A longer course of therapy may be indicated if the woman does not respond to treatment or if she is immunocompromised or has impaired renal function (Davis & Rantell, 2017).

A number of structural and functional changes occur during pregnancy that predispose pregnant women to urinary tract infections. Ureters elongate and are laterally displaced by the gravid uterus. In addition, progesterone, which relaxes smooth muscles, can facilitate hypertrophy of the distal ureters with resulting ureteral stenosis and dilation, especially in the second half of pregnancy. Though the bladder has an increased capacity in pregnancy, it also has a decreased tone because progesterone relaxes the smooth muscle. Estrogen causes the bladder mucosa to become hyperemic and more susceptible to trauma and infection. Additionally, the intravesical pressure may be decreased due to the displacement of the bladder and ureters. With micturation, the pressure may increase with urine regurgitating into the ureters. Therefore, changes in the bladder and ureters and hormonal influences both contribute to the propensity of pregnant women to develop urinary tract infections (Blackburn, 2018). This is significant because a positive association exists between women with urinary tract infections and preterm birth. Treatment for an initial infection in pregnant women includes a 3-day course of nitrofurantoin 100 mg twice a day or cephalexin (Keflex) 250–500 mg orally twice a day. Longer courses of therapy are generally indicated for recurrent infection (Duff & Birsner, 2017). In complicated UTIs, treatment is organism culture specific. For any of these medications, it is important to emphasize completion of the course of treatment.

Upper Urinary Tract Infection (Pyelonephritis)

Pyelonephritis (inflammatory disease of the kidneys) is less common, affecting 1 to 2% of pregnancies, but is more serious than cystitis and is often preceded by a lower UTI (Duff & Birsner, 2017). Women with pyelonephritis during pregnancy are at significantly increased risk of preterm labor, preterm birth, development of acute respiratory distress syndrome, and septic shock (Duff & Birsner, 2017). Acute pyelonephritis has a sudden onset with chills, high temperature of 39.6° to 40.6°C (103° to 105°F), and costovertebral angle tenderness or flank pain, which can be unilateral or bilateral. Nausea and vomiting and general malaise may ensue. With accompanying cystitis, the woman may experience frequency, urgency, and burning with urination.

Edema of the renal parenchyma or ureteritis with blockage and swelling of the ureter may lead to temporary suppression of urinary output. This is accompanied by severe, colicky (spastic, intense) pain, vomiting, dehydration, and ileus of the large bowel. The woman with acute pyelonephritis will generally have significant bacteria in her urine culture, pyuria, and the presence of white blood cell casts.

Pregnant women are frequently hospitalized and started on intravenous (IV) antibiotics. Therapy also includes IV hydration, urinary analgesics such as Pyridium, pain management, and acetaminophen to manage fever. In the case of obstructive pyelonephritis, a blood culture is necessary. The woman is kept on bedrest. If signs of urinary obstruction occur or continue, the ureter may be catheterized to establish adequate drainage. See *Case Study: Benita Cartier*.

Initially an antibiotic such as ceftriaxone is administered IV. A second antibiotic such as gentamicin or aztreonam may be indicated if the woman is critical or if she is at high risk for a resistant organism (Duff & Birsner, 2017). IV therapy should continue until the woman is afebrile for 48 hours. Oral antibiotics are given to complete the 10 to 14 days of therapy (Hurt, 2015). With appropriate drug therapy, the woman's temperature should return to normal, the pain subsides, and the urine shows no bacteria within 2 to 3 days. Follow-up urinary cultures are needed to determine that the infection has been eliminated completely.

CASE STUDY: Benita Cartier

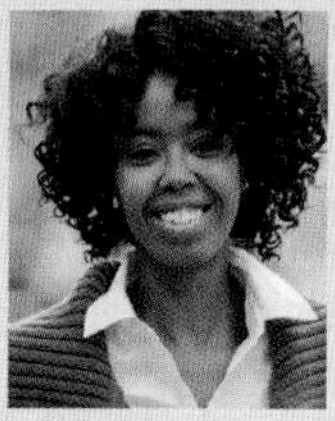

SOURCE: blvdone/Shutterstock.

Benita has a long history of UTIs that are thought to be increased because she has sickle cell trait. As a result, if the urine dip shows any signs of proteinuria or leukocytes, the physician obtains a urinalysis.

Question to Ponder

What urinary-related complications may occur in a woman with a urinary tract infection?

●○● NURSING MANAGEMENT

For the Woman with a Urinary Tract Infection

Nursing Assessment and Diagnosis

During the woman's visit, obtain a medical history, including a sexual history, to determine whether she is at risk for a UTI. Additionally, note any complaints from the woman of painful urination or other urinary difficulties and systemic complaints such as fever, chills, nausea and vomiting, or flank or back pain. A clean-catch urine sample is obtained to evaluate for the presence of bacteriuria.

Nursing diagnoses that may apply to the woman with a UTI include:

- ***Pain, Acute***, related to dysuria, systemic discomforts, flank or back pain secondary to lower or upper urinary tract infection
- ***Knowledge, Deficient***, related to lack of understanding about ways of preventing UTIs related to an expressed desire to avoid recurrence
- ***Fear*** related to the possible long-term effects of the disease

(NANDA-I © 2017)

Nursing Plan and Implementation

Most bacteria enter through the urethra after having spread from the anal area. Therefore, make sure that the woman is aware of good hygiene practices and provide information on other ways to avoid a UTI (Figure 5–5).

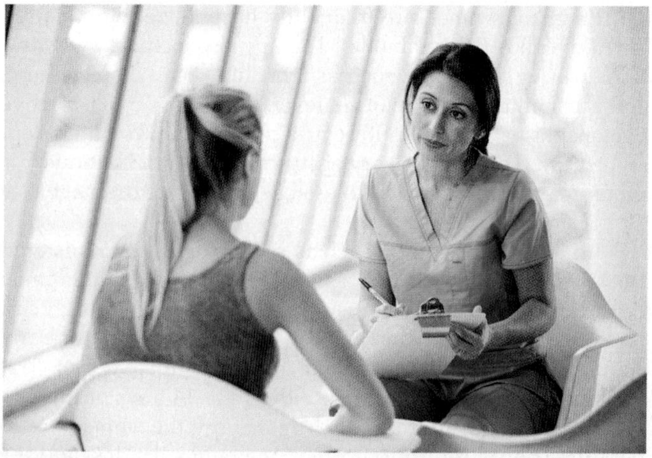

Figure 5–5 **A nurse counsels a woman about measures for preventing urinary tract infection.**

SOURCE: Monkey Business/Fotolia.

Additionally, provide the woman with information to help her recognize the signs and symptoms of a UTI to facilitate early identification and treatment of future infections. Reinforce instructions and answer any additional questions the woman may have regarding the prescribed antibiotic and the reasons for these treatments. UTIs usually respond quickly to treatment, but follow-up clinical evaluation and urine cultures are important. Recurrent urinary tract infection can result from reinfection or relapse. With frequent reinfections, defined as three or more infections in 1 year or two infections within 6 months, long-term prophylaxis may be needed and can decrease the risk of recurrence significantly (Davis & Rantell, 2017).

Health Promotion

Provide women with the following information about measures they can take to avoid cystitis.

- Avoid bladder irritants, such as alcohol, caffeine products, and carbonated beverages.
- Make regular urination a habit; avoid long waits.
- Practice good genital hygiene, including wiping from front to back after urination and bowel movements.
- Be aware that initial, vigorous, or frequent sexual activity may contribute to urinary tract infection.
- Complete medication regimens even if symptoms decrease.
- Do not use medication left over from previous infections.

Clinical Tip

Research indicates that consuming cranberry juice (8-oz, two to three times daily) or cranberry capsules may be useful in preventing UTIs among adults at risk for UTI (Shin, 2014).

Evaluation

Expected outcomes of nursing care include:

- The woman implements self-care measures to help prevent recurrent UTIs as part of her personal routine.
- The woman completes her prescribed course of antibiotic therapy.
- The woman can identify signs of recurrent UTIs or signs and symptoms of worsening urinary symptoms that would require follow-up care.
- The woman's infection is cured.

Focus Your Study

- Vulvovaginal candidiasis (moniliasis), a vaginal infection most often caused by *Candida albicans*, is most common in women who use oral contraceptives, are taking antibiotics, are currently pregnant, are immunosuppressed, or have diabetes mellitus. It is generally treated with intravaginal miconazole or clotrimazole suppositories or fluconazole orally.
- Bacterial vaginosis (BV), a common vaginal infection, is diagnosed by its characteristic fishy odor and by the presence of "clue" cells on a vaginal smear. It is treated with metronidazole.
- Chlamydial infection is difficult to detect in a woman but can result in pelvic inflammatory disease (PID) and infertility. It is treated with antibiotic therapy. It often coexists with gonorrhea.
- Gonorrhea, a common sexually transmitted infection, can be asymptomatic in women initially but can cause PID if not diagnosed early. The treatment of choice is ceftriaxone intramuscularly combined with azithromycin.
- Herpes genitalis, caused by the herpes simplex virus, is a recurrent infection with no known cure. Acyclovir (Zovirax) may reduce the symptoms.
- Syphilis, caused by *Treponema pallidum*, is a sexually transmitted infection that is treatable if diagnosed. The characteristic lesion is the chancre. Syphilis can also be transmitted in utero to the fetus of an infected woman. The treatment of choice is benzathine penicillin G.
- Condylomata acuminata (genital warts) are transmitted by the human papilloma virus (HPV). Treatment is indicated because research has identified approximately 15 HPV genotypes linked with cervical cancer. The treatment chosen depends on the size and location of the warts and the woman's reproductive status. Two vaccines are now available to prevent several types of HPV.
- Pelvic inflammatory disease can be life-threatening and can lead to infertility. The organisms that cause PID most frequently include *C. trachomatis* and *N. gonorrhoeae*. *Mycoplasma genitalium* and bacterial vaginosis (BV) are increasingly being noted as pathogens causing PID.
- Women with an abnormal finding on a pelvic examination will need careful explanation of the finding and techniques of diagnosis and emotional support during the diagnostic period.
- The classic symptoms of a lower urinary tract infection (UTI) are dysuria, urgency, frequency, and sometimes hematuria. Nitrofurantoin, amoxicillin, ampicillin, and cephalexin are used for the treatment of asymptomatic bacteriuria.
- An upper UTI is a serious infection that can permanently damage the kidneys if untreated. Generally the woman is acutely ill and may require supportive therapy as well as antibiotics.

In order to make safe and effective judgments using NANDA-I © 2017 nursing diagnoses, it is essential that nurses refer to the definitions and defining characteristics of the diagnoses used in this text, which can be found in Appendix C.

References

American College of Obstetricians and Gynecologists (ACOG). (2017). *Preventing urinary tract infections: Frequently asked questions.* Retrieved from https://www.acog.org/-/media/Departments/Toolkits-for-Health-Care-Providers/UTI-Toolkit/Preventing-UTIs-PDF_1.pdf?dmc=1&ts=20171017T2229304080

Blackburn, S. (2018). *Maternal, fetal, & neonatal physiology: A clinical perspective* (5th ed.). New York, NY: Saunders Elsevier.

Centers for Disease Control and Prevention (CDC). (2015). Sexually transmitted diseases treatment guidelines, 2015. *Morbidity and Mortality Weekly Report: Recommendations and Reports, 64*(3), 1–136.

Centers for Disease Control and Prevention (CDC). (2016). *Sexually transmitted disease surveillance 2015.* Retrieved from https://www.cdc.gov/std/stats15/std-surveillance-2015-print.pdf

Centers for Disease Control and Prevention (CDC). (2017a). *Pelvic inflammatory disease (PID)—CDC fact sheet.* Retrieved from https://www.cdc.gov/std/pid/stdfact-pid.htm

Centers for Disease Control and Prevention (CDC). (2017b). *Pubic crab lice treatment.* Retrieved from https://www.cdc.gov/parasites/lice/pubic/treatment.html

Davis, C., & Rantell, A. (2017). Lower urinary tract Infections in women. *British Journal of Nursing, Urology Supplement, 26*(9), S12–18.

Duff, P., & Birsner, M. (2017). Maternal and perinatal infection in pregnancy: Bacterial. In S. G. Gabbe, J. R. Niebyl, J. L. Simpson, M. B. Landon, H. L. Galan, E. R. M. Jauniaux, . . . W. A. Grobman (Eds.), *Obstetrics: Normal and problem pregnancies* (7th ed., pp 1130–1146). Philadelphia, PA: Elsevier.

Hurt, K. J. (Ed.). (2015). *Pocket obstetrics and gynecology.* Philadelphia, PA: Wolters Kluwer Health.

Mogha, K. V., & Prajapati, J. B. (2016). Probiotics for treating bacterial vaginosis. *Reviews in Medical Microbiology, 27*(3), 87–94. DOI:10.1097/MRM.0000000000000080

Nasioudis, D., Linhares, I., Ledger, W., & Witkin, S. (2017). Bacterial vaginosis: A critical analysis of current knowledge. *BJOG: An International Journal of Obstetrics and Gynecology, 124*(1), 61–69. DOI:10.1111/1471-0528.14209

Nursing 2016 Drug Handbook (36th ed.). (2016). Philadelphia, PA: Wolters Kluwer.

Shin, C. (2014). The effects of cranberries on preventing urinary tract infections. *Clinical Nursing Research, 23*(1), 54–79.

Stewart, K. I., & Ehsanipoor, R. M. (2015). Genitourinary assessment and renal disease in pregnancy. In C. T. Johnson, J. L. Hallock, J. L. Bienstock, H. E. Fox, & E. E. Wallach (Eds.), *The Johns Hopkins manual of gynecology and obstetrics* (5th ed., pp. 222–227). Philadelphia, PA: Wolters Kluwer.

Sun, M., Huang, Y., Xu, Y., & Cao, Y. (2017). Efficacy of vitamin B complex as an adjuvant therapy for the treatment of complicated vulvovaginal candidiasis: An in vivo and in vitro study. *Biomedicine and Pharmacotherapy, 88*, 770–777. DOI:10.1016/j.biopha.2017.01.001

Vanthuyne, A., & Pittrof, R. (2016). Diagnosis and treatment of pelvic inflammatory disease. *Prescriber, 27*(10), 47–50. DOI:10.1002/psb.1507

Wilson, B. A., Shannon, M. T., & Shields, K. M. (2017). *Nurse's drug guide 2017.* Hoboken, NJ: Pearson.

World Health Organization (WHO). (2017). *Global hepatitis report, 2017.* Retrieved from http://www.who.int/hepatitis/publications/global-hepatitis-report2017/en/

Xie, H. Y., Feng, D., Wei, D. M., Mei, L., Chen, H., Wang, X., & Fang, F. (2017). Probiotics for vulvovaginal candidiasis in non-pregnant women. *Cochrane Database of Systematic Reviews,* Issue 11, Article No. CD010496. DOI:10.1002/14651858.CD010496.pub2

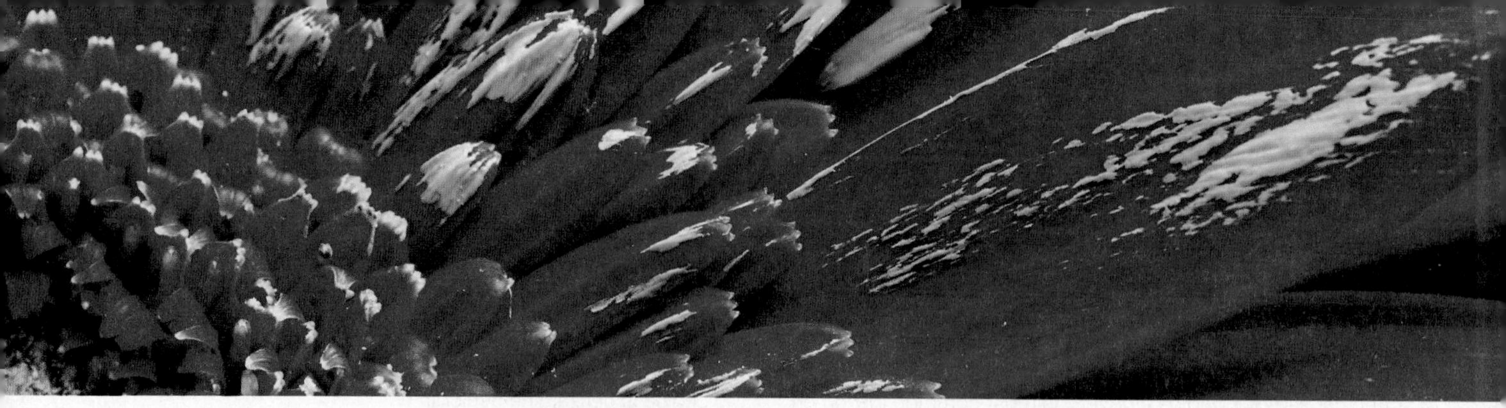

Chapter 6

Women's Health Problems

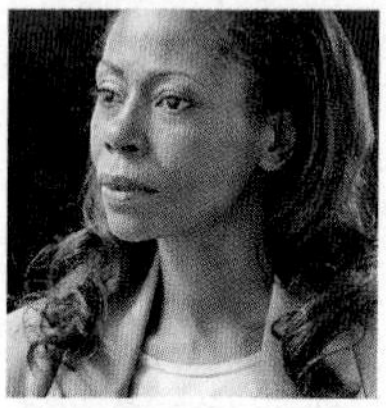

SOURCE: Corbis/ SuperStock.

A friend was turning 42 years old a few months ago and knew that it was time for her annual gynecology exam. She had been putting off having her first mammogram because she had heard stories about how much it hurt. Finally, knowing that her nurse practitioner would ask her if she had gotten a mammogram, she scheduled the test the week before her annual gynecology exam. The mammogram detected a suspicious mass and she had a biopsy that confirmed intraductal carcinoma. She never had a palpable lump; she was not considered high risk for breast cancer; and she was an active, health-conscious woman. It never occurred to her that she could get breast cancer.

Learning Outcomes

6.1 Contrast the common benign and malignant breast disorders.

6.2 Describe the emotional reactions a woman may experience in regard to a diagnosis of breast cancer.

6.3 Identify the implications of an abnormal finding during a pelvic examination.

6.4 Discuss the importance of an annual Pap smear and appropriate follow-up for an abnormal finding.

6.5 Discuss abnormal uterine bleeding and abdominal masses.

6.6 Discuss the signs and symptoms, medical therapy, and implications for fertility of endometriosis.

6.7 Discuss the signs and symptoms, diagnosis criteria, treatment options, and health implications of polycystic ovarian syndrome.

6.8 Compare the signs and symptoms and treatment options of the three forms of pelvic relaxation—cystocele, rectocele, and uterine relaxation.

6.9 Contrast laparoscope-assisted vaginal hysterectomy and abdominal hysterectomy with regard to indications for use and the advantages and disadvantages of each procedure.

6.10 Delineate the psychosocial responses a woman may experience when facing any of the common gynecologic procedures.

6.11 Compare the essential components of fertility with the possible causes of infertility.

6.12 Summarize the indications for the tests and associated treatments that are performed in an infertility workup.

6.13 Relate the physiologic and psychologic effects of infertility on a couple to the nursing management indicated for them.

Healthy People 2020

(C-3) Reduce the female breast cancer death rate

(G-1) Increase the proportion of women with a family history of breast and/or ovarian cancer who receive genetic counseling

(C-15) Increase the proportion of women who receive a cervical cancer screening based on the most recent guidelines

(C-18.2) Increase the proportion of women who were counseled by their providers about Pap tests

(C-4) Reduce the death rate from cancer of the uterine cervix

(MICH-17.1) Reduce the proportion of women ages 18 to 44 years who have impaired fecundity (i.e., a physical barrier preventing pregnancy or carrying a pregnancy to term)

(MICH-17.2) Reduce the proportion of men ages 18 to 44 years who have impaired fecundity

From early childhood through adolescence, the active reproductive years, into menopause and the years beyond, a woman will likely face a variety of gynecologic or urinary problems. Some may be minor, whereas others have the potential to be quite serious, provoking a wide array of physical and psychologic responses. This chapter provides information about selected gynecologic problems that a woman may encounter during her lifetime with an emphasis on problems commonly addressed in community-based settings. Additionally, this chapter explores a particularly troubling reproductive problem, the inability to conceive.

For a detailed discussion of gynecologic cancers, for more detailed information on any of the subjects covered in this chapter, or for more in-depth discussion of gynecologic procedures, please consult a specialized text.

Care of the Woman with a Disorder of the Breast

Throughout her lifetime a woman may experience a variety of breast disorders. Some, like mastitis, which is discussed in Chapter 35, are acute disorders, whereas others, such as fibrocystic breast changes, also known as *benign breast disease (BBD)*, are chronic. This section begins with breast screening techniques and then deals with some of the common breast disorders a woman may experience.

Screening Techniques for the Breasts

Despite their limitations, breast examination and mammography remain the most effective screening techniques available for disorders of the breast.

BREAST EXAMINATION

Like the uterus, the breast undergoes regular cyclic changes in response to hormonal stimulation. Each month, in rhythm with the cycle of ovulation, the breasts become engorged with fluid in anticipation of pregnancy, and the woman may experience sensations of tenderness, lumpiness, or pain. If conception does not occur, the accumulated fluid drains away via the lymphatic network. *Mastodynia* or *mastalgia* (premenstrual swelling and tenderness of the breasts) is common and usually lasts for 3 to 4 days before the onset of menses. Some women may also experience mastalgia at the time of ovulation, about 14 days into her cycle; for other women, the symptoms may persist throughout the month.

After menopause, connective breast tissue atrophies and is replaced by adipose tissue. The breasts lose elasticity and may droop and become pendulous. The recurring breast engorgement associated with ovulation ceases. If hormone therapy (HT) is used to counteract other symptoms of menopause, breast engorgement may resume.

The American College of Obstetricians and Gynecologists (ACOG, 2017a) stresses **breast self-awareness (BSA)**, the need for a woman to be aware of how her breasts normally look and feel. BSA is now being advocated as a good method for detecting breast masses early. Women at high risk for breast cancer are specifically encouraged to be attentive to the importance of early detection through BSA. The change to BSA versus **breast self-examination (BSE)** is secondary to the U.S. Preventive Services Task Force's (2009) recommendation against teaching women breast self-examination based on studies they reviewed that led the task force to believe that BSE did not reduce breast cancer mortality but resulted in additional imaging procedures and biopsies. ACOG (2017a) identifies BSE as one way for a woman to develop self-awareness. The American Cancer Society (ACS, 2017a) does not recommend that BSE be presented to women but does recommend that women be familiar with how their breasts normally appear and feel. The effectiveness of BSE is determined by the woman's ability to perform the procedure correctly, by her knowledge of her own breast tissue, and by the density of her breast tissue. (See *Teaching Highlights: Breast Self-Examination*.)

Clinical breast examination (CBE) by a trained healthcare provider, such as a physician, nurse practitioner, or nurse-midwife, is an essential element of a routine gynecologic examination. ACOG (2017a) recommends CBE every 1 to 3 years for women ages 25 to 39 and annually for women 40 years and older. The ACS (2017a) does not recommend clinical breast examination. In clinical practice, however, many caregivers advocate annual CBE for all women over age 20.

MAMMOGRAPHY

A **mammogram** is a soft-tissue x-ray image of the breast taken without the injection of a contrast medium. It can detect lesions in the breast before they can be felt and has gained wide acceptance as an effective screening tool for breast cancer. Currently, the ACS (2017a) guidelines recommend that women ages 40 to 45 talk with their healthcare provider about when to start screening. By age 45 women should begin annual mammograms and continue to have them until 55 years of age; at that point, a woman should decide whether to continue with annual mammograms or transition to biennial mammograms provided she is in good health (ACOG, 2017a). ACOG's (2017a) recommendations also include starting at 40 years of age and then annually or biennially until the age of 75 years. In addition, the ACS (2017a) now recommends both mammogram and magnetic resonance imaging (MRI) beginning at age 30 in women who are at a high risk for breast cancer due to gene mutations and/or a strong family history of breast cancer and in women who had radiation to the chest between the ages of 10 and 30 years because they often develop breast cancer at a younger age.

The sensitivity of mammography in accurately diagnosing breast cancer increases with age and the presence of a palpable mass. It decreases in accuracy in women with increased breast density. If a lump is found, the mammogram is then followed by an ultrasound for further information on the consistency of the palpable lump. Fine-needle aspiration will follow if the lump in question appears suspicious on imaging. Up to 5% of symptomatic breast cancers are not found with mammogram (Galea, 2016).

Breast sensitivity seems to vary from woman to woman and may be a factor in a woman's reluctance to have a mammogram. To help prevent any discomfort, the nurse can suggest that this x-ray study be scheduled when the woman's breasts are least sensitive, which is about 2 weeks after the onset of menses. In most cases, a mammogram causes feelings of compression but not pain (Figure 6–2). All women should be instructed to refrain from applying lotions, powders, deodorant, or other cosmetic substances to the torso on the day of the exam because the substances may appear as questionable areas on the mammogram and can interfere with accurate interpretation. The risk of radiation exposure with

TEACHING HIGHLIGHTS | Breast Self-Examination

Describe and demonstrate the correct procedure for BSE.

Inspection

The woman should inspect her breasts by standing or sitting in front of a mirror. She should inspect them in three positions: Both arms relaxed at her sides, both arms raised straight over her head, and both hands placed on her hips while she leans forward. Instruct her to note the following:

- ***Size and symmetry of the breasts, and their shape, contours, and direction.*** Have her check for redness or inflammation, rashes, ulceration, or nipple discharge. A blue hue with a marked venous pattern that is focal or unilateral may indicate an area of increased blood supply due to tumor. Symmetric venous patterns are normal.
- ***Thickening or edema.*** Skin edema is seen as thickened skin with enlarged pores ("orange peel"). It may indicate blocked lymph drainage due to a tumor.
- ***Surface of the skin.*** Skin dimpling, puckering, or retraction when the hands are pressed together in front of the chest or against the hips suggests malignancy.
- ***The nipples.*** Note any deviation, flattening, broadening, or recent inversion.

Palpation

The woman should be instructed to palpate her breasts as follows:

- Lie down. Put one hand behind your head. With the other hand, fingers flattened, gently feel your breast. Press lightly (Figure 6–1A).
- Still lying down, check each breast as shown in Figure 6–1B. Follow the arrows shown in the image, moving in an up-and-down pattern, feeling gently for a lump or thickening. Remember to feel all parts of each breast, including the "tail" of tissue near the armpit. Repeat the process on the second breast.
- Now repeat the same process on each breast while sitting up, with your hand still behind your head.
- Squeeze the nipple between your thumb and forefinger. Look for any discharge—clear, bloody, or milky (Figure 6–1C).

Determine whether the client has any questions about her findings during this examination. If she has questions, palpate the area and attempt to identify whether it is normal.

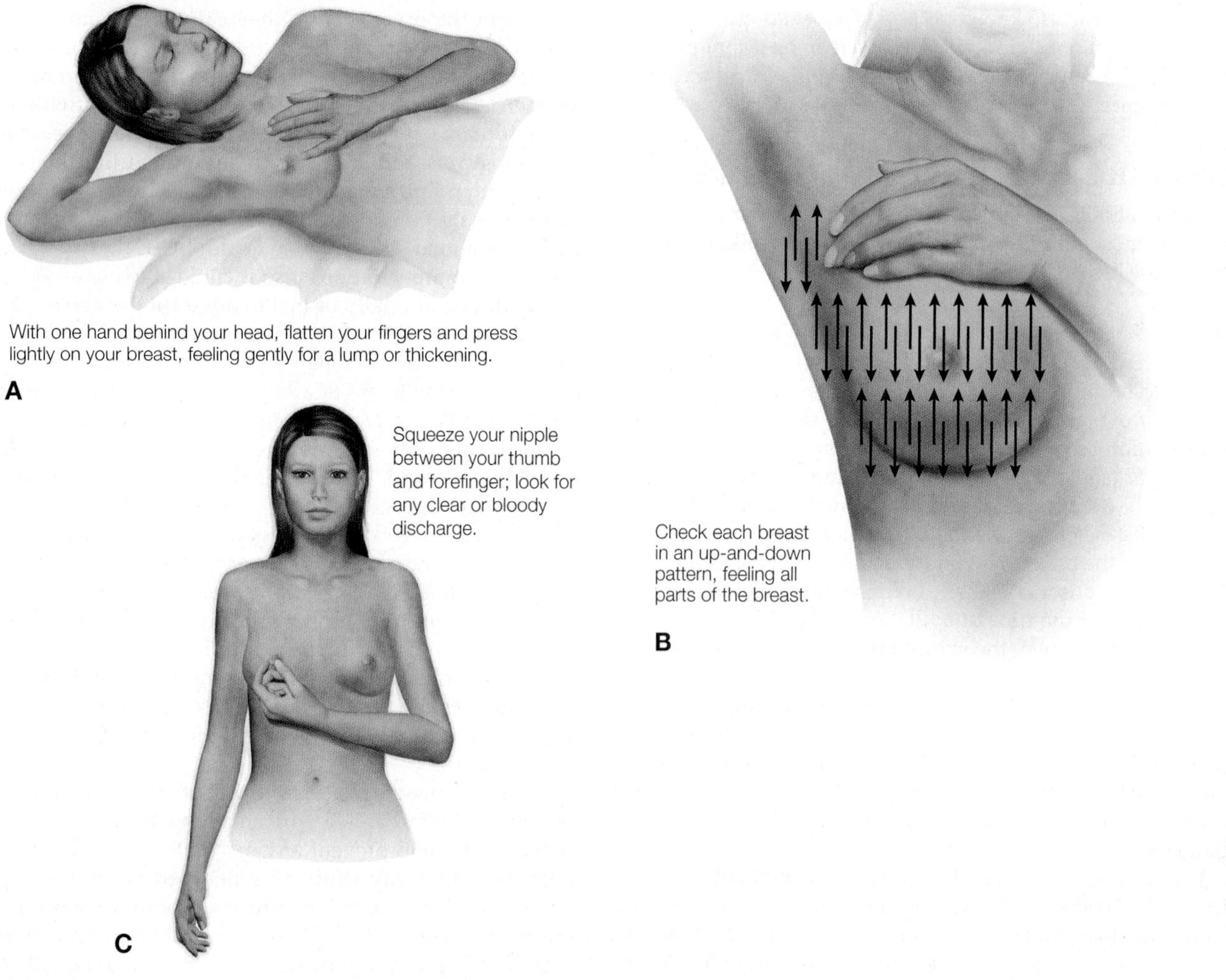

Figure 6–1 Procedure for breast self-examination.

SOURCE: Data from American Cancer Society. (1973). Breast self-examination and the nurse. No. 3408 PB.

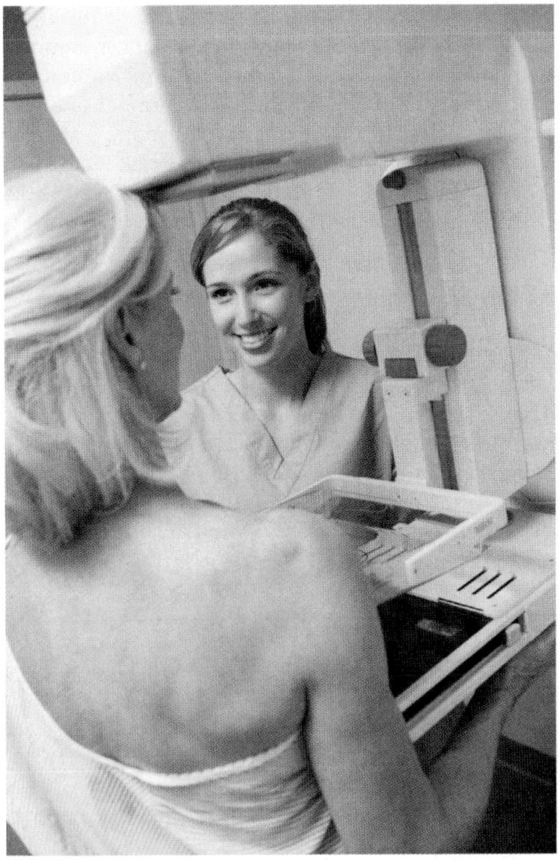

Figure 6–2 Recommended position for mammogram.

SOURCE: Monkey Business/Fotolia.

mammograms is low because strict guidelines are in place to ensure that the equipment is safe and uses the lowest dose of radiation possible.

Benign Breast Conditions

Fibrocystic breast changes, also known as *benign breast disorder (BBD)*, is the most common of the benign breast disorders, accounting for greater than 90% of referrals to breast clinics (Galea, 2016). Fibrocystic changes are the most common type of BBD and are most prevalent in women 20 to 50 years of age. Generally, fibrocystic changes are not a risk factor for breast cancer. In some rare cases, if the change is proliferative and results in hyperplasia or buildup of the cells of the breast ducts, atypia may occur. Fibrocystic changes may produce an asymptomatic mass but more often are accompanied by pain or tenderness and sometimes nipple discharge. Fluctuations in size and rapid appearance or disappearance of breast masses are common. Bilateral, cyclic breast pain is the most common symptom, and the nodularities may be unilateral or bilateral, often in the upper outer quadrants of the breasts.

The woman often reports pain, tenderness, and swelling that is cyclic, worsening in the late luteal phase of the menstrual cycle (just before menses) and improving about 1 to 2 days into the menstrual cycle. Physical examination may reveal only mild signs of irregularity, or the breasts may feel dense, with areas of irregularity and nodularity. Women often refer to this as "lumpiness."

If the woman has a large, fluid-filled cyst, she may experience a localized painful area as the capsule containing the accumulated fluid distends coincident with her cycle. However, if small cysts form, the woman may experience not a solitary tender lump but a diffuse tenderness. Several characteristics help differentiate a cyst from a cancerous lesion. Cysts tend to be mobile and tender and do not cause skin retraction (pulling) in the surrounding tissue, whereas cancerous lesions tend to be fixed and painless and may cause skin retraction.

Mammography, sonography, MRI, palpation, and fine-needle aspiration can be used to confirm fibrocystic breast changes. Often, fine-needle aspiration provides treatment as well as relief from the tenderness or pain. Palpable cysts are often treated conservatively with medical management; however, all discrete masses should have a tissue sample sent for biopsy.

In some cases, a mild analgesic is necessary. Oral contraceptives help alleviate symptoms for the majority of women, but, unfortunately, symptoms tend to recur when the oral contraceptives are discontinued. In severe cases, the hormone inhibitor danazol is often helpful because it suppresses follicle-stimulating hormone (FSH) and luteinizing hormone (LH), resulting in anovulation. However, it can cause several undesirable side effects such as nausea, depression, menstrual irregularities, headaches, and masculinization. Women who do not respond to other treatment approaches may be given a trial of bromocriptine, a prolactin inhibitor.

Methylxanthines (found in caffeine-containing products such as coffee, tea, colas, chocolate, and some medications) and the use of tobacco have been posited to contribute to the development of fibrocystic breast changes and that limiting use of these substances will help decrease fibrocystic changes; however, research has not supported this belief.

Fibroadenoma is a common benign tumor most often seen in women in their teens and early 20s. It is an asymptomatic, mobile, well-defined, painless palpable mass with a rubbery texture. Women with no family history and a simple fibroadenoma are at no greater risk for breast cancer than the general population.

Ultrasound is the best method for imaging women under age 35 with a palpable mass because of the density of their breast tissue. Most women can be observed and followed regularly to detect any changes in the size or appearance of the lump. Some clinicians may prefer surgical excision to prove that it is benign.

The term for nipple discharge not associated with lactation (production of milk for breastfeeding) is **galactorrhea**. Nipple discharge can occur in patients of all ages and races and is generally a nonsignificant finding. Nonclinically significant nipple discharge occurs in women who have fibrocystic changes in the breast, who are using contraceptives, or who are on hormone therapy. Certain medications that are used to treat psychiatric disorders have a side effect of galactorrhea.

The most common types of nipple discharge occur in both breasts, are secreted from several ducts, and vary in color from white to brown. The likelihood of malignancy increases with the presence of a spontaneous discharge arising from a single duct in one breast that is watery or bloody in nature; this warrants further investigation. Mammogram is used initially for evaluation. Ultrasound may be used if the nipple discharge is accompanied by a palpable mass or if positive findings are seen on the mammogram.

Intraductal papillomas are tumors growing in the terminal portion of a duct or, sometimes, throughout the duct system within a section of the breast. Symptoms may include a unilateral mass or a spontaneous, and often bloody, nipple discharge.

The majority of papillomas present as solitary nodules. These small, usually less than 1 cm, ball-like lesions may be detected on mammography but are often nonpalpable. A papilloma is often frightening to the woman because her primary symptom is a discharge from the nipple that may be serosanguineous or brownish-green because of old blood. The location of the papilloma within the duct system and its pattern of growth determine whether nipple discharge will be present. Triple testing (clinical exam plus imaging plus biopsy) is recommended, and if the triple test is negative, the woman is monitored every 6 months by clinical exam. Papillomas are typically benign, but they are generally excised to rule out the possibility of cancer.

Duct ectasia (comedomastitis), an inflammation of the ducts behind the nipple, commonly occurs during or near the onset of menopause and is not associated with malignancy. The condition typically occurs in women who have borne and nursed children. It is characterized by a thick, sticky nipple discharge of various colors and by burning pain, pruritus, and inflammation. Nipple retraction may also be noted, especially in postmenopausal women. Treatment is conservative, with drug therapy aimed at symptomatic relief. The major central ducts of the breast occasionally have to be excised.

Table 6–1 provides a comparison of the most frequently seen benign breast disorders.

Malignant Breast Disease

Breast cancer is the second leading cause of cancer deaths in women. The lifetime risk of women developing breast cancer in the United States is one in eight. Breast cancer accounts for nearly 14% of all cancer deaths in women, surpassed only by lung cancer, which accounts for 25% of cancer deaths in women (ACS, 2017b). In the United States breast cancer is more common in non-Hispanic White women than in women of other races and ethnicities. Breast cancer has a number of modifiable risk factors, such as postmenopausal hormone (estrogen and progesterone) therapy, and nonmodifiable risk factors, such as older age and an inherited mutation of *BRCA1* and *BRCA2* genes (ACS, 2017b). See *Developing Cultural Competence: Breast Cancer Survival Rates*.

Developing Cultural Competence Breast Cancer Survival Rates

African American women have a lower incidence of breast cancer than non-Hispanic White women. Nevertheless, although survival rates for both groups have increased in recent years, in absolute terms they are 11% lower for Black women than for White women (ACS, 2017b).

PREDISPOSING FACTORS

Factors that predispose a woman to breast cancer include (ACS, 2017b):

- Age; incidence increases steadily with age
- Female gender
- History of previous breast cancer, especially early-onset breast cancer
- Having an inherited *BRCA1* or *BRCA2* gene mutation from either parent is the most common cause of hereditary breast

TABLE 6–1 Summary of Benign Breast Disorders

CONDITION	AGE	PAIN	CANCER RISK	NIPPLE DISCHARGE	LOCATION	CONSISTENCY AND MOBILITY	DIAGNOSIS AND TREATMENT
Fibrocystic breast changes	30–50	Yes	Yes, with proliferative disease and atypical hyperplasia	Varies: None at all or may be clear, milky, straw colored, or green	Upper outer quadrant	Multiple lumps occurring bilaterally, influenced by menstrual cycle, nodular	Needle aspiration, Cytology of nipple discharge, observation, biopsy if unresolved mass exists or mammographic changes, sonography
Fibroadenoma	15–25, median age 20	No	No	No, but milky discharge in pregnancy	Nipple or upper outer quadrant along the lateral side	Solid, well defined, sharply delineated, rounded, rubbery, mobile	Mammography, observation, surgical excision
Intraductal papilloma	Menopausal 50–60	Yes, on palpation	Yes, with multiple papillomas	Yes, serous bloody or brownish-green	No specific location	Nonpalpable or small, ball-like, poorly delineated	Pap smear of nipple discharge, mammography ductogram; surgical, excision
Duct ectasia	45–55	Yes, burning and itching around the nipple	No	Yes, in perimenopausal women: Thick, sticky, green, greenish-brown or bloodstained	Mass behind or around the nipple	Poorly circumscribed inflammation, nipple retraction, axillary lymphadenopathy	Pap smear of breast discharge, mammography, drug therapy for symptoms, surgical excision, observation

cancer. Women with *BRCA1* mutations have a lifetime risk of developing breast cancer of 55 to 65%, while women with *BRCA2* mutations have a 45% risk.

- Family history of first-degree relative (mother, sister, or daughter) with breast cancer; risk increases with the number of first-degree relatives with breast cancer
- Long-term, postmenopausal combined estrogen and progestin hormone therapy
- Being overweight or obese after menopause
- Alcohol consumption; risk increases with the amount of alcohol consumed
- No history of pregnancy or first pregnancy after age 30
- Never breastfeeding a child
- Longer reproductive phase (early menarche [before age 12] and/or late menopause [after age 55])
- History of high-dose radiation to the chest between the ages of 10 and 30
- Physical inactivity
- Smoking.

Diagnosis

A malignant neoplasm may originate either in a duct or in the epithelium of the breast lobes. About half of breast cancers originate in the upper outer quadrant and spread or metastasize to the axillary lymph nodes. Common sites of distant metastasis are the lymph nodes, lungs, liver, brain, and bone.

As previously discussed, a cancerous lump may be discovered by the woman herself, by the clinician who palpates or observes an abnormality, or by mammogram. A painless mass or lump is the most important physical symptom of breast cancer. Early detection greatly improves the treatment options available and increases women's long-term survival rates.

Worrisome findings that point to a higher risk of breast cancer include dimpling of the breast tissue, recent or acute nipple inversion, change in breast size or shape, increase of size in breast mass, skin erosion or ulceration, or presence of an axillary lump. Routine mammography screening detects masses 2 to 3 years before clinical appearance. Other diagnostic modalities include fine-needle biopsy, ultrasonography, and MRI. Biopsy is essential for a diagnosis. Once the diagnosis is made and lymph node involvement is evaluated, clinical staging of the disease is determined and a treatment plan that coincides with the stage is initiated.

Clinical Therapy

Once breast cancer is diagnosed, the woman and her physician make treatment decisions together. The decision is based on a consideration of the following factors:

- Stage of cancer
- Optimal treatment for that stage
- Woman's age
- Personal preferences
- Risks and benefits of each treatment protocol.

Most women diagnosed with breast cancer have some form of surgery. The primary goal of the surgery is to remove the cancer from the breast and the lymph nodes, if they are involved. Surgical treatment may consist of *breast-conserving surgery (BCS)* (lumpectomy or partial mastectomy) or *mastectomy* (simple or total), which involves removal of the entire breast. A *modified radical mastectomy* involves the removal of the breast and the axillary lymph nodes but does not include removal of any of the pectoral muscles of the chest wall. Women who undergo mastectomy are generally given the option of having breast reconstruction surgery. This surgery may be done at the time of the mastectomy or delayed until the prescribed chemotherapy and/or radiation is completed.

Lumpectomy, or the removal of the cancerous tissue plus a rim of normal tissue, is a breast-sparing approach that is often used for women with stage I or II breast cancer. It is almost always followed by several weeks of radiation therapy to destroy any remaining cancerous cells. *Sentinel node biopsy* involves the removal of selected lymph nodes, which are tested for cancerous cells. Negative findings reduce the need for full dissection of all the axillary nodes (Harbeck & Gnant, 2017).

Adjunctive therapy for breast cancer includes chemotherapy, radiation, and hormone therapy. Chemotherapy typically involves a combination of drugs known to combat breast cancer. As indicated previously, radiation is often used to destroy remaining cells following surgery, but it may also be used to reduce the size of a cancerous tumor before surgery. This is termed *neoadjuvant therapy*. *Hormone therapy* is based on the knowledge that the hormone estrogen, which is produced by the ovaries, stimulates certain types of breast cancer. Women who have a form of breast cancer that tests positive for estrogen receptors can be given an antiestrogen drug such as tamoxifen or toremifene. Tamoxifen counters the effects of circulating estrogen in the body to reduce the risk that the cancer returns or spreads to another area of the body. It is also used for cancer prevention by women who are at high risk for developing breast cancer. This drug has side effects and women taking it need to be monitored closely. Raloxifine, a selective estrogen receptor modulator (SERM), is used to prevent osteoporosis. However, it was shown to be even more effective than tamoxifen in decreasing the risk of breast cancer in postmenopausal women who were taking it for osteoporosis.

Aromatase inhibitors are drugs that stop the body from making estrogen. These are given to postmenopausal women only and to those whose cancers are estrogen receptor positive (Harbeck & Gnant, 2017). These have been shown to prevent the return of breast cancer and are often given in place of tamoxifen or after the 5-year course of tamoxifen for further prevention. Targeted therapy would include the use of Herceptin, a synthetic antibody protein that targets the growth-promoting protein known as HER2 on cancer cells (ACS, 2017c). Herceptin may be given alone or with chemotherapy. Chemotherapy in early breast cancer consists of taxanes and anthracyclines given singly or together over 4 to 6 months; these may be given pre- and postoperatively (Harbeck & Gnant, 2017). Women with HER2-negative metastatic breast cancer may be treated with endocrine therapy, such as tamoxifen, aromatase inhibitors, fulvestrant, and progestins administered sequentially based on side effects (Harbeck & Gnant, 2017).

Some women prefer a combined approach to treatment that draws on both allopathic and complementary medicine. These women elect to use complementary therapies, such as herbal remedies, therapeutic touch, acupuncture, aromatherapy, and massage, in combination with medical treatments.

When a woman is confronted with a breast cancer diagnosis, she must decide which therapy is worth what personal risk for her. Although prompt treatment is indicated, a second opinion is encouraged. Care of the woman with breast cancer involves a multidisciplinary approach, including a primary care provider, radiotherapist, surgeon, oncologist, and nursing specialists.

Psychologic Adjustment

The emotional feelings a woman experiences can range from fear of the loss of a body part, to fear of the ill effects of treatments, to fear of death and leaving children and family behind. The nurse should encourage the woman to discuss her feelings and concerns, informing her of all procedures, their pros and cons, and alternative options.

The course of adjustment confronting the woman with cancer has been described in four phases: Shock, reaction, recovery, and reorientation. In the *shock* phase, women make statements such as "Everything is unreal" or "I can't understand why this is happening to me." Shock generally extends from the discovery of the lump through the process of diagnosis.

Reaction occurs in conjunction with the initiation of treatment. As treatment begins, the woman is compelled to face what has occurred and begins to take in what has happened. Coping mechanisms become evident during this phase. Reaction coincides with the length of treatment. For many women, radiation treatment or chemotherapy prolongs this period to months. Treatment reinforces the diagnosis of cancer and the immediate consequences of the disease. Denial of breast loss, if a mastectomy is done, and denial of the reality of the illness are common responses by the woman during the periods of diagnosis and treatment. Denial protects the woman, making therapy tolerable.

Recovery begins during convalescence following the completion of medical treatment. Anxiety about her illness diminishes, and the woman looks to the future once more. She turns outward and gradually resumes her former activities. Conversely, depression and social isolation occur if the woman is unable to negotiate the recovery phase successfully.

A woman's family and friends significantly influence her recovery. Women often perceive their partners as their primary source of support. Both members of a couple must adjust to the woman's condition and its implications as well as to the effect of therapy on their sexual intimacy. Difficulties with psychosocial adjustment to breast cancer tend to be similar for women and their partners except in the area of role adjustments, where women have more difficulties. Many hospitals and community agencies sponsor support groups for women with breast cancer. Online support groups are also available and are of particular value to women in rural areas and in areas that lack adequate community support. In addition, the ACS sponsors support groups for cancer survivors and their families. They also have a highly successful program, "Reach to Recovery," for women following surgery.

Reorientation follows recovery and can be challenging. It is accomplished when the woman can acknowledge that breast cancer is part of her life; yet living, for her, has returned to or perhaps exceeded its former fullness and meaning.

"The physician also felt the lump and thickening, and now I'm waiting to have my mammogram. My thoughts and feelings since I first felt the lump have been like a roller coaster. I'm 46 and I'm wondering if this is it. Am I dying? Now? I am afraid as I have not been afraid since one of our children was very ill."

●○● NURSING MANAGEMENT

For the Woman with Breast Cancer

Nursing care of the woman with breast cancer is multidimensional. It involves meeting the educational, psychosexual, and physical needs of the woman and, to a certain extent, those of her family. In meeting these needs, the nurse functions as a caregiver, counselor, educator, liaison, and advocate. You will need to support the woman in her effort to provide self-care. This increases her self-esteem and sense of control. Nursing care changes as the woman progresses from the period of diagnosis to the period of recovery.

Nursing Assessment and Diagnosis

During the period of diagnosis of any breast disease, the woman may be extremely anxious. You can use therapeutic communication to assess the significance the woman places on her breasts; her current emotional status, coping mechanisms used during periods of stress, and knowledge and beliefs about cancer; and other variables that may influence her coping and adjustment.

Assessment is an ongoing process. Sufficient data must be obtained to provide you and other members of the healthcare team with increasing insight into the woman's physical, mental, emotional, and social situation.

Nursing diagnoses that may apply to a woman with a disorder of the breast include :

- ***Knowledge, Readiness for Enhanced,*** related to information about diagnostic procedures for suspected breast cancer related to an expressed wish for information
- ***Anxiety*** related to threat to body image or her life

(NANDA-I © 2017)

Nursing Plan and Implementation

During the prediagnosis period, provide emotional support, clarify misconceptions, encourage the woman to express her anxiety, and urge her to ask questions. Once a diagnosis has been made, ensure that the woman clearly understands her condition, its association to breast malignancy, and treatment options. Locate appropriate resources in the community and encourage the woman to make use of them as she deals with this difficult time. The woman and her partner or support person should discuss the treatment alternatives with her healthcare provider. Nursing advocacy involves supporting the woman's right to make the best treatment decision for her. With your assistance, the woman can explore her fears, clarify her values, and identify the treatment options that would be personally acceptable. Provide psychologic support for the woman with a troublesome diagnosis, supply her with patient education materials, and refer her to professional support groups.

For women who must undergo surgery, nursing care focuses on necessary perioperative interventions. Refer to a medical-surgical nursing textbook for detailed information on these aspects of nursing care.

Health Promotion

Encourage women to take action to reduce modifiable risks for breast cancer. These include:

- Avoiding obesity
- Exercising regularly
- Reducing dietary fat
- Limiting intake of processed meat and red meat
- Limiting alcohol intake (not more than one drink per day).

Women at high risk of breast cancer may choose to begin chemoprevention using tamoxifen or raloxifene. Women at very high risk may consider bilateral prophylactic mastectomy (ACS, 2016).

Evaluation

Expected outcomes of nursing care include:

- The woman is able to discuss her fears, concerns, and questions during the period of diagnosis.
- The diagnosis is made quickly and accurately, and treatment is initiated, if indicated.

Care of the Woman During a Pelvic Examination

In 2017, the U.S. Preventive Services Task Force issued a statement ascertaining that not enough evidence exits to support performing a screening pelvic examination without a specific cause. The impact of this conclusion on routine screening remains to be seen.

Women have a pelvic examination performed for a variety of reasons, ranging from health maintenance to disease diagnosis. Many women perceive the pelvic exam as an uncomfortable and embarrassing procedure. These negative feelings may cause women to delay having yearly gynecologic examinations, and this avoidance may pose a threat to life and health.

A woman's first pelvic examination is especially important because a positive experience can help allay anxiety and make subsequent pelvic exams less threatening. Because the initial pelvic examination is typically done when a young woman is a teenager, nurses should be sensitive to a teen's attitudes and concerns. Teens are often shy about revealing their bodies and may feel very embarrassed by the procedure. Nurses can also help by being alert for atypical responses that might indicate a history of sexual abuse.

To make the pelvic exam less threatening, and hopefully improve the woman's health-seeking behavior, it is important to create a trusting atmosphere and incorporate practices that help the woman maintain a sense of control. Additionally, it is important for the nurse to assist in facilitating a nonjudgmental and safe environment in which the woman can be honest in response to the healthcare providers' inquiries. Some healthcare providers perform what is called an educational pelvic exam. During this type of exam, the woman becomes an active participant and has an opportunity to learn about her body, voice her concerns, and share decisions about her care.

The educational exam includes offering the woman a mirror to watch the procedure, pointing out anatomic parts to her, and positioning and draping her to allow eye-to-eye contact with the practitioner. The woman is encouraged to participate by asking questions and giving feedback. The nurse can assist the woman by encouraging her to relax with specific advice such as "Keep your bottom flat against the table" and "Wiggle your toes if you find yourself beginning to tense your muscles."

Nurse practitioners, certified nurse-midwives, and physicians all perform pelvic examinations. Nurses may assist the practitioner and the woman during the examination. See *Clinical Skill 6–1: Assisting with a Pelvic Examination*.

The pelvic examination consists of three segments: Inspection of the vulva, inspection of the vagina and the cervix via a speculum examination, and palpation of the cervix, uterus, and ovaries via a bimanual examination. Often a Papanicolaou (Pap) smear and sexually transmitted disease testing are obtained during the speculum examination. The Pap smear is discussed in the section on abnormal Pap smear results, later in this chapter. See *Women with Special Needs: Lithotomy Position*.

Women with Special Needs **Lithotomy Position**

Some women are unable to assume the lithotomy position because of deformity or disease. Positioning the woman on her side with knees flexed may allow adequate visualization for pelvic examination.

Vulvar Self-Examination

During the pelvic examination many healthcare providers also provide education about self-examination of the vulva. This procedure, like breast self-awareness (discussed previously), permits early detection of abnormalities, thereby maximizing the possibility of early diagnosis and treatment.

Self-examination of the vulva is simple to perform. The woman is advised to assume a sitting position on a bed or a chair. In good light, she holds a mirror in one hand and uses the other hand to expose the tissues of her perineum while she carefully inspects and palpates the area. Pregnant or obese women may find it easier to inspect this area in a standing position with one foot elevated on a low stool. The woman should report palpable masses, open sores or lesions, and areas of marked tenderness that cannot be attributed to a specific cause such as vigorous intercourse.

Care of the Woman with Vulvitis

The term *vulvitis* refers to an inflammation of the vulva or external female genitalia. Sometimes vulvar irritation is the result of nonpathologic factors such as:

- Frequent douching or use of over-the-counter douches (these are not recommended)
- Feminine deodorant spray
- Detergents, harsh soaps, or bubble bath
- Colored or perfumed toilet paper
- Contraceptive creams, foams, or suppositories
- Condoms, possibly related to a latex or nonoxynol-9 (spermicide) sensitivity
- Dye, such as found in new clothing
- Synthetic clothing, such as nylon pantyhose, underwear, or synthetic slacks that may trap moisture
- Tight clothing, such as jeans
- Some repetitive motion exercise, such as running or biking
- Frequent shaving of the perineum
- Frequent intercourse or intercourse without adequate lubrication
- Deodorant menstrual pads or tampons, or frequent use of menstrual pads or tampons

Clinical Skill 6–1

Assisting with a Pelvic Examination

NURSING ACTION

Preparation

- Ensure that the room is sufficiently warm by checking room temperature and adjusting the thermostat, if necessary. If overhead heat lamps are available, turn them on.
- Explain the procedure to the woman. If she has never had a pelvic examination, show her the equipment to be used as part of the explanation.

Rationale: *Explaining the procedure helps reduce anxiety and increase cooperation.*

- Ask the woman to empty her bladder and to remove clothing below the waist.

Rationale: *An empty bladder promotes comfort during the internal examination.*

- Have padding on the stirrups. If stirrups are not padded, the woman may prefer to leave her shoes on during the procedure.

Rationale: *Stirrups are padded to ease the pressure of the feet against the metal and to decrease the discomfort associated with cold stirrups. If they are not padded, wearing shoes accomplishes the same purpose.*

- Give the woman a disposable drape or sheet to use during the exam. Ask her to sit at the end of the examining table with the drape opened across her lap.
- Position the woman in the lithotomy position with her thighs flexed and abducted. Place her feet in the stirrups. Her buttocks should extend slightly beyond the edge of the examining table.

Rationale: *This position provides the exposure necessary to conduct the examination effectively.*

- Drape the woman with the sheet, leaving a flap so that the perineum can be exposed.

Rationale: *The drape helps preserve the woman's sense of dignity and privacy.*

Equipment and Supplies

- Vaginal specula of various sizes, warmed with water or on a heating pad prior to insertion
- Gloves (*Note:* Sterile gloves may be used in some cases, e.g., pregnant woman with suspected rupture of the membranes.)
- Water-soluble lubricant
- Materials for Pap smear or ThinPrep® Pap test and cultures
- Good light source.

Note: Water-soluble lubricant on the speculum will decrease the patient's discomfort and will not alter cervical cytology results (ACOG, 2016a). It is also used during the bimanual examination.

Procedure: Gloves

1. The examiner dons gloves for the procedure. Explain each part of the procedure as the certified nurse-midwife, nurse practitioner, or physician performs it. Let the woman know that the examiner begins with an inspection of the external genitalia. Speculums vary in size and the examiner will choose the appropriate size specific to the woman. A small amount of water-soluble lubricant is applied to the speculum. The speculum is then inserted to allow visualization of the cervix and vaginal walls and to obtain specimens for testing (e.g., Pap smear). After the speculum is withdrawn the examiner performs a bimanual examination of the internal organs using the fingers of one hand inserted in the woman's vagina while the other hand presses over the woman's uterus and ovaries. The final step of the procedure is generally a rectal examination.
2. Ask the woman to breathe slowly and regularly and to use any method she finds effective in helping her to remain relaxed.

Rationale: *Relaxation helps decrease muscle tension. Bearing down helps open the vaginal orifice and relaxes the perineal muscles.*

3. Let her know when the examiner is ready to insert the speculum and ask her to bear down.
4. After the speculum is withdrawn, lubricate the examiner's fingers prior to the bimanual examination.

Rationale: *Lubrication decreases friction and eases insertion of the examiner's fingers.*

5. After the examiner has completed the examination and moved away from the woman, move to the end of the examination table and face the woman. Cover her with the drape. Apply gentle pressure to her knees and encourage her to move toward the head of the table. Assist her to remove her feet from the stirrups, then offer your hand to her and assist her to sit up.

Rationale: *Assistance is important because the lithotomy position is an awkward one and many women, especially those women who are pregnant, obese, or older, may find it difficult to get out of the stirrups.*

6. Provide her with tissues to wipe the lubricant from her perineum.

Rationale: *Vaginal secretions and lubricant may be discharged from the vagina when the woman sits upright.*

7. Provide the woman with privacy while she dresses. Be sure that she is not dizzy and that she is standing or sitting safely before leaving the room.

Rationale: *Lying supine may cause postural hypotension.*

Clinical Tip

With the examiner's consent (obtained beforehand), offer the woman a hand mirror so that she can watch all or part of the examination. This practice removes the "mystery" from the procedure and enables the woman to become familiar with the appearance of her body.

- Estrogen deprivation due to menopause, surgical menopause, or medication-induced menopause (such as chemotherapy).

Other times, external genital irritation may be the result of inflammation or infection of the vagina or cervix. The irritation results when increased vaginal or cervical secretions flow distally and create inflammation of the vulvar tissues. This condition is called *vulvovaginitis*.

Often it is difficult to differentiate, by symptoms alone, vulvitis from vaginitis. The nurse needs to understand that vulvitis can occur as a distinct entity from vaginitis and that the previously mentioned practices may be significant contributing factors to both.

●○● NURSING MANAGEMENT

For the Woman with Vulvitis

Gather data from the woman to help differentiate behaviors that may cause isolated vulvitis from those that may cause vaginal and cervical inflammation. Once the assessment of vulvitis has been made, you have a crucial role to play in providing education about contributing factors that may have led to the development of vulvitis. In addition, educate the woman about behaviors to avoid, strategies or therapies to improve symptoms, and signs of a worsening condition that require further evaluation.

Care of the Woman with an Abnormal Finding During Pelvic Examination

An abnormal finding resulting from pelvic examination may involve tissues of the vulva, vagina, or cervix; abnormal uterine bleeding; or ovarian or uterine masses.

Vulvar Lesion

The skin of the vulva is subject to diseases and changes, just like skin elsewhere on the body. Because cancer of the vulva may be present in a variety of different types of lesions, it is important that the external genitalia be examined carefully at the time of pelvic examination. A common benign condition of the vulva, atrophic vaginitis, which is caused by a lack of estrogen stimulation to the vulva and vagina, is discussed in Chapter 3.

BARTHOLIN GLAND CYST

Infection of the Bartholin gland resulting in inflammation of the gland itself is a common vulvovaginal lesion. The infection can be caused by a number of different organisms, the most common of which are gonorrhea and staphylococcus. Symptoms include unilateral pain and swelling of the Bartholin gland, ranging from mild to moderate discomfort to severe pain. Treatment involves incision and drainage of the abscess, culture and sensitivity of the discharge, and appropriate antibiotic therapy.

LICHEN SCLEROSUS

Lichen sclerosus is a chronic disorder of the vulva that can occur at any age but is more common in perimenopausal and postmenopausal women. There is a strong link between lichen sclerosus and a variety of autoimmune-related disorders. On examination, lichen sclerosus appears as white papules and plaques, often with a keyhole appearance around the vulva, introitus, and anal area. Diagnosis is made by clinical exam and confirmed by biopsy. Initial treatment includes topical antihistamines while more difficult cases may require high-dose topical steroid cream applied nightly for 6 to 12 weeks and then decreased to once or twice weekly thereafter.

VULVAR VESTIBULITIS

Women with *vestibulitis* experience local irritation and inflammation of the vulvar vestibule, severe pain with vaginal penetration (tampons or intercourse), burning and itching, and sometimes urinary frequency or dysuria. Proposed precipitating factors are numerous and include history of recurrent vaginal infections; use of oral contraceptives, especially at an early age; and exposure to destructive treatments such as trichloroacetic acid. There is some question whether past sexual or physical abuse is a contributing factor. No definitive treatment exists, so therapies are directed at comfort measures to relieve symptoms. Therapies include Burrow soaks, sitz baths, vaginal and introital lubricants such as A&D ointment, topical corticosteroids, topical anesthetics, local interferon injections, oral antifungal medications, oral tricyclic antidepressants such as amitriptyline, physical therapy, biofeedback techniques, and, in severe cases, surgical intervention (Jernigan & Giuntoli, 2015).

VULVAR INTRAEPITHELIAL NEOPLASIA

Cancer of the vulva is increasing in incidence, specifically in women in their 40s (ACOG, 2016b). The woman may present with pruritus, a lump, or a flat lesion or, in the case of most HPV-related lesions, may be relatively asymptomatic. Risk factors include chronic vulvar inflammation, immunosuppression from chronic steroid use, smoking, diabetes, HPV infection or HIV, and history of lower genital tract cancer.

Clinical appearance can vary greatly and depends somewhat on the age of the patient. Diagnosis is made by colposcopic examination and biopsy. Treatment usually involves surgery to remove the lesions and often the tissue surrounding the lesion. Laser ablation or topical imiquimod may be used if vulvar occult (not readily seen) invasion is not a risk.

Cervicitis

Acute inflammation of the cervix is usually the result of infection from *Neisseria gonorrhoeae* or *Chlamydia trachomatis*. It may be caused by other organisms such as *Candida*, *Gardnerella vaginalis*, *Trichomonas*, herpes, staphylococci, or enterococci. Other causes may include use of intravaginal feminine hygiene products, frequent tampon use, frequent intercourse, or presence of a foreign body (such as an intrauterine device [IUD], contraceptive sponge, diaphragm, or tampon).

Symptoms often include a yellowish-white vaginal discharge or copious purulent discharge that is sometimes malodorous, depending on the etiology. **Dyspareunia** (painful intercourse) is a common complaint, with postcoital bleeding and occasional irregular vaginal bleeding. Sometimes there is a sense of pelvic heaviness and urinary symptoms such as urgency, frequency, and burning. Diagnosis and evaluation consist of a clinical pelvic examination, wet-mount smear, cultures, and a Pap smear. Treatment depends on the identified problem. It may include antibiotics to treat positive cultures (see Chapter 5), removal of foreign bodies, and in some instances treatment of nonspecific inflammation with local medication (metronidazole gel or clindamycin cream).

Abnormal Pap Smear Results

Women tend to expect a normal Pap smear report, but various abnormal findings are common. Notification of an abnormal result may cause significant anxiety in the woman. Therefore, results should be provided in a caring manner with an accurate explanation of the findings, reassurance that early detection of a problem allows early intervention, and information about expected further evaluation, treatment, and follow-up. The woman should be encouraged to ask questions and to voice her concerns.

PAP SMEAR

The purpose of the Papanicolaou smear (**Pap smear**) is to screen for the presence of cellular abnormalities by obtaining a sample containing cells from the cervix and the endocervical canal. Precancerous and cancerous conditions, as well as atypical findings and inflammatory changes, can be identified by a colposcopy.

A liquid-based medium Pap smear, now more commonly used than the older, conventional Pap slide, is used to detect cervical cancer. The Pap smear is obtained using a speculum to reveal the cervix. The cervix is visualized and a smear is obtained using a plastic spatula on the surface of the cervix and a cytobrush, which is inserted into the cervical os or opening to obtain cells in the cervical canal. The brush and spatula are swished in the solution to release cells. The specimen is sent to a laboratory where a special processor prepares a slide.

Liquid-based Pap smear preparations have become the method of choice for cervical cancer screening. These types of preparations allow for removal of debris from the sample, such as blood and mucus, thereby increasing the accuracy of the test. Additionally, these preparations allow for HPV screening and for some sexually transmitted infection (STI) screening. The Pap smear is a screening tool. A definitive diagnosis of cervical cancer is made by studying tissue samples obtained by biopsies. See *Professionalism in Practice: Pap Smear Preparation.*

Professionalism in Practice Pap Smear Preparation

Whenever you teach about pelvic examination and Pap smear, be certain that the woman understands that she should avoid having anything in her vagina for 24 hours before the examination—no intercourse, no tampons, no female hygiene products, and no douching—because this might interfere with the accuracy of the test.

In 2012, new guidelines for cervical cancer screening were issued by the U.S. Preventive Services Task Force, the American Cancer Society, and other groups. These guidelines, still current, are found in Table 6–2. It is important to recognize that these recommendations are population-based guidelines reflecting statistical analysis. As such, they are not appropriate for all women. Each woman needs to consult her caregiver about the best approach to screening based on her risk factors, history, preexisting conditions, and signs and symptoms.

THE BETHESDA SYSTEM

The *Bethesda System* (Table 6–3) is a standardized method of reporting cytologic Pap smear findings and is the most widely used method in the United States. It provides a uniform format and classification of terminology based on current understanding of cervical disease.

TABLE 6–2 Screening for Cervical Cancer

POPULATION	TEST AND FREQUENCY
Women under age 21	No screening, with exception of women with HIV and immunocompromised
Women ages 21–29	Screening with cytology alone every 3 years (*Note:* Co-testing for HPV is not recommended for this group because of the high prevalence of HPV.)
Women ages 30–65	Preferred approach: Screen with cytology every 3 years and HPV co-testing every 5 years Acceptable approach: Test with cytology alone every 3 years
Women over 65 years of age who have had adequate prior screening and are not at high risk	Do not screen
Women who have undergone hysterectomy and have no history of high-grade precancer or cervical cancer	Do not screen

SOURCE: Data from American College of Obstetricians and Gynecologists (ACOG). (2016). Cervical cancer screening and prevention (ACOG Committee Opinion No. 168). *Obstetrics and Gynecology, 128*(4), e111–e130; Centers for Disease Control and Prevention (CDC). (2013). Cervical cancer screening guidelines for average-risk women. Retrieved from http://www.cdc.gov/cancer/cervical/pdf/guidelines.pdf

Cervical Abnormalities

Cervical cancer is most common in women who have never been screened (50%) or screened inappropriately (10%) (ACOG, 2016a). An estimated 12,820 new cases of cervical cancer will be diagnosed in 2017 (ACS, 2017b). It is almost always caused by the human papilloma virus (HPV) infection, specifically HPV 16 (55–60%) and HPV 18 (10–15%) (ACOG, 2016a).

Cervical cancer is considered a preventable disease because it is slow-growing, has a lengthy preinvasive state, has inexpensive and available screening programs, and has effective treatment approaches for preinvasive lesions. Factors that place a woman at high risk for cervical cancer include:

- Coitus at an early age (first intercourse before 16 years of age increases the risk of cervical cancer twofold)
- History of multiple sexual partners
- Sex partner with a history of numerous sexual partners
- Exposure to STIs
- History of HPV infection
- History of immunosuppressive therapy (chemotherapy) or immunocompromised state (HIV)
- Long-term oral contraceptive use (greater than 5 years)
- Smoking
- Antenatal exposure to diethylstilbestrol (DES)
- History of dysplasia.

TABLE 6–3 The Bethesda System for Classifying Pap Smears

Specimen Type

Indicate conventional smear (Pap smear) versus liquid based versus other

Specimen Adequacy

Satisfactory for evaluation *(describe presence or absence of endocervical/transformation zone component and any other quality indicators, e.g., partially obscuring blood inflammation)*

Unsatisfactory for evaluation *(specify reason)*

Specimen rejected/not processed *(specify reason)*

Specimen processed and examined, but unsatisfactory for evaluation of epithelial abnormality because of *(specify reason)*

General Categorization (Optional)

Negative for intraepithelial lesion or malignancy

Epithelial cell abnormality; see interpretation/result *(specify squamous or glandular as appropriate)*

Other; see interpretation result *(e.g., endometrial cells in a woman* greater than or equal to *40 years of age)*

Automated Review

If case examined by automated device, specify device and result

Ancillary Testing

Provide a brief description of the test methods and report the result so that it is easily understood by the clinician

Interpretation/Result

Negative for intraepithelial lesion or malignancy (when there is no cellular evidence of neoplasia, state this in the General Categorization above and/or in the Interpretation/Result section of the report, whether or not there are organisms or other nonneoplastic findings)

Organisms:

- *Trichomonas vaginalis*
- Fungal organisms morphologically consistent with *Candida* spp
- Shift in flora suggestive of bacterial vaginosis
- Bacteria morphologically consistent with *Actinomyces* spp.
- Cellular changes associated with herpes simplex virus

Other Nonneoplastic Findings:

(Optional to report; list not inclusive)

Reactive cellular changes associated with:

—Inflammation (includes typical repair)

—radiation

—intrauterine contraceptive device (IUD)

Glandular cells status posthysterectomy

Atrophy

Other

Endometrial cells (in a woman greater than or equal to 40 years of age) *(specify if negative for squamous intraepithelial lesion)*

Epithelial Cell Abnormalities

Squamous Cell

Atypical squamous cells

—of undetermined significance (ASC-US)

—cannot exclude HSIL (ASC-H)

Low-grade squamous intraepithelial lesion (LSIL)

—encompassing HPV/mild dysplasia/CIN-1

High-grade squamous intraepithelial lesion (HSIL)

—encompassing: Moderate and severe dysplasia CIS/CIN-2 and CIN-3

—with features suspicious for invasion *(if invasion is suspected)*

Squamous cell carcinoma

Glandular Cell

Atypical

—endocervical cells *(NOS or specify in comments)*

—endometrial cells *(NOS or specify in comments)*

—glandular cells *(NOS or specify in comments)*

Atypical

—endocervical cells, favor neoplastic

—glandular cells, favor neoplastic

Endocervical adenocarcinoma in situ

Adenocarcinoma

—endocervical

—endometrial

—extrauterine

—not otherwise specified (NOS)

Other Malignant Neoplasms (Specify)

Educational Notes and Suggestions (Optional)

Suggestions should be concise and consistent with clinical follow-up guidelines published by professional organizations (references to relevant publications may be included).

SOURCE: Courtesy of National Cancer Institute.

“Several years ago I was treated for HPV—I got the infection from my husband—and seemed to be doing well. But now I've had some abnormal Pap smears and my doctor is talking about doing a LEEP procedure. I was a virgin when I got married, but my husband wasn't. I've done a lot of reading, and I know how common HPV is, so I guess I can't be too upset. Still, I have to admit that I feel a little nudge of resentment—I'm the one with problems. He is symptom-free.”

The 2014 Bethesda System identifies three categories for premalignant squamous cell lesions:

1. Atypical squamous cells (ASC)
2. Low-grade squamous intraepithelial lesion (LSIL)
3. High-grade squamous intraepithelial lesion (HSIL), which includes CIN 2 (moderate dysplasia) and CIN 3 (severe dysplasia and carcinoma in situ).

The focus of the Pap smear is on the detection of high-grade cervical disease, especially *cervical intraepithelial neoplasia* (CIN). CIN refers to a lesion that may progress to invasive carcinoma (cancer). It is synonymous with the term *dysplasia*. To further support this objective, the ASC category is subdivided into two qualifiers that recognize the importance of detecting HSIL:

- Atypical squamous cells of undetermined significance (ASC-US)
- Atypical squamous cells—cannot exclude HSIL (ASC-H).

The category ASC-H includes those changes that are suggestive of a high-grade lesion but are lacking sufficient criteria for a definitive evaluation and interpretation. An immediate colposcopy is advised because women with this finding have an increased risk of having a moderate to severe lesion.

Colposcopy is the direct, detailed visualization and examination of the cervix. It is done in most gynecologic offices. To do a colposcopy, a speculum is placed in the vagina and the cervix is isolated. A 3% acetic acid solution applied on the cervix causes the abnormal epithelial cells to take on a characteristic white appearance. The colposcope, with its bright light and various color filters, provides a 6 to 40 times magnification of the cervical tissues. Lesions or other abnormalities are identified and documented, and directed biopsies can be obtained at this time, if indicated. Sometimes the biopsy itself can be therapeutic as well as diagnostic if the entire lesion can be removed.

Another cervical cytology result is atypical glandular cells (AGUS), which represents cells that are glandular rather than squamous in origin. These are further subdivided into the following:

- Atypical endocervical cells
- Atypical endometrial cells
- Atypical glandular cells not otherwise specified.

The workup for this type of finding is more aggressive because it may represent a more invasive form of disease, and colposcopy and endometrial sampling are done (Massad et al., 2013).

In women who test HPV positive and negative cytology (normal cells on Pap smear), two options are available (Massad et al., 2013):

- Option I: Repeat the Pap with HPV co-testing in 12 months; if either test is positive, refer for colposcopy; if both tests are negative, return to routine testing
- Option II: Test for HPV 16 or 16/18 genotypes (high-risk types); if positive, refer for colposcopy.

Evaluation of Abnormal Cytology

The following points summarize the primary guidelines for managing women with abnormal cancer screening results (Jeronimo et al., 2016):

- Women with ASC-US: Preferred management is HPV testing; if positive, refer for colposcopy; if negative, repeat HPV co-testing in 3 years. Alternately, cytology can be repeated in 1 year; if negative, return to routine screening; if ASC is the same or greater, refer for colposcopy.
- Women with ASC-H are at greater risk for CIN than women with ASC-US and should be referred directly for colposcopy.
- Women with LSIL and no HPV test or a positive HPV test are referred for colposcopy.
- Women with HSIL can be managed in one of two ways: (1) Immediate loop electrosurgical excision or (2) colposcopy followed by treatment as indicated.
- Women with biopsy-confirmed CIN grade 2 or 3: LOOP excision or ablation of the T-zone of the cervix is indicated.

Endocervical curettage (ECC) may also be done at this time to evaluate for extension into the cervical canal. This involves a scraping of the endocervix from the internal os to the external os to obtain endocervical cells for cytology. Histologic evaluation of tissue biopsies and ECC samples is necessary for a definitive diagnosis.

The woman may experience moderate to severe cramplike pains during and after the biopsy and/or ECC. To help alleviate this discomfort, nurses can advise women to premedicate with 600 mg ibuprofen about 30 minutes before the procedure. A small amount of bleeding, initially bright red and then becoming darker, is normal for up to 2 weeks. Bleeding as heavy as a menstrual period is not normal and should be reported to the woman's healthcare provider.

Surgical Treatment for Abnormal Cytology

Premalignant (precancerous) and malignant (cancerous) lesions are often treated with surgical procedures, varying from simple biopsy of the cervix to radical surgery of the pelvic organs, depending on the diagnosis and extent of the disease. A diagnosis of cancer can only be made after a pathologic evaluation of tissue obtained via biopsy. The goals of management are to exclude the presence of invasive cancer, to determine the extent and distribution of noninvasive cancer, and to provide appropriate treatment.

The treatment of cervical cancer depends on the stage of the disease, which is determined by the extent of its spread to other tissues or structures. Surgical treatment of cervical cancer may include a total abdominal hysterectomy (TAH), bilateral salpingo-oophorectomy (BSO), and bilateral lymphadenectomy (discussed further in the section "Care of the Woman Requiring Gynecologic Surgery"). It may also include radiation therapy and chemotherapy.

LOOP ELECTROSURGICAL EXCISION PROCEDURE

The *loop electrosurgical excision procedure (LEEP)* can be used to treat cervical, vaginal, and vulvar intraepithelial neoplasia. When an abnormal Pap smear and a colposcopic evaluation indicate a premalignant lesion, a small electrically hot wire loop can be used to excise the entire lesion, squamocolumnar junction, and transformation zone (Jeronimo et al., 2016). The cutting effect is created by a steam envelope that develops between the wire loop and the water-laden tissue. This procedure can be performed on an outpatient basis, often in the gynecologic office, under local anesthesia. Complications following LEEP are usually minimal, and it is virtually painless and bloodless. The woman can expect some slight bleeding and possibly a malodorous dark brown discharge for 1 to 2 weeks after the procedure. The woman needs to know that moderate to heavy bleeding would be abnormal and should be reported to her healthcare provider.

CRYOSURGERY

Cryosurgery is used to treat women with a small ectocervical lesion who have a negative ECC and no endocervical gland involvement. A double freezing method is advocated, using nitrous oxide or carbon dioxide to freeze the tissue below –20°C (–4°F), resulting in tissue destruction and necrosis. Cryosurgery is less widely used since the development of LEEP because it scars the cervix, making the transformation zone, or squamocolumnar junction, more difficult to evaluate with future colposcopies. It can easily be done in a gynecologic office or clinic without anesthesia. The woman may experience some mild cramping and should be told to expect a thin, watery, persistent, and sometimes heavy vaginal discharge for up to several weeks as the frozen tissue is sloughed. She should avoid tampon use and sexual intercourse while the discharge is present to minimize further damage to the cervix.

LASER THERAPY

A carbon dioxide (CO_2) laser is used to treat cervical, vaginal, and vulvar intraepithelial lesions. The laser is used when all boundaries of the lesion are visible on colposcopy and when the ECC is negative. The invisible, highly concentrated beam is absorbed by water in the tissues, elevating the temperature in the tissues to above 100°C (212°F). The targeted tissue "boils" and the exploded cells are vaporized, leaving the normal tissue intact. Laser treatment can be done in outpatient or office settings without anesthesia. The woman may experience mild cramping and a slight discharge for 5 to 7 days; however, bleeding is minimal. She should avoid tampon use, intercourse, and douching for 2 weeks; complete healing may take up to 12 weeks. In many clinical settings, laser therapy has become less common with the advent and effective use of LEEP.

CONIZATION

A *cold knife conization (CKC)* of the cervix (also known as a *cone*) is most commonly performed when the entire lesion cannot be visualized by colposcopic examination or when there is a positive ECC sampling. In this procedure, a cone-shaped section of cervical tissue is excised. The width and depth of the tissue removed varies depending on the extent of the lesion. A large amount of normal tissue is removed, as well as the abnormal tissue, and this procedure can often be diagnostic as well as therapeutic if the entire lesion is excised. Conization is usually done under general anesthesia with the woman in a lithotomy position. Immediate postoperative risks include infection and hemorrhage; long-term risks include spontaneous abortion, insufficient cervix, or preterm labor with future pregnancies. A prolonged or profuse menstrual period may occur in two or three cycles following the procedure. Conization is used less frequently today because of the availability of LEEP.

Abnormal Uterine Bleeding

Abnormal uterine bleeding (AUB) is a common gynecologic problem defined as uterine bleeding in the absence of pregnancy that is abnormal in volume, frequency, regularity, or duration. It may be chronic or acute (ACOG, 2017b). Acute AUB is an episode of heavy bleeding that is severe enough to cause concern about blood loss.

A classification system has been developed for the causes of AUB using the acronym PALM-COEIN (ACOG, 2017b). Determining the cause is an essential first step in planning treatment.

Structural causes (PALM) include:

- **P**olyp
- **A**denomyosis
- **L**eiomyoma
- **M**alignancy and hyperplasia.

Nonstructural causes include (COEIN):

- **C**oagulopathy
- **O**vulatory dysfunction
- **E**ndometrial
- **I**atrogenic
- **N**ot otherwise classified.

Systemic diseases that cause AUB include coagulation disorders such as von Willebrand disease, thrombocytopenia, acute leukemia, and advanced liver disease. Medications such as anticoagulants may also play a role.

Evaluation of AUB begins with a thorough history and physical examination including a careful pelvic exam and Pap smear. The diagnosis is made by excluding organic causes, specifically pregnancy, uterine or ovarian pathology, medications, or systemic disease. Based on the information gained, specific laboratory tests such as pregnancy test, liver and renal function tests, thyroid tests, coagulation studies, or prolactin levels may be indicated. Based on the woman's age and findings, other tests that may be indicated include transvaginal ultrasound, saline infusion sonography (SIS), hysteroscopy, MRI, and endometrial biopsy.

The goals of treatment are to control bleeding, prevent or treat anemia, prevent endometrial hyperplasia or cancer, and restore quality of life. Pharmacologic treatment for AUB varies depending on the woman's desire for pregnancy and whether she is premenopausal, perimenopausal, or postmenopausal. Combined oral contraceptives (COCs) are the most common treatment for women who are not actively trying to conceive. COCs help regulate cycles while also providing contraception. Other options include short-term, high-dose estrogen therapy, cyclic progesterone to regulate cycles in women with contraindications to estrogen therapy, tranexamic acid (prevents fibrin degradation to help control bleeding), and the levonorgestrel intrauterine system (LNG-IUS) (see Chapter 4). If conservative measures are not effective, the woman and her provider may consider surgical interventions, such as dilation and curettage (D&C), endometrial ablation, uterine artery embolization, and hysterectomy (ACOG, 2017b).

Dysfunctional uterine bleeding (DUB) is characterized by AUB that does not have a demonstrable organic cause. DUB can occur at any age but is most common at either end of the reproductive age span. Adolescents often experience DUB during the first 2 years following menarche due to hypothalamic immaturity after menarche. Perimenopausal women account for 50% of cases due to waning ovarian function. It is typically treated medically. Surgical intervention is generally limited to cases in which medical therapy is contraindicated or has failed.

Ovarian (Adnexal) Masses

An *adnexal mass* most commonly refers to an ovarian abnormality, but it can also refer to masses found in the fallopian tubes, broad ligament, or bowel, or even a lateral mass of the uterus. Between 70 and 80% of ovarian masses are benign. More than 50% are functional cysts (cysts that develop from ovarian follicles, from the corpus luteum, or from the theca luteum) occurring most commonly in women 20 to 40 years of age. Functional cysts are rare in women who take oral contraceptives.

Ovarian cysts usually represent physiologic variations in the menstrual cycle. Nearly all perimenopausal women have ovarian cysts, and about 15% of postmenopausal women have them. Dermoid cysts (cystic teratomas) comprise 10% of all benign ovarian masses. Cartilage, bone, teeth, skin, or hair can be observed in these cysts. Endometriomas, or "chocolate cysts," are another common type of ovarian mass.

No relationship exists between benign ovarian masses and ovarian cancer. At present, no adequate techniques exist for ovarian cancer screening. Approximately 5% of cancer deaths in women are from ovarian cancer, with an estimated 22,240 new ovarian cancer cases diagnosed in 2017 (ACS, 2017b). More than 14,000 deaths in the United States occur each year as a result of ovarian cancer. Unfortunately, only about 15% of all cases are diagnosed when the cancer is still localized. The 5-year survival rate for women with advanced disease is about 46%; this increases to over 92% if the disease is diagnosed early (ACS, 2017b). Risk factors for ovarian cancer include:

- Increased age
- History of breast cancer
- *BRCA1* or *BRCA2* gene mutations
- Family history of breast or ovarian cancer.

Some cases of ovarian cancer are associated with a mutation in specific genes (*BRCA1* and *BRCA2* genes). It is now possible to identify many of these mutations. These two mutations are inherited in an autosomal dominant pattern, meaning that the gene can come from either parent. Hereditary ovarian cancer tends to occur at a younger age, but the prognosis is generally better. In reality, ovarian cancer is the most fatal of all cancers in women because it is difficult to diagnose and often has spread throughout the pelvis before it is detected. Symptoms are often vague and nonspecific and may include:

- Bloating
- Increased abdominal size
- Difficulty eating
- Abdominal or pelvic pain
- Urinary symptoms (urgency and frequency).

Women who have these symptoms daily for several weeks should see a gynecologist for prompt medical evaluation. The risk of ovarian cancer is decreased significantly by bearing children, taking combined oral contraceptive pills for more than 5 years, or having a tubal ligation.

A woman with an ovarian mass may be asymptomatic; the mass may be noted on a routine pelvic examination. She may experience a sensation of fullness or cramping in the lower abdomen (often unilateral), dyspareunia, irregular bleeding, or delayed menstruation.

Diagnosis is made on the basis of a palpable mass, with or without tenderness, and other related symptoms. Radiography or ultrasonography may be used to assist or confirm the diagnosis.

The woman is frequently kept under observation for a month or two because most cysts will resolve on their own and are harmless. Oral contraceptives may be prescribed for 1 to 2 months to suppress ovarian function. If this regimen is effective, a repeat pelvic examination should yield normal findings. If the mass is still present after 60 days of observation and oral contraceptive therapy, a diagnostic laparoscopy or laparotomy may be considered. Tubal or ovarian lesions, ectopic pregnancy, cancer, infection, or appendicitis must also be ruled out before a diagnosis can be confirmed.

Surgery is not always necessary but will be considered if the mass is larger than 6 to 7 cm in circumference; if the woman is over 40 years of age with an adnexal mass, a persistent mass, or continuous pain; or if the woman is taking oral contraceptives. Surgical exploration is also indicated when a palpable mass is found in an infant, a young girl, or a postmenopausal woman.

Women may need clear explanations about why the initial therapy is observation. A discussion of the origin and resolution of ovarian cysts may clarify this treatment plan. If a surgical treatment removes or impairs the function of one ovary, the woman needs to be assured that the remaining ovary can be expected to take over ovarian functioning and that pregnancy is still possible.

Uterine Masses

Endometrial polyps are pedunculated (growing on a stalk) overgrowths of the endometrium. They can occur as single or multiple growths. Polyps are common and are often accompanied by symptoms of midcycle bleeding or spotting, bleeding or spotting after intercourse, or prolonged bleeding or spotting with menstrual cycles. Polyps are generally benign, but they can coexist with carcinoma of the endometrium in about 10% of postmenopausal women. Treatment is dilation and curettage (D&C) using the hysteroscope for visualization.

Fibroid tumors, or *leiomyomas*, are among the most common benign disease entities in women. By the age of 50, 70% of Caucasian American women and 80% of African American women have fibroids (Rice, Secrist, Woodrow, et al., 2012). Uterine fibroids account for approximately 39% of all hysterectomies (De La Cruz & Buchanan, 2017).

The most common symptoms include pelvic pain, menstrual irregularities, and infertility. Women most often seek treatment for bleeding and pain.

Many uterine fibroids are asymptomatic and require no treatment but 20 to 50% of women do seek treatment. On pelvic examination the woman may have an irregular-shaped, enlarged uterus. Diagnosis is most often made using pelvic ultrasound and MRI. Occasionally, hysterosonography is used for further evaluation (De La Cruz & Buchanan, 2017).

Treatment for uterine fibroids varies and may include:

- Combined oral contraceptives to control heavy menstrual bleeding
- GnRH analogs such as Lupron to reduce the size and subsequent bleeding. These medications carry with them symptoms of menopause such as hot flashes and bone loss and are often used for short-term therapy in perimenopausal women. GnRH analogs may also be used before surgery to reduce the size of the fibroid and decrease complications (De La Cruz & Buchanan, 2017).
- Levonorgestrel intrauterine system (LNG-IUS) for contraception and control of excessive menstrual bleeding by suppression of endometrial growth
- MRI-guided ultrasound, which focuses high-intensity sound waves on the fibroids, resulting in clotting, necrosis, and shrinkage of the tumor
- *Myomectomy*, a surgical procedure to remove the fibroid without removing the uterus, which can preserve or improve fertility
- Uterine artery embolization (UAE), an interventional radiologic procedure in which the uterine arteries are blocked, resulting in diminished blood flow to the uterus and necrosis of the fibroids.

Hysterectomy may be indicated and can be performed laparoscopically or abdominally depending on the size of the uterus.

Endometrial cancer is the most common female genital tract cancer, accounting for approximately 6% of all cancers in women, with an estimated 61,380 new cases in 2017 (National Cancer Institute [NCI], 2017). It has a high rate of cure if detected early, 84% in Caucasian American women and 62% in African American women (ACS, 2017b).

Risk factors for endometrial cancer include (NCI, 2017):

- Increased age *(mean age is 60)*
- Obesity with adult weight gain
- Nulliparity

CASE STUDY: Angelina Newman

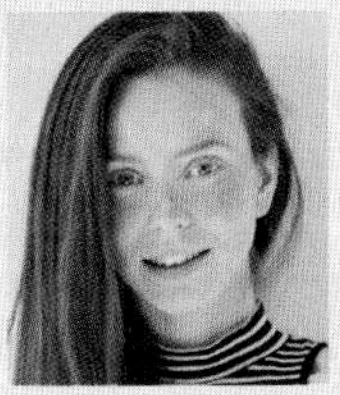

SOURCE: WAYHOME studio/Shutterstock

Angelina presents for her prenatal visit and is informed she has an abnormal Pap smear. The nurse reveals that she had atypical squamous cells of undetermined significance (ASC-US) on her first visit. Angelina becomes very distressed because her sister also had a "something like that" diagnosis and had to have surgery. She becomes tearful and asks if she will lose her baby.

Questions to Ponder

What are the guidelines for the woman who tests positive with ASC-US? What reassurance and explanation would you provide to Angelina at this visit?

- Polycystic ovary syndrome
- Hereditary nonpolyposis colon cancer syndrome (Lynch syndrome)
- Postmenopausal estrogen therapy
- Early menarche or late menopause
- Use of tamoxifen.

The majority of endometrial cancer occurs in postmenopausal women. The hallmark sign is vaginal bleeding in postmenopausal women not treated with hormone therapy (HT). Women may present with vaginal bleeding or have an incidental finding on a Pap smear of atypical endometrial cells. Generally a pelvic ultrasound is done to evaluate the thickness of the endometrium; followed by an endometrial biopsy, which will confirm the suspicion of cancer; and the grade of lesion will be reported with pathology. Hysterectomy is the treatment of choice, often with bilateral salpingo-oophorectomy (removal of both fallopian tubes and ovaries). Depending on the staging of the tumor, radiation therapy, chemotherapy, or hormone suppression therapy may also be indicated.

●○● NURSING MANAGEMENT

For the Woman with an Abnormal Finding During a Pelvic Examination

Only nurses with special training perform pelvic examinations and Pap smears. In most cases, nursing assessment is directed toward evaluating the woman's understanding of the findings and their implications and her psychosocial response.

Provide the woman with accurate information on the etiology of the disorder, its symptoms, and treatment options. Encourage her to report symptoms and keep appointments for follow-up examination and evaluation. The woman needs realistic reassurance if her condition is benign; she may require counseling and effective emotional support if a malignancy is likely. If the management plan includes surgery, she may need support in obtaining a second opinion and making her decision. You can also provide information on available community resources, including support groups.

Care of the Woman with Endometriosis

Endometriosis, a condition characterized by the presence of endometrial tissue outside the uterine cavity, occurs in about 11% of reproductive-age women and 30 to 50% of women with infertility (Alexander, Dupper, & Millard, 2017). Endometriosis has been found almost everywhere in the body, including the vagina, lungs, cervix, central nervous system, and gastrointestinal tract. The most common location, however, is the pelvic cavity. This tissue responds to the hormonal changes of the menstrual cycle and bleeds in a cyclic fashion. The bleeding results in inflammation, scarring of the peritoneum, and formation of adhesions.

Endometriosis may occur at any age after puberty, although it is most commonly diagnosed in women between 20 and 45 years of age and is rare in postmenopausal women. The exact cause of endometriosis is unknown. Proposed causative factors include retrograde menstrual flow, inflammation of the endometrium, hereditary tendency, and a possible immunologic effect.

The most common symptom of endometriosis is pelvic pain, which is often dull or cramping. Usually the pain is related to menstruation itself and is often thought to be dysmenorrhea by the affected woman. However, the pain of dysmenorrhea usually begins right before menses starts and lasts for a day or two, decreasing as prostaglandin levels decrease. Dyspareunia (painful intercourse) may be present due to scarring of the pelvic tissues and organs from the endometrial implants. The condition is often diagnosed when the woman seeks evaluation for infertility. Bimanual examination may reveal a fixed, tender, retroverted uterus and palpable nodules in the cul-de-sac. Diagnosis is confirmed by laparoscopy.

Treatment may be medical, surgical, or a combination of the two. In women with minimal disease and symptoms, treatment includes observation, analgesics, and nonsteroidal anti-inflammatory drugs (NSAIDs). Medical therapies include:

- ***Combined oral contraceptives (COCs)***, which suppress menstruation, can be used in women who do not desire fertility.
- ***Progestins*** such as medroxyprogesterone acetate (MPA) exert an antiendometriotic effect and ultimate atrophy. The medication is administered intramuscularly every 3 months, and the effectiveness of the treatment is evaluated every 3 to 6 months. Side effects may include nausea, weight gain, fluid retention, and breakthrough bleeding.
- ***Danazol*** is a testosterone derivative that suppresses ovulation and causes amenorrhea. It is intended for short-term therapy. Because of adverse effects on lipid metabolism and significant side effects such as weight gain, hirsutism, acne, oily skin, vaginal dryness, hot flashes, reduced libido, voice changes, clitoral enlargement, and decreased breast size, many clinicians have moved away from danazol to other treatment options.
- ***GnRH analogs*** such as nafarelin acetate (given as a metered nasal spray twice daily) and leuprolide acetate (Lupron, given once a month as an intramuscular injection) are

gaining popularity because many women tolerate them better than danazol, and their results in treating endometriosis are comparable. GnRH analogs suppress the menstrual cycle through estrogen antagonism. This may result in the hypoestrogen side effects of hot flashes, vaginal dryness, headache, breast reduction, and loss of bone density. Consequently, the use of GnRH agonists should be limited to 6 months (Woo & Yates, 2015). Calcium, vitamin D, or low-dose combined (estrogen and progesterone) oral contraceptives may be given to decrease bone loss.

In more advanced cases, surgery may be done to remove endometrial implants and break up adhesions. If severe dyspareunia or dysmenorrhea is a symptom, the surgeon may perform a presacral neurectomy to relieve the pain. In advanced cases in which childbearing is not an issue, treatment may be a hysterectomy (removal of the uterus) with bilateral salpingo-oophorectomy (removal of the fallopian tubes and ovaries). See *Complementary Health Approaches: Treatment of Endometriosis*.

●○● NURSING MANAGEMENT

For the Woman with Endometriosis

Nursing Assessment and Diagnosis

Be aware of the common symptoms of endometriosis and elicit an accurate history if a woman mentions these symptoms. If a woman is being treated for endometriosis, assess the woman's understanding of the condition, its implications, and the treatment alternatives.

Nursing diagnoses that may apply to a woman with endometriosis include:

- ***Pain, Acute,*** related to peritoneal irritation secondary to endometriosis
- ***Coping: Family, Compromised,*** related to depression secondary to infertility

  (NANDA-I © 2017)

Nursing Plan and Implementation

Be available to explain the condition, its symptoms, treatment alternatives, and prognosis to the woman. Help the woman evaluate treatment options and make appropriate choices. If the woman begins taking medication, review the dosage, schedule, possible side effects, and any warning signs. Women are often advised to avoid delaying pregnancy because of the risk of infertility. The woman may wish to discuss the implications of this decision on her life choices, relationship with her partner, and personal preferences. You can serve as a nonjudgmental listener and help the woman consider her options. In addition, you can refer the woman to the Endometriosis Association. This group offers women support and education.

Evaluation

Expected outcomes of nursing care include:

- The woman is able to discuss her condition, its implications for fertility, and her treatment options.
- After considering the alternatives, the woman chooses appropriate treatment options.

Care of the Woman with Polycystic Ovarian Syndrome

Polycystic ovarian syndrome (PCOS) is a complex endocrine disorder of ovarian dysfunction that is evidenced by menstrual dysfunction, signs of androgen excess (typically hirsutism, acne), and infertility affecting approximately 7% of women in the United States (De La Luz Nieto, 2017).

The most common clinical signs and symptoms of PCOS include:

- ***Menstrual dysfunction.*** Irregular menses, ranging from total absence of periods (amenorrhea) to intermittent or infrequent periods (oligomenorrhea) are the hallmarks of PCOS. Anovulation is usually a chronic problem with PCOS and may present as a history of menstrual irregularities.
- ***Hyperandrogenism.*** Women with PCOS consistently have elevated serum androgen levels. These elevated androgen levels often lead to clinical manifestations such as hirsutism (excessive hair growth), acne, deepening voice, and increased muscle mass.
- ***Obesity.*** The obesity is generally of the android type, with an increased hip-to-waist ratio.
- ***Hyperinsulinemia.*** Women with PCOS may be insulin resistant. This insulin resistance, characterized by the failure of insulin to enter the cells appropriately, places these women at increased risk for impaired glucose tolerance and type 2 diabetes mellitus (Stewart & Kolp, 2015).
- ***Infertility.*** The majority of women who have been diagnosed with PCOS struggle with some degree of infertility related to anovulation.

Diagnosis of PCOS

PCOS is a diagnosis of exclusion (Stewart & Kolp, 2015). If a woman presents with complaints of hirsutism, menstrual irregularities, acne, difficulty conceiving, and unexplained weight gain, a careful history is taken and a physical examination is performed. A pelvic ultrasound, hemoglobin A1c, lipid panel, and glucose testing (2-hour) are ordered. Several other disorders must be ruled out. Important disorders to consider include

Complementary Health Approaches

Treatment of Endometriosis

Complementary therapies that may play a role in the treatment of endometriosis include (Oyelowo & Johnson, 2018):

- Acupuncture to help with pain control
- Vag Packs (suppositories with vitamins, minerals, and herbs)
- Yoga for relaxation and stress reduction
- Massage
- Traditional Chinese herbal medicine for symptomatic relief
- Spiritual therapies such as prayer, religious rituals, meditation, and support groups.

hyperthyroidism or hypothyroidism, congenital adrenal hyperplasia, Cushing syndrome, hyperprolactinemia, and androgen-producing tumors. Ultrasound examination may reveal polycystic changes in one or both ovaries.

Clinical Therapy

Once PCOS is diagnosed, the goals for treatment should be established. These include:

- Decreasing the effects of hyperandrogenism (hirsutism, acne, etc.)
- Restoring reproductive functioning for women desiring pregnancy
- Protecting the endometrium (increased risk for uterine cancer)
- Reducing long-term risks, specifically type 2 diabetes and cardiovascular disease.

If pregnancy is not an immediate goal, menstrual irregularities can be treated with a COC or cyclic progesterone. COCs help to regulate menstrual cycles; provide a balance between estrogen and progesterone, thereby protecting the endometrium and decreasing the risk of uterine cancer; and may improve acne by inhibiting ovarian androgen production.

Antiandrogens such as spironolactone (Aldactone) may be used to decrease symptoms of androgen excess, including acne and hirsutism. Metformin (Glucophage) improves tissue sensitivity to insulin, inhibits glucose production in the liver, and improves glucose uptake by fat and muscle cells. It improves ovarian function, reduces the degree of hyperandrogenism, restores normal ovulation in women with PCOS, and is associated with an improved ability to lose weight. In addition, lifestyle changes are important. Modifications should include weight loss, regular exercise, balanced diet, and smoking cessation.

If initial approaches to helping a woman with PCOS become pregnant fail, fertility medications as Clomid and FSH/LH injections may be administered followed by assisted reproductive technology (ART), in vitro fertilization, intrauterine insemination, or intracytoplasmic sperm injection. This may be combined with gonadotropin therapy (Oyelowo & Johnson, 2018).

Long-Term Implications

PCOS may increase a woman's risk for developing overt type 2 diabetes, dyslipidemia, hypertension, cardiovascular disease, endometrial cancer, breast cancer, and ovarian cancer. Additionally, and very importantly, the woman with PCOS may struggle with significant emotional responses to this chronic disorder. She will likely face, throughout her lifetime, issues related to body image, infertility, problematic menses, and depression.

●○● NURSING MANAGEMENT

For the Woman with Polycystic Ovarian Syndrome

The nurse plays a vital role in the identification, evaluation, management, and follow-up when caring for a woman with PCOS. Sometimes it is the nurse who puts the bigger picture together, especially in a community health setting where knowledge of PCOS may be lacking. Women with PCOS may present with complaints such as weight gain, excess hairiness, difficult periods, inability to get pregnant, or depression, or express feelings like, "What is wrong with me? Why do I look like this?"

The signs of PCOS, especially hirsutism, negatively impact women's feelings of femininity; they may feel physically inferior and lack self-confidence. You can help women recognize these feelings and find ways to develop a more positive body image. You also play an important role in providing accurate information, education, and counseling for a woman diagnosed with PCOS. Finally, because the woman with PCOS is at great risk for developing long-term complications, you and subsequent nurses can play a key role in follow-up and continuity of care throughout the life of a woman facing this challenging disorder.

Care of the Woman with Pelvic Relaxation

The muscles of the pelvic floor form a supportive layer that prevents the abdominal and pelvic organs from prolapsing or sagging downward into the genital tract. If these muscles are weakened or damaged, a variety of conditions may develop, including cystocele, rectocele, and uterine prolapse.

Cystocele

A **cystocele** is the downward displacement of the bladder, which appears as a bulge in the anterior vaginal wall. Arbitrary classifications of mild to severe are frequently given. Genetic predisposition, childbearing, obesity, and increased age are factors that may contribute to cystocele.

Women with a cystocele commonly show symptoms of stress urinary incontinence (SUI) including loss of urine with coughing, sneezing, laughing, or sudden exertion. The woman may present with complaints of the perception of something "falling out" of her vagina. She may also have urinary retention, problems with sexual dysfunction, or pelvic pressure. If pelvic relaxation is mild, Kegel exercises are helpful in restoring tone(for information on Kegel exercises, see Chapter 13). The exercises involve contracting and relaxing the pubococcygeal muscle. Women have found these exercises helpful before and after childbirth in maintaining vaginal muscle tone. Estrogen may improve the condition of vaginal mucous membranes, especially in menopausal women.

Medications such as Detrol, DetrolLA, Oxytrol, or Sanctura may be used to treat urinary stress incontinence. Vaginal pessaries or rings may be used if surgery is undesirable or impossible or until surgery can be scheduled. Surgery may be considered for cystoceles considered moderate to severe.

The nurse can instruct the woman in the use of Kegel exercises. Providing information on causes and contributing factors and discussing possible alternative therapies greatly assists the woman.

Rectocele

A *rectocele* may develop if the posterior vaginal wall is weakened. The anterior wall of the rectum protrudes forward, ballooning into the vagina, pushing the weakened posterior wall of the vagina into the vaginal lumen. When the woman strains to have a bowel movement, a pocket of rectum develops that traps stool, and constipation results. The harder a woman with rectocele strains, the larger the pocket becomes. To defecate, women with a rectocele may find it necessary to press the tissue between the vagina and rectum, which elevates the rectocele.

Diagnosis is based on history and physical examination. Decisions about treatment are based on the size of the prolapse, the presence and severity of symptoms, and the woman's individual situation including her overall health status. Surgery is often indicated.

Uterine Prolapse

Because the vagina and the uterus are attached to one another, prolapse of the uterine cervix is associated with prolapse of the upper vagina. The extent of the prolapse is determined by the location of the cervix in the vagina. In severe cases the cervix may prolapse below the vaginal introitus. The woman may report a "dragging" sensation in her groin and a backache over the sacrum, which is caused by pulling on the uterosacral ligaments. Typically these sensations are relieved when the woman lies down. Furthermore, with pronounced prolapse, exposure of the moist vaginal walls may cause a sensation of perineal wetness that the woman might mistake for incontinence. As with cystocele, conservative treatment includes the use of topical or systemic estrogen and vaginal pessaries. Surgery for uterine prolapse often involves hysterectomy and repair of the prolapsed vaginal walls.

Care of the Woman Requiring Gynecologic Surgery

Gynecologic surgeries—particularly hysterectomies—are some of the most common surgical procedures being done in the United States. Many new techniques have been developed for treating a variety of gynecologic and reproductive disorders, and controversy remains regarding the high number of procedures being done annually. For these reasons, it is important for the woman and her partner considering medical or surgical management of a given gynecologic problem to be well informed.

There are many components to an informed decision to undergo reproductive tract surgery. Questions that should be addressed include, for example: What are the indications for having the surgery? What are the risks? What is the success rate? Are there other alternative therapies to try before proceeding to surgery? An explanation of the surgical procedure and the reasons it is recommended over other possible therapies should be given to the woman. Effects on childbearing ability and potential impact on sexual desire and performance should be addressed as well as the effects on the general functioning of the body. A discussion of the risks and benefits should be presented, and the risks should include the common risks, the nonserious risks, the rare or unusual complications, and the risk of death.

The question of whether to seek a second opinion about the recommended treatment is somewhat controversial. In the case of elective surgery, different physicians may have very different opinions. A woman and her partner should be encouraged to consult other physicians when there is controversy about a treatment (as in the treatment of early cervical cancer) or when the surgeon is unknown to the woman. A specialist in gynecology is the preferred source for a second opinion. The woman can analyze the information and discuss her concerns with the nurse or physician before signing a written consent acknowledging that the information has been given and authorizing the surgery.

Other concerns that may influence the decision to have reproductive surgery may be categorized as general concerns about surgery and specific concerns related to gynecologic surgery. General concerns may include:

- Fear of general anesthesia because of loss of control or fear of "not waking up"; fear of regional anesthesia because of possible postoperative problems and concern about being awake during surgery
- Fear of death or disability
- Concerns about limitation of normal functioning and dependency during recovery
- Financial coverage for hospitalization and potential financial loss if it is necessary to take extensive time off from work
- Concerns about welfare of family members while undergoing surgery (such as child care, loss of wages, household responsibilities).

Specific concerns related to gynecologic surgery are related to the significance of the reproductive organs for the woman. Surgery to alter or remove reproductive organs may be perceived as a threat to self-concept.

Body image is affected whenever a body part is lost. The degree of mourning for that loss is related to the significance attached to it. Even though there is no outwardly apparent change with a hysterectomy and most other gynecologic procedures, the loss may be felt very strongly. Many women fear postoperative changes such as masculinization, weight gain, loss of sexuality, and permanent loss of the ability to have a child. Reproductive surgery may also be seen as a threat to femininity in any social or cultural group that emphasizes childbearing and motherhood.

Hysterectomy

Hysterectomy is the surgical removal of the uterus. In the United States, it is the most common non–pregnancy-related surgical procedure that women undergo.

Removal of the uterus through an abdominal incision is called a *total abdominal hysterectomy (TAH)*, and removal of both fallopian tubes and ovaries is called a *bilateral salpingo-oophorectomy (BSO)*; when both procedures are done at the same time it is termed a *TAH-BSO*. When the uterus is removed through the vagina it is termed a *total vaginal hysterectomy (TVH)*.

A *laparoscopic-assisted vaginal hysterectomy (LAVH)* may also be used. In this technique, the surgeon inserts the laparoscope through an incision near the umbilicus and uses it to assist with visualization and dissection to facilitate vaginal removal of the uterus. The benefit is that the surgeon can achieve results similar to those of a TAH without a large abdominal incision. Abdominal hysterectomy is generally recommended for cancer of the cervix, endometrium, or ovary; large fibroids; severe endometriosis; chronic pelvic inflammatory disease (PID); and adenomyosis. TAH is preferred when cancer is suspected or confirmed because it permits easier exploration of the abdomen and pelvis to determine the degree and extent of involvement. This approach is also helpful when large uterine masses are present, requiring a larger incision. Disadvantages include more scarring, more postoperative pain, slower recovery, and more problems with bowel function.

Vaginal hysterectomy is generally done for pelvic relaxation, abnormal uterine bleeding, or small fibroids. An anterior and posterior repair of the vaginal walls may also be performed during TVH. Sometimes this repair is done when weakened pelvic supports have displaced one or more of the pelvic organs (such as the urethra, bladder, or rectum), sometimes causing urinary incontinence, constipation, or defecation problems. Advantages include earlier ambulation, less postoperative pain, less anesthesia and operative time, less blood loss, no visible scar, and a shorter hospital stay. This approach is preferred for women if possible but specifically for elderly, obese, or debilitated women who are poor risks for abdominal surgery. The major disadvantage is increased risk of trauma to the bladder.

Removal of the ovaries at the time of hysterectomy remains controversial. In premenopausal women, without evidence of ovarian pathology, the ovaries are generally left to avoid forced surgical menopause. Because of the risk of ovarian cancer, some physicians recommend removal of ovaries in all women over 40 years old who undergo hysterectomy. Still others recommend removal of the ovaries in any woman with a family history of ovarian cancer. In any case, removal of the ovaries is not considered routine, and when a BSO is performed in a premenopausal woman, supplemental estrogen replacement therapy is recommended.

Dilation and Curettage

In the United States, *dilation and curettage (D&C)* is the most frequently performed minor gynecologic procedure. Indications for a D&C may be diagnostic or therapeutic. Diagnostic indications include evaluation for uterine malignancy, infertility evaluation, and investigation of dysfunctional uterine bleeding (DUB). Therapeutic indications include elective abortion, treatment of heavy bleeding, incomplete abortion, dysmenorrhea, and removal of polyps. Sometimes D&C is done after hysteroscopy, which is a procedure that allows visualization of the endometrial cavity and minor surgical procedures. Another procedure that can be done at the time of hysteroscopy is an endometrial ablation, which cauterizes endometrial tissue, preventing regeneration and further bleeding. This procedure is not recommended for women who desire pregnancy, and so a simple D&C may be more appropriate. All of these procedures can be done under general anesthesia, intravenous sedation, and/or regional anesthesia, and most are done as an outpatient procedure.

Uterine Ablation

Uterine ablation is frequently being used to treat abnormal uterine bleeding. Uterine ablation is a procedure using a variety of specialized instruments to destroy the innermost layer of the endometrium. The instruments often involve some type of heat source, such as cautery or a balloon filled with hot water. In most cases, this procedure is done in a day-surgery setting, and it will often immediately follow a hysteroscopy/D&C, if these procedures confirm the diagnosis of simple endometrial hyperplasia. The success rate varies, depending on the device used and the experience of the operator of the device.

Salpingectomy

The unilateral or bilateral removal of the fallopian tube is called a *salpingectomy*. Indications include diseases of the tube, sepsis, malignancy, and ectopic pregnancy of the fallopian tube. Salpingectomy for an ectopic pregnancy is generally an emergency procedure. The developing placental tissue erodes the fallopian tube and can cause rupture and hemorrhage once the tube is completely eroded. This procedure can be done via laparoscopy or via an open abdominal approach.

Oophorectomy

Oophorectomy is the unilateral or bilateral removal of the ovary. Indications include severe PID, malignancy, ectopic pregnancy, and symptomatic ovarian cysts. When both ovaries are removed in a premenopausal woman, abrupt surgical menopause occurs. In this case the woman will experience the same symptoms she might in natural menopause: Decreased libido, decreased vaginal lubrication, hot flashes and/or night sweats, and decreased sensation in the lower vaginal tract. These symptoms can be treated with estrogen replacement.

Vulvectomy

A *simple vulvectomy* is the removal of the labia majora, labia minora, and clitoris. *Radical vulvectomy* is the removal of the entire vulva, including the skin and the fat of the femoral triangle and the pelvic lymph nodes. Skin grafts may be necessary. A simple vulvectomy is performed for leukoplakia and intractable pruritus, whereas a radical procedure is done for malignant disease.

This disfiguring procedure is associated with marked psychosexual disturbances. Most women report decreased sexual arousal levels and low self-image. Sexual activity can be resumed within 3 months; however, significant adjustments will be necessary owing to the loss of sensory perception for foreplay. Stimulation of breasts, thighs, buttocks, or anterior abdominal wall can be suggested.

●○● NURSING MANAGEMENT

For the Woman Undergoing Gynecologic Surgery

Nursing Assessment and Diagnosis

Nursing assessment for all of the previously discussed surgical procedures includes identifying the woman's physiologic, psychosocial, and sexual needs as she approaches her surgery. Additionally, it is important to understand her learning needs about the procedure and its effects. Some factors to consider are the age of the woman, her cultural background and educational level, the attitude of her partner and family, her preoperative status (physically and emotionally), and whether or not this involves a cancer diagnosis. The significance of her reproductive health to her self-image will be reflected in her attitudes about menstruation, childbearing, body image, and sexuality. Many of these procedures have the potential to involve loss, so grieving, anger, sadness, and loss of control are just a few of the feelings the woman may experience.

Nursing diagnoses that may apply to a woman facing gynecologic surgery include:

- ***Knowledge, Deficient***, related to lack of information about preoperative routines, postoperative activities, and expected postoperative changes
- ***Fear*** related to the unknown outcome and long-term implications of the surgery

(NANDA-I © 2017)

Nursing Plan and Implementation

Preoperative teaching may be brief, as in the instance of a simple D&C, or more extensive, as in the instance of hysterectomy. In any case, preoperative teaching should include information about the procedure, expected preparation, type of anesthesia to be used, possible risks and complications, postoperative care routines, and expected recovery time (Figure 6–3).

Routine postoperative care includes monitoring of physiologic responses, emotional responses, and nursing interventions to facilitate physical and emotional well-being specific to the procedure performed. The woman should be aware of potential postoperative complications and when to follow up with her surgeon. Additionally, it is important to discuss those psychosocial issues identified preoperatively, such as support at home, potential for sadness or depression related to the loss she has experienced, and expected sexual and self-image fears. In some instances, it may be necessary to refer the woman to a professional therapist who can help her adjust to these dramatic changes.

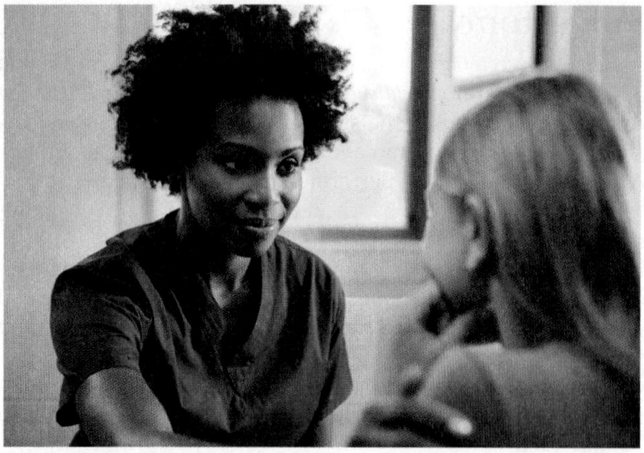

Figure 6–3 **A nurse provides preoperative teaching for a woman who will be undergoing gynecologic surgery.**

SOURCE: Monkey Business Images/Shutterstock.

Evaluation

Expected outcomes of nursing care include:

- The woman can discuss the reasons for her surgery, the alternatives, and the aspects of self-care after surgery.
- The woman has an uneventful recovery without complications.
- The woman feels she is able to ask questions and obtain support.
- The woman participates in decision making about her care.
- The woman is aware of available resources if she has physical or emotional concerns in the postoperative period.

Infertility

Infertility is defined as a failure to achieve a successful pregnancy after 12 months or more of regular, unprotected intercourse (Duke & Christianson, 2015). It has a profound emotional, psychologic, and economic impact on both the affected couple and society. The term **sterility** is applied when there is an absolute factor preventing reproduction. *Subfertility* is used to describe a couple who has difficulty conceiving because both partners have reduced fertility. *Primary infertility* refers to a woman with no prior pregnancies; *secondary infertility* refers to couples who have been unable to conceive after one or more successful pregnancies or who cannot sustain a pregnancy.

In the United States, approximately 15.5% of couples in their reproductive years are infertile (Greil, Slauson-Blevins, Tiemeyer et al., 2016). Public perception is that the incidence of infertility is increasing, but in fact there has been no significant change in the proportion of infertile couples in the United States. What has changed is that the demand for infertility services has increased in recent years because of delayed childbearing in women, an increase in the variety and effectiveness of reproductive technologies, an increase in tubal-related infertility because of sexually transmitted infections, and the relative scarcity of babies available for adoption (Duke & Christianson, 2015).

Essential Components of Fertility

Understanding the elements essential for normal fertility can help the nurse identify the many factors that may cause infertility. The components necessary for normal fertility are correlated with possible causes of deviation in Table 6–4. Infertility can be due to a male factor (30%), a female factor (60%), or either an unknown cause (unexplained infertility) or a problem with both partners (10%) (Duke & Christianson, 2015).

TABLE 6–4 Possible Causes of Infertility

NECESSARY NORMS	DEVIATIONS FROM NORMAL
Female	
Favorable cervical mucus	Cervicitis, cervical stenosis, use of coital lubricants, antisperm antibodies (immunologic response)
Clear passage between cervix and tubes	Myomas, adhesions, adenomyosis, polyps, endometritis, cervical stenosis, endometriosis, congenital anomalies (e.g., septate uterus, diethylstilbestrol [DES] exposure)
Patent tubes with normal motility	PID, peritubal adhesions, endometriosis, IUC, salpingitis (e.g., chlamydia, recurrent STIs), neoplasm, ectopic pregnancy, tubal ligation
Ovulation and release of ova	Primary ovarian failure, polycystic ovarian disease, hypothyroidism, pituitary tumor, lactation, periovarian adhesions, endometriosis, premature ovarian failure, hyperprolactinemia, Turner syndrome
No obstruction between ovary and tubes	Adhesions, endometriosis, PID
Endometrial preparation	Anovulation, luteal phase defect, malformation, uterine infection, Asherman syndrome
Male	
Normal semen analysis	Abnormalities of sperm or semen, polyspermia, congenital defect in testicular development, mumps after adolescence, cryptorchidism, infections, gonadal exposure to x-rays, chemotherapy, smoking, alcohol abuse, malnutrition, chronic or acute metabolic disease, medications (e.g., morphine, aspirin, ibuprofen), cocaine, marijuana use, constrictive underclothing, heat
Unobstructed genital tract	Infections, tumors, congenital anomalies, vasectomy, strictures, trauma, varicocele
Normal genital tract secretions	Infections, autoimmunity to semen, tumors
Ejaculate deposited at the cervix	Premature ejaculation, impotence, hypospadias, retrograde ejaculation (e.g., as can occur with diabetes), neurologic cord lesions, obesity (inhibiting adequate vaginal penetration)

Young couples with no history that is suggestive of reproductive disorders should be referred for infertility evaluation if they have been unable to conceive after at least 1 year of attempting to achieve pregnancy. An earlier workup is indicated in couples with positive history for fertility-lowering disease or advancing maternal age. For women over age 35, it is appropriate to refer the couple after only 6 months of unprotected intercourse without conception or earlier if clinically indicated. See *Genetic Facts: Down Syndrome and Fertility*.

Genetic Facts **Down Syndrome and Fertility**

Approximately half of all women with Down syndrome are fertile and can become pregnant. However, they have a higher incidence of miscarriage, especially as they age, which reduces the incidence of live born offspring with Down syndrome (Stern, Biron, & Moses, 2016). It is estimated that about 35 to 50% of children born to women with Down syndrome will also have trisomy 21 or other developmental disabilities (National Down Syndrome Society, 2018). Information about fertility in men with Down syndrome is limited, although it does appear to be reduced. It is unknown if they are at an increased risk to have offspring with trisomy 21.

Initial Investigation: Physical and Psychosocial Issues

The easiest and least intrusive infertility testing approach is used first. The nurse provides information about the most fertile times to have intercourse during the menstrual cycle. Teaching the couple the signs and timing of ovulation, the most effective times for intercourse within the cycle, and other fertility-awareness behaviors may solve the problem (see *Teaching Highlights: Suggestions for Improving Fertility*). Primary assessment, including a comprehensive history (with a discussion of genetic conditions) and physical examination for any obvious causes of infertility, is done before a costly, time-consuming, and emotionally trying investigation is initiated.

The basic infertility investigation depends on the couple's history and usually includes assessment of ovarian function, cervical mucus adequacy and receptivity to sperm, sperm adequacy, tubal patency, and the general condition of the pelvic organs.

The mutual desire to have children is a cornerstone of many marriages. A fertility problem is a deeply personal, emotion-laden area in a couple's life. The self-esteem of one or both partners may be threatened if the inability to conceive is perceived as a lack of virility or femininity. It is never easy to discuss one's sexual activity, especially when potentially irreversible problems with fertility exist. The nurse can provide comfort to couples by offering a sympathetic ear, a nonjudgmental approach, and appropriate information and instructions throughout the diagnostic and therapeutic process. The first interview should involve both partners and include a comprehensive history and physical examination. Table 6–5 lists the items in a complete infertility physical workup and laboratory evaluation for both partners. A semen analysis is one of the first diagnostic tests done before moving on to more invasive diagnostic procedures involving the woman. Figure 6–4 outlines the couple's history and physical examination data, diagnostic tests usually performed, and healthcare interventions used in cases of infertility.

Assessment of the Woman's Fertility

After a thorough history and physical examination, both partners may undergo tests to identify causes of infertility. A thorough female evaluation includes assessment of the hypothalamic–pituitary axis in terms of ovulatory function, as well as structure and function of the cervix, uterus, fallopian tubes, and ovaries. See Chapter 9 for an in-depth discussion of the female reproductive cycle.

EVALUATION OF OVULATORY FACTORS

Ovulation problems are a common cause of infertility.

Testing For Ovulation

- **Basal body temperature (BBT)** recording is the least expensive method for detecting ovulation, but interpretation of these charts can be complex and have wide variations depending on who is reading them.
- Serum testing is generally used for assessment of ovulatory function in women with irregular menstrual cycles.

TEACHING HIGHLIGHTS | Suggestions for Improving Fertility

- Avoid douching and artificial lubricants (gels, oils, saliva) that can alter sperm motility. Prevent alteration of pH of vagina and introduction of spermicidal agents.
- Promote retention of sperm. The male superior position with female remaining recumbent for at least 20 to 30 minutes after intercourse maximizes the number of sperm reaching the cervix.
- Avoid leakage of sperm. Have the woman elevate her hips with a pillow after intercourse for 20 to 30 minutes to allow liquefaction of seminal fluid and motility of the sperm toward the egg. Avoid getting up to urinate or shower for 1 hour after intercourse.
- Maximize the potential for fertilization. Instruct the couple that it is optimal if sexual intercourse occurs every other day during the fertile period. Because each woman's menstrual cycle varies in length, the fertile period can extend from cycle day (CD) 7 through CD 17. Note CD 1 is considered the first day of actual menstrual flow.
- Avoid emphasizing conception during sexual encounters to decrease anxiety and potential sexual dysfunction.
- Maintain adequate nutrition and reduce stress. Stress reduction techniques and good nutritional habits increase sperm production.
- Explore other methods to increase fertility awareness, such as home assessment of cervical mucus and basal body temperature (BBT) recordings, and use of a home ovulation predictor kit (tests LH surge to time intercourse).
- Consider incorporating culturally appropriate methods to enhance fertility.

TABLE 6–5 Initial Infertility Physical Workup and Laboratory Evaluations

FEMALE	MALE
Physical Examination	**Physical Examination**
Assessment of general health	Assessment of general health
Endocrine evaluation of thyroid	Endocrine evaluation (e.g., presence of gynecomastia)
Optic fundi evaluation for presence of increased intracranial pressure, especially in oligomenorrheal or amenorrheal women (possible pituitary tumor)	Abnormal hair patterns
Reproductive features (including breast and external genital area)	**Urologic Examination**
Physical ability to tolerate pregnancy	Presence or absence of phimosis
Pelvic Examination	Location of urethral meatus
Pap smear	Size and consistency of each testis, vas deferens, and epididymis
Culture for gonorrhea, if indicated	Presence of varicocele
Signs of vaginal infections	**Rectal Examination**
Shape of escutcheon (e.g., does pubic hair distribution resemble that of a male's?)	Size and consistency of the prostate with microscopic evaluation of prostate fluid for signs of infection
Size of clitoris (enlargement caused by endocrine disorders)	Size and consistency of seminal vesicles
Evaluation of cervix: Old lacerations, tears, erosion, polyps, condition and shape of os, signs of infection	**Laboratory Examination**
Bimanual Examination	Complete blood count
Size, shape, position, and motility of uterus	Sedimentation rate, if indicated
Presence of congenital anomalies	Serology
Presence of endometriosis	Urinalysis
Evaluation of adnexa: Ovarian size, cysts, fixations, or tumors	Rh factor and blood grouping
Rectovaginal Examination	Semen analysis
Presence of retroflexed or retroverted uterus	Testicular biopsy, buccal smear, if indicated
Laboratory Examination	Hormonal assays, FSH, LH, prolactin
Complete blood count	
Sedimentation rate, if indicated	
Serology	
Urinalysis	
Rh factor and blood grouping	
Rubella immunoglobulin (IgG)	
FSH level regardless of age and regularity of menstrual cycles	
Other tests as indicated, depending on age and regularity of menstrual cycles	

A mid–luteal phase serum progesterone level should be obtained approximately 1 week before expected menstruation to document ovulation. A progesterone level greater than 3 ng/mL collected between days 19 and 23 for a typical 28-day cycle is evidence of recent ovulation. If the progesterone level is less than 3 ng/mL, an evaluation of anovulation is warranted (Duke & Christianson, 2015). This includes measurement of serum prolactin, TSH, FSH, and assessment for PCOS.

- Over-the-counter urinary ovulation prediction kits are also available. These kits detect LH and predict the timing of the LH surge, which reliably predict ovulation. However, they have false-positive and false-negative rates. Serum confirmation may be useful for clients unable to detect urinary LH surge.
- **Endometrial biopsy (EMB)** provides information about the effects of progesterone produced by the corpus luteum after ovulation and endometrial receptivity. EMB is reliable for determining the presence of ovulation. Histologic evidence of secretory endometrium detected by endometrial biopsy shows ovulation and corpus luteum formation. However, it is not effective for diagnosing luteal phase deficiency.
- **Transvaginal ultrasound** is the method of choice for follicular monitoring of women undergoing induction cycles, for timing ovulation for insemination and intercourse, for retrieving oocytes for in vitro fertilization (IVF), and for monitoring early pregnancy.

EVALUATION OF CERVICAL FACTORS

As ovulation approaches, the ovary increases its secretion of estrogen and produces changes in the cervical mucus. The amount of mucus increases 10-fold. At ovulation, mucus elasticity (spinnbarkeit) increases. Excellent spinnbarkeit exists when the mucus can be stretched 8 to 10 cm or longer. Mucous elasticity is determined by using two glass slides (see Figure 4–1A in Chapter 4) or by grasping some mucus at the external os.

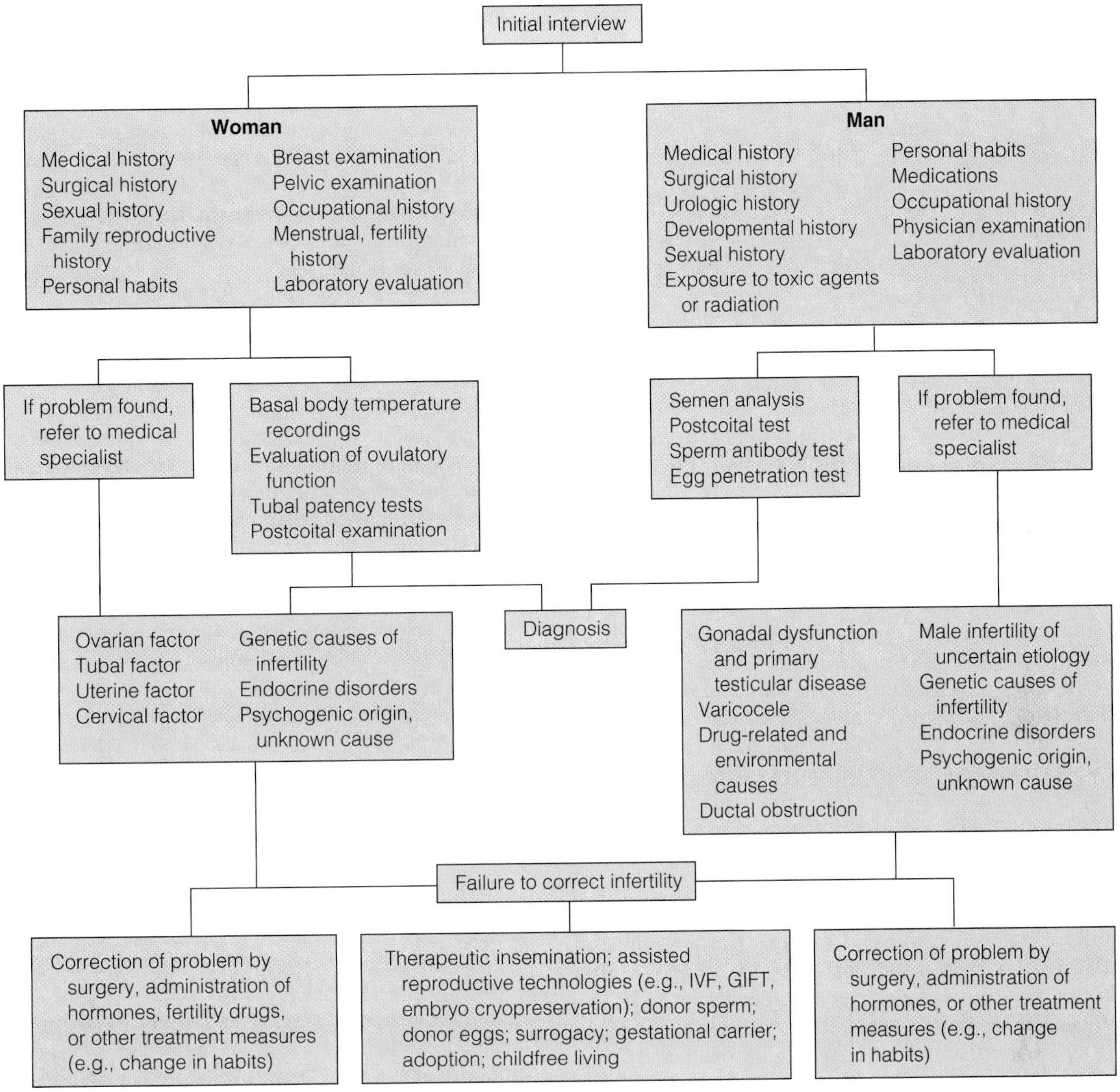

Figure 6–4 **Flowchart for management of the infertile couple.**

The **ferning capacity** (crystallization) (see Figure 4–1B) of the cervical mucus also increases as ovulation approaches. Ferning is caused by decreased levels of salt and water interacting with the glycoproteins in the mucus during the ovulatory period and is thus an indirect indication of estrogen production. To test for ferning, mucus is obtained from the cervical os, spread on a glass slide, allowed to air dry, and examined under the microscope. Within 24 to 48 hours postovulation, rising levels of progesterone markedly decrease the quantity of cervical mucus and increase its viscosity and cellularity. The resulting absence of spinnbarkeit and ferning capacity decreases sperm survival.

To be receptive to sperm, cervical mucus must be thin, clear, watery, profuse, alkaline, and acellular. As shown in Figure 6–5A, the mazelike microscopic mucoid strands align in a parallel manner to allow for easy sperm passage. The mucus is termed inhospitable if these changes do not occur (Figure 6–5B).

Cervical mucus inhospitable to sperm survival can have several causes, some of which are treatable. Cone biopsy, electrocautery, or cryosurgery of the cervix may remove large numbers of mucus-producing glands, creating a "dry cervix" that decreases sperm survival. Intrauterine insemination (IUI) is often the most appropriate therapy to overcome these obstacles. When mucosal hostility to sperm is because of cervical infection, antimicrobial therapy may be effective.

The cervix can also be the site of secretory immunologic reactions in which antisperm antibodies are produced, causing agglutination or immobilization of sperm. The treatment for antisperm antibodies may include IUI of the man's washed sperm to bypass cervical factors.

EVALUATION OF UTERINE STRUCTURES AND TUBAL PATENCY

Uterine abnormalities are a relatively uncommon cause of infertility but should be considered. Tubal patency and uterine structure are usually evaluated by hysterosalpingography or laparoscopy. Other invasive tests used to evaluate only the uterine cavity are hysteroscopy and sonohysterography. Hysteroscopy may be performed earlier in the evaluation if the woman's history suggests the potential for adhesive disease or uterine abnormalities.

Hysterosalpingography. Hysterosalpingography (HSG), or *hysterography*, involves the instillation of a radiopaque substance into the uterine cavity for visualization. In addition, the dye and

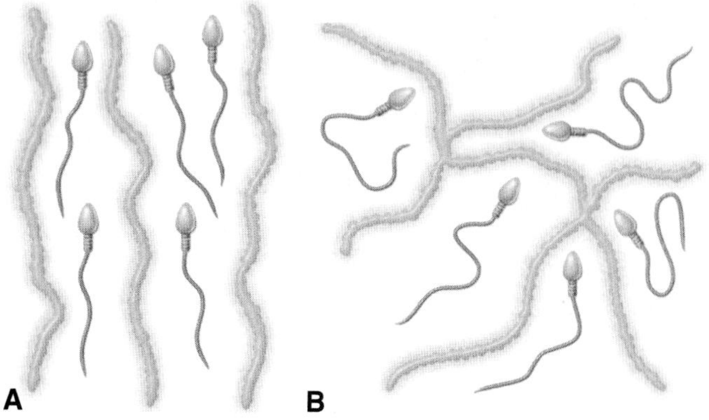

Figure 6–5 **Sperm passage through cervical mucus. A. Appearance at the time of ovulation with channels favoring efficient sperm penetration and migration upward. B. Unfavorable mazelike configuration found at other times during the menstrual cycle.**

injection pressure used in HSG may have a therapeutic effect, causing the flushing of debris, breaking of adhesions, or induction of peristalsis by the instillation of the radiopaque substance.

HSG should be performed in the early follicular phase of the cycle, within 1 week of the end of menses, to avoid interrupting an early pregnancy. This timing also avoids the lush secretory changes in the endometrium that occur after ovulation, which may prevent the passage of the dye through the tubes and present a false picture of obstruction of the entry point of the fallopian tube into the uterus.

Hysteroscopy and Laparoscopy. Hysteroscopy is the definitive method for both diagnosis and treatment of intrauterine pathology (Duke & Christianson, 2015). Hysteroscopy permits evaluation of any areas of suspicion within the uterine cavity or fallopian tubes revealed by the HSG. It can be done in conjunction with a laparoscopy or independently in the office and does not require general anesthesia. A fiberoptic instrument called a *hysteroscope* is placed into the uterus for further evaluation of polyps, fibroids, or structural variations. The newest generation hyperscope allows for minor operative procedures to be performed in the office setting.

Laparoscopy enables direct visualization of the pelvic organs to evaluate endometriosis and pelvic adhesions. It is used only if there is strong clinical suspicion of these conditions or before considering more aggressive treatments with higher risks and/or costs. In routine preanesthesia instructions, the woman is told that she may have some discomfort from organ displacement and shoulder and chest pain caused by gas in the abdomen as a result of distending the peritoneal cavity with carbon dioxide gas in order to visualize the pelvic organs better. Using postoperative pain medication and assuming a supine position may help relieve discomfort caused by any remaining gas.

Assessment of the Man's Fertility

Male infertility can be caused by numerous factors, some of which can be identified and are reversible, such as ductal obstruction and varicocele (an abnormal dilation of scrotal veins). Other identifiable conditions are not reversible, such as bilateral testicular atrophy secondary to viral orchitis and congenital bilateral absence of the vas deferens. Idiopathic male infertility factor occurs when the etiology of an abnormal semen analysis is not identifiable.

If a male infertility factor is present, it is usually defined by the findings of an abnormal semen analysis. A semen analysis of sperm quality, quantity, and motility is the single most important diagnostic study of the male partner. The sample is usually obtained by masturbation after 3 days of abstinence. It should be done early in the couple's evaluation, before invasive testing of the woman. A minimum of two separate analyses is recommended for confirmation.

Sperm analysis provides information about sperm motility and morphology and a determination of the absolute number of spermatozoa present. Although low numbers and motility may indicate compromised fertility, other parameters, such as morphology, motion patterns, and progression, are important prognostic indicators. The quality of sperm decreases with increasing paternal age and may result in chromosomal damage. For example, fathers older than 40 years may be at an increased risk for offspring with chromosomal abnormalities or new gene mutations.

Spermatozoa have been shown to possess intrinsic antigens that can provoke male immunologic infertility. Any disruption in the blood–testes barrier, such as vasectomy reversals, or genital trauma, such as testicular torsion, can lead to the production of antisperm antibodies (ASAs).

Treatment for ASAs is directed toward preventing the formation of antibodies or arresting the underlying mechanism that compromises sperm function. The treatment of choice for clinically significant ASAs is intracytoplasmic sperm injection (ICSI) in conjunction with IVF. If the man's history indicates, he may be referred to a urologist for further testing.

Genetic Facts **Male Fertility**

Genetic factors may affect male fertility. Men with oligospermia (semen with a low concentration of sperm) and nonobstructive azoospermia (impaired or nonexistent sperm production) have an increased risk for chromosomal abnormalities and Y chromosome deletions.

Methods of Infertility Management

Methods of managing infertility include pharmacologic agents, intrauterine insemination (IUI), IVF, and other assisted reproductive techniques. In addition, many couples choose adoption as their preferred response to infertility.

PHARMACOLOGIC AGENTS

The pharmacologic treatment chosen depends on the specific cause of infertility.

Clomiphene Citrate. Oral *clomiphene citrate* (Clomid, Serophene) is often used as first-line therapy for women with normal ovaries, a normal prolactin level, and an intact pituitary gland. It works by binding to estrogen receptors in the hypothalamus and pituitary gland. This blocks the negative feedback of circulating estrogen and stimulates a release of GnRH, LH, and FSH, thereby inducing ovulation (Wilson, Shannon, & Shields, 2017). Ovulation is restored in 70% of women treated with clomiphene, but fewer than half achieve pregnancy (Tredway, Schertz, Bock, et al., 2011).

The antiestrogenic effects of clomiphene may cause a decrease in cervical mucus production and endometrial lining development. Other side effects include vasomotor flushes, abdominal distention and ovarian enlargement secondary to follicular growth (bloating) and multiple corpus luteum formation, pain, soreness, breast discomfort, nausea and vomiting, visual symptoms (spots, flashes), headaches, dryness or loss of hair, and multiple pregnancies.

For the first course of clomiphene citrate, the woman usually takes 50 mg/day orally for 5 days from CD 3 to CD 7 or CD 5 to CD 9. Ovulation should be confirmed to ensure that if continued doses are needed, they are at the lowest possible dose.

The woman should be knowledgeable about side effects and call her healthcare provider if they occur. The antiestrogenic effects of this drug were discussed previously. Although rare, visual disturbances can be permanent and should be treated immediately. When visual disturbances (flashes, blurring, spots) occur, the woman should avoid bright lighting.

Most women who conceive do so within the first six cycles, although the medication can be continued for 12 cycles. An ophthalmologic exam is indicated at regular intervals if clomiphene is continued for more than 1 year (Wilson et al., 2017). Failure to conceive after clomiphene induction is an indication to expand the diagnostic evaluation or to change the overall treatment plan if evaluation is complete.

Gonadotropins. *Human menopausal gonadotropins (hMGs)* are indicated as a first line of therapy for anovulatory infertile women with low to normal levels of gonadotropins (FSH and LH). It is a second line of therapy in women who fail to ovulate or conceive with clomiphene citrate therapy and in women undergoing controlled ovarian stimulation with assisted reproduction.

Gonadotropin therapy requires close observation with serum estradiol levels and ultrasound. Follicle development must be monitored to minimize the risk of multiple pregnancies and to avoid ovarian hyperstimulation syndrome.

SAFETY ALERT!

Ovarian hyperstimulation syndrome (OHSS) is a potentially life-threatening complication of ovulation induction and can, in its most severe form, result in massive ovarian enlargement and multiple cysts, hemoconcentration, and third-space accumulation of fluid. This can lead to renal failure, hypovolemic shock, thromboembolism, acute respiratory distress syndrome, and death.

The daily dose of medication given is titrated based on serum estradiol and ultrasound findings, but usually starts with a dose of 50 to 100 IU daily. Human chorionic gonadotropin (hCG) is used to trigger ovulation once ovarian follicles are mature. The couple is advised to have intercourse 24 to 36 hours after hCG administration and for the next 2 days. Women who elect to undergo ovarian stimulation with gonadotropins have usually passed through all other forms of management without conceiving. Strong emotional support and thorough education are needed because of the numerous office visits and injections that are required. Often the partner is instructed, with return demonstration, to administer the daily injections. The risk of multiple gestations is higher with gonadotropin therapy than with clomiphene citrate therapy.

Letrozole. Originally developed for the treatment of advanced breast cancer in postmenopausal women, letrozole is more commonly being used off label for ovulation induction. This aromatase inhibitor blocks the conversion of androgens to estrogens. When estradiol levels are low, there is less negative feedback on the hypothalamus and pituitary and increased levels of GnRH and FSH to stimulate follicular development. Letrozole can be used in women who experience side effects from or do not respond to clomiphene. Like clomiphene, it is given for 5 consecutive days starting as early as day 3 of the cycle.

Bromocriptine. High prolactin levels may impair the glandular production of FSH and LH or block their action on the ovaries. When hyperprolactinemia accompanies anovulation, the infertility may be treated with bromocriptine (Parlodel). This medication acts directly on the prolactin-secreting cells in the anterior pituitary. It inhibits the pituitary's secretion of prolactin, thus preventing suppression of the secretion of FSH and LH. This restores normal menstrual cycles and induces ovulation by allowing FSH and LH production.

GnRH. *GnRH* is a therapeutic tool for inducing ovulation, but its use is limited to women who have insufficient endogenous release of GnRH or it is used adjunctively with gonadotropin therapy. Pulsatile GnRH therapy is administered by continuous intravenous infusion with a portable infusion pump.

Insulin-Sensitizing Agents. Approximately 80% of anovulatory women have PCOS, causing insulin resistance and hyperinsulinemia. Strategies to induce ovulation include weight loss followed by oral treatment with clomiphene, aromatase inhibitors including letrozole, or gonadotropin therapy. However, hyperinsulinemia may cause these women to be more resistant to treatment. Recently, studies have shown that oral hypoglycemia agents (e.g., metformin and rosiglitazone) can induce ovulation in women with PCOS. Clinical trials are underway to determine the appropriateness of oral hypoglycemic agents with and without clomiphene in the infertility setting.

INTRAUTERINE INSEMINATION

Intrauterine insemination (IUI) has replaced the previously used term *artificial insemination* and involves the depositing of semen at the cervical os or in the uterus by mechanical means. **Donor insemination (DI)** is the current term for the use of sperm from a donor rather than the woman's partner.

IUI is generally indicated for the following:

- Seminal deficiencies as oligospermia (low sperm count), asthenospermia (decreased motility), and teratospermia (low percentage, abnormal morphology)
- Anatomic defects accompanied by inadequate deposition of semen such as hypospadia (a congenital abnormal male urethral opening on the underside of the penis)
- Ejaculatory dysfunction (such as retrograde ejaculation)
- Cases of unexplained infertility
- Some cases of female factor infertility, such as scant or inhospitable mucus, persistent cervicitis, or cervical stenosis.

The couple undergoing genetic counseling may consider assisted reproduction techniques, such as intrauterine insemination using donor sperm (donor insemination [DI]). This alternative is appropriate in several instances; for example, if the man has an autosomal dominant disease, DI would decrease to zero

CASE STUDY: Melissa Bond-James

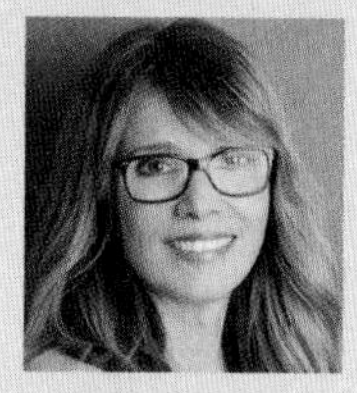

SOURCE: Kinga/ Shutterstock

Melissa presents to her appointment and appears upset. She says that her wife, Nancy, was recently diagnosed with uterine fibroids, and they are worried that a hysterectomy will be recommended for her. Melissa is concerned because Nancy had voiced the possibility of wanting to carry a pregnancy when they expand their family in the future. Melissa asks if there is any procedure available that would enable Nancy's eggs to be retrieved prior to undergoing hysterectomy.

Questions to Ponder

Does Nancy have options for controlling bleeding with a diagnosis of fibroids other than a hysterectomy? How would you explain to Melissa the procedure that can be used to retrieve Nancy's eggs? If Nancy underwent successful donor insemination prior to the hysterectomy, could her embryos later be implanted into Melissa's uterus?

the risk of having an affected child (if the sperm donor is not at risk) because the child would not inherit any genes from the affected parent. If the man is affected with a male sex-linked disorder and does not wish to continue the gene in the family (all his daughters will be carriers), DI would be an alternative to terminating all pregnancies with a female fetus. If the man is a carrier for a balanced translocation and if termination of pregnancy is against family ethics, DI is an appropriate alternative. If both parents are carriers of an autosomal recessive disorder, DI lowers the risk to a very low level or to zero if a carrier test is available. Finally, donor sperm may be appropriate if the family is at high risk for a multifactorial disorder or in cases of azoospermia (absence of sperm), severe oligospermia, or asthenospermia. In the past several years, indications for donor insemination have expanded to include single women or lesbians who want to become pregnant. Some states have specified the parental rights of single women and donors, but most are silent on this issue.

DI has become more complicated and expensive in the past decade because of the need for strict screening and processing procedures to prevent transmission of a genetic defect or sexually transmitted infection to the offspring or recipient. Guidelines have been established and updated by the American Society for Reproductive Medicine (ASRM, 2018) that include mandatory medical (genetic) and infectious disease screening of both donor and recipient, the need for informed consent from all parties, the need to limit the number of pregnancies per donor, and the need for accurate means of record keeping. Finally, because of the risk of transmitting infectious diseases, donated sperm must be frozen and quarantined for 6 months from the time of acquisition, and the donor must be retested before sperm can be released for use.

Numerous factors need to be evaluated before DI is performed. Has every possible effort been made to diagnose and treat the cause of the male infertility? Do tests indicate normal fertility and sperm–ovum transport in the woman? Has the couple had an opportunity to discuss this option with an infertility counselor to explore the issues of secrecy, disclosure, and potential feelings of loss the couple (particularly the male partner) may feel about not having a genetic child? Are there any religious constraints? After making the decision, the couple should allow themselves time to assess further their concerns and explore their feelings individually and together to ensure that this option is acceptable to both. See *Developing Cultural Competence: Infertility Treatments.*

Developing Cultural Competence Infertility Treatments

The acceptance of infertility treatments varies widely around the world. Some belief systems do not allow various treatments because using a fertility treatment is considered interfering with God's design or because the treatment itself is seen as tainted or sinful. For example, artificial reproductive technology in predominantly Muslim countries is accepted and encouraged because adoption is not an accepted solution. However, the approved methods for treating infertility are limited to use of intrauterine insemination using the husband's sperm or IVF involving the fertilization of the wife's ovum by the husband's sperm because the use of donor sperm, egg, or embryo is condemned by Islamic law (Obeisat, Gharaibeh, Owis, et al., 2012).

In Jewish cultures, infertile couples are encouraged to try all possible means to have children, including egg and sperm donation. However, owing to the *Niddah* laws of separation, Orthodox Jewish women are forbidden from engaging in sexual intercourse from the start of their menstruation until 7 days after the end of menses when they immerse themselves in a ritual bath (*mikveh*). Women with unexpected spotting or bleeding must seek the advice of a rabbi or physician, and if uterine bleeding is diagnosed, she may not participate in intercourse for 7 days thereafter (Haimov-Kochman, Adler, Ein-Mor, et al., 2012). For this reason, Jewish law has a significant impact on fertility, particularly for women with irregular and unpredictable cycles. If the infertility is because of a male factor, artificial insemination with sperm from a non-Jewish sperm donor is acceptable because "Jewishness" is conferred through the matriline. IVF and embryo transfer (ET) are also acceptable artificial insemination methods because they do not involve putting sperm into another's wife.

Note: It is unwise to attribute specific attitudes or beliefs to all members of a cultural group. The information in the Developing Cultural Competence boxes offers possible insights into caring for women from different cultural groups.

IN VITRO FERTILIZATION

In vitro fertilization (IVF) is selectively used in cases in which infertility has resulted from tubal factors, mucus abnormalities, male infertility, unexplained infertility, male and female immunologic infertility, and cervical factors. It has an overall success rate of 36.8% (Duke & Christianson, 2015). In IVF, a woman's ovaries are stimulated by a combination of medications, one or more oocytes are aspirated from her ovaries and fertilized in the laboratory, and then are placed into her uterus after normal embryo development has begun. These steps occur over a 2-week period of time, known as an *IVF cycle*. If the procedure is successful, the embryo continues to develop in the uterus, and pregnancy proceeds naturally.

Fertility drugs are used to induce ovulation before the process of IVF begins. Follicular growth is monitored frequently with ultrasound and hormonal assays. Monitoring usually begins around CD 5, and medications are titrated according to individual response. When the follicles have grown to an appropriate size, hCG is given to induce final egg maturation and control the induction of ovulation. Egg retrieval is performed approximately 34 to 36 hours later before ovulation occurs.

In the majority of cases, egg retrieval is performed by a transvaginal approach under ultrasound guidance (Figure 6–6A). It is an outpatient procedure performed with sedation, usually intravenous propofol but occasionally conscious sedation or a regional block is used. A needle guide that helps direct the aspirating needle through the posterior vaginal wall into the follicle is attached to the vaginal ultrasound probe (Figure 6–6B). Many follicles can be aspirated with only one puncture, and the procedure generally lasts no more than 30 minutes. Many physicians use prophylactic antibiotics to reduce the risk of infection from the procedure.

Oocytes are then mixed with spermatozoa in culture medium and fertilization is confirmed about 17 hours later by observing two pronuclei within the zygote (Figure 6–7). After fertilization, the cells will continue to divide exponentially every 12 to 14 hours so that the embryo is approximately eight cells, about 72 hours after retrieval. Many programs will transfer these *cleavage stage* embryos at this time. Some programs wait until day 5 when the embryo is at the *blastocyst stage*, with the theory that better-quality embryos can be transferred at a time when natural implantation would be occurring. After the procedure, the woman is advised to engage in only minimal activity for 12 to 24 hours. To optimize endometrial receptivity, progesterone supplementation is prescribed at the time of oocyte retrieval or embryo transfer to promote implantation and support the early pregnancy.

OTHER ASSISTED REPRODUCTIVE TECHNIQUES

Other assisted reproductive techniques include procedures for transfer of gametes, zygotes, or embryos; cryopreservation of embryos; IVF using donor oocytes; assisted hatching (AH) of the embryo; and use of a gestational carrier.

Gamete intrafallopian transfer (GIFT) involves the retrieval of oocytes by laparoscopy; immediate placement of the oocytes in a catheter with washed, motile sperm; and placement of the gametes into the fimbriated end of the fallopian tube. Fertilization occurs in the fallopian tube as with normal conception (in vivo) rather than in the laboratory (in vitro). The fertilized egg then travels through the fallopian tube to the uterus for implantation as in normal reproduction.

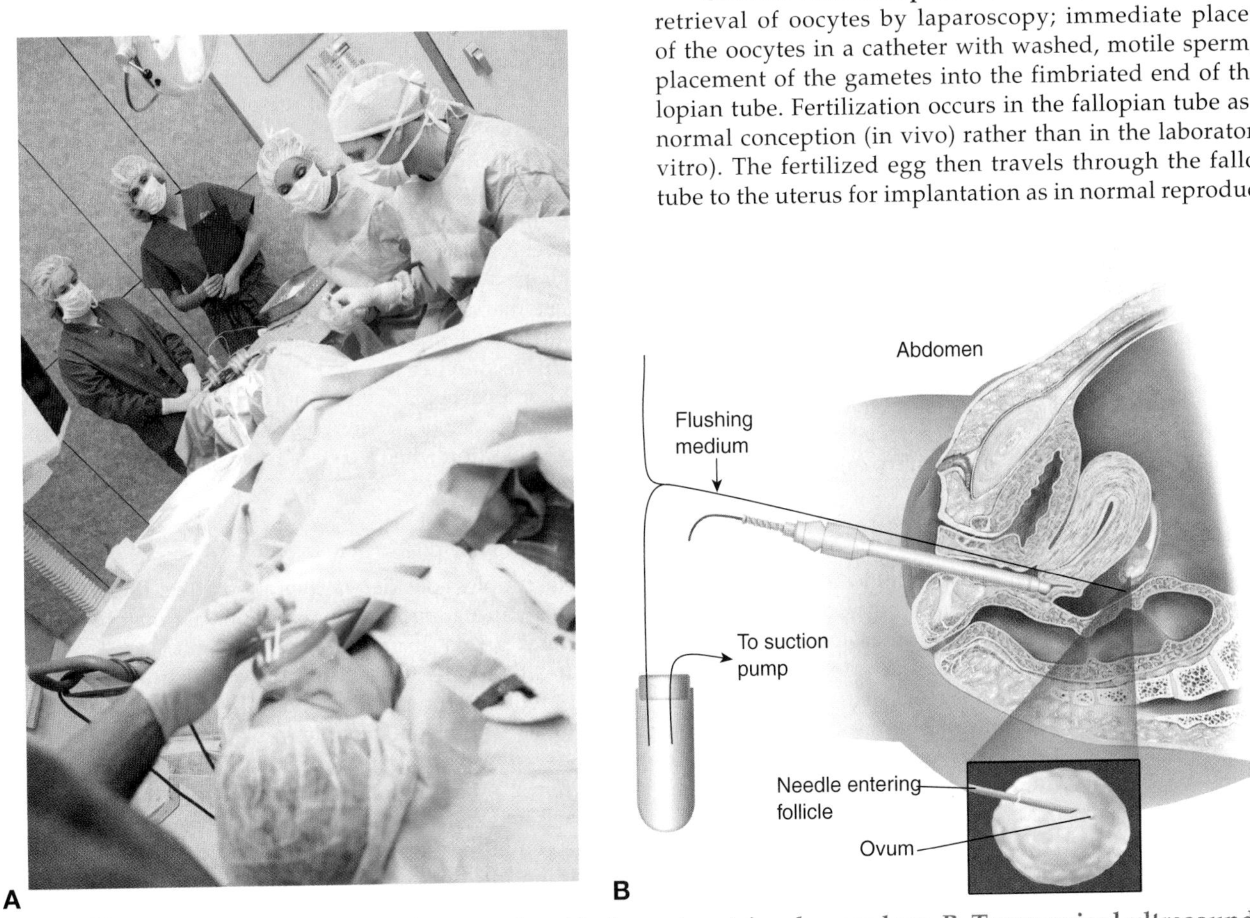

Figure 6–6 **A. Patient undergoing ultrasound-guided oocyte retrieval procedure. B. Transvaginal ultrasound-guided oocyte retrieval.**

SOURCE: A. Cathy Yeulet/123RF.

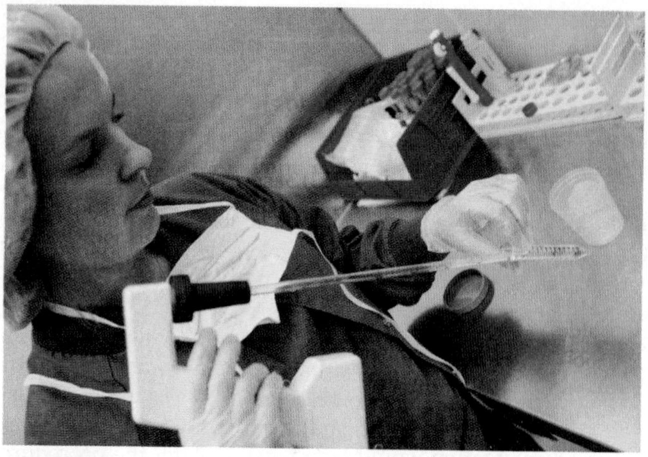

Figure 6–7 **Embryologist processing sample.**

SOURCE: Cathy Yeulet/123RF.

GIFT may be more acceptable than other procedures such as zygote intrafallopian transfer (ZIFT) to adherents of some religions because fertilization does not occur outside the woman's body.

From the GIFT technology evolved procedures such as **zygote intrafallopian transfer (ZIFT)** and **tubal embryo transfer (TET)**. In these procedures, eggs are retrieved and incubated with the man's sperm. However, the eggs are transferred back to the woman's body at a much earlier stage of cell division than in IVF and, as in GIFT, are placed in the fallopian tube or tubes and not the uterus. In TET, the placement is done at the embryo stage. These procedures allow fertilization to be documented, which is not possible with GIFT, and the pregnancy rate is theoretically increased when the fertilized ovum is placed in the fallopian tube.

Assisted hatching (AH), a micromanipulation procedure that creates a small hole in the zona pellicuda, thus increasing the rate of implantation, has proved to be an effective adjunct therapy in IVF. IVF using a gestational carrier allows infertile women who are genetically sound but unable to carry a pregnancy to exercise the option of having their own biologic child. Other technologies involve oocyte donation (women donate ovum to another woman) and cryopreservation of the embryo (embryos are frozen and then thawed at a later date).

PREIMPLANTATION GENETIC DIAGNOSIS

Recent advances in micromanipulation allow a single cell to be removed from the embryo for genetic study. Couples at risk for having a detectable single-gene or chromosomal anomaly may wish to undergo such *preimplantation genetic testing*, called *blastomere analysis* or, more recently, *preimplantation genetic diagnosis* (PGD). PGD is used when one or both genetic parents carry a gene mutation or balanced chromosome rearrangement to determine whether that mutation or unbalanced chromosomal complement has been passed to the oocyte or embryo (Bay et al., 2016). *Preimplantation genetic screening (PGS)* is used when the genetic parents are known or presumed to have normal chromosomes, and their embryos are screened for aneuploidy with the purpose of increasing the likelihood of a viable pregnancy with normal chromosomes. The single cell is obtained from an eight-cell embryo and the genetic content of the cell is examined using polymerase chain reaction or comparative genome hybridization (Bay et al., 2016). Biopsied embryos are examined so that embryos affected with a particular genetic disease or chromosomal abnormality are not placed in the mother. Both PGD and PGS can produce false-positive and false-negative results. Prenatal diagnostic testing to confirm the results is strongly encouraged.

The diagnosis of genetic disorders before implantation provides couples with the option of foregoing the attempt to establish a pregnancy and thereby avoiding a difficult decision about terminating an affected pregnancy. This technology also raises several ethical issues, including:

- Identification of couples at risk. There is a need for criteria that identify couples at risk for diseases that constitute significant hardship and suffering so that "wrongful birth" cases can be avoided.
- Availability of and access to centers providing PGD. Should society provide access for those at risk for genetic transfer of disease but without the financial resources to pay for the services?
- Analysis of blastomeres for sex chromosome testing when a genetic disorder carried on the sex chromosomes is suspected. In X-linked diseases, the only way to prevent the disorder is to select against the blastomere with the Y chromosome.
- Identification of late-onset diseases. The Human Genome Project has aided in the identification of genetic markers for late-onset disease. Couples may wish to choose to implant blastomeres that do not carry these markers.
- Effect on the offspring as a result of removing cells from the embryo.
- Selection for nonmedical reasons and potential concern of eugenics "designer babies."

Sperm Sorting. *Sperm sorting* is a technology designed to select highly motile, morphologically viable sperm to increase the effectiveness of ART (Chinnasamy, Behr, & Demirci, 2016). It may also be used to separate sperm that primarily produce females or those that primarily produce males. Sorted sperm enriched with male- or female-producing sperm is then used for IUI or IVF. This technology is used to increase the likelihood of having a child of a particular gender in couples at risk for an X-linked genetic disorder or for couples interested in family balancing (gender selection when a couple has two or more children of the same gender).

ADOPTION

Infertile couples consider various alternatives for resolving their infertility, and adoption is one option that may be considered at several points during the treatment process. The adoption of a healthy American baby can be difficult and frustrating, often involving long waiting periods, continual setbacks, and high costs. Thus, many couples seek international adoption or consider adopting older children, children with handicaps, or children of mixed parentage because the adoption process in such cases is quicker and more children are available. Nurses in the community can assist couples considering adoption by providing information on community resources for adoption and support through the adoption process. Couples need support if they remain childless, either by choice or circumstance. Informational books, websites such as Childless by Choice, and support groups such as San Francisco RESOLVE's "living without children" are available for couples who remain childless by choice or circumstance.

PREGNANCY AFTER INFERTILITY

The feeling of being infertile does not necessarily disappear with pregnancy. Although there may be initial ecstasy, couples may face a whole new arena of fear and anxiety, and the parents-to-be often do not know where they "fit in." They may feel a great sense of isolation because those who have had no trouble conceiving cannot relate to the physical and emotional pain they endured to achieve the pregnancy. Contact with their past support system of other infertile couples may vanish when peers learn the couple has resolved their infertility. Although the desperation to become pregnant may have superseded the couple's ability to acknowledge their concerns about undergoing various treatments or procedures, questions about the repeated cycle of fertility drugs or the achievement of pregnancy through IVF technology or cryopreservation may now arise. The expectant couple may be very concerned about the potential of these treatments to adversely affect the fetus. Couples may need reassurance throughout the pregnancy to allay these anxieties. Research indicates that during pregnancy and postpartum, depressive symptoms are not associated with conception by IVF despite the psychologic stress women experience because of subfertility and its treatment (Gambadauro, Iliadis, Bränn, et al., 2017).

The nurse can assist couples who conceive after infertility by acknowledging their past experiences of infertility treatment; validating their fears and anxieties as they face childbirth classes, birth, and parenting issues; and providing support and education about what to anticipate physically and emotionally throughout the pregnancy. The nurse can also counsel couples that infertility because of nonstructural causes may correct itself following a successful pregnancy and birth; therefore, postchildbirth contraception counseling may be warranted. These interventions will go a long way toward normalizing the experience for the couple.

RECURRENT PREGNANCY LOSS

Recurrent pregnancy loss (RPL) is a disease distinct from infertility. It is defined as three or more consecutive pregnancy losses; however, the definition is not standardized, as some researchers consider two instead of three losses while others include women with nonconsecutive losses (Cunningham et al., 2018). There are several etiologies, including chromosomal abnormalities and other genetic conditions, uterine abnormalities, maternal medical complications, autoimmune disorders, and thrombotic causes.

●○● NURSING MANAGEMENT

For the Infertile Couple

Infertility therapy taxes a couple's financial, physical, and emotional resources. Treatment can be costly, and insurance coverage is limited. Years of effort and numerous evaluations and examinations may take place before conception occurs, if it occurs at all. In a society that values children and considers them to be the natural result of marriage, infertile couples face a myriad of tensions and discrimination.

Clinic nurses need to be constantly aware of the emotional needs of the couple confronting infertility evaluation and treatment. Often an intact marriage will become stressed with intrusive infertility procedures and treatments. Constant attention to temperature charts and instructions about their sex life from a person outside the relationship naturally affects the spontaneity of a couple's interactions. Tests and treatments may heighten feelings of frustration or anger between partners. The need to share this intimate area of a relationship, especially when one or the other is identified as the "cause" of infertility, may precipitate feelings of guilt or shame. Infertility often becomes a central focus for role identity, especially for women.

The couple may experience feelings of loss of control, feelings of reduced competency and defectiveness, loss of status and ambiguity as a couple, a sense of social stigma, stress on the marital and sexual relationships, and a strained relationship with healthcare providers. The couple will need to recognize and express how infertility affects their lives and grieve the loss of potential children. They then can decide on a plan to manage their infertility (Massey, 2015). The nurse's roles can be summarized as those of counselor, educator, facilitator, and advocate.

Your ability to assess and respond to emotional and educational needs is essential to give infertile couples a sense of control and help them negotiate the treatment process. It is important to use a nursing framework that recognizes the multidimensional needs of the infertile individual or couple within physical, social, psychologic, spiritual, and environmental contexts.

Infertility may be perceived as a loss by one or both partners. Affected individuals have described this as a loss of their relationship with spouse, family, or friends; their health; their status or prestige; their self-esteem and self-confidence; their security; and the potential child. Any one of these losses may lead to depression, but in many cases the crisis of infertility evokes feelings similar to those associated with all these losses (Massey, 2015). Each couple passes through several stages of feelings: Surprise, denial, anger, isolation, guilt, grief, and resolution. The impact of these feelings on the couple and how fast they move into resolution, if ever, may depend on the cause and on the duration of treatment. Each partner may progress through the stages at different rates. Nonjudgmental acceptance and a professional, caring attitude on your part can go far in dissipating the negative emotions the couple may experience while going through these stages. This is also a time to assess the couple's relationship: Are both partners able and willing to communicate verbally and share feelings? Are the partners mutually supportive? The answers to such questions may help to identify areas of strength and weakness and to construct an appropriate plan of care.

Referral to mental health professionals is helpful when the emotional issues become too disruptive in the couple's relationship or life. The couple should be aware of infertility support and education organizations such as RESOLVE (National Infertility Association), which may help meet some of their needs and validate their feelings. Finally, individual or group counseling with other infertile couples can help the couple resolve feelings brought about by their own difficult situation.

Focus Your Study

- With fibrocystic breast changes, the cysts tend to be round, mobile, and well delineated. The woman generally experiences increased discomfort premenstrually.
- Because of the increased risk of breast cancer, women with fibrocystic changes should understand the importance of monthly breast self-awareness (BSA).
- Galactorrhea (nipple discharge not associated with lactation) should be evaluated with cytologic testing.
- Breast cancer affects one in eight women in the United States. Biopsy is essential for a diagnosis, and prompt treatment is critical.
- Vulvitis is an inflammation of the vulva often caused by external irritants such as tight clothing, feminine hygiene products, and some harsh soaps.
- Vulvar lesions range from slight irritation to vulvar cancer. A common vulvar lesion found in postmenopausal women is atrophic vaginitis. All vulvar lesions should be closely evaluated because cancer of the vulva can have various presentations.
- Pap smear screening is recommended for all women 21 years of age and older. Several factors put a woman at high risk for an abnormal Pap: Intercourse at a young age, multiple partners, history of immunotherapy, long-term combined oral contraceptive (COC) use, smoking, and previous history of dysplasia. Human papilloma virus (HPV) is highly associated with abnormal Pap smears and cervical cancer.
- Abnormal uterine bleeding can occur with or without organic pathology. Treatment is geared toward controlling bleeding, preventing anemia, and detecting pathology.
- Endometriosis is a condition in which endometrial tissue occurs outside the endometrial cavity. This tissue bleeds in a cyclic fashion in response to the menstrual cycle. The bleeding leads to inflammation, scarring, and adhesions. The primary symptoms include dysmenorrhea, dyspareunia, and infertility.
- Treatment of endometriosis may be medical, surgical, or a combination of both. For the woman not desiring pregnancy at present, oral contraceptives are used. Women desiring pregnancy are treated with danazol or the gonadotropin-releasing hormone (GnRH) analogs.
- Polycystic ovary syndrome (PCOS) is a disorder of unknown etiology characterized by ovulatory dysfunction, hyperandrogenism, and polycystic ovaries. Women with PCOS often experience infertility, hirsutism, and difficulty controlling their weight. They are at increased risk for type 2 diabetes and cardiovascular disease.
- There are three common forms of pelvic relaxation. A cystocele is a downward displacement of the bladder into the vagina. Often it is accompanied by stress incontinence. Kegel exercises may help restore tone in mild cases. A rectocele is displacement of the rectum into the vagina. Prolapse of the uterus is displacement of the uterine cervix into the vagina.
- Gynecologic surgeries are some of the most common surgical procedures performed in the United States. It is important for the nurse to understand the purpose of the procedure, to know the alternatives to surgery, and to assess the woman's emotional response.
- A couple is considered infertile when they do not conceive after 1 year of unprotected coitus.
- A thorough history and physical of both partners are essential as a basis for infertility investigation.
- General fertility investigations include evaluation of ovarian function, cervical mucus adequacy and receptivity to sperm, sperm number and function, tubal patency, general condition of the pelvic organs, and certain laboratory tests.
- Methods of managing infertility include pharmacologic agents, intrauterine insemination, IVF, and other assisted reproductive techniques. In addition, many couples choose adoption as their preferred response to infertility.
- Medications may be prescribed to induce ovulation, facilitate cervical mucus formation, reduce antibody concentration, increase sperm count and motility, and suppress endometriosis.
- The emotional aspect of infertility may be more difficult for the couple than the testing and therapy.

In order to make safe and effective judgments using NANDA-I © 2017 nursing diagnoses, it is essential that nurses refer to the definitions and defining characteristics of the diagnoses used in this text, which can be found in Appendix C.

References

Alexander, A. G., Dupper, M., & Millard, H. S. (2017). Endometriosis. In M. B. Stephens, F. J. Domino, R. A. Baldor, & J. Golding (Eds.), *The 5-minute clinical consult 2017* (25th ed., pp. 340–341). Philadelphia, PA: Wolters Kluwer.

American Cancer Society (ACS). (2016). *Preventive surgery to reduce breast cancer risk.* Retrieved from https://www.cancer.org/cancer/breast-cancer/risk-and-prevention/preventive-surgery-to-reduce-breast-cancer-risk.html

American Cancer Society (ACS). (2017a). *American Cancer Society recommendations for the early detection of breast cancer.* Retrieved from https://www.cancer.org/cancer/breast-cancer/screening-tests-and-early-detection/american-cancer-society-recommendations-for-the-early-detection-of-breast-cancer.html

American Cancer Society (ACS). (2017b). *Cancer facts and figures: 2017.* Retrieved from https://www.cancer.org/content/dam/cancer-org/research/cancer-facts-and-statistics/annual-cancer-facts-and-figures/2017/cancer-facts-and-figures-2017.pdf

American Cancer Society (ACS). (2017c). *Targeted therapy for breast cancer.* Retrieved from https://www.cancer.org/cancer/breast-cancer/treatment/targeted-therapy-for-breast-cancer.html#written_by

American College of Obstetricians and Gynecologists (ACOG). (2016a). Cervical cancer screening and prevention (ACOG Committee Opinion No. 168). *Obstetrics and Gynecology, 128*(4), e111–e130. DOI:10.1097/AOG.0000000000001708

American College of Obstetricians and Gynecologists (ACOG). (2016b). Management of vulvar intraepithelial neoplasia (ACOG Committee Opinion No. 675). *Obstetrics and Gynecology, 128*(4), e178–e182. DOI:10.1097/AOG.0000000000001713

American College of Obstetricians and Gynecologists (ACOG). (2017a). *Breast cancer risk assessment in average-risk women* (ACOG Practice Bulletin No. 179). Washington, DC: Author. DOI: 10.1097/AOG.0000000000002158

American College of Obstetricians and Gynecologists (ACOG). (2017b). *Management of acute abnormal uterine bleeding in nonpregnant reproductive-aged women* (ACOG Committee Opinion No. 557; issued 2013, reaffirmed 2017). Washington, DC: Author.

American Society for Reproductive Medicine (ASRM). (2018). Third-party reproduction: A guide for patients. Retrieved from https://www.reproductivefacts.org/globalassets/rf/news-and-publications/bookletsfact-sheets/english-fact-sheets-and-info-booklets/third-party_reproduction_booklet_web.pdf

Bay, B., Ingerslev, H. J., Lemmen, J. G., Degn, B., Rasmussen, I. A., & Kesmodel, U. S. (2016). Preimplantation genetic diagnosis: A national multicenter obstetric and neonatal follow-up study. *Fertility and Sterility, 106*(6), 1363–1369.

Chinnasamy, T., Behr, B., & Demirci, U. (2016). Microfluidic sperm sorting device for selection of functional human sperm for IUI application. *Fertility and Sterility, 105*(2S), e17–e18.

Cunningham, F. G., Leveno, K. J., Bloom, S. L., Spong, C., Dashe, J. S., Hoffman, B. L., . . . Sheffield, J. S. (2014). *Williams obstetrics* (24th ed.). New York, NY: McGraw-Hill.

De la Cruz, M. S. D., & Buchanan, E. M. (2017). Uterine fibroids: Diagnosis and treatment. *American Family Physician, 95*(2), 100–107.

De La Luz Nieto, M. (2016). Polycystic ovarian syndrome (PCOS). In M. B. Stephens, F. J. Domino, R. A. Baldor, & J. Golding (Eds.), *The 5-minute clinical consult 2017* (25th ed., pp. 822–823). Philadelphia, PA: Wolters Kluwer.

Duke, C. M. P., & Christianson, M. S. (2015). Infertility and assisted reproductive technologies. In C. T. Johnson, J. L. Hallock, J. L. Bienstock, H. E. Fox, & E. E. Wallach (Eds.), *The Johns Hopkins manual of gynecology and obstetrics* (5th ed., pp. 467–484). Philadelphia, PA: Wolters Kluwer.

Galea, M. (2016). Benign breast disorders. *Surgery (United Kingdom), 34*(1), 19–24. DOI:10.1016/j.mpsur.2015.10.006

Gambadauro, P., Iliadis, S., Bränn, E., & Skalkidou, A. (2017). Conception by means of in vitro fertilization is not associated with maternal depressive symptoms during pregnancy or postpartum. *Fertility and Sterility, 108*(2), 325–332.

Greil, A. L., Slauson-Blevins, K. S., Tiemeyer, S., McQuillan, J., & Shreffler, K. M. (2016). A new way to estimate the potential unmet need for infertility services among women in the United States. *Journal of Women's Health, 25*(2), 133–140.

Haimov-Kochman, R., Adler, C., Ein-Mor, E., Rosenak, D., & Hurwitz, A. (2012). Infertility associated with precoital ovulation in observant Jewish couples: Prevalence, treatment, efficacy and side effects. *Israel Medical Association Journal, 14,* 100–103.

Harbeck, N., & Gnant, M. (2017). Breast cancer. *Lancet, 389*(10074), 1134–1150. DOI:10.1016/S0140-6736(16)31891

Jernigan, A. M., & Giuntoli II, R. L. (2015). Diseases of the vulva and vagina. In C. T. Johnson, J. L. Hallock, J. L. Bienstock, H. E. Fox, & E. E. Wallach (Eds.), *The Johns Hopkins manual of gynecology and obstetrics* (5th ed., pp. 568–583). Philadelphia, PA: Wolters Kluwer.

Jeronimo, J., Castle, P. E., Temin, S., Denny, L., Gupta, V., Kim, J. J., . . . Shastri, S. S. (2016). Secondary prevention of cervical cancer: ASCO resource-stratified clinical practice guideline. *Journal of Global Oncology, 3,* 635–657. DOI:10.1200/JGO.2016.006577

Massad, L. S., Einstein, M. H., Huh, W. K., Katki, H. A., Kinney, W. K., Schiffman, M., . . . Lawson, H. W. (2013). 2012 Updated consensus guidelines for the management of abnormal cervical cancer screening tests and cancer precursors. *Journal of Lower Genital Tract Disease, 17*(5), S1–27.

Massey, M. T. (2015). Managing infertility in primary care. *Practice Nurse, 45*(3), 17–27.

National Cancer Institute (2017). *Endometrial cancer prevention (PDQ®)—Health professional version.* Retrieved from https://www.cancer.gov/types/uterine/hp/endometrial-prevention-pdq

National Down Syndrome Society. (2018). *Sexuality.* Retrieved from https://www.ndss.org/resources/sexuality/

Obeisat, S., Gharaibeh, M. K., Owis, A., & Gharaibeh, H. (2012). Adversities of being infertile: The experience of Jordanian women. *Fertility and Sterility, 98*(2), 444–449.

Oyelowo, T., & Johnson, J. (2018). *A guide to women's health* (2nd ed.). Burlington, MA: Jones & Bartlett Learning.

Rice, K. E., Secrist, J. R., Woodrow, E. L., Hallock, L. M., & Neal, J. L. (2012). Etiology, diagnosis, and management of uterine leiomyomas. *Journal of Midwifery and Women's Health, 57,* 241–247.

Stewart, K. I., & Kolp, L. (2015). Hypoandrogenism. In C. T. Johnson, J. L. Hallock, J. L. Bienstock, H. E. Fox, & E. E. Wallach (Eds.), *The John Hopkins manual of gynecology and obstetrics* (5th ed., pp. 536–545). Philadelphia, PA: Wolters Kluwer.

Stern, S., Biron, D., & Moses, E. (2016). Transmission of trisomy decreases with maternal age in mouse models of Down syndrome, mirroring a phenomenon in human Down syndrome mothers. *BioMed Central Genetics, 17*(1), 105.

Tredway, D., Schertz, J. C., Bock, D., Hemsey, G., & Diamond, M. (2011). Anastrozole vs. clomiphene citrate in infertile women with ovulatory dysfunction: A phase II, randomized, dose-finding study. *Fertility and Sterility, 95*(5), 1720. DOI:10.1016/j.fertnstert.2010.12.064

United States Preventive Services Task Force. (2009). *Screening for breast cancer.* Retrieved from http://www.uspreventiveservicestaskforce.org/uspstf/uspsbrca.htm

United States Preventive Services Task Force. (2014). *Guide to clinical preventive services: Recommendations of the U.S. Preventive Services Task Force.* Retrieved from https://www.uspreventiveservicestaskforce.org/Page/Name/tools-and-resources-for-better-preventive-care

United States Preventive Services Task Force. (2017). *Screening for gynecologic conditions with pelvic examination.* U.S. Preventive Services Task Force Recommendation Statement. *Journal of the American Medical Association, 317*(9), 947–953. DOI:10.1001/jama.2017.0807

Wilson, B. A., Shannon, M. T., & Shields, K. M. (2017). Pearson nurse's drug guide 2018. Hoboken, NJ: Pearson Education, Inc.

Woo, I., & Yates, M. (2015). Menstrual disorders: Endometriosis, dysmenorrhea, and premenstrual dysmorphic disorder. In C. T. Johnson, J. L. Hallock, J. L. Bienstock, H. E. Fox, & E. E. Wallach (Eds.), *The Johns Hopkins manual of gynecology and obstetrics* (5th ed., pp. 503–512). Philadelphia, PA: Wolters Kluwer.

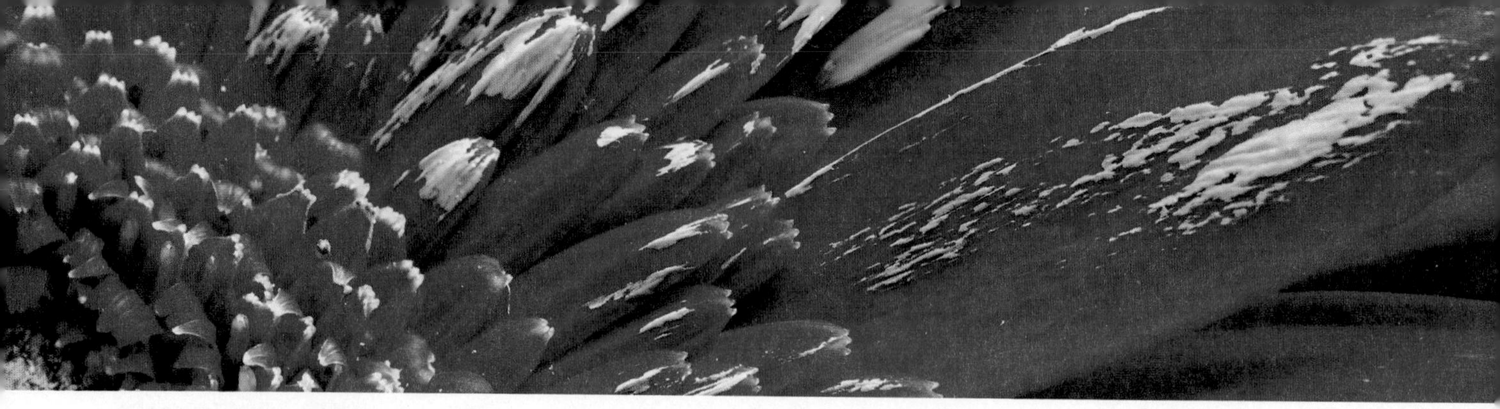

Chapter 7
Social Issues

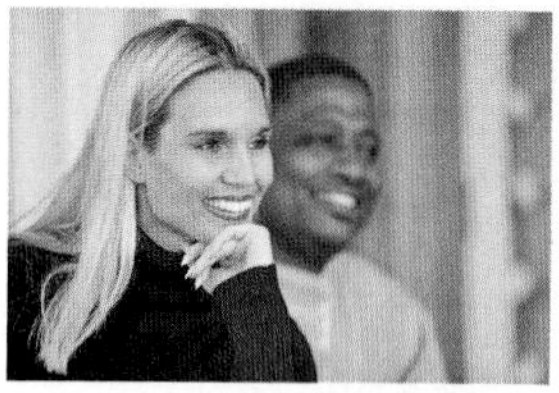

SOURCE: Kablonk/SuperStock.

There has never been a more exciting time for women. Although we face many challenges—work, wage, and role issues; safety in pregnancy and childbearing; and conflict over women's rights—we have never been more active and involved in issues that affect us. Moreover, the men who care about us, and recognize the importance of fairness for all, are beginning to join us in speaking out. Together, people of integrity and vision are making a difference in women's lives.

Learning Outcomes

7.1 Discuss the meaning of the phrase *feminization of poverty* and its impact on women and their families.

7.2 Identify contributing factors that perpetuate the gender wage gap and economic inequality for women.

7.3 Discuss the impact of poverty on women's access to healthcare.

7.4 Describe the implications of the Family and Medical Leave Act (FMLA) of 1993 on maternity and paternity leave and how this has impacted families.

7.5 Identify potential adverse outcomes associated with environmental hazards in the workplace or the home of a woman of childbearing age.

7.6 Specify the factors that commonly contribute to many older women's economic vulnerability.

7.7 Identify the four different types of elder abuse and the detrimental impact they have on older women.

7.8 Discuss possible adverse outcomes that may occur as a result of aging on a woman's health and healthcare.

7.9 Identify the five types of disability and their impact on quality of life for disabled women.

7.10 Explain the implications of various barriers that lesbian, bisexual, and transgender women face and how they can negatively impact healthcare access and outcomes.

7.11 Discuss the cultural and healthcare implications of female genital mutilation.

Healthy People 2020

(EH 17.1) Increase the proportion of pre-1978 housing that has been tested for the presence of lead-based paint

(EH 3.3) Reduce the risk of adverse health effects caused by major sources of airborne toxins

(LGBT-2) Increase the number of states, territories, and the District of Columbia that include questions that identify sexual orientation and gender identity on state-level surveys or data systems

OA-12.1 Increase the number of states and the District of Columbia that collect and make publicly available information on the characteristics of victims, perpetrators, and cases of elder abuse, neglect, and exploitation

In the 21st century, many women in developed nations are creating and experiencing new opportunities for personal and professional growth. Despite these unparalleled opportunities, women, including successful women with stable careers, still struggle daily to overcome some of the following:

- Poverty
- Wage discrimination
- Age discrimination
- Abuse
- Economic and interpersonal effects of disability
- Unequal treatment because of sexual orientation or gender expression
- Lack of paid maternity and paternity leave
- Lack of safe and nurturing daycare for their children.

Every day in their clinical practices, nurses working with women are confronted with these issues and their impact on women's health and well-being. To help nurses better understand their patients' concerns and problems, this chapter addresses some of the serious social issues facing women today.

Social Issues Affecting Women Living in Poverty

For impoverished women, life is a day-by-day struggle fraught with anxiety and hardship.

> "I never thought this would happen to me. Two months after I became pregnant with our second child, it was over. My husband left us. Suddenly, I am the sole support of myself and my children. Since he left I haven't been able to get a job, so I don't have medical insurance or any benefits to help with this pregnancy. Applying for Medicaid has to be one of the most humiliating experiences I have ever had. I'm an intelligent woman with a college degree, and yet I couldn't figure out the forms. I felt so dumb. The lines and the impersonal treatment that you hear about are real. I felt like a number, shuttled from one place to the next. I know they don't do it on purpose; they've heard so many awful stories. Still, it hurt. It will take 6 weeks to qualify for assistance, and by then I will be more than halfway through my pregnancy. What's more, only two doctors here accept Medicaid, and they are clear across town—that means three bus transfers with a 2-year-old in tow. I'm thankful that I can get some help, but it is so hard. I never dreamed I'd be in this position. I just never dreamed."

The Feminization of Poverty

The fact that many more women than men live below the poverty level is reflected in the phrase **feminization of poverty**, which was coined by Diana Pearce in 1993. Increasing numbers of U.S. women and their children are attempting to live on $24,250 or less per year, which is the current income that defines the poverty level for a family of four. In 2015, the number of women living in poverty totaled 16.9 million (National Women's Law Center [NWLC], 2016).

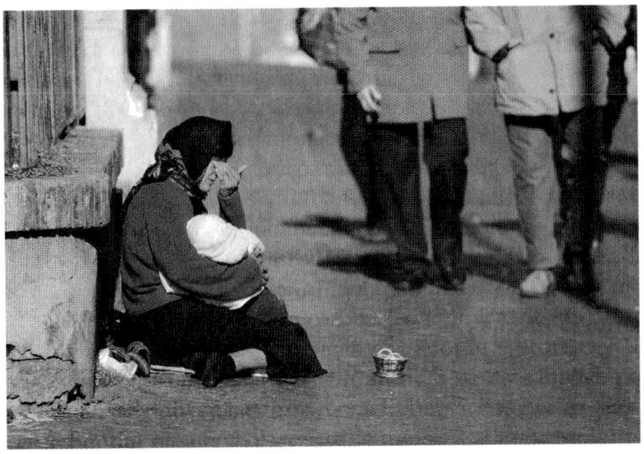

Figure 7–1 Two-thirds of Americans living in poverty are women and children.

SOURCE: Absolut/Fotolia.

Women raising children alone are more likely to be impoverished when compared to single male–headed households or married-couple households. In 2015, 36.5% of the households headed by single mothers lived in poverty (NWLC, 2016). Unmarried women account for 40.2% of all births in the United States (Hamilton, Martin, Osterman, et al., 2015). Single motherhood has been declining since 2008 in groups that have the highest rates of economic instability associated with single motherhood, including women in their teenage years, Black and Hispanic women, and women without college degrees. However, the number of college-educated, unmarried women over the age of 35 choosing to give birth has increased (Miller, 2015). These women have more financial resources and economic stability and are less likely to experience poverty (Miller, 2015). Despite this trend, the majority of single female–headed households continues to be economically disadvantaged and these families are four times more likely to live in poverty compared to families with two parents (Centers for Disease Control and Prevention [CDC], 2016) (Figure 7–1).

Beside relationship status, parental race is one of the leading indicators of poverty in children. In some communities of color, parents may have low education and income levels. In 2016, the poverty rates by race were: African Americans (22%), Hispanics (19.4%), Asian Americans (10.1%), and Caucasian Americans (8.8%) (Federal Safety Net, 2017).

Globally, poverty among women is even more common than in the United States, as women must cope with unique challenges. They typically work more hours than men but are paid less for the same work; they are often expected to bear and raise many children, sometimes in addition to performing work outside the home; they are frequently abused and beaten in their own homes; and they often have few legal rights.

Both globally and in the United States, poverty has been directly linked to a lack of literacy and educational attainment. In many countries, the literacy rate for females is lower than that for males, and education—when available—is more frequently provided for men, even though economic returns on investment in women's education are found to exceed those for men. Also, women who use their skills to increase their income typically invest more in their children's health and education. See *Case Study: Angelina Newman*.

CASE STUDY: Angelina Newman

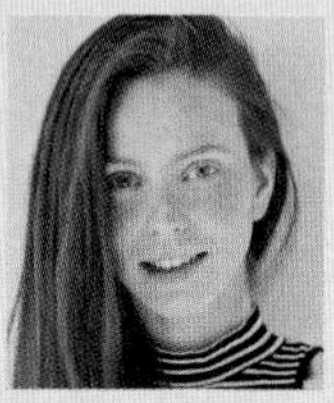

SOURCE: WAYHOME studio/Shutterstock

Angelina, pregnant with her first baby, is a sophomore in high school. She had wanted to attend a four-year college upon graduation, but she realizes her dreams of living in a college dorm and hanging out with new friends are now unlikely. She recently attended a teen pregnancy support group after being referred to the group by the Women, Infant, and Children (WIC) program nutritionist. In the group, the therapist shared that most teenage mothers are limited in their educational opportunities due to financial issues, lack of child care, and inability to support themselves once they give birth. When Angelina presents to her next prenatal appointment she appears down and subdued. She says that she is feeling hopeless and fears she will be unable to support herself and her baby.

Questions to Ponder

What types of support services and resources can you provide to assist her in obtaining financial support and help her maintain enrollment in high school? What resources may enable her to obtain educational or vocational resources after high school?

Economic Effects of Divorce

The highest divorce rates occurred in the 1970s and 1980s and have been decreasing since that time. Divorce rates in general have been difficult to calculate because marriage trends have changed dramatically over the last century. Fewer people are marrying and when individuals do marry, they do so at an older age (National Vital Statistics System, 2015). Multiple factors have contributed to changes in marriage and divorce trends. While the number of working women, career opportunities, shared household responsibilities, and reproductive rights increased, divorce rates have steadily decreased. Individuals marrying later in life have also contributed to a reduction in divorce rates. If the numbers continue on this downward trend, two-thirds of couples that marry will never divorce (Wong, 2014). When divorce does occur, a woman's standard of living generally decreases significantly, whereas a man's increases. This dramatic change in the standard of living is usually associated with the lower earning capacity of women and the fact that women receive custody of their children in most cases.

Shifts in childbearing trends have resulted in higher numbers of single mothers who have never married. Approximately 49% of single mothers never marry, while 51% are separated, divorced, or widowed. It is estimated that approximately 40% of single mothers live in poverty, whereas only approximately 7.6% of married couples live in poverty. Although many single mothers have child support agreements in place, only about one-third receive child support, which averages $430 per month. Single mothers also have higher incidences of being *food insecure*, meaning they rely on food banks, food pantries, and low-income food programs to ensure there is adequate food available for themselves and their children. Poorer families, especially those that are led by single mothers, have less access to child care, educational resources, healthcare, and job opportunities (Single Mother Guide, 2016).

The U.S. Department of Justice and various state agencies have made attempts to decrease the number of noncustodial parents who do not pay child support by enacting the following measures:

- Investigate and prosecute individuals who cross state lines to avoid paying child support.
- Withhold delinquent parents' income tax refunds.
- Mandate that employers report all newly hired employees to state agencies, including reporting to a national directory.
- Enhance state central registries of child support orders with centralized collection and disbursement units.
- Authorize states to garnish wages, seize assets, and revoke driver's and professional licenses.
- Require court-ordered, mandatory community service for individuals who are delinquent in making child support payments. Information about the enforcement program may be found on the DHHS Office of Child Support Enforcement's website.

Despite good intentions, it is estimated that 25% of noncustodial parents pay no child support, while another 30% provide only partial payments (Single Mother Guide, 2016). The determination of an individual's support payment amount is based on a state-mandated calculation that often includes the noncustodial parent's income, number of children, and various other factors. Child support payments can also be reduced if the noncustodial parent suffers a disability or has a change in employment.

Factors Contributing to Poverty for Working Women

Women have steadily increased their participation in the labor force. In the United States, the number of women working outside the home has risen from 5.1 million in 1900, to 18.4 million in 1950, to nearly 73.5 million in 2015 (U.S. Department of Labor, Bureau of Labor Statistics, 2017). Despite women having equal roles, experience, and educational attainment level, it is estimated that women are paid 79 cents for every dollar made by their male counterparts (NWLC, 2016).

Although women's earnings have increased historically, a significant wage discrepancy still exists that is even more profound in women of color. The disparity between men's and women's wages may be attributed to several factors:

- In historically female occupations, such as nursing, teaching, and administrative assistant roles, the pay is much less when compared with male-dominated positions requiring comparable levels of responsibility, skill, and education. When men are employed in these historically female occupations, however, they are often paid more than their female counterparts.
- Women are paid less than men for comparable work in virtually all occupations: In 2015, professional and technical

women earned almost 21% less than their male counterparts (NWLC, 2016).

- Reduced wages, smaller pensions, and lower Social Security benefits at retirement are associated with less time spent in the workforce, which is usually related to a woman's childbearing and childrearing responsibilities over time.

For working divorced or single women with children, the cost of rearing children demands a great portion of their earnings. Due to their lack of social support and partners, working women often miss work because of ill children, which can be negatively perceived by employers. As more enlightened employers strive to accommodate working mothers, it is hoped that women's compensation will increase, which will provide the working mother with more options for child care needs and emergencies.

Public Assistance

The U.S. welfare system was originally designed to provide assistance to those in need, frequently single female heads of households and their children. Unfortunately, the system often failed to provide adequate assistance to raise families above poverty levels and, in many cases, actually provided disincentives for women to work.

The Office of Family Assistance administers federal funding by administering block grants to states to operate their own programs. The largest of these programs is Temporary Assistance for Needy Families (TANF), which was created to provide short-term financial assistance to needy families. States can provide whatever services they choose, as they long as the initiatives are congruent with the four TANF purposes set out in federal law (Center on Budget and Policy Priorities, 2017):

- Provide assistance to needy families so that children may be cared for in their own homes or in the homes of relatives.
- End the dependence of needy parents on government benefits by promoting job preparation, work, and marriage.
- Prevent and reduce the incidence of out-of-wedlock pregnancies and establish annual numerical goals for preventing and reducing the incidence of these pregnancies.
- Encourage the formation and maintenance of two-parent families.

Under TANF, states are granted unprecedented flexibility in designing welfare programs to meet the needs of their recipients, but they must demonstrate measurable results in moving families toward self-sufficiency and work. States may also, under federal law, allow up to 20% of the recipients to exceed established time limits. Although TANF was a productive program when initially introduced, there are now fewer and fewer families reached and the number of families living in poverty or deep poverty has increased, even with this program in place. Policy reformation is needed to provide families with basic needs while at the same time helping them to find productive employment to support independence (Center on Budget and Policy Priorities, 2017).

Homelessness

In 2016, the number of individuals who were homeless continued to fall, although homelessness in the United States remains a significant social issue. This downward trend is likely fueled by the Homeless Emergency Assistance and Rapid Transition to Housing (HEARTH) Act of 2009 that has led to an increase in shelter beds and rehousing options in a federal effort to reduce homelessness. Approximately 564,708 people are homeless on any given night in the United States; of these, 206,286 are members of families (Social Solutions, 2016). Children account for 36% of those who are homeless. Homelessness may be temporary or sporadic; chronic homelessness is found in 15% of people who are homeless. The number of veterans who are homeless account for 6% of the total homeless population (Social Solutions, 2016).

FACTORS CONTRIBUTING TO HOMELESSNESS

A number of factors increase the risk of homelessness:

- Family headed by a single mother
- Lack of housing, mortgage foreclosure
- Job loss, low-paying job, few work opportunities
- Poverty, unstable finances, unforeseen financial emergency
- Substance abuse
- Untreated or undertreated mental illnesses
- Intimate partner violence
- Recent prison release
- Changes and cuts in public assistance programs
- Poor educational attainment
- High number of children
- Lack of social or family support
- Family emergency, death of a family member.

HEALTH RISKS OF WOMEN AND CHILDREN WHO ARE HOMELESS

Women and children who are homeless experience greater health risks and problems than do people in the general population. Malnutrition predisposes them to a variety of respiratory and nutritional disorders. Moreover, a disproportionately high number of women and children who are homeless do not receive preventive healthcare services, such as screening tests and immunizations. Pregnant women who are homeless are more likely to have:

- Lack of or inadequate prenatal care
- Limited access to preventive healthcare
- Poor nutrition and limited access to nutritional food
- Increased incidence of low-birth-weight newborns
- Higher rates of infant mortality
- Higher incidence of substance abuse, including alcohol
- Higher rates of sexually transmitted infections (STIs)
- Higher rates of hepatitis A, B, and C and HIV/AIDS.

HOMELESSNESS IN ADOLESCENCE

The teenage years can be a time of tumultuous family interactions that can sometimes lead adolescents to run away from home. Homelessness in the teen years can be related to disagreements with parents, divorce, parental substance abuse, neglect, and abuse. The majority of runaway teens eventually return to the family home.

Both children and adolescents who are homeless are at risk for the commercial sexual exploitation of children (CSEC). Young teens may find themselves with no other options for survival and may trade sex for food and shelter. Although many are physically and sexually abused, others are forced through intimidation or are falsely offered unconditional love by predators. When their emotional vulnerability is targeted with promises of stability of their basic needs (food and shelter), young people can be pressured or forced to enter the commercial sex industry.

While homelessness creates vulnerability and significant risk factors for physical, psychologic, and sexual abuse, adverse outcomes are increased for lesbian/gay/bisexual/transgender/

questioning/intersex (LGBTQI) adolescents, who have higher rates of physical abuse and sexual assault than heterosexual adolescents who are homeless. LGBTQI teens have higher rates of mental illness and are more likely to engage in unprotected intercourse and unsafe sex practices. These teens often find themselves at risk for hate crimes and are twice as likely to attempt suicide. Support services are less frequently utilized and homelessness persists for many of these youths (National Alliance to End Homelessness, 2017).

Effects of Poverty on Women's Healthcare

The effects of poverty on women's healthcare are extensive.

Medicaid is the major U.S. program providing healthcare to low-income people in four categories: Children, adults in families, older adults, and people who are blind or otherwise disabled. Traditionally, Medicaid has played an important role in financing maternity care, covering the costs of about half of all births in the United States (Whitman, 2016). Despite programs aimed at improving medical care for pregnant women living in poverty, women receiving TANF must apply again for Medicaid services when they become pregnant. Although the specific types of programs available vary by state, TANF recipients are often eligible for programs including the WIC program, nonmedical home visitations for families, and youth development programs aimed at reducing pregnancies in single females. As of 2017, health insurance coverage continued to be a major problem for the poor, despite passage in 2010 of the Patient Protection and Affordable Care Act. The Affordable Care Act, as it is commonly termed, was passed into law with the aim of increasing the quality and affordability of health insurance, lowering the uninsured rate, expanding public and private insurance coverage, and reducing the costs of healthcare for individuals and the government. In 2015, 10.5% of non-elderly Americans did not have health coverage, which equates to over 28.5 million people. While about half of Americans get health insurance coverage through an employer, the rates are declining (Kaiser Family Foundation, 2017). Although the Affordable Health Care Act was designed to provide coverage for all Americans, a percentage of Americans remain uninsured because of the high costs associated with coverage. Many do not make enough income to allow them to purchase insurance, especially in states where Medicaid (a state-funded program) did not expand services. This has led to declines in preventive healthcare. Women who do not receive prenatal care are three times more likely to have low-birth-weight babies, and the incidence of low-birth-weight babies is increasing. Women who receive adequate prenatal care are less likely to develop severe complications, such as preterm labor. Moreover, lack of prenatal care is a risk factor for infant morbidity and mortality.

> **Professionalism in Practice Assisting Impoverished Women**
>
> Nurses can assist impoverished women by working with community groups and organizations and becoming actively involved in the political process. Nurses can use their work experience to present their views to legislators, support various childbearing programs, and alert legislators to legislation that would benefit mothers and families. Nurse researchers can explore medical and social issues related to the impact of poverty on families.

The issue of women and poverty is critical and carries significant implications for the childbearing family, including financial, physical, and psychosocial. Assessing women's financial status is part of the initial family assessment (see Chapter 2). Sparse economic resources may affect the woman's ability to obtain needed medical care, medical supplies, and infant care items, such as diapers or formula. Some families have so few economic resources that acquiring basic necessities, such as clothing, electricity, and water, may be compromised. The nurse should ask questions in a sensitive manner and refer women with insufficient resources to social workers or appropriate agencies. A nurse who is knowledgeable about community resources and who can provide the woman with follow-up contacts and phone numbers provides an immeasurable service to impoverished patients.

Social Issues Affecting Women in the Workplace

In 2016, 72.5% of women with children under the age of 18 were employed outside the home (U.S. Department of Labor, Bureau of Labor Statistics, 2017). As a result of political and social changes that began in the early 1970s, women's career options have expanded dramatically and now include multiple options. Progress has its costs, however, and workforce issues have plagued women in many ways, including:

- Need to balance work and family life
- Emotional stress associated with finding quality affordable child care
- Professional or job-related stress
- Delayed childbearing in order to reach financial and professional stability, which can result in infertility issues and may make bearing her own child impossible for a woman
- Inability to adopt a child because of age limits for prospective adoptive parents.

In contrast, the woman who is a stay-at-home mother may experience stresses and strains of a different nature, such as:

- Economic strain of a single-earner family
- Sacrifice of earnings, retirement savings, and Social Security benefits
- Risk for loneliness and isolation due to lost opportunities for social contact and intellectual stimulation.

Several social issues affect women in the workplace. Key among these are wage discrepancy, maternity/paternity leave issues, discrimination, child care, advocacy, and environmental hazards.

Wage Discrepancy

Gender wage gap inequalities in the past have been associated with:

- Perception that men were the sole breadwinners
- Limited occupations and female-dominated professions
- Acceptance of lower salaries in exchange for flexibility for child care needs and family issues
- Negative perceptions of assertive women in the workplace
- Societal importance focusing on women's appearance rather than intellect
- Lack of opportunities for higher education.

Professionalism in Practice Speaking in Public

Encourage women to advocate publicly for wage equality to ensure that the gender wage gap continues to narrow. Speaking out about issues that affect women, children, and families is an integral part of maternal-child nursing. It is difficult for many nurses to do this, so you should practice with friends and family frequently. Be prepared with accurate information and try various techniques for presenting the information. A friendly, supportive audience will help you get started.

While the gender wage gap continues to be problematic, there are some optimistic signs, namely that younger women entering their career years are less likely to be impacted as much by the gender gap as working women of the past. Women starting careers today are more likely to obtain managerial and professional positions and are more likely to have pursued education beyond high school.

Maternal and Paternal Leave Issues

Combining employment with motherhood has always been challenging. In the past, pregnant women commonly lost benefits, missed out on promotions, or lost their jobs completely. Paternity leave for fathers was unheard of and remains underutilized, even in developed countries.

In 1993, the Family and Medical Leave Act (FMLA) became law. FMLA offers the following protections and benefits to both men and women:

- Twelve weeks of unpaid leave from work following the birth, adoption, or placement of a foster child
- Leave provided for serious illness or the illness of a spouse, child, or parent
- Continued health insurance benefits
- Job security to return to the person's former position or one considered comparable.

Although FMLA has been extremely helpful in expanding maternity and paternity leave options for families, there are limitations:

- FMLA applies only to companies with 50 or more employees.
- Employees must work at least 25 hours per week to be eligible.
- Employees must have been in their position for at least 1 year.

Despite the advances made in this country by the FMLA, parental leave benefits in the United States are meager in comparison with benefits provided in other countries. Paid maternity leave, and often paternity leave, are standard in most European countries and Canada. The United States remains one of the few countries that have no legislation requiring a national *paid* maternity leave program.

Discrimination Against Pregnant Women

Discrimination against pregnant women by employers who cling to false stereotypes about them (that they cannot do their jobs, take more sick leave than other employees, fail to return to work after having given birth, etc.) remains an important women's issue. Every year the Equal Employment Opportunity Commission receives complaints from pregnant women who were turned down for jobs, denied transfers to positions for which they were qualified, or fired unjustly (U.S. Equal Employment Opportunity Commission, 2017). Thus, it is important that pregnant women be aware of their legal rights. The Pregnancy Discrimination Act of 1978 guarantees the following:

- A pregnant woman cannot be denied a job if she is able to perform major job functions.
- The same procedure for using sick leave pay or disability benefits must be used for the pregnant woman as for other employees.
- Employee medical coverage must include pregnancy benefits.
- The woman can use all her maternity benefits without penalty.

When a woman is planning a pregnancy, she should acquire information about pregnancy benefits in her work setting and laws or regulations in the state in which she lives.

"I was thrilled when I found out I was pregnant! Although I had a high-stress job and worked long hours, I rejoiced in the thought of being a mother. As my pregnancy became apparent, my boss started "worrying about me." He feared I could not keep up with my demanding schedule and that the "emotional strain" would be hard on the baby. By the time I reached 28 weeks, I learned that a coworker would be taking over some of my responsibilities, and 2 weeks later I was laid off. My boss felt that my current workload would be too difficult for a "very pregnant woman or a new mother." I immediately started fighting for my right to keep my position. I was the perfect employee previously with flawless evaluations. Sure, there may be legal protection in place, but right now I have no income, am paying high insurance premiums to maintain my health insurance, and am rapidly depleting my savings. I am angry and cry all of the time. I have been diagnosed with depression and am now taking antidepressants. I never missed a minute of work, my performance remained flawless . . . their only complaint, I was pregnant! This should be the happiest time of my life, but instead I'm in counseling and taking Prozac. It's so unfair!"

Child Care

In 1947, only 12% of mothers with small children (under 6 years of age) were employed. By 2016 that percentage had jumped to 60.8% (U.S. Department of Labor, Bureau of Labor Statistics, 2017). Families with younger children are more likely to have mothers who are not in the workforce. In the past, mothers assumed the primary role in childrearing and household chores and duties. Since 2013, the number of families with stay-at-home dads has nearly doubled, with approximately 7.1% of all married fathers in 2016 staying home to care for children while the mother is working outside the home (U.S. Department of Labor, Bureau of Labor Statistics, 2017) (Figure 7–2). Among dual-career families, household chores and spending time with and disciplining children are shared responsibilities; however, planning children's activities and staying home when children are ill are tasks still primarily done by working mothers rather than working fathers (Pew Research Center, 2015).

Today, while the vast majority of children (69%) are raised in two-parent households, the number of single-parent households continues to rise. In 2015, 35% of children were being raised in

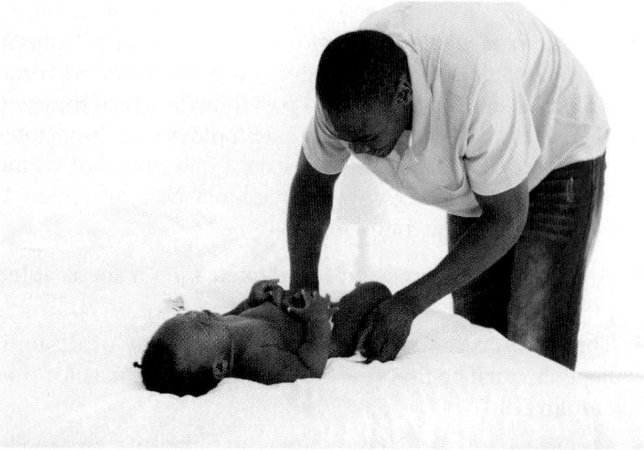

Figure 7–2 **Some women rely on their husbands or partners to provide full-time child care at home while they pursue their careers. The number of families with stay-at-home dads has nearly doubled since 2013.**

SOURCE: Michaeljung/Fotolia.

single-parent households (Pew Research Center, 2015). Those headed by single fathers are far less common and account for only 4% of all U.S. households. An estimated 4% of American children do not live with their parents, including children living with other family members and the 687,000 children annually who are in foster care (Children's Bureau, 2017).

The majority of children living in single-parent households live with mothers. The United States has more single-parent households than any other developed country. It is estimated that approximately one-third of single mothers and their children are living in poverty, compared to approximately 6% of children living in poverty with both parents (Russell & Porter, 2016). Recently, many have noted that marital status alone is not a defining factor in risk factors for families living in poverty. Many women living in poverty are those who have grown up impoverished, live in poor areas with high rates of unemployment and incarceration, and have poor educational attainment. It is unlikely that marriage alone would be a factor that would dramatically impact these families socioeconomically, indicating that identification of parental marital status alone is not as significant an indicator for poverty as once thought (Badger, 2014).

Child care costs in the United States typically consume a large portion of the family budget, especially for those with very young children and those with multiple children. Child care costs account for more than 15% of a two-parent family's income. For single mothers, the cost can be as high as 65% of their salary (Bahney, 2015). Costs vary considerably based on multiple factors:

- ***Geographic location.*** The most affordable child care is in the South and rural areas, whereas the Northeast and urban areas have higher costs.
- ***Age of children.*** Infant care is the most expensive type of child care; cost of care decreases with age and level of supervision needed.
- ***Children with disabilities.*** Cost for children with special needs is more costly and often not accessible in some areas. Lack of qualified caregivers is also a factor that increases cost of care.
- ***Type of facility.*** Child care center, franchised care center, home setting, licensed facility, unlicensed facility.
- ***Educational level of staff.*** Quality child care is an important consideration for families. Indicators associated with high-quality child care include:
  - Low turnover in staffing
  - Caregiver education and training
  - Licensing compliance
  - Smaller class sizes with low student-to-teacher ratios
  - Adequate teacher salaries
  - Age-appropriate curriculum
  - Individualized assessments to determine student placements
  - Warm and nurturing care providers.

Women who have college educations and are working outside of the home are more likely to have the means to enroll their children in high-quality child care centers (Figure 7–3). The quality and availability of care is directly related to a family's economic resources. In impoverished areas, care may be limited and the quality of care and care providers may be inadequate. Male children living in poverty are more likely to be expelled from child care centers; this has a direct correlation to long-term outcomes (Bahney, 2015). The benefits of enrolling children in high-quality child care settings have been studied extensively in the past half century and are associated with the following factors for children (Child Care Services Association, 2017):

- Higher high school graduation rates
- Higher rates of graduation from college with a four-year degree
- Lower rates of juvenile crime
- Lower incidence of adolescent pregnancy
- Older age at time of birth of first child
- Decreased utilization of public assistance programs
- Higher earning potential
- Reduced aggressive behavior
- Higher levels of academic learning ability
- Higher math scores that continue through second grade
- Increases in school readiness
- Improved memory

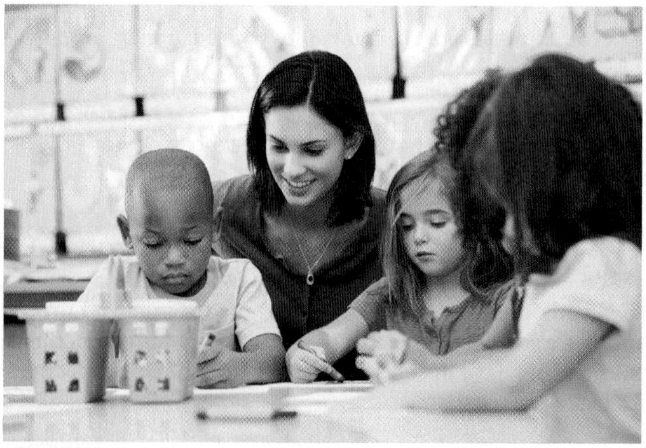

Figure 7–3 **Childhood education centers provide preschoolers with advanced skills for early education and provide care while parents work outside of the home.**

SOURCE: Monkey Business/Fotolia.

- Better language skills
- Higher cognitive, language, social, and developmental scores on objective testing measures.

In contrast, low-quality child care is associated with the following:

- Increased peer arguments
- Higher expulsion rates
- Bullying
- Participation in risky and impulsive behaviors
- Lower cognitive, language, and developmental scores
- Reduced school readiness scores.

Employers and working families are now identifying creative ways to obtain quality child care services, including:

- Use of referral programs
- Creation of on-worksite or near-worksite child care centers
- Employer-sponsored financial assistance programs
- Child care cooperatives with shared educational responsibilities with co-members.

Increasingly common are grandparents and other relatives who assume responsibility for one or more children whose parents are unable to care for them. In the United States, 4.9 million children live with their grandparents (Weinberger, 2016). The most common reasons for grandparents obtaining guardianship of grandchildren include:

- Parental substance abuse—drugs and/or alcohol
- Economic instability
- Parental divorce
- Severe parental mental illness
- Parental loss of custody due to abuse or neglect
- Intimate partner violence
- Parental incarceration
- Parental death or severe disability.

Nurses need to assist families in which grandparents serve as the primary guardians of children. Financial resources are often reduced during the retirement years, making financial hardship a common occurrence. Referrals for TANF, food stamps, low-cost child care programs, and Medicaid may be available. Children with deceased or disabled parents may be eligible for Social Security benefits. Grandparents who have guardianship may also qualify for certain tax benefits, including the Dependency Exemption, Earned Income Tax Credit, Child Tax Credit, Dependent Care Credit, or an Adoption Credit, for those who wish to adopt their grandchildren. State or county mental health services or Medicaid may be a source of support to provide counseling for children dealing with issues related to separation from parents.

Advocacy for Working Women

All women considering employment options—particularly those who must balance work and family responsibilities, including nurses—should inquire about family-friendly policies such as:

- Maternity and paternity leave
- Child care benefits
- Options for alterative working strategies including telecommuting options (Figure 7–4), flex time, flexible work hours, and job sharing

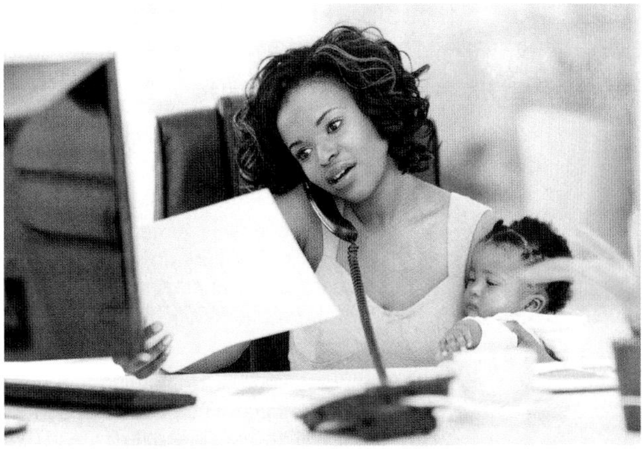

Figure 7–4 Some mothers are able to combine professional careers with motherhood by telecommuting from a home office.

SOURCE: Michaeljung/Fotolia.

- Availability of onsite, affordable daycare
- Specific rooms available for breastfeeding or pumping.

> **Professionalism in Practice Advocating for Working Women**
>
> Nurses can act as advocates for working women by serving as role models, providing positive reinforcement and support, and working actively to establish woman-friendly workplace policies.

Environmental Hazards in the Workplace and at Home

Women in developed countries such as the United States are increasingly exposed to **environmental toxins**, chemical compounds found in air, food, and water the bioaccumulation of which can lead to adverse health effects. Women living in poverty and/or in countries with the greatest amount of air pollution are exposed to more indoor pollutants, lead, pesticides, and allergens (Jeong, Zhou, & Flaws, 2017). Impoverished workers are also more likely to work in occupations where chemical exposure is higher. Women may have additional risk factors that can exacerbate environmental exposures, including adverse living conditions, poor neighborhood environment, psychologic stressors, and poor nutrition (Jeong et al., 2017). There are over 100 chemicals that are considered unsafe and potentially teratogenic in pregnancy, including lead, mercury, toluene, perchlorate, bisphenol A, flame retardants, perfluorinated compounds, organochlorine pesticides, and phthalates (Jeong et al., 2017). Pesticides, fuels, chemicals, and plastics are potential toxins that may be associated with endocrine disruption, which can be linked to childhood cancers, menstrual irregularities, ovulation defects, premature menopause, and infertility, along with alterations in sperm production and quality and male infertility. Chemicals, fuels, plastics, and pesticides, unlike pharmacologic agents, do not undergo robust testing to ensure their safety prior to use and have led to the development of adverse health outcomes and ongoing developmental and adverse reproductive outcomes (Jeong et al., 2017). Toxins of greatest concern include gases that may contaminate indoor air, toxic chemicals found in the work and home environment, and contaminated food sources. See Table 7–1.

TABLE 7–1 Sources and Risks Associated with Common Environmental Toxins

ENVIRONMENTAL TOXIN	COMMON SOURCE	SYSTEMS AFFECTED BY EXPOSURE
Lead	Paint applied prior to 1978, soil, batteries	Developmental, cardiovascular, kidney, brain, hematologic, musculoskeletal, ocular, reproductive (risk for spontaneous abortion, prematurity, low birth weight)
Mercury	Certain fish, (marlin, tuna, shark, swordfish, king mackerel, tilefish), mercury-containing thermometers, fluorescent light bulbs, coal, ore, petroleum, forest fires, volcanic eruptions, contaminated water sources	Developmental, gastrointestinal, neurologic, renal, ocular
Polycarbonates biphenyls (PCBs)	Commercial materials produced prior to 1977, including fluorescent lighting fixtures, electrical appliances containing PCB capacitors, old microscope oil and hydraulic fluids, fish (walleye, bass), soil, certain water and groundwater supplies, indoor air inhalation in older buildings, industrial accidents in older buildings constructed with toxic materials	Developmental, dermal, endocrine, hepatic, immunologic, neurologic
Fluoride	Water, supplements	Dermal, musculoskeletal, ocular, respiratory, neurologic, reproductive (preterm birth, maternal anemia)
Toluene	Paint thinners, industrial chemicals	Neurologic, hepatic, kidney, dermal, ocular, developmental, reproductive (spontaneous abortion)
Tetrachloroethylene (PERC)	Dry cleaning agents, degreasing agents, paint strippers, metal-working cleaning agents, soil, water	Neurologic, dermal, respiratory, ocular Carcinogen
Dichlorodiphenyltrichloroethane (DDT)	Pesticides and insecticides produced prior to 1972, soil, water, predatory birds	Developmental, endocrine, dermal, musculoskeletal, respiratory, ocular, reproductive (preterm birth, lactation problems) Carcinogen
Arsenic	Pesticides, soil, car batteries, ammunition, insecticides, treated wood products, herbicides, groundwater, volcanic ash, ore, glass production, nonferrous metal alloys, and electronic semiconductor manufacturing	Dermal, gastrointestinal, respiratory, hepatic, immunological, kidney, reproductive (genetic alterations) Carcinogen
Chlorpyrifos	Insecticides, acaricide, and miticide produced prior to 2001, crops, water, mice	Developmental, neurologic, autoimmune disorders, learning disabilities, respiratory, reproductive (low birth weight) Carcinogen
Bisphenol A (BPA)	Plastic (BPA) beverage containers, plastic containers, epoxy resins, color developer, receipt paper	Possible reproductive, endocrine, developmental, neurologic, metabolic; banned in infant formula packaging by Environmental Protection Agency in 2012 Carcinogen
Formaldehyde	Wood products, shelving, paneling	
Radon	Rock, soil	
Phthalates	Salt compounds, low levels in some cosmetics	Reproductive
Dioxin	Petroleum impurity	Developmental, neurologic Carcinogen

SOURCE: Data adapted from Jeong, Zhou, & Flaws, 2017.

Clinical Tip

Prenatal screening for potential lead exposure should include questions regarding living in a home with paint that was applied prior to 1978, home renovations that involve floor sanding or other activities that disburse airborne particulate matter, household water supply delivered by older systems that may contain lead pipes, and gardening or working in contaminated soil. Occupational risk factors include the following professions: home renovation, construction, and plumbing. With the current do-it-yourself (DIY) movement, women who refinish older furniture pieces or who use older materials should be counseled appropriately.

Air pollution is a mixture of natural and man-made substances within the air that includes fine particles produced by a combination of the burning of fossil fuels; ground-level ozone, which is contained in smog; and noxious gases such as sulfur dioxide, nitrogen oxides, carbon monoxide, and chemical vapors (National Institute of Environmental Health Sciences, 2017). Indoor air pollution comes from a variety of sources, including:

- Lighted cigarettes
- Burning candles, especially those scented with synthetic chemicals
- Wood-burning stoves
- Kerosene lamps
- Oil-burning furnaces
- Cleaning products
- Paint and varnish

- Cat dander, dust mites, cockroaches
- Mold and mildew
- Synthetic carpet fibers.

Health conditions associated with air pollution include:

- Eye, nose, and throat irritation
- Headaches
- Asthma
- Cardiovascular disease
- Cancer.

There are a variety of potentially harmful chemicals and other toxic substances that women may encounter in their home or work environments. Although there are more than 80,000 chemicals in commercial use, only about 1500 have been tested to determine if they are potential carcinogens.

Nurses should be educated about environmental risk factors, which may vary with geographic location; living conditions or neighborhoods; occupation; water supply source; commercial and residential exposure to chemicals, fumes, and gases; and choices of food consumed by the family. An environmental assessment should check for environmental risk factors or occupational exposure. Recommendations can then be made that will help the woman and her family reduce their risk factors. As research continues to evolve, more chemicals may be identified as being hazardous or carcinogenic. With this in mind, women should strive for a healthy, organically based diet when possible.

Pesticides are a broad category of chemicals used to prevent or treat pests and remove them from the environment. Pesticide exposure can result in a variety of vague symptoms including increased body temperature, eye irritation, headache, dizziness, irritability, nausea and vomiting, epigastric pain, myalgia, pain in the limbs and joints, skin irritation, and sweating. Pesticide exposure can be linked to a variety of adverse health outcomes, including (U.S. National Library of Medicine, 2017):

- Increased risk of cancer
- Nervous system abnormalities
- Birth defects
- Endocrine abnormalities
- Hormonal imbalances
- Liver damage
- Kidney failure.

Banned in the mid-1970s, *organochlorines* (a combination of dioxin, malathion, chlorpyrifos, and lindane) is a chemical pesticide subtype that degrades slowly and remains in the environment for decades. Persistent exposure to organochlorines during the childbearing years has implications for pregnancy and lactation and can cause long-term childhood developmental delays and infertility later in adulthood (U.S. National Library of Medicine, 2017).

Genetic Facts Exposure to Toxins

Environmental factors can impact future generations when people are exposed to toxins. Epigenetic changes in gene expression can occur when a woman is exposed to various environmental toxins. Depending on the agent and exposure, the cell nucleus can be altered at the molecular level and can impact if a gene is expressed or silenced (Stahl, 2017).

The exposure to various biologic and chemical toxins inherent in providing care for sick people constitutes an occupational hazard for nurses. Exposure to toxoplasmosis, rubella, cytomegalovirus, herpes simplex, and hepatitis B may adversely affect pregnancy and fetal outcome. Nurses are at risk for bloodborne illnesses through needlesticks or other high-risk medical procedures. Latex allergy is rapidly becoming a significant problem among healthcare workers, with 5 to 15% demonstrating hypersensitivity symptoms ranging from mild contact dermatitis to severe systemic reactions and anaphylactic shock (American Academy of Allergy, Asthma & Immunology [AAAAI], 2014). See Chapter 14 for a discussion of toxins found in foods.

Professionalism in Practice Safety and Health Resources

Nurses should familiarize themselves with recommendations from the Occupational Safety and Health Administration (OSHA), part of the Department of Labor, which is responsible for creating and enforcing workplace health and safety regulations, and the National Institute for Occupational Safety and Health (NIOSH), which is part of the Department of Health and Human Services and is primarily a research agency. These agencies disseminate information on preventing workplace injury and illness, provide training to occupational safety and health professionals, and investigate potentially hazardous working situations when requested by employers or employees.

Nurses can also utilize the web site of Tox Town, administered by the National Institutes of Health, which provides the most recent data on toxic substances and chemicals. Women, nurses, and all healthcare providers can utilize the site to determine if certain chemicals are dangerous for women and their families.

Social Issues Affecting Older Women

In the United States and other developed nations, women tend to outlive men. Thus, women are overrepresented in the ranks of older people. This phenomenon is referred to as the **feminization of later life**. The Baby Boomer generation (those born between 1946 and 1964) has contributed to unprecedented growth in the population of older adults. According to population experts from the United States Census Bureau, by 2050 the number of people over the age of 65 years will be double the number of children under the age of 5 years. This will represent the first time in history such a crossing of demographics has occurred. As of 2015, 14.9% of the total population in the United States is over the age of 65; by 2050, that number is estimated to be 22.1% (Jeffrey, 2016).

Economic Vulnerability of Older Women

The feminization of later life means that older women are more likely than their male counterparts to be widowed, to live alone, to be disabled, and to be poor. In 2015, 14% of all women over the age of 65 continued to work, with 51.4% working part time. Women over the age of 65 who work full time earn an average of $37,000 annually (Institute for Women's Policy Research [IWPR],

2015). Of all older adults in the United States, women of color have the highest poverty rates. Factors that contribute to the increased economic vulnerability of older women include:

- Women over the age of 65 are far less likely to have a bachelor's degree. Only 19.6% of women compared to 29.9% of men over the age of 65 have obtained a bachelor's degree (IWPR, 2015).
- Women must stretch their financial resources further than men because of their longer life expectancy.
- Historically, women have been economically dependent on men and may have intermittent or nonexistent employment histories.
- Women typically earn less than men and often work in jobs without pension benefits or have only limited benefits.
- Intermittent employment is more common in women, which decreases their Social Security and retirement benefits.
- Women generally have more family caregiving responsibilities than men.
- A husband's long, costly illness and the decrease or loss of his pension following his death can negatively impact a woman's financial resources.
- Because women are living longer, they are more likely to have out-of-pocket medical expenses after the age of 65 (IWPR, 2015).
- Women spend twice as much as men on long-term care expenses (IWPR, 2015).

Elder Abuse

Elder abuse includes any deliberate action, or lack of action, that causes harm to an older adult. It is difficult to determine how many older women in the United States are victims of abuse because perpetrators are usually careful to conceal their behavior, but older women are believed to be more at risk than older men. The incidence of elder abuse in the United States is 7.6 to 10% and continues to rise (National Center on Elder Abuse [NCEA], 2017a).

Five different categories of elder abuse have been recognized: Psychologic abuse, physical abuse (including sexual abuse), neglect (by self or caregiver), financial abuse, and abandonment (Table 7–2). Multiple forms of abuse may occur simultaneously and tend to intensify with time unless intervention occurs. It is imperative, however, that nurses who care for older adults be alert for signs of abuse and take steps to address the problem when it is identified.

Ethics in Action!

How would you respond if an older patient had symptoms of neglect but verbally denied neglect when directly questioned about her care?

Implications of Aging for Women's Health and Healthcare

Older women often face health problems that become more common as people age, such as:

- Hypertension
- Coronary artery disease
- Arthritis
- Diabetes
- Osteoporosis
- Dementia
- Depression.

Heart disease is the leading cause of death for all women age 65 or older (IWPR, 2015). By age 65, half of all women have developed two or more chronic diseases. Women over the age of 65 are also more likely to have breast cancer, mental health issues, and be overweight or obese. Because women live longer than men, older women are more likely to be living alone and without partners to assist them with their care.

Professionalism in Practice Elder Abuse

If you suspect elder abuse is occurring, you should immediately report the case to the county social services office of Adult Protective Services.

TABLE 7–2 Definitions of Elder Abuse

TYPE OF ABUSE	DEFINITION
Physical abuse	Any physical pain or injury that is intentionally inflicted upon an older person by a caregiver or individual who has custody of, or stands in a position of trust with, that person. Sexual assault, physical attacks, unreasonable physical restraint, and prolonged deprivation of food and water all constitute physical abuse.
Financial abuse	Any theft or misuse of an older person's money or property by a caregiver or person in a position of trust.
Neglect	Failure on the part of a caregiver, or any person having custody of an older adult, to provide reasonable care, which is the degree of care that a reasonable person would provide. Reasonable care includes, but is not limited to, assistance with personal hygiene; protection from health and safety hazards; and provision of shelter, food, clothing, health needs, and medical care except in instances when the individual refuses treatment.
Self-neglect	Failure to provide adequate self-care because of inability or inattention.
Psychologic abuse	The intentional infliction of mental suffering on an older adult by a caregiver or person in a position of trust. Psychologic abuse includes, but is not limited to, verbal assaults, threats, humiliation, intimidation, or isolation of the individual.
Abandonment	The desertion of an older adult by any person responsible for the care and custody of that individual, under circumstances in which a reasonable person would continue to provide care.

SOURCE: Data from National Center on Elder Abuse, 2017b.

Unfortunately, older women, particularly those who are poor, face multiple barriers in obtaining adequate healthcare services, including:

- Lack of transportation
- Lack of private health insurance coverage
- Excessive medical costs not covered by Medicare.

Polypharmacy, which means *multiple medicines*, is another common problem in the older adult population. Older women (as well as older men) often have multiple healthcare providers with different specialties who provide pharmacologic intervention. These multiple medications may have an array of side effects and potentially dangerous interactions with each other. Sometimes polypharmacy is justified, but often it is inadvertent because healthcare providers may be unaware that a woman is taking medications prescribed by multiple providers. In addition, the older woman may not know the specific medications she takes. Some older women may also take nutritional supplements, herbs, homeopathic remedies, and over-the-counter medications without the knowledge of their healthcare providers. These supplemental agents can interact with prescription drugs and cause adverse effects.

While most pharmacies utilize electronic monitoring systems, filling prescriptions at various pharmacies or in a pharmacy that does not use an electronic monitoring system can increase the risk of obtaining medications with potential drug interactions. Opioid use has reached epidemic levels in the United States and, as in other age groups, there is a rise of opioid use in the older adult population. In this age group use increased 32% between 2007 and 2012, an increase that is higher than many other age groups. Due to metabolic differences in older adults, the effects of opioids can be more intense and result in confusion, disorientation, memory loss, risk of falls, severely adverse health outcomes, and even death (National Institute on Drug Abuse, 2016). Nurses must advise older patients of the following (Figure 7–5):

- Have all prescriptions filled at one pharmacy.
- Maintain a medication list with the name, dosage, and prescribing practitioner on hand.
- Provide family members or care providers with an updated medication list periodically.

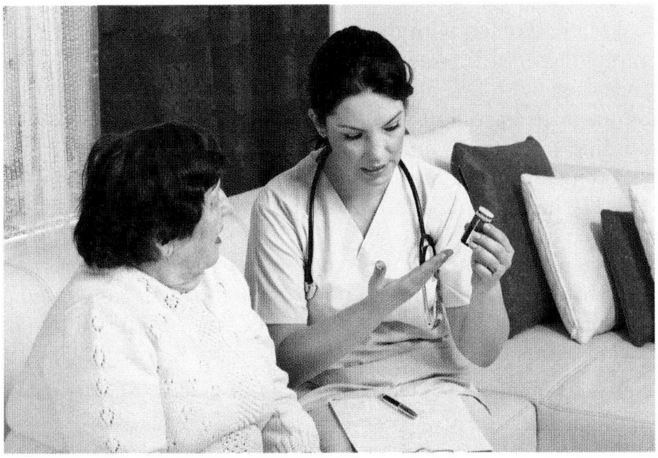

Figure 7–5 **Older women are more likely to have multiple medical conditions that require medication. Careful instructions should be given to prevent medication interactions.**

SOURCE: Gabriel Blaj/Fotolia.

Clinical Tip

Certain drugs can cause cognitive impairment, especially when diminished kidney and liver function is present. Drugs that alter the central nervous system include anticholinergics, antihistamines, antidepressants, anxiolytics, antipsychotics, and antiepileptics. These drugs may cause forgetfulness, confusion, disorientation, and inability to concentrate.

Social Issues Affecting Women with Disabilities

Approximately 27 million U.S. women and girls have some type of mental or physical disability. The most common disabilities in women are arthritis or rheumatism (CDC, 2016). The incidence of disability increases with age.

Definitions of Disability

A **disability** is a chronic physical or mental health problem or impairment that restricts an individual's ability to perform one or more major activities. Whether a given activity is considered major depends on the circumstances and responsibilities of the woman in question. For example, if a middle-aged woman cannot care for her home and children because of a disability, that disability would be considered major. If an elderly woman's disability makes independent self-care impossible, that disability would be considered major. Disabilities may also be categorized as "work" and "severe." *Work disabilities* restrict individuals from employment; a nurse who sustains a back injury that becomes chronic and prevents her from returning to her position as a staff nurse has a work disability. *Severe disabilities* prohibit individuals from performing basic activities of daily living without assistance.

Types of Disabilities

Disabilities are additionally categorized as physical, developmental, learning, neurologic, psychiatric, and sensory. *Developmental disabilities* are defined as a diverse group of severe chronic conditions that are due to mental and/or physical impairments. They include autism, blindness, cerebral palsy, learning disabilities, attention-deficit/hyperactivity disorder (ADHD), stuttering, developmental delays, intellectual disabilities, seizures, and hearing loss and are ongoing and manifest before 22 years of age (CDC, 2016). Developmental disabilities cause limitations in three or more of the following areas: Self-care, receptive and expressive language, learning, mobility, self-direction, ability to live alone, and financial independence. Approximately 13.8% of individuals have some type of developmental disability, and *intellectual disability* is the most common, affecting 6.5 million people in the United States (CDC, 2016) (Figure 7–6).

In the early- to mid-20th century, women with intellectual disabilities were often forced to undergo mandatory, involuntary sterilization. In contemporary society, the need for sexual health education is imperative because some girls and women with intellectual disabilities may face unplanned pregnancies. A number of women with intellectual disabilities are choosing to become pregnant based on their desires to become parents, which is a basic human right.

Pregnancy for a woman with an intellectual disability may result in:

- Late prenatal care enrollment
- Failure to recognize signs and symptoms related to pregnancy

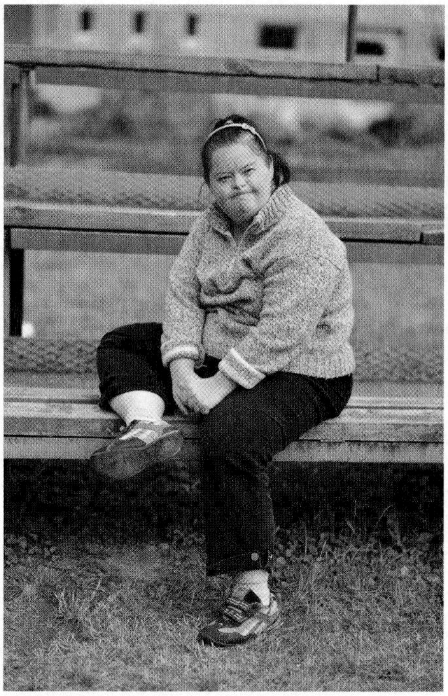

Figure 7–6 **Intellectual disability is the most common developmental disability.**

SOURCE: Marcel Jancovic/Shutterstock.

- Increased pregnancy termination rates
- Request for termination of pregnancy after gestational age limit
- Fear of telling others about pregnancy
- Child Protective Services involvement (25%) (Baum, 2018).

When women with intellectual disabilities do become pregnant, the following interventions should be implemented:

- Additional social support
- Parenting education
- Peer support
- Modifying teaching materials and delivery to meet varying learning needs.

Learning disabilities can inhibit educational attainment and employment. There are various learning disabilities, including:

- Dyslexia (language processing disorder that can hinder reading, writing, spelling, and, rarely, speaking)
- Dyscalculia (a range of learning disabilities involving math processing)
- Dysgraphia (difficulties with spelling, poor handwriting, and ability to put thoughts on paper)
- Dyspraxia (affects motor skill development; often coexists with learning disabilities)
- Executive functioning (difficulties in one's ability to plan, organize, and manage details).

Some women with learning disabilities may also have a co-occurring disorder that can impact learning, such as:

- Visual processing disorder
- Auditory processing disorder
- ADHD
- Autism spectrum disorders.

Common *neurologic disabilities* include spina bifida, cerebral palsy, multiple sclerosis, and Alzheimer disease. Spina bifida, or congenital malformation of the spinal cord, can cause partial paralysis. Multiple sclerosis, which affects a disproportionately high number of women in comparison with men, can cause severe mental and physical disability through degeneration of nerve fibers in the brain and spinal cord. Alzheimer disease causes ongoing, incurable dementia that culminates in death.

Psychiatric disabilities can cause significant impairment and significantly alter an individual's quality of life. Women's rates of depression, anxiety, panic disorders, and phobic disorders are 50% higher than men's. *Sensory disabilities* such as hearing loss and visual impairments can dramatically impair a woman's ability to interact socially and to live independently (Davidson, 2012).

Economic Vulnerability of Women with Disabilities

About 18% of individuals with disabilities are employed, in contrast with 64% of individuals without a disability. It should be noted that there are many different types of disabilities. Individuals with more severe disabilities commonly are impacted to a greater degree than those with less severe disabilities. Severe physical disability, such as in cases where an individual needs assistance with activities of daily living (ADLs), is often associated with greater economic difficulties due to possible limited education, employment and transportation issues, increased needs for healthcare equipment and resources, and the need to hire others to provide assistance. The most common factors related to unemployment among women with disabilities include:

- Lack of education or training
- Transportation issues/barriers
- Access issues for women with physical disabilities
- Need for special accommodations on the job
- Higher residence in rural areas where there are fewer employment options.

Many women with disabilities can only manage part-time employment, which severely restricts their income potential. The Americans with Disabilities Act (ADA) of 1990 was intended to reduce such barriers by mandating modest improvements in building accessibility and forbidding unjustified hiring discrimination against persons with disabilities (CDC, 2016). Although the ADA has brought about some improvements, many barriers to employment still exist.

Even when women with disabilities are able to work and find work, they typically do not earn as much as women who are not disabled. A greater number of disabled women live in poverty compared to men or women without a disability.

Clinical Tip

Most women who rely on Social Security disability benefits live in poverty and have scarce economic resources to afford medical care services. Familiarize yourself with local government assistance programs and nonprofit organizations in your area so that you may be able to offer assistive services.

Violence Against People with Disabilities

Women with disabilities are twice as likely to be victims of domestic violence as nondisabled women. During their lifetimes, 50% of disabled women will experience abuse or violence (Davidson, 2012). Disabled women are often victimized in ways that are specific to their disability and its severity, including:

- Inappropriate power and control by partner or care provider
- Financial abuse if woman has difficulty understanding basic finances
- Withholding care such as removal of hearing aids, refusal to take to the bathroom, removal of wheelchair
- Withholding medical treatment and services, food, and other essentials
- Emotional abuse by labeling woman as a burden.

Women who are disabled have unique challenges that put them at risk for violence along with an inability to obtain resources when violence does occur, which may include:

- Difficulty escaping from or fighting off an attacker
- Physical inability to leave a violent environment
- Communication deficits that make it difficult to report crime, abuse, or violence
- Inability to identify perpetrators due to vision or cognitive impairment
- Lack of understanding that abuse is not warranted or normal
- Fear of identifying care providers as perpetrators
- Lack of accessible shelters for victims of abuse
- Inability to recognize that certain attention represents abuse, neglect, or someone taking advantage of them.

Effects of Disability on Women's Healthcare

Women with disabilities need routine gynecologic care and preventive health education, as do all women, but healthcare services for women who are disabled are often suboptimal. Many women with disabilities report that various barriers prevent them from obtaining routine healthcare services. Overall, women who are disabled receive less preventive care than women without disabilities but have 2.5 times the yearly health expenditures of women without disabilities (Parish, 2013).

An additional problem is that many healthcare providers assume incorrectly that women with severe disabilities are not sexually active. Thus, many women who are disabled are not offered screening for sexually transmitted infections (STIs), education regarding STI/HIV prevention, contraceptive counseling, or preconception counseling. In the past, women with disabilities have not been appropriately screened for cervical cancer, breast cancer, HPV, and HIV (Parish, 2013). Women with intellectual disabilities are more likely to develop osteoporosis and need appropriate screening (Parish, 2013).

Social Issues Affecting Lesbian, Bisexual, and Transgender Women

Various social issues can detract from lesbian, bisexual, and transgender women's quality of life. Although contemporary society is embracing changing views, employment and housing discrimination; discrimination involving marriage, domestic life, and parenting issues; and general social discrimination are still encountered. In addition, lesbian, bisexual, and transgender women may face perceived and actual discrimination on the part of healthcare providers that negatively affects both access to and quality of healthcare.

Employment Discrimination

Employment discrimination is the most frequent complaint the American Civil Liberties Union (ACLU) receives from LGBTQI individuals. By 2016, 22 states and the District of Columbia had passed laws prohibiting employment discrimination based on sexual orientation and gender identity, and three additional states prohibited discrimination based on sexual orientation. In July, 2013, the Employment Non-Discrimination Act (ENDA) passed in the Senate but still has not been approved by the House of Representatives (Human Rights Campaign, 2016).

Employment discrimination is now a well-recognized issue, and the great majority of Fortune 500 companies have enacted antidiscrimination workplace regulations for sexual orientation, while a smaller number of companies has enacted policies related to gender identity (Human Rights Campaign, 2016).

The federal government has also made gains in combatting discrimination with the Don't Ask, Don't Tell Repeal Act of 2010, which now allows military service members to be openly gay or lesbian and serve in the military. The military now recognizes marriage among gay and lesbian service members and in 2016 made acceptance of transgender military members legal as well (Powers, 2016). As of the writing of this text, however, the current state of the decision to let transgender people serve in the military has been called into question.

Marriage Discrimination

In 2015, same-sex marriage became legal in all 50 states when the Supreme Court declared that refusal to marry same-sex couples was unconstitutional. According to Pew Research Center researchers Masci , Brown, and Kiley (2017), a progressive shift in beliefs and an increasing level of support and acceptance in the United States population began decades ago. Same-sex marriage is performed or recognized in 25 other countries and parts of Mexico and is gaining acceptance globally (Pew Research Center, 2017).

Spousal Benefits

Married LGBTQ families now have equality and receive the following benefits:

- Social Security benefits
- Tax return benefits for joint filing

- Estate tax and estate planning benefits
- Estate and gift tax exemptions
- Estate tax portability
- Life estate trusts
- Veteran and military benefits
- Federal employee benefits
- Immigration benefits.

Housing Discrimination

The federal Fair Housing Act prohibits housing discrimination based on race, color, national origin, religion, sex, disability, and familial status (presence of children in household), but has no specific provisions to protect the LGBTQI community. Despite the legalization of same-sex marriage, there have been no changes to the wording of the Fair Housing Act, thus leaving a loophole in which LGBTQI individuals can face discrimination in finding fair and affordable housing. Housing discrimination trends may improve as married couples can now show a combined family income that may provide better housing opportunities, but ongoing research will be needed to see if other discriminatory factors will continue to impact fair housing opportunities.

Parenting Issues

Although lesbian couples have more options to pursue parenting than gay couples, state adoption laws continue to place barriers on parenting for these families. Many lesbian women wish to become parents. For lesbian single women and couples, there are a considerable number of options. For some lesbian women, a partner may already have children from a previous relationship. When a lesbian partner assumes the role of another parent figure, it is known as becoming a *second parent*. All states, except Mississippi, recognize second parent or stepparent adoptions. When a second parent legally adopts the child, then that woman obtains the same legal rights as the biological parent. In some states, second-parent adoptions are only legal if the couple is married or have a civil union or domestic partnership. Although married couples seem to have more legal rights than unmarried couples, struggles for adoption rights and custody issues, should a split occur, remain complicated and undefined in many states.

In states where second-parent or stepparent adoption is not an option for same-sex couples, the second parent has no legal right to the children should the relationship dissolve. For example, in Mississippi, a single LGBTQI individual can legally adopt a child, but the partner is specifically prohibited from adopting the child, meaning there is no legal means to become the legal second parent.

If no biological children are brought into a relationship and a lesbian couple wishes to have children, there are a number of options to achieve parenthood (Figure 7–7):

- One partner undergoes artificial insemination via unknown donor or selected donor sperm.
- One partner becomes pregnant through a prearranged consensual sexual encounter for the purpose of conception.
- Both women jointly adopt a child.
- One woman adopts the child and becomes the legal parent.

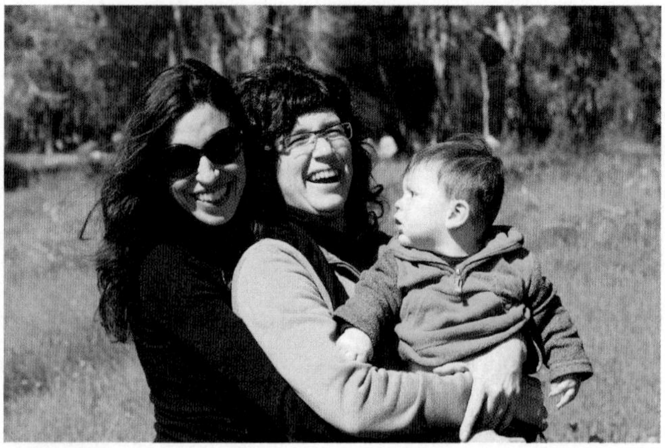

Figure 7–7 Lesbian families face discrimination that more traditional families do not commonly encounter.

SOURCE: Dubova/Shutterstock.

The majority of states have no official rules or regulations on fostering or adopting children based solely on identifying oneself as a LGBTQI family. As of 2018, only California, New Jersey, Rhode Island, and Washington, D.C. had laws in place to prohibit discrimination based on both sexual orientation and gender identity in order to ensure that all potential parents had the legal right to provide care to foster care children or to legally adopt children. An additional five states provided protection against discrimination based on sexual orientation, while 42 states had no policies and were considered "silent," meaning they do not support or oppose the issue. Currently, seven states have laws specifying that placement agencies can refuse to place children with same-sex couples if there is religious opposition (Movement Advancement Project, 2018). As same-sex marriage has become federal law, the rights for LGBTQI families will likely continue to evolve and play a role in upcoming political debate.

Social Barriers

LGBTQI individuals and couples often face discrimination—and even danger. They may be treated inappropriately and be subjected to rude comments. Some continue to be ostracized by business networks, churches, neighbors, and even their own families.

While the number of hate crimes in the United States has declined, hate crimes targeting LGBTQI individuals continue to climb, and they are now the highest recorded group targeted for violence. In 2016, close to 20% of the 6121 reported hate crimes were attributed to an individual's perceived sexual orientation or gender identity (Federal Bureau of Investigation, 2016). While hate crimes against LGBTQI individuals are tracked by the Federal Bureau of Investigation, there are a significant number of hate crimes that are never reported by the victims for fear of retribution, shame, guilt, and the desire for anonymity.

Ethics in Action!

How would you respond to another nurse who is negatively portraying a lesbian woman in labor due to her sexual orientation?

Effects of Discrimination on Lesbian, Bisexual, Transgender, and Intersex Women's Healthcare

Healthy People 2020 recognizes that health disparities continue to exist for the LGBTQI community. Lesbian, bisexual, transgender, and intersex women are at greater risk for health and social disparities, including:

- Increased suicide risk
- Increased risk of homelessness
- Increased incidence of violence
- Increased incidence of obesity
- Increased depression rates due to stigma and lack of social acceptance
- Increased tobacco use
- Higher incidence of alcohol use
- Increased rate of substance abuse disorders
- Lack of screening for female-related cancers (breast cancer and cervical cancer).

Lesbians have historically been at greater risk of adverse health outcomes based on their sexual orientation. In general, women's health services and healthcare practitioners have not shown acceptance of lesbian, bisexual, or transgender status. The common use of questions related to relationship status that excludes options for homosexual women to appropriately identify their sexual orientation and the assumption that all women are in need of contraception for birth control often are cited as reasons that lesbian women may conceal their sexual orientation. Lesbian women's reluctance to disclose their sexual orientation can lower the quality of healthcare they receive. For example, women who do not admit that they live with a same-sex partner will not be screened for domestic violence, which is a routine screening for women in heterosexual relationships.

Transgender women (those who were born as males according to their genitalia) and transgender men (those who were born as females according to their genitalia) both need resources for appropriate care. Transgender women and men and their families face emotional issues related to gender dysphoria. For transgender individuals and their family members and friends, there is often a period of time when others may find it difficult to process their new identity. Transgender women also have issues with hormone therapy and side effects associated with hormones. Transgender men, despite hormone use, who have a uterus, ovaries, and a cervix, are still at risk for female reproductive cancers and require ongoing screening. They may also need education regarding gender confirmation surgeries. Currently, it is not uncommon for transgender persons to have difficulties with health insurance companies refusing to pay for certain benefits. Variations in healthcare coverages are often state-based. Although federal law prohibits discrimination on the basis of gender, insurance companies may still refuse to pay for certain services. It is important for transgender persons to carefully review insurance plans prior to enrolling in certain plans.

Health issues for the intersex community include chromosomal problems, sexual performance and reproductive concerns due to ambiguous genitalia, and the mental health concerns that come with coping with these differences.

Many healthcare providers are unaware of the unique healthcare needs of lesbian, bisexual, transgender, and intersex women who are at increased risk for certain conditions (CDC, 2017). See Table 7–3.

Female Genital Mutilation

Female genital mutilation (FGM), also known as *female genital cutting*, *female circumcision*, and *genital circumcision*, refers to the practice of removing all or parts of a girl's or woman's genitalia for cultural reasons. FGM is a cultural ritual that is performed most commonly in sub-Saharan Africa and to a lesser extent in Asia and the Middle East. The ritual is a deep-rooted cultural practice that is performed for a variety of reasons, including perceived improved hygiene, social acceptance, marriageability, preservation of virginity/reduction of female sexual desire, male sexual pleasure, and religious requirement (UNICEF, 2017). The number of women in the United States who have undergone the procedure is on the rise due to immigration from regions of the world where the procedure is common. Women may feel a sense of shame or embarrassment once the procedure has been performed. It is important for nurses to ask women who have immigrated to the United States if they have had the procedure performed because it has implications for labor and birth, including urinary retention, painful examination/inability to adequately perform cervical examination, difficulty in placing intrauterine pressure catheter or fetal scalp electrode, need for extensive episiotomy and repair, third- or fourth-degree lacerations, and increased risk of cesarean birth (UNICEF, 2017). Some women will request that modifications, such as widening the vaginal opening, be performed after birth. Nearly all of these women will need an episiotomy because severe lacerations will occur with vaginal births. Some women may prefer to have the vaginal opening restored to its prebirth appearance. Because some women may be unable to ask for a revision in front of their husbands, questioning the woman when alone is preferred.

There are varying degrees of mutilation, ranging from complete removal of the external genitalia to complete removal of the clitoris. FGM can cause a variety of health problems, including bleeding, infection, urinary tract infections, urinary strictures, reproductive tract infection, infertility, painful intercourse, and difficulties related to childbearing, including obstructed labor, nonreassuring fetal status, postpartum hemorrhage, and postpartum sepsis. Some families may be offended by language that implies reversing the procedure because this may be viewed as judgmental. Instead, families may be more receptive to the discussion about how a repair after childbirth can be performed that will decrease the risks of medical complications in the future. It is imperative that women understand how the repair will look and that she knows what to expect once it has healed. See *Case Study: Azia Askari*.

TABLE 7–3 Healthcare Needs of Lesbian, Bisexual, Transgender, and Intersex Women

HEALTH CONDITION	RISK FACTORS	SCREENING RECOMMENDATIONS	NURSING INTERVENTION
Heart disease	Obesity, smoking, stress	Perform BMI, dietary recall, smoking history	Dietary counseling; refer to dietician for ongoing weight loss management, smoking-cessation classes, and pharmacologic aids.
Reproductive cancers	Reduced births, breastfeeding, and oral contraceptive pill use, lack of routine Pap and screening mammograms	Regular Pap smears, mammogram screening after 40, smoking history	Assess childbearing plans and discuss parenting options including sperm donation and artificial insemination; encourage breastfeeding if planning a pregnancy; oral contraceptives can be used for gynecological issues such as menorrhea, irregular menses; smoking-cessation counseling and pharmacologic management; advise women that smoking increases risk of cervical cancer.
Anxiety or depression and stress	Social stigma, lack of acceptance of sexual orientation by others, societal stressors, violence, lack of health insurance to cover mental health services	Use formal assessment instruments to diagnose anxiety and depression. Perform a mental health assessment at each visit, assess for intimate partner violence (IPV)	Provide referrals for individual and group counseling; provide psychoeducation for taking any prescribed medications for depression or anxiety; provide community-based resources; assist woman to identify support systems or establish new support system; assist with completing a safety plan should IPV occur. Stress reduction strategies should be taught that may include stretching or exercise, relaxation exercises, yoga, meditation, mindfulness exercises, or relaxing music.
Polycystic ovarian syndrome (PCOS)	Higher rates of PCOS in lesbian women	Hormone levels, menstrual calendar, fertility history, physical examination, assess for abnormal glucose/insulin levels, H-A1C	Advise women of insulin sensitivity and risk of diabetes; encourage exercise program; provide recommended dietary guidelines and help set goal weight; educate woman on medications used to manage PCOS as needed. If fertility desired, advise endocrinology consult. Pharmacologic management may result in improved fertility; infertility consult if pregnancy desired,
Lung cancer	Higher incidence of smoking in lesbian, bisexual, and transgender populations	Smoking history, family history, secondhand smoke exposure, physical exam, chest x-ray if symptomatic. For women ages 55–74 years who have smoked for 30 years and still smoke or who have quit within the past 15 years, perform a low-dose computed tomography. Women with pulmonary symptoms or those who continue to smoke should be screened annually.	Provide smoking-cessation counseling; consider both behavioral and pharmacologic interventions for smoking cessation. Discontinue all smoking and exposure to secondhand smoke.
Alcohol and substance abuse	Higher incidence in lesbian, bisexual, and transgender individuals	Alcohol and substance use/abuse history, review risk factors, previous use, family history of use	Referral to support groups (AA, NA), substance abuse treatment center; alcohol or drug detoxification as needed; counseling, behavioral modifications.
Obesity	Higher incidence in LGBT women, poor dietary habits	Screen for coexisting conditions, HA1C or FBS, screen for PCOS, obtain fitness history, family history, BMI, 24-hour dietary recall	Refer for behavioral interventions, nutritionist, and support groups. Encourage fitness program (such as walking) that includes 2 hours 30 minutes of exercise per week. Provide healthy dietary recommendations including calcium intake, well-balanced diet with limits on salt and fats. Increase healthy grains, lean meats and fish; encourage adequate hydration with water and consumption of organic products when possible.
Sexually transmitted infections (STIs)	Women with multiple sex partners, bisexual women increased risk of HIV	Women are at risk for bacterial vaginosis, candidiasis, herpes, and human papillomavirus infections. Screening tests should be based on past sexual history and presence of symptoms, if any. If high-risk sexual behavior in the past, comprehensive STI screening, including HIV testing, is warranted. Bisexual women have the highest rates of HIV seroconversion (higher than lesbian or heterosexual women).	Safe-sex counseling should include use of a dental dam, avoidance of oral sex during menstruation, handwashing before and after sex, use of latex gloves if cuts on hand are present, avoid oral sex from partner if mouth sores are present, avoid sharing sex toys, use condoms on sex toys if shared use is common practice, avoid activities that can cause bleeding.

CASE STUDY: Azia Askari

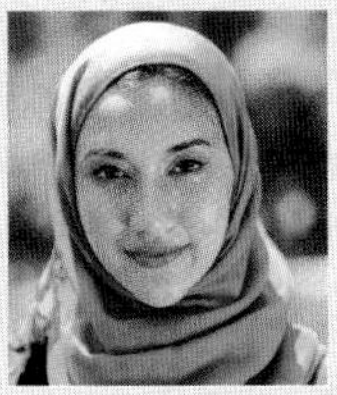

SOURCE: HONGQI ZHANG/123RF

Azia's mother-in-law, Shira, has arrived from Iran to help with the new baby. Shira is distressed after attending a prenatal appointment with her son and daughter-in-law because she learned that Azia has never been cut and is, therefore, considered to be unclean. Shira pleaded with the certified nurse-midwife to perform genital circumcision at the time of birth so that Azia will look more normal and be able to adequately perform sexual activities more culturally appropriate for her husband once she has recovered from childbirth.

Questions to Ponder

How would you engage Shira in a discussion on the ethical aspects of mandating her daughter-in-law undergo this technique after birth at the sole request of her husband's family? How could you, as a nurse, advocate for Azia, who states she is frightened and does not want to undergo the procedure?

Clinical Tip

Whenever possible, a woman who has undergone FGM should be delivered by an experienced practitioner who has skill in performing specific types of genital tract and perineal incisions needed to facilitate birth. Repair of birth-related episiotomies and incisions are best performed by a clinician familiar with the needs of this population.

Focus Your Study

- The number of women living in poverty is increasing. Childbearing women seem to be at particular risk because of current trends in the divorce rate, the frequency with which the mother gains custody of children, and factors in the work environment that make it difficult for women to earn an adequate wage.
- The number of families that are homeless has long-term implications for parents and children.
- Women's wages have always been lower than men's because of demand, education, skills, discrimination, and underlying philosophies that deem women's work less valuable.
- Employee benefits that affect women include maternity leave, paternity leave, and child care. The Family and Medical Leave Act mandates parental leave for childbirth or adoption but applies only to companies with 50 or more employees. Insurance coverage for childbirth varies by company.
- Elder abuse includes physical abuse, financial abuse, neglect, self-neglect, psychologic abuse, and abandonment.
- Older women may face multiple barriers when obtaining healthcare, including transportation difficulties, lack of health coverage, lack of research regarding chronic conditions affecting women, and symptom-specific, rather than holistic, care.
- There are multiple types of disabilities. All have the potential for limiting a woman's quality of life, her ability to care for herself, and the quality of her healthcare.
- Lesbian, bisexual, transgender, and intersex people face various forms of discrimination, some of which can negatively affect their health and healthcare.
- Nurses must provide culturally sensitive care to women who have undergone procedures involving genital mutilation.

References

American Academy of Allergy, Asthma & Immunology. (2014). *Allergy statistics.* Retrieved from http://www.aaaai.org/media/statistics/allergy-statistics.asp#latex_allergy

Badger, E. (2014). *The relationship between single mothers and poverty is not as simple as it seems.* Retrieved from https://www.washingtonpost.com/news/wonk/wp/2014/04/10/the-relationship-between-single-mothers-and-poverty-is-not-as-simple-as-it-seems/?utm_term=.0407f54563d4

Bahney, A. (2014). *Child care is biggest cost for many families.* Retrieved from http://www.forbes.com/sites/annabahney/2015/06/29/child-care-is-biggest-expense-for-a-growing-number-of-families/#3de5b096e8ad

Baum, S. (2018). *Parents with intellectual disabilities.* Retrieved from http://www.intellectualdisability.info/family/articles/parents-with-intellectual-disabilities

Center on Budget and Policy Priorities. (2017). *Policy basics: An introduction to TANF.* Retrieved from http://www.cbpp.org/research/policy-basics-an-introduction-to-tanf

Centers for Disease Control and Prevention (CDC). (2016). *Disability & health: Data & statistics.* Retrieved from http://www.cdc.gov/ncbddd/disabilityandhealth/data.html

Centers for Disease Control and Prevention (CDC) (2017). *Lesbian and bisexual women.* Retrieved from https://www.cdc.gov/lgbthealth/women.htm

Child Care Services Association. (2017). *Child care quality.* Retrieved from http://www.childcareservices.org/fs/finding/child-care-quality

Children's Bureau. (2017). *Trends in foster care and adoption.* Retrieved from https://www.acf.hhs.gov/cb/resource/trends-in-foster-care-and-adoption

Davidson, M. R. (2012). *A nurse's guide to women's mental health.* New York, NY: Springer.

Federal Bureau of Investigation. (2016). *Hate crime statistics: 2016.* Retrieved from http://www.fbi.gov/about-us/cjis/ucr/hate-crime/2016

Federal Safety Net. (2017). *U.S. poverty statistics.* Retrieved from http://federalsafetynet.com/us-poverty-statistics.html

Hamilton, B. E., Martin, J. A., Ostermen, M. J. K., Curtin, S. C., & Matthews, M. A. (2015). Births: Final data for 2014. *National Vital Statistics Reports, 64*(12), 1–61.

Human Rights Campaign. (2016). *Support the Equity Act.* Retrieved from https://www.hrc.org/campaigns/support-the-equality-act

Institute for Women's Policy Research (IWPR). (2015). *The status of women in the states, 2015.* Retrieved from https://iwpr.org/publications/the-status-of-women-in-the-states-2015-full-report

Jeffrey, T. P. (2016). *First time in human history: People 65 and older will outnumber people younger than 5.* Retrieved from http://www.cnsnews.com/news/article/terence-p-jeffrey/first-time-human-history-global-population-over-65-poised-pass

Jeong, C. H., Zhou, C., & Flaws, J. A. (2017). Environmental toxicants and reproduction. In R. G. Farquharson & M. D. Stephenson (Eds.), *Early pregnancy* (2nd ed., pp. 62–67). Cambridge, UK: Cambridge University Press.

Kaiser Family Foundation. (2017). *Key facts about the uninsured population.* Retrieved from http://kff.org/uninsured/fact-sheet/key-facts-about-the-uninsured-population

Masci, D., Brown, A., & Kiley, J. (2017). *5 facts about same sex marriage.* Pew Research Center. Retrieved from http://www.pewresearch.org/fact-tank/2017/06/26/same-sex-marriage

Miller, C. C. (2015). *Single motherhood, in decline overall, rises for women 35 and older.* Retrieved from http://www.nytimes.com/2015/05/09/upshot/out-of-wedlock-births-are-falling-except-among-older-women.html?_r=0

Movement Advancement Project (MAP). (2018). *Foster and adoption laws.* Retrieved from http://www.lgbtmap.org/equality-maps/foster_and_adoption_laws

National Alliance to End Homelessness. (2017). *LGBTQ youth.* Retrieved from https://endhomelessness.org/category/lgbt/

National Center on Elder Abuse (NCEA). (2017a). *Statistics/data.* Retrieved from https://ncea.acl.gov/whatwedo/research/statistics.html#population

National Center on Elder Abuse (NCEA). (2017b). *What is elder abuse?* Retrieved from https://ncea.acl.gov/faq/#faq1

National Institute on Drug Abuse. (2016). *Misuse of prescription drugs.* Retrieved from https://www.niehs.nih.gov/health/topics/agents/air-pollution/index.cfm

National Institute of Environmental Health Sciences. (2017). *Air pollution.* Retrieved from https://www.niehs.nih.gov/health/topics/agents/air-pollution/index.cfm

National Women's Law Center [NWLC]. (2016). *National snapshot: Women & families living in poverty: 2015.* Retrieved from https://nwlc.org/resources/national-snapshot-poverty-among-women-families-2015

National Vital Statistics System. (2015). National marriage and divorce trends. Retrieved from https://www.cdc.gov/nchs/nvss/marriage_divorce_tables.htm

Parish, S. L. (2013). *Preventative health care services for women with developmental disabilities.* Retrieved from http://aadmd.org/sites/default/files/D2%2003%20Parish.pdf

Pew Research Center. (2015). *Raising kids and running a household: How working parents share the load: In close to half of two-parent families, both mom and dad work full time.* Retrieved from http://www.pewsocialtrends.org/2015/11/04/raising-kids-and-running-a-household-how-working-parents-share-the-load

Pew Research Center. (2017). *Gay marriage around the world.* Retrieved from http://www.pewforum.org/2017/08/08/gay-marriage-around-the-world-2013/

Powers, R. (2016). *Policies concerning homosexuals in the US military.* Retrieved from https://www.thebalance.com/policy-concerning-homosexuals-us-military-3347134

Russell, K., & Porter, E. (2016). *Living with one parent.* Retrieved from https://www.nytimes.com/interactive/2016/03/22/business/economy/children-with-single-parent.html?_r=0

Single Mother Guide. (2016). *Single mother statistics.* Retrieved from https://singlemotherguide.com/single-mother-statistics/

Social Solutions. (2016). *2016's shocking homelessness statistics.* Retrieved from http://www.socialsolutions.com/blog/2016-homelessness-statistics/

Stahl, S. M. (2017). *Stahl's essential psychopharmacology: Neuroscientific basis and practical application* (6th ed.). Cambridge, UK: Cambridge University Press.

UNICEF. (2017). *Female genital mutilation/cutting: A statistical overview.* Retrieved from http://unicef.org/media/files/FGCM_Lo_res.pdf

U.S. Department of Labor, Bureau of Labor Statistics. (2017). *Employment characteristics of families summary.* Retrieved from https://www.bls.gov/news.release/pdf/famee.pdf

U.S. Equal Employment Opportunity Commission. (2017). *Pregnancy discrimination.* Retrieved from https://www.eeoc.gov/laws/types/pregnancy.cfm

U.S. National Library of Medicine. (2017). *Tox town: Phthalates.* Retrieved from http://toxtown.nlm.nih.gov/text_version/chemicals.php?id=24

Weinberger, B. Z. (2016). *When grandkids need you to care for them: What are your options?* Retrieved from http://www.huffingtonpost.com/bari-zell-weinberger-esq/grandparents-caring-for-grandchildren_b_11910112.html

Whitman, E. (2016). Bundles of joy?: How new payment models for maternal care could deliver lower costs. *Modern Healthcare.* Retrieved from http://www.modernhealthcare.com/article/20160813/MAGAZINE/308139965

Wong, B. (2014). The truth about divorce is surprisingly optimistic. *Huffington Post.* Retrieved from http://www.huffingtonpost.com/2014/12/02/divorce-rate-declining-_n_6256956.html

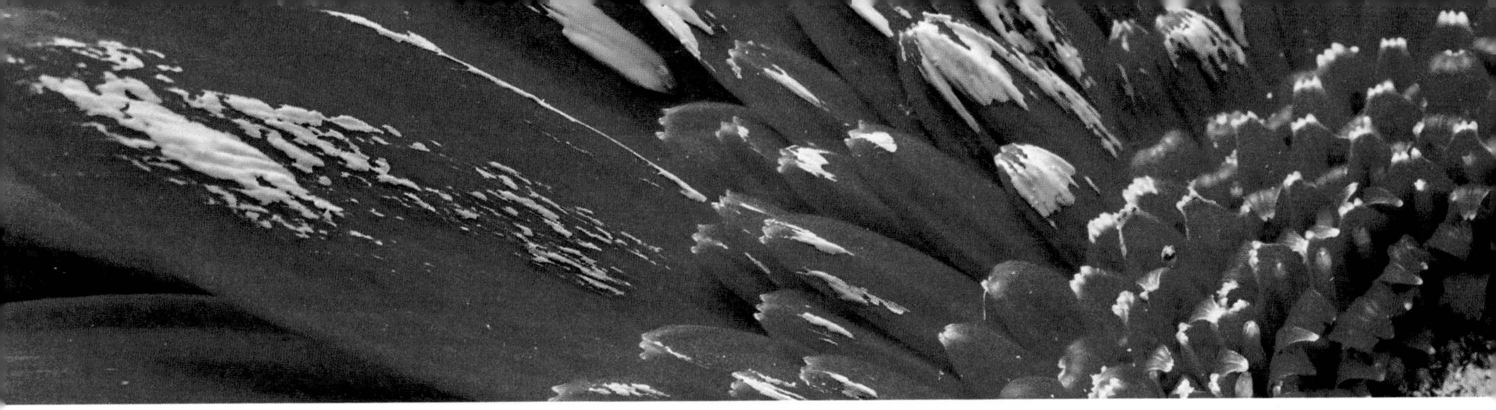

Chapter 8
Violence Against Women

My friends believe I'm living the American dream. My husband has a great job in his company and our life looks ideal. Even if I told them about the occasional slap, the shove, the forced sex, and the angry words, they would probably think it was worth it. Sometimes I think about leaving, but it would mean admitting I failed. I know it doesn't make sense—he does the hitting, but I feel ashamed. I'm not a battered wife; I can't be. My husband just has a quick temper.

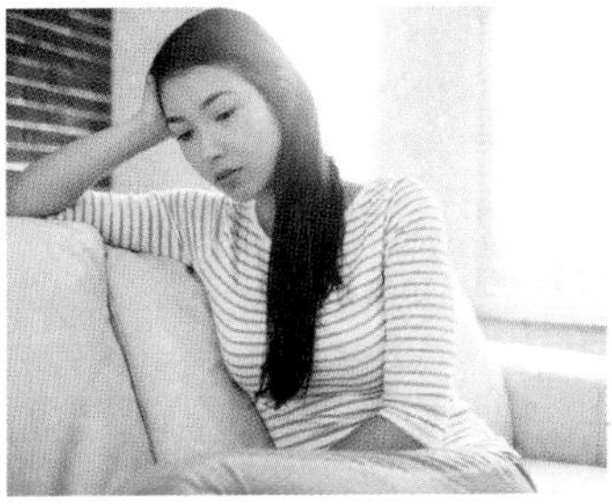

SOURCE: wavebreakmedia/Shutterstock.

Learning Outcomes

- 8.1 Describe the factors that contribute to the occurrence of domestic violence and sexual assault.
- 8.2 Identify factors that contribute to domestic violence.
- 8.3 Identify the phases of the cycle of violence.
- 8.4 Summarize the characteristics of batterers and perpetrators of sexual assault.
- 8.5 Delineate the role of the nurse in caring for women who have experienced partner abuse.
- 8.6 Specify physical and psychologic signs that may indicate a woman is in an abusive relationship.
- 8.7 Describe the needs that women with abusive partners and their children may have beyond the healthcare setting.
- 8.8 Identify the phases of the rape trauma syndrome.
- 8.9 Discuss the nurse's role as patient advocate with domestic violence and sexual assault survivors.
- 8.10 Summarize the procedures for collecting and preserving physical evidence of sexual assault.
- 8.11 Discuss the legal responsibilities of the community to prevent and address violence against women.

Healthy People 2020

(IVP-39) (Developmental) Reduce violence by current or former partners

(IVP-40) (Developmental) Reduce sexual violence

Violence against women is a public health problem that has a negative effect on millions of people in the United States each year. Experts suggest that as many as one in three women will be abused at some time in their lives. Violence affects women of all ages, races, ethnic backgrounds, religions, socioeconomic status, educational level, and sexual orientation. Two of the most common forms of societal violence are domestic violence, also called *intimate partner violence (IPV)* or *relationship violence*, and sexual violence, also called *sexual assault*. Worldwide, 35% of women have experienced intimate partner violence or nonpartner sexual violence at some time in their lives; estimates suggest that 38% of all female murders are committed by an intimate partner (World Health Organization [WHO], 2016).

Although women of all ages are victims of rape/sexual assault, the majority (54%) are between the ages of 18 and 34 (Rape, Abuse & Incest National Network [RAINN], 2016). Sexual assault remains one of the most underreported violent crimes in the United States. In 2015, only an estimated 32.5% of rapes or sexual assaults were reported to the police, making the actual number of victims significantly higher (Truman & Morgan, 2016). Over 72% of victims know their offender; about half of assailants are age 30 or older. Although both men and women can be sexually assaulted, research indicates that approximately 9 out of every 10 rape or sexual assault victims are female (RAINN, 2016).

> **Developing Cultural Competence Intraracial Victimization**
>
> In the United States during 2012–2015, the majority of violent victimizations were *intraracial*, meaning that both the victim and the offender were of the same race. Specifically, White victims' offenders were White in 57% of cases, and Black victims' offenders were Black in 63% of cases (Morgan, 2017).

Rates of victimization are higher among lesbian and bisexual women than among heterosexual women. Partner violence in lesbian/gay/bisexual/transgender/queer/questioning/intersex (LGBTQI) relationships has only recently been recognized as an important social problem. Historically, it has been difficult to gather information on violence within same-sex relationships because the studies have had to rely on small convenience samples of women who are sufficiently open and comfortable with their sexual orientation to participate in a study (Calton, Cattaneo, & Gebhard, 2016).

Although it may be less recognized, older women can also be victims of intimate partner violence. In this age group, psychologic abuse, including yelling, is often the most common type of violence. Research suggests a link between age-related dependency and abuse. Because an older woman may fear for her future without financial support and may even fear nursing home placement, she may be reluctant to report abuse.

In addition to injuries sustained during violent episodes, physical, sexual, and psychologic violence are linked to a number of adverse physical and mental health outcomes. The estimated health-related costs of violence against women exceed $8.3 billion *annually* in the United States. This cost includes medical care, mental health services, and lost productivity (e.g., time away from work) (Centers for Disease Control and Prevention [CDC], 2015a).

Individuals who are controlling of their partners are much more likely to be physically assaultive, sending partners for visits to emergency departments and often leading to future homicides. Healthcare providers can play a critical role in identifying and reducing violence, even in homicide prevention efforts.

Over the past three decades there have been a number of notable changes in healthcare policy and practices aimed at responding to violence against women. *Healthy People 2020*, a national project sponsored by the Office of Disease Prevention and Health Promotion, identifies IPV as a problem crossing racial/ethnic boundaries and socioeconomic strata and cites intervention and prevention for violent behavior as a national priority. Significantly, nursing has played and continues to play a key role in developing and evaluating innovative healthcare practices aimed at identifying and reducing violence against women.

Historic Factors Contributing to Violence Against Women

Violence against women is not new. Throughout history, for thousands of years in patriarchal societies, women have been victims of violence. Within the institution of marriage, wives were considered the property of husbands, subject to their wishes and demands. A husband had the right—even the duty—to "keep her in line," to have sex on demand, even to kill her. Outsiders were expected to "keep out of it"; battering and sexual assault were family matters. The legal status of women has improved over the years in a number of cultures. However, many people still hold to the traditional views of male dominance in marriage or any intimate relationship, which can contribute to the occurrence of domestic violence and sexual assault.

Traditionally, rape outside of marriage was not viewed as an act of a man against a woman, but as an act of aggression against another man—the woman's husband, father, or brother, whoever was considered her "owner."

Worldwide, women today are at great risk. Violence against women and girls is increasingly being used as a weapon of war, stigmatizing, humiliating, and terrifying women and their families. Over the years the United Nations (UN) has passed resolutions that address the need to eliminate all forms of discrimination against women. Resolution 2122, passed in 2013, reaffirms this commitment. Among the issues it addresses, the resolution expresses " . . . *deep concern* at the full range of threats and human rights violations and abuses experienced by women in armed conflict and post-conflict situations, *recognizing* that those women and girls who are particularly vulnerable or disadvantaged may be specifically targeted or at increased risk of violence, and *recognizing* in this regard that more must be done to ensure that transitional justice measures address the full range of violations and abuses of women's human rights . . . ." (United Nations, 2013, p. 2/6). In 2014, the World Health Organization's 67th World Health Assembly adopted a resolution "Strengthening the role of the health system in addressing violence, in particular against women and girls, and against children" (p. 1).

Domestic Violence

Domestic violence, also called *intimate partner violence (IPV)*, is defined as a pattern of coercive behaviors and methods used to gain and maintain power and control by one individual over another in an adult intimate relationship. Domestic violence occurs in relationships in which the partners are dating, living together, married, separated, or divorced. Among heterosexual couples, estimates indicate that in at least 95% of all domestic violence cases the perpetrators are men. Although the perpetrators in female same-sex relationships are women, lesbians who abuse other women may do it for similar reasons to that of heterosexual males.

Domestic violence is staggeringly common. In the United States, nearly one in four women will experience domestic violence (CDC, 2015a). The incidence of domestic violence is highest in females age 18 to 24 and 25 to 34, but it does occur in all age groups and among men (Figure 8–1).

Forms of abuse vary but typically fall into the following categories:

- ***Physical abuse:*** May include acts such as pushing, shoving, slapping, hitting with a fist or object, kicking, choking, threatening with a gun or knife, or using a gun or knife against the woman; may also include forcing alcohol or drug use or denying a partner medical care
- ***Emotional abuse:*** Constant criticism, name calling, unreasonable demands, damaging her relationship with her children and others who matter to her
- ***Sexual abuse:*** Forced sex including vaginal, oral, or anal intercourse; also includes sexually demeaning treatment,

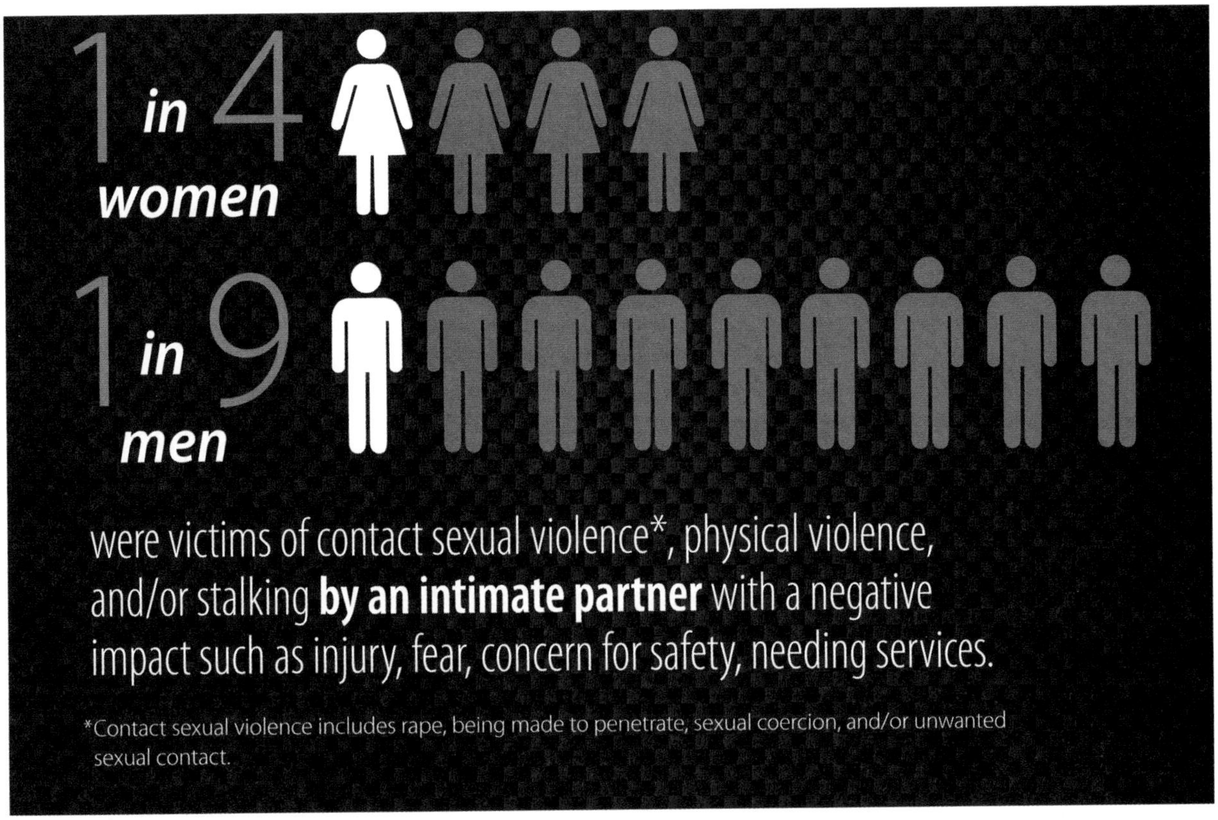

Figure 8–1 **Intimate partner violence is widespread.**

SOURCE: CDC, 2016. Retrieved from https://www.cdc.gov/violenceprevention/pdf/NISVS-infographic-2016.pdf

forced use of objects, or forcing a woman to have sex with someone else against her will

- *Isolation:* Controlling who she sees and where she goes, using jealousy to justify restricting her actions, interfering with her job, forbidding her to see family and friends, limiting her outside involvement
- *Economic abuse:* Preventing her from getting or keeping a job, making her ask for money, controlling her money, destroying her property, making all the financial decisions
- *Coercion threats:* Making and/or carrying out threats to harm her or her family and friends, threatening to commit suicide, pressuring her to drop charges, threatening negative consequences if she does not cooperate with his wishes, pressuring her with gifts, promises, or apologies
- *Intimidation:* Making her afraid through looks and gestures, smashing things, harming pets, displaying weapons, yelling, stalking her, driving recklessly
- *Using others:* Using the children against her, using visitation to harass her, threatening to take the children away from her, using religion to control her
- *Male privilege:* Treating her like a servant, defining rigid men's and women's roles, making all of the decisions or rules in the household
- *Stalking:* Repeated unwanted contact or attention or conduct directed at a specific person that would cause a reasonable person to feel fear.

The power and control wheel shown in Figure 8–2 illustrates how abusers use these tactics in relationships.

Typically, these forms of abuse begin slowly and subtly after some form of commitment, such as engagement, onset of a sexual relationship, marriage, pregnancy, first childbirth, or first

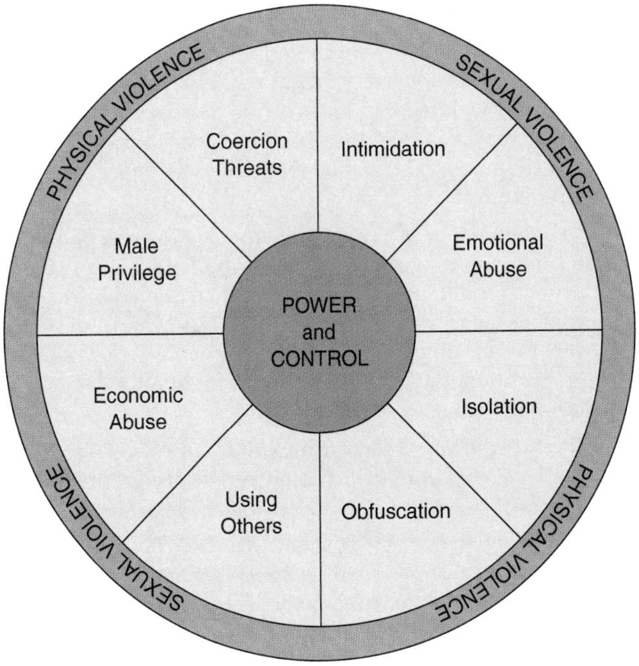

Figure 8–2 **The power and control wheel.**

SOURCE: Adapted from the Domestic Abuse Intervention Project, Duluth, Minnesota.

statement of commitment. Sometimes the woman will not recognize that she is in an abusive relationship.

The consequences of the abuse can be profound. In addition to the physical consequences, which are outlined later in this chapter, a woman may experience adverse psychologic consequences, such as symptoms of posttraumatic stress disorder, depression, antisocial behavior, anxiety, suicidal behavior, low self-esteem, and fear of intimacy. Women sometimes face social consequences as well, including restricted access to services, isolation from social networks, and strained relationships with health providers and employers. Clearly, it is important to understand the factors that contribute to domestic violence and the role of the nurse in caring for women who have experienced battering.

Women with Special Needs Intimate Partner Violence

Women with disabilities are at greater risk of being victimized and of suffering intimate partner violence. Women who rely on their partner for assistance with activities of daily living are at risk for having care withheld and neglect, in addition to physical and mental abuse. They are also at risk for financial abuse. The nurse should provide an extensive intimate partner assessment with the woman without the partner present to determine if abuse is occurring.

Contributing Factors

Domestic violence is a result of the complex and dynamic interaction of social, cultural, political, and psychologic factors. Although none of these factors alone is sufficient to explain why domestic violence occurs, there is substantial research to suggest that the following factors are significantly related to experiences of domestic violence.

- *Childhood experiences:* Children who witness or experience abuse and battering are more likely to become batterers (men) or to be abused (women) in their own relationships. Exposure to domestic violence, however, is not a prerequisite for future abuse. Not all children who witness violence in the home as children find themselves in abusive relationships as adults.
- *Male dominance in the family:* Worldwide, male economic and decision-making authority in the family is one of the strongest predictors of societies that demonstrate high violence against women, including domestic violence. Men raised in patriarchal families (those that encourage traditional gender roles) are more likely to engage in domestic violence.
- *Marital conflict:* Relationships that are characterized by high levels of conflict, including verbal disagreements, are more likely to include the use of violence than are those relationships with lower levels of marital conflict.
- *Unemployment/low socioeconomic status:* Domestic violence occurs in all socioeconomic classes; however, it is more common in families with low incomes and unemployed men. The reasons for this have not yet been determined. It may not be a lack of income, but some other variable related to living in poverty—stress, frustration, feelings of inadequacy in filling the male role of provider, overcrowding, or a lack of community institutions and norms that would create quality community social interactions—that explains this relationship.
- *Traditional definitions of masculinity/hypermasculinity:* Cultures that link definitions of manhood to dominance, toughness, or male honor are more likely to demonstrate violence against women. This may result because socialization into traditional male norms includes telling young boys to be tough, not to shy away from violence, and to hide their feelings, particularly those that are associated with traditional notions of femininity.
- *Internalized homophobia (within lesbian relationships):* A woman with an underdeveloped or unaccepted view of her own sexual identity might engage in violence against her partner. Additionally, a woman who identifies as LGBTQI and who has low self-worth might believe that she deserves to be treated abusively.

Common Myths about Battering and Women with Abusive Partners

Both professionals and the public believe numerous myths about battering and about women with abusive partners. These myths often reinforce misunderstanding of battering, furthering a woman's sense of victimization. Some commonly accepted myths are discussed here.

- ***Battering occurs in a small percentage of the population.*** The statistics on reported cases underrepresent the true incidence. As many as one in four women may be the victim of assault by her partner in her lifetime; however, it is a widely underreported crime.
- ***Women who are abused provoke men to beat them; women push men beyond the breaking point and incite physical violence.*** It is important to recognize that people are individually responsible for their own behavior. Batterers become violent because of their own internal inadequacies, not because of what their partners did or did not do.
- ***Alcohol and drug abuse cause battering.*** Studies do show a relationship between battering incidents and alcohol or drug use by batterers, and many batterers have a history of alcoholism or drug addiction. However, claims that substance abuse *causes* domestic violence are false and only serve to shift the responsibility away from the batterer. Nevertheless, alcohol or drugs may reduce the batterer's inhibitions, increasing the likelihood of violent acts. Battered women sometimes think that the abuse will stop if their partners stop drinking or using drugs. Unfortunately, this usually does not happen.
- ***Battered women can easily leave the situation.*** Leaving is easier said than done. Battered women may still love their partners or husbands and believe the promises of change, rely on them for financial support, and feel their children need a father. They are often isolated by their abusers from family, friends, and agencies that could assist them. Women may also experience a lack of support from family members, friends, and their religious communities. Many women with children have no place to go, and shelters sometimes have long waiting lists. Moreover, battered women are at greatest risk for injury or domestic homicide when they leave their abusers. Women may fear for their safety, their children's safety, and the safety of those who help them.

- ***Domestic violence is a low-income or minority issue.*** Domestic violence occurs among all sectors of society. It happens to women of all socioeconomic statuses, races, ethnicities, and religious faiths.
- ***Battered women will be safer when they are pregnant.*** Battering may occur for the first time during pregnancy or may escalate in intensity if the woman is already being abused. The injury is frequently aimed at the breasts, abdomen, or vagina. Many researchers and advocates believe that batterers are threatened by a pregnancy because the fetus interferes with the abuser's ability to maintain power and control within the relationship.

"Miles hit me for the first time when I was 5 months pregnant. I was stunned. My father never laid a hand on my mother or on any of us. Women who stayed in abusive situations had always appalled me, but suddenly I found myself making excuses for him and rationalizing that he hadn't meant it, that he would never do it again. Three months later he shoved me so hard I fell against an end table. I was pretty bruised, but I didn't go into labor. Somehow I found the courage to call my dad. He came and got me that night. My baby is 3 months old now and Miles keeps calling, telling me how sorry he is and that he loves me. Oh, how I want to believe him when he says he is changed, but I just can't take the chance."

Cycle of Violence

Walker (1984), in an effort to better explain the experience of battered women, developed the theory of the **cycle of violence**, which postulates that battering takes place in a cyclic fashion through three phases.

1. In the *tension-building phase*, the batterer demonstrates power and control. This phase is characterized by anger, arguing, blaming the woman for external problems, and possibly minor battering incidents. As the stress builds and communications break down, the woman often senses growing danger. She may also blame herself for the battering and believe she can prevent the escalation of the batterer's anger by her own actions, hoping that the relationship will somehow change for the better. The length of this phase varies considerably across individual cases, ranging from weeks to years.
2. The *acute battering incident* is typically triggered by some external event or internal state of the batterer. It is an episode of acute violence distinguished by lack of predictability and major destructiveness. The batterer blames the woman for the abuse, and the woman may accommodate him in order to survive, believe that escape is futile, or escape and return when the crisis is over. This is generally the briefest of the three phases, lasting from a few hours to a few days.
3. The *tranquil phase* is also sometimes called the *honeymoon period*. This phase may be characterized by extremely loving, kind, and contrite behaviors by the batterer as he tries to make up with the woman, or it may simply be manifested by an absence of tension and violence. The couple or family is often relieved that the crisis is past, and the woman may accept the batterer's promises and gifts because she is worn down and wants to believe that the violence will not happen again. Without intervention this phase will end at some point, and the cycle of violence will repeat. Over time, the cycle of violence often increases in severity and frequency. See *Case Study: Angelina Newman*.

Characteristics of Batterers

Batterers come from all racial, ethnic, and religious groups and all professions, occupations, and socioeconomic strata. What they have in common are feelings of insecurity, inferiority, powerlessness, and helplessness that conflict with their assumptions of male supremacy. Because they tend to be emotionally immature and aggressive, they have a tendency to express their overwhelming feelings of inadequacy through violence.

Many batterers feel undeserving of their partners, yet they blame and punish the very person they value. Extreme jealousy and possessiveness are the hallmarks of abusers. They characteristically express their ambivalence by alternating episodes of unmerciful beatings with periods of remorse and loving attention. Extremes in behavior and overreacting are typical patterns.

Batterers may be very calculating and select a partner they feel may be vulnerable. Over time they slowly and purposefully isolate the woman, creating a situation of increased dependence. Women often describe their abusive husbands or partners as lacking respect toward women in general, having come from homes where they have witnessed abuse of their mothers or were themselves abused as children, and having a hidden rage that erupts occasionally. Batterers accept conventional "macho" values, yet when they are not angry or aggressive, they may appear childlike, dependent, seductive, manipulative, and in need of nurturing.

Batterers may be well respected in the community. This is important because it is one of the reasons why women are sometimes not believed or taken seriously when they seek support and

CASE STUDY: Angelina Newman

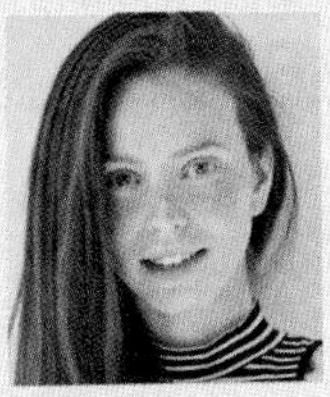

SOURCE: WAYHOME studio/Shutterstock

Angelina and her boyfriend had a physical altercation yesterday evening after he had been drinking beer with his friends. She presents with an edematous lip and it is obvious that she has been crying. Her mother notes this is an isolated incident, "a rough patch," and that she is sure it will never occur again. When you question her, Angelina admits he has pushed her before and even slapped her once at a party.

Question to Ponder

How would you describe the cycle of abuse to Angelina and explain why the violence will likely occur again?

assistance from friends, family members, and other resources. This dual personality of batterers reflects the conflict between their belief that they must live up to their macho image and their feelings of inadequacy and insecurity in the role of husband or provider. Combined with low tolerance for frustration and poor impulse control, the batterers' pervasive sense of powerlessness leads them to strike out at life's inequities by abusing women.

●○● NURSING MANAGEMENT

For the Woman Experiencing Domestic Violence

Increased publicity, public sensitivity, and heightened awareness of domestic violence are encouraging women with abusive partners to seek resources and community assistance. See Figure 8–3. In the past decade, many communities have developed domestic violence programs, shelters, and resources for women with abusive partners. However, the needs of women who have been abused and their children are still insufficiently met.

Women in abusive relationships enter the healthcare system in many different settings. Nurses may see them in the physician's office with minor trauma or in the emergency department with multiple severe injuries. They are frequently seen in obstetric services because battering often begins or escalates during pregnancy. Nurses in psychiatric or mental health services frequently counsel women who have been battered, and community health nurses may find women reporting abuse during home visits. Universal screening is advocated as an effective approach to identify women in such situations, and you must recognize that being so identified requires both caring concern and follow-up practices. In order to help battered women, you need advanced knowledge of the dynamics of battering; assessment skills for recognizing and documenting abuse; and appropriate intervention skills in counseling, safety planning, and referral. Working with women who have been abused is sometimes frustrating, and many healthcare providers feel puzzled when women return to their abusive situations. Understand that you cannot rescue women with abusive partners; women must decide on their own how to handle the situation, which is often incredibly complex and dangerous. Research has shown that women's risks for homicide and additional violence are greatest during separation or attempts at separation. Provide women who have been abused with information that empowers them in decision making and provide critical assistance in safety planning for women and their children.

Nursing Assessment and Diagnosis

Domestic violence often remains unidentified by healthcare providers even though experts and caregivers now advocate universal screening of all female patients at every healthcare encounter.

It is essential to recognize the importance of and need for comprehensive domestic violence education and training for healthcare providers. In addition to factual information about domestic violence and its impact on women's physical, psychologic, and sexual health, comprehensive education and training should include opportunities to practice skill development (e.g., in screening, assessment, empathic listening, diagnosis, planning, and communication across diverse age and ethnic/cultural groups) as well as opportunities to explore one's personal responses, attitudes, and values related to abuse.

You may be hesitant to ask about domestic violence because you presume the woman may be offended by the questions. However, women are rarely offended by questions about abuse, particularly if prefaced by a statement such as, "Because violence is so common in many people's lives, I've begun routinely asking all the women I care for about it." Basic screening questions are useful in identifying women who are experiencing abuse. If a woman responds affirmatively to the questions, ask her to mark the area(s) of injury on a body map. Screening for women experiencing domestic violence must be done privately, with only yourself and the patient present, in a safe and quiet place (Figure 8–4). Reassure the woman that her responses will be kept confidential. Strive for a calm and reassuring tone. Although tone, body language, and other nonverbal signs are important in establishing trusting relationships with all women, be especially aware of these issues in interventions with women from cultural and linguistic minority groups. They may be sensitized to these cues because they have used them as a survival strategy against discrimination and prejudice. See *Case Study: Azia Askari*.

A number of signs that may not be related to a woman's presenting injuries can indicate the possibility that a woman is in a violent relationship. Although no single one of these signs necessarily indicates abuse, the occurrence of several of these signs certainly merits an at-risk diagnosis. Exercise your professional judgment and communicate your conclusions to the woman. Signs that may indicate a woman is in an abusive relationship include:

- ***Neurologic signs:*** Headaches, including headache following trauma or concussion, tension headache, and migraines; dizziness; paresthesias; unexplained stroke from strangulation; hearing loss; detached retina
- ***Gynecologic signs:*** Dyspareunia (painful intercourse), sexually transmitted infections (STIs), frequent vaginal infections, sexual dysfunction, menstrual disorders, pelvic pain
- ***Obstetric signs:*** Late onset of prenatal care, premature labor, low-birth-weight newborn, excessive concern over fetal wellbeing, recurrent therapeutic abortion, recurrent spontaneous abortion
- ***Gastrointestinal signs:*** Dyspepsia, irritable bowel syndrome, globus (sensation of a lump in the throat)
- ***Musculoskeletal signs:*** Arthralgias (painful joints), chronic pain, osteoarthritis, fibromyalgia
- ***Psychiatric signs:*** Anxiety, panic, posttraumatic stress disorder, mood disorders, depression, suicide attempts, somatization, eating disorders, substance abuse, child abuse and neglect
- ***Constitutional signs:*** Fatigue, weight loss, weight gain, multiple somatic complaints, contusions, abrasions, sleep and appetite disturbances, decreased concentration, frequent use of pain medication or tranquilizers
- ***Trauma:*** Any injury to the female organs, extensive accident history, old fractures, sexual trauma
- ***Other signs:*** History of missed appointments or frequently changed appointments; low self-esteem, as seen in the woman's dress, her appearance, and the way she relates to healthcare providers.

When a woman seeks care for an injury, the nurse should be alert to the following cues of abuse:

- Hesitation in providing detailed information about the injury and how it occurred
- Inappropriate affect for the situation
- Defensive injuries
- Delayed reporting of symptoms or of seeking care for injuries

2017

Preventing Intimate Partner Violence

What is intimate partner violence?

Intimate partner violence (IPV) is violence or aggression that occurs in a close relationship. The term "intimate partner" includes current and former spouses and dating partners. IPV can vary in frequency and severity and occurs on a continuum, ranging from one episode that might or might not have lasting impact, to chronic and severe episodes over a period of years.

IPV includes four types of behavior:[1]

- **Physical violence** is when a person hurts or tries to hurt a partner by hitting, kicking, or using another type of physical force.
- **Sexual violence** is forcing or attempting to force a partner to take part in a sex act, sexual touching, or a non-physical sexual event (e.g., sexting) when the partner does not or cannot consent.
- **Stalking** is a pattern of repeated, unwanted attention and contact by a partner that causes fear or concern for one's own safety or the safety of someone close to the victim.
- **Psychological aggression** is the use of verbal and non-verbal communication with the intent to harm another person mentally or emotionally and/or exert control over another person.

Several types of IPV can occur together. IPV is associated with several risk and protective factors. It is connected to other forms of violence, and causes serious health and economic consequences. By using a public health approach that addresses risk and protective factors for multiple types of violence, IPV and other forms of violence can be prevented.[2]

How big is the problem?

IPV is common. It affects millions of people in the U.S. each year. Data from CDC's National Intimate Partner and Sexual Violence Survey (NISVS) indicate:[3]

- Nearly 1 in 4 adult women and approximately 1 in 7 adult men report having experienced severe physical violence from an intimate partner in their lifetime.
- 16% of women and 7% of men have experienced contact sexual violence from an intimate partner (this includes rape, being made to penetrate someone else, sexual coercion, and/or unwanted sexual contact).
- 10% of women and 2% of men report having been stalked by an intimate partner.

IPV starts early and continues throughout the lifespan. An estimated 8.5 million women (7%) in the U.S. and over 4 million men (4%) reported experiencing physical violence, rape (or being made to penetrate someone else), or stalking from an intimate partner in their lifetime and indicated that they first experienced these or other forms of violence by that partner before the age of 18.[3] A nationally representative survey of U.S. high school students also indicates high levels of teen dating violence, a risk factor for IPV in adulthood. Among students who reported dating, 12% of girls and 7% of boys had experienced physical dating violence and 16% of girls and 5% of boys had experienced sexual dating violence in the past 12 months.[4]

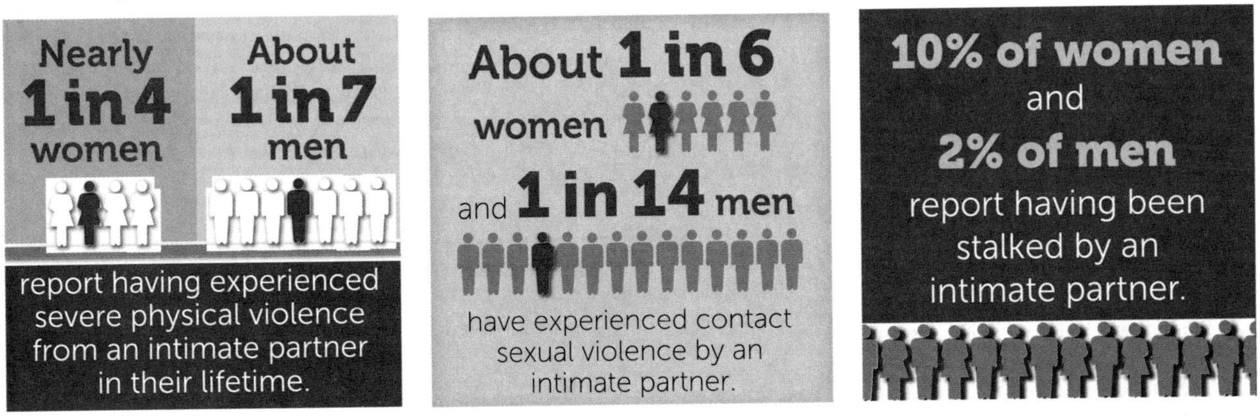

National Center for Injury Prevention and Control
Division of Violence Prevention

Figure 8-3 **Fact Sheet 2017: Preventing intimate partner violence.**

SOURCE: CDC, 2017. Retrieved from https://www.cdc.gov/violenceprevention/pdf/ipv-factsheet.pdf

CASE STUDY: Azia Askari

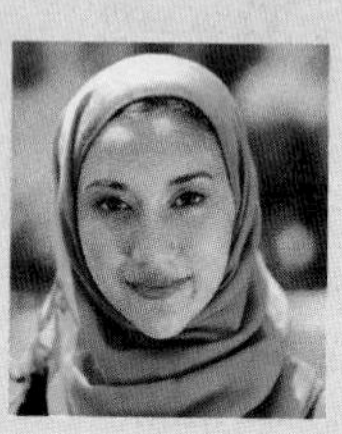

SOURCE: HONGQI ZHANG/123RF

Azia presents for her second prenatal visit and you inform her that, because intimate partner violence is so common, all women are screened in pregnancy. You ask if there is any history of interpersonal violence or if she has ever been hit, slapped, kicked, or hurt by anyone. She becomes very upset that you perceive her husband to be abusive.

Questions to Ponder

How do you reassure her that pregnancy screening is offered to all women? What behaviors are associated with physical and emotional abuse?

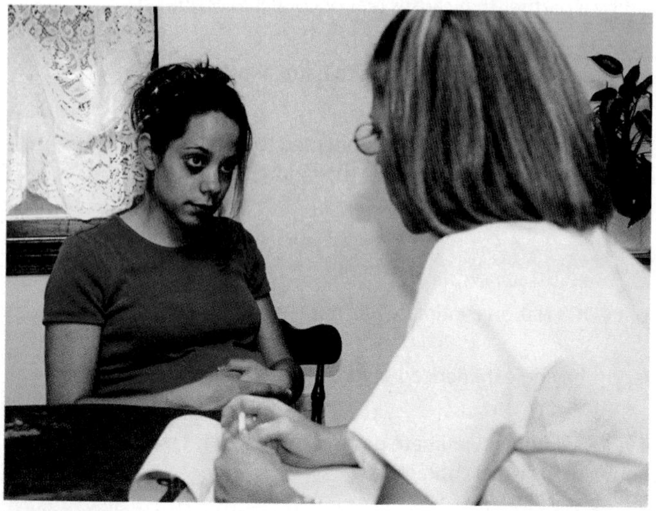

Figure 8–4 **Screening for domestic violence should be done privately.**

- Pattern of injury consistent with abuse, including multiple injury sites involving bruises, abrasions, or contusions to the head (eyes and back of neck), throat, chest, breast, abdomen, or genitals (Nonbattered women's injuries are usually located at one or two sites and on the extremities, such as sprains and strains. Women in abusive relationships may have scars and evidence of old injuries that have healed.)
- Inappropriate explanation for the injuries, such as being "accident prone"
- Vague complaints without accompanying pathology
- Lack of eye contact
- Signs of increased anxiety in the presence of the possible batterer, who frequently does most of the talking or hovers around the woman.

As with the universal screening, if you observe these potential cues, arrange for a private place and speak to the woman alone, with no others present. Encourage the woman to talk about her injuries and home situation by asking, "How did this happen to you?" or by saying, "We often see injuries like yours when a woman has been beaten. Has this happened to you?" When culturally appropriate, it is important to maintain eye contact and avoid excessive note taking. Assure the woman that her privacy will be respected. It is essential that you remain nonjudgmental; create a warm, caring climate conducive to sharing; and demonstrate a willingness to talk about violence. A woman will often interpret your willingness to discuss violence as permission for her to discuss it as well.

"No one had ever asked me about my 'injuries' until I was in the ER one night and the nurse asked me right out if I had been beaten. It gave me real hope to think that people might see what was happening to me."

It is important to gather information about the woman's history of abuse. Help the woman assess whether or not the cycle of violence is becoming more frequent or severe. Determining whether or not there are weapons in the home, and whether or not her batterer has used or threatened to use weapons, might also be warranted. In cases of severe abuse, it is important to address the connection between homicide and domestic violence. Finally, ask about the presence of sexual abuse within the relationship, another factor that indicates severe abuse.

It is equally important, however, that the assessment of the woman who may be experiencing abuse includes information about her strengths and her support system. Strengths may include education, employment history, activities in the home, community involvement, and her ability to cope with past problems. The woman's support system may include her family, friends, neighbors, and community agencies or organizations. It is helpful to consider assessing a woman's strengths in a cultural context. If you are aware of strong values that a particular cultural group holds, then look for opportunities to recognize and affirm those strengths as valuable.

Clinical Tip

In seeking ways to help a woman feel less helpless, consider actually recording a woman's strengths in her medical record and showing her that they are an official part of the record. This action lets her know that you believe that her strengths are as significant as any problems that were noted.

During the assessment phase, begin building a relationship with the woman based on trust, understanding, and advocacy. A woman may feel ashamed and embarrassed about her injuries and her situation. It is important to tell her the purpose of the assessment and to communicate what level of confidentiality she can expect.

In cases in which the woman states she has been beaten, kicked, punched, or attacked but does not identify the assailant, record the extent of injuries (e.g., size, shape, color, location), note the woman's exact words, and describe the incident with a diagnosis of *probable battering*. Full documentation of specific information is critical because you might be called to testify in court or the medical records might be subpoenaed as evidence in legal proceedings such as custody disputes, stay-away/restraining orders, or other civil or criminal proceedings. Moreover, documenting the abuse works to ensure a woman's continuity of care. Those cases in which the woman states she was beaten by a husband or partner may be diagnosed as battering with all evidence recorded, including the woman's statements. In both cases, taking photographs of the injuries can be of great value (Figure 8–5). However, to further protect the woman's confidentiality and safety, it is critical that you or other medical personnel do not refer to domestic violence or abuse on any discharge papers.

When abuse or battering is suspected or determined, formulate nursing diagnoses based on the assessment findings. Nursing diagnoses related to nonphysical components of abuse or battering may include:

- ***Powerlessness, Risk for***, related to feelings of worthlessness secondary to ongoing psychologic partner abuse
- ***Knowledge, Readiness for Enhanced***, related to information about community resources to assist battered women who have expressed desire to learn about alternatives to remaining in an abusive situation

(NANDA-I © 2017)

Nursing Plan and Implementation

A woman who is experiencing abuse needs to reestablish a feeling of control over her world. She needs to regain a sense of predictability by knowing what to expect from her disclosure. Provide the woman with sufficient information about what to expect in terms that she can understand.

Supportive counseling and reassurance are professional skills you will use throughout each phase of the nursing process with a woman who has been battered. Utilize the following guidelines:

- Acknowledge and support the woman for discussing her situation. Reporting abuse is a risk.
- Let the woman work through her story, problems, and situation at her own pace.
- Let the woman know that she is believed and that her feelings are reasonable and normal.
- Anticipate her ambivalence in the love–hate relationship with the batterer. She knows he may be loving and contrite after the incident if she has been through the cycle of violence before.

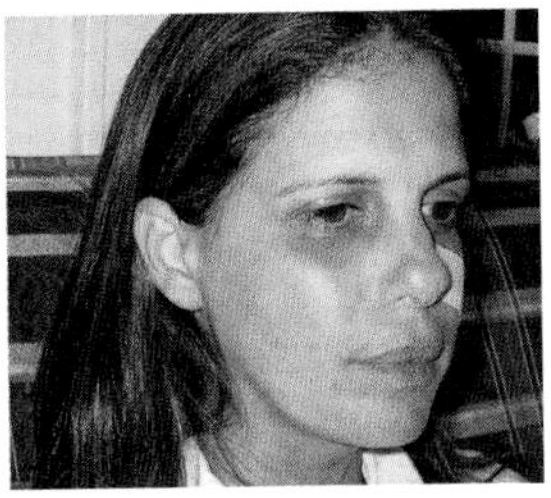

Figure 8–5 When a woman has been battered, it is vital to record all evidence, including photographs.

- Respect the woman's capacity to change and grow when she is ready.
- Assist her in identifying specific problems and support realistic ideas for reducing or eliminating those problems.
- Help clarify the woman's beliefs and myths; provide information to change her false beliefs.
- Stress that no one should be abused and that the abuse is not her fault.

Explore options and resources with the woman, allowing her to make her own decisions. Even advising or encouraging a woman to leave an abusive situation is not always in the woman's best interest; leaving the home is a major decision with long-lasting consequences. The woman may be economically unable to leave the situation, especially if she has young children. If the woman leaves and then later returns home, both husband and wife may become more frustrated, increasing the possibility of further beatings and even homicide. It often takes many interventions before a woman gains enough courage and skill to leave an abusive situation. See *Health Promotion: Developing an Exit Plan*.

Health Promotion Developing an Exit Plan

If the woman returns to an abusive situation, encourage her to develop an exit, or safety, plan for herself and her children, if she has any. As part of the plan, she should:

- Pack a change of clothes for herself and the children, including toilet articles and an extra set of car and house keys stored away from her house with a friend or neighbor.
- Ask a neighbor to call the police if violence begins.
- Have money, identification papers (driver's license, Social Security cards), checkbook, bank account information, other financial records (such as mortgage papers, rent and utility receipts, automobile title, insurance policies and numbers), and information about the children to help her enroll them in school.
- Have a plan for where she will go, regardless of the day or time.
- Identify friends and family who know about the situation and will help her. Ask that she establish a code word for danger with those individuals.
- Have a planned escape route and emergency telephone numbers she can call, including personal numbers, the local police, a phone hotline, and a women's shelter if one is available in the community.

Community-Based Nursing Care

Along with offering emotional support, medical treatment, and counseling, inform any woman who may be in an abusive situation of the services available in the hospital, through agencies, and in the community. Provide the woman with the phone number of any local resources, as well as the number for the National Domestic Violence Hotline (1-800-799-SAFE [7233]).

Specifically, a woman who has been abused may need:

- Medical treatment for injuries
- Temporary shelter to provide a safe environment for herself and her children

- Legal assistance for protection or prosecution of the batterer
- Financial assistance to provide shelter, food, and clothing
- Job training or employment counseling
- Counseling to raise her self-esteem and help her understand the dynamics of domestic violence, or an ongoing support group for herself and her children.

A network of community agencies can meet the numerous, varied needs of women, children, and batterers. An overview of resources available to women with abusive partners and their children is presented in the following sections.

Emergency Department Services

Many women who are experiencing abuse are first seen and diagnosed in the emergency departments (EDs) of their neighborhood hospitals. ED nurses and personnel need to be alert to symptoms of battering, recognize these cues, and encourage women to seek assistance from community agencies. The most innovative and effective domestic violence programs in hospitals and urgent care facilities work collaboratively with domestic violence service agencies, develop a comprehensive community referral network, and work with multidisciplinary intervention teams. Some states require that suspected cases of abuse and battering be reported to the legal authorities or social service agencies. Domestic violence forensic examinations are now available at many large community hospitals, allowing for needed forensic gathering of evidence for possible future legal use by the survivor.

Ethics in Action!

Can there be justification for an abused woman who kills her abusive partner to protect herself or her children?

Shelters

Because domestic violence has been recognized as a major social problem, many community agencies have sought federal and state funds to provide shelters. These shelters differ in the services they provide, depending on the governing body, financial resources and funding agencies, organizational structure, staff qualifications, and range of available community services. Typical shelters provide women in abusive relationships and their children with a room, beds, food, clothing, and other basic necessities. If professional staff is available, the shelter may offer crisis counseling, individual and group counseling, and information about community agencies such as legal aid, welfare, job training, financial and employment agencies, and women's counseling or support groups.

For safety reasons, the location of most shelters is undisclosed, but they can be contacted through a community crisis line. Admission requirements vary from shelter to shelter, so it is wise for you to become familiar with all local shelters and other resources available in case one or more shelters are full and the woman and her children are in need of a safe place to stay.

Living in a shelter may be particularly difficult for older women because of the lack of privacy; accessibility issues related to the physical structure, which may include multiple levels and many stairs; the often chaotic environment because of the number of families with young children; the need for medication support and assistance; and the absence of an age-related support group. Thus, improving accessibility, providing more private space, offering counseling services about starting a new life, and providing assistance with medications and health-related issues are important considerations in supporting older women who have experienced abuse (LeBlanc & Weeks, 2013).

Domestic violence shelters historically have provided services that are primarily heterocentric by assuming the perpetrator of violence is male and that the female victim is heterosexual. This can be a barrier to women who identify as LGBTQI and who seek refuge from an abusive relationship. These services can be improved by providing training for staff, by making sure that the information given is presented in neutral language, and by having an overall mission statement that is LGBTQI friendly (Calton et al., 2016).

Legal Services and Options

During incidents of domestic violence, the woman or her neighbors may summon the police. Domestic violence often occurs on the weekend or in late evening, when most social service agencies are closed; therefore, the police department is one of the first major agencies involved, in addition to those that provide medical services.

Legal options for women with abusive partners vary according to state laws and services. In some states a woman may seek a restraining (or protective) order from the family court or a domestic relations court to protect herself from the batterer. Unfortunately, many abusers violate the restraining/protective order and continue to stalk, harass, intimidate, and abuse their female partners. The case then becomes a criminal matter. Criminal court hearings may result in a fine, probation, or a jail sentence if the batterer is convicted, giving the man a criminal record. The prosecution process is often lengthy and may last more than a year. Divorce is another legal recourse a woman may choose, but divorce takes time and may cause added financial burdens for the woman.

Currently, some communities provide legal advocacy services to help women understand the judicial process, their options within that system, and the possible consequences for the woman, her children, and the batterer.

Professionalism in Practice Legislative Advocacy

Patient advocacy is a nursing responsibility that extends beyond individual nurse–patient relationships. Nurses can follow and become involved in legislative advocacy for issues related to domestic violence and other issues related to women's health through participation in their local and state chapters of the American Nurses Association, by being aware of current issues, by following the progress of specific bills online, by writing to their legislators, and by exercising their right to vote.

Financial Services

Once women who have been in battering relationships leave their homes or seek legal assistance, they usually receive no financial support from their batterers. Without funds, women and their children are at the mercy of community social service agencies, and it usually takes weeks for papers to be processed before any money is forthcoming. Agencies that may provide financial assistance include their county welfare department, federal programs (e.g., Temporary Assistance for Needy Families [TANF]), the United Way, women's support groups, religious organizations, and, possibly, the Salvation Army. There may be other local groups who assist abused women in other ways, such as by providing food or clothing.

Employment Training or Placement

Some women who experience abuse are full-time mothers who may lack advanced education, training, and job experience. Minimal or out-of-date skills and inadequate transportation often make it difficult for these women to obtain employment with an adequate salary. Women who have children must consider where to place them during working hours as well as the added cost of child care. Often, the woman's choice is restricted to accepting welfare or taking a low-paying job. Either choice usually means lowering the standard of living to mere subsistence.

Some women do seek job training if the opportunities are available, but training provides no guarantee of future job placement. A woman may still have to arrange for financial support and child care while obtaining advanced employment skills or an education.

Counseling or Advocacy

Women who have experienced domestic violence may be offered a variety of counseling and advocacy services—such as crisis intervention, short-term individual therapy, group therapy, or peer support groups—over an extended period. Specially trained nurses, social workers, psychologists, mental health specialists, or clergy may provide counseling and therapy.

Evaluation

Expected outcomes of nursing care include:

- The woman receives compassionate, respectful, and individualized medical attention.
- The woman recovers from the physical effects of physical and sexual abuse.
- The woman has the information she needs to make a decision about her future based on thoughtful consideration of alternatives.
- The woman is able to identify culturally appropriate community resources available to her and develops strategies for keeping herself, her children, and her family as safe as possible.
- If the woman chooses to apply for a restraining order or to prosecute her assailant, all necessary documentation is recorded in her medical records, leading to a more successful prosecution.

Sexual Assault

Sexual assault is a broad term that refers to a variety of types of unwanted sexual touching or penetration without consent. **Rape** is forced sexual intercourse as a result of physical force or psychologic coercion. Forced sexual intercourse refers to vaginal, oral, or anal penetration by a body part or by an object.

The rapist may be a stranger, acquaintance, spouse or other relative, or employer. Rape is an act of violence expressed sexually—most commonly, a person's need for power and control acted out against a woman.

Reporting varies by the type of rape or sexual assault. Rapes and sexual assaults committed by strangers are more likely to be reported to the police than rapes and sexual assaults committed by "nonstrangers," including intimate partners, other relatives, and friends or acquaintances. Women injured during a rape incident are also much more likely to report it to the police. No woman of any age, cultural or ethnic background, or socioeconomic status is immune. However, risk factors for sexual assault include (Vrees, 2017):

- Younger than age 25 (up to 80% of reported first sexual assaults)
- Prior assault
- Lesbian or transgender persons
- Military personnel
- Homelessness
- Physical or mental disability
- Use of drugs and alcohol.

Common Myths about Rape

As with domestic violence, many myths about rape exist. These myths can have a negative impact on women who are assaulted and can hinder their ability to receive optimum health care following their attack. Some of the most commonly cited myths include:

- ***Only certain types of women are raped.*** No woman is safe from a rape attempt. Women of all ages, races, ethnicities, classes, religious backgrounds, occupations, ability levels, sexual and gender identities, and appearances are raped.
- ***Men rape women because that is men's nature and biologic role.*** Rape is not universal to all societies and not all men rape women. Generally, violent societies that encourage aggression in boys and men tend to have more reports of sexual violence.
- ***Women who party hard, drink, and do drugs are setting themselves up to be sexually assaulted.*** No one asks for or deliberately "sets herself up" to be sexually violated. The misunderstanding that rape is about sex perpetrates this myth. Rape is sexual violence and a crime of power. Blaming the victim for the crime is not only inappropriate, it serves to excuse the behavior of the perpetrator. Because alcohol and drugs may affect judgment, feelings, and perceptions as well as lower inhibitions, a woman may be in a more vulnerable position when she engages in these activities. However, it is not a crime to wear particular clothes, show naiveté, use poor judgment, or even engage in reckless behavior. The victim's behavior before the crime is irrelevant.
- ***If a woman just relaxes, it will all be over with soon. She might even find it isn't so bad after all.*** Rape is an act of violence in which the perpetrator uses sex as a weapon to control, intimidate, and violate the victim. Rape involves persistent pressure, taking advantage of a person's inability to say "no"; calculated drugging with alcohol or other substances; and/or threats, sometimes against the woman's life, her livelihood, her academic career, even her family members and friends. Many survivors recall being in fear for their lives, even if a weapon was not present.
- ***A rapist is easy to spot in a crowd.*** There is no way to distinguish men who commit sexual assault from men who do not on the basis of race, ethnicity, socioeconomic status, educational level, marital status, or religious background.
- ***Women lie about rape as an act of revenge or guilt.*** According to the Federal Bureau of Investigation, while false allegations of rape do occur, they are the exception, not the rule (McNamara, McDonald, & Lawrence, 2012).

- ***Fighting back incites a rapist to violence.*** Most assailants pick out potential victims they believe may be good targets without a fight. They may even test women nonverbally or verbally before determining whether or not to assault. Both verbal and physical resistance may actually lessen the severity of injury in some instances. Women who recognize that they have options for responding to their assailant are less likely to be paralyzed by fear and more likely to resist. Each incident is unique. Only the targeted person knows her abilities and can assess the assailant's behavior. Evaluating her options realistically may help the survivor understand that submission is also a viable form of self-protection.

Characteristics of Perpetrators

Like their victims, rapists come from all ethnic, racial, and religious backgrounds; socioeconomic statuses; educational levels; and professions. Many rapists are married and engage in regular sexual relationships, both inside and outside of marriage. A substantial number of perpetrators are quite young.

Attitudes toward women do seem to influence who is likely to be a rapist and who is not, especially when it comes to believing that men have a right to sexual access of women. Perpetrators tend to be impulsive and have antisocial tendencies. They may prefer impersonal sex and feel hostility toward women. Additional individual risk factors for perpetration include being male, alcohol and drug use, having friends who are sexually aggressive, an emotionally unsupportive family environment, childhood history of witnessing or experiencing violence, and a belief in societal norms or shared beliefs that support male entitlement and sexual violence.

Types of Rape

Rape has been categorized in different ways, which are not mutually exclusive. Specifically, rape may be categorized according to the rapist's possible motives or purposes for the assault, according to the relationship between the victim and perpetrator, or according to the number of assailants.

- In *power rape*, the purpose of the assault is control or mastery. The assailant uses sexual intercourse to place a woman in a powerless position so that he can feel dominant, potent, and strong. He often believes that his victim enjoys the assault, and he exerts only the amount of force necessary to subdue his victim. Often power rape is a planned stranger attack, but most acquaintance rapes are also power rapes. The vast majority of all rapes are motivated by this need for power and control.
- In *anger rape*, the sexual assault is used to express feelings of rage and to retaliate for what the attacker perceives as wrongs against him. These perceived wrongs most often have nothing to do with the rape victim. Considerable brutality and degradation can characterize this type of rape. Attacks on older women are often a form of anger rape.
- In *sadistic rape*, the assailant has an antisocial personality and delights in torture and mutilation. In this type of rape, the victim and assailant are generally strangers, and the assault is planned. Sadistic rapes cause the most injuries, including homicide.
- In *stranger rape*, the assailant and victim are strangers, and the rape is often a blitz-style attack—sudden and unexpected. The rapist is more likely to use a weapon and threaten violence or murder.
- In **acquaintance rape** or *nonstranger rape*, the assailant is someone with whom the victim has had previous nonviolent interaction. Marital rape and date rape are included in this category. In **date rape**, the male has usually planned to have sex and will do what he feels is necessary if denied.
- In *gang rape*, the rape is used as a reinforcing mechanism for membership in a particular group of men (such as a street gang, fraternity, athletic team, or other known group). Often responding to peer pressure from the group leader, individuals participate in the rape as a means to demonstrate their power by forcing sex on a woman, thus proving their status in the group. Often gang rape can escalate to severe violence as the young men resort to mob mentality.

> “I always knew that rape was a terrifying experience physically but I never really thought about the horror that comes from being helpless and in someone else's control.”

Role of Substances in Sexual Assault

In some cases, a perpetrator uses alcohol or other drugs to sedate his intended victim, leading to incapacitation. This is called *alcohol- or drug-facilitated sexual assault*. While alcohol is the most common and most easily obtained drug, flunitrazepam (Rohypnol), a potent sedative-hypnotic that is legal in 80 countries worldwide but illegal in the United States, has received considerable attention as the "date rape drug of choice" since the late 1990s. Typically, Rohypnol, which dissolves easily and is odorless, is slipped into the drink of an unsuspecting woman. Gamma hydroxybutyrate (GHB), ketamine, MDMA (Ecstasy), clonazepam, and scopolamine have also been identified as date rape drugs that are used to incapacitate a woman. More recently, prescription drugs have been used in combination with alcohol to facilitate many sexual assaults. Because these drugs frequently produce amnesia, the woman may be unable to remember details of her assault, thereby making prosecution more difficult. She may be left uncertain about the perpetrator's identity, the events of the assault, the presence of birth control or a condom, and possible injury or risk for contracting sexually transmitted infections (STIs). See Table 8–1 for indicators of possible drug-facilitated sexual assault.

TABLE 8–1 Indicators of Possible Drug-Facilitated Sexual Assault

- Becoming intoxicated very rapidly, especially after accepting a drink from someone else or drinking a drink she left unattended
- Having just one or two drinks, and then suddenly feeling "very drunk"; feeling more intoxicated than usual after drinking an amount of alcohol she is used to consuming
- Feeling drowsy, dizzy, agitated, weak, confused, or nauseous; experiencing an increased heart rate or blood pressure, slurred speech, or a lack of motor coordination
- Waking up suspecting she may have been raped because of vaginal soreness, finding herself in an unfamiliar place, or other indicators
- Being told that she suddenly appeared drunk, drowsy, dizzy, or confused with impaired motor skills, judgment, and amnesia or partial amnesia

Date Rape and Violence on College Campuses

Statistics indicate that 23.1% of all undergraduate females experience sexual assault or rape through violence, physical force, or incapacitation (RAINN, 2016). Awareness of the prevalence of date rape and violence against women on college campuses has increased significantly in the wake of several high-profile rape cases at American universities. Title IX legislation—best known for its requirement that all colleges and universities that receive federal funds provide equal opportunities for women in athletic programs, facilities, educational programs, and the like—also addresses the issue of sexual harassment and violence against women. Today, campuses have a Title IX compliance officer and are actively working to provide education to students, faculty, and staff about these issues.

Rape Trauma Syndrome

Rape is viewed as a situational crisis, that is, an unanticipated traumatic event that the victim generally is unprepared to handle because it is unforeseen. Following rape, the survivor may experience a cluster of symptoms originally described by Burgess and Holmstrom (1979) as the **rape trauma syndrome**. An additional phase—*integration and recovery*—was later suggested (Holmes, 1998). These four phases are described in Table 8–2. Although the phases of response are listed individually, they often overlap, and individual responses and their duration may vary.

SILENT REACTION

Women who do not report the rape go through the phases of the rape trauma syndrome without using available support systems. Their reasons for keeping silent vary. A woman may be embarrassed, she may accept society's "temptress view" and blame herself, or she may fear retaliation. Her experience may be discovered much later, perhaps when she seeks professional help in resolving a different crisis.

Some women seek medical help for their physical injuries without disclosing that a rape was the cause. The nurse who suspects that a woman has been raped should seek validation through sympathetic questioning.

Sexual Assault as a Cause of Posttraumatic Stress Disorder

Sexual assault survivors may exhibit high levels of **posttraumatic stress disorder (PTSD)**, the same disorder that developed in many of the veterans of the Vietnam War. To be diagnosed as having PTSD, a person must:

- Have been exposed to a traumatic event that triggered feelings of intense fear, horror, or helplessness
- Reexperience the event in recurrent, intrusive thoughts, images, perceptions, and flashbacks
- Persistently avoid stimuli associated with the trauma and demonstrate a generalized "numbing" of responsiveness
- Demonstrate persistent signs of increased arousal, such as exaggerated startle response, difficulty falling asleep, hypervigilance or outbursts of anger, emotional detachment, and sleep disturbances that were not present before the trauma occurred.

PTSD is marked by varying degrees of intensity depending on prior mental health issues and the woman's own resiliency. Among women veterans, the relationship between military sexual trauma (sexual harassment, sexual coercion, sexual assault, and rape) and PTSD is gaining increased attention because research suggests that military sexual trauma is the most significant traumatic event these women experience (Kintzle, Schuyler, Ray-Letourneau, et al., 2015). Fortunately, the issue is gaining increased attention as more women serve in the armed forces.

PTSD is difficult to treat. Because the symptoms keep an individual from addressing the problem, she cannot integrate

TABLE 8–2 Phases of Recovery Following Sexual Assault

PHASE	RESPONSE
Acute (disorganization) phase	Survivor may experience fear, shock, disbelief, desire for revenge, anger, anxiety, guilt, denial, embarrassment, humiliation, helplessness, dependence, self-blame, wide variety of physical reactions, lost or distorted coping mechanisms. She may suppress her emotions or may reveal them by crying, sobbing, or acting tense and restless; may also experience alterations in sleep patterns, such as insomnia, nightmares, or crying out at night.
Outward adjustment (denial) phase	Survivor appears outwardly composed, denying and repressing feelings (e.g., she returns to work, buys a weapon); refuses to discuss the assault; denies need for counseling. She may move to a different residence or may institute security measures, such as installing extra locks or requesting an unlisted telephone number. She may buy a weapon or take a course in self-defense. These activities do not resolve her emotional trauma; they simply push it further into her subconscious.
Reorganization	Survivor must alter her self-concept and resolve her feelings about the rape. She may use emotional distancing; may engage in risky sexual behaviors; may experience sexual dysfunction, phobias, flashbacks, sleep disorders, nightmares, anxiety, difficulty trusting others, eating disorders. She may have a strong urge to talk about or resolve feelings; may seek counseling or remain silent.
Integration and recovery	Time of resolution; survivor begins to feel safe and be comfortable trusting others; places blame on assailant; may become an advocate for others.

the event into her life, and healing is blocked. Recovery depends on empowering the woman to seek to regain control of her life within the context of healing relationships and professional counseling.

Physical Care of the Sexual Assault Survivor

Following a sexual assault, a primary purpose of care is to meet the needs of the survivor. This is accomplished by the following actions:

- Evaluating and treating injuries
- Conducting prompt examinations
- Providing support, crisis intervention, and advocacy
- Providing prophylaxis against STIs
- Assessing for pregnancy risk and discussing treatment options
- Providing follow-up care for medical and emotional needs.

As many as 35% of women who are sexually assaulted sustain injuries. Although often the injuries are minor, more severe physical consequences may also occur (Planty et al., 2013). Sexual assault victims tend to have more medical complaints and to access healthcare services more than those who have not been victimized. Both emotional and physical symptoms manifest themselves in the aftermath of an assault, sometimes immediately and sometimes for a lengthy period following the assault.

Because sexual assault is a crime as well as a traumatic emergency, however, the other purpose of health care is to collect and preserve legal evidence for use in prosecuting the assailant. It is important to note that even though evidence is collected, it does not necessarily mean that the survivor has to prosecute; the survivor always has the right to reconsider her decisions.

Unfortunately, in many communities the treatment of a woman immediately following a sexual assault has been almost as traumatic as the assault itself. It may be characterized by victim blaming and insensitive and prying care. To address this concern, many emergency departments have developed a *Sexual Assault Response Team (SART)*. This team is composed of law enforcement and prosecution professionals, forensic examiners and/or healthcare providers, and victim advocates. The goal of the team is to establish programs and evaluation protocols of those programs in order to provide effective care to sexual assault survivors and their families. A *forensic nurse examiner (FNE)*, formally known as a sexual assault nurse examiner (SANE), is often the healthcare provider who completes the sexual assault exam when a patient presents reporting sexual assault. Research suggests that more cases progress through the criminal justice system when an FNE program is available than in communities without one (Vrees, 2017).

Professionalism in Practice Start by Believing

Start by Believing is a public awareness campaign begun in 2015 by End Violence Against Women International, an organization focused on improving the criminal justice system's response to sexual assault. Start by Believing (2017) urges us not to doubt or blame but to believe victims of sexual assault and provide help as they attempt to heal. April 6, 2016, was the first "Start by Believing" Day.

DETAILED HISTORY

Obtaining a detailed history is an essential first step in acquiring necessary medical and forensic data, but it can also be a therapeutic tool if done in a sensitive, caring way. Because a sexual assault survivor may appear calm and normal when first seen, caregivers may underestimate her needs, but it is essential that she receive immediate attention. Immediately after the woman has received any necessary emergency medical care, the nurse takes an explicit history of the event in the woman's own words to aid in evidence collection and examination of injuries. This focuses on the *who* (identity of assailant), *what* (characteristics of the assault), *when* (time of the assault), *with what* (any weapons, other objects, contraceptive methods such as condom used), and *how* (specific details of the assault) (Vrees, 2017). Many agencies use a standardized forensic chart containing a history flow sheet to record information obtained. The nurse should use a nonjudgmental approach and must avoid leading or coaching the woman. It is also important to keep in mind that sexual assault survivors have to tell their history multiple times. A patient may encounter up to 20 people during the initial reporting of the assault (police officers, detectives, ED registration, triage nurse, triage tech, ED nurse, ED physician, victim's advocate, and FNE, to name a few).

COLLECTION OF EVIDENCE

The collection of evidence may, in itself, be traumatic for the woman. It is valuable to have someone available to provide support and act as an advocate. This person may be a family member or close friend, a victim's advocate from a local community organization or police department, or another nurse. An interpreter should also be provided, if necessary.

The woman should receive a thorough explanation of the procedures to be carried out and should sign an informed consent form. It must be clearly communicated to the patient that she has the right to take a break or stop the evidence collection at any point during the process. This helps give control back to the patient, which is the first step to healing.

A careful examination of the entire body is necessary. Vaginal and rectal examinations are performed, along with a complete physical examination for trauma. Any lacerations or abrasions of the perineal, vaginal, or anal tissue are noted. A colposcope with photographic capability can be used to document injuries to the genitalia.

An important legal concept when dealing with rape survivors is the need to preserve the *chain of evidence*, meaning that all physical evidence and specimens must remain in the hands of a professional until they are turned over to a police officer. Most agencies have special sexual assault kits that contain all necessary supplies for collecting and labeling evidence.

Clothing. Each piece of clothing and foreign material dislodged from clothing is marked, placed in an individual paper bag, sealed, and labeled.

Swabs of Stains and Secretions. Swabs of body stains and secretions are analyzed for saliva, semen, or sperm. The absence of sperm, however, does not signify that no sexual assault has occurred. Many assailants do not ejaculate because of sexual dysfunction, or they may use a condom. Because victims are often forced to commit fellatio, oral swabs are also examined for semen.

Hair and Scrapings. Clippings or swabs of the woman's fingernails are examined for blood or tissue from the assailant. Approximately 20 to 25 hairs are pulled from her head to analyze the root structure and identify foreign hairs. Her pubic hair is also combed to check for loose hairs that may have been transferred from the rapist.

Blood and Urine Samples. If there is a concern that the assault was drug-facilitated, blood and urine samples may be collected to determine if any foreign substance is in the patient's system. Blood samples are useful if a patient presents within 24 hours of the assault, and urine may be collected up until 96 hours, although that protocol may differ between states. It is crucial to document a thorough medication history from the patient, including vitamins, prescribed medications, and illicit drugs. This should be done in a nonjudgmental manner, as most patients will be hesitant to admit to voluntary illicit drug use prior to the assault for fear that will place blame in their direction. Additional blood may be drawn or a urine sample given for a pregnancy test if the woman indicates that she wants to take emergency contraception (see discussion in Chapter 4) to prevent pregnancy. She has to have a negative pregnancy test to receive the medication.

Photographs. Photographs should be taken of injured areas, if possible. Before taking any photos, the healthcare provider should ask the woman to sign an informed consent form.

PREVENTION OF SEXUALLY TRANSMITTED INFECTIONS

Among women who have been sexually assaulted, trichomoniasis, bacterial vaginosis, gonorrhea, and chlamydia are the most frequently diagnosed STIs. The decision to test for specific STIs should be made on an individual basis (CDC, 2015b). Following a sexual assault, preventive therapy is recommended. This includes a single dose of ceftriaxone intramuscularly, a single oral dose of azithromycin, and a single oral dose of metronidazole or tinidazole (CDC, 2015b). Women who have not been previously vaccinated against hepatitis B should receive postexposure hepatitis B vaccination, with follow-up doses at 1 to 2 months and 4 to 6 months following the initial dose. In addition, female survivors between the ages of 9 and 26 years of age should be given the HPV vaccine if they have not previously received it (CDC, 2015b). If the individual chooses not to receive prophylactic antibiotic treatment, the nurse should encourage her to be seen by her caregiver in 2 weeks for assessment for any STIs.

If the assailant's HIV status is not known, consideration should be given to offering postexposure prophylaxis (PEP) with HIV antiretroviral medications. If PEP is considered, consultation with an HIV specialist is advised (CDC, 2015b).

PREVENTION OF PREGNANCY

The woman is questioned about her menstrual cycle and contraceptive practices. If she is at risk for pregnancy and a pregnancy test is negative, she should receive information about her treatment options. Women of different ages, social, cultural, and religious/spiritual backgrounds will have diverse feelings about acceptable treatment options. The nurse needs to be sensitive and nonjudgmental when discussing various reproductive health services. If the woman wishes, emergency contraception is provided. (See Chapter 4 for further discussion.)

●○● NURSING MANAGEMENT

For the Woman Who Has Been Sexually Assaulted

Sexual assault survivors frequently enter the healthcare system by way of the ED; thus nurses are often the first to provide services to them. Because the nurse's values, attitudes, and beliefs will necessarily affect the competence and focus of the care, if you work with survivors you must understand your own attitudes and beliefs about sexual assault and sexual assault survivors and resolve any conflicts that may exist to ensure nonjudgmental patient support.

In addition to examining your attitudes and beliefs, you must be mindful of the potential for increased complexity of treatment with sexual assault survivors who are members of different ethnic or cultural backgrounds. Being aware of potential cultural differences is important when discussing future courses of action available.

Nursing Assessment and Diagnosis

Policies for admitting and examining sexual assault survivors vary among institutions, but clinical guidelines and protocols for the healthcare of sexual assault victims have been issued by many national medical agencies to create consistency in treatment in healthcare facilities across the United States. A woman who has been assaulted is under great stress and needs the sensitive care of professionals who are aware of her special needs. The first priority is creating a safe, secure environment. Professionals should gather admission information from the victim in a quiet, private room and reassure the woman that she is not alone, will not be abandoned, and is safe from a second attack.

A full mental status examination should be performed, both for the purpose of planning care and as possible courtroom evidence. Scrupulous documentation is essential because the victim's medical record is often used in the courtroom to verify her testimony if the rapist is prosecuted.

Examples of nursing diagnoses that may apply to the sexual assault victim include:

- *Fear* related to invasion of personal space secondary to assault
- *Powerlessness* related to inability to regain sense of control secondary to assault

(NANDA-I © 2017)

Nursing Plan and Implementation

Table 8–3 outlines the general nursing actions that are appropriate during each of the phases of recovery. It is imperative that control be returned to the woman as quickly as possible. When feasible, the woman should decide on the sequence of forensic events, such as pulling her own hair (head and pubic), having blood drawn after clothes are collected rather than before, and so forth. In this way you can help her deal with her crisis in small, manageable increments. Encourage the woman to express her feelings and reassure her that anger and fear are normal, appropriate responses. Avoid using terms such as *alleged* when gathering information (Vrees, 2017). Address expressed or unexpressed guilt by assuring the woman that the sexual assault was not her fault.

By explaining the general health or forensic examination and the sequence of events in the ED, you can alleviate the patient's anxiety related to fear of the unknown. Throughout the experience, act as the survivor's advocate, providing support without usurping decision making. You need not agree with all the survivor's decisions, but you should respect and defend her right to make them. A victim also has the right to have a victim advocate, family member, or friend with her throughout the examination process.

The family members or friends on whom the survivor calls also need nursing care. Like those of the victim, the reactions of the family will depend on the values to which they ascribe. Some family members or partners may blame the survivor for the

TABLE 8–3 Nursing Actions Appropriate to Phases of Recovery Following Rape

PHASE OF RECOVERY	NURSING ACTIONS
Acute phase	Create a safe environment. Explain the sequence of events in the healthcare facility. Allow the woman to grieve and express her feelings. Provide care for significant others.
Outward adjustment phase	Provide advocacy and support at the level requested by the woman. Provide assistance to significant others.
Reorganizational phase	Establish a trusting relationship. Assist the woman to understand her role in the assault. Clarify and enhance the woman's feelings. Assist the woman in planning for her future.
Integration and recovery	Acknowledge the victim's success in overcoming trauma; support advocacy efforts.

sexual assault and feel angry with her for not having been more careful. They may also incorrectly view the assault as a sexual act rather than as an act of violence. They may feel personally wronged or attacked and see the survivor as being devalued or unclean. Their reactions may compound the victim's crisis. By spending some time with family members before their first interaction with the survivor, you can reduce their anxiety and help them examine and reconcile their feelings, sparing the woman further trauma. In most cases, you should contact and/or refer them to a sexual assault advocate who can help them address their needs. Hospital-based advocates, if available, should be called to the ED to provide support services.

Community-Based Nursing Care

As the woman enters the reorganization phase, she usually feels a strong urge to discuss and resolve her feelings about herself and her assailant. During this phase, the victim may benefit from talking with a specially trained sexual assault advocate or counselor.

Information and support, provided by qualified nurses or other service providers, are valuable tools in helping the sexual assault victim come to terms with her attack and its impact on her life. It is important for the provider to help the woman realize that the sexual assault was not her fault. The fault always lies with the perpetrator. With the provider/advocate, the woman explores her thoughts and feelings about self-care and celebrates her victories. It is important to emphasize that the loss of control that occurred during the assault was temporary and that she *does* have control over other aspects of her life.

Local high schools, colleges, or rape awareness groups may offer courses in preventive strategies. Because sexual assault is a considerable risk for any woman, courses in what to do during and after an attack and how family members and friends can support a survivor are also helpful. Table 8–4 provides general guidelines for helping victims of sexual assault. Nurses who have completed additional education and are thoroughly prepared are well qualified to initiate or participate in preventive instruction.

> **Professionalism in Practice** **Remaining Nonjudgmental**
>
> Strive to listen and respond nonjudgmentally. Allowing your own beliefs to interfere with care can make the difference in a victim's readiness to disclose the full details of her assault and to begin the recovery process. Hindering that ability is detrimental to the mental health of the woman and can decrease the possibility of identifying a sex offender.

Sexual Assault Advocacy and Information

Most sexual assault crisis centers operate 24 hours a day, 7 days a week. Their services are invaluable. Properly trained advocates and counselors can help the victim regain control early in the crisis. Many sexual assault crisis centers offer free services to victims or can refer them to qualified counselors within the community. Information on STIs and pregnancy alternatives may also be obtained from these centers. In addition, there are many internet resources that provide information for survivors and their family members and friends as well as for professionals seeking information about how to better assist victims of sexual assault.

Evaluation

Expected outcomes of quality nursing care include:

- The woman receives prompt, compassionate, respectful, and individualized medical attention.
- The woman recovers from the physical effects of the sexual assault.
- The woman is able to verbalize her recognition that sexual assault is a crime of violence expressed sexually.
- The woman is able to identify culturally appropriate community resources available to her as she works to adjust psychologically to the assault.
- The woman makes a decision about whether to prosecute her assailant.
- If a victim decides to prosecute her assailant, all necessary forensic evidence will have been collected, leading to a more successful investigation and prosecution.

Prosecution of the Assailant

Legally, sexual assault, like any criminal action, is considered a crime against the state rather than against the victim. Therefore,

TABLE 8–4 General Guidelines for Helping Victims of Sexual Assault

- Believe the victim—one of the greatest fears of sexual assault survivors is that they will not be believed.
- Listen and be patient—let the person talk and tell the story at her or his own pace.
- Reinforce the fact that the sexual assault was not the victim's fault.
- For recent assaults, encourage the victim to report the assault and preserve evidence.
- Encourage the person to seek medical attention.
- Suggest seeking counseling and other support services.
- Help the victim to organize her or his thoughts, but let the survivor make her or his own decision on how to proceed.
- Take care of yourself—assisting a friend or family member can be stressful. Set aside time for yourself so that you don't feel overwhelmed by the survivor's problems.
- Acknowledge your limits and realistically identify your abilities to assist the survivor.

SOURCE: Data from General Guidelines for Helping Victims of Sexual Assault. George Mason University Office of Sexual Assault Services.

prosecution of the assailant is a community responsibility in which the prosecuting attorney will act on the victim's behalf. The victim, however, must initiate the process by reporting the crime and pressing charges against her assailant.

Many sexual assault survivors who have gone through the judicial process refer to it as a "second rape"—and sometimes a more damaging one. The victim must identify the assailant and repeat the details of the assault. Delays can further frustrate the victim and increase her fear. Publicity may intensify her feelings of humiliation, and if the perpetrator is released on bail pending trial, she may fear retaliation.

During the trial itself, cross-examination by the defendant's attorney can be a severely degrading and intimidating experience for the victim. The defense attorney may try to discredit her testimony, causing a second victimization. Fortunately, rape shield laws are quite common, and nearly every state prohibits the publicizing of a victim's sexual history. Moreover, despite the difficulties of prosecution, many victims feel a sense of justice in taking their case to court.

The nurse involved with any sexual assault victim needs to be aware of the judicial sequence to anticipate rising tension and frustration in the victim and her support system. They will need consistent, effective support at this crucial time.

Responding to Violence Against Women: Vicarious Trauma

Vicarious trauma, or secondary trauma effect, can occur as a result of working with people who are trauma victims. It refers to a gradual internal transformation that can negatively affect commitment to one's work, reduce any sense of accomplishment, and lead to a questioning of personal belief systems. *Burnout* is similar to vicarious trauma but is more severe. Symptoms may include exhaustion, depression, apathy, depersonalization, loss of compassion, and cynicism. Nurses who treat and assist domestic violence and sexual assault survivors should be aware of this phenomenon so that they are able to periodically assess the effect of their work on their lives. When the lives of nurses—and indeed of all healthcare professionals—are balanced and there is equal time for self, family, friends, work, play, and rest, they are better able to provide compassionate and sensitive health care.

Sex Trafficking

Sex trafficking refers to "the recruitment, harboring, transportation, provision, or obtaining of a person, through force, fraud, or coercion, for the purpose of commercial sex" (Nurse Practitioners in Women's Health [NPWH], 2017, p. 8). *Domestic minor sex trafficking (DMST)*, a subset of the problem, refers specifically to the engagement of minors (less than 18 years of age). DMST also refers to sexual acts in which a child is the victim of sexual exploitation for remuneration to survive, including, for example, money, shelter, food, or clothing (Goldberg, Moore, Houck, et al., 2017).

In 2000 the U.S. Trafficking Victims Protection Act (TVPA) was passed to address this issue. The TPVA actually updated the post–Civil War slavery statutes that guaranteed freedom from involuntary servitude and slavery. The act has been reauthorized several times. Unfortunately, the TPVA is narrow in scope and only provides assistance to undocumented immigrant women who are victims of severe forms of trafficking and to girls under age 18 (Bromfield, 2016).

Females at highest risk of sex trafficking include those who are young, have limited education, engage in drug use, live in extreme poverty, or have a history of abuse in their families. Adolescent runaways are especially vulnerable. Women who are victims of trafficking often suffer long-term physical and mental health problems including unintended pregnancies, poor dentition because of malnutrition, sexually transmitted infections, depression, and PTSD (NPWH, 2017).

Nurses need to be alert to signs that a woman or girl may be in an exploitive situation. Often these are similar to the signs of domestic violence. These may include submissive behavior and evidence of being controlled; vague answers to questions about history; discrepancies between the clinical presentation of an injury and the patient's explanation of how the injury occurred; delay in seeking treatment for an injury; signs of physical abuse; depression, substance abuse, or PTSD; recurrent STIs; genital or rectal trauma; and history of repeat miscarriages or abortion (NPWH, 2017).

Sex trafficking is a complex, international issue, one that impacts multiple fields and disciplines including nursing, medicine, social work, law, and criminal justice, to name a few. Efforts are required at the micro level to address the specific needs of victims of trafficking. Efforts are also needed at the macro level to address the social, economic, cultural, and policy issues that allow this practice to continue (Edwards & Mika, 2016).

Focus Your Study

- Domestic violence is very common. Nearly one in four women will experience violence at the hands of an intimate partner during her lifetime.
- Batterers use psychologic, physical, and sexual abuse to maintain power and control in abusive relationships.
- Battering occurs in a cyclic pattern called the cycle of violence, which increases in frequency and severity over time.
- Women in abusive relationships who belong to cultural and linguistic minority communities and immigrant women face additional barriers when attempting to access services. The nurse must work to provide culturally aware and competent care.
- Nurses are in an excellent position to intervene and assist women with abusive partners by recognizing their cues, diagnosing their problems appropriately, and understanding the complex dynamics of the battering family. The nurse provides information about available culturally appropriate community resources, medical attention, and emotional support.
- Estimates suggest that the majority of sexual assaults are not reported to the police. Rapes and sexual assaults committed by strangers are more likely to be reported to the police than rapes or sexual assaults committed by nonstrangers, including intimate partners, other relatives, and friends or acquaintances.
- Rape is an act of violence acted out sexually. Most sexual assaults are expressions of a need for power and control.
- Following sexual assault, the victim will usually experience an assortment of symptoms known as rape trauma syndrome. Recent research also links the effects of rape to posttraumatic stress disorder. Nursing actions to assist rape victims are encompassed in the roles of healthcare provider, advocate, and educator.
- Nurses inform the woman of the sequence of events involved in providing her care and developing the chain of evidence and support the victim's decisions.
- Widespread education is needed to abolish societal myths surrounding domestic violence and sexual assault.
- Sex trafficking is a complex problem that requires a multidisciplinary approach. Nurses need to be aware of signs of sex trafficking, which are often similar to those exhibited by women who are victims of domestic violence.

In order to make safe and effective judgments using NANDA-I © 2017 nursing diagnoses, it is essential that nurses refer to the definitions and defining characteristics of the diagnoses used in this text, which can be found in Appendix C.

References

American College of Obstetricians and Gynecologists (ACOG). (2012). *Intimate partner violence* (ACOG Committee Opinion No. 518). Washington, DC: Author.

Bromfield, N. F. (2016). Sex slavery and sex trafficking of women in the United States: Historical and contemporary parallels, policies, and perspectives in social work. *Affilia, 31*(1), 129–139.

Burgess, A. W., & Holmstrom, L. L. (1979). *Rape: Crisis and recovery.* Englewood Cliffs, NJ: Prentice Hall.

Calton, J. M., Cattaneo, L. B., & Gebhard, K. T. (2016). Barriers to help seeking for lesbian, gay, bisexual, transgender, and queer survivors of intimate partner violence. *Trauma, Violence, and Abuse, 17*(5), 585–600.

Catalano, S. (2012). *Intimate partner violence, 1993–2010.* Retrieved from http://www.bjs.gov/content/pub/pdf/ipv9310.pdf

Centers for Disease Control and Prevention (CDC). (2015a). *Intimate partner violence: Consequences.* Retrieved from http://www.cdc.gov/violenceprevention/intimatepartnerviolence/consequences.html

Centers for Disease Control and Prevention (CDC). (2015b). *2015 sexually transmitted diseases treatment guidelines.* Retrieved from https://www.cdc.gov/std/tg2015/default.htm

Edwards, L., & Mika, K. M. (2016). Advancing the efforts of the macro-level social work response against sex trafficking. *International Social Work, 60*(3), 695–706.

Goldberg, A. P., Moore, J. L., Houck, C., & Barron, C. E. (2017). Domestic minor sex trafficking patients: A retrospective analysis of medical presentation. *Journal of Pediatric and Adolescent Gynecology, 30*(1), 109–115.

Holmes, M. M. (1998). The clinical management of rape in adolescents. *Contemporary OB/GYN, 43*(5), 62–78.

Kintzle, S., Schuyler, A. C., Ray-Letourneau, D., Ozuna, S. M., Munch, C., Xintarianos, E., Hasson, A. M., & Castro, C. A. (2015). Sexual trauma in the military: Exploring PTSD and mental health care utilization in female veterans. *Psychological Services, 12*(4), 394–401.

LeBlanc, K., & Weeks, L. (2013). Are transition houses equipped to meet the needs of women in midlife and older? *Journal of Family Violence, 28*(6), 535–545.

McNamara, J., McDonald, S., & Lawrence, J. (2012). False allegations of adult crimes. *Journal of Forensic Science, 57* (3), 643–646.

Morgan, R. E. (2017). Race and Hispanic origin of victims and offender, 2012–2015. Retrieved from https://www.bjs.gov/content/pub/pdf/rhovo1215.pdf

Nurse Practitioners in Women's Health (NPWH). (2017). Position statement: Human sex trafficking. *Women's Healthcare: A Clinical Journal for NPs, 5*(2), 1–16.

Planty, M., Langton, L., Krebs, C., Berzofsky, M., & Smiley-McDonald, H. (2013). *Female victims of sexual violence, 1994–2010.* U. S. Department of Justice Special Report. Retrieved from http://www.bjs.gov/content/pub/pdf/fvsv9410.pdf

Rape, Abuse & Incest National Network (RAINN). (2016). *Victims of sexual violence: Statistics.* Retrieved from https://www.rainn.org/statistics/victims-sexual-violence

Start by Believing. (2017). *Start by Believing: Take Action.* Retrieved from http://www.startbybelieving.org/home

Truman, J., & Morgan, R. E. (2016). *Criminal victimization, 2015.* Retrieved from https://www.bjs.gov/content/pub/pdf/cv15.pdf

United Nations. (2013). *United Nations Security Council Resolution 2122 (2013).* Retrieved from http://www.un.org/en/ga/search/view_doc.asp?symbol=S/RES/2122(2013)

Vrees, R. A. (2017). Evaluation and management of female victims of sexual assault. *Obstetrical and Gynecological Survey, 72*(1), 39–53.

Walker, L. (1984). *The battered woman syndrome.* New York, NY: Springer.

World Health Organization (WHO). (2014). *World Health Assembly adopts a historic resolution that addresses violence against women and girls.* Retrieved from http://www.who.int/reproductivehealth/topics/violence/en

World Health Organization (WHO). (2016). Fact sheet: Violence against women. Retrieved from http://www.who.int/mediacentre/factsheets/fs239/en/

Human Reproduction

Part III

Chapter 9

Reproductive Physiology, Conception, and Fetal Development

My friends tease me when I say this, but I know the moment my daughter was conceived. My husband and I had both been so busy at work, but we finally went away for a long weekend together. It was wonderful—we got back some of the magic as we took long walks and talked and talked. Until that weekend, whenever we discussed having children it was always "maybe someday." On the second night we decided to skip the birth control for the first time ever. Our lovemaking seemed so special that evening, a true reflection of the emotional closeness we had recaptured. I never went back to using birth control after that weekend, but I am convinced that Jennifer is the result of that night together!

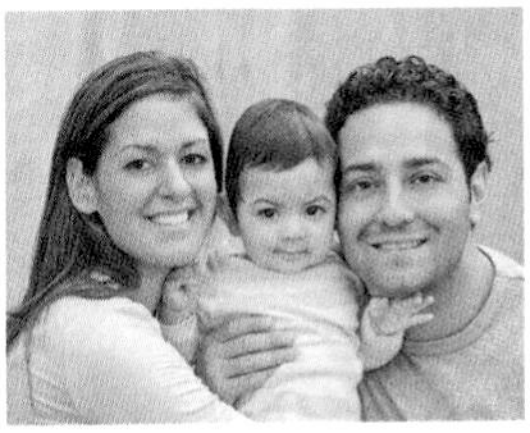

SOURCE: Blend Images/SuperStock.

Learning Outcomes

9.1 Discuss the significance of specific female reproductive structures during pregnancy and childbirth.

9.2 Summarize the actions of the hormones that affect reproductive functioning.

9.3 Identify the two phases of the ovarian cycle and the changes that occur in each phase.

9.4 Describe the phases of the uterine (menstrual) cycle, their dominant hormones, and the changes that occur in each phase.

9.5 Identify the structures and functions of the male reproductive system.

9.6 Compare the processes by which ova and sperm are produced.

9.7 Analyze the components of the process of fertilization as to how each may affect conception.

9.8 Summarize the processes that occur during the cellular multiplication and differentiation stages of intrauterine development and their effects on the structures that form.

9.9 Compare the factors and processes by which fraternal (dizygotic) and identical (monozygotic) twins are formed.

9.10 Describe the development, structure, and functions of the placenta and umbilical cord during intrauterine life (embryonic and fetal development).

9.11 Summarize the significant changes in growth and development of the fetus at 4, 6, 12, 16, 20, 24, 28, 32, 36, and 40 weeks' gestation.

9.12 Identify the factors that influence congenital malformations of the organ systems and the resulting congenital malformations.

Healthy People 2020

(MICH-14) Increase the proportion of women of childbearing potential with daily intake of at least 400 mcg of folic acid from fortified foods or dietary supplements

Understanding childbearing requires more than understanding sexual intercourse or the process by which the female and male sex cells unite. The nurse must also become familiar with the structures and functions that make childbearing possible and the phenomena that initiate it. This chapter considers the anatomy and physiology of the female and male reproductive systems and explores the processes involved in conception and fetal development—the basis of human uniqueness.

Female Reproductive System

The female reproductive system consists of the external and internal genitals and accessory organs of the breasts. Because you have already studied anatomy and physiology, refer to that textbook for specific function and structure, which will only be referred to in this chapter.

External Genitals

The appearance of the external genitalia varies greatly among women. Heredity, age, race, and the number of children a woman has borne influence the size, color, and shape of her external organs.

The female external genitals, called the **vulva**, include the following structures (Figure 9–1):

- Mons pubis
- Labia majora
- Labia minora (converge near the anus forming the *fourchette)*
- Clitoris
- Urethral meatus and opening of the paraurethral (Skene) glands
- Vaginal vestibule (vaginal orifice, vulvovaginal (Bartholin) glands, hymen, and fossa navicularis)
- Perineal body.

Although they are not true parts of the female reproductive system, the urethral meatus and perineal body are considered part of the external genitals because of their proximity and relationship to the vulva.

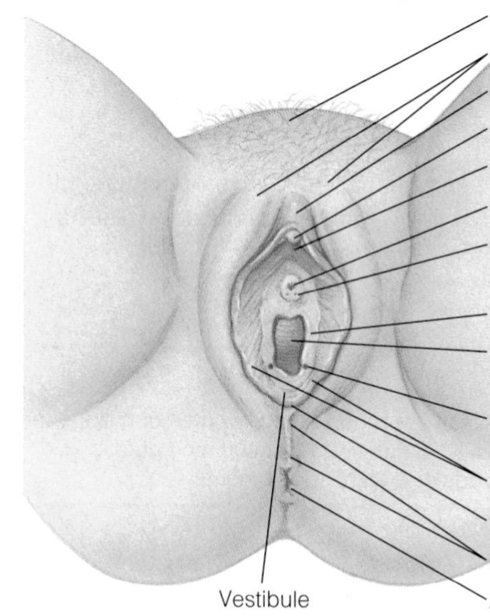

Figure 9–1 **Female external genitals, longitudinal view.**

Female Internal Reproductive Organs

The female internal reproductive organs—the vagina, uterus, fallopian tubes, and ovaries—are target organs for estrogenic hormones, and they play a unique part in the reproductive cycle (Figure 9–2). Certain internal reproductive organs can be palpated during vaginal examination and assessed with various instruments.

VAGINA

The **vagina** is a muscular and membranous tube that connects the external genitals with the uterus (see Figure 9–2). It extends from the vulva to the uterus in a position nearly parallel to the plane of the pelvic brim. The vagina is often referred to as the *birth canal* because it forms the lower part of the axis through which the fetus must pass during birth.

In the upper part of the vagina, which is called the *vaginal vault*, there is a recess or hollow around the cervix (the distal end of the uterus). This area is called the vaginal fornix. Because the walls of the vaginal vault are very thin, various structures can be palpated through them, including the uterus, a distended bladder, the ovaries, appendix, cecum, colon, and ureters. The upper fourth of the vagina is separated from the rectum by the pouch of Douglas (sometimes referred to as the cul-de-sac of Douglas), which is posterior to the cervix.

When a woman lies on her back after intercourse, the space in the fornix permits the pooling of semen. The collection of a large number of sperm near the cervix at or near the time of **ovulation** (the discharge of a mature ovum from an ovary) in the woman increases the chances of pregnancy.

The walls of the vagina are covered with ridges, or *rugae*, crisscrossing each other. These rugae allow the vaginal tissues to stretch enough for the fetus to pass through during childbirth as well as stretch for accommodation during coitus.

During a woman's reproductive life, the vaginal environment is normally acidic (pH 4 to 5). Secretion from the vaginal epithelium provides a moist environment. The acidic environment is maintained by a symbiotic relationship between lactic acid–producing bacilli (Döderlein bacillus or *Lactobacillus*) and the vaginal epithelial cells. These cells contain glycogen, which is broken down by the bacilli into lactic acid. The amount of glycogen is regulated by the ovarian hormones. During pregnancy and increased vascularity, vaginal secretions are markedly increased and may be mistaken for amniotic fluid (Cunningham et al., 2018).

The vagina has the following functions:

- To serve as the passageway for sperm during coitus and for the fetus during birth
- To provide passage for the menstrual blood flow from the uterine endometrium to the outside of the body.

UTERUS

The **uterus** is a hollow, muscular, thick-walled organ shaped like an upside-down pear (Figure 9–3). It is level with or slightly below the brim of the pelvis with the external opening of the cervix (the external os) about the level of the ischial spines. The uterus of a nulligravid (never been pregnant) mature woman weighs about 60 g and weighs more in a woman who has been pregnant. The nulligravid uterus measures approximately 6 to 8 cm in length and measures approximately 9 to 10 cm in multiparous women (Cunningham et al., 2018).

The uterus is divided into two major parts: An upper triangular portion called the **corpus**, or uterine body, and a lower cylindrical portion called the *cervix* (see Figure 9–2). The corpus

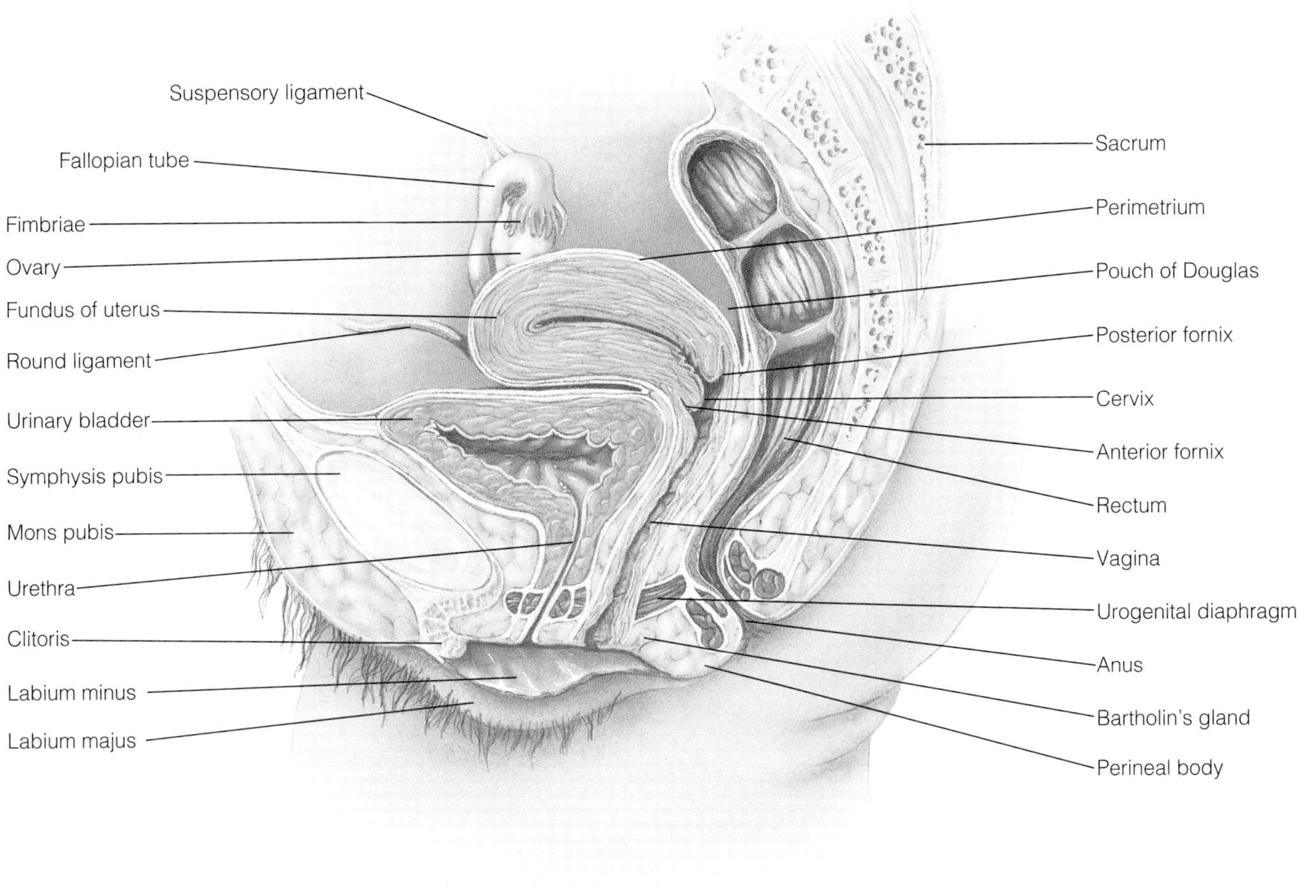

Figure 9–2 **Female internal reproductive organs.**

comprises the upper two-thirds of the uterus and is composed mainly of a smooth muscle layer (myometrium). The lower third is the cervix, or neck. The rounded uppermost portion of the corpus that extends above the points of attachment of the fallopian tubes is called the **fundus**. The elongated portion of the uterus where the fallopian tubes enter is called the **cornua**.

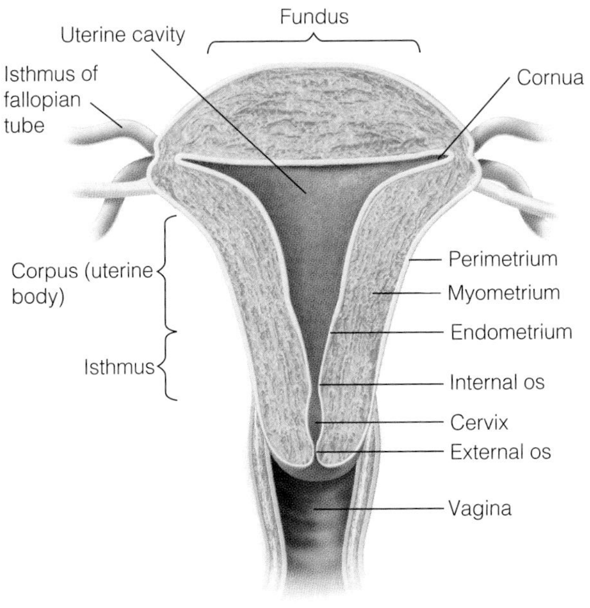

Figure 9–3 **Structures of the uterus.**

The **isthmus** is that portion of the uterus between the internal cervical os and the endometrial cavity. The isthmus is about 6 mm above the uterine opening of the cervix (the internal os), and it is in this area that the uterine lining changes into the mucous membrane of the cervix; it joins the corpus to the cervix. The isthmus takes on importance in pregnancy because it becomes the lower uterine segment. At birth, this thin lower segment, situated behind the bladder, is the site for lower-segment cesarean births (see Chapter 25).

The blood supplies to the uterus are extensive (Figure 9–4). The uterus is innervated entirely by the autonomic nervous system. Efferent sympathetic motor nerves are believed to cause vasoconstriction and muscular contraction. Even without an intact nerve supply, the uterus can contract adequately for birth. Thus, for example, hemiplegic women have adequate uterine contractions. Pain of uterine contractions is carried to the central nervous system by the 11th and 12th thoracic nerve roots. Pain from the cervix and upper vagina passes through the ilioinguinal and pudendal nerves. The motor fibers to the uterus arise from the 7th and 8th thoracic vertebrae. Because the sensory and motor levels are separate, epidural anesthesia can be used during labor and birth.

The function of the uterus is to provide a safe environment for fetal development. The uterine lining is cyclically prepared by steroid hormones for implantation of the embryo, a process known as **nidation**. Once the embryo is implanted, the developing fetus is protected until it is expelled.

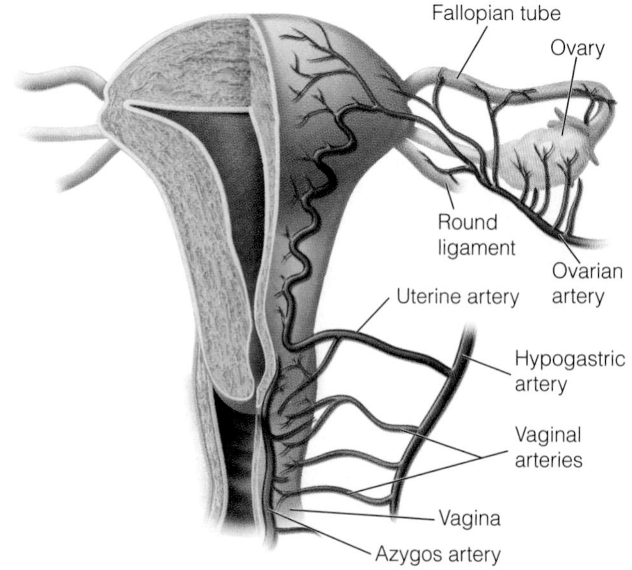

Figure 9–4 Blood supply to the vagina, ovary, uterus, and fallopian tube.

Both the body of the uterus and the cervix are changed permanently by pregnancy. The uterine body never returns to its prepregnant size, and the external os changes from a circular opening of about 3 mm to a transverse slit with irregular edges.

Uterine Corpus. The uterine corpus is made up of three layers. The outermost layer is the *serosal layer*, or **perimetrium**, which is composed of peritoneum. The middle layer is the *muscular uterine layer*, or **myometrium**. This muscular uterine layer is continuous with the muscle layer of the fallopian tubes and with that of the vagina. This characteristic helps the organs present a unified reaction to various stimuli—ovulation, orgasm, or the deposit of sperm in the vagina. These muscle fibers also extend into the ovarian, round, and cardinal ligaments and minimally into the uterosacral ligaments, which helps explain the vague but disturbing pelvic "aches and pains" reported by many pregnant women.

The myometrium has three distinct layers of uterine (smooth) involuntary muscles (Figure 9–5). The outer layer, found mainly over the fundus, is made up of longitudinal muscles that cause the descent of the fetus, which places pressure on the cervical fibers, leading to cervical effacement and delivery of the fetus. The thick middle layer is made up of interlacing muscle fibers in figure-eight patterns that assist the longitudinal fibers in expelling the fetus. These muscle fibers surround large blood vessels, and their contraction produces a hemostatic action (a tourniquet-like action on blood vessels to stop bleeding after birth). The inner muscle layer consists of circular fibers that form sphincters at the fallopian tube attachment sites and at the internal os. The internal os sphincter inhibits the expulsion of the uterine contents during pregnancy but relaxes in labor as cervical dilatation occurs. An incompetent cervical os can be caused by a torn, weak, or absent sphincter at the internal os. The sphincters at the fallopian tubes prevent menstrual blood from flowing backward into the fallopian tubes from the uterus.

Although each layer of muscle has been discussed as having a unique function, it must be remembered that the uterine musculature works as a whole. The uterine contractions of labor are responsible for the dilatation of the cervix and provide the major force for the passage of the fetus through the pelvic and vaginal canal at birth.

The innermost layer of the uterine corpus is the *mucosal layer*, or **endometrium**, which is composed of a single layer of columnar epithelium, glands, and stroma. From menarche to menopause, the endometrium undergoes monthly renewal and degeneration in the absence of pregnancy. As it responds to a governing hormonal cycle and prostaglandin influence as well, the endometrium varies in thickness from 0.5 to 5 mm.

The glands of the endometrium produce a thin, watery, alkaline secretion that keeps the uterine cavity moist. This endometrial milk not only helps sperm travel to the fallopian tubes but also nourishes the developing embryo before it implants in the endometrium.

The blood supply to the endometrium is unique. In the myometrium, the radial arteries branch off from the arcuate arteries at right angles. Once inside the endometrium, they become the basal arteries supplying the zona basalis (a layer of the endometrium) and ultimately become the coiled arteries supplying the zona functionalis (also part of the endometrium). The basal arteries are not sensitive to cyclic hormonal control; hence, the zona basalis portion remains intact and is the site of new endometrial tissue generation. The coiled arteries are extremely sensitive to cyclic hormonal control. Their response is alternate relaxation and constriction during the ischemic, or terminal, phase of the menstrual cycle. These differing responses allow for part of the endometrial tissue to remain intact while other endometrial tissue is shed during menstruation.

When pregnancy occurs and the endometrium is not shed, the reticular stromal cells surrounding the endometrial glands become the decidual cells of pregnancy. The stromal cells are highly vascular, channeling a rich blood supply to the endometrial surface.

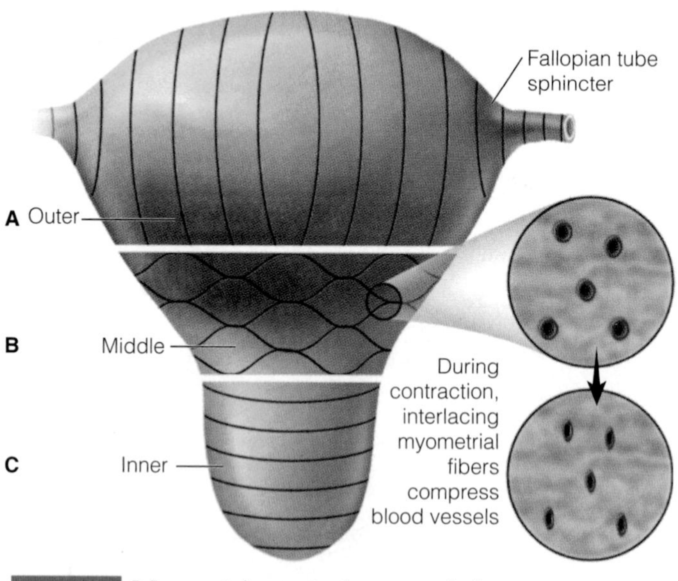

Figure 9–5 Myometrium uterine muscle layers placement and function. A. Outer layer (longitudinal muscles) suited to expel fetus. B. Middle layer (interlacing muscle fibers in a figure-eight pattern) surround and constrict blood vessels to stop bleeding. C. Inner layer (circular muscle fibers form sphincters at fallopian tubes and internal os) to prevent backflow of menstrual blood into fallopian tubes and cervical dilatation during labor/delivery.

Cervix. The distal end of the uterus is called the **cervix**. It meets the body of the uterus at the internal os and descends about 2.5 cm to connect with the vagina and ends at the external os (see Figure 9–2 and Figure 9–4). Thus, it provides a protective portal for the body of the uterus. The cervix is divided by its line of attachment into the vaginal and supravaginal areas. The cervical canal appears rosy red and is lined with columnar ciliated epithelium, which contains mucus-secreting glands. Elasticity is the chief characteristic of the cervix. Its ability to stretch is due to the high fibrous and collagenous content of the supportive tissues and also to the vast number of folds in the cervical lining.

The cervical mucus has three functions:

- To provide lubrication for the vaginal canal
- To act as a bacteriostatic agent
- To provide an alkaline environment to shelter deposited sperm from the acidic vaginal secretions. (At ovulation, cervical mucus is clearer, thinner, and more alkaline than at other times.)

FALLOPIAN TUBES

The two **fallopian tubes**, also known as *oviducts* or *uterine tubes*, arise from each side of the uterus and reach almost to the side of the pelvis, where they turn toward the ovaries (Figure 9–6). Each tube is approximately 8 to 13.5 cm long. A short section of each fallopian tube is inside the uterus; its opening into the uterus is 1 mm in diameter. The fallopian tubes link the peritoneal cavity with the uterus and vagina. This linkage increases a woman's vulnerability to disease processes in the pelvis.

Each fallopian tube may be divided into three parts: The isthmus, the ampulla, and the infundibulum or fimbria. The fallopian tube isthmus is straight and narrow, with a thick muscular wall and an opening (lumen) 2 to 3 mm in diameter (Cunningham et al., 2018). It is the site of tubal ligation (a surgical procedure to prevent pregnancy; see Chapter 4).

Next to the isthmus is the curved **ampulla**, which comprises the outer two-thirds of the tube. Fertilization of the secondary oocyte by a spermatozoon usually occurs here. The ampulla ends at the **fimbria**, which is a funnel-like enlargement with many moving fingerlike projections (fimbriae) reaching out to the ovary. The longest of these, the *fimbria ovarica*, is attached to the ovary to increase the chances of intercepting the ovum as it is released.

The wall of the fallopian tube is made up of four layers. The *peritoneum* covers the tube. The *subserous* layer contains the blood and nerve supply, and the muscular layer is responsible for the peristaltic movement of the tube. The *mucosal* layer, next to the muscular layer, is composed of ciliated and nonciliated cells, with the number of ciliated cells more abundant at the fimbria. Nonciliated cells secrete a protein-rich, serous fluid that nourishes the ovum. The constantly moving tubal cilia propel the ovum toward the uterus. This ciliary action is needed to assist the tube's muscular layer peristalsis. Any malformation or malfunction of the tubes could result in infertility, ectopic pregnancy, or even sterility.

A well-functioning tubal transport system involves active fimbriae close to the ovary, peristalsis of the tube created by the muscular layer, ciliated currents beating toward the uterus, and the proximal contraction and distal relaxation of the tube caused by different types of prostaglandins.

The fallopian tubes have three functions:

- Provide transport for the ovum from the ovary to the uterus (transport through the fallopian tubes varies from 3 to 4 days)
- Provide a site for fertilization
- Serve as a warm, moist, nourishing environment for the ovum or zygote (a fertilized egg).

OVARIES

The **ovaries** are two almond-shaped glandular structures just below the pelvic brim. One ovary is located on each side of the pelvic cavity. Their size varies among women and according to the stage of the menstrual cycle. Each ovary weighs 6 to 10 g and is 1.5 to 3 cm wide, 2 to 5 cm long, and 1 to 1.5 cm thick. The ovaries of girls are small, but they become larger after puberty and then decrease in size following menopause. They also change in appearance from smooth-surfaced, dull white organs to pitted gray organs as the woman ages. The pitting appearance on their surface is the result of scarring after ovulation. Each ovary is maintained in place by the ovarian, broad, and infundibulopelvic ligaments (see Figure 9–7). The ovarian ligament is at the upper border of the round ligament and can alter the position of the ovary so that it can help the fimbria of the fallopian tube "catch" the ovum. The infundibulopelvic ligament suspends and supports the ovary.

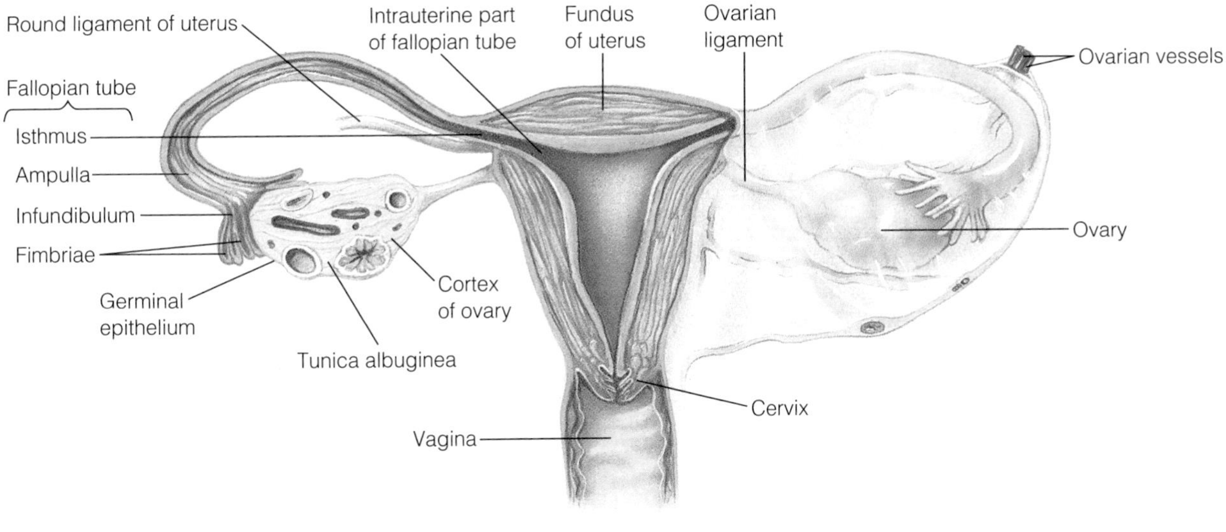

Figure 9–6 **Fallopian tube and ovaries.**

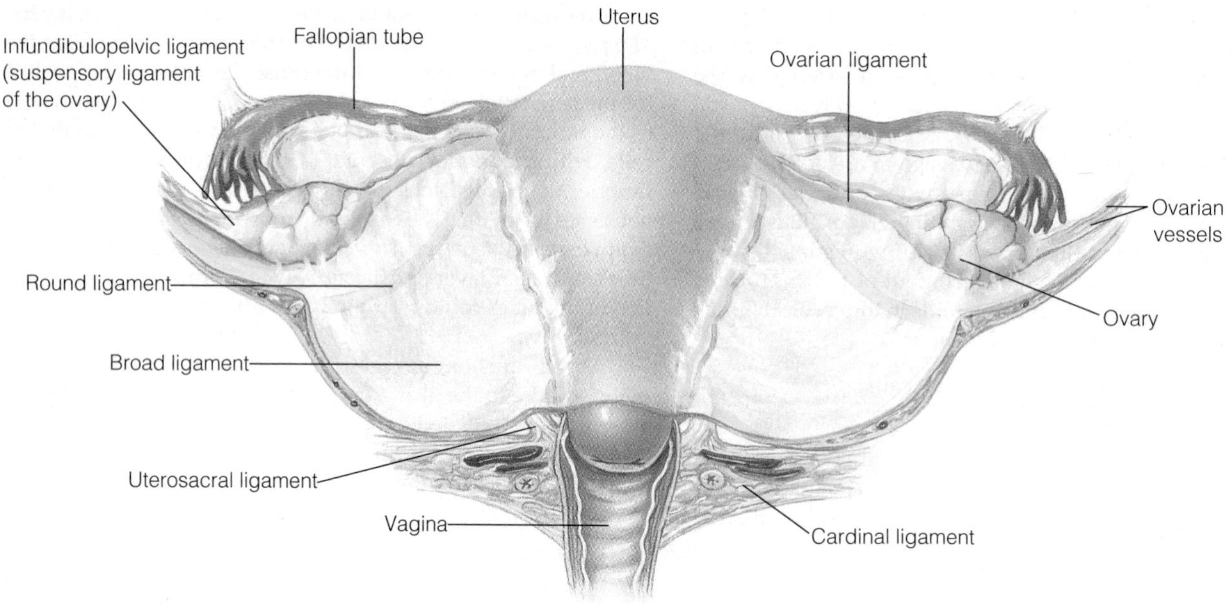

Figure 9–7 **Uterine ligaments.**

There is no peritoneal covering for the ovaries. Although this lack of covering assists the mature ovum to erupt, it also allows easier spread of malignant cells from cancer of the ovaries. A single layer of cuboidal epithelial cells, called the *germinal epithelium*, covers the ovaries. The ovaries are composed of three layers: The tunica albuginea, the cortex, and the medulla. The *tunica albuginea* is dense and dull white and serves as a protective layer. The *cortex* is the main functional part, containing ova, graafian follicles, corpora lutea, degenerated corpora lutea (corpora albicantia), and degenerated follicles. The *medulla* is completely surrounded by the cortex and contains the nerves and the blood and lymphatic vessels.

The ovaries are the primary source of two important hormones: The estrogens and progesterone, which are discussed later in the chapter.

BONY PELVIS

The female bony pelvis has two unique functions:

- To support and protect the pelvic contents
- To form the relatively fixed axis of the birth passage.

Because the pelvis is so important to childbearing, its structures should be understood clearly. See Chapter 12 for a discussion of pelvic assessment and Chapter 19 for information on pelvic types as they relate to labor and birth.

Breasts

The **breasts**, or *mammary glands*, considered accessories of the reproductive system, are specialized sebaceous glands. They are conical and symmetrically placed on the sides of the chest. The greater pectoral and anterior serratus muscles underlie each breast. Suspending the breasts are fibrous tissues, called *Cooper ligaments*, which extend from the deep fascia in the chest outward to just under the skin covering the breast. The left breast is frequently larger than the right. In different racial groups breasts develop at slightly different levels in the pectoral region of the chest.

In the center of each mature breast is the **nipple**, a protrusion about 0.5 to 1.3 cm in diameter. The nipple is composed mainly of erectile tissue, which becomes more rigid and prominent during the menstrual cycle, sexual excitement, pregnancy, and lactation. The nipple is surrounded by the heavily pigmented ring of skin called the **areola**, 2.5 to 10 cm in diameter. Both the nipple and areola are roughened by small papillae called *tubercles of Montgomery*. As a baby suckles, these tubercles secrete a fatty substance that helps lubricate and protect the nipple.

The breasts are composed of glandular, fibrous, and adipose tissue. The glandular tissue consists of acini, or alveoli (Figure 9–8), which are arranged in a series of 15 to 24 lobes separated from each other by adipose and fibrous tissue. Each lobe is made up of several lobules, which are made up of many grapelike clusters of alveoli around tiny ducts. The lining of these ducts secretes the various components of milk. The ducts from several lobules share common openings, called *nipple pores*, that open on the surface of the nipple. The smooth muscle of the nipple causes erection of the nipple on contraction.

The biologic function of the breasts is to:

- Provide nourishment and protective maternal antibodies to newborns and infants through the lactation process
- Be a source of pleasurable sexual sensation.

Female Reproductive Cycle

The **female reproductive cycle (FRC)** is composed of the ovarian cycle, during which ovulation occurs, and the menstrual cycle, during which menstruation occurs. These two cycles take place simultaneously (Figure 9–9).

Effects of Female Hormones

Menstruation is an orderly process under neurohormonal control. Each month, multiple oocytes mature, with one rupturing from the ovary and entering the fallopian tube. The ovary, vagina, uterus, and fallopian tubes are major target organs for female hormones.

The ovaries produce mature gametes and secrete hormones. Ovarian hormones include the estrogens, progesterone, and testosterone. The ovary is sensitive to **follicle-stimulating hormone (FSH)** and **luteinizing hormone (LH)**. The relative

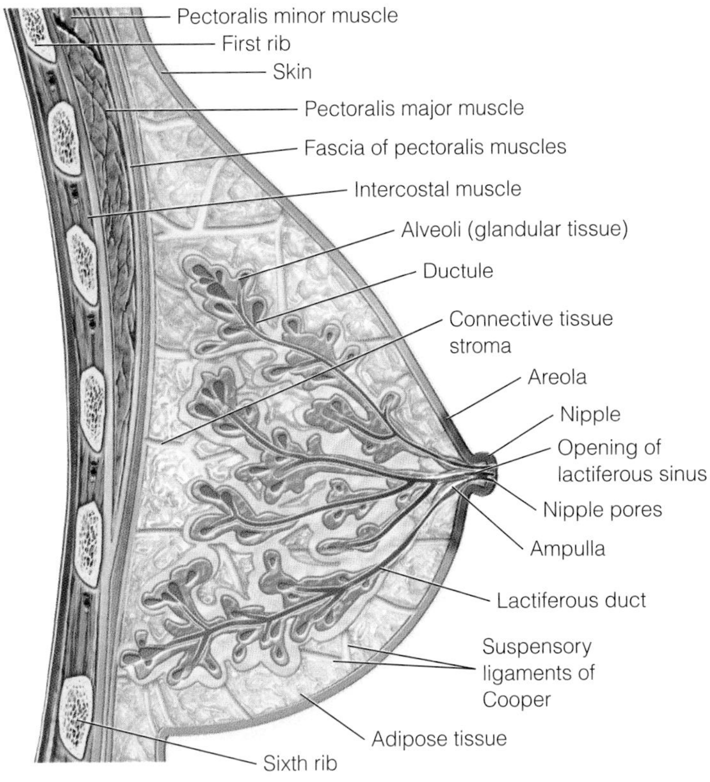

Figure 9–8 **Anatomy of the breast.**

proportions of these hormones control the events of both ovarian and menstrual cycles and thus are responsible for the cyclic changes that allow pregnancy to occur.

ESTROGENS

Estrogens are hormones that are associated with those characteristics contributing to "femaleness," including breast alveolar lobule growth and duct development. They also assist in the maturation of the ovarian follicles and cause the endometrial mucosa to proliferate following menstruation. The amount of estrogens is greatest during the proliferative (follicular or estrogenic) phase of the menstrual cycle. Estrogens cause the uterus to increase in size and weight because of increased glycogen, amino acids, electrolytes, and water. Blood supply is expanded as well. Under the influence of estrogens, myometrial contractility increases in both the uterus and the fallopian tubes, and uterine sensitivity to oxytocin increases. Estrogens inhibit FSH production and stimulate LH production. The major estrogenic effects are due primarily to three estrogens: Estrone, β-estradiol, and estriol, with β-estradiol being the major estrogen.

The ovaries secrete the largest amounts of estrogens; however, the adrenal cortex (extraglandular sites) produces minute amounts of estrogens in nonpregnant women and the fat cells produce a secondary estrogen.

Estrogens have effects on many hormones and other carrier proteins, such as contributing to the increased amount of protein-bound iodine in pregnant women and women who use oral contraceptives containing estrogen.

PROGESTERONE

Progesterone is secreted by the corpus luteum and is found in greatest amounts during the secretory (luteal or progestational) phase of the menstrual cycle. Progesterone is often called the *hormone of pregnancy* because its effects on the uterus allow pregnancy to be maintained. Under the influence of progesterone the following occur:

- Vaginal epithelium proliferates
- Cervix secretes thick, viscous mucus
- Breast glandular tissue increases in size and complexity
- Breasts prepare for lactation
- Temperature rises about 0.3°C to 0.6°C (0.5°F to 1.0°F), which accompanies ovulation and persists throughout the secretory phase of the menstrual cycle.

PROSTAGLANDINS

Prostaglandins (PGs) are hormones produced by the cells of the endometrium. The two primary types of prostaglandins are groups E and F. Generally, PGE relaxes smooth muscles and is a potent vasodilator; PGF is a potent vasoconstrictor and increases the contractility of muscles and arteries. Although their primary actions seem antagonistic, their basic regulatory functions in cells are achieved through an intricate pattern of reciprocal events.

Prostaglandin production increases during follicular maturation, is dependent on gonadotropins, and seems to be critical to follicular rupture. Extrusion of the ovum, resulting from follicular swelling and increased contractility of the smooth muscle in the theca layer of the mature follicle, is thought to be caused by $PGF_{2\alpha}$. Significant amounts of PGs are found in and around the follicle at the time of ovulation.

Neurohormonal Basis of the Female Reproductive Cycle

The female reproductive cycle is controlled by complex interactions between the nervous and endocrine systems and their target tissues. These interactions involve the hypothalamus, anterior pituitary, and ovaries.

The hypothalamus secretes **gonadotropin-releasing hormone (GnRH)** to the pituitary gland in response to signals received from the central nervous system. This releasing hormone is often called *follicle stimulating hormone–releasing hormone (FSHRH)* or *luteinizing hormone–releasing hormone (LHRH)* (Blackburn, 2018). In response to GnRH, the anterior pituitary secretes the gonadotropic hormones FSH and LH.

FSH is primarily responsible for the maturation of the ovarian follicle. As the follicle matures, it secretes increasing amounts of estrogen, which enhance the development of the follicle. (This estrogen is also responsible for the rebuilding/proliferation phase of the endometrium after it is shed during menstruation.)

Final maturation of the follicle will not come about without the action of LH. The anterior pituitary's production of LH increases 6-fold to 10-fold as the follicle matures. The peak production of LH can precede ovulation by as much as 10 to 12 hours (Blackburn, 2018). LH is also responsible for "luteinizing" the increase in production of progesterone by the granulosa cells of the follicle. As a result, estrogen production declines and progesterone secretion continues. Thus, estrogen levels fall a day before ovulation; tiny amounts of the hormones inhibin and progesterone are in evidence (Blackburn, 2018). Ovulation takes place following the very rapid growth of the follicle—as the sustained high level of estrogen diminishes and progesterone secretion begins.

The ruptured follicle undergoes rapid change, complete luteinization is accomplished, and the mass of cells becomes the **corpus luteum**. The lutein cells secrete large amounts of progesterone with smaller amounts of estrogen. (Concurrently,

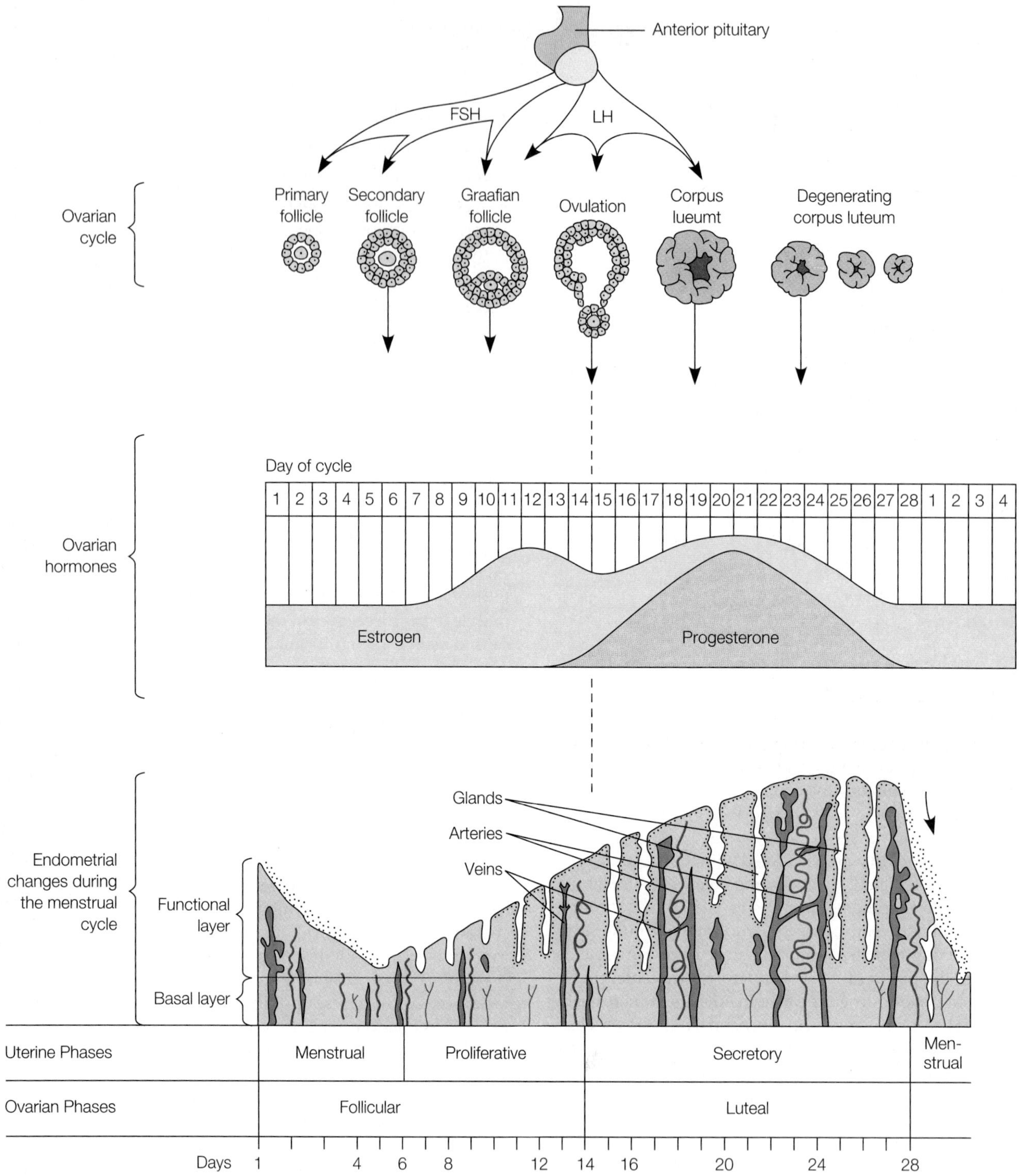

Figure 9–9 Female reproductive cycle: Interrelationships of hormones with the three phases of the uterine cycle and the two phases of the ovarian cycle in an ideal 28-day cycle.

the excessive amounts of progesterone are responsible for the secretory phase of the uterine cycle.) On day 7 or 8 following ovulation, the corpus luteum begins to involute, losing its secretory function. The production of both progesterone and estrogen is severely diminished. The anterior pituitary responds with increasingly large amounts of FSH; a few days later, LH production begins. New follicles become responsive to another ovarian cycle and begin maturing.

OVARIAN CYCLE

The ovarian cycle has two phases: The *follicular phase* (days 1 to 14) and the *luteal phase* (days 15 to 28 in a 28-day cycle). Figure 9–10 depicts the changes that the follicle undergoes during the ovarian cycle. In women whose menstrual cycles vary, usually it is only the length of the follicular phase that varies because the luteal phase is of fixed length (Blackburn, 2018; Cunningham et al., 2018). During the follicular phase, the

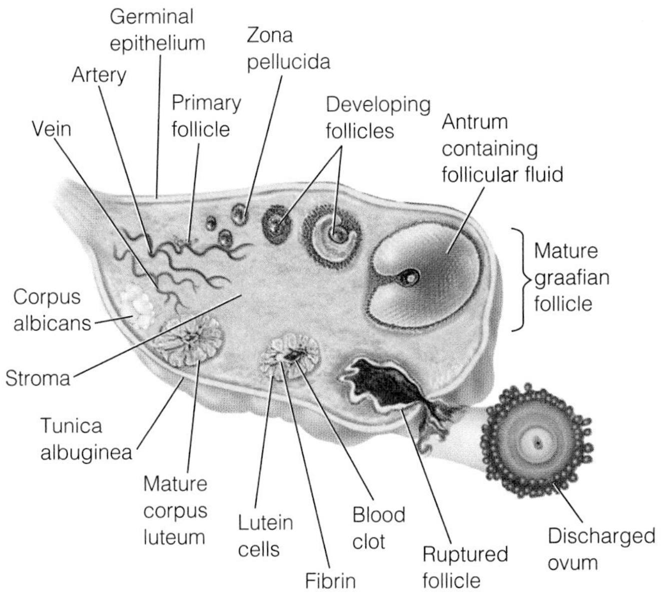

Figure 9–10 **Various stages of development of the ovarian follicles.**

immature follicle matures as a result of FSH. Within the follicle, the oocyte grows.

A mature **graafian follicle** appears about the 14th day under dual control of FSH and LH. It is a large structure, measuring about 5 to 10 mm, and produces increasing amounts of estrogen. In the mature graafian follicle, the cells surrounding the fluid-filled antral cavity are called *granulosa cells*. The mass of granulosa cells surrounding the oocyte and follicular fluid is called the *cumulus oophorus*. In the fully mature graafian follicle, the zona pellucida, a thick elastic capsule, develops around the oocyte. Just before ovulation, the mature oocyte completes its first meiotic division (see a description of meiosis later in the chapter). As a result of this division, two cells are formed: A small cell called a *polar body* and a larger cell called the *secondary oocyte*. The secondary oocyte matures into the ovum.

As the graafian follicle matures and enlarges, its walls thin and it travels outward to the surface of the ovary. This surface has a blister-like protrusion 10 to 15 mm in diameter, where the secondary oocyte, polar body, and follicular fluid are pushed out. The ovum is discharged near the fimbria of the fallopian tube and is pulled into the tube to begin its journey toward the uterus (see Figure 9–6).

In some women, ovulation is accompanied by midcycle pain, known as *mittelschmerz*. This pain may be caused by a thick tunica albuginea or by a local peritoneal reaction to the expelling of the follicular contents. Vaginal discharge may increase during ovulation, and a small amount of blood (midcycle spotting) may be discharged as well.

The body temperature increases about 0.3°C to 0.6°C (0.5°F to 1°F) 24 to 48 hours after the time of ovulation. It remains elevated until the day before menstruation begins. There may be an accompanying sharp basal body temperature drop just before the increase. These temperature changes are useful clinically to determine the approximate time ovulation occurs (Blackburn, 2018).

Generally, the ovum takes several minutes to travel through the ruptured follicle to the fallopian tube opening. The contractions of the tube's smooth muscle and its ciliary action propel the ovum through the tube. The ovum remains in the ampulla, where, if it is fertilized, cleavage can begin. The ovum is thought to be fertile for only 6 to 24 hours. It reaches the uterus 72 to 96 hours after its release from the ovary.

The luteal phase begins when the ovum leaves its follicle. Under the influence of LH, the corpus luteum develops from the ruptured follicle. Within 2 or 3 days the corpus luteum becomes yellowish and spherical and increases in vascularity. If the ovum is fertilized and implants in the endometrium, the fertilized egg begins to secrete **human chorionic gonadotropin (hCG)**, which is needed to maintain the corpus luteum. If fertilization does not occur, within about a week after ovulation, the corpus luteum begins to degenerate, eventually becoming a connective tissue scar called the *corpus albicans*. With degeneration comes a decrease in estrogen and progesterone. This allows for an increase in LH and FSH, which triggers the hypothalamus.

Uterine (Menstrual) Cycle

Menstruation is cyclic uterine bleeding in response to cyclic hormonal changes. Menstruation occurs when the ovum is not fertilized and begins about 14 days after ovulation (in an ideal 28-day cycle) in the absence of pregnancy. The menstrual discharge, also referred to as the *menses* or *menstrual flow*, is composed of blood mixed with cervical and vaginal secretions, bacteria, mucus, leukocytes, and other cellular debris. The menstrual discharge is dark red and has a distinctive odor.

Menstrual parameters vary greatly among individuals. Generally, menstruation occurs every 29 days but varies from 21 to 35 days. Some women normally have longer cycles, which can skew standard calculations of the estimated date of birth (EDB) when they become pregnant. Emotional and physical factors such as illness, excessive fatigue, stress or anxiety, and rigorous exercise programs can alter the cycle interval. Certain environmental factors such as temperature and altitude may also affect the cycle. The duration of menses is from 2 to 8 days, with the blood loss averaging 25 to 60 mL and the loss of iron averaging 0.5 to 1 mg daily.

A review of the endometrium and its arterial blood supply will provide further understanding of the menstrual process (Figure 9–11). Blood flow from the spiral arterioles in the superficial endometrium is reduced, leading to a lack of blood and oxygen, which in turn produces tissue death (necrosis) and discharge of the superficial endometrium (menses). At the same time, the straight arterioles provide the basal endometrium with sufficient blood flow to maintain this layer of the endometrium and the endometrial glands (or seeds) that are responsible for the generation of the endometrium in the next female reproductive or menstrual cycle (see Figure 9–9). Bleeding is controlled by vasospasm of the straight basal arterioles, resulting in coagulative necrosis at the vessel tips (Cunningham et al., 2018).

The uterine (menstrual) cycle has three phases: The menstrual phase, proliferative phase, and secretory phase. Menstruation occurs during the *menstrual phase*. Some endometrial areas are shed, whereas others remain. Some of the remaining tips of the endometrial glands begin to regenerate. The endometrium is in a resting state following menstruation. Estrogen levels are low, and the endometrium is 1 to 2 mm deep. During this part of the cycle the cervical mucus is scanty, viscous, and opaque.

The *proliferative phase* begins when the endometrial glands enlarge, becoming twisted and longer, in response to increasing amounts of estrogen. The blood vessels become prominent and dilated, and the endometrium increases in thickness 6-fold to 8-fold. This gradual process reaches its peak just before ovulation. The cervical mucus becomes thin, clear, watery, and more alkaline, making the mucus more favorable to spermatozoa. As ovulation nears, the cervical mucus shows increased elasticity (see Figure 4–1A) and its pH increases from below 7 to 7.5 at the time of ovulation.

The *secretory phase* follows ovulation. The endometrium, under estrogenic influence, undergoes slight cellular growth.

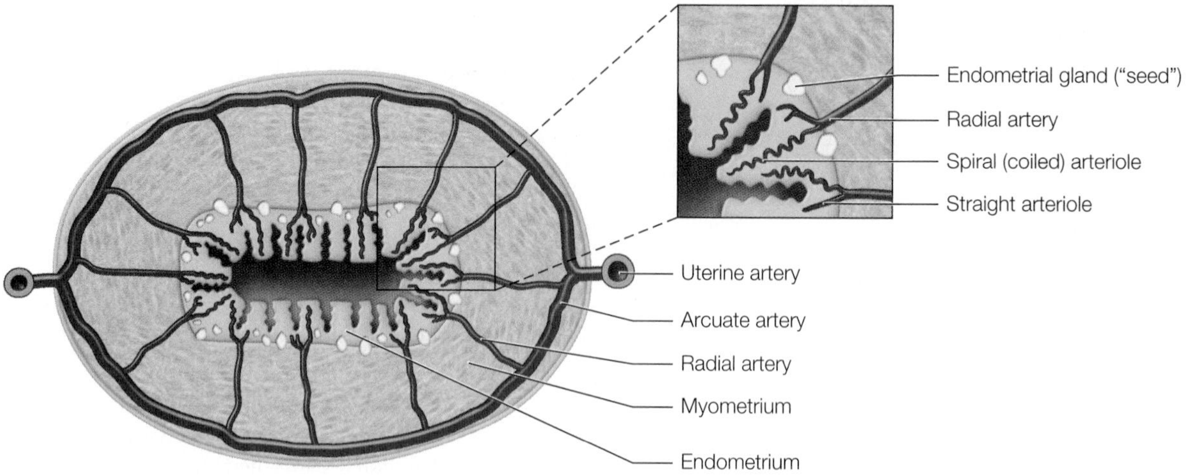

Figure 9–11 **Blood supply to the endometrium (cross-sectional view of the uterus).**

Progesterone, however, causes such marked swelling and growth that the epithelium is warped into folds (Figure 9–12). The amount of tissue glycogen increases. The glandular epithelial cells begin to fill with cellular debris, become twisted, and dilate. The glands secrete small quantities of endometrial fluid in preparation for a fertilized ovum. The vascularity of the entire uterus increases greatly, providing a nourishing bed for implantation. If implantation occurs, the endometrium, under the influence of progesterone, continues to develop and become even thicker (implantation is discussed later in the chapter).

If fertilization does not occur, the *menstrual phase* (days 27–28) begins. The corpus luteum begins to degenerate and, as a result both estrogen and progesterone levels fall. Extensive vascular changes also occur. Small blood vessels rupture, and the spiral arteries constrict and retract, causing a deficiency of blood in the endometrium, which becomes pale. Then there is escape of blood into the stromal cells of the uterus. The menstrual flow (days 1–6) begins, thus beginning the menstrual cycle again. After menstruation the basal layer remains, so that the tips of the glands can regenerate the new functional endometrial layer. See *Key Facts to Remember: Summary of the Female Reproductive Cycle.*

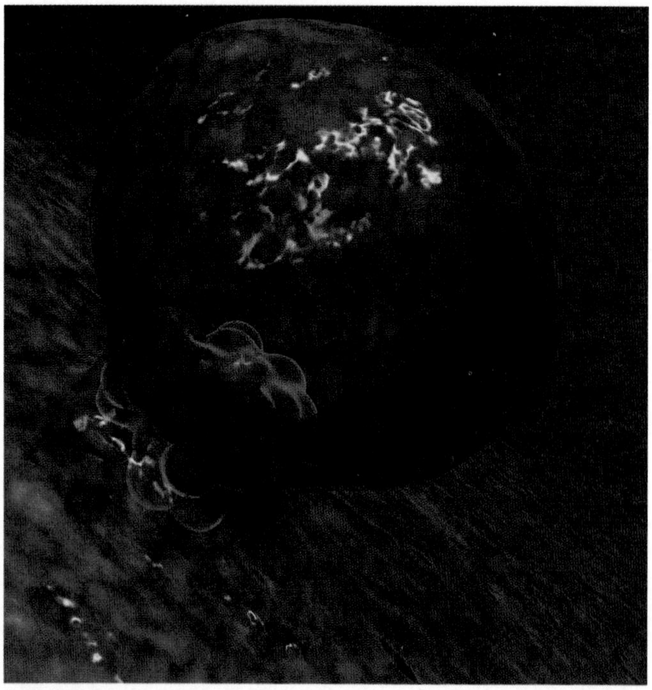

A

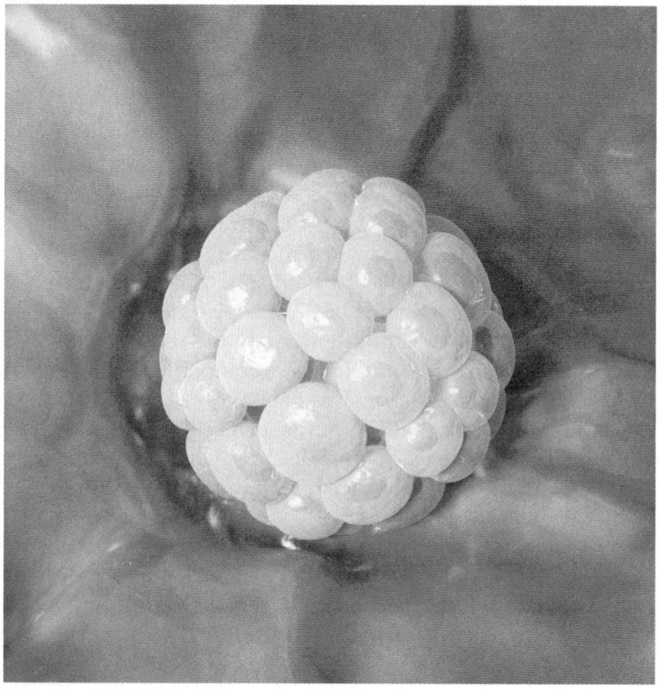

B

Figure 9–12 **Scanning electron micrographs of the uterine lining during the secretory phase of the uterine cycle and at the time of blastocyst implantation. A. A blastocyst begins implanting in the wall of the uterus. B. Light micrograph (LM) of an 11-day-old implantation site in the human endometrium (uterine lining) showing bilaminar embryo, amnion, and surrounding placental trophoblasts. Magnification unknown.**

SOURCE: **A**. Stocktrek Images, Inc./Alamy Stock Photo; **B**. David Mack/Science Source.

Key Facts to Remember
Summary of the Female Reproductive Cycle

Ovarian Cycle

- *Follicular phase* (days 1–14): Primordial follicle matures under influence of FSH and LH up to the time of ovulation.
- *Luteal phase* (days 15–28): Ovum leaves follicle; corpus luteum develops under LH influence and produces high levels of progesterone and low levels of estrogen.

Menstrual Cycle

- *Menstrual phase* (days 1–6): Estrogen levels are low.
  Cervical mucus is scant, viscous, and opaque.
  Endometrium is shed.
- *Proliferative phase* (days 7–14): Endometrium and myometrium thickness increases.
  Estrogen peaks just before ovulation.
  Cervical mucus at ovulation is clear, thin, watery, and alkaline; it is more favorable to sperm and has increased elasticity on microscopic exam.
  Just before ovulation, body temperature may drop slightly, then at ovulation basal body temperature increases 0.3° to 0.6°C (0.5° to 1.0°F).
  Mittelschmerz and/or midcycle spotting may occur.
- *Secretory phase* (days 15–26): Estrogen drops sharply, and progesterone dominates.
  Vascularity of entire uterus increases.
  Tissue glycogen increases, and the uterus is made ready for implantation.
- *Menstrual phase begins* (days 27–28): Both estrogen and progesterone levels drop.
  Spiral arteries undergo vasoconstriction.
  Endometrium becomes pale; blood vessels rupture.
  Blood escapes into uterine stromal cells, gets ready to be shed.

Male Reproductive System

The primary reproductive functions of the male genitals are to produce and transport the male sex cells (sperm) through and eventually out of the genital tract into the female genital tract. The male reproductive system consists of the external and internal genitals (Figure 9–13).

External Genitals

The two external reproductive organs are the penis and the scrotum.

PENIS

The **penis** is an elongated, cylindrical structure consisting of a body, termed the *shaft*, and a cone-shaped end called the *glans*. A circular fold of skin arises just behind the glans and covers it. Known as the *prepuce*, or *foreskin*, it is frequently removed by the surgical procedure of circumcision (see Chapter 28). The primary reproductive function of the penis is to deposit sperm in the female vagina during sexual intercourse so that fertilization of the ovum can occur.

SCROTUM

The *scrotum* is a pouchlike structure that hangs in front of the anus and behind the penis. Inside the scrotum are two lateral compartments. Each compartment contains a testis with its related structures.

The function of the scrotum is to protect the testes and the sperm they produce by maintaining a temperature lower than that of the body. Spermatogenesis will not occur if the testes fail to descend and thus remain at body temperature. Because it is sensitive to touch, pressure, temperature, and pain, the scrotum defends against potential harm to the testes.

Male Internal Reproductive Organs

The male internal reproductive organs include the gonads (testes or testicles), a system of ducts (epididymis, vas deferens, ejaculatory duct, and urethra), and accessory glands (seminal vesicles, prostate gland, bulbourethral glands, and urethral glands) (see Figure 9–13).

TESTES

The **testes**, a pair of oval glandular organs contained in the scrotum (Figure 9–14), have two primary functions:

- To serve as the site of spermatogenesis
- To produce **testosterone**, the most prevalent and potent of the testicular hormones.

SEMEN

The male ejaculate, **semen** or *seminal fluid*, is made up of spermatozoa and the secretions of all the accessory glands. The seminal fluid transports viable and motile sperm to the female reproductive tract. Effective transportation of sperm requires adequate nutrients, an adequate pH (about 7.5), a specific concentration of sperm to fluid, and an optimal osmolarity.

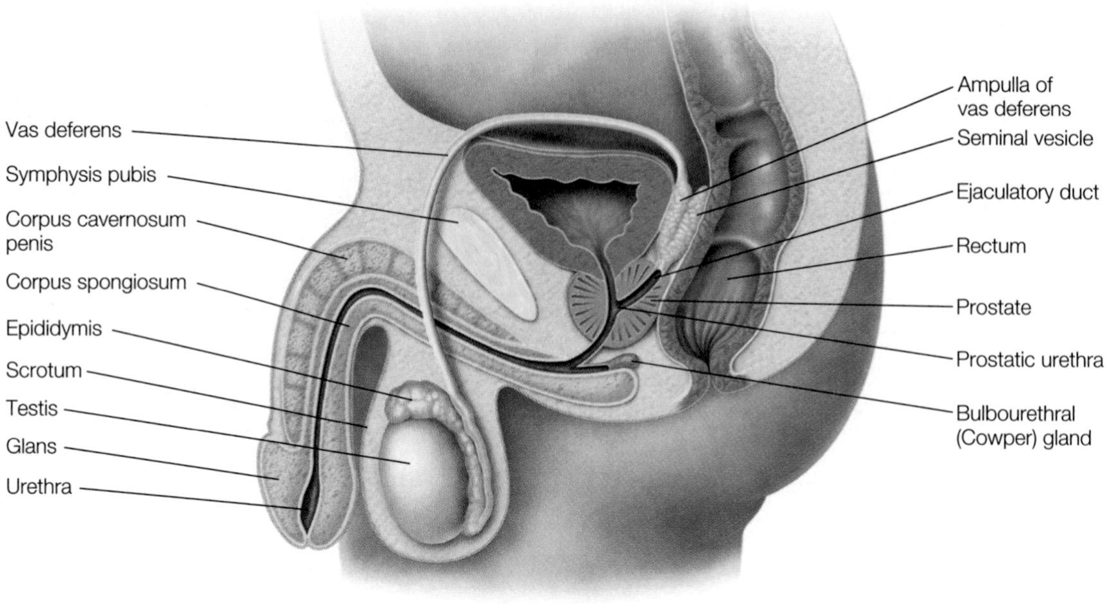

Figure 9–13 **Male reproductive system, sagittal view.**

See *Key Facts to Remember: Summary of Male Reproductive Organ Functions*.

Key Facts to Remember
Summary of Male Reproductive Organ Functions

- The penis deposits sperm in the female vagina during sexual intercourse so that fertilization of the ovum can occur.
- The testes house seminiferous tubules and the gonads in the scrotum.
- Seminiferous tubules contain sperm cells in various stages of development and undergoing meiosis.
- Sertoli cells nourish and protect spermatocytes (phase between spermatids and spermatozoa).
- Leydig cells are the main source of testosterone.
- Epididymides provide an area for the sperm to become motile and fertile and a reservoir for mature spermatozoa.
- The vas deferens connects the epididymis with the prostate gland and then connects with ducts from the seminal vesicle to become an ejaculatory duct.
- Ejaculatory ducts provide a passageway for semen and seminal fluid into the urethra.
- Seminal vesicles secrete yellowish fluid rich in fructose, prostaglandins, and fibrinogen. This provides nutrition that increases motility and fertilizing ability of sperm. Prostaglandins also aid fertilization by making the cervical mucus more receptive to sperm.
- The prostate gland secretes thin, alkaline fluid containing calcium, citric acid, and other substances. Alkalinity counteracts acidity of ductus and seminal vesicle secretions.
- Bulbourethral (Cowper) glands secrete alkaline, viscous fluid into semen, aiding in neutralization of acidic vaginal secretions.
- The urethral glands (Littre glands) are tiny mucus-secreting glands and their secretions are added to those of the bulbourethral glands.

Conception and Fetal Development

Chromosomes

Human (body) cells contain within their nuclei threadlike bodies known as **chromosomes**, which are composed of strands of deoxyribonucleic acid (DNA) and protein.

Every somatic (body) cell in the human body contains 46 chromosomes, referred to as the **diploid number of chromosomes**. These are divided into 23 pairs. There are 22 pairs of similar cells in both males and females, called *autosomes*, and one pair of sex chromosomes (XX in females, XY in males). One chromosome of each pair is contributed by the individual's mother, and the other is contributed by the father. *Genes* are regions in the DNA strands that contain coded information used to determine the unique characteristics—or *traits*—of an individual. Genes in the autosomes determine such traits as hair color or blood type, whereas genes in the sex chromosomes determine the individual's gender. Reproductive genetics is discussed in greater detail in Chapter 10.

Cellular Division

Each human begins life as a single cell called a fertilized ovum or **zygote**. This single cell reproduces itself, and in turn each new cell also reproduces itself in a continuing process. The new cells are similar to the cells from which they came. Cells are reproduced either by mitosis or meiosis, two different but related processes.

MITOSIS

Mitosis results in the production of diploid body (somatic) daughter cells, which are exact copies of the original cell. Daughter cells have the same diploid number of chromosomes (46) and the same genetic makeup as the cell from which they came. Mitosis makes growth and development possible, and in mature individuals it is the process by which our body cells continue to divide and replace themselves.

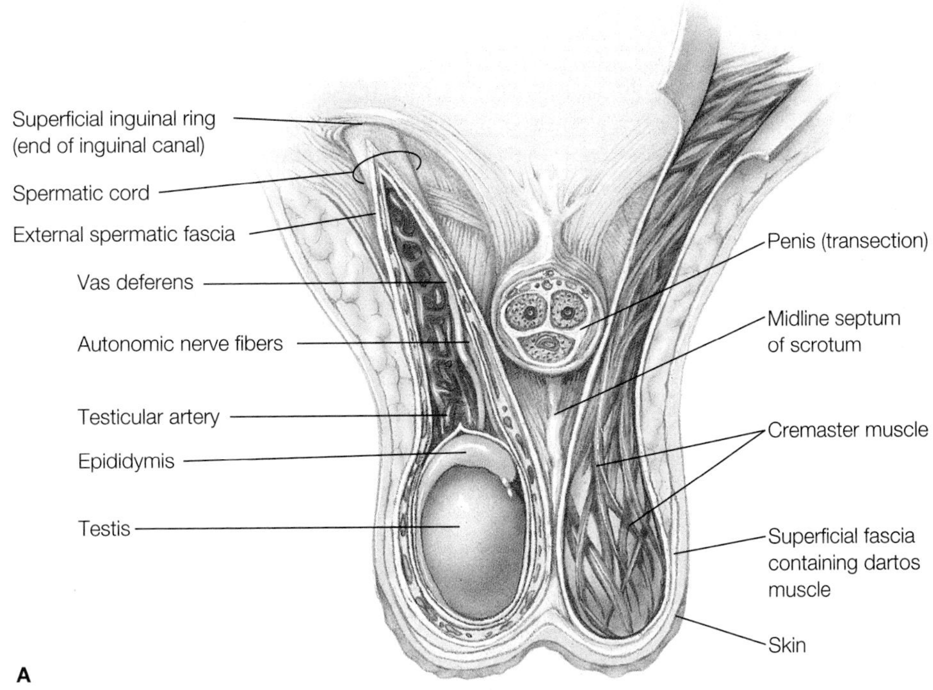

MEIOSIS

Meiosis is a special type of cell division by which diploid cells give rise to **gametes** (sperm and ova). These cells are different from other somatic (body) cells because they contain half the genetic material of the parent cell—only 23 chromosomes—the **haploid number of chromosomes**.

Meiosis consists of two successive cell divisions. In the first division, the chromosomes replicate. Next, a pairing takes place between homologous chromosomes (Sadler, 2015). Instead of separating immediately, as in mitosis, the similar chromosomes become closely intertwined. At each point of contact, there is a physical exchange of genetic material between the chromatids (arms of the chromosomes). New combinations are provided by the newly formed chromosomes; these combinations account for the wide variation of traits, such as hair or eye color. The cell divides, forming two daughter cells, each with 23 double-structured chromosomes—the same amount of DNA as a normal somatic cell. In the second division, cell division occurs, resulting in the formation of four cells, each containing 23 single chromosomes, the haploid number of chromosomes. These daughter cells contain only half the DNA of a normal somatic cell (Sadler, 2015).

The process of meiosis is important for the following reasons:

- It maintains the *constancy of the chromosome number* from one generation to the next by reducing the chromosome number from diploid to haploid, thereby producing haploid gametes.
- It allows random assortment of *maternal and paternal chromosomes* between the gametes.
- It relocates segments of maternal and paternal chromosomes by the *crossing-over of chromosome segments*, which "shuffles" the genes and produces a recombination of genetic material.

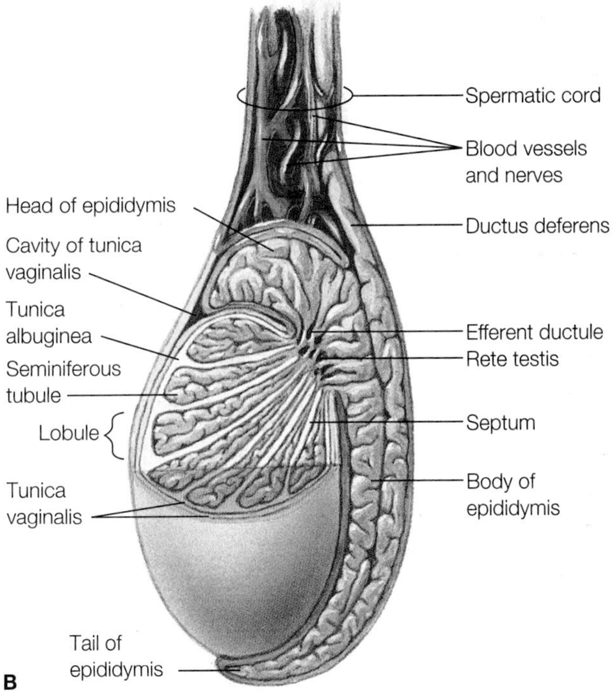

Figure 9–14 **The testes. A. External view. B. Sagittal view showing interior anatomy.**

Mutations may occur during the second meiotic division if two of the chromatids do not move apart rapidly enough when the cell divides. The still-paired chromatids are carried into one of the daughter cells and eventually form an extra chromosome. This condition is referred to as an *autosomal nondisjunction* (chromosomal mutation) and is harmful to the offspring that may result should fertilization occur. Another type of chromosomal mutation can occur if chromosomes break during meiosis. If the broken segment is lost, the result is a shorter chromosome; this is known as a *deletion*. If the broken segment becomes attached to another chromosome, a harmful mutation called a *translocation* is the result. The effects of nondisjunction and translocation are described in Chapter 10. See *Key Facts to Remember: Comparison of Mitosis and Meiosis*.

Key Facts to Remember
Comparison of Mitosis and Meiosis

MITOSIS

Purpose

Produces cells for growth and tissue repair. Cell division characteristic of all somatic cells.

Cell Division

One-stage cell division

Number of Daughter Cells

Two daughter cells identical to the mother cell, each with the diploid number (46 chromosomes)

MEIOSIS

Purpose

Produces reproductive cells (gametes). Reduction of chromosome number by half (from diploid [46] to haploid [23]), so that when fertilization occurs the normal diploid number is restored. Introduces genetic variability.

Cell Division

Two-stage reduction

Number of Daughter Cells

Four daughter cells, each containing one-half the number of chromosomes of the mother cell, or 23 chromosomes. Nonidentical to original cell.

Gametogenesis

Meiosis occurs during **gametogenesis**, the process by which germ cells or gametes (ovum and sperm) are produced. These cells contain only half the genetic material of a typical body cell. The gametes must have a haploid number (23) of chromosomes so that when the female gamete (egg or ovum) and the male gamete (sperm or spermatozoon) unite to form the **zygote** (fertilized ovum), the normal human diploid number of chromosomes (46 chromosomes)—half from the mother and half from the father—is reestablished.

OOGENESIS

Oogenesis is the process that produces the female gamete, called an ovum (egg). The ovaries begin to develop early in the fetal life of the female, and all the ova that the female will produce in her lifetime are present at birth. The ovary gives rise to oogonial cells, which develop into oocytes. Meiosis (cell replication by division) begins in all oocytes before the female fetus is born but stops before the first division is complete and remains in this arrested phase until puberty. During puberty the mature primary oocyte continues through the first meiotic division in the graafian follicle of the ovary.

The first meiotic division produces two cells of unequal size with different amounts of cytoplasm but with the same number of chromosomes. One of these cells is the *secondary oocyte* and the other is a minute *polar body*. Both the secondary oocyte and the first polar body contain 22 double-structured autosomal chromosomes and one double-structured sex chromosome (X).

At the time of ovulation, the second meiotic division begins immediately and proceeds as the oocyte moves down the fallopian tube. Division is again not equal, and the secondary oocyte moves into the metaphase stage of cell division, where its meiotic division is arrested until and unless the oocyte is fertilized.

When the secondary oocyte completes the second meiotic division after fertilization, the result is a mature ovum with the haploid number of chromosomes and virtually all the cytoplasm. In addition, the second polar body (also haploid) forms at this time (Figure 9–15A). The first polar body has now also divided, producing two additional polar bodies. Thus, when meiosis is completed, four haploid cells have been produced: Three small polar bodies, which eventually disintegrate, and one ovum (Sadler, 2015).

SPERMATOGENESIS

During puberty, the germinal epithelium in the seminiferous tubules of the testes begins the process of **spermatogenesis**, which produces the male gametes (sperm). The diploid spermatogonium replicates before it enters the first meiotic division, during which it is called the *primary spermatocyte*. During this first meiotic division, the spermatogonium replicates and forms two haploid cells termed *secondary spermatocytes*, each of which contains 22 double-structured autosomal chromosomes and either a double-structured X sex chromosome or a double-structured Y sex chromosome. During the second meiotic division, they divide to form four spermatids, each with the haploid number of chromosomes (Figure 9–15B). The spermatids undergo a series of changes during which they lose most of their cytoplasm and become sperm (spermatozoa). The nucleus becomes compacted into the head of the sperm, which is covered by a cap called an *acrosome* that is, in turn, covered by a plasma membrane. A long tail is produced from one of the centrioles.

The Process of Fertilization

Fertilization is the process by which a sperm fuses with an ovum to form a new diploid cell, or zygote. The zygote begins life as a single cell with a complete set of genetic material, 23 chromosomes from the mother's ovum and 23 chromosomes from the father's sperm for a total of 46 chromosomes. The following events lead to fertilization.

PREPARATION FOR FERTILIZATION

The mature ovum and spermatozoon have only a brief time to unite. Ova are considered fertile for about 12 to 24 hours after ovulation. Sperm can survive in the female reproductive tract for 48 to 72 hours but are believed to be healthy and highly fertile for only about the first 24 hours.

The ovum's cell membrane is surrounded by two layers of tissue. The layer closest to the cell membrane is called the *zona pellucida*. It is a clear, noncellular layer whose thickness influences the fertilization rate. Surrounding the zona pellucida is a ring of elongated cells, called the *corona radiata* because they radiate from

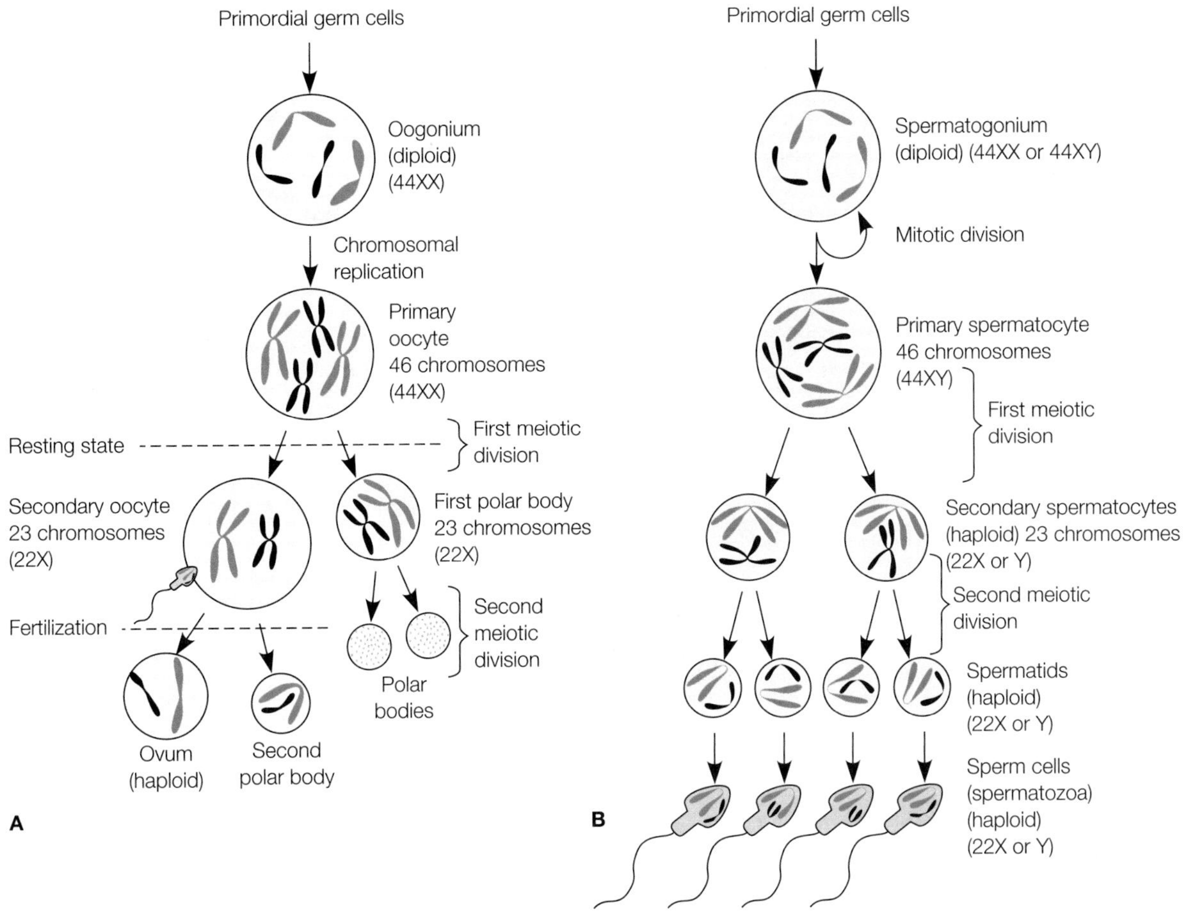

Figure 9–15 Gametogenesis involves meiosis within the ovary and testis. A. During meiosis, each oogonium produces a single haploid ovum once some cytoplasm moves into the polar bodies. B. Each spermatogonium, in contrast, produces four haploid spermatozoa.

the ovum like the gaseous corona around the sun. These cells are held together by hyaluronic acid. The ovum has no power of movement of its own. During ovulation, high estrogen levels increase peristalsis within the fallopian tubes, which helps move the ovum through the tube toward the uterus. The high estrogen levels also cause a thinning of the cervical mucus, easing passage of the sperm through the cervix, into the uterus, and up the fallopian tube.

The process of fertilization usually takes place in the ampulla (outer third) of the fallopian tube. In a single ejaculation, the male deposits approximately 200 to 500 million spermatozoa in the vagina, of which only about 1000 sperm actually reach the ampulla (Sadler, 2015). Fructose in the semen, secreted by the seminal vesicles, is the energy source for the sperm. The spermatozoa propel themselves up the female tract by the flagellar movement of their tails. Transit time from the cervix into the fallopian tube can be from as short as 30 minutes to as long as 6 days (Sadler, 2015). Prostaglandins in the semen may increase uterine smooth muscle contractions, which help transport the sperm. The fallopian tubes have a dual ciliary action that facilitates movement of the ovum toward the uterus and movement of the sperm from the uterus toward the ovary.

The sperm must undergo two processes before fertilization can occur: Capacitation and the acrosomal reaction. **Capacitation** is the removal of the plasma membrane and glycoprotein coat overlying the spermatozoa's acrosomal area and the loss of seminal plasma proteins. If the glycoprotein coat is not removed, the sperm will not be able to fertilize the ovum (Sadler, 2015). Capacitation occurs in the female reproductive tract (aided by uterine enzymes) and is thought to take about 7 hours. Sperm that undergo capacitation take on three characteristics: (1) the ability to undergo the acrosomal reaction, (2) the ability to bind to the zona pellucida, and (3) the acquisition of hypermotility.

The **acrosomal reaction** follows capacitation. The acrosome caps of the sperm surrounding the ovum release their enzymes (hyaluronidase, a protease called *acrosin*, and trypsin-like substances) and thus break down the hyaluronic acid that holds the elongated cells of corona radiata, the outer layer of the ovum, together (Sadler, 2015). About a thousand acrosomes must rupture to clear enough hyaluronic acid for even a single sperm to penetrate the ovum successfully.

At the moment of penetration by a fertilizing sperm, the zona pellucida undergoes a reaction that prevents additional sperm from entering a single ovum (Blackburn, 2018). This is known as the *block to polyspermy*. This cellular change is mediated by release of materials from the cortical granules, organelles found just below the ovum's surface, and is called the *cortical reaction* (Figure 9–16).

THE MOMENT OF FERTILIZATION

After the sperm enters the ovum, a chemical signal prompts the secondary oocyte to complete the second meiotic division, forming the nucleus of the ovum and ejecting the second polar

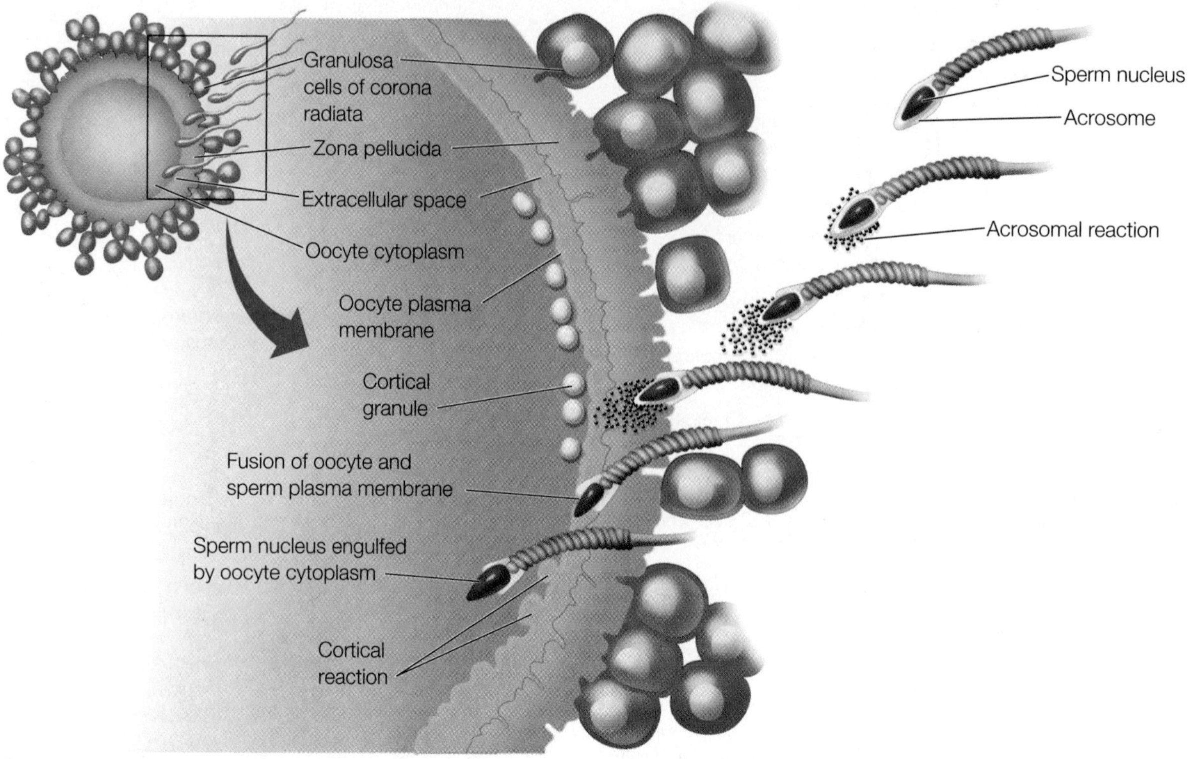

body. Then the nuclei of the ovum and sperm swell and approach each other. The true moment of fertilization occurs as the nuclei unite. Their individual nuclear membranes disappear, and their chromosomes pair up to produce the diploid zygote. Because each nucleus contains a haploid number of chromosomes (23), this union restores the diploid number (46). The zygote contains a new combination of genetic material that results in an individual different from either parent and from anyone else.

At the moment of fertilization, the sex of the zygote is determined. The two chromosomes (the sex chromosomes) of the 23rd pair—either XX or XY—determine the sex of an individual. X chromosomes are larger and bear more genes than Y chromosomes. Females have two X chromosomes, and males have an X and a Y chromosome. The mature ovum produced by oogenesis can have only one type of sex chromosome—an X—while spermatogenesis produces two sperm with an X chromosome and two sperm with a Y chromosome. When each gamete contributes an X chromosome, the resulting zygote is female. When the ovum contributes an X chromosome and the sperm contributes a Y, the resulting zygote is male. The sex of the new child is determined by the father. As discussed in Chapter 10, certain traits are termed *sex-linked* because they are controlled by the genes on the X sex chromosome. Two examples of sex-linked traits are color blindness and hemophilia.

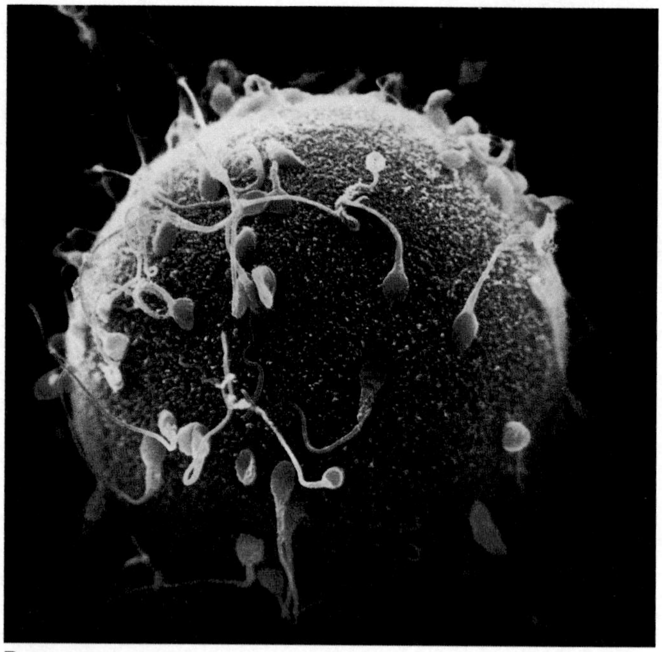

Figure 9–16 Sperm penetration of an ovum. A. The sequential steps of oocyte penetration by a sperm are depicted moving from top to bottom. B. Scanning electron micrograph of human sperm surrounding a human oocyte (750×). The smaller spherical cells are granulosa cells of the corona radiata.

SOURCE: B. Phillips D/Photo Researchers/Getty Images.

Preembryonic Stage

The first 14 days of human development, starting on the day the ovum is fertilized (conception), are referred to as the *preembryonic stage*, or the *stage of the ovum*. Development after fertilization can be divided into two phases: Cellular multiplication and cellular differentiation. These phases are characterized by rapid cellular multiplication and differentiation and the establishment of the primary germ layers and embryonic membranes. Synchronized development of both the endometrium and embryo is a prerequisite for implantation to succeed (Moore, Persaud, & Torchia, 2016). These phases and the process of implantation (nidation), which occurs between them, are discussed next.

CELLULAR MULTIPLICATION

Cellular multiplication begins as the zygote moves through the fallopian tube toward the cavity of the uterus. This transportation takes 3 days or more and is accomplished mainly by a very weak fluid current in the fallopian tube resulting from the beating action of the ciliated epithelium that lines the tube.

The zygote now enters a period of rapid mitotic divisions called **cleavage**, during which it divides into two cells, four cells, eight cells, and so on. These cells, called *blastomeres*, are so small that the developing cell mass is only slightly larger than the original zygote. The blastomeres are held together by the zona pellucida, which is under the corona radiata. The blastomeres will eventually form a solid ball of 12 to 32 cells called the **morula** (Moore et al., 2016).

As the morula enters the uterus, two things happen: The intracellular fluid in the morula increases, and a central cavity forms within the cell mass. Inside this cavity is an inner solid mass of cells called the **blastocyst**. The outer layer of cells that surround the cavity and have replaced the zona pellucida is the **trophoblast**. Eventually, the trophoblast develops into one of the embryonic membranes, called the *chorion*. The blastocyst develops into a double layer of cells called the *embryonic disc*, from which the embryo and the amnion (embryonic membrane) will develop. The journey of the fertilized ovum to its destination in the uterus is illustrated in Figure 9–17.

Early pregnancy factor (EPF), an immunosuppressant, is secreted by the trophoblastic cells. EPF appears in the maternal serum within 24 to 48 hours after fertilization and forms the basis of a pregnancy test during the first 10 days of development (Moore et al., 2016).

IMPLANTATION (NIDATION)

While floating in the uterine cavity, the blastocyst is nourished by the uterine glands, which secrete a mixture of lipids, mucopolysaccharides, and glycogen. The trophoblast attaches itself to the surface of the endometrium for further nourishment. The most frequent site of attachment is the upper part of the posterior uterine wall (see Figure 9–17). Between days 7 and 10 after fertilization, the zona pellucida disappears, and the blastocyst implants itself by burrowing into the uterine lining and penetrating down toward the maternal capillaries until it is completely covered (Moore et al., 2016). The blastocyst will orient itself so that the embryonic pole is closest to the endometrial lining. The lining of the uterus thickens below the implanted blastocyst, and the cells of the trophoblast grow down into the thickened lining, forming processes called *chorionic villi*.

Under the influence of progesterone, the endometrium increases in thickness and vascularity in preparation for implantation and nourishment of the ovum. After implantation, the endometrium is called the *decidua*. The portion of the decidua that covers the blastocyst is called the **decidua capsularis**, the portion directly under the implanted blastocyst is the **decidua basalis**, and the portion that lines the rest of the uterine cavity is the **decidua vera (parietalis)** (see Figure 9–17, inset). The maternal part of the placenta develops from the decidua basalis, which contains large numbers of blood vessels. The chorionic villi (discussed shortly) in contact with the decidua basalis will form the fetal portion of the placenta.

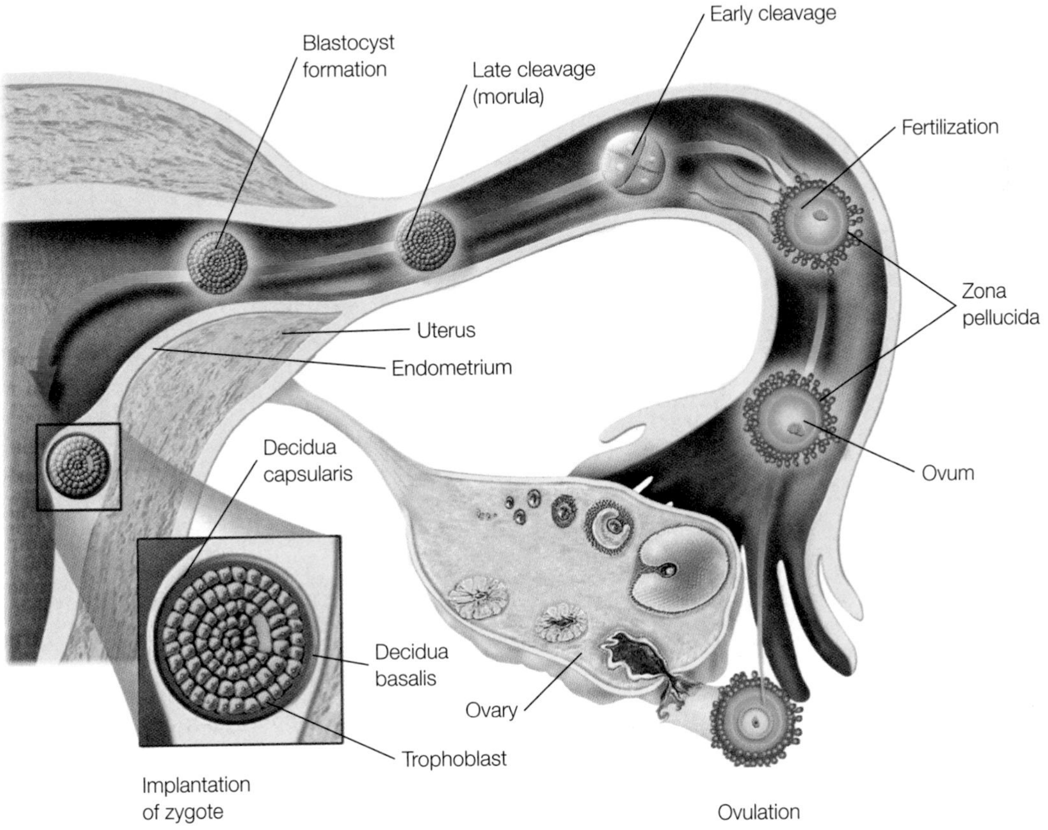

Figure 9–17 **During ovulation, the ovum leaves the ovary and enters the fallopian tube. Fertilization generally occurs in the outer third of the fallopian tube. Subsequent changes in the fertilized ovum from conception to implantation are depicted.**

CELLULAR DIFFERENTIATION

Primary Germ Layers. About 10 to 14 days after conception, the homogenous mass of blastocyst cells differentiates into the primary germ layers. These layers—the **ectoderm, mesoderm,** and **endoderm**—are formed at the same time as the embryonic membranes. All tissues, organs, and organ systems will develop from these primary germ cell layers (Figure 9–18). See Table 9–1. For example, differentiation of the endoderm results in the formation of the epithelium lining the respiratory and digestive tracts (Figure 9–19).

Embryonic Membranes. The **embryonic membranes** (the chorion and amnion) begin to form at the time of implantation (Figure 9–20). These membranes protect and support the embryo as it grows and develops inside the uterus. The first and outermost membrane to form is the **chorion**. This thick membrane develops from the trophoblast and has many fingerlike projections, called *chorionic villi*, on its surface. These chorionic villi can be used for early genetic testing of the embryo at 8 to 11 weeks' gestation by chorionic villi sampling (CVS) (see Chapter 16). As the pregnancy progresses, the villi begin to degenerate, except for those just under the embryo, which grow and branch into depressions in the uterine wall, forming the fetal portion of the placenta. By the fourth month of pregnancy, the surface of the chorion is smooth except at the place of attachment to the uterine wall.

The second membrane, the amnion, originates from the ectoderm, a primary germ layer, during the early stages of embryonic development. The **amnion** is a thin protective membrane that contains amniotic fluid. The space between the amniotic membrane and the embryo is the *amniotic cavity*. This cavity surrounds the embryo and yolk sac, except where the developing embryo (germ layer disc) attaches to the trophoblast via the umbilical cord. As the embryo grows, the amnion expands until it comes in contact with the chorion. These two slightly adherent membranes form the fluid-filled amniotic sac, also called **bag of waters (BOW)**, which protects the floating embryo.

Amniotic Fluid. The primary functions of **amniotic fluid** are to:

- Act as a cushion to protect the fetus against mechanical injury
- Help control the temperature of the embryo/fetus (relies on the mother to release heat)
- Permit symmetric external growth and development of the embryo/fetus
- Prevent adherence of the embryo/fetus to the amnion (decreases chance of amniotic band syndrome) to allow freedom of movement so that the embryo/fetus can change position (flexion and extension), thus aiding in musculoskeletal development
- Allow the umbilical cord to be relatively free of compression
- Act as an extension of fetal extracellular space (hydropic fetuses/neonates have increased amniotic fluid)
- Act as a wedge during labor.

Additionally, amniotic fluid can be used for analysis to determine fetal health and maturity.

Amniotic fluid is slightly alkaline and contains albumin, urea, uric acid, creatinine, lecithin, sphingomyelin, bilirubin, fat, fructose, leukocytes, proteins, epithelial cells, enzymes, and fine hair called **lanugo**. The amount of amniotic fluid at 10 weeks is about 30 mL and increases to 210 mL at 16 weeks (Cunningham et al., 2018). After 28 weeks the volume ranges from 700 to 1000 mL. The amniotic fluid volume changes little until 36-38 weeks, after which it decreases dramatically (Blackburn, 2018; Mattson & Smith, 2016). As the pregnancy continues, the fetus influences the volume of amniotic fluid by swallowing the fluid, excreting lung fluid, and excreting urine into the amniotic fluid. Abnormal variations in amniotic fluid volume can be classified as *oligohydramnios* (less than 400 mL of amniotic fluid) and *hydramnios* (more than 2000 mL or an amniotic fluid index greater than 97.5 percentile for the corresponding gestational age). Hydramnios is also called *polyhydramnios*. Chapter 23 discusses

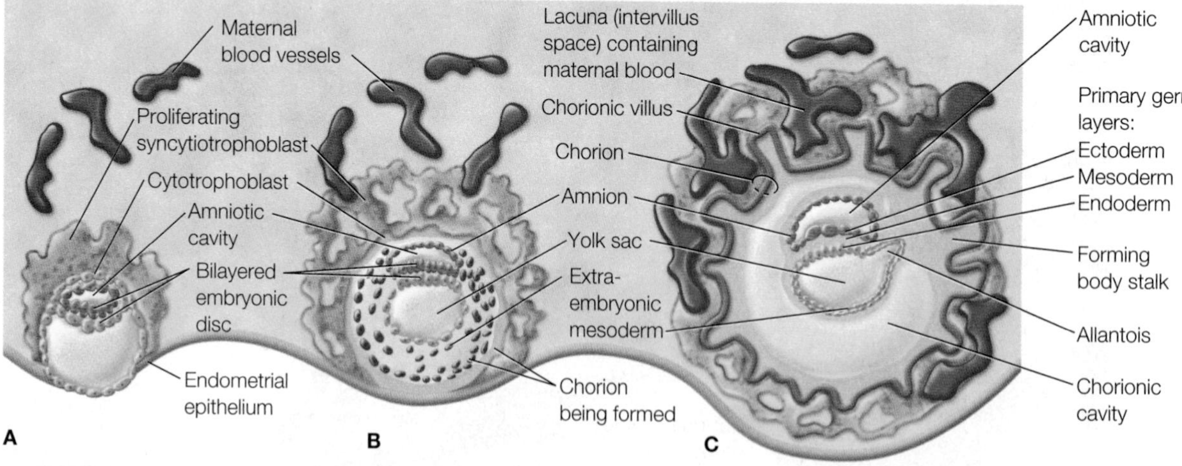

Figure 9–18 **Formation of primary germ layers. A. Implantation of a 7½-day blastocyst in which the cells of the embryonic disc are separated from the amnion by a fluid-filled space. The erosion of the endometrium by the syncytiotrophoblast is ongoing. B. Implantation is completed by day 9, and extraembryonic mesoderm is beginning to form a discrete layer beneath the cytotrophoblast. C. By day 16, the embryo shows all three germ layers, a yolk sac, and an allantois (an outpouching of the yolk sac that forms the structural basis of the body stalk, or umbilical cord). The cytotrophoblast and associated mesoderm has become the chorion, and chorionic villi are developing.**

TABLE 9–1 Derivation of Body Structures from Primary Cell Layers

ECTODERM	MESODERM	ENDODERM
Epidermis	Dermis	Respiratory tract epithelium
Sweat glands	Wall of digestive tract	Epithelium (except nasal), including pharynx, tongue, tonsils, thyroid, parathyroid, thymus, tympanic cavity
Sebaceous glands	Kidneys and ureter (suprarenal cortex)	Lining of digestive tract
Nails	Reproductive organs (gonads, genital ducts)	Primary tissue of liver and pancreas
Hair follicles	Connective tissue (cartilage, bone, joint cavities)	Urethra and associated glands
Lens of eye	Skeleton	Urinary bladder (except trigone)
Sensory epithelium of internal and external ear, nasal cavity, sinuses, mouth, anal canal	Muscles (all types)	Vagina (parts)
Central and peripheral nervous systems	Cardiovascular system (heart, arteries, veins, blood, bone marrow)	
Nasal cavity	Pleura	
Oral glands and tooth enamel	Lymphatic tissue and cells	
Pituitary gland	Spleen	
Mammary glands		

alterations in amniotic fluid volume. Figure 9–21 summarizes the major pathways of exchange.

After 23 to 25 weeks' gestation, the fetal kidneys are the major source of fluid that enters the amniotic sac. Abnormalities of fetal urine production can result in changes in amniotic fluid volume. For example, with obstruction of urine outflow, as in Potter syndrome, oligohydramnios develops. Conversely, Bartter syndrome results in fetal diuresis and hydramnios. The fetal lungs are also significant contributors to amniotic fluid. Fetal breathing movements are associated with the bidirectional flow of fluid through the trachea. This outflow of lung and tracheal fluid is used as the basis for amniotic fluid tests of fetal lung maturity.

The major mechanism by which amniotic fluid is removed in the last half of the pregnancy is fetal swallowing, which occurs mostly during periods of fetal breathing movements. In pregnancy, when the fetus does not swallow normal amounts of amniotic fluid (as in esophageal atresia and anencephalus), hydramnios will result. A potential route of amniotic fluid removal is by the transmembranous pathway, that is, the movement of fluid across the amniochorion and into the maternal circulation within the

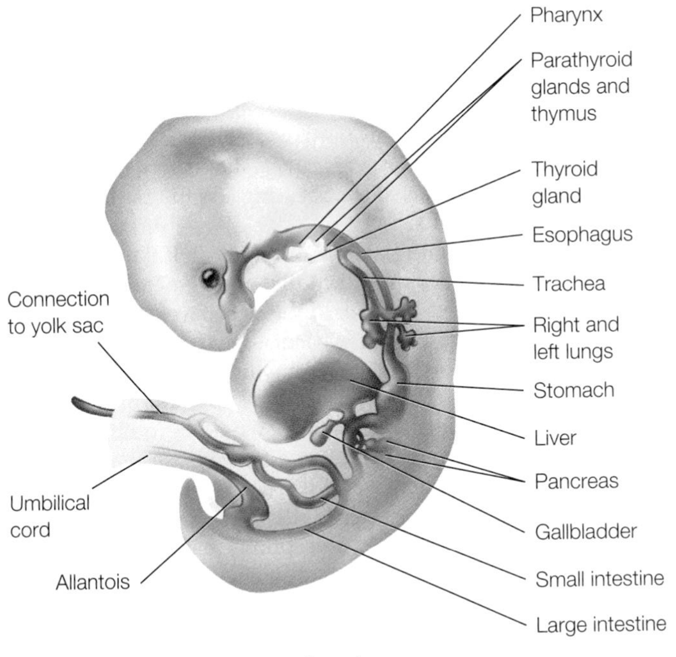

Figure 9–19 Endoderm differentiates to form the epithelial lining of the digestive and respiratory tracts and associated glands.

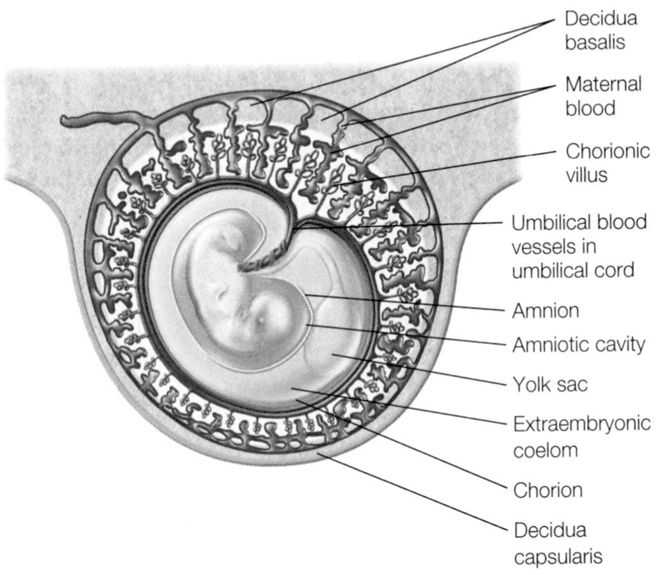

Figure 9–20 Early development of primary embryonic membranes. At 4½ weeks, the decidua capsularis (placental portion enclosing the embryo on the uterine surface) and decidua basalis (placental portion encompassing the elaborate chorionic villi and maternal endometrium) are well formed. The chorionic villi lie in blood-filled intervillous spaces within the endometrium. The amnion and yolk sac are well developed.

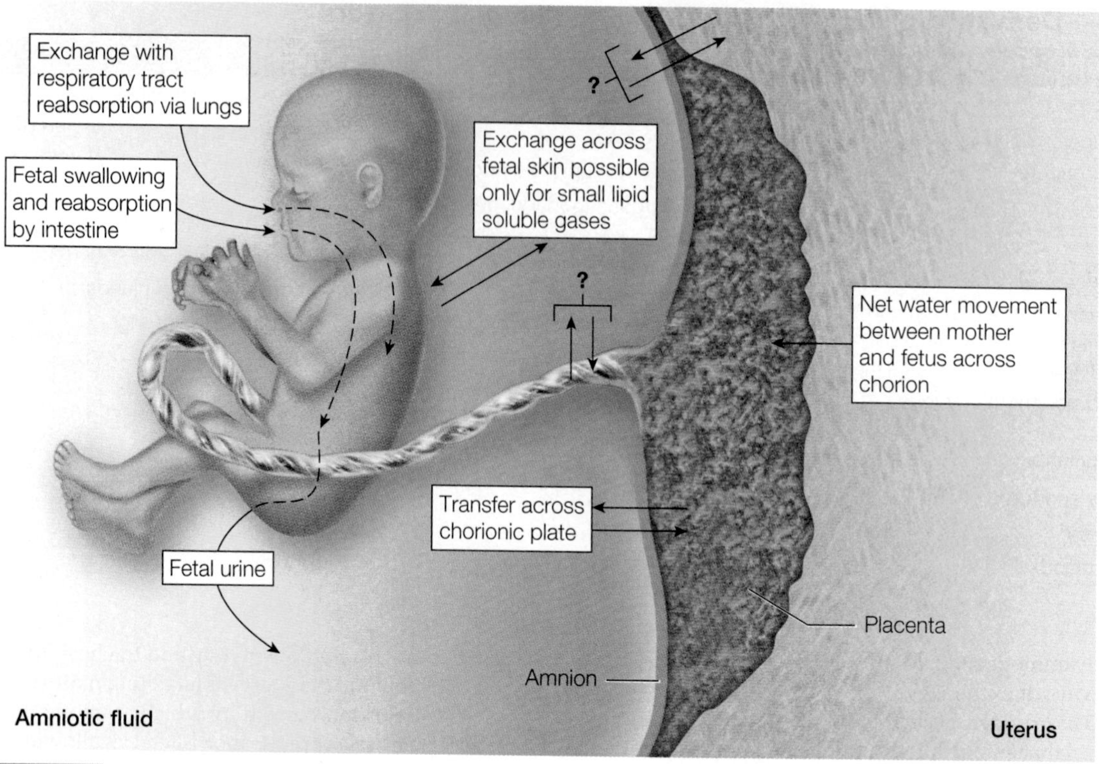

Figure 9–21 **Summary of the significant pathways of water and solute exchange between the amniotic fluid and fetus.**

uterine wall. Another major regulator of amniotic fluid volume and composition is the intramembranous pathway. This pathway causes amniotic water and/or solutes to be absorbed by the fetal blood that perfuses the fetal surface of the placenta.

Yolk Sac. In humans the yolk sac is small and functions only in early embryonic life. It develops as a second cavity in the blastocyst, about day 8 or 9 after conception, and forms primitive red blood cells during the first 6 weeks of development until the embryo's liver takes over the process. As the embryo develops, the yolk sac is incorporated in the umbilical cord, where it can be identified as a degenerate structure after birth.

Umbilical Cord. As the placenta is developing, the **umbilical cord** is also being formed from the mesoderm and is covered by the amnion (Blackburn, 2018). The *body stalk*, which attaches the embryo to the yolk sac, contains blood vessels that extend into the chorionic villi. The body stalk fuses with the embryonic portion of the placenta to provide a circulatory pathway from the chorionic villi to the embryo. As the body stalk elongates to become the umbilical cord, the vessels in the cord decrease to one large vein and two smaller arteries. About 1% of umbilical cords have only two vessels, an artery and a vein; this condition may be associated with congenital malformations, primarily of the renal, cardiovascular, and gastrointestinal systems (Sadler, 2015). A specialized connective tissue known as **Wharton jelly** surrounds the blood vessels in the umbilical cord (Moore et al., 2016). This tissue, plus the high blood volume pulsating through the vessels, prevents compression of the umbilical cord in utero. The umbilical cord has no sensory or motor innervation, so cutting the cord after birth is not painful. At term (37 to 42 weeks' gestation), the average cord is 2 cm (0.8 in.) across and about 55 cm (22 in.) long. The cord can attach itself to the placenta at various sites. Central insertion into the placenta is considered normal. (Chapter 23 discusses the various attachment sites.)

Umbilical cords appear twisted or spiraled. This is most likely caused by fetal movement. A true knot in the umbilical cord rarely occurs; if it does, the cord is usually long (Blackburn, 2018). More common are so-called "false knots" caused by the folding of cord vessels. A *nuchal cord* exists when the umbilical cord encircles the fetal neck.

Twins

Twinning normally occurs in approximately 33 in 1000 live births in the United States (Gabbe et al., 2017). The current rate of twinning is attributed to delayed childbearing and the use of artificial reproductive treatments.

Twins may be either fraternal or identical. If they are fraternal (nonidentical), they are dizygotic, which means they arise from two separate ova fertilized by two separate spermatozoa (Figure 9–22A). There are two placentas, two chorions, and two amnions; however, the placentas sometimes fuse and look as if they are one. Despite their birth relationship, fraternal twins are no more similar to each other than they would be to siblings born singly. They may be the same sex or different sexes.

Dizygotic twinning increases with maternal age up to about 35 years and then decreases abruptly. The chance of dizygotic twins increases with parity, in conceptions that occur in the first 3 months of a relationship, and with increased coital frequency. The chance of dizygotic twinning decreases during periods of malnutrition and during winter and spring for women living in the northern hemisphere. Studies indicate that dizygotic twins tend to occur in certain families, perhaps because of genetic factors that result in elevated serum gonadotropin levels, leading to double ovulation (Moore et al., 2016). Fraternal (dizygotic) twins have been reported to occur more often among Black than among

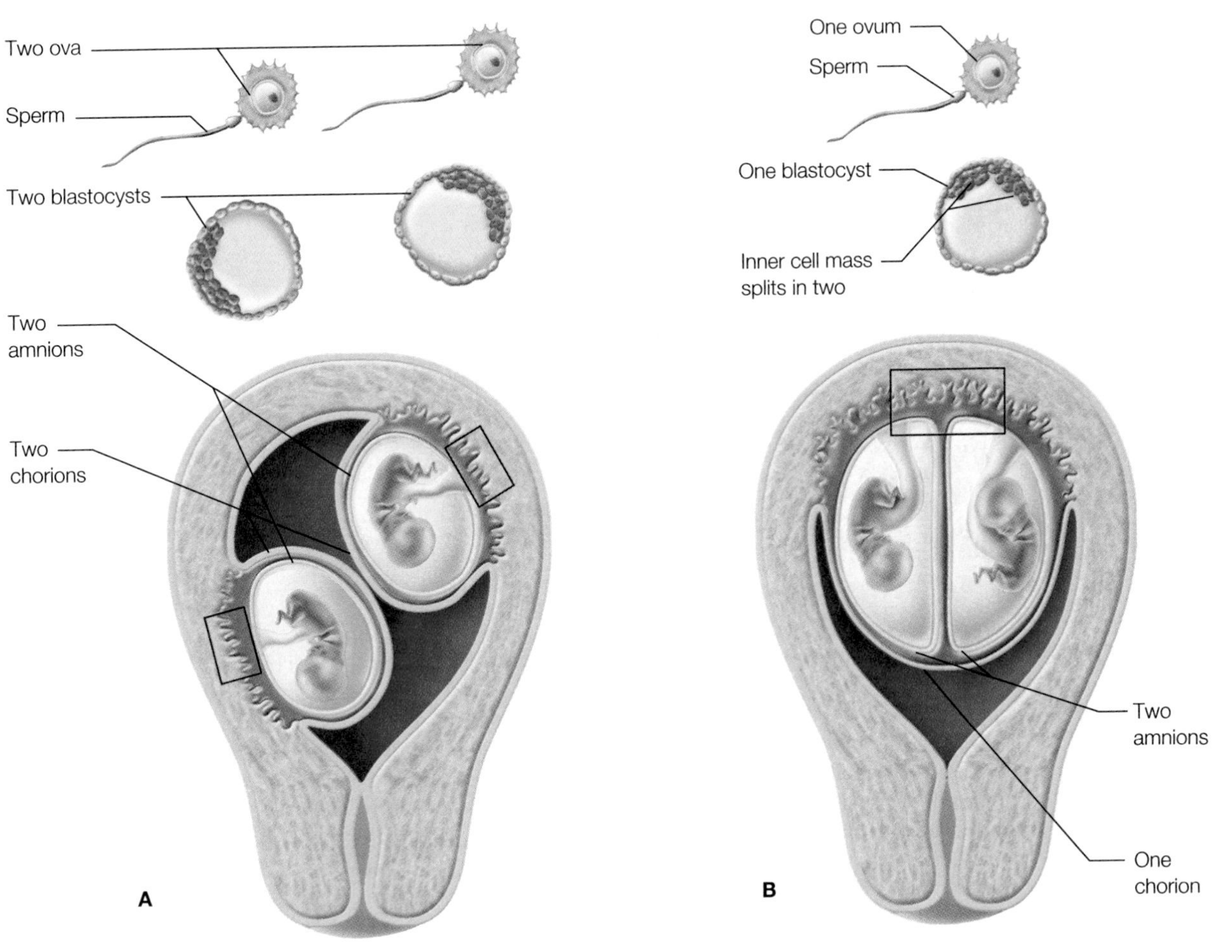

Figure 9–22 A. Formation of fraternal twins. (Note separate placentas.) B. Formation of identical twins.

White women and more often among White women than among women of Asian origin (Moore et al., 2016). Among all groups, as parity (having given birth to a viable baby) increases, so does the chance for multiple births.

Identical, or monozygotic, twins develop from a single fertilized ovum. They are of the same sex and have the same phenotype (appearance). Identical twins usually have a common placenta (see Figure 9–22B). Monozygosity is not affected by environment, race, physical characteristics, or fertility.

Monozygotic twins originate from division of the fertilized ovum at different stages of early development, after the zygote consists of thousands of cells. Complete separation of the cellular mass into two parts is necessary for twin formation. The number of amnions and chorions present depends on the timing of the division.

- If division occurs within 4 days of fertilization (before the inner cell mass and chorion are formed), two embryos, two amnions, and two chorions will develop. This dichorionic-diamniotic situation occurs about 25% of the time, and there may be two distinct placentas or a single fused placenta.
- If division occurs about 4 to 8 days after fertilization (when the inner cell mass is formed and the chorion cells have differentiated but those of the amnion have not), two embryos develop with separate amnion sacs. These sacs will eventually be covered by a common chorion; thus there will be a monochorionic-diamniotic placenta.
- If the amnion has already developed approximately 8 to 12 days after fertilization, division results in two embryos with a common amnion sac and a common chorion (monochorionic-monoamniotic placenta) (Cunningham et al., 2018). This type occurs rarely.

Monozygotic twinning is considered a random event and occurs in approximately 3 to 4 per 1000 live births (Gabbe et al., 2017). The survival rate of monozygotic twins as a group is 10% lower than that of dizygotic twins, and congenital anomalies are more prevalent. Both twins may have the same malformation.

Development and Functions of the Placenta

The **placenta** is the means of metabolic and nutrient exchange between the embryonic and maternal circulations. Placental development and circulation do not begin until the third week of embryonic development. The placenta develops at the site where the developing embryo attaches to the uterine wall. Expansion of the placenta continues until about 20 weeks, when it covers about half the inside of the uterus. After 20 weeks' gestation, the placenta becomes thicker but not wider. At 40 weeks' gestation, the placenta is about 15 to 20 cm (5.9 to 7.9 in.) in diameter and 2.5 to 3 cm (1 to 1.2 in.) in thickness. It weighs approximately 400 to 600 g (14 to 21 oz).

The placenta has two parts: The maternal portion and the fetal portion. The maternal portion consists of the decidua basalis and its circulation. Its surface is red and fleshlike (often called *Dirty Duncan*) (Figure 9–23). The fetal portion consists of the chorionic villi and their circulation. The fetal surface of the placenta

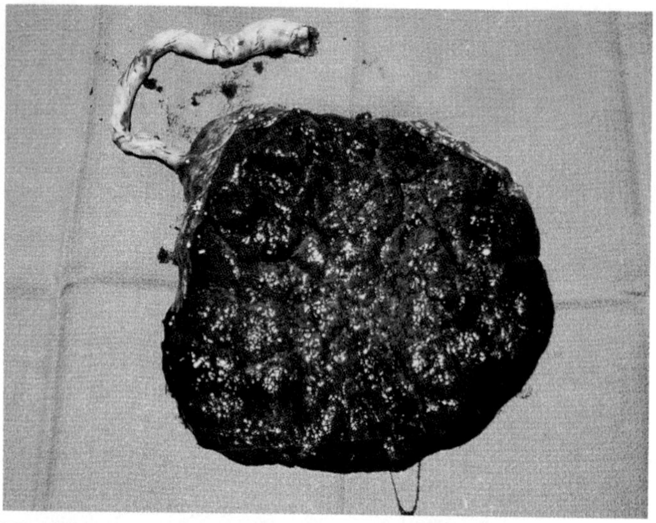

Figure 9–23 **Maternal side of placenta (Dirty Duncan).**

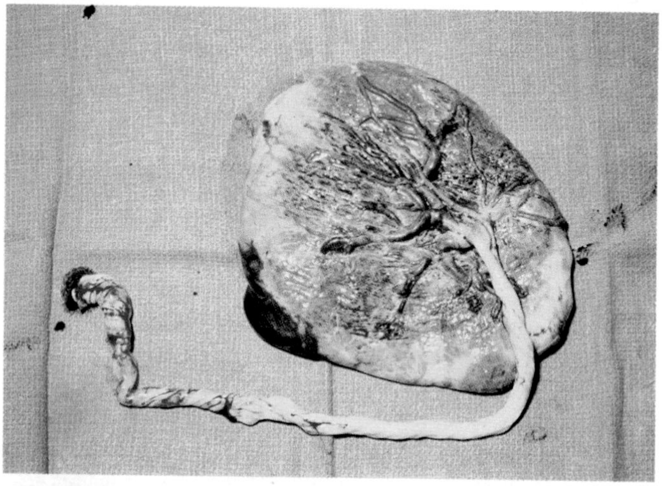

Figure 9–24 **Fetal side of placenta (Shiny Schultze).**

is covered by the amnion, which gives it a shiny, gray appearance (often called *Shiny Schultze*) (Figure 9–24).

Development of the placenta begins with the chorionic villi. The trophoblastic cells of the chorionic villi form spaces in the tissue of the decidua basalis. These spaces fill with maternal blood, and the chorionic villi grow into these spaces. As the chorionic villi differentiate, two trophoblastic layers appear: An outer layer called the *syncytium* (consisting of syncytiotrophoblasts) and an inner layer known as the *cytotrophoblast*. The cytotrophoblast thins out and disappears at about the fifth month, leaving only a single layer of syncytium covering the chorionic villi. The syncytium is in direct contact with the maternal blood in the intervillous spaces. It is the functional layer of the placenta and secretes the placental hormones of pregnancy.

A third, inner layer of connective mesoderm develops in the chorionic villi, forming *anchoring villi*. These anchoring villi eventually form the *septa* (partitions) of the placenta. These septa divide the mature placenta into 15 to 20 segments called **cotyledons** (subdivisions of the placenta made up of anchoring villi and decidual tissue). In each cotyledon, the *branching villi* form a highly complex vascular system that allows compartmentalization of the uteroplacental circulation. The exchange of gases and nutrients takes place across these vascular systems.

Exchange of substances across the placenta is minimal during the first 3 to 5 months of development because the villous membrane is initially too thick, which limits its permeability. As the villous membrane thins, the placental permeability increases until about the last month of pregnancy, when permeability begins to decrease as the placenta ages. In the fully developed placenta, fetal blood in the villi and maternal blood in the intervillous spaces are separated by three to four thin layers of tissue.

PLACENTAL CIRCULATION

After implantation of the blastocyst, the cells differentiate into fetal cells and trophoblastic cells. The proliferating trophoblast successfully invades the decidua basalis of the endometrium, first opening the uterine capillaries and later opening the larger uterine vessels. The chorionic villi are an outgrowth of the blastocystic tissue. As these villi continue to grow and divide, the fetal vessels begin to form. The intervillous spaces in the decidua basalis develop as the endometrial spiral arteries are opened.

The completion of the maternal–placental–fetal circulation occurs about 17 days after conception, when the embryonic heart begins functioning (Moore et al., 2016). By the end of the fourth week, embryonic blood is circulating between the embryo and the chorionic villi. In the intervillous spaces, maternal blood supplies oxygen and nutrients to the embryonic capillaries in the villi. The placenta has begun to function as a means of metabolic exchange between embryo and mother. Waste products and carbon dioxide diffuse into the maternal blood. By 14 weeks the placenta is a discrete organ. It has grown in thickness as a result of growth in the length and size of the chorionic villi and accompanying expansion of the intervillous space.

The cotyledons of the maternal surface contain branches of a single placental mainstream villus, allowing for some compartmentalization of the uteroplacental circulation. Each cotyledon is a vascular unit containing branching vessels that are distributed throughout a particular lobule and partially separated from other lobules by the cotyledon's thin septal partitions. As previously discussed, the cytotrophoblast thins out and disappears after the fifth month.

In the fully developed placenta's umbilical cord, fetal blood flows through the two umbilical arteries to the capillaries of the villi, and oxygen-enriched blood flows back through the umbilical vein to the fetus (Figure 9–25). Late in pregnancy, a soft blowing sound (*funic souffle*) can be heard over the area of the umbilical cord of the fetus. The sound is synchronous with the fetal heartbeat and the flow of fetal blood through the umbilical arteries.

Maternal blood, rich in oxygen and nutrients, moves from the arcuate artery to the radial artery to the uterine spiral arteries and then spurts into the intervillous spaces. These spurts are produced by the maternal blood pressure. The spurt of blood is directed toward the chorionic plate, and as the blood flow loses pressure, it becomes lateral (spreads out). Fresh blood continually enters and exerts pressure on the contents of the intervillous spaces, pushing blood toward the exits in the basal plate. Blood is then drained through the uterine and other pelvic veins. A *uterine souffle* is also heard in the latter months of pregnancy. This uterine souffle, which is timed precisely with the mother's pulse and heard just above the mother's **symphysis pubis** (the fibrocartilaginous joint between the pelvic bones), is caused by the augmented blood flow entering the dilated uterine arteries.

Braxton Hicks contractions (see Chapter 11) are intermittent, painless uterine contractions that may occur every 10 to 20 minutes and occur more frequently near the end of pregnancy.

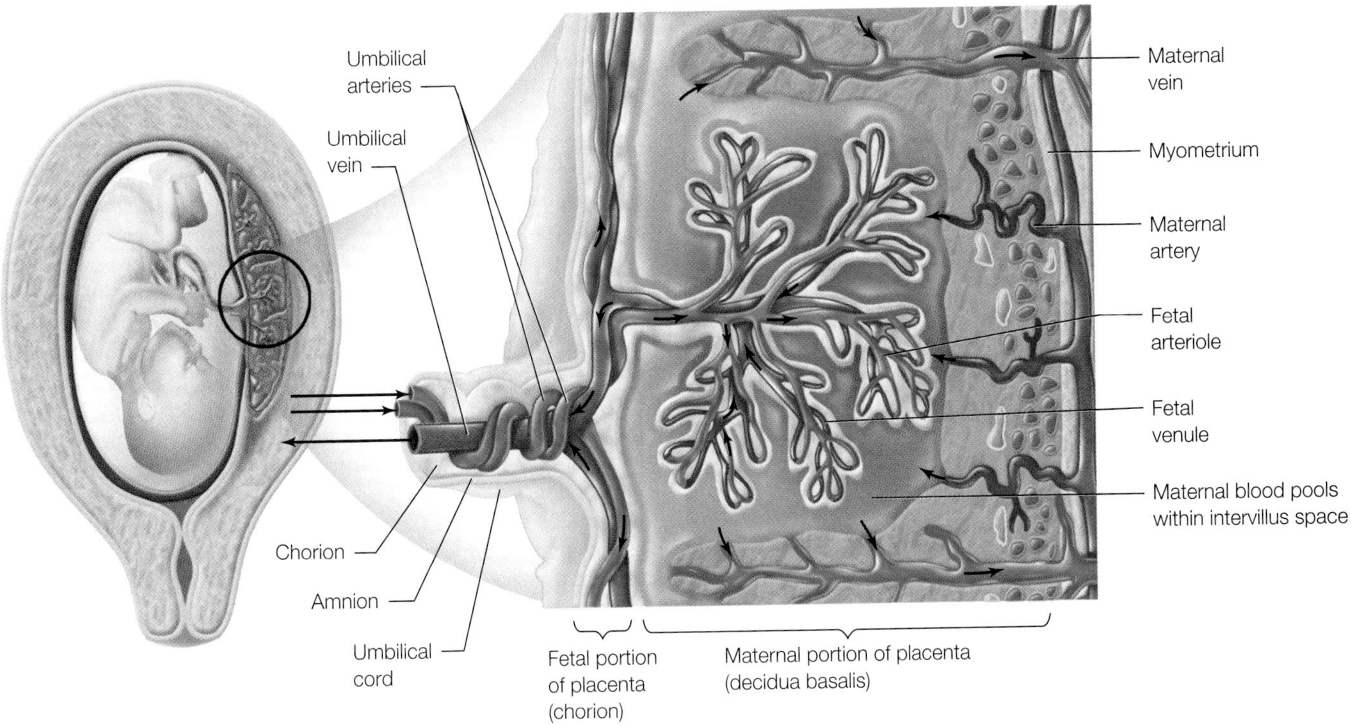

Figure 9–25 **Vascular arrangement of the placenta. Arrows indicate the direction of blood flow. Maternal blood flows through the uterine arteries to the intervillous spaces of the placenta and returns through the uterine veins to maternal circulation. Fetal blood flows through the umbilical arteries into the villous capillaries of the placenta and returns through the umbilical vein to the fetal circulation.**

These contractions are believed to facilitate placental circulation by enhancing the movement of blood from the center of the cotyledon through the intervillous space. Placental blood flow is thought to be enhanced when the woman is lying on her side because the venous return from the lower extremities is not compromised.

PLACENTAL FUNCTIONS

Placental exchange functions occur only in those fetal vessels that are in intimate contact with the covering syncytial membrane. The syncytium villi have brush borders containing many microvilli, which greatly increase the exchange rate between maternal and fetal circulation (Sadler, 2015).

The placental functions, many of which begin soon after implantation, include fetal respiration, nutrition, and excretion. To carry out these functions, the placenta is involved in metabolic and transfer activities. In addition, it has endocrine functions and special immunologic properties (see discussion later in this section).

Metabolic Activities. The placenta performs several essential metabolic activities:

- Produces glycogen, cholesterol, and fatty acids continuously for fetal use and hormone production
- Produces numerous enzymes required for fetoplacental transfer such as sulfatase, which enhances excretion of fetal estrogen precursors, and insulinase, which increases the barrier to insulin
- Breaks down certain substances, such as epinephrine and histamine
- Stores glycogen and iron.

Transport Functions. The placental membranes actively control the transfer of a wide range of substances by a variety of transport mechanisms.

- *Simple diffusion* moves substances from an area of higher concentration to an area of lower concentration. Substances that move across the placenta by simple diffusion include water, oxygen, carbon dioxide, electrolytes (sodium and chloride), anesthetic gases, and drugs. Insulin and steroid hormones originating from the adrenal glands and thyroid hormones also cross the placenta but at a very slow rate. The rate of oxygen transfer across the placental membrane is greater than that allowed by simple diffusion, indicating that oxygen is also transferred by some type of facilitated diffusion. Unfortunately, many substances of abuse, such as cocaine and heroin, cross the placenta via simple diffusion.
- *Facilitated transport* involves a carrier system to move molecules from an area of greater concentration to an area of lower concentration. Molecules such as glucose, galactose, and some oxygen are transported by this method. The glucose level in the fetal blood is ordinarily 20 to 30% lower than the glucose level in the maternal blood because glucose is being metabolized rapidly. This in turn causes rapid transport of additional glucose (facilitated by insulin) from the maternal blood into the fetal blood.
- *Active transport* can work against a concentration gradient, allowing molecules to move from areas of lower concentration to areas of higher concentration. Amino acids, calcium, iron, iodine, water-soluble vitamins, and glucose are transferred across the placenta this way. The measured amino acid content of fetal blood is greater than that of maternal blood, and calcium and inorganic phosphate occur in greater

concentration in fetal blood than in maternal blood (Blackburn, 2018; Mattson & Smith, 2016).

Other modes of transport also exist. *Pinocytosis* is important for transferring large molecules, such as albumin and gamma globulin. Materials are engulfed by amoeba-like cells forming plasma droplets. *Hydrostatic* and *osmotic pressures* allow the bulk flow of water and some solutes. Fetal red blood cells pass into the maternal circulation through breaks in the placental membrane, particularly during labor and birth. Certain cells, such as maternal leukocytes, and microorganisms, such as viruses (e.g., HIV, which causes AIDS) and the bacterium *Treponema pallidum*, which causes syphilis, can also cross the placental membrane under their own power (Moore et al., 2016). Some bacteria and protozoa infect the placenta by causing lesions and then entering the fetal blood system.

Reduction of the placental surface area, as with *abruptio placentae* (partial or complete premature separation of a normally implanted placenta), will lessen the area that is functional for exchange. Placental diffusion distance also affects exchange. In conditions such as diabetes and placental infection, edema of the villi increases the diffusion distance, thus increasing the distance the substance has to be transferred.

Blood flow alteration changes the transfer rate of substances, the ratio of blood on each side of the placenta, and the binding and dissociation abilities of carrier molecules in the blood. Decreased intervillous space blood flow is seen during labor and with certain maternal disease conditions such as hypertension. Mild fetal hypoxia increases the umbilical blood flow, but severe hypoxia results in decreased blood flow.

As the maternal blood picks up fetal waste products and carbon dioxide, it drains back into the maternal circulation through the veins in the basal plate. Fetal blood is hypoxic by comparison; therefore, it attracts oxygen from the mother's blood. Affinity for oxygen also increases as the fetal blood gives up its carbon dioxide, which decreases its acidity.

Endocrine Functions. The placenta produces hormones that are vital to survival of the fetus. These include human chorionic gonadotropin (hCG), human placental lactogen (hPL), relaxin, inhibin, and two steroid hormones, estrogen and progesterone.

The hormone hCG is similar to luteinizing hormone (LH) and prevents the normal involution of the corpus luteum at the end of the menstrual cycle. If the corpus luteum stops functioning before the 11th week of pregnancy, spontaneous abortion occurs. The hCG also causes the corpus luteum to secrete increased amounts of estrogen and progesterone.

After the 11th week, the placenta produces enough progesterone and estrogen to maintain pregnancy. In the male fetus, hCG also exerts an interstitial cell–stimulating effect on the testes, resulting in the production of testosterone. This small secretion of testosterone during embryonic development causes male sex organs to grow. The hormone hCG may play a role in the trophoblast's immunologic capabilities (ability to exempt the placenta and embryo from rejection by the mother's system). This hormone is used as a basis for pregnancy tests (for discussion of pregnancy tests, see Chapter 11).

The hormone hCG is present in maternal blood serum 8 to 10 days after fertilization, just as soon as implantation has occurred, and is detectable in maternal urine at the time of the missed menses. Chorionic gonadotropin reaches its maximum level at 50 to 70 days' gestation and then begins to decrease as placental hormone production increases.

Progesterone is a hormone essential for pregnancy. It increases the secretions of the fallopian tubes and uterus to provide appropriate nutritive matter for the developing morula and blastocyst. It also appears to aid in ovum transport through the fallopian tube. Progesterone causes decidual cells to develop in the uterine endometrium, and it must be present in high levels for implantation to occur. Progesterone also decreases the contractility of the uterus, thus preventing uterine contractions from causing spontaneous abortion.

Before hCG stimulation, the production of progesterone by the corpus luteum reaches a peak about 7 to 10 days after ovulation. Implantation occurs at about the same time as this peak. At 16 days after ovulation, the production of progesterone reaches a level between 25 and 50 mg per day and continues to rise slowly in subsequent weeks. After 11 weeks, the placenta (specifically, the syncytiotrophoblast) takes over the production of progesterone and secretes it in tremendous quantities, reaching levels of more than 250 mg per day late in pregnancy.

By 7 weeks, the placenta produces more than 50% of the estrogens in the maternal circulation. *Estrogens* serve mainly a proliferative function, causing enlargement of the uterus, breasts, and breast glandular tissue. Estrogens also have a significant role in increasing vascularity and vasodilation, particularly in the villous capillaries, near the end of pregnancy. Placental estrogens increase markedly toward the end of pregnancy to as much as 30 times the daily production in the middle of a normal monthly menstrual cycle. The primary estrogen secreted by the placenta (estriol) is different from that secreted by the ovaries (estradiol). The placenta secretes mainly estriol, whereas the ovaries secrete primarily estradiol. The placenta cannot synthesize estriol by itself. Essential precursors such as dehydroepiandrosterone sulfate (DHEA-S) are provided by the fetal adrenal glands, processed by the fetal liver, and transported to the placenta for the final conversion to estrone, estradiol, and estriol (Blackburn, 2018).

The hormone hPL (human placental lactogen; sometimes referred to as human chorionic somatomammotropin, or hCS) is similar to human pituitary growth hormone; hPL stimulates certain changes in the mother's metabolic processes. These changes ensure that more protein, glucose, and minerals are available for the fetus. Secretion of hPL can be detected by about 4 weeks.

Relaxin acts to quiet the myometrium, facilitates the decidual reaction, remodels collagen, softens the cervix, and softens ligaments and cartilage in the skeletal system (Blackburn, 2018). Inhibin, another glycoprotein, is produced by the trophoblast. In combination with the sex steroids, inhibin decreases the secretion of follicle-stimulating hormone from the pituitary gland, thereby stopping ovulation during the pregnancy.

Immunologic Properties. The placenta and embryo are transplants of living tissue within the same species and, therefore, are considered *homografts*. Unlike other homografts, the placenta and the embryo appear exempt from immunologic reaction by the host. Most recent data suggest that the placental hormones (progesterone and hCG) suppress cellular immunity during pregnancy. One theory posits that chorionic villi syncytiotrophoblastic tissue is immunologically inert. The chorionic villi may lack major histocompatibility (MHC) antigens and thus do not evoke rejection responses. It does, however, protect against antibody formation. Extravillous trophoblast (EVT) cells, which invade the uterine decidas, have human leukocyte antigen G (HLA-G), which is not readily recognized by sensitized T lymphocytes and natural killer cells (Cunningham et al., 2018).

Development of the Fetal Circulatory System

The circulatory system of the fetus has several unique features that, by maintaining the blood flow to the placenta, provide the fetus with oxygen and nutrients while removing carbon dioxide and other waste products.

Most of the blood supply bypasses the fetal lungs because they do not carry out respiratory gas exchange. The placenta assumes the function of the fetal lungs by supplying oxygen and allowing the fetus to excrete carbon dioxide into the maternal bloodstream. Figure 9–26 shows the fetal circulatory system. The blood from the placenta flows through the umbilical vein, which enters the abdominal wall of the fetus at the site that, after birth, is the umbilicus (belly button). As umbilical venous blood approaches the liver, a small portion of the blood enters the liver sinusoids, mixes with blood from the portal circulation, and then enters the inferior vena cava via hepatic veins. Most of the umbilical vein's blood flows through the **ductus venosus** directly into the inferior vena cava, bypassing the liver. This blood then enters the right atrium, passes through the **foramen ovale** into the left atrium, and pours into the left ventricle, which pumps it into the aorta. Some blood returning from the head and upper extremities by way of the superior vena cava is emptied into the right atrium and passes through the tricuspid valve into the right ventricle. This blood is pumped into the pulmonary artery, and a small amount passes to the lungs and provides nourishment only. The larger portion of blood passes from the pulmonary artery

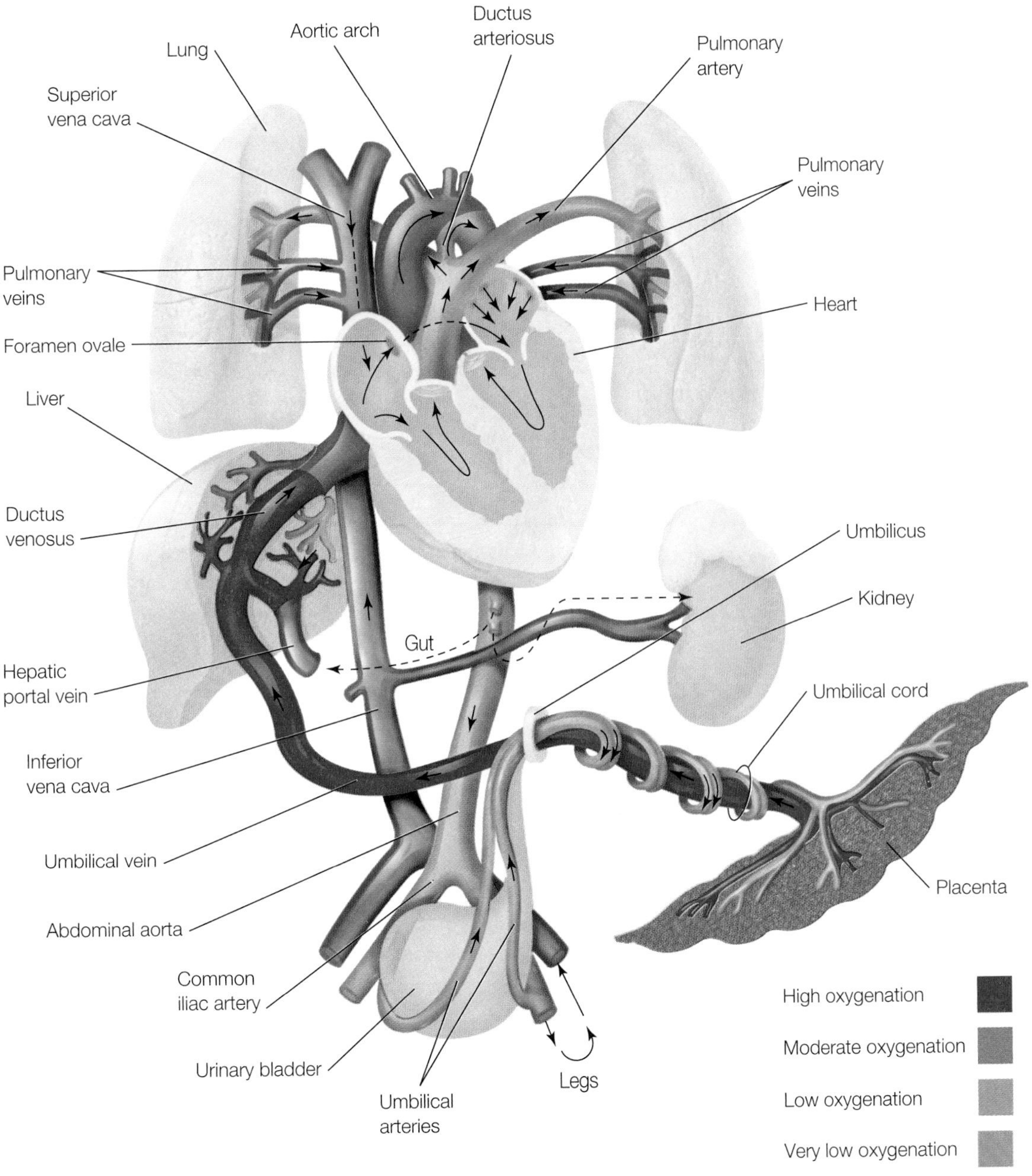

Figure 9–26 **Fetal circulation. Blood leaves the placenta and enters the fetus through the umbilical vein. After circulating through the fetus, the blood returns to the placenta through the umbilical arteries. The ductus venosus, the foramen ovale, and the ductus arteriosus allow the blood to bypass the fetal liver and lungs.**

through the **ductus arteriosus** into the descending aorta, bypassing the lungs. Finally, blood returns to the placenta through the two umbilical arteries, and the process is repeated.

The fetus receives oxygen via diffusion from the maternal circulation because of the gradient difference of Po_2 of 50 mmHg in maternal blood in the placenta to a Po_2 of 30 mmHg in the fetus. At term, the fetus receives oxygen from the mother's circulation at a rate of 20 to 30 mL/min (Sadler, 2015). Fetal hemoglobin facilitates obtaining oxygen from the maternal circulation because it carries as much as 20 to 30% more oxygen than adult hemoglobin.

Fetal circulation delivers the highest available oxygen concentration to the head, neck, brain, and heart (coronary circulation) and a lesser amount of oxygenated blood to the abdominal organs and the lower body. This circulatory pattern leads to cephalocaudal (head-to-tail) development in the fetus.

Embryonic and Fetal Development

Pregnancy is calculated to last an *average* of 10 lunar months: 40 weeks, or 280 days. This period of 280 days is calculated from the beginning of the last normal menstrual period to the time of birth. Many obstetric units in the United States and Australia use a combination of menstrual dates and ultrasonographic dates to perform this calculation. Estimated date of birth (EDB), sometimes referred to as the *estimated date of delivery (EDD)*, is usually calculated by this method. Most fetuses are born within 10 to 14 days of the calculated date of birth. The fertilization age (or postconception age) of the fetus is calculated to be *about* 2 weeks less, 266 days (38 weeks) or 9½ calendar months. The latter measurement is more accurate because it measures time from the fertilization of the ovum, or conception. See Chapter 12 for a detailed discussion of due date determination, including Nägele's rule.

The basic events of organ development in the embryo and fetus are outlined in Table 9–2. The time periods used are **postconception age periods** (period of time calculated from the time of fertilization of the ovum). During the period from fertilization to the end of the embryonic period (8 weeks), age is often expressed in days but can be given in weeks. During the fetal period (9th week until birth), age is given in weeks (Moore et al., 2016). The National Institute for Health and Clinical Excellence (2017) guidelines state that the crown–rump length (CRL) should be used to determine gestational age; if the CRL is greater than 84 mm, the head circumference (HC) should be used instead. After about 12 weeks, the crown–heel length (CHL) may also be measured.

In review, human development follows three stages. The preembryonic stage just discussed consists of the first 14 days

TABLE 9–2 Timeline of Organ System Development in the Embryo and Fetus

AGE: 2–3 WEEKS	
Length: 2 mm (0.08 in.) CRL **Nervous system:** Groove forms along middle back as cells thicken; neural tube forms from closure of neural groove **Cardiovascular system:** Beginning of blood circulation; tubular heart begins to form during third week **Gastrointestinal system:** Liver begins to function	**Genitourinary system:** Formation of kidneys begins **Respiratory system:** Nasal pits form **Endocrine system:** Thyroid tissue appears **Eyes:** Optic cup and lens pit form; pigment in eyes **Ears:** Auditory pit is now enclosed structure
AGE: 4 WEEKS	
Length: 4–6 mm (0.16–0.24 in.) CRL **Weight:** 0.4 g (0.014 oz) **Nervous system:** Anterior portion of neural tube closes to form brain; closure of posterior end forms spinal cord **Musculoskeletal system:** Noticeable limb buds	**Cardiovascular system:** Tubular heartbeats at 28 days, and primitive red blood cells circulate through fetus and chorionic villi **Gastrointestinal system:** Mouth: formation of oral cavity; primitive jaws present; esophagotracheal septum begins division of esophagus and trachea **Digestive tract:** Stomach forms; esophagus and intestine become tubular; ducts of pancreas and liver forming
AGE: 5 WEEKS	
Length: 8 mm (0.32 in.) CRL **Weight:** Only 0.5% of total body weight is fat (to 20 weeks) **Nervous system:** Brain has differentiated and cranial nerves are present	**Musculoskeletal system:** Developing muscles have innervation **Cardiovascular system:** Atrial division occurs
AGE: 6 WEEKS	
Length: 12 mm (0.47 in.) CRL **Musculoskeletal system:** Bone rudiments present; primitive skeletal shape forms; muscle mass begins to develop; ossification of skull and jaws begins **Cardiovascular system:** Chambers present in heart; groups of blood cells can be identified	**Gastrointestinal system:** Oral and nasal cavities and upper lip form; liver begins to form red blood cells **Respiratory system:** Trachea, bronchi, and lung buds present **Ears:** Formation of external, middle, and inner ear continues **Sexual development:** Embryonic sex glands appear
AGE: 7 WEEKS	
Length: 18 mm (0.71 in.) CRL **Cardiovascular system:** Fetal heartbeats can be detected **Gastrointestinal system:** Mouth: Tongue separates; palate folds. Digestive tract: Stomach attains final form **Genitourinary system:** Separation of bladder and urethra from rectum	**Respiratory system:** Diaphragm separates abdominal and thoracic cavities **Eyes:** Optic nerve forms; eyelids appear, thickening of lens **Sexual development:** Differentiation of sex glands into ovaries and testes begins

AGE: 8 WEEKS

Length: 2.5–3.0 cm (0.98–1.2 in.) CRL

Weight: 2 g (0.07 oz.)

Musculoskeletal system: Digits form; further differentiation of cells in primitive skeleton; cartilaginous bones show first signs of ossification; development of muscles in trunk, limbs, and head; some movement of fetus now possible

Cardiovascular system: Development of heart essentially complete; fetal circulation follows two circuits—four extraembryonic and two intraembryonic; heartbeat can be heard with Doppler at 8–12 weeks

Gastrointestinal system: Mouth: Completion of lip fusion. Digestive tract: Rotation in midgut; anal membrane perforates.

Ears: External, middle, and inner ear assume final forms

Sexual development: Male and female external genitals appear similar until end of ninth week

AGE: 10 WEEKS

Length: 5–6 cm (1.97–2.36 in.) CRL

Weight: 14 g (0.49 oz.)

Nervous system: Neurons appear at caudal end of spinal cord; basic divisions of brain present

Musculoskeletal system: Fingers and toes begin nail growth

Gastrointestinal system: Mouth: Separation of lips from jaw; fusion of palate folds

Digestive tract: Developing intestines enclosed in abdomen

Genitourinary system: Bladder sac forms

Endocrine system: Islets of Langerhans differentiate

Eyes: Eyelids fuse closed; development of lacrimal duct

Sexual development: Males: Production of testosterone and physical characteristics between 8 and 12 weeks

AGE: 12 WEEKS

Length: 8 cm (3.15 in.) CRL; 11.5 cm (4.53 in.) CHL

Weight: 45 g (1.59 oz)

Musculoskeletal system: Clear outlining of miniature bones (12–20 weeks); process of ossification establishes throughout fetal body; appearance of involuntary muscles in viscera

Gastrointestinal system: Mouth: Completion of palate

Digestive tract: Appearance of muscles in gut; bile secretion begins; liver is major producer of red blood cells

Respiratory system: Lungs acquire definitive shape

Skin: Pink and delicate

Endocrine system: Hormonal secretion from thyroid; insulin present in pancreas

Immunologic system: Appearance of lymphoid tissue in fetal thymus gland

AGE: 16 WEEKS

Length: 13.5 cm (5.3 in.) CRL; 15 cm (5.9 in.) CHL

Weight: 200 g (7 oz)

Musculoskeletal system: Teeth begin to form hard tissue that will become central incisors

Gastrointestinal system: Mouth: Differentiation of hard and soft palate

Digestive tract: Development of gastric and intestinal glands; intestines begin to collect meconium

Genitourinary system: Kidneys assume typical shape and organization

Skin: Appearance of scalp hair; lanugo present on body; transparent skin with visible blood vessels; sweat glands develop

Eyes, ears, and nose: Formed

Sexual development: Sex determination possible

AGE: 18 WEEKS

Musculoskeletal system: Teeth begin to form hard tissue (enamel and dentine) that will become lateral incisors

Cardiovascular system: Fetal heart tones audible with fetoscope at 16–20 weeks

AGE: 20 WEEKS

Length: 19 cm (7.5 in.) CRL; 25 cm (9.84 in.) CHL

Weight: 435 g (15.34 oz) (6% of total body weight is fat)

Nervous system: Myelination of spinal cord begins

Musculoskeletal system: Teeth begin to form hard tissue that will become canines and first molars; lower limbs are of final relative proportions

Gastrointestinal system: Fetus actively sucks and swallows amniotic fluid; peristaltic movements begin

Skin: Lanugo covers entire body; brown fat begins to form; vernix caseosa begins to form

Immunologic system: Detectable levels of fetal antibodies (IgG type)

Blood formation: Iron is stored and bone marrow is increasingly important

AGE: 24 WEEKS

Length: 23 cm (9.06 in.) CRL; 28 cm (11.02 in.) CHL

Weight: 780 g (1.72 lb)

Nervous system: Brain looks like mature brain

Musculoskeletal system: Teeth are beginning to form hard tissue that will become the second molars

Respiratory system: Respiratory movements may occur (24–40 weeks); nostrils reopen; alveoli appear in lungs and begin production of surfactant; gas exchange possible

Skin: Reddish and wrinkled; vernix caseosa present

Immunologic system: IgG levels reach maternal levels

(continued)

TABLE 9–2 Timeline of Organ System Development in the Embryo and Fetus *(continued)*

AGE: 28 WEEKS	
Length: 27 cm (10.63 in.) CRL; 35 cm (13.8 in.) CHL **Weight:** 1200–1250 g (2.65–2.76 lb) **Nervous system:** Begins regulation of some body functions **Skin:** Adipose tissue accumulates rapidly; nails appear; eyebrows and eyelashes present	**Eyes:** Eyelids open (26–29 weeks) **Sexual development:** Males: Testes descend into inguinal canal and upper scrotum
AGE: 32 WEEKS	
Length: 31 cm (12.2 in.) CRL; 38–43 cm (15.0–17.0 in.) CHL **Weight:** 2000 g (4.4 lb) **Nervous system:** More reflexes present	
AGE: 36 WEEKS	
Length: 35 cm (13.78 in.) CRL; 42–48 cm (16.5–18.9 in.) CHL **Weight:** 2500–2750 g (5.5–6.1 lb) **Musculoskeletal system:** Distal femoral ossification centers present **Skin:** Pale; body rounds, lanugo disappears, hair fuzzy or woolly; few sole creases; sebaceous glands active and helping to produce vernix caseosa (36–40 weeks)	**Ears:** Earlobes soft with little cartilage **Sexual development:** Males: Scrotum small and few rugae present; descent of testes into upper scrotum to stay (36–40 weeks) Females: Labia majora and minora equally prominent
AGE: 38–40 WEEKS	
Length: 40 cm (15.75) CRL; 48–52 cm (18.9–20.5 in.) CHL **Weight:** 3000–3600 g+ (6.6–7.9 lb+) (16% of total body weight is fat) **Resspiratory system:** At 38 weeks, lecithin–sphingomyelin (L/S) ratio approaches 2:1 (indicates decreased risk of respiratory distress from inadequate surfactant production if born now)	**Skin:** Smooth and pink; vernix present in skinfolds; moderate to profuse silky hair; lanugo on shoulders and upper back; nails extend over tips or digits; creases cover sole **Ears:** Earlobes firmer because of increased cartilage **Sexual development:** Males: Rugous scrotum Females: Labia majora well developed and minora small or completely covered

Note: Age refers to postfertilization or postconception age. Measurements are an average.

SOURCES: Data from Moore et al., 2016; Sadler, 2015.

of development after the ovum is fertilized; the embryonic stage covers the period from day 15 until approximately the end of the eighth week postconception; and the fetal stage extends from the end of the eighth week until birth.

EMBRYONIC STAGE

The stage of the **embryo** starts on day 15 (beginning of the third week after conception) and continues until approximately 8 weeks or until the embryo reaches a CRL of 3 cm (1.2 in.). This length is usually reached about 56 days after fertilization (the end of the eighth gestational week). During the embryonic stage, tissue differentiates into essential organs, and the main external features develop (Figure 9–27). The embryo is most vulnerable to *teratogens* during this period. These are discussed in more depth later in the chapter.

Three Weeks. In the third week, the embryonic disc becomes elongated and pear-shaped, with a broad cephalic end and a narrow caudal end. The ectoderm has formed a long cylindrical tube called the notochord for brain and spinal cord development. The gastrointestinal tract, created from the endoderm, appears as another tubelike structure communicating with the yolk sac. The most advanced organ is the heart. At 3 weeks, a single tubular heart forms just outside the body cavity of the embryo.

Four to Five Weeks. During days 21 to 32, *somites*, a series of mesodermal blocks, form on either side of the embryo's midline. The vertebrae that form the spinal column will develop from these somites. Before 28 days, arm and leg buds are not visible, but the tail bud is present. The pharyngeal arches—which will form the lower jaw (mandibular arch), hyoid bone, and cartilage of the larynx—develop at this time. The pharyngeal pouches appear now; these pouches will form the Eustachian tube and cavity of the middle ear, the tonsils, and the parathyroid and thymus glands. The primordia of the ear and eye are also present (Figure 9–28). By the end of 28 days, the tubular heart is beating at a regular rhythm and pushing its own primitive blood cells through the main blood vessels.

During the fifth week, the optic cups and lens vesicles of the eye form and the nasal pits develop. Partitioning in the heart occurs with the dividing of the atrium. The embryo has a marked C-shaped body, accentuated by the rudimentary tail and the large head folded over a protuberant trunk (Figure 9–29). By day 35, the arm and leg buds are well developed with paddle-shaped hand and foot plates. The heart, circulatory system, and brain show the most advanced development. The brain has differentiated into five areas, and 10 pairs of cranial nerves are recognizable.

Six Weeks. At 6 weeks, the head structures are more highly developed, and the trunk is straighter than in earlier stages. The upper and lower jaws are recognizable, and the external nares are well formed. The trachea has developed, and its caudal end is bifurcated for beginning lung formation. The upper lip has formed, and the palate is developing. The ears are developing

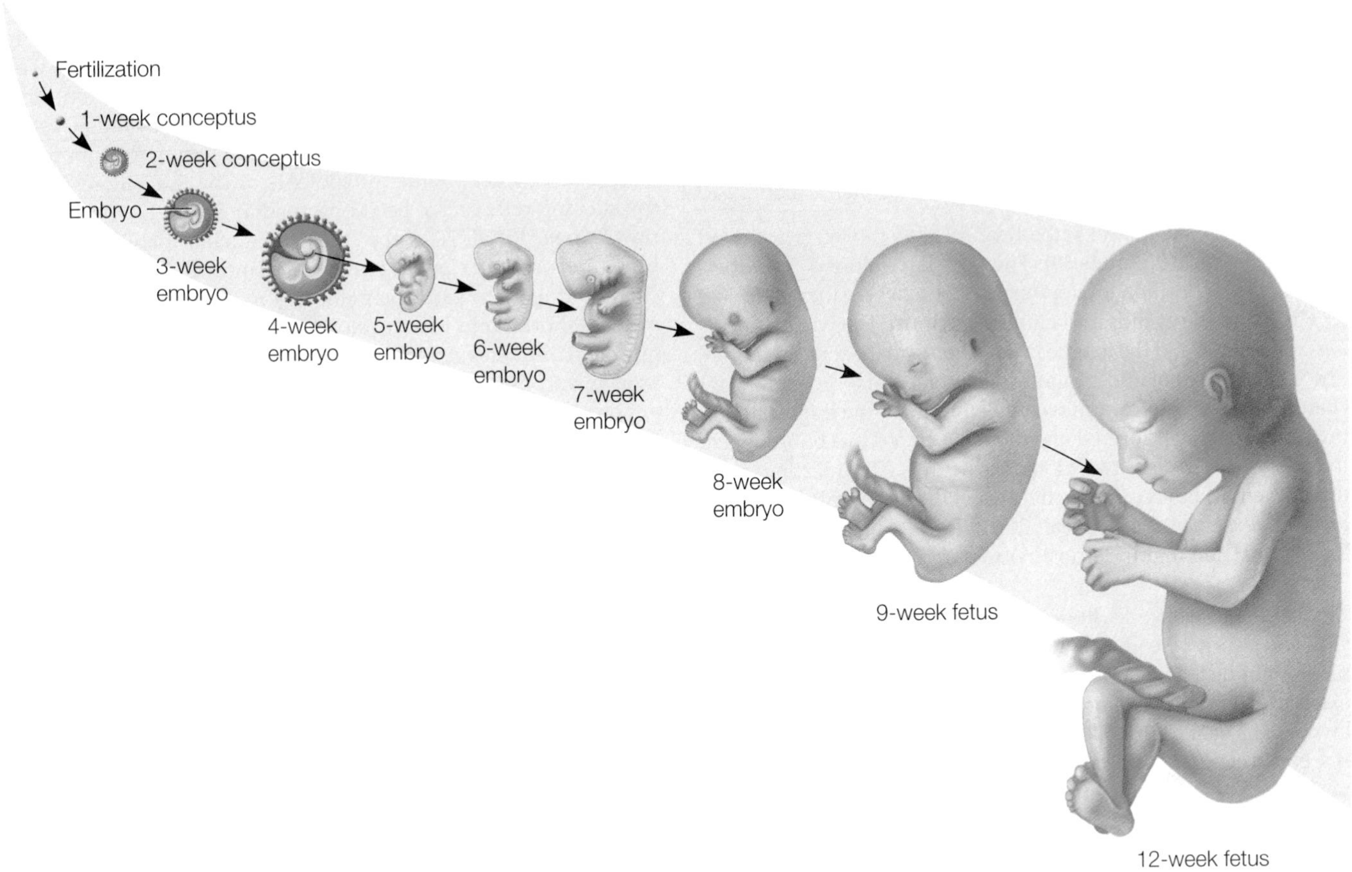

Figure 9–27 The human conceptus from fertilization to the early fetal stage. The embryonic stage begins in the third week after fertilization; the fetal stage begins in the ninth week.

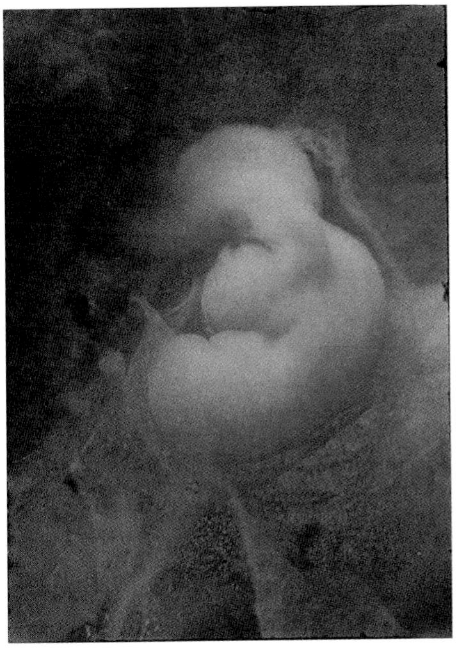

Figure 9–28 The embryo at 4 weeks. Pharyngeal arches, pharyngeal pouches, and primordia of the ear and eye are present.

SOURCE: Petit Format/Science Source.

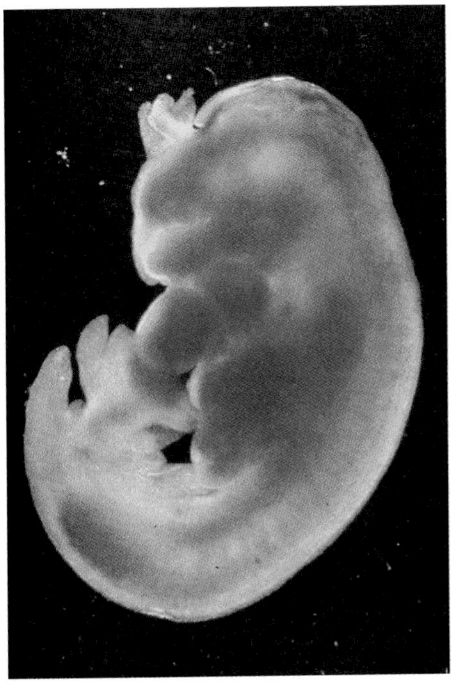

Figure 9–29 The embryo at 5 weeks. The embryo has a marked C-shaped body and a rudimentary tail.

SOURCE: Professor Pietro M. Motta/Science Source.

rapidly. The arms have begun to extend ventrally across the chest, and both arms and legs have digits, although they may still be webbed. There is a slight elbow bend in the arm, which is more advanced in development than the leg. Beginning at this stage the prominent tail will recede. The heart now has most of its definitive characteristics, and fetal circulation begins to be established. The liver begins to produce blood cells.

Seven Weeks. At 7 weeks, the head of the embryo is rounded and nearly erect (Figure 9–30). The eyes have shifted from their original lateral position to a forward location, where they are closer together, and the eyelids are beginning to form. The palate is nearing completion, and the tongue is developing in the formed mouth. The gastrointestinal and genitourinary tracts undergo significant changes during the seventh week. Before this time the rectal and urogenital passages formed one tube that ended in a blind pouch; they now separate into two tubular structures. The intestines enter the extraembryonic coelom in the area of the umbilical cord (called *umbilical herniation*) (Moore et al., 2016). The beginnings of all essential external and internal structures are present.

Eight Weeks. At 8 weeks, the embryo is approximately 3 cm (1.2 in.) CRL and clearly resembles a human being (Figure 9–31). Facial features continue to develop. The eyelids begin to fuse. Auricles of the external ears begin to assume their final shape, but they are still set low (Moore et al., 2016). External genitals appear, but the embryo's sex is not clearly identifiable. The rectal passage opens with the perforation of the anal membrane. The circulatory system through the umbilical cord is well established. Long bones are beginning to form, and the large muscles are now capable of contracting.

FETAL STAGE

By the end of the eighth week, the embryo is sufficiently developed to be called a **fetus**. Every organ system and external structure that will be found in the full-term newborn is present. The remainder of gestation is devoted to refining structures and perfecting function.

Nine to Twelve Weeks. By the end of the ninth week, the fetus reaches a CRL of 5 cm (2 in.) and weighs about 14 g (0.5 oz). The head is large and comprises almost half of the entire size of the fetus (Figure 9–32). At 12 weeks, the fetus reaches an 8-cm (3.2-in.) CRL and weighs about 45 g (1.6 oz). The face is well formed, with the nose protruding, the chin small and receding, and the ears acquiring a more adult shape. The eyelids close at about the 10th week and will not begin to reopen until about the 26th to 29th week. Some movements of the lips suggestive of the sucking reflex have been observed at 3 months. Tooth buds now appear for all 20 of the child's first teeth (baby teeth). The limbs are long and slender with well-formed digits. The fetus can curl the fingers toward the palm and make a tiny fist. The legs are still shorter and less developed than the arms. The urogenital tract completes its development, well-differentiated genitals appear, and the kidneys begin to produce urine. Red blood cells are produced primarily by the liver. Spontaneous movements of the fetus occur. Fetal heart tones (the sound of the heartbeat) can be ascertained by electronic devices between 8 and 12 weeks. The heart rate is 120 to 160 beats per minute.

Thirteen to Sixteen Weeks. This is a period of rapid growth. At 13 weeks, the fetus weighs 55 to 60 g (1.9 to 2.1 oz) and is about 9 cm (3.5 in.) CRL. Lanugo, or fine hair, begins to develop, especially on the head. Blood vessels are clearly visible beneath transparent skin. More muscle tissue and body skeleton have developed, which hold the fetus more erect (Figure 9–33). Active movements are present—the fetus stretches and exercises its arms and legs. It makes sucking motions, swallows amniotic fluid, and produces meconium in the intestinal tract. Bronchial tubes are branching out in the primitive lungs, and sweat glands are developing. The liver and pancreas now begin production of their appropriate secretions. By the beginning of week 16, skeletal ossification is clearly identifiable.

Twenty Weeks. The fetus doubles its CRL and now measures about 19 cm (7.5 in.). Fetal weight is between 435 and 465 g (15.3 and 16.4 oz). Lanugo covers the entire body and is especially prominent on the shoulders. Subcutaneous deposits of brown fat, which has a rich blood supply, make the skin a little less transparent. Nipples now appear over the mammary glands. The head may be covered with fine, "woolly" hair, and the eyebrows and

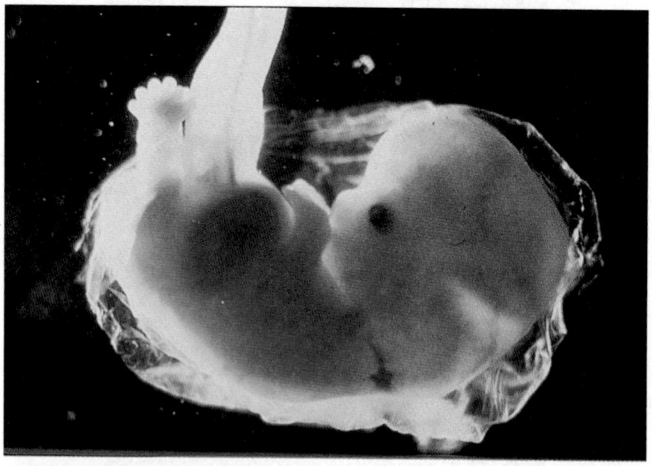

Figure 9-30 The embryo at 7 weeks. The head is rounded and nearly erect. The eyes have shifted forward and are closer together, and the eyelids begin to form.

SOURCE: Petit Format/Science Source.

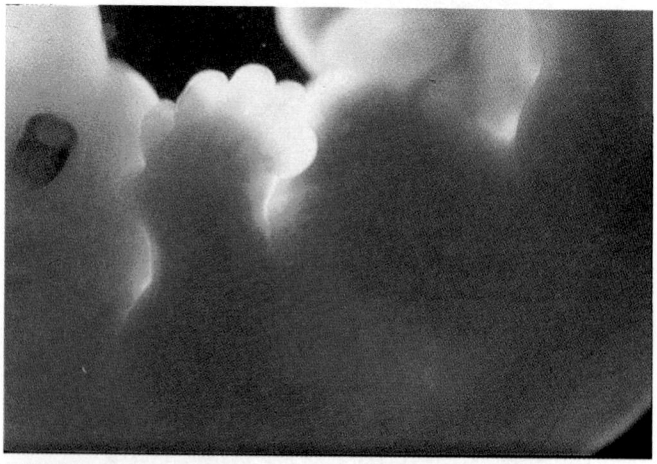

Figure 9-31 The embryo at 8 weeks. Although only 3 cm CRL, the embryo clearly resembles a human being. Facial features continue to develop.

SOURCE: Science Pictures Ltd./Science Source.

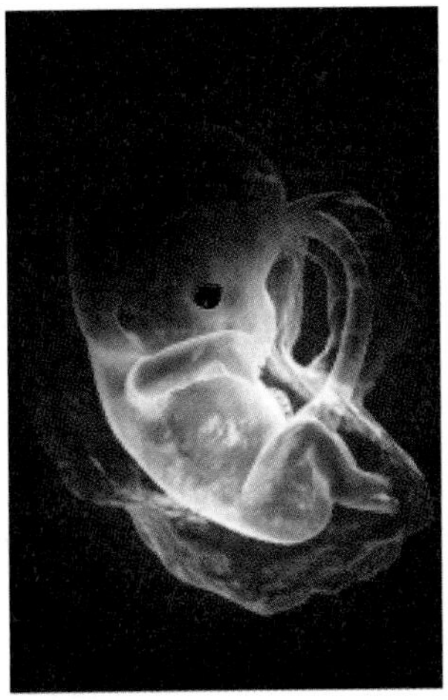

Figure 9–32 **The fetus at 9 weeks. Every organ system and external structure is present.**

SOURCE: MedicalRF.com/Getty Images.

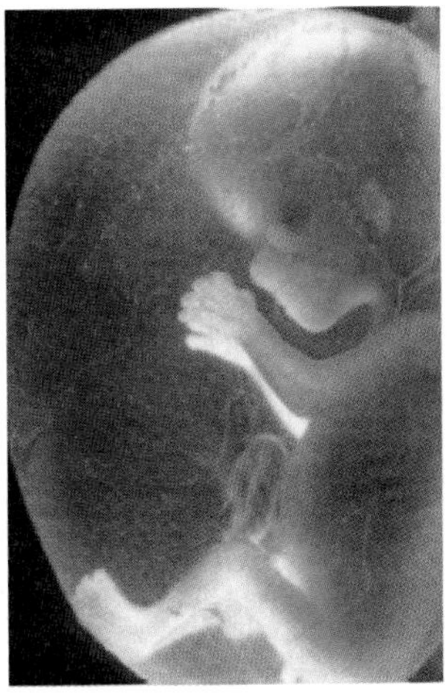

Figure 9–33 **The fetus at 14 weeks. During this period of rapid growth, the skin is so transparent that blood vessels are visible beneath it. More muscle tissue and body skeleton have developed, and they hold the fetus more erect.**

SOURCE: Claude Edelmann/Science Source.

eyelashes are beginning to form (Figure 9–34). Nails are present on both fingers and toes. Muscles are well developed, and the fetus is active. Fetal movement, known as *quickening*, is felt by the mother. The fetal heartbeat is audible through the fetoscope. Quickening and fetal heartbeat can help in validating the EDB.

Twenty-Four Weeks. The fetus at 24 weeks reaches a CHL of 28 cm (11.02 in.) and weighs about 780 g (1.72 lb). The hair on the head is growing long, and eyebrows and eyelashes have formed. The eyes are structurally complete and will soon open. The fetus has a reflex hand grip (grasp reflex) and, by the end of 6 months, a startle reflex. Skin covering the body is reddish and wrinkled, with little subcutaneous fat. Skin on the hands and feet has thickened, with skin ridges on the palms and soles forming distinct footprints and fingerprints. The skin over the entire body is covered with a protective cheeselike fatty substance, called **vernix caseosa**, secreted by the sebaceous glands. The alveoli in the lungs are just beginning to form.

Twenty-Five to Twenty-Eight Weeks. At about 25 weeks, the fetal skin is still red, wrinkled, and covered with vernix caseosa. The brain is developing rapidly, and the nervous system is complete enough to provide some degree of regulation of body functions. The eyelids open and close under neural control. The fetus has nails on both fingers and toes. If the fetus is a male, the testes begin to descend into the scrotal sac. Even though the lungs are still physiologically immature, they are sufficiently developed to provide gas exchange. A fetus born at this time will require immediate and prolonged intensive care to survive and then to decrease the risk of major handicap. The fetus at 28 weeks is about 27 cm (10.6 in.) CRL or 35 to 38 cm (13.8 to 15.0 in.) CHL and weighs 1200 to 1250 g (2.65 lb to 2.75 lb).

Twenty-Nine to Thirty-Two Weeks. At 30 weeks, the pupillary light reflex is present (Moore et al., 2016). The fetus is gaining weight from an increase in body muscle and fat and weighs about 2000 g (4 lb 6.5 oz) with a CRL of 31 cm (12.4 in.) or CHL of about 38 to 43 cm (15 to 17 in.) by 32 weeks of age. The central nervous system (CNS) has matured enough to direct rhythmic breathing movements and partially control body temperature. However, the lungs are not yet fully mature. Bones are now fully developed but are soft and flexible. The fetus begins storing iron, calcium, and phosphorus. In males, the testicles may be located in the scrotal sac but are often still high in the inguinal canals.

Thirty-Five to Thirty-Six Weeks. The fetus is beginning to get plump with less-wrinkled skin covering the deposits of subcutaneous fat. Lanugo hair is beginning to disappear, and the nails reach the edge of the fingertips. By 35 weeks, the fetus has a firm grasp

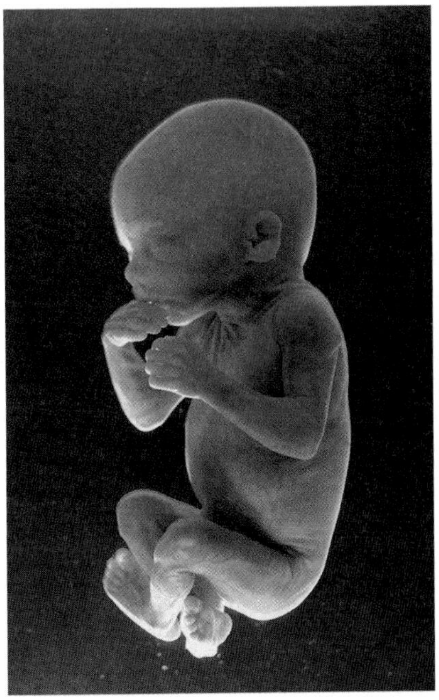

Figure 9–34 **The fetus at 20 weeks. The fetus weighs approximately 435 to 465 g (15.3 to 16.4 oz) and measures about 19 cm (7.5 in.). Subcutaneous deposits of brown fat make the skin less transparent. "Woolly" hair may cover the head, and nails have developed on the fingers and toes.**

SOURCE: James Stevenson/Science Source.

and exhibits spontaneous orientation to light. By 36 weeks of age, the weight is usually 2500 to 2750 g (5 lb 12 oz to 6 lb 11.5 oz), and the CHL of the fetus is about 42 to 48 cm (16.5 to 18.9 in.) or the CRL is about 35 cm (13.78 in.). A baby born at this time has a good chance of surviving but may require some special care, especially if there is intrauterine growth restriction.

Thirty-Eight to Forty Weeks. The fetus is now considered full term. The CHL varies from 48 to 52 cm (18.9 to 20.5 in.) or CRL of 40 cm (15.75 in.), with males usually longer than females. Males also usually weigh more than females. The weight at term is about 3000 to 3600 g (6.6 lb to 7.9 lb) and varies in different ethnic groups. The skin is pink and has a smooth, polished look. The only lanugo left is on the upper arms and shoulders. The hair on the head is no longer woolly but is coarse and about 1 inch long. Vernix caseosa is present, with heavier deposits remaining in the creases and folds of the skin. The body and extremities are plump, with good skin turgor, and the fingernails extend beyond the fingertips. The chest is prominent but still a little smaller than the head, and mammary glands protrude in both sexes. In males, the testes are in the scrotum or palpable in the inguinal canals.

As the fetus enlarges, amniotic fluid diminishes to about an average of 500 mL, and the fetal body mass fills the uterine cavity (Mattson & Smith, 2016). The fetus assumes what is called its *position of comfort*, or lie. The head is generally pointed downward, following the shape of the uterus (and also possibly because the head is heavier than the feet). The extremities and often the head are well flexed. After 5 months, feeding patterns, sleeping patterns, and activity patterns become established, so the fetus at term has its own body rhythms and individual style of response. See *Key Facts to Remember: Embryonic and Fetal Development: What Parents Want to Know* for important developmental milestones. For a detailed discussion of each body system's transition to full functioning in the newborn, see Chapter 26.

Key Facts To Remember

Embryonic and Fetal Development: What Parents Want to Know

4 weeks	The fetal heart begins to beat.
8 weeks	All body organs are formed.
8–12 weeks	Fetal heart tones can be heard by ultrasound Doppler device.
16 weeks	Baby's sex can be seen.
	Although thin, the fetus looks like a baby.
20 weeks	Heartbeat can be heard with fetoscope.
	Mother feels movement (quickening).
	Baby develops a regular schedule of sleeping, sucking, and kicking.
	Hands can grasp.
	Baby assumes a favorite position in utero.
	Vernix (lanolin-like covering) protects the body, and lanugo (fine hair) keeps oil on skin.
	Head hair, eyebrows, and eyelashes present.
24 weeks	Weighs 780 g (1 lb 10 oz).
	Activity is increasing.
	Fetal respiratory movements begin.
	Baby makes sucking movements.
28 weeks	Eyes begin to open and close.
	Baby can breathe at this time.
	Surfactant needed for breathing at birth is formed.
	Baby is two-thirds its final length.
32 weeks	Baby has fingernails and toenails.
	Subcutaneous fat is being laid down.
	Baby appears less red and wrinkled.
38+ weeks	Baby fills total uterus.
	Baby gets antibodies from mother.

Factors Influencing Embryonic and Fetal Development

Factors that may affect embryonic development include the quality of the sperm or ovum from which the zygote was formed, the genetic code established at fertilization, and the adequacy of the intrauterine environment. If the environment is unsuitable before cellular differentiation occurs, all the cells of the zygote are affected. The cells may die, which causes spontaneous abortion, or growth may be slowed, depending on the severity of the situation. When differentiation is complete and the fetal membranes have formed, an injurious agent has the greatest effect on those cells undergoing the most rapid growth. Thus, the time of injury is critical in the development of anomalies.

Because organs are formed primarily during embryonic development, the growing organism is considered most vulnerable to hazardous agents during the first months of pregnancy. All agents (e.g., drugs, viruses, or radiation) that can cause development of abnormal structures in an embryo are referred to as **teratogens**. It is important to remember that the effects of teratogens depend on the (1) maternal and fetal genotype, (2) stage of development when exposure occurs, and (3) dose and duration of exposure of the agent. Potential teratogens can cause malformations of the heart, limbs, eyes, and other organ systems as early as 3 weeks postconception (Moore et al., 2016). Chapter 13 discusses the effects of specific teratogenic agents on the developing fetus.

Adequacy of the maternal environment is also important during the periods of rapid embryonic and fetal development. Maternal nutrition can affect brain and neural tube development. The period of maximum brain growth and myelination begins with the fifth lunar month before birth and continues into adulthood. Amino acids, glucose, and fatty acids are considered to be the primary dietary factors in brain growth. A subtle type of damage that affects the associative capacity of the brain, possibly leading to learning disabilities, may be caused by nutritional deficiency at this stage. Studies in Tunisia showed that babies of mothers who were pregnant during the observance of Ramadan (the ninth month of the Islamic calendar) and practiced the required strict fasting for 29 to 30 days had reduced birth weight, head circumference, ponderal index, and placental weight (van Bilsen, Savitri, Amelia, et al., 2017). Similar results were found in studies of pregnant women fasting during Ramadan in Saudi Arabia.

SAFETY ALERT!

Vitamins and folic acid supplements taken before conception can reduce the incidence of neural tube defects.

Poor maternal nutrition may also predispose babies who are small or disproportionate at birth to the development of adult coronary heart disease, hypertension, and diabetes (Moore et al., 2016). Maternal nutrition is discussed in depth in Chapter 14.

Another prenatal influence on the intrauterine environment is maternal hyperthermia associated with sauna baths or hot tub use. Studies of the effects of maternal hyperthermia during the first trimester have raised concern about possible spontaneous abortion, central nervous system (CNS) defects, and failure of neural tube closure. Cigarette smoking during pregnancy (see Chapter 13) is a well-established cause of intrauterine growth restriction (IUGR) (Moore et al., 2016). Maternal substance abuse and viral illnesses also affect the intrauterine environment (see Chapters 17 and 30).

Focus Your Study

- The female reproductive system consists of the ovaries, where female germ cells and female sex hormones are formed; the fallopian tubes, which capture the ovum and allow transport to the uterus; the uterus, which is the implantation site for the fertilized ovum (blastocyst); the cervix, which is a protective portal for the body of the uterus and the connection between the vagina and the uterus; and the vagina, which is the passageway from the external genitals to the uterus and provides for discharge of menstrual products to the outside of the body.
- The female reproductive cycle may be described in terms of the ovarian cycle, during which ovulation occurs, and the menstrual cycle, during which menstruation occurs. These two cycles take place simultaneously and are under neurohormonal control.
- The ovarian cycle has two phases: The follicular phase and the luteal phase. During the follicular phase, the primordial follicle matures under the influence of FSH and LH until ovulation occurs. The luteal phase begins when the ovum leaves the follicle and the corpus luteum develops under the influence of LH. The corpus luteum produces high levels of progesterone and low levels of estrogen.
- The menstrual cycle has three phases: Menstrual, proliferative, and secretory. Menstruation is characterized by degeneration of the corpus luteum, decreases in both estrogen and progesterone levels, constriction of the spiral arteries, and escape of blood into the stromal cells of the endometrium. Then begins the actual shedding of the endometrial lining, when estrogen levels are low. The proliferative phase begins when the endometrial glands begin to enlarge under the influence of estrogen and cervical mucosal changes occur; the changes peak at ovulation. The secretory phase follows ovulation and, influenced primarily by progesterone, the uterus increases its vascularity to make ready for possible implantation.
- The male reproductive system consists of the testes, where male germ cells and male sex hormones are formed; a series of continuous ducts through which spermatozoa are transported outside the body; accessory glands that produce secretions important to sperm nutrition, survival, and transport; and the penis, which serves as the reproductive organ of intercourse.
- Mitosis is the process by which additional somatic (body) cells are formed. It provides growth and development of the organs and replacement of body cells.
- Meiosis produces cells called gametes (ova and sperm) that are necessary for reproduction of the species. It occurs during gametogenesis (oogenesis and spermatogenesis) and consists of two successive cell divisions (reduction division), which produce a gamete with 23 chromosomes (22 chromosomes and 1 sex chromosome)—the haploid number of chromosomes.
- Gametes must have a haploid number (23) of chromosomes so that when the female gamete (ovum) and the male gamete (spermatozoon) unite to form the zygote, the normal human diploid number of chromosomes (46) is reestablished.
- An ovum is considered fertile for about 12 to 24 hours after ovulation, and the sperm is believed to be capable of fertilizing the ovum for about 24 hours after it is deposited in the female reproductive tract.
- Fertilization usually takes place in the ampulla (outer third) of the fallopian tube. Both capacitation and the acrosomal reaction must occur for the sperm to fertilize the ovum. Capacitation is the removal of the plasma membrane, which exposes the acrosomal covering of the sperm head. The acrosomal reaction is the deposit of hyaluronidase in the corona radiata, which allows the sperm head to penetrate the ovum.
- Sex chromosomes are referred to as X and Y. Females have two X chromosomes, and males have an X and a Y chromosome. Y chromosomes are carried only by the sperm. To produce a female child, both the mother and the father contribute an X chromosome. To produce a male child, the mother contributes an X chromosome and the father contributes a Y chromosome.
- Intrauterine development first proceeds via cellular multiplication in which the zygote undergoes rapid mitotic division called cleavage. As a result of cleavage, the zygote divides and multiplies into cell groupings called blastomeres, which are held together by the zona pellucida. The blastomeres will eventually become a solid ball of cells called the morula. When a cavity forms in the morula cell mass, the inner solid cell mass is called the blastocyst.
- Implantation usually occurs in the upper part of the posterior uterine wall when the blastocyst burrows into the uterine lining.
- After implantation, the endometrium is called the decidua. Decidua capsularis is the portion that covers the blastocyst. Decidua basalis is the portion that is directly under the blastocyst. Decidua vera is the portion that lines the rest of the uterine cavity.
- Embryonic membranes are called the amnion and the chorion. The amnion is formed from the ectoderm and is a thin protective membrane that contains the amniotic fluid and the embryo. The chorion is a thick membrane that develops from the trophoblast and encloses the amnion, embryo, and yolk sac.

- Amniotic fluid cushions the fetus against mechanical injury, controls the embryo's temperature, allows symmetric external growth, prevents adherence to the amnion, and permits freedom of movement.
- Primary germ layers will give rise to all tissues, organs, and organ systems. The three primary germ cell layers are the ectoderm, endoderm, and mesoderm.
- The umbilical cord contains two umbilical arteries, which carry deoxygenated blood from the fetus to the placenta, and one umbilical vein, which carries oxygenated blood from the placenta to the fetus. The umbilical cord has a central insertion into the placenta. Wharton jelly, a specialized connective tissue, prevents compression of the umbilical cord in utero.
- Twins are either dizygotic (fraternal) or monozygotic (identical). Dizygotic twins arise from two separate ova fertilized by two separate spermatozoa. Monozygotic twins develop from a single ovum fertilized by a single spermatozoon.
- The placenta, which develops from the chorionic villi and the decidua basalis, has two parts. The maternal portion, consisting of the decidua basalis, is red and flesh-looking; the fetal portion, consisting of chorionic villi, is covered by the amnion and appears shiny and gray. The placenta is made up of 15 to 20 segments called cotyledons.
- The placenta serves metabolic functions, endocrine functions (production of human placental lactogen [hPL], human chorionic gonadotropin [hCG], estrogen, and progesterone), and immunologic functions. It acts as the fetus' respiratory organ, is an organ of excretion, and aids in the exchange of nutrients.
- Fetal circulation is a specially designed circulatory system that provides for oxygenation of the fetus while bypassing the fetal lungs.
- Stages of fetal development include the preembryonic stage (the first 14 days of human development starting at fertilization), the embryonic stage (from day 15 after fertilization, or the beginning of the third week, until approximately 8 weeks after conception), and the fetal stage (from 8 weeks until birth at approximately 38 weeks postconception).
- Significant events that occur during the embryonic stage are that at 4 weeks the fetal heart begins to beat and at 6 weeks fetal circulation is established.
- The fetal stage is devoted to refining structures and perfecting function. Review Table 9–2 for significant developments during the fetal stage.
- The embryo is particularly vulnerable to teratogenesis during the first 8 weeks of cell differentiation and organ system development. Effects of teratogens depend on the (1) maternal and fetal genotype, (2) stage of development when exposure occurs, and (3) dose and duration of exposure of the agent.

References

Blackburn, S. T. (2018). *Maternal, fetal, & neonatal physiology: A clinical perspective* (5th ed.). St. Louis, MO: Saunders.

Cunningham, F. G., Leveno, K. J., Bloom, S. L., Spong, C. Y., Dashe, J. S., Hoffman, B. L., . . . Sheffield, J. S. (2018). *Williams obstetrics* (25th ed.). New York, NY: McGraw-Hill.

Gabbe, S. G., Niebyl, J. L. R., Simpson, J. L., Landon, M. B., Galan, H. L., Jauniaux, E. R. M., . . . & Grobman, W. A. (2017). *Obstetrics: Normal and problem pregnancies* (7th ed.). Philadelphia, PA: Saunders/Elsevier.

Mattson, S., & Smith, J. E. (2016). *Core curriculum for maternal-newborn nursing* (5th ed.). St. Louis, MO: Elsevier.

Moore, K. L., Persaud, T. V. N., & Torchia, M. G. (2016). *The developing human: Clinical oriented embryology* (10th ed.). Philadelphia, PA: Saunders/Elsevier.

National Institute for Health and Clinical Excellence (NICE). (2014). *Antenatal care: Routine care for the healthy pregnant woman.* Retrieved from http://www.nice.org.uk/CG62

Sadler, T. W. (2015). *Langman's medical embryology* (13th ed.). Philadelphia, PA: Lippincott Williams & Wilkins.

U.S. Department of Health and Human Services. (2011). *Healthy People 2020 topics & objectives.* Retrieved from http://www.healthypeople.gov/2020/topicsobjectives2020/default.aspx

Van Bilsen, L. A., Savitri, A. I., Amelia, D., Baharuddin, M., Grobbee, E., & Uiterwaal, C. S. P. M. (2017). Predictors of Ramadan fasting during pregnancy. *Journal of Epidemiology and Global Health. 6,* 267–275. DOI: 10.1016/j.jegh.2016.06.002

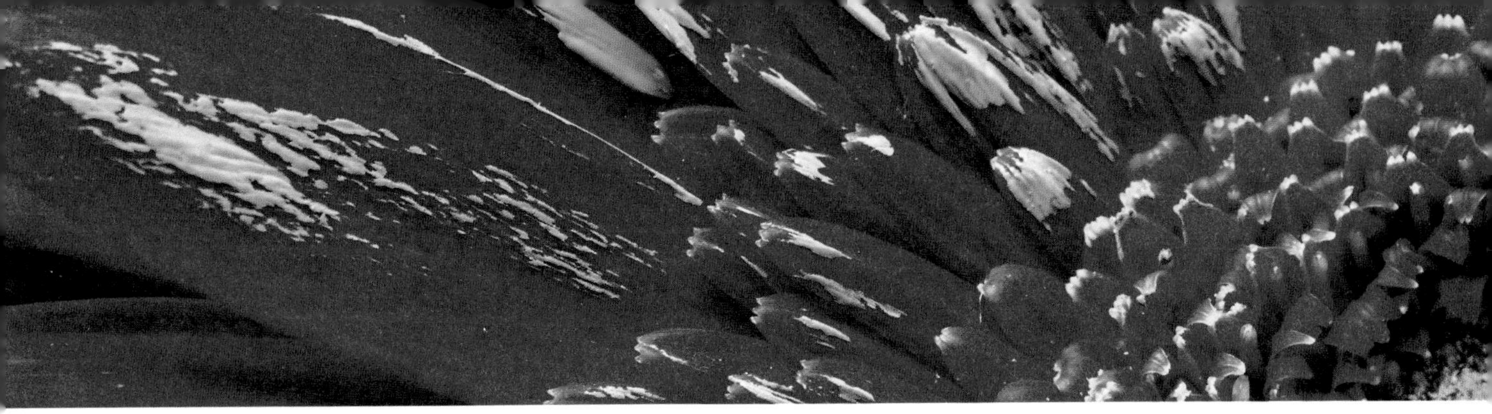

Chapter 10

Reproductive Genetics

It took me 3 years to conceive my daughter, Nina, but everything seemed normal. When she was 4 months old, her pediatrician became worried about her low muscle tone and the fact that she wasn't meeting her milestones, so we were referred to a specialist. When Nina was 6 months old, she was diagnosed with spinal muscular atrophy (SMA). My husband and I were both confirmed to be carriers of the genetic mutation that causes SMA. I had never heard of SMA before. How was I supposed to know we were at risk? Nina is now 14 months old and a blessing, but she requires 24-hour nursing care and her life will be significantly shortened because of her condition. Despite our history of infertility, I am unexpectedly pregnant. There is a 25% chance this baby also has SMA, and I plan to have prenatal diagnosis. My husband and I don't know how we'll handle the results, but we know we need the information as soon as possible.

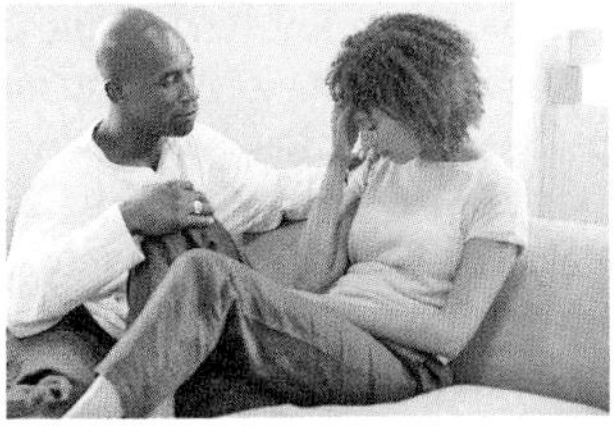

SOURCE: Ian Cook/Image Source/SuperStock.

Learning Outcomes

10.1 Identify the characteristics of autosomal dominant, autosomal recessive, X-linked (sex-linked) recessive, and multifactorial inheritance disorders.

10.2 Compare prenatal and postnatal diagnostic procedures used to determine the presence of genetic disorders.

10.3 Identify couples who may benefit from preconceptual genetic counseling and testing, including those with special reproductive concerns.

10.4 Examine the emotional impact on a couple experiencing the birth of a baby with a genetic disorder.

10.5 Describe the nurse's roles as counselor, educator, and advocate for the family undergoing genetic evaluation, counseling, and treatment.

Healthy People 2020

(MICH-1.6) Reduce the rate of fetal and infant deaths due to birth defects

(MICH-26) Reduce the proportion of children diagnosed with a disorder through newborn blood spot screening who experience developmental delay requiring special education services

For most couples, pregnancy and childbirth usually take their normal course and a healthy baby is born. This chapter explores issues of families who face the risk of bearing babies with genetic problems.

Genetic Disorders

The desired and expected outcome of any pregnancy is the birth of a healthy, "perfect" baby. Parents experience grief, fear, and anger when they discover that their baby has been born with a defect or a genetic disease. Such an abnormality may be evident prenatally, at birth, or may not appear for some time. The baby may have inherited a disorder from one parent or both, creating guilt and strife within the family.

Regardless of the type or scope of the problem, parents will have many questions: "What did I do?" "What caused it?" "How do I cope with it?" "Will it happen again?" As our society's knowledge and understanding of genetics and genomic health increases, the role of professional nurses has been expanded to address the needs of patients and families. Graduates of nursing programs are now expected to understand the impact of genetic disease, construct and utilize family history tools, provide patient education, and anticipate genetic counseling referral needs (Camak, 2016). Nurses must understand the basics of genetics to appropriately identify individuals and families at risk for genetic diseases in themselves or their offspring.

Chromosomes and Chromosomal Analysis

All hereditary material is carried on tightly coiled strands of deoxyribonucleic acid (DNA) known as **chromosomes**. The chromosomes carry the *genes*, the functional unit of inheritance. All *somatic* (*body*) *cells* contain 46 chromosomes, which is the *diploid* number; the sperm and egg (gametes [reproductive cells]) contain half as many (23) chromosomes, or the *haploid* number. There are 23 pairs of homologous chromosomes (a matched pair of chromosomes, one inherited from each parent). Twenty-two of the pairs are known as *autosomes* (non–sex chromosomes), and one pair is the sex chromosome, X and Y. A normal female has a 46, XX chromosome constitution, and the normal male, 46, XY (Figure 10–1 and Figure 10–2).

The **karyotype**, or pictorial analysis of an individual's chromosomes, is usually obtained from specially treated and stained peripheral blood lymphocytes. Placental tissue or amniotic fluid can be obtained prenatally and sent for karyotyping of the fetus.

Chromosome abnormalities are not uncommon in a fetus and often result in miscarriage early in pregnancy. However, approximately 1 in 150 live births involves some type of chromosomal abnormality that results in a broad range of clinical presentations including birth defects or developmental disabilities (American College of Obstetricians and Gynecologists Committee on Genetics & the Society for Maternal Fetal Medicine Publications Committee [ACOG & SMFM], 2016a). Chromosome abnormalities can occur in either the autosomes or the sex chromosomes and can be divided into two categories: Abnormalities of number and abnormalities of structure. Even small alterations in chromosomes can cause problems, especially those associated with delayed growth and development. Some of these abnormalities can also be passed on to other offspring. Thus, in some cases, chromosomal analysis is appropriate even if clinical manifestations are mild.

ABNORMALITIES OF CHROMOSOME NUMBER

Abnormalities of chromosome number are most commonly seen as trisomies, monosomies, and mosaicism. In all three cases, the abnormality is most often caused by *nondisjunction*, a failure of paired chromosomes to separate during cell division. If nondisjunction occurs in either the sperm or the egg before fertilization, the resulting zygote (fertilized egg) will have an abnormal chromosome makeup in all of the cells (trisomy or monosomy). If nondisjunction occurs after fertilization, the developing zygote will have cells with two or more different chromosome makeups, evolving into two or more different cell lines (mosaicism).

Trisomies are the product of the union of a normal gamete (egg or sperm) with a gamete that contains an extra chromosome. The individual will have 47 chromosomes and be *trisomic* (have three copies of the same chromosome) for whichever chromosome is extra. Down syndrome (trisomy 21) is the most common trisomy abnormality seen in live born children (Figure 10–3). The presence of the extra chromosome 21 produces distinctive clinical features, mild to moderate intellectual disability, and a variety of physical health concerns (Figure 10–4). Advances in medical science and early intervention services have improved the quality of life and life expectancy of individuals with Down syndrome.

The other two common trisomies are trisomy 18 (Figure 10–5) and trisomy 13 (Figure 10–6). See Table 10–1. The prognoses for both trisomy 18 and 13 are extremely poor. Most children (70%) die within the first 3 months of life as a result of complications related to respiratory and cardiac abnormalities (Nelson, Rosella, Mahant, et al., 2016; Pierce, 2014). However, 10% survive beyond the first year of life; therefore, the family needs to plan for the possibility of long-term care of a medically fragile infant and for family support.

Monosomies occur when a normal gamete unites with a gamete that is missing a chromosome. In this case, the individual will have only 45 chromosomes and is said to be *monosomic*.

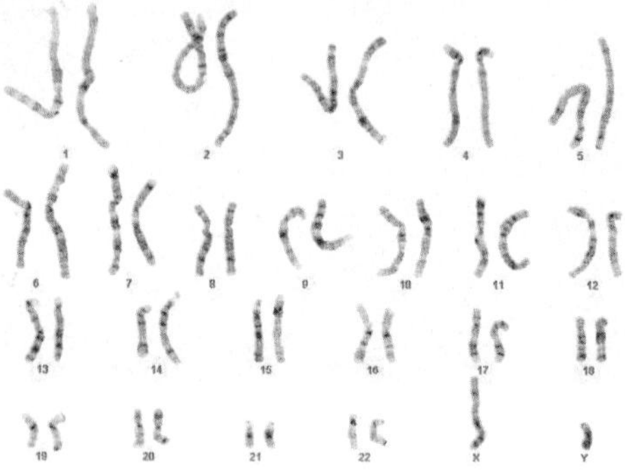

Figure 10–2 **Normal male karyotype.**

SOURCE: Susan Olson, PhD, Oregon Health & Science University Knight Diagnostic Laboratories.

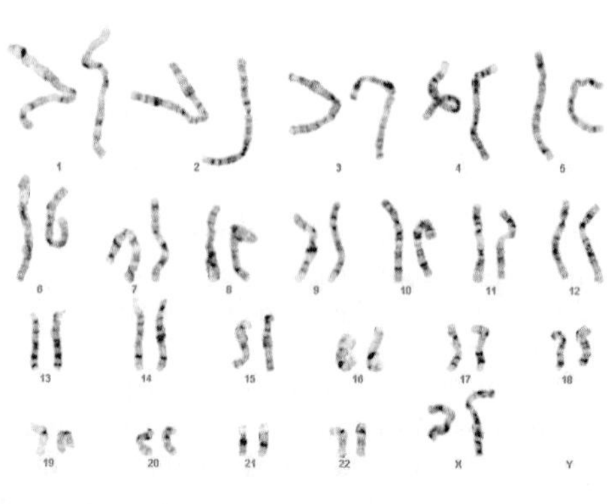

Figure 10–1 **Normal female karyotype.**

SOURCE: Susan Olson, PhD, Oregon Health & Science University Knight Diagnostic Laboratories.

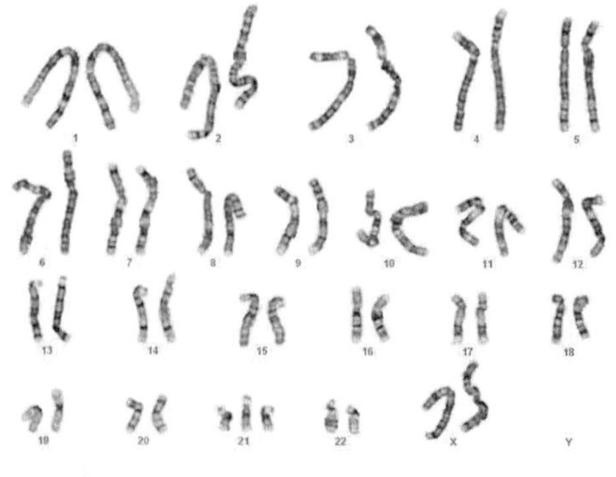

Figure 10–3 **Karyotype of a female who has trisomy 21, Down syndrome. Note the extra chromosome 21.**

SOURCE: Susan Olson, PhD, Oregon Health & Science University Knight Diagnostic Laboratories.

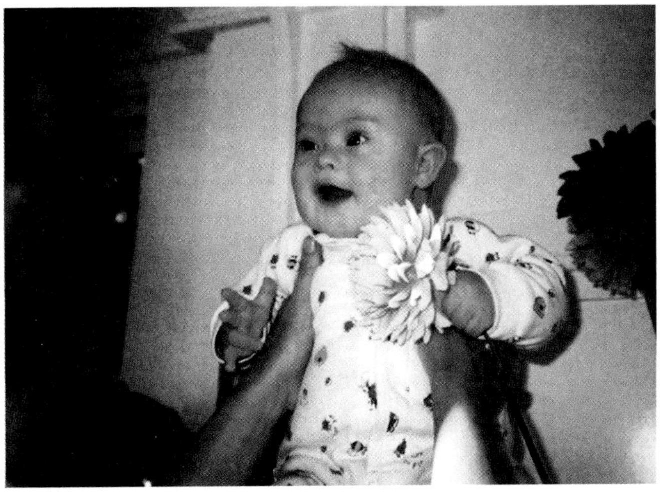

Figure 10–4 A boy with Down syndrome.

SOURCE: Michele Davidson.

Monosomy of the sex chromosomes (e.g., 45,X) is compatible with life while monosomy of an entire autosomal chromosome is not.

Polyploidies occur when there are extra sets of chromosomes rather than a single chromosome that may be missing or extra. Instead of the normal diploid number there may be three sets totaling 69 chromosomes (known as *triploidy*) or four sets of each chromosome totaling 92 (known as *tetraploidy*). Some types of triploidy can result in a partial hydatiform mole, which has a small risk for gestational trophoblastic disease and choriocarcinoma. Tetraploidy usually results in an anembryonic pregnancy (also called *blighted ovum*). Polyploidy accounts for 5 to 10% of all first-trimester miscarriage and are generally not considered compatible with live birth.

A

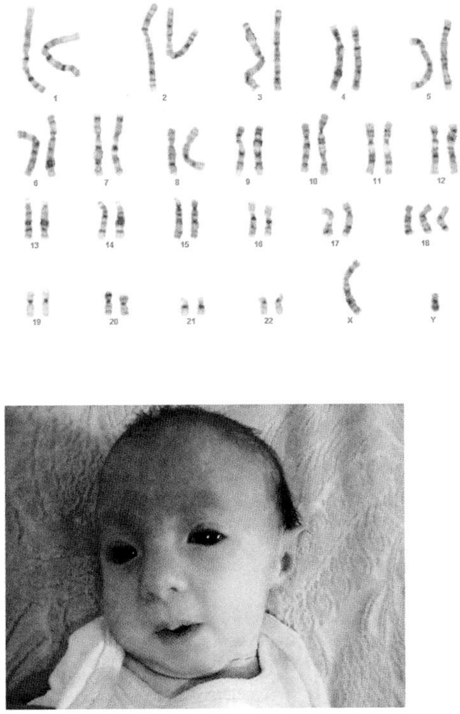

B

Figure 10–5 A. Karyotype of a male who has trisomy 18. B. Infant girl with trisomy 18.

SOURCE: A. Susan Olson, PhD, Oregon Health & Science University Knight Diagnostic Laboratories. **B.** OHSU Department of Obstetrics & Gynecology.

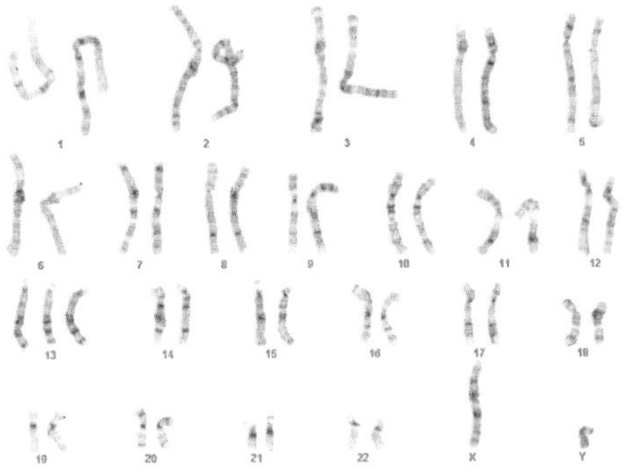

Figure 10–6 Karyotype of a male with trisomy 13.

SOURCE: Susan Olson, PhD, Oregon Health & Science University Knight Diagnostic Laboratories.

Mosaicism occurs after fertilization and results in an individual with two different cell lines, each having a different chromosomal number. This error in mitosis, when a cell does not split evenly into two, results in some cells having the normal number of 46 chromosomes and other cells having an extra #21 chromosome or having 47 chromosomes. Mosaicism tends to be more common in the sex chromosomes.

NUMERICAL ABNORMALITIES OF THE SEX CHROMOSOME

To better understand abnormalities of the sex chromosomes, the nurse should know that in females, at an early embryonic stage, one of the two normal X chromosomes becomes inactive. This phenomenon is called *X-inactivation* or *lyonization*. The inactive X chromosome forms a dark-staining area known as the *Barr body*, or sex chromatin body. The typical female has one Barr body because one of her two X chromosomes has been inactivated. The typical male has no Barr bodies because he has only one X chromosome.

The most common sex chromosome abnormalities are Turner syndrome in females (45,X with no Barr bodies present) (Figure 10–7) and Klinefelter syndrome in males (47,XXY with one Barr body present). See Table 10–1 for clinical descriptions of these abnormalities.

ABNORMALITIES OF CHROMOSOME STRUCTURE

Abnormalities of chromosome structure involve only parts of the chromosome and can occur in the form of translocation, deletions, duplications, or inversions. It is estimated that 1 in 375 newborns has a structural chromosome abnormality (Norton, Scoutt, & Feldstein, 2017).

A *translocation* is the transfer of a segment of one chromosome to another chromosome. There are two types of translocations: Reciprocal and Robertsonian. *Reciprocal translocations* occur between two nonhomologous chromosomes and usually leave the total chromosomal number unchanged. They are relatively common (found in 1 in 600 newborns) and, because there is no deletion or duplication of chromosome material, are considered to be *balanced*. Individuals with a balanced reciprocal translocation generally do not have any health concerns related to the rearrangement. However, they can have offspring with an *unbalanced* translocation, in which there is chromosome material deleted or duplicated. An unbalanced translocation can lead to pregnancy loss, congenital anomalies, intellectual disability, or other health concerns.

Translocations that involve two acrocentric chromosomes (chromosomes 13, 14, 15, 21, and 22) that fuse near the centromere regions with loss of the short (p) arms are called *Robertsonian translocations*. An individual with a balanced Robertsonian

TABLE 10–1 Chromosomal Syndromes

SYNDROME	CHARACTERISTICS
Trisomy 21 (Down Syndrome)	
Secondary nondisjunction or unbalanced translocation involving chromosome 21 (see Figure 10–3 and Figure 10–4) *Incidence:* Average 1 in 700 live births; incidence variable with age of woman	• ***Central nervous system (CNS):*** Mild to moderate intellectual disability; hypotonia at birth • ***Head:*** Flattened occiput; depressed nasal bridge; upward slant to the eyes; epicanthal folds; white specking of the iris (Brushfield spots); protrusion of the tongue; high, arched palate; low-set ears • ***Hands:*** Broad, short fingers; abnormalities of finger and foot; dermal ridge patterns (dermatoglyphics); single transverse palmar crease • ***Other:*** Congenital heart disease (50%)
Trisomy 18	
Incidence: 1 in 4000 live births (see Figure 10–5)	• ***CNS:*** Intellectual disability; severe hypotonia • ***Head:*** Prominent occiput; low-set ears; corneal opacities; ptosis (drooping of eyelids) • ***Hands:*** Third and fourth fingers overlapped by second and fifth fingers; abnormal dermatoglyphics; syndactyly (webbing of fingers) • ***Other:*** Congenital heart defects (> 90%); renal abnormalities; single umbilical artery; gastrointestinal tract abnormalities; rocker-bottom feet; cryptorchidism; various malformations of other organs
Trisomy 13	
Incidence: 1 in 8000 live births (see Figure 10–6)	• ***CNS:*** Intellectual disability; severe hypotonia; seizures; anatomic defects of the brain (holoprosencephaly) in 60% • ***Head:*** Microcephaly; microphthalmia and/or coloboma (keyhole-shaped pupil); malformed ears; aplasia of external auditory canal; micrognathia (abnormally small lower jaw); cleft lip and palate • ***Hands:*** Polydactyly (extra digits); abnormal posturing of fingers; abnormal dermatoglyphics • ***Other:*** Congenital heart defects (80%); hemangiomas; gastrointestinal tract defects; various malformations of other organs
22Q11.2 Deletion Syndrome	
Deletion of long arm of chromosome 22 Also called *velocardiofacial* or *DiGeorge syndrome* *Incidence:* 1 in 3000 live births	• ***CNS:*** Learning differences or mild intellectual disability • ***Head:*** Palatal anomalies (70%), characteristic facial features • ***Other:*** Congenital heart disease (75%)
45,X (Monosomy X, Turner Syndrome)	
Incidence: 1 in 300 to 7000 live female births (see Figure 10–7)	• ***CNS:*** No intellectual impairment; some perceptual difficulties • ***Head:*** Low hairline; webbed neck • ***Trunk:*** Short stature; cubitus valgus (increased carrying angle of arm); excessive nevi (congenital discoloration of skin due to pigmentation); broad chest with widely spaced nipples • ***Other:*** Fibrous streaks in ovaries; underdeveloped secondary sex characteristics; primary amenorrhea; infertility; renal anomalies; coarctation of the aorta
47,XXY (Klinefelter syndrome)	
Incidence: 1 in 1000 live male births	• ***CNS:*** Increased risk for learning disabilities, ADHD, autism spectrum disorder • ***Trunk:*** Occasional gynecomastia (abnormally large male breasts); abnormal body proportions (long legs, short trunk, shoulder equal to hip size) • ***Other:*** Small, firm testes; underdeveloped secondary sex characteristics; reduced fertility/infertility

translocation will have 45 chromosomes, including the translocation chromosome, which is made up of the long arms of two chromosomes (Figure 10–8). For example, the two most common Robertsonian translocations are 13q14q (the long arm of one chromosome 13 is fused to the long arm of one chromosome 14) and 14q21q. The translocation involving 13q and 14q is found in about 1 person out of 1300 and is the most common chromosome rearrangement in humans. Individuals with Robertsonian translocations are at risk of having offspring with unbalanced translocations. This may lead to pregnancy loss or live born offspring with trisomy 13 or trisomy 21. Structural abnormalities also include *duplications* or *deletions* of chromosomal material.

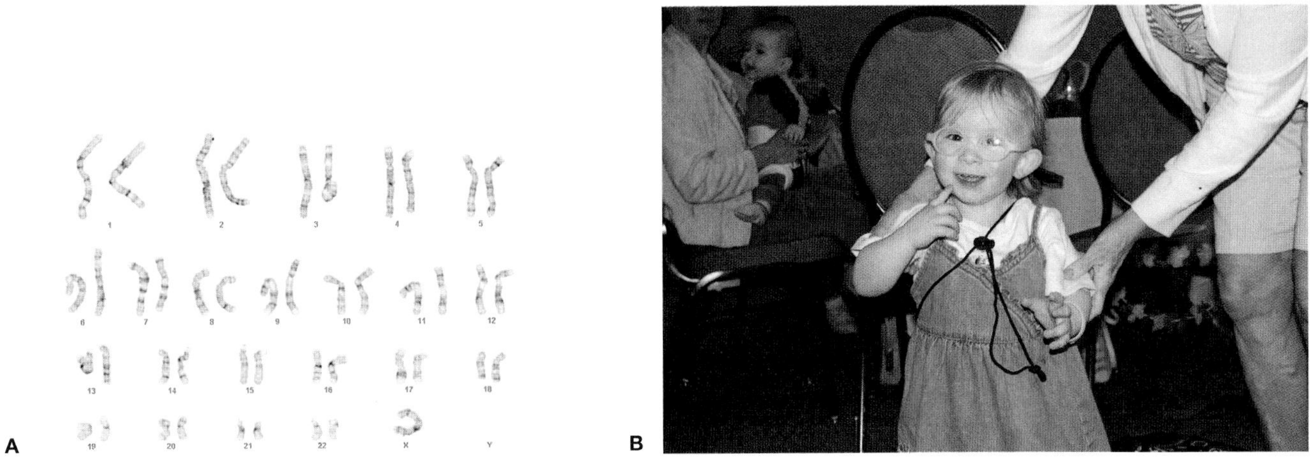

Figure 10–7 A. Karyotype of a female with Turner syndrome. B. Toddler girl with Turner syndrome.

SOURCE: A. Susan Olson, PhD, Oregon Health & Science University Knight Diagnostic Laboratories. **B.** Turner Syndrome Society. Copyright © by Cindy Scurlock. Used by permission of Cindy Scurlock.

Any portion of a chromosome may be lost or added, generally leading to some adverse effect. Many types of duplications and deletions have been described, such as 22q11.2 deletion syndrome (see Table 10–1).

Chromosomal Analysis Techniques. Several techniques can be used to determine if a chromosome abnormality is present. This includes traditional G-banded karyotype, *fluorescence in situ hybridization (FISH)*, and *chromosomal microarray analysis (CMA)*. FISH analysis uses fluorescent-labeled probes to identify the number of specific chromosome regions present in a sample, with results available more rapidly than a karyotype. Some chromosome abnormalities are too minute to detect with standard karyotype. These chromosome abnormalities, known as *microdeletions* and *microduplications*, can be detected by specific FISH probes or by the use of *chromosomal microarray (CMA)*. CMA is a technology that compares a patient's DNA with that of a normal control individual and detects not only aneuploidies and large structural changes

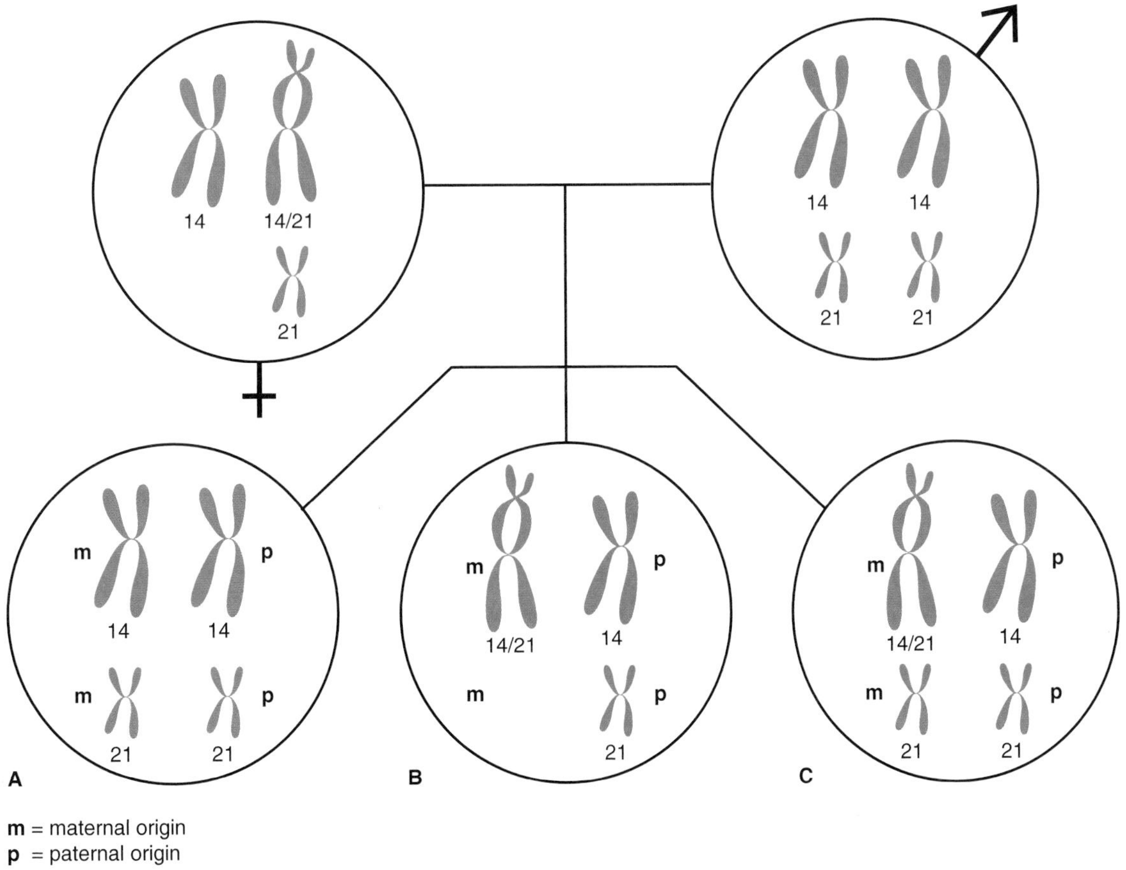

Figure 10–8 Diagram of various types of offspring when the mother has a balanced translocation between chromosomes 14 and 21 and the father has a normal arrangement of chromosomal material. A. Normal offspring. B. Balanced translocation carrier. C. Unbalanced translocation. Child has Down syndrome.

across the genome, but also submicroscopic duplications, deletions, and unbalanced rearrangements in genes. Because of the advantages over traditional karyotyping, CMA has become a first-line test for chromosome analysis, particularly in those with congenital malformations and intellectual disabilities (Bornstein et al., 2016).

Modes of Inheritance

Many inherited diseases are produced by an abnormality in a single gene or pair of genes. In such instances the chromosomes are grossly normal because the defect is at the gene level. Some of these gene abnormalities can be detected by technologies such as DNA sequencing and other biochemical assays.

There are two major categories of inheritance: **Mendelian (single-gene) inheritance** and **non-Mendelian (multifactorial) inheritance**. Each single-gene trait is determined by a pair of genes working together. These genes are responsible for the observable expression of the traits (e.g., brown eyes, dark skin), referred to as the **phenotype**. The total genetic makeup of an individual is referred to as the **genotype** (pattern of the genes on the chromosomes).

One of the genes for a trait is inherited from the mother; the other is from the father. Individuals who have two identical genes at a given locus are considered to be *homozygous* for that trait. Individuals are considered to be *heterozygous* for a particular trait when they have two different alleles (alternate forms of the same gene) at a given locus on a pair of homologous chromosomes.

The best known modes of single-gene inheritance are autosomal dominant, autosomal recessive, and X-linked (sex-linked).

AUTOSOMAL DOMINANT INHERITANCE

A person is said to have an autosomal dominantly inherited disorder if the disease trait is heterozygous; that is, the abnormal gene overshadows the normal gene of the pair to produce the trait. The genetic condition may be familial, meaning it was passed to an individual from one of his or her parents; or it may be the result of a *de novo* (new) mutation that occurred during meiosis of the egg or sperm that created the individual, and he or she is the first and only affected person in the family. In autosomal dominant inheritance, the following occurs:

- An affected individual may have an affected parent. The family **pedigree** (graphic representation of a family tree) can show multiple generations having the disorder.
- Affected individuals have a 50% chance of passing on the abnormal gene to each of their children (Figure 10–9).
- Males and females are equally affected, and a father can pass the abnormal gene on to his son. This is an important principle when distinguishing autosomal dominant disorders from X-linked disorders.
- Autosomal dominant inherited disorders have varying degrees of presentation. This is an important factor when counseling families concerning these disorders. Although a parent may have a mild form of the disease, the child may have a more severe form.

Some autosomal dominant conditions have differences in their expression and can lead to difficulties in diagnosis. These differences in expression are known as reduced penetrance, variable expressivity, and pleiotropy. *Penetrance* is the possibility that a gene will have any phenotypic expression at all. When an individual with the genetic trait for a condition fails to express features of the disorder, the gene is said to show reduced penetrance. *Expressivity* is the severity of expression of the phenotype. When the severity of the condition differs in people who have the same genotype, the phenotype is said to have variable expressivity. When a single abnormal gene produces diverse phenotypic effects, such as which organ systems are affected and which symptoms occur, the expression is said to be *pleiotropic*.

AUTOSOMAL RECESSIVE INHERITANCE

In an autosomal recessively inherited disorder, the individual must have two abnormal genes to be affected. A *carrier* is an individual who is heterozygous for the abnormal gene and clinically does not show any signs of the genetic disorder. It is not until two carriers mate and pass on the same abnormal gene that affected children may appear. In autosomal recessive inheritance, the following occurs:

- An affected individual can have clinically normal parents, but both parents are generally carriers of the abnormal gene (Figure 10–10).
- In the case where both parents are carriers, each pregnancy has a 25% chance of resulting in an affected child.
- If the child of two carrier parents is clinically normal, there is a two-thirds chance that the child is a carrier of the gene.

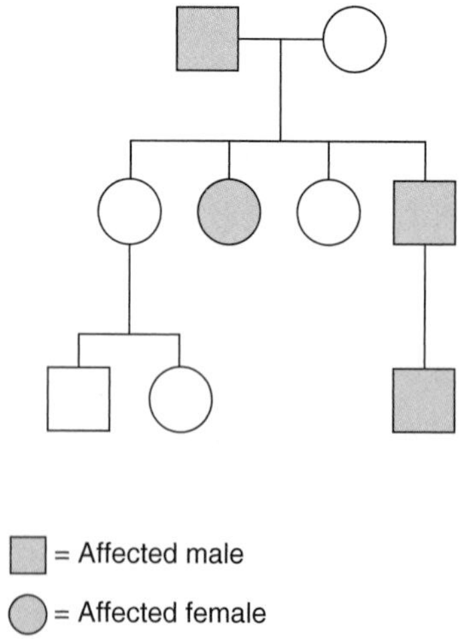

Figure 10–9 Autosomal dominant pedigree. One parent is affected. Statistically, 50% of offspring will be affected, regardless of sex.

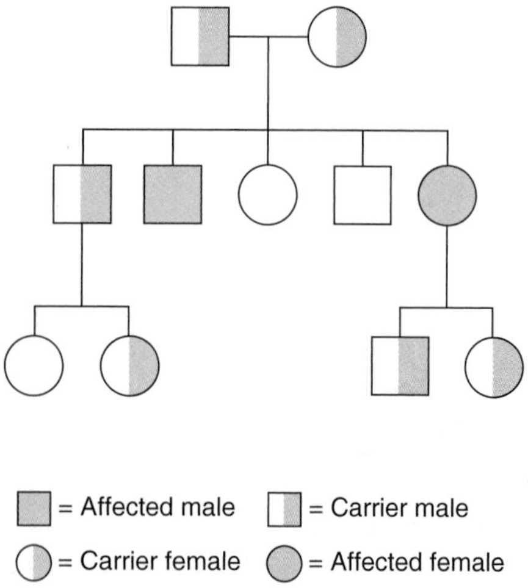

Figure 10–10 Autosomal recessive pedigree. Both parents are carriers. Statistically, 25% of offspring will be affected, regardless of sex.

- Both males and females are equally affected.
- There is an increased risk for autosomal recessive conditions in couples with consanguinity (mating of blood relatives). See *Developing Cultural Competence: Consanguineous Marriages*.

Some of the more common autosomal recessive inherited disorders are cystic fibrosis, phenylketonuria (PKU), sickle cell disease, spinal muscular atrophy (SMA), and many metabolic disorders.

Developing Cultural Competence Consanguineous Marriages

In the United States, marriage between related individuals is generally taboo. There is a concern that a child conceived by people who are related by blood may have an increased risk for autosomal recessive disorders and poor pregnancy outcome (Kapurubandara, Melov, Shalou, et al., 2016). In many other cultures, marriage of first cousins and others who are related by blood is acceptable and even common. In several Middle Eastern cultures, consanguineous marriage, generally between cousins, is common. Reasons for consanguineous marriage include "increase family links," "they knew each other and everything would be clear before marriage," "customs and traditions," and "less cost."

Note: It is unwise to attribute specific attitudes or beliefs to all members of a cultural group. The information in the Developing Cultural Competence boxes offers possible insights into caring for women from different cultural groups.

X-LINKED RECESSIVE INHERITANCE

X-linked, or sex-linked, disorders are those for which the abnormal gene is carried on the X chromosome. An X-linked recessive disorder is manifested in a male who carries the abnormal gene on his only X chromosome and is considered *hemizygous* for the condition. Approximately two-thirds of the time, the mother of a male with an X-linked disorder will be a carrier. Most carrier females (known as *heterozygous females*) do not have symptoms of the condition. However, in some X-linked conditions heterozygous females can manifest symptoms of the disorder due to skewed X chromosome inactivation (*lyonization*), but the symptoms tend to be milder and have later onset. In X-linked recessive inheritance, the following occurs:

- There is no male-to-male transmission. Affected males are related through the female line (Figure 10–11).
- There is a 50% chance that a carrier mother will pass the abnormal gene to each of her sons, who will thus be affected. There is a 50% chance that a carrier mother will pass the normal gene to each of her sons, who will thus be unaffected.
- There is a 50% chance that a carrier mother will pass the abnormal gene to each of her daughters, who become carriers.
- Fathers affected with an X-linked disorder cannot pass the disorder to their sons, but all their daughters become carriers of the disorder. They are known as *obligate carriers*.

Some of the more common X-linked recessive disorders are hemophilia, Duchenne muscular dystrophy, and some forms of color blindness.

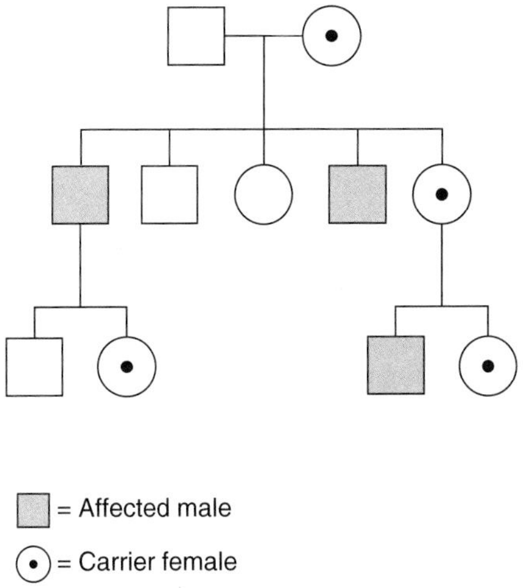

Figure 10–11 X-linked recessive pedigree. The mother is the carrier. Statistically, 50% of male offspring will be affected, and 50% of female offspring will be carriers.

X-LINKED DOMINANT INHERITANCE

X-linked dominant disorders are rare, the most common being vitamin D–resistant rickets. When X-linked dominance does occur, the pattern is similar to X-linked recessive inheritance except that heterozygous females can also be affected. In X-linked dominant inheritance, there is no male-to-male transmission. Affected fathers will have affected daughters but no affected sons. Some types of X-linked dominant disorders are so severe that they can be lethal in utero or in the newborn period in hemizygous males (e.g., Rett syndrome or severe forms of otopalataldigital [OPD] syndrome).

TRINUCLEOTIDE REPEAT DISORDERS

Some genetic disorders are caused by a phenomenon known as *anticipation*. Anticipation occurs when a trinucleotide repeat expands during meiosis, resulting in a gene passed from generation to generation with a larger and larger number of triplet repeats. A larger number of repeats is associated with phenotypic expression of the condition; typically, the larger the number of repeats, the more severe the condition. More than a dozen diseases are known to result from triplet repeat expansion, including autosomal dominant disorders such as Huntington disease and myotonic dystrophy, as well as Friedreich ataxia, an autosomal recessive disorder.

Ethics in Action!

Huntington disease is an autosomal dominant with three nucleotides (CAG) repeats that increase with each generation. This leads to an ethical challenge. Does the patient want to know of this inheritance, because it eventually leads to disease presentation and worsens with every generation as there are expanded repeats each generation? Should the patient have children? Should IVF with preimplantation genetic diagnosis (PGD) be advised?

Fragile X syndrome is an X-linked recessive disorder that exhibits anticipation. This condition is the most common form of inherited intellectual disability, second only to Down syndrome. The *FMRI gene* is responsible for making *fragile X mental retardation protein (FMRP)*, which facilitates communication between nerve cells in the brain. It is caused by an increased number of CGG trinucleotide repeats in the

FMR1 gene DNA, located at a "fragile site" on the long arm of the X chromosome. This mutation affects how the body makes FMRP; it causes the body to make only a little bit or none of the protein, which can cause the symptoms of Fragile X. The normal number of these three nucleotides (CGG) repeats is up to 60. Individuals with a repeat number ranging between 60 and 200 have a *premutation* allele, meaning that the copy number can increase during maternal (but not paternal) meiosis. If the CGG repeat number increases to over 200, the individual (particularly hemizygous males) can have fragile X syndrome. Approximately one-third of females with over 200 CGG repeats will be affected with fragile X syndrome, one-third will have mild developmental or learning disabilities, and one-third will have no symptoms at all.

MULTIFACTORIAL INHERITANCE

Many common congenital malformations do not follow a clear pattern of Mendelian inheritance. Examples include cleft palate, heart defect, spina bifida, dislocated hips, clubfoot, and pyloric stenosis. They are generally caused by an interaction of many genes and environmental factors and are considered to have *multifactorial* or *polygenic* inheritance. In multifactorial inheritance, the following occurs:

- The risk of recurrence depends on the incidence of the disorder and is greatest among close relatives. It decreases with distance of relationship but is highest when multiple family members are affected.
- The malformations may vary from mild to severe but the more severe the defect, the greater number of causative genes and the higher the risk for relatives.
- There is often unequal sex incidence with a higher risk for relatives of a patient of the sex in which the condition is less common. For example, pyloric stenosis is more common in males, and brothers of an affected female are at higher risk than brothers of an affected male.

Although most congenital malformations are multifactorial, a careful family history should always be taken because, occasionally, cleft lip and palate, certain congenital heart defects, and other malformations can also be inherited as autosomal dominant or recessive traits. Other disorders thought to be within the multifactorial inheritance group are diabetes, hypertension, some heart diseases, and mental illness.

Prenatal Diagnostic Tests

Every pregnancy has a 3 to 5% risk of resulting in a neonate with a birth defect, chromosome abnormality, genetic disease, or developmental disability. Family-planning counseling has become a major responsibility of professional nurses. To be effective counselors, nurses need to have the most current knowledge available concerning prenatal testing options. In light of the philosophy of preventive healthcare, information on what data can be obtained prenatally should be made available to all couples who are expecting a baby or who are contemplating pregnancy. Appropriate counseling should occur before any prenatal screening or diagnostic testing is done as it is essential that the couple be completely informed of the known or potential risks. The reasons to accept or decline testing can be very personal and nurses should strive to support their patients' decision making without passing judgment. Sometimes following **prenatal diagnosis** (detection of anatomic and physiologic problems in the fetus before birth) a couple may decide to interrupt the pregnancy. Even when termination is not an option, prenatal diagnosis can give parents an opportunity to prepare for the birth of a child with special needs, to contact other families with children with similar problems, to work with specialists to develop a treatment plan, and to contact support services before the birth.

Screening and invasive diagnostic testing for chromosome abnormalities should be available to all women regardless of maternal age (ACOG & SMFM, 2016b). Women should be counseled regarding the differences between screening and invasive diagnostic testing. Screening tests are designed to gather information about the risk that the pregnancy could have specific chromosome abnormalities or open spina bifida. Prenatal diagnostic techniques, such as amniocentesis and chorionic villus sampling (CVS) (discussed later in the chapter), obtain cells from the pregnancy to rule out or diagnose a chromosome abnormality or certain genetic disorders and are associated with a small risk of pregnancy complications, including miscarriage.

GENETIC ULTRASOUND

Ultrasound may be used to assess the fetus for genetic or congenital problems. With ultrasound, one can visualize the fetal head for abnormalities in size, shape, and structure. (For a detailed discussion of ultrasound technology, see Chapter 16.) Craniospinal defects (anencephaly, microcephaly, hydrocephalus), gastrointestinal malformations (omphalocele, gastroschisis), renal malformations (dysplasia or obstruction), and skeletal malformations (caudal regression, conjoined twins) are only some of the disorders that can be diagnosed in utero by ultrasound. Screening by ultrasound for congenital anomalies is generally done at 18 to 22 weeks of gestation, when fetal structures have completed development.

First-trimester screening for chromosome abnormalities is widely available by measuring the fetal nuchal translucency between 11 and 13 weeks. The nuchal translucency is a fluid-filled space at the back of the fetal neck. An increased amount of fluid is associated with an increased risk for chromosome abnormalities, birth defects, genetic syndromes, and poor pregnancy outcome—the larger the nuchal translucency, the higher the risk for abnormalities. The nuchal translucency should only be measured by a specifically trained sonographer or physician.

MATERNAL SERUM SCREENING

Measuring specific hormones and proteins in the maternal serum during the first and/or second trimester can determine the risk for Down syndrome, trisomy 18, or open spina bifida. In the first trimester, the nuchal translucency measurement is often added to improve the detection rate for Down syndrome and trisomy 18. Detection and false-positive rates differ depending on the type of screening test that is performed and may also differ depending on the laboratory that performs the screening. The gestational age window for the various types of tests also differs. Examples of maternal serum screening tests include the quadruple marker screen, first-trimester screening with nuchal translucency, and combined first- and second-trimester screening, often referred to as the *sequential screen* or the *integrated screen*. (For more information about these tests, see Chapter 16.)

PRENATAL CELL-FREE DNA SCREENING

Also known as *noninvasive prenatal testing* (*NIPT*) or *noninvasive prenatal screening (NIPS)*, prenatal cell-free DNA testing screens for specific fetal chromosome abnormalities by measuring circulating **cell-free DNA (cfDNA)** (DNA that circulates in a person's blood or plasma) in maternal blood. Approximately 3 to 13% of the circulating DNA in a woman's plasma is derived from the placenta and can be detected as early as 9 to 10 weeks of gestation. All laboratories offering cfDNA screening assess risk for Down syndrome, trisomy 18, and trisomy 13. Some laboratories also offer screening for sex chromosome abnormalities and other rare aneuploidies (Gregg, Skotko, Benkendorf, et al., 2016).

Clinical Tip

Nurses counseling patients about cfDNA screening should be aware of which conditions are screened for by their laboratory as well as the sensitivity and specificity quoted for each condition.

Although cfDNA screening is the most sensitive screening option for Down syndrome, trisomy 18, and trisomy 13, it is not meant to replace diagnostic testing such as chorionic villus sampling (CVS) or amniocentesis. False-positive and false-negative results are possible and patients should not take irreversible action based on screening results alone. Limitations of cfDNA screening include lack of data on twin gestations or pregnancies with a vanishing twin and concern for no-call results (test failures) and false-positive results due to maternal or placental mosaicism. Patients with abnormal, no-call, or complex results, or those with other factors suggestive of a chromosome abnormality, should receive genetic counseling and be given the option of standard confirmatory diagnostic testing (Gregg et al., 2016). There are several commercial laboratories currently offering cfDNA screening, each with their own name brand.

GENETIC AMNIOCENTESIS

A major method of prenatal diagnosis is genetic amniocentesis (Figure 10–12A). This procedure obtains amniotic fluid containing amniocytes from the developing fetus for chromosome analysis, biochemical testing, or other genetic testing. A genetic amniocentesis is generally performed between 15 and 16 weeks' gestation, although it can be performed later, up to about 20 weeks. Early amniocentesis (before 14 weeks' gestation) is not recommended due to the increased risk for complications. The risk for major complications, including infection and procedure-related pregnancy loss, is thought to be less than 0.1 to 0.3% if performed by experienced healthcare providers (ACOG & SMFM, 2016a). Additional risks, although rare, include failure to obtain adequate sample, culture failure, and maternal cell contamination. See Chapter 16 for a discussion of the amniocentesis procedure and *Clinical Skill 16–2: Assisting During Amniocentesis*.

CHORIONIC VILLUS SAMPLING

Chorionic villus sampling (CVS) is a technique that obtains chorionic villi tissue (cytotrophoblast) from the placenta either transabdominally or transcervically depending on the location of

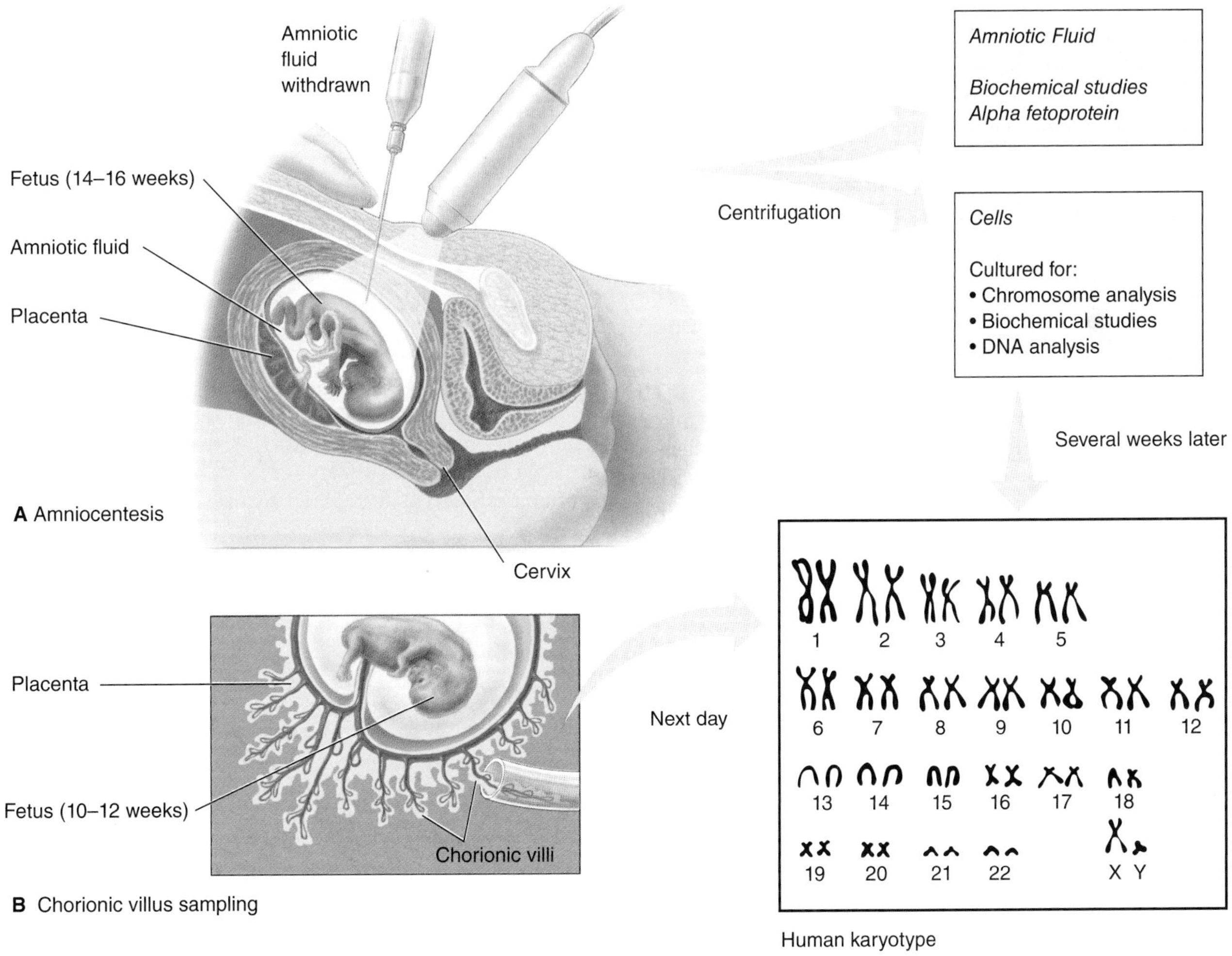

Figure 10–12 A. Genetic amniocentesis for prenatal diagnosis is typically done between 15 and 20 weeks' gestation. B. Chorionic villus sampling is done from week 10 through week 13 of gestation, and the cells are cultured and karyotyped.

the placenta (Figure 10–12B). The diagnostic capability is similar to that of amniocentesis, although placental mosaicism occurs in 0.83% of all cases, prompting further testing and follow-up (Mardy & Wapner, 2016). However, diagnostic information is available earlier in gestation as the procedure can be performed at 10 to 13 weeks' gestation. The risk for minor complications, such as vaginal spotting or bleeding, may occur in up to 32% of patients undergoing transcervical CVS (lower if the procedure is performed transabdominally), but the risk of major complications such as infection and procedure-related pregnancy loss is estimated to be less than 0.5% (ACOG & SMFM, 2016a). Like amniocentesis, rare additional risks include failure to obtain adequate sample, culture failure, and maternal cell contamination. Limb-reduction defects have been associated with CVS, although the risk is not increased over the general population if the procedure is performed after 10 weeks' gestation. See Chapter 16 for a discussion of the CVS procedure.

Although ACOG and SMFM guidelines state that all women should be offered invasive prenatal diagnosis, common indications for genetic amniocentesis or CVS include:

- ***Maternal age 35 or older:*** The risk of having a live-born baby with a chromosome problem increases with maternal age. For example, the risk for any chromosome abnormality at delivery for a 35-year-old woman is approximately 1 in 200 (0.5%), but increases to 1 in 20 (5%) by age 45 (ACOG & SMFM, 2016a). See *Case Study: Melissa Bond-James*.
- ***Previous pregnancy with a chromosomal abnormality:*** Couples who have had a pregnancy with a chromosome abnormality have approximately a 1% recurrence risk or their age-related risk, whichever is higher.
- ***Parent with a balanced translocation:*** These couples are at an increased risk to have conceptions with an unbalanced translocation. Depending on the chromosomes involved in the translocation, there may be an increased risk for pregnancy loss or a viable offspring with congenital anomalies and/or intellectual disability. For example, a woman who carries a balanced 14:21 translocation has a risk of approximately 10 to 15% that her children will have Down syndrome; if the father is a carrier, there is a 2 to 5% risk.
- ***Mother carrying an X-linked disease:*** For families in which the woman is a known or possible carrier of an X-linked disorder, such as Duchenne muscular dystrophy or hemophilia A or B, the risk of having an affected male fetus is 50%. Amniocytes can be cultured for DNA testing to determine if the fetus is affected.
- ***Both parents carrying an autosomal recessive disease:*** When both parents are carriers of an autosomal recessive disease, there is a 25% risk in *each pregnancy* that the fetus will be affected. Amniocytes can be cultured for DNA testing to determine if the fetus is affected.
- ***Family history of neural tube defects:*** Genetic amniocentesis is available to couples at risk for neural tube defects such as spina bifida or anencephaly. The diagnosis is made by measuring amniotic fluid alpha-fetoprotein (AFP) and a neurotransmitter called *acetylcholinesterase*. Neural tube defects are usually multifactorial traits.
- ***Fetus with major or minor anomalies on ultrasound:*** Major structural anomalies or minor markers associated with an increased risk for chromosome abnormalities or other genetic disorders may be diagnosed by ultrasound. Depending on the ultrasound finding, patients may benefit from genetic testing by amniocentesis.
- ***Women with positive serum screening results, including cell-free DNA screening (cfDNA):*** Because these are screening tests, confirmatory testing through amniocentesis or CVS is indicated to confirm or rule out a diagnosis.

PERCUTANEOUS UMBILICAL BLOOD SAMPLING

Percutaneous umbilical blood sampling (*PUBS*) is a technique in which blood is obtained from the umbilical cord during pregnancy. Obtaining fetal blood cells allows for rapid diagnosis of chromosome abnormalities, infection, or workup and transfusion for fetal anemia. Under ultrasound guidance, a needle is inserted into the fetal umbilical vein and blood is withdrawn for testing. Blood or medications can also be infused for treatment. The risk for pregnancy complications, including fetal bradycardia or intrauterine fetal demise, is higher than with CVS or amniocentesis (3%), although many of these pregnancies are already at very high risk due to hydrops (Bigelow et al., 2016).

PRODUCTS OF CONCEPTION TESTING

It is estimated that half of all recognized miscarriages and 5% of stillbirths are due to a cytogenetic abnormality (ACOG & SMFM, 2016a). Chromosome analysis can be performed on products of conception (POCs) obtained after a miscarriage, termination of pregnancy, or delivery of a stillborn fetus. Because karyotype requires metaphase cells, there is a high incidence of culture failure after miscarriage or fetal demise. Chromosomal microarray is often preferred as it does not require cultured cells, although

CASE STUDY: Melissa Bond-James

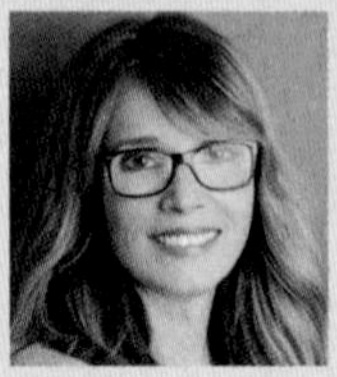

SOURCE: Kinga/Shutterstock

Melissa and her wife, Nancy, underwent donor insemination (DI) to achieve pregnancy. They have no intention of terminating their pregnancy if there is a genetic defect, but they are concerned that Melissa is at a higher risk due to her age, and Melissa is considering undergoing genetic testing.

Questions to Ponder

Why are women over the age of 35 at a greater risk for genetic anomalies in their fetuses? What diagnostic procedure(s) should the nurse anticipate needing to provide patient education and counseling for Melissa and Nancy?

it is less likely to detect certain types of polyploidies (Ozawa et al., 2016).

> "When the nurse on the mother-baby unit first told me the doctors were concerned my son had Down syndrome, I was shocked. I had had a blood test for Down syndrome earlier in the pregnancy and was told the results were normal, plus there were never any concerns on my ultrasounds. I called my OB and found out that my blood test results were below the cut-off and not considered abnormal, but my risk was four times higher than expected for a woman my age. No one had explained that to me during pregnancy; they just told me my results were normal. I think if I had known I was at an increased risk, I may have asked to speak with a high-risk pregnancy doctor or even considered an amniocentesis. I wouldn't have ended the pregnancy, but I think I would have been better prepared emotionally for my son's birth."

●○● NURSING MANAGEMENT

For the Woman with Possible Risk Factors for Genetic Disorders

During annual exams and other clinical appointments, interview all women of childbearing age to determine if there is any family history or other risk factors for genetic disorders. Collection of family history information is one of the most important parts of genetic assessment and can provide a unique opportunity to connect to patients (Mahon, 2016). The National Society of Genetic Counselors (NSGC) has developed standardized criteria for the graphic presentation of family history information known as a *genetic pedigree* (Figure 10–13). Nurses should be competent in their ability to construct and utilize a genetic pedigree to develop a potential plan of care, educate patients, and assess the need for genetic counseling referral (Camak, 2016).

A three-generation pedigree can assess if couples are at risk for having offspring with inherited disorders and should include medical history information such as current ages, age at death and cause of death, age at diagnosis of medical conditions or genetic disease, other relevant health information regarding significant medical problems or surgeries, relationships between siblings and children (differentiating between half or full), pregnancy complications with gestational age noted (e.g., miscarriage, stillbirth, termination of pregnancy), history of infertility, ethnic background/country of origin, and whether or not there is consanguinity (noting how they are related by blood). There are several "red flags" suggestive of a genetic condition or predisposition to an inherited disease that might be identified, and these patients should be encouraged to consider genetic counseling before discontinuation of contraception. Due to improvements in medical care, advances in the understanding of genetics, and progress in reproductive technologies, many women with genetic conditions are able to achieve pregnancy. These women will require a multidisciplinary approach from preconception through the postpartum period including careful counseling regarding genetic condition–associated risks during pregnancy, risk assessment for offspring, and maternal medical management (ACOG, 2017). See *Key Facts to Remember: Couples Who May Benefit from Preconceptual or Prenatal Genetic Counseling.*

Genetic Evaluation

Depending on the outcome of genetic counseling or for other factors, a couple may opt to undergo genetic evaluation. The following sections discuss methods of genetic evaluation.

Key Facts To Remember

Couples Who May Benefit from Preconceptual or Prenatal Genetic Counseling

- Women age 35 or over at time of birth
- Couples in which one member has a balanced chromosome translocation
- Personal or family history of known or suspected genetic disorder (e.g., cystic fibrosis, hemophilia A or B, Duchenne muscular dystrophy)
- Couples with a previous pregnancy or child with a chromosomal abnormality
- Couples in which one or both partners are known carriers for a recessive genetic disorder
- Personal or family history of birth defects and/or global developmental disabilities
- Ethnic groups at increased risk for specific disorders (see *Developing Cultural Competence: Genetic Screening Recommendations for Various Ethnic Groups*)
- Couples with a history of two or more first-trimester spontaneous abortions
- Women with an abnormal maternal serum screening test including cell-free DNA screening
- Women with a teratogenic risk secondary to an exposure or maternal health condition (e.g., diabetes, seizure disorder)

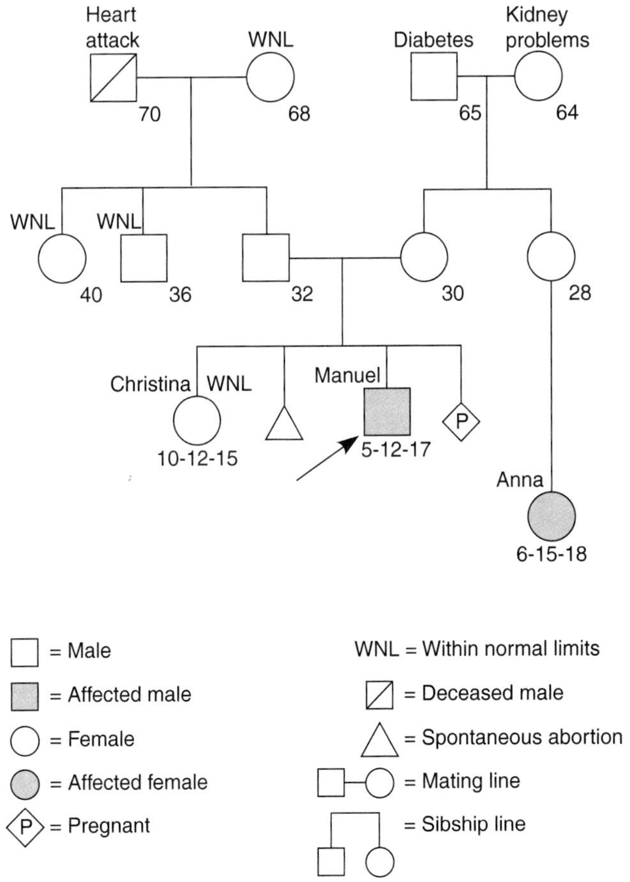

Figure 10–13 Screening pedigree. Arrow indicates the nearest family member affected with the disorder being investigated. Numbers refer to the ages or birth dates of family members.

Professionalism in Practice Prenatal Screening

- Remember that prenatal screening and diagnosis are an optional part of routine prenatal care and women have the right to decline.
- Present options to patients using a nondirective manner. *Nondirective counseling* is a technique designed to allow patients to talk through their options and reach the decision that is best for themselves or their families with a minimum of direction from the person serving as their counselor.
- Give patients accurate, up-to-date information about the various prenatal screening and diagnostic testing options. Remain impartial and do not recommend any specific course of action.
- Be aware of the language you use when discussing these options with patients. For example, in discussing prenatal screening for Down syndrome, terms such as *handicapped* or *retarded* should be replaced with *developmentally disabled.* Use the words *risk for*, or consider using the terms *chance of* or *possibility of.*

Ethics in Action!

The Human Genome Project has had significant implications for the identification and management of inherited disorders. However, concerns have been voiced about ethical considerations with genetic testing. What guidelines are needed to protect children and families so that genetic testing does not lead to discrimination in future employment or health insurance? Who should be tested for genetic diseases, and who should have access to the results? Is the Genetic Information Nondiscrimination Act (GINA) of 2008 enough to protect individuals from genetic discrimination in health insurance and employment?

CARRIER SCREENING FOR RECESSIVE DISORDERS

Carrier screening (genetic testing to see if a person is a carrier for specific autosomal recessive diseases) for individual conditions based on severity, race or ethnicity, prevalence, carrier frequency, and detection rates have been considered part of prenatal care for many years. It is generally agreed that conditions should be relatively severe in nature or show evidence that early detection can impact treatment and outcome. Currently, many professional societies recommend screening for specific conditions depending on assessment of ancestry (see *Developing Cultural Competence: Genetic Screening Recommendations for Various Ethnic Groups*). Ethnicity-based carrier screening requires patients to correctly assess their racial/ethnic background, which impacts the detection rates and residual risks for the disorders on the panel. In addition, national organizations appear to differ on the conditions recommended for screening (Haque et al., 2016). For example, ACOG recommends panethnic cystic fibrosis carrier screening, whereas the American College of Medical Genetics (ACMG) recommends both cystic fibrosis and spinal muscular atrophy carrier screening (Haque et al., 2016).

Newer technology allows for efficient screening of a large number of conditions simultaneously and has prompted the development of *expanded carrier screening (ECS)* panels. These panels include additional conditions for which carrier screening in the general population is not currently recommended but may provide more comprehensive screening for our increasingly multiethnic society. With ECS, all individuals are offered screening for the same set of conditions regardless of race or ethnicity. These panels can contain screening for more than 100 autosomal recessive genetic conditions, although some conditions on the panel may be inherited in an X-linked or autosomal dominant manner. Although it may not be practical to fully educate patients about each condition on the panel, individuals receiving pretest counseling should be aware that some of the conditions have varying degrees of severity that may not be predicted based on genetic testing alone. Patients should also be aware that the disease prevalence, detection rates, and residual risk estimations may not be reliable because of rarity of the conditions on the panel and that screening panels may change over time (Edwards et al., 2015).

Residual risk is an important concept for both patients and healthcare providers to understand as negative results reduce the likelihood that an individual is a carrier of a particular condition but cannot eliminate it. Nurses caring for families in which one member of the couple is a known carrier of an autosomal recessive disorder but the other member has tested negative should be aware of the remaining, or residual, risk for affected offspring. Pretest and posttest genetic counseling is an important component of any carrier screening program.

PREIMPLANTATION GENETIC TESTING

Couples who have difficulty conceiving a child may turn to assisted reproductive technologies (ART) such as in vitro fertilization (IVF), in which a woman's ovaries are stimulated by a combination of medications, one or more oocytes are aspirated from her ovaries and fertilized in the laboratory, and then they are placed into her uterus after normal embryo development has begun.

Recent advances in micromanipulation allow a small number of cells to be removed from the embryo prior to implantation for genetic studies. **Preimplantation genetic diagnosis (PGD)** is a term used when a pregnancy is at risk for a detectable single gene disorder or chromosome abnormality and testing is performed to determine whether that mutation or unbalanced chromosomal complement has been passed to the embryo. *Preimplantation genetic screening (PGS)* is a term used when the embryos are screened for aneuploidy with the purpose of increasing the likelihood of a viable pregnancy with normal chromosomes. PGS is most often recommended when there is advanced maternal age, recurrent miscarriage, repeated IVF implantation failure, previous pregnancy with aneuploidy, and severe male factor infertility (Garcia-Herrero et al., 2016).

A PGD/PGS cycle requires several steps such as ovarian stimulation, follicular aspiration, oocyte retrieval, intracytoplasmic injection of processed sperm, culture of fertilized oocytes until biopsy can be performed, testing of the biopsied cells, and, finally, transfer of a genetically normal embryo. There are several strategies for biopsy including polar body biopsy, blastomere biopsy of day 3 embryos, and blastocyst biopsy of day 5 embryos. Blastocyst biopsy appears to be the preferred method as it allows for a large quantity of cells (4–10) to be removed from the extra-embryonic trophectoderm. This leaves the inner cell mass that will become the fetus untouched and increases the accuracy by testing a larger number of cells. The entire PGD/PGS cycle can take several weeks. Results of genetic screening or testing on the preimplantation embryos vary from 24 hours to up to 2 weeks. Sometimes unaffected embryos may still be transferred during the required biologic window of time

Developing Cultural Competence Genetic Screening Recommendations for Various Ethnic Groups

BACKGROUND OF POPULATION AT RISK	DISORDER	CARRIER SCREENING	PRENATAL DIAGNOSIS
Ashkenazi Jewish, French-Canadian, Cajun	Tay-Sachs disease	Serum hexosaminidase A levels or DNA mutation analysis	Chorionic villus sampling (CVS) or amniocentesis for hexosaminidase A assay or DNA mutation analysis
Ashkenazi Jewish	Cystic fibrosis, Canavan disease, familial dysautonomia, several other disorders	DNA mutation analysis	CVS or amniocentesis for DNA mutation analysis
African; Hispanic from Caribbean, Central America, or South America; Middle Eastern; Egyptian; Asian Indian	Hemoglobinopathies, particularly sickle cell disease	Hemoglobin electrophoresis	CVS or amniocentesis for DNA mutation analysis
Greek, Italian	Hemoglobinopathies, particularly beta-thalassemia	Mean corpuscular volume less than 80%; confirmatory hemoglobin electrophoresis	CVS or amniocentesis for DNA mutation analysis
Southeast Asian (Vietnamese, Laotian, Cambodian), Filipino	Hemoglobinopathies, particularly alpha-thalassemia	Mean corpuscular volume less than 80%; confirmatory hemoglobin electrophoresis	CVS or amniocentesis for DNA mutation analysis or gene deletion studies
Caucasian (northern European, Celtic population), Ashkenazi Jewish	Cystic fibrosis	DNA mutation analysis	CVS or amniocentesis for DNA mutation analysis

without the need for cryopreservation ("fresh" transfer), but often the embryos are cryopreserved using a process called *vitrification* and transferred during a subsequent cycle ("frozen" transfer) (Garcia-Herrero et al., 2016). Both PGD and PGS can produce false-positive and false-negative results and prenatal diagnostic testing to confirm the results is recommended once a pregnancy is achieved. PGD and PGS raise several ethical issues, including:

- *Identification of couples at risk.* There is a need for criteria that identify couples at risk for diseases that constitute significant hardship and suffering. Should all IVF centers offer, or require that patients undergo, expanded carrier screening or other genetic testing prior to treatment?
- *Availability of and access to centers providing PGD.* Should society provide access for those at risk for genetic transfer of disease but without the financial resources to pay for the services?
- *Analysis of embryos for sex chromosome testing when a genetic disorder carried on the sex chromosomes is suspected.* In X-linked diseases, this may mean selecting against the embryo with the Y chromosome.
- *Identification of late-onset disease or cancer predisposition.* Couples may wish to choose to implant embryos that do not carry these markers.
- *Effect of removing cells from the embryo, including possible destruction of the embryo or effect on the offspring.*
- *Selection for nonmedical reasons and potential concern of eugenics and "designer babies."*

Ethics in Action!

How do you respond to a couple requesting preimplantation genetic testing for family balancing or gender selection? What if the couple faces significant societal pressure and stigma based on cultural values?

See *Developing Cultural Competence: Iraqi Childbirth Customs.*

Developing Cultural Competence Iraqi Childbirth Customs

"My sister, she did not have baby for very, very long time, you see. This is very sad where I am from [Iraq]. Her husband's family wanted him to leave her and we so feared he would. Then my sister became pregnant and it was very nice, we all so happy, you see. Then I learned my sister birthed a baby girl and I cried and cried for a week. My mother cried, too, so sad all this time no baby come and then finally to have a girl. I still feel sad for her."

Source: Excerpt from author's interview with an Iraqi woman on childbirth customs in Iraq

POSTNATAL DIAGNOSIS

Questions concerning genetic disorders (cause, treatment, and prognosis) are most often first discussed in the newborn nursery or during the baby's first few months of life. When a child is born with anomalies, has a stormy neonatal period, or does not progress as expected, a genetic evaluation may be warranted. Accurate diagnosis and an optimal treatment plan includes a complete and detailed history to determine whether the problem is prenatal (congenital), postnatal, or familial in origin; a thorough physical and dysmorphology examination by a trained clinical geneticist; and laboratory analysis, which may include various forms of genetic testing.

Referral. A referral to an outpatient genetics clinic or genetic counselor is advised for newborns/infants and children with major or minor congenital abnormalities, dysmorphic features, global developmental disabilities, autism spectrum disorder with intellectual disability, known inherited conditions including metabolic disorders, and known or suspected chromosome abnormalities.

Initial Session. During the initial session, the genetic counselor gathers additional information about the pregnancy, the affected child's growth and development, and the family members' understanding of the problem. The counselor also elicits information concerning ethnic background and family origin. Many genetic disorders are more common among certain ethnic groups or in particular geographic areas. (See *Developing Cultural Competence: Genetic Screening Recommendations for Various Ethnic Groups.*)

Generally, the child is given a physical examination by a physician who has trained as a clinical geneticist. Other family members may also be examined. If any laboratory tests, such as chromosomal analysis, genetic testing, metabolic studies, or viral titers, are indicated, they are performed at this time.

Follow-Up Counseling. When all the data have been carefully examined and analyzed, the family may return for a follow-up visit. At this time the parents are given all the information available, including:

- Medical facts
- Diagnosis
- Probable course of the disorder and any available management
- Inheritance pattern for this particular family
- Risk of recurrence and the options or alternatives for dealing with recurrence.

See *Professionalism in Practice: Prenatally and Postnatally Diagnosed Conditions Awareness Act.*

Professionalism in Practice Prenatally and Postnatally Diagnosed Conditions Awareness Act

The Prenatally and Postnatally Diagnosed Conditions Awareness Act (S.1810) was signed into law in 2008. This law requires that medical providers give parents accurate, updated, and scientific information regarding their child's diagnosis, prognosis, treatment, and life expectancy. Many states are also implementing similar laws for licensed physicians and nurses. Nurses are often an important source of information and support when a prenatal or postnatal diagnosis of a genetic condition or birth defect is made and should be aware of both state and federal laws.

●○● NURSING MANAGEMENT

For the Family Undergoing Genetic Evaluation and Counseling

The nurse has a key role in preventing recurrence. One cannot expect a couple who has just learned that their child has a birth defect or genetic condition to take in any information concerning future risks. However, the couple should never be kept from genetic counseling for so long that they conceive another affected child because of lack of information. Genetic counseling is the process of helping people understand and adapt to the medical, psychologic, and familial implications of genetic contributions to disease (National Society of Genetic Counselors [NSGC], 2016). After genetic counseling, the nurse with the appropriate knowledge of genetics is in an ideal position to help families review what has been discussed during the sessions and to answer any additional questions they might have. When working with a family undergoing genetic counseling, you may wish to attend the counseling sessions. Because you have already established a rapport with the couple, you can act as a liaison between the family and the genetic counselor. Hearing directly what the genetic counselor says helps you clarify issues for the family, which in turn helps them formulate questions. See *Key Facts to Remember: Nursing Responsibilities in Genetic Evaluation and Counseling.*

Key Facts To Remember

Nursing Responsibilities in Genetic Evaluation and Counseling

- Identify families at risk for genetic problems.
- Determine how the genetic problem is perceived and what information is desired before proceeding.
- Assist families in acquiring accurate information about the specific problem.
- Act as liaison between the family and the genetic counselor.
- Assist the family in understanding and dealing with information received.
- Provide information on support groups.
- Aid families in coping with the diagnosis.
- Provide information about known genetic factors.
- Ensure continuity of nursing care to the family.

Nurses are ideally situated to educate parents about *newborn screening* as they often perform the screening and are key in implementing follow-up and quality improvement initiatives (Hom & Martin, 2016). The United States Department of Health and Human Services (2017) has implemented a Recommended Universal Screening Panel (RUSP) of 34 core conditions and 26 secondary conditions to serve as a helpful guide for states performing newborn screening. Core conditions are those that newborn screening is specifically designed to identify. A disorder is classified as a core condition if it has a specific and sensitive test available to identify it, has well-understood health outcomes, has an available and effective treatment, and could impact future reproductive decisions for the family. The core conditions on the RUSP include several metabolic disorders, hemoglobinopathies, cystic fibrosis, severe combined immunodeficiencies, congenital hypothyroidism, congenital adrenal hyperplasia, hearing loss, and critical congenital heart disease. Secondary conditions are those that are detected incidentally or when confirmatory testing for a core condition is performed.

Because newborn screening is generally a state-level program, it is your responsibility to know what conditions are screened for in your state and what methods are used. By understanding why screening is important, how it is performed, recommendations for follow-up for positive screens, and the limitations of screening, you can advocate for families and improve early detection for babies born with significant medical conditions. Most states require that a nurse or other healthcare professional obtain a few drops of blood from the baby's heel and place it on a specialized filter paper to be sent to a laboratory for analysis. Hearing is assessed by automated auditory brainstem response (AABR) or otoacoustic emissions (OE), in which sounds (tones or clicks) are played through small earphones and responses are automatically measured. Screening for critical congenital heart disease (CCHD) is performed using pulse oximetry. To find out more about newborn screening in your state, visit the website of *Baby's First Test*, which is funded by the Health Resource and Service Administration (HRSA) of the U.S. Department of Health and Human Services (2018). See Chapter 28 for more detailed information on newborn screening.

Focus Your Study

- In autosomal dominant disorders, an affected parent has a 50% chance of having an affected child. Such disorders equally affect both males and females. The characteristic presentation will vary in each individual with the gene. Some of the common autosomal dominant inherited disorders are Huntington disease, polycystic kidney disease, and neurofibromatosis (von Recklinghausen disease).
- Autosomal recessive disorders are characterized by both parents being carriers; each offspring has a 25% chance of having the disease, a 25% chance of not being affected, and a 50% chance of being a carrier. Males and females are equally affected. Some autosomal recessive inheritance disorders are cystic fibrosis, phenylketonuria (PKU), galactosemia, sickle cell disease, Tay-Sachs disease, and most metabolic disorders.
- X-linked recessive disorders are characterized by no male-to-male transmission; effects limited to males; a 50% chance that a carrier mother will pass the abnormal gene to her sons; a 50% chance that her daughters will be carriers; and a 100% chance that daughters of affected fathers will be carriers. Common X-linked recessive disorders are hemophilia, some forms of color blindness, and Duchenne muscular dystrophy.
- Multifactorial inheritance disorders include cleft lip and palate, spina bifida, dislocated hips, clubfoot, and pyloric stenosis.
- Some genetic conditions that can currently be diagnosed prenatally are neural tube and cranial defects, renal malformations, hemophilia, fragile X syndrome, thalassemia, cystic fibrosis, and many inborn errors of metabolism such as Tay-Sachs disease. This list expands daily as new technology allows more conditions to be detected.
- The chief tools of prenatal diagnosis are ultrasound, maternal serum screening, cell-free DNA screening, amniocentesis, chorionic villus sampling, and percutaneous umbilical blood sampling.
- Based on sound knowledge about common genetic problems, the nurse should prepare the family for counseling and act as a resource person during and after the counseling sessions. Many nurses with advanced training are entering the field of genetic counseling.

References

American College of Obstetricians and Gynecologists (ACOG) Committee on Genetics (2015, reaffirmed 2017). Identification and referral of maternal genetic conditions in pregnancy (ACOG Committee Opinion No. 643). *Obstetrics & Gynecology, 126*(4), e49–51.

American College of Obstetricians and Gynecologists (ACOG) Committee on Genetics and the Society for Maternal Fetal Medicine Publications Committee. (2016a). Prenatal diagnostic testing for genetic disorders (Practice Bulletin No.162). *Obstetrics & Gynecology, 127*(5), 976–978.

American College of Obstetricians and Gynecologists (ACOG) Committee on Genetics and the Society for Maternal Fetal Medicine Publications Committee. (2016b). Screening for fetal aneuploidy (Practice Bulletin No.163). *Obstetrics & Gynecology, 127*(5), 976–981.

Bigelow, C. A., Cinelli, C. M., Little, S. E., Benson, C. B., Frates, M. C., & Wilkins-Haug, L. E. (2016). Percutaneous umbilical blood sampling: Current trends and outcomes. *European Journal of Obstetrics & Gynecology and Reproductive Biology, 200*, 98–101. DOI: 10.1016/j.ejogrb.2016.02.038

Bornstein, E., Berger, S., Cheung, S. W., Maliszewski, K. T., Patel, A., Pursley, A. N., . . . Divon, M. Y. (2016). Universal prenatal chromosomal microarray analysis: Additive value and clinical dilemmas in fetuses with normal karyotypes. *American Journal of Perinatology, 34*(4), 340–348. DOI:10.1055/s-0036-1586501

Camak, D. J. (2016). Increasing importance of genetics in nursing. *Nurse Education Today, 44*, 86–91. DOI: 10.1016/j.nedt.2016.05.018

Edwards, J. G., Feldman, G., Goldberg, J., Gregg, A. R., Norton, M. E., Rose, N. C., . . . Watson, M. S. (2015). Expanded carrier screening in reproductive medicine—points to consider. *Obstetrics & Gynecology, 125*(3), 653–662.

Garcia-Herrero, S., Cervero, A., Mateu, E., Mir, P., Poo, M. E., Rodrigo, L., . . . Rubio, C. (2016). Genetic analysis of human preimplantation embryos. *Current Topics in Developmental Biology, 120*, 421–447.

Gregg, A. R., Skotko, B. G., Benkendorf, J. L., Monaghan, K. G., Bajaj, K., Best, R. G., . . . Watson, M. S. (2016). Noninvasive prenatal screening for fetal aneuploidy, 2016 update: A position statement of the American College of Medical Genetics and Genomics. *Genetics in Medicine, 18*(10), 1056–1065. DOI:10.1038/gim.2016.97

Haque, I. S., Lazarin, G. A., Kang, P., Evans, E. A., Goldberg, J. D., & Wapner, R. J. (2016). Modeled fetal risk of genetic diseases identified by expanded carrier screening. *Journal of the American Medical Association, 316*(7), 734–742.

Hom, L. A., & Martin, G. R. (2016). Newborn critical congenital heart disease screening using pulse oximetry: Nursing aspects. *American Journal of Perinatology, 33*(11), 1072–1075.

Kapurubandara, S., Melov, S., Shalou, E., & Alahakoon, I., (2016). Consanguinity and associated perinatal outcomes, including stillbirth. *Australian and New Zealand Journal of Obstetrics and Gynaecology, 56*(6), 599–604. DOI:10.1111/ajo.12493

Mahon, S. M. (2016). The three-generation pedigree: A critical tool in cancer genetics care. *Oncology Nursing Forum, 43*(5), 655–660.

Mardy, A., & Wapner, R. (2016). Confined placental mosaicism and its impact on confirmation of NIPT results. *American Journal of Medical Genetics Part C, 172C*, 118–122.

National Society of Genetic Counselors (NSGC). (2016). *Students and prospective genetic counselors: What is genetic counseling?* Retrieved from https://www.nsgc.org/page/frequently-asked-questions-students#what

Nelson, K. E., Rosella, L. C., Mahant, S., & Guttmann, A. (2016). Survival and surgical interventions for children with trisomy 13 and 18. *Journal of the American Medical Association, 316*(4), 420–428. DOI: 10.1001/jama.2016.9819

Norton, M. E., Scoutt, L. M., & Feldstein, V. A. (2017). *Callen's ultrasonography in obstetrics and gynecology* (6th ed.). Philadelphia, PA: Elsevier.

Ozawa, N., Sago, H., Matsuoka, K., Maruyama, T., Migita, O., Aizu, Y., & Inazawa, J. (2016). Cytogenetic analysis of spontaneously discharged products of conception by array-based comparative genomic hybridization. *SpringerPlus*, *5*, 874.

Pierce, B. A. (2014). *Genetics: A conceptual approach* (5th ed.). New York, NY: W. H. Freeman.

U.S. Department of Health and Human Services, Advisory Committee on Heritable Disorder in Newborns and Children. (2017). *Recommendations to HHS Secretary with responses.* Retrieved from https://www.hrsa.gov/advisory-committees/heritable-disorders/recommendations-reports/index.html

U.S. Department of Health and Human Services. (2018). *Baby's First Test.* Retrieved from http://www.babysfirsttest.org

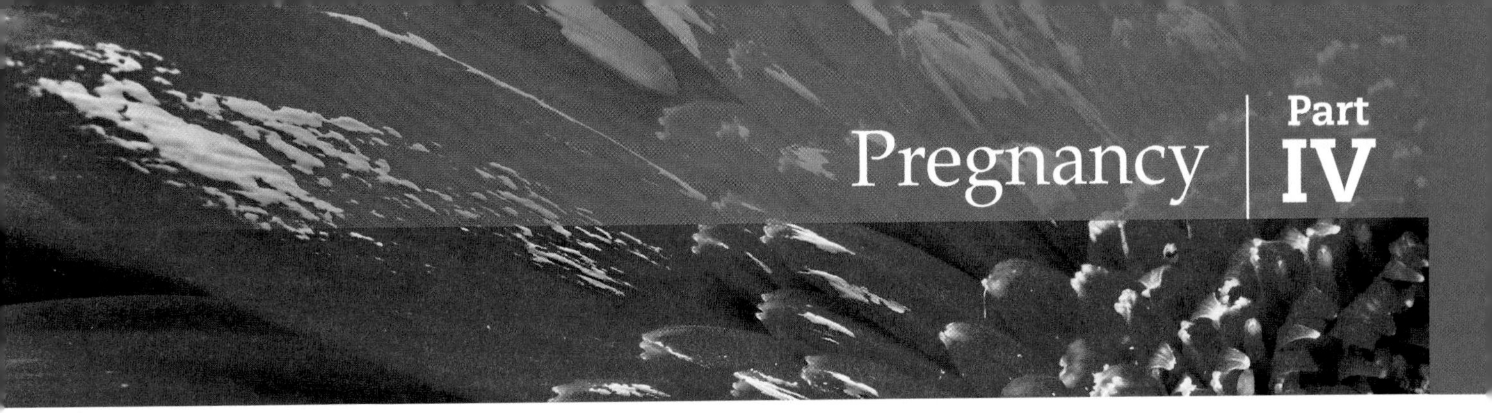

Chapter 11

Physical and Psychologic Changes of Pregnancy

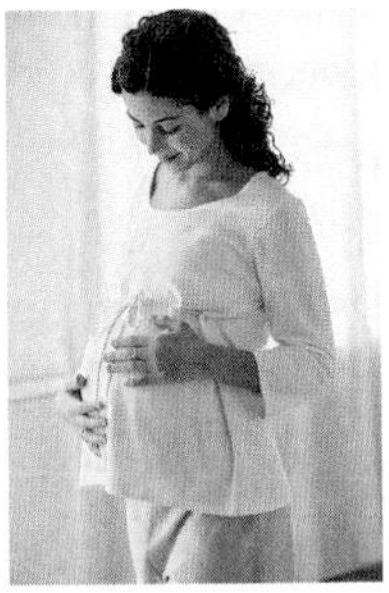

SOURCE: Blend Images/SuperStock.

The atmosphere of approval in which I was bathed—even by strangers on the street, it seemed—was like an aura I carried with me. . . . This is what women have always done.

—Adrienne Rich, *Of Woman Born*

Learning Outcomes

11.1 Identify the anatomic and physiologic changes that occur during pregnancy.

11.2 Relate the physiologic and anatomic changes that occur in the body systems during pregnancy to the signs and symptoms that develop in the woman.

11.3 Compare subjective (presumptive), objective (probable), and diagnostic (positive) changes of pregnancy.

11.4 Contrast the various types of pregnancy tests.

11.5 Discuss the emotional and psychologic changes that commonly occur in a woman, her partner, and her family during pregnancy.

11.6 Summarize cultural factors that may influence a family's response to pregnancy.

Healthy People 2020

MICH-6 Reduce maternal illness and complications due to pregnancy (complications during hospitalized labor and delivery)

MICH-10 Increase the proportion of pregnant women who receive early and adequate prenatal care

MICH-13 (Developmental) Increase the proportion of mothers who achieve a recommended weight gain during their pregnancies

Through modern technology and highly evolved research methods, we know a great deal about how pregnancy occurs and what happens to the fetus and the woman's body during gestation. No matter how much we learn about pregnancy and the changes that occur in the woman and in the developing fetus, it never ceases to amaze us. First, it is nothing short of a miracle that the union of two microscopic entities—an ovum and a sperm—can produce a living being. Second, the woman's body must undergo extraordinary physical changes to sustain a pregnancy. A pregnant woman's body changes in size and shape, and all her organ systems modify their functions to create an environment that protects and nurtures the growing fetus.

Pregnancy is divided into three trimesters, each approximately a 3-month period. Each trimester has its own predictable developments in both the fetus and the mother. This chapter describes both obvious and subtle physical and psychologic changes caused by pregnancy. It also discusses the various cultural factors that can affect a woman's well-being during pregnancy. Subsequent chapters build on this information in describing effective approaches to planning and providing care.

Anatomy and Physiology of Pregnancy

The changes that occur in the pregnant woman's body are caused by several factors. Many changes are the result of hormonal influences, some are caused by the growth of the fetus inside the uterus, and some are a result of the mother's physical adaptation to the changes that are occurring.

Reproductive System

Some of the most dramatic changes of pregnancy occur in the reproductive organs.

UTERUS

The changes in the uterus during pregnancy are phenomenal. Before pregnancy the uterus is a small, almost solid, inverted, fist-sized, pear-shaped organ weighing about 70 g (2.5 oz). At the end of pregnancy it weighs approximately 1100 g (2.4 lb). Its capacity increases from 10 to 5000 mL (5 L) or more (Cunningham, Leveno, Bloom, et al., 2018).

The enlargement of the uterus is primarily a result of an increase in size (hypertrophy) of the preexisting myometrial cells. Only a limited increase in cell number (hyperplasia) occurs. The amount of fibrous tissue between the muscle bands increases markedly, which adds to the strength and elasticity of the muscle wall.

The uterine walls become considerably thicker during the first few months of pregnancy than during the nonpregnant state. The initial changes are stimulated by increased estrogen and progesterone levels and not by mechanical distention (enlargement) by the fetus, placenta, and amniotic fluid. In general, the uterus enlarges more around the placental insertion site and in the upper portion of the uterus, the *fundus* (Cunningham et al., 2018). After approximately the third month, the uterine contents begin to exert intrauterine pressure. The myometrial hypertrophy continues during the first few months of pregnancy. Then the musculature begins to distend, resulting in a thinning of the muscle wall to a thickness of 1 to 2 cm at term (38 through 41 weeks of gestation). The ease of palpating the fetus through the abdominal wall attests to this thinning.

The circulatory requirements of the uterus increase as the uterus enlarges and the fetus and placenta develop. The size and number of the blood and lymphatic vessels within the uterine layers increase greatly. By the end of pregnancy, one-sixth of the total maternal blood volume is contained within the vascular system of the uterus.

Braxton Hicks contractions—irregular, generally painless contractions of the uterus—occur intermittently throughout pregnancy. They may be felt through the abdominal wall beginning about the fourth month of pregnancy. These contractions help stimulate the movement of blood through the intervillous spaces of the placenta. In late pregnancy as these contractions increase in frequency, they can become uncomfortable and may be confused with true labor contractions.

Clinical Tip

Beginning early in pregnancy, have the woman feel her uterus periodically so that she becomes familiar with the size and the way it feels. As her pregnancy progresses she then will be more likely to identify Braxton Hicks contractions and preterm labor should it occur.

CERVIX

Estrogen stimulates the glandular tissue of the cervix, which increases in cell number and becomes hyperactive. The endocervical glands occupy about half the mass of the cervix at term, as compared with a small fraction in the nonpregnant state. They secrete thick, sticky mucus that accumulates and forms the **mucous plug**, which seals the endocervical canal and prevents the ascent of microorganisms or other substances into the uterus. This plug is expelled when cervical dilatation begins. The hyperactive glandular tissue also causes an increase in the normal physiologic mucorrhea, at times resulting in a profuse discharge. Increased vascularization causes both the softening of the cervix (**Goodell sign**) and a blue-purple discoloration of the cervix (**Chadwick sign**). Increased vascularization is a result of hypertrophy and engorgement of the vessels below the growing uterus.

OVARIES

The ovaries cease ovum production during pregnancy. Many follicles develop temporarily but never to the point of maturity. The cells lining these follicles, called theca cells, become active in hormone production and have been called the interstitial glands of pregnancy.

During early pregnancy human chorionic gonadotropin (hCG) maintains the corpus luteum, which persists and produces hormones until about weeks 6 to 8 of pregnancy. The corpus luteum secretes progesterone to maintain the endometrium until the placenta produces enough progesterone to maintain the pregnancy; then the corpus luteum disintegrates slowly.

VAGINA

The vaginal epithelium undergoes hypertrophy, increased vascularization, and hyperplasia during pregnancy. As with the cervical changes, these changes are estrogen induced and result in a thickening of mucosa, a loosening of connective tissue, and an increase in vaginal secretions. The secretions are thick, white, and acidic (pH 3.5 to 6). The acid pH plays a significant role in preventing infections. However, it also favors the growth of yeast organisms, resulting in moniliasis, a common vaginal infection during pregnancy.

As in the uterus, the smooth muscle cells of the vagina hypertrophy, with an accompanying loosening of the supportive connective tissue. By the end of pregnancy, the vaginal wall and perineal body have become sufficiently relaxed to permit distention of the tissues and passage of the baby.

Because the blood flow to the vagina increases, it may show the same bluish-purple color (Chadwick sign) seen in the cervix.

BREASTS

Soon after the woman first misses her menstrual period, estrogen- and progesterone-induced changes occur in the mammary glands. Increases in breast size and nodularity are the result of glandular hyperplasia and hypertrophy in preparation for lactation. By the end of the second month, superficial veins are prominent, nipples are more erectile, and pigmentation of the areola is obvious. Pigmentation tends to be more pronounced in women with dark complexions. Hypertrophy of Montgomery follicles is noted within the primary areola. **Striae** (purplish stretch marks that slowly turn silver after childbirth) may develop as the pregnancy progresses. Breast changes are often most noticeable in the woman who is pregnant for the first time.

Colostrum, an antibody-rich, yellow secretion, may be expressed manually by the 12th week and may leak from the breasts during the last trimester of pregnancy. Colostrum gradually converts to mature milk during the first few days following childbirth.

Respiratory System

Pulmonary function is modified throughout pregnancy. Pregnancy induces a small degree of hyperventilation as the tidal volume (amount of air breathed with ordinary respiration) increases by 30 to 40% (Antony, Racusin, Aagaard, et al., 2017). In addition, progesterone decreases airway resistance, permitting a 15 to 20% increase in oxygen consumption to meet the increased needs of the mother as well as those of the fetus and placenta. The vital capacity (maximum amount of air that can be moved in and out of the lungs with forced respiration) increases slightly, while lung compliance (elasticity) and pulmonary diffusion remain constant. The diaphragm is elevated and the subcostal angle is increased as a result of pressure from the enlarging uterus. This change causes the rib cage to flare with a decrease in the vertical diameter and increases in the anteroposterior and transverse diameters. The circumference of the chest may increase by as much as 6 cm (Cunningham et al., 2018). The increase compensates for the elevated diaphragm, and there is no significant loss of intrathoracic volume. Breathing changes from abdominal to thoracic as pregnancy progresses. Overall, pulmonary function is not impaired by pregnancy. Many women experience an increased awareness of the need to breathe, however, starting early in pregnancy. Actual lung disease may be aggravated by pregnancy because of the increased need for oxygen by the woman and her fetus.

Nasal stuffiness and congestion, referred to as rhinitis of pregnancy, are not uncommon. Epistaxis (nosebleeds) may also occur. They are primarily the result of estrogen-induced edema and vascular congestion of the nasal mucosa.

Cardiovascular System

The growing uterus exerts pressure on the diaphragm, pushing the heart upward and to the left and rotating it forward. This lateral displacement makes the heart appear somewhat enlarged on x-ray examination. A systolic murmur can be heard in 90% of pregnant women, and the first and third heart sounds are louder.

Blood volume progressively increases throughout pregnancy, beginning in the first trimester, and increases rapidly until about 30 to 34 weeks, then plateaus until birth at about 40 to 50% above nonpregnant levels. This increase is due to increases in both plasma and erythrocytes (Antony et al., 2017). No increase occurs in pulmonary capillary wedge pressure or in central venous pressure despite the increase in blood volume. This is due to decreases in both systemic vascular resistance and pulmonary vascular resistance, which enable the circulation to adapt to higher blood volume while maintaining normal vessel pressures. Cardiac output begins to increase early in pregnancy and peaks at 25 to 30 weeks' gestation at 30 to 50% above prepregnant levels. It generally remains elevated in the third trimester.

During pregnancy, organ systems receive additional blood flow according to their increased workload. Thus, blood flow to the uterus, placenta, and breasts increases, whereas hepatic and cerebral flow remains unchanged.

The pulse rate frequently increases during pregnancy, although the amount varies from almost no increase to an increase of 10 to 15 beats per minute. The blood pressure decreases slightly during pregnancy, reaching its lowest point during the second trimester. The blood pressure then gradually increases during the third trimester and is near prepregnant levels at term (when the baby is due).

The femoral venous pressure slowly rises as the uterus exerts increasing pressure on return blood flow. There is an increased tendency toward stagnation of blood in the lower extremities, with a resulting dependent edema and tendency toward varicose vein formation in the legs, vulva, and rectum late in pregnancy. In addition to the effects of increased femoral venous pressure, a reduction of plasma colloid osmotic pressure resulting from a reduction in plasma albumin further maintains the presence of fluid in the extravascular space. The pregnant woman becomes more prone to develop postural hypotension because of the increased blood volume in the lower extremities.

During pregnancy the enlarging uterus may put pressure on the vena cava when the woman is supine, resulting in **supine hypotensive syndrome**, or **vena caval syndrome**, also called *aortocaval compression*, because the enlarging uterus may press on the aorta and its collateral circulation as well. This pressure interferes with returning blood flow and produces a marked decrease in blood pressure with accompanying dizziness, pallor, and clamminess, which can be corrected by having the woman lie on her left side (Figure 11–1).

Hemoglobin and hematocrit levels drop in early to mid-pregnancy as a result of pregnancy-associated hemodilution (Antony et al., 2017). The total erythrocyte volume increases by about 25%. This increase is necessary to transport additional oxygen required to support the growth of the fetus during pregnancy. The increase in plasma volume averages approximately 50%. Because the plasma volume increase (50%) is greater than the erythrocyte increase even in women who take supplemental iron (30%), the hematocrit decreases slightly (Antony et al., 2017). This decrease is sometimes referred to as **physiologic anemia of pregnancy**, also called *pseudoanemia*.

Iron is necessary for hemoglobin formation, and hemoglobin is the oxygen-carrying component of erythrocytes. Thus, the increase in erythrocyte levels results in an increased need for iron by the pregnant woman. The American College of Obstetricians and Gynecologists (ACOG, 2015) recommendation for an iron supplement during pregnancy is 27 mg of iron daily. This can be found in most prenatal supplements. Women who were diagnosed with anemia prior to pregnancy may require more iron supplementation.

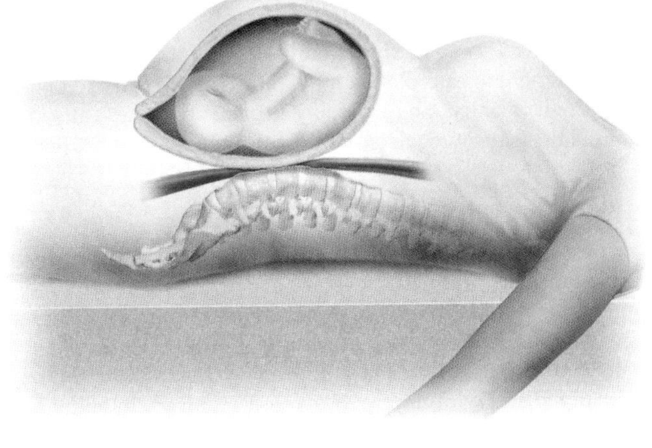

Figure 11–1 **Vena caval syndrome. The gravid uterus compresses the vena cava when the woman is supine. This reduces the blood flow returning to the heart and may cause maternal hypotension.**

Leukocyte production equals or is slightly greater than the increase in blood volume. The average cell count is 5600 to $12{,}200/mm^3$. In normal labor, the total white blood count could be as high as $20{,}000/mm^3$ to $30{,}000/mm^3$. Although the exact cause of the leukocytosis is not known, this increase is a normal finding (Antony et al., 2017).

The platelet count does not change much in pregnancy, but the plasma fibrinogen has been known to increase by as much as 50%. The increased fibrinogen accounts for the nonpathologic rise of the sedimentation rate. Although the blood clotting time of the pregnant woman does not differ significantly from that of the nonpregnant woman, blood factors VII, VIII, IX, and X are increased so that pregnancy becomes a somewhat hypercoagulable state. These changes, coupled with venous stasis in late pregnancy, place the pregnant woman at increased risk of developing venous thrombosis.

Gastrointestinal System

Many of the discomforts of pregnancy are attributed to changes in the gastrointestinal system. Nausea and vomiting during the first trimester are sometimes associated with the hCG secreted by the implanted blastocyst and with a change in carbohydrate metabolism that occurs in early pregnancy. Peculiarities of taste and smell are common and can further aggravate gastrointestinal discomfort. Gum tissue may become hyperemic and softened and may bleed when only mildly traumatized. The secretion of saliva may increase or become excessive (ptyalism).

During the second half of pregnancy, numerous gastrointestinal symptoms are attributable to the pressure of the growing uterus and smooth muscle relaxation due to elevated progesterone levels. The intestines are moved laterally and posteriorly and the stomach superiorly. Heartburn (pyrosis) is caused by the reflux of acidic secretions from the stomach into the lower esophagus as a result of relaxation of the cardiac sphincter. Gastric emptying time and intestinal motility are delayed, leading to frequent complaints of bloating and constipation, which can be aggravated by the smooth muscle relaxation and increased electrolyte and water reabsorption in the large intestine. Hemorrhoids frequently develop if constipation is a problem or, in the second half of pregnancy, from pressure on vessels below the level of the uterus.

Only minor liver changes occur with pregnancy. Plasma albumin concentrations and serum cholinesterase activity decrease with normal pregnancy as with certain liver diseases.

The emptying time of the gallbladder is prolonged during pregnancy as a result of smooth muscle relaxation from progesterone. Hypercholesterolemia may follow, and it can predispose the woman to gallstone formation. Pruritus (itching) caused by retained bile salts may also occur (Cunningham et al., 2018).

Urinary Tract

During the first trimester, the growing uterus puts pressure on the bladder, producing urinary frequency until the second trimester, when the uterus becomes an abdominal organ. Near term, when the presenting part engages in the pelvis, pressure is again exerted on the bladder. This pressure can impair the drainage of blood and lymph from the hyperemic bladder, rendering it more susceptible to infection and trauma. The bladder, normally a convex organ, becomes concave from the external pressure, and its capacity is greatly reduced.

Dilation of the kidneys and ureter may occur, most frequently on the right side above the pelvic brim, because of the lie of the uterus. This dilation is accompanied by elongation and curvature of the ureter. There appears to be no single factor accounting for this anatomic variation; instead, a combination of ureteral atonia and hypoperistalsis, probably caused by pressure from the enlarging fetus with some progesterone effects, seems to be involved. The presence of amino acids and glucose in the urine in conjunction with the tendency toward ureteral atonia and stasis of urine in the ureters may increase the risk of urinary tract infection.

The glomerular filtration rate (GFR) and renal plasma flow (RPF) increase early in pregnancy. The GFR rises by as much as 50% by the beginning of the second trimester and remains elevated until birth. RPF increases by about 80% before the first trimester has ended and decreases somewhat during the third trimester (Cunningham et al., 2018). The mechanism for these rises remains unclear.

An increased renal tubular reabsorption rate compensates for the increased glomerular activity. Amino acids and water-soluble vitamins are excreted in greater amounts than in the nonpregnant woman. Glycosuria is not uncommon or necessarily pathogenic during pregnancy but is merely a reflection of the kidneys' inability to reabsorb all of the glucose filtered by the glomeruli. However, pregnancy can be diabetogenic, so the possibility of diabetes mellitus cannot be disregarded.

The increased renal function during pregnancy results in an increased clearance of urea and creatinine and in a lowering of the blood urea and nonprotein nitrogen values. Because of this, measurement of creatinine clearance provides an accurate test of renal functioning during pregnancy.

Skin and Hair

Changes in skin pigmentation commonly occur during pregnancy. These changes are thought to be stimulated by increased estrogen, progesterone, and α-melanocyte-stimulating hormone levels.

Pigmentation of the skin increases primarily in areas that are already hyperpigmented: The areolae, the nipples, the vulva, the perianal area, and the linea alba. The linea alba refers to the midline of the abdomen from the pubic area to the umbilicus and above. During pregnancy increased pigmentation may cause this area to darken. It is then referred to as the **linea nigra** (Figure 11–2). Some women also develop facial **chloasma**, also called *melasma gravidarum*, the "mask of pregnancy." This is an irregular pigmentation of the cheeks, forehead, and nose that occurs in many women during pregnancy and is accentuated by sun exposure. Similar changes may occur in women who are taking oral contraceptives. Facial chloasma is more prominent in dark-haired women and is occasionally disfiguring. Fortunately, it fades or at least regresses soon after birth when the hormonal influence of pregnancy has stopped.

Striae, or stretch marks, are reddish, wavy, depressed streaks that may occur over the abdomen, breasts, and thighs as pregnancy progresses. They are caused by reduced connective tissue strength due to elevated adrenal steroid levels.

Vascular spider nevi may develop on the chest, neck, face, arms, and legs. They are small, bright-red elevations of the skin radiating from a central body. They may be caused by increased subcutaneous blood flow in response to increased estrogen levels. This condition is of no clinical significance and disappears after pregnancy ends.

The rate of hair growth may decrease during pregnancy, and the number of hair follicles in the resting or dormant phase also decreases. After birth the number of hair follicles in the resting phase increases sharply, and the woman may notice increased shedding of hair for 1 to 4 months. Practically all hair is replaced within 6 to 12 months, however.

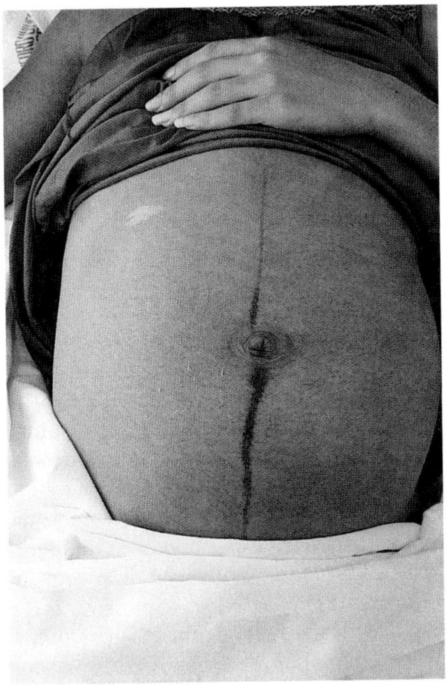

Figure 11–2 Linea nigra.

Finally, the sweat and sebaceous glands are frequently hyperactive during pregnancy. Some women may notice heavy perspiration, night sweats, and/or the development of acne even if they have never experienced these symptoms before.

Musculoskeletal System

No demonstrable changes occur in the teeth of the pregnant woman. No demineralization takes place. The fairly common occurrence of dental caries during pregnancy has led to the myth "a tooth for every pregnancy." The dental caries that may accompany pregnancy is likely to be caused by inadequate oral hygiene and dental care.

The sacroiliac, sacrococcygeal, and pubic joints of the pelvis relax in the later part of pregnancy, presumably as a result of hormonal changes. This often causes a waddling gait. A slight separation of the symphysis pubis can often be demonstrated on radiologic examination.

As the pregnant woman's center of gravity gradually changes, the lumbodorsal spinal curve is accentuated, and the woman's posture changes (Figure 11–3). This posture change compensates for the increased weight of the uterus anteriorly and frequently results in low backache. Late in pregnancy, aches in the neck, shoulders, and upper extremities may occur because of shoulder slumping and anterior flexion of the neck accompanying the lumbodorsal lordosis. Paresthesias of the extremities may occur late in pregnancy as a result of pressure on peripheral nerves.

Often, pressure of the enlarging uterus on the abdominal muscles causes the rectus abdominis muscle to separate, producing *diastasis recti*. If the separation is severe and muscle tone is not regained postpartum, subsequent pregnancies will not have adequate support, and the woman's abdomen may appear pendulous.

Central Nervous System

Pregnant women frequently describe decreased attention, concentration, and memory during and shortly after pregnancy, but few studies have explored this phenomenon. Changes occur in the walls of the blood vessels that do predispose a woman to aneurysm rupture. Also during pregnancy there is a fivefold increase in the risk of subarachnoid hemorrhage (Antony et al., 2017).

Eyes

Two changes generally occur in the eyes during pregnancy. First, intraocular pressure decreases, probably as a result of increased vitreous outflow. Second, a slight thickening of the cornea occurs, which is generally attributed to fluid retention (Antony et al., 2017). Although these changes are not readily perceived, some pregnant women experience difficulty wearing previously comfortable contact lenses. The change in the corneas generally disappears by 6 weeks postpartum.

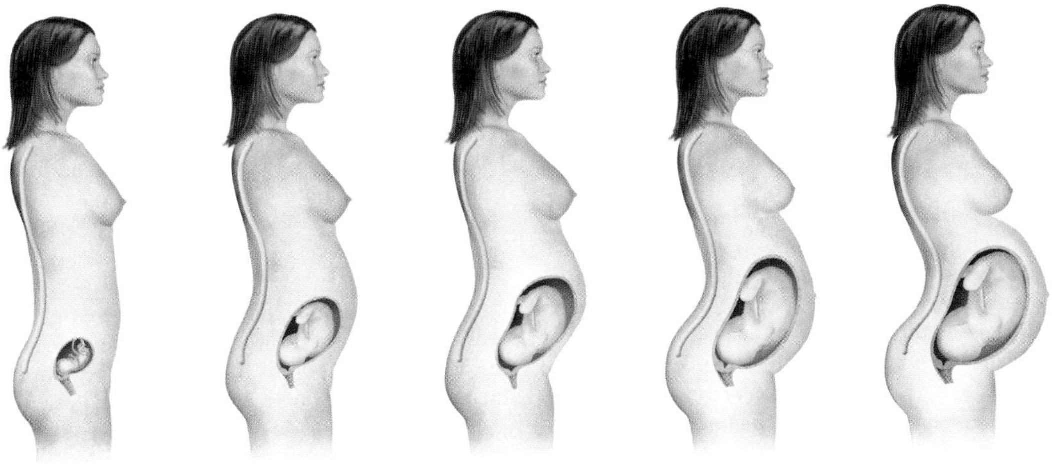

Figure 11–3 Postural changes during pregnancy. Note the increasing lordosis of the lumbosacral spine and the increasing curvature of the thoracic area.

Metabolism

Most metabolic functions accelerate during pregnancy to support the additional demands of the growing fetus and its support system. The expectant mother must meet her own tissue replacement needs, those of the fetus, and those preparatory for labor and lactation. No other event in life induces such profound metabolic changes.

WEIGHT GAIN

Growth of the uterus and its contents, growth of the breasts, and increases in intravascular fluids account for most of the weight gain in pregnancy. In addition, extra water, fat, and protein are stored; these are usually called *maternal reserves*.

The recommended total weight gain during pregnancy for a woman of normal weight before pregnancy is 11.5 to 16 kg (25 to 35 lb); for women who were overweight before becoming pregnant, the recommended gain is 6.8 to 11.5 kg (15 to 25 lb). Women who are obese are advised to limit weight gain to 5 to 9 kg (11 to 20 lb). Women who are underweight are advised to gain 12.7 to 18.1 kg (28 to 40 lb) (Institute of Medicine [IOM], 2009). Weight may decrease slightly during the first trimester because of nausea and vomiting and food intolerances of early pregnancy. The lost weight is soon regained, and the IOM (2009) recommends that a normal-weight woman gain 0.5 to 2 kg (1.1 to 4.4 lb) during the first trimester, followed by an average gain of about 0.45 kg (1 lb) per week during the last two trimesters.

ACOG (2016) supports the IOM recommendations and recommends that healthcare providers determine a woman's body mass index (BMI) at the initial prenatal visit. Individualized care and clinical judgment should then be used to determine the appropriate weight gain. See Chapter 14 for more information.

Clinical Tip

It is important to educate the patient on weight gain and diet throughout the entire pregnancy.

WATER METABOLISM

Increased water retention is a basic chemical alteration of pregnancy. Several interrelated factors cause this phenomenon. The increased level of steroid sex hormones affects sodium and fluid retention. The lowered serum protein also influences the fluid balance, as do the increased intracapillary pressure and permeability. The extra water is needed for the products of conception—the fetus, placenta, and amniotic fluid—and the mother's increased blood volume, interstitial fluids, and enlarged organs.

NUTRIENT METABOLISM

The fetus makes its greatest protein and fat demands during the second half of gestation, doubling in weight in the last 6 to 8 weeks. The increased protein retention that begins in early pregnancy is initially used for hyperplasia and hypertrophy of maternal tissues, such as the uterus and breasts. Protein must also be stored during pregnancy to maintain a constant level within the breast milk and to avoid depletion of maternal tissues.

Fats are more completely absorbed during pregnancy, resulting in a marked increase in the serum lipids, lipoproteins, and cholesterol and decreased elimination through the bowel. Fat deposits in the fetus increase from about 2% at midpregnancy to almost 12% at term. The excess nitrogen and lipidemia are considered to be a preparation for lactation. In addition, the woman's body switches from glucose metabolism to lipid metabolism once glucose from food intake has been used up. This leads to an increased tendency to develop ketosis between meals and overnight.

The demand for carbohydrate increases, especially during the last two trimesters. Intermittent glycosuria is not uncommon during pregnancy. When it is not accompanied by a rise in blood sugar levels, glycosuria is a physiologic entity secondary to the increased glomerular filtration rate. Fasting blood sugar levels tend to fall slightly, returning to more normal levels by the sixth postpartum month. The oral glucose tolerance test shows no change with pregnancy.

The possibility of diabetes must not be overlooked during pregnancy. Plasma levels of insulin increase during pregnancy (probably because of hormonal changes that cause increased tissue resistance), and rapid destruction of insulin takes place within the placenta. Insulin production must be increased by the mother during the second trimester, and any marginal pancreatic function quickly becomes apparent. The woman with diabetes often experiences increased exogenous insulin demands during pregnancy. See Care of the Woman with Diabetes in Chapter 17 for detailed information.

For a detailed discussion of nutrient, vitamin, and mineral metabolism, see Chapter 14.

Endocrine System

The endocrine system and its hormones support pregnancy in many ways.

THYROID GLAND

Pregnancy influences the thyroid gland's size and activity. Often a palpable change is noted, which represents an increase in vascularity and hyperplasia of glandular tissue. Total serum thyroxine (T_4) increases in early pregnancy, plateaus at about 18 weeks, and then continues at that level throughout the remainder of pregnancy. The level of free serum T_4 rises slightly in early pregnancy and then returns to normal after the first trimester. Thyroid-stimulating hormone (TSH) levels decrease (Cunningham et al., 2018). Increased thyroxine-binding capacity is evidenced by an increase in serum protein-bound iodine (PBI), probably due to the increased levels of circulating estrogens.

The basal metabolic rate (BMR) increases by as much as 20 to 25% during pregnancy. The increased oxygen consumption is due primarily to fetal metabolic activity.

PARATHYROID GLAND

The concentration of the parathyroid hormone and the size of the parathyroid glands increase, paralleling the fetal calcium requirements. Parathyroid hormone concentration reaches its highest level of approximately twofold between 15 and 35 weeks of gestation, returning to a normal or even subnormal level before childbirth.

PITUITARY GLAND

During pregnancy, the pituitary gland enlarges somewhat, but it returns to normal size after birth. There is no significant change in the posterior lobe of the gland, although the anterior lobe increases in weight with each successive pregnancy.

Pregnancy is made possible by the hypothalamic stimulation of the anterior pituitary hormones: Follicle-stimulating hormone (FSH), which stimulates follicle growth within the ovary, and luteinizing hormone (LH), which affects ovulation. Pituitary stimulation prolongs the corpus luteal phase of the ovary, which maintains the secretory endometrium for development of the pregnancy.

Two additional pituitary hormones, thyroid-stimulating hormone and adrenotropin, alter maternal metabolism to support the pregnancy. Prolactin, also an anterior pituitary secretion, is responsible for initial lactation. Its levels increase 10-fold during pregnancy and then, somewhat surprisingly, decrease after childbirth, even in breastfeeding women. (Continued lactation depends on the suckling of the baby.)

The posterior pituitary contains the mechanism for the release of oxytocin and vasopressin, which exert oxytocic, vasopressor, and antidiuretic effects. The main effects of oxytocin are the promotion of uterine contractility and the stimulation of milk ejection from the breasts. Vasopressin causes vasoconstriction, which results in increased blood pressure; it also has an antidiuretic effect and plays an important role in the regulation of water balance. Vasopressin secretion is controlled by changes in plasma osmolarity and blood volume.

ADRENAL GLANDS

Little structural change occurs in the adrenal glands during a normal pregnancy. Estrogen-induced increases in the levels of circulating cortisol result primarily from lowered renal excretion. The circulating cortisol levels regulate carbohydrate and protein metabolism. A normal level resumes 1 to 6 weeks' postpartum.

The adrenal glands secrete increased levels of aldosterone by the early part of the second trimester. The levels of secretion are even more elevated in the woman on a sodium-restricted diet. This increase in aldosterone in a normal pregnancy may be the body's protective response to the increased sodium excretion associated with progesterone (Cunningham et al., 2018).

PANCREAS

The pregnant woman has increased insulin needs. The islets of Langerhans are stressed to meet this increased demand, and a latent deficiency may become apparent during pregnancy, producing symptoms of gestational diabetes. See Care of the Woman with Diabetes in Chapter 17 for more information.

HORMONES IN PREGNANCY

Several hormones are required to maintain pregnancy. Most of these are produced initially by the corpus luteum; production is then assumed by the placenta.

Human Chorionic Gonadotropin. The trophoblast secretes hCG in early pregnancy. This hormone stimulates progesterone and estrogen production by the corpus luteum to maintain the pregnancy until the placenta is developed sufficiently to assume that function.

Human Placental Lactogen. Also called human chorionic somatomammotropin (hCS), human placental lactogen (hPL) is produced by the syncytiotrophoblast. This hormone is an antagonist of insulin; it increases the amount of circulating free fatty acids for maternal metabolic needs and decreases maternal metabolism of glucose to favor fetal growth.

Estrogen. Secreted originally by the corpus luteum, estrogen is produced primarily by the placenta as early as the seventh week of pregnancy. Estrogen stimulates uterine development to provide a suitable environment for the fetus. It also helps to develop the ductal system of the breasts in preparation for lactation.

Progesterone. Progesterone, also produced initially by the corpus luteum and then by the placenta, plays the greatest role in maintaining pregnancy. It maintains the endometrium and also inhibits spontaneous uterine contractility, thus preventing early spontaneous abortion due to uterine activity. In addition, progesterone helps develop the acini and lobules of the breasts in preparation for lactation.

Relaxin. Relaxin is detectable in the serum of a pregnant woman by the time of the first missed menstrual period. Relaxin inhibits uterine activity, diminishes the strength of uterine contractions, aids in the softening of the cervix, and has the long-term effect of remodeling collagen. Its primary source is the corpus luteum, but small amounts are believed to be produced by the placenta and uterine decidua throughout pregnancy.

PROSTAGLANDINS IN PREGNANCY

Prostaglandins (PGs) are lipid substances that can arise from most body tissues but occur in high concentrations in the female reproductive tract and are present in the decidua during pregnancy. The exact functions of PGs during pregnancy are still unknown, although it has been proposed that they are responsible for maintaining reduced placental vascular resistance. Decreased PG levels may contribute to hypertension and preeclampsia. Prostaglandins are also believed to play a role in the complex biochemistry that initiates labor, although their specific functions are still being defined.

Signs of Pregnancy

Many of the changes women experience during pregnancy are used to diagnose the pregnancy itself. They are called the subjective (or presumptive) changes, the objective (or probable) changes, and the diagnostic (or positive) changes of pregnancy.

Subjective (Presumptive) Changes

The subjective changes of pregnancy are the symptoms the woman experiences and reports. They can be caused by other conditions (Table 11–1) and, therefore, cannot be considered proof of pregnancy. The following can be diagnostic clues when other signs and symptoms of pregnancy are also present.

- *Amenorrhea* is the earliest symptom of pregnancy. In a healthy woman whose menstrual cycles are regular, missing one or more menstrual periods leads to the consideration of pregnancy.
- *Nausea and vomiting of pregnancy* (*NVP*) are experienced by almost half of all pregnant women during the first 3 months of pregnancy and may be the result of elevated human chorionic gonadotropin (hCG) levels and changed carbohydrate metabolism. Further research is being conducted to determine other causes for nausea and vomiting. The woman may feel merely a distaste for food or may suffer extreme vomiting, which may be accompanied by dehydration and ketosis. Because these symptoms frequently occur in the early part of the day and disappear within a few hours, they are commonly called **morning sickness**. In reality, symptoms may occur at any time. This gastrointestinal disturbance usually appears about 6 weeks after the first day of the last menstrual period (LMP) and usually disappears spontaneously 6 to 12 weeks later, although it may be prolonged in some instances. Research suggests that women who experience NVP often have a more favorable pregnancy outcome than those who do not (Antony et al., 2017).

TABLE 11–1 Differential Diagnosis of Pregnancy—Subjective Changes

SUBJECTIVE CHANGES	POSSIBLE ALTERNATIVE CAUSES
Amenorrhea	Endocrine factors: Early menopause; lactation; thyroid, pituitary, adrenal, ovarian dysfunction
	Metabolic factors: Malnutrition, anemia, climatic changes, diabetes mellitus, degenerative disorders, long-distance running
	Psychologic factors: Emotional shock, fear of pregnancy or sexually transmitted infection, intense desire for pregnancy (pseudocyesis), stress
	Obliteration of endometrial cavity by infection or curettage
	Systemic disease (acute or chronic), such as tuberculosis or malignancy
Nausea and vomiting	Gastrointestinal disorders
	Acute infections such as encephalitis
	Emotional disorders such as pseudocyesis or anorexia nervosa
Urinary frequency	Urinary tract infection
	Cystocele
	Pelvic tumors
	Urethral diverticula
	Emotional tension
Breast tenderness	Premenstrual tension
	Chronic cystic mastitis
	Pseudocyesis
	Hyperestrogenism
Quickening	Increased peristalsis
	Flatus ("gas")
	Abdominal muscle contractions
	Shifting of abdominal contents

“I believed that nausea and vomiting would only occur in the morning because everyone called it morning sickness. I soon realized that it could occur any time of the day or night. I couldn't eat my favorite foods because they made me sick. I could not even brush my teeth without feeling nauseated. I was relieved when I started my second trimester and the nausea ended!”

- *Excessive fatigue* may be noted within a few weeks after the first missed menstrual period and may persist throughout the first trimester.
- *Urinary frequency* is experienced during the first trimester as the enlarging uterus exerts pressure on the bladder. The increased vascularization and pelvic congestion that occur in each pregnancy can also cause frequent voiding. This symptom decreases during the second trimester, when the uterus is an abdominal organ, but reappears during the third trimester, when the presenting part descends into the pelvis.
- *Changes in the breasts* are frequently noted in early pregnancy. Some women report significant breast changes even before missing their first menses. Engorgement of the breasts due to the hormone-induced growth of the secretory ductal system results in the subjective symptoms of tenderness and tingling, especially of the nipple area. The veins also become more visible and form a bluish pattern beneath the skin in fair-skinned women.
- **Quickening**, or the mother's perception of fetal movement, occurs about 18 to 20 weeks after the LMP in a primigravida (a woman who is pregnant for the first time) but may occur as early as 16 weeks in a multigravida (a woman who has been pregnant more than once). Quickening is a fluttering sensation in the abdomen that gradually increases in intensity and frequency.

Clinical Tip

Some women suggest that it is easiest to imagine the fluttering associated with quickening by letting the outer tips of the eyelashes brush a finger and then imagining that same sensation deep inside the abdomen.

Objective (Probable) Changes

An examiner can perceive the objective changes that occur in pregnancy. They are more diagnostic than the subjective symptoms. However, their presence does not offer a definite diagnosis of pregnancy (Table 11–2).

- *Changes in the pelvic organs* caused by increased vascular congestion are the only physical signs detectable within the first 3 months of pregnancy. These changes are noted on pelvic examination. There is a softening of the cervix, called Goodell sign. Chadwick sign is the deep red to purple or bluish coloration of the mucous membranes of the cervix, vagina, and vulva due to increased vasocongestion of the pelvic vessels. **Hegar sign** is a softening of the isthmus of the uterus, the area between the cervix and the body of the uterus, which occurs at 6 to 8 weeks of pregnancy. This area may become so soft that on a bimanual exam there seems to be nothing between the cervix and the body of the uterus

TABLE 11–2 Differential Diagnosis of Pregnancy—Objective Changes

OBJECTIVE CHANGES	POSSIBLE ALTERNATIVE CAUSES
Changes in pelvic organs	Increased vascular congestion
Goodell sign	Estrogen-progestin oral contraceptives
Chadwick sign	Vulvar, vaginal, cervical hyperemia
Hegar sign	Excessively soft walls of nonpregnant uterus
Uterine enlargement	Uterine tumors
Braun von Fernwald sign	Uterine tumors
Piskacek sign	Uterine tumors
Enlargement of abdomen	Obesity, ascites, pelvic tumors
Braxton Hicks contractions	Hematometra; pedunculated, submucous, and soft myomas
Uterine souffle	Large uterine myomas, large ovarian tumors, or any condition with greatly increased uterine blood flow
Pigmentation of skin	Estrogen-progestin oral contraceptives
Chloasma (melasma)	Melanocyte hormonal stimulation
Linea nigra	
Nipples/areola	
Abdominal striae	Obesity, pelvic tumor
Ballottement	Uterine tumors/polyps, ascites
Pregnancy tests	Increased pituitary gonadotropins at menopause, choriocarcinoma, hydatidiform mole
Palpation for fetal outline	Uterine myomas

(Figure 11–4). *Ladin sign* is a soft spot anteriorly in the middle of the uterus near the junction of the body of the uterus and cervix (Figure 11–5A). **McDonald sign** is an ease in flexing the body of the uterus against the cervix. The uterus assumes an irregular globular shape during the early months of pregnancy. Irregular softening and enlargement at the site of implantation, known as *Braun von Fernwald sign*, occurs about the fifth week (Figure 11–5B). Occasionally an almost tumorlike, asymmetric enlargement occurs, called *Piskacek sign* (Figure 11–5C). Generalized enlargement and softening of the body of the uterus are present after the eighth week of pregnancy. The fundus of the uterus is palpable just above the symphysis pubis at approximately 10 to 12 weeks' gestation and at the level of the umbilicus at 20 to 22 weeks' gestation (Figure 11–6).

- *Enlargement of the abdomen* during the childbearing years is usually regarded as evidence of pregnancy, especially if the enlargement is progressive and is accompanied by continuing amenorrhea. It is generally more pronounced in a woman whose abdominal musculature has lost some of its tone because of previous childbirth.
- *Braxton Hicks contractions*, as mentioned earlier, are irregular, ordinarily painless contractions that occur at irregular intervals throughout pregnancy but can be palpated most commonly after week 28. As the woman approaches the end of the pregnancy, these contractions often become more uncomfortable and are then called *false labor*.
- *Uterine souffle* may be heard when auscultating the abdomen over the uterus. It is a soft blowing sound at the same rate as the maternal pulse and is due to the increased uterine vascularization and the blood pulsating through the placenta. It is sometimes confused with the *funic souffle*, which is a soft blowing sound of blood pulsating through the umbilical arteries. The funic souffle is at the same rate as the fetal heart rate.
- *Changes in pigmentation of the skin* and the *appearance of abdominal striae* are common manifestations in pregnancy. Facial melasma (chloasma) occurs in varying degrees after week 16. The pigmentation of the nipple and areola may

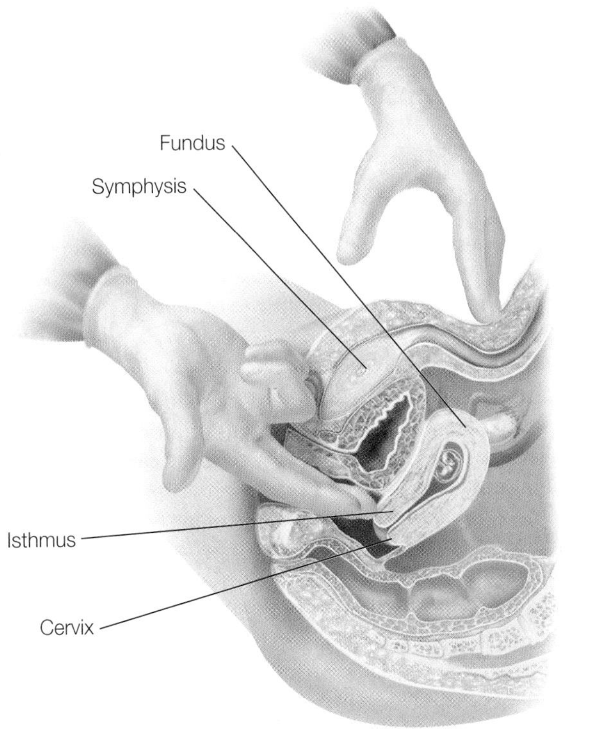

Figure 11–4 **Hegar sign, a softening of the isthmus of the uterus, can be determined by the examiner during a vaginal examination.**

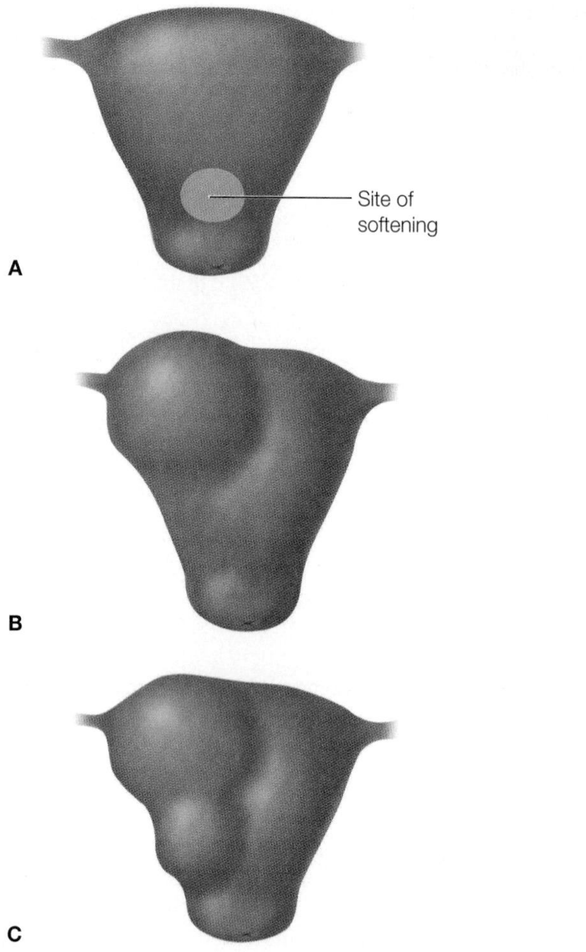

Figure 11-5 **Early uterine changes of pregnancy. A. Ladin sign: A soft spot anteriorly in the middle of the uterus near the junction of the body of the uterus and the cervix. B. Braun von Fernwald sign: Irregular softening and enlargement at the site of implantation. C. Piskacek sign: A tumorlike asymmetric enlargement.**

darken, especially in primigravidas and dark-haired women. The Montgomery glands of the areola may become enlarged. The skin in the midline of the abdomen may develop a pigmented line, the linea nigra (see Figure 11–2). As pregnancy progresses, striae appear on the abdomen and buttocks.

- *Fetal outline* may be identified by palpation in many pregnant women after 24 weeks of gestation, becoming easier to distinguish as term approaches. **Ballottement** is the passive fetal movement elicited by pushing up against the cervix with two fingers. This pushes the fetal body up and, as it falls back, the examiner feels a rebound.
- *Pregnancy tests* are based on analysis of maternal blood or urine for the detection of hCG, the hormone secreted by the trophoblast. These tests are not considered positive signs of pregnancy because conditions other than pregnancy can cause elevated levels of hCG.

CLINICAL PREGNANCY TESTS

A variety of assay techniques are available to detect hCG in either blood serum or urine during early pregnancy. Companies

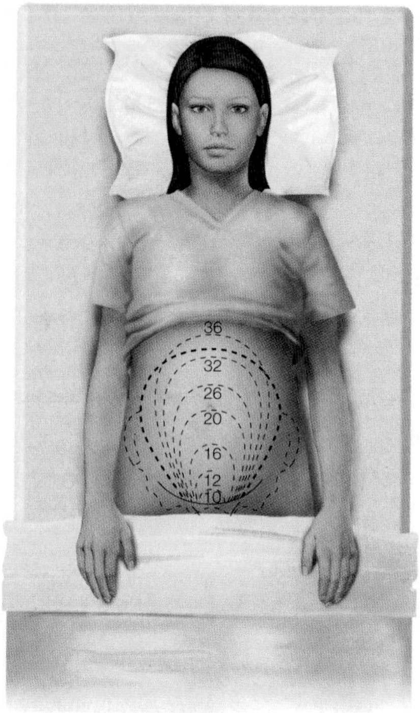

Figure 11-6 **Approximate height of the fundus at various weeks of pregnancy.**

that manufacture pregnancy tests provide instructions for performance and interpretation of the test as well as test accuracy. Studies have demonstrated that some pregnancy test diagnostic sensitivities and specificities may be greater than 97% accurate (Greene, Schmidt, Kamer, et al., 2013).

Several pregnancy tests are available, including:

- *β-subunit radioimmunoassay (RIA)* uses an antiserum with specificity for the β-subunit of hCG in blood plasma. This test may not only detect pregnancy but also detect an ectopic pregnancy or trophoblastic disease.
- *Enzyme-linked immunosorbent assay (ELISA)* uses a substance that results in a color change after binding. This assay, which may be done on urine or blood, is sensitive and quick. It can detect hCG levels as early as 7 to 9 days after ovulation and conception, which is 5 days before the first missed period.
- *Fluoroimmunoassay (FIA)* uses an antibody tagged with a fluorescent label to detect serum hCG. The test, which takes about 2 to 3 hours to perform, is extremely sensitive and is used primarily to identify and follow hCG concentrations.

OVER-THE-COUNTER PREGNANCY TESTS

Home pregnancy tests (HPTs) are available over the counter at a reasonable cost. These enzyme immunoassay tests are quite sensitive and detect even low levels of hCG in urine. Home pregnancy tests are convenient, provide privacy, and allow women to diagnose pregnancy prior to visiting a provider.

Multiple brands and types of HPTs are available, which differ in use and instructions. The false-positive rate of these tests is quite low but can also occur in certain situations such as early pregnancy loss, protein in the urine, or the presence of background hCG production. False-negative results are more common and more concerning and should be followed up in the presence of pregnancy symptoms. False-negative results typically occur when the test is completed too early or too late. If the results are negative, the woman should repeat the test in 1 week if she has not started her menstrual period; at that time the test may become positive.

Diagnostic (Positive) Changes

The diagnostic signs of pregnancy are completely objective, cannot be confused with pathologic states, and offer conclusive proof of pregnancy.

- *Fetal heartbeat* can be detected with an electronic Doppler device as early as weeks 10 to 12. Auscultation of the abdomen may reveal sounds other than that of the fetal heart. The maternal pulse, emanating from the abdominal aorta, may be unusually loud, or a uterine souffle may be heard.
- *Fetal movement* is actively palpable by a trained examiner after about 20 weeks' gestation. The movements vary from a faint flutter in the early months to more vigorous movements late in pregnancy.
- *Visualization of the fetus* by transvaginal ultrasound confirms a pregnancy. The gestational sac can be observed by 4 to 5 weeks' gestation (2 to 3 weeks after conception). After 6 weeks fetal heart movement can usually be noted (Cunningham et al., 2018).

Psychologic Response of the Expectant Family to Pregnancy

Pregnancy is a developmental challenge, a turning point in a family's life accompanied by stress and anxiety whether the pregnancy is desired or not. Pregnancy confirms one's biological capabilities to reproduce. It is evidence of one's participation in sexual activity and as such is an affirmation of one's sexuality. For beginning families, pregnancy is the transition period from childlessness to parenthood. If the pregnancy terminates in the birth of a child, the couple enters a new stage of their life together, one that is irreversible and characterized by awesome responsibilities.

The expectant couple may be unaware of the physical, emotional, and cognitive states peculiar to pregnancy. The couple may anticipate no problem from such a normal event as pregnancy and, therefore, may be confused and distressed by new feelings and behaviors that are generally considered normal.

If the expectant woman is married or has a stable partner, she no longer is only a mate but also must assume the role of mother. Her partner, whether a man or a woman, will also assume a parenting role. Career goals and mobility may be altered or thwarted for one or both partners. Each partner begins to see the other in a different light. Their relationship takes on a different meaning to them and within the larger family and community. With each pregnancy, routines and family dynamics are altered, requiring readjustment and realignment.

If a pregnant woman is without a stable partner, she will still experience changes in role identity and psychobiological maturation. She must deal alone with the role changes, fears, and adjustments of pregnancy or seek support from family and friends. She also faces the reality of planning for the future as a single parent. Even if the pregnant woman plans to relinquish her baby, she must still deal with the adjustments of pregnancy. She is no longer a separate individual; she must consider the needs of another being who depends on her totally, at least during the pregnancy. This adjustment can be especially difficult without a good support system.

In most pregnancies—whether of a mother with a supportive partner, a single mother, or a relinquishing mother—finances are an important consideration. Traditional lore relegates to the father the role of primary breadwinner, and, indeed, finances are often a very real concern for fathers and partners who are the primary breadwinners. However, in today's society even pregnant women with stable partners recognize the financial impact of a child and may feel concern about financial issues. For the single mother, finances may be a major source of concern.

Decisions about financial matters need to be made at this time. Will the woman work during the pregnancy and return to work after the baby is born? Who will provide child care if she works? Decisions may also need to be made about the division of tasks within the home. Any differences of opinion must be discussed openly and resolved so that the family can meet its members' needs.

The couple must face the realities of labor and birth. Many nonparents have little idea what labor entails. Their information is frequently based on contacts with visual or print media and on experiences related to them by family members or friends, and these tales are often fraught with myths and exaggerations. Classes in prepared childbirth can help them address this lack of information or misinformation.

Labor is threatening in many respects. Pain, disfigurement, disruption of bodily function, and even death are potential threats for the woman. The partner faces the threat of the woman's disfigurement, impairment of her health, or her death. Both fear that the baby may be ill or disfigured. The expectant couple is subject to anxiety during this period because no one can provide total reassurance about the outcome.

Pregnancy can be viewed as a developmental stage with its own distinct developmental tasks. It can be a time of support or conflict for a couple, depending on the amount of adjustment each is willing to make to maintain the family's equilibrium. Family dynamics are an important factor in adjusting to pregnancy. Family strengths include the ability of the couple to talk about issues that are important to them, to resolve conflicts and make compromises, and to seek and receive assistance and support from loved ones.

During pregnancy, the woman and her partner plan together for the first child's arrival, collecting information on how to be parents. At the same time, each continues to participate in some separate activities with friends or family members. The availability of social support is an important factor in psychosocial well-being during pregnancy. Most pregnant women turn to their partners as their primary source of social support. In addition, the broader social network is often a major source of advice for the pregnant woman. However, evidence indicates that both sound and unsound information is given.

The expectant mother and her partner both face significant changes during pregnancy and must deal with major psychosocial adjustments (Table 11–3). Other family members, especially other children of the woman or couple and the grandparents-to-be, must also adjust to the pregnancy.

In late pregnancy, the concerns of expectant fathers/partners tend to focus most on the health of the unborn child and the safety of the mother. The concerns of expectant mothers center on the health of the baby and their ability to handle labor and birth. Couples typically agree on the primary concern, the health of the unborn child. Nurses can use this focus as a springboard for discussing other concerns. A woman worries about how she will handle labor and birth but has little concern for her own safety; the father/partner's expression of fear for her safety can be seen as evidence that the individual cares enough to worry about her.

TABLE 11–3 Parental Reactions to Pregnancy

FIRST TRIMESTER	SECOND TRIMESTER	THIRD TRIMESTER
	Mother's Reactions	
Informs partner secretively or openly. Feels ambivalent toward pregnancy, anxious about labor and responsibility of child. Is aware of physical changes; daydreams of possible miscarriage. Develops special feelings for and renewed interest in her own mother, with formation of a personal identity.	Remains regressive and introspective; projects all problems with authority figures onto partner; may become angry if she perceives partner's lack of interest as a sign of weakness. Continues to deal with feelings as a mother; shops for nursery furniture as something concrete to do. May experience anxiety or, alternately, may be extremely lackadaisical and wait until ninth month to look for furniture and clothes for baby. Feels movement and is aware of fetus and incorporates it into herself. Dreams that partner will be killed; telephones him often for reassurance. Experiences more distinct physical changes; sexual desires may increase or decrease.	Experiences more anxiety and tension, with physical awkwardness. Feels much discomfort and insomnia from physical condition. Prepares for birth, assembles layette; picks out names. Dreams often about misplacing baby or not being able to give birth; fears birth of deformed baby. Feels ecstasy and excitement; has spurt of energy during last month.
	Father's Reactions	
Differ according to age, parity, desire for child, economic stability. Acceptance of pregnant woman's attitude or complete rejection and lack of communication. Is aware of his sexual feelings; may develop more or less sexual arousal. Accepts, rejects, or resents mother-in-law. May develop new hobby outside of family as sign of stress.	If he can cope, will give her extra attention she needs; if he cannot cope, will develop a new time-consuming interest outside of home. May develop a creative feeling and a "closeness to nature." Many become involved in pregnancy and buy or make furniture. Feels for movement of baby, listens to heartbeat, or remains aloof, with no physical contact. May have fears and fantasies about being pregnant himself; may become uneasy with this feminine aspect in himself. May react negatively if partner is too demanding; may become jealous of physician and of physician's importance to partner and her pregnancy.	Adapts to alternative methods of sexual contact. Becomes concerned over financial responsibility. May show new sense of tenderness and concern, treats partner like doll. Daydreams about child as if older and not newborn; dreams of losing partner. Renewed sexual attraction to partner. Feels he is ultimately responsible for whatever happens.

This response may allow the mother to depend on her partner more during the vulnerable time of late pregnancy and birthing. Sharing such views gives the father/partner a chance to express love and concern for mother and child, encouraging the development of stronger marital and parental relationships.

For some couples, pregnancy is more than a developmental stage; it is a crisis. *Crisis* can be defined as a disturbance or conflict in which the individual cannot maintain a state of equilibrium. Pregnancy can be considered a *maturational crisis* because it is a common event in the normal growth and development of the family. During such a crisis, the individual or family is in disequilibrium. The period of disequilibrium and disorganization is marked by abortive attempts to solve the perceived problems. If the crisis is not resolved, it will result in maladaptive behaviors in one or more family members and possible disintegration of the family. Families who are able to resolve a maturational crisis successfully will return to normal functioning and can even strengthen the bonds in the family relationship.

Mother

Pregnancy is a condition that alters body image and also necessitates a reordering of social relationships and changes in roles of family members. The way a particular woman meets the stresses of pregnancy is influenced by her emotional makeup, her sociologic and cultural background, and her acceptance or rejection of the pregnancy. However, many women manifest similar psychologic and emotional responses during pregnancy, including ambivalence, acceptance, introversion, mood swings, and changes in body image.

INTENDEDNESS

Many pregnancies are unintended, but not all unintended pregnancies are unwanted. For some women, an unintended pregnancy has more psychologic and social advantages than disadvantages. It provides purpose and direction to life and allows a woman to test the devotion and love of her partner and family. Nevertheless, an unintended pregnancy may be a risk factor for depression. Higher levels of depression were found in women who reported more negative responses to pregnancy, who believed that their pregnancies had greater consequences, and who experienced more symptoms, especially in the third trimester (Jessop, Craig, & Ayers, 2014). It is important for health-care providers to identify depression and make referrals as necessary so women get the support they need to reduce stress and enhance resiliency.

AMBIVALENCE

Many women commonly experience feelings of ambivalence during early pregnancy. This ambivalence may be related to feelings that the timing is somehow wrong; worries about the need to modify existing relationships or career plans; fears about assuming a new role; unresolved emotional conflicts with the woman's own mother; and fears about pregnancy, labor, and birth. Research indicates that women who are ambivalent about pregnancy are generally younger, less likely to have been pregnant previously, and more likely to have been a victim of sexual violence, to have experienced pregnancy coercion, to have unhealthy behaviors such as smoking, and to have psychologic risk factors. They are also more likely to experience stress and depression during pregnancy (Patel, Laz, & Berenson, 2015). Indirect expressions of ambivalence include complaints about considerable physical discomfort, prolonged or frequent depression, significant dissatisfaction with changing body shape, excessive mood swings, and difficulty in accepting the life changes resulting from the pregnancy.

Such feelings may be even more pronounced if the pregnancy is unintended or unwanted. Women who view their pregnancy as unwanted are more likely to delay prenatal care and to experience complications. The support and opinion of the woman's current partner, even if he is not the father of the child, have a major impact on the acceptance of the pregnancy. Financial and emotional support from the partner is essential to the woman's positive attitude. Involving the partner in the prenatal care may help promote a supportive attitude. During the early months, the pregnant woman may consider the possibility of a therapeutic abortion if the pregnancy is unwanted. In the event of religious conflicts about induced abortion, the woman may experience feelings of guilt about her thoughts or may tend to focus on the possibility of spontaneous abortion (miscarriage). Even when the pregnancy is planned, thoughts of abortion and miscarriage arise. Concurrently, the pregnant woman may feel guilty for having such negative thoughts and may worry that in some way these thoughts will harm the baby.

ACCEPTANCE

Acceptance of pregnancy is influenced by many factors. Lower acceptance tends to be related to an unplanned pregnancy and greater evidence of fear and conflict. The woman carrying an unplanned pregnancy tends to experience more physical discomfort and depression. When a pregnancy is well accepted, the woman demonstrates feelings of happiness and pleasure in the pregnancy. She experiences less physical discomfort and shows a high degree of tolerance for the discomforts associated with the third trimester.

First Trimester. During the first trimester, evidence of pregnancy is often limited to amenorrhea and to the word of the caregiver that the pregnancy test was positive. Unless the woman has the opportunity to see the gestational sac during an ultrasound, her baby may not seem real. Consequently, she may tend to focus on herself and her pregnancy. She may experience one or more of the early symptoms of pregnancy, such as breast tenderness or morning sickness, which are unsettling and at times unpleasant. In an effort to verify her condition, a woman may become minutely conscious of changes in her body that could validate the pregnancy.

Second Trimester. The second trimester is relatively tranquil. Morning sickness generally passes, the threat of spontaneous abortion diminishes, and the woman begins to accept the reality of her pregnancy. It is not unusual for an enthusiastic primigravida to don maternity clothes at the beginning of this trimester even when it is not truly necessary. The clothing serves as a verification of her pregnant state.

The highlight of the second trimester is quickening, which generally occurs about weeks 16 to 20 or midway through the pregnancy. Actual perception of fetal movement helps the woman think of her baby as a real person, and she generally becomes excited about the pregnancy even if earlier she was not.

As quickening and her altered physical appearance confirm her pregnant state, the woman adjusts to the idea of change and begins to prepare for her new role and her new set of relationships—with her partner and family, the child-to-be and other children, friends, and loved ones. When the pregnancy is well accepted, the woman takes pleasure in the sensations of pregnancy and attempts to picture her baby in order to know him or her better. She may seek out other women who are pregnant or have recently given birth. She feels well, is excited, and may exhibit the "glow" so often attributed to pregnant women.

Third Trimester. The third trimester combines a sense of pride with anxiety about labor and birth. During this time, the special prerogatives of pregnancy may be most marked. As her protruding abdomen proclaims her advanced pregnancy, the woman may find that others become more solicitous, that a chair may be offered in a crowded room, that others may carry her parcels. The woman may actually need this help, she may simply enjoy the attention as a privilege of pregnancy, or she may reject it if she fears that such gestures indicate she is helpless.

During the final trimester, physical discomforts again increase, and adequate rest becomes a necessity. The woman makes final preparation for the baby and may spend long periods considering names for the child. During this time she worries more about the health and safety of her unborn child and may have concerns that she will not behave well during childbirth.

The woman may feel vulnerable to rejection, loss, or insult. She may worry about a variety of things and may withdraw into the security and quiet of her home. Toward the end of this period many women report bursts of energy in which they vigorously clean and organize their homes ("nesting").

INTROVERSION

Introversion, or turning in on oneself, is a common occurrence in pregnancy. An active, outgoing woman may become less interested in previous activities and more concerned with needs for rest and time alone. This concentration of attention permits the woman to plan, adjust, adapt, build, and draw strength in preparation for her child's birth. As she becomes more aware of herself, her partner may feel she is being overly sensitive. Her partner may perceive her introversion and passivity as exclusionary and may in turn become unable to interact with her, either verbally or physically, or to provide the affection, support, and consideration she requires. This change may result in disequilibrium and stress for the entire family. It is essential that the couple work together to establish new, mutually acceptable patterns of response to overcome these blocks to communication.

Fantasies about the unborn child are quite common among pregnant women. However, the themes of the fantasies (baby's appearance, gender, traits, impact on parents, and so forth) vary by trimester and also differ between women pregnant for the first time and women who already have children.

MOOD SWINGS

Throughout pregnancy, the emotions of many women are characterized by mood swings, from great joy to deep despair. Frequently, the woman will become tearful with little apparent cause. When asked why she is crying, she may find it difficult or impossible to give a reason. The situation may be extremely unsettling for the partner, causing feelings of confusion and inadequacy, and the partner may react by withdrawing and ignoring the problem. Because the pregnant woman needs increased love and affection, she may perceive this reaction as unloving and nonsupportive. Once the couple understands that this behavior is characteristic of pregnancy, it becomes easier for them to deal with it more effectively—although it will be a source of stress to some extent throughout pregnancy.

CHANGES IN BODY IMAGE

Pregnancy produces marked changes in a woman's body within a relatively short time. With these changes, women also experience changes in body image. The degree of this change is related to a certain extent to personality factors, social network responses, and attitudes toward pregnancy. Changes in body image are normal but can be very stressful for the pregnant woman. Explanation and discussion of the changes may help both the woman and her partner deal with the stress associated with this aspect of pregnancy.

> “I'm due in 2 weeks and I can't wait. These last few weeks have been hard on my self-image. I can't see my feet anymore and I feel awkward and lumbering, not graceful at all.”

PSYCHOLOGIC TASKS OF THE MOTHER

Rubin (1984) identified four major tasks that the pregnant woman undertakes to maintain her intactness and that of her family and at the same time incorporate her new child into the family system. These tasks form the basis for a mutually gratifying relationship with her baby:

1. ***Ensuring safe passage through pregnancy, labor, and birth.*** The pregnant woman feels concern for both her unborn child and herself. She seeks competent maternity care to provide a sense of control. She may also seek knowledge from literature, observation of other pregnant women and new mothers, and discussion with others. The pregnant woman also seeks to ensure safe passage by engaging in self-care activities related to diet, exercise, alcohol consumption, and so forth. In the third trimester, as her movements slow and her body mass increases, she becomes aware of external threats in the environment—a toy on a stair, the awkwardness of an escalator—that pose a threat to her intactness and represent hazards to be overcome. She may worry if her partner is late or if she is home alone. Sleep becomes difficult, and she begins to long for the baby's birth, even though it, too, is frightening.
2. ***Seeking of acceptance of this child by others.*** The birth of a child alters a woman's primary support group, her family, and her secondary affiliative groups. The family generally makes the transition, and the woman slowly and subtly alters her secondary network to meet the needs of her pregnancy. In this adjustment the woman's partner is the most important figure. The partner's support and acceptance influence her completion of her maternal tasks and the formation of her maternal identity. If there are other children in the home, the mother also works to ensure their acceptance of the coming child. Accepting the coming change in exclusive relationships—woman and partner or mother and first child—can be stressful, and the woman will often work to maintain some special time with her partner or older child. Achieving social acceptance of the child and of herself as mother may be more difficult for the adolescent mother or single woman. The child to come is not always wanted, and the woman often must direct her energies to changing this situation.
3. ***Seeking of commitment and acceptance of self as mother to the child (binding-in).*** During the first trimester, the child remains a rather abstract concept. With quickening, however, the child begins to become a real person, and the mother begins to develop bonds of attachment. The mother experiences the movement of the child within her in an intimate, exclusive way, and out of this experience bonds of love form. This possessive love increases her maternal commitment to protect her fetus now and after her child is born.
4. ***Learning to give of oneself on behalf of one's child.*** Childbirth involves many acts of giving. The man "gives" a child to a woman; she in turn "gives" a child to the man. Life is given to a baby; a sibling is given to older children of the family. The woman begins to develop a capacity for self-denial and learns to delay immediate personal gratification to meet the needs of another. Baby showers and baby gifts are acts of giving that help the mother's self-esteem while also helping her acknowledge the separateness and needs of the coming baby.

Father

In the past, the expectant father was often viewed as a "bystander" or observer of his partner's pregnancy. He was necessary for conception, for bill paying, and for providing male guidance as his child matured. This view has changed, and the father of today is expected to fulfill the role of nurturing, caring, involved parent as well as provider. In response to societal pressures, the influence of the feminist movement, and the economic pressures that result in more women employed outside the home, shared parenting and breadwinning have become more commonplace. Many men have actively sought to be more involved in the experience of childbirth and parenting.

Initially, expectant fathers may feel pride in their virility, which pregnancy confirms, but they may also have many of the same ambivalent feelings as expectant mothers (Kowlessar, Fox, & Wittkowski, 2015). The extent of ambivalence depends on many factors, including the father's relationship with his partner, his previous experience with pregnancy, his age, his economic stability, and whether the pregnancy was planned.

In adjusting to his role, the expectant father must first deal with the reality of the pregnancy and then struggle to gain recognition as a parent from his partner, family, friends, coworkers, society—and from his baby as well. The expectant mother can help her partner be a participant and not merely a helpmate to her if she has a definite sense of the experience as *their* pregnancy and *their* baby and not her pregnancy and her baby.

The expectant father must establish a fatherhood role, just as the woman develops a motherhood role. Fathers who are most successful at this task generally like children, are excited about the prospect of fatherhood, are eager to nurture a child, and have confidence in their ability to be a parent. Barriers to a father's involvement may exist if there is an unhealthy relationship between the father and mother or if the father has a lack of understanding of what is involved in having a child. Fathers may have a lack of understanding of their role if they came from a dysfunctional family, if they lacked positive role models, or if there was a general lack of education available (Alio, Lewis, Scarborough, et al., 2013). In general, the expectant father faces psychologic stress as he makes the transition from nonparent to parent or from parent of one to parent of two or more. Sources of stress include financial issues, unexpected events during pregnancy, concern that the baby will not be healthy and normal, worry about the pain the partner will experience in childbirth, and his role during labor and birth. Other sources of stress for expectant fathers include concern over the changing relationship with their partners, diminished sexual responsiveness in their partners or in themselves, change in relationships with their families or male friends, and their ability to parent.

The role of the father is crucial both prenatally and postnatally. Healthcare providers need to encourage and welcome the father's involvement during the pregnancy. It is important to educate fathers about the role they can play in promoting healthy child development and how they can best support the mother during pregnancy to enhance healthy outcomes.

FIRST TRIMESTER

After the initial excitement of the announcement of the pregnancy to friends and relatives and receipt of their congratulations, an expectant father may begin to feel left out of the pregnancy. He is also often confused by his partner's mood changes and perhaps bewildered by his responses to her changing body. He may resent the attention given to the woman and the need to change their relationship as she experiences fatigue and a decreased interest in sex.

During this time, his child is a "potential baby." Fathers often picture interacting with a child of 5 or 6 rather than a newborn. Even the pregnancy itself may seem unreal until the woman shows more physical signs.

SECOND TRIMESTER

The second trimester is a time of growing acceptance as the man sees evidence of pregnancy in his partner's bodily changes. He begins to develop an emotional attachment to their baby and to feel part of the pregnancy process (Kowlessar et al., 2015). His involvement may increase as he watches and feels fetal movement and listens to the fetal heartbeat during a prenatal visit. For many men, seeing the fetus during an ultrasound is an important experience in accepting the reality of pregnancy. Like expectant mothers, expectant fathers need to confront and resolve some of their conflicts about the parenting they received. A father needs to sort out which behaviors of his own father he wants to imitate and which he wants to avoid (Kowlessar et al., 2015).

> “I was excited about the chance to be the kind of father who was involved and available. However, I also wanted to provide adequately for my child, support my wife, and still have time to do the things I loved to do. I was surprised by how excited my father was about becoming a grandfather. He even talked to me about the regrets he had about not being around as I was growing up. I think the experience will help to bring my dad and me closer as he tries to be a good grandfather and I understand more about his struggles as a father.”

The anxiety of the father-to-be is lessened if both parents agree on the support role the man is to assume during pregnancy and on his projected paternal role. For example, if both see his role as that of breadwinner, the man's stress is low. However, if the man views his role as that of breadwinner and the woman expects him to be actively involved in preparations and child care, his stress increases.

The woman's appearance begins to alter at this time, too, and men react differently to the physical change. For some it decreases sexual interest; for others it may have the opposite effect. Both partners experience a multitude of emotions, and it continues to be important for them to communicate and accept each other's feelings and concerns. In situations in which the expectant mother's demands dominate the relationship, the expectant father's resentment may increase to the point that he is spending more time at work, involved in a hobby, or with his friends. The behavior is even more likely if the expectant father did not want the pregnancy and/or if the relationship was not a good one before the pregnancy.

THIRD TRIMESTER

During the third trimester, the man redefines himself as a father and begins to visualize doing things with his child. In essence he recognizes that he is leaving his old life behind and needs to rethink his own values and priorities (Kowlessar et al., 2015).

If the couple have communicated their concerns and feelings to one another and grown in their relationship, the third trimester is a special and rewarding time. A more clearly defined role evolves at this time for the expectant father, and it becomes more obvious how the couple can prepare together for the coming event. They may become involved in childbirth education classes and make concrete preparations for the arrival of the baby, such as shopping for a crib, car seat, and other equipment. If the expectant father has developed a detached attitude about the pregnancy before this time, however, it is unlikely that he will become a willing participant even though his role becomes more obvious.

Concerns and fears may recur. Many men are afraid of hurting the unborn baby during intercourse or become concerned about labor and birth. Also he may wonder what kind of parents he and his partner will be.

COUVADE

The term **couvade** traditionally referred to the observance of certain rituals and taboos by the male to signify the transition to fatherhood. This observance affirms his psychosocial and biophysical relationship to the woman and child. These taboos may have taken specific form—for example, the man may have been forbidden to eat certain foods or carry certain weapons before and immediately after the birth. More recently, the term has been used to describe the unintentional development of physical symptoms, such as fatigue, increased appetite, difficulty sleeping, depression, headache, or backache by the partner of the pregnant woman. Men who demonstrate couvade syndrome tend to have a higher degree of paternal role preparation and be involved in more activities related to this preparation.

Partners of Lesbian Mothers

The motivations for pregnancy for lesbian couples are similar to those of heterosexual couples but the process of becoming parents is complex, with more obstacles to overcome including the basic decision as to which woman will become the biological parent. In negotiating their relationship, the lesbian couple needs to determine the language they will use in referring to the nonbiological or nonbirth mother. Terms such as co-parent, social mother, other mother, or second parent are often used (Pharris, Bucchio, Dotson, et al, 2016).

For the nonbirth parent, transitioning to parenthood can be challenging. She is not able to contribute biologically and is at risk legally unless an adoption process is completed. The lesbian couple may have made decisions about having both parents' names on the birth certificate or for the nonbiological parent to adopt the baby. However, legal options vary from state to state and the vast majority of states do not provide for the nonbiological parent to adopt her partner's child (McKelvey, 2014). The couple needs to have a clear understanding of their legal options and their preferences with regard to the role of the nonbiological parent.

Early research on the perinatal experiences of nonbirth lesbian mothers determined that these women felt "like everyone else but not quite" (Erlandsson, Linder, & Haggstrom-Nordin, 2010, p. 100). Nonbiological parents want to be supportive but often feel unwelcomed and misunderstood in their families of origin and in healthcare settings. The pervasive emotion identified is a feeling of "otherness" coupled with the desire to be acknowledged as an equal and legitimate parent (Wojnar & Katzenmeyer, 2014). In essence, they seek to receive the same respect shown to fathers throughout pregnancy and birth. However, nonbirth mothers often feel at the mercy of healthcare providers, who set the tone for how they are viewed and treated (McKelvey, 2014).

A shared last name is often an important element for the nonbirth mother. It helps the family be identified as a cohesive unit and enables the nonbirth mother to be recognized as a parent by healthcare providers (McKelvey, 2014).

A strong support group is helpful during the pregnancy and beyond, but it may not be readily available. Fortunately, today the needs of lesbian couples are being identified and addressed more effectively. Nurses can play an important role in identifying resources and sharing information with lesbian couples.

Siblings

The introduction of a new baby into the family is often the beginning of sibling rivalry. Sibling rivalry results from children's fear of change in the security of their relationships with their parents. Some of the behaviors demonstrating feelings of sibling rivalry may even be directed toward the mother during the pregnancy as she experiences more fatigue and less patience with her toddler, for example. Parents who recognize the situation early in pregnancy and begin constructive actions can help minimize the problems of sibling rivalry.

Preparation of the young child begins several weeks before the anticipated birth and is designed according to the age and experience of the child. Because they do not have a clear concept of time, young children should not be told too early about the pregnancy. From the toddler's point of view "several weeks" is an extremely long time. The mother may let the child feel the baby moving in her uterus, explaining that this is "a special place where babies grow." The child can help the parents prepare the baby's room, perhaps by putting baby clothes in drawers.

Consistency is important in dealing with young children. They need reassurance that certain people, special things, and familiar places will continue to exist after the new baby arrives. The crib is an important though transient object in a child's life. If it is to be given to the new baby, the parents should thoughtfully help the child adjust to this change. Any move from crib to bed or from one room to another should precede the baby's birth by several weeks or more. If the new baby is to share a room with siblings, the parents must discuss this with the older child or children.

Some parents advocate co-sleeping or bed sharing (one or both parents sleeping with their baby or young child), and so the crib is less of an issue. Co-sleeping, which is common in many non-Western cultures, is increasing in the United States even though it is not recommended. It is discussed further in Chapter 34.

If the child is ready for toilet training, it is most effectively done several months before or after the baby's arrival. Parents should know that the older, toilet-trained child may regress to wetting or soiling because he or she sees the new baby getting attention for such behavior. The older, weaned child may want to drink from the breast or bottle again after the new baby comes. If the new mother anticipates these behaviors, they will be less frustrating during her early postpartum days.

During the pregnancy, older children should be introduced to a new baby for short periods to get an idea of what a new baby is like. This introduction dispels fantasies that the new arrival will be big enough to be a playmate. Pregnant women may also find it helpful to bring their children to a prenatal visit after they have been told about the expected baby. The children are encouraged to become involved in prenatal care and to ask any questions they may have. They are also given the opportunity to hear the baby's heartbeat, either with a stethoscope or with the Doppler. This helps make the baby more real to them. Reminiscing about their birth by viewing videos or looking at pictures may also be helpful.

If siblings are school-age children, the pregnancy should be viewed as a family affair; thus, it is important to tell older children about the baby before telling friends and extended family. Teaching about the pregnancy should be based on the child's level of understanding and interest. Overeager parents may go into lengthier and more in-depth responses than the child is able to understand. Some children are more curious than others. Books at their level of understanding can be made available in the home. Involvement in family discussions, encouragement to feel fetal movement, and an opportunity to listen to the fetal heart supplement the learning process and help make the school-age child feel part of the pregnancy. Sibling preparation classes assist in the transition process for both parents and children (see Chapter 13). After attending the classes, children often exhibit less anxiety and increased ability to express their feelings.

It is important to set realistic expectations about the baby's normal behavior including sleeping, eating, and crying. Ask for the older child's support and help so they feel involved with the baby's care. It may also be helpful to identify the benefits of being the older child and all the things older children can do such as playing with friends, watching videos, and going to the playground.

Older children or adolescents may appear to have a sophisticated knowledge base, but it may be intermingled with many misconceptions. Thus, the parents should make opportunities to discuss their concerns and should involve the children in preparation for the new baby.

Even after the birth, siblings need to feel that they are part of a family affair. Changes in hospital regulations allowing siblings to be present at the birth or to visit their mother and the new baby facilitate this process. Participation in special programs for siblings may help in this process. On arrival at home, siblings can share in "showing off" the new baby.

Sibling preparation for the arrival of a new baby is essential, but other factors are equally important. These include the amount of parental attention focused on the new arrival, the amount of parental attention given the older child after the birth of the baby, and parental skill in dealing effectively with regressive and/or aggressive behavior.

Grandparents

The first relatives told about a pregnancy are usually the couple's parents, the expectant grandparents. Although relationships with parents can be very complex, the expectant grandparents often become increasingly supportive of the expectant couple, even if conflicts previously existed. But it can be difficult for even sensitive grandparents to know how deeply to become involved in the childrearing process.

Grandparents can be an important source of comfort and support for prospective and new parents. They are now being included more frequently in the birthing process and immediate postpartum period (Figure 11–7).

Because grandparenting can occur over a wide expanse of years, people's response to this role can vary considerably. Younger grandparents leading active lives may not demonstrate as much interest as the young couple would like. In other cases, expectant grandparents may give advice and gifts unsparingly. For grandparents, conflict may be related to the expectant couple's need to feel in control of their lives, or it may stem from events that signal changing roles in the grandparents' own lives (e.g., retirement, financial concerns, menopause, or death of a friend). Some parents of expectant couples may already be grandparents with a developed style of grandparenting. This influences their response to the pregnancy.

Childbearing and childrearing practices are very different for today's childbearing couple. It helps family cohesiveness for young couples to share with interested grandparents what today's practices are and why they feel they are effective. At the same time, it is important for young couples to listen to any differences expectant grandparents want to explain. When grandparents give advice, it helps to remember that they care. When their recommendations seem effective, it is significant to the expectant grandparents that young couples do listen and follow their advice. Occasionally a grandparent may give advice that is inaccurate or no longer current practice. In such cases, it may be necessary to tactfully explain why the advice is not being followed.

Occasionally, young couples feel they are receiving more advice than they can tolerate. Too often they perceive parents' suggestions as criticizing their ability to prepare adequately for the childbearing process—and later as criticizing their care of the newborn. It is useful for the young couple to discuss the problem and agree on a plan of action. Prior to bringing the baby home, the role of the grandparents needs to be clarified to ensure a comfortable situation for all.

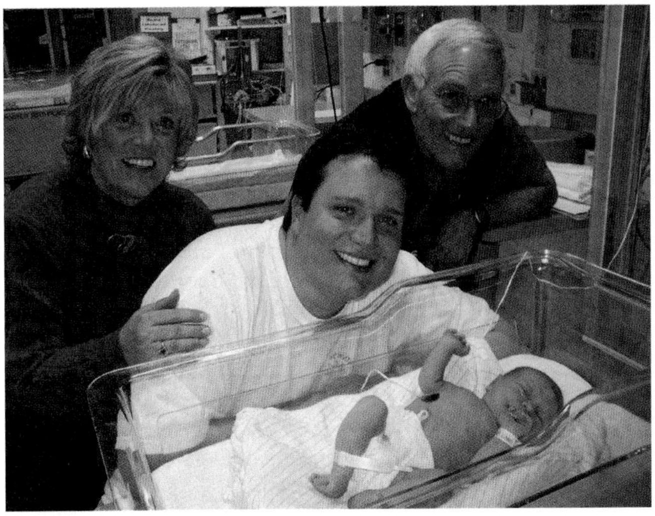

Figure 11–7 **These grandparents and their son, the baby's father, enjoy a moment with their first grandson.**

SOURCE: Michele Davidson.

In some areas, classes for grandparents provide information about changes in birthing and parenting practices. These classes help familiarize grandparents with new parents' needs and may offer suggestions for ways in which the grandparents can support the childbearing woman or couple.

Cultural Values and Pregnancy

A universal tendency exists to create ceremonial rituals and rites around important life events. Thus pregnancy, childbirth, marriage, and death are often tied to rituals. The rituals, customs, and practices of a group are a reflection of the group's values. In many developed countries such as the United States, Canada, England, France, and Germany, populations are becoming more and more ethnically diverse as the number of immigrants continues to grow. Research indicates that the experiences they have had in their country of origin shape their expectations of pregnancy and birth (Benza & Liamputtong, 2014). Thus, it is not realistic or appropriate to assume that people who are new to a country or area will automatically abandon their ways and adopt the practices of the dominant culture. Consequently, the identification of cultural values is useful in planning and providing culturally sensitive care. See *Case Study: Azia Askari.*

It is important to identify the main beliefs, values, and behaviors that relate to pregnancy and childbearing. This

CASE STUDY: Azia Askari

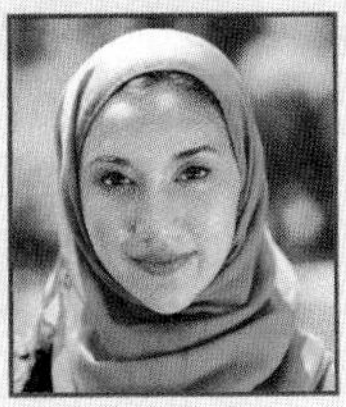

SOURCE: HONGQI ZHANG/123RF

Azia presents for a routine prenatal care appointment accompanied by her mother-in-law, Shira. An interpreter is present at the visit to translate. Azia begins to tell you she fatigues easily and hesitantly reveals that she is more emotional and stressed this pregnancy. Shira scolds her and tells her it is her job to maintain calmness for her baby. She appears agitated that her daughter-in-law confides this information to you.

Questions to Ponder

How can you provide reassurance, support, and appropriate education while respecting the cultural values of Azia's native ancestry? Why is it important to consider cultural values when addressing psychosocial issues in pregnancy?

includes information about ethnic background, amount of affiliation with the ethnic group, patterns of decision making, religious preferences, language, communication style, and common etiquette practices. Once this information is gathered, the nurse can then plan and provide care that is appropriate and responsive to the family's needs. These topics are discussed in detail in Chapter 2.

The *National Standards for Culturally and Linguistically Appropriate Services in Health and Health Care*, the CLAS Standards, developed in 2000 by the Office of Minority Health within the U.S. Department of Health and Human Services, provided a blueprint for advancing and sustaining culturally and linguistically appropriate services. Revised and updated, the national CLAS standards also provide tools for health professionals including nurses (U.S. Department of Health and Human Services, Office of Minority Health, 2016). Additional guidelines and resources are available from The Joint Commission and from professional organizations such as the American Nurses Association and the Transcultural Nursing Society.

Developing Cultural Competence: Providing Effective Prenatal Care to Families of Different Cultures summarizes the key actions a nurse can take to become more culturally aware.

Developing Cultural Competence Providing Effective Prenatal Care to Families of Different Cultures

Nurses who are interacting with expectant families from a different culture or ethnic group can provide more effective, culturally sensitive nursing care by doing the following:

- Examine critically their own cultural beliefs.
- Identify personal biases, attitudes, stereotypes, and prejudices.
- Make a conscious commitment to respect and study the values and beliefs of others.
- Use sensitive, current language when describing others' cultures.
- Learn the rituals, customs, and practices of the major cultural and ethnic groups with whom they have contact.
- Include cultural assessment and assessment of the family's expectations of the healthcare system as a routine part of prenatal nursing care.
- Incorporate the family's cultural and spiritual practices into prenatal care as much as possible.
- Foster an attitude of respect for and cooperation with alternative healers and caregivers whenever possible.
- Provide for the services of an interpreter if language barriers exist.
- Learn the language (or at least several key phrases) of at least one of the cultural groups with whom they interact.
- Recognize that ultimately it is the woman's right to make her own healthcare choices.
- Evaluate whether the patient's healthcare beliefs have any potential negative consequences for her health.

Source: Data from Spector, 2017.

Focus Your Study

- Virtually all systems of a woman's body are altered in some way during pregnancy. Blood pressure decreases slightly during pregnancy. It reaches its lowest point in the second trimester and gradually increases to near normal levels in the third trimester. The enlarging uterus may exert pressure on the vena cava when the woman lies supine, causing a drop in blood pressure. This is called vena caval syndrome or supine hypotension.
- A physiologic anemia may occur during pregnancy because the total plasma volume increases more than the total number of erythrocytes. This produces a drop in the hematocrit.
- The glomerular filtration rate increases during pregnancy. Glycosuria may be caused by the body's inability to reabsorb all the glucose filtered by the glomeruli.
- Changes in the skin include the development of chloasma; linea nigra; darkened nipples, areolae, and vulva; striae; and spider nevi.
- Insulin needs increase during pregnancy. A woman with a latent deficiency state may respond to the increased stress on the islets of Langerhans by developing gestational diabetes mellitus.
- The subjective (presumptive) signs of pregnancy are those symptoms experienced and reported by the woman, such as amenorrhea, nausea and vomiting, fatigue, urinary frequency, breast changes, and quickening.
- The objective (probable) signs of pregnancy can be perceived by the examiner but may be caused by conditions other than pregnancy.
- The diagnostic (positive) signs of pregnancy can be perceived by the examiner and can be caused only by pregnancy.
- During pregnancy the expectant woman may experience ambivalence, acceptance, introversion, emotional lability, and changes in body image.

- Rubin (1984) identified four developmental tasks for the pregnant woman: (1) ensuring safe passage through pregnancy, labor, and birth; (2) seeking acceptance of this child by others; (3) seeking commitment and acceptance of self as mother to the child; and (4) learning to give of oneself on behalf of one's child.
- Fathers, partners, and same-sex spouses also face a series of adjustments as they accept their new role.
- Siblings of all ages require assistance in dealing with the birth of a new baby.
- Cultural values, beliefs, and behaviors influence a couple's response to childbearing and the healthcare system.
- A cultural assessment should focus on factors that will influence the practices of the childbearing family with regard to their health needs.

References

Alio, A. P., Lewis, C. A., Scarborough, K., Harris, K., & Fiscella, K. (2013). A community perspective on the role of fathers during pregnancy: A qualitative study. *BMC Pregnancy and Childbirth, 13*(60), 1–11.

American College of Obstetricians and Gynecologists (ACOG). (2013). *Weight gain during pregnancy* (ACOG Committee Opinion No. 548). Retrieved from https://www.acog.org/Resources_And_Publications/Committee_Opinions/Committee_on_Obstetric_Practice/Weight_Gain_During_Pregnancy

American College of Obstetricians and Gynecologists (ACOG). (2015). *Nutrition during pregnancy.* Retrieved from https://www.acog.org/Patients/FAQs/Nutrition-During-Pregnancy

Antony, K. M., Racusin, D. A., Aagaard, K., & Dildy III, G. A. (2017). Maternal physiology. In S. G. Gabbe, J. R. Niebyl, J. L. Simpson, M. B. Landon, H. L. Galan, E. R. M. Jauniaux, D. A. Driscoll, V. Berghella, & W. A. Grobman (Eds.), *Obstetrics: Normal and problem pregnancies* (7th ed.). Philadelphia, PA: Elsevier.

Benza, S., & Liamputtong, P. (2014). Pregnancy, childbirth and motherhood: A meta-analysis of the lived experiences of immigrant women. *Midwifery, 30*, 575–584.

Cunningham, F. G., Leveno, K. J., Bloom, S. L., Dashe, J., Hoffman, B. L., Casey, B. M., & Spong, C. Y. (2018). *Williams obstetrics* (25th ed.). New York, NY: McGraw-Hill Education.

Erlandsson, K., Linder, H., & Haggstrom-Nordin, E. (2010). Experiences of gay women during their partners' pregnancy and childbirth. *British Journal of Midwifery, 18*(2), 99–103.

Greene, D. N., Schmidt, R. L., Kamer, S. M., & Grenache, D. G. (2013). Limitations in qualitative point of care hCG tests for detecting early pregnancy. *Clinica Chimica Acta, 415*, 317–321.

Institute of Medicine (IOM). (2009). *Weight gain during pregnancy: Reexamining the guidelines.* Washington, DC: National Academies Press.

Jessop, D. C., Craig, L., & Ayers, S. (2014). Applying Leventhal's self-regulatory model to pregnancy: Evidence that pregnancy-related beliefs and emotional responses are associated with maternal health outcomes. *Journal of Health Psychology, 19*(9), 1091–1102.

Kowlessar, O., Fox, J. R., & Wittkowski, A. (2015). The pregnant male: A metasynthesis of first-time fathers' experiences of pregnancy. *Journal of Reproductive and Infant Psychology, 33*(2), 106–127.

McKelvey, M. M. (2014). The other mother: A narrative analysis of the postpartum experiences on nonbirth lesbian mothers. *Advances in Nursing Science, 37*(2), 101–116.

Patel, P. R., Laz, T. H., & Berenson, A. B. (2015). Patient characteristics associated with pregnancy ambivalence. *Journal of Women's Health, 24*(1), 37–41.

Pharris, A., Bucchio, J., Dotson, C., & Davidson, W. (2016). Supporting lesbian couples during pregnancy. *International Journal of Childbirth Education, 31*(3), 23–24.

Rubin, R. (1984). *Maternal identity and the maternal experience.* New York, NY: Springer.

Spector, R. (2017). *Cultural diversity in health and illness* (9th ed.). Boston, MA: Pearson.

U. S. Department of Health and Human Services. (2013). *Healthy people 2020.* https://www.healthypeople.gov/2020

U.S. Department of Health and Human Services, Office of Minority Health. (2016). The National CLAS Standards. Retrieved from https://minorityhealth.hhs.gov/omh/browse.aspx?lvl=2&lvlid=53

Wojnar, D. M., & Katzenmeyer, A. (2014). Experiences of preconception, pregnancy, and new motherhood for lesbian nonbiological mothers. *Journal of Obstetric, Gynecologic and Neonatal Nursing, 43*(1), 50–60.

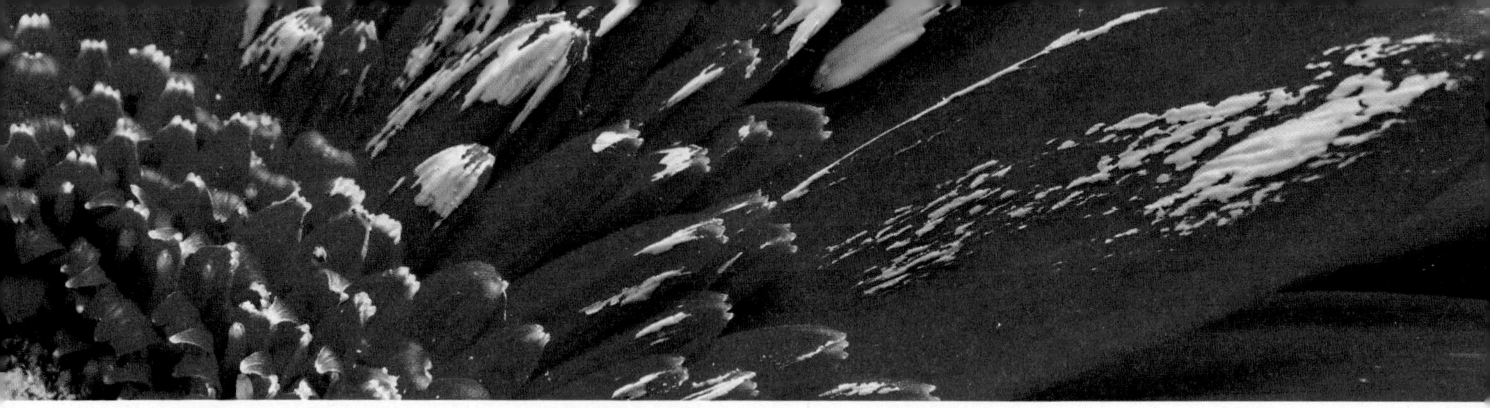

Chapter 12

Antepartum Nursing Assessment

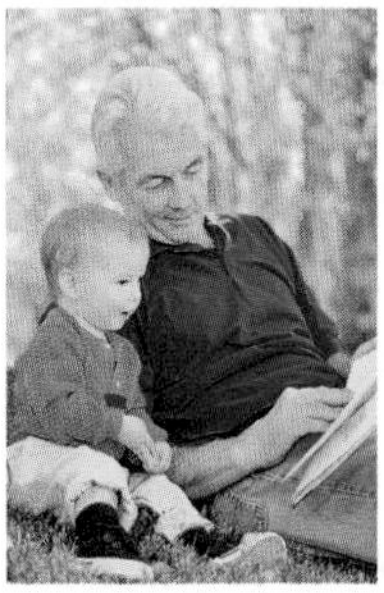

SOURCE: Steve Smith/SuperStock.

From the father of one of the book authors: The father of the late 1950s . . . Main objective: Get your wife to the hospital on time. Check her in and find the father's waiting lounge. You won't be needed until the baby is born. Fathers are really useless at this time. Try not to be nervous. Coffee is available. Lots of coffee.

More coffee, pacing, no sleep, waiting for word. What a drain on the father. . . . The baby finally comes. "It's a beautiful, healthy baby girl. Mother and baby are doing fine. You can see them now, but only for 5 minutes." What a relief. The pressure is finally off. Isn't nature wonderful?

Today's father, my grandson. Attends most of the prenatal visits. Schooled in Lamaze. Drives his wife to the birthing center. Coaches her through her labor. Helps her push. His digital camera is ready. The baby is born. He cuts the cord. He sends e-mail and pictures of the baby to everyone. Isn't nature wonderful?

Learning Outcomes

12.1 Summarize the essential components of a prenatal history.

12.2 Define common obstetric terminology found in the history of maternity patients.

12.3 Predict the normal physiologic changes one would expect to find when performing a physical assessment on a pregnant woman.

12.4 Calculate the estimated date of birth using the common methods.

12.5 Describe the essential measurements that can be determined by clinical pelvimetry.

12.6 Summarize the results of the major screening tests used during the prenatal period in the assessment of the prenatal patient.

12.7 Relate the danger signs of pregnancy to their possible causes.

12.8 Relate the components of the subsequent prenatal history and assessment to the progress of pregnancy and the nursing care of the prenatal patient.

Healthy People 2020

(MICH-5) Reduce the rate of maternal mortality

(MICH-6) Reduce maternal illness and complications due to pregnancy (complications during hospitalized labor and delivery)

(MICH-8) Reduce low birth weight (LBW) and very low birth weight (VLBW)

(MICH-9) Reduce preterm births

(MICH-10) Increase the proportion of pregnant women who receive early and adequate prenatal care

(MICH-11) Increase abstinence from alcohol, cigarettes, and illicit drugs among pregnant women

MCH-13 Increase the proportion of mothers who achieve a recommended weight gain during their pregnancies

MICH-25 Reduce the occurrence of fetal alcohol syndrome (FAS)

The RN may complete many areas of prenatal assessment. Advanced practice nurses such as certified nurse-midwives (CNMs) and nurse practitioners are able to perform complete antepartum assessments. The primary roles of a nurse in an office or prenatal clinic are to counsel, educate, and meet the psychologic needs of the expectant family and perform other nursing care functions and assessments. This chapter focuses on the prenatal assessments completed initially and at subsequent visits to provide optimum care for the childbearing family.

Initial Patient History

The course of a pregnancy depends on a number of factors, including the past pregnancy history (if this is not a first pregnancy), prepregnancy health of the woman, presence of disease/illness states, family history, emotional status, and past health care. Ideally, antenatal care is a continuation of established care that the woman has been receiving to ensure a status of health outside of pregnancy. For some women, however, this may be the only healthcare that they have received in many years. One important method of determining the adequacy of a woman's prepregnancy care is by completing a thorough history.

Definition of Terms

The following terms are used in recording the obstetric history of maternity patients:

- **Antepartum:** Time between conception and onset of labor, usually used to describe the period during which a woman is pregnant; used interchangeably with *prenatal*.
- **Intrapartum:** Time from onset of labor until the birth of the baby and placenta.
- **Postpartum:** Time from birth until the woman's body returns to an essentially prepregnant condition, typically about 6 weeks.
- **Gestation:** The number of weeks since the first day of the last menstrual period (LMP) in a pregnancy.
- **Abortion:** Birth that occurs before 20 weeks' gestation or the birth of a fetus-newborn who weighs less than 500 g (Cunningham et al., 2018). An abortion (ab) may occur spontaneously or it may be induced by medical or surgical means. If induced, it is often called a *therapeutic abortion*.
- **Term:** The American College of Obstetrics and Gynecology (ACOG, 2015a) recommends that the label *term* no longer be used. Instead, the following definitions are preferred:
    - **Early term:** Extending from 37 0/7 weeks through 38 6/7 weeks' gestation
    - **Full term:** Extending from 39 0/7 weeks through 40 6/7 weeks' gestation
    - **Late term:** Extending from 41 0/7 weeks through 41 6/7 weeks' gestation
    - **Postterm:** 42 0/7 weeks and beyond
- **Preterm labor** *(premature labor)*: Labor that occurs after 20 weeks but before the completion of 37 weeks of gestation (Cunningham et al., 2018).
- **Postterm labor:** Labor that occurs after 42 weeks of gestation.
- **Gravida:** A pregnant woman; any pregnancy, regardless of duration, including present pregnancy.
- **Nulligravida:** A woman who has never been pregnant.
- **Primigravida:** A woman who is pregnant for the first time.
- **Multigravida**: A woman who is in her second or any subsequent pregnancy.
- **Para**: A woman who has given birth after 20 weeks' gestation, regardless of whether the baby is born alive or dead.
- **Nullipara**: A woman who has not given birth at more than 20 weeks' gestation.
- **Primipara**: A woman who has had one birth at more than 20 weeks' gestation, regardless of whether the baby is born alive or dead.
- **Multipara**: A woman who has had two or more births at more than 20 weeks' gestation.
- **Stillbirth:** A fetus born dead after 20 weeks' gestation.

The terms *gravida* and *para* refer to pregnancies, not to the fetus. Thus, traditionally, twins, triplets, and other multiple fetuses are counted as one pregnancy and one birth. This approach is confusing because it fails to identify the number of children a woman may actually have. Consequently, to provide more comprehensive data, a detailed approach is now used by many healthcare team members. A useful acronym for remembering the system is ***TPAL*** (King et al., 2015).

- *T:* Number of term births the woman has experienced (number of babies born at 37 0/7 weeks' gestation or beyond)
- *P:* Number of *preterm* births (births after 20 weeks' but before 37 0/7 weeks' gestation, whether living or stillborn)
- *A:* Number of pregnancies ending in either spontaneous or therapeutic *abortion* (before 20 weeks' gestation)
- *L:* Number of currently *living* children to whom the woman has given birth.

The following examples delineate the differences between the two systems.

1. Jean Sanchez has one child born at 39 weeks' gestation and became pregnant for a second time. The second pregnancy ended in a miscarriage at 15 weeks' gestation. Using the *traditional approach* her obstetric history would be recorded as "gravida 2 para 1 ab 1." Using the *detailed approach*, her obstetric history would be recorded as "gravida 2 para 1011."
2. Tracy Hopkins is pregnant for the fourth time. At home she has a child who was born at full term. Her second pregnancy ended at 10 weeks' gestation. She then gave birth to twins at 35 weeks. Using the *traditional approach*, her obstetric history would be recorded as "gravida 4 para 2 ab 1." Using the *detailed approach*, her obstetric history would be recorded as "gravida 4 para 1113."

To avoid confusion, it is best for practicing nurses to clarify the recording system used at their facilities.

Clinical Tip

In general, it is best to avoid an initial discussion of a woman's gravida and para in front of her partner. It is possible that the woman had a previous pregnancy that she has not mentioned to her partner and revealing the information could violate her right to privacy.

Patient Profile

The patient's history is a screening tool that identifies factors that can affect the course of a pregnancy. For optimal prenatal care, the nurse should obtain the following information for each maternity patient at the initial prenatal assessment:

1. *Current pregnancy*
   - First day of last menstrual period (LMP). Is this a sure date or uncertain? Within days? Does she know the last month of menses? Do her cycles normally occur every 28 days, or do her cycles tend to be longer or shorter? Does she have monthly menses? Was the LMP normal in duration and bleeding? Was she using any form of contraception?
   - Presence of cramping, bleeding, or spotting since LMP
   - Woman's opinion about time when conception occurred and when the baby is due. Was she charting her cycles?
   - Woman's attitude toward pregnancy (Is pregnancy planned or unplanned? Wanted?)

     Note: It is important to realize that an unplanned pregnancy is not always unwanted. Approximately 50% of pregnancies in the United States are unplanned.
   - Date of positive pregnancy test; date of negative pregnancy test
   - Any pregnancy discomforts since LMP, such as nausea and vomiting, urinary frequency, fatigue, breast tenderness, constipation, fever, headaches
   - Spontaneous conception? Infertility treatments?
2. *Past pregnancies*
   - Number of pregnancies
   - Number of abortions, spontaneous or therapeutic
   - Number of living children
   - History of previous pregnancies: Length of pregnancy, length of labor and birth, type of birth (vaginal, forceps or vacuum-assisted birth, cesarean), location of birth, healthcare provider, gestational age at time of birth, type of anesthesia/analgesia used (if any), woman's perception of the experience, complications (antepartum, intrapartum, postpartum)
   - Neonatal status of previous children: Apgar scores, birth weights, general development, complications, feeding method (breast, formula, or both). If breastfed, how long?
   - Loss of a child (miscarriage, elective or medically indicated abortion, stillbirth, neonatal death, relinquishment, death after the neonatal period). Cause of loss? What was the experience like for her? What coping skills helped? How did the father/partner, if involved, respond?
   - Blood type and Rh factor (If Rh negative, was Rh immune globulin received after birth/miscarriage/abortion?)
   - Prenatal education classes, resources (books, websites); knowledge about pregnancy, childbirth, and parenting.
3. *Gynecologic history*
   - Date of last Pap smear; result? History of abnormal Pap results? Colposcopy? Loop electrosurgical excision procedure (LEEP)? Human papillomavirus (HPV)?
   - Previous infections: Vaginal, cervical, pelvic inflammatory disease (PID), sexually transmitted
   - Previous surgery (uterine, ovarian)
   - Age of menarche
   - Regularity, frequency, and duration of menstrual flow
   - History of dysmenorrhea
   - History of infertility
   - Sexual history
   - Contraceptive history (If hormonal method was used, did pregnancy immediately follow cessation of method? If not, how long after? When was contraception last used?)
4. *Current medical history*
   - Weight (prepregnancy and current), height, body mass index (BMI) (determine recommended weight gain)
   - Blood type and Rh factor
   - General health, including nutrition (dietary practices or problems such as vegetarianism, lactose intolerance, food allergies), regular exercise program (type, frequency, duration), monthly breast self-exams; eye exam; date of last dental exam
   - Any medication use (nonprescription, homeopathic, or herbal medications); medications taken since LMP?
   - Previous or present use of alcohol, tobacco, or caffeine (if yes, ask about amounts consumed each day); planning cessation?
   - Illicit drug use or abuse (specific drugs such as cocaine, crack, marijuana, methamphetamines); planning cessation?
   - Drug or food allergies, latex allergy or sensitivities: What type of reaction?
   - Potential teratogenic insults to this pregnancy, such as viral infections, medications, x-ray examinations, surgery, or cats in the home (source of toxoplasmosis)
   - Presence of chronic disease conditions, such as diabetes, hypertension, asthma, cardiovascular disease, renal problems, or thyroid disorders
   - Infections or illnesses since LMP (flu, measles)
   - Record of immunizations (especially rubella); up to date?
   - Presence of any abnormal signs/symptoms.
5. *Past medical history*
   - Childhood diseases (varicella)
   - Past treatment for any disease condition (Any hospitalizations? Major accidents?)
   - Surgical procedures
   - Presence of bleeding disorders or tendencies
   - Blood transfusion history? Will she accept blood transfusion?
6. *Family medical history*
   - Presence of diabetes, cardiovascular disease, hypertension, hematologic disorders, tuberculosis, thyroid disease, cancer
   - Occurrence of multiple births
   - History of congenital diseases or deformities
   - History of mental illness
   - Occurrence of cesarean births and cause, if known
   - Cause of death of deceased parents or siblings.
7. *Genetic history (patient, father of child [FOC], and both families)*
   - Thalassemia, neural tube defect, congenital heart defect, Down syndrome, Tay-Sachs disease, Canavann disease, sickle cell disease or trait, hemophilia or other blood disorders, muscular dystrophy, cystic fibrosis, Huntington chorea, intellectual disability/autism, other genetic disorder
   - Recurrent pregnancy loss or stillbirth.
8. *Religious/cultural history*
   - Does the woman wish to specify a religious preference on her chart? Does she have any spiritual beliefs or practices that might influence her healthcare or that of her child,

such as prohibition against receiving blood products, dietary considerations, or other practices?
- What practices are important to maintain her spiritual well-being?
- Are there practices in her culture or that of her partner that might influence her care or that of her child?

9. *Occupational history*
   - Occupation
   - Physical demands (Does she stand all day, or are there opportunities to sit and elevate her legs? Does she do any heavy lifting?)
   - Exposure to lead, chemicals, or other harmful substances
   - Opportunity for regular meals and breaks for nutritious snacks
   - Provision for maternity or family leave.
10. *Birth father's physical history*
   - Presence of genetic conditions or diseases in him or in his family history
   - Age
   - Significant health problems
   - Blood type and Rh factor
   - Immunizations up to date.
11. *Father's/partner's social history*
   - Occupation
   - Educational level; methods by which he or she learns best
   - Current tobacco use, drug use, and alcohol intake
   - Thoughts/feelings regarding pregnancy.

   Note: It is important to be aware that different partner situations exist (married/unmarried couple, single parent, LGBTQ couple). It is important to understand the woman's current relationship situation early on in pregnancy.

12. *Personal information about the woman (social history)*
   - Age
   - Relationship status (Married? Birth father involved? Partner's level of involvement [if partner is not the birth father]?)
   - Educational level; methods by which she learns best
   - Race or ethnic group (to identify need for prenatal genetic screening or counseling)
   - Housing; stability of living conditions
   - Economic level
   - Intimate partner violence (IPV): Any history of emotional or physical deprivation or abuse of herself or children. (Does she experience any abuse in her current relationship? Has she been hit, slapped, kicked, or hurt within the past year or since she has been pregnant? Is she afraid of her partner or anyone else? If yes, of whom is she afraid?) *Note:* Ask these questions when the woman is alone.
   - History of emotional/mental health disorder (depression in general, postpartum depression, anxiety)
   - Support systems/postpartum support
   - Personal preferences about the birth (expectations of both the woman and her partner, presence of others, and so on)
   - Plans for care of child following birth; plans for circumcision if the baby is male
   - Feeding method for the baby (breast milk, formula, or both).

Ethics in Action!

A patient in your practice has finally disclosed to you after repeated IPV screenings that her husband is physically abusive to her. You practice in a state where you are covered by the IPV mandatory reporting law, but your patient has asked you to not report as she is scared for her life. How do you respond to this situation?

Obtaining Data

In many settings, nurses use standardized charting forms to obtain the necessary data for the initial prenatal visit. The questionnaire developed by the American College of Obstetricians and Gynecologists (ACOG), the Antepartum Record and Postpartum Form, is commonly used in many clinical settings. The form allows for complete documentation from the first visit through the postpartum period, including patient education/plans, birth information, discharge details, and postpartum clinic visits.

SAFETY ALERT!

Because some medications may pose a risk to the fetus if taken during pregnancy, it is crucial to develop a list of all the medications the pregnant woman is currently taking as well as those she took from conception to the initial prenatal visit. This includes prescribed, over-the-counter, illicit, and herbal preparations. Because the woman may not always know when she became pregnant, you may need to give her a time frame (e.g., "In the last 3 months") depending on how far along she is in her pregnancy when she first presents for care. (See discussion of classification system for medications taken during pregnancy in Chapter 13.)

The nurse can review the questionnaire and obtain further information in a direct interview with the patient. This allows the pregnant woman to expand or clarify her responses to questions and allows the nurse to gather additional information or clarify data provided. The initial interview provides the nurse and the woman the opportunity to begin developing a healthy relationship. The expectant partner should be encouraged to attend the initial and subsequent prenatal visits. The partner is often able to contribute information to the history and may use this opportunity to ask questions and express concerns that may be of particular importance to him or her. See *Case Study: Angelina Newman*.

"I didn't know what to expect when I went for my first prenatal visit. I'm clean now and wanted to be honest, but I was afraid they would treat me differently if I told them about some of the really dumb things I did in high school—the drinking, the marijuana, the sex, and stuff. I really liked the nurse-midwife who was taking care of me, so I decided to be straight with her—for the baby's sake, you know. She was great about everything and really made me feel okay."

Prenatal Risk-Factor Screening

A highly significant part of the prenatal assessment is screening for risk factors. **Risk factors** are any findings that have been shown to have potential negative effects on pregnancy outcomes

CASE STUDY: Angelina Newman

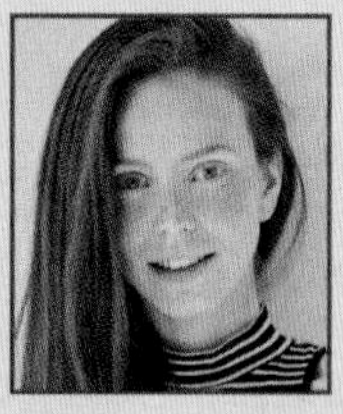

SOURCE: WAYHOME studio/Shutterstock

Angelina presents for a routine antepartum visit with her boyfriend and her mother. You begin to obtain the assessment and note that the young woman's mother is providing all of the information for the maternal assessment.

Question to Ponder

Why is it important for you to advocate for Angelina to answer questions on her own and be the primary historian of her prenatal care?

either for the woman or her unborn child. Often risk factors can be identified during the initial prenatal assessment, while others may be detected during subsequent visits through subjective and objective data collection. Risk-identified counseling has the ability to impact maternal behavior positively and reduce psychosocial risk in pregnancy.

All risk factors do not threaten the pregnancy to the same degree and some factors, such as chronic illness (hypertension, thyroid disease), cannot be modified to decrease the risk. The nurse needs to be aware of potential risk factors and the impact that they might have on the pregnancy. It is possible that a pregnancy may begin as low risk and change to high risk because of current or developed risk factors. Risk is also assessed during the intrapartum and postpartum periods. Ideally, the initial risk assessment should occur prior to pregnancy when changes can be made to decrease risks during pregnancy.

Table 12–1 identifies the major prenatal risk factors currently recognized. The table describes potential maternal and fetal/neonatal implications should the risk be present in the pregnancy. In addition to the factors listed, the perinatal health team also needs to evaluate psychosocial factors, including ethnic background, occupation, education, financial status, environment including living arrangements and location, and the woman's and her family's concept of health, which might influence her attitude toward seeking health care. Women's health status and risk are continually evaluated at every healthcare team encounter.

Initial Prenatal Assessment

The initial prenatal assessment focuses on the woman holistically by considering physical, cultural, and psychosocial factors that influence her health. The establishment of the nurse–patient relationship will help the woman evaluate the health team and also provide the nurse with a basis for developing an atmosphere that is conducive to interviewing, support, and education. Because many women are excited and anxious at the first antepartum visit, the initial psychosocial-cultural assessment is of a general nature. See *Women with Special Needs: Assessing Care Needs During Pregnancy*.

As part of the initial psychosocial-cultural assessment the nurse discusses with the woman any religious, cultural, or socioeconomic factors that may influence the woman's expectations of the childbearing experience. It is especially helpful if the nurse is familiar with common practices of various religious and cultural groups who reside in the community. Gathering the data in a tactful, caring way can help make the childbearing woman's experience a positive one and provides opportunity for a partnership in care to develop. Cultural considerations are discussed in Chapter 13. See *Developing Cultural Competence: Using Cultural Information Effectively*.

Women with Special Needs Assessing Care Needs During Pregnancy

During the initial assessment, the woman with a disability should be questioned to determine her current level of functioning and the degree of assistance she normally requires in her everyday routine. This assists the healthcare team in planning care and interventions that may be needed. Care needs may change during pregnancy and warrant ongoing assessments of the woman's level of functioning.

Developing Cultural Competence Using Cultural Information Effectively

During prenatal assessment, it is important for nurses to avoid stereotyping women based on race, culture, or ethnicity. Women who have immigrated may not understand the pregnancy, labor, and birth culture of the United States and can feel frightened or overwhelmed by recommended medical interventions. Nurses have an obligation to be aware of other cultures and develop a culturally sensitive plan of care to meet the needs of the childbearing woman and her family (Spector, 2017).

After the history is obtained, the nurse prepares the woman for the physical examination. The physical examination begins with assessment of vital signs followed by the head-to-toe examination with the pelvic examination completed last. It is important for the nurse or caregiver to provide anticipatory guidance and reassurance when completing the physical exam because this may be the patient's first gynecologic examination. See *Professionalism in Practice: Physical Exams and Scope of Practice*.

TABLE 12–1 Prenatal High-Risk Factors

FACTOR	MATERNAL IMPLICATIONS	FETAL/NEONATAL IMPLICATIONS
Social-Personal		
Low income level/low educational level	Insufficient antenatal care or late antenatal care ↑ risk preterm birth Poor nutrition ↑ risk of preeclampsia	Low birth weight Prematurity Intrauterine growth restriction (IUGR)/small for gestational age (SGA)
Poor diet	Inadequate nutrition/inadequate weight gain Poor weight gain ↑ risk preterm labor/birth ↑ risk anemia ↑ risk preeclampsia	Fetal malnutrition Prematurity IUGR/SGA
Living at high altitude	↑ hemoglobin	Prematurity IUGR ↑ hemoglobin (polycythemia)
Multiparity greater than 3	↑ risk antepartum or postpartum hemorrhage	Anemia Fetal death
Weight less than 45.5 kg (100 lb)	Poor nutrition Cephalopelvic disproportion Prolonged labor	IUGR Hypoxia associated with difficult labor and birth
Weight greater than 91 kg (200 lb)	↑ risk hypertension ↑ risk cephalopelvic disproportion ↑ risk diabetes	↓ fetal nutrition/perfusion ↑ risk macrosomia
Age younger than 16	Poor nutrition Insufficient/late antenatal care ↑ risk preeclampsia ↑ risk cephalopelvic disproportion	Low birth weight ↑ fetal demise
Age older than 35	↑ risk preeclampsia ↑ risk cesarean birth Psychosocial issues	↑ risk congenital anomalies ↑ chromosomal abnormalities
Smoking one pack/day or more	↑ risk hypertension ↑ risk cancer	↓ placental perfusion → ↓ O_2 and nutrients available Low birth weight IUGR/SGA Preterm birth
Use of illicit drugs	↑ risk poor nutrition ↑ risk of infection with intravenous (IV) drugs ↑ risk HIV, hepatitis C ↑ risk abruptio placentae	↑ risk congenital anomalies ↑ risk low birth weight Neonatal withdrawal Lower serum bilirubin
Excessive alcohol consumption	↑ risk poor nutrition Possible hepatic effects with long-term consumption	↑ risk fetal alcohol syndrome (FAS)
Preexisting Medical Disorders		
Diabetes mellitus	↑ risk preeclampsia, hypertension Episodes of hypoglycemia and hyperglycemia ↑ risk cesarean birth	Low birth weight Macrosomia Neonatal hypoglycemia ↑ risk congenital anomalies ↑ risk respiratory distress syndrome

(continued)

TABLE 12–1 Prenatal High-Risk Factors *(continued)*

FACTOR	MATERNAL IMPLICATIONS	FETAL/NEONATAL IMPLICATIONS
Preexisting Medical Disorders *(continued)*		
Cardiac disease	Cardiac decompensation Further strain on mother's body ↑ maternal death rate	↑ risk fetal demise ↑ perinatal mortality
Anemia: Hemoglobin less than 11 g/dL; hematocrit less than 32%	Low energy level Decreased oxygen-carrying capacity	Fetal death Prematurity Low birth weight
Hypertension	↑ vasospasm ↑ risk central nervous system (CNS) irritability ↑ risk convulsions ↑ risk cerebrovascular accident (CVA) ↑ risk renal damage	↓ placental perfusion ↓ low birth weight Preterm birth
Thyroid disorder	↑ infertility	↑ spontaneous abortion
Hypothyroidism	↓ basal metabolic rate (BMR), goiter, myxedema ↑ risk miscarriage ↑ risk preterm labor/birth ↑ risk preeclampsia	↑ risk congenital goiter ↑ risk IUGR/SGA ↑ risk anemia ↑ risk stillbirth
Hyperthyroidism	↑ risk postpartum hemorrhage ↑ risk preeclampsia Danger of thyroid storm	Intellectual disability (cretinism) ↑ incidence congenital anomalies ↑ IUGR/SGA ↑ neonatal hyperthyroidism
Renal disease (moderate to severe)	↑ risk renal failure	↑ risk IUGR/SGA ↑ risk preterm birth
Diethylstilbestrol (DES) exposure	↑ Infertility, spontaneous abortion ↑ cervical insufficiency ↑ risk breech presentation	↑ risk preterm birth
Obstetric Considerations		
Previous Pregnancy		
Stillborn	↑ emotional/psychologic distress	↑ risk IUGR/SGA ↑ risk preterm birth
Recurrent abortion	↑ emotional/psychologic distress	↑ risk abortion
Cesarean birth	↑ possibility repeat cesarean birth Risk of uterine rupture	↑ risk preterm birth ↑ risk respiratory distress
Rh or blood group sensitization		↑ risk erythroblastosis fetalis Hydrops fetalis Neonatal anemia Kernicterus Hypoglycemia
Current Pregnancy		
Large for gestational age (LGA)	↑ risk cesarean birth ↑ risk gestational diabetes ↑ risk operative birth	↑ risk birth injury Hypoglycemia
Gestational diabetes mellitus	↑ risk operative birth ↑ risk preeclampsia ↑ risk extensive lacerations ↑ risk primary pulmonary hypertension (PPH) ↑ risk shoulder dystocia	Macrosomia Hyperbilirubinemia ↑ risk birth injury

FACTOR	MATERNAL IMPLICATIONS	FETAL/NEONATAL IMPLICATIONS
***Current Pregnancy* (continued)**		
Rubella (first trimester)		Congenital heart disease Cataracts Nerve deafness Bone lesions Prolonged virus shedding
Rubella (second trimester)		Hepatitis Thrombocytopenia
Toxoplasmosis Cytomegalovirus		Retinochoroiditis Convulsions, coma, microcephaly IUGR Encephalopathy
Herpesvirus type 2	Severe discomfort Concern about possibility of cesarean birth, fetal infection	Neonatal herpesvirus type 2 Hepatitis with jaundice Neurologic abnormalities
Syphilis	↑ incidence abortion	↑ fetal demise Congenital syphilis
Urinary tract infection	↑ risk preterm labor Uterine irritability	↑ risk preterm birth
Abruptio placentae and placenta previa	↑ risk hemorrhage Bed rest Extended hospitalization	Fetal/neonatal anemia Intrauterine hemorrhage ↑ fetal demise
Preeclampsia/eclampsia	See hypertension	↓ placental perfusion ↑ low birth weight
Multiple gestation	↑ risk postpartum hemorrhage ↑ risk gestational diabetes ↑ risk preeclampsia ↑ risk placenta previa ↑ risk cesarean birth ↑ risk cord prolapse	↑ risk preterm labor/birth ↑ risk stillbirth ↑ risk fetal demise ↑ risk IUGR/SGA ↑ risk malpresentation ↑ risk stillbirth
Elevated hematocrit (greater than 41%)	Increased viscosity of blood	Fetal death rate five times normal rate
Spontaneous premature rupture of membranes	↑ risk uterine infection	Preterm birth Fetal demise

Professionalism in Practice Physical Exams and Scope of Practice

Increasing numbers of nurses, such as certified nurse-midwives and other advanced practice nurses, are educationally prepared to perform physical examinations. The nurse who has not yet fully developed these specific assessment skills obtains the woman's vital signs, explains the procedures to allay apprehension, positions her for examination, and assists the examiner as necessary. Each nurse is responsible for operating at expected professional standards within his or her skill level, educational preparation, state nurse practice act, and knowledge base.

Before the examination, the woman should provide a clean urine specimen for screening. When her bladder is empty, the patient will be more comfortable during the pelvic examination, and the examiner can palpate the pelvic organs more easily. After the woman has emptied her bladder, the nurse asks her to disrobe and gives her a gown and sheet or some other protective covering to provide modesty, comfort, and warmth.

Clinical Tip

Gloves are worn for procedures that involve contact with body fluids such as drawing blood for laboratory work, handling urine specimens, and conducting pelvic examinations. Because of the increased incidence of latex allergies, it is becoming more common for latex-free gloves to be used. It is important to inquire about latex allergies with any patient before beginning the exam.

Thoroughness and a systematic procedure are the most important considerations when performing the physical portion of an antepartum examination (see *Assessment Guide: Initial Prenatal Assessment*). To promote completeness, the assessment

ASSESSMENT GUIDE | Initial Prenatal Assessment

Physical Assessment/Normal Findings	Alterations and Possible Causes*	Nursing Responses to Data†
Vital Signs		
Blood Pressure (BP): Less than or equal to 120/80 mmHg	High BP (chronic hypertension; renal disease; gestational hypertension, apprehension; preeclampsia if initial assessment not done until after 20 weeks' gestation)	BP of 120–139/80–89 is considered prehypertensive. BP greater than 140/90 requires immediate consideration; establish woman's BP; refer to healthcare provider if necessary. Assess woman's knowledge about high BP; counsel on self-care and medical management.
Pulse: 60–100 beats/min; rate may increase 10 beats/min during pregnancy	Increased pulse rate (excitement or anxiety, dehydration, infection, cardiac disorders)	Count for 1 full minute; note irregularities. Evaluate temperature, increase fluids.
Respirations: 12–20 breaths/min (or pulse rate divided by 4); pregnancy may induce a degree of hyperventilation; thoracic breathing predominant	Marked tachypnea or abnormal patterns	Assess for respiratory disease.
Temperature: 36.2°C–37.6°C (97°F–99.6°F)	Elevated temperature (infection)	Assess for infection process or disease state if temperature is elevated; refer to healthcare provider.
Weight		
Depends on body build	Weight less than 45 kg (100 lb) or greater than 91 kg (200 lb); rapid, sudden weight gain (preeclampsia)	Evaluate need for nutritional counseling; obtain information on eating habits, cooking practices, food regularly eaten, food avoided, food allergies, income limitations, need for food supplements, pica and other abnormal food habits. Note initial weight to establish baseline for weight gain throughout pregnancy. Determine body mass index (BMI) and recommended weight gain for pregnancy.
Skin		
Color: Consistent with racial background; pink nail beds	Pallor (anemia); bronze, yellow (hepatic disease; other causes of jaundice)	Tests to perform: Complete blood count (CBC), bilirubin level, urinalysis, and blood urea nitrogen (BUN).
	Bluish, reddish, mottled; dusky appearance or pallor of palms and nail beds in dark-skinned women (anemia)	If abnormal, refer to healthcare provider.
Condition: Absence of edema (slight edema of lower extremities is normal during pregnancy)	Edema (preeclampsia, normal pregnancy changes); rashes, dermatitis (allergic response)	Counsel on relief measures for slight edema. Initiate preeclampsia assessment; refer to healthcare provider.
Lesions: Absence of lesions	Ulceration (varicose veins, decreased circulation)	Further assess circulatory status; refer to healthcare provider if lesion is severe.
Spider nevi common in pregnancy	Petechiae, multiple bruises, ecchymosis (hemorrhagic disorders; abuse)	Evaluate for bleeding or clotting disorder. Provide opportunities to discuss abuse if suspected.
	Change in size or color (carcinoma)	Refer to healthcare provider.
Moles		
Pigmentation: Pigmentation changes of pregnancy include linea nigra, striae gravidarum, melasma		Assure woman that these are normal manifestations of pregnancy and explain the physiologic basis for the changes.
Café-au-lait spots	Six or more (Albright syndrome or neurofibromatosis)	Consult with healthcare provider.

Physical Assessment/Normal Findings	Alterations and Possible Causes*	Nursing Responses to Data†
Nose		
Character of Mucosa: Redder than oral mucosa; in pregnancy nasal mucosa is edematous in response to increased estrogen, resulting in nasal stuffiness (rhinitis of pregnancy) and nosebleeds	Olfactory loss (first cranial nerve deficit)	Counsel woman about possible relief measures for nasal stuffiness and nosebleeds (epistaxis); refer to healthcare provider for olfactory loss.
Mouth		
May note hypertrophy of gingival tissue because of estrogen	Edema, inflammation (infection); pale in color (anemia)	Assess hematocrit for anemia; counsel regarding dental hygiene habits. Refer to healthcare provider or dentist if necessary. Routine dental care appropriate during pregnancy.
Neck		
Nodes: Small, mobile, nontender nodes	Tender, hard, fixed, or prominent nodes (infection, carcinoma)	Examine for local infection; refer to healthcare provider.
Thyroid: Small, smooth, lateral lobes palpable on either side of trachea; slight hyperplasia by third month of pregnancy	Enlargement or nodule tenderness (hyperthyroidism, hypothyroidism, carcinoma)	Test to perform: Thyroid-stimulating hormone (TSH). Listen over thyroid for bruits, which may indicate hyperthyroidism. Question woman about dietary habits (iodine intake). Ascertain history of thyroid problems; refer to healthcare provider.
Chest and Lungs		
Chest: Symmetric, elliptic, smaller anteroposterior (AP) than transverse diameter	Increased AP diameter, funnel chest, pigeon chest (emphysema, asthma, pulmonary disease)	Evaluate for emphysema, asthma, pulmonary disease.
Ribs: Slope downward from nipple line	More horizontal (pulmonary disease) Angular bumps Rachitic rosary (vitamin C deficiency)	Evaluate for pulmonary disease. Evaluate for fractures. Consult healthcare provider. Consult nutritionist.
Inspection and Palpation: No retraction or bulging of intercostal spaces (ICS) during inspiration or expiration; symmetric expansion	ICS retractions with inspirations, bulging with expiration; unequal expansion (respiratory disease)	Do thorough initial assessment. Refer to healthcare provider.
Tactile fremitus	Tachypnea, hyperpnea (respiratory disease)	Refer to healthcare provider.
Percussion: Bilateral symmetry in tone	Flatness of percussion, which may be affected by chest wall thickness	Evaluate for pleural effusions, consolidations, or tumor.
Low-pitched resonance of moderate intensity	High diaphragm (atelectasis or paralysis), pleural effusion	Refer to healthcare provider.
Auscultation: Upper lobes—bronchovesicular sounds above sternum and scapulas; equal expiratory and inspiratory phases	Abnormal if heard over any other area of chest	Refer to healthcare provider.
Remainder of Chest: Vesicular breath sounds heard; inspiratory phase longer (3:1)	Rales, rhonchi, wheezes; pleural friction rub; absence of breath sounds; bronchophony, egophony, whispered pectoriloquy	Refer to healthcare provider.

(continued)

ASSESSMENT GUIDE | Initial Prenatal Assessment *(continued)*

Physical Assessment/Normal Findings	Alterations and Possible Causes*	Nursing Responses to Data†
Breasts		
Supple: Symmetric in size and contour; darker pigmentation of nipple and areola; may have supernumerary nipples, usually 5–6 cm below normal nipple line	"Pigskin" or orange-peel appearance, nipple retractions, swelling, hardness (carcinoma); redness, heat, tenderness, cracked or fissured nipple (infection)	Discuss value of regular self-examination; instruct woman how to examine her breasts (see Chapter 6).
Axillary nodes nonpalpable or pellet sized	Tenderness, enlargement, hard node (carcinoma); may be visible bump (infection)	Refer to healthcare provider for evaluation of abnormal breast findings. Plan ultrasound/mammogram/magnetic resonance imaging (MRI) of breasts.
Pregnancy Changes: **1.** Size increase noted primarily in first 20 weeks. **2.** Become nodular. **3.** Tingling sensation may be felt during first and third trimester; woman may report feeling of heaviness. **4.** Pigmentation of nipples and areolae darkens. **5.** Superficial veins dilate and become more prominent. **6.** Striae seen in multiparas. **7.** Tubercles of Montgomery enlarge. **8.** Colostrum may be present after 12th week. **9.** Secondary areola appears at 20 weeks, characterized by series of washed-out spots surrounding primary areola. **10.** Breasts less firm, old striae may be present in multiparas.		Discuss normalcy of changes and their meaning with the woman. Teach and/or institute appropriate relief measures. Encourage use of supportive, well-fitting brassiere.
Heart		
Normal rate, rhythm, and heart sounds	Enlargement, thrills, thrusts, gross irregularity or skipped beats, gallop rhythm, or extra sounds (cardiac disease)	Complete an initial assessment. Explain normal pregnancy-induced changes. Refer to healthcare provider, if indicated.
Pregnancy Changes: **1.** Palpitations may occur due to sympathetic nervous system disturbance. **2.** Short systolic murmurs that increase in held expiration are normal due to increased volume.		
Abdomen		
Normal appearance, skin texture, and hair distribution; liver nonpalpable; abdomen nontender	Muscle guarding (anxiety, acute tenderness); tenderness, mass (ectopic pregnancy, inflammation, carcinoma)	Assure woman of normalcy of diastasis. Provide initial information about appropriate prenatal and postpartum exercises. Evaluate woman's anxiety level. Refer to healthcare provider.
Pregnancy Changes: **1.** Purple striae may be present (or silver striae on a multipara) as well as linea nigra. **2.** Diastasis of the rectus muscles late in pregnancy.		

Physical Assessment/Normal Findings	Alterations and Possible Causes*	Nursing Responses to Data†
3. Size: Flat or rotund abdomen; progressive enlargement of uterus due to pregnancy. 10–12 weeks: Fundus slightly above symphysis pubis. 16 weeks: Fundus halfway between symphysis and umbilicus. 20–22 weeks: Fundus at umbilicus. 28 weeks: Fundus three finger breadths above umbilicus. 36 weeks: Fundus just below ensiform cartilage.	Size of uterus inconsistent with length of gestation (intrauterine growth restriction [IUGR], multiple pregnancy, fetal demise, incorrect estimated date of birth [EDB], abnormal amniotic fluid, hydatidiform mole)	Reassess menstrual history regarding pregnancy dating. Evaluate increase in size using McDonald method. Use ultrasound to establish diagnosis.
4. Fetal heart rate: 110–160 beats/ min may be heard with Doppler at 10–12 weeks' gestation; may be heard with fetoscope at 17–20 weeks.	Failure to hear fetal heartbeat with Doppler (fetal demise, hydatidiform mole)	Refer to healthcare provider. Administer pregnancy tests. Use ultrasound to establish diagnosis.
5. Fetal movement palpable by a trained examiner after the 18th week.	Failure to feel fetal movements after 20 weeks' gestation (fetal demise, hydatidiform mole)	Refer to healthcare provider.
6. Ballottement: During fourth to fifth month fetus rises and then rebounds to original position when uterus is tapped sharply.	No ballottement (oligohydramnios)	Refer to healthcare provider.
Extremities		
Skin warm, pulses palpable, full range of motion; may be some edema of hands and ankles in late pregnancy; varicose veins may become more pronounced; palmar erythema may be present	Nonpalpable or diminished pulses (arterial insufficiency); marked edema (preeclampsia)	Evaluate for other symptoms of heart disease; initiate follow-up if woman mentions that her rings feel tight. Discuss prevention and self-treatment measures for varicose veins; refer to healthcare provider, if indicated.
Spine		
Normal Spinal Curves: Concave cervical, convex thoracic, concave lumbar	Abnormal spinal curves; flatness, kyphosis, lordosis	Refer to healthcare provider, if indicated.
In pregnancy, lumbar spinal curve may be accentuated	Backache	May have implications for administration of spinal anesthetics; see Chapter 22 for relief measures.
Shoulders and iliac crests should be even	Uneven shoulders and iliac crests (scoliosis)	Refer very young women to healthcare provider; discuss back-stretching exercise with older women.
Reflexes		
Normal and symmetric	Hyperactivity, clonus (preeclampsia)	Evaluate for other symptoms of preeclampsia.
Pelvic area		
External Female Genitals: Normally formed with female hair distribution; in multiparas, labia majora loose and pigmented; urinary and vaginal orifices visible and appropriately located	Lesions, genital warts, hematomas, varicosities, inflammation of Bartholin's glands; clitoral hypertrophy (masculinization)	Explain pelvic examination procedure. Encourage woman to minimize her discomfort by relaxing her hips. Provide privacy.
Vagina: Pink or dark pink, vaginal discharge odorless, nonirritating; in multiparas, vaginal folds smooth and flattened; may have episiotomy scar	Abnormal discharge associated with vaginal infections	Obtain vaginal discharge sample. Provide understandable verbal and written instructions about treatment for woman and partner, if indicated.

(continued)

ASSESSMENT GUIDE | Initial Prenatal Assessment *(continued)*

Physical Assessment/Normal Findings	Alterations and Possible Causes*	Nursing Responses to Data†
Cervix: Pink color; os closed except in multiparas, in whom os admits fingertip	Eversion, reddish erosion, nabothian or retention cysts, cervical polyp; granular area that bleeds (carcinoma of cervix); lesions (herpes, human papillomavirus [HPV]); presence of string or plastic tip from cervix (intrauterine device [IUD] in uterus)	Provide woman with a hand mirror and identify genital structures for her; encourage her to view her cervix if she wishes. Refer to healthcare provider, if indicated. Advise woman of potential serious risks of leaving an IUD in place during pregnancy; refer to healthcare provider for removal.
Pregnancy Changes:		
1–4 weeks' gestation: Enlargement in anteroposterior diameter		
4–6 weeks' gestation: Softening of cervix (Goodell sign); softening of isthmus of uterus (Hegar sign); cervix takes on bluish coloring (Chadwick sign)	Absence of Goodell sign (inflammatory conditions, carcinoma)	Refer to healthcare provider.
8–12 weeks' gestation: Vagina and cervix appear bluish violet in color (Chadwick sign)	Fixed (pelvic inflammatory disease [PID]); nodular surface (fibromas)	Refer to healthcare provider.
Uterus: Pear shaped, mobile; smooth surface		
Ovaries: Small, walnut shaped, nontender (ovaries and fallopian tubes are located in the adnexal areas)	Pain on movement of cervix (PID); enlarged or nodular ovaries (cyst, tumor, tubal pregnancy, corpus luteum of pregnancy)	Evaluate adnexal areas; refer to healthcare provider. Plan ultrasound to evaluate mass.
Pelvic Measurements		
Internal Measurements: 1. Diagonal conjugate at least 11.5 cm (see Figure 12–7)	Measurement below normal	Vaginal birth may not be possible if deviations are present. However, a diagnosis of cephalopelvic disproportion is not suspected unless the woman fails to progress during labor or the fetus fails to descend (King et al., 2015).
2. Obstetric conjugate estimated by subtracting 1.5 cm from diagonal conjugate	Disproportion of pubic arch	
3. Inclination of sacrum	Abnormal curvature of sacrum	
4. Motility of coccyx; external intertuberosity diameter greater than 8 cm	Fixed or malposition of coccyx	
Anus and Rectum		
No lumps, rashes, excoriation, tenderness; cervix may be felt through rectal wall	Hemorrhoids, rectal prolapse; warts (HPV infection); nodular lesion (carcinoma)	Counsel about appropriate prevention and relief measures; refer to healthcare provider for further evaluation.
Laboratory Evaluation		
Hemoglobin: 12–16 g/dL; women residing in areas of high altitude may have higher levels of hemoglobin	Less than 11 g/dL in the first trimester, less than 10.5 g/dL in the second trimester, and less than 11 g/dL in the third trimester (anemia) (West, Hark, & Catalano, 2017)	Hemoglobin less than 12 g/dL requires nutritional counseling; less than 11 g/dL requires iron supplementation.
ABO and Rh Typing: Normal distribution of blood types	Rh negative	If Rh negative, check for presence of anti-Rh antibodies. Check blood type of father of child; if he is Rh positive, discuss with woman the need for Rh immune globulin administration at 28 weeks, management during the intrapartum period, and possible need for Rh immune globulin after childbirth. (See Chapter 18.)

Physical Assessment/Normal Findings	Alterations and Possible Causes*	Nursing Responses to Data†
Complete Blood Count (CBC)		
Hematocrit: 38–47% physiologic anemia (pseudoanemia) may occur	Marked anemia or blood dyscrasias	Perform CBC and Schilling differential cell count.
Red Blood Cells (RBCs): 4.2–5.4 million/microliter		
White Blood Cells (WBCs): 5000–12,000/microliter	Presence of infection; may be elevated in pregnancy and with labor	Evaluate for other signs of infection.
Differential Neutrophils: 40–60% Bands: up to 5% Eosinophils: 1–3% Basophils: up to 1% Lymphocytes: 20–40% Monocytes: 4–8%		
First-trimester aneuploidy screening (testing to detect conditions related to abnormal chromosome number): If nuchal translucency (NT) testing is available, offer first-trimester screening for Down syndrome using nuchal translucency and serum markers (PAPP-A and free β-hCG). Normal range.	Increased nuchal translucency, elevated β-hCG, and reduced PAPP-A (Down syndrome, trisomy 18, trisomy 13, Turner syndrome)	If findings are positive, genetic counseling and diagnostic testing using chorionic villus sampling (CVS) or second-trimester amniocentesis are offered.
Integrated screening: Combines first-trimester aneuploidy screening results with second-trimester quad screen to detect aneuploidy and neural tube defects; may be used in areas in which NT testing is not available. (See discussion in *Assessment Guide: Subsequent Prenatal Assessment Guide*.)		
Syphilis Tests: Serologic tests for syphilis (STS), complement fixation test, venereal disease research laboratory (VDRL) test—nonreactive	Positive reaction STS—tests may have 25–45% incidence of biologic false-positive results; false results may occur in individuals who have acute viral or bacterial infections, hypersensitivity reactions, recent vaccinations, collagen disease, malaria, or tuberculosis	Positive results may be confirmed with the fluorescent treponemal antibody-absorption (FTA-ABS) test; all tests for syphilis give positive results in the secondary stage of the disease; antibiotic tests may cause negative test results. Refer to healthcare provider for treatment.
Gonorrhea Culture: Negative	Positive	Refer for treatment.
Urinalysis (u/a): Normal color, specific gravity; pH 4.6–8	Cloudy appearance (infection; pus or tissue); abnormal color (porphyria, hemoglobinuria, bilirubinemia): Alkaline urine (metabolic alkalemia, *Proteus* infection, old specimen)	Repeat u/a; refer to healthcare provider.
Negative for protein, red blood cells, white blood cells, casts	Positive findings (contaminated specimen, UTI, kidney disease)	Repeat u/a; urine culture with sensitivities if bacteria detected; refer to healthcare provider.
Glucose: Negative (small degree of glycosuria may occur in pregnancy)	Glycosuria (low renal threshold for glucose, diabetes mellitus)	Assess blood glucose level; test urine for ketones.
Rubella Titer: Hemagglutination-inhibition (HAI) test—1:10 or above indicates woman is immune	HAI titer less than 1:10	Immunization will be given postpartum. Instruct woman whose titers are less than 1:10 to avoid children who have rubella. Educate regarding prevention measures and need for immunization after birth.

(continued)

ASSESSMENT GUIDE | Initial Prenatal Assessment *(continued)*

Physical Assessment/Normal Findings	Alterations and Possible Causes*	Nursing Responses to Data†
Hepatitis B Screen for hepatitis B surface antigen (HbsAg): Negative	Positive	If positive, refer to physician. Neonates born to women who test positive are given hepatitis B immune globulin soon after birth followed by first dose of hepatitis B vaccine.
HIV Screen: Negative	Positive	Refer to healthcare provider.
Illicit Drug Screen: Offered to all women who have positive verbal screen; negative	Positive	Refer to healthcare provider.
Sickle-Cell Screen for Patients of African Descent: Negative	Positive; test results would include a description of cells	Refer to healthcare provider.
Pap Smear: If indicated because woman is due for the test; negative	Test results that show abnormal cells with negative or positive high-risk HPV	Refer to healthcare provider. Discuss with the woman the meaning of the findings and the importance of follow-up. Plan colposcopy, if indicated by results.
Cultural Assessment	**Variations to Consider***	**Nursing Responses to Data†**
Determine the woman's fluency in written and oral English.	Woman may be fluent in language other than English.	Work with a knowledgeable translator to provide information and answer questions.
How does she prefer to be addressed? Nickname?	Some women prefer informality; others prefer to use titles.	Address the woman according to her preference. Maintain formality in introducing yourself if that seems preferred.
Determine customs and practices regarding prenatal care:		
• Are there certain practices she expects to follow when she is pregnant?	Practices are influenced by individual preference, cultural expectations, or religious beliefs. Some women believe that they should perform certain acts related to sleep, activity, or clothing.	Honor a woman's practices and provide for specific preferences unless they are contraindicated because of safety. Have information printed in the language of different cultural groups that live in the area.
• Are there any activities she cannot do while she is pregnant?	Some women have restrictions or taboos they follow related to work, activity, sexual, environmental, or emotional factors.	
• Are there certain foods she is expected to eat or avoid while she is pregnant? Determine whether she has lactose intolerance or food allergies.	Foods are an important cultural factor. Some women may have certain foods they must eat or avoid; many women have lactose intolerance and have difficulty consuming sufficient calcium.	Respect the woman's food preferences, help her plan an adequate prenatal diet within the framework of her preferences, and refer to a dietitian, if necessary.
• Is the caregiver's gender of concern to her?	Some women are comfortable only with a female caregiver.	Arrange for a female caregiver if it is the woman's preference.
• What amount or type of partner involvement in her pregnancy does she expect or want? This includes her mother, other family members, and friends.	A woman may not want her partner involved in the pregnancy. For some the role falls to the woman's mother or a female relative or friend.	Respect the woman's preferences about her partner or husband's involvement; avoid imposing personal values or expectations.
• What type of support and counseling resources are available to her?	Some women seek advice from family members, *curanderas*, tribal healers, or religious leaders.	Respect and honor the woman's sources of support.
Psychologic Status		
Excitement and/or apprehension, ambivalence	Marked anxiety (fear of pregnancy diagnosis, fear of medical facility or providers)	Establish lines of communication. Active listening is useful. Establish trusting relationship. Encourage woman to take active part in her care.
	Apathy; display of anger with pregnancy diagnosis	Establish communication and begin counseling. Use active listening techniques.

Physical Assessment/Normal Findings	Alterations and Possible Causes*	Nursing Responses to Data†
Educational Needs		
May have questions about pregnancy or may need time to adjust to reality of pregnancy		Establish educational, supporting environment that can be expanded throughout pregnancy.
Support System		
Can identify at least two or three individuals with whom woman is emotionally intimate (partner, parent, sibling, friend)	Isolated (no telephone, unlisted number); cannot name a neighbor or friend whom she can call on in an emergency; does not perceive parents as part of her support system	Institute support system through community groups. Help woman to develop trusting relationship with healthcare professionals.
Family Functioning		
Emotionally supportive Communications adequate Mutually satisfying Cohesiveness in times of trouble	Long-term problems or specific problems related to the pregnancy, potential stressors within the family, pessimistic attitudes, unilateral decision making, unrealistic expectations of the pregnancy or child	Help identify the problems and stressors, encourage communication, and discuss role changes and adaptations. Refer to counseling, if indicated.
Economic Status		
Source of income is stable and sufficient to meet basic needs of daily living and medical needs	Limited prenatal care; poor physical health; limited use of healthcare system; unstable economic status	Discuss available resources for health maintenance and the birth. Institute appropriate referral for meeting expanding family's needs (food stamps, WIC [a federally funded nutrition program for women, infants, and children], and so forth)
Stability of Living Conditions		
Adequate, stable housing for expanding family's needs	Crowded living conditions; questionable supportive environment for newborn	Refer to appropriate community agency. Work with family on self-help ways to improve situation.

* Possible causes of alterations are identified in parentheses.

†This column provides guidelines for further assessment and initial intervention.

guide is organized into three columns that address the areas to be assessed, the variations or alterations that may be observed, and nursing responses to the data. The nurse should be aware that certain organs and systems are assessed concurrently with other systems during the physical portion of the examination. Nursing interventions based on assessment of the normal physical and psychosocial changes, as well as the cultural influences associated with pregnancy and patient teaching and counseling needs that have been mutually defined, are discussed further in Chapter 13.

Determination of Due Date

Childbearing families are generally eager to know the "due date," or the date around which childbirth will occur. Determination of the due date should be attempted at the initial visit. It is important to have an accurate due date because it drives all aspects of care in the prenatal period. Historically, the due date has been called the *estimated date of confinement (EDC)* or *estimated date of delivery*. In keeping with a view that emphasizes the normality of the process, we have chosen to refer to the due date as the **estimated date of birth (EDB)** throughout this text.

To calculate EDB, it is essential to know the first day of the woman's LMP. The LMP is sometimes not known because some women have episodes of irregular bleeding or amenorrhea or they may fail to keep track of their menstrual cycles. Thus, other techniques also help determine how far along a woman is in her pregnancy, that is, how many weeks' gestation she is. Other techniques that can be used include evaluating uterine size, establishing when quickening occurs (or occurred), using early ultrasound (US), and auscultating the fetal heart rate with a Doppler device or ultrasound. An early ultrasound should be obtained if a precise LMP is not available to help establish an accurate EDB. Fetal measurements determined by ultrasound are used to identify the gestational age at the time of the imaging and they are compared with the LMP dating to finalize the EDB. See *Evidence-Based Practice: Estimating Gestational Age*.

EVIDENCE-BASED PRACTICE | Estimating Gestational Age

Clinical Question

What are the best diagnostic estimates to use in estimating gestational age accurately?

The Evidence

Ninety-one percent of preterm births occur in low- and middle-income countries. Globally, prematurity is the leading cause of mortality in children less than 5 years of age. The evidence is strong that ultrasound dating in early pregnancy is the most accurate method of estimating gestational age. Maternal recall of last menstrual period (LMP) is useful, but is less reliable in low-literacy populations. In low- and middle-income settings in the developing world, ultrasound may be inaccessible, and mothers may wait until late in their pregnancy to seek antenatal care.

Other measures of gestational age use a combination of neurologic and physical signs to create a score that is not dependent upon timing and technology. A systematic review by Lee et al. (2017) sought to identify individual neonatal signs or clinical scores that can be used to ascertain the gestational age of babies without access to ultrasound. Sixty-six articles were included in the final review. Taken together, these studies included thousands of babies and their mothers. This type of large review of research studies represents the strongest level of evidence for practice.

The review identified 18 assessments that have been used for gestational estimation. The assessments are completed upon the neonate's birth to determine appropriate care regimens. The most accurate was the Dubowitz score, which was accurate within 2.6 weeks. It includes assessment of a variety of superficial and neurological signs. However, feasibility remains a concern. The Dubowitz score requires assessment of multiple neonatal characteristics, and its complexity requires training and time to conduct the evaluation (Lee et al., 2017).

Best Practice

When ultrasound is unavailable for gestational dating, the Dubowitz score can provide the most accurate assessment of whether a neonate is preterm. This is particularly important in developing countries that may lack access to technology. However, its use requires training and practice to ensure its maximal accuracy is achieved.

Clinical Reasoning

What are the nursing implications of accurately dating the gestational age of a neonate? What are the potential issues associated with inaccurate dating?

NÄGELE'S RULE

The most common method of determining the EDB is by **Nägele's rule**. To use this method, begin with the first day of the LMP, subtract 3 months, and add 7 days. The following is an example of Nägele's rule:

First day of LMP	July 20
Subtract 3 months	– 3 months
	April 20
Add 7 days	+ 7 days
EDB (of the next year)	April 27
It is simpler to change the months to numeric terms:	
July 20 becomes	07 / 20
Subtract 3 months	– 3
	04 / 20
Add 7 days	+ 7
EDB (of the next year)	04 / 27

A gestation calculator or "wheel" permits the caregiver to calculate the EDB even more quickly (Figure 12–1).

Nägele's rule can be a fairly accurate determiner of EDB if a woman has a history of menses every 28 days, has an accurate LMP, and was not utilizing hormonal contraception prior to conception. Some women, however, may have cycles that last from 35 to 40 days in length, which will cause ovulation to be delayed by several days. Ovulation usually occurs 14 days before the onset of the next menses, not 14 days after the previous menses. In cases of unsure LMP, irregular menstrual cycles, breastfeeding women, amenorrhea, or hormonal contraception use, an ultrasound is done to visualize the gestational sac and obtain measurements of the embryo/fetus to determine EDB. (See the discussion of ultrasound in Chapter 16.)

Thus, Nägele's rule, although helpful, is not always accurate. It is of no use in calculating EDB for the following:

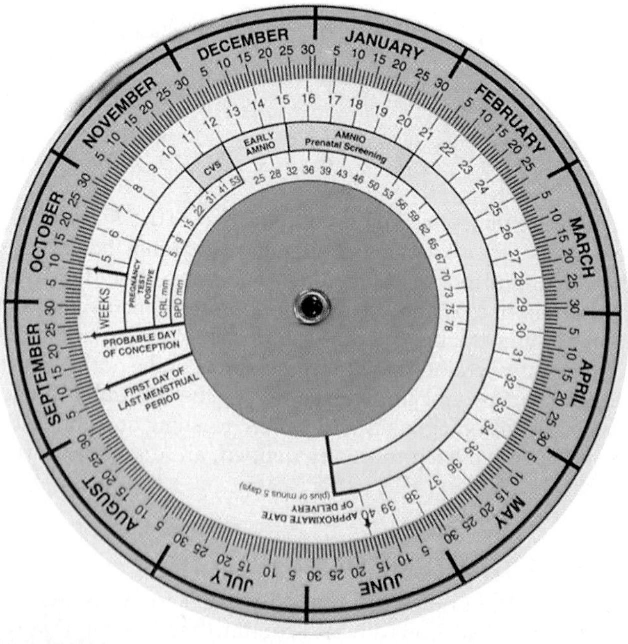

Figure 12–1 **The EDB wheel can be used to calculate the due date. To use it, place the arrow labeled "first day of last period" on the date of the woman's LMP. Then read the EDB at the arrow labeled 40. In this case, the LMP is September 8 and the EDB is June 17.**

- Women with markedly irregular periods that include 1 or more months of amenorrhea
- Women who have amenorrhea but are ovulating and conceive while breastfeeding
- Women who conceive before regular menstruation is established following discontinuation of oral contraceptives or termination of a pregnancy.

An estimation of EDB can be made using other subjective and objective findings such as fundal height, uterine size, auscultation of fetal heart tones, and timing of quickening. In addition to these assessments, an ultrasound should be completed as early as possible to confirm the EDB.

Uterine Assessment

PHYSICAL EXAMINATION

The initial physical examination is done at the patient's first prenatal visit to evaluate for potential health concerns but also to evaluate uterine size to assist with dating the pregnancy. The exam could occur in the first, second, or third trimester depending on when the woman seeks care initially. It becomes much more difficult to accurately evaluate uterine size as the pregnancy progresses in obese women, in multiple gestations, or if uterine fibroids are present.

FUNDAL HEIGHT

Fundal height is an evaluation/screening tool that may be used as an indicator of uterine size, although this method is less accurate late in pregnancy. A tape measure is used to measure the distance in centimeters from the top of the symphysis pubis over the curve of the abdomen to the top of the uterine fundus (McDonald method) (Figure 12–2).

Fundal height in centimeters correlates well with weeks of gestation between 22 weeks and 36 weeks. At 26 weeks' gestation, for example, fundal height is probably about 26 cm. Typically, ±2 cm is considered normal. To be most accurate, fundal height should be measured by the same examiner each time.

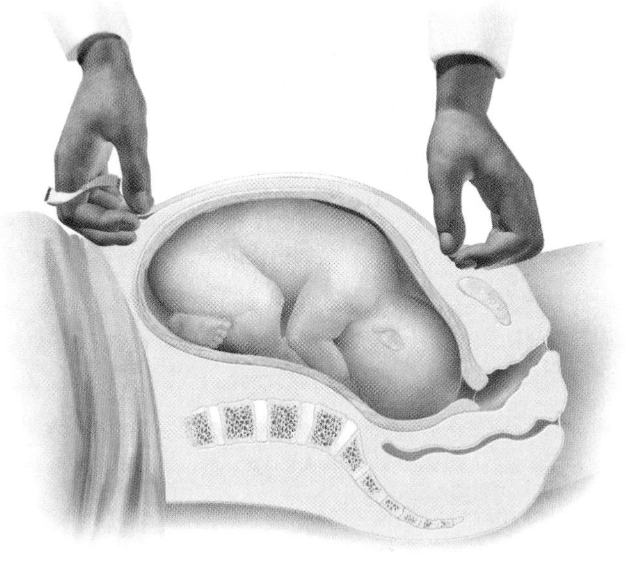

Figure 12–2 **A cross-sectional view of fetal position when the McDonald method is used to assess fundal height.**

Maternal position (trunk elevation, knee flexion) may influence fundal height measurement. If the woman is very tall or very short, fundal height may also differ. In the third trimester, variations in fetal weight and position decrease the accuracy of fundal height measurements. This method of assessment in pregnancy can be quite inaccurate in the following situations:

- Obese women (because of difficulty palpating the fundus accurately)
- Women with uterine fibroids (because uterine size may be distorted)
- Women who develop hydramnios (because the excess fluid increases uterine size, leading the examiner to conclude the fetus is larger than it is).

Clinical Tip

The woman should empty her bladder before measuring fundal height. A full bladder may impact the accuracy of the measurement.

A lag in the progression of fundal height from visit to visit may indicate intrauterine growth restriction (IUGR), or oligohydramnios, and a sudden increase in height may indicate the presence of twins, hydramnios, or a large-for-gestational-age (LGA) fetus. Abnormal fundal height measurements should be assessed by ultrasound to determine possible cause.

Assessment of Fetal Development

QUICKENING

Fetal movements felt by the mother or perception of life—*quickening*—may give some indications that the fetus is nearing 20 weeks' gestation. Quickening may be experienced between 16 and 22 weeks' gestation, so this is not a completely accurate method to date a pregnancy. Because multiparous women have experienced quickening before, they often report fetal movement earlier than a primigravida does.

Clinical Tip

Early fetal movement may be described by the mother as feeling butterfly movements, gas, flicking sensations, or bubbles.

FETAL HEARTBEAT

The ultrasonic Doppler device (Figure 12–3) is the primary tool for assessing fetal heartbeat. It may detect fetal heartbeat at about 10 to 12 weeks' gestation. The normal range for fetal heart tones (FHT) is 110–160. An ultrasound should be completed if the nurse is unable to auscultate between 10 and 12 weeks because there may be a discrepancy of EDB, twins, or a missed abortion.

ULTRASOUND

In the first trimester, transabdominal ultrasound can detect a gestational sac as early as 4 to 5 weeks after the LMP, fetal heart activity by 6 to 7 weeks, and fetal breathing movements by 10 to 11 weeks of pregnancy. Crown-to-rump measurements can be made to assess fetal age from 4 days until about 12 weeks (until the fetal head can be visualized clearly). Biparietal diameter (BPD) measurements can be made by approximately 12 to 13 weeks and

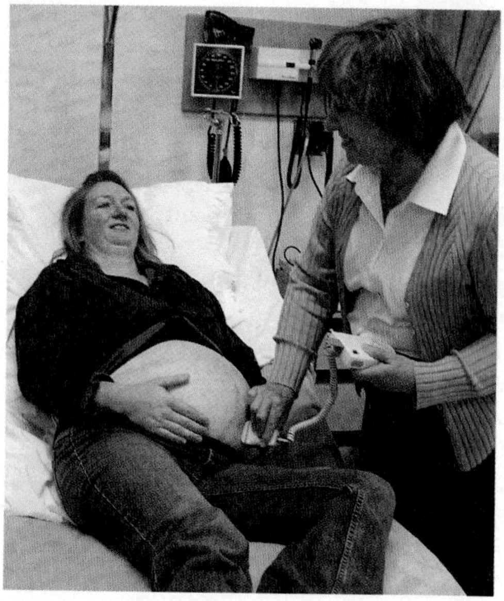

Figure 12–3 **Listening to the fetal heartbeat with a Doppler device.**

SOURCE: Michele Davidson.

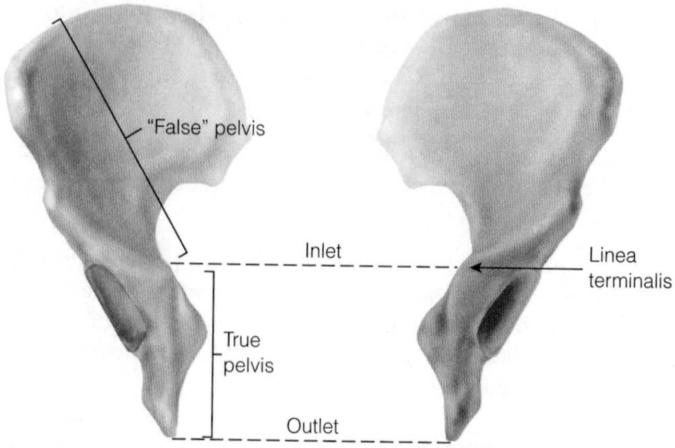

Figure 12–4 **Female pelvis. The false pelvis is the shallow cavity above the inlet; the true pelvis is the deeper portion of the cavity below the inlet and consists of the inlet, cavity (midpelvis), and outlet.**

are most accurate between 14 and 26 weeks, when rapid growth in biparietal diameter occurs. The BPD predicts EDB within 7 to 10 days. (See Chapter 16 for an in-depth discussion of ultrasound scanning of the fetus.)

> "I went with my wife to her prenatal visit, which included an ultrasound. I was not only able to hear the heartbeat of my first child, I was also able to see the baby. What an experience! Seeing my baby on the screen really made everything a reality for me!"

Assessment of Pelvic Adequacy

By performing a series of assessments and measurements, the examiner assesses the pelvis vaginally to determine whether the size and shape are adequate for a vaginal birth. This procedure, called *clinical pelvimetry*, is typically performed by physicians and advanced practice nurses during the pelvic exam. Clinical pelvimetry should not be used to determine if a patient is appropriate to attempt a vaginal birth. All women should be allowed a trial of labor despite clinical pelvimetry findings. Nevertheless, in developing countries where a contracted pelvis is more common, clinical pelvimetry continues to play an important role in prenatal assessment (King et al., 2015).

PELVIC CAVITY

The pelvic cavity is divided into the false pelvis and the true pelvis (Figure 12–4). The **false pelvis** is the portion above the pelvic brim, or linea terminalis, and serves to support the weight of the enlarged pregnant uterus and direct the presenting fetal part into the true pelvis below.

The **true pelvis** is the portion that lies below the pelvic brim. The bony circumference of the true pelvis is made up of the sacrum, coccyx, and innominate bones and represents the bony limits of the birth canal. The relationship of the fetal head to the true pelvic cavity is of paramount importance. The size and shape of the true pelvis must be adequate for normal fetal passage during labor and at birth. The true pelvis consists of three parts: The inlet, the pelvic cavity, and the outlet. Each part has distinct measurements that aid in evaluating the adequacy of the pelvis for childbirth. Measurement techniques are discussed in the following sections. Maternal pelvis types are discussed in the Critical Factors in Labor section in Chapter 19. The effects of inadequate or abnormal pelvic diameters on labor and birth are discussed in Chapter 24.

Pelvic Inlet. The **pelvic inlet** is the upper border of the true pelvis and is typically round in the female. The size and shape of the pelvic inlet are determined by assessing three anteroposterior diameters: The diagonal conjugate, obstetric conjugate, and conjugate vera, or true conjugate (Figure 12–5). Other diameters are the transverse (approximately 13.5 cm) and the oblique (averages 12.75 cm).

The **diagonal conjugate** extends from the subpubic angle to the middle of the sacral promontory and is typically 12.5 cm. To measure the diagonal conjugate, the distance from the lower

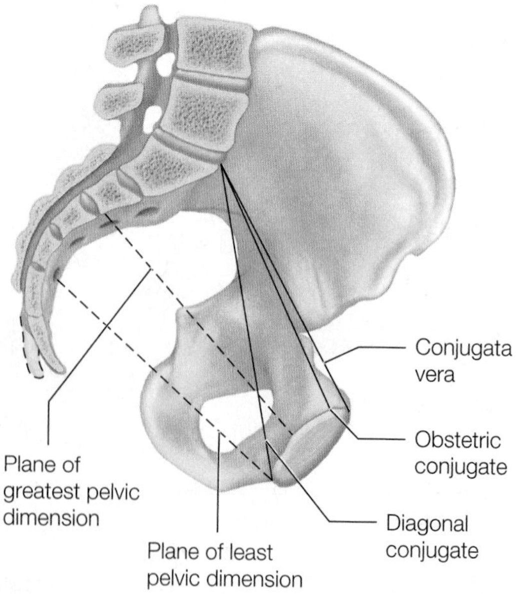

Figure 12–5 **Anteroposterior diameters of the pelvic inlet and their relationship to the pelvic planes.**

border of the symphysis pubis to the sacral promontory, the examiner inserts a gloved hand into the vagina with index and middle finger extended. The thumb remains extended outside the vagina. The examiner then attempts to reach from the lower border of the symphysis pubis to the sacral promontory with the middle finger. The clinician should determine the length of the finger before attempting this. The diagonal conjugate can then be measured by marking the place where the proximal part of the hand makes contact with the pubis (Figure 12–6A). The examiner measures the distance (which normally measures at least 11.5 cm).

The **obstetric conjugate** is the smallest and thus the most important anteroposterior diameter through which the fetus must pass. It extends from the middle of the sacral promontory to the upper inner point on the symphysis. Because it cannot be measured manually (but only by X-ray examination), it is estimated by subtracting 1.5 cm from the length of the diagonal conjugate. It should measure 10 cm or more in order for an average-size baby (7.5 to 8 lb) to pass through without difficulty. The **true conjugate** extends from the upper border of the symphysis pubis to the middle of the sacral promontory. It can be determined by subtracting 1 cm from the diagonal conjugate.

An additional measurement, the transverse diameter, helps determine the shape of the inlet. The **transverse diameter** is the largest diameter of the inlet and is measured by using the linea terminalis as the point of reference.

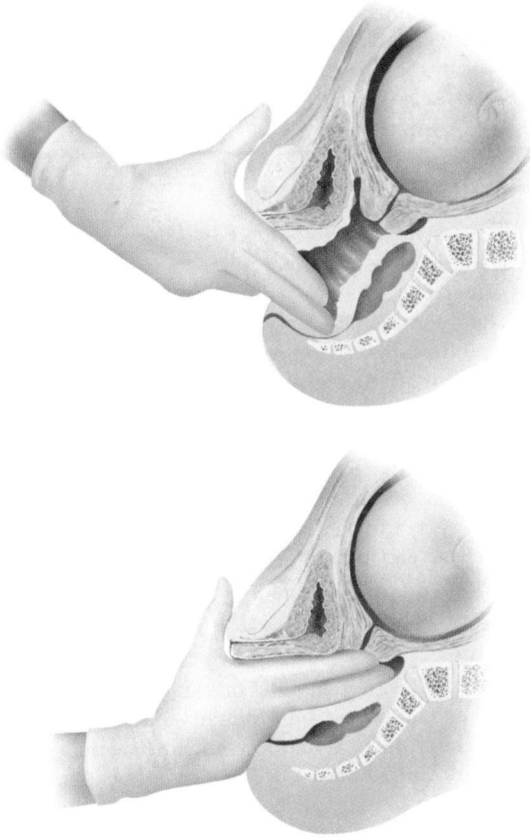

A

B

Figure 12–6 Manual measurement of inlet and outlet. A. Estimation of the diagonal conjugate, which extends from the lower border of the symphysis pubis to the sacral promontory. B. Estimation of the anteroposterior diameter of the outlet, which extends from the lower border of the symphysis pubis to the tip of the sacrum.

Midpelvis of the Pelvic Cavity. The *midpelvis* is a curved canal with a longer posterior than anterior wall. During labor, the descent of the fetal head into the true pelvis can be described by station, and the midpelvis and ischial spines serve to mark zero station (Cunningham et al., 2018). (See Chapter 19 for further discussion.) A change in the lumbar curve can increase or decrease the pelvic inclination and can influence the progress of labor because the fetus has to adjust itself to this curved path as well as to the different diameters of the true pelvis.

Important midpelvic measurements include the plane of least dimension, or midplane (anteroposterior diameter, normally 11.5 to 12 cm; posterior sagittal diameter, 4.5 to 5 cm; and transverse diameter [interspinous], 10 cm). It is shown in Figure 12–5. The planes of the midpelvis cannot be accurately measured by clinical examination. An evaluation of adequacy is made based on the prominence of the ischial spines and degree of convergence of the side walls.

Location of the sacrospinous ligament, a firm ridge of tissue, makes location of the ischial spines easier. When this ligament is located, the examiner should run the fingers along it laterally toward the anterior portion of the pelvis. The spines may range from a small, firm bump like the knuckle of a finger (termed *not encroaching*) to a very prominent bone (called *encroaching*).

The sacrosciatic notch should admit two fingers. A wide notch means that the sacrum curves posteriorly, giving the anteroposterior diameter of the midpelvis a greater length. A narrow notch indicates a decreased diameter. The width of the sacrosciatic notch is more accurately evaluated through X-ray examination but can be estimated through vaginal exam. The length of the sacrospinous ligament is measured by tracing the ligament from its origin on the ischial spines to its insertion on the sacrum. It is usually 4 cm, or two to three finger breadths long.

The capacity of the cavity can be assessed by sweeping the fingers down the side walls bilaterally to evaluate the shape of the pelvic side walls. They may be termed *convergent* (closer together at the outlet than the inlet, like a funnel), *divergent* (side walls farther apart at the outlet, which typically means the pubic arch will have a wide angle), or *straight* (normal finding). The curvature, inclination, and hollowness of the sacrum help indicate the capacity of the posterior pelvis. It is estimated digitally by palpating the sacrococcygeal junction and by inching up toward the promontory. The examiner then estimates the hollowness of the sacrum. A flat or shallow sacrum has less room; a hollow sacrum is considered normal. The plane of greatest pelvic dimensions represents the largest portion of the pelvic cavity and has no obstetric significance.

Pelvic Outlet. The **pelvic outlet** is at the lower border of the true pelvis. The size of the pelvic outlet can be determined by assessing the *transverse diameter*. The anteroposterior diameter of the pelvic outlet increases during birth as the presenting part pushes the coccyx posteriorly at the mobile sacrococcygeal joint. Decreased mobility, a large fetal head, and/or a forceful birth can cause the coccyx to break. As the baby's head emerges, the long diameter of the head (occipital frontal) parallels the long diameter of the outlet (anteroposterior).

The transverse diameter (*bi-ischial* or *intertuberous*) extends from the inner surface of one ischial tuberosity to the other. It is the shortest diameter of the pelvic outlet and becomes even shorter if the woman has a narrowed pubic arch. The pubic arch has great importance because the baby must pass under it during birth. If it is narrow, the baby's head may be pushed backward toward the coccyx, making the extension of the head difficult. This situation, known as *outlet dystocia*, may require the use of

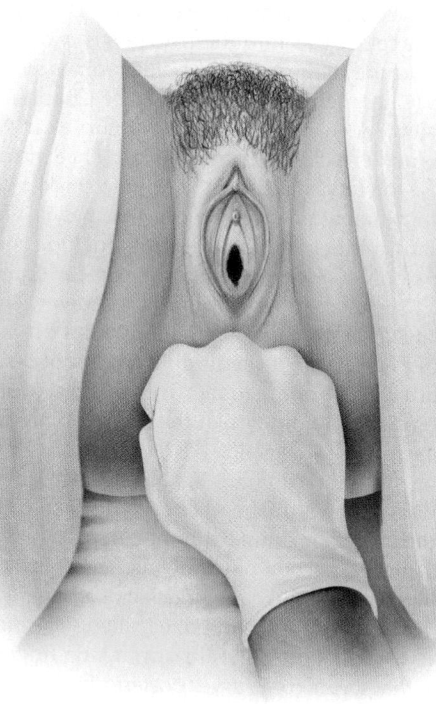

Figure 12–7 **Use of a closed fist to measure the outlet. Most examiners know the distance between their first and last proximal knuckles. If they do not, they can use a measuring device.**

forceps or a cesarean birth. The shoulders of a large baby may also get stuck under the pubic arch, making birth more difficult.

The anteroposterior diameter of the pelvic outlet (9.5 to 11.5 cm), which extends from the lower border of the symphysis pubis to the tip of the sacrum, can be measured digitally (Figure 12–6B). The transverse diameter of the outlet is measured by placing the fist between the ischial tuberosities. It usually measures 8 to 10 cm (Figure 12–7). The posterior sagittal diameter, the third important outlet diameter, normally measures at least 7.5 cm.

The mobility of the coccyx is determined by pressing down on it with the forefinger and middle finger during the initial vaginal examination. An immobile coccyx can decrease the diameter of the outlet.

The subpubic angle is estimated by palpating the bony structure externally with two fingers placed side by side at the border of the symphysis (Figure 12–8A). It should be 85 to 90 degrees. The angle is probably less if the examiner cannot separate his or her fingers.

The length and shape of the pubic rami affect the transverse diameter of the outlet. The pubic ramus is expected to be short and concave inward, as opposed to straight and long.

The height and inclination of the symphysis pubis are measured, and the contour of the pubic arch is estimated. Excessively long or angulated bone structure shortens the diameter of the obstetric conjugate. Height can be determined by placing the index finger of the gloved hand up to the superior border of the symphysis (Figure 12–8B). The examiner should measure the length of the first phalanx of the index finger (normally about 2.5 cm). Inclination can be determined by externally placing one finger on the top of the symphysis while the internal finger palpates the internal margin (Figure 12–8C). An imaginary line is drawn between the fingers, and the angle is estimated.

A posterior inclination with the lower border of the pubis slanting inward decreases the anteroposterior diameter. The anteroposterior sagittal diameter is the most significant diameter of the outlet because it is the shortest diameter through which the fetus must pass. The examiner uses two fingers to determine the contour of the pubic arch. This provides information on the width of the angle at which these bones come together (Figure 12–8D). The pubic arch has obstetric importance; if it is narrow, the fetus's head may be pushed backward toward the coccyx, making extension of the fetal head difficult, which may lengthen the second stage of labor.

Screening Tests

Many screening tests are routinely performed or offered during pregnancy, either at the initial prenatal visit or at specified times during pregnancy. Tests completed at the initial visit include a Pap smear, if indicated, complete blood count, HIV screening, rubella titer, ABO and Rh typing, urine culture, and hepatitis B screen, as well as testing for sexually transmitted infections such as syphilis, HIV, chlamydia, and gonorrhea. The urine is screened for abnormal findings initially and at each prenatal visit, if indicated.

Hemoglobin electrophoresis should be performed in women of African, Southeast Asian, and Mediterranean decent to evaluate for sickle cell disease and types of thalassemia. Prenatal screening for cystic fibrosis has been a routine screening offered to all pregnant women for over a decade. To avoid redundant testing, caregivers should determine whether the woman was screened for cystic fibrosis during a previous pregnancy. See *Genetic Facts: Thalassemia.*

Genetic Facts **Thalassemia**

Thalassemias are inherited blood disorders characterized by less hemoglobin and fewer red blood cells in the body than normal. Hemoglobin is the substance in red blood cells that allows them to carry oxygen. Thus, low hemoglobin and fewer red blood cells may cause anemia, leaving the patient fatigued and weak. With mild thalassemia, the patient may not need treatment. But more severe forms of the disorder require regular blood transfusions.

The type of thalassemia depends on the number of gene mutations an individual inherits from the parents and which part of the hemoglobin molecule is affected by the mutations. The more mutated genes, the more severe the thalassemia.

A tuberculin test (either PPD or QuantiFERON®-TB Gold) should also be completed on women who are considered to be high risk. High-risk populations include women who were not born in the United States, women who have had a known exposure to tuberculosis, and healthcare workers who care for patients with tuberculosis. Women who have not received varicella immunization or report a negative disease history should also be evaluated for varicella immunity. If they do not have documented immunity, plans should be made for the woman to be immunized after pregnancy.

Screening for gestational diabetes mellitus (GDM) is typically completed between 24 and 28 weeks' gestation and early testing completed in the first or early second trimester in women

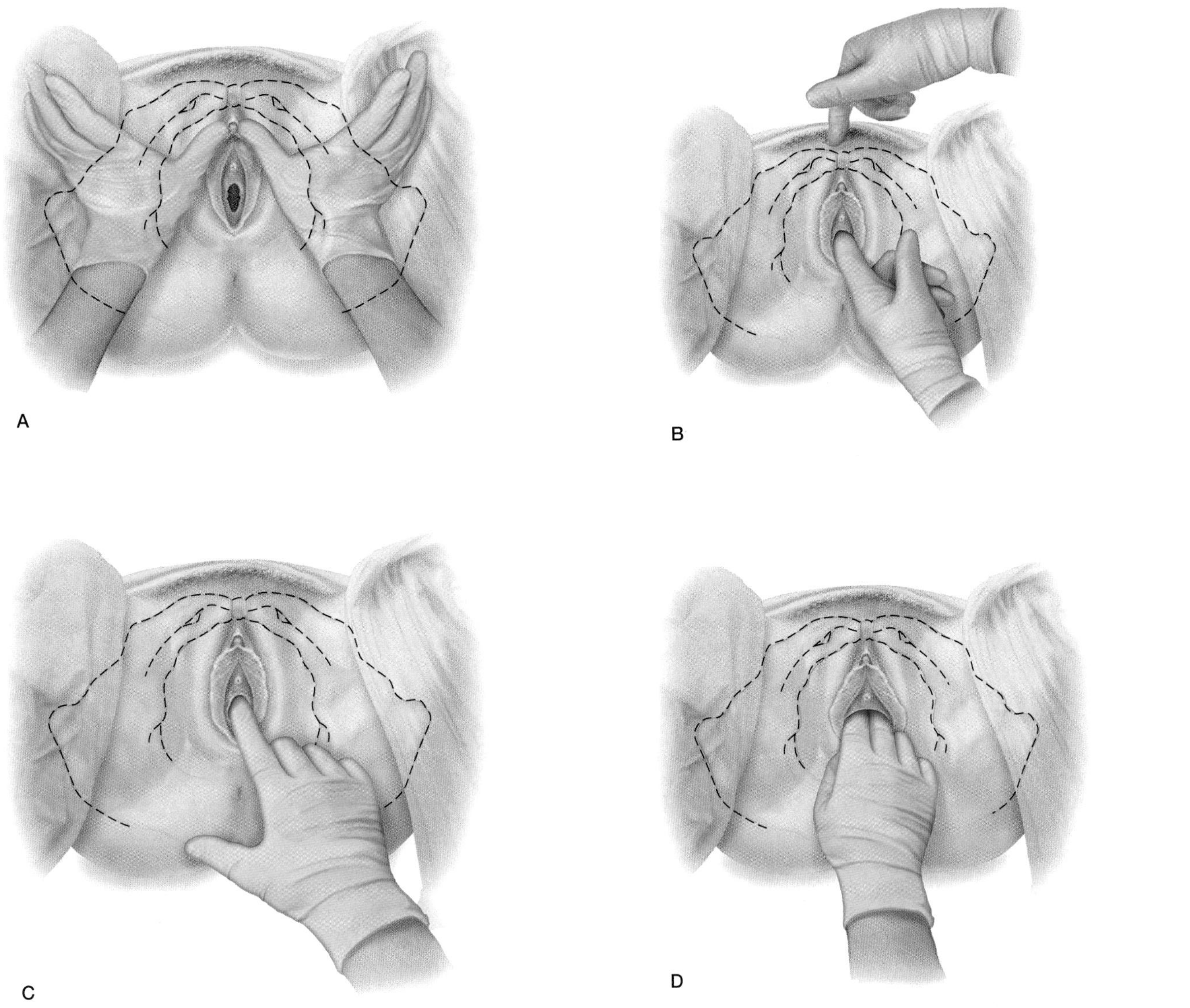

Figure 12–8 **Evaluation of the outlet. A. Estimation of the subpubic angle. B. Estimation of the length of the pubic ramus. C. Estimation of the depth and inclination of the pubis. D. Estimation of the contour of the subpubic angle.**

with risk factors (history of GDM, family history of DM). Two approaches are available:

1. One-step approach: Using 75-g oral glucose tolerance test (OGTT)
2. Two-step approach: Initial nonfasting test using a 50-g 1-hour glucose screen followed by a 3-hour 100mg OGTT if initial testing is positive.

The American Academy of Pediatrics (AAP) and ACOG (2017) together recommend the two-step approach (for a discussion of DM/GDM, see Chapter 17). The American Diabetes Association (2018) recommends that pregnant women at average risk should be screened at 24 to 28 weeks' gestation using either approach. A hemoglobin or hematocrit is also completed at this time to evaluate for iron deficiency anemia.

Group B streptococcus (GBS) can cause serious problems for a newborn. Consequently, rectal and vaginal swabs of the mother are taken at 35 to 37 weeks' gestation to screen for the bacteria. Women with GBS in the urine at any time during the pregnancy are considered to be positive and do not need a culture completed. GBS passed on to the newborn is discussed in more detail in Chapter 28.

Ethics in Action!

How do you counsel a woman who responds to your discussion of GBS screening with this response: "I am not going to complete the screening as I think it is very unlikely that I am a carrier, and I have concerns about taking antibiotics during pregnancy."

Additional tests are completed in the event of pathologic findings or known disease states. For example, a woman with known chronic hypertension should have evaluation of serum creatine, electrolytes, uric acid, liver enzymes, platelet count, and urine protein (dipstick or quantification such as 24-hour urine) early in pregnancy to establish baseline levels for evaluation of superimposed preeclampsia later in pregnancy (AAP & ACOG, 2017). Women with hypothyroidism also have thyroid-stimulating hormone (TSH) evaluated regularly throughout the pregnancy and medication adjustments made accordingly.

SCREENING FOR FETAL ANEUPLOIDY (TRISOMY) AND NEURAL TUBE DEFECTS

All pregnant women, regardless of age or risk factors, should be offered screening or diagnostic testing for fetal chromosome anomolies (*aneuploidy*) including Down syndrome, trisomy 18, trisomy 13, and Turner syndrome (ACOG, 2016). First-trimester screening is available at many centers using ultrasound assessment of the thickness of the fetal nuchal fold (called *nuchal translucency* [NT]) combined with serum screening for *free β-hCG* and for *pregnancy-associated plasma protein A (PAPP-A)*.

Clinical Tip

Screening for aneuploidy should be presented as an informed choice. The decision to proceed with screening is a personal choice and stems from one's values, beliefs, and interests. The nurse should be knowledgeable about the options available for screening and next steps if an abnormal result occurs.

The *quadruple screen (quad screen)* is a safe, useful screening test performed on the mother's serum between weeks 15 and 25 of pregnancy. The test is used to detect levels of specific serum markers—alpha-fetoprotein (AFP), human chorionic gonadotropin (hCG), unconjugated estriol (UE), and inhibin-A (a placental hormone). This test is typically completed if a woman enters prenatal care beyond the first trimester screening window.

It is important for healthcare professionals to provide parents with factual information about the results of tests that detect chromosomal defects or fetal anomalies including the false-positive and detection rates and the implications of the findings. Families should be made aware of the next steps, including available diagnostic testing if a positive screening result occurs. Parents then need to decide on a course of action if a fetal anomaly is confirmed. See Chapter 16 for a full discussion of fetal assessment.

Subsequent Patient History

At subsequent prenatal visits the nurse continues to gather data about the course of the pregnancy to date and the woman's responses to it. The nurse also asks about the following:

- Adjustment of the support person and of other children, if any, in the family
- Preparations the family has made for the new baby
- Discomfort, especially the kinds of discomfort that are often seen at specific times during a pregnancy
- Physical changes that relate directly to the pregnancy, such as fetal movement
- Exposure to contagious illnesses
- Medical treatments and therapies prescribed for nonpregnancy problems since the last visit
- Consumption of prescription or over-the-counter medications, herbal supplements, alcohol, nicotine, or illicit drugs that were not prescribed as part of the woman's prenatal care
- Use of complementary and alternative therapies
- Danger signs of pregnancy and signs of preterm labor
- Intimate partner violence.

Ethics in Action!

How do you respond to a woman who reports that she has continued to drink wine regularly during pregnancy even though you counseled her about the risks of alcohol for the fetus at her first prenatal visit?

Danger signs and signs of preterm labor that a woman should report immediately are discussed during the initial prenatal visit and reviewed at each subsequent prenatal visit (Figure 12–9). Many caregivers also provide printed information on the subject written in lay terms. Table 12–2 identifies the danger signs of pregnancy and possible causes for each. See *Key Facts to Remember: Signs of Preterm Labor*.

Key Facts To Remember
Signs of Preterm Labor

- Painful menstrual-like cramps
- Dull low backache
- Suprapubic pain or pressure
- Pelvic pressure or heaviness
- Change in character or amount of vaginal discharge (bloody, thinner, thicker)
- Diarrhea
- Uterine contractions felt every 10 minutes for 1 hour
- Leaking of water from vagina

The interchange between the nurse and woman will be facilitated if it takes place in a friendly, trusting environment. The nurse should give the woman sufficient time to ask questions and to voice concerns. If the nurse provides the time and demonstrates genuine interest, the woman will feel more at ease bringing up questions that she may believe are silly or concerns that she has been afraid to verbalize. The nurse who has an accurate

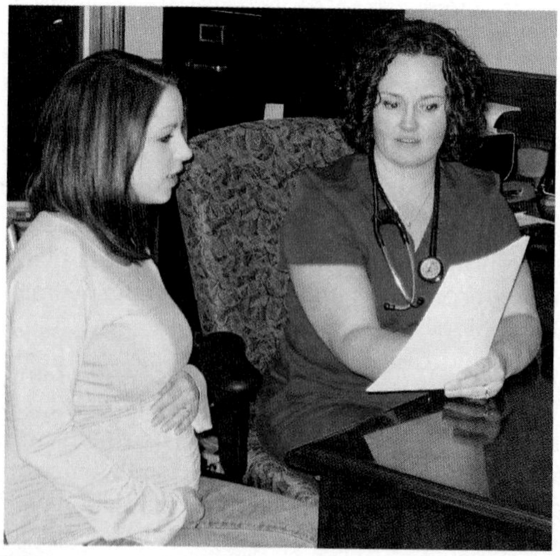

Figure 12–9 **The nurse reviews the danger signs in pregnancy at the initial prenatal visit and at each subsequent visit.**

SOURCE: Patricia A. Wieland Ladewig.

TABLE 12–2 Danger Signs in Pregnancy

The woman should report the following danger signs immediately	
DANGER SIGN	**POSSIBLE CAUSE**
Sudden gush of fluid from vagina	Premature rupture of membranes
Vaginal bleeding	Abruptio placentae, placenta previa Lesions of cervix or vagina "Bloody show" Cervical, vaginal infection Friable cervix (irritation of cervix) from intercourse, infection, or pregnancy
Abdominal pain	Premature labor, abruptio placentae
Temperature above 38.3°C (101°F) and chills	Infection
Dizziness, blurring of vision, double vision, spots before eyes	Hypertension, preeclampsia
Persistent nausea and vomiting	Hyperemesis gravidarum
Severe headache	Hypertension, preeclampsia
Edema of hands or face	Preeclampsia
Seizures or convulsions	Preeclampsia, eclampsia
Epigastric pain	Preeclampsia, ischemia in major abdominal vessel
Dysuria	Urinary tract infection
Absent or decreased fetal movement	Maternal medication, obesity, fetal death, fetal distress

understanding of all the changes of pregnancy is most able to answer questions and provide information.

The nurse should be sensitive to religious, spiritual, cultural, and socioeconomic factors that may influence a family's response to pregnancy as well as to the woman's expectations of the healthcare system. The nurse can avoid stereotyping simply by asking each woman about her expectations for the antepartum period. Although many women's responses may reflect what are thought to be traditional norms, other women will have decidedly different views or may have expectations that represent a blending of beliefs or cultures.

Clinical Tip

Encourage the woman and her partner to bring a list of questions or concerns to subsequent prenatal visits. This helps ensure that the needs and concerns of the woman and her family are addressed.

Subsequent Prenatal Assessment

During the prenatal period, it is essential that the nurse begin assessing the developing readiness of the woman and her partner to take on the responsibilities of parenthood successfully. Table 12–3 identifies areas for assessment and provides some sample questions the nurse might use to obtain necessary information. If the woman's responses are primarily negative, the nurse can plan interventions for the prenatal and postpartum periods.

Depression during and after pregnancy is a common problem, one that is gaining increased attention worldwide. The challenges of pregnancy and motherhood can be overwhelming for women experiencing perinatal depression. Postpartum depression impacts the entire family. Babies of depressed women are at increased risk for their social-emotional development, cognitive development, behavioral development, and physical health to be negatively impacted. It is recommended (ACOG, 2015b; Meschino, Philipp, Israel, et al., 2016) that all women be screened during the prenatal period for depression and anxiety using a validated screening tool, despite a lack of evidence that supports a true benefit in this activity. It is important that nurses have the ability to provide the avenues to treatment and follow-up.

During the subsequent antepartum assessments, most women demonstrate ongoing psychologic adjustment to pregnancy and ever-improving coping skills. However, some women may exhibit signs of psychologic problems. These signs may include one or more of the following:

- Increasing anxiety
- Depression or feelings of sadness
- Inability to establish communication
- Inappropriate responses or actions
- Denial of pregnancy
- Inability to cope with stress
- Intense preoccupation with the sex of the baby
- Failure to acknowledge quickening
- Failure to plan and prepare for the baby (e.g., living arrangements, clothing, feeding methods)
- Indications of substance abuse.

If the woman's behavior indicates possible psychologic problems, the nurse should provide ongoing support and counseling and also refer the woman to appropriate professionals, as indicated.

The woman's individual needs and the assessment of her risks should determine the frequency of subsequent visits. Generally, the recommended frequency of prenatal visits is as follows:

- Every 4 weeks for the first 28 weeks of gestation
- Every 2 weeks until 36 weeks' gestation
- After week 36, every week until childbirth.

Assessment Guide: Subsequent Prenatal Assessment provides a systematic approach to the regular physical examinations the pregnant woman should undergo for optimal prenatal care and a model for evaluating both the pregnant woman and the expectant partner, if he or she is involved in the pregnancy.

Clinical Tip

When assessing blood pressure, use a BP cuff of the appropriate size and have the pregnant woman sit up with her arm resting on a table so that her arm is at the level of her heart. Women should sit for 5 minutes before taking a BP reading and be instructed to uncross their legs, relax, and not talk during the evaluation. Expect a decrease in her blood pressure from baseline during the second trimester because of normal physiologic changes. The BP will gradually return to normal during the third trimester.

TABLE 12–3 Guide to Prenatal Assessment of Parenting

AREAS ASSESSED	SAMPLE QUESTIONS
I. Perception of complexities of mothering	
A. Desires baby for itself ***Positive:*** **1.** Feels positive about pregnancy ***Negative:*** **1.** Wants baby to meet own needs such as someone to love her, someone to get her out of unhappy home	**1.** "Was this pregnancy planned or a surprise?" **2.** "How do you feel about being pregnant?"
B. Expresses concern about impact of mothering role on other roles (wife, career, school) ***Positive:*** **1.** Realistic expectations of how baby will affect job, career, school, and personal goals **2.** Interested in learning about child care ***Negative:*** **1.** Feels pregnancy and baby will make no emotional, physical, or social demands on self **2.** Has no insight that mothering role will affect other roles or lifestyle	**1.** "What do you think it will be like to take care of a baby?" **2.** "How do you think your life will be different after you have your baby?" **3.** "How do you feel this baby will affect your job, career, school, and personal goals?" **4.** "How will the baby affect your relationship with your partner?" **5.** "Have you done any reading, babysitting, or caring for other children (siblings, cousins)?"
C. Gives up routine habits because "not good for baby" ***Positive:*** **1.** Quits smoking, improves eating habits	
II. Attachment	
A. **Strong feelings regarding sex of baby. Why?** ***Positive:*** **1.** Verbalizes positive thoughts about the baby ***Negative:*** **1.** Baby will be like negative aspects of self and partner	**1.** "Why do you prefer a certain sex?" (Is reason inappropriate for a baby?) **2.** Note comments patient makes about baby not being normal and why patient feels this way.
B. Interested in data regarding fetus (e.g., growth and development, heart tones) ***Positive:*** **1.** As above ***Negative:*** **1.** Shows no interest in fetal growth and development, quickening, and fetal heart tones **2.** Expresses negative feelings about fetus by rejecting counseling regarding nutrition, rest, hygiene	
C. Fantasies about baby ***Positive:*** **1.** Follows cultural norms regarding preparation **2.** Time of attachment behaviors appropriate to her history of pregnancy loss ***Negative:*** **1.** Bonding conditional depending on sex, age of baby, and/or labor and birth experience **2.** Woman considers only own needs when making plans for baby **3.** Exhibits no attachment behaviors after critical period of previous pregnancy **4.** Failure to follow cultural norms regarding preparation	**1.** "What did you think or feel when you first felt the baby move?" **2.** "Have you started preparing for the baby?" **3.** "What do you think your baby will look like—what age do you see your baby at?" **4.** "How would you like your new baby to look?"
III. Acceptance of child by significant others	
A. Acknowledges acceptance by significant other of the new responsibility inherent in child ***Positive:*** **1.** Acknowledges unconditional acceptance of pregnancy and baby by significant others **2.** Partner accepts new responsibility inherent with child **3.** Timely sharing of experience of pregnancy with significant others	**1.** "How does your partner feel about this pregnancy?" **2.** "How does your family feel?" **3.** "What do your friends think?" **4.** "Does your partner have a preference regarding the baby's sex? Why?" **5.** "How does your partner feel about being a parent?" **6.** "What do you think he/she will be like as a parent?"

AREAS ASSESSED	SAMPLE QUESTIONS
Negative: **1.** Significant others not supportively involved with pregnancy **2.** Conditional acceptance of pregnancy depending on gender, race, age of baby **3.** Decision making does not take in needs of fetus (e.g., spends food money on new car) **4.** Takes no/little responsibility for needs of pregnancy, woman/fetus	**7.** "What do you think he/she will do to help you with child care?" **8.** "Have you and your partner talked about how the baby might change your lives?" **9.** "Who have you told about your pregnancy?"
B. Concrete demonstration of acceptance of pregnancy/ baby by significant others (e.g., baby shower, significant other involved in prenatal education) ***Positive:*** **1.** Baby shower **2.** Significant other attends prenatal class with patient	**1.** Note if partner attends clinic with patient (degree of interest; e.g., listens to heart tones). **2.** "Does your partner plan to be with you during labor and birth?" **3.** "Is your partner contributing financially?"
IV. Ensures physical well-being	
A. Concerns about having normal pregnancy, labor and birth, and baby ***Positive:*** **1.** Preparing for labor and birth, attends prenatal classes, interested in labor and birth **2.** Aware of danger signs of pregnancy **3.** Seeks and uses appropriate health care (e.g., time of initial visit, keeps appointments, follows through on recommendations) ***Negative:*** **1.** Denies signs and symptoms that might suggest complications of pregnancy **2.** Verbalizes extreme fear of labor and birth—refuses to talk about labor and birth **3.** Misses appointments, fails to follow instructions, refuses to attend prenatal classes	**1.** "What have you heard about labor and birth?" **2.** "How are you planning to prepare for labor, birth, parenting (reading, classes, friends, family)? **3.** Note data about patient's reaction to prenatal class.
B. Family/patient decisions reflect concern for health of mother and baby (e.g., use of finances, time) ***Positive:*** **1.** As above	

Note: When "Negative" is not listed in a section, the reader may assume that negative is the absence of positive responses.

SOURCE: Data from the Minneapolis Health Dept., Minneapolis, MN.

ASSESSMENT GUIDE | Subsequent Prenatal Assessment

Physical Assessment/Normal Findings	Alterations and Possible Causes*	Nursing Responses to Data†
Vital Signs		
Temperature: 36.2°C–37.6°C (97°F–99.6°F)	Elevated temperature (infection)	Evaluate for signs of infection. Refer to healthcare provider.
Pulse: 60–100 beats/min; rate may increase 10 beats/min during pregnancy	Increased pulse rate (anxiety, cardiac disorders)	Note irregularities. Assess for anxiety, stress, dehydration, infection. Refer to healthcare provider.
Respiration: 12–20 breaths/min	Marked tachypnea or abnormal patterns (respiratory disease)	Refer to healthcare provider.
Blood Pressure: Less than or equal to 120/80 (falls in second trimester)	BP of 120–139/80–89 is considered prehypertensive. Greater than 140/90 or increase of 30 mm systolic and 15 mm diastolic (preeclampsia)	Assess for edema, proteinuria, and hyperreflexia. Refer to healthcare provider. Schedule appointments more frequently.

(continued)

ASSESSMENT GUIDE | Subsequent Prenatal Assessment *(continued)*

Physical Assessment/Normal Findings	Alterations and Possible Causes*	Nursing Responses to Data†
Weight Gain		
Prepregnant weight based on body mass index (BMI): Normal BMI: Total recommended weight gain 11.5–16 kg (25–35 lb)		
First Trimester: 1.6–2.3 kg (3.5–5 lb)	Inadequate weight gain (poor nutrition, nausea, intrauterine growth restriction [IUGR])	Discuss appropriate weight gain.
Second Trimester: 5.5–6.8 kg (12–15 lb)	Excessive weight gain (excessive caloric intake, edema, preeclampsia)	Provide nutritional counseling. Assess for presence of edema or anemia. Refer to dietitian as needed.
Third Trimester: 5.5–6.8 kg (12–15 lb)		
Edema		
Small amount of dependent edema, especially in last weeks of pregnancy	Marked edema in hands, face, legs, and feet (preeclampsia)	Identify any correlation between edema and activities, blood pressure, or proteinuria: Refer to healthcare provider, if indicated.
Uterine Size		
See *Assessment Guide: Initial Prenatal Assessment* for normal changes during pregnancy	Unusually rapid growth (multiple gestation, hydatidiform mole, hydramnios, miscalculation of estimated date of birth [EDB])	Evaluate fetal status. Determine height of fundus. Use diagnostic ultrasound.
Fetal Heartbeat		
110–160 beats/min Funic souffle	Absence of fetal heartbeat after 20 weeks' gestation (maternal obesity, fetal demise)	Evaluate fetal status.
Laboratory Evaluation		
Hemoglobin: 12–16 g/dL Pseudoanemia of pregnancy	Less than 11 g/dL (anemia)	Provide nutritional counseling. Hemoglobin is repeated at 7 months' gestation. Women of Mediterranean heritage need a close check on hemoglobin because of the possibility of thalassemia.
Quad Marker Screen: Blood test performed at 15–21 weeks' gestation. Evaluates four factors—maternal serum alpha-fetoprotein (MSAFP), unconjugated estriol (UE), human chorionic gonadotropin (hCG), and inhibin-A: Normal levels	Elevated MSAFP (neural tube defect, underestimated gestational age, multiple gestation); lower than normal MSAFP (Down syndrome, trisomy 18); higher than normal hCG and inhibin-A (Down syndrome); lower than normal UE (Down syndrome)	Offered to all pregnant women. If quad screen abnormal, further testing such as ultrasound or amniocentesis is offered.
Indirect Coombs Test done on Rh-negative women: Negative (done at 28 weeks' gestation)	Rh antibodies present (maternal sensitization has occurred)	If Rh negative and unsensitized, Rh immune globulin given (see Chapter 18). If Rh antibodies present, Rh immune globulin not given; fetus monitored closely for isoimmune hemolytic disease.
50-g 1-hour glucose screen (done between 24 and 28 weeks' gestation)	Plasma glucose level greater than 130–140 (gestational diabetes mellitus [GDM])	Refer for a diagnostic 100-g oral glucose 3-hour tolerance test. Discuss implications of GDM if diagnosis is made. Refer to healthcare provider.
Urinalysis: See *Assessment Guide: Initial Prenatal Assessment* for normal findings	See *Assessment Guide: Initial Prenatal Assessment* for deviations	Urinalysis and culture are completed at initial visit and at subsequent visits as indicated.

Physical Assessment/Normal Findings	Alterations and Possible Causes*	Nursing Responses to Data†
Protein: Negative	Proteinuria, albuminuria (contamination by vaginal discharge, urinary tract infection, preeclampsia)	Obtain dipstick urine sample. Refer to healthcare provider if deviations are present.
Glucose: Negative ***Note:*** Glycosuria may be present due to physiologic alterations in glomerular filtration rate and renal threshold.	Persistent glycosuria (diabetes mellitus)	Refer to healthcare provider.
Screening for Group B Streptococcus (GBS): Rectal and vaginal swabs obtained at 35–37 weeks' gestation for all pregnant women	Positive culture (maternal carrier)	Explain maternal and fetal/neonatal risks (see Chapter 18). Refer to healthcare provider for therapy.
Cultural Assessment	**Variations to Consider***	**Nursing Responses to Data†**
Determine the mother's (and family's) attitudes about the sex of the unborn child.	Some women have no preference about the sex of the child; others do. In many cultures, boys are especially valued as firstborn children.	Provide opportunities to discuss preferences and expectations; avoid a judgmental attitude to the response.
Ask about the woman's expectations of childbirth. Will she want someone with her for the birth? Whom does she choose? What is the role of her partner?	Some women want their partner present for labor and birth; others prefer a female relative or friend.	Provide information on birth options but accept the woman's decision about who will attend.
	Some women expect to be separated from their partner once labor begins.	
Ask about preparations for the baby. Determine what is customary for the woman.	Some women may have a fully prepared nursery; others may not have a separate room for the baby.	Explore reasons for not preparing for the baby. Support the mother's preferences and provide information about possible sources of assistance if the decision is related to a lack of resources.
Expectant Mother		
Psychologic Status	Increased stress and anxiety	Encourage woman to take an active part in her care.
First Trimester/Period of Adjustment: Incorporates idea of pregnancy; may feel ambivalent or anxious, especially if she must give up desired role; usually looks for signs of verification of pregnancy, such as increase in abdominal size or fetal movement	Inability to establish communication; inability to accept pregnancy; inappropriate response or actions; denial of pregnancy; inability to cope	Establish lines of communication. Discuss and provide anticipatory guidance regarding normalcy of feelings and actions. Establish a trusting relationship. Counsel as necessary. Refer to appropriate professional as needed.
Second Trimester/Period of Radiant Health: Baby becomes more real to woman as abdominal size increases and she feels movement; she begins to turn inward, becoming more introspective		
Third Trimester/Period of Watchful Waiting: Begins to think of baby as separate being; may feel restless, uneasy, and may feel that time of labor will never come; remains self-centered and concentrates on preparing place for baby. Fears well-being for herself and baby		

(continued)

ASSESSMENT GUIDE | Subsequent Prenatal Assessment *(continued)*

Physical Assessment/Normal Findings	Alterations and Possible Causes*	Nursing Responses to Data†
Educational Needs		
Self-Care Measures and Knowledge About the Following: Health promotion; Breast care; Hygiene; Rest; Exercise; Nutrition; Relief measures for common discomforts of pregnancy; Danger signs in pregnancy (see Table 12–2); Signs of preterm labor (see *Key Facts to Remember: Signs of Preterm Labor*)	Inadequate information	Provide information and counseling.
Sexual Activity: Woman knows how pregnancy affects sexual activity	Lack of information about effects of pregnancy and/or alternative positions during sexual intercourse	Provide counseling.
Preparation for Parenting: Appropriate preparation	Lack of preparation (denial, failure to adjust to baby, unwanted child)	Counsel. If lack of preparation is due to inadequacy of information, provide information.
Preparation for Childbirth		If couple chooses particular technique, refer to classes.
Patient Aware of the Following: **1.** Prepared childbirth techniques **2.** Normal processes and changes during childbirth	Continued abuse of drugs and alcohol; denial of possible effect on self and baby	Encourage prenatal class attendance. Educate woman during visits based on current physical status. Provide reading list for more specific information.
3. Problems that may occur as a result of drug and alcohol use and of smoking		Review danger signs that were presented on initial visit.
Woman has met other physician or nurse-midwife who may be attending her birth in the absence of primary caregiver	Introduction of new individual at birth may increase stress and anxiety for woman and partner	Introduce woman to all members of group practice.
Impending Labor ***Patient Knows Signs of Impending Labor:*** **1.** Uterine contractions that increase in frequency, duration, and intensity **2.** Bloody show **3.** Expulsion of mucous plug **4.** Rupture of membranes	Lack of information	Provide appropriate teaching, stressing importance of seeking appropriate medical assistance.
Expectant Father/Partner		
Psychologic Status		
First Trimester: May express excitement over confirmation of pregnancy and, if father, of his virility; concerns move toward providing for financial needs; energetic, may identify with some discomforts of pregnancy and may even exhibit symptoms	Increasing stress and anxiety; inability to establish communication; inability to accept pregnancy diagnosis; withdrawal of support; abandonment of the mother	Encourage expectant partner to come to prenatal visits. Establish line of communication. Establish trusting relationship.

Physical Assessment/Normal Findings	Alterations and Possible Causes*	Nursing Responses to Data†
Second Trimester: May feel more confident and be less concerned with financial matters; may have concerns about woman's changing size and shape, her increasing introspection		Counsel. Let expectant partner know that it is normal to experience these feelings.
Third Trimester: May have feelings of rivalry with fetus, especially during sexual activity; may make changes in physical appearance and exhibit more self-interest; may become more energetic; fantasizes about child but usually imagines older child; fears mutilation and death of woman and child		Include expectant partner in pregnancy activities as he or she desires. Provide education, information, and support. Increasing numbers of expectant partners are demonstrating desire to be involved in many or all aspects of prenatal care, education, and preparation.

*Possible causes of alterations are identified in parentheses.

†This column provides guidelines for further nursing assessment and initial intervention.

Focus Your Study

- A complete history forms the basis of prenatal care and is reevaluated and updated as necessary throughout the pregnancy.
- The initial prenatal assessment is a careful and thorough physical examination and cultural and psychosocial assessment designed to identify variations and potential risk factors.
- Laboratory tests completed at the initial visit, such as a complete blood count, ABO and Rh typing, urinalysis/culture, Pap smear, chlamydia culture, gonorrhea culture, rubella titer, and various blood screens (such as rapid plasma reagin [RPR], HIV, and hepatitis B) provide information about the woman's health during early pregnancy and also help detect potential problems.
- The estimated date of birth (EDB) can be calculated using Nägele's rule. Using this approach, one begins with the first day of the last menstrual period, subtracts 3 months, and adds 7 days. A "wheel" may also be used to calculate the EDB.
- Accuracy of the EDB may be evaluated by physical examination to assess uterine size, measurement of fundal height, and ultrasound. Perception of quickening and auscultation of fetal heartbeat are also useful tools in confirming the gestation of a pregnancy.
- The diagonal conjugate is the distance from the lower posterior border of the symphysis pubis to the sacral promontory. The obstetric conjugate is estimated by subtracting 1.5 to 2 cm from the length of the diagonal conjugate.
- As part of the assessment of the pelvic cavity (midpelvis), the prominence of the ischial spines is assessed, the sacrosciatic notch and the length of the sacrospinous ligament are measured, and the shape of the pelvic side walls is evaluated. Finally, the hollowness of the sacrum is determined.
- The anteroposterior diameter of the pelvic outlet is determined, the mobility of the coccyx is assessed, the suprapubic angle is estimated, and the contour of the pubic arch is evaluated to assess the adequacy of the pelvic outlet.
- The nurse begins evaluating the woman psychosocially during the initial prenatal assessment. This assessment continues and is modified throughout the pregnancy.
- Cultural and ethnic beliefs may strongly influence the woman's attitudes and apparent cooperation with care during pregnancy.

References

American Academy of Pediatrics (AAP) & American College of Obstetricians and Gynecologists (ACOG). (2017). *Guidelines for perinatal care* (8th ed.). Elk Grove Village, IL: Author.

American College of Obstetricians and Gynecologists (ACOG). (reaffirmed, 2015a). *Definition of term pregnancy* (ACOG Committee Opinion No. 579). Washington, DC: Author.

American College of Obstetricians and Gynecologists (ACOG). (2015b). *Screening for perinatal depression* (ACOG Committee Opinion No. 630). Washington, DC: Author.

American College of Obstetricians and Gynecologists (ACOG). (2016). *Prenatal diagnostic testing for genetic disorders* (ACOG Practice Bulletin No. 162). Washington, DC: Author.

American Diabetes Association (ADA). (2018). Standards of medical care in diabetes–2018. *Diabetes Care, 41*(Suppl. 1), S1–S143.

Baisch, M. J., Carey, L. K., Conway, A. E., & Mounts, K. O. (2010). Perinatal depression: A health marketing campaign to improve screening. *Nursing for Women's Health, 14*(1), 18–33.

Cunningham, F. G., Leveno, K. J., Bloom, S. L., Dashe, J., Hoffman, B. L., Casey, B. M., & Spong, C. Y. (2018). *Williams obstetrics* (25th ed.). New York, NY: McGraw-Hill Education.

King, T. L., Brucker, M. C., Kriebs, J. M., Fahey, J. O., Gegor, C. L., & Varney, H. (2015). *Varney's midwifery* (5th ed.). Burlington, MA: Jones & Bartlett Learning.

Lee, A. C., Panchal, P., Folger, L., Whelan, H., Whelan, R., Rosner, B., Blencowe, H., & Lawn, J. E. (2017). Diagnostic accuracy of neonatal assessment for gestational age determination: A systematic review. *Pediatrics, 140*(6), 1–26.

Meschino, S., Philipp, D., Israel, A., & Vigod, S. (2016). Maternal-infant mental health: Postpartum group intervention. *Archives of Women's Mental Health, 19*, 243–251.

Spector, R. (2017). *Cultural diversity in health and illness* (9th ed.). Boston, MA: Pearson.

West, E. H., Hark, L., & Catalano, P. M. (2017). Nutrition during pregnancy. In S. G. Gabbe, J. R. Niebyl, J. L. Simpson, M. B. Landon, H. L. Galan, E. R. M. Jauniaux, D. A. Driscoll, V. Berghella, & W. A. Grobman (Eds.), *Obstetrics: Normal and problem pregnancies* (7th ed., pp. 122–135). Philadelphia, PA: Elsevier.

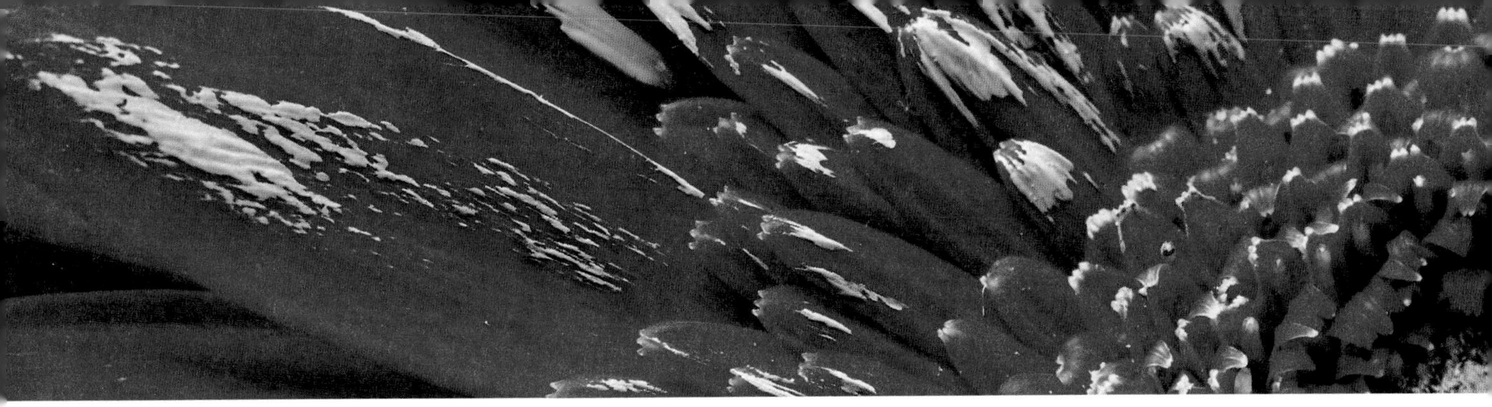

Chapter 13
The Expectant Family: Needs and Care

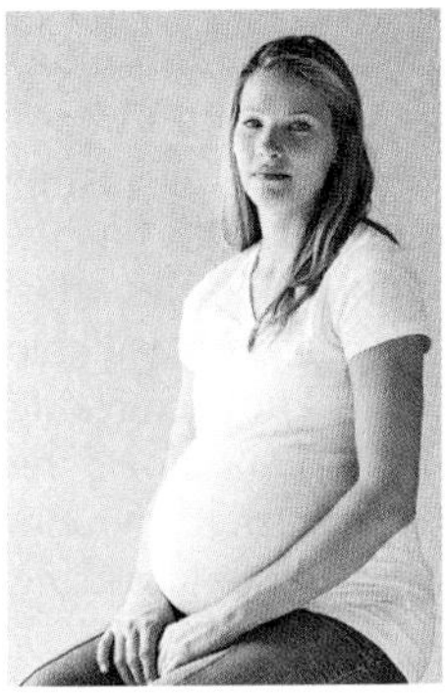

SOURCE: RubberBall/SuperStock.

I am so excited about this pregnancy. I had a miscarriage last year, so this time the first few months were stressful, but all has gone smoothly. The nursery is ready for our daughter (yes, we did find out it's a girl!), our parents are ready to become grandparents for the first time, and I look forward to seeing my feet again!

Learning Outcomes

13.1 Describe the significance of using the nursing process to promote health in the woman and her family during pregnancy.

13.2 Describe actions the nurse can take to help maintain the well-being of the expectant father or partner and siblings during a family's pregnancy.

13.3 Discuss the significance of cultural considerations in managing nursing care during pregnancy.

13.4 Identify information that expectant parents may need to assist them in making the best decisions possible about issues related to pregnancy, labor, and birth.

13.5 Explain the basic goals of childbirth education in providing care to expectant couples and their families.

13.6 Identify the common discomforts of pregnancy and their causes.

13.7 Summarize appropriate measures to alleviate the common discomforts of pregnancy.

13.8 Delineate self-care actions a pregnant woman and her family can take to maintain and promote well-being during each trimester of pregnancy.

13.9 Identify some of the concerns that an expectant couple may have about sexual activity.

Healthy People 2020

(MICH-10) Increase the proportion of pregnant women who receive early and adequate prenatal care

(MICH-21) Increase the proportion of infants who are breastfed

(MICH-11) Increase abstinence from alcohol, cigarettes, and illicit drugs among pregnant women

From the moment a woman finds out that she is pregnant, she faces a future marked by dramatic changes. Her appearance will be altered. Her relationships will change. She will experience a variety of unique physical changes throughout the pregnancy. Even her psychologic state will be affected. In coping with these changes, she needs to make adjustments in her daily life.

Her family must also adjust to the pregnancy. Roles and responsibilities of family members will change as the woman's ability to perform certain activities changes. They too must adapt psychologically to the situation.

Nurses caring for pregnant women need a clear understanding of pregnancy and the changes it brings if they are to be effective in managing nursing care. They also need a clear understanding of the importance of a family-centered approach to care, which is based on the concept that a hospital can provide professional services to mothers, fathers, and babies in a home-like environment that enhances the integrity of the family unit. Family-centered care is discussed in detail in Chapter 1.

With this in mind, Chapter 11 provides a database for the nurse by presenting material related to the normal physical, psychologic, social, and cultural changes of pregnancy. Chapter 12 then uses that database to begin a discussion of nursing management by focusing on patient assessment. This chapter further addresses nursing management as it relates to the needs of the expectant woman and her loved ones and includes some of the decisions a childbearing family must consider, such as the choice of a care provider, type of prenatal care, childbirth preparation, birth setting, and labor support.

Nursing Care During the Prenatal Period

The nursing process is a valuable tool in providing care during the months of pregnancy.

Nursing Diagnoses

The nurse may see a pregnant woman only once every 4 to 6 weeks during the first several months of her pregnancy. To ensure continuity of care, therefore, a written care plan that incorporates assessment data, nursing diagnoses, and patient goals is essential.

Anticipate that, for many women with a low-risk pregnancy, certain nursing diagnoses will be made more frequently than others. Nursing diagnoses will, of course, vary from woman to woman and according to the time in the pregnancy. Examples of common nursing diagnoses include:

- ***Constipation*** related to the physiologic effects of pregnancy
- ***Sexuality Pattern, Ineffective***, related to discomfort during late pregnancy
- ***Nausea*** related to the physiologic changes of pregnancy

(NANDA-I © 2017)

After formulating an appropriate diagnosis, the nurse establishes related goals to guide the nursing plan and interventions.

Nursing Plan and Implementation

Once nursing diagnoses have been identified, the next step is to establish priorities of nursing care. Sometimes priorities of care are based on the most immediate needs or concerns perceived by the woman. For example, during the first trimester, a woman is probably not ready to hear about labor and birth because she is likely to have more immediate concerns, such as nausea or sexual intimacy with her partner.

At other times priorities may develop as a result of findings during a prenatal visit. For example, the nurse may stress the need for frequent rest periods for a woman who is showing signs of preeclampsia (a pregnancy complication discussed in Chapter 18). However, the woman may feel well physically and find it difficult to accept the nurse's emphasis on rest. It is the responsibility of medical and nursing professionals to help the woman and her family understand the significance of a problem and to plan appropriate interventions to deal with it.

The intervention methods most used by nurses in caring for the expectant woman and her family are communication techniques and teaching–learning strategies. These intervention methods are often used in groups, such as early pregnancy classes and childbirth education classes, but the nurse in the prenatal setting also applies these techniques with individuals.

COMMUNITY-BASED NURSING CARE

Prenatal care, especially for women with low-risk pregnancies, is community based, typically in a clinic or private office. The healthcare community recognizes the value of providing a primary care nurse in these settings to coordinate care for each childbearing family. The nurse in a clinic or health maintenance organization (HMO) may be the only source of continuity for the woman, who may see a different physician or certified nurse-midwife (CNM) at each visit. The nurse can be extremely effective in working with the expectant family by answering their questions; providing them with complete information about pregnancy, appropriate prenatal self-care measures, and community resources or referral agencies; and supporting the healthcare activities of the woman and her family. Communities often have a wealth of services and educational opportunities available for pregnant women and their families, and the knowledgeable nurse can help the woman access these services. This allows the family to assume equal responsibility with healthcare providers in working toward their common goal of a positive childbearing experience.

Throughout the prenatal period the nurse provides informal and formal teaching to the childbearing family designed to help the family carry out self-care when appropriate and to report changes that may indicate a possible health problem. The teaching is most effective if timed to coincide with the woman's (couple's) readiness and needs (Table 13–1). The nurse also provides anticipatory guidance to help the family plan for changes that will occur following childbirth. See *Health Promotion: Anticipatory Guidance for the Postpartum Period*.

Home Care. Home care can be of benefit to any pregnant woman, but it is especially effective in removing barriers for women who have difficulty accessing health care. These barriers may include lack of locally available healthcare facilities, problems with transportation to the facility, or schedule conflicts with available appointment times because of employment hours or family responsibilities.

Health Promotion Anticipatory Guidance for the Postpartum Period

Anticipatory guidance helps the expectant couple identify and discuss issues that could be sources of postpartum stress. Issues to be addressed beforehand may include the sharing of baby and household chores, help in the first few days after childbirth, options for babysitting to allow the mother (and couple) some free time, the mother's return to work after the baby's birth, and sibling rivalry. Couples resolve these issues in different ways, but postpartum adjustment tends to be easier for couples who agree on the issues beforehand than for couples who do not confront and resolve these issues.

TABLE 13–1 Topics for Patient Teaching During Pregnancy

All Three Trimesters
- Discomforts of pregnancy
- Nutrition and weight gain
- Sexual activity
- Sibling preparation

First Trimester
- Attitude toward pregnancy
- Exercise and rest
- Smoking; use of alcohol and other drugs
- Traveling
- Fetal growth and development
- Danger signals associated with spontaneous abortion
- Employment
- Early pregnancy classes

Second Trimester
- Concerns related to changes in body
- Fetal growth and development
- Fetal movement
- Clothing
- Care of skin and breasts
- Beginning preparation for care of the newborn (equipment and room)
- Decisions about newborn/infant feeding

Third Trimester
- Exercise and rest
- Traveling
- Danger signals
- Preparation for labor and birth
- Completion of preparation in home for new baby
- Decisions about the newborn (circumcision, method of feeding, and so forth)
- Decision making for the early postpartum period
- Education about psychologic and physical expectations in the early postpartum period

In-home nursing assessments vary according to the scope of practice of the nurse and include current history and those screening procedures typically completed in an office or clinic: Vital signs, weight, urine screen, physical activity, and dietary intake. Advanced practice nurses can also assess reflexes, perform tests of fetal well-being, and even do cervical examinations. Once the assessments are completed, the nurse can determine the level of follow-up home care or telephone contact needed.

A prenatal home care visit or phone contact can also be useful for women who anticipate a short inpatient stay after childbirth. At the prenatal contact, the nurse explains the postpartum program and answers any questions the woman or her family has.

Although the use of home care for women with uncomplicated pregnancies is growing, it is most often used for women with prenatal complications that can be managed without hospitalization if effective nursing assessment and care are provided in the home (see Chapters 17 and 18).

Care of the Pregnant Woman's Family

Relieving the expectant woman's discomforts, maintaining her physical health, and providing anticipatory guidance are important parts of nursing management. In addition, the nurse helps meet the needs of the woman's family to better maintain the harmony and integrity of the family unit. The nurse does this by providing support and prenatal education. If the nurse is effective, family members may gain greater problem-solving ability, self-esteem, self-confidence, and ability to participate in health care.

Care of the Father or Partner

Although the father of the baby is generally present, his presence cannot be assumed. If he is not a part of the family structure, it is important to assess the woman's support system to determine which significant persons in her life will play a major role during this childbearing experience. The following information also applies to a same-sex spouse or partner.

When the father/partner is part of the family or support system, providing anticipatory guidance is a necessary part of any plan of care. The individual may need information about the anatomic, physiologic, and emotional changes that occur during pregnancy and postpartum, the couple's sexuality and sexual response, and the reactions that may be experienced. The father/partner may wish to express feelings about breastfeeding versus formula-feeding, the sex of the child, and other topics. If it is culturally acceptable to the couple and personally acceptable to the father/partner, the nurse refers the couple to expectant parents' classes. These classes provide valuable information about pregnancy and childbirth using a variety of teaching strategies such as discussion, films, demonstrations with educational models, and written handouts. Some classes even give the father/partner the opportunity to get a "feel" for pregnancy by wearing a pregnancy simulator (Figure 13–1).

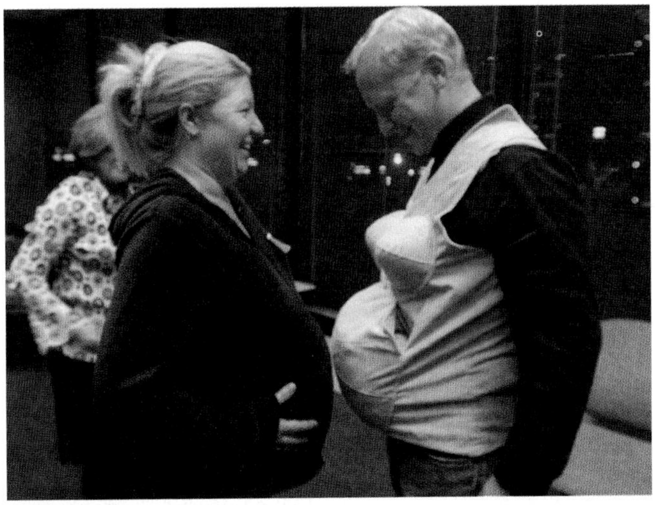

Figure 13–1 **The Empathy Belly is a pregnancy simulator that allows males and females to experience some of the symptoms of pregnancy. The "belly," which weighs 33 lb, produces symptoms such as shortness of breath, bladder pressure, shift in the center of gravity with resulting waddling gait, increased lordosis and backache, and fatigue. It can also simulate fetal kicking movements.**

SOURCE: ZUMA Press, Inc./Alamy Stock Photo.

The nurse assesses the father's or partner's intended degree of participation during labor and birth and knowledge of what to expect. If the couple prefers that the father's or partner's participation be minimal or restricted, the nurse supports their decision and does not try to impose personal values. Research indicates that expectant fathers have more positive feelings about the father role when they feel supported by a health professional (Urso, 2016). The non-birth mother or co-mother in a lesbian relationship, on the other hand, sometimes feels at the mercy of healthcare providers and unrecognized as the "other mother" by staff and healthcare professionals during the birthing process (Wojnar & Katzenmeyer, 2014). It is important for nurses to recognize that the support of a health professional is important for co-mothers as well.

Care of Siblings and Other Family Members

In the plan for prenatal care, the nurse considers the effect of the pregnancy on any other children the couple may have. For example, the nurse may initiate a discussion about the ambivalence that older children may feel about the pregnancy. Parents who are unprepared for the older child's feelings of anger, jealousy, and rejection may respond inappropriately in their confusion and surprise. The nurse emphasizes that open communication between parents and children (or acting out feelings with a doll if the child is too young to verbalize) helps children master their feelings and may prevent them from hurting the baby when they are unsupervised. Children may feel less neglected and more secure if they know that their parents are willing to listen to their expressions of sadness or to help with their anger and aggressiveness.

Parents may be encouraged to bring their children to antepartum visits. Seeing what is involved and listening to the fetal heartbeat may make the pregnancy more real to siblings. Many agencies also provide sibling classes geared to different ages and levels of understanding.

Relationship changes with in-laws should be addressed as well as the woman's or couple's expectations of the grandparents. Although some grandparents are eager to assist with child care by babysitting, others are not (Figure 13–2). The parents should also give some thought to the best ways of dealing with possible conflicts with the grandparents over childrearing approaches.

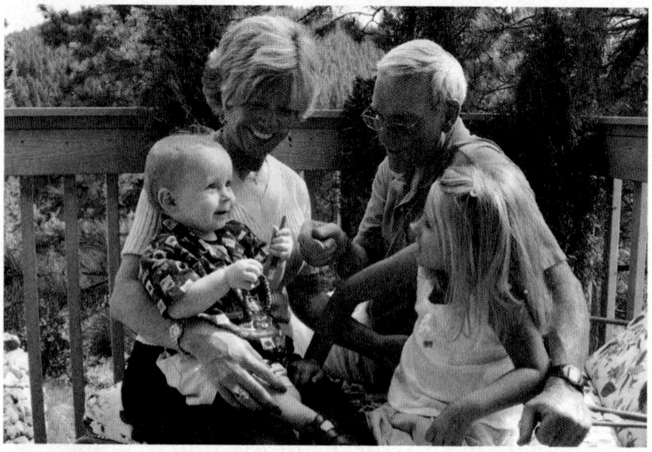

Figure 13–2 Grandparents can offer nurturing and guidance to their grandchildren, not to mention lots of fun.

SOURCE: Patricia A. Wieland Ladewig.

Cultural Considerations in Pregnancy

As discussed in Chapter 2, the increasingly diverse population in the United States, Canada, and other countries around the world requires a more inclusive approach—culturally competent care—to the delivery of care to people who belong to diverse and multicultural groups. The cultural competence approach allows care providers to include patients' cultural backgrounds in their care; this approach, however, does not examine the role of individual experience in people's health-related values, beliefs, and behaviors. The concept of *cultural humility* has been proposed as a more suitable goal in multicultural education. Cultural humility focuses on the process of intercultural exchange, paying explicit attention to clarifying the healthcare professional's values and beliefs through self-reflection and self-critique—in other words, identifying the caregiver's own biases; additionally, it incorporates the characteristics of both the healthcare professional and the patient into a mutually beneficial and balanced relationship (Baptiste, Foronda, Reinholdt, et al., 2016). Being open to cultural differences and learning from patients about their beliefs, values, and practices helps caregivers build relationships based on similarities.

By assessing each woman individually, the cultural humility approach removes the need to know the cultural features of every diverse group. Consequently, prenatal care should always include a discussion that clarifies each woman's health-related values and beliefs.

This conversation allows the nurse to adapt to the specific healthcare needs of each perinatal patient. Using the nursing process, the nurse can then formulate a transcultural nursing diagnosis that is focused on the cultural beliefs of the specific woman. The nursing diagnosis should reflect cultural sensitivity and build on the strengths of the patient.

A major goal of transcultural nursing is to understand and assist people of different cultural groups with their healthcare needs. Culturally sensitive nurses recognize that each childbearing family, shaped by culture and life experience, has expectations of both its members and the healthcare system during pregnancy and birth.

Pregnancy and childbirth are recognized as special events in virtually all cultures. Additionally, specific actions during pregnancy are often determined by cultural beliefs. These beliefs can be divided into three types (AWHONN, Mattson, & Smith, 2015):

- *Prescriptive beliefs or requirements*, which describe expected behaviors
- *Restrictive beliefs*, which are stated negatively and limit behaviors
- *Taboo beliefs*, which refer to specific supernatural consequences.

These activities are viewed as having the potential to impact the outcome of the pregnancy either positively or negatively. Table 13–2 describes activities that are encouraged (prescriptive) or forbidden (restrictive) or taboo by specific cultures. The table is not meant to be all-inclusive but rather to offer a few examples of cultural activities that may be important to some patients during the prenatal period.

TABLE 13–2 Cultural Beliefs and Practices During Pregnancy

These are a few examples of cultural beliefs and practices related to pregnancy. It is important not to make assumptions about a patient's beliefs because cultural norms vary greatly within a culture and from generation to generation. The nurse should observe the patient carefully and take the time to ask questions. Patients will benefit greatly from the nurse's increased awareness of their cultural beliefs and practices.

BELIEF OR PRACTICE	NURSING CONSIDERATION
Home Remedies	
Pregnant women of Native American background may use herbal remedies. An example is the dandelion, which contains a milky juice in its stem believed to increase breast milk flow in mothers who choose to breastfeed (Spector, 2017). Patients of Chinese descent may drink ginseng tea for faintness after childbirth or as a sedative when mixed with bamboo leaves. Some people of African heritage may use self-medication for pregnancy discomforts—for example, laxatives to prevent or treat constipation (Purnell, 2014).	Find out what medications and home remedies your patient is using, and counsel your patient regarding overall effects. It is common for individuals to avoid telling healthcare workers about home remedies; the patient may feel this will be judged unfavorably. Phrase your questions in a sensitive, accepting way. In some cases, you might want to suggest remedies that may be more effective—for example, eating high-fiber foods to reduce constipation. If the home remedy is not harmful, there is no reason to ask a patient to discontinue this practice.
Nutrition	
Some women of Italian background may believe that it is necessary to satisfy desires for certain foods in order to prevent congenital anomalies. Also, they may believe that they must eat food that they smell, or else the fetus will move "inside," which will result in a miscarriage. Pregnant women of Vietnamese descent are considered to be in a weak, cold state and must correct this by eating and drinking hot foods during the first trimester (Purnell, 2014). So, too, people of Ethiopian descent may believe that unfulfilled cravings may cause miscarriage (Spector, 2017).	Discuss the patient's beliefs and practices in regard to nutrition during pregnancy. Obtain a diet history from the patient. Discuss the importance of a well-balanced diet during pregnancy with consideration of the patient's cultural beliefs and practices.
Alternative Healthcare Providers	
Pregnant women of Mexican background may choose to seek out the care of a *partera* (midwife) for prenatal and intrapartum care. A partera speaks their language, shares a similar culture, and can care for pregnant women at home or in a birthing center instead of a hospital. Some people in Hispanic American communities may use the *curandero*, the holistic folk healer. The curanderos are believed to have received their gift from God and may use herbs or prescribe over-the-counter medications (Spector, 2017).	Discuss the variety of choices of healthcare providers available to the pregnant woman. Contrast the benefits and risks of different settings for prenatal care and birth. Provide reassurance that the goal of healthcare during pregnancy and birth is a healthy outcome for mother and baby with respect for the specific cultural beliefs and practices of the patient.
Exercise	
Pregnant women of Korean descent may work hard toward the end of pregnancy to increase the chances of giving birth to a small baby (Purnell, 2014). Some people of European, African, and Mexican descent believe that reaching over the head during pregnancy can harm the baby.	Ask your patient whether there are any activities she is afraid to do because of the pregnancy. Assure her that reaching over her head will not harm the baby and evaluate other activities regarding their effect on the pregnancy.
BELIEF OR PRACTICE	**NURSING CONSIDERATION**
Spirituality	
Navajo Native Americans are aware of the mind–soul connection and may try to follow certain practices to have a healthy pregnancy and birth. Practices could include focus on peace and positive thoughts as well as certain types of prayers and ceremonies. A traditional healer may assist them (Purnell, 2014). Some people of European background may tend to pay more attention to spirituality in their life to alleviate fears and ensure a safe birth.	Encourage the use of support systems and spiritual aids that provide comfort for the mother.
Birth Rituals	
In certain countries such as Algeria, Brazil, China, and Korea the father is usually not present at birth. In Japan a new mother may be confined for up to 100 days, while in Bangladesh the new mother remains indoors for up to 40 days. In Iran, Iraq, and Greece amulets may be placed on the baby or crib (Spector, 2017).	Recognize the importance of birth practices that are part of a family's tradition and honor these practices when possible.

Note: It is unwise to attribute specific attitudes or beliefs to all members of a cultural group. The information in this table offers possible insights into caring for women from different cultural groups.

Developing Cultural Competence Pregnant Women of African American Heritage

In caring for pregnant women of African American heritage, it may be helpful to consider the following general points (Purnell, 2014):

- Some African American pregnant women may be guided by their extended family into common practices such as geophagia, the ingestion of dirt or clay, which is believed to alleviate mineral deficiencies. This practice has implications for the focus of teaching a nurse offers.
- Many African American families are matriarchal. Women are respected and heeded in decision making and often stress good behavior and firm parenting with their children, especially to keep them safe in dangerous situations.
- Three-generation extended families are common, and the grandmother is often highly respected for her wisdom. She may play a critical role in the care of the children.
- Certain taboos may exist, such as the belief in the necessity to avoid taking pictures during pregnancy to prevent stillbirths. Some women of African American heritage may also believe that the purchase of baby clothing or supplies can result in a stillbirth. Thus, they may appear to be unprepared for the arrival of the baby.

Note: It is unwise to attribute specific attitudes or beliefs to all members of a cultural group. The information in the Developing Cultural Competence boxes offers possible insights into caring for women from different cultural groups.

In working with patients of another culture, the healthcare professional should be as open as possible to other beliefs. If certain activities are not harmful, there is no need to impose one's beliefs and practices on a patient. See *Professionalism in Practice: Providing Culturally Sensitive Care.* If the activities are proving to be harmful, the nurse can consult or work with someone within the culture or someone aware of the cultural beliefs and values to see whether the patient's behavior can be modified (Figure 13–3). See *Nursing Care Plan: Language Barriers at First Prenatal Visit.*

Professionalism in Practice Providing Culturally Sensitive Care

In providing effective, culturally sensitive care, nurses can use the following strategies:

- Take actions that help break down language barriers.
- Ask the patient what she or he believes caused the illness.
- Integrate folk treatments and Western medicine as much as possible.
- Enlist the family caretaker and others as needed.
- Respect the patient's beliefs
- Provide printed materials in the patient's language.

Childbearing Decisions

Childbearing decisions are decisions parents face about their childbirth preferences and experiences. A method that has assisted many couples in making these choices is called a birth plan. In the **birth plan**, prospective parents identify aspects of the childbearing experience that are most important to them. (A sample birth plan is presented in Figure 13–4.) The birth plan helps identify available options and becomes a tool for communication among the expectant parents, the healthcare providers, and the healthcare professionals at the birth setting.

The birth plan also helps pregnant women and couples set priorities. Using the plan, they identify areas that they want to incorporate in their own birth experience. Then they can take the birth plan to a visit with their physician/CNM or other healthcare provider and use it in discussing and comparing their wishes with the philosophy and beliefs of the healthcare provider. It is imperative that the couple discuss their preferences at a prenatal visit before labor. Sometimes couples may include requests that need clarification. For example, if the couple states they do not want any external monitoring, the provider needs to explain that intermittent monitoring could be provided but that eliminating all monitoring during labor could jeopardize both the mother and the fetus. Possible obstetric interventions that may be needed should also be part of the birth plan. The couple can also take the birth plan to the birth setting and use it as a basis for communicating their wishes during the childbirth experience.

Today, pregnant women and couples have many more choices. Some of these are explored in Table 13–3. Although most birth experiences are close to the desired experience, at times expectations cannot be met. This may be because of the unavailability of some choices in the community or unexpected problems during pregnancy or birth. While maternal satisfaction is highest when a planned cesarean birth or vaginal birth is achieved, it is important for nurses to help expectant parents keep sight of what is realistic for their situation.

Healthcare Provider

One of the first decisions facing expectant parents is the selection of a healthcare provider. The nurse working with the woman's primary care provider assists them by explaining the various options and outlining what can be expected from each. A thorough understanding of the differences of educational preparation, skill level, practice style, and general philosophy and characteristics of practice of certified nurse-midwives, obstetricians, family practice physicians, and lay midwives is essential. The nurse can encourage expectant parents to investigate the healthcare provider's credentials, basic and special education and training, fee schedule, and availability to new patients; this is often accomplished by telephoning the healthcare provider's office.

The nurse can also help the woman/couple develop a list of interview questions for their first visit to an obstetrical healthcare provider. These could include:

- Who is in practice with you, or who covers for you when you are unavailable?
- At what point after admission do you come to the hospital or birth setting to provide support?
- How do your partners' philosophies compare to yours?
- How do you feel about my partner, other support person, or other children coming to the prenatal visits?

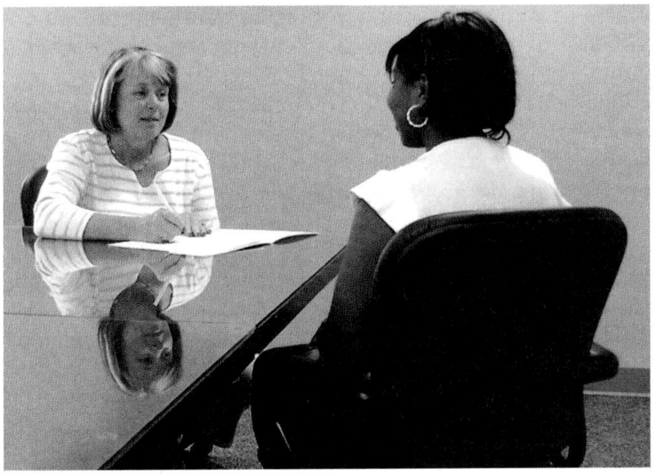

Figure 13–3 The culturally competent nurse respects the culture and values of the pregnant woman.

SOURCE: Patricia A. Wieland Ladewig.

- Do you offer centering (group care) or individual prenatal care visits?
- What weight gain do you recommend and why?
- What are your feelings about (fill in special desires for the birth event, such as different positions assumed during labor, avoidance of an episiotomy, induction of labor, other people present during the birth, pain control measures, breastfeeding immediately after the birth, no separation of newborn and parents following birth, and so on)?
- If a cesarean birth is necessary, can my partner be present?
- What are your feelings regarding complementary treatments during labor (herbs to augment labor, use of acupressure/massage/hypnosis, use of oils for perineal massage, and so on)?

Expectant parents also need to discuss the qualities they want in a healthcare provider for the newborn. They may want to visit several pediatric healthcare providers before the birth to select someone who will meet their needs and those of their child.

Nursing Care Plan: Language Barriers at First Prenatal Visit

1. Nursing Diagnosis: *Health Maintenance, Ineffective*, related to alteration in verbal and written communication skills (NANDA-I © 2017)

Goal: Patient will demonstrate understanding of health information received during prenatal visits.

INTERVENTION	RATIONALE
• If no interpreter is available, refer to posters with pictures to explain routine care and procedures during the prenatal examination.	• Posters put words into verbal images and are helpful in communicating information.
• Provide handouts and brochures about prenatal care in the woman's native language.	• Translated handouts provide information that the patient can refer to at home. This reinforces information discussed during the visit and helps the family understand what the woman will experience during the pregnancy and at each visit.
• Use teaching models to demonstrate procedures. Teaching models may include plastic pelvis, knitted uterus, fetal model, breast model, birth control devices, ultrasound equipment, and so forth.	• Visual aids help to communicate information during the examination.
• Schedule an interpreter for subsequent prenatal visits.	• If a family member (preferably not the patient's child) cannot translate the health information to the patient, an independent translator is essential to ensure that information is accurately provided. When an interpreter is used (especially a family member), the nurse should be sure that the interpreter is translating information received from the woman and not simply answering the questions for her.
• Refer the woman to prenatal classes taught in her own language, if available.	• Prenatal classes taught in the woman's language enable her to receive health information that is easily understood, which will prove a better understanding of what she should expect during pregnancy, birth, and postpartum. Prenatal classes may also provide a social outlet for patients.
• Involve other members of the healthcare team in planning and providing care.	• Cultures vary in language, nonverbal expression, dietary habits, use of time, spatial expectations, and so forth. Use of medication and blood products may also be influenced by cultural beliefs. Social workers who are familiar with the patient's cultural beliefs, for example, may help the patient adjust to different healthcare practices while providing suggestions to ensure prenatal care that is more in line with the woman's cultural beliefs. Dietitians may help the woman plan meals that are aligned with her cultural practices while meeting the nutritional needs of pregnancy.

EXPECTED OUTCOME: Effective communication occurs. The patient will gain an understanding of basic prenatal information as evidenced by using hand gestures, by pointing to pictures on posters and translated phrases on handouts, and through an interpreter, if one is available.

Sample Birth Plan

Choice
- Care provider:
  - Certified nurse-midwife
  - Obstetrician
  - Family physician
  - Lay midwife
- Birth setting:
- Hospital:
  - Birthing room
  - Delivery room
- Birth center
- Home
- Support during labor and birth:
  - Partner present
  - Doula present
- During labor:
  - Ambulate as desired
  - Shower if desired
  - Wear own clothes
  - Use hot tub
  - Use own rocking chair
  - Have perineal prep
  - Have enema
- Water birth
- Electronic fetal monitor
- Membranes:
  - Rupture naturally
  - Amniotomy if needed
- Labor stimulation if needed
- Medication:
  - Identify type desired
- Fluids or ice as desired
- Music during labor and birth
- Massage
- Therapeutic touch
- Healing touch

Choice
- Position during birth:
  - On side
  - Hands and knees
  - Kneeling
  - Squatting
  - Birthing chair
  - Birthing bed
  - Other:
- Family present (sibs)
- Filming of birth (videotaping)
- Photography of birth
- Leboyer
- Episiotomy
- No sterile drapes
- Partner to cut umbilical cord
- Hold baby immediately after birth
- Breastfeed immediately after birth
- No separation after birth
- Save the placenta
- Collect cord blood for banking
- Newborn care:
  - Eye treatment for the baby
  - Vitamin K injection
  - Heptovac injection
  - Breastfeeding
  - Formula feeding
  - Pacifier use
  - Glucose water
  - Circumcision
- Postpartum care:
  - Short stay
  - 48-hour stay after vaginal birth
  - Home visits after discharge
  - Home doula
- Other:

Figure 13–4 **Birth plan for childbirth choices. The columns list various choices that the couple may consider during their childbirth experience. Once the couple has considered each of the choices, they can circle the items they desire.**

Professionalism in Practice Referrals

The nurse provides referrals to appropriate providers, hospitals, and clinics as needed to ensure that the woman receives competent, professional healthcare.

Prenatal Care Services

The nurse can assist expectant parents in obtaining the type of prenatal care services that are most appropriate for their personal needs. Most practitioners offer individual prenatal care services in which the woman or the woman and her family attend a clinic or office visit on a regular basis depending on her stage of pregnancy. Recently, the concept of **centering**, or group prenatal care, has become popular.

When empowering women to choose health-promoting behaviors, it may be helpful to consider a relatively new, innovative model for prenatal care called *Centering Pregnancy*. Centering Pregnancy integrates the three major components of care—health assessment, education, and support—into a unified program providing complete prenatal care to women within a group setting. This model replaces the traditional one-on-one visits in an examination room with a healthcare provider. Instead, group meetings are held where mothers-to-be and their partners receive care and education and form a sense of community with other group members. It is discussed in more detail later in this chapter.

Patients begin meeting in small groups at 12 to 16 weeks' gestation and continue to meet monthly for the first 4 months and biweekly as their due dates approach. Each group session begins with the expectant mothers taking their own blood pressure, monitoring weight gain, checking urine samples, and recording data on medical charts under their provider or nurse's guidance. The provider then reviews each group member's information and completes any further assessments that are indicated. After all assessments are completed, the group members convene in a circle to discuss topics such as nutrition, fetal development, common discomforts of pregnancy and possible remedies, exercise, relaxation, labor and birth procedures, parenting and relationship issues, contraception, and baby care (DeCesare & Jackson, 2015). Both mothers and fathers report an increased investment in the pregnancy and self-care after attending group sessions.

Birth Setting

The nurse can help expectant parents choose a birth setting by suggesting they tour facilities and talk with nurses there as well as talk with friends or acquaintances who are recent parents. Questions that may be asked of new parents include:

- What kind of support did you receive during labor? Was it what you wanted?
- How was your labor support person treated?
- Were you allowed to take an active role in decision making throughout the birth process?
- If you had a doula, was her role respected? Was she welcome in the birth setting?
- Was your birth plan respected? Did you share it with the facility before the birth? If something did not work, why do you think there were problems?
- Did the nurse offer suggestions regarding comfort measures?
- Did the healthcare team provide emotional support?
- How were medications handled during labor? Were you comfortable with this?
- Were siblings welcomed in the birth setting? At the birth? After the birth?
- Did you feel you were given ample time to spend with your baby immediately after childbirth?
- Was the nursing staff helpful after the baby was born? Did you receive self-care and newborn care information? Was it in a usable form? Did you have a choice about what information you got? Did they let you decide what information you needed?
- Did you feel your choice of feeding method was supported?

The nurse helps expectant parents understand the array of choices available to them. The nurse can encourage them to consider options early in the pregnancy to allow time for talking with other parents and touring facilities.

TABLE 13–3 Benefits and Risks of Some Consumer and Medical Decisions During Pregnancy, Labor, and Birth

ISSUE	BENEFITS	RISKS
Breastfeeding	• No additional expense • Contains maternal antibodies • Decreases incidence of infant otitis media, vomiting, and diarrhea; hospitalizations during the first year of life; and allergies • Easier to digest than formula • Immediately after birth, promotes uterine contractions and decreases incidence of postpartum hemorrhage • Promotes maternal-infant bonding	• Transmission of maternal infections to newborn, such as HIV • Irregular ovulation and menses can cause false sense of security and nonuse of hormonal contraceptives • Increased nutritional requirement in mother

Ambulation during labor	• Comfort for laboring woman
	• May assist in labor progression by
	  • Stimulating contractions
	  • Allowing gravity to help descent of fetus
	  • Giving sense of independence and control
		• Cord prolapse with rupture of membranes unless engagement has occurred
		• Birth of baby in undesirable locations (hallways, outdoors, waiting area)
		• Inability to monitor fetal heart rate (FHR) unless telemetry unit available

Electronic fetal monitoring	• Helps evaluate fetal well-being • Helps identify fetal stress • Useful in diagnostic testing • Helps evaluate labor progress	• Supine postural hypotension • Intrauterine perforation (with internal uterine pressure device) • Infection (with internal monitoring) • Decreases personal interaction with mother because of attention paid to the machine • Mother is unable to ambulate or change her position freely
Whirlpool (jet hydrotherapy)	• Increased relaxation • Decreased anxiety • Stimulation of labor • Pain relief • Slight decrease in blood pressure (BP) • Increased diuresis • Decreased incidence of vacuum and forceps births • Increased pain threshold • Higher satisfaction with birth • Decreased use of pain medication for women in active labor (King, Brucker, Kriebs, et al., 2015)	• May slow contractions if used before active labor is established • Possible risk of infection if membranes are ruptured • Slight increase in maternal temperature and pulse in tub • Hypothermia • Increases fetal heart rate (FHR) by 10–20 beats/min
Analgesia	• Maternal relaxation facilitates labor	• All drugs reach the fetus in varying degrees and with varying effects
Episiotomy	• Decreases irregular tearing of perineum • Easier to repair for practitioner	• Increased pain after birth and for 1–3 months following birth • Dyspareunia • Infection • Increased frequency of third- and fourth-degree lacerations (Cunningham et al., 2018)

> “What I've seen time and again is that the technology of the hospital overwhelms patients' natural instincts; they are intimidated, afraid of appearing stupid or clumsy or sentimental in a surrounding that seems too efficient and immaculate and intelligent.”
>
> — A midwife's story

Nurses involved in childbirth education need to include the concept of individuality when providing information to expectant parents about the process of childbirth and their own pattern of coping. The wave of the future in childbirth education is to encourage women to incorporate their natural responses into coping with the pain of labor and birth. Alternative self-care activities should be explored with the expectant

EVIDENCE-BASED PRACTICE | Interventions to Reduce Childbirth Fear in Pregnant Women

Clinical Question

Can education and psychological support reduce the fear of childbirth in healthy pregnant women?

The Evidence

Fear of the process of childbirth has been linked to adverse maternal outcomes, including high rates of surgical birth, mental health issues, and increased postpartum depression. Many women with childbirth fear may request surgical birth if they perceive their fears have not been addressed. These researchers used a randomized trial to test an antenatal intervention of psychological support and education delivered by nurse-midwives. More than 1,400 women were included in the study population. Randomized trials with large sample sizes form a strong level of evidence.

The intervention was a telephone education counseling intervention that reviewed the woman's current expectations and feelings regarding fear of childbirth. The nurse supported the expression of feelings and provided a framework for women to identify and work through the elements of childbirth that they found frightening. The intervention focused on helping the mother develop situational supports for the birth and a plan for dealing with the childbirth experience that gave the mother control over her birth process. The women who received the intervention reported lower levels of fear and higher levels of self-efficacy and sense of control (Toohill et al., 2014). These mothers also had fewer depression symptoms and requested surgical birth with less frequency.

Best Practice

Prenatal psychologic support and education may reduce the fear of childbirth among women. Improving antenatal emotional well-being has a myriad of positive benefits and may result in an optimal childbirth experience. Providing this support leads to fewer requests for surgical births.

Clinical Reasoning

What are some of the ways that the nurse can help the mother gain a sense of control over the birth process? What might be some of the benefits of reduced childbirth fear for the mother and for the provider?

couple to identify preferences. See Chapter 19 for further discussion of childbirth education.

Clinical Tip

Call the birthing facilities in your community and inquire about what choices are available in each facility so that you can answer expectant parents' questions.

Labor Support Person

Some of the first formal childbirth preparation classes were patterned after a book titled *Husband-Coached Childbirth* by Dr. Robert Bradley (2008), which was originally published in 1965. Since that time, husbands and partners of expectant women have been very involved in acting as "coaches" or support persons during childbirth classes, labor, and birth. Although some husbands/partners welcome the role and look forward to providing emotional and physical support, others do not. Some may become anxious and fearful. These feelings can be related to past experiences and/or cultural factors. In these situations, the nurse provides encouragement and support to both the woman and her support person. Women who had continuous intrapartum support were less likely to have intrapartum analgesia, to have an operative birth, or to report dissatisfaction with their childbirth experiences (Donna, 2011). A woman's satisfaction with childbirth is directly affected by the relationship with the healthcare provider, the support she received from caregivers, personal expectations, and her involvement with decision making. Clearly, the role of the nurse cannot be overestimated.

For centuries, women have been serving and assisting other women in childbirth. The role of the **doula** has evolved out of this need for companionship and special support during the birthing journey. *Doula* is a Greek word that means "woman's servant." In the birthing environment, a doula is a companion who provides support but does not perform any clinical tasks. The doula provides *labor support*, which includes emotional, physical, and informational support, and acts as an advocate for the woman and her family by verbalizing their wishes to the nurses and physicians/CNMs. Continuous labor support facilitates birth, enhances the mother's memory of the experience, strengthens mother–newborn bonding, increases breastfeeding success, and significantly reduces many forms of medical intervention, including cesarean birth and the use of analgesia, anesthesia, vacuum extraction, and forceps (Donna, 2011). A doula may also be trained to provide support and care during the postpartum period. Later postpartum benefits for the mother include increased

Developing Cultural Competence Female Relatives as Caregivers

In most Middle Eastern countries, childbirth is exclusively attended to by women. A woman in labor is most commonly surrounded by female relatives and friends and men are not expected to be involved. In Jordan, for example, many Muslims believe that a woman who is pregnant is responsible for her soul and that of her unborn child, and at doomsday God will ask her about it. Once she is pregnant, her mother and mother-in-law and women around her will provide the physical and psychologic advice and support she needs (Bawadi & Al-Hamdan, 2016).

Note: It is unwise to attribute specific attitudes or beliefs to all members of a cultural group. The information in the Developing Cultural Competence boxes offers possible insights into caring for women from different cultural groups.

bonding/interaction with the newborn and decreased symptoms of depression. The doula may accompany the childbearing couple on a volunteer basis or may be paid a fee by the family. Another support person who has been involved in labor and birthing is a *monitrice*. *Monitrice* is a French word that refers to a specially trained nurse who provides assessment, nursing care, and support. The role of *monitrice* is not common in the United States.

Siblings at Birth

Some couples decide to have their other children present at the birth. Children who will attend a birth can be prepared through books, audiovisual materials, models, discussion, and sibling classes.

It is imperative that the child has his or her own support person or coach whose sole responsibility is tending to the needs of that child during the labor and birth experience. The support person should be familiar to the child, warm, sensitive, flexible, knowledgeable about the birth process, and comfortable with sexuality and birth. This person must be prepared to explain to the child what is happening and to intervene when necessary. The support person should be prepared and willing to leave the birthing room at any time, should that be the child's desire. The support person for the child should assume responsibility for providing distractions such as trips to the cafeteria, visits to the nursery window, outdoor walks, and other age-appropriate activities.

Children should be given the option of relating to the birth in whatever manner they choose as long as it is not disruptive. Children should understand that it is their own choice to be there and that they may stay or leave the room as they choose. To help children recognize their needs and desires, the nurse may wish to elicit exactly what they expect from the experience. Children need to feel free to ask questions and express feelings.

Allowing children to participate in the arrival of their sibling engenders the desire to nurture "our" baby, as opposed to jealousy and rivalry directed at "Mom's" baby. The mother does not disappear mysteriously into the hospital and return with a demanding outsider. Instead, the family attending the birth together finds a new opportunity for closeness and growth by sharing in the birth of a new member.

Classes for Family Members During Pregnancy

Childbirth classes are routinely taught by certified childbirth educators (CBEs or CCEs). These are individuals who have received specific educational preparation related to pregnancy, labor, birth, and postpartum/newborn care and issues. Many CBEs are also registered nurses; however, nursing education is not required. The majority of the certification programs do, however, require witnessing a minimum number of births.

The CBE should consider elements developed by authoritative organizations such as the Coalition for Improving Maternity Services (CIMS) when developing their own philosophy of childbirth for their classes. The "Mother-Friendly Childbirth Initiative" was created in 1996 by CIMS, a national alliance of more than 50 childbirth organizations and many prominent individuals. The coalition's mission is to promote a wellness model of maternity care that will improve birth outcomes and substantially reduce costs. The philosophic cornerstones of mother-friendly care are (CIMS, 2016):

- Normalcy of the birthing process
- Empowerment of the mother
- Autonomy to make informed decisions based on accurate and up-to-date information
- Do no harm
- Responsibility of caregivers to provide high-quality care.

Prenatal education programs provide important opportunities to share information about pregnancy, childbirth, coping mechanisms, and choices available for the woman and her support person. Studies have shown that prepared childbirth education programs can have a beneficial effect on performance in labor and birth. The prenatal period should be used to expose the prospective parents to up-to-date, evidence-based information about the following topics:

- Labor and birth
- Pain relief
- Obstetric complications and procedures
- Breastfeeding
- Normal newborn care
- Postpartum adjustment.

The content of each class is generally directed by the overall goals of the program. For example, specific classes may address the following subjects:

- Gestational changes and fetal development
- Childbirth choices available today
- Preparation of the mother for pregnancy and birth
- Preparation for cesarean birth or for vaginal birth after cesarean
- Preparation for couples who desire an unmedicated birth
- Preparation of the grandparents or siblings for the birth
- Newborn care and safety
- Self-care during the postpartum period.

The nurse who knows the types of prenatal programs available in the community can direct expectant parents to programs that meet their special needs and learning goals.

From the expectant parents' point of view, class content is best presented in chronology with the pregnancy. It is important that the classes begin by identifying the parents' needs, goals, and learning styles. Although both parents expect to learn breathing and relaxation techniques and baby care, fathers usually expect facts and mothers expect coping strategies. Women's goals commonly include gaining information, reducing anxiety/increasing confidence, having their partner present and involved, and having a positive emotional experience in childbirth. Classes that provide an environment supportive of practicing newly learned techniques and the freedom to ask questions and receive explanations are beneficial in helping class participants obtain these goals (Figure 13–5). By the end of the class, parents should feel that they will be able to make appropriate and informed decisions. Classes may be divided into early and late classes so specific needs can be addressed.

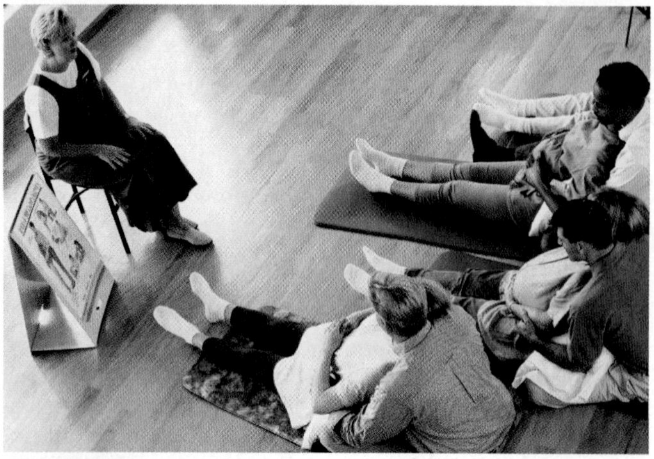

Figure 13–5 **In a group setting with a nurse-instructor, expectant parents share information about pregnancy and childbirth.**

SOURCE: Purestock/Getty Images.

Education of the Family Having a Cesarean Birth

Cesarean birth is an alternative method of birth that now accounts for 32% of births in the United States (Martin et al., 2017). Consequently, although the need for a cesarean is not often known in advance, more and more childbirth preparation classes are integrating content on cesarean birth into the curriculum.

Class content should cover what the parents can expect to happen during a cesarean birth, what they might feel, and what choices are available. All pregnant women and couples should be encouraged to discuss with their physician/CNM the progression of events if a cesarean birth becomes necessary. Cesarean birth and repeat cesarean birth are discussed in detail in Chapter 25.

When expectant parents are anticipating a repeat cesarean birth, they have time to plan and prepare. Many birthing units provide preparation classes for repeat cesarean birth. Parents who have had previous negative experiences need an opportunity to describe what contributed to their feelings. They should be encouraged to identify what they would like to change and to list interventions that would make the experience more positive. Those who have had positive experiences require reassurance that their needs and desires will be met in a similar manner. All parents should be encouraged to air any fears or anxieties.

Often a woman facing a repeat cesarean is concerned about postoperative pain. She needs reassurance that subsequent cesarean births are often less painful than the first. In addition, planned cesarean births involve less fatigue than unplanned procedures because they are not preceded by a long, strenuous labor. Providing this information will help the woman cope more effectively with stressful stimuli, including pain.

Preparation for Parents Desiring Trial of Labor After Cesarean Birth

Trial of labor after cesarean birth (TOLAC) was previously termed *vaginal birth after cesarean (VBAC)* and is discussed in detail in Chapter 25. Parents who have had a cesarean birth and are now anticipating a vaginal birth have unique needs. Because they may have unresolved questions and concerns about the last birth, it is helpful to begin the series of classes with an informational session. The nurse can supply information about the criteria necessary to attempt a trial of labor and identify decisions to be made regarding the birth experience. Some childbirth educators suggest that parents prepare two birth plans: One for vaginal birth and one for cesarean birth. Preparing birth plans seems to give parents some sense of control over the birth experience and tends to increase the positive aspects of the experience.

Breastfeeding Programs

Programs offering information on breastfeeding are increasing. For decades, a primary source of information has been La Leche League. Information can also be obtained from lactation consultants, peer counselors, labor and postpartum nurses, birthing centers, hospitals, and health clinics. Online support groups can also be an important resource for breastfeeding mothers. Breastfeeding is discussed in detail in Chapter 29.

Rates of breastfeeding in the United States are well below the *Healthy People 2020* objective of 81.9% (U.S. Department of Health and Human Services [HHS], 2013). *Healthy People 2020* has set goals not only for increasing the rate of breastfed newborns and infants, but also for increasing the availability of worksite lactation support programs to encourage mothers to continue breastfeeding following their return to work.

Classes and support groups typically include information about the following topics:

- Advantages and challenges of breastfeeding
- Techniques and positioning
- Methods of breast pumping and milk storage
- How to involve the father or partner in the feeding process, such as having him or her bring the baby to the mother for feedings, burp the baby between or after feedings, or rock the baby back to sleep
- Ways of successfully breastfeeding and returning to work.

Sibling Preparation: Adjustment to a Newborn

The birth of a new sibling is a significant event in a child's life. Positive adjustment can be enhanced by attendance at formal sibling preparation classes (Figure 13–6). Typically, the classes are attended by children ages 3 to 12 years. Children younger than 3 tend to have shorter attention spans and may have difficulty participating in the class; however, many facilities will allow younger children to attend, especially if an older sibling is enrolled in the class. These classes can assist with decreasing sibling rivalry and reducing children's anxiety. They help children feel that they are part of the birthing process. The classes also enable parents to identify children's concerns related to the new baby. They provide a means to facilitate communication and explore children's feelings. They also provide basic information about pregnancy, childbirth, and the characteristics and behavior of newborns. The classes usually focus on:

- Reducing anxiety in the child
- Providing opportunities for the child to express feelings and concerns
- Encouraging realistic expectations of the newborn
- Teaching the older child to be an active participant in the baby's care by showing how to safely hold the newborn, feed and burp the baby, or even change diapers.

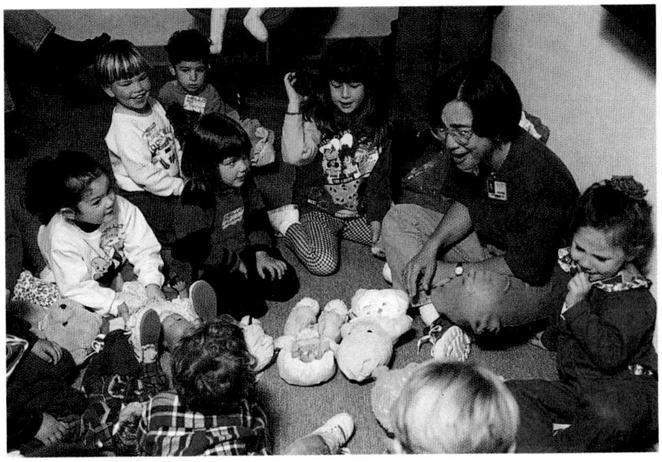

Figure 13–6 **It is especially important that siblings be well prepared when they are going to be present at the birth. However, even siblings who will not be present at the birth can benefit from information about childbirth and the new baby ahead of time.**

Typically, parents and their children attend the class together. Many activities are devised to help each child feel special. Time is usually allotted at the end of the class for talking with parents about coping skills and providing hints about dealing with sibling jealousy. Class content typically includes care and behavior of new babies, a practice session holding anatomically correct dolls, changing diapers, and a tour of the "bedroom" and the nursery where Mom and baby will stay. Many times, a newborn is held up at the nursery window so the children can see a "real baby." Some facilities give the children a special gift for attendance or a trip to the cafeteria for a special treat. In addition, parents may wish to take advantage of books and videos designed to help children prepare for a new sibling (Figure 13–7).

Classes for Grandparents

Grandparents are an important source of support and information for prospective and new parents. They are now being included in the birthing process more frequently. Prenatal programs for grandparents can address current roles, transitioning to a new role, beliefs regarding childbirth, and ways to support the new family unit. Grandparents can also benefit from educational information, such as the benefits of breastfeeding, and updates on baby care, such as proper sleep positions for baby and when to introduce foods. If they plan to be integral members of the labor and birth team, they will need information about providing support to the mother.

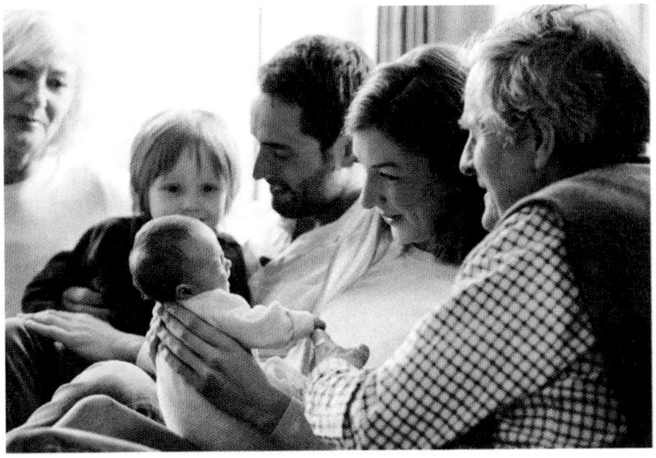

Figure 13–7 **A properly prepared "big brother" and enthusiastic grandparents greet the newest member of the family.**

SOURCE: Monkey Business/Shutterstock.

Relief of the Common Discomforts of Pregnancy

Healthcare professionals often refer to the common discomforts of pregnancy as minor discomforts. These discomforts, however, are not minor to the pregnant woman.

Most of the discomforts of pregnancy are a result of physiologic and anatomic changes and are fairly specific to either the first trimester or to the second and third trimesters.

Clinical Tip

At each prenatal visit, focus your teaching on changes or possible discomforts the woman might encounter during the coming month and the next trimester. If the pregnancy is progressing normally, spend a few minutes describing her baby at this stage of development.

First Trimester

The dramatic hormonal changes of the first trimester account for many of the discomforts experienced in this period. These discomforts tend to abate by the beginning of the fourth month of pregnancy.

NAUSEA AND VOMITING

Nausea and vomiting of pregnancy (NVP) are early, common symptoms occurring in 50 to 80% of pregnant women (ACOG, 2018). These symptoms appear sometime after the first missed menstrual period and usually cease by the fourth missed menstrual period. Some women develop an aversion only to specific foods. Many experience nausea on arising in the morning, and others experience nausea only in the evening.

The exact cause of NVP is unknown but is believed to be multifactorial. The elevation of human chorionic gonadotropin (hCG) is often cited as a major factor because it begins to be present in the body at about the time symptoms of morning sickness usually begin, and hCG levels are subsiding when the discomfort of nausea and vomiting usually ends. In addition, elevated estrogen levels, relaxation of the smooth muscle of the stomach, changes in carbohydrate metabolism, fatigue, and emotional factors may also play a role in the development of NVP.

Health Promotion. Treatment of nausea and vomiting is not always successful, but the symptoms can be reduced. To decrease the potential for development of *hyperemesis gravidarum* (severe nausea and vomiting that causes dehydration and weight loss), prompt treatment is important.

The nurse needs to assess the onset, frequency, duration, and severity of symptoms and actual nutritional intake to be helpful in suggesting methods of relief or necessary medical care. Physical assessment of the woman should include particular attention to skin color, texture, and turgor as well as vital signs and bowel sounds. For some women, simply avoiding the odor of certain foods or other conditions that precipitate the problem may relieve nausea. If nausea occurs most frequently during early morning, the woman may find it helpful to eat dry crackers or toast before arising and to rise from bed slowly. Rising slowly and avoiding sudden position changes throughout the day may also help prevent nausea due to hypotensive episodes. In addition, the nurse can suggest that the woman avoid brushing her teeth right after eating because this, too, may trigger vomiting. Generally, it is helpful to eat small meals every 2 to 3 hours during the day and to avoid greasy or highly seasoned foods. Food may be salted to taste. The salt increases the palatability of the food and replaces any chloride lost when the woman vomits hydrochloric acid from the stomach. Eating dry meals and taking all liquids, including soups, between meals may help some women by avoiding overdistention of the stomach. Sudden changes in blood sugar levels can be avoided if the small meals are high in low-fat protein or complex carbohydrates. Some women find that slowly sipping herbal tea (peppermint, chamomile, or spearmint) or a carbonated beverage helps reduce nausea.

In addition to common self-care measures, certain complementary or alternative therapies may be useful. For example, many women find that acupressure applied to pressure points in the wrists is helpful (Figure 13–8).

Ginger has long been used as a traditional remedy for treating nausea and vomiting associated with early pregnancy. Ginger is available in a variety of forms, including fresh or dried root, capsules, tea, candy, cookies, crystals, inhaled powdered ginger, and sugared ginger. It has few side effects when taken in small doses (National Center for Complementary and Integrative Health [NCCIH], 2015). Some women find pyridoxine (vitamin B_6) helpful. Diclegis, a combination of pyridoxine 10 mg plus doxylamine succinate 10 mg, was approved by the Food and Drug Administration (FDA) in 2013 specifically for the treatment of NVP (Fantasia, 2014). Antihistamine H_1-receptor antagonists such as dimenhydrinate, benzamides such as trimethobenzamide, and phenothiazines such as prochlorperazine are considered to be safe and effective for treating refractory cases. In very severe cases, methylprednisolone, a steroid, may be used with caution after 10 weeks' gestation but strictly as a last resort because of potential risk to the fetus and to avoid serious maternal adverse effects. (American College of Obstetricians and Gynecologists [ACOG], 2018).

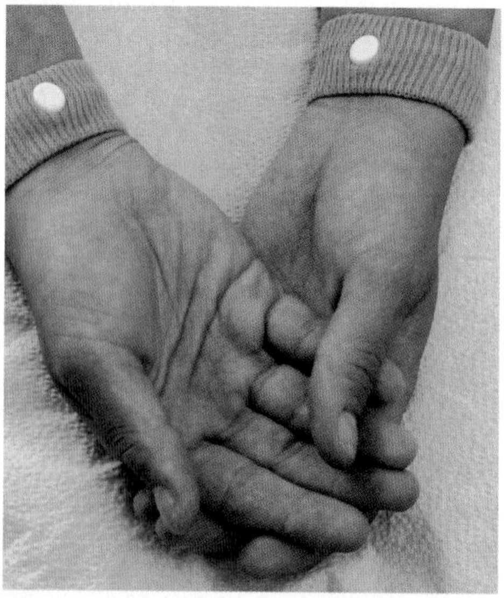

Figure 13–8 **Acupressure wristbands are sometimes used to help relieve nausea during early pregnancy.**

The nurse should advise the woman to contact her care provider if she vomits more than once per day or shows signs of dehydration, such as dry mouth, decreased amounts of highly concentrated urine, or decreased skin turgor. In such cases, the physician/CNM may order antiemetics. However, antiemetics should be avoided if at all possible during the first trimester because of the danger of teratogenic effects on embryo development.

Nausea and vomiting symptoms generally decrease by the 16th week of pregnancy. If they do not, hyperemesis gravidarum, which occurs in 0.3 to 2% of pregnancies, must be considered. Hyperemesis symptoms include weight loss, dehydration, and nutrition imbalance and may require hospitalization (Johnson, Hallock, Bienstock, et al., 2015).

URINARY FREQUENCY

Urinary frequency, a common discomfort of pregnancy, occurs early in pregnancy and again during the third trimester because of the pressure of the enlarging uterus on the bladder. Although the glomerular filtration rate increases in pregnancy, it does not cause a significant increase in urine output. Urinary frequency is considered normal during the first and third trimesters; however, the nurse should advise the woman to contact her healthcare provider if she experiences any signs of bladder infection such as painful urination (dysuria), burning with voiding, or blood in the urine (hematuria).

Health Promotion. There are no methods of decreasing the frequency of urination in pregnancy. Fluid intake should never be decreased to prevent frequency. The woman should be encouraged to maintain an adequate fluid intake of at least 2000 mL per day. She should also be encouraged to empty her bladder frequently (approximately every 2 hours while awake).

Frequent bladder emptying helps decrease the incidence of leakage of urine and also reduces the risk of developing a urinary tract infection (UTI). Because frequency often results in several trips to the bathroom each night, it is important to remind the woman to consider safety factors in the home, such as a clear path to the bathroom and the use of a nightlight. The woman who leaks urine may choose to wear pantyliners during the day. Pantyliners should be changed as soon as they become damp to avoid perineal excoriation and to avoid contamination of the perineum from the rectal area if the pads move back and forth while walking. Tightening of the pubococcygeus muscle, which supports internal organs and controls voiding, can help maintain good perineal tone. This procedure, known as the Kegel exercise, is discussed later in this chapter.

FATIGUE

Marked fatigue, often out of proportion to the woman's normal pattern, is so common in early pregnancy that it is considered a presumptive sign of pregnancy. It is aggravated if the woman has to arise several times each night because of urinary frequency. Typically, it resolves soon after the end of the first trimester.

Health Promotion. Scheduling activities to allow for napping is helpful. Women should be encouraged to use every opportunity available to rest, including going to bed earlier in the evening. The woman's partner needs to understand that the fatigue is normal and will subside. The partner can be encouraged to assume more home responsibilities to support the woman and enable her to rest.

BREAST TENDERNESS

Sensitivity of the breasts occurs early and continues throughout the pregnancy. Increased levels of estrogen and progesterone contribute to the soreness and tingling felt in the breasts and to the increased sensitivity of the nipples.

Health Promotion. A well-fitting, supportive bra gives the most relief for this discomfort. The qualities of a properly supportive bra are discussed in *Breast Care* later in this chapter.

INCREASED VAGINAL DISCHARGE

Increased whitish vaginal discharge, called **leukorrhea**, is common in pregnancy. It occurs as the result of hyperplasia of vaginal mucosa and increased production of mucus by the endocervical glands. In addition, the increased acidity of the secretions encourages the growth of *Candida albicans*, and the woman is thus more susceptible to monilial vaginitis.

Health Promotion. Cleanliness is important in preventing excoriation and vaginal infections. Daily bathing is adequate; douching is avoided during pregnancy. The woman should avoid nylon underpants and pantyhose because they retain heat and moisture in the genital area; absorbent cotton underpants should be worn to help prevent problems. The nurse can advise the pregnant woman to report any change in vaginal discharge, any irritation in the perineal area, and intense vaginal itching. These changes frequently indicate vaginal infections.

NASAL STUFFINESS AND EPISTAXIS

Once pregnancy is well established, elevated estrogen levels may produce edema of the nasal mucosa, resulting in nasal stuffiness, nasal discharge, and obstruction (rhinitis of pregnancy). *Epistaxis* (nosebleed) may also result.

Health Promotion. Cool air vaporizers and normal saline nose drops may be helpful. However, the problem is often unresponsive to treatment. Women experiencing these problems find it difficult to sleep and may resort to medicated nasal sprays and decongestants to relieve the problem. Such interventions may provide relief initially but can actually increase the nasal stuffiness over time. The use of any medication in pregnancy should be avoided, if possible.

PTYALISM

Ptyalism is a rare discomfort of pregnancy in which excessive, often bitter, saliva is produced. Its cause has not been established (King et al., 2015). Effective treatments are limited.

Health Promotion. Using astringent mouthwashes, chewing gum, or sucking on hard candy may minimize the problem of ptyalism. Many women also choose to carry tissues or a small towel to spit into when necessary.

Second and Third Trimesters

It is difficult to classify discomforts as specifically occurring in the second or third trimester because their timing varies because of individual variations in women. The symptoms discussed in this section usually do not appear until the third trimester in primigravidas but may occur earlier with each succeeding pregnancy.

HEARTBURN (PYROSIS)

Heartburn is the regurgitation of acidic gastric contents into the esophagus. It creates a burning or irritating sensation in the esophagus and radiates upward, sometimes leaving a bad taste in the mouth. As many as four-fifths of women experience heartburn in the third trimester (King et al., 2015). Heartburn appears to be primarily a result of the displacement of the stomach by the enlarging uterus. The increased production of progesterone in pregnancy, decreases in gastrointestinal motility, and relaxation of the cardiac (esophageal) sphincter also contribute to heartburn.

Health Promotion. Heartburn is aggravated by overeating, ingesting fatty and fried foods, and lying down soon after eating. The woman should, therefore, avoid these situations. The woman should be encouraged to drink an adequate amount of fluid (8 to 10 8-oz glasses) each day and to eat smaller, more frequent meals to accommodate the decreased size of her stomach. Good posture is important because it allows more room for the stomach to function. Some women choose complementary and alternative therapies to relieve their heartburn (see Chapter 2 for more information about alternative therapies).

Liquid forms of low-sodium antacids are often most effective in providing relief. However, many women prefer chewable over-the-counter antacid tablets. The nurse should advise women that antacids containing aluminum may cause constipation, and antacids containing magnesium can cause diarrhea. The nurse should also let women know that they should avoid sodium bicarbonate (baking soda) and Alka-Seltzer because they may lead to electrolyte imbalance.

If maternal heartburn is severe, not relieved by antacids, and accompanied by gastrointestinal reflux, an antisecretory agent (H_2 blocker) such as ranitidine (Zantac), cimetidine (Tagamet), or omeprazole (Losec) may be helpful. To date they have not been linked with an excessive risk of birth defects.

ANKLE EDEMA

Most women experience ankle edema in the last part of pregnancy because of the increasing difficulty of venous return from the lower extremities. Prolonged standing or sitting and warm weather increase the edema. It is also associated with varicose veins. Ankle edema becomes a concern only when accompanied by hypertension or proteinuria or when the edema is not postural in origin.

Health Promotion. The aggravating conditions just mentioned should be avoided. If the woman has to sit or stand for long periods, frequent dorsiflexion of her feet will help contract muscles, thereby squeezing the fluid back into circulation. The pregnant woman should not wear tight garters or other restrictive bands around her legs. During rest periods, the woman should elevate her legs and hips as described in the following section on varicose veins.

VARICOSE VEINS

Varicose veins are a result of weakening of the walls of veins or faulty functioning of the valves. Poor circulation in the lower extremities predisposes the woman to varicose veins in the legs and thighs, as does prolonged standing or sitting. The weight of the gravid uterus on the pelvic veins aggravates the development of varicosities in the legs and pelvic area by preventing good venous return. Increased maternal age, excessive weight gain, a large fetus, heredity, and multiple gestation can all contribute to the problem. Symptoms may range from mildly unpleasant cosmetic effects to chronic pain and superficial thrombophlebitis.

Vulvar varicosities may also be a problem in pregnancy, although they are less common. Varicosities in the vulva and perineum cause aching and a sense of heaviness.

Surgical correction of varicose veins is not generally recommended during pregnancy (Cunningham et al., 2018). The woman should be aware that treatment might be needed after pregnancy because the problem will be aggravated by a succeeding pregnancy.

Health Promotion. Regular exercise, such as swimming, cycling, or walking, promotes venous return, which helps prevent varicosities. Avoiding factors that contribute to venous stasis is also helpful. The pregnant woman should avoid standing or sitting for prolonged periods. She should also avoid crossing her legs at the knees because of the pressure on her veins. She should not wear garters or hosiery with constricting bands, such as knee-high hose. However, supportive hose or elastic stockings may be extremely helpful. Supportive hose should be put on in the morning and should be washed daily with soap and warm water to help retain elasticity.

The pregnant woman should be encouraged to elevate her legs level with her hips when she sits. She can enhance comfort by supporting the entire leg rather than simply propping her feet up on a stool, which may lead to hyperextension of the knees. The woman who sits or stands for long periods should walk around frequently to promote venous return to the heart. She can also be encouraged to dorsiflex her feet, hold the position for 3 seconds, then release, with 8 to 10 repetitions several times each day. Venous return is most effectively promoted if the woman lies down with her feet elevated several times a day. To avoid difficulty related to pressure of the uterus on the vena cava, the woman can lie with her legs elevated on pillows and a pillow placed under one hip to displace the uterus to one side (Figure 13–9).

Wearing one of the foam rubber commercial products that is placed across the perineum and held in place by a sanitary pad–type belt can provide support for vulvar varicosities (Cunningham et al., 2018). Elevation of only the legs aggravates vulvar varicosities by creating stasis of blood in the pelvic area. Therefore, it is important that the pelvic area also be elevated to promote venous drainage into the trunk of the body. More than one firm pillow under the hips may be needed to accomplish this elevation. Near the end of pregnancy, this position may be extremely awkward; the woman may best relieve uterine pressure on the pelvic veins by resting on her side. Blocks may also be placed under the foot of her bed to elevate it slightly.

FLATULENCE

Flatulence results from decreased gastrointestinal motility, leading to delayed emptying, and from pressure on the large intestine by the growing uterus. Air swallowing may also contribute to the problem.

Health Promotion. The woman should be advised to avoid gas-forming foods and to chew her food thoroughly. Regular bowel habits and exercise can also decrease flatulence.

HEMORRHOIDS

Hemorrhoids are varicosities of the veins in the lower end of the rectum and anus. During pregnancy, the gravid uterus presses on the veins and interferes with venous circulation. As the pregnancy progresses, the straining that accompanies constipation can contribute to the development of hemorrhoids.

Hemorrhoids may not bother some women until the second stage of labor, when the hemorrhoids appear as they push just before birth. Hemorrhoids that occur in pregnancy or at birth usually become asymptomatic after the early postpartum period.

Symptoms of hemorrhoids include itching, swelling, pain, and bleeding. Internal hemorrhoids are located above the anal sphincter and are responsible for bleeding, usually with defecation. They are not usually painful unless they protrude from the anus. External hemorrhoids are located outside the anal sphincter. They are not usually the source of bleeding or pain; however, thrombosis of the hemorrhoids can occur, and in that case they become extremely painful. The thrombosis may resolve itself in 24 hours, or the physician can treat it by incising and evacuating the blood clot. Women who have hemorrhoids before pregnancy frequently experience more difficulties with them during pregnancy.

Health Promotion. Relief can be achieved by gently and carefully reinserting the hemorrhoids. The woman lies on her side or in the knee-to-chest position. She places some lubricant on her finger and presses against the hemorrhoids, pushing them inside. She holds them in place for 1 to 2 minutes and then gently withdraws her finger. The anal sphincter should then hold them inside the rectum. The woman will find it especially helpful if she can then maintain a side-lying (Sims) position for a time, so this procedure is best done before bed or before a daily rest period.

Avoiding constipation is important in preventing or relieving the discomfort of hemorrhoids. Relief measures for existing hemorrhoid symptoms include ice packs, use of topical ointments and anesthetic agents, and warm soaks.

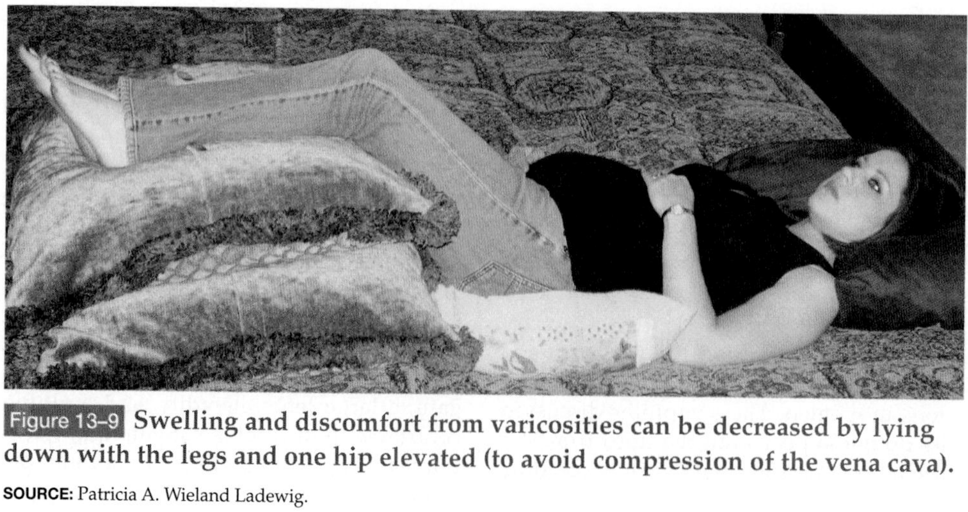

Figure 13–9 Swelling and discomfort from varicosities can be decreased by lying down with the legs and one hip elevated (to avoid compression of the vena cava).

SOURCE: Patricia A. Wieland Ladewig.

The woman should contact her healthcare provider if the hemorrhoids become hardened and noticeably tender to touch. Rectal bleeding that is more than spotting following defecation should also be reported.

CONSTIPATION

Constipation is common is pregnancy. Changes that predispose the woman to constipation include general bowel sluggishness caused by increased progesterone and steroid metabolism; displacement of the intestines, which increases with the growth of the fetus; and oral iron supplements, which most pregnant women need.

Health Promotion. Increased fluid intake (at least 2000 mL/day), adequate roughage or bulk in the diet, regular bowel habits, and adequate daily exercise can often maintain good bowel function in women who have not had previous problems. The addition of dietary fiber, from food sources or from products such as Metamucil, or surface active agents, such as Colace, can also decrease constipation. Some women find it helpful to drink a warm beverage or glass of prune juice in the morning. Women should leave sufficient time following breakfast so that the natural action of the body will produce defecation.

In severe or preexisting cases of constipation, the woman may need a mild laxative, stool softeners, or suppositories as recommended by her caregiver.

BACKACHE

Nearly 70% of women experience lower backache during pregnancy (King et al., 2015). Backache is due primarily to the increased curvature of the lumbosacral vertebrae that occurs as the uterus enlarges and becomes heavier. Circulating steroid hormones cause a softening and relaxation of pelvic joints, contributing to the problem. If the woman does not learn how to correct this curvature, the strain on the muscles and ligaments will cause backache. Low backache can occur at any point during pregnancy.

Health Promotion. An exercise called the pelvic tilt can help restore proper body alignment. As the anterior pelvis is tilted upward, the curvature of the back is automatically decreased, relieving much of the discomfort. There are many exercises that can be done by the pregnant woman to relieve symptoms of low back pain. See *Exercises to Prepare for Childbirth* later in this chapter.

The use of proper posture and good body mechanics throughout pregnancy is important. The pregnant woman should avoid bending over to lift or pick up items from the floor. The strain is felt in the muscles of the back. Leg muscles should be used to do the work instead. The woman can keep her back straight by bending her knees to lower her body into a squatting position (Figure 13–10). She should place her feet 12 to 18 inches apart to maintain body balance. When lifting a heavy object, such as a child, she should place one foot flat on the floor, slightly in front of the other foot, and lower herself to the other knee. The object is held close to her body for lifting. This same principle of keeping the back straight and bending the knees applies when the woman sits down or gets out of a chair. Work heights that require constant bending can contribute to backache and should be adjusted as necessary.

A pendulous abdomen contributes to backache by increasing the curvature of the spine. Women may utilize maternity support belts to decrease low back pain in pregnancy, despite inadequate evidence to conclude that wearing them is effective. The use of a supportive maternity girdle is discussed later in this chapter, as is the role of high-heeled shoes in increasing the lumbosacral curvature.

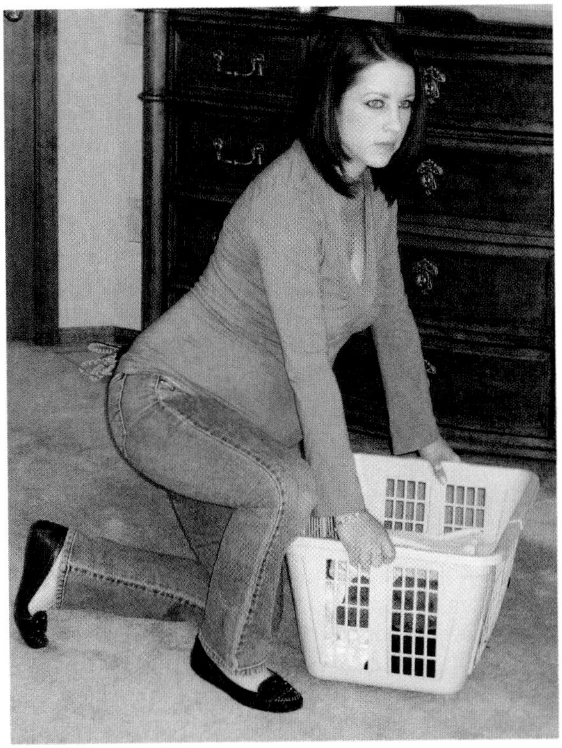

Figure 13–10 **When picking up objects from floor level or lifting objects, the pregnant woman must use proper body mechanics.**

SOURCE: Patricia A. Wieland Ladewig.

LEG CRAMPS

Leg cramps are painful muscle spasms in the gastrocnemius muscles. They occur most frequently at night after the woman has gone to bed but may occur at other times. Extension of the foot can often cause leg cramps. The nurse should warn the pregnant woman not to extend the foot during childbirth preparation exercises or during rest periods.

Health Promotion. The woman can achieve immediate relief of the muscle spasm by stretching the muscle. With the woman lying on her back, another person can press the woman's knee down to straighten her leg while pushing her foot toward her leg (Figure 13–11). The woman may also stand and put her foot flat on the floor. Massage and warm packs can be used to alleviate discomfort from leg cramps. Stretching exercises before bedtime may help prevent leg cramps.

FAINTNESS

Many pregnant women occasionally feel faint, especially in warm, crowded areas. Faintness is caused by a combination of changes in the blood volume and postural hypotension due to venous pooling of blood in the dependent veins. Sudden change of position or standing for prolonged periods can cause this sensation, and fainting can occur.

Health Promotion. The nurse should first be certain that the pregnant woman understands the symptoms of faintness. These include slight dizziness, a "swirling" or "floating" sensation,

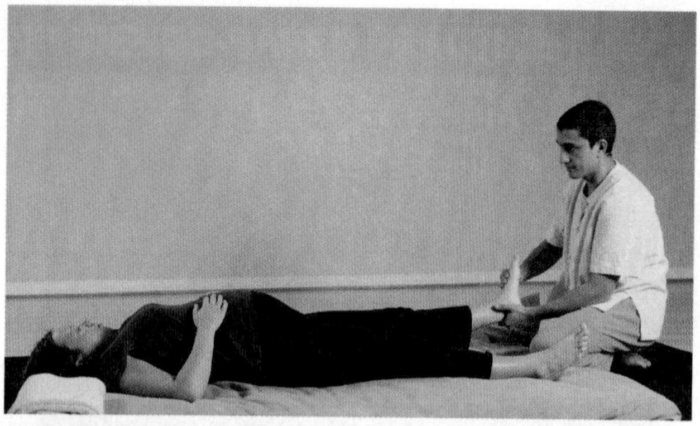

Figure 13–11 **The expectant father can help relieve the woman's painful leg cramps by flexing her foot and straightening her leg.**

SOURCE: Yanik Chauvin/Shutterstock.

and a decreased ability to hear or focus attention. If a woman feels faint from prolonged standing or from being in a warm, crowded room, she should sit down and lower her head between her knees. If this procedure does not help, the woman should be assisted to an area where she can lie down and get fresh air. When arising from a resting position, she should move slowly. Women whose jobs require standing in one place for long periods should march in place regularly to increase venous return from the legs.

SHORTNESS OF BREATH

Shortness of breath occurs as the uterus rises into the abdomen and causes pressure on the diaphragm. This problem worsens in the last trimester as the enlarged uterus presses directly on the diaphragm, decreasing vital capacity. The primigravida experiences considerable relief from shortness of breath in the last few weeks of pregnancy, when **lightening** occurs, and the fetus and uterus move down into the pelvic cavity. Because the multigravida does not usually experience lightening until labor, shortness of breath will continue throughout her pregnancy.

Health Promotion. During the day, sitting straight in a chair and using proper posture when standing help provide relief. If distress is great at night, the woman can sleep propped up in bed with several pillows behind her head and shoulders.

DIFFICULTY SLEEPING

From 12 weeks of pregnancy into the postpartum period, sleep disturbances are common. The pregnant woman may have difficulty falling asleep or she may wake up throughout the night, resulting in fewer overall hours of sleep. Although the pregnant woman may experience difficulty sleeping for many of the same psychologic reasons as the nonpregnant woman, many physical factors also contribute to this problem. The enlarged uterus may make it difficult to find a comfortable position for sleep, and an active fetus may aggravate the problem. The other discomforts of pregnancy such as urinary frequency, shortness of breath, and leg cramps may also be contributing factors.

Health Promotion. The nurse should conduct a thorough assessment of the sleep habits of the pregnant woman and offer information about habits and activities that help promote restful sleep. The pregnant woman may find it helpful to drink a warm (caffeine-free) beverage before bed and may benefit from a soothing backrub given by her partner or a family member. Pillows may be used to provide support for her back, between her legs, or for her upper arm when she lies on her side. Relaxation techniques may also help. The woman should avoid caffeine products, stimulating activity, and sleeping medication.

RESTLESS LEG SYNDROME

Approximately 15 to 25% of pregnant women develop *restless leg syndrome (RLS)*, also called *Willis-Ekborn disease (WED)*, particularly in the second half of pregnancy. RLS is characterized by the need to move the legs and tingling or other sensations in the calves, usually as the woman falls asleep (Picchietti et al., 2015).

Health Promotion. RLS has been associated with iron deficiency anemia, prolonged immobility (traveling in an airplane or car), and inactivity. Moderate-intensity, low-impact exercise may be indicated. Iron supplements may also decrease leg restlessness if anemia is present. Carbidopa/levodopa orally at bedtime may be considered for the treatment of severe cases (Picchietti et al., 2015). See *Case Study: Benita Cartier*.

ROUND LIGAMENT PAIN

As the uterus enlarges during pregnancy, the round ligaments stretch, hypertrophy, and lengthen as the uterus rises up in the abdomen. Round ligament pain is attributed to this stretching.

Health Promotion. The woman may feel concern when she first experiences round ligament pain because it is often intense and causes a "grabbing" sensation in the lower abdomen and inguinal area. The nurse should warn women of this possible discomfort. Few treatment measures really alleviate this discomfort, but understanding the cause will help decrease anxiety. Once

CASE STUDY: Benita Cartier

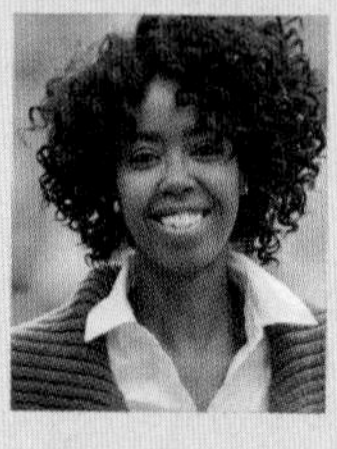

SOURCE: blvdone/Shutterstock

Benita is seeing you for her 24-week routine visit and notes she is having issues with shortness of breath, feeling faint, and inability to keep her legs still while trying to sleep. Her friend has restless leg syndrome, and Benita feels she also has the same signs. She notes she had these issues in a mild form in her previous pregnancy, but now with the additional physical strain of caring for her daughter, the symptoms are more difficult to control. Benita tells you her husband is now doing longer flights in his new job, which takes him out of town more than in her previous pregnancy.

Questions to Ponder

What interventions can you suggest to help control or reduce Benita's symptoms? Do any of these symptoms warrant further medical testing to rule out complications associated with pregnancy?

the caregiver has ascertained that the cause of the discomfort is not related to a medical complication such as appendicitis or gallbladder disease, the woman may find that a heating pad applied to the abdomen brings some relief. She may also benefit from bringing her knees up on her abdomen.

CARPAL TUNNEL SYNDROME

Carpal tunnel syndrome (CTS), characterized by numbness and tingling of the hand near the thumb, is confirmed by neurophysiologic testing. It is caused by compression of the median nerve in the carpal tunnel of the wrist. The syndrome is commonly bilateral but may be more pronounced in the dominant hand and is characterized by numbness, tingling, or burning in the fleshy part of the palm near the thumb. The syndrome is aggravated by repetitive hand movements, such as typing/keyboarding, and may disappear following birth. Treatment involves splinting, avoiding aggravating movements, and in severe cases injecting steroids into the carpal tunnel. Surgery is indicated in severe cases.

Health Promotion. Although the condition is not preventable, the woman should be advised to avoid aggravating activities and use her splint as directed.

See *Key Facts to Remember: Self-Care Measures for Common Discomforts of Pregnancy*.

Key Facts To Remember

Self-Care Measures for Common Discomforts of Pregnancy

Discomfort	Influencing Factors	Self-Care Measures
FIRST TRIMESTER		
Nausea and vomiting	Increased levels of human chorionic gonadotropin Changes in carbohydrate metabolism Emotional factors Fatigue	Avoid odors or causative factors. Eat dry crackers or toast before arising in morning. Have frequent, small meals. Avoid greasy or highly seasoned foods. Take dry meals with fluids between meals. Drink carbonated beverages.
Urinary frequency	Pressure of uterus on bladder in both first and third trimesters	Void when urge is felt. Increase fluid intake during the day. Decrease fluid intake *only* in the evening to decrease nocturia.
Fatigue	Specific causative factors unknown May be aggravated by nocturia due to urinary frequency	Plan time for a nap or rest period daily. Go to bed earlier. Seek family support and assistance with responsibilities so that more time is available to rest.
Breast tenderness	Increased levels of estrogen and progesterone	Wear well-fitting, supportive bra.
Increased vaginal discharge	Hyperplasia of vaginal mucosa and increased production of mucus by the endocervical glands due to the increase in estrogen levels	Promote cleanliness by daily bathing. Avoid douching, nylon underpants, and pantyhose; cotton underpants are more absorbent; powder can be used to maintain dryness if not allowed to cake.
Nasal stuffiness and nosebleed (epistaxis)	Elevated estrogen levels	May be unresponsive, but cool-air vaporizer may help; avoid use of nasal sprays and decongestants.
Ptyalism (excessive, often bitter salivation)	Specific causative factors unknown	Use astringent mouthwashes, chew gum, or suck hard candy. Carry tissues or a small towel to spit into when necessary.
SECOND AND THIRD TRIMESTERS		
Heartburn (pyrosis)	Increased production of progesterone, decreasing gastrointestinal motility and increasing relaxation of cardiac sphincter, displacement of stomach by enlarging uterus, thus regurgitation of acidic gastric contents into the esophagus	Eat frequent, small meals. Use low-sodium antacids. Avoid overeating, fatty, and fried foods; lying down after eating; and sodium bicarbonate.
Ankle edema	Prolonged standing or sitting Increased levels of sodium due to hormonal influences Circulatory congestion of lower extremities Increased capillary permeability Varicose veins	Practice frequent dorsiflexion of feet when prolonged sitting or standing is necessary. Elevate legs when sitting or resting. Avoid tight garters or restrictive bands around legs.
Varicose veins	Venous congestion in the lower veins that increases with pregnancy Hereditary factors (weakening of walls of veins, faulty valves) Increased age and weight gain	Elevate legs frequently. Wear supportive hose. Avoid crossing legs at the knees, standing for long periods, garters, and hosiery with constrictive bands.

(continued)

Key Facts To Remember (*continued*)

Discomfort	Influencing Factors	Self-Care Measures
Hemorrhoids	Constipation (see following discussion) Increased pressure from gravid uterus on hemorrhoidal veins	Avoid constipation. Apply ice packs, topical ointments, anesthetic agents, warm soaks, or sitz baths; gently reinsert into rectum as necessary.
Constipation	Increased levels of progesterone, which cause general bowel sluggishness Pressure of enlarging uterus on intestine Iron supplements Diet, lack of exercise, and decreased fluids	Increase fluid intake, fiber in the diet, and exercise. Develop regular bowel habits. Use stool softeners as recommended by physician.
Backache	Increased curvature of the lumbosacral vertebrae as the uterus enlarges Increased levels of hormones, which cause softening of cartilage in body joints Fatigue Poor body mechanics	Use proper body mechanics. Practice the pelvic-tilt exercise. Avoid uncomfortable working heights, high-heeled shoes, lifting heavy loads, and fatigue.
Leg cramps	Imbalance of calcium/phosphorus ratio Increased pressure of uterus on nerves Fatigue Poor circulation to lower extremities Pointing the toes	Practice dorsiflexion of feet to stretch affected muscle. Evaluate diet. Apply heat to affected muscles. Arise slowly from resting position.
Faintness	Postural hypotension Sudden change of position causing venous pooling in dependent veins Standing for long periods in warm area Anemia	Avoid prolonged standing in warm or stuffy environments. Evaluate hematocrit and hemoglobin.
Dyspnea	Decreased vital capacity from pressure of enlarging uterus on the diaphragm	Use proper posture when sitting and standing. Sleep propped up with pillows for relief if problem occurs at night.
Flatulence	Decreased gastrointestinal motility leading to delayed emptying time Pressure of growing uterus on large intestine Air swallowing	Avoid gas-forming foods. Chew food thoroughly. Get regular daily exercise. Maintain normal bowel habits.
Carpal tunnel syndrome	Compression of median nerve in carpal tunnel of wrist Aggravated by repetitive hand movements	Avoid aggravating hand movements. Use splint as prescribed. Elevate affected arm.

Health Promotion During Pregnancy

The pregnant woman is faced with the important responsibility of maintaining her health not only for her sake but also for the sake of her fetus. Nurses can help promote maternal and fetal well-being by providing expectant couples with accurate and complete information about health behaviors that can affect pregnancy and childbirth. Some women prefer to gather their own information. The nurse can refer these women to a variety of sources, including the National Women's Health Information Center, which is sponsored by the U.S. Public Health Service's Office on Women's Health.

Fetal Activity Monitoring

Many caregivers encourage pregnant women to monitor their unborn child's well-being by regularly assessing fetal activity beginning at 28 weeks' gestation. Vigorous fetal activity generally provides reassurance of fetal well-being, whereas a marked decrease in activity or cessation of movement may indicate possible fetal compromise requiring immediate evaluation. Sound, drugs, cigarette smoking, fetal sleep state, blood glucose levels, and time of day affect fetal activity. At times, a healthy fetus may be minimally active or inactive. See Chapter 16 for an in-depth discussion of maternal–fetal activity monitoring and *Teaching Highlights: What to Tell the Pregnant Woman About Assessing Fetal Activity.*

Breast Care

Whether the pregnant woman plans to formula-feed or breastfeed her baby, proper support of the breasts is important to promote comfort, retain breast shape, and prevent back strain, particularly if the breasts become large and pendulous. The sensitivity of the breasts in pregnancy is also relieved by good support.

A well-fitting, supportive bra has the following qualities:

- The straps are wide and do not stretch (elastic straps soon lose their tautness because of the weight of the breasts and frequent washing).
- The cup holds all breast tissue comfortably.

- The bra has tucks or other devices that allow it to expand, thus accommodating the enlarging chest circumference.
- The bra supports the nipple line approximately midway between the elbow and shoulder. At the same time, the bra is not pulled up in the back by the weight of the breasts.

Cleanliness of the breasts is important, especially as the woman begins producing colostrum. Colostrum that crusts on the nipples should be removed with warm water. The woman planning to breastfeed should not use soap on her nipples because of its drying effect.

Some women have flat or inverted nipples. True nipple inversion, which is rare, is usually diagnosed during the initial antepartum assessment. Occasionally, a nipple appears inverted at all times. In other cases, the nipple appears normal initially, but pressure on the areola with the examiner's thumb and finger causes the nipple to retract. The normal or flat nipple protrudes when this is done (Figure 13–12). Breast shields designed to correct inverted nipples can be effective, but some women gain little or no benefit from them.

More information on breastfeeding can be found on the websites of La Leche League, the American Academy of Pediatrics, the National Organization of Mothers of Twins Club, and other breastfeeding-focused sites.

Clothing

Traditionally, maternity clothes have been constructed with fuller lines to allow for the increase in abdominal size during pregnancy. Skirts and slacks have soft elastic waistbands and a stretchable panel over the abdominal area. However, maternity wear has changed in recent years and now also includes clothes that are more fitted, with little attempt to hide the pregnant abdomen. Maternity clothing is expensive, however, and is worn for a relatively short time. Women can economize by sharing clothes with friends, sewing their own garments, or buying used maternity clothing.

High-heeled shoes aggravate back discomfort by increasing the curvature of the spine. They should not be worn if the woman experiences backache or problems with her balance. Shoes should fit properly and feel comfortable.

Bathing

Daily bathing is important because of the increased perspiration and mucoid vaginal discharge that occurs during pregnancy. Practices related to cleansing the body are often influenced by cultural norms; thus, a pregnant woman may choose to cleanse only some portions of her body daily or may elect to take a daily shower or tub bath. Caution is needed during tub baths because balance becomes a problem as pregnancy advances. Rubber tub mats and handgrips are valuable safety devices. Moreover, vasodilation due to the warm water may cause the woman to experience some faintness when she attempts to get out of the tub. Thus, she may require assistance, especially in the third trimester. To avoid introducing infection, tub baths are contraindicated in the presence of vaginal bleeding or when the membranes are ruptured. During the first trimester, pregnant women should avoid hyperthermia associated with the use of a hot tub or whirlpool bath, such as a Jacuzzi, because it may increase the risk for neural tube defects. The American Academy of Pediatrics (AAP) and ACOG (2017) recommend that, if a pregnant woman uses a hot tub, she should limit her time in it to 10 minutes and should avoid submerging her head, arms, shoulders, and upper chest so there is less surface area exposed to heat.

Employment

Pregnant women who have no complications can usually continue to work until they go into labor (AAP & ACOG, 2017). However, pregnant women who are employed in jobs that require prolonged standing, strenuous physical activity, and/or use of industrial machines and those who experience other adverse environmental factors in the workplace may be at increased risk of poor pregnancy outcomes; thus, the risk factors should be modified as necessary (Gregory, Ramos, & Jauniaux, 2017).

Major deterrents to employment during pregnancy include fetotoxic hazards in the environment, excessive physical strain, overfatigue, and medical- or pregnancy-related complications. In the last half of pregnancy, occupations involving balance should be adjusted to protect the mother.

Fetotoxic hazards in the environment are always a concern to the expectant couple. If the pregnant woman or the woman contemplating pregnancy is working in industry, she should contact her company physician or nurse about possible hazards in her work environment and should do her own reading and research on environmental hazards as well. Similarly, the father can seek information about hazards in his workplace that might affect his sperm, if he has not already done this before conception.

Travel

If medical or pregnancy complications are not present, there are no restrictions on travel. Because of the risk of venous stasis and thromboembolism, the woman should be advised to avoid prolonged sitting during plane or car travel. Car travel should be limited to 6 hours per day and the pregnant woman needs frequent opportunities to get out of the car and walk. A good

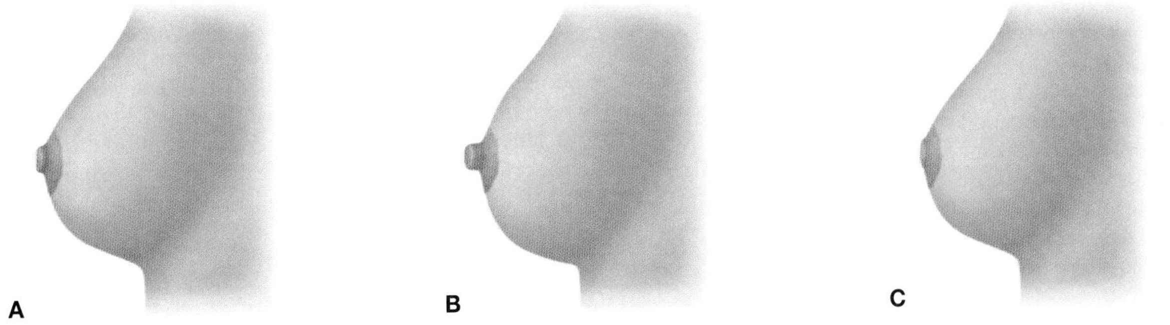

Figure 13–12 A. When not stimulated, normal and inverted nipples often look alike. B. When stimulated, the normal nipple protrudes. C. When stimulated, the inverted nipple retracts. However, great variation exists; in some women, for example, one or both nipples always appear inverted, even when not stimulated.

pattern to follow is to stop every 2 hours and walk around for approximately 10 minutes (Gregory et al., 2017). A pregnant woman should use a seat belt, specifically a properly positioned three-point restraint. She should wear both lap and shoulder belts. The lap belt should fit snugly and be positioned under the abdomen and across the upper thighs. The shoulder belt should be positioned snugly between the breasts. Seat belts play an important role in preventing fetal and maternal mortality and morbidity with subsequent fetal death (Cunningham et al., 2018). Fetal death in car accidents is also caused by placental separation (abruptio placentae) as a result of uterine distortion. Use of the shoulder belt decreases the risk of traumatic flexion of the woman's body, thereby decreasing the risk of placental separation. Thus, it is clearly important for nurses to provide information about car safety early in the prenatal period.

Currently, occasional flying is considered safe in the absence of any obstetric or medical complications (AAP & ACOG, 2017). However, those women who have medical or obstetric complications—such as poorly controlled diabetes, sickle cell disease, or preeclampsia—and those women with placental abnormalities or who are at risk for preterm birth are advised to avoid flying during pregnancy. Before flying, the pregnant woman should check with her particular airline to see if it has any travel restrictions. Most airlines permit pregnant women to fly up to 36 weeks' gestation. Some airlines restrict international travel earlier in pregnancy; others may require documentation of gestation (AAP & ACOG, 2017). Prior to embarking on any extended travel, the woman may wish to obtain a copy of her medical records as a precautionary measure.

To avoid the development of phlebitis or blood clots while flying, pregnant women should drink plenty of fluids to avoid dehydration and hemoconcentration; avoid caffeinated beverages, which act as diuretics, and smoking, which causes vasoconstriction; and wear support hose. They should also walk about the plane periodically and change positions frequently. Because of the risk of unexpected turbulence and the subsequent risk for trauma, pregnant women should wear their seat belts at all times while seated (Cunningham et al., 2018). The availability of medical care at her destination is an important consideration for the near-term woman who travels. Women who have medical or obstetric conditions that might require emergency care or could be exacerbated by travel are not advised to travel (AAP & ACOG, 2017).

Activity and Rest

Exercise during pregnancy helps maintain maternal fitness and muscle tone, leads to improved self-image, increases energy, improves sleep, relieves tension, helps control weight gain, promotes regular bowel function, and is associated with improved postpartum recovery. Exercise also improves symptoms of depression during pregnancy (Shivakumar, 2015). Preliminary findings suggest that women who exercised during pregnancy had a reduced risk of both small-for-gestational age (SGA) and large-for-gestational-age (LGA) newborns, but further research is needed (Kuhrt, Hezelgrave, & Shennan, 2015). Normal participation in exercise can continue throughout an uncomplicated pregnancy and is encouraged.

Exercise may play a role in the prevention of maternal and fetal complications (Kuhrt et al., 2015). For women who are morbidly obese, exercise may assist in the prevention of gestational diabetes. Exercise is also recommended by the American Diabetes Association (2018) to assist in glycemic control for women with gestational diabetes. Before beginning an exercise program, a pregnant woman should check with her physician/CNM. A pregnant woman who is already in an exercise program can discuss her degree of participation with her caregiver. If a woman has not been physically active before her pregnancy, she should gradually increase her exercise period. However, maximum benefit of exercise for pregnant women is derived for those who have been physically fit before conception. See *Teaching Highlights: Exercise Guidelines for the Pregnant Woman*.

The woman should check with her physician/CNM about taking part in strenuous sports. ACOG (2015) recommends that women avoid sky diving; scuba diving; hot yoga; activities with a high risk for falling, such as downhill skiing, water skiing, gymnastics, off-road cycling, surfing, and horseback riding; and those activities that have a high risk of blunt trauma, such as ice hockey, soccer, boxing, and basketball. Absolute contraindications to exercise include (AAP & ACOG, 2017):

- Rupture of the membranes
- Preeclampsia-eclampsia
- Cervical insufficiency (cerclage)
- Persistent vaginal bleeding in the second or third trimesters
- Multiple gestation at risk for preterm labor
- Preterm labor in the current pregnancy
- Placenta previa after 26 weeks' gestation
- Chronic medical conditions that might be negatively impacted by vigorous exercise such as significant heart disease or restrictive lung disease.

Warning signs during exercise include (ACOG, 2015):

- Chest pain
- Vaginal bleeding
- Regular, painful uterine contractions
- Leakage of amniotic fluid
- Calf pain or swelling
- Dizziness, headache, dyspnea before exertion, and muscle weakness.

The woman should stop exercising if any of these symptoms occur and modify her exercise program. If the symptoms persist, the woman should contact her healthcare provider.

Adequate rest in pregnancy is important for both physical and emotional health. Women need more sleep throughout pregnancy, particularly in the first and last trimesters, when they tire easily. Without adequate rest, pregnant women have less resilience.

Finding time to rest during the day may be difficult for women who work outside the home or have small children. The nurse can help the expectant mother examine her daily schedule to develop a realistic plan for short periods of rest and relaxation.

Sleeping becomes more difficult during the last trimester because of the enlarged abdomen, increased frequency of urination, and greater activity of the fetus. Finding a comfortable position becomes difficult for the pregnant woman. Figure 13–13 shows a position most pregnant women find comfortable. Progressive relaxation techniques similar to those taught in prepared childbirth classes can help prepare the woman for sleep.

Exercises to Prepare for Childbirth

Certain exercises help strengthen muscle tone in preparation for birth and promote more rapid restoration of muscle tone after birth. Many body-conditioning exercises for pregnancy are taught; a few of the more common ones are discussed here.

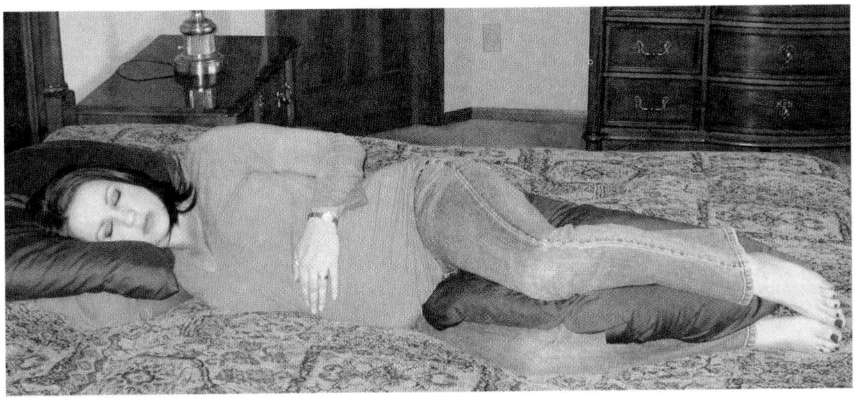

Figure 13–13 Position for relaxation and rest as pregnancy progresses.

SOURCE: Patricia A. Wieland Ladewig.

TEACHING HIGHLIGHTS | Exercise Guidelines for the Pregnant Woman

- Moderate-intensity exercise for at least 20 to 30 minutes per day on most, if not all, days of the week is recommended (ACOG, 2015).
- A moderate, rhythmic exercise routine involving large muscle groups such as swimming, cycling, or brisk walking is best. Other safe exercises include low-impact aerobics and modified yoga or Pilates (ACOG, 2015).
- Women who were regular exercisers before pregnancy and who have uncomplicated pregnancies should be able to continue high-intensity programs such as running, jogging, racquet sports, and strength training without untoward effects, while women who were sedentary before pregnancy should begin a gradually increasing exercise program (ACOG, 2015).
- After the first trimester, women should avoid exercising in the supine position. In most pregnant women, the supine position is associated with decreased cardiac output. Because uterine blood flow is reduced during exercise as blood is shunted from the visceral organs to the muscles, the remaining cardiac output is further decreased. Similarly, women should also avoid standing motionless for prolonged periods.
- Light muscle strength training using light weights (or resistance bands) and more repetitions done once or twice per week helps improve overall fitness and does not negatively affect the fetus.
- Because decreased oxygen is available for aerobic exercise during pregnancy, women should modify the intensity of their exercise based on their symptoms, should stop when they become fatigued, and should avoid exercising to the point of exhaustion.
- As pregnancy progresses and the woman's center of gravity changes, especially in the third trimester, she should avoid exercises in which the loss of balance could pose a risk to her or her fetus. Similarly, the woman should avoid any type of exercise that has a high potential for physical contact such as basketball, soccer, and ice hockey because it could result in trauma to the woman or her fetus.
- A normal pregnancy requires an additional 300 kcal per day. Women who exercise regularly during pregnancy should be careful to ensure that they consume an adequate diet (ACOG, 2015).
- To augment heat dissipation, especially during the first trimester, pregnant women who exercise should wear appropriate clothing and shoes, including a supportive bra, ensure adequate hydration, and avoid prolonged overheating.
- The woman should be advised to warm up and stretch to help prepare the joints for activity and cool down with a period of mild activity to help restore circulation and avoid pooling of blood.
- As a result of the cardiovascular changes of pregnancy, heart rate is not an accurate indicator of the intensity of exercise for pregnant women. If a pregnant woman is unable to talk or feels unable to breathe, then the exercise effort is too high.

The **pelvic tilt**, or pelvic rocking, helps prevent or reduce back strain and strengthens abdominal muscle tone. To do the pelvic tilt, the pregnant woman lies on her back and puts her feet flat on the floor. This bent position of the knees helps prevent strain and discomfort. She decreases the curvature in her back by pressing her spine toward the floor. With her back pressed to the floor, the woman tightens her buttocks and abdominal muscles as she tucks in her buttocks. The pelvic tilt can also be performed on hands and knees (Figure 13–14), while sitting in a chair, or while standing with the back against a wall. The body alignment achieved when the pelvic tilt is correctly done should be maintained as much as possible throughout the day.

Clinical Tip

Doing the pelvic tilt on hands and knees may aggravate back strain. Teach women with a history of minor back problems to do the pelvic tilt only in the standing position.

ABDOMINAL EXERCISES

A basic exercise to increase abdominal muscle tone is tightening abdominal muscles with each breath. It can be done in any position, but it is best learned while the woman lies supine. With knees

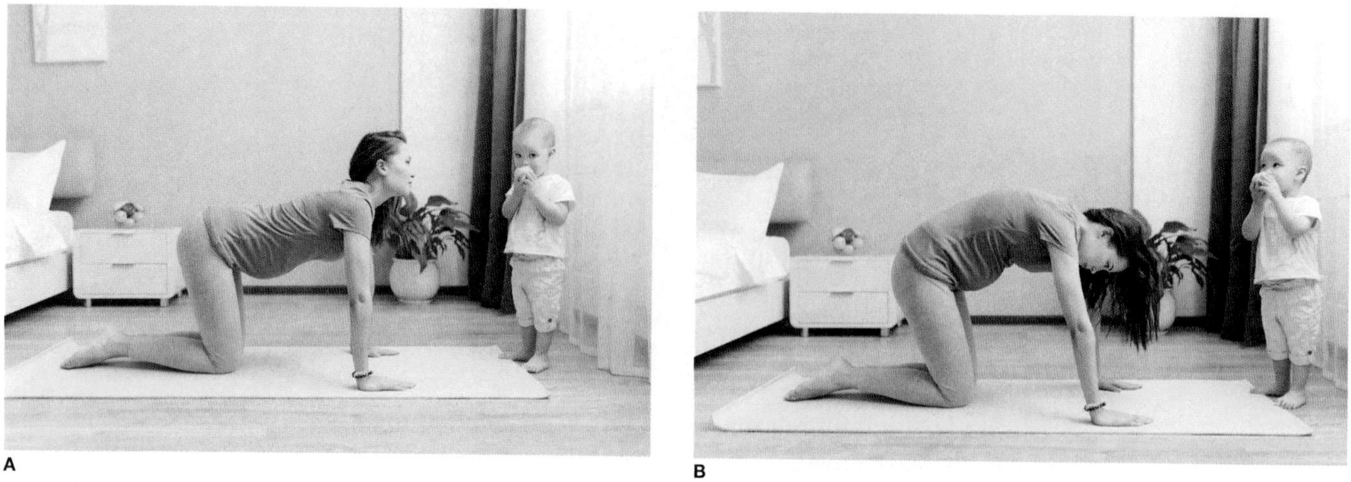

A B

Figure 13–14 **When the pelvic tilt is done on hands and knees, the starting position is back flat and parallel to the floor, hands below the head, and knees directly below the buttocks. A. For the first part of the tilt, head is up, neck is long and separated from the shoulders, buttocks are up, and pelvis is thrust back, allowing the back to drop and release on an inhaled breath. B. The next part of the tilt is done on a long exhalation, allowing the pregnant woman to arch her back, drop her head loosely, push away from her hands, and draw in the muscles of her abdomen to strengthen them. Note that in this position the pelvis and buttocks are tucked under, and the buttock muscles are tightened.**

SOURCE: UvGroup/Shutterstock.

flexed and feet flat on the floor, the woman expands her abdomen and slowly takes a deep breath. As she slowly exhales, she gradually pulls in her abdominal muscles until they are fully contracted. She relaxes for a few seconds and then repeats the exercise.

Partial sit-ups strengthen abdominal muscle tone and are done according to individual comfort levels, if there is no preexisting diastasis recti (a condition in which the large abdominal muscles separate). When doing a partial sit-up, the woman lies on the floor as just described. The exercise is done with the knees bent and the feet flat on the floor to avoid undue strain on the lower back. She stretches her arms toward her knees as she slowly pulls her head and shoulders off the floor to a comfortable level. (If she has poor abdominal muscle tone, she may not be able to pull up very far.) She then slowly returns to the starting position, takes a deep breath, and repeats the exercise. To strengthen the oblique abdominal muscles, she repeats the process but stretches the left arm to the side of her right knee, returns to the floor, takes a deep breath, and then reaches with the right arm to the left knee.

These exercises can be done approximately five times in a sequence, and the sequence can be repeated several times during the day as desired. It is important that the woman do the exercises slowly to prevent muscle strain and overtiring. If the woman does have diastasis recti, isometric abdominal exercises can be done instead.

PERINEAL EXERCISES

Perineal muscle tightening, also referred to as **Kegel exercises**, strengthens the pubococcygeus muscle and increases its elasticity (Figure 13–15). This muscle helps support the pelvic organs, including the uterus and bladder. A strong pubococcygeus

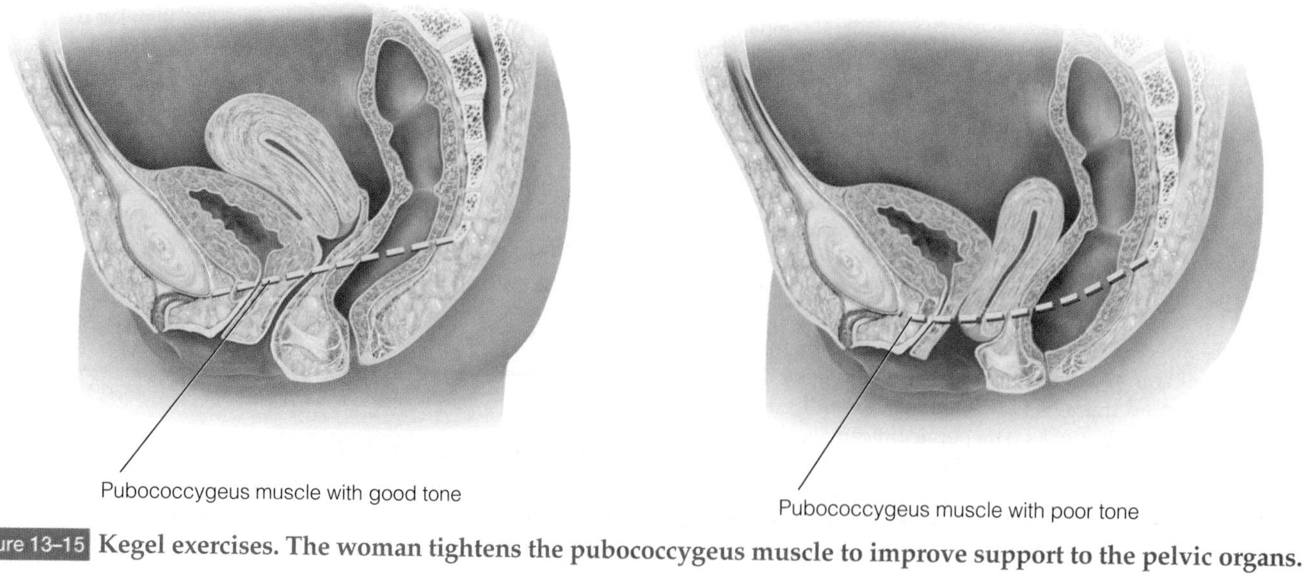

Figure 13–15 **Kegel exercises. The woman tightens the pubococcygeus muscle to improve support to the pelvic organs.**

muscle helps prevent stress incontinence, cystocele, rectocele, and uterine prolapse in women following childbirth.

The woman can feel the specific muscle group to be exercised by stopping urination midstream. However, doing Kegel exercises while urinating is discouraged because this practice has been associated with urinary stasis and urinary tract infection.

Childbirth educators sometimes use the following technique to teach Kegel exercises. They tell the woman to think of her perineal muscles as an elevator. When she relaxes, the elevator is on the first floor. To do the exercises, she contracts, bringing the elevator to the second, third, and fourth floors. She keeps the elevator on the fourth floor for a few seconds, and then gradually relaxes the area. If the exercise is properly done, the woman does not contract the muscles of the buttocks and thighs.

Kegel exercises can be done at almost any time. Some women use ordinary events—for instance, stopping at a red light—as a cue to remember to do the exercise. Others do Kegel exercises while waiting in a checkout line, talking on the telephone, or watching television.

INNER-THIGH EXERCISE

The pregnant woman should assume a cross-legged sitting position whenever possible. This "tailor sit" stretches the muscles of the inner thighs in preparation for labor and birth (Figure 13–16).

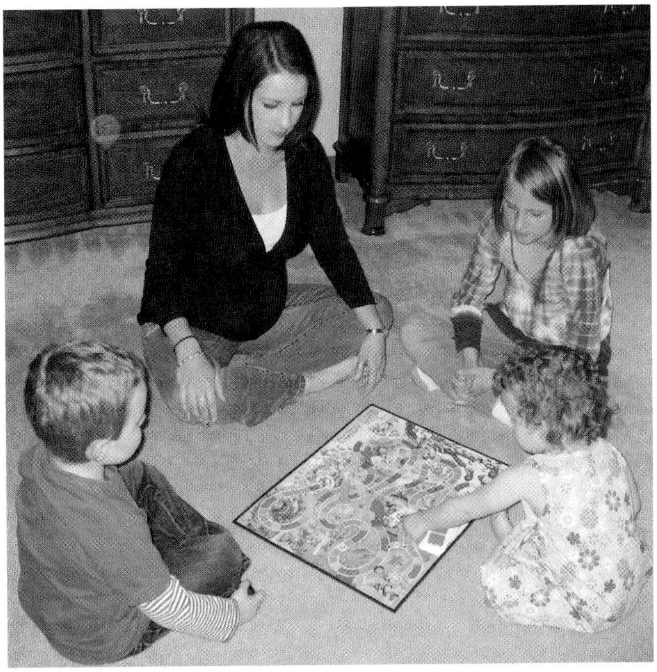

Figure 13–16 **To help prepare her inner thigh muscles for labor and birth, the pregnant woman should assume a cross-legged sitting position whenever possible during the day.**

SOURCE: Patricia A. Wieland Ladewig.

Sexual Activity

As a result of the physiologic, anatomic, and emotional changes of pregnancy, the couple usually has many questions and concerns about sexual activity during pregnancy. Often these questions are about possible injury to the baby or the woman during intercourse and about changes in the desire each partner feels for the other.

In a healthy pregnancy, there is no medical reason to limit sexual activity. However, intercourse is contraindicated if the pregnancy is vulnerable because of the diagnosis of threatened spontaneous abortion, placenta previa, or the risk of preterm labor (Cunningham et al., 2018).

The expectant mother may experience changes in sexual desire and response. Often these are related to the various discomforts that occur throughout pregnancy. During the third trimester, interest in coitus may again decrease as the woman becomes more uncomfortable and fatigued. In addition, shortness of breath, painful pelvic ligaments, urinary frequency, and decreased mobility may lessen sexual desire and activity. If they are not already using them, the couple should consider coital positions other than male superior, such as side-by-side, female superior, and vaginal rear entry.

Sexual activity does not have to include intercourse. Cuddling, kissing, and being held can satisfy many of the nurturing and sexual needs of the pregnant woman. The warm, sensual feelings that accompany these activities can be an end in themselves. Her partner, however, may choose to masturbate for satisfaction.

Many factors in pregnancy can affect the sexual desires of men. These include the previous relationship with the partner, acceptance of the pregnancy, attitudes toward the partner's change of appearance, and concern about hurting the expectant mother or baby. Some men find it difficult to view their partners as sexually appealing while they are adjusting to the concept of her as a mother. Other men feel their partner's pregnancy is arousing and experience feelings of increased happiness, intimacy, and closeness.

The expectant couple should be aware of their changing sexual desires, the normality of these changes, and the importance of communicating these changes to each other so that they can make nurturing adaptations. The nurse has an important role in addressing the sexuality concerns of the expectant couple. The couple must feel free to express concerns about sexual activity, and the nurse must be able to respond and give anticipatory guidance in a comfortable manner. See *Teaching Highlights: Sexual Activity During Pregnancy*.

Dental Care

It is important for the pregnant woman to maintain good dental care during pregnancy, including regular brushing and flossing and scheduled cleanings. Dental work is safe throughout pregnancy and any medically indicated dental treatment can be undertaken (AAP & ACOG, 2017). Ideally, a woman should have a dental examination as part of preconception planning. If that does not occur, the pregnant woman is encouraged to have a dental checkup early in her pregnancy. She should inform her dentist of her pregnancy so that she is not exposed to teratogenic substances. Dental x-rays are permitted during pregnancy as long as the woman's abdomen is shielded with a lead apron and a leaded thyroid collar is used (AAP & ACOG, 2017).

Immunizations

Ideally, women of childbearing age should receive immunizations prior to becoming pregnant to avoid unnecessary fetal exposure. All women of childbearing age need to be fully aware of the risks of receiving specific immunizations if pregnancy is possible. Expectant women, especially those who intend to travel internationally, should be aware of the immunizations that are contraindicated during pregnancy. Immunizations with attenuated live viruses, such as rubella vaccine, should not be given in pregnancy because of the possible teratogenic effect of the live virus. The most current recommendations on vaccines related to pregnancy can be obtained from the Centers

TEACHING HIGHLIGHTS | Sexual Activity During Pregnancy

In starting a discussion about sexual activity during pregnancy, universal statements that give permission, such as "Many couples experience changes in sexual desire during pregnancy. What kinds of changes have you experienced?" are often effective.

In your teaching, explain the following points to the woman and her partner:

- The pregnant woman may experience changes in desire during the course of pregnancy. During the first trimester, discomforts such as nausea, fatigue, and breast tenderness may make intercourse less desirable for many women. In the second trimester, as symptoms decrease, desire may increase. In the third trimester, discomfort and fatigue may lead to decreased desire in the woman.
- Men may notice changes in their level of desire, too. This may be related to feelings about their partner's changing appearance, their belief about the acceptability of sexual activity with a pregnant woman, or concern about hurting the woman or fetus. Some men find the changes of pregnancy erotic; others must adjust to the notion of their partners as mothers.
- The woman may notice that orgasms are much more intense during the last weeks of pregnancy and may be followed by cramping.
- Because of the pressure of the enlarging uterus on the vena cava, the woman should not lie flat on her back for intercourse after about the fourth month. If the couple prefers that position, a pillow should be placed under her right hip to displace the uterus. Alternative positions such as side-by-side, female superior, or vaginal rear entry may become necessary as her uterus enlarges.
- Sexual activities that both partners enjoy are generally acceptable. It is not advisable for couples who favor anal sex to go from anal penetration to vaginal penetration because of the risk of introducing *Escherichia coli* into the vagina.
- Alternative methods of expressing intimacy and affection such as cuddling, holding and stroking each other, and kissing may help maintain the couple's feelings of warmth and closeness. If the man feels desire for further sexual release, his partner may help him masturbate to ejaculation, or he may prefer to masturbate in private.
- Sexual intercourse is contraindicated once the membranes are ruptured or if bleeding is present. Women with a history of preterm labor may be advised to avoid intercourse because the oxytocin that is released with orgasm stimulates uterine contractions and may trigger preterm labor. Because oxytocin is also released with nipple stimulation, fondling the breasts may also be contraindicated in those cases.
- Stress the importance of open communication so that the couple feels comfortable expressing their feelings, preferences, and concerns. Deal with any specific questions about the physical and psychologic changes that the couple may have.

for Disease Control and Prevention website. Recommendations for immunizations during pregnancy are summarized in Table 13–4.

Ethics in Action!

In a situation where a vaccine is necessary but in limited supply, should pregnant women and their unborn fetuses be given precedence over the general population for vaccination?

Complementary Health Therapies

As discussed in Chapter 2, many women use complementary health therapies—such as homeopathy, herbal medicine (phytomedicine), acupressure, acupuncture, biofeedback, therapeutic touch, massage, and chiropractic—as part of an integrative approach to their healthcare regimens.

The use of herbal medicine requires careful consideration. It is important to note that herbs are considered to be dietary supplements and are not regulated by the FDA as prescription or over-the-counter drugs are. In particular, pregnant women need to avoid certain categories of herbs such as abortifacient (abortion-inducing) herbs, herbs that induce menstruation, nervous system stimulants, stimulant laxatives, and others. In general, it is best to advise pregnant women not to ingest any herbs, except ginger, during the first trimester of pregnancy.

For a reliable source of information about herbs and other alternative options, consumers or healthcare providers can access the National Center for Complementary and Integrative Health (NCCIH) website and the Office of Dietary Supplements website.

Nurses are in a unique position to bridge the gap between conventional therapies and complementary and alternative therapies. As patient advocates, nurses are able to provide patients with information needed to make informed decisions about their health and health care. Utilizing a nonjudgmental approach, the nurse should inquire about the use of complementary or alternative therapies as part of routine antepartum assessment. It is important that nurses working with pregnant women and their families develop a general understanding of the more commonly used therapies to be able to answer questions and provide resources as needed. See Chapter 2 for an in-depth discussion of this topic.

"I think I am like a lot of women. I have read up on complementary health approaches and during my pregnancy I have used the ones that make the most sense to me. The acupressure wrist bands definitely helped with my nausea as did the ginger I took. I found a massage therapist who specializes in massage for pregnant women, and lately I have been having regular massages. I love how they help me feel!"

Teratogenic Substances

Substances that adversely affect the normal growth and development of the fetus are called **teratogens**. Many of these effects are readily apparent at birth, but others may not be identified for years.

Medications are perhaps the most well-documented teratogens, but other factors can also harm the fetus, including certain infections such as rubella, syphilis, herpes virus type 2,

TABLE 13–4 Recommendations for Immunization Before, During, and After Pregnancy

VACCINE	BEFORE PREGNANCY	DURING PREGNANCY	AFTER PREGNANCY	TYPE OF VACCINE
Tdap (Tetanus, diphtheria, and pertussis [whooping cough])	May be recommended; it is better to vaccinate during pregnancy when possible	Yes, during *each* pregnancy	Yes, immediately post-partum, if Tdap never received during lifetime; it is better to vaccinate during pregnancy	Toxoid/inactivated
Td	May be recommended	May be recommended but Tdap is preferred	May be recommended	Toxoid
Hepatitis A	May be recommended	May be recommended	May be recommended	Inactivated
Hepatitis B	May be recommended	May be recommended	May be recommended	Inactivated
Meningococcal	May be recommended	Base decision on risk versus benefit; inadequate data for specific recommendation	May be recommended	Inactivated
Pneumococcal	May be recommended	Base decision on risk versus benefit; inadequate data for specific recommendation	May be recommended	Inactivated
HPV	May be recommended (through 26 years of age)	No	May be recommended (through 26 years of age)	Inactivated
MMR	May be recommended; once received, avoid conception for 4 weeks	No	May be recommended	Live
Varicella	May be recommended; once received, avoid conception for 4 weeks	No	May be recommended	Live

SOURCE: Centers for Disease Control and Prevention (CDC). (2016). *Maternal vaccination*. Retrieved from www.cdc.gov/vaccines/pregnancy/downloads/immunizations-preg-chart.pdf

toxoplasmosis, and cytomegalovirus (CMV). The harmful effects of other substances, such as some pesticides or exposure to x-rays in the first trimester of pregnancy, have also been documented. During pregnancy, women need to have adequate information available and a realistic perspective on potential environmental hazards. Factors that are suspected to be hazardous to the general population should be avoided, if possible.

MEDICATIONS

The use of medications during pregnancy, including prescriptions, over-the-counter drugs, and herbal remedies, is of great concern because maternal drug and chemical exposure is associated with birth defects. Many pregnant women need medication for therapeutic purposes, such as the treatment of infections, allergies, or other pathologic processes. Known teratogenic agents are not prescribed and usually can be replaced by medications considered safe. Even when a woman is highly motivated to avoid taking any medications, she may have taken potentially teratogenic medications before her pregnancy was diagnosed, especially if she had an irregular menstrual cycle.

The greatest potential for gross abnormalities in the fetus occurs during the first trimester of pregnancy, when fetal organs are first developing. The classic period of teratogenesis in a woman with a 28-day cycle extends from day 31 after the last menstrual period (17 days after fertilization) to day 71 (57 days after fertilization) (Niebyl, Weber, & Biggs, 2017). Many factors influence teratogenic effects, including the specific identity and dose of the teratogen, the state of embryo development, and the genetic sensitivity of the mother and fetus. For example, the commonly prescribed acne medication isotretinoin (Accutane) is associated with a high incidence of spontaneous abortion and congenital malformations if taken early in pregnancy. Valproic acid, an anticonvulsant, is associated with an increased risk of neural tube defects and cleft lip.

In some cases, the relationship between a medication and its teratogenic effects is unclear; the medication may be an appropriate choice in the latter portion of pregnancy but not a first-line option in the first trimester. In such cases, the healthcare provider should discuss the potential risks and benefits with the woman.

Formerly drugs were classified in categories A, B, C, D, and X, with category X indicating that the demonstrated fetal risks clearly outweigh any possible benefit. In 2014, the FDA amended its regulations governing the labeling of prescription drugs and biologic products for women who are pregnant or lactating. These regulations became effective in June 2015. According to the new requirements, three categories have been specified (Food and Drug Administration [FDA], 2014):

- ***Pregnancy.*** If the drug is absorbed systemically, labeling must include a risk summary of adverse developmental outcomes that includes data from all relevant sources including human, animal, and/or pharmacologic information. The labeling must also contain relevant information to help healthcare providers counsel women about the use of the drug during pregnancy. In addition, if there is a pregnancy exposure registry for the drug, the labeling should include a specific statement to that effect followed by contact information needed to obtain information about the registry or to enroll.
- ***Lactation.*** For drugs that are absorbed systemically, labeling must include a summary of the risks of using a drug when the woman is lactating. To the extent that information is available, the summary should include relevant information

about the drug's presence in human milk, the effects of the drug on milk production, and the effects of the drug on the breastfed child.

- ***Females and males of reproductive potential.*** This section must include information when human or animal data suggest drug-associated effects on fertility. It should also specify when contraception or pregnancy testing is required or recommended, such as before, during, or after the drug therapy.

Although the first trimester is the critical period for teratogenesis, some medications are known to have teratogenic effects when taken in the second and third trimesters. For example, tetracycline taken in late pregnancy is commonly associated with staining of teeth in children and has been shown to depress skeletal growth, especially in preterm newborns. Sulfonamides taken in the last few weeks of pregnancy are known to compete with bilirubin attachment of protein-binding sites, increasing the risk of jaundice in the newborn (Niebyl et al., 2017).

Pregnant women should avoid all medication—prescribed, homeopathic, or over the counter—if possible. If a medication is necessary during pregnancy, the benefits must clearly outweigh the risks. If no alternative exists, it is wisest to select a well-known medication rather than a newer drug whose potential teratogenic effects may not be known. When possible, the oral form of the drug should be used, and it should be prescribed in the lowest possible therapeutic dose for the shortest time possible. Finally, the healthcare provider should carefully consider the multiple components of the medication.

The nurse should remind the woman of the need to check with her healthcare provider about medications or herbs she was taking when pregnancy occurred and about any nonprescription drugs she is contemplating using. Any medication with possible teratogenic effects must be avoided.

TOBACCO

In the United States, smoking during pregnancy is one of the most significant, modifiable causes of poor pregnancy outcomes. It is associated with an increased risk of spontaneous abortion, intrauterine growth restriction, low birth weight, preterm birth, perinatal mortality, placenta previa, abruptio placentae, and premature rupture of membranes. Smoking, both during pregnancy and afterward, is also associated with an increased risk of sudden infant death syndrome (SIDS) (Niebyl et al., 2017).

The ingredients in cigarette smoke, such as carbon monoxide, nicotine, lead, and cotinine, are toxic to the fetus. Carbon monoxide decreases availability of oxygen to maternal and fetal tissue, while nicotine decreases uteroplacental blood flow to the fetus (Cunningham et al., 2018).

In response to public health education campaigns in the United States, smoking during pregnancy has decreased significantly. In fact, approximately 46% of women who smoke quit during pregnancy. Unfortunately, 50 to 60% of women who quit smoking during their pregnancy resume smoking within a year after birth (ACOG, 2017). This finding suggests that although women are aware of the potential impact of smoking on the fetus, they may be less knowledgeable about the effects of passive smoke on the baby.

Pregnancy may be a difficult time to stop smoking, but the nurse can encourage the pregnant woman to reduce the number of cigarettes she smokes each day. Studies demonstrate that any decrease in smoking during pregnancy improves fetal outcome, and researchers continue to explore approaches designed to help women quit smoking. ACOG (2017) suggests a 5- to 15-minute intervention with women who smoke fewer than 20 cigarettes a day to be most effective. This program and other programs encourage healthcare providers to use the five As:

- *Ask* about tobacco use.
- *Advise* to quit smoking.
- *Assess* willingness to quit.
- *Assist* in attempt to quit.
- *Arrange* for follow-up care.

The nurse can play an important role in counseling women about the importance of smoking cessation during pregnancy and can be actively involved in offering smoking cessation programs.

If smoking cessation efforts are not successful in pregnant women who smoke more than 20 cigarettes per day, the healthcare provider might consider prescribing nicotine replacement therapy (NRT), which is available as gum, lozenge, patch, nasal spray, or inhaler. This approach, while somewhat controversial, delivers less nicotine than cigarettes and avoids exposure to the other substances found in tobacco smoke (Niebyl et al., 2017). Medications such as bupropion and varenicline have been approved for smoking cessation therapy in the general population, but their safety in pregnancy has not been demonstrated, and they both have FDA product warnings about the risk of psychiatric symptoms and suicide associated with their use (Niebyl et al., 2017).

Many educational resources are available for healthcare providers and consumers on smoking-cessation programs through organizations such as the American Lung Association, the March of Dimes, the American Cancer Society, and Healthy Mothers, Healthy Babies.

ALCOHOL

Alcohol is now considered one of the primary teratogens in the Western world. Fetuses of women who are heavy drinkers are at increased risk for developing **fetal alcohol syndrome (FAS)**. Currently FAS, characterized by growth restriction, behavioral disturbances, craniofacial abnormalities, and brain, cardiac, and spinal defects, is a major preventable cause of intellectual disability in the United States. See Chapter 30 for further discussion of FAS in the newborn.

The effects of moderate consumption of alcohol during pregnancy are unclear. Research suggests an increased incidence of lowered birth weight and some neurologic effects, such as attention-deficit disorder. Evidence suggests that the risk of teratogenic effects increases proportionately with increased average daily intake of alcohol. Although an occasional drink during pregnancy does not carry any documentable risk, no safe level of drinking during pregnancy has been identified (Niebyl et al., 2017).

Alcohol passes the placental barrier within minutes after consumption, with fetal blood alcohol levels becoming equivalent to maternal blood alcohol levels. The effects of alcohol consumption vary according to the stage of fetal development. During the first trimester, alcohol probably alters embryonic development; throughout pregnancy, alcohol may interfere with cell division and growth; in the third trimester, the time of most rapid brain growth, alcohol may alter CNS development and contribute to growth retardation (Cunningham et al., 2018). The risk of neurologic damage decreases with the cessation of heavy drinking in the third trimester. Decreased consumption of alcohol in midpregnancy is associated with a lower incidence of growth restriction.

Assessment of alcohol intake is a chief part of each woman's medical history, with questions asked in a direct, nonjudgmental manner. All women of childbearing age who are sexually active and not using an effective method of birth control should be advised of the teratogenic effect of alcohol.

Because the most profound impact of alcohol occurs in the first weeks after conception, however, nurses and other healthcare providers will see the most dramatic decrease in the effects of alcohol during pregnancy by increasing their teaching efforts in the period before conception. If heavy consumption is involved, women should be referred early to an alcoholic treatment program. Because the drug disulfiram (Antabuse), which is often used in the treatment of alcoholism, is a suspected teratogen, a woman in such a program should inform her counselor if she becomes pregnant.

CAFFEINE

While studies continue, current research reveals no evidence that moderate levels of caffeine are linked to birth defects, spontaneous abortions, or preterm birth. Until more definitive data is available, nurses should advise women of common sources of caffeine, including coffee, tea, colas, and chocolate, and suggest they limit their caffeine intake to about 200 mg/day (Niebyl et al., 2017). The average cup of brewed coffee has 100 mg, a cup of tea has 50 mg, a regular cola drink has up to 40 mg, and a normal-sized chocolate bar has up to 50 mg.

Evaluation

Throughout the antepartum period, evaluation is an essential part of effective nursing care. As nurses ask questions of the pregnant woman and her family or make observations of physical changes, they are evaluating the results of previous interventions. In evaluating the effectiveness of the interventions, the nurse should not be afraid to try creative solutions if they are logical and carefully thought out. This is especially important in dealing with families from other cultures. If a practice is important to a woman and not harmful, the culturally competent nurse will not discourage it.

In completing an evaluation, the nurse must also recognize situations that require referral for further evaluation. For example, a woman who has gained 4 lb in 1 week probably does not require counseling about nutrition; she needs further assessment for preeclampsia. The nurse who has a sound knowledge of theory will recognize this and act immediately.

The ongoing and cyclic nature of the nursing process is especially evident in the prenatal setting. Throughout the course of pregnancy nurses can use certain criteria to determine the quality of care provided. In essence, nursing care has been effective if the following have been met:

- The common discomforts of pregnancy are quickly identified and are relieved or lessened effectively.
- The woman is able to discuss the physiologic and psychologic changes of pregnancy.
- The woman implements appropriate self-care measures, if they are indicated, during pregnancy.
- The woman avoids substances and situations that pose a risk to her well-being or that of her child.
- The woman seeks regular prenatal care.

Focus Your Study

- Providing anticipatory guidance about childbirth, the postpartum period, and childrearing is a primary responsibility of the nurse caring for women in an antepartum setting.
- The nurse assesses the expectant father's or partner's knowledge level and intended degree of participation and then works with the couple to help ensure a satisfying experience.
- Culturally based practices and taboos may have a major impact on the childbearing family.
- Childbearing decisions include selecting the healthcare provider, birth setting, support persons, and whether to include siblings in the birth experience.
- Prenatal education programs vary in their goals, content, leadership techniques, and method of teaching.
- Prenatal classes may be offered early or late in the pregnancy. The class content varies depending on the type of class and the individual offering it. Expectant parents tend to want information in chronologic sequence with the pregnancy.
- Breastfeeding programs in the prenatal period offer encouragement, practical instruction, and resources for the breastfeeding family.
- Siblings are now included in the whole birthing process, and classes for them are available from many sources.
- Grandparents have unique information needs that are addressed in grandparents' classes.
- The common discomforts of pregnancy occur as a result of physiologic and anatomic changes. The nurse provides the woman with information about self-care activities aimed at reducing or relieving discomfort.
- To make appropriate self-care choices and ensure healthful habits, a pregnant woman requires accurate information about a range of subjects from exercise to sexual activity, from bathing to immunization.
- Maternal assessment of fetal activity keeps the woman "in touch" with her fetus and provides ongoing assessment of fetal status.
- Teratogenic substances are substances that adversely affect the normal growth and development of the fetus.
- A pregnant woman should avoid taking nonessential medications or using over-the-counter preparations during pregnancy.
- Evidence confirms that smoking or consuming alcohol during pregnancy may be harmful to the fetus.

In order to make safe and effective judgments using NANDA-I © 2017 nursing diagnoses, it is essential that nurses refer to the definitions and defining characteristics of the diagnoses used in this text, which can be found in Appendix C.

References

American Academy of Pediatrics (AAP) and the American College of Obstetricians and Gynecologists (ACOG). (2017). *Guidelines for perinatal care* (8th ed.). Elk Grove Village, IL: Author.

American College of Obstetricians and Gynecologists (ACOG). (2015). *Physical activity and exercise during pregnancy and the postpartum period* (ACOG Committee Opinion No. 267). Washington, DC: Author.

American College of Obstetricians and Gynecologists (ACOG). (2017). *Smoking cessation during pregnancy* (ACOG Committee Opinion No. 721). Washington, DC: Author.

American College of Obstetricians and Gynecologists (ACOG). (2018). *Nausea and vomiting of pregnancy* (ACOG Practice Bulletin No. 189). Washington, DC: Author.

American Diabetes Association. (2018). Standards of medical care in diabetes—2018. *Diabetes Care, 41*(S1), S1–S143.

AWHONN, Mattson, S., & Smith, J. E. (2015). *Core curriculum for maternal-newborn nursing.* (5th ed.). St. Louis, MO: Elsevier.

Baptiste, D. L., Foronda, C., Reinholdt, M. M., & Ousman, K. (2016). Cultural humility: A concept analysis. *Journal of Transcultural Nursing, 27*(3), 210–217.

Bradley, R. A. (2008). *Husband-coached childbirth* (5th ed.). New York: Bantam.

Bawadi, H. A., & Al-Hamdan, Z. (2016). The cultural beliefs of Jordanian women during childbearing: Implications for nursing care. *International Nursing Review, 64*(2), 187–194.

Coalition for Improving Maternity Services (CIMS). (2016). *Mother-friendly childbirth initiative.* Retrieved from http://www.motherfriendly.org/MFCI

Cunningham, F. G., Leveno, K. J., Bloom, S. L., Bloom, S. L., Dashe, J. S., Hoffman, B. L., Casey, B. M., & Spong, C. Y. (2018). *Williams obstetrics* (25th ed.). New York, NY: McGraw-Hill.

DeCesare, J. Z., & Jackson, J. R. (2015). Centering pregnancy: Practical tips for your practice. *Archives of Gynecology and Obstetrics, 291*(3), 499–507.

Donna, S. (2011). *Promoting normal birth: Research, reflections and guidelines.* Chester-le-Street, UK: Fresh Heart Publishing.

Fantasia, H. C. (2014). A new pharmacologic treatment for nausea and vomiting of pregnancy. *Nursing for Women's Health, 18*(1), 73–77.

Food and Drug Administration (FDA). (2014). *Content and format of labeling for human prescription drug and biological products: Requirements for pregnancy and lactation labeling.* Retrieved from https://s3.amazonaws.com/public-inspection.federalregister.gov/2014-28241.pdf

Gregory, K. D., Ramos, D. E., & Jauniaux, E. R. M. (2017). Preconception and prenatal care. In S. G. Gabbe, J. R. Niebyl, J. L. Simpson, M. B. Landon, H. L. Galan, E. R. M. Jauniaux, D. A. Driscoll, V. Berghella, & W. A. Grobman (Eds.), *Obstetrics: Normal and problem pregnancies* (7th ed., pp. 102–122). Philadelphia, PA: Elsevier.

Johnson, C. T., Hallock, J. L., Bienstock, J. L., Fox, H. E., & Wallach, E. E. (2015). *The John Hopkins manual of gynecology and obstetrics* (5th ed.). Philadelphia, PA: Wolters Kluwer.

King, T. L., Brucker, M. C., Kriebs, J. M., Fahey, J. O., Gegor, C. L., & Varney, H. (2015). *Varney's midwifery* (5th ed.). Burlington, MA: Jones & Bartlett Learning.

Kuhrt, K., Hezelgrave, N. L., & Shennan, A. H. (2015). Exercise in pregnancy. *The Obstetrician and Gynaecologist, 17,* 281–287.

Martin, J. A., Hamilton, B. E., Osterman, M. J. K., Driscoll, A. K., & Mathews, T. J. (2017). Births: Final data for 2015. *National Vital Statistics Reports, 66*(1), 1–70.

National Center for Complementary and Integrative Health (NCCIH). (2015). *Herbs at a glance: Ginger.* Retrieved from http://nccih.nih.gov/health/ginger

Niebyl, J. R., Weber, R. J., & Briggs, G. G. (2017). Drugs and environmental agents in pregnancy and lactation: Teratology, epidemiology. In S. G. Gabbe, J. R. Niebyl, J. L. Simpson, M. B. Landon, H. L. Galan, E. R. M. Jauniaux, . . . W.A. Grobman (Eds.), *Obstetrics: Normal and problem pregnancies* (7th ed., pp. 136–159). Philadelphia, PA: Elsevier.

Picchietti, D. L., Hensley, J. G., Bainbridge, J. L., Lee, K. A., Manconi, M., McGregor, J. A., . . . Walters, A. S. (2015). Consensus clinical practice guidelines for the diagnosis and treatment of restless leg syndrome/ Willis-Ekborn disease during pregnancy and lactation. *Sleep Medicine Reviews, 22,* 64–77.

Purnell, L. D. (2014). *Guide to culturally competent health care* (3rd ed.). Philadelphia, PA: F.A. Davis.

Shivakumar, G. (2015). Exercise improves depressive symptoms during pregnancy. *BJOG: An International Journal of Obstetrics and Gynaecology, 122*(1), 63.

Spector, R. E. (2017). *Cultural diversity in health and illness* (9th ed.). Hoboken, NJ: Pearson.

Toohill, J., Fenwick, J., Gamble, J., Creedy, D., Bulst, A., Turkstra, E., & Ryding, E. (2014). A randomized controlled trial of a psycho-education intervention by midwives in reducing childbirth fear in pregnancy women. *Birth, 41*(4), 384–395.

United States Department of Health and Human Services (HHS). (2013). *Healthy People 2020.* Retrieved from http://www.healthypeople.gov/2020

Urso, P. P. (2016). Expectant fathers in training: Effective educational approaches for use by childbirth educators. *International Journal of Childbirth Education, 31*(3), 37–39.

Wojnar, D. M., & Katzenmeyer, A. (2014). Experiences of preconception, pregnancy, and new motherhood for lesbian nonbiological mothers. *Journal of Obstetric, Gynecologic and Neonatal Nursing, 43*(1), 50–60.

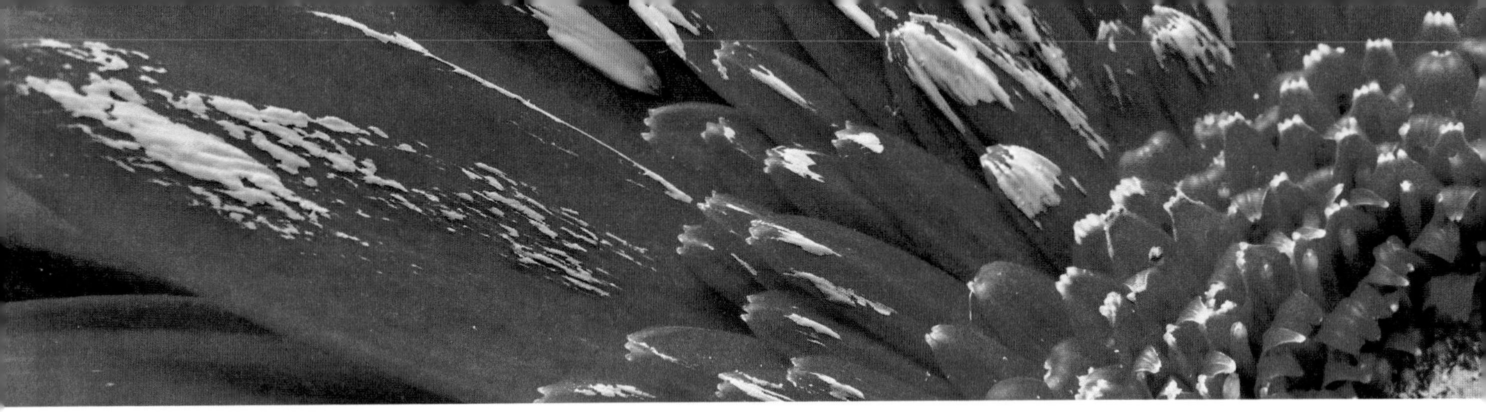

Chapter 14
Maternal Nutrition

I'm trying to be very careful about what I eat. I've had more salads and fresh fruit than I can remember. Sometimes, though, I get a "cookie attack" and indulge myself. My husband says I should eat oatmeal cookies so I could feel that my cravings were nutritionally sound!

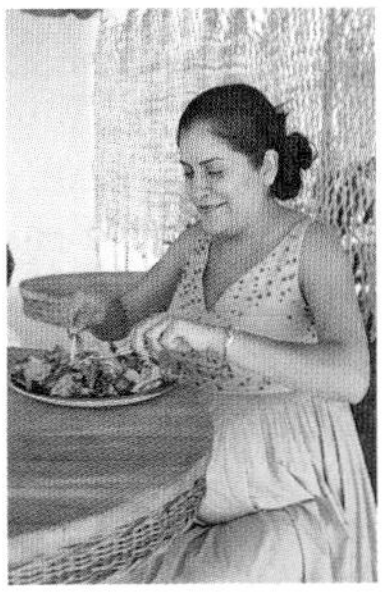

SOURCE: Anne Ackermann/Exactstock/SuperStock.

Learning Outcomes

14.1 Describe the recommended levels of weight gain during pregnancy.

14.2 Explain the significance of specific nutrients in the diet of the pregnant woman.

14.3 Compare nutritional needs during pregnancy, the postpartum period, and lactation with nonpregnant requirements.

14.4 Plan adequate prenatal vegetarian diets based on the nutritional requirements of pregnancy.

14.5 Explain the ways in which various physical, psychosocial, and cultural factors can affect nutritional intake and status in the nursing care management of pregnant women.

14.6 Compare recommendations for weight gain and nutrient intakes in the pregnant adolescent with those for the mature pregnant adult.

14.7 Describe basic factors a nurse should consider when offering nutritional counseling to a pregnant adolescent.

14.8 Compare nutritional counseling issues for breastfeeding and formula-feeding mothers.

Healthy People 2020

(MICH-16.5) Increase the proportion of women delivering a live birth who had a healthy weight prior to pregnancy

(MICH-14) Increase the proportion of women of childbearing potential with intake of at least 400 mcg of folic acid from fortified foods or dietary supplements

A woman's nutritional status before and during pregnancy can significantly influence her own health and that of her unborn child. In most prenatal clinics and offices, nurses provide nutritional counseling directly or work closely with dietitians in providing any necessary nutritional assessment and teaching.

This chapter focuses on the nutritional needs of a normal pregnant woman. Special sections consider the nutritional needs of the pregnant adolescent and the woman after birth.

Many factors influence a woman's ability to achieve good prenatal nutrition, including:

- ***General nutritional status before pregnancy.*** Good prenatal nutrition is the result of proper eating throughout life, not just during pregnancy, although pregnancy may motivate a woman to improve poor eating habits. Nutritional deficits at conception and during the early prenatal period may influence the outcome of the pregnancy.

- *Maternal age.* An expectant adolescent must meet the nutritional needs for her own growth in addition to the nutritional needs of pregnancy.
- *Maternal parity.* A mother's nutritional needs and the outcome of her pregnancy are influenced by the number of pregnancies she has had and by the intervals between them.

A mother's nutritional status does affect her fetus. Factors influencing fetal well-being are interrelated, but nutrient deficiencies alone can produce measurable effects on cell and organ growth of the developing fetus. Fetal growth occurs in three overlapping stages:

1. Growth by increase in cell number
2. Growth by increase in cell number and cell size
3. Growth by increase in cell size alone.

The nutritional problems that interfere with cell division may have permanent consequences. If the nutritional insult occurs when cells are mainly enlarging, the changes are usually reversible when normal nutrition resumes.

Growth of fetal and maternal tissues requires increased quantities of nutrients. These are listed in the **dietary reference intakes (DRIs)**, a set of reference values used to plan and assess nutrient intakes of healthy people, which includes specific allowances for pregnant and lactating women developed jointly by the United States and Canada (Table 14–1). The DRIs distinguish between pregnant women and pregnant adolescents because of the greater nutrient needs of the adolescent. DRIs are subdivided into the **recommended dietary allowance (RDA) and adequate intake (AI)**. An RDA is the daily dietary intake that is considered sufficient to meet the nutritional requirements of nearly all individuals in a specific life stage and gender group. An AI is a value cited for a nutrient when the data are not sufficient to calculate an estimated average requirement.

Maternal Weight

Maternal weight gain during pregnancy is an important factor in a pregnant woman's overall health and well-being, both during pregnancy and following childbirth.

Prepregnancy Weight

Prepregnancy weight is an important factor for both mothers and their babies. Women who are underweight before pregnancy, especially younger adolescents, have a higher risk of giving birth to a low-birth-weight neonate than women who begin pregnancy at normal weight for height. Being overweight or obese during pregnancy puts women at risk for gestational diabetes, hypertension, and preeclampsia, as well as complications during labor and birth. Babies of women who are obese may be at a higher risk of preterm birth, injuries during labor, and becoming obese themselves as they age.

Maternal Weight Gain

Maternal weight gain is an important factor in fetal growth and in newborn birth weight. An adequate weight gain over time indicates an adequate caloric intake. It does not, however, ensure that the woman has a sufficient nutrient intake. The diet may not be of high enough nutritional quality even though its caloric content supports the recommended weight gain. The pregnant woman must maintain the nutritional quality of her diet as her weight gain progresses.

Weight gain, even in women with a healthy pregnancy outcome, tends to be quite variable. Optimal weight gain depends on the woman's weight for height (*body mass index [BMI]*) and her prepregnant nutritional state. The Institute of Medicine (IOM, 2009) recommends weight gain in terms of optimum ranges based on prepregnant BMI, and the American College of Obstetricians and Gynecologists (ACOG, 2015b) supports these recommendations. The IOM recommendations for total weight gain during pregnancy are:

Underweight woman, BMI less than 18.5	12.5–18 kg (28–40 lb)
Normal-weight woman, BMI 18.5–24.9	11.5–16 kg (25–35 lb)
Overweight woman, BMI 25–29.9	7–11.5 kg (15–25 lb)
Obese woman, BMI over 30	5–9.1 kg (11–20 lb)

Research indicates that setting more restrictive weight gain limitations for overweight and obese women do not pose a threat of harm to the mother or fetus as long as the fetus is growing normally

TABLE 14–1 Dietary Reference Intakes for Nonpregnant, Pregnant, and Lactating Females

	AGE	VITAMIN A (MCG/D)	VITAMIN D (IU)	VITAMIN E (MG/D α-TOCOPHEROL)	VITAMIN K (MCG/D)	VITAMIN C (MG/D)	THIAMINE (MG/D)	RIBOFLAVIN (MG/D)	NIACIN (MG/D)
Females	9–13 years	600	600	11	60*	45	0.9	0.9	12
	14–18 years	700	600	15	75*	65	1.0	1.0	14
	19–30 years	700	600	15	90*	75	1.1	1.1	14
	31–50 years	700	600	15	90*	75	1.1	1.1	14
	51+ years	700	600	15	90*	75	1.1	1.1	14
Pregnancy	≤18 years	750	600	15	75*	80	1.4	1.4	18
	19–30 years	770	600	15	90*	85	1.4	1.4	18
	31–50 years	770	600	15	90*	85	1.4	1.4	18
Lactation	≤18 years	1200	600	19	75*	115	1.4	1.6	17
	19–30 years	1300	600	19	90*	120	1.4	1.6	17
	31–50 years	1300	600	19	90*	120	1.4	1.6	17

SOURCE: Based on Institute of Medicine, 2010.

Note: All values on chart are Recommended Dietary Allowances (RDAs) except those denoted by *, which are Adequate Intakes (AIs).

(ACOG, 2015b). When weight gain is within a healthy range, the risk of problems during pregnancy, labor, and birth is low.

The pattern of weight gain during pregnancy is also important. For example, inadequate prenatal weight gain during the second trimester is closely associated with reduced birth weight in the newborn. For women of normal weight, assuming a gain of 0.5 to 2 kg (1.1 to 4.4 lb) during the first trimester, the recommended gain during the second and third trimesters is 0.45 kg (1 lb) per week. The rate of weight gain in the second and third trimesters needs to be slightly higher for underweight women and slightly lower for overweight women (IOM, 2009). A maternal weight gain of 1.5 lb per week has been suggested for normal-weight women during the second half of a twin pregnancy.

The average maternal weight gain is distributed as follows:

5 kg (11 lb)	Fetus, placenta, amniotic fluid
0.9 kg (2 lb)	Uterus
1.8 kg (4 lb)	Increased blood volume
1.4 kg (3 lb)	Breast tissue
2.3 to 4.5 kg (5 to 10 lb)	Maternal stores

The prevalence of obesity in the United States has increased dramatically over the past 25 years. In the United States, almost 32% of women of childbearing age (20 to 39 years) are obese. When the overweight and obese categories are combined, that percentage increases to 58.5% (ACOG, 2018). Pregnant women who are obese are at risk for many pregnancy complications including gestational diabetes mellitus (GDM), preeclampsia, and cesarean birth, and their fetuses are at increased risk for congenital anomalies, stillbirth, prematurity, macrosomia, and childhood obesity. Thus, it is recommended that these women receive counseling on strategies to move toward and to remain at a healthful weight prior to conceiving (ACOG, 2018).

Because of the association between maternal weight gain and pregnancy outcome, most caregivers pay close attention to weight gain during pregnancy (Figure 14–1). Weight gain charts can be useful in monitoring the rate of weight gain over time. If a significant deviation from the anticipated pattern occurs, the cause should be determined and appropriate interventions planned with the woman.

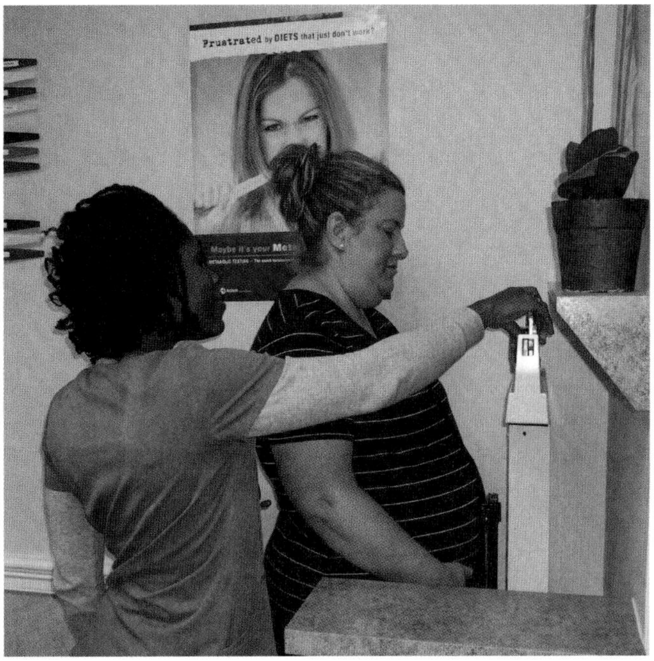

Figure 14–1 It is important to monitor a pregnant woman's weight over time.

SOURCE: Michele Davidson.

As mentioned earlier, weight gain alone does not guarantee adequate nutrition. A diet may be high in energy (calories) but low in vitamins, minerals, or complex carbohydrates and protein. All pregnant women should include a variety of nutrient-rich foods each day to ensure they are meeting the nutritional needs of both themselves and their babies. An online tool (choosemyplate.gov) that can help expectant women customize an eating plan based on age, weight, height, physical activity, and gestation stage is offered by the U.S. Department of Health and Human Services and the U.S. Department of Agriculture (USHHS & USDA, 2015) (Figure 14–2).

VITAMIN B_6 (MG/D)	FOLATE (MCG/D)	VITAMIN B_{12} (MCG/D)	CALCIUM (MG/D)	PHOSPHORUS (MG/D)	MAGNESIUM (MG/D)	IRON (MG/D)	ZINC (MG/D)	SELENIUM (MCG/D)
1.0	300	1.8	1300	1250	240	8	8	40
1.2	400	2.4	1300	1250	360	15	9	55
1.3	400	2.4	1000	700	310	18	8	55
1.3	400	2.4	1000	700	320	18	8	55
1.5	400	2.4	1200	700	320	8	8	55
1.9	600	2.6	1300	1250	400	27	12	60
1.9	600	2.6	1000	700	350	27	11	60
1.9	600	2.6	1000	700	360	27	11	60
2.0	500	2.8	1300	1250	360	10	13	70
2.0	500	2.8	1000	700	310	9	12	70
2.0	500	2.8	1000	700	320	9	12	70

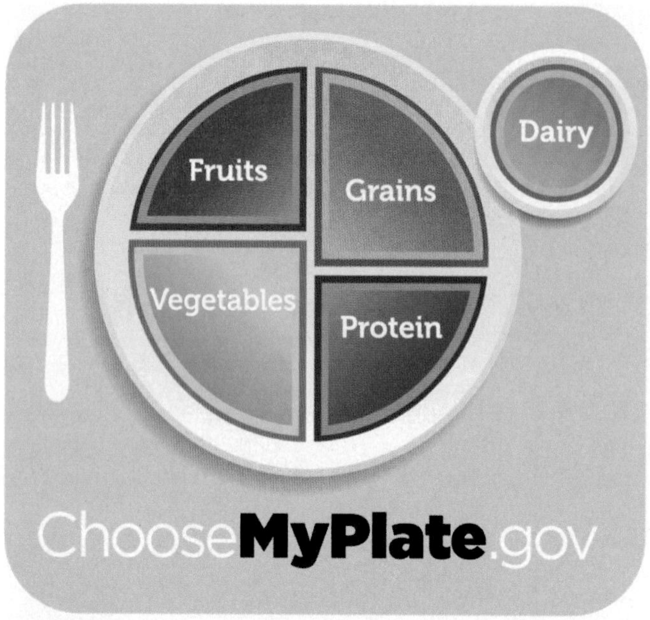

Figure 14–2 **MyPlate identifies the basic food groups and provides guidance about healthful eating. Fruits and vegetables are emphasized, in addition to whole grains, proteins, and dairy. Including healthy fats from fish, nuts, and vegetable oils is encouraged, as is limiting fats like butter, margarine, shortening, and lard. Limiting amounts of added sugars is also recommended.**

SOURCE: U.S. Department of Agriculture.

The pregnant woman can obtain most of the recommended nutrients by eating a well-balanced diet each day. The basic food groups and recommended amounts during pregnancy and lactation are presented in Table 14–2.

Clinical Tip

Consider factors that may cause variations in weight. Weight varies with time of day, amount of clothing, inaccurate scale adjustment, or weighing error. Consequently, do not overemphasize a single weight but pay attention to the pattern of weight gain.

Nutritional Requirements

The requirements for calories and almost all nutrients increase during pregnancy, although the amount of increase varies with each nutrient. These increases reflect the additional requirements of both the mother and the developing fetus (see Table 14–1). See *Women with Special Needs: Additional Nutrients*.

Women with Special Needs Additional Nutrients

Women with spasticity, such as those with cerebral palsy or spinal cord injuries, need additional nutrients because they use a large number of calories daily. Additional food sources should include healthy choices of nutrient-dense foods. Non-weight-bearing women are also more prone to osteoporosis and bone mineral density loss and should receive supplemental calcium and Vitamin D.

Calories

The term ***calorie (cal)*** stands for the amount of heat required to raise the temperature of 1 gram of water 1 degree Celsius. The **kilocalorie (kcal)** is equivalent to 1000 cal and is the unit used to express the energy value of food.

The dietary reference intakes for total energy indicate that energy requirements do not change during the first trimester. During the second and third trimesters, pregnant women should consume an extra 300 kcal per day. Weight gains should be monitored regularly, and dietary recommendations should be individualized to help the pregnant woman meet her caloric needs.

Prepregnant weight, height, maternal age, activity, and health status all affect caloric requirements. Women who are underweight may require additional calories, whereas women who are overweight or obese may need fewer calories. See *Teaching Highlights: Helping the Pregnant Woman Add 300 kcal to Her Diet* for basic nutritional information and suggestions for increasing caloric intake.

Carbohydrates

Carbohydrates provide the body's primary source of energy as well as fiber necessary for proper bowel functioning. If the carbohydrate intake is not adequate, the body uses protein for energy. Protein then becomes unavailable for growth needs. In addition, protein breakdown leads to ketosis. Ketosis can be a problem, especially in women with diabetes, because of glycosuria, reduced alkaline reserves, and lipidemia.

The carbohydrate and caloric needs of the pregnant woman increase, especially during the last two trimesters. Carbohydrate intake promotes weight gain and growth of the fetus, placenta, and other maternal tissues. Grains such as breads, cereals, pastas, and brown rice, dairy products, fruits, and vegetables all contain carbohydrates.

Protein

During pregnancy, the woman needs increased amounts of protein to provide amino acids for fetal development, blood volume expansion, and growth of other maternal tissues, such as the breasts and uterus. Protein also contributes to the body's overall energy metabolism. Pregnant women require 71 g of protein, compared to 46 g for the nonpregnant woman (West, Hark, & Catalano, 2017). The quality of dietary protein is as important as the total amount consumed. The quality is determined by the complex of amino acids that makes up the protein. Plant proteins can meet a woman's protein needs; however, more of a given protein may be needed as animal proteins are of higher quality (see later discussion of vegetarianism).

To obtain high-quality protein in the diet, it is best to eat a variety of foods. Animal products—such as lean meats, fish, poultry, eggs, and low-fat dairy products—are sources of high-quality protein. Good sources of plant proteins include beans, soy products, lentils, nuts, and nut butters. Table 14–3 provides information on the protein content of common foods.

Women who have allergies to milk, who have lactose intolerance, or who practice vegetarianism may find fortified soy or rice milks or almond milk acceptable alternatives to dairy.

Fat

Fats are valuable sources of energy for the body. Fats are more completely absorbed during pregnancy, resulting in a marked increase in serum lipids, lipoproteins, and cholesterol and

TABLE 14–2 Daily Food Plan for Pregnancy and Lactation

FOOD GROUP	NUTRIENTS PROVIDED	FOOD SOURCE	RECOMMENDED DAILY AMOUNT DURING PREGNANCY	RECOMMENDED DAILY AMOUNT DURING LACTATION
Dairy products	Protein; riboflavin; vitamins A, D, and others; calcium; phosphorus; zinc; magnesium	Milk—whole, 2%, low-fat, skim, dry, buttermilk Cheeses—hard, semisoft, cottage Yogurt—plain, low-fat Soybean milk—canned, dry	Four (8 oz) cups (five for teenagers) used plain or with flavoring, in shakes, soups, puddings, custards, cocoa Calcium in 1 cup milk equivalent to 1½ cups cottage cheese, 1½ oz hard or semisoft cheese, 1 cup yogurt, 1½ cups ice cream (high in fat and sugar)	Four (8 oz) cups (five for teenagers); equivalent amount of cheese, yogurt, and so forth
Meat and meat alternatives	Protein; iron; thiamine, niacin, and other vitamins; minerals	Beef, pork, veal, lamb, poultry, animal organ meats, fish, tofu; eggs; legumes; nuts, seeds, peanut butter, grains in proper vegetarian combination (vitamin B_{12} supplement needed)	Three servings (one serving = 2 oz), combination in amounts necessary for same nutrient equivalent (varies greatly)	Two servings
Grain products, whole grain or enriched	B vitamins; iron; whole grain also has zinc, magnesium, and other trace elements; provides fiber	Breads and bread products such as cornbread, muffins, waffles, hotcakes, biscuits, dumplings, cereals, pastas, rice	Six to 11 servings daily: One serving = one slice bread, ¾ cup or 1 oz dry cereal, ½ cup rice or pasta	Same as for pregnancy
Fruits and fruit juices	Vitamins A and C; minerals; raw fruits for roughage	Citrus fruits and juices, melons, berries, all other fruits and juices	Two to four servings (one serving for vitamin C): One serving = one medium fruit, ½–1 cup fruit, 4 oz orange or grapefruit juice	Same as for pregnancy
Vegetables and vegetable juices	Vitamins A and C; minerals; provides roughage	Leafy green vegetables; deep yellow or orange vegetables such as carrots, sweet potatoes, squash, tomatoes; green vegetables such as peas, green beans, broccoli; other vegetables such as beets, cabbage, potatoes, corn, lima beans	Three to five servings (one serving of dark green or deep yellow vegetables for vitamin A): One serving = ½–1 cup vegetables, two tomatoes, one medium potato	Same as for pregnancy
Fats	Vitamins A and D; linoleic acid	Butter, cream cheese, fortified table spreads; cream, whipped cream, whipped toppings; avocado, mayonnaise, oil, nuts	As desired in moderation (high in calories): One serving = 1 tbsp butter or enriched margarine	Same as for pregnancy
Sugar and sweets		Sugar, brown sugar, honey, molasses	Occasionally, if desired	Same as for pregnancy
Desserts		Nutritious desserts such as puddings, custards, fruit whips, and crisps; other rich, sweet desserts and pastries	Occasionally, if desired	Same as for pregnancy
Beverages		Coffee, decaffeinated beverages, tea, bouillon, carbonated drinks	As desired, in moderation	Same as for pregnancy
Miscellaneous		Iodized salt, herbs, spices, condiments	As desired	Same as for pregnancy

Note: The pregnant woman should eat regularly, three meals a day, with snacks of fruit, vegetables, low-fat dairy, or whole grains between meals, if desired. (More frequent but smaller meals are also recommended.) Four to six (8 oz) glasses of water and a total of 8 to 12 (8 oz) cups total fluid intake should be consumed daily. Water is an essential nutrient.

TEACHING HIGHLIGHTS Helping the Pregnant Woman Add 300 kcal During Pregnancy

- The notion of "eating for two" may result in overeating. Emphasize the relatively small increase in calories necessary during pregnancy.
- The additional 300 kcal/day recommended during pregnancy can be achieved by adding two milk servings and one serving of meat or alternative.
- MyPlate is designed to represent the food groups needed to make a balanced diet. Following MyPlate recommendations, women should aim to have half their plate consist of fruits and vegetables, make at least half their grains whole grains, and choose fat-free or low-fat (1%) milk, yogurt, and cheese. Women are encouraged to drink water rather than sugary drinks and to compare the sodium content of foods and choose foods that are lower in sodium (USHHS & USDA, 2015). A balanced diet includes:
  - ***Grains:*** Six to 11 servings (one serving = 1 slice bread, ½ hamburger roll, 1 oz dry cereal, 1 tortilla, ½ cup pasta, rice, grits)
  - ***Fruits:*** Two to four servings; one should be a good source of vitamin C (one serving = 1 medium-sized piece of fruit, ½ cup juice)
  - ***Vegetables:*** Three to five servings (one serving = 1 cup raw vegetable, 1 cup green leafy vegetable, ½ cup cooked vegetable)
  - ***Dairy:*** Two to three servings (one serving = 1 cup milk or yogurt, 1½ oz hard cheese (cheddar, mozzarella, parmesan, or Swiss), 2 cups cottage cheese, 1 cup pudding made with milk)
  - ***Meats and alternatives:*** 5 to 5½ ounces/day; 1 ounce includes 1oz cooked lean meat, poultry, or fish; 1 egg; ½ oz nuts (12 almonds, 24 pistachios); ½ oz seeds; ¼ cup cooked legumes (kidney, lima, garbanzo, or soybeans, split peas)
  - Not all foods that are nutritionally equivalent have the same number of calories; it is important to consider that when making food choices
- Consider using low-fat milk, lean cuts of meat, or fish broiled or baked instead of fried.
- Foods can be combined. For example, 1 cup spaghetti with a 2-oz meatball would count as 1 serving of meat, ¾ cup spaghetti = 1 grain, and ¼ cup tomato sauce = ½ serving of vegetable.
- Use a calorie-counting guide to compare the calories in a variety of foods that are equivalent, such as 2 oz beef and 2 oz fish or 1 cup low-fat milk and 1 cup whole milk.

decreased elimination of fat through the bowel. Fat deposits in the fetus increase from about 2% at midpregnancy to almost 12% at term. The U.S. Dietary Guidelines recommend that about 20 to 35% of total daily caloric intake should be from dietary fat, of which only 10% should be saturated fat (USDHHS & USDA, 2015).

Essential fatty acids are important for the development of the central nervous system of the fetus. Of particular interest are the omega-3 fatty acids and their derivatives, eicosapentaenoic acid (EPA) and docosahexaenoic acid (DHA). EPA supports the heart and immune system, while DHA supports brain, eye, and central nervous system development. Dietary sources of EPA and DHA are naturally occurring in oily fish (see information on fish consumption under *Mercury in Fish* later in this chapter). Plant sources of omega-3 fatty acids include soybean oil, canola oil, flaxseeds and their oil, and walnuts.

Minerals

The woman can increase minerals needed for the growth of new tissue during pregnancy by improving mineral absorption and increasing mineral intake.

CALCIUM AND PHOSPHORUS

Calcium and phosphorus are involved in the mineralization of fetal bones and teeth, energy and cell production, and acid–base buffering. Calcium is absorbed and used more efficiently during pregnancy. Some additional calcium and phosphorus are required early in pregnancy, but most of the fetus's bone calcification occurs during the last 2 to 3 months. Teeth begin to form at about 8 weeks' gestation and are formed by birth. The 6-year molars begin to calcify just before birth. Additional calcium is stored in the maternal skeleton as a reserve for lactation.

TABLE 14–3 Amount of Protein in Common Foods

FOOD	PROTEIN (G)
Dairy Products	
Milk, 8 oz	8
Cheese: Cheddar, Swiss, and so forth, 1 oz	7
Cottage cheese, ¼ cup	7
Meat and Meat Alternatives	
Meat, fish, poultry, 1 oz	7
Egg, 1	7
Cooked dry beans and peas, ½ cup	7
Cooked soybeans, ½ cup	11
Tofu, raw, ½ cup	10
Peanut butter, 2 tbsp	7
Peanuts (3 tbsp), cashews/almonds (5 tbsp)	7
Breads and Cereals	
Bread, 1 slice	2
Buns, biscuits, muffins, 1	2
Cooked cereals and grains, ½ cup	2
Breakfast cereal, 1 oz	2
Vegetables and Fruits	
Vegetables, ½ cup	0.5–1
Fruits and juices, ½ cup	0.5
Miscellaneous	
Soy milk, 8 oz	6.6

The identified adequate intake for calcium for the pregnant or lactating woman 19 years of age or older is 1000 mg per day; it is 1300 mg/day for pregnant women under age 19. If calcium intake is not adequate, fetal needs will be met at the mother's expense by demineralization of maternal bone. Food is the preferred source of calcium because food provides other nutrients as well. A diet that includes 4 cups of milk or an equivalent dairy alternative (see Table 14–4) and a variety of other foods will provide sufficient calcium. Smaller amounts of calcium are supplied by legumes, nuts, dried fruits, and dark green leafy vegetables (such as kale, broccoli, collard greens, and beet greens). It is important to remember that some of the calcium in beet greens, spinach, and Swiss chard is bound with oxalic acid, which makes it less available to the body. Larger amounts of these foods need to be consumed if they are substituted for dairy sources of calcium (see Table 14–4).

The recommended dietary allowance (RDA) for phosphorus does not change from that of a nonpregnant woman age 19 or older: 700 mg per day. Similarly, for females age 18 and younger it remains stable at 1250 mg per day. Phosphorus is readily supplied through calcium- and protein-rich foods, especially milk, eggs, and meat.

IODINE

Iodine is an essential part of the thyroid hormone thyroxine. Inorganic iodine is excreted in the urine during pregnancy. Enlargement of the thyroid gland may occur if iodine is not replaced by adequate dietary intake or additional supplement. Iodine deficiency is the most widespread nutritional cause of impaired brain development. This can result in cretinism and lesser degrees of intellectual disability.

A woman can meet the iodine requirement of 220 mcg per day by using iodized salt. Seafood is also a good source of iodine. Plant sources vary because they reflect the iodine content of the soil in which they grow. When sodium is restricted, the physician may prescribe an iodine supplement.

SODIUM

Sodium is essential for proper metabolism and the regulation of fluid balance. Sodium intake in the form of salt is never entirely curtailed during pregnancy, even when hypertension or preeclampsia is present. The woman can obtain moderate sodium intake by using fresh food lightly seasoned to taste during cooking. The use of extra salt at the table should be avoided. Salty foods, such as potato chips, ham, sausage, and sodium-based seasonings, can be eliminated to avoid excessive intake.

TABLE 14–4 Food Sources of Calcium

FOOD	CALCIUM
Milk 1%, 8 oz	305 mg
Cheddar cheese, 1.5 oz	287 mg
Fruit yogurt, lowfat, 8 oz	383 mg
American cheese, pasteurized, 2 oz	387 mg
Soy milk, 8 oz*	383 mg
Tofu, ½ cup	434 mg
Figs, 1 cup	300 mg
Orange juice, calcium-fortified, 8 oz	349 mg
Mustard spinach, raw, 1 cup	315 mg
Sardines, canned in oil, 3 oz	325 mg
Almonds, 4 oz	300 mg

SOURCE: Data from U.S. Department of Health and Human Services & U. S. Department of Agriculture, 2015.

*Amounts may vary with brand; be sure to check label.

ZINC

Zinc is involved in protein metabolism and the synthesis of deoxyribonucleic acid (DNA) and ribonucleic acid (RNA). It is essential for normal fetal growth and development as well as milk production during lactation. Zinc deficiency may cause symptoms such as growth retardation, impaired immune response, delayed wound healing, and mental lethargy. The RDA during pregnancy for women age 19 and older is 11 mg per day. This increases to 12 mg during lactation. Best sources of zinc are meats, shellfish, and poultry. Good sources include whole grains and legumes.

MAGNESIUM

Magnesium is essential for cellular metabolism and structural growth. The RDA for pregnancy is 350 mg for women 19 to 30 years of age and 360 mg for women 31 to 50 years of age. Good sources include milk, whole grains, dark green vegetables, nuts, and legumes.

IRON

Iron requirements increase during pregnancy because of the growth of the fetus and placenta and the expansion of maternal blood volume. Anemia in pregnancy is mainly caused by low iron stores, although it may also result from inadequate intake of other nutrients, such as vitamins B_6 and B_{12}, folic acid, ascorbic acid, copper, and zinc. Women with poor diet histories, frequent conceptions, or records of prior iron depletion are particularly at risk.

Iron deficiency anemia is generally defined as a decrease in the oxygen-carrying capacity of the blood. This significantly reduces the hemoglobin per deciliter of blood, the volume of packed red cells per deciliter of blood (hematocrit), or the number of erythrocytes. Iron deficiency anemia is associated with an increased risk of preterm birth, low-birth-weight newborns, and maternal and infant mortality. It can also have a negative impact on normal fetal/neonatal brain development (West et al., 2017).

Fetal demands for iron further contribute to symptoms of anemia in the pregnant woman. The fetal liver stores iron, especially during the third trimester. The baby will need this stored iron during the first 4 months of life to compensate for the normally inadequate levels of iron in breast milk and non-iron-fortified formulas.

To prevent anemia, the woman must balance iron requirements and intake. Doing so is a problem for nonpregnant women and a greater one for pregnant women. Although the rate of absorption increases during pregnancy, it is still important to select foods high in iron to increase the daily intake. Lean meats, dark green leafy vegetables, eggs, and whole-grain and enriched breads and cereals are the foods usually depended on for their iron content. Other iron sources include dried fruits, legumes, shellfish, and molasses.

Iron absorption is generally higher for animal products than for vegetable products. However, the woman may enhance absorption of iron from nonmeat sources by combining them with meat or a food rich in vitamin C. In addition, the use of iron-fortified foods is a cost-effective and efficient way to increase iron intake.

The RDA for iron during pregnancy is 27 mg/day, but this intake is almost impossible to achieve through diet alone. Thus, in the second and third trimesters the pregnant woman should take a daily supplement of 30 mg elemental iron (West et al., 2017). Unfortunately, iron supplements often cause gastrointestinal discomfort, especially if taken on an empty stomach. Taking the iron supplement after a meal may help reduce this discomfort. Iron supplements may also cause constipation, so an adequate fluid intake is important.

Vitamins

Vitamins are organic substances necessary for life and growth. They are found in small amounts in specific foods and generally cannot be synthesized by the body in adequate amounts.

Vitamins are grouped according to their solubility. Those that dissolve in fat are A, D, E, and K; those soluble in water include vitamin C and the B-complex vitamins. An adequate intake of all vitamins is essential during pregnancy; however, several are required in larger than normal amounts to fulfill specific needs.

A balanced diet generally provides necessary vitamins without the need for supplementation. Despite this, many people who are concerned about nutrition have become involved in the practice of taking exceptionally large doses—megadoses—of vitamins. However, in vitamin therapy more is not necessarily better. Megadoses of vitamins, especially vitamins A, D, C, and B_6, have been documented to have a negative effect on the fetus. Furthermore, excessive intake of one vitamin may interfere with the body's use of another vitamin. For example, excessive intake of vitamin C may block the body's use of vitamin B_{12}. Consequently, although it is important to meet the recommended dietary allowances of vitamins during pregnancy, megadoses are best avoided.

FAT-SOLUBLE VITAMINS

The fat-soluble vitamins A, D, E, and K are stored in the liver and thus are available should the dietary intake become inadequate. They are not excreted in the urine, so excessive consumption of these vitamins, particularly vitamins A and D, can lead to toxicity. Symptoms of fat-soluble vitamin toxicity include nausea, gastrointestinal upset, dryness and cracking of the skin, and loss of hair.

Vitamin A. Vitamin A is involved in the growth of epithelial cells, which line the entire gastrointestinal tract and compose the skin. Vitamin A plays a role in the metabolism of carbohydrates and fats. The body cannot synthesize glycogen in the absence of vitamin A, and the body's ability to handle cholesterol is also affected. In addition, the protective layer of tissue surrounding nerve fibers does not form properly if vitamin A is lacking. Probably the best-known function of vitamin A is its effect on vision in dim light. A person's ability to see in the dark depends on the eye's supply of retinol, a form of vitamin A. In this manner, vitamin A prevents night blindness. Vitamin A is associated with the formation and development of healthy eyes in the fetus.

If maternal stores of vitamin A are adequate, the overall effects of pregnancy on the woman's vitamin A requirements are not remarkable. The blood serum level of vitamin A decreases slightly in early pregnancy, rises in late pregnancy, and falls before the onset of labor. Thus, the RDA for vitamin A is 770 mcg per day for pregnant women age 19 and older.

Deficiencies of vitamin A are not common in the United States. Among the poor of developing countries, vitamin A deficiency is a major cause of preventable childhood blindness and an important factor in morbidity and mortality from infection, especially among pregnant women and children. Although routine supplementation with vitamin A is not recommended, supplementation with 5000 international units is indicated for women whose dietary intake may be inadequate, such as strict vegetarians and recent emigrants from countries where deficiency of vitamin A is endemic.

Rich plant sources of vitamin A include deep green and yellow or deep orange vegetables and some fruits; animal sources include liver, egg yolk, cream, butter, fortified margarine, and milk.

Vitamin D. Vitamin D is best known for its role in the absorption and utilization of calcium and phosphorus in skeletal development. To supply the needs of the developing fetus, the pregnant woman should have a vitamin D intake of 600 international units (IU) (15 mcg) per day.

Main food sources of vitamin D include fortified milk, margarine, butter, liver, and egg yolks. Drinking a quart of vitamin D–fortified milk daily provides the vitamin D needed during pregnancy. Vitamin D is also obtained through the synthesis of sunlight on the skin. During the winter months, however, women who live in northern latitudes are at risk for limited sun exposure, as are women who routinely wear sun protection including high-SPF products and protective clothing. Vitamin D deficiency is more common than previously recognized. While universal screening for vitamin D deficiency is not currently recommended, women at risk (vegetarians, women with limited sun exposure, ethnic and racial groups with dark skin) may be screened. If a deficiency is identified, a daily dose of 1000 to 2000 international units is safe (ACOG, 2015a).

Excessive intake of vitamin D is not usually a result of eating but of taking high-potency vitamin preparations. Overdoses during pregnancy can cause hypercalcemia, or high blood calcium levels, because of withdrawal of calcium from the skeletal tissue. Symptoms of toxicity include excessive thirst, loss of appetite, vomiting, weight loss, irritability, and high blood calcium levels.

Vitamin E. The major function of vitamin E, or tocopherol, is as an antioxidant. Vitamin E takes on oxygen, thus preventing other nutrients from undergoing chemical changes. For example, vitamin E helps spare vitamin A by preventing its oxidation in the intestinal tract and the tissues. It decreases the oxidation of polyunsaturated fats, thus helping to retain the flexibility and health of the cell membrane. In protecting the cell membrane, vitamin E affects the health of all cells in the body.

Vitamin E is also involved in certain enzymatic and metabolic reactions. It is an essential nutrient for the synthesis of nucleic acids required in the formation of red blood cells in the bone marrow. Vitamin E is beneficial in treating certain types of muscular pain and intermittent claudication, in surface healing of wounds and burns, and in protecting lung tissue from the damaging effects of smog. These functions may help explain the abundant claims and cures attributed to vitamin E, many of which have not been scientifically proved.

The newborn's need for vitamin E has been widely recognized. Human milk provides adequate vitamin E, whereas cow's milk is lower in vitamin E content. Deficiency symptoms of vitamin E are related to long-term inability to absorb fats. In humans, malabsorption problems exist in cases of cystic fibrosis, liver cirrhosis, postgastrectomy, obstructive jaundice, pancreatic problems, and sprue (chronic malabsorption syndrome).

The recommended intake of vitamin E is unchanged at 15 mg per day. Vitamin E is widely distributed in foodstuffs, especially vegetable fats and oils, whole grains, greens, and eggs. Excessive intake of vitamin E has been associated with abnormal coagulation in the newborn.

Vitamin K. Vitamin K, or menadione as used synthetically in medicine, is an essential factor for the synthesis of prothrombin; its function is thus related to normal blood clotting. Synthesis occurs in the intestinal tract by the *Escherichia coli* normally inhabiting the large intestine. However, the body's need for vitamin K is not totally met through synthesis. Green leafy vegetables and liver are excellent sources. The adult requirement for vitamin K, 90 mcg per day, does not increase during pregnancy.

Intake of vitamin K is usually adequate in a well-balanced prenatal diet. Secondary problems may arise if an illness results in malabsorption of fats or if antibiotics are used for an extended period. Antibiotics inhibit vitamin K synthesis by destroying intestinal *E. coli*.

WATER-SOLUBLE VITAMINS

Water-soluble vitamins are excreted in the urine. Only small amounts are stored, so there is little protection from dietary inadequacies. Thus, adequate amounts must be ingested daily. During pregnancy, the concentration of water-soluble vitamins in the maternal serum falls, whereas high concentrations are found in the fetus.

Vitamin C. The requirement for vitamin C (ascorbic acid) is increased in pregnancy from 75 to 85 mg per day. The major function of vitamin C is to aid the formation and development of connective tissue and the vascular system. Ascorbic acid is essential to the formation of collagen, which binds cells together. If the collagen begins to disintegrate because of lack of ascorbic acid, cell functioning is disturbed, and cell structure breaks down, causing muscular weakness, capillary hemorrhage, and eventual death. These are symptoms of scurvy, the disease caused by vitamin C deficiency. Newborns of women who have taken megadoses of vitamin C may experience a rebound form of scurvy.

Maternal plasma levels of vitamin C progressively decline throughout pregnancy, with values at term being about half those at midpregnancy. It appears that ascorbic acid concentrates in the placenta; levels in the fetus are 50% or more above maternal levels.

A nutritious diet should meet the pregnant woman's needs for vitamin C without additional supplementation. Common food sources of vitamin C include citrus fruit, tomatoes, cantaloupe, strawberries, potatoes, and broccoli and other leafy green vegetables. Ascorbic acid is readily destroyed by water and oxidation. Therefore, foods containing vitamin C should have limited exposure to air, heat, and water during storage and cooking.

The B Vitamins. The B vitamins include thiamine (B_1), riboflavin (B_2), niacin, folic acid, pantothenic acid, vitamin B_6, and vitamin B_{12}. These vitamins serve as vital coenzyme factors in many reactions, such as cell respiration, glucose oxidation, and energy metabolism. Consequently, the quantities needed invariably increase as caloric intake increases to meet the metabolic and growth needs of the pregnant woman.

- ***Thiamine.*** Required amount increases from the prepregnant level of 1.1 mg per day to 1.4 mg per day. Sources include pork, liver, milk, potatoes, enriched breads, and cereals.
- ***Riboflavin.*** Deficiency is manifested by *cheilosis* (fissures and cracks of the lips and the corners of the mouth) and other skin lesions. During pregnancy, women may excrete less riboflavin and still require more because of increased energy and protein needs. An additional 0.3 mg per day, to 1.4 mg per day, is recommended for pregnant women age 19 and older. Sources include milk, liver, eggs, enriched breads, and cereals.
- ***Niacin.*** Requirements increase by 4 mg per day during pregnancy to 18 mg. Sources of niacin include meat, fish, poultry, liver, whole grains, enriched breads, cereals, and peanuts.
- ***Folic acid (folate).*** Required for normal growth, reproduction, and lactation, **folic acid** prevents the macrocytic, megaloblastic anemia of pregnancy, which is seldom found in the United States, but does occur. An inadequate intake of folic acid has been associated with neural tube defects (NTDs) (e.g., spina bifida, anencephaly). Although these defects are considered multifactorial, research indicates that most of these birth defects could be prevented if folic acid supplementation recommendations were followed. Specifically the Centers for Disease Control and Prevention and the U.S. Public Health Service recommend that *all* women of childbearing age (15 to 45 years) consume 400 mcg of folic acid daily because half of all U.S. pregnancies are unplanned and NTDs occur very early in pregnancy (3 to 4 weeks after conception), before most women realize they are pregnant (CDC, 2016). The best food sources of folates are fresh green leafy vegetables, liver, peanuts, and whole-grain breads and cereals. Folic acid can be made inactive by oxidation, ultraviolet (UV) light, and heating. It can easily be lost during improper storage and cooking. To prevent unnecessary loss, foods should be stored covered to protect them from light, cooked with only a small amount of water, and not overcooked.
- ***Pantothenic acid.*** No allowance has been set during pregnancy, but 5 mg per day is considered a safe, adequate intake. Sources include meats, egg yolk, legumes, and whole-grain cereals and breads.
- ***Vitamin B_6 (pyridoxine).*** Associated with amino acid metabolism, thus a higher-than-average protein intake requires increased pyridoxine intake. The RDA during pregnancy is 1.9 mg per day, an increase of 0.6 mg over the allowance for nonpregnant women. Generally, the slightly increased need can be supplied by dietary sources, which include wheat germ, yeast, fish, liver, pork, potatoes, and lentils.
- ***Vitamin B_{12} (cobalamin).*** Plays a role in the synthesis of DNA and red blood cells and is important in maintaining the myelin sheath of nerve cells. Vitamin B_{12} is the cobalt-containing vitamin found only in animal sources. Women of reproductive age rarely have a vitamin B_{12} deficiency. Vegans (see later discussion of vegetarianism) can develop a deficiency, however, so it is essential that their dietary intake be supplemented with this vitamin. A deficiency may also be due to a congenital inability to absorb vitamin B_{12}, resulting in pernicious anemia; however, infertility is a complication of this type of anemia. Occasionally, vitamin B_{12} levels decrease during pregnancy but increase again after birth. The RDA during pregnancy is 2.6 mcg per day, an increase of 0.2 mcg.

Clinical Tip

In eliciting a pregnant woman's health history, keep in mind the fact that many women are consuming over-the-counter vitamin, mineral, and food supplements. Thus, it is important to ask about the use of any over-the-counter supplements to help avoid potentially harmful excess intakes.

Fluid

Water is essential for life and is found in all body tissues. It is necessary for many biochemical reactions. It also serves as a lubricant, acts as a medium of transport for carrying substances in and out of the body, and aids in the regulation of body temperature. A pregnant woman should consume at least 8 to 12 (8 oz) glasses of fluid each day, of which 4 to 6 glasses should be water. Other beverages such as juices and milk can contribute water as well as other nutrients to the diet. Sodas and diet sodas should be used in moderation because they do not contribute to the nutritional value of the diet. Caffeinated beverages also have a diuretic effect, which may be counterproductive to increasing fluid intake.

Vegetarianism

Vegetarianism is the dietary choice of many people for religious, health, ethical, and economic reasons. Well-planned vegetarian diets are nutritionally adequate and appropriate for all stages of life, including pregnancy. Vegetarian diets offer numerous health benefits and may help prevent certain diseases. There are several types of vegetarians, and dietary practices vary among the types. **Lacto-ovo-vegetarians** include milk, dairy products, and eggs in their diet. **Lacto-vegetarians** include dairy products but no eggs. **Vegans** are strict vegetarians who will not eat any food from animal sources.

Appropriate meal planning for vegetarian or vegan diets ensures that a pregnant woman obtains necessary nutrients to promote the growth and development of the fetus. Supplementation may be recommended for those who have difficulty meeting the recommended amounts of folic acid, iron, vitamin B_{12}, or calcium through food sources. Protein needs increase slightly for vegans because of the lower-quality protein sources ingested when animal proteins are excluded. Adequate dietary protein can be obtained by consuming a varied diet with adequate caloric intake and plant-based proteins. Consuming an assortment of plant proteins throughout the day such as beans and rice, peanut butter on whole-grain bread, and whole-grain cereal with soy milk, ensures that the expectant mother obtains all essential amino acids. Protein and amino acid supplements are not recommended and are unnecessary in well-planned diets. Obtaining sufficient calories to achieve adequate weight gains can be difficult because vegan diets tend to be higher in fiber and, therefore, filling. Low prepregnancy weight and optimum pregnancy weight gains are often a problem. Supplementation with energy-dense foods helps provide increased energy intake to prevent the body from using protein for caloric needs.

Although vegan diets may be lower in some vitamins and minerals naturally occurring in animal foods, a varied diet including fortified foods can usually meet the nutritional needs of a pregnant woman. Vitamin B_{12}, iron, calcium, and zinc are of particular concern, and emphasizing the use of fortified foods containing these nutrients is advised. A guide to vegetarian food groups is provided in Table 14–5.

Factors Influencing Nutrition

It is important to consider the many factors that affect a patient's nutrition. What are the age, lifestyle, dietary practices, and culture of the pregnant woman? What food beliefs and habits does she have? What a person eats is also determined by availability, economics, and symbolism. These and other factors influence the expectant mother's acceptance of the nurse's intervention.

Common Discomforts of Pregnancy

Gastrointestinal functioning can be altered at times during pregnancy, resulting in discomforts such as nausea and vomiting, heartburn, and constipation. Although these changes can be uncomfortable for the woman, they are seldom a major problem. These discomforts and dietary modifications that may provide relief are discussed in Chapter 13.

Complementary and Alternative Therapies

While the use of some herbal, botanical, and alternative therapies may seem like a natural and safe alternative to some individuals, the pregnant consumer should take caution. Few clinical trials exist that have examined the safety of supplements and herbs during pregnancy. Many herbs are considered safe for use in pregnancy. Other herbs could pose a risk. Pregnant women should be advised to consult reputable sources such as the National Center for Complementary and Integrative Health website about these therapies and should also speak with their healthcare providers to determine the safety of such products or therapies.

TABLE 14–5 Vegetarian Food Groups

FOOD GROUP	MIXED DIET	LACTO-OVO-VEGETARIAN	LACTO-VEGETARIAN	VEGAN
Grain	Bread, cereal, rice, pasta	Bread, cereal, rice, pasta	Bread, cereal, rice, pasta	Bread, cereal, rice, pasta
Fruit	Fruit, fruit juices	Fruit, fruit juices	Fruit, fruit juices	Fruit, fruit juices
Vegetable	Vegetables, vegetable juices	Vegetables, vegetable juices	Vegetables, vegetable juices	Vegetables, vegetable juices
Dairy and dairy alternatives	Milk, yogurt, cheese	Milk, yogurt, cheese	Milk, yogurt, cheese	Fortified soy milk, rice milk, and other dairy-free milks
Meat and meat alternatives	Meat, fish, poultry, eggs, legumes, tofu, nuts, nut butters	Eggs, legumes, tofu, nuts, nut butters	Beans, legumes, tofu, nuts, nut butters	Beans, legumes, tofu, nuts, nut butters

Use of Artificial Sweeteners

Foods and beverages that contain nonnutritive sweeteners are increasingly available. Nonnutritive sweeteners are safe for use during pregnancy and include acesulfame potassium (Sweet One), aspartame (NutraSweet, Equal), saccharin (Sweet N Low, Sugar Twin), sucralose (Splenda), stevia (Truvia, PureVia, Sun Crystals), and advantame (Food and Drug Administration [FDA], 2016b). As with other foods, moderation should be exercised in using nonnutritive sweeteners because calorie-free foods and beverages may displace other nutritious foods and beverages.

Energy Drinks

Energy drinks, such as Monster Energy, Red Bull, and 5-Hour Energy, used to boost performance and delay fatigue have become increasingly popular in recent years. These beverages are soft drinks with ingredients such as caffeine, ginseng, guarana, taurine, and sugar added to provide stimulation and increase energy. Because they are classified as dietary supplements and not food, they are not subject to the same regulations and monitoring as food. The caffeine content of energy drinks can be as high as 300 mg (equivalent to about three average cups of brewed coffee) and accounts for most of the health risks associated with their intake. Excessive intake of energy drinks can cause a variety of symptoms including hypertension, palpitations, anxiety, headache, agitation, tremors, seizures, and altered mental state. Pregnant women who consume high levels of caffeine are at increased risk for late miscarriage, stillbirths, and small-for-gestational-age newborns (Breda et al., 2014). Pregnant women are advised to use energy drinks cautiously and include the drink's caffeine content in calculating daily caffeine intake in order to stay within the recommended level, which is 200 mg/day (Niebyl, Weber, & Briggs, 2017).

Mercury in Fish

Fish and shellfish provide protein, healthy omega-3 fats, and many vitamins and minerals, but nearly all contain traces of mercury. Although this is not a concern for most people, some fish and shellfish contain higher levels of mercury than others, and mercury can pose a threat to the unborn baby or a young child.

SAFETY ALERT!

Women who are pregnant or who may become pregnant, breastfeeding mothers, and young children should not eat swordfish, shark, tilefish, or king mackerel because these fish contain high levels of methyl mercury. Mercury crosses the placenta, as well as the blood–brain barrier, and exposure to the developing fetal brain can have a negative effect on cognitive functioning.

Many pregnant women are aware of the mercury warning and far less aware of the important nutritional value of fish, especially fish high in docosahexaenoic acid (DHA). However, a strong body of evidence supports the nutritional value of fish during pregnancy. Thus, pregnant women need to be encouraged to eat at least 8 oz and up to 12 oz/week (two average meals) of a variety of shellfish and fish that are lower in mercury (U.S. Department of Agriculture [USDA], 2015). Commonly eaten fish and shellfish that are low in mercury and higher in omega-3s include salmon, herring, trout, sardines, pollack, and mussels. Albacore (white) tuna has more mercury than canned light tuna; therefore, only 6 oz/week of albacore tuna is recommended (USDA, 2015).

Foodborne Illnesses

Salmonella and *Listeria monocytogenes* are two bacteria that pose a threat to expectant mothers and their fetuses. To avoid *Salmonella*, pregnant women should avoid eating or tasting foods that may contain raw or undercooked eggs, including raw dough, cake batter, homemade eggnog, homemade dressings, ice cream, or hollandaise sauce.

L. monocytogenes is found in refrigerated, ready-to-eat foods such as unpasteurized milk and dairy products, meat, poultry, and seafood. To prevent listeria infection (listeriosis), pregnant women should be advised to do the following (Food and Drug Administration [FDA], 2016a):

- Maintain refrigerator temperature at 40°F (4°C) or below and the freezer at 0°F (–18°C).
- Refrigerate or freeze prepared foods, leftovers, and perishables within 2 hours after eating or preparation. Discard food left out at room temperature for longer than 2 hours.
- Do not eat hot dogs and luncheon meats unless they are reheated until they are steaming hot.
- Avoid soft cheeses such as feta, brie, Camembert, blue-veined cheeses, queso fresco, and queso blanco (a soft cheese often used in Hispanic cooking) unless the label clearly states that they are made with pasteurized milk.
- Do not eat refrigerated patés or meat spreads or foods that contain raw (unpasteurized) milk; do not drink unpasteurized milk.
- Avoid eating refrigerated smoked seafood such as salmon, trout, cod, tuna, or mackerel unless it is in a cooked dish such as a casserole. Canned or shelf-stable patés, meat spreads, and smoked seafood are considered safe to eat.

Lactase Deficiency (Lactose Intolerance)

Some individuals have difficulty digesting milk and dairy products. This condition, known as **lactase deficiency** or **lactose intolerance**, results from an inadequate amount of the enzyme lactase, which breaks down the milk sugar lactose into smaller digestible substances.

Lactase deficiency is a common condition affecting millions in the United States. Some ethnic and racial populations are more affected than others and include African Americans, Hispanic Americans, American Indians, and Asian Americans. People who are not affected are mainly of Northern European heritage. Symptoms may include abdominal distention, discomfort, nausea and vomiting, loose stools, and cramps.

When counseling pregnant women who might be intolerant of milk and milk products, the nurse should be aware that tolerances vary among individuals, and even a partial serving of milk or dairy products can produce symptoms. Milk in cooked form, such as custard, is sometimes tolerated, as are cultured or fermented dairy products such as buttermilk, some cheeses, kefir, and yogurt. Lactase deficiency need not be a problem for pregnant women because the enzyme is available over the counter in tablets or drops. In addition, specially treated cow's milk is now available in most large grocery stores.

Cultural, Ethnic, and Religious Influences

Cultural, ethnic, and religious backgrounds determine one's experiences with food and influence food preferences and habits (Figure 14–3). People of different nationalities are accustomed to eating foodstuffs available in their country of origin and prepared in a manner consistent with the customs and traditions of their ethnic and cultural group. In addition, the laws of certain religions allow particular foods, prohibit others, and direct the preparation and serving of meals. (See *Developing Cultural Competence: Dietary Practices to Protect Health.*)

Developing Cultural Competence Dietary Practices to Protect Health

Dietary practices to protect health vary across the world but many are practiced to maintain health and prevent illness. Following are a few examples (Spector, 2017):

- The kosher diet followed by many Jewish people forbids the eating of pork products and shellfish. In addition, according to kosher dietary rules, meat and dairy products should not be mixed and eaten at the same meal.
- Many Muslims also avoid pork products and the meats that are eaten must be *halal* or approved by Islamic law.
- Among some traditional Chinese people, "thousand-year-old" eggs (preserved eggs that take about 4 to 5 weeks to prepare) are viewed as health promoting and are eaten with rice.
- In some Italian, Greek, or Native American homes garlic or onions may be eaten, worn on the body, or hung in the home to prevent illness.
- In some Hispanic homes foods must be balanced between those that are considered to be *hot* and those that are considered to be *cold*.

Note: It is unwise to attribute specific attitudes or beliefs to all members of a cultural group. The information in the Developing Cultural Competence boxes offers possible insights into caring for women from different cultural groups.

In each culture, certain foods have symbolic significance. Generally, these symbolic foods are related to major life experiences such as birth, death, or developmental milestones. Although generalizations have been made about the food practices of ethnic and religious groups, there are many variations. Food customs will differ among groups in various regions of the same country, among families within local regions, and among individuals within the same family. The extent to which the use of traditional ethnic foods and customs is continued is affected by the recency of immigration, the extent of exposure to other cultures, and the availability, quality, and cost of the traditional foods.

When working with a pregnant woman from any ethnic background, the nurse needs to understand the cultural influences on the woman's eating habits and to identify beliefs she may have about food and pregnancy (Figure 14–4). Talking with the patient can enable the nurse to determine the level of influence that traditional food customs exert. Only then can the nurse provide dietary advice in a manner that is meaningful to the woman.

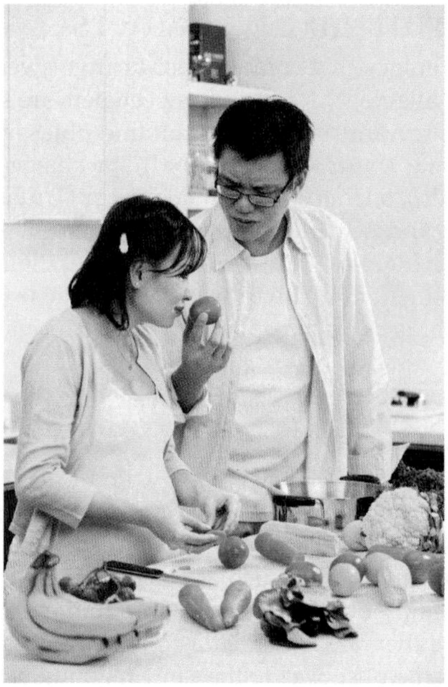

Figure 14–3 **Cultural factors affect food preferences and habits.**

SOURCE: Arto/Fotolia.

Psychosocial Factors

The sharing of food has long been a symbol of friendliness, warmth, and social acceptance in many cultures. Food is also symbolic of motherliness; that is, taking care of the family and feeding them well are part of the traditional mothering role. Some foods and food-related practices are associated with status. Certain items may be prepared "just for company." Other foods are served only on special occasions or holidays.

Socioeconomic level may be a determinant of nutritional status. Poverty-level families are unable to afford the same foods that higher-income families can. Thus, pregnant women with low incomes are frequently at risk for inadequate intake of nutrients.

Knowledge about the basic components of a balanced diet is essential. Often educational level is related to economic status, but even people on very limited incomes can prepare well-balanced meals if their knowledge of nutrition is adequate.

The expectant woman's attitudes and feelings about her pregnancy may influence her nutritional status. For example, food may be used as a substitute for the expression of emotions such as anger or frustration or as a way of expressing feelings of joy. The woman who is depressed or who does not wish to be pregnant may manifest these feelings by loss of appetite or by an overindulgence of certain foods.

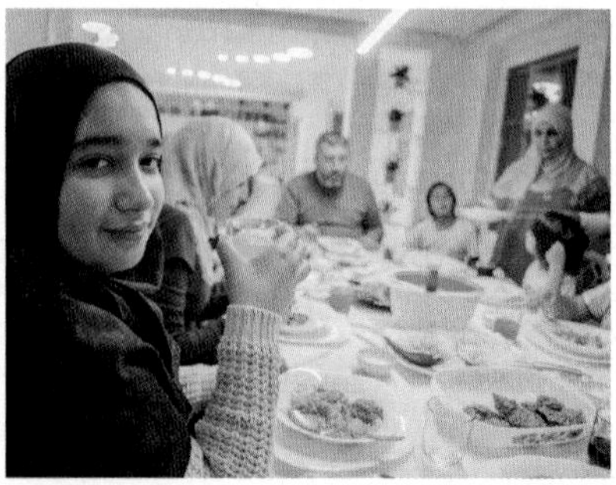

Figure 14–4 **Shared meals are an important part of family life and food preferences are often influenced by the family's culture.**

SOURCE: Zurijeta/Shutterstock

Eating Disorders

Two serious eating disorders, anorexia nervosa and bulimia nervosa, affect millions of men and women, although they develop most commonly in adolescent girls and young women. These psychologic disorders can have a major impact on a pregnant woman's physiologic and emotional well-being.

Anorexia nervosa is characterized by an extreme fear of weight gain and fat. People with this problem have distorted body images and perceive themselves as fat even when they are extremely underweight. Their dietary intake is very restrictive in both variety and quantity. They may also engage in excessive exercise to prevent weight gain.

Bulimia nervosa is characterized by bingeing (secretly consuming large quantities of food in a short period) and purging. Self-induced vomiting is the most common method of purging; laxatives and/or diuretics may also be used. Individuals with bulimia often maintain normal or near-normal weight for their height, so it is difficult to know whether bingeing and purging occur.

Women with anorexia nervosa often do not become pregnant because of the physiologic changes that affect their reproductive systems. Women with bulimia can become pregnant. Their self-induced vomiting may produce many of the same complications as hyperemesis gravidarum (see Chapter 18).

Women with eating disorders who become pregnant are at risk for a variety of complications. The consequences of the restricting, bingeing, and purging behaviors characteristic of eating disorders can result in a lack of nutrients available for the fetus. Other risks to the mother and baby include miscarriage, low birth weight, premature birth, and even perinatal mortality and birth defects. Pregnancy can be an especially difficult time for the woman with an eating disorder, even if she has long desired a child. For someone who already struggles with eating and body image, the consumption of additional food and the expectations that she will gain additional weight can result in feelings of fear, anxiety, depression, and guilt. Postpartum depression may also affect more women with a history of eating disorders than pregnant women without a prior history of eating concerns. When working with a pregnant woman with an eating disorder, education and individualized meal plans can help the woman increase her dietary intake while maintaining a sense of control.

The treatment needs of a woman with an eating disorder can best be met by a team approach that includes medical, nutritional, and psychiatric practitioners who are familiar with eating disorders. The pregnant woman with an eating disorder needs to be closely monitored and supported throughout her pregnancy to help ensure the best possible outcome.

> "I developed anorexia during my sophomore year in college. My parents were shocked when they saw me at Thanksgiving and, fortunately, they got me some help. For the past several years I have maintained my weight in the low normal range and feel OK about it. Now I am expecting my first child. It is so difficult to think of gaining 25 to 30 pounds, but I am working very hard to eat properly for my baby. I have reconnected with my therapist so that I can be sure I keep my head on straight about the importance of good nutrition. I don't think people realize how tough eating disorders are to overcome, but I will *not* jeopardize my child—I just won't!"

Pica

Pica is the persistent craving and eating of substances such as soil or clay (*geophagia*), powdered laundry starch or corn starch (*amylophagia*), soap, baking powder, ice (*pagophagia*), freezer frost, burned matches, paint, or ashes that are not ordinarily considered edible or nutritionally valuable. Most women who eat such substances do so only during pregnancy.

Iron deficiency anemia is the most common concern with pica. The ingestion of laundry starch or certain types of clay may contribute to iron deficiency by replacing iron-containing foods from the diet or by interfering with iron absorption. Women with pica that involves eating ice or freezer frost often have poor weight gain because of lack of appetite, whereas the ingestion of starch may be associated with excessive weight gain. The ingestion of large quantities of clay could fill the intestine and cause fecal impaction. Lead levels should be checked in women who may have eaten peeling paint.

Assessment for pica is an important part of a nutritional history. However, women may be embarrassed about their cravings or reluctant to discuss them for fear of criticism. It is helpful if the nurse uses a nonjudgmental approach and explains the possible harmful effects. Some women are able to switch to eating nonfat powdered milk instead of laundry starch and frozen fruit pops instead of ice. Others find that sucking on hard lemon or mint candies helps decrease the craving.

Nutritional Care of the Pregnant Adolescent

Nutritional care of the pregnant adolescent is of particular concern to healthcare professionals. Many adolescents are nutritionally at risk because of a variety of complex and interrelated emotional, social, and economic factors that may adversely affect dietary intake. Important nutrition-related factors to assess in pregnant adolescents include low prepregnant weight, low weight gain during pregnancy, younger age with regard to menarche, smoking, excessive prepregnant weight, excessive weight gain, anemia, unhealthy lifestyle (drugs, alcohol use), chronic disease, and history of an eating disorder.

Pregnant teens are advised to follow the adult recommendations for weight gain based on their BMI. In the United States about 17% of adolescent girls are obese and they face the same risks during pregnancy that adult women face (West et al., 2017). Research indicates that, like their adult counterparts, pregnant teens who gain excessive weight are at increased risk for a cesarean birth, macrosomia, and preeclampsia, as well as for postpartum weight retention (Beaudrot, Elchert, & DeFranco, 2016).

The nutritional needs of adolescents are generally determined by using the dietary references intakes (DRI) for nonpregnant teenagers (ages 11 to 14 or 15 to 18) and adding nutrient amounts recommended for all pregnant women (see Table 14–1). If she is mature (more than 4 years since menarche), the pregnant adolescent's nutritional needs approach those reported for pregnant adults. However, adolescents who become pregnant less than 4 years after menarche are at high biologic risk because of their physiologic and anatomic immaturity. They are more likely than older adolescents to still be growing, which can impact the fetus's development. Thus, young adolescents (age 14 and under) need to gain more weight than older adolescents (18 years and older) to produce babies of equal size.

In determining the optimal weight gain for the pregnant adolescent, the nurse adds the recommended weight gain for an adult pregnancy to that expected during the postmenarchal year in which the pregnancy occurs. If the teenager is underweight, additional weight gain is recommended to bring her to a normal weight for her height.

Specific Nutrient Concerns

Caloric needs of pregnant adolescents vary widely. Major factors in determining caloric needs include whether growth has been completed and the physical activity level of the individual. Figures as high as 50 kcal/kg have been suggested for young, growing teens who are very active physically. A satisfactory weight gain usually confirms an adequate caloric intake.

An inadequate iron intake is a major concern with the adolescent diet. Iron needs are high for the pregnant teen because of the requirement for iron by the enlarging maternal muscle mass and blood volume. Iron supplements—providing 30 to 60 mg of elemental iron—are indicated.

Calcium is another nutrient that demands special attention from pregnant adolescents. Inadequate intake of calcium is frequently a problem in this age group. Adequate calcium intake is needed to support normal growth and development of the fetus as well as growth and maintenance of calcium stores in the adolescent. Inadequate calcium has been associated with maternal hypertension and preeclampsia. An extra serving of dairy products is usually recommended for teenagers. Calcium supplementation is indicated for teens with an aversion to or intolerance of milk unless they consume other dairy products or significant calcium sources.

Because folic acid plays a role in cell reproduction, it is also an important nutrient for pregnant teens. As previously indicated, a supplement is often suggested for pregnant females, whether adult or adolescent.

Other nutrients and vitamins must be considered when evaluating the overall nutritional quality of the teenager's diet. Nutrients that have frequently been found to be deficient in this age group include zinc and vitamins A, D, E, and B_6. Eating a wide variety of foods—especially fresh and lightly processed foods—is helpful in obtaining adequate amounts of trace minerals, fiber, and other vitamins.

Dietary Patterns

Healthy adolescents often have irregular eating patterns. Many skip breakfast, and most tend to be frequent snackers (Figure 14–5). Teens rarely follow the traditional three-meals-a-day pattern; their day-to-day intake often varies drastically; and they eat food combinations that may seem bizarre to adults. Despite this, adolescents usually achieve a better nutritional balance than most adults would expect.

In assessing the diet of the pregnant adolescent, the nurse should consider the eating pattern over time, not simply a single day's intake. This pattern is critical because of the irregularity of most adolescent eating patterns. Once the pattern is identified, counseling can be directed toward correcting deficiencies.

“My mom is so cool. She has hung in with me throughout this pregnancy even though I know she feels bad about it—she thinks my life will be harder, and I guess she is right. She is really working to make sure that I eat right so that I have a healthy baby, but instead of nagging, she has turned this into something we are doing together. We have taken a couple of cooking classes and experimented with different recipes. Last week we made some healthy but great snacks and I brought them to my friend Cary's birthday party. Those snacks just disappeared!”

Counseling Issues

A positive approach to nutritional counseling for the pregnant adolescent is more effective than a negative one. The nurse must be ready to suggest nutrient-dense foods that pregnant teens can choose in many places and at any time. If an adolescent's family member does most of the meal preparation, it may be useful to include that person in the discussion if the adolescent agrees. Involving the expectant father in counseling may be beneficial.

The pregnant teenager will soon become a parent, and her understanding of nutrition will influence not only her well-being but also that of her child. However, teens tend to live in the present, and counseling that stresses long-term changes may be less effective than more concrete approaches. Messages should emphasize that the pregnant teen is eating for her health and that of the baby and should focus on foods themselves rather than on nutrients. In many cases, classes with other teens are effective. Clinics and schools often offer classes and focused activities designed to address this topic. In a group atmosphere,

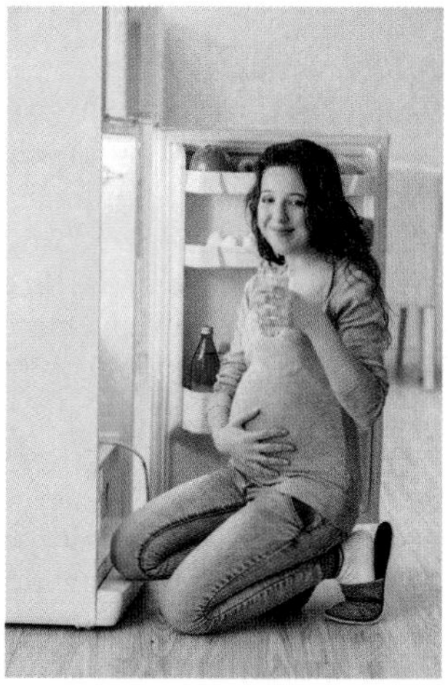

Figure 14–5 It is important to help teens understand the importance of a well-balanced diet.

SOURCE: Elnur Amikishiyev/123RF

CASE STUDY: Angelina Newman

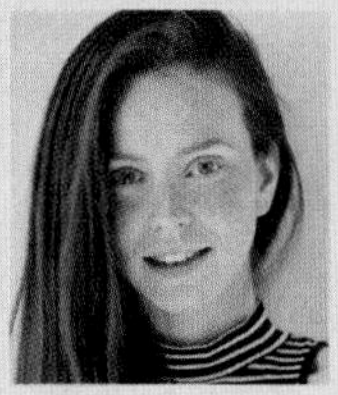

SOURCE: WAYHOME studio/Shutterstock

Angelina presents to her 27th-week visit with her boyfriend. You note from the EMR that her overall weight gain is 4.5 pounds since she began prenatal care at 7 weeks. At that time, she said that she had lost 6 to 8 pounds prior to her initial visit due to nausea and vomiting. At this visit, she expresses her desire to keep her weight down so she will be able to attend prom and get back to her prepregnancy weight as soon as possible after birth.

Questions to Ponder

Based on her age and insufficient weight gain, what nutritional education would you provide to her? How would you determine the ideal amount of weight this young woman should gain during her pregnancy?

adolescents often work together to plan adequate meals including foods that are their special favorites. See *Case Study: Angelina Newman*.

Postpartum Nutrition

Nutritional needs will change following the birth. Nutrient requirements will vary depending on whether the mother decides to breastfeed. An assessment of postpartum nutritional status is necessary before the nurse provides nutritional guidance.

Postpartum Nutritional Status

Postpartum nutritional status is determined primarily by assessing the new mother's weight, hemoglobin and hematocrit levels, clinical signs, and dietary history.

After birth, there is a weight loss of approximately 4.5 to 5.4 kg (10 to 12 lb). Additional weight loss will be most rapid during the first few weeks after birth as the uterus returns to normal size, tissue fluids are released, and maternal blood volume returns to normal. The mother's weight will then begin to stabilize. Weight loss may also be affected by lactation. Individual weight loss of women who breastfeed will vary but tends to be greater than that of women who do not, if breastfeeding continues for at least 6 months.

The rate of postpartum weight loss is influenced by many factors. Some women approach their prepregnancy weight several weeks after birth; most approach this weight about 6 months later. The amount of weight gained during pregnancy is a major determinant of weight loss after childbirth. Generally, women who gain excessive weight during pregnancy are more likely to sustain a weight gain 1 year following childbirth, putting them at increased risk of long-term overweight or obesity.

It is important to evaluate the mother's current weight, ideal weight for her height, weight before pregnancy, and weight before the birth. Women who are interested in weight reduction should be referred to a dietitian or nutritionist. Hemoglobin and erythrocyte values vary after birth, but they should return to normal levels within 2 to 6 weeks. Hematocrit levels should rise gradually because of hemoconcentration as extracellular fluid is excreted. The hematocrit is usually checked at the postpartum visit to detect any anemia. Mothers can be encouraged to eat a diet high in iron. Iron supplements are generally prescribed for 2 to 3 months following birth to replenish supplies depleted by pregnancy.

The nurse assesses any clinical symptoms the new mother may be experiencing. Food cravings and aversions typically drop significantly during the postpartum period and do not usually pose a problem. However, constipation is a common problem following birth. The nurse can encourage the woman to maintain a high fluid intake to keep the stool soft. Dietary sources of fiber and physical exercise are also helpful in preventing constipation.

The nurse obtains specific information on diet and eating habits directly from the woman. Visiting the mother during mealtimes provides an opportunity for unobtrusive nutritional assessment. Which foods has a woman selected? Has she avoided fruits and vegetables? Is her diet nutritionally sound? A comment focusing on a positive aspect of her meal selection may initiate a discussion of nutrition.

The dietitian should be informed about any woman whose cultural or religious beliefs require specific foods. Appropriate meals can then be prepared for her. The nurse may also refer women with unusual eating habits or numerous questions about food or nutrition to a dietitian. In all cases, the nurse should provide literature on nutrition so that the woman will have a source of appropriate information at home.

During the childbearing years the risk for obesity becomes especially problematic for women. Consequently, it is critical to use the postpartum period to change behaviors and help promote effective weight management in women.

Nutritional Care of Formula-Feeding Mothers

After birth, the formula-feeding mother's dietary requirements return to prepregnancy levels (see Table 14–1). If the mother has a good understanding of nutritional principles, it is sufficient to advise her to reduce her daily caloric intake by about 300 kcal and to return to prepregnancy levels for other nutrients.

If the mother has a poor understanding of nutrition, this is an opportunity to teach her the basic principles and the importance of a well-balanced diet. Her eating habits and dietary practices will eventually be reflected in the diet of her child.

If the mother has gained excessive weight during pregnancy (or perhaps was overweight before pregnancy), referral to a dietitian or nutritionist is appropriate. Weight reduction diets to meet nutritional needs and food preferences can be designed. Weight loss goals of 1 to 2 lb (0.45 to 0.9 kg) per week are usually suggested.

In addition to learning how to meet her own nutritional needs, the new mother will usually be interested in learning how to provide for her baby's nutritional needs. A discussion of newborn/infant feeding, which includes topics such as selecting newborn/infant formulas, formula preparation, and vitamin and mineral supplementation, is appropriate and generally well received.

Nutritional Care of Breastfeeding Mothers

Nutrient needs increase during breastfeeding. Table 14–1 lists the dietary reference intakes (DRIs) during breastfeeding for specific nutrients. Table 14–2 includes a daily food guide for lactating women. A few key nutrients need further discussion.

CALORIES

One of the most important factors in the breastfeeding woman's diet is calories. An inadequate caloric intake can reduce milk volume. However, milk quality generally remains unaffected. The breastfeeding mother should increase her caloric intake by 200 kcal over the pregnancy requirements (i.e., a 500-kcal increase from her prepregnancy requirement). This results in a total of about 2500 to 2700 kcal per day for most women.

Depending on her own dietary preferences, the breastfeeding mother can use the MyPlate food guide to assess her dietary intake. She should strive to include a variety of foods from each food group. Her caloric intake needs to provide enough energy to sustain lactation. After her weight stabilizes several weeks following childbirth, weight loss should not exceed more than 1 lb per week.

PROTEIN

An adequate protein intake is essential while breastfeeding because protein is an important component of breast milk. An intake of 65 g per day during the first 6 months of breastfeeding and 62 g per day thereafter is recommended. As in pregnancy, it is important that the woman consume adequate nonprotein calories to prevent the use of protein as an energy source.

CALCIUM

Calcium is also an important nutrient in milk production, and increases over nonpregnancy needs are expected. Requirements during breastfeeding remain the same as requirements during pregnancy: 1000 mg per day. An inadequate intake of calcium from food sources necessitates the use of calcium supplements.

IRON

Iron needs during lactation are not substantially different from those of nonpregnant women because iron is not a principal component of breast milk. However, as previously mentioned, continued supplementation of the mother for 2 to 3 months after parturition is advisable to replenish maternal stores depleted by pregnancy.

FLUIDS

Liquids are especially important during lactation because inadequate fluid intake may decrease milk volume. The recommended fluid intake of 8 to 10 (8-oz) glasses daily can be met by the consumption of water, juices, milk, and soups.

"For me, the hardest part of breastfeeding was drinking enough fluids. I am not a big water person and they told me to go easy on caffeine beverages. Once I started adding a slice of lemon to my water, I found it a lot easier. My baby is 13 months old now and I have stopped breastfeeding, but I still drink the water with lemon. I think I have developed a good new habit!"

Counseling Issues

In addition to counseling mothers on how to meet their increased nutrient needs during breastfeeding, nurses should discuss a few issues related to newborn/infant feeding. For example, many mothers are concerned about how specific foods they eat will affect their babies during breastfeeding. Generally, there are no foods the nursing mother must avoid except those to which she might be allergic. Occasionally, however, some breastfeeding mothers find that their babies are affected by certain foods. Onions, turnips, cabbage, chocolate, spices, and seasonings are commonly listed as offenders. The best advice to give the breastfeeding mother is to avoid those foods she suspects cause distress in her baby. For the most part, however, she should be able to eat any nourishing food she wants without fear that her baby will be affected. For further discussion of successful newborn/infant feeding, see Chapter 29.

●○● NURSING MANAGEMENT

For the Pregnant Woman Desiring Optimum Nutrition

Nursing Assessment and Diagnosis

Nutritional status must be assessed in order to plan an optimal diet with each woman. Gather data by consulting the woman's chart and by interviewing her. Obtain information about the following:

- The woman's height and weight and her weight gain during pregnancy
- Pertinent laboratory values, especially hemoglobin and hematocrit
- Clinical signs that have possible nutritional implications, such as constipation, anorexia, or heartburn
- Diet history to determine the woman's views on nutrition as well as her specific nutrient intake.

Obtain a diet history by asking the woman to complete a 24-hour diet recall, in which she lists everything consumed in the previous 24 hours, including foods, fluids, and any supplements. At least 3 days of diet recalls should be done to compensate for daily variations. Diet may also be evaluated using a food frequency questionnaire. The questionnaire lists common categories of foods and asks the woman how frequently in a day (or week) she consumes foods from the list. Common categories include vegetables, fruits, milk or cheese, meat or poultry, fish, desserts or sweets, coffee or tea, and alcoholic beverages. This method may not be completely reliable because it requires the individual to be accurate about her intake.

During the data-gathering process, take the opportunity to discuss important aspects of nutrition in the context of the family's needs and lifestyle. Also seek information about psychologic, cultural, and socioeconomic factors that may influence food intake.

Clinical Tip

When completing a diet history, nurses who are effective communicators remember that it is as important to identify the foods a woman avoids as it is to determine which foods she eats.

Once the data are obtained, begin to analyze the information, formulate appropriate nursing diagnoses, and develop patient goals. For a woman during the first trimester, the nursing diagnosis may be *Nutrition, Imbalanced: Less than Body Requirements, related to nausea and vomiting* (NANDA-I © 2017). In many cases the diagnosis may be related to excessive weight gain. In such cases the diagnosis might be *Overweight, Risk for, related to excessive calorie intake* (NANDA-I © 2017). Although these diagnoses are broad, be specific in addressing issues such as inadequate intake of nutrients such as iron, calcium, or folic acid; problems with nutrition because of a limited food budget; problems related to physiologic alterations, such as anorexia, heartburn, or nausea; and behavioral problems related to excessive dieting, anorexia nervosa, or bulimia. In some instances, the diagnosis *Knowledge, Readiness for Enhanced, related to nutrition* (NANDA-I © 2017) may seem most appropriate, especially if the woman asks for information about nutrition.

Nursing Plan and Implementation

After the nursing diagnosis is made, you can plan an approach to correct any nutritional deficiencies or improve the overall quality of the diet.

In counseling the pregnant woman, avoid "talking down" or "preaching" to her. Present information in a clear, logical way, using appropriate language but avoiding jargon. Examples are often helpful in clarifying material. Answer all questions appropriately and clearly.

When a person requires nutritional counseling, a dietary change is usually necessary. However, change is often difficult. Counseling will be more effective if you understand the woman's values and explain the needed change in a way that is meaningful to her. Because the pregnant woman must follow the plan, it should be developed in cooperation with her, be suitable for her socioeconomic level and background, and be based on reasonable, achievable goals. See *Health Promotion: Optimizing Maternal–Fetal Health*.

Health Promotion Optimizing Maternal–Fetal Health

- Achieve appropriate weight gain based on prepregnancy weight and BMI.
- Participate in regular physical activity (at least 150 minutes of moderate, safe activity per week, which may be divided into 30-minute segments 5 days per week or even smaller 10-minute segments).
- Consume a variety of healthy foods that form the basic food groups, including fruits, vegetables, grains, proteins, and dairy using MyPlate as a guideline.
- Consume 8 to 12 ounces of fish high in omega-3 fatty acids weekly.
- Take appropriate vitamin and mineral supplements.
- Consume caffeine in moderation.
- Avoid alcohol, tobacco, and other harmful substances.
- Follow safe food-handling practices.

SOURCE: Data from the American College of Obstetricians and Gynecologists (ACOG). (2015). *Nutrition during pregnancy*. Patient Education Pamphlet AP001. Washington, DC: Author; ACOG. (2016). *Exercise during pregnancy*. ACOG Publication No. 119. Washington, DC: Author.

Ethics in Action!

How do you respond to a woman who severely limits her nutrient and caloric intake despite counseling about the importance of a nutritious diet for her health and that of her fetus because she is concerned about gaining weight?

The following example demonstrates one way you can implement a plan with a patient based on the nursing diagnosis.

Nursing Diagnosis: *Nutrition, Imbalanced: Less than Body Requirements, related to low intake of calcium* (NANDA-I © 2017)

Patient goal: The woman will increase her intake of calcium to the DRI level.

Implementation:

1. Plan with the woman additional milk or dairy products that she can reasonably add to the diet (specify amounts).
2. Encourage the use of other calcium sources, such as leafy green vegetables and legumes.
3. Plan for the addition of powdered milk in cooking and baking.
4. If none of the above is realistic or acceptable, consider the use of calcium supplements.

Most families can benefit from guidance about food purchasing and preparation. Advise women to plan food purchases thoughtfully by preparing menus and a grocery list before shopping. It is also helpful to advise patients to monitor sales, compare brands, and be selective when purchasing "convenience" foods, which tend to be expensive. Other techniques for keeping food costs down without jeopardizing quality include buying food in season, using bulk foods when appropriate, using whole-grain or enriched products, buying lower-grade eggs (grading has no relation to the egg's nutritional value but indicates color of the shell and delicacy of flavor), and avoiding fancy grades of food and foods in elaborate packaging.

Community-Based Nursing Care

Food is a significant portion of a family's budget and meeting nutritional needs may be a challenge for families on limited incomes. Community-based services offered through clinics, local agencies, schools, and volunteer organizations are effective in addressing these needs. Increasingly, nurses play an important role in managing such community-based services, especially those services focusing on patient education. In addition, most communities offer special assistance to qualifying families to meet their nutritional needs. The Supplemental Nutrition Assistance Program (SNAP), formerly referred to as the Food Stamp Program, provides an electronic benefit transfer or EBT card, which is similar to a debit card, for participating households whose net monthly income is below a specified level. This card can be used to purchase food for the household each month.

The Special Supplemental Nutrition Program for Women, Infants, and Children (WIC) is designed to assist low-income pregnant, postpartum, or breastfeeding women and their children under 5 years of age. To be eligible, applicants must meet income guidelines (income at or below 185% of the U.S. poverty level), meet state residency requirements, and be individually determined to be nutritionally at risk by a healthcare professional (Food and Nutrition Service, 2016). The program provides food assistance, nutrition education, and referrals to healthcare providers. The food distributed—including dried beans and peas, peanut butter, eggs, cheese, milk, fortified adult and infant cereals, juice, and iron-fortified infant formula—is designed to provide good sources of iron, protein, and certain vitamins for individuals with an inadequate diet. Participation in the WIC program during pregnancy and infancy is associated with a reduced risk of infant death. In addition, the WIC program is credited with helping reduce the incidence of low birth weight in newborns and in decreasing the incidence of anemia in the infants and young children of low-income families.

Evaluation

Once a plan has been developed and implemented, you and the patient may wish to identify ways of evaluating its effectiveness. Evaluation may involve keeping a food journal, writing out weekly menus, returning weekly for weighing, and the like. If anemia is a special problem, periodic hematocrit assessments are also indicated.

Women with serious nutritional deficiencies are referred to a dietitian. You can then work closely with the dietitian and the patient to improve the pregnant woman's health by modifying her diet.

Focus Your Study

- Maternal weight gains averaging 11.5 to 16 kg (25 to 35 lb) for a normal-weight woman are associated with the best reproductive outcomes.
- If the diet is adequate, folic acid and iron are the only supplements generally recommended during pregnancy.
- Women should not restrict caloric intake to reduce weight during pregnancy.
- Pregnant women should be encouraged to eat regularly and to eat a wide variety of foods, especially fresh and lightly processed foods.
- Taking megadoses of vitamins during pregnancy is unnecessary and potentially dangerous.
- Pregnant women who eat vegetarian diets should place special emphasis on obtaining ample proteins, calories, calcium, iron, vitamin D, vitamin B_{12}, and zinc through food sources or supplementation if necessary.
- Pregnant women should avoid eating fish such as swordfish, shark, tilefish, or king mackerel, which contain high levels of mercury, and should limit their intake of fish that are lower in mercury.
- Food safety and sanitation should be a priority when preparing and storing food; foods that are known to cause foodborne illness should be avoided during pregnancy.
- Evaluation of physical, psychosocial, and cultural factors that affect food intake is essential before the nurse can determine nutritional status and plan nutritional counseling.
- Adolescents who become pregnant less than 4 years after menarche have higher nutritional needs and are considered to be at high biologic risk.
- Weight gains during adolescent pregnancy must accommodate recommended gains for a normal pregnancy plus necessary gains due to growth.
- After childbirth, the formula-feeding mother's dietary requirements return to prepregnancy levels.
- Breastfeeding mothers require an additional 200 calories above pregnancy intake and increased fluid intake to maintain ample milk volume.

In order to make safe and effective judgments using NANDA-I © 2017 nursing diagnoses, it is essential that nurses refer to the definitions and defining characteristics of the diagnoses used in this text, which can be found in Appendix C.

References

American College of Obstetricians and Gynecologists (ACOG). (2014). *Ethical issues in the care of the obese woman* (Committee Opinion No. 600). Washington, DC: Author.

American College of Obstetricians and Gynecologists (ACOG). (2015a). *Vitamin D: Screening and supplementation during pregnancy* (Committee Opinion No. 495). Washington, DC: Author.

American College of Obstetricians and Gynecologists (ACOG). (2015b). *Weight gain during pregnancy* (Committee Opinion No. 548, issued 2013, reaffirmed 2015.). Washington, DC: Author.

American College of Obstetricians and Gynecologists (ACOG). (reaffirmed 2018). *Obesity in pregnancy* (ACOG Practice Bulletin No. 156, issued 2015, reaffirmed 2018). Washington, DC: Author.

Beaudrot, M. E., Elchert, J. A., & DeFranco, E. A. (2016). Influence of gestational weight gain and BMI on cesarean delivery risk in adolescent pregnancies. *Journal of Perinatology, 36,* 612–617.

Breda, J. J., Whiting, S. H., Encarnação, R., Norberg, S., Jones, R., Reinap, M., & Jewell, J. (2014). Energy drink consumption in Europe: A review of the risks, adverse health effects, and policy options to respond. *Frontiers in Public Health.* Retrieved from http://dx.doi.org/10.3389/fpubh.2014.00134

Centers for Disease Control and Prevention (CDC). (2016). *Folic acid: Recommendations.* Retrieved from http://www.cdc.gov/ncbddd/folicacid/recommendations.html

Food and Drug Administration (FDA). (2016a). *Food safety for moms-to-be: While you're pregnant—listeria.* Retrieved from http://www.fda.gov/Food/FoodborneIllnessContaminants/PeopleAtRisk/ucm083320.htm

Food and Drug Administration (FDA). (2016b). *How sweet it is: All about sugar substitutes.* Retrieved from http://www.fda.gov/forconsumers/consumerupdates/ucm397711.htm

Food and Nutrition Service. (2016). *WIC eligibility requirements.* Retrieved from http://www.fns.usda.gov/wic/wic-eligibility-requirements

Institute of Medicine (IOM). (2009). *Weight gain during pregnancy: Reexamining the guidelines.* Retrieved from https://www.ncbi.nlm.nih.gov/pubmed/20669500

Institute of Medicine (IOM). (2010). *Dietary reference intakes (DRIs): Recommended dietary allowances and adequate intakes, vitamins and elements.* Washington, DC: Food and Nutrition Board, Institute of Medicine, National Academies.

Niebyl, J. R., Weber, R. J., & Briggs, G. G. (2017). Drugs and environmental agents in pregnancy and lactation: Teratology, epidemiology. In S. G. Gabbe, J. R. Niebyl, J. L. Simpson, M. B. Landon, H. L. Galan, E. R. M. Jauniaux, . . . W.A. Grobman (Eds.), *Obstetrics: Normal and problem pregnancies* (7th ed., pp.136–159). Philadelphia, PA: Elsevier.

Spector, R. E. (2017). *Cultural diversity in health and illness* (9th ed.). Hoboken, NJ: Pearson.

U.S. Department of Agriculture (USDA). (2015). *Eating fish while you are pregnant or breastfeeding.* Retrieved from https://www.choosemyplate.gov/moms-food-safety-fish

U.S. Department of Health and Human Services & U.S. Department of Agriculture (USHHS & USDA). (2015). *Dietary guidelines for Americans, 2015–2020* (8th ed.). Retrieved from http://health.gov/dietaryguidelines/2015/guidelines

West, E. H., Hark, L., & Catalano, P. M. (2017). Nutrition during pregnancy. In S. G. Gabbe, J. R. Niebyl, J. L. Simpson, M. B. Landon, H. L. Galan, E. R. M. Jauniaux, . . . W. A. Grobman (Eds.), *Obstetrics: Normal and problem pregnancies* (7th ed., pp.122–135). Philadelphia, PA: Elsevier.

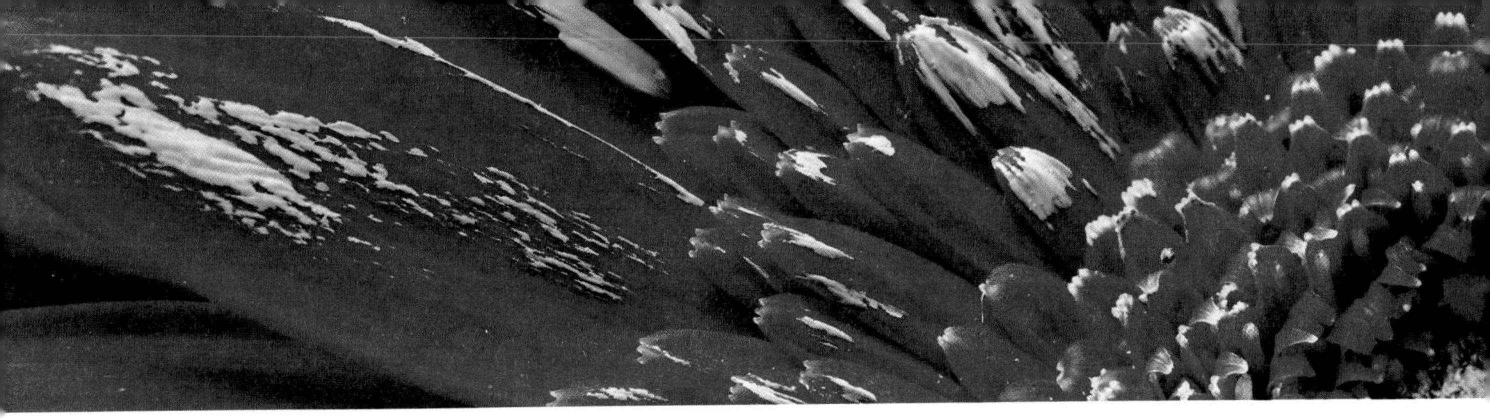

Chapter 15

Pregnancy in Selected Populations

Life is strange. I am 38 years old and 7 months pregnant with my first son. I am also the doting grandmother of a beautiful 3-month-old boy. I had my daughter when I was 16. My husband and I are excited about this baby, but it is disconcerting to realize that my son and grandson will be in the same grade in school.

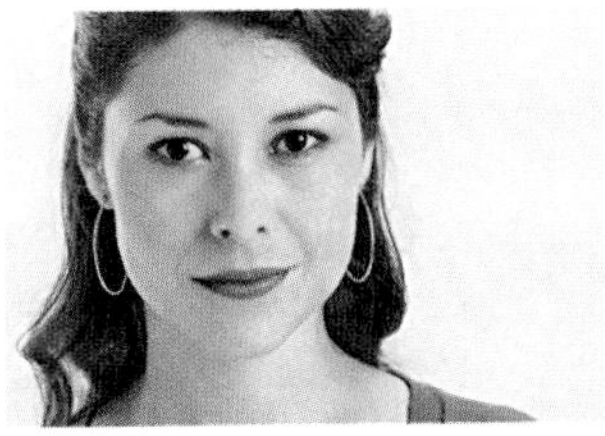

SOURCE: Hola Images/Alamy Stock Photo.

Learning Outcomes

15.1 Describe the scope of the problem and the impact of adolescent pregnancy.

15.2 Identify the physical, psychologic, and sociologic risks a pregnant adolescent faces.

15.3 Delineate the characteristics of the fathers of children of adolescent mothers.

15.4 Discuss the possible reactions of the adolescent's family and social network to her pregnancy.

15.5 Describe successful community approaches to prevention of adolescent pregnancy.

15.6 Identify factors that have contributed to the increased incidence of pregnancy in women over 35 years of age.

15.7 Summarize the nursing care needs of an expectant woman over age 35.

15.8 Discuss general healthcare risks that a woman with a significant chronic physical disability might face during pregnancy.

15.9 Identify the key needs of a pregnant woman with an intellectual disability.

Healthy People 2020

(FP-8) Reduce pregnancies among adolescent females

(FP-9) Increase the proportion of adolescents aged 17 years and under who have never had sexual intercourse

(FP-12) Increase the proportion of adolescents who received formal instruction on reproductive health topics before they were 18 years old

While pregnancy is a normal process, for certain women it carries increased risk. This is especially true for adolescents, pregnant women over age 35, and women with physical and/or mental disabilities. This chapter focuses on their needs and care.

Adolescent Pregnancy

In the United States teenage childbearing has declined steadily over the last few decades. In 2016, the birth rate (number of births per 1000 women) for adolescents ages 15 to 19 fell to 20.3, a historic low level, specifically the lowest rate reported in over half a century (Hamilton, Martin, Osterman, et al., 2017). See Figure 15–1. Equally significant, these declines occurred for all race and Hispanic origin groups. These declines cannot be attributed to an increase in the incidence of abortion because the number of abortions has decreased as the number of pregnancies has decreased. However, this steady decline may be attributed to improvements in contraceptive technology coupled with increased educational and labor market opportunities for women (Kearney & Levine, 2015). From a public policy perspective, research indicates that the expansion of family planning services through income-based

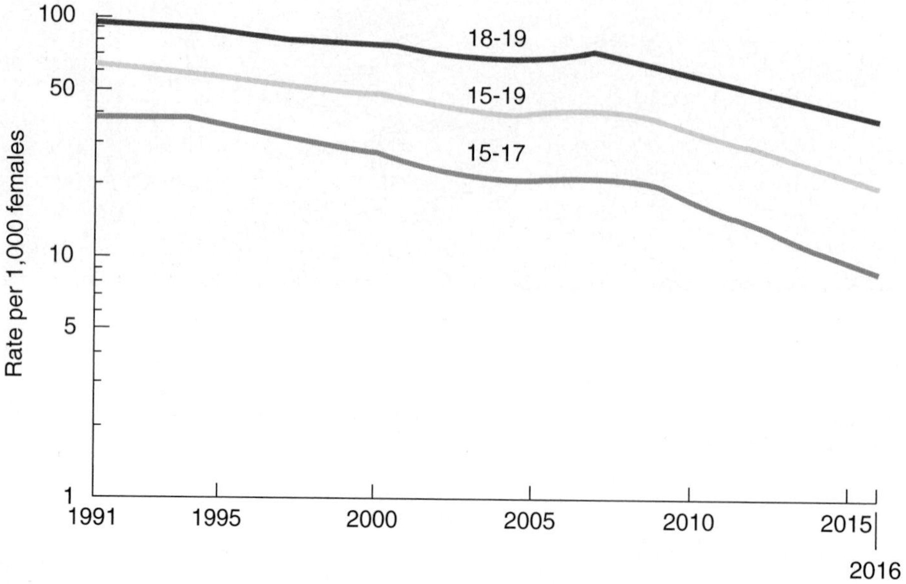

Figure 15–1 **Birth rates for teenagers ages 15–19 by age group: United States, final 1991–2015 and provisional 2016.**

Note: Rates are plotted on a logarithmic scale.

SOURCE: *NCHS, National Vital Statistics System. Retrieved from* https://www.cdc.gov/nchs/data/vsrr/report002.pdf

waivers to the Medicaid program and falling welfare benefit levels have also had a small impact (12.6%) on the total decline in teen birth rates (Kearney & Levine, 2015).

During the past decade there has not been a significant change in the overall proportion of teens who are sexually active. The decline in the birth rate of U.S. teenagers seems to be primarily attributable to improvements in their access to and use of contraceptives (Lindberg, Santelli, & Desai, 2016). Improved comprehensive sex education programs, messages in the media, the AIDS crisis, and a shift in fertility patterns as more women delay marriage may also be factors (Boonstra, 2014).

Even with this recent decline in adolescent pregnancies, the U.S. teenage birth rate remains one of the highest of any industrialized nation (exceeded only by Bulgaria's [41.7] and Romania's [35.2]), almost twice as high as that of Canada (14.1) and six times as high as that of the Netherlands (4.8) (Ventura, Hamilton, & Mathews, 2014). Although levels of sexual activity are similar among teens in the United States and in Europe, European teens are more likely to use contraceptives and to choose the most effective methods. Thus, their pregnancy rates are significantly lower (Guttmacher Institute, 2017).

Overview of the Adolescent Period

Developmentally, teens undergo many physical and psychosocial changes during the adolescent period.

PHYSICAL CHANGES

Puberty—that period during which an individual becomes capable of reproduction—is a maturational process that can last from 1.5 to 6 years. The major physical changes of puberty include a growth spurt, weight change, and the appearance of secondary sexual characteristics. **Menarche**, or the time of the first menstrual period, usually occurs in the last half of this maturational process, with the average age between 12 and 13. The initial menstrual cycles are usually irregular and often anovulatory, although not always. Thus, contraception is important for all sexually active adolescents.

PSYCHOSOCIAL DEVELOPMENT

Many authorities have described the developmental tasks of adolescence, based on a variety of classic theories. The following are major developmental tasks of this period (Steinberg, 2017):

- Developing a sense of identity
- Gaining autonomy and independence
- Developing intimacy in a relationship
- Developing comfort with one's own sexuality
- Developing a sense of achievement.

Resolution of these tasks is a developmental process that occurs over time. Although average ages for the completion of tasks have been identified, these ages are somewhat arbitrary and are affected by many factors, including culture, religion, and socioeconomic status.

In **early adolescence** (ages 14 and under), teens still see authority in their parents. However, they begin the process of gaining independence from the family by spending more time with friends. Conformity to peer group standards is important. Adolescents in this phase are very egocentric and are concrete thinkers, with only a minimal ability to see themselves in the future or to foresee the consequences of their behavior. Teens perceive their locus of control as external; that is, their destinies are controlled by others such as parents and school authorities.

Middle adolescence (ages 15 to 17 years) is the time for challenging; experimenting with drugs, alcohol, and sex are common avenues for rebellion. Middle adolescents seek independence and turn increasingly to their peer groups. They begin to move from concrete thinking to formal operational thought, but they are not yet able to anticipate the long-term implications of all their actions. These years are often a time of great turmoil for the family as the adolescent struggles for independence and challenges the family's values and expectations.

In **late adolescence** (ages 18 to 19 years) teens are more at ease with their individuality and decision-making ability. They can think abstractly and anticipate consequences. Late adolescents are capable of formal operational thought. They learn to solve problems, to conceptualize, and to make decisions. These abilities help them see themselves as having control, which leads to the ability to understand and accept the consequences of their behavior.

Factors Contributing to Adolescent Pregnancy

A number of things may be contributive to adolescent pregnancy, including socioeconomic, cultural, behavioral, and psychosocial factors. See *Evidence-Based Practice: Risk Factors for Adolescent Pregnancy*.

SOCIOECONOMIC AND CULTURAL FACTORS

Poverty is a major risk factor for adolescent pregnancy. Adolescents who do not have access to middle-class opportunities tend to maintain their pregnancies because they see pregnancy as their only option for adult status. Then, too, the lack of economic opportunity and the social marginalization that comes with poverty may contribute to hopelessness about the future and the ability to achieve desired or valued outcomes (Fedorowicz, Hellerstedt, Schreiner, et al., 2014).

In the United States, the adolescent birth rate is higher among African American teens and Hispanic teens than among White teens. To some degree, the higher teenage pregnancy rate in these groups reflects the impact of poverty because a disproportionately high number of African American and Hispanic youths live in poverty (Yoost, Hertweck, & Barnett, 2014).

Social connections are a significant factor in preventing teen pregnancy. Teens from warm, nurturing families who value future accomplishments and are engaged in academic pursuits are less likely to engage in risky sexual behavior (Kogan et al., 2013). Teens with future goals (i.e., college or job) tend to use birth control more consistently compared with other teens; if they become pregnant, they are also more likely to have abortions.

The younger the teen when she first gets pregnant, the more likely she is to have another pregnancy in her teens. Just over one-third (35%) of adolescents who have had an abortion or recent birth become pregnant again within 2 years (Baldwin & Edelman, 2013). The likelihood of repeat pregnancies increases when the teen is living with her sexual partner and has dropped out of school. Daughters of adolescent mothers are 22% more likely to become teen mothers themselves as compared to their peers (TeenHelp.com, 2016).

Developing Cultural Competence Impact of Education on Marriage and Childbearing

Throughout the world, the higher a woman's educational level, the more likely she is to delay marriage and childbirth.

Internationally, female adolescents who are married are more likely to welcome a pregnancy in countries in which Islam is the predominant religion, where large families are desired, where social change is slow in coming, and where most childbearing occurs within marriage. Early pregnancy is less desired in countries in which the reverse is true.

HIGH-RISK BEHAVIORS

Developmentally, adolescents, especially younger ones, are not yet able to foresee the consequences of their actions. As a result, they may have a sense of invulnerability that leads to the mistaken idea that harm will not befall them. This sense of invulnerability may also result in an overly optimistic view of the risks associated with their actions.

Among American adolescents there is great peer pressure to become sexually active during the teen years. Premarital sexual activity is commonplace, and teenage pregnancy is more socially

EVIDENCE-BASED PRACTICE | Risk Factors for Adolescent Pregnancy

Clinical Question

What are risk factors for adolescent pregnancy in vulnerable populations?

The Evidence

Unplanned pregnancy for an adolescent can result in a host of adverse outcomes for both mother and baby. These risks are even higher among vulnerable populations. Two research studies focused on identifiable risk factors in specific vulnerable populations in an effort to target preventive efforts effectively. Researchers conducted an integrated literature review of 18 research studies that identified risk factors for teen pregnancy among African American adolescents. A second study used a predictive model to study risk factors among nearly 300 adolescents in the child welfare system/foster homes. Taken together, these studies form a strong basis of evidence. Lee, Cintron, and Kocher (2014) found that five major factors contributed to adolescent pregnancy among African American youth: Substance use, gender roles, peer influences, parental involvement, and level of knowledge about sexual health. Of these, substance use was also a predictive factor for teens in the welfare system, but in this population, delinquency was also a risk factor (Hefrich & McWey, 2014). In the latter study, the timing of pregnancy was also identified; pregnancy occurred, on average, within 3 years of a predictive event.

Best Practice

Knowing specific predictive factors for a population enables the development of risk-specific educational programs for the prevention of adolescent pregnancy. These data suggest that supports need to be wide-reaching and include reducing substance abuse, encouraging parental involvement, and integration of peer support into interventions.

Clinical Reasoning

How can the nurse determine risk factors of teen pregnancy for a specific population? How can parents and peers be involved in adolescent pregnancy prevention programs?

acceptable today than it was in the past. Research indicates that young people have sex for the first time around age 17, although 44% of unmarried females and 49% of unmarried males ages 15 to 19 have had sexual intercourse (Guttmacher Institute, 2017). Sexual innuendo permeates every aspect of the popular media, but issues of sexual responsibility are commonly ignored.

Texting is a form of flirting and social behavior that has become commonplace among teens and young adults. Of particular note is the current blend of "sex and text," called *sexting*, in which teens and young adults share semi-nude or nude pictures of themselves or others using cell phones, websites, and social media networks. Sexting is associated with an increased likelihood of being sexually active and of engaging in risky sexual behavior such as using drugs and alcohol before sex and having unprotected sex. Individuals in a romantic relationship are more likely to engage in sexting (Klettke, Hallford, & Mellor, 2014).

High-risk sexual behaviors including multiple partners and lack of contraceptive use are of concern. Research indicates that young people 15 to 24 years of age account for half of all new cases of sexually transmitted infections (STIs) and that among sexually active female teens, one in four has an STI such as chlamydia or human papillomavirus (HPV) (Centers for Disease Control and Prevention [CDC], 2016). This is particularly worrisome because many STIs, including human immunodeficiency virus (HIV), are asymptomatic. Thus, apparently healthy young people who are infected may not have a reason to seek healthcare.

Statistics have demonstrated an increased use of condoms among the adolescent population, with 68% of females ages 15 to 19 and 80% of males using condoms during their first sexual intercourse, probably because of the tremendous educational efforts related to HIV infection (Guttmacher Institute, 2017). Adolescents, however, remain inconsistent contraceptive users. Many teens lack accurate and adequate knowledge about contraceptive options. This is a common topic of sex education programs; nevertheless, debate continues about the appropriateness of such programs in schools. Proponents advocate early sex education to provide teens with the knowledge they need to avoid unwanted pregnancy and the risk of STIs. Opponents feel that sex education is the responsibility of parents and worry that sex education in the schools will promote sexual activity. However, a review of research on comprehensive sex education reveals that it does not increase initiation of sexual activity at an earlier age. In fact, it helps delay the start of sexual activity, increases condom or contraceptive use, reduces the number of sexual partners and the frequency of sex, and reduces sexual risk taking (Boonstra, 2014). Other factors affecting the use of contraception include access or availability, cost of supplies, and concern about confidentiality.

PSYCHOSOCIAL FACTORS

Pregnancy desire tends to be higher among teens who are older, who were younger when they became sexually active, who are in a short-term relationship (which may be romanticized and intense), and who have greater perceived stress in their lives (Sipsma, Ickovics, Lewis, et al., 2011).

Family dysfunction and poor self-esteem are also major risk factors for adolescent pregnancy. Some young teenagers deliberately plan to get pregnant. A female adolescent may use pregnancy for various subconscious or conscious reasons: To punish her parents, to escape from an undesirable home situation, to gain attention, or to feel that she has someone to love and someone who loves her. Pregnancy may also be an adolescent's form of acting out. For others, pregnancy marks an important milestone that leads to enhanced maturity, better decision making, and healthier behaviors (Herrman & Nandakumar, 2012).

Evidence suggests that teens who have a history of sexual abuse, physical abuse, or neglect are more likely to give birth as a teenager than those who have not been maltreated (Garwood, Gerassi, Jonson-Reid, et al., 2015; Herrman, 2014). Teenage pregnancy can also result from an incestuous relationship. In the very young adolescent, incest or sexual abuse should be suspected as a possible cause of pregnancy. More teens who become pregnant, compared with teens who have never been pregnant, have been physically, emotionally, or sexually abused. In fact, maltreatment of any kind is a high-risk contributor to early teen pregnancy. Teenage pregnancy could also be caused by other nonvoluntary sexual experiences such as acquaintance rape.

Risks to the Adolescent Mother

The pregnant teen faces physical, psychologic, and sociologic risks that can profoundly impact her in both short-term and long-term ways.

PHYSIOLOGIC RISKS

Adolescents older than 15 years who receive early, thorough prenatal care are at no greater risk during pregnancy than women older than age 20. Unfortunately, adolescents often begin prenatal care later in pregnancy than other age groups. Thus, risks for pregnant adolescents include preterm births, low-birth-weight newborns, cephalopelvic disproportion, iron deficiency anemia, and preeclampsia and its sequelae. In the adolescent age group, prenatal care is the critical factor that most influences pregnancy outcome.

Teenagers ages 15 to 19 have a high incidence of STIs, including herpesvirus, syphilis, and gonorrhea. The incidence of chlamydial infection is also increased in this age group. The presence of such infections during a pregnancy greatly increases the risk to the fetus. Other problems seen in adolescents are cigarette smoking and drug use. By the time pregnancy is confirmed, the fetus may already have been harmed by these substances.

PSYCHOLOGIC RISKS

The major psychologic risk to the pregnant adolescent is the interruption of her developmental tasks. Adding the tasks of pregnancy to her own developmental tasks creates a huge amount of psychologic work, the completion of which will affect the adolescent's and her newborn's futures. Table 15–1 suggests typical behaviors of the adolescent when she becomes aware of her pregnancy. In reviewing these behaviors, the nurse should realize that other factors may influence individual response.

SOCIOLOGIC RISKS

Being forced into adult roles before completing adolescent developmental tasks causes a series of events that may result in prolonged dependence on parents, lack of stable relationships with the opposite sex, and lack of economic and social stability. Many teenage mothers have their schooling interrupted or drop out of school. Research indicates that teen mothers are less likely to graduate from high school and to enroll in and finish college. In fact, only 38% of teenage mothers age 15 to 17 earn a high school diploma and by age 30 only 1.5% of women who gave birth as adolescents have earned a college degree (TeenHelp.com, 2016). In addition, teenage mothers are more likely to have big families and more likely to be single. Lack of education in turn reduces the quality of jobs available and leads to more tenuous employment and increased poverty. In addition, research reveals that 80% of unmarried adolescent mothers become welfare dependent (TeenHelp.com, 2016).

TABLE 15–1 Initial Reaction to Awareness of Pregnancy

AGE	ADOLESCENT BEHAVIOR	NURSING IMPLICATIONS
Early adolescent (14 years and younger)	Fears rejection by family and peers. Enters healthcare system with an adult, most likely mother (parents still seen as locus of control). Value system closely reflects that of parents, so teen turns to parents for decisions or approval of decisions. Pregnancy probably not a result of intimate relationship. Self-conscious about normal adolescent changes in body. Self-consciousness and low self-esteem likely to increase with rapid breast enlargement and abdominal enlargement of pregnancy.	Be nonjudgmental in approach to care. Focus on needs and concerns of adolescent, but if parent accompanies daughter, include parent in plan of care. Encourage both to express concerns and feelings regarding pregnancy and options: Abortion, maintaining pregnancy, adoption. Be realistic in discussing implications of each option. During physical exam of adolescent, respect increased sense of modesty. Explain in simple and concrete terms physical changes that are produced by pregnancy versus puberty. Explain each step of physical exam in simple and concrete terms.
Middle adolescent (15–17 years)	Fears rejection by peers and parents. Unsure of whom to confide in. May seek confirmation of pregnancy on own with increased awareness of options and services, such as over-the-counter pregnancy kits and Planned Parenthood. If in an ongoing, caring relationship with partner (peer), may choose him as confidant. Economic dependence on parents may determine if and when parents are told. Future educational plans and perception of parental support or lack of support are significant factors in decision regarding termination or maintenance of the pregnancy. Possible conflict between parental and own developing value system.	Be nonjudgmental in approach to care. Reassure the adolescent that confidentiality will be maintained. Help adolescent identify significant individuals in whom she can confide to help make a decision about the pregnancy. Be aware of state laws regarding requirement of parental notification if abortion intended. Also be aware of state laws regarding requirements for marriage: Usually, minimum age for both parties is 18; 16- and 17-year-olds are, in most states, allowed to marry only with consent of parents. Encourage adolescent to be realistic about parental response to pregnancy.
Late adolescent (18–19 years)	Most likely to confirm pregnancy on own and at an earlier date due to increased acceptance and awareness of consequences of behavior. Likely to use pregnancy kit for confirmation. Relationship with father of baby, future educational plans, and personal value system are among significant determinants of decision about pregnancy.	Be nonjudgmental in approach to care. Reassure the adolescent that confidentiality will be maintained. Encourage adolescent to identify significant individuals in whom she can confide. Refer to counseling as appropriate. Encourage adolescent to be realistic about parental response to pregnancy.

Some pregnant adolescents choose to marry the father of the baby, who may also be a teenager. Unfortunately, most adolescent marriages end in divorce. This fact should not be surprising because pregnancy and marriage interrupt the adolescents' childhood and basic education. Lack of maturity in dealing with an intimate relationship also contributes to marital breakdown.

Dating violence is often an issue for teens. When surveyed, 10.3% of adolescents reported some level of physical dating violence and 10.4% experienced some form of sexual dating violence ranging from touching to forced intercourse (Kann et al., 2014). The violence increases in pregnant teens. However, research suggests that this number is significantly lower than reality because teens are far less likely to report intimate partner violence than are adults.

The increased incidence of maternal complications, preterm birth, and low-birth-weight babies among teen mothers also affects society because many of these mothers are on welfare. The need for increased financial support for good prenatal care and nutritional programs remains critical.

In the United States, the results of teenage childbearing cost taxpayers $9.4 billion annually (Ventura et al., 2014). Much of this cost comes from Medicaid, state health department maternal care clinics, federal monies for Aid to Families with Dependent Children programs, the Supplemental Nutrition Assistance Program (SNAP), and direct payments to healthcare providers.

Table 15–2 identifies the early adolescent's response to the developmental tasks of pregnancy. Middle and older adolescents respond differently, reflecting their progression through developmental tasks. In addition to her maturational level, the amount of nurturing the pregnant adolescent receives is a critical factor in the way she handles pregnancy and motherhood.

Risks for the Child

Children of adolescent parents are at a disadvantage in many ways because teens are not developmentally or economically prepared to be parents. In general, children of teenage mothers are found to be at a developmental disadvantage compared with children whose mothers were older at the time of their birth. Many factors contribute to these differences, especially the adverse socioeconomic conditions many teenage mothers face. These factors result in high rates of family instability and behavior problems. In addition, these children do not do as well in school, are less likely to complete high school, and are more likely to be involved in delinquent activity, to become sexually active earlier, and to become an adolescent parent. This may reflect the social environment, specifically the reality that adolescent mothers are more likely than adult mothers to be single and poor (Steinberg, 2017). Children born to adolescent mothers also have higher rates of abuse and neglect (Ouaknine, 2016).

Partners of Adolescent Mothers

Over the past 40 years the proportion of adolescent births fathered by adult men has decreased, although teen mothers in poor, recently immigrated populations are especially likely to

TABLE 15–2 The Early Adolescent's Response to the Developmental Tasks of Pregnancy

STAGE	DEVELOPMENTAL TASKS OF PREGNANCY	EARLY ADOLESCENT'S RESPONSE TO PREGNANCY	NURSING IMPLICATIONS
First trimester	Pregnancy confirmation. Seeks early prenatal care as a confirmation tool. Begins to evaluate her diet and general health habits. Initial ambivalence common. Usually supportive partner.	May delay confirmation of pregnancy until late first trimester or later. Reasons for delay may include lack of awareness that she is pregnant, fear of confiding in anyone, and/or denial. Rapid enlargement and sensitivity of breasts are embarrassing and frightening to early adolescents—may be perceived as changes of puberty. If confiding in mother, may be experiencing family turmoil in response to pregnancy.	Explain physiologic changes of pregnancy versus those associated with puberty. Explain that ambivalence is normal with any pregnancy, but recognize it as a much greater concern with adolescent pregnancy. Emphasize need for good nutrition as important for her well-being as much as baby's (prevention of preeclampsia and anemia). Use simple explanations and lots of audiovisual aids. Have adolescent listen to fetal heart rate with Doppler.
Second trimester	Changes in physical appearance begin, and fetal movement is experienced, causing pregnancy to be experienced as a reality. Begins wearing maternity clothes to accommodate the physical changes. As a result of quickening, she perceives her fetus as a real baby and begins preparing for the maternal role and new relationships with her partner and members of her family.	Some teenagers may delay validation of pregnancy until now, with family turmoil occurring at this time. Abdominal enlargement and quickening may be perceived as loss of control over body image. May try to maintain prepregnant weight and wear restrictive clothing to control and conceal changing body. Becomes dependent on her own mother for support. Egocentric; unable to develop a maternal role at this time.	Continue to discuss importance of good nutrition and adequate weight gain as noted above. Discuss ways of wearing common teenage clothing (large sweatshirts, blouses) to promote comfort but preserve adolescent image to some degree. Discuss plans being made for baby, continued educational plans, and role of teen's parents. Explain physiologic changes of pregnancy versus those associated with puberty. Explain that ambivalence is normal with any pregnancy, but recognize it as a much greater concern with adolescent pregnancy.
Third trimester	At end of second trimester, begins to view fetus as separate from self. Buys baby clothes and supplies. Prepares a place for the baby. Realistic about what baby is like. Prepares to give birth to baby. Anxiety increases as labor and birth approach and has concerns about well-being of fetus.	May focus on "wanting it to be over." May have trouble individuating fetus. May have fantasies, dreams, or nightmares about childbirth. Natural fears of labor and birth greater than with older primigravida. Probably has not been in a hospital, and may associate this with negative experiences.	Assess whether adolescent is preparing for baby by buying supplies and preparing a place in the home. Childbirth education is important. Provide hospital tour. Assess for discomforts of pregnancy, such as heartburn and constipation. Adolescent may be uncomfortable mentioning these and other problems.

have older partners. On average, the age difference between teenage mothers and their partners is about 2 to 3 years (Steinberg, 2017). Adolescent males tend to become sexually active at an earlier age than females, and they have more sexual partners in their teenage years. When the father is an adolescent, he too has uncompleted developmental tasks for his age group and is no better prepared psychologically than his female counterpart to deal with the consequences of pregnancy. Teenage fathers are relatively more likely to have problems with school, self-esteem, drugs, alcohol, work, and aggression. They are also more likely to have been born to an adolescent father (Steinberg, 2017). Adolescent fatherhood may lead to a decrease in the years of schooling the male receives and it increases the rate of cohabitation and early marriage.

In general, adolescent males tend to view an unintended pregnancy as negative because of the impact on their aspirations, life goals, and current freedoms. Attitudes toward teen pregnancy tend to be more favorable among adolescent men of lower socioeconomic status and/or lower educational level (Lohan, Cruise, O'Halloran, et al., 2010).

The adolescent who attempts to assume his responsibility as a father faces many of the same psychologic and sociologic risks as the adolescent mother. The mother and father are generally from similar socioeconomic backgrounds and have similar educational levels.

Although they may not be married, many adolescent couples have meaningful relationships. The male partners may be very involved in the pregnancy and may be present for the birth. In situations in which the adolescent father wants to assume some responsibility, healthcare providers should support him in his decision. It is also important to ensure that the pregnant adolescent has the opportunity to decide for herself whether she wants the father to participate in her healthcare.

Biological fathers are included on birth certificates far more frequently today than in the past. This inclusion helps ensure the fathers' rights and encourages them to meet their responsibilities to their children. In addition, legal paternity gives children access to military and Social Security benefits and to medical information about their fathers. In some situations, the pregnant adolescent may not want to identify or contact the father of the baby, and the male may not readily acknowledge paternity. Those situations include rape, exploitative sexual relations, incest, and casual sexual relations. If healthcare providers suspect any of the first three causes, further investigation into the situation is important for the well-being of the pregnant adolescent, and referral to other resources should be made as appropriate.

Even if the adolescent father has been included in the healthcare of the young woman throughout the pregnancy, it is not unusual for her to want her mother as her primary support person during labor and birth. Younger adolescents are especially likely to choose their mothers for this role. It is important to support the pregnant adolescent's wishes and to acknowledge and support the adolescent father's wishes as appropriate.

Father love is an important predictor of a child's well-being. Children whose fathers are involved and loving are more likely to have healthy self-esteem, do well in school, and avoid drug use and criminal activity than those children with fathers who are uninvolved (Kirven, 2014). Therefore, it behooves healthcare professionals to do what they can to support the efforts of adolescent fathers to be effective.

As a part of counseling, the nurse should assess the young man's stressors, his support systems, his plans for involvement in the pregnancy and childbearing, and his future plans. He should be referred to social services for counseling about his educational and vocational future. When the father is involved in the pregnancy, the young mother feels less deserted, more confident in her decision making, and better able to discuss her future.

Reactions of Family and Social Network to Adolescent Pregnancy

The reactions of families and support groups to adolescent pregnancy vary widely. In families that foster children's educational and career goals, adolescent pregnancy is often a shock. Anger, shame, and sorrow are common reactions. The majority of pregnant adolescents from these families are likely to choose abortion, with the exception of teens whose cultural and religious beliefs prevent them from seeking abortions.

In populations in which adolescent pregnancy is more prevalent and more socially acceptable, family and friends may be more supportive of the adolescent parents. In many cases the teen's friends and mother are present at the birth. The expectant parents may also have friends who are already teen parents. Some male partners of these adolescent mothers see pregnancy and the birth of a baby as signs of adult status and increased sexual prowess—a source of pride.

The mother of the pregnant adolescent is usually among the first to be told about the pregnancy. She typically becomes involved with decision making, especially with the young adolescent, about issues such as maintaining the pregnancy, abortion, and dealing with the father-to-be and his family.

Once the pregnant adolescent decides how to proceed, it is often her mother who helps her access healthcare, and her mother's support is essential if the teen self-image is to grow to include the notion of herself as "mother" (Turnage & Pharris, 2013). If the pregnancy is maintained, the mother may participate in prenatal care and classes and can be an excellent source of support for her daughter. She should be encouraged to participate if the mother–daughter relationship is positive. If the baby's father is involved in the pregnancy, he and the pregnant adolescent's mother may be able to work together to support the teenage mother. The nurse can update the pregnant adolescent's mother on current childbearing practices to clarify any misconceptions she might have. During labor and birth, the mother may be a key figure for her daughter, offering reassurance and instilling confidence in the teen.

The younger the adolescent when she gives birth, the more she needs her mother's support. Children of adolescent parents experience more negative outcomes, including more aggressive behavior at a younger age, when the adolescent is in constant conflict with her mother and becomes less involved in parenting.

“Miranda left for college last September. She was just 18, and I thought she had the world in front of her. At Thanksgiving she came home to tell us she was 4 months pregnant and planned to keep the baby even though she and Adam had broken up and he wanted no part of fatherhood. She finished the semester then moved back home to attend a state college near us. Emma was born 2 days after her mom finished the spring semester. Now Miranda's life is a juggling act—part-time job, part-time school, full-time mom. We help all we can. I am so sorry that my daughter has lost out on so much, but I am proud of the woman she has become.”

●○● NURSING MANAGEMENT

For the Adolescent Mother-to-Be

Nursing Assessment and Diagnosis

In working with adolescents, remember that oftentimes the nurse is the first contact with the healthcare system that the adolescent has. Then, too, many adolescents have never before accessed healthcare without a parent. Establish a knowledge base to plan interventions for the adolescent mother-to-be and family. Areas of assessment include history of family and personal physical health, developmental level and impact of pregnancy, and emotional and financial support. Also assess the family and social support network and the father's degree of involvement in the pregnancy.

As with all pregnant women, it is important to have information on the teen's general physical health. This may be the first time the adolescent has ever provided a health history. Consequently, it may be helpful to ask specific questions and give examples if the young woman appears confused about a question. The teen's mother may be best able to answer questions about family history because the adolescent is often unaware of this information.

The following areas should be assessed:

- Family and personal health history
- Medical history
- Menstrual history
- Obstetric and gynecologic history
- Substance abuse history.

It is important to assess the maturational level of each person. The adolescent's development level and the impact of pregnancy are reflected in the degree of recognition of the realities and responsibilities involved in teenage pregnancy and parenting. Also assess the teen mother's self-concept (including body image), her relationship with the significant adults in her life, her attitude toward her pregnancy, and her coping methods in the situation, as well as the teen's knowledge of, attitude toward, and anticipated ability to care for the coming baby. Ask specifically about dating violence. Teens are not likely to reveal dating violence unless they are asked about it.

The socioeconomic status of the pregnant adolescent often places the baby at risk throughout life, beginning with conception. It is essential to assess family and social support systems, as well as the extent of financial support available.

The nursing diagnoses applicable to pregnant women in general apply to the pregnant adolescent. Other nursing diagnoses are influenced by the adolescent's age, support systems, socioeconomic situation, health, and maturity. Examples of nursing diagnoses specific to the pregnant adolescent may include:

- ***Nutrition, Imbalanced: Less than Body Requirements***, related to poor eating habits
- ***Self-Esteem, Situational Low, Risk for***, related to unanticipated pregnancy

(NANDA-I © 2017)

Planning and Implementation

Community-Based Nursing Care

If pregnancy occurs, early, thorough prenatal care is the strongest and most critical determinant for reducing risk for the adolescent mother and her newborn. The nurse needs to understand the special needs of the adolescent mother to meet this challenge successfully.

Many new and innovative community-based programs have evolved to provide care for high-risk patients and their partners throughout the childbearing experience and beyond. Nurses in community-based agencies can help adolescents access the healthcare system as well as social services and other support services (e.g., food banks and the Special Supplemental Nutrition Program for Women, Infants, and Children [WIC]). These nurses are also involved extensively in counseling and patient teaching.

Teaching adolescents in groups according to their ages is often more effective for learning. In addition, many teens prefer teaching aids that are visual and that they can handle, such as realistic fetal models. Pregnant teens with low reading levels tend to prefer handouts and posters that have visual interest, short sentences, bulleted items, and white space.

Issue of Confidentiality

Most states have passed legislation that confirms the right of some minors to assume the rights of adults; they are then called **emancipated minors**. An adolescent may be considered emancipated if he or she is self-supporting and living away from home, married, pregnant, a parent, or in the military. Even if a minor has not become formally "emancipated," all 50 states permit confidential testing and treatment for sexually transmitted infections (STIs) but only 26 states and the District of Columbia explicitly permit all minors to consent to contraception without a parent's knowledge or consent; 20 states permit minors to consent to contraception in certain circumstances (Guttmacher Institute, 2018). Currently 37 states and the District of Columbia explicitly allow some minors to consent to prenatal care; of that group, 32 states allow all minors to give consent; 13 states have no relevant law or policy (Guttmacher Institute, 2018). Thirty states explicitly allow minors to give consent for their children's medical care; the remaining 20 states have no policy (Guttmacher Institute, 2018). See *Professionalism in Practice: Emancipated Minors.*

> **Professionalism in Practice Emancipated Minors**
>
> It is important to remember that if a pregnant minor is considered emancipated, she has the right and responsibility to consent to healthcare for herself and later for her child. She is entitled to respect and confidentiality in her dealings with healthcare providers. Only with her consent can other adults, including her parents, be included in communication.

Development of a Trusting Relationship with the Pregnant Adolescent

The first visit to the clinic or caregiver's office may make the young woman feel anxious and vulnerable. Making this first experience as positive as possible for the young woman will encourage the adolescent to return for follow-up care and to cooperate with her healthcare providers and will help her recognize the importance of healthcare for her and her baby (Figure 15–2). Developing a trusting relationship with the pregnant adolescent is essential. Honesty, respect, and a caring attitude promote self-esteem.

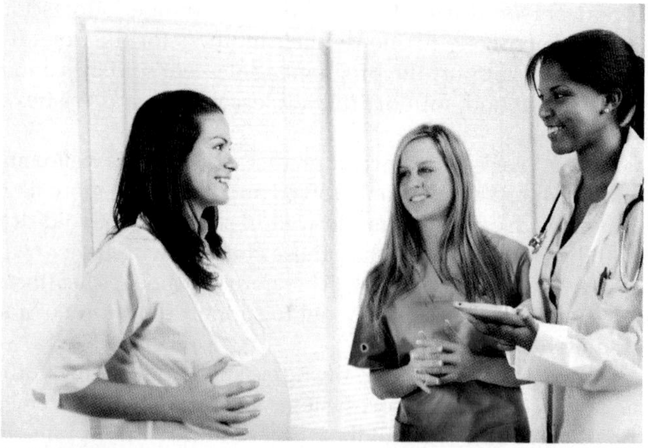

Figure 15–2 Nurses must work to develop a trusting relationship with a pregnant teen.

SOURCE: Pablocalvog/Fotolia.

> **Clinical Tip**
>
> During the initial pelvic examination, with the consent of the examiner, offer the teen a handheld mirror. A mirror is helpful in enabling the young woman to see her cervix, thus educating her about her anatomy. It also gives her an active role in the examination if she so desires.

Depending on the adolescent's age, this may be her first pelvic examination, an anxiety-provoking experience for any woman. Provide explanations during the procedure. A gentle and thoughtful examination technique will help the young woman to relax.

Promotion of Self-Esteem and Problem-Solving Skills

Assist the adolescent in her decision making and problem solving so that she can proceed with her developmental tasks and begin to assume responsibility for her life and that of her newborn. Many adolescents are not aware of the legally available options for handling an unplanned pregnancy. In an open, nonjudgmental way, without imposing personal values, educate the teen about her alternatives: Terminating the pregnancy, maintaining the pregnancy and parenting the baby, or relinquishing the baby for adoption. The nurse can also provide information about community resources available to help with each alternative. Once the teen has decided on a course of action, healthcare providers should respect her decision and support her efforts to achieve her goals. See *Case Study: Angelina Newman*.

Adolescents who choose to terminate a pregnancy cite reasons such as economic hardship or interference with school or a career. Teens most often involve their parents and their partners in the decision. Their involvement does not always indicate that they support the adolescent's decision. Research, however, indicates that a significant portion of pregnant teens report pressure from their mother, partner, or other family member to consider terminating the pregnancy. Teens are similar to adults in how

CASE STUDY: Angelina Newman

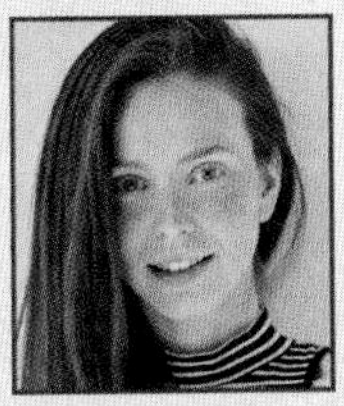

SOURCE: WAYHOME studio/Shutterstock

Angelina has recently become increasingly concerned about how she will support herself and her baby. Her long-term goals involve attending college and becoming a teacher. Her extended family members have urged her to consider adoption as an alternative to raising the baby herself. Her cousin is a social worker and has told her that it could be difficult to afford college, work a full-time job, and be active in raising the baby. Her mother and father have told her she can live at home with the baby, but they can't really help her out with child care as they both work. Her boyfriend has become less reassuring about their relationship since she has become less involved with attending parties and hanging out with friends once she learned she was pregnant. Angelina is beginning to talk about the possibility of adoption for her baby.

Questions to Ponder

What resources would you provide to Angelina as she is considering adoption? What are the potential emotional aspects of relinquishing a baby for adoption?

they experience abortion. They expect to feel a range of emotions and believe they are prepared to cope with them after the abortion (Ralph, Gould, Baker, et al., 2014).

If the adolescent chooses to continue her pregnancy, describe what she can expect over the prenatal period and provide an explanation and rationale for each procedure as it occurs. This overview fosters the adolescent's understanding and gives her some control.

Early adolescents tend to be egocentric and oriented to the present. They may not think it is important that their health and habits affect the fetus. Thus, it is often helpful to emphasize how these practices affect the teens themselves. Early adolescents also need help in problem solving and in visualizing the future so they can plan effectively.

Middle adolescents are developing the ability to think abstractly and can recognize that actions may have long-term consequences. They may not yet have acquired assertive communication skills, however, and may be reluctant to ask questions. Therefore, ask teens directly if they have questions. Middle adolescents can absorb more detailed health teaching and apply it.

Late adolescents can usually think abstractly, plan for the future, and function in a manner comparable to older pregnant women. They can also handle complex information and apply it.

Promotion of Physical Well-Being

Baseline weight and blood pressure measurements are valuable in assessing weight gain and predisposition to preeclampsia (Figure 15–3). Encourage the adolescent to take part in her care by measuring and recording her own weight. Use this time as an opportunity for assisting the young woman in problem solving. Encourage her to ask herself the following questions: "Have I gained too much or too little weight?" "What influence does my diet have on my weight?" "How can I change my eating habits?"

Introduce the subject of nutrition during measurement of baseline and subsequent hemoglobin and hematocrit values. Because the adolescent is at risk for anemia, she needs education about the importance of iron in her diet. Indeed, basic education about nutrition is a critical component of care for pregnant teens. See *Concept Map: Anemia in Pregnancy*.

Preeclampsia is the most prevalent medical complication of pregnant adolescents. Blood pressure readings of 140/90 mmHg are not acceptable as the determinant of preeclampsia in adolescents. Young women ages 14 to 20 years without evidence of high blood pressure usually have diastolic readings between 50 and 66 mmHg. Gradual increases from the prepregnant diastolic readings, along with excessive weight gain, must be evaluated as precursors to preeclampsia. Establishment of baseline readings is one reason early prenatal care is vital to management of the pregnant adolescent.

Adolescents have an increased incidence of STIs. The initial prenatal examination should include gonococcal and chlamydial cultures; wet-mount prep for *Candida*, *Trichomonas*, and *Gardnerella*; and tests for syphilis. Although today's teens are knowledgeable about HIV/AIDS, they know much less about other STIs, especially with regard to symptoms and risk reduction, so education is important. If the adolescent's history indicates that she is at increased risk for HIV, she should be given information about it and offered HIV screening.

Discuss substance abuse with the adolescent. It is important to review the risks associated with the use of tobacco, caffeine, drugs, and alcohol. The young woman should be aware of how these substances affect both her and her fetus's development.

Ongoing care should include the same assessments that an older pregnant woman receives. Pay special attention to evaluating fetal growth by determining when quickening occurs and by measuring fundal height, fetal heart rate, and fetal movement. If there is a question of size–date discrepancy by 2 cm either way when assessing fundal height, an ultrasound is warranted to

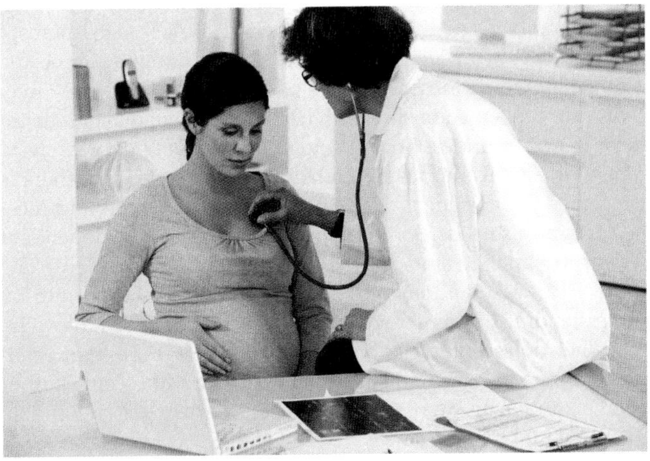

Figure 15–3 **The nurse carefully assesses this pregnant teen.**

SOURCE: Auremar/Fotolia.

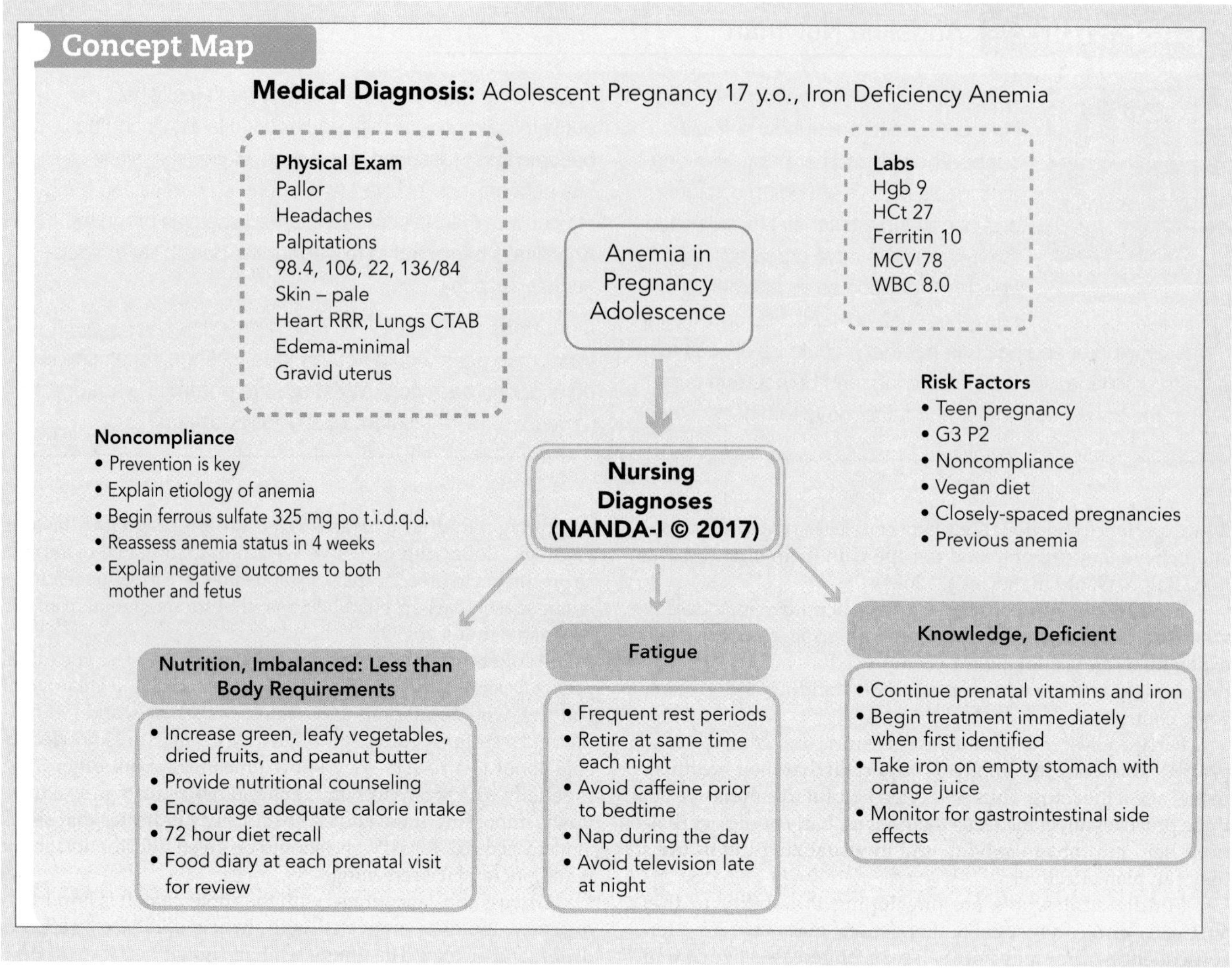

establish fetal age so that instances of intrauterine growth restriction can be detected early. See *Evidence-Based Practice: Estimating Gestational Age* in Chapter 12.

Promotion of Family Adaptation

Assess the family situation during the first prenatal visit and find out the level of involvement the adolescent wants from each of her family members and the father of the child, as well as her perception of their present support. If the mother and daughter agree, the mother should be included in the patient's care. Pregnancy may change a teen's relationship with her mother from one of antagonism to one of understanding and empathy. The opportunity to renew or establish a positive relationship with their mothers is welcomed by most teens. Help the teen's mother assess and meet her daughter's needs. Some adolescents become more dependent during pregnancy, and some become more independent. The mother can ease and encourage her daughter's self-growth by understanding how best to respond to and support the adolescent.

The adolescent's relationship with her father is also affected by her pregnancy. Provide information to the adolescent's father and encourage his involvement to whatever degree is acceptable to both daughter and father.

The father of the adolescent's baby should not be forgotten in promoting the family's adaptation to the pregnancy. He should be included in prenatal visits, classes, health teaching, and the birth itself to the extent that he wishes and that is acceptable to the teenage mother. He should also have the opportunity to express his feelings and concerns and to have his questions answered.

Most childbirth educators believe that prenatal classes with other teens are best, even though they can be challenging to teach (Figure 15–4). The pregnant teen may be accompanied by her

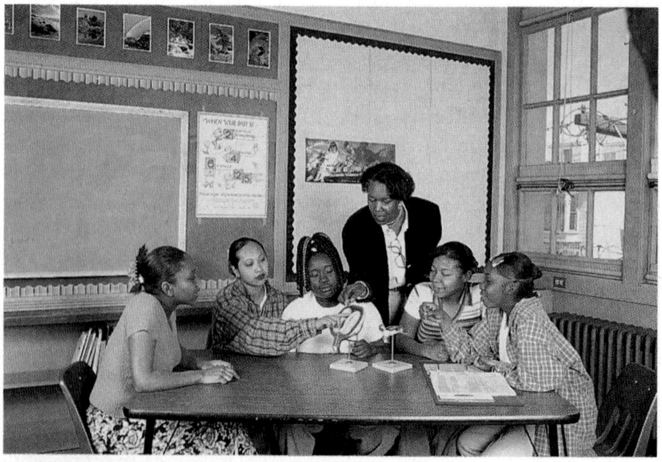

Figure 15–4 Prenatal classes for adolescents. Young adolescents may benefit from prenatal classes designed for them.

mother, her boyfriend, or her girlfriends. Those who bring girlfriends may bring a different one each time, and giggling and side conversations may occur. Such activity reflects the short attention span of the teen and is fairly typical.

Goals for prenatal classes may include some or all of the following:

- Providing anticipatory guidance about pregnancy
- Preparing participants for labor and birth
- Helping participants identify the problems and conflicts of teenage pregnancy and parenting
- Promoting increased self-esteem
- Providing information about available community resources
- Helping participants develop adaptive coping skills.

To keep the attention of adolescent participants in childbirth preparation classes, it is important to use a variety of teaching strategies including audiovisual aids, demonstrations, and games. Although parenting topics are sometimes included in prenatal classes for adolescents, teens may not retain the information because they tend to be present oriented. Parenting skills are crucial, but adolescents generally are not ready to learn about these skills until birth makes the newborn—and thus parenting—a reality. See *Health Promotion: Education: What Schools Can Do*.

Health Promotion **Education: What Schools Can Do**

- School systems attempt to meet prenatal education needs in many ways. The most effective method appears to be mainstreaming the pregnant adolescent in academic classes with her peers and adding classes appropriate to her needs during pregnancy and postpartum.
- Classes about growth and development beginning with the newborn and early infancy periods can help teenage parents to develop realistic expectations of their babies and may help decrease child abuse.
- Vocational guidance in this setting is also beneficial as pregnant teens plan for their futures.

Hospital-Based Nursing Care

As mentioned earlier, the adolescent's mother is often present during the teen's labor and birth. The father of the baby may also be involved. Close girlfriends may arrive soon after the teen is admitted. At admission, ask the teen who will be her primary support person in labor and whom she wants involved in the labor and birth. This information may also be included on her prenatal record. The adolescent in labor has the same care needs as any pregnant woman. However, she may require more sustained care. Be readily available and answer questions simply and honestly, using lay terminology. Also help the adolescent's support people understand their roles in assisting the teen. If the father of the baby is involved, encourage him, at his own level of comfort, to play an active role in all phases of the birth process, perhaps by supporting the teen's relaxation techniques, feeding her ice chips, timing her contractions, and coaching her with her breathing. Recommend hand-holding, back rubs, and supportive touching.

As part of discharge planning, ensure that the teen is aware of community resources available to assist her and her family. Postpartum classes, especially with peers, can be particularly beneficial. Such classes address a variety of topics, including postpartum adaptation; newborn, infant, and child development; and parenting skills.

Discharge Teaching: Contraception

During the postpartum period, most teens do not foresee that they will become sexually active in the near future and are often adamant that they will not become pregnant again for a long time. However, the statistics demonstrate a different reality. Consequently, predischarge teaching should include information about the resumption of ovulation and the importance of contraception.

Several safe and effective contraceptive options are available for adolescents. Condoms are by far the most common method of contraception among teens and, when used consistently and correctly, they offer the added advantage of protection against STIs. Increasingly, experts are recommending a dual approach to prevent pregnancy and STIs—a condom combined with a second method of contraception.

The American Academy of Pediatrics (AAP, 2014) has issued a policy statement on contraception for adolescents that advises caregivers to recommend contraceptive methods that require the least individual adherence, specifically, long-acting reversible contraception (LARC) such as progestin implants and intrauterine contraceptives (IUCs), followed by Depo-Provera (DMPA), combined oral contraceptives (COCs), and other hormone-based approaches including the vaginal ring, transdermal patch, and progestin-only pills.

The Society for Adolescent Health and Medicine (SAHM, 2017) has also issued a position statement urging that healthcare providers work to increase knowledge of, access to, and use of long-acting reversible contraceptives (LARCs) among teens and young adults as an effective method of contraception. The SAHM points out that LARCs are highly effective methods and have a lower failure rate than oral contraceptives and condoms, the most popular methods of contraceptives used by teens.

The LARCs Implanon and Nexplanon are both single-rod implants that may be left in place for 3 years. They are highly effective. DMPA is convenient for teens because it is easy to use. However, it does require an injection every 13 weeks.

IUC, another LARC, is now considered to be a safe, first-line contraceptive choice for adolescents. Research indicates that IUCs do not increase the adolescent's risk of pelvic inflammatory disease (PID) or affect her fertility (AAP, 2014), and the levonorgestrel-releasing intrauterine system (LNG-IUS) can be beneficial in teens by reducing heavy menstrual bleeding and alleviating symptoms of dysmenorrhea.

COCs are a popular method of contraception among teenage girls, especially long term, and have few contraindications; however, they do require individual adherence. Extended or continuous-cycle pills are an option for teens who prefer amenorrhea.

SAFETY ALERT!

Nurses need to be certain that adolescents who are prescribed combined oral contraceptives (COCs) clearly understand the correct use, possible complications, warning signs, and implications of missed pills. They should also be aware that some medications, such as certain antibiotics, decrease the effectiveness of COCs.

Evaluation

Expected outcomes of nursing care include:

- A trusting relationship is established with the pregnant adolescent.
- The adolescent is able to use her problem-solving abilities to make appropriate choices.

- The adolescent follows the recommendations of the healthcare team and receives effective healthcare throughout her pregnancy, the birth, and the postpartum period.
- The adolescent, her partner (if he is involved), and their families are able to cope successfully with the effects of the pregnancy.
- The adolescent is able to discuss pregnancy, prenatal care, and childbirth.
- The adolescent develops skill in child care and parenting.

Prevention of Adolescent Pregnancy

At the individual level, balanced and realistic sexual education, which includes information on both abstinence and contraception, can delay teens' onset of sexual activity, increase the use of contraception by sexually active teens, and reduce the number of their sexual partners. The AAP (2014) policy statement on contraception for adolescents addresses the role of healthcare providers in working with adolescents. The statement stresses the importance of encouraging abstinence while also providing counseling on risk-reduction approaches, including the use of latex condoms for every act of sexual intercourse. It points out that latex condoms also help reduce the transmission of STIs. In addition, the statement emphasizes the need to ensure ready access to contraceptive services and appropriate follow-up.

In 2012, AAP issued a policy statement supporting the availability of emergency contraception (EC) and recommending that both male and female teens should be counseled about emergency contraception as part of routine anticipatory guidance about safe sex and family planning. In 2013 the Food and Drug Administration (FDA) approved the Plan B One-Step emergency contraceptive for use by all women of childbearing potential without any age restrictions, thereby giving teens access to EC. At the national level, the Power to Decide (formerly the National Campaign to Prevent Teen and Unplanned Pregnancy [NCPTUP]; 2018b), a private, nonprofit organization made up of a broad spectrum of religious, political, social, human services, health, and academic organizations, envisions three major goals (Power to Decide, 2018b) to achieve by 2026:

1. Reduce teenage pregnancy rates by 50%.
2. Reduce unplanned pregnancies by 25% among women 18 to 29 years of age.
3. Reduce socioeconomic and racial/ethnic disparities in teen and unplanned pregnancies by 50%.

The Association of Women's Health, Obstetric and Neonatal Nurses (AWHONN) is one of the many professional organizations that joined this group and made a commitment to focus on adolescent pregnancy prevention. Not surprisingly, the Power to Decide has found that adolescent pregnancy is a multifaceted problem with no easy answers. The best approaches are local ones based on strong, community-wide involvement with a variety of programs directed at the multiple causes of the problem.

A problem in local communities continues to be conflict among different groups about how to approach adolescent pregnancy prevention. Most teens and adults believe that teens should be strongly encouraged to avoid having sex until they have completed high school, but both groups also favor providing young people with information about both abstinence and contraception. Nevertheless, some parents favor an abstinence-only approach. No evidence to date supports the effectiveness of this approach and it may have the unintended consequence of deterring teens from using contraceptives, thereby increasing the risk of STIs or unintended pregnancy (Boonstra, 2014). Most Americans support providing education in junior and senior high schools with information about protection against unplanned pregnancy and STIs. Evidence suggests that comprehensive programs that support both abstinence and the use of contraceptives and condoms have a positive effect in delaying or reducing sexual activity or in increasing the use of condoms or other contraceptives (Boonstra, 2014).

The Power to Decide's task forces have identified characteristics shared by all successful programs, regardless of the type of offering or community. Effective adolescent pregnancy prevention programs are evidence-based, long term, and intensive. They also involve adolescents in program planning, include good role models from the same cultural and racial backgrounds, and focus on the adolescent male.

Power to Decide has identified a list of recommendations for parents that are designed to help teens avoid pregnancy (see *Key Facts to Remember: Recommendations for Parents to Help Their Teens Avoid Pregnancy*). Nurses can use this information when working with parents (Power to Decide, 2018a).

Key Facts To Remember
Recommendations for Parents to Help Their Teens Avoid Pregnancy

- Parents should be clear about their own sexual attitudes and values in order to communicate clearly with children.
- Parents need to talk with their children about sex early and often and be specific in the discussions.
- Parents should supervise and monitor their children and teens with well-established rules, expectations, curfews, and standards of behavior.
- Parents should know their children's friends and their families.
- Parents need to clearly discourage early dating as well as frequent and steady dating.
- Parents should take a strong stand against allowing a daughter to date a much older boy; similarly, they should not allow a son to develop an intense relationship with a much younger girl.
- Parents need to help children set goals for their future and have options that are more attractive than early pregnancy and childrearing.
- Parents should show their children that they value education and take school performance seriously.
- Parents need to monitor what their children are reading, listening to, and watching.
- It is especially important for parents to build a strong, loving relationship with their children from an early age by showing affection clearly and regularly, spending time with them doing age-appropriate activities, building children's self-esteem, and having meals together as a family often.

Care of Expectant Parents Over Age 35

Today an increasing number of women are choosing to have their first baby after age 35. In fact, in 2015, birth rates rose for women age 30 to 44 and declined for women under age 30 (Hamilton et al., 2017). Many factors have contributed to this trend, including:

- The availability of effective birth control methods
- The expanded roles and career options available for women
- The increased number of women getting advanced education, pursuing careers, and delaying parenthood until they are established professionally
- The increased incidence of later marriage and second marriage
- The high cost of living, which causes some young couples to delay childbearing until they are more financially secure
- The increased availability of specialized reproductive technologies, which may help women previously considered infertile.

There are advantages to having a first baby after age 35. Single women or couples who delay childbearing until they are older tend to be well educated and financially secure. Usually their decision to have a baby was deliberately and thoughtfully made (Figure 15–5). Because of their greater life experiences, they also are more aware of the realities of having a child and what it means to have a baby at their age. Many of the women have experienced fulfillment in their careers and feel secure enough to take on the added responsibility of a child. Some women are ready to make a change in their lives and want to stay home with a new baby. Those who plan to continue working typically can afford good child care.

Medical Risks

In the United States and Canada, the risk of death has declined dramatically during the past 30 years for women of all ages. However, the risk of maternal death is higher for women over age 35 and even higher for women age 40 and older. These women are more likely to have chronic medical conditions that can complicate a pregnancy. Preexisting medical conditions such as hypertension or diabetes probably play a more significant role than age in maternal well-being and the outcome of pregnancy. In addition, the rate of multiple gestation, miscarriage, stillbirth, preterm birth, low birth weight, and perinatal morbidity and mortality is higher in women over age 35 (Grotegut, Chisholm, Johnson, et al., 2014). Nevertheless, while the risk of pregnancy complications is higher in women over age 35 who have a chronic condition such as hypertension or diabetes or who are in poor general health, the risks are much lower than previously believed for physically fit women without preexisting medical problems (Cunningham et al., 2014).

Because of advances in reproductive technology, the number of women over age 45 who give birth is increasing, although these women still constitute a very small percentage of overall births. While these women have a higher risk of complications than their younger counterparts, the absolute rate of stillbirth or perinatal death is still low (less than 10 per 1000) if they are healthy and free of preexisting disease. Thus, for most, the outcome of pregnancy is positive (Cakmak, Aygun, Kucukoduk, et al., 2016).

The risk of conceiving a child with Down syndrome does increase with age, especially over age 35 (see *Genetic Facts: Incidence of Down Syndrome Increases with Maternal Age*). The American College of Obstetricians and Gynecologists (ACOG, 2016) recommends that all pregnant women, regardless of age, be offered screening for Down syndrome, ideally at the first prenatal visit. A quadruple screening to detect Down syndrome and trisomy 18 is often used. It is performed early in the second trimester, typically between 15 and 22 6/7 weeks (ACOG, 2016). Noninvasive analysis of cell-free DNA (cfDNA) is also available for prenatal diagnosis early in the first trimester and has great potential as a screening method, although currently ACOG recommends conventional screening approaches for low-risk women. Alternatively, first-trimester ultrasound assessment of the thickness of fetal nuchal folds (nuchal translucency [NT]), combined with serum screens of free beta-human chorionic gonadotropin (β-hCG) and pregnancy-associated plasma protein A (PAPP-A), may be used in the detection of Down syndrome, trisomy 18, and trisomy 13. If the screening results are not in the normal range, follow-up testing using ultrasound is often indicated (ACOG, 2016). Chapter 16 discusses fetal assessment in detail.

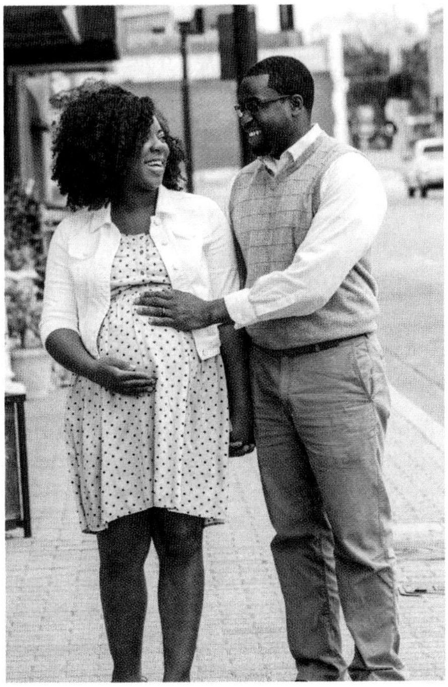

Figure 15–5 For many older couples, the decision to have a child may be very rewarding.

SOURCE: pixelheadphoto digitalskillet/Shutterstock.

Genetic Facts Incidence of Down Syndrome Increases with Maternal Age

MATERNAL AGE	INCIDENCE
Age 21	1 in 1700
Age 25	1 in 1200
Age 30	1 in 900
Age 35	1 in 350
Age 38	1 in 200
Age 40	1 in 100
Age 45	1 in 30
Age 49	1 in 10

SOURCE: National Down Syndrome Society, 2018.

Advanced paternal age is associated with adverse fetal and neonatal outcomes. It is also linked to increased risk of miscarriage and obstetric complications, as well as certain childhood cancers such as leukemia in offspring (Mok, Antonsen, Pedersen, et al., 2017). Additionally, advanced paternal age increases the risk for autism spectrum disorders (Andersen & Urhoj, 2017). See *Case Study: Melissa Bond-James.*

CASE STUDY: Melissa Bond-James

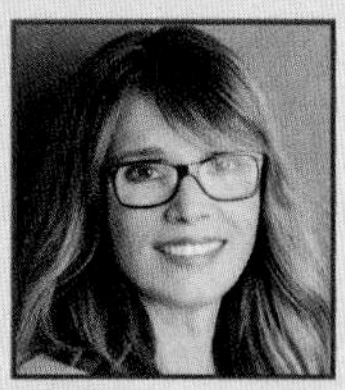

SOURCE: Kinga/ Shutterstock

Melissa presents for her 28 week prenatal visit and learns that her 1-hour glucola was 148. The CNM advises her she will need to complete a 3-hour glucose tolerance test. Melissa is concerned and tells the nurse she is conscientious about her diet, limits her sugar intake, and has no history of diabetes in her family. The nurse explains that advanced maternal age can increase the risk of gestational diabetes.

Questions to Ponder

How would you respond when Melissa asks what other conditions are more likely to occur in women over the age of 35? Discuss these conditions and modifiable risk factors that could reduce Melissa's risk profile.

Special Concerns of Expectant Parents Over Age 35

No matter what their age, most expectant parents have concerns about the well-being of the fetus and their ability to parent. Expectant parents over age 35 often have additional concerns about their age, especially the closer they are to age 40. Some couples are concerned about whether they will have enough energy to care for a new baby. Of greater concern is their ability to deal with the needs of the child as they age.

The financial concerns of the older couple are usually different from those of the younger couple. The older couple is generally more financially secure, but when their "baby" is ready for college, the older couple may be close to retirement and might not have the means to provide for their child. The older couple may also be forced to face their own mortality. Certainly the realization of one's mortality is not uncommon in midlife, but older expectant parents may confront the issue earlier as they consider what will happen as their child grows.

Older couples facing pregnancy in a late or second marriage or after therapy for infertility may find themselves somewhat isolated socially. They may feel different because they are often the only couple in their peer group expecting their first baby. In fact, many of their peers are likely to be parents of adolescents or young adults and may be grandparents as well.

Older couples who already have children may respond quite differently to learning that the woman is pregnant, depending on whether the pregnancy was planned or unexpected. Other factors influencing their response include their children's, family's, and friends' attitudes toward the pregnancy; the impact on their lifestyle; and the financial implications of having another child. Sometimes couples who had previously been married to other mates will choose to have a child together. *Blended families* are formed when "her" children, "his" children, and "their" children come together as a new family group.

Healthcare professionals may treat older expectant parents differently than they would a younger couple. They may offer older women more medical procedures, such as amniocentesis and ultrasound, than younger women. They may also discourage an older woman from using a birthing room or birthing center even if she is healthy because her age is considered to put her at risk.

The woman who has delayed pregnancy may be concerned about the limited amount of time that she has to bear children. When pregnancy does not occur as quickly as she had hoped, the older woman may become increasingly anxious as time slips away on her "biological clock." When an older woman becomes pregnant but has a spontaneous abortion, her grief for the loss of her unborn child is exacerbated by anxiety about her ability to conceive again in the time remaining to her.

"I didn't think I would marry but then I met Lars and fell hard. I was 38 and he was 43, a widower with no children. We both really wanted a baby, so here I am 39 and pregnant. Prenatal tests don't indicate any problems with our baby, a girl. I pray all goes well."

●○● NURSING MANAGEMENT

For the Pregnant Woman Over Age 35

Nursing Assessment and Diagnosis

In working with a woman in her late 30s or 40s who is pregnant, make the same assessments as are indicated in caring for any woman who is pregnant. Assess physical status, the woman's understanding of pregnancy and its changes, the couple's attitudes about the pregnancy and their expectations of the impact a baby will have on their lives, their health teaching needs, the degree of support the woman has, and her knowledge of newborn/infant care.

The nursing diagnoses applicable to pregnant women in general apply to pregnant women over age 35. Examples of other nursing diagnoses that may apply include:

- ***Decisional Conflict*** related to unexpected pregnancy
- ***Anxiety*** (moderate) related to uncertainty about fetal well-being

(NANDA-I © 2017)

Planning and Implementation

Once an older couple has made the decision to have a child, respect and support the couple in this decision. As with any patient, discuss risks, identify concerns, and promote strengths. Do not make the woman's age an issue. It is helpful in promoting a sense of well-being to treat the pregnancy as normal unless the woman has specific health risks.

As the pregnancy continues, identify and discuss concerns the woman may have related to her age or to specific health problems. The older woman who has made a conscious decision to become pregnant often has carefully thought through potential problems and may actually have fewer concerns than a younger woman or one with an unplanned pregnancy.

Childbirth education classes are important in promoting adaptation to the event of childbirth for expectant parents of any age. However, older expectant parents often feel uncomfortable in classes in which most of the participants are much younger. Consequently, classes for expectant parents over age 35 are now available in many communities.

Women who are over age 35 and having their first baby tend to be better educated than other healthcare consumers. These women frequently know the kind of care and services they want and may be assertive in their interactions with the healthcare system. You should not be intimidated by these patients and you should not assume that anticipatory guidance and support are not needed. Instead, support the couple's strengths and be aware of their individual needs.

In working with older expectant couples or an older single woman, be sensitive to special needs. A particularly difficult issue these women face is the possibility of bearing an unhealthy child or a child with a genetic disorder. As discussed previously, screening tests are available to assess for Down syndrome. Because of the risk of Down syndrome in these families, amniocentesis is often suggested or may be indicated if screening results are not in the normal range.

For couples who agree to amniocentesis, the first few months of pregnancy are a difficult time. Amniocentesis cannot be done until week 14 of pregnancy, and the chromosomal studies take roughly 2 weeks to complete. Their fear that the fetus is at risk may delay the successful completion of the psychologic tasks of early pregnancy.

You can support couples who decide to have amniocentesis by providing information and answering questions about the procedure and by providing comfort and emotional support during the amniocentesis. If the results indicate that the fetus has Down syndrome or another genetic abnormality, ensure that the couple has complete information about the condition, its range of possible manifestations, and its developmental implications.

Evaluation

Expected outcomes of nursing care include:

- The woman and her partner are knowledgeable about the pregnancy and express confidence in their ability to make appropriate healthcare choices.
- The expectant parents (and their children) are able to cope with the pregnancy and its implications for the future.
- The woman receives effective healthcare throughout her pregnancy and during birth and the postpartum period.
- The woman and her partner develop skills in child care and parenting.

Care of the Pregnant Woman with Special Needs

Approximately 163,700 women with a chronic physical disability (CPD) that causes them to need assistance with activities of daily living (ADL) become pregnant each year (Iezzoni, Yu, Wint, et al., 2014).

Chronic physical disabilities may include mobility difficulties that involve upper or lower extremities, arthritis, vision or hearing problems, disorders such as multiple sclerosis or cerebral palsy, heart or lung problems, and a variety of diseases. These numbers are predicted to increase because dramatic improvements in medical care are enabling women born with a CPD and those who acquire them through accident or illness to live into their childbearing years and beyond. Moreover, changes in societal attitudes have led to a decrease in stigmatization of disability, and civil rights laws such as the Americans with Disabilities Act provide increased support and acceptance for women with disabilities who seek motherhood. In addition, technologically sophisticated maternity and newborn care has made positive pregnancy outcomes more likely (Iezzoni, Wint, Smeltzer, et al., 2014).

Collectively, women with disabilities have often been discouraged from becoming mothers. Research suggests that these women often perceive themselves as "perennial outsiders" who are automatically categorized as high risk because of their disability (Walsh-Gallagher, McConkey, Sinclair, et al., 2013).

For women with CPD, the decision to become pregnant is influenced by a variety of personal, biologic, and social factors. Three factors are significant (LaPierre, Zimmerman, & Hall, 2017):

- The personal importance of pregnancy and motherhood
- The feasibility of pregnancy and raising a child in light of the woman's health condition, finances, support, and available resources
- The costs of pregnancy including the physical risks (including death), genetic issues, dangers for the fetus of maternal medications, and potential impact of the woman's disability on the child's future quality of life.

Women with an intellectual or developmental disability (IDD) may also become pregnant and have special needs for teaching and support. Among these women there is a high incidence of unplanned pregnancy, and they often seek prenatal care late. Typically they have lower reading and comprehension levels and are at a disadvantage when presented with complex information. Healthcare providers may perceive the pregnancy negatively, and the woman may experience lack of social support and anxiety (Potvin, Brown, & Cobigo, 2016).

Women with IDD have a higher incidence of preterm birth and of preeclampsia, longer hospital stays, and a higher rate of cesarean births when compared to other women. In addition, their babies are more likely to have low birth weight (Parish, Mitra, Son, et al., 2015). Women with intellectual disabilities are also at increased risk of intervention by social services, which may result in the removal of the newborns from their custody.

A family-centered approach is designed to optimize the childbearing experience of *all* women by providing a high quality, individualized experience that builds on the strength of each woman rather than perceived limitations. Ideally, this begins with preconception counseling so that the woman is in optimal health before conception. The woman and her family should be advised of potential health concerns and given information about their management.

During pregnancy, professional support and a team effort are essential. The woman needs to have a sense that she is empowered to make her healthcare decisions and that she has a good degree of control over the experience. In many cases, care at a tertiary-level facility is important to an optimal outcome.

NURSING MANAGEMENT

For the Woman with a Disability

Nursing Assessment and Diagnosis

In addition to the assessments made for all pregnant women, nursing assessment of a woman with a disability needs to be condition specific. These assessments will vary depending on the extent of the woman's disability. A discussion of every possible disability is beyond the scope of this text. Some general principles are provided here.

A woman with a mobility disorder, especially if it is extensive, as in the case of a spinal cord injury, needs careful assessment. Be alert for commonly occurring complications associated with her condition such as hypotension, bradycardia, pulmonary complications, pressure ulcers, bladder infection, gastroesophageal reflux disease (GERD), deep vein thrombosis, stool impaction, anemia, and autonomic dysreflexia (a rapid increase in blood pressure in response to a noxious stimulus such as catheterization or uterine contractions below the level of the spinal cord lesion) (Sweis & Biller, 2017). Weight gain and changes in the woman's center of gravity may increase the risk for falls. In addition, the woman may be unaware of preterm labor and thus faces the possibility of an unattended birth.

Assess the woman with an intellectual disability for her level of understanding of instructions and printed materials. Determine her awareness of the signs of complications and of the onset of labor. Also evaluate her level of support from her partner and family members. Nursing diagnoses that may apply include:

- ***Dysreflexia, Autonomic***, related to a spinal cord injury
- ***Skin Integrity, Risk for Impaired***, related to decreased or absent mobility
- ***Knowledge, Deficient***, related to a documented learning disability

(NANDA I © 2017)

Nursing Plan and Implementation

Women with a disability involving a lower extremity (e.g., amputation, spinal cord injury, and so forth) may need assistance in issues involving mobility such as transferring to an examination table or bed. Typically, they will have adaptive equipment. Women who use wheelchairs may find that additional weight late in pregnancy may interfere with their ability to propel their chairs (Figure 15–6). Thus, it is important that the woman avoid excessive weight gain and regularly perform range-of-motion exercises.

During labor assist the woman to change position periodically to avoid dependent edema. Be alert for signs of respiratory distress, deep vein thrombosis, and autonomic dysreflexia. Provide necessary adaptive equipment. Women with a loss of sensation in the lower extremities may find it difficult or impossible to push effectively and consequently have an increased incidence of cesarean birth. Women with upper extremity disorders may need assistance with, for example, position change or holding the newborn. Assist with breastfeeding as necessary.

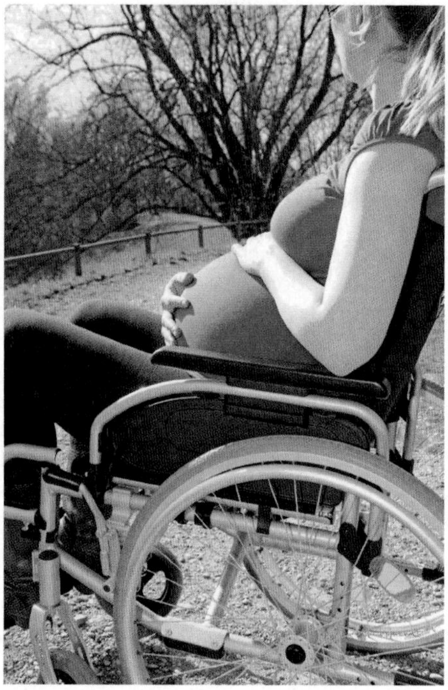

Figure 15–6 **Pregnant woman with a lower extremity disability.**

SOURCE: RioPatuca Images/Fotolia.

The most important need of pregnant women with intellectual disabilities is for information that is timely, accessible, and understandable. They often find that information available for the general population is too difficult to understand. To address this need, easy-to-understand information should be available. It is also helpful for caregivers to allow extra consultation time and good communication aids. This might include videotaping or audiotaping information so the woman can refer to it as needed.

Evaluation

Expected outcomes of nursing care include:

- The expectant woman is able to cope with the pregnancy and its implications for the future.
- The woman receives effective healthcare throughout her pregnancy and during birth and the postpartum period.

Focus Your Study

- Many factors contribute to the high teenage pregnancy rate, including earlier age of first sexual intercourse, lack of knowledge about conception, lack of easy access to contraception, lessened stigma associated with adolescent pregnancy in some populations, poverty, early school failure, and early childhood sexual abuse.
- Physical risks of adolescent pregnancies include preterm births, low-birth-weight newborns, cephalopelvic disproportion, iron deficiency anemia, and preeclampsia and its sequelae.
- Factors affecting an adolescent's response to pregnancy include her degree of achievement of the developmental tasks of adolescence (which can be closely associated with age) as well as cultural, religious, and socioeconomic factors.
- Nurses working with pregnant adolescents face many challenges, including safeguarding the patient's confidentiality, winning her trust, and helping to build her sense of self-esteem.

- Often the adolescent has little understanding of pregnancy, childbirth, or parenting. Consequently, education is a primary responsibility of the nurse.
- Adolescent pregnancy prevention programs should be multifaceted, target males as well as females, and involve community-wide approaches.
- Childbirth among women over age 35 is becoming increasingly common. It poses fewer health risks than previously believed and offers advantages for the woman or couple who makes this choice.
- A major risk for the older expectant couple relates to the increased incidence of Down syndrome in children born to women over age 35. Screening tests and amniocentesis can provide information as to whether the fetus has Down syndrome. The couple can then decide whether they wish to continue the pregnancy.
- Common risks of a pregnant woman with a mobility disorder include pressure ulcers, bladder infection, gastroesophageal reflux disease (GERD), deep vein thrombosis, stool impaction, anemia, and autonomic dysreflexia.
- The most pressing needs of a woman with an intellectual disability who becomes pregnant are accurate information appropriate to her level of understanding and consistent emotional support.

In order to make safe and effective judgments using NANDA-I © 2017 nursing diagnoses, it is essential that nurses refer to the definitions and defining characteristics of the diagnoses used in this text, which can be found in Appendix C.

References

American Academy of Pediatrics (AAP). (2012). Policy statement: Emergency contraception. *Pediatrics*, 130(6), 1174–1180.

American Academy of Pediatrics (AAP). (2014). Policy statement: Contraception for adolescents. *Pediatrics*, 134(4), e1244–e1256.

American College of Obstetricians and Gynecologists (ACOG). (2016). *Screening for fetal aneuploidy* (Practice Bulletin No. 163). Washington, DC: Author.

Andersen, A. N., & Urhoj, S. K. (2017). Is advanced paternal age a health risk for the offspring? *Fertility and Sterility*, 107(2), 312–318.

Baldwin, M. K., & Edelman, A. B. (2013). The effect of long-acting reversible contraception on rapid repeat pregnancy in adolescents: A review. *Journal of Adolescent Health*, 52(4, Suppl,), S47–S53.

Boonstra, H. D. (2014). What is behind the declines in teen pregnancy rates? *Guttmacher Policy Review*, 17(3), 1–21.

Cakmak, C. F., Aygun, C., Kucukoduk, S., & Bek, Y. (2016). Maternal and neonatal outcomes in advanced maternal age: A retrospective cohort study. *Journal of Maternal–Fetal and Neonatal Medicine, 29,* 1–5.

Centers for Disease Control and Prevention (CDC). (2016). *Sexually transmitted disease surveillance 2015.* Atlanta, GA: U.S. Department of Health and Human Services.

Cunningham, F. G., Leveno, K. J., Bloom, S. L., Spong, C. Y., Dashe, J. S., Hoffman, B. L., . . . Sheffield, J. S. (2014). *Williams obstetrics* (24th ed.). New York, NY: McGraw-Hill.

Fedorowicz, A. R., Hellerstedt, W. L., Schreiner, P. J., & Bolland, J. M. (2014). Associations of adolescent hopelessness and self-worth with pregnancy attempts and pregnancy desire. *American Journal of Public Health, 104*(8), e133–e140.

Food and Drug Administration. (FDA). (2013). *FDA approves Plan B One-Step emergency contraceptive for use without prescription for all women of child-bearing potential.* Retrieved from https://www.accessdata.fda.gov/drugsatfda_docs/nda/2013/021998Orig1s002.pdf

Garwood, S. K., Gerassi, L., Jonson-Reid, M., Plax, K., & Drake, B. (2015). More than poverty: The effect of abuse and neglect on teen pregnancy risk. *Journal of Adolescent Health, 57*(2), 164–158.

Grotegut, C. A., Chisholm, C. A., Johnson, L. N., Brown, H. L., Heine, R. P., & James, A. H. (2014). Medical and obstetric complications among pregnant women aged 45 and older. *Plos One, 9*(4), e96237.

Guttmacher Institute. (2017). *Fact sheet: Adolescent sexual and reproductive health.* Retrieved from https://www.guttmacher.org/fact-sheet/american-teens-sexual-and-reproductive-health

Guttmacher Institute. (2018). *An overview of minors' consent laws.* Retrieved from https://www.guttmacher.org/state-policy/explore/overview-minors-consent-law

Hamilton, B. E., Martin, J. A., Osterman, M. J. K., Driscoll, A. K., & Rosen, L. M. (2017). Births: Provisional data for 2016. *Vital Statistics Rapid Release,* Report No.2. Hyattsville, MD: National Center for Health Statistics.

Hefrich, C., & McWey, L. (2014). Substance use and delinquency: High-risk behaviors as predictors of teen pregnancy among adolescents involved with the child welfare system. *Journal of Family Issues, 35*(10), 1322–1338.

Herrman, J. W. (2014). Adolescent girls who experience abuse or neglect are at an increased risk of teen pregnancy. *Evidence Based Nursing, 17*(3), 79.

Herrman, J. W., & Nandakumar, R. (2012). Development of a survey to assess adolescent perceptions of teen parenting. *Journal of Nursing Measurement, 20*(1), 3–20.

Iezzoni, L. I., Wint, A. J., Smeltzer, S. C., & Ecker, J. L. (2014). Effects of disability on pregnancy experiences among women with impaired mobility. *Acta Obstetricia et Gynecologica Scandinavica, 94*(2), 133–140.

Iezzoni, L. I., Yu, J, Wint, A. J., Smeltzer, S. C., & Ecker, J. L. (2014). General health, health conditions, and current pregnancy among U.S. women with and without chronic physical disabilities. *Disability and Health Journal, 7,* 181–188.

Kann, L., Kinchen, S., Shanklin, S. L., Flint, K. H., Hawkins, J., Harris, W. A., . . . Zaza, S. (2014). Youth risk behavior surveillance—United States, 2013. *MMWR Surveillance Summaries, 63*(4), 1–172.

Kearney, M. S., & Levine, P. B. (2015). Investigating recent trends in the U.S. teen birth rate. *Journal of Health Economics, 41,* 15–29.

Kirven, J. (2014). Helping teen dads obtain and sustain parental success. *International Journal of Childbirth Education, 29*(2), 85–88.

Klettke, B., Hallford, D. J., & Mellor, D. J. (2014). Sexting prevalence and correlates: A systematic literature review. *Clinical Psychology Review, 34*(1), 44–53.

Kogan, S. M., Cho, J., Allen, K., Lei, M., Beach, S. R. H., Gibbons, F. X., . . . Brody, G. H. (2013). Avoiding adolescent pregnancy: A longitudinal analysis of African-American youth. *Journal of Adolescent Health, 53,* 14–20.

LaPierre, T. A., Zimmerman, M. K., & Hall, J. P. (2017). "Paying the price to get there": Motherhood and the dynamics of pregnancy deliberations among women with disabilities. *Disability and Health Journal, 10,* 419–425.

Lee, Y., Cintron, A., & Kocher, S. (2014). Factors related to risky sexual behaviors and effective STI/HIV and pregnancy intervention programs for African American adolescents. *Public Health Nursing, 31(5),* 414–427.

Lindberg, L., Santelli, J., & Desai, S. (2016). Understanding the decline in adolescent fertility in the United States, 2007–2012. *Journal of Adolescent Health, 59*(5), 577–583.

Lohan, M., Cruise, S., O'Halloran, P., Alderdice, F., & Hyde, A. (2010). Adolescent men's attitudes in relation to pregnancy and pregnancy outcomes: A systematic review of the literature from 1980–2009. *Journal of Adolescent Health, 47,* 327–345.

Mok, P. L. H., Antonsen, S., Pedersen, C. B., & Webb, R. T. (2017). Younger or older parental age and risk of suicidality, premature death, psychiatric illness, and criminality in offspring. *Journal of Affective disorders, 208* 15, 130–138.

National Down Syndrome Society. (2018). *Down syndrome: Does Down syndrome run in families?* Retrieved from https://www.ndss.org/about-down-syndrome/down-syndrome

Ouaknine, B. (2016). *Consequences of teen pregnancy options: Keeping the baby.* Retrieved from https://www.teenhelp.com/teen-pregnancy/consequences-of-teen-pregnancy-options/

Parish, S. L., Mitra, M., Son, E., Bonardi, A., Swoboda, P. T., & Igdalsky, L. (2015). Pregnancy outcomes among U.S. women with intellectual and developmental disabilities. *American Journal on Intellectual and Developmental Disabilities, 120*(5), 433–443.

Potvin, L. A., Brown, H. K., & Cobigo, V. (2016). Social support received by women with intellectual and developmental disabilities during pregnancy and childbirth: An exploratory qualitative study. *Midwifery, 37*, 57–64.

Power to Decide. (2018a). *Ten tips for parents to help their children avoid teen pregnancy.* Retrieved from https://powertodecide.org/sites/default/files/resources/primary-download/10tips_final.pdf

Power to Decide. (2018b). *What we do: FAQs.* Retrieved from https://powertodecide.org/what-we-do/information/faqs

Ralph, L., Gould, H., Baker, A., & Foster, D. G. (2014). The role of parents and partners in minors' decisions to have an abortion and anticipated coping after abortion. *Journal of Adolescent Health, 54*, 428–434.

Sipsma, H. L., Ickovics, J. R., Lewis, J. B., Ethier, K. A., & Kershaw, T. S. (2011). Adolescent pregnancy desire and pregnancy incidence. *Women's Health Issues, 21*(2), 110–116.

Society for Adolescent Health and Medicine (SAHM). (2017). Position statement: Improving knowledge about, access to, and utilization of long-acting reversible contraception among adolescents and young adults. *Journal of Adolescent Health, 60*(4), 472–474.

Steinberg, L. (2017). *Adolescence* (11th ed.). New York, NY: McGraw-Hill.

Sweis, R., & Biller, J. (2017). Systemic complications of spinal cord injury. *Current Neurology and Neuroscience Reports, 17*(2), 8–17.

TeenHelp.com. (2016). *Teen pregnancy statistics.* Retrieved from https://www.teenhelp.com/teen-pregnancy/teen-pregnancy-statistics/

Turnage, B. F., & Pharris, A. D. (2013). Supporting the pregnant adolescent. *International Journal of Childbirth Education, 28*(4), 72–76.

Ventura, S. J., Hamilton, B. E., & Mathews, T. J. (2014). National and state patterns of teen births in the United States, 1940–2013. *National Vital Statistics Reports, 63*(4), 1–34.

Walsh-Gallagher, D., McConkey, R., Sinclair, M., & Clarke, R. (2013). Normalising birth for women with a disability: The challenges facing practitioners. *Midwifery, 29*(4), 294–299.

Yoost, J. L., Hertweck, S. P., & Barnett, S. N. (2014). The effect of an educational approach to pregnancy prevention among high-risk early and late adolescents. *Journal of Adolescent Health, 55*(2), 222–227.

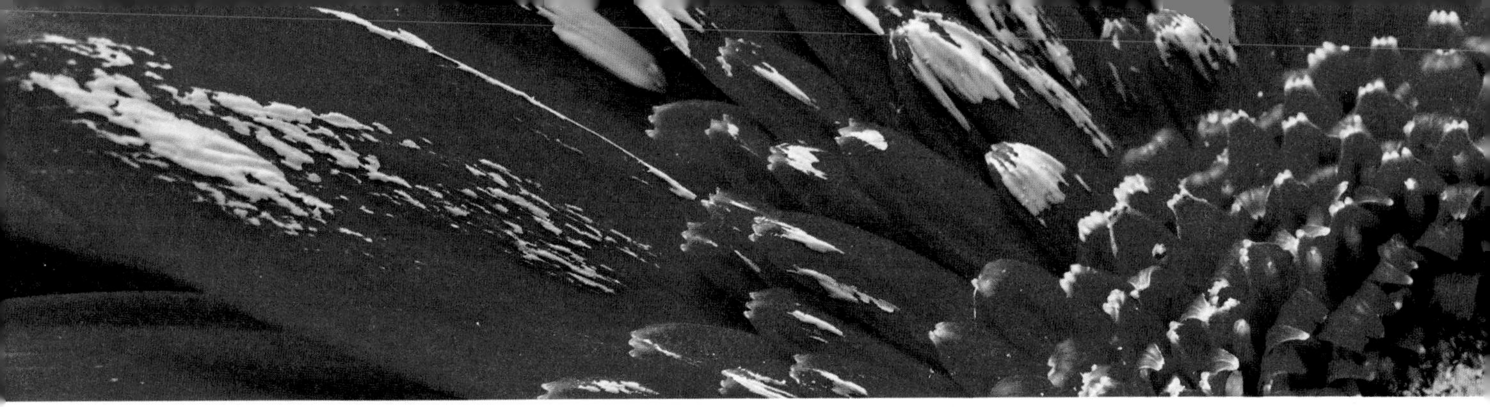

Chapter 16
Assessment of Fetal Well-Being

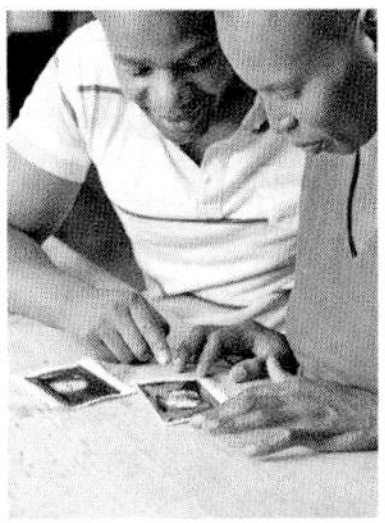

My first pregnancy was very complicated, and I hoped for a healthy baby throughout, but my baby did not survive. This experience made us very reserved and anxious through our next pregnancy, as we could only do so much to ensure the well-being of our baby. The testing options and technology we used did provide some comfort beyond feeling the baby move because we could see the baby on ultrasound and hear the heartbeat.

SOURCE: Gallo Images/SuperStock.

Learning Outcomes

16.1 Describe the various psychologic responses to antenatal testing.

16.2 Identify indications and interpret findings for ultrasound examinations performed in the first trimester.

16.3 Describe the procedures used in the first trimester to confirm fetal viability.

16.4 Delineate the use of ultrasound in the second trimester to assess fetal life, number, presentation, anatomy, age, and growth.

16.5 Identify pertinent information to be discussed with the woman regarding her own assessment of fetal activity and methods of recording fetal activity.

16.6 Identify the indications for ordering a nonstress test for compromised or at-risk fetuses or maternal at-risk pregnancies.

16.7 Compare the indications and procedures used when conducting a nonstress test, a contraction stress test, the biophysical profile, and the collection of an amniotic fluid index.

16.8 Explain the purposes of the sequential screen, quad screen, and cell-free DNA testing and the implications of abnormal values.

16.9 Contrast the use of amniocentesis and chorionic villus sampling in detecting a fetus with a chromosomal disorder.

16.10 Discuss fetal fibronectin and transvaginal ultrasound measurement of cervical length as predictors of preterm labor.

16.11 Discuss how the lecithin/sphingomyelin ratio of the amniotic fluid and phosphatidylglycerol (PG) can be used to assess fetal lung maturity.

While every mother wishes for an uneventful pregnancy and a healthy baby, some women experience maternal complications during pregnancy. The Centers for Disease Control and Prevention (CDC, 2016b) has termed **severe maternal morbidity (SMM)** as "maternal morbidity includ(ing) physical and psychologic conditions that result from or are aggravated by pregnancy and have an adverse effect on a woman's health" (para 1). It is estimated that 65,000 women annually are affected by SMM, with the numbers steadily rising (CDC, 2016b). In addition, approximately 3% of all newborns are born with a birth defect from either a genetic or environmental influence, and 10% of all newborns are born prematurely, before 37 completed weeks. Newborns born prior to 32 weeks are at a significant risk for long-term disabilities and death (CDC, 2016a). Premature birth represents the greatest risk of neurologic injury and disability. Antenatal fetal assessment techniques discussed in this chapter are designed to identify a fetus at risk; however, a perfect pregnancy outcome can never be predicted or guaranteed.

The United States spends more on healthcare expenditures than any other country in the world, yet it continues to have a higher infant mortality rate than many other industrialized countries (Central Intelligence Agency, 2016). Reproductive technologies significantly raise the cost of health care. These technologic advances are not without risks; therefore, prevention of perinatal morbidity must always be a primary goal. The decision to use the tests discussed in this chapter is made by the childbearing family only after careful reflection regarding possible outcomes, management options, testing limitations, and personal ethics and cultural beliefs. Practitioners and nurses assist families in analyzing the risks versus the benefits.

Psychologic Reactions to Antenatal Testing

Little has been written about the psychologic impact of antenatal diagnostic testing on childbearing families; however, maternal anxiety occurs in women when undergoing prenatal testing procedures. Çakar, Tari Kasnakoglu, Ökem, et al., (2016) studied pregnant women undergoing invasive prenatal testing and found that 60% of those women suffered from anxiety, but the women who received prenatal education experienced less anxiety. Nurses often play a key role not only in teaching families about various testing options, but also in providing clarity and emotional support to the woman and her family undergoing antenatal testing. To decrease anxiety and alleviate fear for the woman and her family, the nurse provides clear, concise explanations of possible results from testing and management options after the testing has been completed. See Box 16–1 for sample nursing approaches to pretest teaching. Generally, normal results alleviate the family's anxiety; however, equivocal or positive results, indicating the necessity of additional testing, require ongoing counseling of the woman and her family members.

Clinical Tip

Families undergoing fetal testing experience a wide range of emotions based on personal expectations, past experiences, fears, and cultural norms. Encouraging the family to verbalize concerns, ask questions, and express any apprehensions or fears can help put the family at ease.

The use and safety of ultrasound examination has been documented for decades. Obstetrical ultrasound performed in the second or third trimester is effective in identifying multiple gestation, gestational age, fetal anomalies, placental disorders, maternal structural abnormalities, amniotic fluid volume, fetal presentation and position, and fetal well-being. Women should be counseled appropriately before undergoing antenatal testing, including ultrasonography, in order to minimize shock and confusion if adverse findings are reported. When more invasive testing is recommended, it may evoke fear and anxiety in the woman and her partner as they consider the reason for the test, the risk to the fetus and woman during the test, and the implications of the test results. All testing should be presented as optional and only performed when the woman so desires (van Schendel et al., 2016).

●○● NURSING MANAGEMENT

For the Woman Undergoing Antenatal Testing

Nurses in a variety of settings have an opportunity to specialize in and provide care to families undergoing antenatal testing. You will serve as a vital link between the woman and the physician or certified nurse-midwife (CNM). Thus, you will need to present easy-to-understand information, encourage the family to ask questions and voice concerns, and provide follow-up care, including interpreting results, arranging for additional testing, answering questions, and supporting the woman and her family emotionally.

Nursing Assessment and Diagnosis

Nursing assessment begins with a history of the present prenatal course and identifying possible indications for a particular

BOX 16–1

Sample Nursing Approaches to Pretest Teaching

Assess whether the woman knows the reason the screening or diagnostic test is being offered or recommended. *Examples:*

"What has your doctor/nurse-midwife told you about this test?"

"Sometimes tests are done for many different reasons. Can you tell me why you are having this test?"

"What is your understanding about what the test will show?"

Provide an opportunity for questions. *Examples:*

"What questions do you have about the test?"

"What things about the test are unclear to you?"

Explain the test procedure, paying particular attention to any preparation the woman needs to do prior to the test. *Example:*

"The test that has been ordered for you is designed to . . . " (Add specific information about the particular test. Give the explanation in simple language.)

Validate the woman's understanding of the preparation. *Example:*

"Tell me what you will have to do to get ready for this test."

Give permission for the woman to continue to ask questions if needed. *Example:*

"I'll be with you during the test. If you have any questions at any time, please don't hesitate to ask."

diagnostic test. Examples may include identifying family medical/genetic history, advanced maternal age, previous history of a child with a birth defect, or the presence of a particular maternal medical condition. Assess the woman's and her family's understanding of the indication for testing, the test itself, and the presence of any psychosociocultural factors that may influence the teaching or learning process. During the test and afterward, complete needed assessments to monitor the status of the woman and her fetus.

The primary nursing diagnoses are directed toward providing information about the screening or diagnostic test and minimizing any risks to the woman and her unborn child. Examples of nursing diagnoses that may be applicable include:

- *Knowledge, Readiness for Enhanced,* related to fetal assessment testing due to an expressed desire to understand its purpose, benefits, risks, and alternatives
- *Fear* related to the risks of a specific test or possible unfavorable test results
- *Attachment, Risk for Impaired,* because of high-risk label attached to the pregnancy
- *Anxiety* related to the potential outcomes or unfavorable test results.

(NANDA-I © 2017)

Nursing Plan and Implementation

Direct the nursing plan of care toward each specific nursing diagnosis. Provide needed and desired information about the screening or diagnostic test. Be an advocate for the expectant woman by helping her clarify questionable areas and obtain needed information. You may be able to anticipate the woman's greatest concerns and fears. When the woman is not able to verbalize questions, assist her by providing information that answers questions that other women have had. For example, many women undergoing amniocentesis (a procedure used for genetic diagnosis that is discussed in detail later in the chapter) fear pain during the procedure. Inform the woman that she will feel pressure during the insertion of the needle and may feel subsequent cramping, which can last for several hours. Provide information about the procedure itself and follow-up monitoring to evaluate fetal well-being.

It is important to realize that women react differently to pregnancy and testing. Your role is to remain nonjudgmental and to offer individualized support when needed. Establishing a trusting relationship increases the possibility that a woman will talk freely and share her concerns and emotional needs with you. If possible, coordinate services the woman may need, such as community resources for financial, psychologic, or social support.

Nurses working in community clinics have an integral role in performing fetal surveillance tests throughout the antepartum period. They may find themselves not only performing some of these tests, such as nonstress tests, but also performing comprehensive assessments of the woman's health, family dynamics, and living situation. Community health nurses often have a more accurate understanding of the woman's physical resources, such as the adequacy of living conditions, proximity to healthcare resources, and availability of public transportation. Often you will have the most contact with the pregnant woman. Because of this, you are in an excellent position to provide anticipatory guidance, reiterate teaching provided by the woman's healthcare provider, and monitor her current plan of care. Approach each encounter with calmness, compassion, and honesty.

Evaluation

Evaluate the understanding of antepartum testing procedures by the woman and her family. Determining if the family understands the indication for follow-up testing is imperative. Assess whether the teaching methods used are effective for that family. Evaluation should include both physical and psychologic factors. In addition, determine if adequate resources, such as social support and physical resources, are available for the pregnant woman. Women from different cultures may need additional support because they may encounter language and other cultural barriers (Spector, 2017).

Ultrasound

Ultrasound has become one of the most commonly used diagnostic and screening tools in pregnancy and provides a critical role in the practice of obstetrics. Because ultrasound is used widely to assess fetal well-being in all three trimesters, it is also discussed within this framework later in the chapter.

Ultrasound is a diagnostic procedure that uses high-frequency sound waves exceeding 20,000 cycles per second, greater than what the human ear can hear, to produce an image that varies based on the density of the structure under the transducer. The reflected energy creates a small electrical voltage that is displayed on the screen. Very dense components, such as bone, appear white on the screen, whereas soft tissues appear gray and fluid appears black (Norton, 2016). Instruments used in ultrasonography operate at 2 to 10 megahertz (MHz). The higher the frequency of the sound, the shallower the depth of penetration but the better the resolution of the image produced. Ultrasound uses a device called a *transducer* to turn the sound waves into electrical signals.

Transducers can be used either transabdominally (Figure 16–1), operating at 3 to 5 MHz, or transvaginally (Figure 16–2), operating at 5 to 10 MHz (Norton, 2016). These transducers and their use are described fully later in the chapter.

Ultrasound can be used to produce images called *sonograms* in several different ways. In motion mode (M mode), the reflected echo generates a moving display. This is how fetal cardiac activity is seen. Brightness modulation (B mode) converts the signals

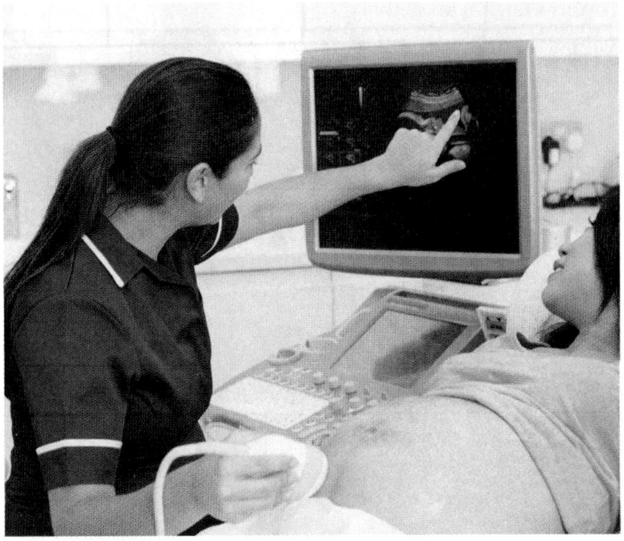

Figure 16–1 **Ultrasound scanning permits visualization of the fetus in utero.**

SOURCE: Monkey Business Images/Shutterstock.

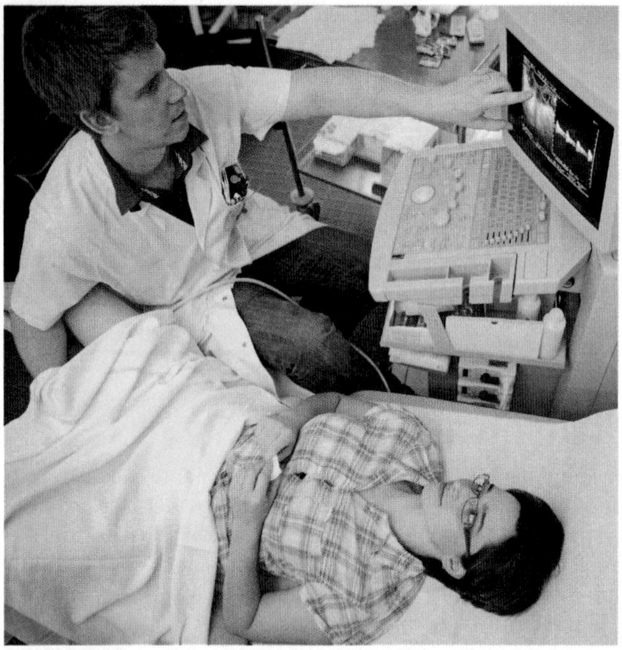

Figure 16–2 **Transvaginal ultrasound.**

SOURCE: CHASSENET/BSIP SA/Alamy Stock Photo.

into varying degrees of brightness and produces a two-dimensional image. Three-dimensional ultrasound uses algorithms to vary opacity, transparency, and depth to project an image. This allows curved structures such as the fetal face and body to be viewed (Figure 16–3).

Extent of Ultrasound Exams

Ultrasound examinations are classified as standard or basic, limited (identifying only certain components), or specialized (sometimes referred to as detailed) (Norton, 2016). A *limited ultrasound examination* may be used to address a specific question or determine specific information. The procedure can do the following:

- Determine fetal presentation before or during labor
- Locate the placenta
- Confirm fetal heart activity
- Estimate amniotic fluid volume

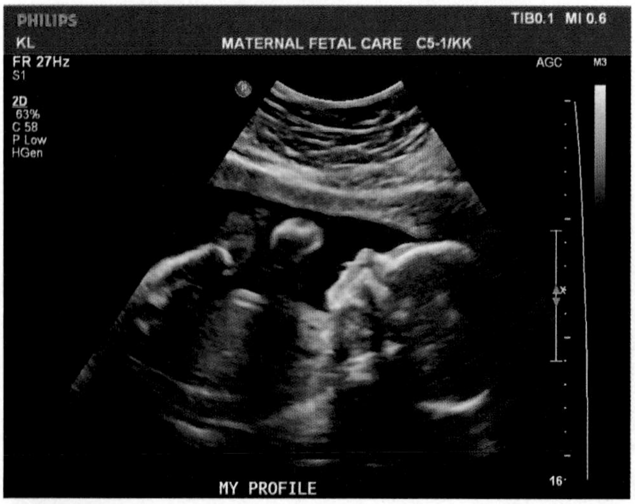

Figure 16–3 **Ultrasound of the face and body of a fetus.**

SOURCE: Craig London

- Diagnose multiple gestation
- Evaluate interval growth
- Evaluate the cervix
- Guide amniocentesis.

A *standard ultrasound examination* is performed during the second or third trimester and includes an evaluation of:

- Fetal presentation
- Fetal number
- Amniotic fluid volume
- Placental position
- Cardiac activity
- Fetal biometry
- Anatomic survey.

A standard ultrasound should also attempt to evaluate the maternal cervix and the uterus and ovaries when feasible.

A *specialized (detailed) ultrasound examination* is performed when an anomaly is suspected, and the components of the exam are determined by the expert conducting the examination. These components may include fetal Doppler, biophysical profile, fetal echocardiogram, amniotic fluid assessment, or additional biometric studies (Norton, 2016).

Methods of Ultrasound Scanning

The two most common methods of ultrasound scanning are *transabdominal* and *transvaginal* scanning (Figure 16–1 and Figure 16–2). The two methods are compared in Table 16–1.

Clinical Tip

In preparation for a transabdominal ultrasound exam, the woman is advised to drink 1 to 1.5 quarts of water approximately 2 hours before the examination, and she is asked to refrain from emptying her bladder. If the bladder is not sufficiently filled, she is asked to drink 3 to 4 (8 oz) glasses of water and is rescanned 30 to 45 minutes later.

Indications for Ultrasound

Ultrasound examinations should be performed by licensed medical practitioners, including nurses, following published standards and guidelines. The American College of Obstetricians and Gynecologists (ACOG, 2014) endorses the use of obstetrical ultrasound to obtain the following data:

- Estimation of gestational age
- Evaluation of cervical insufficiency
- Evaluation of fetal growth or fetal well-being
- Evaluation of vaginal bleeding
- Determination of fetal presentation
- Evaluation of abdominal or pelvic pain
- Suspected multiple gestation
- Significant discrepancy between uterine size and clinical date
- Evaluation of pelvic mass or uterine abnormality
- Examination of suspected hydatidiform mole
- Adjunct to special procedures including amniocentesis, cervical cerclage placement, or external cephalic version
- Evaluation for premature rupture of the membranes or premature labor

TABLE 16–1 Comparison of Transvaginal and Transabdominal Ultrasound

FACTORS	TRANSVAGINAL	TRANSABDOMINAL
Transducer location	Vaginal insertion with lubricant placed over protective probe cover	Abdominal placement with transducer gel spread over abdomen
Maternal positioning	Lithotomy with buttocks at end of examination table with drape over legs and abdomen	Semi-Fowler with drape over abdomen
Status of bladder	Empty bladder	Full bladder
Structures visualized	Gestational sac, presence or absence of a yolk sac or embryo, crown–rump length (CRL) for accurate gestational age dating, presence of cardiac activity, fetal number, maternal anatomy (uterus, cervix, and adnexal structures)	Vagina, cervix, bladder
Timing	First trimester; may be used throughout pregnancy to assess cervical status	Second and third trimesters; may be used in first trimester if bleeding is noted
Source of discomfort (if any)	Pressure from movement of probe, pushing	Bladder distension, pressure from pushing on abdomen, shortness of breath, hypotension, dizziness
Comfort measures	Offer for woman to insert probe herself, advise her to report discomfort	Use wedge to place woman in a semi-tilted position to increase blood flow; allow her to empty small amount of urine if she voices discomfort
Purpose	Facilitate chorionic villus sampling (CVS), identify serial cervical insufficiency: Cervical length and cervical funneling (a cone-shaped indentation in the cervical os)	Amniocentesis, routine fetal assessment of anatomy

- Evaluation of suspected fetal death
- Evaluation of suspected ectopic pregnancy
- Evaluation of suspected amniotic fluid abnormalities
- Evaluation of suspected placental abruption
- Evaluation of abnormal biochemical markers
- Follow-up evaluation of fetal anomaly
- Follow-up evaluation of placental location for suspected placenta previa
- Evaluation of those with history of previous congenital anomaly
- Evaluation of fetal condition in late presentation for prenatal care
- To assess findings that may increase the risk of chromosomal abnormalities
- To screen for fetal anomalies.

Assessment of Fetal Well-Being in the First Trimester

The first trimester represents a crucial time for establishing fetal viability and determining an accurate gestational age. Ultrasound can be used during the first trimester to help determine certain characteristics, including some chromosomal disorders. There are a variety of methods that the practitioner can use to determine fetal well-being in early pregnancy.

Viability

Viability, or the potential for the pregnancy to result in a live neonate, is the first issue to consider in pregnancy. A positive urine pregnancy test does not confirm viability, but represents the presence of beta human chorionic gonadotropin hormone. This hormone becomes present in the bloodstream when the developing embryo implants into the uterus at approximately 10 to 14 days after conception has occurred (Gabbe, Niebyl, Simpson, et al., 2017). Bleeding is the most common symptom associated with performing a first-trimester ultrasound. Previous fetal loss, unknown last menstrual period (LMP), and dating and size discrepancy are other indicators for performing a first-trimester ultrasound examination. Bleeding can also be associated with a nonviable pregnancy in cases of spontaneous abortion (miscarriage) and ectopic (tubal) or extrauterine pregnancy. Serial quantitative beta hCG testing, progesterone-level testing, and ultrasound can be used to distinguish a normally developing fetus from an ectopic pregnancy, which, if undiagnosed, carries a high rate of maternal morbidity.

QUANTITATIVE BETA HCG TESTING

Beta human chorionic gonadotropin (beta hCG) is a product of the trophoblast or placenta and is a very accurate marker of the presence of pregnancy and placental health. Beta hCG is detectable in the blood serum of approximately 5% of pregnant women by 8 days after conception and in virtually all pregnancies by 11 days. The level in the serum approximately doubles every 2 days in the first 10 days of pregnancy, peaking at 60 to 90 days after conception (Gabbe et al., 2017) (Table 16–2). In early pregnancy, the doubling of two quantitative beta hCG levels drawn 48 hours apart serves as an excellent test of the viability of the pregnancy. Conversely, if the beta hCG level remains stable or falls over 48 hours, a miscarriage or ectopic pregnancy should be suspected. See Chapter 18 for a discussion of beta hCG testing in ectopic pregnancy.

Although not routine in all pregnancies, serologic evaluation in the first trimester should be done for women with the following indicators:

- History of spontaneous abortion
- History of ectopic pregnancy

TABLE 16–2 Approximate Beta hCG Values in Pregnancy

GESTATIONAL AGE (WEEKS)	BETA HCG VALUES (MILLI–INTERNATIONAL UNITS/ML)
1–2	16–156
2–3	101–4870
3–4	1110–31,500
4–5	2560–82,300
5–6	23,100–151,000
6–7	27,300–233,000
7–11	20,900–291,000
11–16	6140–103,000
16–21	4720–80,100
21–39	2700–78,100

- Risk of ectopic pregnancy (intrauterine device in place, previous pelvic inflammatory disease, or reversal of a tubal sterilization)
- Vaginal bleeding (more than spotting)
- Conception through assisted reproductive methods.

The 48 hours between the beta hCG tests can be an extremely anxious time for the couple. To offer effective counseling, the nurse must understand the information these tests provide, as well as their limitations. For example, the woman may not know why she must wait 48 hours for a repeat blood test. The nurse needs to allow time for the woman and her partner, if present, to express their anxiety and fears. False reassurances should not be offered. Instead, attention is directed toward helping them cope with the inherent uncertainty that occurs while the exams are being completed and until a definitive diagnosis can be made.

PROGESTERONE-LEVEL TESTING

Progesterone is secreted in early pregnancy by the corpus luteum until approximately 8 weeks' gestation, at which point the placenta begins to manufacture its own progesterone. Low levels of progesterone are associated with spontaneous abortions and ectopic pregnancies (Gabbe et al., 2017). Although progesterone levels are not routinely tested in early pregnancy, they can be assessed by performing a simple blood test when there is a history of spontaneous abortions or bleeding in early pregnancy. Progesterone levels above 25 ng/mL are typically associated with normally developing intrauterine pregnancies. Progesterone levels that are below 5 ng/mL typically indicate a nonviable fetus. Levels between 5 ng/mL and 25 ng/mL are inconclusive. Approximately 10% of women have progesterone levels below 25 ng/mL (Gabbe et al., 2017). In many settings it is the nurse who notifies the healthcare provider if levels are low. The healthcare provider, in conjunction with the woman's desires, bases the decision of whether or not to supplement progesterone during early pregnancy on current progesterone levels, past history of spontaneous abortions, and/or presence of spotting or vaginal bleeding. However, supplementing with progesterone also has the potential of prolonging an inevitable nonviable pregnancy. Transvaginal ultrasound is often used in combination with hCG and progesterone level testing to determine viability of a pregnancy. Low progesterone levels can be treated by giving the woman progesterone either orally or via vaginal suppositories or intramuscular injection. This indication for supplementation is warranted only throughout the first trimester. After 12 gestational weeks, supplements are not needed because the placenta will make adequate progesterone levels (Gabbe et al., 2017).

ULTRASOUND

The sonographic landmarks (presence of gestational sac, cardiac motion, embryo development) of normal early pregnancy, detected by transvaginal ultrasound, are very predictable. Up to about 4½ to 5 weeks of gestation, before the appearance of a gestational sac, only the endometrial stripe can be seen in the uterus. The gestational sac at first appears empty and may be confused with the pseudogestational sac of ectopic or extrauterine pregnancy. The presence of an *intradecidual sign* provides clarity. An intradecidual sac appears prior to a gestational sac and is an echogenic focus that appears as a straight line. This markedly thickened decidua is located on the uterine cavity wall and is present until 8 weeks of gestation (Norton, 2016). Presence of this sign with no gestational sac warrants a repeat ultrasound examination, in which, after 1 to 2 weeks, the gestational sac should be visualized.

A true gestational sac is associated with beta hCG levels of 1800 milli–International Units/mL if the sonogram is being done transvaginally and 6500 milli–International Units/mL if the sonogram is being done transabdominally. At approximately 5½ weeks, the yolk sac, a small round structure sometimes resembling a "double ring," is visible within the gestational sac. It is an embryonic structure, so its appearance provides strong evidence supporting the presence of an intrauterine pregnancy (Norton, 2016). At 6 to 6½ weeks, the embryo itself becomes visible, and shortly thereafter cardiac activity is detectable (Posner, 2013). During the ultrasound examination, the gestational sac and embryo (crown–rump length [CRL]) are measured to determine gestational age (Figure 16–4).

GESTATIONAL AGE

Determination of an accurate expected date of birth (EDB) early in pregnancy is essential for evaluating well-being throughout the pregnancy. Labor contractions (rhythmic tightening and relaxing of the uterine muscles during labor; see Chapter 19 for a full discussion) that may be perfectly normal at 37 weeks could be a problem if they occur prior to 34 weeks. Conversely, a 40-week pregnancy inadvertently thought to be 42 weeks may

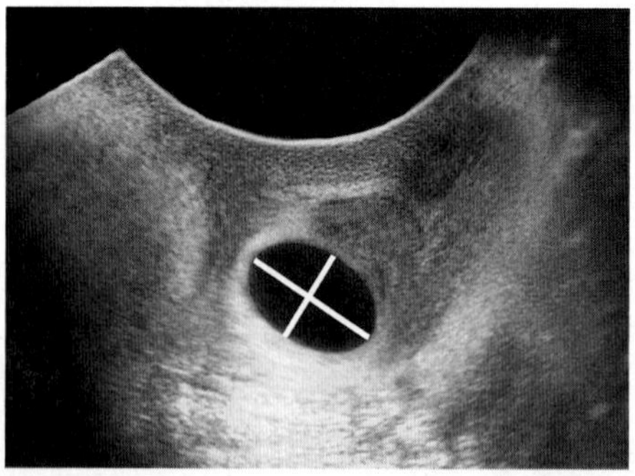

Figure 16–4 Measurement of the gestational sac. The ultrasound shows the uterus; the blackened oval area is the gestational sac. The fluid in the gestational sac does not generate echoes from the ultrasound and thus appears dark in contrast to the uterine tissue surrounding it. The lines through the gestational sac represent measurements that are taken.

result in an unnecessary and risk-laden induction of labor. Much of the physician's or midwife's efforts are aimed at determining the most accurate EDB possible. Traditional means of establishing an EDB are documenting a reliable last menstrual period (LMP) from the woman, measuring uterine size, noting the date of the first audible fetal heart tones, and noting the date of quickening (the first recognized fetal movement). A definite and normal LMP established early in pregnancy is considered the most reliable indicator of an EDB (Norton, 2016). Problems occur if the woman cannot recall her LMP, if her menstrual cycles were extremely irregular, if she was lactating, if she was using hormonal contraception, or if she had bleeding in early pregnancy.

An early transvaginal or abdominal sonogram is indicated when there is a need to establish an accurate gestational age. When dating a pregnancy using ultrasound:

- Crown–rump length is considered most accurate for 6- to 12-week gestational periods (plus or minus 3 to 5 days) (Figure 16–5).
- For example, if the EDB based on a 10-week sonogram is September 9, it is reasonable to expect that date determined by LMP is accurate from September 4 through September 14.
- After 12 weeks' gestation, femur length, abdominal circumference, and biparietal diameter are the most accurate markers for dating ± 7 to 14 days (Figure 16–6).

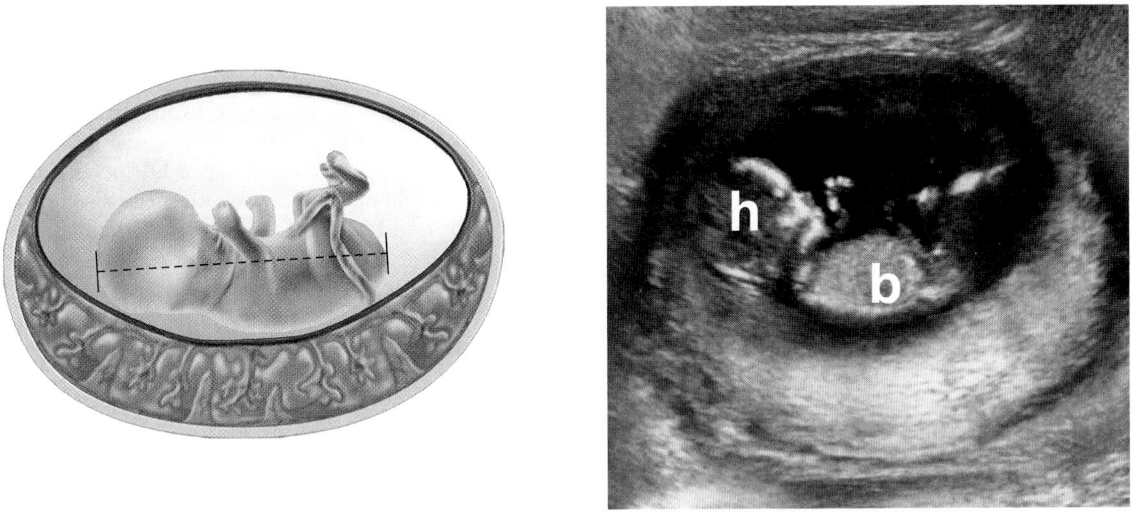

A B

Figure 16–5 **Measurement of the crown–rump length. A. Schematic diagram. Dotted line shows the measurement from the top of the fetal crown (head) to the bottom of the rump (buttocks). B. Ultrasound scan of the pregnant uterus, showing the longest length of a 9-week fetus. The head (h) can be differentiated from the body (b), but the internal anatomy cannot be clearly distinguished.**

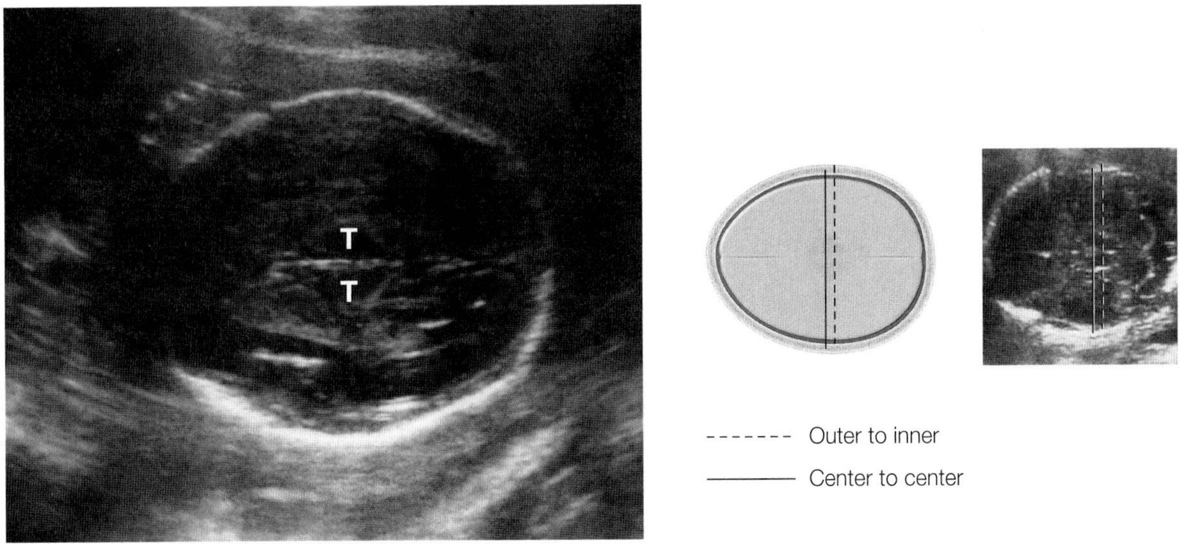

A B

Figure 16–6 **Measurement of the biparietal diameter. A. Ultrasound transaxial image of the fetal head, taken with the thalami (T) imaged in the midline, equidistant from the temporoparietal tables of the calvarium. B. Diagram and image showing the leading edge (outer) to the leading edge (inner) measurements of the fetal head, taken at the level of the thalami.**

- For example, if the EDB is October 1, estimated by a second-trimester sonogram, the reasonable date of birth can be from September 16 through October 14.
- After 26 weeks' gestation, fetal growth rates are less uniform, making ultrasound an inappropriate means of determining gestational age. In the third trimester, ultrasound can estimate an EDB with plus or minus 14 to 21 days of accuracy. See Table 16–3.

Clinical Tip

Although practices may vary, most practitioners do not change a due date based on the second-trimester sonogram unless there is a discrepancy of greater than 11 to 14 days from the LMP.

Determining an accurate EDB based on a first-trimester ultrasound can be extremely important later in pregnancy should there become a size–date discrepancy. It assists the physician or midwife in diagnosing intrauterine growth restriction (to be discussed later in this chapter).

Genetic Screening Options

First-trimester single screening tests include nuchal translucency measurement, serum-free β-hCG, or total human chorionic gonadotropin (hCG) along with pregnancy-associated plasma protein A analyte levels (PAPP-A). These tests are performed between 11 weeks and 0 days and 13 weeks and 6 days to determine if a fetus is at risk for a chromosomal disorder, such as Down syndrome (trisomy 21), trisomy 13, and trisomy 18. The ultrasound assesses the accumulation of fluid between the posterior cervical spine and the overlying skin in the fetal neck, known as the **nuchal fold**. If the nuchal fold is greater than 3 mm, the incidence of Down syndrome is increased (ACOG, 2016). The test is performed in conjunction with a maternal serum blood test measuring the biochemical markers PAPP-A and free beta hCG. The combination of blood testing and the ultrasound screening test is 82 to 87% accurate for detecting Down syndrome (ACOG, 2016).

Cell-free DNA (cfDNA) testing is a noninvasive maternal serum blood test that extracts fetal DNA from maternal circulation with a 98% detection rate for fetal trisomy 21 and lower detection rates for trisomies 13 and 18. It can be performed any time after 10 gestational weeks (ACOG, 2016). Cell-free DNA testing can also determine fetal sex and the presence of a Rh-positive fetus in a Rh-negative mother, as well as detect some paternally derived autosomal dominant genetic abnormalities (ACOG, 2016). If an abnormal test result is obtained, the mother is referred for genetic counseling and offered invasive diagnostic testing, such as chorionic villus sampling (CVS) or amniocentesis (ACOG, 2016).

Assessment of Fetal Well-Being in the Second Trimester

Many women undergo first-trimester screening and also have additional testing that occurs during the second trimester. The **integrated test** includes the first-trimester combined test, nuchal translucency testing, PAPP-A, and second-trimester maternal serum testing—also known as the **quadruple screen (quad screen)**, which measures AFP, uE3, beta hCG, and inhibin A—to calculate the risk of having an affected fetus. When the integrated test is used, the woman receives the first-trimester screening between 10 weeks and 13-6/7 weeks, followed by the quad screen between 15 and 22 weeks, although optimal testing time is 16 to 18 weeks (ACOG, 2016). The integrated test approach requires two separate testing intervals, but is 96% accurate in detecting trisomy 21. **Contingent screening** is based on, or contingent on, first-trimester results. If first-trimester results are negative, no additional testing is pursued. If first-trimester results are indeterminate, second-trimester testing is offered. If first-trimester results are positive, diagnostic testing is offered. Some women may decline diagnostic testing, but may wish to pursue additional screening tests, such as the cfDNA testing.

Stepwise screening is a screening approach in which women identified at highest risk after first-trimester screening are offered diagnostic testing or cfDNA testing. As the testing comes back, women with abnormal values will continue to obtain the more invasive testing options and decide what additional testing they wish to pursue. Women with results that indicate the risk of aneuploidy is lower than the laboratory-derived positive screening cutoff are also offered stepwise screening. These women then have the quad screen performed at 16 to 18 weeks. The detection rate for stepwise screening is 91 to 93% (ACOG, 2016).

Ultrasonographic Screening

The second trimester is considered by many to be the most advantageous time for basic obstetric ultrasound for several reasons, including:

- Uniformity of fetal growth allows biometric measurements that provide an accurate estimation of gestational age.
- Large volume of amniotic fluid relative to the fetal size allows for excellent images of fetal anatomy.
- Fetal anatomy can be visualized in extreme detail, allowing confirmation of normal anatomy.

TABLE 16–3 Parameters for Estimating Gestational Age

SOURCE OF EVIDENCE	WHEN OBTAINED	ESTIMATED ACCURACY
In vitro fertilization	At conception	Less than 1 day
Ultrasound measurement of crown–rump length	6–10 weeks	3 days
Clinical measurement of normal uterus	Less than 12 weeks	7 days
Ultrasound measurement of biparietal diameter	Less than 20 weeks	7 days
Ultrasound measurement of biparietal diameter	20–26 weeks	10 days
Ultrasound measurement of biparietal diameter	26–30 weeks	14–21 days
Ultrasound measurement of biparietal diameter	Greater than 30 weeks	21–28 days

Clinical Tip

The ideal time for the second-trimester basic sonogram is 18 to 24 weeks. Sonograms done at 20 to 22 weeks may be easier to perform and less likely to require an additional scan than one done at 18 weeks; however, if lethal anomalies are identified and elective termination is a consideration, later examinations reduce options.

A standard (comprehensive) second-trimester sonogram provides the following information about the fetus, placenta, and uterine conditions:

- Fetal life
- Fetal number
- Fetal presentation
- Presence of abnormal heart rate or rhythm
- Evaluation of fetal anatomy
- Gestational age and growth
- Amniotic fluid volume
- Placental localization, including relationship to cervical os
- Umbilical cord, including the number of vessels present
- Uterine anatomy.

In addition, multiple gestations should be assessed for chorionicity, amnionicity, comparison of fetal sizes, the amount of amniotic fluid on each side of the membrane, and fetal genitalia if visible (Gabbe et al., 2017).

FETAL LIFE

Presence of cardiac motion confirms fetal life. If gestational age has already been established and fetal heart tones have been visualized with an ultrasound or heard with a Doppler in the first trimester, then absence of cardiac motion in the second trimester is consistent with fetal demise.

FETAL NUMBER

The second trimester is an ideal time to identify **multiple gestation** or the number of fetuses in the uterus. The number of placentas and their location can also be noted at this point.

FETAL PRESENTATION

Fetal presentation on a second-trimester ultrasound can be obtained but has no clinical significance because large amounts of amniotic fluid and small fetal size result in frequent presentation changes at this stage of pregnancy.

FETAL ANATOMY SURVEY

A systematic examination of the fetal parts is conducted to identify possible abnormalities. Components of this examination include the fetal parts discussed in the following sections.

Head. The skull should be symmetrical with the cranium, ossified, and intact. The ventricular system (passageways within the brain) is evaluated. The choroids should appear symmetrical. The choroid plexuses are found within the ventricles of the brain and in the subarachnoid space around the brain and spinal cord and produce cerebral spinal fluid. Choroid cysts, if noted, are usually benign but have been associated with chromosomal abnormalities in 1% of fetuses (Gabbe et al., 2017). The nuchal fold thickness should be measured because thickening of the nuchal fold, the skin at the base of the fetal skull, has also been associated with certain chromosomal abnormalities.

The most dramatic abnormality diagnosed by ultrasound is anencephaly (a neural tube defect in which a portion of the fetal brain is missing). It is abnormal not to see the bony structures of the skull above the orbits of the eye after 14 weeks' gestation. The skull is brightly echogenic (appearing white because of its increased density) and is easily visualized. Failure to see the skull should alert the experienced examiner to the possibility of anencephaly (Gabbe et al., 2017).

Spine. The spine is examined both sagittally and coronally for the presence of a sac or an outward splaying of the vertebrae laminae, suggestive of a possible spinal cord defect such as spina bifida.

Thorax and Heart. A transverse plane of the fetal thorax provides valuable information about the size, shape, and symmetry of the chest. The size, location, and axis of the heart are also evaluated. A four-chambered view of the heart should demonstrate ventricles and atria of approximately equal size and an intact intraventricular septum. The heart occupies one-quarter to one-third of the chest cavity on transverse image. The lungs should have a homogenous appearance. The diaphragm should be imaged. Chest size is correlated with lung size.

Abdomen. The bladder, stomach, and kidneys should all be visualized. The fetal stomach and bladder can be seen on ultrasound by 14 weeks. Persistent failure to visualize the fetal stomach can be due to various fetal abnormalities, the most common being esophageal atresia. Mild dilation of the renal pelvis of less than 10 mm is rarely progressive and usually physiologic (Gabbe et al., 2017). The abdominal wall should be visualized and intact. A transverse image of the umbilical cord should reveal a three-vessel cord with a visible insertion site of the umbilical cord where it enters the placental tissue.

Extremities. The femur is the only bone routinely measured on the basic ultrasound. If the length seems abnormal, a more comprehensive exam is performed to compare it with the lengths of the other long bones. The upper extremities and the presence of hands and feet are also documented.

GESTATIONAL AGE AND GROWTH

The Hadlock method uses an average of measures of the biparietal diameter, head circumference, abdominal circumference, and femur length to estimate gestational age (Figures 16–7 to Figure 16–10). Comparison of measures made at intervals to standardized measures can be used to estimate fetal growth.

AMNIOTIC FLUID VOLUME

Amniotic fluid volume (AFV) changes with gestational age. In general, a subjective assessment of amniotic fluid volume as decreased, normal, or increased is adequate during the second-trimester examination. The **amniotic fluid index (AFI)** is another method of reporting fluid volume and is calculated by dividing the maternal abdomen into four quadrants with the umbilicus as the reference point. The deepest vertical pocket of fluid in each quadrant is then measured, and these four measurements are summed to calculate the AFI.

PLACENTA LOCATION

The placenta's appearance, location, and relationship to the cervical os should be evaluated to assess for the possible complication

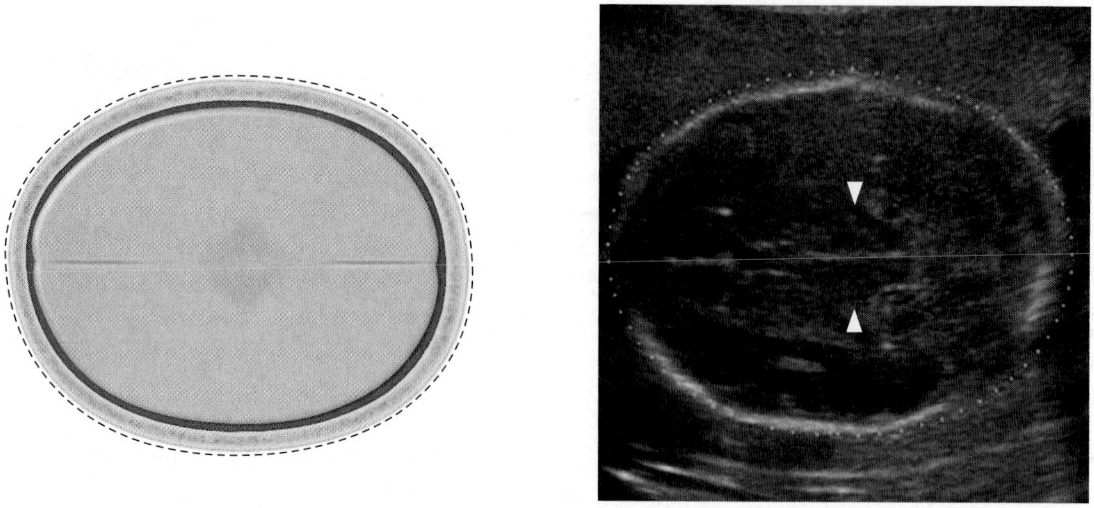

A B

Figure 16–7 Measurement of the head circumference. A. Diagram showing a dotted line outlining the head, which indicates the correct place to make a circumference measurement. B. Ultrasound transaxial scan showing the thalami (arrowheads), positioned in midline. A dotted line created by the digitizer outlines the correct parameter, just outside of the hyperechoic calvarium to obtain a circumference measurement.

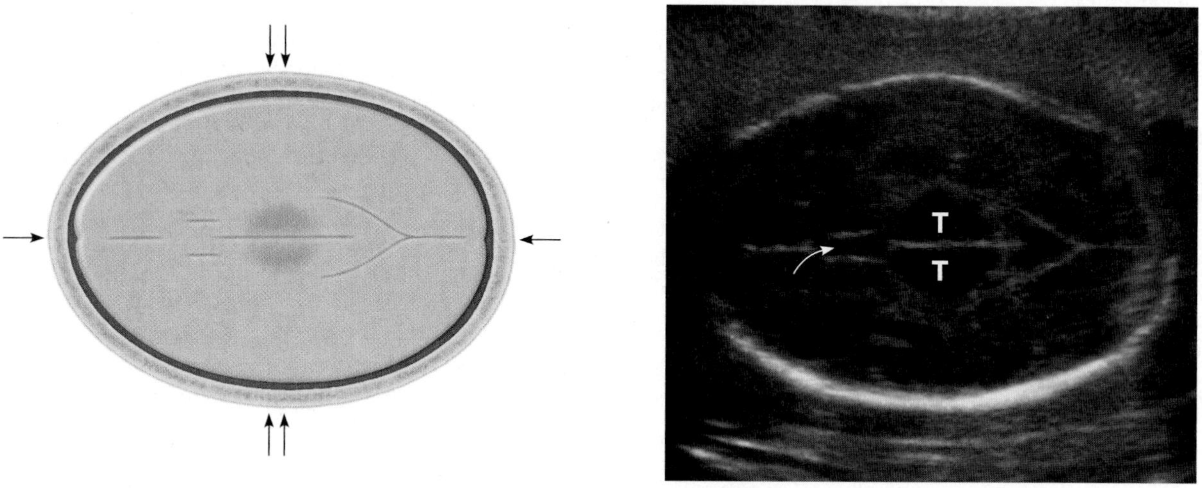

A B

Figure 16–8 Measurement of the cephalic index. A. The biparietal diameter (double arrows) and fronto-occipital diameter (single arrows) are both taken outer edge to outer edge. A ratio of the two gives the cephalic index. B. Ultrasound transaxial scan of the fetal head of the thalami (T) and cavum septi pellucidi (curved arrow).

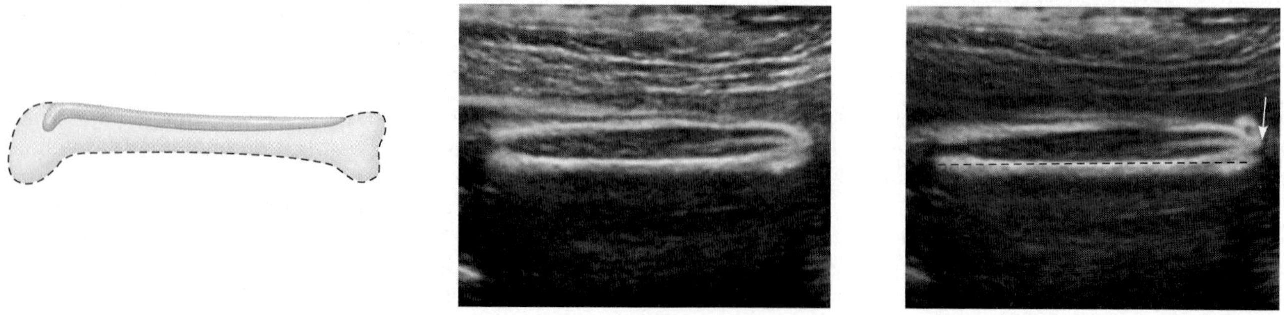

A B C

Figure 16–9 Measurement of the femur length. A. Schematic diagram. B. Ultrasound image. The hyperechoic line is in the ossified lateral margin of the femoral diaphysis. The ends of the bone are the epiphyseal cartilages that have not yet calcified and are therefore hypoechoic. C. The hyperechoic diaphysis is measured from one end to the other, denoted by the cursors and a dotted line. The "distal femoral point" (see arrow) is a nonossified extension of the distal epiphyseal cartilage. It should be included in the measurement.

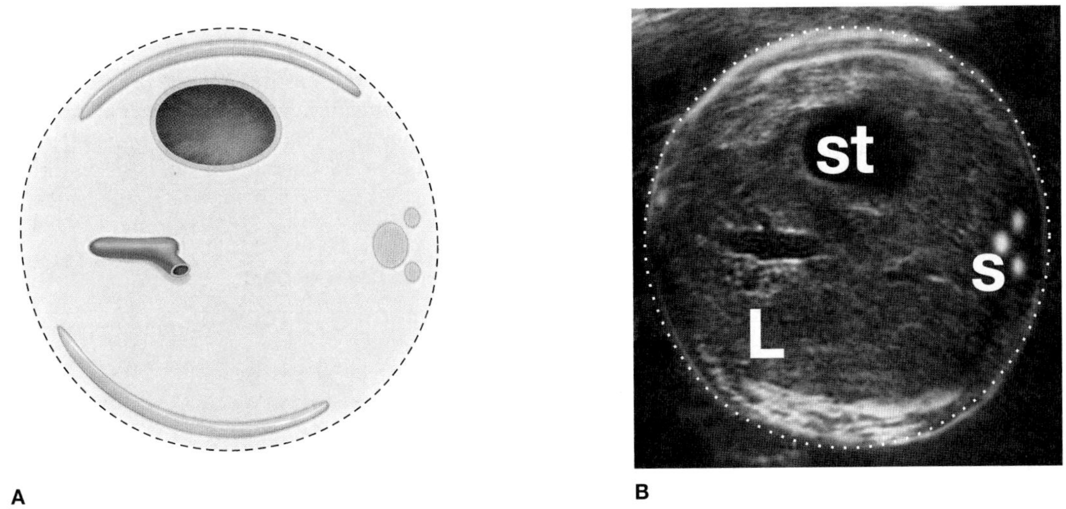

Figure 16–10 Measurement of the abdominal circumference. A. Diagram showing the abdominal circumference as a dotted line traced at the outer margin of the abdomen. B. Ultrasound transaxial image showing the umbilical portion of the left portal vein (arrowheads) correctly positioned within the liver and equidistant from the lateral walls. (S, spine; L, liver; st, stomach.) A dotted line, created by a digitizer, outlines the outer margins of the abdomen, the correct place to obtain an abdominal circumference measurement.

of placenta previa. Placental positions that are noted by sonogram in early pregnancy may not correlate well with the location at the time of birth. Factors such as the woman's position during the assessment or overdistention of the bladder may give a false-positive diagnosis of placenta previa. Therefore, a possible low-lying placenta or placenta previa that is identified on a second-trimester ultrasound must be confirmed by a follow-up sonogram in the third trimester (Gabbe et al., 2017).

SURVEY OF UTERINE ANATOMY

The uterus is assessed to examine maternal anatomy and identify any uterine defects or abnormalities. Adnexal (ovarian) masses or cysts may be noted. Uterine myomas (fibroids) are common and must be noted and monitored because they may grow more quickly in pregnancy, affecting the growth and well-being of the fetus or causing overdistention of the uterus, leading to preterm labor or birth (Gabbe et al., 2017). Ultrasound may also be used to measure both cervical length and dilatation of the internal cervical os. A shortened cervix and a dilated internal os noted by ultrasound can be predictive of preterm birth. However, false-positive results using this technique can be common because the degree of effacement or dilatation can be inaccurate. Some practitioners will schedule weekly transvaginal ultrasounds to measure cervical length beginning at 20 weeks for women with a history of preterm labor or cervical insufficiency and for women with a *cervical cerclage* in place (a suture placed in the cervix; see Chapter 23 and Figure 23–3) (Gabbe et al., 2017).

Assessment of Fetal Well-Being in the Third Trimester

Various maternal and prenatal conditions warrant antenatal testing during the third trimester. The type of testing performed is determined by the specific condition and the choice of the healthcare provider.

Conditions Warranting Fetal Surveillance

There are several indications for surveillance of fetal well-being in the third trimester. The following maternal and prenatal conditions require regular assessment:

Maternal Conditions

- Hypertensive disorders
- Diabetes mellitus
- Chronic renal disease
- Cyanotic heart disease
- Systemic lupus erythematosus
- Hyperthyroidism (poorly controlled)
- Antiphospholipid syndrome
- Hemoglobinopathies

Prenatal Conditions

- Preeclampsia
- Gestational diabetes
- Decreased fetal movement
- Oligohydramnios
- Hydramnios
- Intrauterine growth restriction
- Postterm pregnancy
- Isoimmunization (moderate to severe)
- Previous fetal demise
- Multiple gestation
- Known fetal anomaly
- Abnormal biochemical test results.

Fetal Movement Assessment

Fetal movement count, also called *fetal movement assessment*, is an acceptable, noninvasive, cost-effective method of fetal surveillance in both high- and low-risk pregnancies. Fetal movement is monitored by the woman on a daily basis, typically beginning at 28 weeks, at a time when the fetus is usually the most active. The Cardiff Count-to-Ten method is frequently used by women to count fetal movements on a daily basis as they go about their normal activities (Figure 16–11). The woman should feel fetal movement at least 10 times in 12 hours, and many women will feel 10 fetal movements in much less time, perhaps as little as 2 hours. Another method is the Daily Fetal Movement Record (DFMR), in which the woman lies on her side in a comfortable position and counts the number of movements until she reaches a minimum

Sample Cardiff Count–to–Ten scoring card

Month: __________ Week of gestation at beginning of month: __________

	9:00 AM	9:30	10:00	10:30	11:00	11:30	12:00 PM	12:30	1:00	1:30	2:00	2:30	3:00	3:30	4:00	4:30	5:00	5:30	6:00	6:30	7:00	7:30	8:00	8:30	9:00
1																									
2																									
3																									
4																									
5																									
6																									
7																									
8																									
9																									
10																									
11																									
12																									
13																									
14																									
15																									
16																									
17																									
18																									
19																									
20																									
21																									
22																									
23																									
24																									
25																									
26																									
27																									
28																									
29																									
30																									
31																									

Figure 16–11 An adaptation of the Cardiff Count-to-Ten scoring card for fetal movement assessment.

of three movements within a 1-hour period. With both methods, concern arises if the count is not reached within the specified time periods. Reduced fetal activity could be indicative of a fetal or placental issue and warrants further assessment.

Monitoring fetal movement serves as an indirect measure of fetal central nervous system integrity and function. The coordination of whole-body movement in the fetus requires complex neurologic control. For this reason, clinicians generally agree that vigorous fetal movement provides reassurance of fetal well-being and oxygenation. A reduction in activity is often associated with complications of chronic rather than acute nonreassuring fetal status as the compromised fetus decreases its oxygen requirements by reducing activity. Documented cessation of activity warns of the possibility of preterm birth, asphyxia, intrauterine growth restriction, and fetal death (Gabbe et al., 2017). It is these observations that provide the rationale for utilizing fetal movement counting as a means of antepartum fetal surveillance. See *Women with Special Needs: Women with Paralysis*.

Women with Special Needs **Women with Paralysis**

Women with paralysis often warrant intermittent fetal surveillance since they are unable to feel fetal movement or premature contractions. These women are at risk for unattended birth since they cannot perceive their contractions. Their partner or care provider should be trained to palpate contractions and observe for fetal movement on a regular basis.

There is considerable variation in fetal movement that depends on the individual and the gestational age of the fetus. Fetal movement first begins to occur as early as 7 weeks, although the movements are too fine to be perceived until approximately 16 weeks for a multiparous woman and up to 20 weeks for those who are primiparous. Muscle tone is limited before 28 weeks' gestation and fetal movements change in number and strength as pregnancy progresses (Polin, Abman, Rowitz, et al., 2016). Certain substances such as tobacco, drugs, alcohol, and caffeine have been shown to affect fetal movements, but usually reverse after drug clearance. Fetal rest–sleep cycles during which minimal or no movement may occur for up to 40 minutes is considered normal.

SAFETY ALERT!

Lack of fetal movement can be an indication of chronic placental insufficiency or even fetal death; thus, the woman should be advised how to handle nonreassuring findings. The woman should call her healthcare provider, and if advised she should come in for testing. The need to retain a sense of calm is imperative for the mother who is transporting herself to the medical setting for these tests.

It is important to provide patient education so women understand the importance of completing the fetal movement assessment and appropriate documentation on a daily basis. Contact information for questions and who to call with abnormal findings is imperative and should be given to each woman at 28 weeks' gestation. The expectant woman should be instructed to call the healthcare provider if at any time she is concerned about a decrease in fetal movement from the fetus's usual daily pattern. After 28 weeks, if fewer than the expected movements are perceived by the pregnant woman, further fetal surveillance tests, such as the nonstress test, may be used to assess fetal well-being. See *Teaching Highlights: What to Tell the Pregnant Woman About Assessing Fetal Activity*.

TEACHING HIGHLIGHTS | What to Tell the Pregnant Woman About Assessing Fetal Activity

- Explain that fetal movements are first felt around 18 weeks of gestation, but some women may not feel fetal movement until 25 weeks. This is called *quickening*. From that time, the fetal movements get stronger and easier to detect. A slowing or stopping of fetal movement may be an indication that the fetus needs some attention and evaluation. The mother's perception of decreased fetal movement is sufficient in most cases. Formal tracking of fetal movement does not lead to improved outcomes in low-risk pregnancies but may have value in high-risk situations.
- Describe the procedures and demonstrate how to assess fetal movement. Sit beside the woman and show her how to place her hand on the fundus to feel fetal movement. Advise the woman to keep a daily record of fetal movements beginning at about 28 weeks of gestation.
- Explain the procedure for the Cardiff Count-to-Ten method:
    1. Beginning at the same time each day, have the woman place an X on the Cardiff card (Figure 16–11) for each fetal movement she perceives during normal everyday activity until she has recorded 10 of them.
    2. Movement varies considerably, but the woman should feel fetal movement at least 10 times in 12 hours, and many women will feel 10 fetal movements in much less time, possibly 2 hours or less.
- Explain the procedure for the Daily Fetal Movement Record (DFMR) method:
    1. The woman should begin counting at about the same time each day, after taking food.
    2. She should lie quietly in a side-lying position.
    3. The woman should feel at least three fetal movements within 1 hour.
- Instruct the woman to contact her care provider in the following situations:
    1. Using the Cardiff method: If there are fewer than 10 movements in 12 hours.
    2. Using the DFMR method: If there are fewer than three movements in 1 hour.
    3. Both methods: If overall the fetus's movements are slowing, and it takes much longer each day to note the minimum number of movements in the specified time period, and if there are no movements in the morning.
- Whichever method she is using, encourage the woman to complete her fetal movement record daily and to bring it with her during each prenatal visit. Assure her that the record will be discussed at each prenatal visit and that questions may be addressed at that time if desired.
- Provide the woman with a name and phone number in case she has further questions.

Nonstress Test

The **nonstress test (NST)** has become a widely accepted method of evaluating fetal status. This test involves using an external electronic fetal monitor to obtain a tracing of the fetal heart rate (FHR) and observation of acceleration of the FHR with fetal movement. The test is based on the knowledge that the fetus is normally active throughout pregnancy and that fetal activity will result in acceleration of the FHR when the normal fetus moves. Accelerations of the FHR imply an intact central and autonomic nervous system that is not being affected by intrauterine hypoxia. FHR acceleration in response to fetal movement is, therefore, an accepted sign of fetal health. It must be noted, however, that a nonreactive NST is not diagnostic of fetal compromise. In other words, failure to provide evidence of fetal health does not indicate that the fetus is in trouble. The advantages of the NST include:

- Quick and easy to perform
- Inexpensive
- Easy to interpret
- Can be performed in an outpatient setting
- No known side effects.

The disadvantages include:

- Can be difficult to obtain a suitable tracing
- Results are influenced by fetal sleep cycle
- Extended monitoring may be required
- Maternal obesity, excessive fetal movement, hydramnios, and other factors can make the test difficult to perform.

Fetal age must be considered in the use and evaluation of NSTs. The central nervous system (parasympathetic and sympathetic nervous systems) of the fetus is not sufficiently mature to allow frequent accelerations of the heart rate when fetal movement occurs until 30 to 32 weeks of gestation. Acceleration patterns are directly affected by gestational age. The acme of acceleration is 15 beats per minute or more above the baseline rate. The acceleration lasts 15 seconds or longer for less than 2 minutes in fetuses at or beyond 32 weeks (Figure 16–12). There must be at least two accelerations within a 20-minute period. Before 32 weeks, accelerations are defined as having an acme of 10 beats per minute or more for 10 seconds or longer (Cunningham et al., 2014). One study examined FHR pattern changes that occurred with advancing gestational age. Mean baseline FHR, signal loss, and fetal movement all decreased in advancing gestational age (Cunningham et al., 2014).

The NST can be used as an assessment tool in any pregnancy but is especially useful in the presence of diabetes, preeclampsia, intrauterine growth restriction, spontaneous rupture of the membranes, multiple gestation, postdates, and other high-risk pregnancy conditions. These conditions can lead to a decline in uteroplacental functioning, which can result in decreased oxygenation to the fetus and eventual asphyxia. Testing intervals may vary, depending on the condition of the mother and fetus and recommendations of various experts. Most clinicians test twice weekly for high-risk patients and once a week for other conditions (Cunningham et al., 2014).

PROCEDURE FOR PERFORMING A NONSTRESS TEST

The NST can be performed in an inpatient or outpatient setting. Women are advised to eat prior to the test and abstain from cigarette smoking for at least 2 hours prior to the exam. The woman is placed in semi-Fowler position with a small pillow or blanket under the right hip to displace the uterus to the left. The FHR is monitored by the placement of an electronic fetal monitor (see discussion in Chapter 20). Either one or two belts are placed around the woman's abdomen. One belt holds the ultrasound transducer to record the FHR and the other holds a tocodynamometer that detects uterine or fetal movement. The FHR is usually monitored for 20 minutes, but monitoring may be extended to 40 minutes if it appears the fetus is in a sleep cycle. The woman is often requested to record each fetal movement by the use of self-operated markers. See *Clinical Skill 16–1: Performing a Nonstress Test.*

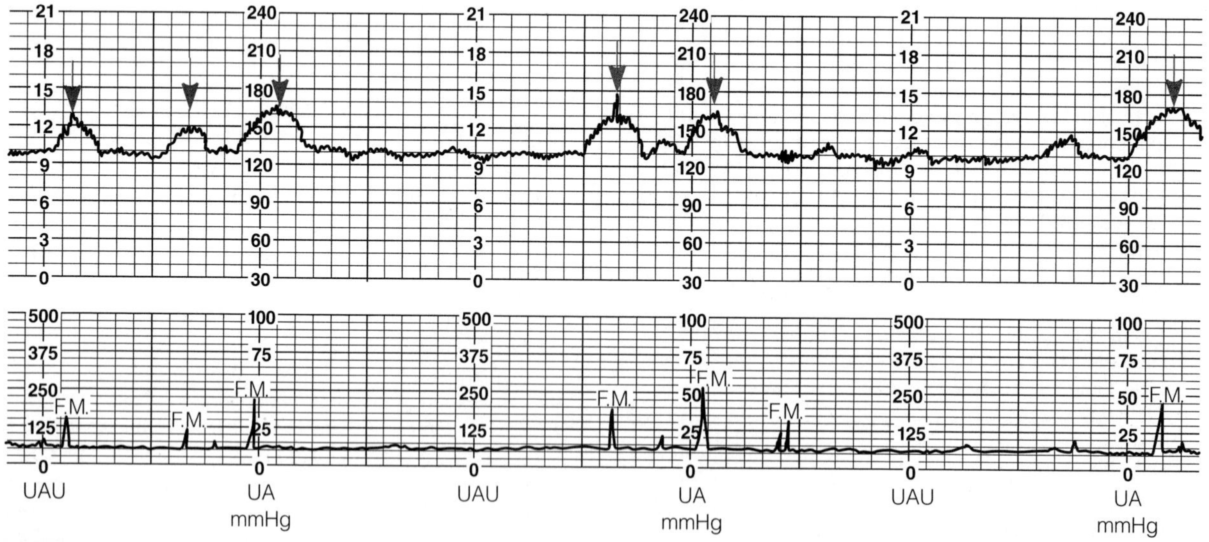

Figure 16–12 Example of a reactive nonstress test (NST). Accelerations of 15 beats/min lasting 15 seconds with each fetal movement (FM). Top of strip shows fetal heart rate (FHR); bottom of strip shows uterine activity tracing. Note that FHR increases (above the baseline) at least 15 beats and remains at that rate for at least 15 seconds before returning to the former baseline.

Clinical Skill 16–1

Performing a Nonstress Test

NURSING ACTION

Preparation

- Explain the procedure, the information it provides, and the process for completing the test.
- Ask the woman if she has recently eaten or smoked cigarettes.

Rationale: *The test should be performed after the woman has eaten. Cigarette smoking can adversely affect the test results, so the woman should be counseled to avoid smoking prior to testing.*

- Ask the woman to void.

Rationale: *The procedure will take at least 20 minutes to complete and the woman will need to remain in semi-Fowler or a side-lying position and will be unable to void without interrupting the testing procedure.*

Equipment and Supplies

External fetal monitor with a monitoring strip

Blood pressure cuff

Procedure

1. Place the woman in a semi-Fowler position with a small pillow or towel placed under her right hip after she has voided.
2. Place the ultrasound transducer from the external fetal monitor on the woman's abdomen over the FHR (typically over the fetal back or chest just below the neck) so a tracing can be obtained on the monitoring strip.
3. If the FHR is not consistently recorded on the monitoring strip, adjust the ultrasound transducer until an adequate reading is obtained.

Rationale: *Fetal or maternal movement can cause an inconsistency in the FHR on the monitoring strip. Multiple adjustments may be needed to obtain consistency in recording the FHR.*

4. Place the tocodynamometer (pressure transducer) on the woman's abdomen over the uterine fundus.

Rationale: *Contractions are best detected when the device is directly placed on the uterine fundus.*

5. Obtain baseline measurements, including blood pressure, fetal activity, variations in the FHR during fetal movement, and contractions, for 20 minutes.

Rationale: *Baseline measurements provide a reference for normal maternal and fetal assessment parameters.*

6. Perform the test for 20 minutes but it may be extended up to 40 minutes.

Rationale: *Testing may be extended for the additional 20 minutes if the fetus is in a sleep cycle.*

7. Give the woman a handheld marker to indicate when she feels fetal movement.

Rationale: *Fetal movement is accompanied by an increase in the FHR in the healthy fetus. Lack of FHR accelerations may be an indication of uteroplacental perfusion problems.*

8. Interpret the results as reactive or nonreactive.

Rationale: *A reactive NST has two or more fetal heart accelerations within a 20-minute period. The FHR acceleration must be at least 15 beats per minute above baseline for at least 15 seconds from baseline to baseline. A nonreactive NST is one that lacks sufficient FHR accelerations over a 40-minute period (Cunningham et al., 2014).*

9. Explain the results to the woman and relate information from the healthcare provider regarding further management needs or additional follow-up that is needed.

Rationale: *The nurse is the key communicator in providing information regarding the test results and their meaning to the woman.*

10. Document baseline maternal and fetal assessment information that was obtained before and during the test. The results of the test should be documented along with information regarding how the information was reported to the healthcare provider. The specific name of the healthcare provider and date and time should be recorded. Any additional orders and instructions to the patient should be documented. Verbalization of understanding of the test results by the woman should be documented along with her understanding of follow-up instructions and future appointments.

INTERPRETATION OF THE NST

NSTs are categorized as either reactive or nonreactive. The most common definition of a reactive (normal) test is that there are two or more fetal heart accelerations within a 20-minute period, with or without fetal movement discernible by the woman. The FHR acceleration must be at least 15 beats/min above the baseline and last 15 seconds from baseline to baseline. A nonreactive (abnormal) NST is one that lacks sufficient FHR accelerations over a 40-minute period (Figure 16–13) (Cunningham et al., 2014). Again, it is important to take into account the gestational age of the fetus. Both fetal movement and the amplitude of the FHR accelerations increase with gestational age.

Spontaneous decelerations of the FHR, known as variable decelerations, that occur during the testing period must also be noted. Variable decelerations may be observed in up to 50% of NSTs. Variable decelerations, if nonrepetitive and brief (less than 30 seconds), do not indicate fetal compromise nor the need for obstetric intervention (Cunningham et al., 2014). In contrast, repetitive variable decelerations (at least three in 20 minutes), even if mild, have been associated with an increased risk of cesarean birth for fetal intolerance. The prognosis for decelerations lasting 1 minute or longer is even more ominous (Cunningham et al., 2014). It is the responsibility of the nurse performing this test to consult the physician or midwife for further evaluation of

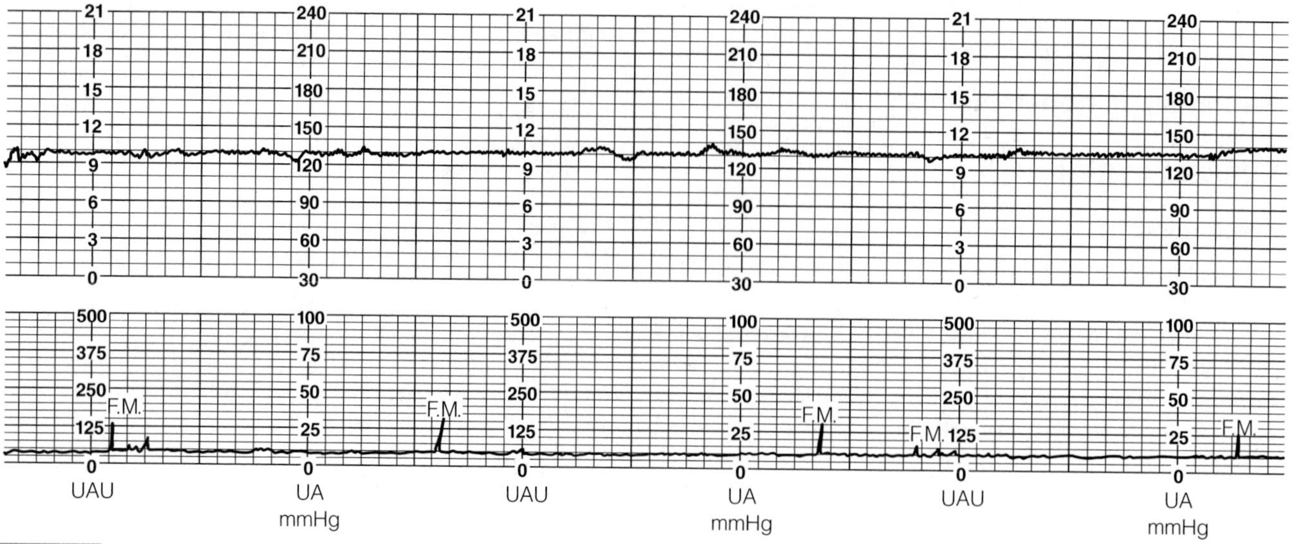

Figure 16–13 **Example of a nonreactive NST. There are no accelerations of FHR with fetal movement (FM). Baseline FHR is 130 beats/min. The tracing of uterine activity is on the bottom of the strip.**

fetal status if there is any question concerning the reactivity of the test or the presence of repetitive decelerations.

CLINICAL MANAGEMENT

The clinical management of a woman following an NST may vary. If the NST is reactive after 20 minutes, the test is concluded and the woman is rescheduled for further testing as indicated by the condition of, or risk factors present for, the mother and/or fetus. Testing may be performed weekly or twice weekly if warranted by maternal or fetal risk factors. Any significant deterioration in the maternal medical status requires fetal reevaluation regardless of the amount of time that has elapsed since the last test (Cunningham et al., 2014).

NURSING MANAGEMENT

For the Woman Undergoing a Nonstress Test

It is important to ensure that the woman understands the indications for the NST, the equipment used, and the procedure prior to beginning the test. Position the woman and apply the electronic fetal monitor. Monitor maternal blood pressure during the NST to determine whether hypotension is present. Administer the NST (you may or may not interpret the results) and report the findings to the provider and the patient. Use this opportunity to assess learning needs concerning the importance of fetal movement and provide information and teaching.

Contraction Stress Test

The **contraction stress test (CST)** is a means of evaluating the respiratory function (oxygen and carbon dioxide exchange) of the placenta. It enables the healthcare team to identify the fetus at risk for intrauterine asphyxia by observing the response of the FHR to the stress of uterine contractions (spontaneous or induced). During contractions, intrauterine pressure increases. Blood flow to the intervillous space of the placenta is reduced momentarily, thereby decreasing oxygen transport to the fetus. A healthy fetus usually tolerates this reduction well and maintains a steady heart rate. If the placental reserve is insufficient, fetal hypoxia, depression of the myocardium, and a decrease in FHR occur.

In many areas, the CST has given way to the biophysical profile. CST is still used in areas where the availability of other technology is reduced (such as during night shifts) or limited (such as at small community hospitals, rural areas, or birthing centers). It may also be used as an adjunct to other forms of fetal assessment. Often, a nurse will document CST results as part of her assessment if the criteria for a CST are met; however, they are rarely ordered in standard practice due to the wide availability of ultrasound technology.

SAFETY ALERT!

Because CST is contraindicated in cases of third-trimester bleeding from placenta previa, marginal abruptio placentae or unexplained vaginal bleeding, previous cesarean with classical incision (vertical incision in the fundus of the uterus), premature rupture of the membranes, cervical insufficiency, cerclage in place, anomalies of the maternal reproductive organs, history of preterm labor (if being done before term), or multiple gestation, the need to obtain a complete and comprehensive patient history prior to starting the test is imperative.

CONTRACTION STRESS TEST PROCEDURE

The critical component of the CST is the presence of uterine contractions. They may occur spontaneously (which is unusual before the onset of labor), or they may be induced (stimulated) with oxytocin (Pitocin) administered intravenously (also known as an oxytocin challenge test [OCT]). A natural method of obtaining oxytocin is through the use of breast stimulation (via either nipple self-stimulation or application of an electric breast pump); the posterior pituitary produces oxytocin in response to stimulation of the breasts or nipples (Cunningham et al., 2014).

An electronic fetal monitor is used to provide continuous data about the fetal heart rate and uterine contractions. After a 15-minute baseline recording of uterine activity and FHR, the tracing is evaluated for evidence of spontaneous contractions. If three spontaneous contractions of good quality and lasting 40 to 60 seconds occur in a 10-minute window, the results are evaluated, and the test is concluded. If no contractions occur or they are insufficient for interpretation, oxytocin is administered intravenously or breast self-stimulation or application of an electric breast pump is done to produce contractions of good quality. (See Chapter 25 for more information on nursing management of oxytocin induction.) The CST should be conducted only in a setting where tocolytic medications are available if a hypersystole pattern occurs or if labor is stimulated from the test.

INTERPRETATION OF CST RESULTS

The CST is classified as follows:

- ***Negative.*** A negative CST shows three contractions of good quality lasting 40 or more seconds in 10 minutes without evidence of late decelerations (Figure 16–14). This is the desired result. It implies that the fetus can handle the hypoxic stress of uterine contractions.
- ***Positive.*** A positive CST shows repetitive persistent late decelerations with more than 50% of the contractions (Figure 16–15). This is not a desired result. The hypoxic stress of the uterine contraction causes a slowing of the FHR. The pattern will not improve and will most likely get worse with additional contractions.
- ***Equivocal or suspicious.*** An equivocal or suspicious test has nonpersistent late decelerations or decelerations associated with tachysystole (contraction frequency of every 2 minutes or duration lasting longer than 90 seconds). When this test result occurs, more information is needed.

CLINICAL APPLICATION

A negative CST implies that the placenta is functioning normally, fetal oxygenation is adequate, and the fetus will probably be able to withstand the stress of labor. If labor does not occur in the ensuing week, further testing is done.

A positive CST with a nonreactive NST presents evidence that the fetus will not likely withstand the stress of labor.

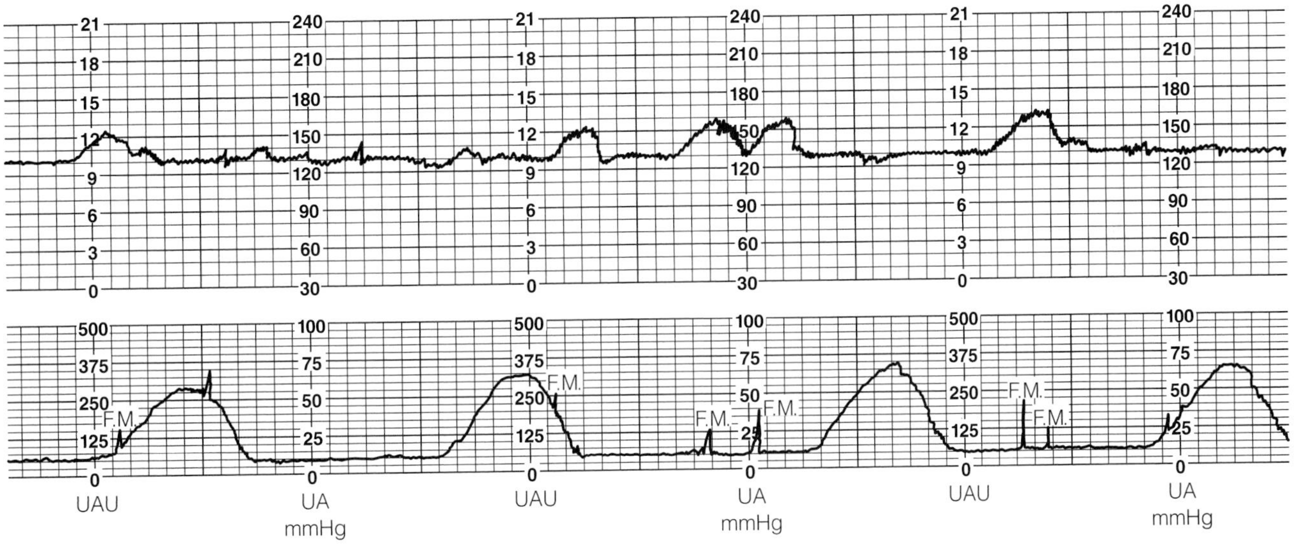

Figure 16–14 **Example of a negative CST (and reactive NST). The baseline FHR is 130 beats/min with acceleration of FHR of at least 15 beats/min lasting 15 seconds with each fetal movement (FM). Uterine contractions recorded on the bottom half of the strip indicate three contractions in 8 minutes.**

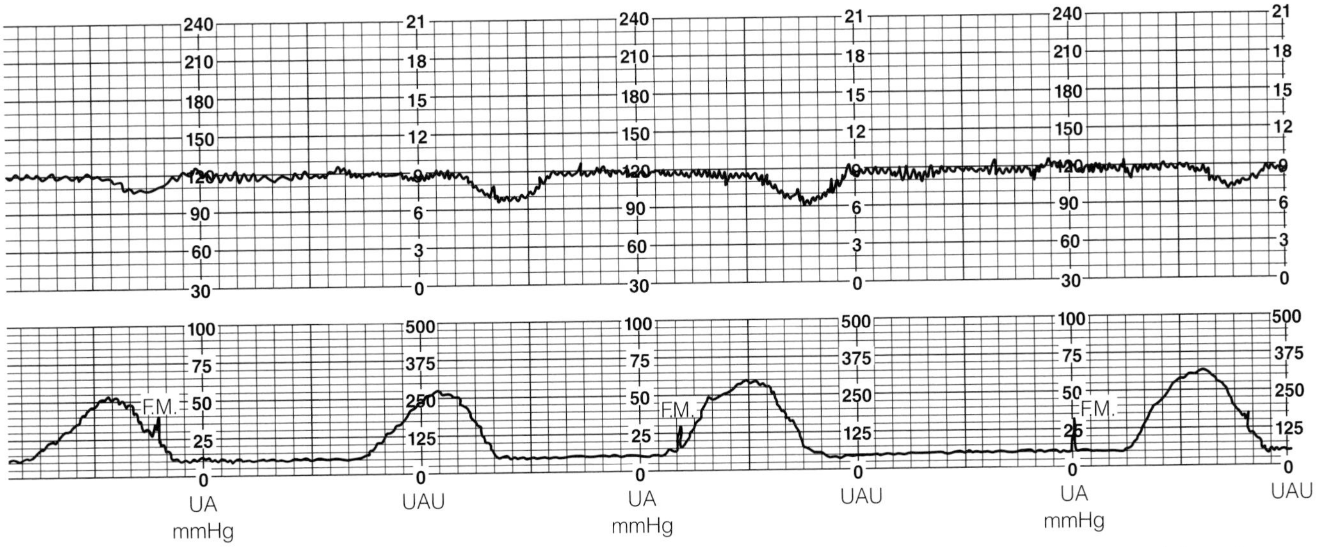

Figure 16–15 **Example of a positive contraction stress test (CST). Repetitive late decelerations occur with each contraction. Note that there are no accelerations of FHR with three fetal movements (FM). The baseline FHR is 120 beats/min. Uterine contractions (bottom half of strip) occurred four times in 12 minutes.**

A positive CST may be able to identify compromised fetuses earlier than a nonreactive NST because of the stimulated interruption of intervillous blood flow (Cunningham et al., 2014). Although a negative CST is reliable in predicting fetal status, a positive result needs to be verified, such as with a biophysical profile.

Amniotic Fluid Index

Assessment of amniotic fluid volume is based on the rationale that decreased uteroplacental perfusion may lead to diminished fetal renal blood flow, decreased urination, and, ultimately, **oligohydramnios** (decreased amniotic fluid volume). Fetal urine output and fetal swallowing are the major determinants of amniotic fluid volume. Oligohydramnios may be the result of diminished urinary output caused by fetal hypoxemia. The resulting placental insufficiency may cause hypoxia and hence oligohydramnios. Therefore, assessment of long-term uteroplacental function may be performed by evaluating amniotic fluid volume (Cunningham et al., 2014). Some poor pregnancy outcomes, such as intrauterine growth restriction, postterm pregnancy, and nonreassuring fetal status in labor, have been associated with abnormalities of amniotic fluid volume. See *Clinical Skill 20–2: Assessing for Amniotic Fluid.*

An amniotic fluid index (AFI) value of 5 or less serves as a red flag that some type of further assessment or management decision is needed (Cunningham et al., 2014). The gestational age of the fetus and the composite maternal condition may influence management decisions, leading to additional testing, induction of labor, or cesarean birth.

Biophysical Profile

The **biophysical profile (BPP)** represents an assessment of five fetal biophysical variables:

- FHR acceleration
- Fetal breathing
- Fetal movements
- Fetal tone
- Amniotic fluid volume.

The first criterion is assessed with the NST. The other variables are assessed by ultrasound scanning. By combining these five assessments, the BPP helps to identify the compromised fetus and confirm the healthy fetus. The test is complete when all the variables have been adequately assessed and should conclude within 30 minutes. Tests that are not completed in 30 minutes are considered abnormal (Bakay, Varolan, Yazgan, et al., 2016). See *Evidence-Based Practice: Completing the Fetal Biophysical Profile.*

Indications for the biophysical profile include those situations in which the NST and CST would be done. Assessment of these fetal biophysical activities is most useful in the evaluation of women who experience decreased fetal movement (who might subsequently have a nonreactive NST) and in the management of intrauterine growth restriction, preterm labor, gestational diabetes, hypertensive disorders, postterm pregnancies, and premature rupture of the membranes (PROM) (Bakay et al., 2016).

The two most important components of the BPP are the NST and the amniotic fluid volume index. The NST reflects the intactness of the nervous system, and the AFI reflects kidney perfusion. A normal AFI indicates that shunting has not occurred and that the fetal kidneys are adequately functioning. Reactive NST and normal fluid therefore reflect fetal well-being.

Specific criteria for normal and abnormal assessments are delineated in Table 16–4. Normal variables are each assigned a score of 2, and abnormal variables a score of 0 (zero). Thus, the highest score possible for a normal fetus is 10.

Clinicians suggest that management not be based solely on BPP scores. Biophysical activities of the fetus that develop first are the last to disappear when all activities are arrested because of asphyxia (Bakay et al., 2016). Those that are the last to develop are the most sensitive to hypoxia, and their disappearance can

EVIDENCE-BASED PRACTICE | Completing the Fetal Biophysical Profile

Clinical Question

Does the amount of ambient illumination change the time needed to complete the fetal biophysical profile?

The Evidence

It has been demonstrated that external stimuli can affect the behavior of a fetus without affecting the actual assessment results. In particular, fetal activity has been demonstrated to be more responsive and, therefore, more quickly measured when external stimuli such as light and sound are applied. Using adjustments to light in the sonography suite has been posed as a possible means to reduce the time needed to complete a fetal biophysical profile. Typically, fetal ultrasound studies are performed in a darkened room to improve visualization for the sonographer. It has not been documented whether this increases the time required to conduct the profile. These researchers set out to determine whether adjusting ambient light during a biophysical profile could improve efficiency by shortening the time required for the exam and reduce the number of low scores. Reducing false low scores could reduce costs, avoid unnecessary procedures, lower parental anxiety, and possibly lead to fewer preterm deliveries. Said et al. (2017) conducted a randomized trial with a large sample size to determine if there was a difference in time for completion and actual scores between darkened and ambient-light environments. Studies of this type with large samples comprise strong evidence for practice.

After studying more than 350 sonographic exams in which ambient light was compared to those in darkened rooms, there was no difference in the time needed to complete the profile; both took a little over 6 minutes. No difference was found in total or individual profile scores of the fetuses in this study. These findings were independent of the mother's body mass. There was no evidence that any level of lighting affected the outcome of the exam (Said et al., 2017).

Best Practice

Using ambient light as opposed to a darkened room is completely optional and has no effect on exam time or outcome. The comfort of the examiner and the ability to visualize the elements of the biophysical profile should be the key determinants. Mothers can be counseled that there is no need for increased light during a sonogram.

Clinical Reasoning

What might be the physiologic mechanisms that cause the fetus to respond to external stimuli during an examination? What alterations in the environment have the potential to affect the time to complete a biophysical profile accurately?

TABLE 16–4 Criteria for Normal and Abnormal Assessments of the BPP

COMPONENT	NORMAL (SCORE = 2)	ABNORMAL (SCORE = 0)
Fetal breathing movements	Greater than or equal to one episode of rhythmic breathing lasting greater than or equal to 30 sec within 30 min	Less than 30 sec of breathing in 30 min
Gross body movements	Greater than or equal to three discrete body or limb movements in 30 min (episodes of active continuous movement considered as single movement)	Less than or equal to two movements in 30 min
Fetal tone	Greater than or equal to one episode of extension of a fetal extremity with return to flexion, or opening or closing of hand	No movements or extension/flexion
Reactive fetal heart rate Nonstress test	Greater than or equal to two accelerations of greater than or equal to 15 beats/min for greater than or equal to 15 sec in 20–40 min	Zero or one acceleration in 20–40 min
Amniotic fluid volume	At least one pocket of amniotic fluid of at least 2 cm AFI ≥5	Less than one pocket of amniotic fluid measuring less than 2 cm

be noted first. For example, fetal tone (exhibited by flexion of the extremities) is the first activity to develop and the last activity to cease during asphyxia. Other activities in the normal developmental sequence are fetal movement, followed by fetal breathing, and then reactivity of the FHR. Therefore, FHR reactivity is the most sensitive to hypoxia (Bakay et al., 2016). One of the first indications of fetal compromise is a nonreactive NST. Table 16–5 outlines BPP test interpretation and the recommended management (Bakay et al., 2016).

Modified Biophysical Profile

The biophysical profile is labor intensive and expensive. It requires a person trained in ultrasonic visualization of the fetus. In addition, studies have shown that when the four dynamic ultrasound variables are normal, the probability of encountering an abnormal (nonreactive) NST is exceedingly small (Bakay et al., 2016). For these reasons, a modified biophysical profile has been developed. This test consists of an NST and a measurement of the amniotic fluid index (AFI), both of which reflect long-term uteroplacental function. The functioning of the placenta is important because a poorly functioning placenta (placental dysfunction) may result in diminished fetal renal perfusion, leading to oligohydramnios. The amniotic fluid volume assessment can therefore be used to evaluate long-term uteroplacental function. A modified BPP is considered normal if the AFV is greater than 5 cm and if the NST is reactive. The test is abnormal if either the NST is nonreactive or the AFI is 5 or less. The frequency of this test is the same as with the standard BPP.

TABLE 16–5 Biophysical Profile Test Interpretation and Recommended Management

TEST SCORE	INTERPRETATION	PERINATAL MORTALITY WITHIN 1 WEEK WITHOUT INTERVENTION	MANAGEMENT
10/10	Normal nonasphyxiated fetus	Less than 1/1000	No fetal indication for intervention; repeat test weekly except in patient with diabetes and pregnancies that are postterm (twice weekly)
8/10 (normal fluid)	Risk of fetal asphyxia extremely rare	Less than 1/1000	Same as above
8/8 if no NST done			
8/10 (abnormal fluid)	Chronic fetal asphyxia suspected	89/1000	Induce birth
6/10	Possible fetal asphyxia	89/1000	If amniotic fluid volume abnormal, induce birth If normal fluid at greater than 36 weeks with favorable cervix, induce birth If repeat test less than or equal to 6, induce birth If repeat test greater than 6, observe and repeat per protocol
4/10	Probable fetal asphyxia	91/1000	Repeat testing same day; if BPP score less than or equal to 6, induce birth
2/10	Almost certain fetal asphyxia	125/1000	Induce birth
0/10	Certain fetal asphyxia	600/1000	Induce birth

Doppler Flow Studies

Doppler flow studies are used in high-risk pregnancies to determine placental functioning and the velocity of blood flow in the vessels. An ultrasound beam, like that provided by the pocket Doppler (a handheld ultrasound device), is used to measure either arterial or venous blood flow. The signal that is reflected off the red blood cells moving within the vessels and the subsequent "picture" (waveform) that is received look like a series of waves. The highest-velocity peak of the waves is the systolic measurement, and the lowest point is the diastolic velocity. Multiple factors can affect the readings of velocity testing including proximity to the placenta, consistency of testing site on the umbilical cord, and selection of the artery being measured. Abnormal Doppler velocity findings are associated with increases in perinatal deaths. Examples of these waveforms are displayed in Figure 16–16 and Figure 16–17.

The use of Doppler velocimetry studies combined with the modified biophysical profile has yielded higher sensitivity in detecting adverse perinatal outcomes than either study performed alone (Bakay et al., 2016). Doppler velocimetry studies can examine either the arterial waveforms or venous parameters. The arterial waveforms provide data on vascular resistance which can be altered from structural changes in the vascular system itself or in changes in the vascular tone. Several measurement techniques can be used to assess arterial blood flow resistance. Increased blood flow resistance results in a reduction in end-diastolic velocity, which results in elevated values in all of the measurement techniques commonly used. The *cerebroplacental ratio (CPR)* is used to detect abnormal blood flow in fetuses with intrauterine growth restriction and late-onset, small-for-gestational-age fetuses to detect fetal-placental and uteroplacental dysfunction, although the accuracy of the test decreases after 34 gestational weeks. Normal CPR findings should be greater than 1.

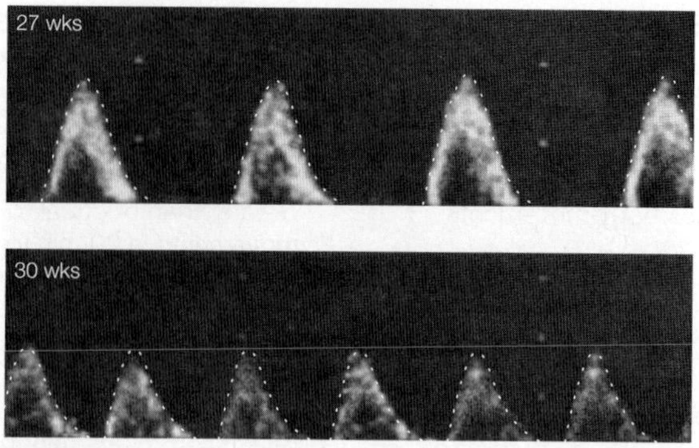

Figure 16–17 **Two examples of abnormal umbilical artery velocity waveforms taken from a patient with intrauterine growth restriction.**

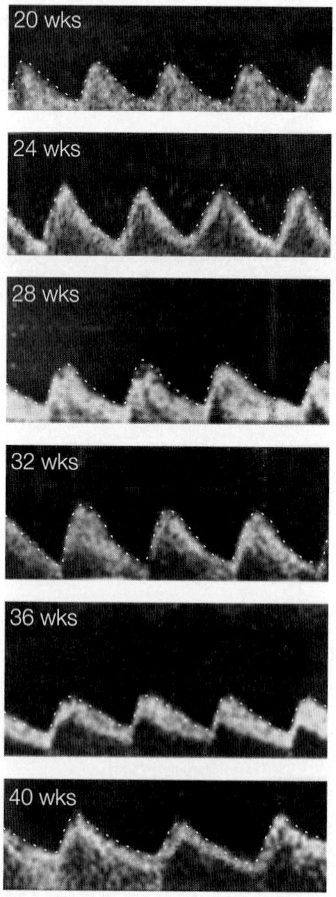

Figure 16–16 **Serial studies of the umbilical artery velocity waveforms in a normal pregnancy from one patient.**

Blood flow velocity can also be measured by the *systolic-to-diastolic (S/D) ratio*. The S/D ratio normally decreases as the fetus nears term. This phenomenon reflects the decreasing resistance of placental and umbilical vasculature to allow for greater umbilical blood flow to meet the needs of a growing fetus. The S/D ratio is considered abnormal if it is elevated above the 95th percentile for gestational age or reversed after 18 to 20 weeks of gestation (Gabbe et al., 2017).

The *resistance index (RI)* is another technique used to evaluate blood flow resistance. If the RI is greater than .58, it is considered abnormal and indicates alteration in perfusion and an increased risk of adverse perinatal outcomes. The *pulsatility index (PI)* has the smallest measurement error but has a narrower window of normal values. In Doppler flow studies, the absence of reversed end-diastolic flow signifies increased impedance and is uniquely associated with intrauterine growth restriction and a higher perinatal mortality rate.

A decrease in fetal cardiac output or an increase in resistance of placental vessels will reduce umbilical artery blood flow. Doppler velocimetry is best used when intrauterine growth restriction is diagnosed or late-term SGA is suggested, whether it occurs as an idiopathic process (cause unknown) or in the presence of hypertension or preeclampsia (Gabbe et al., 2017). No benefit has been demonstrated for umbilical artery velocimetry for other high-risk conditions such as postterm pregnancy, diabetes, systemic lupus erythematosus, or antiphospholipid antibody syndrome. Also, it has not been shown to be of value as a screening test for detecting fetal compromise in the general obstetric population (Gabbe et al., 2017).

Evaluation of Placental Maturity

Placental maturity is evaluated by a grading process that uses ultrasound to measure the changes in the basal layer, chorionic plate, and intervening placental substance. A grade of 0 through III is assigned (grade III is the most mature, showing extensive calcifications) (Figure 16–18). Placentas with multiple calcifications are less likely to function as adequately as those with lower grades. Certain factors can cause a placenta to mature, including maternal smoking, postterm pregnancy, and certain maternal conditions, such as preeclampsia and gestational diabetes. Placental grade may be used to correlate with other findings; however, placental grade alone does not dictate management of a pregnancy (Gabbe et al., 2017).

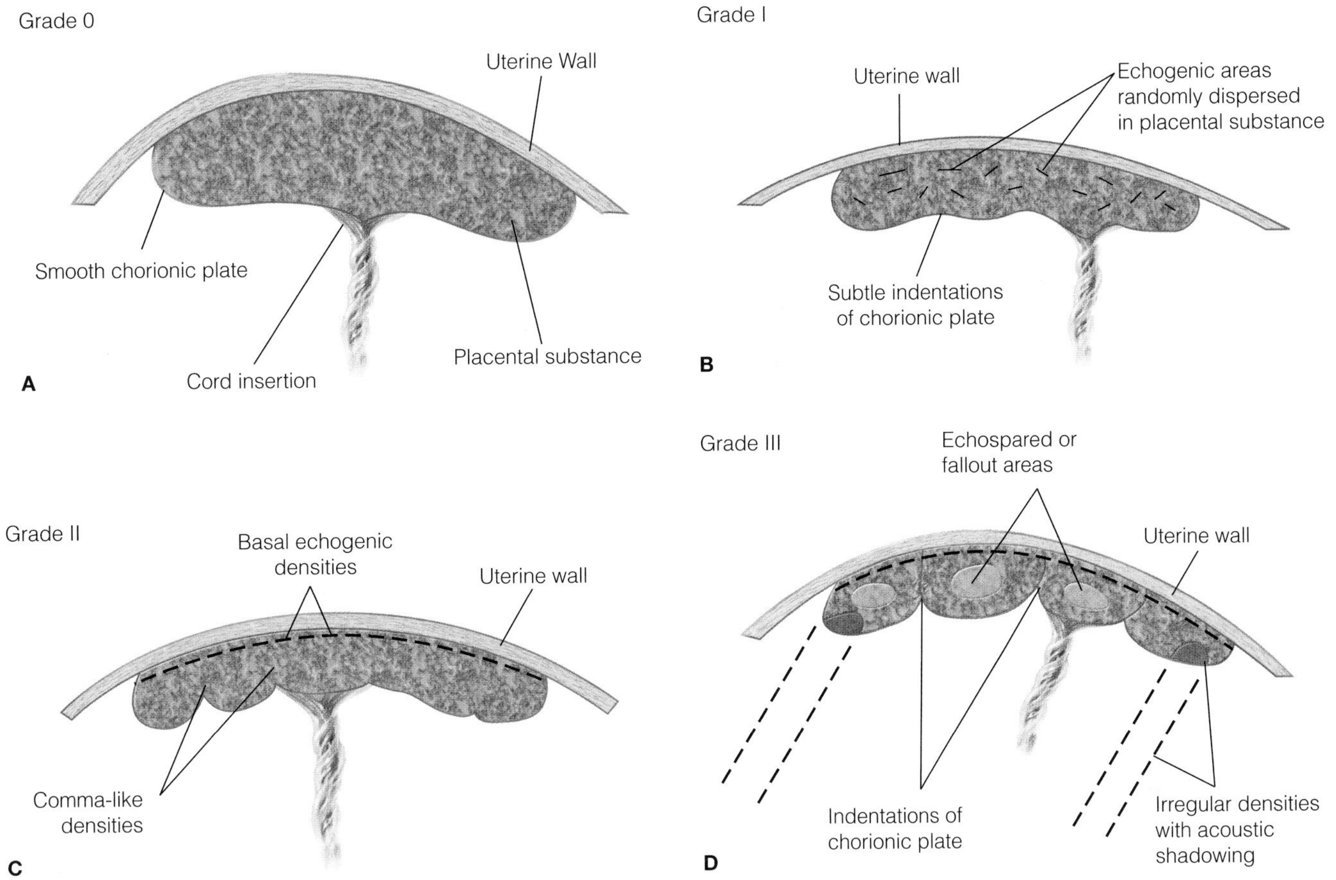

Figure 16–18 **Placental grading. A. Diagram showing the ultrasonic appearance of a grade 0 placenta. B. Diagram showing the ultrasonic appearance of a grade I placenta. C. Diagram showing the ultrasonic appearance of a grade II placenta. D. Diagram showing the ultrasonic appearance of a grade III placenta.**

Estimation of Fetal Weight

Estimating the fetal weight in the third trimester of pregnancy is an important aspect of fetal assessment. Particularly, findings of the fetal weight at either end of the spectrum—inadequate fetal growth or excessive fetal growth—are critical risk factors for alterations in fetal well-being.

Intrauterine growth restriction (IUGR), also known as *inadequate fetal growth,* is a term used to describe any fetus that falls below the 10th percentile in ultrasonic estimation of weight at a given gestational age. Other terms to describe the small fetus include *low birth weight* and *small for gestational age (SGA).* IUGR may or may not be associated with prematurity.

The etiology of IUGR can be separated into either fetoplacental or maternal origin. Fetoplacental etiologies include infections, genetic abnormalities, and placental abnormalities. Maternal etiologies stem from reduced uteroplacental blood flow associated with hypertension, poor maternal weight gain, poor nutrition, substance use such as tobacco or medications, anemia, or chronic illness (Gabbe et al., 2017).

If a fetus is suspected to have IUGR, management includes careful surveillance of the fetus with NSTs, BPPs, and continuous assessment of growth through sonography. As previously discussed, Doppler velocimetry is indicated to monitor vascular functioning. In addition to regular fetal surveillance, women with IUGR are instructed to do daily fetal movement assessments (previously discussed) and to maintain bed rest. If growth ceases altogether or nonreassuring fetal factors occur (nonreassuring FHR patterns), abnormal AFV or low BPP scores occur, or increases in end diastolic flow or absent or reversed end diastolic velocity is identified, immediate birth is warranted.

Macrosomia (excessive fetal growth) is defined as weight greater than 4000 to 4500 g (8 lb 13 oz to 9 lb 14 oz). If a fetus is suspected to be macrosomic, the management of the labor and birth is carefully evaluated to prevent birth-related complications such as *shoulder dystocia* (an intrapartum event that occurs when the baby's head has been delivered, but the shoulders remain wedged behind the mother's pubic bone, causing a difficult birth of the baby with potential for maternal or fetal injury).

The diagnosis of fetal macrosomia is imprecise. The accuracy of estimated fetal weight using ultrasound biometry and that obtained with clinical palpation by the healthcare provider have yielded similar results in fetuses that range from 2500 to 4000 grams; however, both techniques decrease in accuracy in fetuses above 4000 grams (Nahum, 2014). Clinical palpation of the fetus is done using a Leopold maneuver. The clinician places both hands on the uterus and traces the fetal outline, moving his or her hands down along the sides of the maternal abdomen. With macrosomic fetuses, estimating fetal weight is not advised, but this technique can alert the examiner to excessive fetal size and the fetus's position in utero (see Chapter 20 and Figure 20–4). Measuring the fundal height (measured in centimeters with a tape measure from the symphysis pubis to the fundus of the uterus) is another tool in estimating fetal growth. Recent research shows that weight estimations are best achieved when the mother is compared to a similar demographic population (Nahum, 2014). Experienced providers may also ask the woman to provide her own estimate of the fetal weight if she has had a previous birth, based on how big she perceives the baby to be in comparison to her last pregnancy.

The greatest risk factor for macrosomic fetuses is birth trauma due to shoulder dystocia. When macrosomia is present, a potential shoulder dystocia should be anticipated if the woman is giving birth vaginally. The woman should be positioned in the McRoberts position (legs flexed and pulled back toward her shoulders; see Figure 24–12) with the head of the bed lowered. A stool should be available in the event that suprapubic pressure is needed. If a macrosomic fetus is anticipated, the presence of other nursing staff and the neonatal resuscitation team can save time and provide needed assistance. If the physician/CNM requests suprapubic pressure, the nurse applies pressure directly over the symphysis pubis to aid in dislodging the fetal shoulder (see Chapter 24). Having the woman get on all fours is also an acceptable first step to releasing the shoulder (Gabbe et al., 2017).

SAFETY ALERT!

Fundal pressure should never be applied for a macrosomic fetus or a fetus that is believed to have shoulder dystocia. Fundal pressure is known to further wedge the shoulder underneath the pubic bone and may worsen the clinical situation.

Women who are undergoing a *trial of labor after cesarean (TOLAC)* should be counseled on the risks of shoulder dystocia when macrosomia is suspected. In addition, a macrosomic fetus may decrease the likelihood of a successful *vaginal birth after cesarean (VBAC)*, especially if the previous cesarean birth was performed for cephalopelvic disproportion (CPD) (see Chapter 24). Although macrosomia is not a contraindication to a trial of labor, a TOLAC without a previous vaginal birth when the fetus is macrosomic increases the risk of uterine rupture (Gabbe et al., 2017).

Other Diagnostic Tests

Birth defects, defined as structural abnormalities in the neonate present at birth, are the leading cause of infant mortality and a major contributor to infant morbidity in the United States. It is estimated that 1 in 33 babies are born with a birth defect (CDC, 2016a). Birth defects account for one in five infant deaths in the United States annually. Birth defects affect 8 million children worldwide and affect 6 to 7% of all babies born each year. Some birth defects are not identified until later in childhood. It is estimated that by school age, 12 to 14% of children will be identified as having a birth defect. In the United States, 150,000 babies are born with major structural birth defects each year (CDC, 2016a). Infant mortality due to birth defects has not declined as rapidly as overall infant mortality. It has been estimated that approximately 20% of all birth defects are due to gene mutations, and 10% are due to nutritional deficits or exposure to teratogens such as environmental toxins, drugs, chemicals, or radiation. About 70% of all birth defects remain unexplained (CDC, 2016a).

Rapidly developing technologies of biochemical markers and ultrasonography aid in the prenatal diagnosis of fetal anomalies and genetic disorders. Some of the better-known genetic tests that offer screening options for women in early pregnancy include the first-trimester single screening tests along with the second-trimester integrated screening tests (discussed previously), which include the quadruple screen, cfDNA testing, and the penta screen. Contingent and stepwise sequential screening approaches (discussed previously) also provide screening options for women in early to midpregnancy. Diagnostic follow-up with amniocentesis or chorionic villi diagnostic testing is also available. As discussed in Chapter 10, conditions that can be diagnosed prenatally include trisomies 21, 18, and 13, spina bifida and anencephaly, cystic fibrosis, and some familial conditions (Gabbe et al., 2017).

Maternal Serum Alpha-Fetoprotein

Alpha-fetoprotein (AFP) is a fetal protein that is excreted from the fetal yolk sac during the first 6 weeks of pregnancy. The production of AFP is then taken over by the fetal liver as the pregnancy progresses. AFP levels can be high or low, with each having different implications for the fetus. If the fetus has a neural tube defect (NTD), the AFP levels will be elevated. The incidence of NTDs is one in 2853 births and is the most common birth defect in the United States (CDC, 2016a). NTDs can range from *anencephaly* (absence of a portion of the fetal brain, which is incompatible with extrauterine life) to *spina bifida* (an incomplete closure of the vertebral arch that may allow protrusion of the meningeal tissue, spinal cord, or nerve roots through the opening on the spinal cord, and which is associated with lower extremity paralysis, incontinence, and developmental delay).

QUADRUPLE CHECK

Maternal serum alpha-fetoprotein (MSAFP) is a component of the screening test, the "quadruple check," that utilizes the multiple markers, including AFP, hCG, diameric inhibin-A, and estriol, to screen pregnancies for NTD, trisomy 21 (Down syndrome), and trisomy 18. This testing has been largely replaced by first-trimester screening; however, for women who begin prenatal care in the second trimester after the cutoff date for first-trimester screening, the quadruple check remains a viable option. Screening can be performed between 15 and 22 weeks' gestation (16 to 18 weeks yields the most accurate results) (ACOG, 2016). It is currently recommended that all pregnant women be offered aneuploidy screening. See Chapter 10 for a discussion of chromosomal testing and analysis.

The emergence of first-trimester screening techniques have changed the use of MSAFP testing in recent years. The quadruple screen often follows first-trimester screening because the ability to screen for NTDs cannot be performed prior to 15 weeks. Second-trimester ultrasound along with MSAFP testing provide more conclusive and accurate findings than MSAFP testing alone and includes nuchal translucency screening. The penta screen is another screening tool that can be used for women in the second trimester and includes hyperglycosylated hCG (also known as invasive trophoblast antigen) in addition to the quad screen. This test is not routinely used and its accuracy is not known due to its limited use in practice (ACOG, 2016).

Universal screening should be offered to all women because 90% of NTD cases occur in women with no risk factors. MSAFP screening detects approximately 81% of neural tube defects. Most causes of NTDs are unknown; however, risk factors include a previous fetus with an NTD, maternal age less than 20 or greater than 35 years, primiparity or grandmultiparity, low socioeconomic status with nutritional deficiencies, English or Irish ancestry, and inadequate folic acid intake (Gabbe et al., 2017).

The MSAFP is the first marker used in the quadruple check. Most laboratories use a cutoff of 2 to 2.5 multiples of the mean (MoM) of AFP to define a test result as abnormally high. The lower the cutoff, the greater the detection rate but also the higher the false-positive rate. Levels of 2.5 to 3.5 MoM are considered indiscriminate because both normal and abnormal fetuses typically test within this zone. Levels greater than 3.5 MoM are outside the normal distribution and are at high risk for a neural tube defect. Using a cutoff of 2 to 2.5 MoM would yield a 90% detection rate, resulting in 3 to 5% of positive screens with a 2 to 6% false-positive rate (ACOG, 2016). The majority of women with an elevated MSAFP do not have affected fetuses. In 90 to 95% of the group with an elevated MSAFP, the elevation is caused by other variables, such as incorrect gestational age, more than one fetus, other fetal anomalies such as gastroschisis (a hole in the abdominal wall that allows the abdominal contents to protrude outside the body), or fetal death (Gabbe et al., 2017).

In the past, the quadruple screen has also been used to screen for trisomy 21 (Down syndrome), which is the most common chromosomal abnormality found in live births, and for trisomy 18, which is less common, but usually results in death of the infant within the first year of life (see Chapter 10). Because of the use of more accurate earlier screening tools, the use of the quadruple screen to detect potential trisomies is no longer used, except in women who have presented for prenatal care after 14 gestational weeks.

Abnormal test results are generally defined as a calculated Down syndrome risk of 1 in 270 or 1 in 200 (depending on the laboratory). Women who have abnormal results are counseled about these risks and offered a diagnostic test such as amniocentesis, which is considered to be greater than 99% accurate in the diagnosis of chromosomal anomalies.

Screening tests require patient education and counseling to avoid confusion and undue stress. A key point for the nurse to understand and reinforce to the patient is that the MSAFP and the quadruple check are screening tests and are *not* diagnostic. The nurse has an important role in educating the woman about various aspects of these tests. The importance of an accurate gestational age determination before taking the test cannot be overstated. A miscalculated gestational age may result in the incorrect interpretation of the MSAFP level, causing extreme stress to the woman and her family. In addition, further testing is required. An elevation of the MSAFP requires recalculation with an accurate gestational age and repeat test, and a low MSAFP may require an amniocentesis. The nurse also educates the patient on the importance of proper timing of the MSAFP. As stated earlier, the ideal time for screening is between 16 and 18 weeks. False positives can occur with tests done either before or after this window.

All healthcare providers should be sensitive to the ethical issues that these screening tests present to the childbearing family. What benefit would knowing the results of an abnormal MSAFP provide? If the fetus has an NTD, the family and healthcare provider can use this information before the birth to choose the appropriate birth site or birth type (a fetus with an NTD would need to be born in a tertiary care center where immediate care could be given to the neonate if needed). Knowing a fetus has Down syndrome would not necessarily change an obstetric decision about birth method or site, but it would give the family time for psychologic preparation, a chance to talk with social services and support groups, or the opportunity to opt for termination of the pregnancy.

Amniocentesis

Amniocentesis is a procedure used for genetic diagnosis. A sterile needle (under ultrasound guidance) is inserted into the uterine cavity through the maternal abdomen so a small amount of amniotic fluid can be removed, and genetic testing is performed. Amniocentesis is performed ideally between 15 and 16 weeks' gestation, when the proportion of viable and nonviable cells are the greatest and the uterus is accessible abdominally, but it can be performed later (Milunsky & Milunsky, 2015).

Amniocentesis can make chromosomal and biochemical determinations (enzyme analysis, AFP measurement for neural tube defects, blood typing, or cytogenetic, metabolic, or other DNA testing) and can validate abnormalities detected by ultrasound. Later in pregnancy, from about 30 to 39 weeks' gestation, amniocentesis may be done for lung maturity studies, such as lecithin/sphingomyelin ratio, the presence of phosphatidylglycerol and phosphatidylcholine, and surfactant/albumin ratio (see discussion later in this chapter) (Gabbe et al., 2017).

INDICATIONS FOR AMNIOCENTESIS

The following conditions are commonly considered indications for amniocentesis:

- Pregnant women who will be 35 years of age or older on their due dates. The risk of having a baby with a chromosomal problem such as Down syndrome increases with the age of the woman (see Chapter 10).
- Couples who already have had a child with a birth defect or have a family history of certain chromosomal birth defects.
- Pregnant women with other abnormal screening or genetic test results.

PROCEDURE FOR PERFORMING AMNIOCENTESIS

Amniocentesis is done on an outpatient basis but needs to be performed near a birthing area in case acute nonreassuring fetal status is encountered. The pregnant woman should be placed in a left lateral tilt position by placing a wedge under her right hip to prevent hypotension during the procedure. Although a local anesthesia can be used, most women do not find it beneficial and report that the pain is much less than anticipated. Discomfort during the procedure appears to be increased when needle insertion occurs in the lower two-thirds of the uterus (Gabbe et al., 2017).

The abdomen is scanned by ultrasound to locate the placenta, the fetus, and an adequate pocket of fluid. The needle insertion site is of the utmost importance because the fetus, placenta, umbilical cord, bladder, and uterine arteries must all be avoided (Figure 16–19). The importance of locating the placenta cannot be stressed enough, especially in cases of Rh isoimmunization, in which trauma to the placenta increases fetal–maternal transfusion and worsens the isoimmunization (see Chapter 18). If the amniocentesis is being performed in the last few weeks of pregnancy, the fetus may occupy what appears to be all the available space in the uterus, and there is a normal decrease in the amount of amniotic fluid; however, with the aid of ultrasound, fluid can be located. The amniocentesis is then done before the fetus has the opportunity to move.

After the abdomen is scanned, the abdominal skin is cleansed with povidone-iodine (Betadine) or other antiseptic. The woman is given the option of a local anesthetic for the insertion site. A 22-gauge spinal needle is inserted into the uterine cavity. Generally, fluid immediately flows into the needle. The first few drops are discarded to reduce the risk of maternal cell contamination; a syringe is then attached to the needle, and the fluid is aspirated (Figure 16–20).

Clinical Tip

During and after the procedure have the woman lie in a left lateral tilt to ensure adequate placental perfusion.

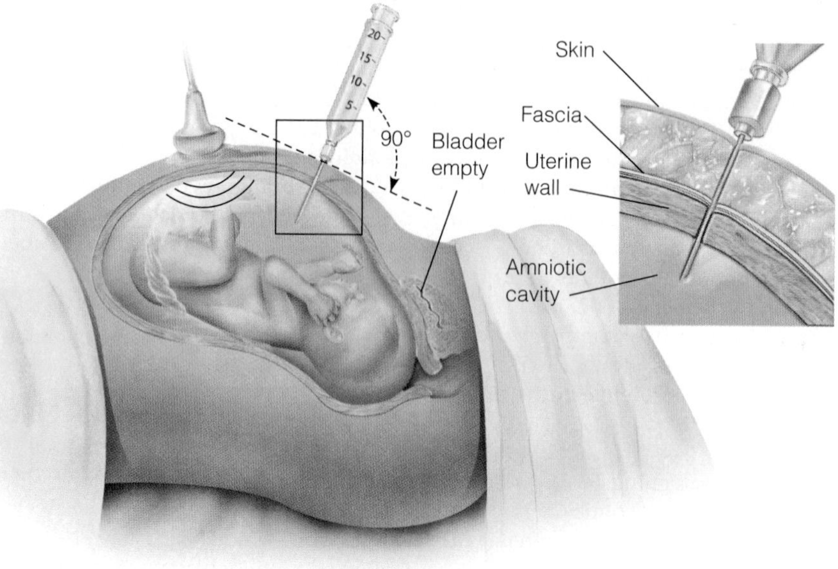

Figure 16–19 **Amniocentesis. The woman is usually scanned by ultrasound to determine the placental site and to locate a pocket of fluid. As the needle is inserted, three levels of resistance are felt when the needle penetrates the skin, fascia, and uterine wall. When the needle is placed within the amniotic cavity, amniotic fluid is withdrawn.**

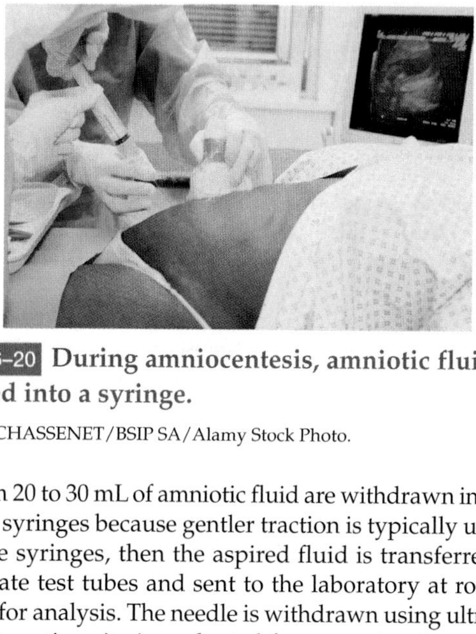

Figure 16–20 **During amniocentesis, amniotic fluid is aspirated into a syringe.**

SOURCE: CHASSENET/BSIP SA/Alamy Stock Photo.

From 20 to 30 mL of amniotic fluid are withdrawn into 10 mL or 20 mL syringes because gentler traction is typically used with these size syringes, then the aspired fluid is transferred to the appropriate test tubes and sent to the laboratory at room temperature for analysis. The needle is withdrawn using ultrasound, and the insertion site is evaluated for streaming (movement of fluid), which would indicate bleeding into the amniotic fluid. The FHR is monitored for 20 to 30 minutes to assess fetal well-being. If the woman's vital signs and the FHR are normal, she is allowed to leave (see *Clinical Skill 16–2: Assisting During Amniocentesis*) (Milunsky & Milunsky, 2015).

Rh-negative women are given Rh immune globulin after amniocentesis, provided that they are not already sensitized.

RISKS/SIDE EFFECTS

Minor complications are infrequent and may include transient vaginal spotting, cramping, amniotic fluid leakage, and chorioamnionitis. Needle injuries to the fetus are rare with the standardized use of ultrasound guidance. Fetal loss rate prior to 24 weeks' gestation is 0.11% (Milunsky & Milunsky, 2015). When amniocentesis is performed prior to 14 weeks' gestation, there is a higher rate of complications due to the lack of membrane fusion to the uterine wall, which makes the puncture of the sac difficult, and the fact that there is less fluid to withdraw (Milunsky & Milunsky, 2015). Failure to obtain an adequate sample occurs in less than 1% of all procedures. A repeat test can be performed the same day; however, if this test also fails, a 7-day waiting period is suggested. Failure to obtain an adequate sample is more common in inexperienced physicians and those who perform less than 50 procedures annually. Most obstetricians now refer women to a perinatologist for testing purposes (Milunsky & Milunsky, 2015). See *Case Study: Melissa Bond-James*.

CASE STUDY: Melissa Bond-James

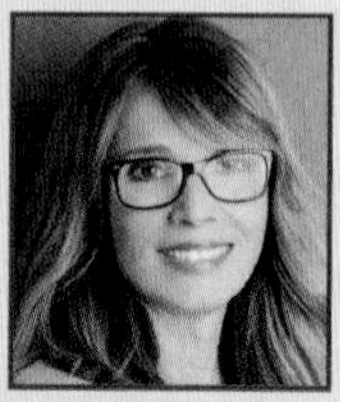

SOURCE: Kinga/ Shutterstock

Melissa and her wife, Nancy, have been counseled on an increased risk of genetic anomalies related to Melissa's maternal age (40 years old). While they have decided they would not terminate the pregnancy if a genetic anomaly was identified, Nancy feels earlier knowledge would allow them to emotionally grieve if the baby has any issues.

Melissa underwent first-trimester screening and her blood levels and ultrasound findings were all within normal limits. She has no family history of genetic disorders.

Question to Ponder

What factors would you discuss with the couple regarding the benefits and possible dangers of amniocentesis specifically related to Melissa's risk factors and current test results from earlier screenings?

Clinical Skill 16–2

Assisting During Amniocentesis

NURSING ACTION

Preparation

- Explain the procedure and the indications for it and reassure the woman.
- Determine whether an informed consent form has been signed. If not, verify that the woman's doctor has explained the procedure and ask her to sign a consent form.

Rationale: *It is the physician's responsibility to obtain informed consent. The woman's signature indicates her awareness of the risks and gives her consent to the procedure.*

Equipment and Supplies

22-gauge spinal needle with stylet
10- and 20-mL syringes
1% lidocaine (Xylocaine)
Povidone-iodine (Betadine)
Three 10-mL test tubes with tops (laboratory will specify color of tubes to use)

Rationale: *Multiple test tubes of fluid should be sent in case contamination occurs.*

Procedure: Sterile Gloves

1. Obtain baseline vital signs including maternal blood pressure (BP), pulse, respirations, temperature, and fetal heart rate (FHR) before procedure begins.
2. Monitor BP, pulse, respirations, and FHR every 15 minutes during procedure.

Rationale: *Baseline information is essential to detect any changes in maternal or fetal status that might be related to the procedure.*

3. The physician uses real-time ultrasound to determine the location of the placenta and to locate a pocket of amniotic fluid. Provide gel for the ultrasound and assist with the procedure as needed.
4. Cleanse the woman's abdomen with antiseptic solution.

Rationale: *Cleansing the abdomen before needle insertion helps decrease the risk of infection.*

5. The physician dons gloves, inserts the needle into the identified pocket of fluid (see Figure 16–19), and withdraws a sample. The first syringe is discarded since it is more likely to contain maternal cells.
6. Obtain the test tubes from the physician. Label the tubes with the woman's correct identification labels and send to the lab with the appropriate lab slips.
7. Monitor the woman and reassess her vital signs.
   - Determine the woman's BP, pulse, respirations, and the FHR.
   - Assess needle insertion site for fluid leakage.
   - Palpate the woman's fundus to assess for uterine contractions.
   - Monitor her using an external fetal monitor for 20 to 30 minutes after the amniocentesis.
   - Determine a treatment course to counteract any supine hypotension and to increase venous return and cardiac output.

Rationale: *Monitoring maternal and fetal status postprocedure provides information about response to the procedure and helps detect any complications such as inadvertent fetal puncture.*

8. Assess the woman's blood type and determine any need for Rh immune globulin.
9. Administer Rh immune globulin if indicated (see *Clinical Skill 18–2: Intramuscular Administration of Rh Immune Globulin*).

Rationale: *To prevent Rh sensitization in an Rh-negative woman, Rh immune globulin is administered prophylactically involving amniocentesis.*

10. Instruct the woman to report any of the following changes or symptoms to her primary caregiver:
    - Unusual fetal hyperactivity or, conversely, any lack of fetal movement
    - Vaginal discharge—either clear drainage or bleeding
    - Uterine contractions or abdominal pain
    - Fluid leakage from needle insertion site
    - Fever or chills.

Rationale: *These are signs of potential complications and require further evaluation.*

11. Encourage the woman to engage only in light activities for 24 hours and to increase her fluid intake.

Rationale: *Decreased maternal activity helps decrease uterine irritability and increase uteroplacental circulation. Increased fluid intake helps replace amniotic fluid through the uteroplacental circulation.*

12. Complete the EMR. Record the type of procedure, the date and time, and the name of the physician who performed the procedure. Also record the maternal-fetal response, disposition of the specimen, and discharge teaching. Maternal vital signs, including level of discomfort, should be recorded. The FHR, presence of contractions, bleeding, and fluid leakage should be documented as well as abnormal symptoms that need to be reported to the physician.

NURSING MANAGEMENT

For the Woman Undergoing Amniocentesis

Assist the physician during the amniocentesis (see *Clinical Skill 16–2: Assisting During Amniocentesis*). In addition, support the woman undergoing amniocentesis. Reassure the woman that the pain is usually less than expected. Encourage relaxation techniques, including deep breathing, guided imagery, or other desired complementary therapies, such as aromatherapy. Women are usually apprehensive about the procedure as well as about the information that will be obtained. The physician explains the procedure before the woman signs the consent form. As it is being performed, the woman may need additional emotional support. She may become anxious during the procedure. She may also become lightheaded, nauseated, and diaphoretic from lying on her back with a heavy uterus compressing the abdominal vessels, so it is important to have her in a lateral tilt with a wedge placed under her right hip. Provide support to the woman by further clarifying the physician's instructions or explanations, by relieving the woman's physical discomfort when possible, and by responding verbally and physically to the woman's need for reassurance.

Chorionic Villus Sampling

Much like amniocentesis, **chorionic villus sampling (CVS)** is a procedure that is used to detect genetic, metabolic, and DNA abnormalities, in this case by obtaining a placental biopsy. CVS involves obtaining a small sample (5 to 40 mg) of chorionic villi from the edge of the developing placenta. CVS is performed in some medical centers for first-trimester diagnosis after at least 9 completed weeks of gestation (usually between 10 and 12 weeks) (Gabbe et al., 2017). Villi in the chorion frondosum, present from 8 to 12 weeks' gestation, are believed to reflect fetal chromosome, enzyme, and DNA content, thereby permitting earlier diagnosis than can be obtained by amniocentesis.

RISKS AND BENEFITS OF CVS

The woman should be aware of the risks and benefits of CVS. There is a spontaneous abortion risk of 0.22%, which is double the amniocentesis risk. Fetal limb reduction defects (a portion of a finger or a toe is missing) have been reported, thus the test is not recommended prior to 9 completed weeks of gestation (Milunsky & Milunsky, 2015).

Additional risks of CVS include failure to obtain tissue, rupture of the membranes, leakage of amniotic fluid, vaginal spotting or bleeding, chorioamnionitis, intrauterine infection, maternal tissue contamination of the specimen, oromandibular defects, and Rh isoimmunization. Rh-negative women are given Rh immune globulin to cover the risk of immunization from the procedure (Milunsky & Milunsky, 2015).

Like amniocentesis, CVS can detect fetal karyotype, hemoglobinopathies (e.g., sickle cell disease and alpha and some beta thalassemias), phenylketonuria, alpha antitrypsin deficiency, Down syndrome, Duchenne muscular dystrophy, and factor IX deficiency. Early sex determination can be made so that pregnancies with a male fetus that would be affected in X-linked disorders can be identified (Gabbe et al., 2017). Because NTDs are not diagnosed by this test, all mothers undergoing CVS should be offered MSAFP screening at 15 to 20 weeks' gestation. A major disadvantage of the earlier testing (CVS) is that if a woman later has an abnormal MSAFP test indicating an increased risk of NTDs, she may then have to undergo an amniocentesis, thus again putting the fetus at risk with an additional invasive procedure.

One of the greatest advantages to a woman undergoing this procedure is earlier diagnosis and decreased waiting time for results. Whereas amniocentesis is typically performed at 15 to 16 weeks' gestation, CVS can be performed as early as 10 weeks. The CVS results are obtained in 24 hours if the direct preparation method is used and in 7 to 10 days when tissue culture is used. Earlier diagnosis may relieve many of the personal, social, and psychologic concerns of families, particularly if therapeutic abortion is being considered. There may be less emotional stress involved with having an abortion at an earlier stage of gestation. First-trimester abortions are also easier to perform, require less time, and are less costly.

PROCEDURE FOR CVS

Before CVS, an ultrasound is done to determine placental location, uterine position (retroverted or anteverted), and presence of intervening structures (i.e., bowel, blood vessels). Various types of equipment can be used to aspirate chorionic villi from the placenta.

After counseling regarding diagnosis and procedure techniques, preliminary bloodwork may be obtained. Prior to the procedure, the woman is asked to drink fluids to fill her bladder because displacement of an anteverted uterus by a full bladder may aid in positioning the uterus for catheter insertion. Ultrasound is used to determine uterine position, cervical position, gestational sac size, and crown–rump length measurement and to identify the area of placental formation and cord insertion.

For the transcervical CVS the woman is placed in lithotomy position, the vulva is cleansed with povidone-iodine solution (Betadine), and a sterile speculum is inserted into the vagina. The vaginal vault and cervix are cleansed with the same solution to decrease contamination from the vagina into the uterus. The anterior lip of the cervix is sometimes grasped with a tenaculum to aid in straightening anteflexion of the uterus. The catheter (or cannula) is slowly inserted under ultrasound guidance through the endocervix to the sampling site at the extra-amniotic placental edge (outside the gestational sac). The obturator is withdrawn from the catheter. A 30-mL syringe, containing 3 to 4 mL of tissue culture medium with heparin, is attached, and a sample of villi is aspirated by using a pressure of 20 to 30 mL. The contents of the syringe are flushed into a petri dish containing nutrient medium, and the villi are inspected microscopically and prepared for cell culture. (See Figure 10–12B in Chapter 10.)

For the transabdominal sampling, the woman is placed in the supine position. After the skin is cleansed with Betadine and local anesthesia is given, an 18- or 20-gauge needle is inserted percutaneously through the maternal abdominal wall and uterine myometrium. The tip of the needle is advanced into the long axis of the chorion frondosum under ultrasound guidance. Chorionic villi are obtained by repeated, rapid aspirations of the syringe containing tissue culture medium and heparin.

A CVS result indicating normal chromosomal configuration in the first trimester does not ensure a healthy newborn. Routine prenatal care and appropriate follow-up are needed. Follow-up ultrasound and lab evaluation of each pregnancy must be done after performance of this procedure to evaluate fetal status. Further neonatal follow-up studies are necessary to evaluate the long-term effects of this technique.

NURSING MANAGEMENT

For the Woman Undergoing CVS

Before the test, ascertain the woman's understanding of CVS, its uses, the procedure, and the possible results. Provide opportunities for questions and act as her advocate when additional questions or concerns are raised. Complete all assessments following the procedure, including monitoring for vaginal bleeding or fluid leakage, excessive cramping, and basic maternal vital signs.

Support the woman or couple and encourage them to express any feelings and fears regarding the procedure and also regarding the decision-making process if abortion is being considered. The supportive role continues if abortion is chosen, even though you may not be present for the procedure. It is important that support be provided following the procedure by the nurse who established a relationship with the couple previously.

Fetal Fibronectin

Fetal fibronectin (fFN) is a glycoprotein produced by the trophoblast and other fetal tissues. The absence of cervicovaginal fFN between 20 and 34 weeks' gestation provided the basis for fetal fibronectin testing on high-risk women at risk for preterm birth in the past. While the negative predictive value of the test is 99.5%, the positive predictive value is only 12.7%. As a result, ACOG no longer recommends using fFN as a routine screening tool for women with possible preterm labor. A meta-analysis of six clinical trials indicated that fFN testing was not associated with a reduction in preterm births or improvement in perinatal outcomes, but did lead to significantly higher costs related to additional screening tests and hospitalization costs (Berghella & Saccone, 2016). Fetal fibronectin testing can produce false-positive readings related to vaginal examinations, sexual intercourse within the previous 24 hours, some vaginal creams, transvaginal ultrasound examinations, and some vaginal medications.

Evaluation of Fetal Lung Maturity

In managing the woman and fetus at risk, the physician is constantly faced with the possibility of having to induce the birth of the baby before term and before the onset of labor. There are many indications for early induction of labor, including repeat cesarean birth, premature rupture of the membranes, diabetes, hypertensive disorders, trauma, and placental insufficiency. Unfortunately, the most common cause of perinatal mortality is prematurity, especially in neonates weighing 1000 g or less, with the three highest etiologies being respiratory failure, infection, and congenital anomalies (Furdon, 2016). The birth of a baby with immature pulmonary function frequently results in respiratory distress syndrome (RDS), previously called *hyaline membrane disease (HMD)* (see Chapter 31).

Because gestational age, birth weight, and the rate of development of organ systems do not necessarily correspond, it may be necessary to determine the lung maturation of the fetus by amniotic fluid analysis before elective childbirth. In these cases, amniocentesis is performed and concentrations of certain phospholipids in the amniotic fluid are measured. In many cases, birth of the baby can be delayed until the lungs show maturity and administration of corticosteroids can be considered. Most fetal lung maturity testing is done in fetuses less than 32 weeks' gestation (Gillen-Goldstein, MacKenzie, & Funai, 2016).

LECITHIN/SPHINGOMYELIN RATIO

The alveoli of the lungs are lined by a substance called **surfactant**, which is composed of phospholipids. Surfactant lowers the surface tension of the alveoli during extrauterine respiratory exhalation. By lowering the alveolar surface tension, surfactant stabilizes the alveoli, and a certain amount of air always remains in the alveoli during expiration (Gabbe et al., 2017). When a newborn with mature pulmonary function takes his or her first breath, a tremendously high pressure is needed to open the lungs. Upon breathing out, the lungs do not collapse, and about half the air in the alveoli is retained. A neonate born too early, when synthesis of surfactant is incomplete, is unable to maintain lung stability, resulting in underinflation of the lungs and development of RDS.

Fetal lung maturity can be assessed by determining the ratio of two components of surfactant—lecithin and sphingomyelin. Early in pregnancy the lecithin concentration in amniotic fluid is less than that of sphingomyelin (0.5:1 at 20 weeks), resulting in a low **lecithin/sphingomyelin (L/S) ratio**. At about 30 to 32 weeks' gestation, the amounts of the two substances become equal (1:1). The concentration of lecithin begins to exceed that of sphingomyelin, and at 35 weeks the L/S ratio is 2:1. When at least two times as much lecithin as sphingomyelin is found in the amniotic fluid, RDS is very unlikely (Gillen-Goldstein et al., 2016). Clinical outcomes, including respiratory distress and other respiratory disorders, should be correlated in individual institutions before specific ratios indicating pulmonary maturity are accepted. Newborns of mothers with diabetes are an exception to this finding and have a high incidence of false-positive results (i.e., the L/S ratio is thought to indicate lung maturity, but after birth the baby develops RDS). Although the same ratios are used, it is important to remember that even when newborns of mothers with diabetes are term (greater than 37 weeks' gestational age), delayed lung maturation can occur because the high blood sugars interfere with biochemical development. A delay in lung maturation has also been found in babies whose mothers have nonhypertensive renal disease and isoimmunization (Gillen-Goldstein et al., 2016).

Some types of chronic intrauterine fetal stress cause an acceleration of lung maturation in the fetus. Prolonged rupture of the membranes (over 24 hours) results in acceleration of lung maturation by approximately 1 week and therefore has a protective effect. Although the L/S ratio is the most universally used test for evaluating pulmonary maturity, the results are not accurate when blood or meconium contaminates the amniotic fluid.

The L/S ratio remains a cumbersome and labor-intensive test despite numerous changes to the original technique. Moreover, improper handling can affect results. For these reasons, many institutions are looking to other fetal lung maturity tests that are being developed.

PHOSPHATIDYLGLYCEROL

Phosphatidylglycerol (PG) is the second most abundant phospholipid in surfactant. PG appears after 35 weeks' gestation and increases in amount until term. In instances of diabetes complicated by premature rupture of the membranes, vascular disease, or severe preeclampsia, PG may be present before 35 weeks' gestation. PG is not measured in specific concentrations; rather, the mere presence of this substance is associated with very low risk of RDS, and the absence of PG is associated with the development of RDS. Mature levels are reported as positive, meaning lung maturity is likely, whereas negative results indicates lung maturity is unlikely.

PG determination is also useful in blood-contaminated specimens. Because PG is not present in blood or vaginal fluids, its presence in a vaginal specimen is reliable for indicating lung maturity.

In recent years, lung maturity has been most frequently assessed by a combination of L/S ratio and PG. Lung maturity can be confirmed in most pregnancies if PG is present in conjunction with an L/S ratio of 2:1.

LAMELLAR BODY COUNTS

Lamellar body counts (LBCs) are concentrated phospholipids that are produced by the type II alveoli cells and are representative of stored surfactant. As the fetal lungs mature, the LBCs rise. Testing of LBCs offers some advantages over other forms of testing because the tests are accurate among women with diabetes. Testing can be performed more quickly than L/S ratio and PG testing and is more cost effective, more objective, and less labor and technique intensive (Gillen-Goldstein et al., 2016). LBCs can be falsely elevated if blood contamination occurs, although meconium passage has little implications for testing. Amniotic fluid LBC greater than 50,000/mcL is predictive of fetal lung maturity. Amniotic fluid LBC less than 15,000/mcL is suggestive of fetal lung immaturity and increased risk of neonatal RDS. When values are greater than 30,000 mcL and less than 50,000 mcL, L/S ratio testing may be performed to ensure accuracy in determining fetal lung maturity status.

Optical density at 650 nm is an indirect measure of LBCs that can be obtained by measuring increases in opalescence, which results from increases in lamellar bodies. Optical density readings greater than 0.15 are associated with lung maturity (Gillen-Goldstein et al., 2016).

The *foam stability index (FSI)* is a measure that assesses total surfactant activity. "Ethanol is added to a sample of amniotic fluid to eliminate the effects of nonsurfactant factors on foam formation. The mixture is then shaken and will generate a stable ring of foam if surfactant is present. The FSI is calculated by utilizing serial dilutions of ethanol to quantitate the amount of surfactant present" (Gillen-Goldstein et al., 2016, para 12). Values greater than 47 are considered positive and are associated with fetal lung maturity. Limitations of this technique include false results related to blood or meconium contamination (Gillen-Goldstein et al., 2016).

NURSING MANAGEMENT

For the Woman Undergoing Testing for Fetal Lung Maturity

In women whose amniotic membranes are prematurely ruptured, a vaginal specimen is obtained for analysis. Assist the physician/CNM by gathering appropriate supplies. Typically, a sterile speculum, a light source, a sterile syringe or a nasogastric tube, and appropriate collection tubes are needed. Position the woman for the speculum exam while providing information about the collection process. Place the woman in a lithotomy position and place her legs in stirrups. If stirrups are not available, a bedpan can be placed upside down and the woman positioned with her buttocks on the bedpan to facilitate collection of the vaginal fluid. The physician/CNM gathers vaginal secretions with a syringe and places the specimen in a collection tube.

In women undergoing early birth for medical indications (uncontrolled preeclampsia or eclampsia or uncontrolled diabetes) when the amniotic membranes are intact, evaluation of fetal lung maturity may be obtained through amniocentesis. See previous discussion regarding nursing management for the woman undergoing amniocentesis. See *Key Facts to Remember: Summary of Screening and Diagnostic Tests.*

KEY FACTS TO REMEMBER

Summary of Screening and Diagnostic Tests

Goal	Test	Timing
To validate the pregnancy	Ultrasound: Gestational sac volume	5–6 weeks after last menstrual period (LMP) by transvaginal ultrasound
To determine how advanced the pregnancy is	Ultrasound: Crown–rump length	6–10 weeks' gestation
	Ultrasound: Biparietal diameter, femur length, abdomen circumference	13–40 weeks' gestation
To identify normal growth of the fetus	Ultrasound: Biparietal diameter	Most useful from 20 to 30 weeks' gestation
	Ultrasound: Head/abdomen ratio	13–40 weeks' gestation
	Ultrasound: Estimated fetal weight	About 24–40 weeks' gestation
To detect congenital anomalies and problems	Nuchal translucency testing	11–13 weeks' gestation
	Ultrasound	18–40 weeks' gestation
	Chorionic villus sampling	10–12 weeks' gestation
	Amniocentesis	15–16 weeks' gestation ideal, but can be performed after 16 weeks
	First-trimester combination screening test	11–13 weeks' gestation
	Quadruple test	Generally 15–22 weeks' gestation (16–18 weeks' most accurate)
	Cell-free DNA (cfDNA)	After 10 weeks' gestation
To localize the placenta	Ultrasound	Usually in third trimester or before amniocentesis
To assess fetal status	Biophysical profile	Approximately 28 weeks to birth
	Maternal assessment of fetal activity	Approximately 28 weeks to birth
	Nonstress test	Approximately 28 weeks to birth
	Contraction stress test	After 28 weeks
To diagnose cardiac problems	Fetal echocardiography	Second and third trimesters
To assess fetal lung maturity	Amniocentesis	Timing for these five tests:
	L/S ratio	Up to 39 weeks, but most commonly performed at less than 32 weeks (ACOG, 2017)
	Phosphatidylglycerol	
	Lamellar body counts	
	Optical density at 650 nm	
To obtain more information about breech presentation	Ultrasound	Just before labor is anticipated or during labor

Focus Your Study

- Nurses often play a key role not only in teaching families about various testing procedures, but also in providing clarity and emotional support to the woman and her family undergoing antenatal testing.
- Ultrasound offers a valuable means of assessing intrauterine fetal growth because the growth can be followed over a period of time. It is noninvasive and painless, allows the practitioner to study the gestation serially, is nonradiating to both the woman and her fetus, and to date has shown no known harmful effects.
- Using ultrasound, the gestational sac may be detected as early as 5 or 6 weeks after the last menstrual period. Measurement of the crown–rump length in early pregnancy is most useful for accurate dating of a pregnancy. The most important and frequently used ultrasound measurements in the second trimester are biparietal diameter, head circumference, abdominal circumference, and femur length.
- Maternal assessment of fetal activity is very useful as a screening procedure in evaluation of fetal status.
- A nonstress test (NST) measures fetal heart rate (FHR) during fetal activity; FHR normally increases in response to fetal activity. The desired result is a reactive test.
- A contraction stress test (CST) provides a method for observing the response of the FHR to the stress of uterine contractions. The desired result is a negative test.
- A fetal biophysical profile (BPP) includes five fetal variables (breathing movement, body movement, tone, amniotic fluid volume, and FHR reactivity). It assesses the fetus at risk for intrauterine compromise.
- Aneuploidy screening includes first-trimester single test screening (nuchal translucency and PAPP-A and beta hCG); stepwise sequential, integrated, or contingent screening; cell-free DNA testing; or quadruple screening of AFP, hCG, diameric inhibin-A, and estriol.
- Amniocentesis can be used to obtain amniotic fluid for testing. A variety of tests is available to evaluate the presence of disease, genetic conditions, and fetal maturity.
- Chorionic villus sampling (CVS) is a procedure that obtains fetal karyotype in the first trimester. It is used to diagnose hemoglobinopathies (e.g., sickle cell disease and alpha and some beta thalassemias), phenylketonuria, alpha antitrypsin deficiency, Down syndrome, Duchenne muscular dystrophy, and factor IX deficiency.
- The lecithin/sphingomyelin (L/S) ratio of the amniotic fluid can be used to assess fetal lung maturity. The presence of phosphatidylglycerol (PG) may also provide information about fetal lung maturity.
- Lamellar body counts (LBCs) testing can be used as a predictive indicator for predicting respiratory distress syndrome (RDS) in preterm newborns. Optical density at 650 nm is an indirect measure of LBCs.

In order to make safe and effective judgments using NANDA-I © 2017 nursing diagnoses, it is essential that nurses refer to the definitions and defining characteristics of the diagnoses used in this text, which can be found in Appendix C.

References

American College of Obstetricians and Gynecologists (ACOG). (2007, reaffirmed 2011). *Screening for fetal chromosomal abnormalities* (ACOG Practice Bulletin No. 77). Washington, DC: Author.

American College of Obstetricians and Gynecologists (ACOG). (2009, reaffirmed 2014). *Ultrasonography in pregnancy* (ACOG Practice Bulletin No. 101). Washington, DC: Author.

American College of Obstetricians and Gynecologists (ACOG). (2016). *Screening for fetal aneuploidy* (ACOG Practice Bulletin No 163). Washington, DC: Author.

Bakay, K., Varolan, A., Yazgan, A., Akyol, A., & Davas, I. (2016). Comparison of modified biophysical profile with Doppler ultrasonographic analysis in determining fetal well-being in the third trimester. *Gynecology Obstetrics and Reproductive Medicine, 19*(2).

Berghella, V., & Saccone, G. (2016). Fetal fibronectin testing for prevention of preterm birth in singleton pregnancies with threatened preterm labor: A systematic review and meta-analysis of randomized controlled trials. *American Journal of Obstetrics and Gynecology, 215*(4), 431–438. DOI: 10.1016/j.ajog.2016.04.038

Çakar, M., Tari Kasnakoglu, B., Ökem, Z. G., Okuducu, Ü., & Beksaç, M. S. (2016). The effect of different information sources on the anxiety level of pregnant women who underwent invasive prenatal testing. *Journal of Maternal, Fetal, and Neonatal Medicine, 29*(23), 3843–3847. DOI: 10.3109/14767058.2016.1149560

Centers for Disease Control and Prevention (CDC). (2016a). *Birth defects: Data & statistics.* Retrieved from http://www.cdc.gov/ncbddd/birthdefects/data.html

Centers for Disease Control and Prevention (CDC). (2016b). *Severe maternal morbidity in the United States.* Retrieved from http://www.cdc.gov/reproductivehealth/maternalinfanthealth/severematernalmorbidity.html

Central Intelligence Agency (CIA). (2016). *The World Factbook.* Retrieved from https://www.cia.gov/library/publications/the-world-factbook/rankorder/2091rank.html

Cunningham, F. G., Leveno, K. J., Bloom, S. L., Spong, C. Y., Dashe, J., Hoffman, B. L., . . . Sheffield, J. S. (2014). *Williams obstetrics* (24th ed.). New York, NY: McGraw-Hill.

Furdon, S.A. (2016). *Prematurity.* Medscape. Retrieved from http://emedicine.medscape.com/article/975909-overview

Gabbe, S. G., Niebyl, J. R., Simpson, J. L., Landon, M. B., Galan, H., Jauniaux, E. R. M., . . . Grobman, W. A. (2017). *Normal and problem pregnancies* (7th ed.). Philadelphia, PA: Elsevier.

Gillen-Goldstein, J., MacKenzie, A. P., & Funai, E. F. (2016). *Assessment of fetal lung maturity.* Up-to-Date.

Retrieved from https://www.uptodate.com/contents/assessment-of-fetal-lung-maturity

Milunsky, A., & Milunsky, J. M. (2015). *Genetic disorders and the fetus: Diagnosis, prevention, and treatment* (7th ed.). Philadelphia, PA: Wiley-Blackwell.

Nahum, G. G. (2014). *Estimating fetal weight.* Emedicine. Retrieved from http://emedicine.medscape.com/article/262865-overview#a8

Norton, M. E. (2016). *Callen's ultrasonography in obstetrics and gynecology* (6th ed.). Boston, MA: Elsevier.

Polin, R., Abman, S., Rowitch, D., & Benitz, W. (2016). *Fetal and neonatal physiology* (5th ed.). Boston, MA: Elsevier.

Posner, G. (2013). *Oxorn-Foote: Human labor and birth* (6th ed.). Columbus, OH: McGraw-Hill.

Said, H., Gupta, S., Vricella, L., Wand, K., Nguyen, T., & Gross, G. (2017). Effect of ambient light on the time needed to complete a fetal biophysical profile: A randomized controlled trial. *European Journal of Obstetrics & Gynecology and Reproductive Biology, 217*, 59–65.

Spector, R. E. (2017). *Cultural diversity in health and illness* (9th ed.). Hoboken, NJ: Pearson.

van Schendel, R. V., Page-Christiaens, G. C., Beulen, L., Bilardo, C. M., de Boer, M. A., . . . & Dutch NIPT Consortium. (2016). Trial by Dutch laboratories for evaluation of non-invasive prenatal testing. Part II—Women's perspectives. *Prenatal Diagnosis, 36*(12), 1091–1098. DOI: 10.1002/pd.4941

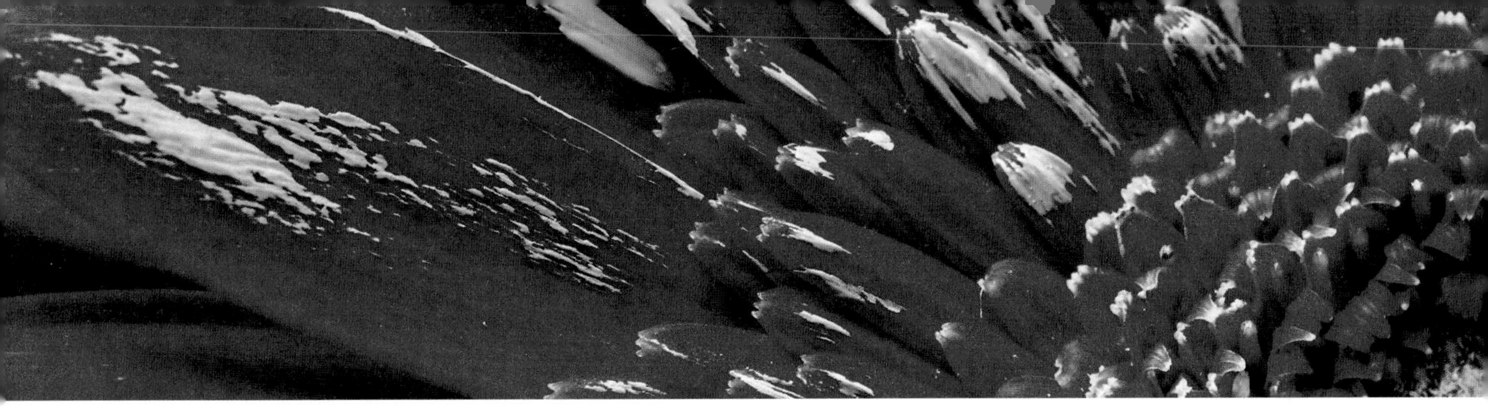

Chapter 17

Pregnancy at Risk: Pregestational Problems

I had gestational diabetes with my first pregnancy. After a week or two of trial and error, I knew what worked for me and what didn't and was able to keep my blood glucose levels within normal ranges using just diet and exercise. I kept track of every meal, snack, exercise, and sugar count in a diary—a little OCD perhaps, but it helped me stick to what worked. No complications for me or my baby.

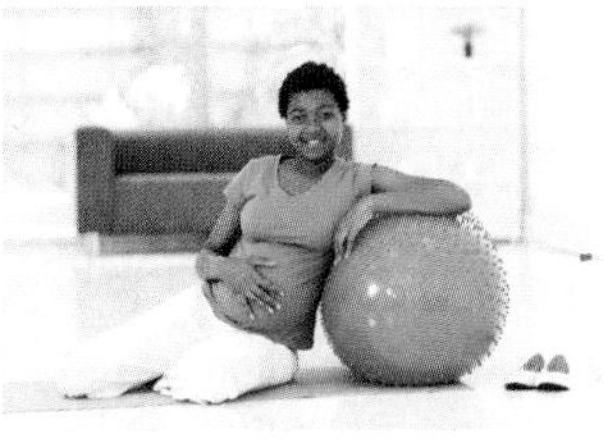

SOURCE: Michaeljung/Fotolia.

Learning Outcomes

17.1 Discuss the pathology, treatment, and nursing care of pregnant women with diabetes.

17.2 Discriminate among the four major types of anemia associated with pregnancy with regard to signs, treatment, implications for pregnancy, and nursing care.

17.3 Summarize the effects of alcohol and illicit drugs on the childbearing woman and her fetus/newborn.

17.4 Explain the possible implications of maternal psychologic factors and disorders in caring for the childbearing family.

17.5 Discuss AIDS, including care of the pregnant woman with HIV/AIDS, neonatal implications, ramifications for the childbearing family, and nursing care.

17.6 Describe the effects of various heart disorders on pregnancy, including their implications for nursing care.

17.7 Compare the effects of selected gestational medical conditions on pregnancy.

Healthy People 2020

(MICH-1.1) Reduce the rate of fetal deaths at 20 or more weeks of gestation

(MICH-15) Reduce the proportion of women of childbearing potential who have low red blood cell folate concentrations

(MICH-11) Increase abstinence from alcohol, cigarettes, and illicit drugs among pregnant women

Pregnancy is biologically, physiologically, and psychologically stressful, even for healthy women. For women with preexisting (pregestational) conditions, it may be life-threatening. For these women, pregestational counseling is especially important to identify early interventions designed to diminish the adverse effects of pregnancy on both the mother and fetus. In some cases, interventions before conception may be critical.

Prenatal care is aimed toward identification, assessment, and care management of women whose pregnancies are at risk because of potential or existing complications. This chapter focuses on women with pregestational medical disorders and their possible effects on the outcome of pregnancy.

Care of the Woman with Diabetes Mellitus

Diabetes mellitus (DM), an endocrine disorder of carbohydrate metabolism, results from inadequate production or utilization of insulin.

Normal Glucose Homeostasis

After consumption of a meal, the body metabolizes carbohydrates into glucose. Insulin, produced by the beta cells of the islets of Langerhans in the pancreas, lowers blood glucose levels by enabling the glucose to move from the blood into muscle and liver cells, where it is stored as glycogen. When several hours have passed since a meal, falling blood glucose levels stimulate the pancreas to release glucagon, which in turn stimulates breakdown of liver glycogen stores into glucose, which is returned to the bloodstream. Glucagon can also stimulate the synthesis of glucose directly from amino acids in stored body proteins.

Carbohydrate Metabolism in Normal Pregnancy

Carbohydrate metabolism is affected early in pregnancy by a rise in serum levels of estrogen, progesterone, and other hormones. These hormones stimulate maternal insulin production and increase tissue response to insulin; therefore, anabolism (building-up) of glycogen stores in the liver and other tissues occurs.

In the second half of pregnancy, the woman demonstrates prolonged hyperglycemia and hyperinsulinemia (increased secretion of insulin) following a meal. Although the mother is producing more insulin, placental secretion of human placental lactogen (hPL) and prolactin (from the decidua) as well as elevated levels of cortisol (an adrenal hormone) and glycogen cause increased maternal peripheral resistance to insulin. This resistance helps ensure that there is a sustained supply of glucose available for the fetus. This glucose is transported across the placenta to the fetus, who uses it as a major source of fuel. Maternal amino acids are also actively transported by the placenta from the mother to her fetus. These amino acids are used by the fetus for protein synthesis and as a source of energy. In addition to ensuring that glucose is available to the fetus, the increased maternal resistance to insulin also means that the pregnant woman has a lower peripheral uptake of glucose to meet her own needs. This results in a catabolic (destructive) state during fasting periods (e.g., during the night and after meal absorption). Because increasing amounts of circulating maternal glucose are being diverted to the fetus, maternal fat is metabolized (lipolysis) during fasting periods much more readily than in a nonpregnant person. This process is called *accelerated starvation*. Ketones may be present in the urine as a result of lipolysis.

The delicate system of checks and balances that exists between glucose production and glucose use is stressed by the growing fetus, who derives energy from glucose taken from the mother and by maternal resistance to the insulin her body produces. This stress is referred to as the diabetogenic effect of pregnancy. Thus, any preexisting disruption in carbohydrate metabolism is augmented by pregnancy, and any diabetic potential may precipitate gestational diabetes mellitus.

Pathophysiology of Diabetes Mellitus

In diabetes mellitus, the pancreas does not produce sufficient amounts of insulin to allow necessary carbohydrate metabolism and/or there is a diminished tissue response to insulin. With inadequate amounts of insulin or defects in insulin action, glucose cannot enter the cells but remains circulating in the blood. The body cells become energy depleted while the blood glucose level remains elevated. Fats and proteins in the body tissues are then oxidized by the cells as a source of energy. This results in wasting of fat and muscle tissue of the body, negative nitrogen balance due to protein breakdown, and ketosis due to fat metabolism. The strong osmotic force of the glucose concentration in the blood pulls water from the cells into the blood, which results in cellular dehydration. The high level of glucose in the blood eventually spills over into the urine, producing glycosuria. Osmotic pressure of the glucose in the urine prevents reabsorption of water into the kidney tubules, causing extracellular dehydration.

These pathologic developments cause the following four cardinal signs and symptoms of diabetes mellitus:

1. ***Polyuria (frequent urination):*** Results because water is not reabsorbed by the renal tubules because of the osmotic activity of glucose
2. ***Polydipsia (excessive thirst):*** Caused by dehydration from polyuria
3. ***Weight loss:*** Due to the use of fat and muscle tissue for energy; seen in *insulin-dependent diabetes*, also called *type 1 diabetes*
4. ***Polyphagia (excessive hunger):*** Caused by tissue loss and a state of starvation that results from the inability of the cells to utilize the blood glucose

Diagnosis of diabetes is based on the presence of clinical symptoms and laboratory tests showing elevated glucose levels in the blood, glycosuria, and ketoacidosis.

Classification of Diabetes Mellitus

The primary classification of diabetes is based on cause and includes four main categories (American Diabetes Association [ADA], 2018):

1. Type 1 diabetes develops because of β-cell destruction and generally results in an absolute insulin deficiency
2. Type 2 diabetes, the most common form, results from a combination of an insulin secretory defect and increased insulin resistance
3. Gestational diabetes mellitus
4. Other specific types resulting from genetic defects, drug-induced diabetes, endocrine disorders, and other causes.

Gestational diabetes mellitus (GDM) is defined as glucose intolerance of variable severity with onset or first recognition during the second or third trimester of pregnancy (ADA, 2018). Diagnosis of GDM is important because even mild diabetes increases the risk of perinatal morbidity and mortality. Furthermore, many women with GDM progress over time to overt type 2 diabetes mellitus. *Note:* Gestational diabetes mellitus is not a preexisting/pregestational condition. It is included here, however, because many of the issues to consider in caring for a woman with GDM are similar to those involved in caring for a woman with preexisting DM.

Influence of Pregnancy on Diabetes

Pregnancy can affect diabetes significantly because the physiologic changes of pregnancy can drastically alter insulin requirements. Pregnancy may also accelerate the progress of vascular disease secondary to diabetes. Pregnancy can affect diabetes in the following ways:

- DM may be more difficult to control during pregnancy because insulin requirements are changeable.
- Insulin need frequently decreases early in the first trimester. Levels of human placental lactogen (hPL), an insulin antagonist, are low; fetal needs are minimal; and the woman may be consuming less food because of nausea and vomiting.

- Nausea and vomiting may cause dietary fluctuations, which can increase the risk of hypoglycemia.
- Insulin requirements usually begin to rise late in the first trimester as glucose use and glycogen storage by the woman and fetus increase. As a result of placental maturation and production of hPL and other hormones, insulin requirements may double or quadruple by the end of pregnancy.
- As pregnancy progresses, the renal threshold for glucose decreases, resulting in glucosuria.
- There is an increased risk of ketoacidosis, which may occur at lower serum glucose levels in the pregnant woman with diabetes than in the nonpregnant woman with diabetes.
- The vascular disease that accompanies DM may progress during pregnancy.
- Hypertension may occur.
- Nephropathy may result from renal blood vessel impairment.
- Retinopathy may develop from occlusion of the microscopic blood vessels of the eye.
- Increased energy needs during labor may require more insulin to balance intravenous glucose.
- After delivery of the placenta, insulin requirements usually decrease abruptly with loss of hPL in the maternal circulation.

Influence of Diabetes on Pregnancy Outcome

The pregnancy of a woman who has diabetes carries a higher risk of complications, especially perinatal mortality and congenital anomalies. The risk has been reduced by the recent recognition of the importance of tight metabolic control if these levels can be obtained without excessive hypoglycemia.

MATERNAL RISKS

Maternal health problems in diabetic pregnancy have been greatly reduced by the team approach to preconception planning and early prenatal care and by the increased emphasis on maintaining tight control of blood glucose levels. The prognosis for the pregnant woman with gestational, type 1, or type 2 diabetes that has not resulted in significant vascular damage is positive. However, diabetic pregnancy still carries higher risks for complications than normal pregnancy. It is also important to note that the risk of developing diabetes later in life is increased in women with GDM (American College of Obstetricians and Gynecologists [ACOG], 2018).

Hydramnios (also called *polyhydramnios*) is an increase in the volume of amniotic fluid and occurs in 3 to 32% of pregnant women with diabetes (Johnson & Milio, 2015). It is thought to be primarily a result of excessive fetal urination because of fetal hyperglycemia.

Preeclampsia-eclampsia occurs more often in diabetic pregnancies, especially when diabetes-related vascular changes already exist. The ADA (2018) recommends that a low-dose aspirin (60–150 mg/day) be prescribed for all pregnant women with type 1 or type 2 diabetes beginning in the second trimester and continuing until childbirth to decrease the risk of preeclampsia.

Hyperglycemia due to insufficient amounts of insulin can lead to *ketoacidosis* as a result of the increase in ketone bodies (which are acidic) in the blood released when fatty acids are metabolized. Ketoacidosis usually develops slowly, but it may develop more rapidly in the pregnant woman because of the hyperketonemia associated with accelerated starvation in the fasting state. The tendency for higher postprandial glucose levels because of decreased gastric motility and the contrainsulin effects of hPL also predispose the woman to ketoacidosis. If the ketoacidosis is not treated, it can lead to coma and death of both mother and fetus.

Another risk to the pregnant woman with diabetes is *dystocia* (difficult labor), caused by fetopelvic disproportion if fetal macrosomia exists. The pregnant woman with diabetes is also at increased risk for recurrent monilial vaginitis and urinary tract infections because of increased glycosuria, which contributes to a favorable environment for bacterial growth. If untreated, asymptomatic bacteriuria can lead to pyelonephritis, a serious kidney infection.

Pregnancy can worsen *retinopathy* in women with diabetes. Good control of blood glucose levels and the use of laser photocoagulation (a treatment used to prevent retinal hemorrhage when the retina shows changes in the blood vessels) are indicated to minimize the risk of the negative effects of pregnancy. Hence, women with preexisting diabetes should have a baseline exam by an ophthalmologist prior to pregnancy or in the first trimester and should then be monitored throughout pregnancy as needed based on the degree of retinopathy (ADA, 2018).

FETAL-NEONATAL RISKS

Many of the problems of the newborn result directly from high maternal plasma glucose levels. In the presence of severe maternal ketoacidosis, the risk of fetal death increases dramatically.

The incidence of *congenital anomalies* in diabetic pregnancies is 6 to 10% and is the major cause of death for babies of mothers with diabetes. This is due primarily to maternal hyperglycemia. When euglycemia is maintained and a normal HbA_1c is present from conception through the first trimester, there is no increase in the incidence of congenital anomalies (Johnson & Milio, 2015). The anomalies often involve the heart, central nervous system (CNS), and skeletal system. Septal defects, coarctation of the aorta, and transposition of the great vessels are the most common heart lesions seen. CNS anomalies include hydrocephalus, meningomyelocele, and anencephaly. One anomaly, *sacral agenesis*, appears only in newborns of mothers with diabetes. In sacral agenesis, the sacrum and lumbar spine fail to develop and the lower extremities develop incompletely. To reduce the incidence of congenital anomalies, preconception counseling and strict diabetes control before conception and in the early weeks of pregnancy are indicated.

Characteristically, newborns of mothers with uncontrolled diabetes are large for gestational age (LGA) as a result of high levels of fetal insulin production stimulated by the high levels of glucose crossing the placenta from the mother. Sustained fetal hyperinsulinism and hyperglycemia ultimately lead to excessive growth, called **macrosomia**, and deposition of fat. If born vaginally, the macrosomic neonate is at increased risk for birth trauma such as fractured clavicle or brachial plexus injuries due to shoulder dystocia. To prevent such injuries, women should be counseled about the option of scheduling cesarean birth if birth weight is expected to exceed 4500 g (ACOG, 2018).

After birth, the umbilical cord is severed, thus the generous maternal blood glucose supply is eliminated. However, continued islet cell hyperactivity leads to excessive insulin levels and depleted blood glucose (hypoglycemia) in 2 to 4 hours after birth in the neonate. Macrosomia can be significantly reduced by tight maternal blood glucose control.

Newborns of mothers with diabetes with vascular involvement may demonstrate *intrauterine growth restriction (IUGR)*. This occurs because vascular changes in the mother decrease the efficiency of placental perfusion, and the fetus is not as well sustained in utero.

Respiratory distress syndrome (RDS) appears to result from inhibition, by high levels of fetal insulin, of some fetal enzymes necessary for surfactant production. *Polycythemia* in the newborn is due primarily to the diminished ability of glycosylated hemoglobin in the mother's blood to release oxygen. *Hyperbilirubinemia* is a result of the inability of immature liver enzymes to metabolize the increased bilirubin resulting from the polycythemia. *Hypocalcemia*, characterized by signs of irritability or even tetany, may occur. The cause of these low calcium levels in newborns of mothers with diabetes is not known.

Clinical Therapy

Gestational diabetes is more common than pregestational diabetes. DM occurs in about 7% of all pregnancies in the United States and of these cases, 86% are related to GDM (ACOG, 2018). Therefore, screening for its detection is a standard part of prenatal care. If diabetes is suspected, further testing is undertaken for diagnosis.

DETECTION AND DIAGNOSIS OF GESTATIONAL DIABETES

All pregnant women should have their risk of diabetes assessed at the first prenatal visit. Women at high risk (non-Caucasian, prior history of GDM or birth of an LGA neonate, marked obesity [body mass index (BMI) greater than 30], diagnosis of polycystic ovarian syndrome, hypertension, presence of glycosuria, or a strong family history of type 2 DM) should be tested for diabetes at the first prenatal visit (ADA, 2018).

Various screening approaches may be used. An HbA_{1c} level equal to or greater than 6.5% would be considered diagnostic, as would a fasting plasma glucose level equal to or greater than 126 mg/dL or a 2-hour plasma glucose level equal to or greater than 200 mg/dL during an oral glucose tolerance test (OGTT) (see following discussion). Women determined to have diabetes at this visit should be diagnosed as having overt diabetes and not GDM (ADA, 2018).

Two approaches to prenatal screening are currently available and performed at 24 to 28 weeks' gestation for all pregnant women not previously diagnosed with overt DM (ADA, 2018):

1. ***Two-step approach:*** Recommended by a National Institutes of Health (NIH) Consensus Conference and ACOG (ACOG, 2018). ACOG supports this approach because of "... the lack of evidence that the use of the one-step 75-g, 2-hour OGTT to diagnose GDM leads to clinically significant improvements in maternal or newborn outcomes ..." (ACOG, 2018, p. e52), but would lead to a significant increase in health care costs (ACOG, 2018).
   - ***Step 1.*** The woman is given a non-fasting, 50-g, 1-hour OGTT. The oral glucose load can be given at any time of the day with no requirement for fasting. One hour later plasma glucose is measured. If plasma glucose levels are elevated (equal to or greater than 130, 135, or 140 mg/dL, depending on the laboratory used), a 100-g, 3-hour glucose test is done (ADA, 2018).
   - ***Step 2.*** To do the 100-g, 3-hour OGTT, the woman eats an unrestricted diet, consuming at least 150 g of carbohydrates per day for at least 3 days before her scheduled test. She then ingests a 100-g oral glucose solution in the morning after an overnight fast. Plasma glucose is measured fasting and at 1, 2, and 3 hours. Gestational diabetes is diagnosed if *two or more* of the following values are met or exceeded (ADA, 2018):

Fasting	95 mg/dL
1 hour	180 mg/dL
2 hours	155 mg/dL
3 hours	140 mg/dL

2. ***One-step approach:*** Recommended by the International Association of Diabetes and Pregnancy Study Groups (IADPSG; 2010). ADA supports this approach, which is the method that has been adopted internationally (ADA, 2018).
   - ***Step 1.*** In the morning, following an overnight fast, the woman ingests a 75-g oral glucose solution. Plasma glucose levels are determined fasting and at 1 and 2 hours. Gestational diabetes is diagnosed if any *one* of the following values are equaled or exceeded:

Fasting	92 mg/dL
1 hour	180 mg/dL
2 hours	153 mg/dL

LABORATORY ASSESSMENT OF LONG-TERM GLUCOSE CONTROL

Glycosylated hemoglobin (HbA_{1c}) is a laboratory test that loosely reflects glucose control over the previous 4 to 8 weeks. It measures the percentage of glycohemoglobin in the blood. Glycohemoglobin, or HbA_{1c}, is the hemoglobin to which a glucose molecule is attached. Because glycosylation is a rather slow and essentially irreversible process, the test is not reliable for screening for gestational diabetes or for close daily control. However, in women with known pregestational DM, abnormal HbA_{1c} values correlate directly with the frequency of spontaneous abortion and fetal congenital anomalies. Consequently, women with preexisting diabetes who plan to become pregnant should work to achieve HbA_{1c} levels at target levels (less than 6.5%) without significant hypoglycemia (ADA, 2018).

Antepartum Management of Diabetes Mellitus

The major goals of medical care for a pregnant woman with diabetes—whether gestational or pregestational—are to maintain a physiologic equilibrium of insulin availability and glucose utilization during pregnancy and to ensure an optimally healthy mother and newborn. To achieve these goals, good prenatal care using a team approach is a top priority. Education of the woman and her partner and their active involvement in managing her care are essential for a good outcome.

The woman with gestational diabetes may find the diagnosis shocking and upsetting. She needs clear explanations about the actions she can take with regard to diet, weight gain, and exercise and the therapy that may be indicated to ensure a good outcome. The nurse-educator plays a major role in this counseling.

The woman with pregestational diabetes needs to understand changes she can expect during pregnancy; thus, she should receive such teaching in preconception counseling. At the initial prenatal visit, height, weight, and vital signs are assessed along with a thorough assessment of thyroid and cardiac function. Special attention is given to dating the pregnancy. Women should be screened for diabetic neuropathy, and a funduscopic examination is done to detect any retinopathy. In some cases, the woman may be referred to an ophthalmologist for further evaluation (ADA, 2018).

DIETARY REGULATION

The pregnant woman with diabetes needs to increase her caloric intake by about 300 kilocalories (kcal) per day. In general, women need approximately 30 kcal/kg of ideal body weight (IBW) during the first trimester and 35 to 36 kcal/kg IBW during the second and third trimesters. If ketonuria develops or the woman complains of hunger, the number of calories may be increased. Dietary guidelines are similar for women with gestational and pregestational diabetes. Approximately 33 to 40% of the kilocalories should come from complex carbohydrates, 20% from protein, and 40% from fats (ACOG, 2018). The food is divided among three meals and two to three snacks. A prebedtime snack may be indicated to prevent hypoglycemia at night. Management should focus on food choices for appropriate weight gain, normoglycemia, and absence of ketones.

Because it is so important that the pregnant woman follow these guidelines, a nutritionist works out meal plans based on the woman's lifestyle, culture, and food preferences and teaches her food exchanges so she can vary and plan her own meals. It is possible to control GDM with diet alone. Daily food records, weekly weight checks, and regular ketone testing can assist in identifying an individual's energy requirements in order to help avoid the need for insulin therapy.

GLUCOSE MONITORING

Glucose monitoring is an essential part of diabetes management for determining the need for insulin and assessing glucose control. Many physicians have the woman come in for a weekly assessment of her fasting glucose levels and one or two postprandial levels. In addition, frequent self-monitoring of glucose levels is paramount in maintaining good glucose control. Self-monitoring is discussed later in the chapter.

INSULIN ADMINISTRATION

Whether the woman with gestational diabetes needs additional insulin (over her own body production) depends on how well her blood glucose levels can be maintained by diet alone. Individuals with pregestational diabetes usually have type 1 diabetes, requiring insulin administration. Whether the patient has gestational or pregestational diabetes, semi-synthetic human insulin or an insulin analog such as lispro or aspart should be used. Insulin is given either in multiple injections or by continuous subcutaneous infusion. Multiple injections are used more commonly and with excellent results. Most women will need a mixture of intermediate and regular insulin.

A three-dose approach is often used: (1) a combination of intermediate-acting insulin and short-acting insulin or an analog taken before breakfast, (2) short-acting insulin or analog at dinner, and (3) an intermediate-acting insulin at bedtime. Some women require a four-injection approach with a small dose of a short-acting insulin or analog before lunch (Landon, Catalano, & Gabbe, 2017).

Oral hypoglycemics, including metformin and glyburide, have been found to be effective during pregnancy, although they do cross the placenta and have not been approved by the FDA for this indication. To date, insulin continues to be the first-line therapy recommended by the ADA (ACOG, 2018; ADA, 2018). Metformin is considered a reasonable alternative therapy for women who are reluctant to use insulin or in cases in which the healthcare provider believes the woman would be unable to safely administer insulin. Glyburide has been increasingly used for GDM but ACOG states that it should not be recommended as a first-choice treatment because ". . . in most studies, it does not yield equivalent outcomes to insulin or metformin" (ACOG, 2018, p. e55).

EVALUATION OF FETAL STATUS

Information about the well-being, maturation, and size of the fetus is important for planning the course of the pregnancy and the timing of birth. See *Key Facts to Remember: Fetal Surveillance by Weeks of Gestation.*

Key Facts To Remember

Fetal Surveillance by Weeks of Gestation

Weeks of Gestation	Fetal Surveillance
8–10	Ultrasound crown–rump measurement for estimated date of birth (EDB)
16–18	Maternal serum alpha fetoprotein
18–20	Targeted ultrasound examination
20–22	Fetal echocardiogram
24	Begin ultrasounds for assessment of fetus and fetal growth
28	Ultrasound for growth; begin daily fetal movement counting
32	Ultrasound for growth
32	Twice-weekly nonstress tests; fetal surveillance should be initiated earlier in pregnancies complicated by IUGR, hypertension, nephropathy, ketoacidosis, pyelonephritis, preeclampsia, and poor compliance
36	Ultrasound for growth
37–39	Consider birth if there is poor compliance or clinical concern for fetal well-being
39	Childbirth

NOTE: Some physicians may order *fetal biophysical profiles* (ultrasound evaluation of fetal well-being in which fetal breathing movements, fetal activity, reactivity, muscle tone, and amniotic fluid volume are assessed) as part of an ongoing evaluation of fetal status.

Intrapartum Management of Diabetes Mellitus

During the intrapartum period, medical therapy includes:

- ***Timing of birth.*** Most women with diabetes are able to give birth at term after spontaneous labor, thereby decreasing the risk of respiratory distress in the newborn. Induction of labor may be indicated prior to 39 weeks for women with worsening hypertension or nonreassuring fetal status. When the estimated fetal weight is 4500g or more, the woman should be counseled about the risks and benefits of a scheduled cesarean birth (ACOG, 2018).
- ***Labor management.*** The degree of prenatal maintenance of normal maternal glucose levels (euglycemia) and the maintenance of maternal euglycemia during labor are important in preventing neonatal hypoglycemia. Maternal insulin requirements often decrease dramatically during labor. Consequently, maternal glucose levels are measured every 1 to 2 hours during the active phase of labor to determine insulin need (Figure 17–1). The primary goal in controlling maternal glucose levels during the intrapartum period is to prevent neonatal hypoglycemia (ADA, 2018). Long-acting insulin should be reduced or stopped, and regular insulin

should be used to meet most or all of the woman's identified needs. Often two intravenous lines are used, one with a 5% dextrose solution and one with a saline solution. The saline solution is then available if a bolus is needed or for piggybacking insulin. Insulin clings to the plastic intravenous bag and tubing. To ensure that the woman receives the desired dose, the intravenous tubing must be flushed with insulin before the prescribed amount is added. During the second stage of labor and the immediate postpartum period, the woman may not need additional insulin. The intravenous insulin is discontinued at the end of the third stage of labor.

Postpartum Management of Diabetes Mellitus

Maternal insulin requirements fall significantly postpartum because the levels of hPL, progesterone, and estrogen fall after placental separation and their anti-insulin effect ceases, resulting in decreased blood glucose levels. The mother with preexisting diabetes may require little or no insulin, and her insulin dosage is usually managed with a sliding scale. Then, reestablishment of insulin needs based on blood glucose testing is necessary. Diet and exercise levels must also be redetermined.

Women with GDM seldom need insulin during the postpartum period. If elevated glucose levels develop, oral antihyperglycemic agents may be tried if the woman is not breastfeeding. The woman should be reassessed 4 to 12 weeks' postpartum with a 75-g OGTT to determine whether her glucose levels are normal. If the levels are normal, she should be reassessed every 1 to 3 years thereafter. The frequency of testing is determined by the presence of other risk factors such as family history or BMI (ADA, 2018).

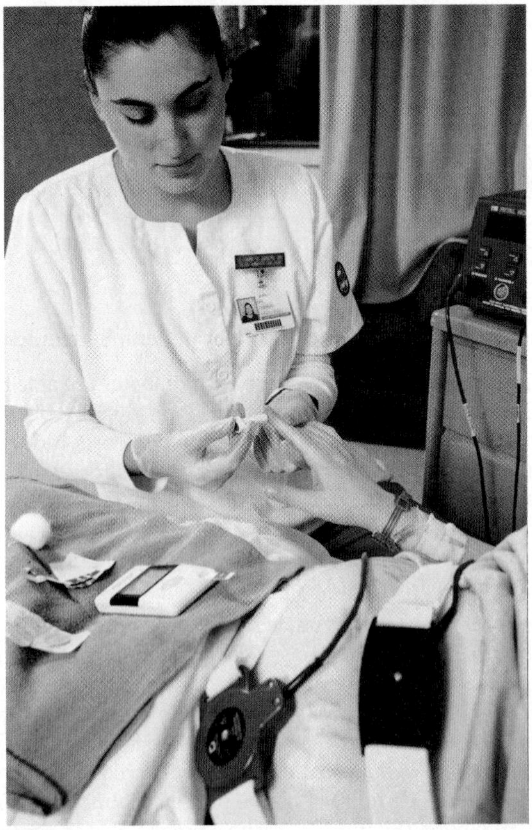

Figure 17–1 **During labor, the nurse closely monitors the blood glucose levels of the woman with diabetes mellitus.**

Breastfeeding is encouraged, but the nurse needs to remember that insulin requirements do decrease with breastfeeding, so a prenursing snack may be indicated (Miller, Mamilly, Fourtner, et al., 2017). The composition of breast milk is not altered by diabetes, and babies of mothers with diabetes gain weight appropriately. The lactating mother with diabetes often has a sense of well-being and diminished insulin needs even while increasing caloric intake. Caloric needs increase during lactation to 500 to 800 kcal above prepregnant requirements. Insulin must be adjusted according to individual needs. Home blood glucose monitoring should continue for the person with insulin-dependent diabetes.

Diabetic control and the establishment of parent–child relationships in light of neonatal needs are the priorities of this period. If her newborn must be cared for in a special care nursery because of hypoglycemia or other complications, the mother needs support and information about the baby's condition. Every effort must be made to provide as much contact as possible between the parents and their newborn.

The woman and her partner should receive information on family planning. Barrier methods of contraception (diaphragm and condom) used with spermicide and long-acting reversible contraceptives (LARCs), such as intrauterine devices and the contraceptive implant, are safe and effective for women with insulin-dependent diabetes. There continues to be insufficient evidence for use of combined oral contraceptives (COCs) by women with diabetes because of the risk of vascular disease (Lauring, Lehman, Deimling, et al., 2016). Many physicians who prescribe low-dose COCs to women with diabetes restrict them to women who have no vascular disease and who do not smoke. The progesterone-only pill may also be used, as may Depo-Provera.

> "It's hard to realize that I have gestational diabetes and to know that it increases my chances of getting diabetes later. My grandmother had diabetes, so I always thought of it as an old person's disease. All the fingersticks, watching my diet, and keeping track has taken some getting used to. I'll be glad when our baby is born and I can put this behind me, at least for now."

●○● NURSING MANAGEMENT

For the Woman with Diabetes Mellitus or Gestational Diabetes Mellitus

The *Nursing Care Plan* for a woman with diabetes mellitus summarizes nursing management.

Nursing Assessment and Diagnosis

Whether diabetes has been diagnosed before pregnancy occurs or the diagnosis is made during pregnancy (GDM), careful assessment of the disease process and the woman's understanding of diabetes are important. Thorough physical examination—including assessment for vascular complications, any signs of infectious conditions, and urine and blood testing for glucose—is essential at the first prenatal visit. Follow-up visits are usually scheduled twice a month during the first two trimesters and weekly during the last trimester.

Assessment also yields vital information about the woman's ability to cope with the combined stress of pregnancy and

Nursing Care Plan: The Woman with Diabetes Mellitus

1. Nursing Diagnosis: *Nutrition, Imbalanced: Less Than Body Requirements*, related to poor carbohydrate metabolism (NANDA-I © 2017)

Goal: Patient will maintain adequate nutrition throughout pregnancy.

INTERVENTION	RATIONALE
• Emphasize importance of regular prenatal visits for assessment of weight gain, controlled blood sugar, fetal heart tones, urine ketones, and fundal height measurement.	• Regular follow-up and assessment of weight, blood sugar levels, fetal heart tones, urine ketones, and fundal height will promote a healthy pregnancy and outcome as well as allow for modifications in the treatment regimen, if necessary.
• Coordinate care with a dietitian to assist patient in meal planning and educate patient on the daily caloric needs of pregnancy.	• A daily intake of high-quality foods promotes fetal growth and controls maternal glucose levels.
• Instruct patient on signs and symptoms of hyperglycemia: Polyphagia, nausea, hot flashes, polydipsia, polyuria, fruity breath, abdominal cramps, rapid deep breathing, headache, weakness, drowsiness, and general malaise. Instruct patient on signs and symptoms of hypoglycemia: Hunger; clammy skin; irritability; slurred speech; seizures; tachycardia; headache; pallor; sweating; disorientation; shakiness; blurred vision; and, if untreated, coma or convulsions.	• Maintaining a euglycemic state throughout pregnancy aids in preventing diabetic complications and promotes a positive pregnancy outcome.
• Instruct patient on management of hyperglycemia and hypoglycemia.	
• Include family members in meal planning.	• Gives the family member a sense of involvement and an understanding of the importance of adequate nutrition in pregnancy.

EXPECTED OUTCOME: The patient will maintain adequate nutrition as evidenced by adequate weight gain, normal blood sugar levels, reassuring fetal heart rate, verbalization of understanding of personal treatment regimen, and appropriate fetal growth and development during pregnancy.

2. Nursing Diagnosis: *Injury, Risk for*, to the fetus related to possible complications associated with altered tissue perfusion secondary to maternal diagnosis of diabetes mellitus (NANDA-I © 2017)

Goal: Uncomplicated birth of a healthy newborn.

INTERVENTION	RATIONALE
• Assess fetal heart tones for reassuring variability and accelerations.	• Reassuring fetal heart rate variability and accelerations are interpreted as adequate placental oxygenation.
• Instruct mother on how to lie in a left recumbent position after eating and record how many fetal movements she feels in an hour.	• Three or more fetal kick counts in an hour is considered a reassuring fetal status.
• **Collaborative:** Perform nonstress tests, oxytocin challenge test (OCT)/contraction stress test (CST) as determined by physician.	• Fetal surveillance testing assesses fetal well-being and adequate placental perfusion.
• Prepare patient for frequent ultrasound assessments.	• Ultrasonography is indicated in the first trimester to confirm gestational age and then repeated regularly to evaluate fetal well-being per physician's orders.
• Assist physician with biophysical profile assessment.	• Helps ensure fetal well-being and a positive fetal outcome.

EXPECTED OUTCOME: The fetus will exhibit signs of adequate tissue perfusion as evidenced by positive fetal activity, reassuring fetal heart rate patterns, a reactive nonstress test, a biophysical profile score between 8 and 10, and a negative CST.

(continued)

Nursing Care Plan: The Woman with Diabetes Mellitus (*continued*)

3. Nursing Diagnosis: *Knowledge, Readiness for Enhanced*, about the effects of blood sugar on pregnancy related to an expressed desire to maintain stable blood glucose levels (NANDA-I © 2017)

Goal: The patient and her family will verbalize the importance of maintaining blood sugar within prescribed ranges during pregnancy.

INTERVENTION	RATIONALE
• Assess the patient and family's cognitive level and develop a teaching strategy that will facilitate learning at that level.	• Behavior changes occur when teaching strategies are appropriate for the patient and family's cognitive level.
• Teach blood glucose monitoring, insulin administration, and predicted insulin needs throughout pregnancy and then have patient and family members repeat the discussion.	• Basic understanding of the relationship between blood sugar levels and how insulin needs change throughout pregnancy will foster compliance with prescribed regimen.
• Emphasize the importance of maintaining a healthy diet and exercise program during pregnancy. Encourage patient and family to develop a sample diabetic diet and exercise regimen that is appropriate for pregnancy while present in the clinic or hospital and evaluate for appropriateness.	• Involves the patient and her family members in the planning of her care, and the evaluation process promotes cooperation, positive reinforcement, and a time for modifications of regimen, if necessary.
• Emphasize the importance of prenatal care for the purpose of maternal and fetal surveillance.	• Frequent prenatal visits allow for modifications in regimen and promote a healthy pregnancy outcome.

EXPECTED OUTCOME: The patient and family members will verbalize understanding of the effects of blood sugar fluctuations on pregnancy as evidenced by asking questions and seeking health information when necessary. The patient adheres to personal treatment regimen throughout pregnancy.

4. Nursing Diagnosis: *Infection, Risk for*, related to increased levels of glucose in urine (NANDA-I © 2017)

Goal: The patient will have no urinary tract infections (UTIs) during pregnancy.

INTERVENTION	RATIONALE
• Encourage patient to utilize preventive measures to prevent UTIs: Increasing intake of water and low-sugar cranberry juice, wearing cotton underwear, wiping perineum from front to back, voiding frequently, and voiding before and immediately after sexual intercourse.	• Utilizing preventive measures decreases the likelihood of patient acquiring a UTI.
• Instruct patient on the signs and symptoms of UTIs: Urinary frequency, dysuria, cloudy urine, hematuria, lower back pain, and foul-smelling urine.	• Patient will be aware of signs and symptoms of UTIs and report to physician for immediate intervention.
• **Collaborative:** Instruct patient on how to obtain a clean-catch urine sample and send to laboratory for culture and sensitivity per physician's orders.	• A clean-catch urine sample will contain bacteria if a UTI is present.
• Administer prescribed antibiotic therapy and teach patient about medication, adverse effects, and appropriate dosage.	• Antibiotic therapy is the appropriate treatment for a UTI. Compliance increases when a patient fully understands medication regimen.
• Encourage patient to drink 8 to 10 glasses of water each day.	• Increased fluid intake assists in flushing bacteria out of the urinary tract system.

EXPECTED OUTCOME: **Patient will remain free of UTIs during pregnancy as evidenced by verbalizing and complying with appropriate preventive measures, increasing fluid intake, and identifying negative urine samples during prenatal visits.**

Nursing Care Plan: The Woman with Diabetes Mellitus (*continued*)

5. Nursing Diagnosis: *Anxiety* related to unfamiliarity with diagnosis (NANDA-I © 2017)

Goal: The patient expresses less anxiety.

INTERVENTION	RATIONALE
• Assess patient's level of anxiety (mild—1, moderate—2, or severe—3) and have patient verbalize causes of anxiety.	• Verbalization of anxiety provokers encourages expression of feelings and questions.
• Share information on diabetes care such as nutrition, exercise, and glucose control in a clear and concise manner.	• Accurate information gives the patient a sense of control and comfort.
• Instruct patient on anxiety-reducing techniques such as imagery, breathing exercises, and massage used in pregnancy.	• Gives patient the tools necessary for decreasing anxiety.
• Refer patient to a diabetes support group.	• A support group allows patients with similar problems to express concerns and share information with each other.

EXPECTED OUTCOME: The patient demonstrates appropriate coping strategies as evidenced by utilizing resources efficiently and verbalizing feelings of anxiety and the ways to deal with them.

diabetes and her ability to follow a recommended regimen of care. Determine the woman's knowledge about diabetes and self-care before formulating a teaching plan.

Nursing diagnoses that may apply to the pregnant woman with diabetes mellitus include:

- *Overweight, Risk for*, related to imbalance between intake and available insulin
- *Injury, Risk for*, related to possible complications secondary to hypoglycemia or hyperglycemia
- *Family Processes, Interrupted*, related to the need for hospitalization secondary to GDM.

(NANDA-I © 2017)

Nursing Plan and Implementation

Prepregnancy counseling should be delivered in a culturally sensitive manner by a nurse and a physician using a team approach. The goal is for the woman to achieve optimal glycemic control (HbA_1c less than 6.5) through medication management, diet, and exercise. The woman may also need to be evaluated for comorbidities, which may include an ophthalmologic evaluation, electrocardiographic study, and urine collection for creatinine clearance and protein excretion. Tight glucose control is important in preventing fetal congenital anomalies. If the diabetes is of recent onset without vascular complications, the outcome of pregnancy should be good, provided that glucose levels are controlled.

Community-Based Nursing Care

In some cases, women with preexisting or gestational diabetes may need to be stabilized in the hospital and necessary teaching for self-care begun. After discharge, ongoing teaching and supervision of pregnant women with diabetes is carried out by nurses in clinics, community agencies, and the women's homes. Communication between the community-based nurse and the woman's prenatal care team is extremely important to help the woman achieve her target glucose goals.

Effective Insulin Use

Ensure that both the woman and her partner understand the purpose of the insulin, the types of insulin the woman is to use, the number of doses she is to receive daily, and the correct procedure for its administration. Instruct the woman's partner about insulin administration in case it should be necessary for the partner to give it. For some highly motivated women whose glucose levels are not well controlled with multiple injections, the continuous insulin infusion pump may improve glucose control.

Teach the woman how and when to monitor her blood sugar, the desired range of blood sugar levels, and the importance of good glycemic control (Figure 17–2). Most women use a glucose meter because it provides a more accurate reading. Teach the patient to follow the manufacturer's directions exactly; to wash hands thoroughly before puncturing her finger; and to touch the blood droplet, not her finger, to the test pad on the strip.

With a blood glucose meter, an electronic eye measures the blood sugar and a digital reading is given. The blood droplet should cover the test pad because uncovered portions are read as low sugar. The glucose meter is a portable pocket-sized device that is more accurate than the visual, color-comparison method. Some meters are able to store and recall a specified number of readings, which helps ensure the accuracy of recorded results.

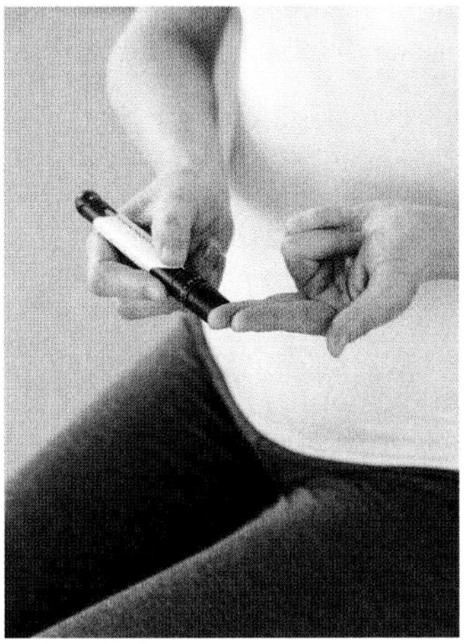

Figure 17–2 As she was taught, this pregnant woman regularly monitors her blood glucose at home.

CLINICAL TIP

When teaching a pregnant woman to do her own blood glucose testing, have gloves available and put them on if it becomes necessary to help the woman obtain a blood sample. The woman does not need to wear gloves during the procedure.

Also be sure to wear gloves when doing fingersticks for blood glucose levels, when testing the urine for ketones, when starting an IV for insulin therapy, or when drawing blood for other laboratory tests.

The following information about finger puncture can be offered to the patient:

- Various spring-loaded devices are available that make puncturing easier.
- Hanging the arm down for 30 seconds increases blood flow to the fingers.
- Warming the hands under running water increases blood flow to them.
- The sides of fingers should be punctured instead of the ends because the ends contain more pain-sensitive nerves.

Patients with diabetes need to keep a record of each blood sugar reading as a guide for management. Specific record sheets are available for this purpose and should be brought to each visit.

Planned Exercise Program

Exercise is encouraged for the woman's overall well-being. If she is used to a regular exercise program, encourage her to continue. Advise her to exercise after meals (when blood sugar levels are high), to wear diabetic identification, to carry a simple sugar such as hard candy (because of the possibility of exercise-induced hypoglycemia), to monitor her blood glucose levels regularly, and to avoid injecting insulin into an extremity that will soon be used during exercise.

If she has not been following a regular exercise plan, encourage her to begin gradually. Because exercise can alter metabolism, the woman's blood glucose should be well controlled before she begins an exercise program. Women with GDM should not use unusual, strenuous, and excessive exercise in an attempt to reduce glucose levels.

Health Promotion Education

Using the information gained during the nursing assessment of the pregnant woman with diabetes, provide appropriate teaching to the woman and her family so that the woman can meet her own healthcare needs as much as possible.

- ***Glucose monitoring.*** Home blood glucose monitoring is the most accurate and convenient way to determine insulin dose and assess control. Women with GDM typically measure their blood glucose four times a day (fasting and 1 to 2 hours after meals), while women with preexisting diabetes may monitor their blood more frequently. The diabetic team will establish the timing of testing. Women are encouraged to maintain blood sugar in the normal ranges as follows: Fasting (before eating or taking insulin), less than 95 mg/dL; 2 hours after each meal, less than 120 mg/dL (ADA, 2018).
- ***Symptoms of abnormal blood glucose levels.*** The pregnant woman with diabetes must recognize symptoms of changing glucose levels—whether hypoglycemia or hyperglycemia accompanied by ketoacidosis—and take appropriate action by immediately checking her capillary blood glucose level. Hypoglycemia may develop fairly rapidly. Symptoms include sweating, periodic tingling, disorientation, shakiness, pallor, clammy skin, irritability, hunger, headache, and blurred vision. If the pregnant woman's blood glucose is less than 60 mg/dL, she should drink 4 ounces of fruit juice or 5 to 6 ounces of a regular soft drink (not diet/low calorie); or eat seven to eight pieces of hard candy; or eat 1 tablespoon of sugar or jelly. She should then wait 15 minutes and recheck blood glucose (Joslin Diabetes Center, 2017). Many people overtreat their symptoms by continuing to eat, which can cause rebound hyperglycemia.

Advise the woman to carry a snack at all times and have other fast sources of glucose (simple carbohydrates such as hard candy) on hand so that she can treat an insulin reaction when other items are not available. Teach family members how to inject glucagon in the event that food does not work or is not feasible, for instance, in the presence of severe morning sickness. The woman will need a prescription for a glucagon kit.

Hyperglycemia and ketoacidosis typically develop more slowly and tend to occur more commonly during the second half of pregnancy. Because most problems for the fetus are related to maternal hyperglycemia, this is a serious situation. Symptoms include polyuria, polydipsia, dry mouth, fatigue, nausea, hot flushed skin, rapid deep breathing, abdominal cramps, acetone breath, headache, drowsiness, depressed reflexes, oliguria or anuria, stupor, or coma. Hyperglycemia is treated with insulin.

- ***Smoking.*** Smoking has harmful effects on the maternal vascular system and the developing fetus and is contraindicated for both pregnancy and diabetes.
- ***Travel.*** Insulin can be kept at room temperature while traveling. Insulin supplies should be kept with the traveler and not packed in the baggage. On international flights, most airlines can supply special meals if notified a few days before departure. If meals are not scheduled to be served, the woman should ensure that she has adequate food before boarding the airplane. The woman needs to wear a diabetic identification bracelet or necklace. In addition, the woman should check with her physician for any instructions or advice before leaving.
- ***Support groups.*** Many communities have diabetes support groups or education classes, which can be helpful to women with newly diagnosed diabetes.
- ***Cesarean birth.*** Chances for a cesarean birth increase if the pregnant woman has diabetes because of the risk of fetal macrosomia and shoulder dystocia. This possibility should be anticipated; enrollment in cesarean birth preparation classes may be suggested. Many hospitals offer classes and information is available through other organizations. The couple may prefer simply to discuss cesarean birth with the nurse and their obstetrician and read some books on the topic.

Hospital-Based Nursing Care

Hospitalization may become necessary during the pregnancy to evaluate blood glucose levels and adjust insulin dosages. In such cases, monitor the woman's status and continue to provide teaching so that the woman is knowledgeable about her condition and its management.

SAFETY ALERT!

Insulin is a high-risk medication that carries significant potential risks. Like all medications, nurses should use two patient identifiers, administer it at the correct time, and monitor the patient afterward. Nurses should have documented knowledge about insulin administration and demonstrate competency in administering, storing, and handling it and in the key assessments and findings indicated for maternity patients receiving insulin.

During the intrapartum period, it is important to have a clear understanding about the impact of labor on the woman's condition. Carefully monitor the woman's status, maintain her intravenous fluids, be alert for signs of hypoglycemia, and provide the care indicated for any woman in labor. If a cesarean birth is indicated, provide appropriate care as described in Chapter 25. See *Key Facts to Remember: Gestational Diabetes and Diabetes Mellitus*.

Key Facts To Remember
Gestational Diabetes Mellitus and Diabetes Mellitus

- Gestational diabetes mellitus (GDM) refers to a carbohydrate intolerance that develops during pregnancy. If untreated, the risk of perinatal morbidity and mortality increases.
- All pregnant women should be screened for GDM.
- Women with GDM are often treated with diet therapy and regular exercise; in some cases insulin or an insulin analog is necessary.
- Women with pregestational DM require careful management. Their long-term glucose control is best assessed by determining the percentage of glycohemoglobin, or HbA_1c, in the blood. The target level is less than 6.5%.
- To maintain normal glucose levels, women with pregestational DM typically receive doses of regular insulin or an insulin analog such as lispro before each meal and a dose of a longer-acting insulin or analog at bedtime.
- During labor, insulin requirements may decrease dramatically and require careful monitoring. The goal is to avoid neonatal hypoglycemia.

Evaluation

Expected outcomes of nursing care include:

- The woman is able to discuss her condition and its possible impact on her pregnancy, labor and birth, and postpartum period.
- The woman participates in developing a healthcare regimen to meet her needs and follows it throughout her pregnancy.
- The woman avoids developing hypoglycemia or hyperglycemia.
- The woman gives birth to a healthy newborn.
- The woman is able to care for her newborn.

Care of the Woman with Anemia

During pregnancy, *anemia* is defined as hemoglobin less than 11 g/dL. Anemia indicates inadequate levels of hemoglobin (Hb) in the blood. Race, altitude, smoking, nutrition, and medications can affect the normal limits of hemoglobin. The lower limit of normal tends to be higher for women who smoke and those who live at higher altitudes because their bodies require a greater quantity of red blood cells to maintain their tissue oxygen levels.

The common anemias of pregnancy are due either to insufficient hemoglobin production related to nutritional deficiency in iron or folic acid during pregnancy or to hemoglobin destruction in inherited disorders, specifically sickle cell disease and thalassemia.

Iron Deficiency Anemia

Dietary iron is needed to synthesize hemoglobin. Because hemoglobin is necessary to transport oxygen, a deficiency of iron may affect the body's transport of oxygen.

Iron deficiency anemia is the most common medical complication of pregnancy and affects one in four pregnancies (ACOG, 2015). Approximately 200 mg of iron will be conserved because of the functional amenorrhea of pregnancy, but a pregnant woman needs approximately 1000 mg more iron intake during the pregnancy. Between 300 and 400 mg of iron is transferred to the fetus; 500 mg is needed for the increased red blood cell mass in the woman's own increased circulating blood volume; another 100 mg is needed for the placenta; and about 280 mg is needed to replace the 1 mg of iron lost daily through feces, urine, and sweat.

The greatest need for increased iron intake occurs in the second half of pregnancy. When the iron needs of pregnancy are not met, maternal hemoglobin falls below 11 g/dL. Serum ferritin levels, indicating iron stores, are below 12 mg/L.

Many women begin pregnancy in a slightly anemic state. In pregnancy, mild anemia can rapidly become more severe; therefore, it needs immediate treatment.

MATERNAL RISKS

The woman with iron deficiency anemia may be asymptomatic, but she is more susceptible to infection, may tire easily, and has an increased chance of perinatal infection, preeclampsia, and bleeding (Abu-Ouf & Jan, 2015). In addition, even minimal blood loss during birth may be poorly tolerated. Healing of an episiotomy or an incision may be delayed. If the anemia is severe (Hb less than 6 g/dL), cardiac failure may ensue.

FETAL-NEONATAL RISKS

There is evidence of increased risk of low birth weight, prematurity, stillbirth, and neonatal death in babies of women with severe iron deficiency (maternal Hb less than 6 g/dL). The newborn is not iron deficient at birth because of active transport of iron across the placenta, even when maternal iron stores are low. However, these babies do have lower iron stores and are at increased risk for developing iron deficiency during infancy.

CLINICAL THERAPY

The first goal of healthcare is to prevent iron deficiency anemia. If it occurs, the goal is to return low iron and hemoglobin levels to normal. To prevent anemia, experts recommend that all pregnant women start on 30 mg/day of iron supplements daily beginning at the first prenatal visit (ACOG, 2015). This amount is contained in most prenatal vitamins. In addition, the woman should be encouraged to eat an iron-rich diet. To prevent constipation, the most common side effect of iron supplementation, a stool softener may be necessary.

If anemia is diagnosed, the dosage should be increased to 60 to 120 mg per day of iron. If the woman remains anemic after 1 month of therapy, further evaluation is indicated. With a twin pregnancy, a larger dose is needed. If a large dose of oral iron causes vomiting, diarrhea, or constipation, or if the anemia is discovered late in pregnancy, parenteral iron may be needed.

●○● NURSING MANAGEMENT

For the Pregnant Woman with Anemia

Nursing Assessment and Diagnosis

The main presenting symptom of iron deficiency anemia may be fatigue. Nutritional history usually gives evidence of poor dietary intake of iron. Determine, as well, whether there is a history of anemia in a prior pregnancy. Physical examination reveals pallor of skin and conjunctiva. Laboratory studies reveal low hemoglobin values (below 11 g/dL), low hematocrit (less than 35%), low serum ferritin levels (less than100 mg/dL), and possibly microcytic and hypochromic red blood cells (a late finding).

Nursing diagnoses that may apply to a pregnant woman with iron deficiency anemia include:

- ***Nutrition, Imbalanced: Less Than Body Requirements, Risk for***, related to inadequate intake of iron-containing foods
- ***Constipation***, related to daily intake of iron supplements.

(NANDA-I © 2017)

Nursing Plan and Implementation

Stress to the woman the importance of an iron-rich diet and of iron supplements during pregnancy. Supplements are indicated because dietary sources cannot meet the extra requirements. Teach the woman to take iron tablets with vitamin C (e.g., orange juice) to increase absorption. Iron absorption is reduced by 40 to 50% if the tablets are taken with meals. However, gastrointestinal upset is more likely if they are taken on an empty stomach. The patient may tolerate the iron better if she starts with small doses and gradually increases the dosage over several days. Inform her that her stool will turn black and may be more formed. Also advise her to keep the tablets out of the reach of children because ingestion may be fatal to a young child.

Evaluation

Expected outcomes of nursing care include:

- The woman is able to identify the risks associated with iron deficiency anemia during pregnancy.
- The woman takes her iron supplements as recommended.
- The woman's Hb levels remain normal or return to normal during her pregnancy.

Folic Acid Deficiency Anemia

Folate deficiency is the most common cause of megaloblastic anemia during pregnancy, affecting between 1 and 4% of pregnant women in the United States. It is more prevalent with twin pregnancies.

Folic acid is needed for deoxyribonucleic acid (DNA) and ribonucleic acid (RNA) synthesis and cell duplication. In its absence, immature red blood cells fail to divide, become enlarged (megaloblastic), and are fewer in number. Even more significantly, an inadequate intake of folic acid has been associated with neural tube defects (NTDs) (spina bifida, anencephaly, meningomyelocele) in the fetus or newborn. With the tremendous cell multiplication that occurs in pregnancy, an adequate amount of folic acid is crucial. However, increased urinary excretion of folic acid and fetal uptake can rapidly result in folic acid deficiency.

CLINICAL THERAPY

Diagnosis of folic acid deficiency anemia may be difficult and it is usually not detected until late in pregnancy or the early puerperium. This is because serum folate levels normally fall as pregnancy progresses. Women with true folic acid deficiency anemia often present with nausea and vomiting and anorexia. Hemoglobin levels as low as 3 to 5 g/dL may be found. Typically, the blood smear reveals that the newly formed erythrocytes are macrocytic.

Folic acid deficiency during pregnancy is prevented by a daily supplement of 0.4 mg (400 mcg) of folate. Treatment of deficiency consists of 1-mg folic acid supplement. Because iron deficiency anemia almost always coexists with folic acid deficiency, the woman also needs iron supplements.

NURSING MANAGEMENT

For the Pregnant Woman with Folic Acid Deficiency Anemia

Help the pregnant woman avoid folate deficiency by teaching her food sources of folic acid and cooking methods for preserving folic acid. The best sources are fresh leafy green vegetables, orange juice, other citrus fruits and juices, red meats, fish, poultry, and legumes. As much as 50 to 90% of folic acid can be lost by cooking in large volumes of water. Microwave cooking destroys more folic acid than conventional cooking.

All women of childbearing age (15 to 45 years) should consume at least 0.4 mg of folic acid every day. A daily supplement is recommended because the typical diet does not provide this level (American Academy of Pediatrics [AAP] & American College of Obstetricians and Gynecologists [ACOG], 2017). This recommendation is important because half of all U.S. pregnancies are unplanned and NTDs occur very early in pregnancy (3 to 4 weeks after conception), before most women realize they are pregnant. Nurses can play a crucial role in helping young women become aware of this important recommendation.

Sickle Cell Disease

Sickle cell disease (SCD) is a recessive autosomal disorder in which the normal adult hemoglobin, hemoglobin A (HbA), is abnormally formed. This abnormal hemoglobin is called *hemoglobin S (HbS)*. The abnormal red cells break down, causing anemia, which is characterized by acute, recurring episodes of tissue, abdominal, and joint pain. Individuals with the disorder are homozygous for the sickle cell gene. They inherit from each parent an allele causing an amino acid substitution in the two beta protein chains in the hemoglobin molecule. Heterozygous individuals are carriers for sickle cell trait (SCT) but are usually asymptomatic. One of the beta protein chains formed in their hemoglobin is normal; the other has the amino acid substitution. See *Genetic Facts: Sickle Cell Disease*.

HbS causes the red blood cells to be sickle or crescent shaped. In conditions of low oxygenation, normal hemoglobin is soluble, but HbS becomes semisolid and distorts the red blood cell shape. These erythrocytes easily interlock and clog capillaries, particularly in organs characterized by slow flow and high oxygen extraction, such as the spleen, bone marrow, and placenta. This phenomenon, called *sickling*, varies in frequency depending on the amount of the HbS in the red blood cells (there is seldom a crisis with levels below 40%) and other hemoglobin factors. Diagnosis is confirmed by hemoglobin electrophoresis

Genetic Facts **Sickle Cell Disease**

- Sickle cell disease (SCD) occurs primarily in people of African descent and occasionally in people of Southeast Asian or Mediterranean origin (e.g., Greek, Italian, Middle Eastern, and Turkish).
- Approximately one in 12 African Americans has sickle cell trait and one in every 300 African American newborns has some form of sickle cell disease (Hathaway, 2016).
- Couples should be screened to evaluate their sickle cell status. If both partners have either sickle cell trait or sickle cell disease, genetic counseling is warranted.

or a test to induce sickling in a blood sample. Prenatal diagnosis and newborn screening for sickle cell disease are important components of perinatal care.

MATERNAL RISKS

Women with sickle cell trait have a good prognosis for pregnancy if they have adequate nutrition and prenatal care. They are, however, at increased risk for nephritis, bacteriuria, and hematuria and tend to become anemic.

Women with sickle cell disease have considerably more risk during pregnancy. Low oxygen pressure—caused by high temperature, dehydration, infection, or acidosis, for example—may precipitate a vaso-occlusive crisis. The crisis produces sudden attacks of pain that may be general or localized in bones or joints, lungs, abdominal organs, or the spinal cord. The pain is due to ischemia in the tissues from occluded capillaries. Vaso-occlusive crises occur more often in the second half of pregnancy.

Maternal mortality due to sickle cell disease is rare. Complications include anemia requiring blood transfusion, infections, and emergency cesarean births. Acute chest syndrome, congestive heart failure, or acute renal failure may also occur.

FETAL-NEONATAL RISKS

The incidence of fetal death during and immediately following a maternal attack has decreased greatly in recent years. Prematurity and IUGR are associated with sickle cell disease. Fetal death is believed to be due to sickling attacks in the placenta (Hathaway, 2016).

CLINICAL THERAPY

Because the woman with sickle cell disease maintains her hemoglobin levels by intense erythropoiesis, additional folic acid supplements (4 mg/day) are required. Maternal infection should be treated promptly because dehydration and fever can trigger sickling and crisis. Vaso-occlusive crisis is best treated by a perinatal team in a medical center. Proper management requires close observation and evaluation of all symptoms. The term *sickle cell crisis* should be applied only after all other possible causes for the pain are excluded.

Rehydration with intravenous fluids; administration of oxygen, antibiotics, and analgesics; and monitoring of fetal heart rate are important aspects of therapy. Antiembolism stockings may be used postpartum.

If vaso-occlusive crisis occurs during labor, the previous therapies are instituted and the woman is kept in a left lateral position. Oxytocics may be used if needed to promote labor. Episiotomy and outlet forceps may be recommended to shorten the second stage of labor.

Several antisickling agents are being researched, and in the future sickle cell crisis may be prevented.

●○● NURSING MANAGEMENT

For the Pregnant Woman with Sickle Cell Disease

Nursing Assessment and Diagnosis

The woman with sickle cell disease usually relates a history of frequent illnesses and recurrent abdominal and joint pain and is found to be extremely anemic. The woman may appear undernourished and have long, thin extremities. Ulcers are often present on her ankles. Anemia may be severe.

A diagnosis of sickle cell disease is confirmed by hemoglobin electrophoresis or a test to induce sickling in a blood sample. Assess the woman for infection, which is associated with one-third of sickle cell crises in adults. Infections most often seen during pregnancy or postpartum are pneumonia, urinary tract infections, puerperal endomyometritis, and osteomyelitis.

Assess fetal status during a crisis by electronic fetal monitoring. During labor, assess the woman's vital signs frequently and initiate continuous fetal heart rate monitoring. Compatible blood should be available for transfusion. Oxygen is administered, if necessary. Assess the woman for joint pain and other signs of sickle cell crisis.

Nursing diagnoses that might apply to the pregnant woman with sickle cell disease include:

- ***Pain, Acute***, related to the effects of sickle cell crisis
- ***Knowledge, Readiness for Enhanced***, about the need to avoid exposure to infection related to the risk of triggering a sickle cell crisis.

(NANDA I © 2017)

Nursing Plan and Implementation

The nursing goal for a pregnant woman with sickle cell disease is to provide effective health teaching to help prevent a sickle cell crisis, improve the anemia, and prevent infection. Teach the woman to increase hydration, use good hygiene, avoid people with infections, seek immediate treatment for infection, and take folic acid supplements (Figure 17–3). As stated earlier, folic acid is important because of its role in red blood cell production; therefore, folic acid supplements are essential. Bedrest is sometimes recommended to decrease the chance of preterm labor. Other nursing interventions are aimed at facilitating the medical therapy and alleviating anxiety through support and education.

Evaluation

Expected outcomes of nursing care include:

- The woman is able to describe her condition and identify its possible impact on her pregnancy, labor and childbirth, and postpartum period.
- The woman takes appropriate healthcare measures to avoid a sickle cell crisis.
- The woman gives birth to a healthy baby.
- The woman and her caregivers quickly identify and successfully manage any complications that arise.

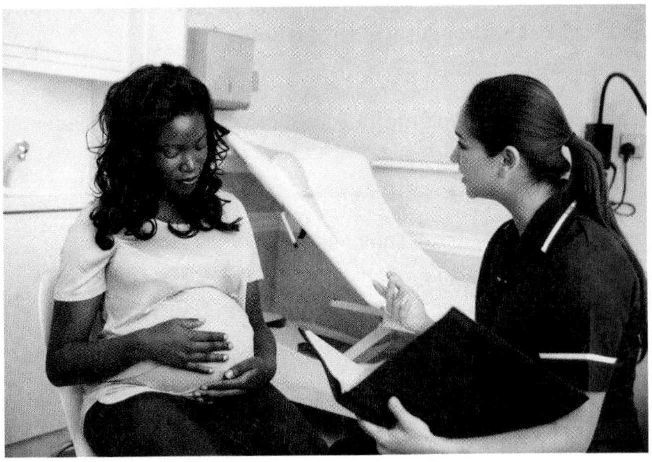

Figure 17–3 **Health teaching is an important part of nursing care for the pregnant woman with sickle cell disease.**

SOURCE: Monkey Business Images/Shutterstock.

Thalassemia

The thalassemias are a group of autosomal recessive disorders characterized by a defect in the synthesis of the alpha or beta chains in the hemoglobin molecule. The one most frequently encountered in the United States is β-thalassemia. Symptoms are caused by the shortened lifespan of the red blood cells, which result in active erythropoiesis in the liver, spleen, and bones. This produces hepatosplenomegaly and, sometimes, bony malformations. The thalassemias are seen most often in persons from Greece, Italy, or southern China and are also known as *Mediterranean anemia* and *Cooley anemia*. Early identification of thalassemia and preventive management avoid missed diagnosis and unnecessary treatment for iron deficiency anemia (Petrakos, Andriopoulos, & Tsironi, 2016). Prenatal genetic diagnosis is now available for this disorder.

If the woman is heterozygous for β-thalassemia, half of the beta chains are formed normally. This is β-thalassemia minor, or β-thalassemia trait. Mild anemia is usually the only symptom.

Persons born homozygous for the disease have β-thalassemia major. Because newborns have fetal hemoglobin (HbF), which does not have beta chains, no symptoms are present for several months. Once infants with β-thalassemia major start producing adult-type hemoglobin (HbA), they develop severe anemia and are dependent on transfusions from which they eventually develop iron overload. Iron chelation therapy must be instituted soon after chronic transfusions are begun because excess iron damages the liver and heart.

When women with β-thalassemia major maintain a proper chelation therapy, they may prevent fertility issues from developing and have a good chance of becoming pregnant. They are also found to have a much longer life expectancy than those who do not maintain chelation therapy, living into their 50s (Cooley's Anemia Foundation, 2017).

MATERNAL–FETAL-NEONATAL RISKS

The woman with β-thalassemia minor has mild anemia with small (microcytic) red cells. This mild anemia must be distinguished from iron deficiency anemia because a woman with β-thalassemia minor should not receive iron therapy unless she is also deficient in iron. A woman with iron deficiency anemia typically has low serum iron and serum ferritin levels, whereas the woman with β-thalassemia minor has normal levels. Pregnancy is rare in women with β-thalassemia major. If it does occur, the woman generally has severe anemia, needs transfusion therapy, and is at risk for congestive heart failure.

CLINICAL THERAPY

Folic acid supplements are indicated for women with thalassemia, but iron supplements are not given. Those with thalassemia intermedia and thalassemia major may need frequent transfusions, however, chelation therapy is often discontinued during pregnancy because of a lack of data on the effect on the fetus. Women with thalassemia should also avoid exposure to infections and seek treatment promptly if an infection develops. Their care is similar to that of women with sickle cell disease.

The woman with thalassemia needs to understand her disease and the possibility of transmitting it to her offspring, thus genetic counseling may be helpful. These patients have lived with thalassemia since childhood but may have questions about its effect on pregnancy outcome and their own prognosis.

Genetic Facts β-Thalassemia

- β-thalassemia is an autosomal recessive disorder characterized by a defect in the synthesis of the alpha or beta chains in the hemoglobin molecule.
- β-thalassemia minor varies in degree of severity from extremely mild (*minima*) anemia, which results in a relatively smooth pregnancy, to a more symptomatic form (*intermedia*).
- Pregnant women with the intermedia and major forms of thalassemia are generally cared for by a perinatologist and cardiologist in a facility that can accommodate high-risk pregnancies.

Care of the Pregnant Woman with a Substance Use Disorder

Perinatal incidence of substance use disorders by pregnant women is highly variable because of the reluctance of women to disclose use. Among pregnant women 15 to 44 years of age in the United States, 5.4% are illicit drug users, compared to 11.4% of nonpregnant women in the same age group. However, the rate of illicit drug use varies significantly by age: 14.6% among pregnant teens 15 to 17 years of age, 8.6% among women 18 to 25 years of age, and 3.2% among women 26 to 44 years of age (Substance Abuse and Mental Health Services Administration [SAMHSA], 2014).

Drugs that are commonly misused include tobacco, alcohol, cocaine, marijuana, amphetamines, barbiturates, hallucinogens, club drugs, prescription opioids, heroin, and other narcotics. Tobacco is discussed in detail in Chapter 13 as a teratogenic substance. For a discussion of the nonmedical abuse of pain relievers and tranquilizers, readers are referred to pharmacology textbooks.

Table 17–1 identifies common addictive drugs and their effects on the fetus and newborn.

Because women of childbearing age (15 to 44 years of age) make up a substantial proportion of the drug-using population, the problem has major significance for women and children. In testimony to these statistics is the increasing number of drug-exposed babies being born throughout the United States. The use of drugs during pregnancy, particularly in the first trimester, may adversely affect the health of the woman and the growth and development of her fetus. Women who abuse substances typically do not seek prenatal care until late in their pregnancies. They may be noncompliant or they may present in labor with no history of prenatal care. When they do seek care early, physicians and nurses typically use a screening tool to ask the women about drug and alcohol use. One such tool is entitled Screening, Brief Intervention, and Referral to Treatment (SBIRT) (Wright, Terplan, Ondersma, et al., 2016).

When asked, women may deny use of illegal substances out of fear, shame, or a reluctance to be confronted with the need to stop using the substance in question. Although some clinics perform routine or random drug screens, the patient should be informed that a drug screen is being performed and how the results will be provided to them.

Clinical Tip

Keep in mind that approximately 1 of 10 women in the United States, regardless of socioeconomic status or ethnic background, is currently abusing a substance. If you consider that possibility with every woman, you will ask the important questions about drug use and be alert for signs of substance abuse.

TABLE 17–1 Possible Effects of Selected Drugs of Abuse/Addiction on the Fetus and Newborn

MATERNAL DRUG	EFFECT ON FETUS/NEWBORN
Depressants	
Alcohol	Intellectual disability, microcephaly, midfacial hypoplasia, cardiac anomalies, intrauterine growth restriction, potential teratogenic effects, fetal alcohol syndrome, fetal alcohol effects
Narcotics	
Heroin	Withdrawal symptoms, known as neonatal abstinence syndrome (NAS), include tremors, irritability, sneezing, vomiting, fever, diarrhea, abnormal respiratory function, and potential seizure activity
Methadone	With abrupt maternal termination of the drug, severe withdrawal symptoms can include preterm labor, rapid labor, placental abruption, nonreassuring fetal status, and meconium aspiration. Neonates may present with NAS and be small for gestational age
Barbiturates	
Phenobarbital	Withdrawal symptoms Fetal growth restriction
Tranquilizers	
Diazepam (Valium)	Withdrawal symptoms
Antianxiety Drugs	
Lithium	Congenital anomalies
Stimulants	
Amphetamines (Benzedrine)	Low birth weight, withdrawal symptoms
Cocaine	Cerebral infarctions, microcephaly, learning disabilities, poor state organization, decreased interactive behavior, central nervous system anomalies, cardiac anomalies, genitourinary anomalies, sudden infant death syndrome (SIDS)
Nicotine (half to one pack cigarettes/day)	Increased rate of spontaneous abortion, increased incidence of placental abruption, small for gestational age, small head circumference, decreased length, SIDS, attention-deficit/hyperactivity disorder in school-age children
Psychotropics	
PCP ("angel dust")	Withdrawal symptoms Impaired neurologic development
Marijuana	Smoking cannabis during pregnancy is linked to lower birth weight in the offspring (Committee on the Health Effects of Marijuana, 2017)

Providing prenatal care to women with substance use disorders presents multiple dilemmas and challenges to clinicians. However, pregnancy represents a period in most women's lives when they recognize the need for and are receptive to caring and responsive interventions. By optimizing the prenatal experience for these women, maternal-fetal outcomes can be improved and the groundwork laid for the ongoing therapeutic services that are needed to maintain the health and well-being of the mother and child (Jones, Deppen, Hudak, et al., 2014).

A woman with a substance use disorder who seeks prenatal care may not voluntarily reveal her addiction, so caregivers should be alert for a history or physical signs that suggest substance abuse (Table 17–2).

Alcohol

Alcohol is a central nervous system depressant and a potent teratogen. Based on self-reports, 9.4% of pregnant women age 15 to 44 reported using alcohol in the past month and 2.3% among pregnant women meet the criteria for binge drinking (SAMSHA, 2014; Wisner, Sit, Bogan, et al., 2017).

Chronic abuse of alcohol can undermine maternal health by causing malnutrition (especially folic acid and thiamine deficiencies), bone marrow suppression, increased incidence of infections, and liver disease. As a result of alcohol dependence, the woman may have withdrawal seizures in the intrapartum period as early as 12 to 48 hours after she stops drinking. Delirium tremens may

TABLE 17–2 Possible Signs of Substance Abuse

History
- History of vague or unusual medical complaints
- Family history of alcoholism or other addiction
- History of childhood physical, sexual, or emotional abuse
- History of cirrhosis, pancreatitis, hepatitis, gastritis, sexually transmitted infections, or unusual infections such as cellulitis or endocarditis
- History of high-risk sexual behavior
- Psychiatric history of treatment and/or hospitalization

Physical Signs
- Dilated or constricted pupils
- Inflamed nasal mucosa
- Evidence of needle "track marks" or abscesses
- Poor nutritional status
- Slurred speech or staggering gait
- Odor of alcohol on breath

Behavioral Signs
- Memory lapses, mood swings, hallucinations
- Pattern of frequently missed appointments
- Frequent accidents, falls
- Signs of depression, agitation, euphoria
- Suicidal gestures

occur in the postpartum period, and the newborn may suffer withdrawal syndrome.

The effects of alcohol on the fetus may result in a group of signs referred to as fetal alcohol spectrum disorders (FASD). The syndrome has characteristic physical and mental abnormalities that vary in severity and combination. (See discussion in Chapter 30.) There is no final answer as to how much alcohol a woman can safely drink during pregnancy. Consequently, the expectant woman should avoid alcohol completely (U.S. Department of Health and Human Services [HHS], 2017). It is essential that nurses and other healthcare providers advise women about the dangers associated with drinking while pregnant.

Ethics in Action!

How do you respond to a woman who continues to drink alcohol during pregnancy despite the risk for her fetus?

The nursing staff in the maternal-newborn unit must be aware of the manifestations of alcohol abuse so that they can prepare for the patient's special needs. Care includes the use of sedative medications—oral benzodiazepines such as chlordiazepoxide (Librium), lorazepam (Ativan), or diazepam (Valium)—which are also available intravenously, to decrease neurologic irritability and tremors and assist with medical withdrawal (Wisner et al., 2017). Seizure precautions, intravenous fluid therapy for hydration, thiamine replacement, and preparation for an addicted newborn are also part of care. Although high doses of sedatives and analgesics may be necessary for the woman, caution is advised because these can cause fetal depression.

Breastfeeding is generally not contraindicated, although alcohol is excreted in breast milk. Excessive alcohol consumption may intoxicate the baby and inhibit the maternal letdown reflex. Discharge planning for the alcohol-addicted mother and newborn should be correlated with the social service department of the hospital.

Cocaine/Crack

Cocaine acts at the nerve terminals to prevent the reuptake of dopamine and norepinephrine, which in turn results in vasoconstriction, tachycardia, and hypertension. Placental vasoconstriction decreases blood flow to the fetus.

Cocaine is usually taken in three ways: Snorting, smoking, and intravenous (IV) injection. *Crack* is a form of freebase cocaine that is made up of baking soda, water, and cocaine mixed into a paste and microwaved to form a rock. The rock can then be smoked. Many women, especially those in low-income areas, favor this form of the drug over other forms because it is cheaper and readily available. In addition, smoking crack leads to a quicker, more intense high because the drug is absorbed through the large surface area of the lungs.

The onset of effects of cocaine occurs rapidly, but the euphoria lasts only about 30 minutes. Irritability, depression, pessimism, fatigue, and a strong desire for more cocaine usually follow this profound euphoria and excitement. This pattern often leads the user to take repeated doses to sustain the effect. Cocaine metabolites may be present in the urine of a pregnant woman for up to 4 to 7 days following use.

Because cocaine is an illegal substance, many women are reluctant to volunteer information about their drug use. The nurse who is familiar with the woman may recognize subtle signs of cocaine use, including mood swings and appetite changes, and withdrawal symptoms such as depression, irritability, nausea, lack of motivation, and psychomotor changes.

Major adverse maternal effects of cocaine use include seizures and hallucinations, pulmonary edema, respiratory failure, and cardiac problems. Women who use cocaine have an increased incidence of spontaneous first-trimester abortion, abruptio placentae, IUGR, preterm birth, and stillbirth (National Institute on Drug Abuse [NIDA], 2016).

Fetal exposure to cocaine increases the risk of IUGR, microcephaly, altered brain development, shorter body length, congenital anomalies, and neurobehavioral abnormalities (Forray & Foster, 2015). Newborns exposed to cocaine in utero may have neurobehavioral disturbances, marked irritability, an exaggerated startle reflex, labile emotions, and an increased risk of sudden infant death syndrome. (See Chapter 30 for further discussion.)

Exposed babies are found to have more feeding difficulties than those who are not exposed. These difficulties may be related to some extent to the babies' behaviors but have also been found to be related to maternal behaviors. Cocaine-using mothers were found to be less flexible, less engaged, and less responsive to their babies' feeding cues. Nursing interventions that help mothers interpret newborn/infant feeding cues and optimize the mother–child relationship should be emphasized. Hyperactivity and short attention span have been noted in toddlers prenatally exposed to opiates, and older exposed children have demonstrated memory and perceptual problems (Behnke & Smith, 2013). Cocaine does cross into the breast milk and may cause such symptoms in the breastfeeding newborn/infant as extreme irritability, vomiting, diarrhea, dilated pupils, and apnea. Thus, women who continue to use cocaine following childbirth should avoid breastfeeding.

Marijuana

Marijuana is used widely among women, and although it remains illegal in the majority of states, its use is expected to increase as more states legalize it. A 2017 review of the state of the evidence concluded that smoking marijuana during pregnancy is linked to lower birth weight in the offspring, but that the relationship between smoking marijuana during pregnancy and other childhood outcomes is unclear (Committee on the Health Effects of Marijuana, 2017). The impact of heavy marijuana use on pregnancy is difficult to evaluate because of the variety of social factors that may influence the impact of marijuana itself. Nevertheless, smoking of any type—be it tobacco or marijuana—poses a risk during pregnancy and is best avoided (World Health Organization [WHO], 2014).

MDMA (Ecstasy)

MDMA (methylenedioxymethamphetamine), a derivative of amphetamine better known as Ecstasy or Molly, is the most commonly used of a group of drugs referred to as *club drugs*, so called because they have become popular among adolescents and young adults who frequent dance clubs and "raves." Other club drugs include flunitrazepam (Rohypnol), gamma hydroxybutyrate (GHB), and ketamine hydrochloride. Phencyclidine (PCP) and lysergic acid diethylamide (LSD) are sometimes classified as club drugs as well.

Ecstasy has been widely perceived as "safe" because of a relatively low incidence of adverse reactions. However, adverse responses are very unpredictable. MDMA is taken by mouth usually in tablet form. Its effects last for about 3 to 6 hours. MDMA use is appealing because it produces euphoria and feelings of empathy for others (hence its other name, "hug drug"). Short-term adverse effects include clouded thinking, agitation, disturbed behavior, sweating, dry mouth, increased heart rate, muscle spasms including jaw clenching, and hyperthermia (elevated temperature). The most common significant adverse effects occur when people take multiple doses in one night (called "stacking"). These effects include hyperthermia, hyponatremia (low blood sodium), hypertension, cardiac arrhythmias, and kidney failure (NIDA, 2017). Deaths have occurred among users. Repeated use of Ecstasy is associated with mood, sleep, and anxiety disorders; memory deficits; increased impulsiveness; and attention problems, which may last for up to 2 years following cessation of use.

Data about the fetal and neonatal effects are sparse. The DAISY Study (Drugs and Infancy Study, 2003–2008) followed a group of women who reported MDMA use during pregnancy and evaluated their infants through 2 years of age. They found that infants whose mothers reported heavier MDMA use during pregnancy had motor delays from 4 months to 2 years of age that were not attributable to other drug or lifestyle factors (Singer, Moore, Min, et al., 2016).

Prescription Opioids and Heroin

Prescription use of opioids such as oxycodone and hydrocodone (opioid use disorder [OUD]) has increased dramatically in recent years. Data indicate that 0.9% of pregnant women between the ages of 15 and 44 misused opioids in the past month. While this is lower than among non-pregnant women in the same age group (2.6%), it resulted in an annual average of about 21,000 women per month (Smith & Lipari, 2017). The incidence of OUD during pregnancy is estimated to be four per 1000 births (SAMHSA, 2018).

Opioid misuse, whether of prescribed medications or illicit substances such as heroin, can disrupt fetal development at any stage of pregnancy. Concurrently as the incidence of OUD has increased, so, too, has the incidence of neonatal abstinence syndrome (NAS), which has more than doubled, increasing from 1.2 cases per 1000 hospital births to 3.4 (Wisner et al., 2017).

Women who misuse opioids during pregnancy have an increased rate of abnormal placental implantation, abruptio placentae, preterm labor, premature rupture of the membranes (PROM), meconium staining, and maternal obstetric complications (Smith & Lipari, 2017; Wisner et al., 2017). The fetus is at risk for IUGR, preterm birth, low birth weight, meconium aspiration, and fetal distress (Wisner et al., 2017).

Heroin is an illicit opioid. It is a central nervous system (CNS) depressant narcotic that alters perception and produces euphoria. Heroin is an addictive drug that is generally administered intravenously, although it may also be sniffed/snorted or smoked. Pregnancy in women who use heroin is considered high risk because of the associated increased incidence of poor nutrition, iron deficiency anemia, and preeclampsia-eclampsia (see Chapter 18). Heroin users also have a higher incidence of sexually transmitted infection because many must rely on prostitution to support their drug habits. They are also at increased risk of HIV infection because they may use nonsterile needles or share needles when administering the drug (Figure 17–4).

The fetus of a woman who is addicted to heroin is at increased risk for preterm birth, IUGR, and withdrawal symptoms (NAS) after birth, such as restlessness; lack of habituation; shrill, high-pitched cry; irritability; fist sucking; vomiting; and seizures. Signs of withdrawal usually appear within 72 hours and may last for several days (Wang, 2014). These behaviors may interfere with successful maternal–newborn attachment and increase the potential for parenting problems or abuse in an already high-risk mother (Behnke & Smith, 2013).

Methadone is the most commonly used drug in the treatment of women who are dependent on prescription opioids and heroin.

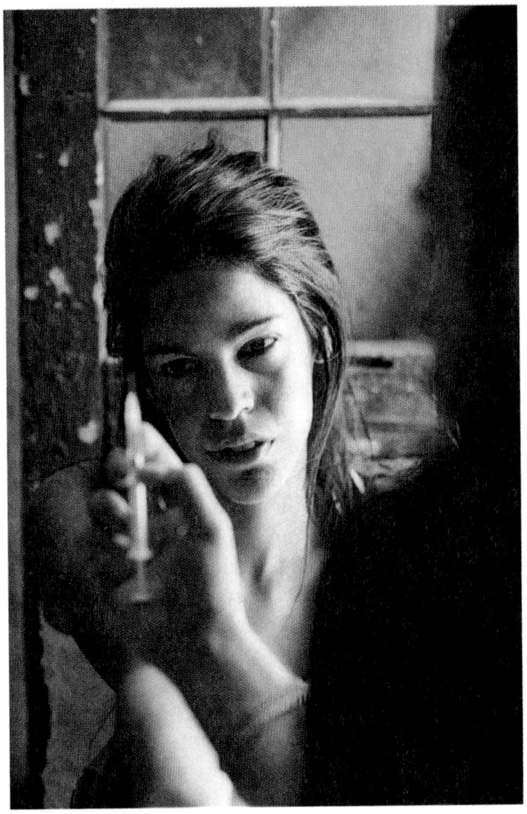

Figure 17–4 The use of illicit drugs puts the pregnant woman and her unborn child at increased risk for a variety of complications.

SOURCE: Diego Cerva/Fotolia.

Methadone blocks withdrawal symptoms and the craving for street drugs. Dosage should be individualized to achieve the most therapeutic level for the mother during pregnancy. Methadone does cross the placenta, and fetal exposure in utero may result in NAS in the newborn. Buprenorphine (Subutex), a partial opioid agonist, is a safe and acceptable alternative to methadone in treating opioid-dependent mothers. In fact, research suggests that neonates born following buprenorphine therapy require less morphine and have a shorter hospital stay than babies born to mothers on methadone therapy (NIDA, 2018).

Clinical Therapy

Antepartum care of the substance-abusing woman involves medical, socioeconomic, and legal considerations. The use of a team approach allows for the comprehensive management necessary to provide safe labor and childbirth for the woman and her fetus.

The management of drug addiction may include hospitalization as necessary to initiate detoxification. "Cold turkey" withdrawal is not advisable during pregnancy because of potential risk to the fetus. Maintenance and support therapy are best individualized to the woman's history and condition.

Urine screening may also be done regularly throughout pregnancy if the woman is known or suspected to be abusing drugs. This testing is helpful in identifying the type and amount of drug being abused and in providing objective feedback to the woman. Screening strategies should include maternal informed consent before screening. Healthcare providers need to stay abreast of their state laws requiring consent for screening in pregnancy to ensure they are in compliance.

●○● NURSING MANAGEMENT

For the Pregnant Woman with Substance Use Disorders

Nursing Assessment and Diagnosis

Nurses and other healthcare providers should make it a practice to screen all pregnant women for substance use disorders. Several simple screening tools are available. In addition to screening, be alert for clues in the history or appearance of the woman that suggest substance abuse (refer to Table 17–2). If abuse is suspected, ask direct questions, beginning with less threatening questions about the use of tobacco, caffeine, and over-the-counter medications. Then progress to questions about alcohol consumption and finally to questions focusing on past and current use of illicit drugs. Being matter-of-fact and nonjudgmental in approach is more likely to elicit honest responses.

Nursing assessment of the woman who is known to abuse substances focuses on her general health status, with specific attention to nutritional status, susceptibility to infections, and evaluation of all body systems. Also assess the woman's understanding of the impact of substance abuse on herself and her pregnancy. Some women are reluctant to discuss their substance abuse; others are quite open about it. Once a relationship of trust is established, it will be easier to gain information to use in planning the woman's ongoing care.

Nursing diagnoses that may apply to the woman practicing substance abuse include:

- *Nutrition, Imbalanced: Less Than Body Requirements*, related to inadequate food intake secondary to substance abuse
- *Infection, Risk for*, related to use of inadequately cleaned syringes and needles secondary to IV drug use
- *Health Maintenance, Ineffective*, related to a lack of information about the impact of substance abuse on the fetus.

(NANDA-I © 2017)

Nursing Plan and Implementation

Preventing substance abuse during pregnancy is the ideal nursing goal and is best accomplished through education. Unfortunately, many women who abuse substances do not receive regular health care and may not seek care until far along in their pregnancies or at the onset of labor.

Your role in providing prenatal care for the woman who has a substance use disorder focuses on ongoing assessment and patient teaching. To provide care that is truly effective, maintain a nonjudgmental, nonpunitive, positive attitude when caring for these women. It is also useful to be aware of substances that are commonly abused in their communities and the signs and symptoms that characterize abuse of these substances.

Provide information about the relationship between substance abuse and existing health problems and the implications for the woman's unborn child. If possible, discuss strategies to help the woman quit (addiction treatment programs, 12-step programs, individual counseling) and suggest a referral for more in-depth assessment by a specialist. If feasible, make an appointment while the woman is in the office or clinic. Also be aware of treatment options available for women who lack financial resources. Finally, make a follow-up appointment to see the woman again after her drug or alcohol assessment. By establishing a relationship of trust and support, the woman's cooperation may be gained.

Preparation for labor and birth should be part of the prenatal planning. Fear, tension, or discomfort may be relieved through psychologic support and careful explanation of the labor process. If pain medication is necessary, it should not be withheld, however, because the notion that it will contribute to further addiction is not correct. Preferred methods of pain relief include the use of psychoprophylaxis and regional or local anesthetics, such as pudendal block and local infiltration. These techniques decrease the risk of additional fetal respiratory depression. Immediate intensive care should be available for the newborn who may have respiratory depression, be small for gestational age (SGA), and be premature. For care of the addicted newborn, see Chapter 30.

Postpartum follow-up and referral are essential and may include home visits. Follow-up requires careful coordination with community agencies and may involve public health nurses and social workers.

Evaluation

Expected outcomes of nursing care include:

- The woman is able to describe the impact of her substance use on herself and her unborn child.
- The woman successfully gives birth to a healthy baby.
- The woman agrees to cooperate with referral to social services (or other appropriate community agency) for follow-up care after discharge.

Care of the Woman with a Psychologic Disorder

An estimated 17.9% of adults age 18 or older reported mental illness in 2015 (Center for Behavioral Health Statistics and Quality, 2016). **Psychologic disorders** are characterized by alterations in thinking, mood, or behavior. Although many such disorders can affect labor and birth, only the most common are discussed here. Because an in-depth discussion of psychologic disorders is beyond the scope of this text, students are encouraged to consult a mental health nursing textbook for further reference. Postpartum psychologic disorders are discussed in Chapter 35. See Table 17–3 for a summary of the maternal implications of psychologic disorders.

Maternal Implications

Depression, a common disorder that affects many pregnant women, often goes undiagnosed or untreated. Estimates suggest that one in seven women will have a perinatal depressive episode during pregnancy or 12 months postpartum. Research findings are mixed, but women with depression may be more likely to have a preterm birth, a small-for-gestational-age newborn, or a low-birth-weight newborn (ACOG, 2016).

Depression can reduce the woman's ability to concentrate or process information being provided by healthcare team members (Figure 17–5). Untreated depression can lead to poor self-care, inadequate nutrition, self-medication, poor maternal–infant bonding, and maternal suicide (ACOG, 2016). The labor process may feel overwhelming to a woman with depression, and she may feel hopelessness about the outcome of her labor. However, she may not be able to articulate these feelings and may appear irritable or withdrawn.

Women with *bipolar disorder* experience the symptoms of depression during the depressive phase. A pregnant woman

TABLE 17–3 Maternal Implications of Psychologic Disorders

PSYCHOLOGIC DISORDER	MATERNAL IMPLICATION
Generalized anxiety disorder	Anxiety related to the birth process or medical interventions
Bipolar disorder	Depressive or manic symptoms during labor
Depression	Withdrawn behavior, physical fatigue due to insomnia, crying spells, sadness, hopelessness, feelings of guilt, lack of interest in baby, thoughts of suicide, headaches during pregnancy
Obsessive–compulsive disorder	Ritualistic behaviors or thoughts, difficulty focusing on directions
Panic disorder	Intense fear or sense of panic related to birth process
Phobias	May have specific fear related to an individual(s) or a procedure or place
Posttraumatic stress disorder	Repressed memories may be triggered during labor, causing intense anxiety, fear, and emotional distress
Schizophrenia	Typically starts in the late 20s and early 30s. May have hallucinations or delusions, lack of sense of present events, high risk for suicide

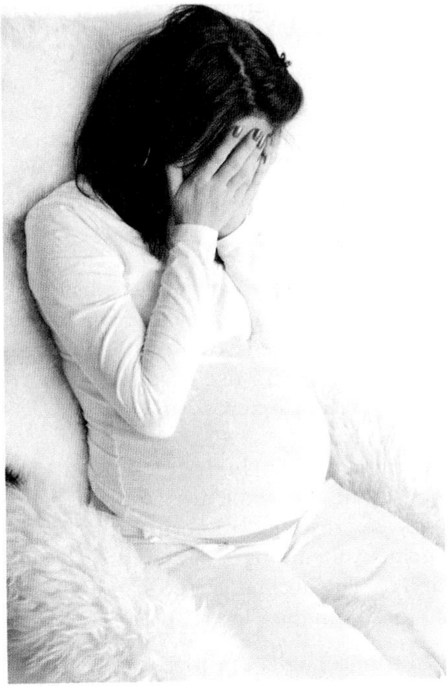

Figure 17–5 A depressed pregnant woman may be inarticulate and appear withdrawn.

SOURCE: Gladskikh Tatiana/Shutterstock.

experiencing a manic episode may engage in behaviors that are dangerous to herself or her fetus, including alcohol or drug use, reckless driving, driving without a seat belt, and unprotected sexual intercourse. If labor occurs during a manic phase, the woman may be hyperexcitable and exhibit poor judgment.

"As a nurse-midwife, all of the women I care for are special, but Karen was one person I will never forget. Karen was diagnosed with bipolar disorder with psychotic episodes that became uncontrolled in pregnancy as a result of discontinuing her medication. In labor, she arrived in a manic state. Her speech was excessively fast-paced, and she rocked in her bed violently throughout the labor. We ensured her physical safety throughout the labor, monitored her contractions and the baby as infrequently as possible, and provided continuous encouragement. At one point, Karen was adamant everyone must "get low" and sit on the floor to facilitate fetal descent. Although it did not seem rational to us, we did sit on the floor. Remarkably, her anxiety dramatically decreased and the sense of control she felt enabled her to focus and 15 minutes later, she pushed her baby out. At her 6-week postpartum visit, Karen was back on medication and enjoying her new role as a mother."

Anxiety disorders include a cluster of diagnoses such as panic disorder, obsessive–compulsive disorder (OCD), posttraumatic stress disorder (PTSD), general anxiety disorder (GAD), and other specific phobias. These disorders can cause a wide range of symptoms in both pregnant and laboring women. For example, women with OCD may need to repeat specific rituals as a means of coping, while women with PTSD may experience flashbacks and avoidance behaviors. Anxiety may cause the laboring woman to experience physical symptoms such as chest pain, shortness of breath, faintness, fear, or even terror. In general, laboring women with psychologic disorders tend to exhibit the behaviors characteristic of their disorders, but these behaviors may be somewhat exaggerated because of the intense emotions that are evoked in the women's memories. Women with a past history of abuse, including physical and sexual abuse, are often fearful of losing control.

Schizophrenia is the most disabling of the psychologic disorders. It is often difficult to treat schizophrenia in pregnant women because many of the medications are teratogenic and, therefore, contraindicated. Women with uncontrolled schizophrenia may have difficulty managing emotions, interacting with the healthcare team, or thinking clearly. The woman's behavior may be dramatically inappropriate, or she may simply be withdrawn. Women with schizophrenia are at risk for medication-related congenital malformations. Specifically, antipsychotics can cause cardiovascular defects. These women have an increased incidence of preterm birth, low birth weight, small for gestational age, placental abnormalities, and antenatal hemorrhage.

Clinical Therapy

The goal of clinical therapy is to provide strategies that will help decrease the woman's anxiety (as well as that of her partner), keep her oriented to reality, and promote optimal functioning during pregnancy and while in labor. Pharmacologic measures such as sedatives, analgesics, or antianxiety medications are determined on an individual basis following careful assessment.

●○● NURSING MANAGEMENT

For the Pregnant Woman with a Psychologic Disorder

Use therapeutic communication and sharing of information to allay anxiety for both the woman and her support person during each prenatal visit and during labor and childbirth. Consistency in her care enables the woman to adjust to new experiences and begin to establish a relationship with her caregivers.

Nursing Assessment and Diagnosis

Research suggests that perinatal mood and anxiety disorders are often underdetected in clinical practice unless a formal screening program is in place (Brockington, Butterworth, & Glangeaud-Freudenthal, 2017). At the first prenatal visit, begin the assessment by reviewing the woman's background. Factors such as age, marital and socioeconomic status, culture, methods of coping, support system, and understanding of the labor process contribute to the woman's psychologic response to pregnancy and birth. It is important to ask all women if they have ever been diagnosed with a psychologic disorder. If the woman has, ask her if she is currently receiving any treatment, including medications or psychotherapy. Also ask if she has ever had a psychiatric hospitalization or if she has ever had thoughts of hurting herself or others.

This same attention to detail is important when the woman goes into labor. The prenatal record should be reviewed for additional information regarding any psychiatric illnesses. During labor, assess the woman for objective cues indicating a psychologic disorder. Monotone replies and/or a flat affect may indicate depression. Women with schizophrenia may lack orientation to person, time, and place. Objective cues indicating acute anxiety or signs of a panic attack include tachycardia and hyperventilation.

As labor progresses, remain alert to the woman's verbal and nonverbal behavioral responses to the pain and anxiety. The woman who is too quiet and compliant, is disoriented, is agitated and seems uncooperative, or is experiencing acute anxiety symptoms may require further appraisal for psychologic disorders. Also observe for nonverbal cues, including tense posture, clenched hands, or pain out of context to the stage of labor. Recognizing the impact of fatigue on pain and anxiety is another important nursing responsibility. Assess which coping mechanisms have been effective for the woman in the past.

Nursing diagnoses that may apply to the woman with a psychologic disorder include:

- ***Anxiety*** related to stress of the labor process, unfamiliar environment, and unknown caregivers
- ***Fear*** related to unknown outcome of labor and invasive medical procedures
- ***Coping, Ineffective***, related to increased anxiety and stress.

(NANDA-I © 2017)

Planning and Implementation

The primary nursing interventions center on providing support to the pregnant woman and her partner or family. During labor, families that have had the opportunity to attend prenatal classes may benefit from encouragement as they employ some of the coping techniques they have learned. If the woman begins to lose her ability to cope or her orientation to reality, she can be helped to regain control and orientation by the following measures:

- Ensure that the woman's external environment is free from excessive stimuli.
- Maintain consistency in care providers to the extent possible.
- Encourage her to identify and to use coping mechanisms that work well for her.
- Identify and reduce the source of distress, if possible.
- Acknowledge the woman's fears, pain, and other symptoms.
- Orient the woman to person, place, and time (repeatedly, if necessary) by statements such as "Janine, I am Tony Martinez and I am your nurse. It is Tuesday and you are in the birthing center because you are in labor now."
- Offer methods to promote relaxation and comfort.
- Provide clear but succinct information about the labor process, medical procedures, the environment, simple breathing exercises, and relaxation techniques.
- Employ a calm, caring, confident, and nonjudgmental approach.
- Provide frequent attention and therapeutic interaction.

Your ability to help the woman and her partner cope with the stress of labor is directly related to the rapport already established with them. Some women with severe psychologic disorders may have excessive symptoms during their labor and birth. Although providing emotional support is imperative, care of these women should focus on maintaining a safe environment and ensuring maternal and fetal well-being. Pharmacologic interventions may be necessary for excessive symptoms.

Evaluation

Anticipated outcomes of nursing care include:

- The woman experiences a decrease in physiologic and psychologic stress and an increase in physical and psychologic comfort.
- The woman remains oriented to person, time, and place.
- The woman uses effective coping mechanisms to manage her stress and anxiety in labor.
- The woman is able to verbalize feelings about her labor.
- The woman's and her family's fear is decreased.

Care of the Woman with HIV

AIDS (*acquired immune deficiency syndrome*), caused by the virus known as **HIV** (*human immunodeficiency virus*), is one of today's major health concerns. By 2016, an estimated 973,846 adults and adolescents in the United States were living with HIV infection (Centers for Disease Control and Prevention [CDC], 2017b). Male adults and adolescents are still the largest group of infected individuals (81%). The rate of infection in 2016 for adult and adolescent males was 24.3 per 100,000 population; the rate for females was 5.4 per 100,000. Infection attributed to male-to-male sexual contact and male-to-male sexual contact *and* IV drug use accounted for 70% of diagnosed infections, while heterosexual contact accounted for 24% (CDC, 2017b).

Of the estimated 2322 children less than 13 years of age living with HIV/AIDS in the United States, the vast majority of infections were attributed to perinatal transmission (CDC, 2017a). Fortunately, the number of new pediatric AIDS cases is declining rapidly. The decline is associated with the following recommendations from the CDC (2017a):

1. Universal counseling about the risks of HIV transmission from mother to fetus for all women who are pregnant or planning to get pregnant
2. Recommended opt-out HIV screening of all pregnant women during each pregnancy (*opt-out* means that the woman is told that HIV testing is part of routine prenatal screening unless she chooses not to have the test)
3. Repeat HIV testing in the third trimester in areas with high HIV prevalence rates, for HIV-negative individuals with high-risk behaviors, and for individuals with unknown HIV status at the time of labor
4. Immediate antiretroviral therapy (ART) as soon as HIV is diagnosed because the earlier HIV is diagnosed and treated,

the more effective ART will be at preventing transmission and improving health outcomes for both the woman and her baby

5. Immediate antiretroviral prophylaxis for HIV-positive pregnant women in labor and their babies following birth.

Pathophysiology of HIV/AIDS

HIV found in blood, semen, vaginal fluid, and breast milk has been implicated in disease transmission, although the virus has been isolated in urine, tears, cerebrospinal fluid, lymph nodes, brain tissue, and bone marrow. HIV affects specific T cells, thereby decreasing the body's immune responses. This makes the affected person susceptible to opportunistic infections such as *Pneumocystis jirovecii*, which causes severe pneumonia, candidiasis, cytomegalovirus, tuberculosis, and toxoplasmosis.

Once infected with the virus, the individual develops antibodies that can be detected with an antigen/antibody assay that can potentially identify HIV infection as early as 14 to 28 days after exposure and differentiates between HIV-1 and HIV-2 antibodies. If the antigen/antibody assay is nonreactive, this is a negative HIV test and no further testing is needed. If the antigen/antibody assay is reactive, then a second assay is used to differentiate HIV-1 from HIV-2 antibodies. If antibodies are reactive for either type, then this is a positive HIV test result. If the antigen/antibody is reactive and the antibody differentiation assay is negative or indeterminant, then further testing is warranted to rule out acute infection. Acute HIV infection can be ruled out with an HIV nucleic acid test (NAT) such as an HIV RNA PCR (HIV viral load) (CDC, 2014). See *Developing Cultural Competence: Variations in the Prevalence Rates of HIV Infections.*

Maternal Risks

Recent advances and availability of antiretroviral therapy (ART) have led HIV-positive women who adhere to their ART to consider pregnancy because of their increased life expectancy. If pregnancy is considered, priorities should focus on maintaining the health of the mother before, during, and after the pregnancy, preventing transmission to a potentially seronegative father, and preventing mother-to-child transmission. Reproductive-assisted technology is one possibility along with further interventions, including cesarean birth, to reduce the risk of transmission to the fetus. Perinatal medical case management during pregnancy can help the woman to achieve HIV suppression during pregnancy and she should continue in HIV care for 1 year postpartum (Anderson, Momplaisir, Corson, et al., 2017).

Developing Cultural Competence Variations in the Prevalence Rates of HIV Infections

The prevalence rates per 100,000 of individuals living with HIV/AIDS infection vary significantly among races and ethnic groups in the United States. At the end of 2016, the rates were 43.6 for Blacks/African Americans, 17.0 for Hispanics/Latinos, 12.9 for persons of multiple races, 10.2 for American Indians/Alaska Natives, 8.5 for Native Hawaiians/other Pacific Islanders, 5.5 for Asian Americans, and 5.2 for Whites/Caucasian Americans (CDC, 2017b).

NOTE: *It is unwise to attribute specific attitudes or beliefs to all members of a cultural group. The information in the Developing Cultural Competence boxes offers possible insights into caring for women from different cultural groups.*

For women who have not had access to ART or who have not followed their plan of care, AIDS-defining symptoms that are more common in women than men include wasting syndrome, esophageal candidiasis, and herpes simplex virus disease. Kaposi sarcoma is rare in women. Non-AIDS-defining gynecologic conditions, such as vaginal *Candida* infections and cervical pathology, are prevalent among women at all stages of HIV infection.

Fetal-Neonatal Risks

HIV transmission can occur during pregnancy and through breast milk; however, it is believed that the majority of all infections occur during labor and birth. For HIV-infected pregnant women who receive no prophylactic medication, the rate of transmission to the newborn is about 25%. However, if an HIV-infected pregnant woman receives prophylactic antiretroviral therapy throughout pregnancy, labor, and birth and provides ART medications to her baby for 4 to 6 weeks, the risk of mother-to-child transmission of HIV can be 1% or less (CDC, 2017a). In some cases, cesarean birth at 38 weeks' gestation before rupture of membranes may be indicated to prevent transmission. After childbirth the HIV-positive woman can prevent HIV transmission to her baby by not breastfeeding and by not prechewing her baby's food (CDC, 2017a). Treatment of newborns of mothers who are HIV-infected is discussed in Chapter 30.

Clinical Therapy

Early knowledge of a woman's HIV status is important for her well-being and that of her child. Thus, the CDC screening guidelines for pregnant women state that HIV screening should be emphasized as a routine part of all prenatal care. To this end, the recommendation that all pregnant women should be tested for HIV has been strengthened while continuing to ensure that testing of pregnant women and their babies is voluntary and informed (Panel on Treatment of Pregnant Women with HIV Infection and Prevention of Perinatal Transmission [hereafter Panel], 2017). Initial testing is done using an enzyme-linked immunosorbent assay (ELISA) and confirmed with the Western blot test or immunofluorescence assay (IFA). A woman who tests positive should be counseled about the implications of the diagnosis for herself and her fetus to ensure an informed reproductive choice. See *Evidence-Based Practice: Antenatal Exposure to HIV Risk Factors.*

Combination antiretroviral therapy (cART) is the treatment of choice for all HIV-infected pregnant women to reduce the rate of perinatal transmission and optimize the health of the mother. The combination antiretroviral therapy contains at least three drugs, consistent with the principles of treatment for nonpregnant adults. To provide infant pre-exposure prophylaxis, at least one of the ARV drugs should provide high transplacental transmission to the fetus (Panel, 2017). It is essential that the pregnant woman understand the importance of adhering to the drug regimen throughout her pregnancy. (*Note:* The discussion of specific ART and cART medications is beyond the scope of this text.)

Women with HIV should be evaluated and treated for other sexually transmitted infections and for conditions occurring more commonly in women with HIV, such as tuberculosis, cytomegalovirus, toxoplasmosis, and cervical dysplasia. Women with HIV infection with no history of hepatitis B should receive the hepatitis vaccine, which is not contraindicated prenatally, as well as the pneumococcal vaccine and an annual flu shot. In addition to routine prenatal laboratory tests, a platelet count and a complete blood count with differential should be obtained at the first prenatal visit and repeated each trimester to identify anemia, thrombocytopenia, and leukopenia, which are associated both with HIV infection and with antiretroviral therapy. Screening for diabetes is also important in this population.

EVIDENCE-BASED PRACTICE | Antenatal Exposure to HIV Risk Factors

Clinical Question

How many pregnant women acquire risk factors for HIV exposure during the antenatal period? Could these women benefit from pre-exposure prophylaxis?

The Evidence

Incidental perinatal transmission of HIV occurs most often during birth and breastfeeding. Although the standard of care is to test for HIV during initial antenatal assessment, infection can occur later in pregnancy. Repeat HIV testing prior to birth is recommended for at-risk women, but this is inconsistently achieved. As a result, babies are exposed to the virus by a mother unaware she has acquired the disease. This study undertook an estimation of the proportion of women who are at increased risk of HIV acquisition during pregnancy and who could benefit from pre-exposure prophylaxis. The authors conducted a retrospective cohort study with more than 1600 subjects in a large, urban medical center (Fruhauf & Coleman, 2017). This type of population study forms a strong level of evidence for public health application.

Based on standards set by the Centers for Disease Control and Prevention, 10% of the women were at increased risk of HIV acquisition during pregnancy. These women would have been eligible for pre-exposure prophylaxis. Of these, 7% were discovered to be at risk in the early stages of pregnancy, but 3% acquired risk after the second trimester. The risk factor that increased most frequently was the acquisition of a sexually transmitted disease (Fruhauf & Coleman, 2017). Pharmacologic prophylaxis is available for these women and has been shown to be safe during pregnancy.

Best Practice

This study underscores the need for repeated risk assessment and physiologic testing during pregnancy. Women may acquire HIV at any time, and so risk factors should be assessed continuously and prophylaxis offered when risk increases. The consequences of late-trimester HIV acquisition are serious for mother and baby alike. Mothers at risk should be encouraged to use prophylaxis as directed and can be reassured that the medication will not affect their baby's health.

Clinical Reasoning

How often should risk factors for diseases be assessed during pregnancy? How might candidates for preventive measures be identified?

The woman with HIV should also be assessed regularly for serologic changes that indicate the disease is progressing. This is determined by plasma HIV RNA levels and the $CD4^+$ T lymphocyte cell count, which provides the number of helper T4 cells. When $CD4^+$ counts fall to $200/mm^3$ or lower, opportunistic infections such as *P. jirovecii* pneumonia are more likely to develop, and prophylaxis may need to be instituted (Panel, 2017).

Prenatal care focuses on monitoring for early signs of complications, such as weight loss or fever. The woman is asked about signs of vaginal infection; her lungs are auscultated for signs of pneumonia; and her lymph nodes, liver, and spleen are palpated for signs of enlargement.

A woman with HIV who is on ART/cART is at increased risk for preterm birth. However, the clear benefits of ART/cART far outweigh the risk (Panel, 2017). The fetus is monitored closely and may require weekly nonstress tests, serial ultrasounds to detect IUGR, and biophysical profiles to determine fetal well-being (see Chapter 16). Invasive procedures such as amniocentesis are avoided when possible to prevent the contamination of a noninfected fetus.

In addition to the medical priorities of care, understanding the woman's emotional and social situation is important. Utilizing tools to screen for depression and intimate partner violence (IPV) will help the multidisciplinary team identify other needed supports to ensure that comprehensive care is provided. Postpartum contraception should be discussed prenatally so that the woman is able to have a plan in place when she gives birth and to reduce the likelihood of a future unintended pregnancy.

Intrapartum care is similar to that for all pregnant women, although strict adherence to standard precautions is crucial to avoid nosocomial infection. To prevent exposure of an uninfected fetus to HIV during labor and birth, invasive procedures such as vaginal examinations following rupture of the membranes, fetal scalp electrode monitoring, fetal scalp sampling, and vacuum extraction should be done only after carefully evaluating the risks and benefits.

Scheduled cesarean birth is indicated for women with HIV RNA levels greater than 1000 copies/mL and for women with unknown HIV RNA levels near the time of birth whether they are on antiretroviral therapy or not. Intravenous (IV) zidovudine is also indicated at this time and is initiated 3 hours before the scheduled operative birth. IV zidovudine is not necessary intrapartally for women on an ART regimen whose HIV RNA is less than or equal to 50 copies/mL. Scheduled cesarean birth performed solely to prevent perinatal transmission is *not* routinely recommended in women receiving ART with HIV RNA levels less than or equal to 1000 copies/mL (Panel, 2017). Women should be informed of the risks associated with cesarean birth. If cesarean birth is indicated for prevention of perinatal transmission of HIV, the risks to a woman should be balanced with potential benefits expected for the neonate.

Women who are HIV positive are at increased risk for complications such as postpartum infection, poor wound healing, and infections of the genitourinary tract. They need careful monitoring and appropriate therapy by physicians knowledgeable about treating individuals with HIV.

●○● NURSING MANAGEMENT

For the Pregnant Woman Who Is HIV Positive

Nursing Assessment and Diagnosis

A woman who tests positive for HIV may be asymptomatic or may present with any of the following signs or symptoms: Fatigue, anemia, malaise, progressive weight loss, lymphadenopathy, night sweats, diarrhea, fever, neurologic dysfunction, cell-mediated immunodeficiency, and evidence of Kaposi sarcoma (purplish, reddish-brown lesions, either externally or internally).

If a woman tests HIV positive or is involved in a relationship or an activity that places her at high risk, assess the woman's knowledge level about the disease, its implications for her and her fetus, and self-care measures the woman can take.

Examples of nursing diagnoses that might apply to an HIV-positive pregnant woman include:

- ***Knowledge, Readiness for Enhanced***, regarding information about HIV/AIDS related to its long-term implications for the woman and her unborn child
- ***Infection, Risk for***, related to altered immunity secondary to HIV/AIDS
- ***Family Processes, Interrupted***, related to the implications of a positive HIV test in one of the family members.

(NANDA-I © 2017)

> "I've been a nurse for 40 years now, and I've never seen anything change nursing practice more than HIV/AIDS has. Nursing students today will take standard precautions for granted because they won't know any other way, but I can remember when we could touch more freely. I remember drying a newborn and stroking him—my hands warm against his skin. I remember a time when people didn't think twice before trying to stop bleeding or give other first aid at an accident scene. I know this way is safer, but a part of me mourns what we have lost."

Nursing Plan and Implementation

Community-Based Nursing Care

Nurses need to help women understand that HIV/AIDS can be a treatable disease. HIV infection can be avoided if women avoid sharing IV drug needles and practice safe sex, including insisting that their sex partners wear a latex condom for each act of intercourse.

A detailed drug and sexual history of each prenatal patient is the first step in perinatal HIV/AIDS prevention. All women should be offered HIV counseling. The following are counseling guidelines for HIV testing:

- Discuss HIV testing during the normal prenatal assessment, explaining that HIV testing is recommended for all pregnant women and that they will receive an HIV test as part of the routine panel unless the woman declines (opt-out testing). No woman should be tested without her knowledge, but no written consent is required.
- Assure the woman of confidentiality, explaining the difference between anonymity and confidentiality.
- Provide an environment that is private, comfortable, and nonjudgmental.
- Provide the woman with information about HIV/AIDS, including pathophysiology, mode of transmission of HIV, high-risk behaviors, and methods of decreasing transmission, such as practicing safe sex and not sharing needles.
- Provide posttest counseling, if possible. A negative test means that no HIV antibodies were found; it does not ensure that the woman has not been infected with the virus because antibodies may not be detected for 6 weeks to 6 months after exposure.
- Offer supportive follow-up if test results are positive. This includes an explanation of the implications for the woman and her unborn child as well as the value of antiretroviral therapy, recommended medical therapy, follow-up of sex partners, transmission prevention, discussion of immediate posttest plans, and referral to appropriate psychologic and educational services.
- Tell the woman not to donate blood or blood products and not to share toothbrushes, razors, and other implements that could be contaminated with blood.

This information can be overwhelming to the woman who is HIV positive and should be provided orally and in writing. She will need more than one counseling session to absorb the information. The initial reaction may be one of shock or denial, so it is important to allow her a little time to think and to give her empathy and support. Stress that being HIV positive does not mean that the woman has AIDS but that she can transmit the virus to others (by sexual contact, sharing IV drug needles, and donating blood) and to her fetus during pregnancy or childbirth or by breastfeeding. Antiretroviral therapy is now able to prolong life expectancy for HIV-positive individuals who adhere to their treatment plans and maintain as healthy a lifestyle as possible (Panel, 2017).

In monitoring the asymptomatic HIV-positive pregnant woman, be alert for nonspecific symptoms such as fever, weight loss, fatigue, persistent candidiasis, diarrhea, cough, skin lesions, and behavior changes. Laboratory findings—such as decreased hemoglobin, hematocrit, and T4 lymphocytes; elevated erythrocyte sedimentation rate (ESR); and abnormal complete blood count, differential, and platelets—may indicate complications or progression of the disease.

Education about optimal nutrition and maintenance of wellness are important and should be reviewed frequently with the woman.

Hospital-Based Nursing Care

Nursing Care Plan: The Woman with HIV Infection summarizes essential nursing management during the antepartum, intrapartum, and postpartum periods. Also see *Key Points: Caring for a Pregnant Woman with HIV Infection.*

SAFETY ALERT!

In 1987, the CDC stated that the increasing prevalence of HIV/AIDS and the risk of exposure faced by healthcare workers are significant enough that *precautions should be taken with all patients* (not only those with known HIV infection), especially when dealing with blood and body fluids. These precautions are called *standard precautions* and continue to be used for all patient care.

Protocols have been established for postexposure treatment of caregivers who experience a needlestick or exposure to the body fluids of a person with HIV or a person whose HIV status is not known. The effectiveness of such therapy, using a combined drug approach, depends on starting therapy rapidly. Thus such exposure should be reported immediately.

Health Promotion Education

The psychologic implications of HIV/AIDS for the childbearing family are staggering.

- The woman is faced with the knowledge that she and her newborn, if infected, have a decreased life expectancy. If her baby is not infected, she must face the possibility that others will raise her child. She must also face the reality that she can only hope to lengthen her life by carefully following an expensive, exacting medical regimen.

NURSING CARE PLAN: The Woman with HIV Infection

1. Nursing Diagnosis: *Infection, Risk for*, related to inadequate defenses (leukopenia, suppressed inflammatory response) secondary to HIV-positive status (NANDA-I © 2017)

Goal: Patient will remain free of opportunistic infection during the course of pregnancy.

INTERVENTION	RATIONALE
• Obtain a complete health history and physical examination during first prenatal visit.	• A complete health history will help determine risk factors for the development of opportunistic infections, and a physical examination will assist in identifying any underlying problem symptoms or illnesses that may compromise the pregnancy or complicate the treatment of HIV.
• Educate the woman as to the signs and symptoms of infection.	• Early recognition of signs and symptoms of infection will allow for immediate treatment, which may decrease the severity of the infection. Signs and symptoms of infection include fever, weight loss, fatigue, persistent candidiasis, diarrhea, cough, and skin lesions (Kaposi sarcoma and hairy leukoplakia in the mouth).
• Obtain nutritional history and monitor weight gain at each prenatal visit.	• The HIV-infected woman needs to maintain optimal nutritional intake. A compromised nutritional status may affect maternal and fetal well-being. Depleted reserves of protein and iron may decrease the patient's ability to fight infection, thereby making her more susceptible to opportunistic infections.
• **Collaborative:** Monitor the absolute $CD4^+$ T lymphocyte count, erythrocyte sedimentation rate (ESR), complete blood count (CBC) with differential, and hemoglobin and hematocrit (H & H) as indicated.	• Laboratory results provide information about the woman's immune system and the potential for disease progression. Opportunistic infections are more likely to occur when the $CD4^+$ T lymphocyte count drops below a level of 200/mm^3. ESR can rise above 20 mm/hr with anemia and with acute and chronic inflammation. CBC with differential and platelet count helps identify anemia, thrombocytopenia, and leukopenia. H & H can also identify anemia.

EXPECTED OUTCOME: Patient will remain free of opportunistic infection as evidenced by $CD4^+$ T lymphocyte count within normal limits; no complaints of chills, fever, or sore throat; normal weight gain throughout pregnancy.

2. Nursing Diagnosis: *Health Maintenance, Ineffective*, related to a lack of information about HIV/AIDS and its long-term implications for the woman, her unborn child, and her family (NANDA-I © 2017)

Goal: The patient and her family will verbalize the importance of following her medication regimen and of regular prenatal care.

INTERVENTION	RATIONALE
• Assess the patient's and family's level of understanding of HIV infection, its modes of transmission, and the long-term implications.	• Knowledge of the woman's (and her family's) level of understanding about her HIV infection forms a starting point for further health teaching.
• Explain the risks of mother-to-child transmission of HIV infection.	• In untreated women the risk of transmission is 25%. That risk can be reduced to 1% or less with the use of antiretroviral therapy throughout pregnancy, labor, and birth; the use of cesarean birth when indicated; and formula-feeding rather than breastfeeding.
• Describe ART. Include the regimen prescribed, its purposes, and the procedures for taking it.	• ART approaches vary based on the health status of the individual woman and whether she is currently on ART. Generally it includes IV ZDV during labor through birth and therapy for the baby for 6 weeks following birth.
• Discuss signs the woman should be alert for, including fever, fatigue, weight loss, cough, skin lesions, and behavior changes.	• These symptoms may indicate that the woman is developing symptomatic loss, persistent candidiasis, diarrhea, and HIV infection.

EXPECTED OUTCOME: Woman will actively seek information about her condition, her treatment regimen, and her pregnancy and will cooperate with her caregivers.

NURSING CARE PLAN: The Woman with HIV Infection (*continued*)

3. Nursing Diagnosis: *Family Processes, Dysfunctional*, related to the implications of positive maternal HIV status on fetal-neonatal well-being and long-term family functioning (NANDA-I © 2017)

Goal: Family is able to manage stressors related to the maternal diagnosis.

INTERVENTION	RATIONALE
• Assess ability and readiness of family to learn about HIV and its long-term implications.	• Readiness is a key element in the teaching–learning process.
• Provide woman and her family with accurate, reliable information about her diagnosis, its prognosis for her and for her baby, and the immediate and long-term implications for her care.	• Fear and anxiety will lessen when the woman and her family understand her health status and the implications of the HIV diagnosis and can then plan for the future.
• Assess interactions between the woman and her family. Be alert for potentially destructive behaviors.	• If the HIV diagnosis was not expected, the couple may have to deal with issues of blame, concerns about mortality, and worries about the status of the baby. If the HIV diagnosis was known, concerns may focus on fetal-neonatal well-being. In either case, negative responses can lead to destructive behaviors.
• Assist family in realistically identifying the needs of the woman and family unit.	• Once needs are identified realistically, it is possible to plan interventions to meet the needs.
• **Collaborative:** Explore available community resources and family support systems.	• Because HIV is a long-term condition, the family may require ongoing assistance.

EXPECTED OUTCOME: Family members actively participate in the treatment plan, are involved in planning for labor and birth in light of a positive HIV status, and are able to express unresolved feelings about the diagnosis.

- The couple must deal with the impact of the illness on the partner, who may or may not be infected, and on other children. The woman and her family may feel fearful, helpless, angry, and isolated.
- It is essential to provide complete, accurate information about the condition, transmission prevention, and ways of coping using language that is well understood by the woman and her partner.
- Ensure that the woman is referred to a comprehensive program that includes social services, psychologic support, and appropriate health care.

Key Facts To Remember

Caring for a Pregnant Woman with HIV Infection

- Following initial infection, antibodies usually become detectable within about 6 to 12 weeks, but it may take 6 months or longer. *Despite this, the woman is infected and infectious.*
- HIV infection is spread primarily through sexual contact, through exposure to contaminated blood, and (perinatally) from infected mother to child.
- Many women who are HIV positive are asymptomatic and may be unaware they have the infection. *Standard precautions are indicated in caring for all pregnant women.*
- A pregnant woman found to be HIV positive should receive prenatal counseling about the possible implications of HIV for the fetus so that she can make an informed choice about continuing her pregnancy. Her choice should be supported.
- During pregnancy, caregivers should be alert to nonspecific symptoms such as weight loss and fatigue, which may indicate progression of HIV disease.
- The incidence of vertical transmission of HIV infection from mother to baby has decreased significantly because of the administration of ART to the mother prenatally and during labor and to the newborn for a specified period following birth.
- Invasive procedures during the intrapartum period increase the risk of exposure to HIV for the fetus (who may be uninfected) and should be undertaken only after carefully weighing the advantages and risks.
- The cardinal rule in caring for pregnant women, and indeed for any patient, is: *If it's wet and it's not yours, use protection when handling it.*

Evaluation

Expected outcomes of nursing care include:

- The woman discusses the implications of her positive HIV antibody screen (or diagnosis of AIDS), its implications for herself and her unborn child, the method of transmission, and treatment options.
- The woman uses information about referral to social services (or other agency) for follow-up assistance and counseling.
- The woman begins to verbalize her feelings about her condition and its implications in an atmosphere she finds supportive.

Care of the Woman with Heart Disease

A healthy woman with a normal heart has adequate cardiac reserve to adjust easily to the demands of pregnancy. The woman with heart disease, however, has decreased cardiac reserve, making it more difficult for her heart to accommodate the larger workload of pregnancy.

Cardiovascular diseases were the leading cause of pregnancy-related deaths in the United States from 2011 to 2013 at 15.5%, followed by noncardiovascular diseases (14.5%), infection or sepsis (12.7%), hemorrhage (11.4%), and cardiomyopathy (11.0%) (CDC, 2017c).

Because of expanded diagnostic, medical, and surgical interventions, many women with congenital heart disease have reached childbearing age and now represent about 4% of all pregnancies. In addition to congenital heart disease, the most common pregnancy complications are arrhythmias and heart failure (Canobbio et al., 2017). The pathology found in pregnant women with heart disease varies with the type of disorder. The conditions occurring most often are discussed here.

Congenital Heart Defects

Congenital heart defects most often seen in pregnant women include tetralogy of Fallot, atrial septal defect, ventricular septal defect, patent ductus arteriosus, and coarctation of the aorta.

For women with congenital heart disease, the impact of pregnancy depends on the specific defect. If the heart defect has been surgically repaired and no evidence of heart disease remains, the woman may undertake pregnancy with confidence. Women with chronic cyanosis are at increased risk for complications and so are their fetuses. A few conditions, such as Eisenmenger syndrome, pulmonary hypertension, uncorrected coarctation of the aorta, severe symptomatic aortic stenosis, and certain types of Marfan syndrome, carry such great risk of complications and death that they can be considered contraindications (Canobbio et al., 2017).

Rheumatic Heart Disease

Rheumatic heart disease has declined rapidly in the last four decades because of prompt identification of pharyngeal infections caused by group A β-hemolytic streptococcus and the availability of penicillin for treatment. Rheumatic fever, which may develop in untreated streptococcal infections, is an inflammatory connective tissue disease that can involve the heart, joints, central nervous system (CNS), skin, and subcutaneous tissue. When the heart is affected, mitral valve stenosis is the most common and serious lesion. Aortic valve involvement, manifested by aortic insufficiency, is the second most common problem. The tricuspid and pulmonic valves are rarely affected.

The increased blood volume of pregnancy, coupled with the pregnant woman's need for increased cardiac output, stresses the heart of a woman with mitral valve stenosis. She may develop dyspnea, orthopnea, and pulmonary edema and is at increased risk for congestive heart failure (CHF). Even the woman who has no symptoms at the onset of pregnancy is at risk for CHF.

Mitral Valve Prolapse

Mitral valve prolapse (MVP) is usually an asymptomatic condition commonly found in women of childbearing age. The condition is more common in women than in men and seems to be inherited. In MVP, the mitral valve leaflets tend to prolapse into the left atrium during ventricular systole because the chordae tendineae that support them are long and thin. As a result, some mitral regurgitation may occur. On auscultation a midsystolic click and a late systolic murmur are heard.

Women with MVP usually tolerate pregnancy well and the prognosis is excellent. Most women require assurance that they can continue with normal activities. A few women experience symptoms such as palpitations, chest pain, and dyspnea, which are usually due to arrhythmias. They are often treated with propranolol hydrochloride (Inderal). Limiting caffeine intake also helps decrease palpitations.

Marfan Syndrome

Marfan syndrome is an autosomal dominant disorder of connective tissue in which there may be serious cardiovascular involvement, usually aortic dissection or rupture. Women with aortic roots greater than 40mm may be advised to delay pregnancy until after repair or root replacement. Women with minimal cardiac involvement and an aortic root less than 40mm are believed to have better outcomes in pregnancy. In women with Marfan syndrome who were not diagnosed before pregnancy and therefore not managed accordingly, the risk of aortic dissection is fivefold greater than in the nonpregnant state. A pregnant woman with Marfan syndrome needs very careful cardiovascular assessment and counseling about her prognosis for pregnancy. Beta-blockers are generally used to prevent aortic dilation from progressing (Roman et al., 2016). Because of its inheritance pattern, there is a 50% chance that the disease will be passed on to offspring.

Peripartum Cardiomyopathy

Peripartum cardiomyopathy is a relatively rare but serious dysfunction of the left ventricle that occurs toward the end of pregnancy or in the first 5 months postpartum in a woman with no previous history of heart disease. The mortality rate is as high as 25 to 50% (Deen et al., 2017). The cause is unknown, thus it is diagnosed after excluding other possible causes of heart disease and pulmonary failure.

The symptoms are related to CHF: Dyspnea, orthopnea, chest pain, palpitations, weakness, and edema. The condition usually presents with anemia and infection; consequently, treatment focuses on underlying abnormalities. Digitalis, diuretics, vasodilators, anticoagulants, sodium restriction, and strict bedrest are often part of the treatment. Peripartum cardiomyopathy may resolve with bedrest as the heart gradually returns to normal size. Preconception counseling is strongly encouraged prior to a subsequent pregnancy because the disease tends to recur.

Clinical Therapy

The primary goal of clinical therapy is early diagnosis and ongoing treatment of the woman with cardiac disease. Auscultation of heart sounds along with a good history and physical are the first steps to diagnosis. Echocardiogram, chest x-ray, electrocardiogram, and sometimes cardiac catheterization may be necessary for establishing the type and severity of the heart disease.

The severity of heart disease can also be determined by the individual's ability to perform ordinary physical activity. A number of professional groups, including those in the United States, Canada, and Europe, have created guidelines for assessing the risk of pregnancy for women with adult congenital heart disease. The modified World Health Organization (WHO) Risk Classification of Cardiovascular Disease and Pregnancy is frequently used clinically to assess risk. It is summarized as follows (Deen et al., 2017; Thorne, MacGregor, & Nelson-Piercy, 2006):

- **WHO-I** Low risk of maternal mortality and morbidity; limited cardiology follow-up required; includes conditions such as uncomplicated or mild pulmonary stenosis and successfully repaired simple lesions such as patent ductus arteriosus (PDA)
- **WHO-II** Small increase in risk; includes conditions such as unoperated atrial septal defect (ASD), ventricular septal defect (VSD), repaired tetralogy of Fallot (TOF), and most arrhythmias
- **WHO-III** Significantly increased risk requiring expert cardiac and obstetric care; includes conditions such as cyanotic heart disease, mechanical valves, systemic right ventricle, and other complex congenital heart disease
- **WHO-IV** Very high risk of maternal mortality; pregnancy contraindicated; if pregnancy occurs, termination may be discussed; includes conditions such as pulmonary hypertension, severe mitral stenosis, severe symptomatic aortic stenosis, severe coarctation of the aorta

Another tool for assessing functional capacity for those with cardiac disease has been standardized by the Criteria Committee of the New York Heart Association (1994). See Table 17–4.

Ethics in Action!

Your patient is a woman with cardiovascular disease risk classification WHO-III or WHO-IV who longs to give birth to a child. How can you help her weigh the health risks and implications of pregnancy for herself, her partner, and the potential child, who may lose his or her mother to disease?

Women in classes I and II usually experience a normal pregnancy and have few complications, whereas those in classes III and IV are at risk for more severe complications, which may affect both maternal and fetal outcomes. Preconception counseling is important for these women to optimize maternal and fetal outcomes.

Because anemia increases the work of the heart, it should be diagnosed early and treated. Infection also increases the cardiac workload, so even minor infections should be treated thoroughly. To reduce the risk of pyelonephritis, monthly screening for asymptomatic bacteriuria is indicated, with antibiotic therapy as needed.

As pregnancy progresses, it is important to minimize cardiac workload and promote tissue perfusion. Depending on the specific lesion, the woman's activity and weight gain may need to be limited.

DRUG THERAPY

Besides the iron and vitamin supplements prescribed during pregnancy, the pregnant woman with heart disease may need additional drug therapy to maintain health. Antibiotic prophylaxis is not indicated for uncomplicated vaginal or cesarean birth unless infection is suspected. If the woman develops coagulation problems, the anticoagulant heparin may be used. Heparin offers the greatest safety to the fetus because it does not cross the placenta. The thiazide diuretics and furosemide (Lasix) may be used to treat congestive heart failure if it develops. Digitalis glycosides and common antiarrhythmic drugs may be used to treat cardiac failure and arrhythmias. These agents do cross the placenta but have no reported teratogenic effect; however, they are classified by the FDA as a category "C," which indicates that they have not been adequately studied to establish their safety in pregnancy (Canobbio et al., 2017).

LABOR AND CHILDBIRTH

Spontaneous natural labor with adequate pain relief is usually recommended for patients in classes I and II. Special attention should be given to the prompt recognition and treatment of any signs of heart failure (Figure 17–6). Those in classes III and IV may need to be hospitalized before onset of labor for cardiovascular stabilization. They may also require invasive cardiac monitoring during labor.

Vaginal birth with low-dose regional analgesia (epidural) is recommended for women with adequate cardiac output with the

TABLE 17–4 Severity of Heart Disease by Functional Capacity

CLASS	FUNCTIONAL CAPACITY
I	Asymptomatic. No limitation of physical activity.
II	Slight limitation of physical activity. Asymptomatic at rest; symptoms occur with ordinary physical activity.
III	Marked limitation of physical activity. Comfortable at rest but symptomatic during less-than-ordinary physical activity.
IV	Inability to carry on any physical activity without discomfort. Even at rest the person experiences symptoms of cardiac insufficiency or anginal pain; discomfort increases with any physical activity.

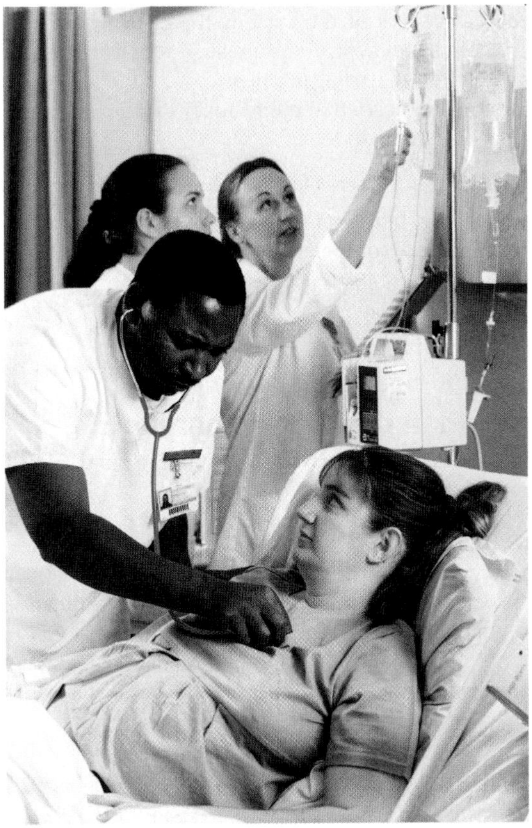

Figure 17–6 When a woman with heart disease begins labor, the nursing students and instructor caring for her monitor her closely for signs of congestive heart failure.

use of forceps or vacuum assistance if necessary to limit maternal pushing. The regional analgesia helps decrease maternal cardiac output and oxygen demand by reducing pain and related maternal anxiety. Cesarean birth is usually used only if fetal or maternal indications exist, not on the basis of heart disease alone.

●○● NURSING MANAGEMENT
For the Pregnant Woman with Heart Disease

Nursing Assessment and Diagnosis

Assess the stress of pregnancy on the functional capacity of the heart during every antepartum visit. Note the category of functional capacity assigned to the woman; take the woman's pulse, respirations, and blood pressure and compare them to the normal values expected during pregnancy and to the woman's previous values. Determine the woman's activity level, including rest, and any changes in the pulse and respirations that have occurred since previous visits. Identify and evaluate other factors that would increase strain on the heart. These might include anemia, infection, anxiety, lack of support system, and household and career demands.

The following symptoms, if they are progressive, are indicative of CHF, the heart's signal of its decreased ability to meet the demands of pregnancy:

- Cough (frequent, with or without hemoptysis)
- Dyspnea (progressive, upon exertion)
- Edema (progressive, generalized, including extremities, face, eyelids)
- Heart murmurs (heard on auscultation)
- Palpitations
- Rales (auscultated in lung bases).

Progressiveness of the cycle is the critical factor because some of these same symptoms are seen to a minor degree in a pregnancy without cardiac problems.

Nursing diagnoses that might apply to the pregnant woman with heart disease include:

- ***Cardiac Output, Decreased,*** resulting in easy fatigability
- ***Gas Exchange, Impaired,*** related to pulmonary edema secondary to cardiac decompensation
- ***Fear*** related to the effects of the maternal cardiac condition on fetal well-being.

(NANDA-I © 2017)

Nursing Plan and Implementation

Nursing care is directed toward maintaining a balance between cardiac reserve and cardiac workload.

Antepartum Period

The priority of nursing actions varies according to the severity of the disease process and the individual needs of the woman as determined by nursing assessment. The woman and her family should thoroughly understand her condition and its management and should recognize signs of potential complications. This will increase their understanding and decrease anxiety. When you provide explanations, use printed material, and offer frequent opportunities to ask questions and discuss concerns, the woman is better able to meet her own healthcare needs and seek assistance appropriately.

As part of health teaching, explain the purposes of the dietary and activity changes that are required. A diet is instituted that is high in iron, protein, and essential nutrients but low in sodium, with adequate calories to ensure normal weight gain. Such a diet best meets the nutrition needs of the patient with cardiac disease. Excessive weight gain is avoided because it taxes the heart. To help preserve her cardiac reserves, the woman may need to restrict her activities. In addition, 8 to 10 hours of sleep and frequent daily rest periods are essential. Encourage the woman to rest in the side-lying position to promote optimal placental perfusion. Because upper respiratory infections may tax the heart and lead to decompensation, the woman must avoid contact with sources of infection and report symptoms of infection immediately.

During the first half of pregnancy, the woman is seen approximately every 2 weeks to assess cardiac status. During the second half of pregnancy, the woman may be seen more often. These assessments are especially important between weeks 28 and 30, when the blood volume reaches maximum amounts. If symptoms of cardiac decompensation occur, prompt medical intervention is indicated to correct the cardiac problem.

Intrapartum Period

Labor and birth exert tremendous stress on the woman and her fetus. This stress could be fatal to the fetus of a woman with cardiac disease because the fetus may be receiving an inadequate oxygen and blood supply. Thus the intrapartum care of a woman with cardiac disease is aimed at reducing the amount of physical exertion and accompanying fatigue.

Evaluate maternal vital signs frequently to determine the woman's response to labor. A pulse rate greater than 100 beats per minute or respirations greater than 24 per minute may indicate beginning cardiac decompensation, especially if accompanied by dyspnea, and require further evaluation. Auscultate the woman's lungs frequently for rales and carefully observe for other signs of developing decompensation.

To ensure cardiac emptying and adequate oxygenation, encourage the laboring woman to assume either a semi-Fowler position with lateral tilt or side-lying position with her head and shoulders elevated. Oxygen by mask, diuretics to reduce fluid retention, sedatives and analgesics, prophylactic antibiotics, and digitalis may also be used as indicated by the woman's status.

Remain with the woman to support her. It is essential to keep the woman and her family informed of labor progress and management plans and to collaborate with them to fulfill their wishes for the birth experience as much as possible. Maintain an atmosphere of calm to lessen the anxiety of the woman and her family.

Continuous electronic fetal monitoring is used to provide ongoing assessment of the fetus's response to labor. To prevent overexertion and the accompanying fatigue, encourage the woman to sleep and relax between contractions and provide her with emotional support and encouragement. During pushing, encourage the woman to continue breathing and use shorter, more moderate pushing (see Chapter 21), with complete relaxation between pushes. Monitor vital signs closely during the second stage.

Postpartum Period

The postpartum period is a significant time for the woman with cardiac disease. As extravascular fluid returns to the bloodstream for excretion, cardiac output and blood volume increase. This physiologic adaptation places great strain on the heart and may lead to decompensation, especially in the first 48 hours postpartum.

To detect any possible problems, the woman may remain in the hospital longer than the low-risk woman postpartum. Monitor her vital signs frequently and assess for signs of decompensation. Keep her in the semi-Fowler or side-lying position, with her head and shoulders elevated, and have her begin a gradual, progressive activity program. Appropriate diet and stool softeners facilitate bowel movement without undue strain.

Postpartum, give the woman opportunities to discuss her birth experience and help her deal with any feelings or concerns that cause her distress. Encourage maternal–newborn attachment by providing frequent opportunities for the mother to interact with her child.

Because there is no evidence that cardiac output is compromised during lactation, the only concern about breastfeeding for women with cardiovascular disease is related to medications that the mother may be taking. These must be evaluated for their ability to pass into the milk and for any effect of the drug on lactation. Assist the breastfeeding mother to a comfortable side-lying position with her head moderately elevated or to a semi-Fowler position. To conserve the mother's energy, position the newborn at the breast and be available to burp the baby and reposition him or her at the other breast. Encourage family members to provide the new mother with support and assistance as needed to help her avoid becoming fatigued.

In addition to providing the normal postpartum discharge teaching, stress that follow-up for the new mother is imperative. Moreover, ensure that the woman and her family understand the signs of possible problems resulting from her heart disease or from other postpartum complications. For women with heart disease, postpartum complications such as hemorrhage, thromboembolism, anemia, and infection pose a real threat and may even precipitate heart failure.

Plan with the woman an activity schedule that is gradual, progressive, and appropriate to her needs and home environment. Provide appropriate health teaching, including information about resumption of sexual activity and contraception. Visiting nurse or homemaker assistance referrals may be necessary, depending on the woman's status.

Evaluation

Expected outcomes of nursing care include:

- The woman is able to discuss her condition and its possible impact on her pregnancy, labor and birth, and the postpartum period.
- The woman participates in developing an appropriate health-care regimen and follows it throughout her pregnancy.
- The woman gives birth to a healthy baby.
- The woman does not develop congestive heart failure, thromboembolism, or infection.
- The woman is able to identify signs and symptoms of possible postpartum complications.
- The woman is able to care effectively for her newborn.

Other Medical Conditions and Pregnancy

A woman with a preexisting medical condition should be aware of the possible impact of pregnancy on her condition, as well as the impact of her condition on the outcome of her pregnancy. Table 17–5 discusses some of the less common medical conditions that might impact pregnancy.

TABLE 17–5 Less Common Medical Conditions and Pregnancy

BRIEF DESCRIPTION	MATERNAL IMPLICATIONS	FETAL-NEONATAL IMPLICATIONS
Asthma		
An obstructive lung condition that is the most common respiratory disease found in pregnancy, complicating approximately 8% of all pregnancies (Whitty & Dombrowski, 2017). Typical symptoms include wheezing, dyspnea, and episodic coughing. A severe asthmatic attack may require hospitalization. It is managed by long-term comprehensive drug therapy to prevent airway inflammation, combined with drug treatment to manage attacks or exacerbations. Patient education focuses on triggers (such as cold air, dust, smoke, exercise, food additives), methods of prevention, and treatment options.	The severity of asthma may improve, worsen, or remain unchanged during pregnancy. The mechanisms associated with these variations remain undefined; however, poor asthma control is associated with increased maternal and neonatal complications, most likely from poor adherence to the treatment regimen. Maternal complications include preeclampsia, growth restriction, and preterm birth. Asthma management during labor and birth focuses on maintenance of adequate hydration and analgesia as well as continuing asthma medications.	With appropriate asthma therapy, most women can breathe easily, have a normal pregnancy, and give birth to a healthy baby. Preterm birth and intrauterine growth restriction are more common among the babies of women who have asthma (Whitty & Dombrowski, 2017). The goal of therapy is to prevent maternal exacerbations because even a mild exacerbation can cause severe hypoxia-related complications in the fetus. If an exacerbation occurs, it should be managed in the same way as for a nonpregnant woman because the asthma drugs used are less of a threat to the fetus than a serious asthma attack.
Epilepsy		
Chronic disorder characterized by seizures; may be idiopathic or secondary to other conditions, such as head injury, metabolic and nutritional disorders such as phenylketonuria (PKU) or vitamin B_6 deficiency, encephalitis, neoplasms, or circulatory interferences. Treated with anticonvulsants.	Vast majority of pregnancies in women with seizure disorders are uneventful and have an excellent outcome. Women with more frequent seizures before pregnancy may have exacerbations during pregnancy, but this may be related to nausea and vomiting, lack of cooperation with drug regimen, or sleep deprivation. During pregnancy the woman should continue to be treated with the medication that best controls her seizures. Folic acid therapy should be started prior to conception, if possible. Folic acid and vitamin D are indicated throughout pregnancy (Ban et al., 2015).	Certain anticonvulsant medications are associated with increased incidence of congenital anomalies, especially cleft lip and heart defects, although the incidence has decreased in recent years. The lowest dose of a single effective medication is the goal of treatment to decrease the potential for fetal anomalies (Ban et al., 2015). Multiple medications and valproic acid should also be avoided for women planning pregnancy when possible.

(continued)

TABLE 17–5 Less Common Medical Conditions and Pregnancy *(continued)*

BRIEF DESCRIPTION	MATERNAL IMPLICATIONS	FETAL-NEONATAL IMPLICATIONS
Hepatitis B		
Caused by the hepatitis B virus (HBV), it is a major, growing health problem. Groups at risk include those from areas with a high incidence (primarily developing countries), illegal intravenous (IV) drug users, prostitutes, homosexuals, those with multiple sex partners, or occupational exposure to blood, although many infected people have no identifiable source of infection. HBV transmission is bloodborne, primarily sexually and perinatally transmitted. Because of the dramatic increase and the difficulty of vaccinating high-risk individuals before they become infected, the CDC now recommends (1) testing all pregnant women for the presence of hepatitis B surface antigen and prophylactic treatment for all babies born to women who are HBsAg positive or whose status is unknown; (2) routine newborn/infant vaccination; (3) vaccination of children and adolescents through age 18 years who have not been vaccinated; (4) vaccination of unvaccinated adults who are at risk for hepatitis B (SMFM, 2016).	Estimates suggest 0.7–0.9% of pregnant women have chronic hepatitis B in the United States (Society for Maternal-Fetal Medicine [SMFM], 2016). Hepatitis B does not usually affect the course of pregnancy. However, chronic HBV carriers have a great potential for infecting others when exposure to blood and body fluids occurs. In addition, chronic carriers may develop long-term sequelae, such as chronic liver disease and liver cancer. It is now recommended that all pregnant women be tested for the presence of hepatitis B surface antigen (HBsAg). A woman who is negative may be given the hepatitis vaccine.	Perinatal transmission most often occurs at or near the time of childbirth. In fact, women who are positive for HBsAg have almost a 90% chance of transmitting HBV to their newborn at birth (Bernstein, 2017). More important, the risk of becoming a chronic carrier of HBV is inversely related to the age of the individual at the time of initial infection. Therefore, babies infected perinatally have the highest risk of becoming chronically infected if not treated. Recommendations now include routine vaccination of all neonates born to HBsAg-negative women and immunoprophylaxis to all newborns of HBsAg-positive women (SMFM, 2016). Within 12 hours of birth, babies born to women with HBV infection should receive hepatitis B immune globulin and the first dose of the HBV vaccine series. The second and third doses of vaccine should be administered at ages 1 and 6 months, respectively (American Academy of Pediatrics [AAP], 2015).
Hyperthyroidism (Thyrotoxicosis)		
Enlarged, overactive thyroid gland; increased T_4:thyroxine-binding globulin (TBG) ratio and increased basal metabolic rate (BMR). Symptoms include muscle wasting, tachycardia, excessive sweating, and exophthalmos. Treatment by antithyroid drug propylthiouracil (PTU) while monitoring free T_4 levels. Surgery is indicated only if drug intolerance exists.	Mild hyperthyroidism is not dangerous. Increased incidence of preeclampsia and postpartum hemorrhage if not well controlled. Serious risk related to thyroid storm characterized by high fever, tachycardia, sweating, and congestive heart failure. Now occurs rarely. When diagnosed during pregnancy, may be transient or permanent.	Neonatal thyrotoxicosis is rare. Even low doses of antithyroid drug in mother may produce a mild fetal-neonatal hypothyroidism; higher dose may produce a goiter or mental deficiencies. Fetal loss not increased in euthyroid women. If untreated, rates of abortion, intrauterine death, and stillbirth increase. Breastfeeding contraindicated for women on antithyroid medication because it is excreted in the milk (may be tried by woman on low dose if neonatal T_4 levels are monitored).
Hypothyroidism		
Characterized by inadequate thyroid secretions (decreased T_4:TBG ratio), elevated thyroid-stimulating hormone (TSH), lowered BMR, and enlarged thyroid gland (goiter). Symptoms include lack of energy, excessive weight gain, cold intolerance, dry skin, and constipation. Treated by thyroxine replacement therapy.	Long-term replacement therapy usually continues; 20 to 30% of pregnant women need an increase in their thyroxine dose in the second half of pregnancy (Mestman, 2017). Serial ultrasounds are done to monitor fetal growth; nonstress tests are not necessary in well-controlled disease but are considered beginning at 32 to 34 weeks' gestation in cases of poorly controlled disease (De Groot et al., 2012).	If mother untreated, fetal complications include IUGR, congenital cretinism, and stillbirth. When the mother is adequately treated, the newborn is usually free of thyroid dysfunction (Johnson & Milio, 2015). Therefore, newborns are screened for T_4 level. Mild TSH elevations present little risk because TSH does not cross the placenta.
Maternal Phenylketonuria (PKU) (Hyperphenylalaninemia)		
Inherited recessive single-gene anomaly causing a deficiency of the liver enzyme needed to convert the amino acid phenylalanine to tyrosine, resulting in high serum levels of phenylalanine. Brain damage and intellectual disability occur if not treated early.	Low phenylalanine diet is mandatory before conception and during pregnancy. The woman should be counseled that her children will either inherit the disease or be carriers, depending on the zygosity of the father for the disease. Treatment at a PKU center is recommended.	Risk to fetus if maternal treatment not begun preconception. In untreated women there is increased incidence of intellectual or developmental disabilities, microcephaly, congenital heart defects, and growth retardation (Camp et al., 2014).

TABLE 17–5 Less Common Medical Conditions and Pregnancy *(continued)*

BRIEF DESCRIPTION	MATERNAL IMPLICATIONS	FETAL-NEONATAL IMPLICATIONS
Multiple Sclerosis (MS)		
Chronic autoimmune demyelinating disease characterized by destruction of the myelin sheath of nerve fibers. The condition occurs primarily in young adults, more commonly in females, and is marked by periods of remission; progresses to marked physical disability in 10 to 20 years.	Relapse rate is reduced during the second and third trimester but increased during the 3 months following birth. Rest is important; help with child care should be planned. Uterine contraction strength is not diminished, but because sensation is frequently lessened, labor may be almost painless.	MS does not appear to have any significant effect on fetal outcomes. A child with one parent with MS has a 2–2.5% risk of developing the disease. This risk is low but is a 20-fold increase from that of the general population. However, it is not usually considered a reason to avoid pregnancy (Gerard & Samuels, 2017).
Rheumatoid Arthritis (RA)		
Chronic autoimmune disease characterized by chronic symmetric inflammatory arthritis of the joints. It is more common in females than in males. Symptoms include fatigue, low-grade fever, pain and swelling of joints, morning stiffness, pain on movement. Treated with salicylates, physical therapy, and rest. Corticosteroids used cautiously if not responsive to above.	Usually there is remission of rheumatoid arthritis symptoms during pregnancy, often with a relapse postpartum. Anemia may be present due to blood loss from salicylate therapy. Mother needs extra rest, particularly to relieve weight-bearing joints, but needs to continue range-of-motion exercises. If in remission, may stop medication during pregnancy.	Pregnancy is usually uneventful for women with RA, with no increased risk for preterm birth or fetal loss. However, certain antirheumatic medications are associated with increased risk. Methotrexate and leflunomide are absolutely contraindicated (Carpenter & Branch, 2017).
Systemic Lupus Erythematosus (SLE)		
Chronic systemic autoimmune collagen disease that primarily affects women of childbearing age; characterized by exacerbations and remissions; symptoms range from characteristic rash to inflammation and pain in joints, fever, nephritis, depression, cranial nerve disorders, and peripheral neuropathies.	SLE during pregnancy needs to be actively managed with careful surveillance of blood pressure, proteinuria, and placental blood flow. SLE medications may be necessary to control exacerbations and lupus flare-ups. Preeclampsia, prematurity, and fetal growth restriction are common complications. Pregnancy outcomes are better if the woman delays conception until she has been free of serious disease activity for 6 months and her medications are well regulated. Women with severe disease may be counseled to avoid pregnancy (Yang et al., 2014).	Increased incidence of caesarean birth, postpartum hemorrhage, and blood transfusion. Women with SLE are more at risk for preterm birth, IUGR, and fetal loss. The incidence of neonatal lupus erythematosus (NLE) is low and is related to transplacental transfer of antibodies (Carpenter & Branch, 2017). Neonatal lupus is characterized by a photosensitive skin rash, thrombocytopenia, neutropenia, or anemia, all of which resolve by about 6 months of age. Complete congenital heart block is the most serious complication of SLE, typically diagnosed in utero. It is associated with an overall mortality rate of 20% (Carpenter & Branch, 2017). When diagnosed, the mother is given corticosteroids that cross the placenta and decrease fetal heart inflammation.
Tuberculosis (TB)		
A major health problem, approximately one-third of the world's population (more than 2 billion people) carries the TB bacteria. Worldwide, TB is one of the top killers of women. Infection is caused by *Mycobacterium tuberculosis*; inflammatory process causes destruction of lung tissue, increased sputum, and coughing. Associated primarily with poverty and malnutrition, 80% of new cases are found in developing countries primarily in Asia and Africa. In the United States the majority of cases occur in foreign-born people. More than 75% of these individuals were born in just 15 countries (WHO, 2016). Treated with isoniazid and either ethambutol or rifampin, or both.	The incidence of pregnancy complications may be higher in women with TB. TB skin test screening is recommended for women in high-risk groups (healthcare workers; foreign-born women from countries with a high TB risk; women who have had known contact with infectious person; those who are HIV infected, alcoholics, or illicit drug users; women living or working in homeless shelters; prisoners and detainees (WHO, 2016). If TB is inactive due to prior treatment, isoniazid therapy is delayed until the postpartum period unless the woman is HIV positive, has close contact with a person with active TB, or has had a skin test convert to positive within the last 2 years. For those women, isoniazid is started during pregnancy. Women with active TB are treated with isoniazid, rifampin, and ethambutol during pregnancy (AAP, 2015). Extra rest and limited contact with others are required until disease becomes inactive.	Women with TB have a higher rate of spontaneous abortion, suboptimal weight gain, and preterm labor; there is also an increased incidence of neonatal mortality and low birth weight. Congenital TB is a rare complication of in utero infection, but the risk of postnatal transmission to the newborn is higher (AAP, 2015). If maternal TB is inactive, the mother may breastfeed and care for her newborn. If TB is active, the newborn should not have direct contact with the mother until she is noninfectious. Isoniazid crosses the placenta, but most studies show no teratogenic effects. Rifampin crosses the placenta. Possibility of harmful effects is still being studied.

Focus Your Study

- Almost any health problem that a person can have when not pregnant can coexist with pregnancy. Some problems, such as anemias, may be exacerbated by pregnancy. Others, such as collagen disease, may go into temporary remission with pregnancy. Regardless of the health problem, careful health care is needed throughout pregnancy to improve the outcome for mother and fetus.
- The diagnosis of high-risk pregnancy can shock an expectant couple. Providing emotional support, teaching about the condition and prognosis, and educating for self-care are important nursing measures that help the patient cope.
- The key point in the care of the pregnant woman with diabetes is scrupulous maternal plasma glucose control. This is best achieved by home blood glucose monitoring, multiple daily insulin injections, regular exercise, and a careful diet. To reduce incidence of congenital anomalies and other problems in the newborn, the woman should be euglycemic (have a normal blood glucose) throughout the pregnancy. Women with diabetes, even more than most other patients, need to be educated about their conditions and involved with their own care.
- Anemia indicates inadequate levels of hemoglobin (Hb) in the blood. Anemia is defined as hemoglobin less than 12 g/dL in nonpregnant women and less than 11 g/dL in pregnant and postpartum women. Iron deficiency anemia is the most common form of anemia. Other anemias include folic acid deficiency, sickle cell disease, and thalassemia.
- Substance abuse (either drugs or alcohol) not only is detrimental to the mother's health but also may have profound lasting effects on the fetus.
- HIV infection, which is transmitted via blood and body fluids, may also be transmitted transplacentally to the fetus. Currently, there is no definitive therapy for HIV/AIDS. Nurses should employ blood and body fluid precautions (standard precautions) in caring for all women to avoid potential spread of infection.
- Cardiac disease during pregnancy requires careful assessment, limitation of activity, and knowing and reporting signs of impending cardiac decompensation by both patient and nurse.
- Worldwide, more women die from TB than from any other infection. Most cases are concentrated in developing countries.

In order to make safe and effective judgments using NANDA-I © 2017 nursing diagnoses, it is essential that nurses refer to the definitions and defining characteristics of the diagnoses used in this text, which can be found in Appendix C.

References

Abu-Ouf, N. M., & Jan, M. M. (2015). The impact of maternal iron deficiency and iron deficiency anemia on child's health. *Saudi Medical Journal, 36*(2), 146–149.

American Academy of Pediatrics (AAP). (2015). *Red book: 2015 Report of the Committee on Infectious Diseases* (30th ed.). Elk Grove Village, IL: Author.

American Academy of Pediatrics (AAP) & American College of Obstetricians and Gynecologists (ACOG). (2017). *Guidelines for perinatal care* (8th ed.). Elk Grove Village, IL: American Academy of Pediatrics.

American College of Obstetricians and Gynecologists (ACOG). (2008, reaffirmed 2015). *Anemia in pregnancy* (ACOG Practice Bulletin No. 95). Washington, DC: Author.

American College of Obstetricians and Gynecologists (ACOG). (2015, reaffirmed 2016). *Screening for perinatal depression* (ACOG Committee Opinion No. 630). Washington, DC: Author.

American College of Obstetricians and Gynecologists (ACOG). (2018). *Gestational diabetes mellitus* (ACOG Practice Bulletin No. 190). Washington, DC: Author.

American Diabetes Association (ADA). (2018). Standards of medical care in diabetes—2018. *Diabetes Care, 41*(Suppl. 1), S1–172.

Anderson, E. A., Momplaisir, F. M., Corson, C., & Brady, K. A. (2017). Assessing the impact of perinatal HIV case management on outcomes along the HIV care continuum for pregnant and postpartum women living with HIV, Philadelphia 2005–2013. *AIDS and Behavior, 21*(9), 2670–2681. DOI: 10.1007/s10461-017-1714-9

Ban, L., Fleming, K. M., Doyle, P., Smeeth, L., Hubbard, R. B., Fiaschi, L., & Tata, L. J. (2015). Congenital anomalies in children of mothers taking antiepileptic drugs with and without periconceptional high dose folic acid use: A population-based cohort study. *Public Library of Science, 10*(7), e0131130. DOI: 10.1371/journal.pone.0131130

Behnke, M., & Smith, V. C. (2013). Prenatal substance abuse: Short- and long-term effects on the exposed fetus. *Pediatrics, 131*(3), e1009–1024.

Bernstein, H. B. (2017). Maternal and perinatal infection in pregnancy. In S. G. Gabbe, J. R. Niebyl, J. L. Simpson, M. B. Landon, H. L. Galan, E. R. M. Jauniaux, . . . W. A. Grobman (Eds.), *Obstetrics: Normal and problem pregnancies* (7th ed., pp. 1099–1129). Philadelphia, PA: Elsevier.

Brockington I., Butterworth, R., & Glangeaud-Freudenthal, N. (2017). An international position paper on mother-infant (perinatal) mental health, with guidelines for clinical practice. *Archives of Women's Mental Health, 20*(1), 113–120. DOI: 10.1007/s00737-016-0684-7

Camp, K. M., Parisi, M. A., Acosta, P. B., Berry, G. T., Bilder, D. A., Blau, N., . . . Young, L. M. (2014). Phenylketonuria scientific review conference: State of the science and future research needs. *Molecular Genetics and Metabolism, 112*, 87.

Canobbio, M. M., Warnes, C. A., Aboulhosn, J., Connolly, H. M., Khanna, A., Koos, B. J., . . . Stout, K.; American Heart Association Council on Cardiovascular and Stroke Nursing; Council on Clinical Cardiology; Council on Cardiovascular Disease in the Young; Council on Functional Genomics and Translational Biology; & Council on Quality of Care and Outcomes Research. (2017). Management of pregnancy in patients with complex congenital heart disease: A scientific statement for healthcare professionals from the American Heart Association. *Circulation, 135*(8), e50–e87.

Carpenter, J. R., & Branch, D. W. (2017). Collagen vascular diseases in pregnancy. In S. G. Gabbe, J. R. Niebyl, J. L. Simpson, M. B. Landon, H. L. Galan, E. R. M. Jauniaux, . . . W. A. Grobman (Eds.), *Obstetrics: Normal and problem pregnancies* (7th ed., pp. 981–997). Philadelphia, PA: Elsevier.

Center for Behavioral Health Statistics and Quality. (2016). *Key substance use and mental health indicators in the United States: Results from the 2015 national survey on drug use and health* (HHS Publication No. SMA 16-4984, NSDUH Series H-51). Retrieved from http://www.samhsa.gov/data

Centers for Disease Control and Prevention (CDC). (2014). *Laboratory testing for the diagnosis of HIV infection: Updated recommendations.* Retrieved from https://stacks.cdc.gov/view/cdc/23447/cdc_23447_DS1.pdf

Centers for Disease Control and Prevention (CDC). (2017a). *HIV among pregnant women, infants, and children.* Retrieved from https://www.cdc.gov/hiv/group/gender/pregnantwomen/index.html

Centers for Disease Control and Prevention (CDC). (2017b). *HIV surveillance report, 2016; Vol. 28.* Retrieved from https://www.cdc.gov/hiv/pdf/library/reports/surveillance/cdc-hiv-surveillance-report-2016-vol-28.pdf

Centers for Disease Control and Prevention (CDC). (2017c). *Pregnancy mortality surveillance system.* Retrieved from https://www.cdc.gov/reproductivehealth/maternalinfanthealth/pmss.html

Committee on the Health Effects of Marijuana. (2017). *The health effects of cannabis and cannabinoids: Current state of evidence and recommendations for research.* Washington, DC: National Academies Press.

Cooley's Anemia Foundation. (2017). *Thalassemia.* Retrieved from www.thalassemia.org/thalassemia-more-information/

Criteria Committee of the New York Heart Association. (1994). *Nomenclature and criteria for diagnosis of diseases of the heart and great vessels* (9th ed.). Dallas, TX: American Heart Association.

Deen, J., Chandrasekaran, S., Stout, K., & Easterling, T. (2017). Heart disease in pregnancy. In S. G. Gabbe, J. R. Niebyl, J. L. Simpson, M. B. Landon, H. L. Galan, E. R. M. Jauniaux, . . . W. A. Grobman (Eds.), *Obstetrics: Normal and problem pregnancies* (7th ed., 803–827). Philadelphia, PA: Elsevier.

De Groot, L., Abalovich, M., Alexander, E. K., Amino, N., Barbour, L., Cobin, R. H., . . . Sullivan, S. (2012). Management of thyroid dysfunction during pregnancy and postpartum: An endocrine society clinical practice guideline. *Journal of Clinical Endocrinology and Metabolism, 97*, 2543.

Forray, A., & Foster, D. (2015) Substance use in the perinatal period. *Current Psychiatry Reports, 17*(11), 91.

Fruhauf, T., & Coleman, J. (2017) A missed opportunity for U.S. perinatal human immunodeficiency virus elimination. *Obstetrics and Gynecology, 130*(4), 703–709.

Gerard, E. E., & Samuels, P. P. (2017). Neurologic disorders in pregnancy. In S. G. Gabbe, J. R. Niebyl, J. L. Simpson, M. B. Landon, H. L. Galan, E. R. M. Jauniaux, . . . W. A. Grobman (Eds.), *Obstetrics: Normal and problem pregnancies* (7th ed., pp. 1030–1056). Philadelphia, PA: Elsevier.

Hathaway, A. R. (2016). Sickle cell disease in pregnancy. *Southern Medical Journal, 109*(9), 554–556.

International Association of Diabetes and Pregnancy Study Groups (IADPSG) Consensus Panel. (2010). International Association of Diabetes and Pregnancy Study Groups recommendations on the diagnosis and classification of hyperglycemia in pregnancy. *Diabetes Care, 33*(3), 676–683.

Johnson, C. T., & Milio, L. A. (2015). Endocrine disorders of pregnancy. In C. T. Johnson, J. L. Hallock, J. L. Bienstock, H. E. Fox, & E. W. Wallach, (Eds.), *The Johns Hopkins manual of gynecology and obstetrics* (5th ed., pp. 176–197). Philadelphia, PA: Wolters Kluwer.

Jones, H. E., Deppen, K., Hudak, M. L., McClelland, C., Sahin, L., Starer, J., . . . Creanga, A. A. (2014). Clinical care for opioid-using pregnant and postpartum women: The role of obstetric providers. *Journal of Obstetrics and Gynecology*, (4), 302–310.

Joslin Diabetes Center. (2017). *How to treat a low blood glucose.* Retrieved from http://www.joslin.org/info/how_to_treat_a_low_blood_glucose.html

Landon, M. B., Catalano, P. M., & Gabbe, S. G. (2017). Diabetes mellitus complicating pregnancy. In S. G. Gabbe, J. R. Niebyl, J. L. Simpson, M. B. Landon, H. L. Galan, E. R. M. Jauniaux, . . . & W. A. Grobman (Eds.), *Obstetrics: Normal and problem pregnancies* (7th ed., pp. 862–897). Philadelphia, PA: Elsevier.

Lauring, J. R., Lehman, E. B., Deimling, T. A., Legro, R. S., & Chuang, C. H. (2016). Combined hormonal contraception use in reproductive-age women with contraindications to estrogen use. *American Journal of Obstetrics and Gynecology, 215*(3), 330, e1–7.

Mestman, J. H. (2017). Thyroid and parathyroid diseases in pregnancy. In S. G. Gabbe, J. R. Niebyl, J. L. Simpson, M. B. Landon, H. L. Galan, E. R. M. Jauniaux, . . . W. A. Grobman (Eds.), *Obstetrics: Normal and problem pregnancies* (7th ed., pp. 921–937). Philadelphia, PA: Elsevier.

Miller, D., Mamilly, L., Fourtner, S., & Rosen-Carole, C. (2017). Breastfeeding an infant or young child with insulin-dependent diabetes. *Breastfeeding Medicine: The Official Journal of the Academy of Breastfeeding Medicine, 12*, 72–76.

National Institute on Drug Abuse [NIDA]. (2016). *Substance use while pregnant and breastfeeding.* Retrieved from https://www.drugabuse.gov/publications/research-reports/substance-use-in-women/substance-use-while-pregnant-breastfeeding

National Institute on Drug Abuse [NIDA]. (2017). *MDMA (Ecstasy) abuse.* Retrieved from https://www.drugabuse.gov/publications/research-reports/mdma-ecstasy-abuse/can-mdma-use-during-pregnancy-harm-the-baby

National Institute on Drug Abuse [NIDA]. (2018). *Heroin.* Retrieved from https://www.drugabuse.gov/publications/research-reports/heroin/how-does-heroin-abuse-affect-pregnant-women

Panel on Treatment of Pregnant Women with HIV Infection and Prevention of Perinatal Transmission. (2017). *Recommendations for use of antiretroviral drugs in pregnant women with HIV infection and interventions to reduce perinatal HIV transmission in the United States.* Retrieved from https://aidsinfo.nih.gov/contentfiles/lvguidelines/PerinatalGL.pdf

Petrakos, G., Andriopoulos, P., & Tsironi, M. (2016). Pregnancy in women with thalassemia: Challenges and solutions. *International Journal of Women's Health, 8*, 441–451. DOI: 10.2147/IJWH.S89308

Roman, M. J., Pugh N. L., Hendershot, T. P., Devereux, R. B., Dietz, H., Holmes, K., . . . Silberbach, M. (2016). Aortic complications associated with pregnancy in Marfan syndrome: The NHLBI national registry of genetically triggered thoracic rtic aneurysms and cardiovascular conditions (GenTAC). *Journal of the American Heart Association, 11*, 5(8).

Singer, L. T., Moore, D. G., Min, M. O., Goodwin, J., Turner, J. J., Fulton, S., & Parrott, A. C. (2016). Motor delays in MDMA (ecstasy) exposed infants persist to 2 years. *Neurotoxicology and Teratology, 54*, 22–28.

Smith, K., & Lipari, R. (2017). *Women of childbearing age and opioids.* Retrieved from https://www.samhsa.gov/data/sites/default/files/report_2724/ShortReport-2724.pdf

Society for Maternal-Fetal Medicine (SMFM). (2016). Hepatitis B in pregnancy screening, treatment, and prevention of vertical transmission. *American Journal of Obstetrics and Gynecology, 214*(1), 6–14.

Substance Abuse and Mental Health Services Administration (SAMHSA). (2014). *Results from the 2013 National Survey on Drug Use and Health: Summary of national findings* (NSDUH Series H-48, DHHS Publication No. SMA 14-4863). Rockville, MD: Author.

Substance Abuse and Mental Health Services Administration (SAMHSA). (2018). *Clinical guidance for treating pregnant and parenting women with opioid use disorder and their infants* (DHHS Publication No. SMA 18-5054). Rockville, MD: Author.

Thorne, S., MacGregor, A., & Nelson-Piercy, A. (2006). Risk of conception and pregnancy in heart disease. *Heart, 92*, 1520–1529.

U.S. Department of Health and Human Services. (2017). *You're pregnant: Now what?* Retrieved from https://www.womenshealth.gov/pregnancy/youre-pregnant-now-what/staying-healthy-and-safe

Wang, M. (2014). Perinatal drug abuse and neonatal withdrawal. *eMedicine.* Retrieved from http://emedicine.medscape.com/article/978492-overview

Whitty, J. E., & Dombrowski, M. P. (2017). Respiratory diseases in pregnancy. In S. G. Gabbe, J. R. Niebyl, J. L. Simpson, M. B. Landon, H. L. Galan, E. R. M. Jauniaux, . . . W. A. Grobman (Eds.), *Obstetrics: Normal and problem pregnancies* (7th ed., pp. 828–849). Philadelphia, PA: Elsevier.

Wisner, K. L., Sit, D. K. Y., Bogen, D. L., Altemus, M., Pearlstein, T. B., Svikis, D. S., . . . Miller, E. S. (2017). Mental health disorders and behavioral health disorders in pregnancy. In S. G. Gabbe, J. R. Niebyl, J. L. Simpson, M. B. Landon, H. L. Galan, E. R. M. Jauniaux, . . . W. A. Grobman (Eds.), *Obstetrics: Normal and problem pregnancies* (7th ed., pp. 1147–1172). Philadelphia, PA: Elsevier.

World Health Organization (WHO). (2014). *Guidelines for the identification and management of substance use and substance use disorders in pregnancy.* Retrieved from http://apps.who.int/iris/bitstream/10665/107130/1/9789241548731_eng.pdf

World Health Organization (WHO). (2016). *Global tuberculosis report, 2016.* Retrieved from http://apps.who.int/iris/bitstream/10665/250441/1/9789241565394-eng.pdf?ua=1

Wright, T. E., Terplan, M., Ondersma, S. J., Boyce, C., Yonkers, K., Chang, G., & Creanga, A. A. (2016). The role of screening, brief intervention, and referral to treatment in the perinatal period. *Journal of Obstetrics and Gynecology, 215*(5), 539–547.

Yang, H., Liu, H., Xu, D., Zhao, L., Wang, Q., Leng, X., . . . Zhang, X. (2014). Pregnancy-related systemic lupus erythematosus: Clinical features, outcome and risk factors of disease flares—A case control study. *Public Library of Science, 9*(8), e104375. DOI: 10.1371/journal.pone.0104375

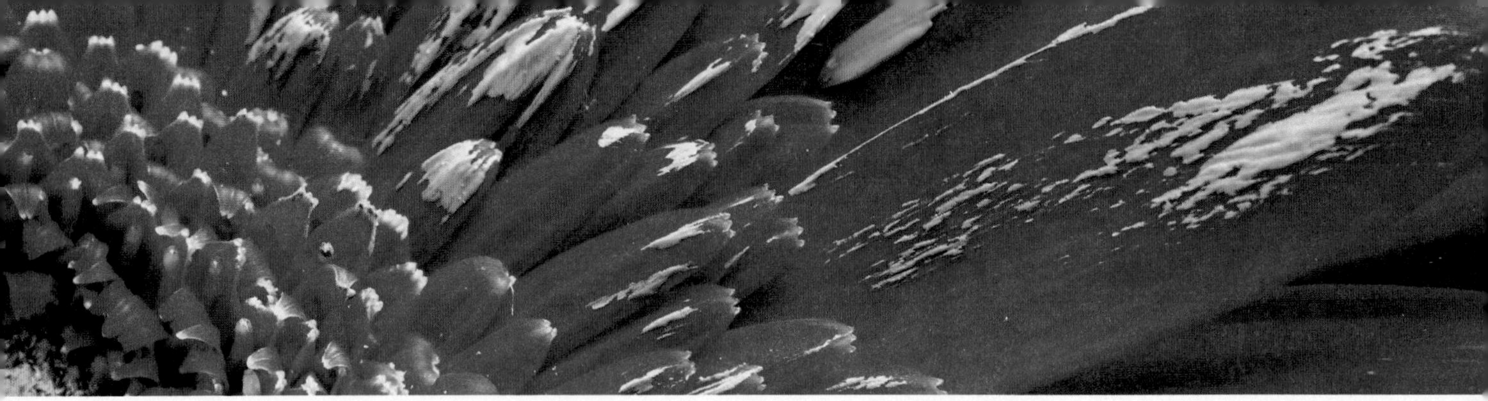

Chapter 18

Pregnancy at Risk: Gestational Onset

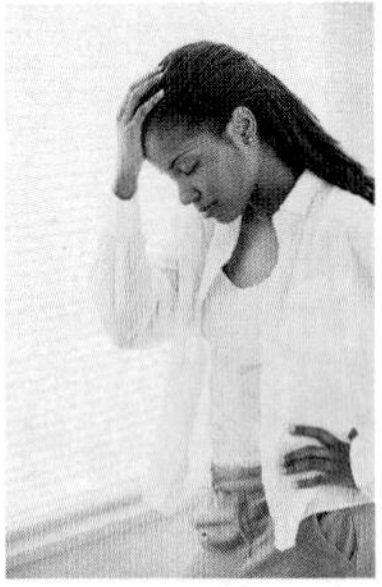

SOURCE: Blend Images/SuperStock.

I had taken more than a year to conceive and was so excited when my home pregnancy test turned positive. My husband was with me when I called my family. I could hardly breathe with the excitement of the moment. Five weeks later, I was in an ambulance speeding to a medical center equipped to save my life. My ectopic pregnancy had not yet been diagnosed when it ruptured at home. I underwent surgery to remove my tube and the pregnancy that was contained within. Afterward, I was dazed and debilitated. For weeks I focused on my recovery rather than my loss. How ironic that I was fully confronted with the reality of my loss on what would have been my due date when in the mail I received a package of samples congratulating me on the birth of my new baby.

—Kristin, R.N.

Learning Outcomes

18.1 Delineate the bleeding problems associated with pregnancy.

18.2 Contrast the etiology, medical therapy, and nursing interventions for the various bleeding problems associated with pregnancy.

18.3 Discuss the medical therapy and nursing care of a woman with hyperemesis gravidarum.

18.4 Describe the maternal and fetal-neonatal risks, clinical manifestations, and nursing care of a pregnant woman with a hypertensive disorder.

18.5 Contrast the effects of various infections on the pregnant woman and her unborn child.

18.6 Summarize the risks and implications of surgical procedures performed during pregnancy.

18.7 Relate the impact of major trauma during pregnancy to the nursing care of the woman and her fetus.

18.8 Discuss the needs and care of the pregnant woman who suffers from intimate partner violence.

18.9 Explain the cause and prevention of hemolytic disease of the fetus and newborn (HDFN) secondary to Rh incompatibility.

18.10 Compare Rh incompatibility to ABO incompatibility with regard to occurrence, treatment, and implications for the fetus/newborn.

Healthy People 2020

(MICH-6) Reduce maternal illness and complications due to pregnancy (complications during hospitalized labor and delivery)

(MICH-5) Reduce the rate of maternal mortality

(BDBS-18.4) Reduce the proportions of persons who develop adverse events due to alloimmunization among persons with hemoglobinopathies

Pregnancy is usually a normal, uncomplicated experience. In some cases, however, problems arise during pregnancy that place the woman and her fetus at risk. Regular prenatal care serves to detect these potential complications quickly so that effective care can be provided. This chapter focuses on problems that primarily occur during pregnancy, those with a *gestational onset*. (Conditions such as diabetes and anemia, which may occur prior to pregnancy or develop during pregnancy, are discussed in Chapter 17.)

Care of the Woman at Risk Because of Bleeding During Pregnancy

During the first and early second trimesters of pregnancy the major cause of bleeding is **abortion**. Broadly, this is the expulsion of the products of conception before the age of viability, defined by the CDC and the World Health Organization as "pregnancy termination or loss before 20 weeks' gestation or with a fetus delivered weighing <500 g" (Cunningham et al., 2018, p. 346). Other complications that can cause bleeding in the first half of pregnancy (up to 20 weeks' gestation) are ectopic pregnancy, gestational trophoblastic disease, and trauma. In the second half of pregnancy, particularly in the third trimester, the two major causes of bleeding are placenta previa and abruptio placentae, although trauma should also be considered. Table 18–1 summarizes causes of bleeding by trimester of pregnancy.

General Principles of Nursing Intervention

Vaginal bleeding during pregnancy is relatively common and may or may not indicate a problem. Vaginal bleeding that does not threaten the pregnancy includes implantation bleeding, bleeding after sexual intercourse when tiny capillaries on the highly vascular cervix are disrupted, or bleeding from some vaginal or cervical lesions. Bleeding that occurs past the time of implantation and that is from the uterus is always suspicious. Pregnant women are advised to report any vaginal spotting or bleeding because it is not possible to know the cause or prognosis without further evaluation. Therefore, it is often the nurse's responsibility to make the initial assessment of bleeding. In general, the following nursing measures should be implemented for pregnant women being evaluated for bleeding:

- Monitor blood pressure and pulse frequently. The frequency is determined by the extent of the bleeding and the stability of the woman's condition.
- Observe the woman for indications of shock, such as changing vital signs, pallor, clammy skin, perspiration, dyspnea, or restlessness.
- Count and weigh pads to assess amount of bleeding over a given time period; save any tissue or clots expelled.
- Assess fetal heart tones with a Doppler if pregnancy is 12 weeks' gestation or beyond unless the loss is inevitable and hearing the heartbeat will only cause the mother more grief.
- Prepare for intravenous (IV) therapy. There may be standing orders to start IV therapy on women who are actively bleeding.
- Obtain an order to type and cross-match for blood if there is evidence of significant blood loss.
- Obtain an order for an obstetric ultrasound to confirm presence of the pregnancy in the uterus, location of the placenta, and viability of the fetus.
- Prepare equipment for examination and a possible intrauterine procedure: Good light source, sterile gloves, sterile speculum, ring forceps, curette, suction, and maintain NPO status.
- Have oxygen therapy available.
- Collect and organize all data, including antepartum history, onset of bleeding episode, any associated pain, laboratory studies (hemoglobin, hematocrit, Rh status, and beta-human chorionic gonadotropin [β-hCG] levels).
- Assess coping mechanisms and support system of the woman in crisis. Give emotional support to enhance her coping abilities by continuous, sustained presence, by clear explanation of procedures, and by communicating her status to her family. Most important, prepare the woman for possible fetal loss. Assess her expressions of anger, denial, guilt, depression, or self-blame.
- Assess the family's response to the situation.

Spontaneous Abortion (Miscarriage)

Abortion is the medical term used to describe both spontaneous and elective interruptions of a pregnancy. **Miscarriage** is a lay term applied to spontaneous abortion.

Overall, the incidence of spontaneous abortion ranges from 11 to 22%, 80% of which occur within the first 12 weeks. Over 50% of these early spontaneous miscarriages will be due to chromosomal abnormalities (Cunningham et al., 2018). Other causes of spontaneous abortion include teratogenic drugs, faulty implantation due to abnormalities of the female reproductive tract, a weakened cervix, placental abnormalities, chronic maternal diseases (autoimmune disorders, kidney disease), endocrine imbalances (thyroid disease, diabetes, obesity), and maternal infections (Simpson & Jauniaux, 2017). In late spontaneous abortion (greater than 13 weeks), the cause is usually a maternal factor, for example, cervical insufficiency or maternal disease. (See Chapter 23 for discussion of cervical insufficiency.) In all cases, vaginal bleeding is usually the number one sign/symptom.

Spontaneous abortion is generally extremely distressing to the couple desiring a child. Chances for carrying the next pregnancy to term after one spontaneous abortion are as good as they are for the general population. Thereafter, however, chances of successful pregnancy decrease with each succeeding and consecutive abortion with the same partner. Following two to three consecutive losses, a woman and her partner should be evaluated by a genetic counselor.

TABLE 18–1 Pregnancy-Related Bleeding by Trimester

FIRST TRIMESTER (0 TO 12 6/7 WEEKS' GESTATION)	SECOND TRIMESTER (13 TO 27 6/7 WEEKS' GESTATION)		THIRD TRIMESTER (28 WEEKS' GESTATION TO BIRTH)
	Less than 20 weeks	**More than 20 weeks**	
Early spontaneous abortion	Late spontaneous abortion	Preterm labor	Preterm labor
Induced abortion	Induced abortion	Trauma (abdominal, genital)	Labor
Ectopic pregnancy	Gestational trophoblastic disease	Placentation problems: Previa; abruptio	Trauma (abdominal, genital)
Gestational trophoblastic disease	Trauma (abdominal, genital)		Placentation problems: Previa; abruptio
Trauma: Uterine, cervical, vaginal			
Cervical friability (easy to bleed)			

CLASSIFICATION

Abortions are subdivided into criteria as described in Table 18–2.

CLINICAL THERAPY

One of the more reliable indicators of a threatened spontaneous abortion is the presence of pelvic cramping and backache. These symptoms are usually absent in bleeding caused by polyps or ruptured cervical blood vessels.

Vaginal bleeding occurs in almost one-fourth of first-trimester pregnancies. Of these, approximately half will result in subsequent miscarriage (Cunningham et al., 2018). Several days of spotting or light bleeding associated with pain may also increase the chance of miscarriage. Painless spotting or light bleeding for a day or two does not increase the risk of miscarriage above the risk for women with no bleeding.

Evaluations to help determine the cause of vaginal bleeding include a speculum examination to determine the presence of cervical polyps or cervical erosion, ultrasound scanning for the presence of a gestational sac or a fetal crown–rump length (CRL) with cardiac activity, and serial β-hCG levels. Presence of a fetal heartbeat on ultrasound provides a high likelihood of the pregnancy continuing. Laboratory determination of a positive β-hCG level can confirm a pregnancy, but because the level falls slowly after fetal death, it cannot confirm a live embryo/fetus. If necessary, serial β-hCG serum levels should be compared for a rise or decline every 48 hours. Hemoglobin and hematocrit levels are obtained to assess blood loss. Blood is typed and cross-matched for possible replacement needs.

Although there is no evidence that supports the value of restricting physical activity, the therapy prescribed for the pregnant woman with bleeding often includes bedrest and abstinence from coitus. If bleeding persists and abortion is imminent or incomplete, the woman may be hospitalized, IV therapy or blood transfusions may be started to replace fluid, and dilation and curettage (D&C) and/or suction evacuation is performed to remove the remainder of the products of conception. If the woman is Rh negative and not alloimmunized, Rh immune globulin (e.g., RhoGAM) is given within 72 hours. (See discussion of Rh alloimmunization later in this chapter.)

TABLE 18–2 Classification of Abortions and Defining Characteristics

TYPE OF ABORTION	DEFINING CHARACTERISTICS
Clinically silent abortion, "silent miscarriage," chemical pregnancy	Loss of a pregnancy after implantation, evidence of a positive pregnancy test, but no clinical recognition via ultrasound. The woman often experiences this as a late-timed menses.
Early abortion	Abortion that occurs during the first trimester.
Late abortion	Abortion that occurs before 20 weeks' gestation or 500 grams, but after 12 6/7 weeks.
Elective abortion	Interruption of a pregnancy per choice of the woman; often called *therapeutic abortion (TAB).*
Therapeutic abortion (TAB)	Interruption of a pregnancy for the health of the woman.
Spontaneous abortion	Natural expulsion of the pregnancy from a woman's body.
Threatened abortion (Figure 18–1A)	Unexplained vaginal bleeding, cramping, or backache. Bleeding may persist for days. The cervix is closed and no tissue has been expelled.
Inevitable or imminent abortion (Figure 18–1B)	Vaginal bleeding and intense cramping as the internal cervical os dilates. There is possible rupture of membranes and expulsion of tissue.
Complete abortion	Expulsion of the entire pregnancy. The uterus is contracted and the cervical os may be closed.
Incomplete abortion (Figure 18–1C)	Expulsion of part of the pregnancy, but the placenta may be retained. The internal cervical os is dilated. Due to continued bleeding, a surgical procedure is often required to evacuate the uterus completely.
Missed abortion	The dead fetus is not expelled. Uterine growth ceases, breast changes regress, and the woman may report a brownish vaginal discharge. The cervix is closed. Diagnosis is made based on history, pelvic examination, and a drop in serum β-hCG levels and is confirmed by ultrasound revealing a fetus without a heartbeat. If the fetus is retained beyond 4 weeks, fetal autolysis (breakdown of cells or tissue) may result in the release of thromboplastin, and disseminated intravascular coagulation may develop. Medical or surgical evacuation of the uterus may be necessary.
Empty sac (preferred term), anembryonic pregnancy, blighted ovum	Ultrasound confirmation of a pregnancy without a fetus; the fetus stopped developing very early or never developed. This scenario may be associated with a *molar* pregnancy.
Recurrent pregnancy loss (RPL), formerly called *habitual abortion*	Early abortions that occur *consecutively* in two or three pregnancies with the same male partner/sperm donor.
Septic abortion	There is presence of infection; may occur with prolonged and unrecognized rupture of the membranes, pregnancy with an intrauterine device in utero, or attempts by inadequately prepared individuals to terminate a pregnancy. Septic abortion is less common since the availability of legal abortion.

SOURCE: Data from Simpson & Jauniaux, 2017.

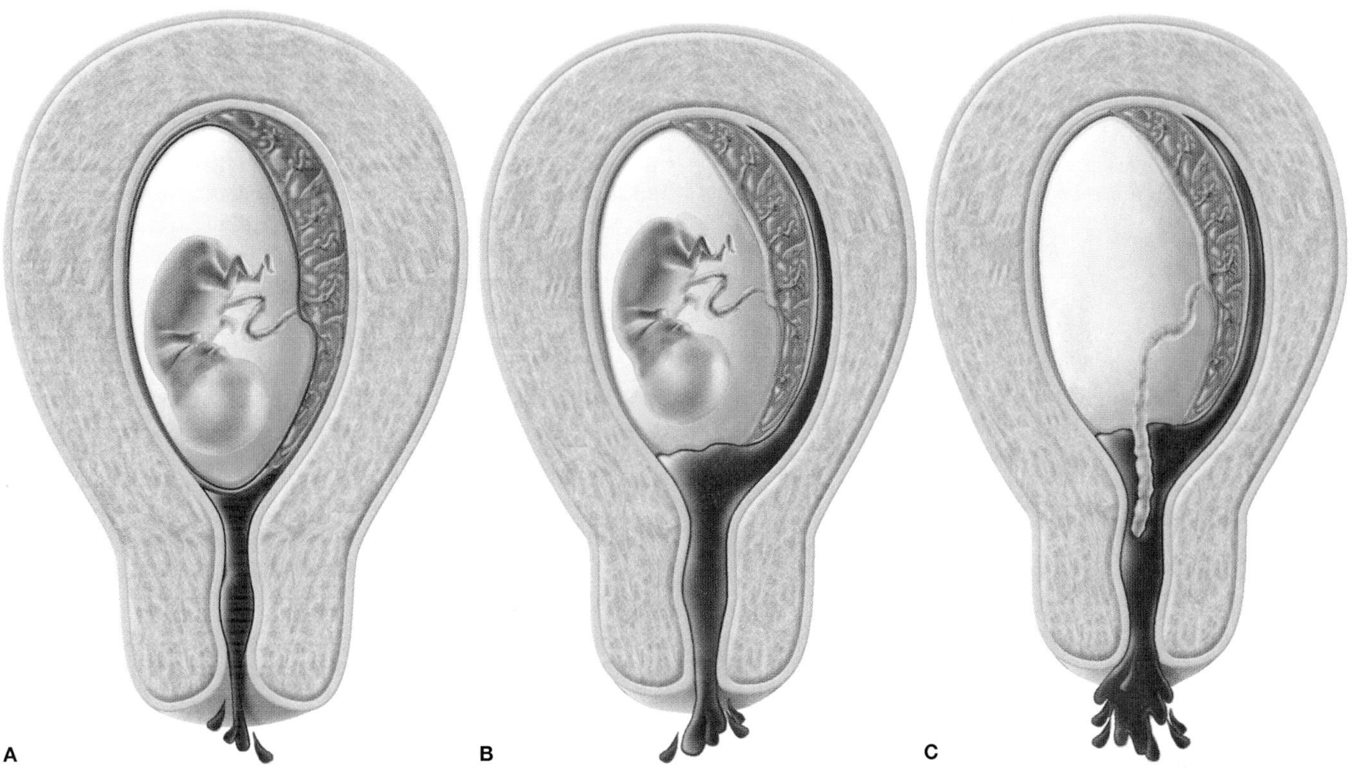

Figure 18–1 Types of spontaneous abortion. A. Threatened. The cervix is not dilated, and the placenta is still attached to the uterine wall, but some bleeding occurs. B. Imminent. The placenta has separated from the uterine wall, the cervix has dilated, and the amount of bleeding has increased. C. Incomplete. The embryo/fetus has passed out of the uterus; however, the placenta remains.

In missed abortions, the products of conception are usually expelled spontaneously. If this does not occur within 1 month to 6 weeks after fetal death, an intervention may be necessary. Medical management with misoprostol or surgical management with D&C and/or suction is offered if the pregnancy is in the first trimester. Beyond 12 weeks' gestation, dilation and evacuation or induction of labor by IV oxytocin and intra-amniotic prostaglandin $F_{2\alpha}$, intravaginal prostaglandin E_2, or misoprostol (a synthetic prostaglandin E_1 analog) may be required to expel the dead fetus.

NURSING MANAGEMENT

For the Woman Experiencing Spontaneous Abortion

Nursing Assessment and Diagnosis

Assess the amount and appearance of any vaginal bleeding and monitor the woman's vital signs and degree of discomfort. Identify the woman's blood type, Rh factor, and antibody status to determine the need for Rh immune globulin. If the pregnancy is 10 to 12 weeks or more, fetal heart rate should be assessed by Doppler unless the loss is inevitable. Also assess the responses of the woman and her family to this crisis and evaluate their coping mechanisms and ability to comfort each other.

Nursing diagnoses that may apply include:

- *Childbearing Process, Ineffective,* related to inability to carry fetus to term
- *Fear* related to the risk of pregnancy loss
- *Fluid Volume: Risk for Deficient,* related to excessive bleeding secondary to spontaneous abortion

(NANDA-I © 2017)

Nursing Plan and Implementation

Community-Based Nursing Care

If a woman in her first trimester of pregnancy begins cramping or spotting and the bleeding is not heavy, she may be evaluated on an outpatient basis. An important aspect of nursing care is providing emotional support for women who are undergoing a miscarriage or who have aborted spontaneously. Couples who approached the pregnancy with feelings of joy and a sense of expectancy now feel grief, sadness, and possibly anger.

Because many women, even with planned pregnancies, feel some ambivalence initially, guilt is a common emotion. The woman may harbor negative feelings about herself, ranging from lowered self-esteem resulting from a belief that she is lacking the ability to reproduce or is otherwise abnormal in some way, to a notion that the abortion may be a punishment for some wrongdoing.

Invaluable psychologic support can be offered to the woman and her family by encouraging them to verbalize their feelings. Reflective listening gives the woman an opportunity to express and explore her feelings. Take cues from questions the woman asks, discuss the grief cycle, and provide resources. Referrals can help the woman and her family find ways to deal with their loss. If the woman has older children, she may need guidance on how to help them understand and cope with what has occurred. Commemorating the pregnancy and the fetus as a "baby" is helpful in validating the significance of the loss. The grieving period following a spontaneous abortion usually lasts 6 to 24 months. Many couples can be helped during this period by an organization or support group established for parents who have lost a fetus or newborn.

Developing Cultural Competence Culture and Response to Fetal Loss

Remember that individual responses to fetal loss following miscarriage may vary greatly and may be influenced by ethnic or cultural norms.

- Miscarriage may be viewed in many ways. For example, it may be seen as a punishment from God, as the result of the "evil eye" or of a hex or curse by an enemy, or as a natural part of life.
- When grieving over a pregnancy loss, women from some cultures and ethnic groups may show their emotions freely, crying and wailing, whereas other women may hide their feelings behind a mask of stoicism.
- In some cultures, the woman's partner is her primary source of support and comfort. In others, the woman turns to her mother or close female relatives for comfort.
- Avoid stereotyping women according to culture. Individual responses are influenced by many factors, including the degree of assimilation into the dominant culture and degree of attachment to the pregnancy.

Note: It is unwise to attribute specific attitudes or beliefs to all members of a cultural group. The information in the Developing Cultural Competence boxes offers possible insights into caring for women from different cultural groups.

"I was stunned by the depth of loss I felt following my miscarriage when I was 2½ months along. It didn't seem possible that I had already become so emotionally attached to the baby I carried. Afterward I was surprised by the number of women I knew who shared stories of their own miscarriages and confirmed that the emotions I was feeling were normal, if painful."

The physical pain of the cramps and the amount of bleeding may be more severe than a couple anticipates, even when they are prepared for the possibility of a miscarriage. Be aware that couples feel unprepared for their first experience of spontaneous abortion. Offer support in dealing with the physical experience by explaining why the discomfort is occurring and by offering analgesics for pain relief.

Hospital-Based Nursing Care

A D&C with suction is performed if the woman experiences an incomplete or missed abortion. This can be performed on an outpatient basis, and, barring any complications, the woman can return home a few hours after the procedure with instructions for self-care. A woman who is Rh negative and not alloimmunized (has a negative antibody screen) should be given Rh immune globulin before discharge.

Throughout the procedure, monitor the woman's physical status and provide emotional support. Answer any questions the woman or her partner may have and provide referrals to community agencies for grief support or family planning options as needed.

Health Promotion

If the woman had a D&C, someone should remain with her for the first 12 to 24 hours. Instruct the woman to report to her healthcare provider all episodes of heavy bleeding, fever, chills, foul-smelling vaginal discharge, or abdominal tenderness. The woman who experiences a pregnancy loss requires information about possible causes of the loss and the chances of recurrence with a future pregnancy. She may also require information about the grief process so she is prepared for it when she goes home. In addition, provide information about available resources, including support groups to help her cope with her feelings related to the loss of the pregnancy. The woman's partner or a family member should be included in the educational process when possible to assist him or her in personal grief work, as well as to provide tools to help support the woman through the loss.

Evaluation

Expected outcomes of nursing care include:

- The woman is able to explain spontaneous abortion, the treatment measures employed in her care, and long-term implications for future pregnancies.
- The woman suffers no complications or unforeseen complications are mitigated early.
- The woman and her partner are able to begin verbalizing their grief and to recognize that the grieving process can last months.

Pregnancy of Unknown Location

Pregnancy of unknown location (PUL) is the term used when a pregnant woman undergoes an ultrasound without a definitive finding of either an intrauterine pregnancy or an ectopic pregnancy. It is not a diagnosis but is considered an interim finding and every effort should be made to determine the correct diagnosis (American College of Obstetricians and Gynecologists [ACOG], 2018c). It occurs in 8 to 31% of early pregnancies (Fields & Hathaway, 2016).

Ectopic Pregnancy

Ectopic pregnancy (EP), also called *extrauterine pregnancy* or *tubal pregnancy*, is the implantation of a fertilized ovum in a site other than the endometrial lining of the uterus. It may result from a number of different causes. Risk factors for ectopic pregnancy include tubal damage caused by pelvic inflammatory disease (PID) from a sexually transmitted infection or mixed bacterial infection; previous pelvic or tubal surgery; endometriosis; previous ectopic pregnancy; presence of an intrauterine device (IUD); high levels of progesterone, which can alter the motility of the egg in the fallopian tube; congenital anomalies of the tube; use of ovulation-inducing drugs; primary infertility; smoking; and advanced maternal age. Symptoms of an EP begin between 6 and 8 weeks' gestational age (after the last menstrual period). Ectopic pregnancy occurs in about 0.5 to 1.5% of pregnancies in the United States and accounts for 3% of all pregnancy-related deaths (Cunningham et al., 2018). See *Evidence-Based Practice: Ectopic Pregnancy*.

An ectopic pregnancy can implant in the fallopian tube, ovary, peritoneal cavity, cervix, or uterine cornua (Figure 18–2) and occurs when the fertilized ovum is prevented or slowed in its journey down the fallopian tube to the endometrial cavity. About 95% of all EPs implant in various portions of the fallopian tube; 70% implant in the ampulla of the tube (Cunningham et al., 2018). A tubal EP is usually resolved by medical or surgical treatment by the end of the first trimester (12 6/7 gestational weeks), hopefully before the fallopian tube ruptures. Although rare, EPs can proceed to later gestations if implanted in the abdominal cavity.

EVIDENCE-BASED PRACTICE | Ectopic Pregnancy

Clinical Question

What is best practice in diagnosing and treating an ectopic pregnancy?

The Evidence

An ectopic pregnancy is one that occurs outside the uterine cavity. The most common site for an ectopic pregnancy is in the fallopian tube. If these pregnancies progress to the point of rupture, they account for significant morbidity and even maternal death. Suspicion of an ectopic pregnancy, then, is considered a medical emergency. If detected early, ectopic pregnancy can be effectively treated with surgical or pharmacological intervention. More than half of women who receive a diagnosis of ectopic pregnancy do not have any known risk factors. Those at highest risk are those with a previous ectopic pregnancy, damaged fallopian tubes, ascending pelvic infection, or prior pelvic or fallopian tube surgery. Contrary to a widely held belief, women who use an IUD for contraception are at a *lower risk* of ectopic pregnancy because of the effectiveness of this contraceptive method. However, if a woman with an IUD in place becomes pregnant, more than half will have an ectopic pregnancy. No other contraceptive methods have been associated with extrauterine pregnancy (ACOG, 2018c).

The American College of Obstetricians and Gynecologists (2018c) reviewed the evidence related to the diagnosis and treatment of ectopic pregnancy and updated their existing practice guidelines. This type of guideline, created by a professional medical organization evaluating and integrating evidence from randomized trials, systematic reviews, and the opinions of clinical experts, is the strongest evidence for practice.

Every sexually active reproductive-age woman who presents with abdominal pain and bleeding should be screened for pregnancy, regardless of whether she believes she is pregnant. Rupture of an ectopic pregnancy can occur very early in a pregnancy, even before the woman suspects she is pregnant. If a woman is pregnant and presents with an acute abdomen, including severe pain of unknown origin, the minimum diagnostic evaluation is a transvaginal ultrasound evaluation and confirmation of pregnancy through serum hCG-level measurement. However, serum hCG alone cannot be used to diagnose an ectopic pregnancy. The absence of a possible gestational sac on ultrasound examination in the presence of a positive hCG measurement strongly suggests a nonviable gestation. In 50 to 70% of these cases, these findings are consistent with ectopic pregnancy (ACOG, 2018c).

Treatment of a confirmed ectopic pregnancy that has not ruptured may be via laparoscopic surgery or intramuscular administration of methotrexate. Both treatments are safe and effective. The decision for surgical or medical management is guided by clinician assessment as well as patient-informed choice. Surgical management is required if the patient is experiencing hemodynamic instability, symptoms of a ruptured ectopic mass, or signs of intraperitoneal bleeding (ACOG, 2018c).

Best Practice

Women who present with acute abdominal pain and bleeding should be screened for pregnancy. If hCG levels are elevated, then a transvaginal ultrasound is indicated to determine if an ectopic pregnancy exists. An ectopic pregnancy constitutes a medical emergency, as rupture of the fallopian tubes is associated with significant morbidity and mortality. Best practice in treatment of ectopic pregnancy includes laparoscopic surgery or administration of methotrexate. Women suffering from ectopic pregnancy can be counseled that both treatments are safe and effective (ACOG, 2018c).

Clinical Reasoning

What elements of a nursing history could raise suspicion about the potential for an ectopic pregnancy? What questions should be asked of every woman who presents with acute abdominal pain?

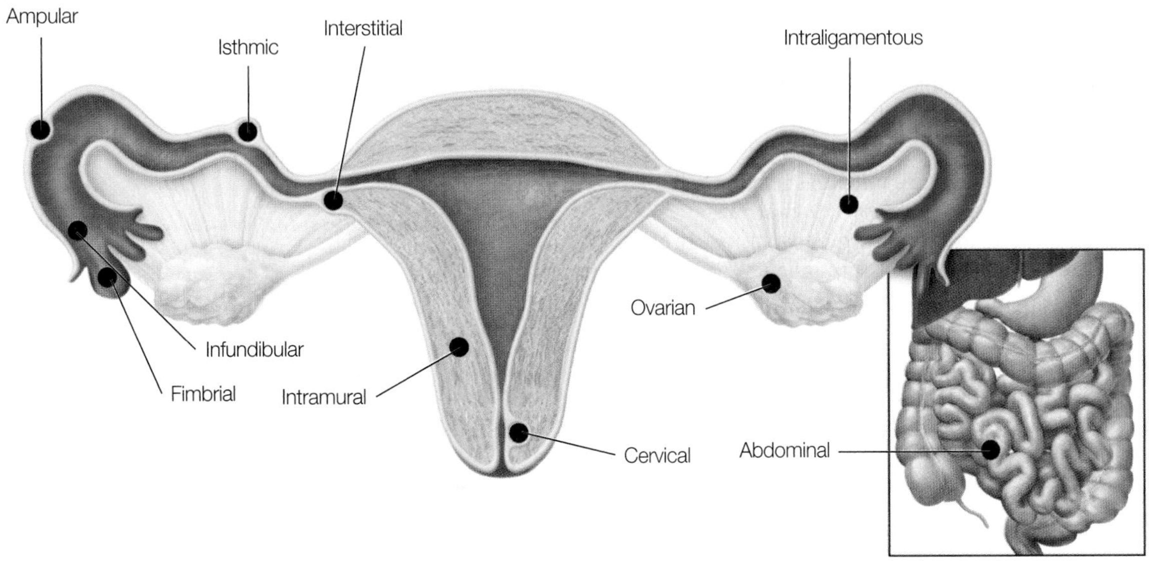

Figure 18–2 Various implantation sites in ectopic pregnancy. The most common site is within the fallopian tube, hence the name *tubal pregnancy*.

Initially, the expected symptoms of pregnancy may be present, specifically, amenorrhea, breast tenderness, and nausea. The hormone β-hCG is present in the blood and urine. With an ectopic implantation, the trophoblastic cells grow into the adjacent tissue, often the tubal wall, and arterial vessels. The faulty implantation of the placenta causes fluctuation of hormone levels. Hormones first stimulate the endometrial lining of the uterus to grow, but fluctuation in levels cannot support the endometrium and vaginal bleeding ensues. When the embryo outgrows this space, the tube ruptures and there is bleeding into the abdominal cavity. The woman may experience one-sided lower abdominal pain or diffuse lower abdominal pain and vasomotor disturbances such as fainting or dizziness. In about 50% of cases, referred right shoulder pain occurs from blood irritating the subdiaphragmatic phrenic nerve. In many instances, however, the symptoms are not obvious (Cunningham et al., 2018).

Physical examination usually reveals adnexal (area over each ovary and fallopian tube) tenderness. An adnexal mass is palpable 50% of the time. With bleeding into the abdominal cavity, pelvic examination is very painful, and a mass of blood may be palpated in the lower abdomen. Bleeding is slow and chronic, and the abdomen gradually becomes rigid and very tender. Laboratory tests may reveal low hemoglobin and hematocrit levels and rising leukocyte levels. In a normal pregnancy, β-hCG levels rise at least 35% and may double every 48 to 72 hours from 4 to 6 weeks' gestation and then peak at 10 weeks' gestation. Ectopic pregnancies are associated with β-hCG levels that do not rise as expected. Serial β-hCG serum levels are typically drawn every 2 to 3 days for comparison until the diagnosis of an intrauterine or extrauterine/ectopic pregnancy is confirmed by ultrasound.

CLINICAL THERAPY

It is important to differentiate an ectopic pregnancy from other disorders with similar clinical presenting pictures. Consideration must be given to possible spontaneous abortion, ruptured corpus luteum cyst, appendicitis, salpingitis, torsion of the ovary, ovarian cysts, and urinary tract infection.

The following measures are used to establish the diagnosis of ectopic pregnancy and assess the woman's status:

- A careful assessment of menstrual history, particularly the last menstrual period (LMP), is completed.
- A pelvic exam is performed to identify any abnormal pelvic masses and tenderness.
- Laboratory testing is completed: Serial β-hCG levels every 24 to 72 hours, complete blood count (CBC), type and Rh factor, antibody screen.
- Transvaginal ultrasound is the initial test of choice to detect an intrauterine pregnancy or an adnexal mass (ACOG, 2018c). Confirming an intrauterine pregnancy nearly always eliminates the diagnosis of ectopic pregnancy.
- Serial measurements of serum β-hCG values are taken, which should increase significantly every 2 to 3 days. Women with an ectopic pregnancy often have serial serum hCG values that increase more slowly than expected with a viable intrauterine pregnancy (Mensah & Yates, 2015).
- Laparoscopic intervention may be necessary for both diagnosis and treatment.

Treatment may be medical or surgical. Medical treatment with intramuscular methotrexate can be offered if the woman is stable, has a confirmed diagnosis (or strong clinical suspicion) of ectopic pregnancy, an unruptured mass, and no absolute contraindications to methotrexate administration (ACOG, 2018c).

Methotrexate is a folic acid antagonist that interferes with the proliferation of rapidly dividing cells such as trophoblastic cells. It is administered intramuscularly (IM) in one of three ways (ACOG, 2018c):

1. Single-dose regimen—50 mg/m^2 IM
2. Two-dose regimen—50 mg/m^2 IM administered on days 1 and 4
3. Fixed multiple-dose regimen—1 mg/kg methotrexate IM administered on days 1, 3, 5, and 7 plus 0.1 mg/kg leucovorin IM on days 2, 4, 6, and 8.

The multidose regimen is far more care intensive and is reserved for patients who present with high levels of β-hCG.

When methotrexate is administered on an outpatient basis, the woman is monitored for increasing abdominal pain and serial β-hCG values are evaluated for declining levels. β-hCG values are assessed on day 4 and day 7. If β-hCG levels do not decrease at least 15% from day 4 to day 7 after the initial injection, an additional dose of methotrexate is given (in the one-dose or two-dose regimen) or surgical intervention may be necessary (ACOG, 2018c).

If surgery is indicated and the woman desires future pregnancies, a laparoscopic linear salpingostomy will be performed to gently evacuate the ectopic pregnancy and preserve the tube. If the tube is ruptured or if future childbearing is not an issue, laparoscopic salpingectomy (removal of the tube) is performed. If the woman is in shock and unstable, an abdominal incision will be made (laparotomy). During surgery, the most important risk to be considered is potential hemorrhage. Bleeding must be controlled, and intravascular replacement therapy should be on hand. The Rh-negative, nonalloimmunized woman is given prophylactic Rh immune globulin.

●○● NURSING MANAGEMENT

For the Woman with an Ectopic Pregnancy

Nursing Assessment and Diagnosis

When the woman with a suspected ectopic pregnancy is admitted to the hospital, assess the appearance and amount of vaginal bleeding. Monitor vital signs, particularly blood pressure and pulse, for evidence of developing shock.

It is important to assess the woman's emotional status and coping abilities and to evaluate the couple's informational needs. If surgery is necessary, perform the ongoing assessments appropriate for any pre/postoperative patient, especially maintaining a status of NPO.

Nursing diagnoses that may apply for a woman with an ectopic pregnancy include:

- ***Childbearing Process, Ineffective***, related to inability to carry fetus to term
- ***Fear*** related to the risk of pregnancy loss
- ***Pain, Acute***, related to abdominal cramping secondary to threatened abortion
- ***Fluid Volume: Risk for Deficient***, related to excessive bleeding secondary to spontaneous abortion

(NANDA-I © 2017)

Nursing Plan and Implementation

Community-Based Nursing Care

Women with ectopic pregnancy are often seen initially in a clinic or office setting. Be alert to the possibility of ectopic pregnancy if a woman presents with complaints of abdominal pain and lack of menses for 1 to 2 months. Once an initial evaluation is complete, if no ultrasound is available, the woman should be referred to a facility where ultrasound is available. The nurse plays an important role in monitoring the woman's condition and providing patient education.

A woman with a confirmed ectopic pregnancy who meets the criteria for methotrexate administration is followed as an outpatient. Advise the woman that some abdominal pain is common following the injection but it is generally mild and lasts only 24 to 48 hours. More severe pain might indicate treatment failure and should be evaluated. The woman should also report heavy vaginal bleeding, dizziness, or tachycardia. In addition, the need to return for follow-up serial β-hCG levels every 48 to 72 hours should be stressed. Nausea from the treatment is expected.

For all women treated for ectopic pregnancy, a follow-up phone call in between office visits may be especially welcome. It gives the woman the opportunity to ask any questions she may have. In addition, the phone call can give you the opportunity to assist the woman in dealing with her grief.

Hospital-Based Nursing Care

Once a diagnosis of ectopic pregnancy is made and surgery is scheduled, start an IV as ordered and begin preoperative teaching. Report signs of developing shock to the physician immediately and initiate interventions. If the woman is experiencing severe abdominal pain, administer appropriate analgesics and evaluate their effectiveness.

Health Promotion

Teaching is an important part of nursing care. The woman may want her condition and various procedures explained. She may need instruction about measures to prevent infection, symptoms to report (pain, bleeding, fever, chills), and her follow-up visit. The woman needs to understand that she is at increased risk of ectopic pregnancy with a subsequent pregnancy. Thus it is important for her to seek early pregnancy confirmation and access to prenatal care.

The woman and her family will need emotional support during this difficult time. Their feelings and responses to this crisis will probably be similar to those that occur in cases of spontaneous abortion. As a result, similar nursing actions are required.

Evaluation

Expected outcomes of nursing care include:

- The woman is able to explain ectopic pregnancy, treatment alternatives, and implications for future childbearing.
- The woman and her caregivers detect possible complications early and manage them appropriately.
- The woman and her partner are able to begin verbalizing their loss and recognize that the grieving process usually lasts several months.

Gestational Trophoblastic Disease

Gestational trophoblastic disease (GTD), a collection of disorders, is often referred to as a *molar pregnancy* (*mole* means growth of cells). It is the pathologic proliferation of trophoblastic cells (the trophoblast is the outermost layer of embryonic cells). In the United States, the incidence is approximately 1 in 1000 to 1 in 1500 pregnancies and includes molar pregnancies with chorionic villi (complete and partial) and nonmolar neoplasms without chorionic villi (choriocarcinoma, placental site trophoblastic tumor, epitheliod trophoblastic tumor) (Salani & Copeland, 2017).

Hydatidiform mole (molar pregnancy) is a condition in which a proliferation of trophoblastic cells results in the formation of an abnormal placenta characterized by *hydropic* (fluid-filled) grapelike clusters. The significance of this disease for the woman is the loss of the pregnancy and the possibility, though remote, of the development of pregnancy cancer, called *choriocarcinoma*.

Molar pregnancies are classified into two types, complete and partial. Little is known about the cause of either type, but some of the pathophysiology has been clarified.

The *complete mole* develops from an anuclear ovum that contains no maternal genetic material, an "empty" egg. In most cases, a haploid sperm, 23X, fertilizes this anuclear egg and duplicates before the first cell division (diploidy). The conceptus then contains in its cells a 46, XX chromosomal set of only paternal origin (Ngan et al., 2015). The hydropic vesicles that form from the chorionic villi are avascular in the complete mole. No embryonic or fetal tissue or membranes are found. Choriocarcinoma is more commonly associated with the complete mole (Ngan et al., 2015).

The *partial mole* usually has a triploid karyotype, that is, 69 chromosomes. Most often, a normal ovum with 23 chromosomes is fertilized by two sperm (dispermy) or by a sperm that has failed to undergo the first meiosis and therefore contains 46 chromosomes. Unlike the complete mole, identifiable fetal parts may be present.

CLINICAL THERAPY

Diagnosis of hydatidiform mole is often suspected in the presence of the following signs:

- Vaginal bleeding is almost universal with molar pregnancies and may occur as early as the fourth week or as late as the second trimester. It is often brownish, "like prune juice," because of liquefaction of the uterine clot, but it may be bright red.
- Anemia occurs frequently because of the loss of blood.
- Hydropic vesicles may be passed and, if so, are diagnostic (Figure 18–3). With a partial mole, the vesicles are often smaller and may not be noticed by the woman. Hydropic vesicles have a "skinned grape" appearance.

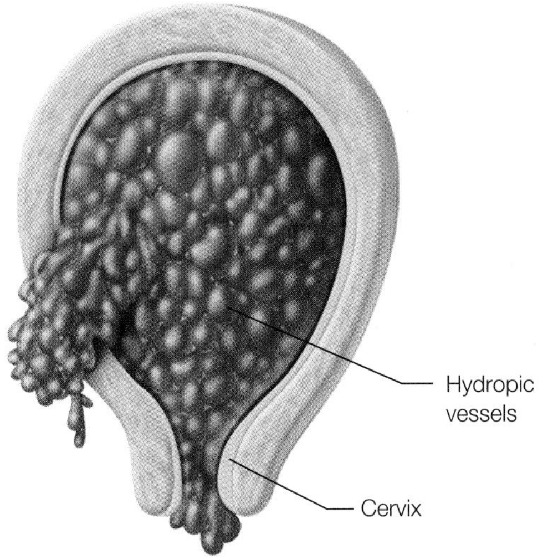

Figure 18–3 Hydatidiform mole. A common sign is vaginal bleeding, often brownish (the characteristic "prune juice" appearance) but sometimes bright red. In this figure, some of the hydropic vessels are being passed. This occurrence is diagnostic for hydatidiform mole.

- Uterine enlargement greater than expected for gestational age is a classic sign with complete moles, present in about 50% of cases. In the remainder of cases, the uterus is appropriate or small for gestational age. Enlargement is due to the proliferating trophoblastic tissue and to a large amount of clotted blood.
- Absence of fetal heart sounds in the presence of other signs of pregnancy is a classic sign of molar pregnancy. (Only rarely has a viable fetus been born in a partial molar pregnancy.)
- Markedly elevated serum β-hCG levels (hundreds of thousands) may be present because of continued secretion by the proliferating trophoblastic tissue.
- Very low levels of α-fetoprotein in the maternal serum (MSAFP) are found because there is no fetus.
- Hyperemesis gravidarum may occur, probably as a result of the high β-hCG levels.
- Preeclampsia (discussed shortly) may be seen, especially if the molar pregnancy continues into the second trimester. Because preeclampsia is a disease of late pregnancy, if symptoms occur in the first half of pregnancy, molar pregnancy must be considered.

Complete and partial hydatidiform molar pregnancies are usually diagnosed in the first trimester with transvaginal ultrasound and serial β-hCG serum levels that are higher than expected for a normal pregnancy. Therapy begins with dilation of the cervix and suction evacuation of the molar pregnancy and curettage of the uterus to remove all fragments of the placenta. Rh immune globulin is administered to nonalloimmunized women who are Rh negative.

Complications associated with hydatidiform mole that require medical recognition and therapy include:

- Anemia (related to blood loss)
- Hyperthyroidism (related to excessive stimulation of the thyroid gland from β-hCG)
- Infection, usually seen with late diagnosis and spontaneous abortion of the molar pregnancy
- Disseminated intravascular coagulation (DIC)
- Trophoblastic embolization of the lung, usually seen after molar evacuation of a significantly enlarged uterus (this creates a cardiorespiratory emergency)
- Ovarian cysts, which may be small or large enough to displace the uterus (due to excessive β-hCG stimulation)

Because of the risk of choriocarcinoma, the woman treated for hydatidiform mole should receive extensive follow-up. Follow-up care includes a baseline chest x-ray to detect lung metastasis and a physical examination, including a pelvic examination. Approaches to ongoing monitoring vary somewhat. Typically, serum β-hCG levels are monitored weekly until negative results are obtained three consecutive times, then monthly for 6 to 12 months (ACOG, 2016a; Ngan et al., 2015). The woman should avoid pregnancy during this time because the elevated β-hCG levels associated with a new pregnancy will cause confusion as to whether a choriocarcinoma cancer has developed. If, after a year of monitoring, the β-hCG serum levels have remained negative without a subsequent pregnancy intervening, a couple may be assured that a normal pregnancy can be anticipated, with a low risk of recurring hydatidiform mole.

If β-hCG levels plateau for 3 consecutive weeks, or should the levels rise, pregnancy must be ruled out. If the woman is not pregnant, she should be evaluated for metastatic disease and treated appropriately (ACOG, 2016a; Ngan et al., 2015).

●○● NURSING MANAGEMENT

For the Woman with Gestational Trophoblastic Disease

Nursing Assessment and Diagnosis

It is important for nurses involved in antepartum care to be aware of symptoms of hydatidiform mole and observe for them at each antepartum visit. The classic symptoms used to diagnose molar pregnancy are found more frequently with the complete mole than with the partial mole. The partial mole may be difficult to distinguish from a missed abortion before evacuation of the uterus.

When the woman is hospitalized for evacuation of the molar pregnancy, monitor vital signs and vaginal bleeding for evidence of hemorrhage, and determine whether abdominal pain is present. Assess the woman's emotional state and coping ability.

Nursing diagnoses that may apply to a woman with a hydatidiform mole include:

- *Childbearing Process, Ineffective*, related to becoming pregnant but not carrying a fetus
- *Fear* related to the risk of development of a gestational cancer
- *Knowledge, Readiness for Enhanced*, related to an expressed desire to understand the need for regular monitoring of β-hCG levels and the long-term implications of the disease

(NANDA-I © 2017)

Nursing Plan and Implementation

Community-Based Nursing Care

If a molar pregnancy is diagnosed, it is important to support the family as they deal with their grief about the loss of a pregnancy. Healthcare counselors, the hospital chaplain, or their own clergy may be of assistance in helping them deal with this loss.

Hospital-Based Nursing Care

When the woman is hospitalized for evacuation of the molar pregnancy, explain that the curettage procedure is necessary. Although the physician is responsible for providing this explanation, the woman and her partner may have many questions and concerns. Discuss their concerns with them and clarify any areas of confusion or misunderstanding.

Typed and cross-matched blood must be available for surgery because of previous blood loss and the potential for hemorrhage. Oxytocin is administered to keep the uterus contracted and prevent hemorrhage. In addition, acute renal failure, a syndrome of rapid onset, may occur when significant hemorrhage results in absolute loss of intravascular fluid volume. Following surgery, carefully observe the woman's urinary output, watch for further signs of bleeding, and assess for any signs of infection.

If the woman is Rh negative and not alloimmunized, she is given prophylactic Rh immune globulin. (See discussion on Rh alloimmunization later in this chapter.) The woman needs to know the importance of all follow-up visits for 1 year. Advise her to use highly effective contraception (preferably a long-acting reversible contraception [LARC] method) for 1 year to delay becoming pregnant again until completion of the follow-up program.

Evaluation

Expected outcomes of nursing care include:

- The woman has a smooth recovery following successful evacuation of the molar pregnancy.
- The woman is able to explain GTD, its treatment, follow-up, and long-term implications for pregnancy.
- The woman and her partner are able to begin verbalizing their grief at the loss of their anticipated child.
- The woman is able to discuss the importance of follow-up assessment and indicates her willingness to cooperate with the regimen.

Care of the Woman with Hyperemesis Gravidarum

Hyperemesis gravidarum is a relatively rare condition in which nausea and vomiting are so severe that they affect hydration and nutritional status (ACOG, 2018b). Dehydration, electrolyte imbalances, acidosis, weight loss, ketonuria, and, possibly, hepatic and renal damage are attributable to hyperemesis.

Hyperemesis occurs more frequently in nulliparous women, adolescents, women with a multiple gestation, women with increased body weight, pregnancies complicated by GTD, women whose fetuses have congenital abnormalities, women with a mother or sister who experienced hyperemesis, and women with a history of hyperemesis in a previous pregnancy (ACOG, 2018b).

The cause of hyperemesis during pregnancy is still unclear, but it has been suggested that β-hCG plays a role. Higher levels of estradiol have also been implicated (ACOG, 2018b). Other mechanisms that may relate to hyperemesis are displacement of the gastrointestinal tract, hypofunction of the anterior pituitary gland and adrenal cortex, abnormalities of the corpus luteum, and psychologic factors. Recent studies suggest a correlation between hyperemesis and *Helicobacter pylori* infection, a common cause of gastric and duodenal ulcers (Niemeijer et al., 2014).

In severe cases, hyperemesis causes dehydration, which leads to fluid–electrolyte imbalance and alkalosis from the loss of hydrochloric acid. More prolonged vomiting can result in loss of predominantly alkaline intestinal juices and the occurrence of acidosis. Hypovolemia from dehydration and decreased urine output leads to hypotension and increased pulse rate, with increased hematocrit and blood urea nitrogen levels. Severe potassium loss (hypokalemia) interferes with the ability of the kidneys to concentrate urine and disrupts cardiac functioning. Starvation causes muscle wasting and severe protein and vitamin deficiencies. Jaundice, hyperpyrexia, and peripheral neuritis may develop. If inadequately or incorrectly treated, complications such as Wernicke encephalopathy, esophageal rupture, pneumothorax, acute tubular necrosis, or even maternal death may occur (ACOG, 2018b).

The diagnostic criteria for hyperemesis include a history of intractable vomiting in the first half of pregnancy, dehydration, ketonuria, and a weight loss of 5% of prepregnancy weight.

Clinical Therapy

The goals of treatment include controlling vomiting, correcting dehydration, restoring electrolyte balance, and maintaining adequate nutrition. It may be beneficial to avoid environmental triggers such as odors (perfume, chemicals, food, smoke), stuffy rooms, heat, humidity, noise, and visual or physical motion, brushing teeth after a meal, and not getting enough rest. Frequent, small meals of high-carbohydrate, low-fat content may be helpful. Carbonated or sour beverages taken in small quantities between meals also appear to help. (See *Complementary Health Approaches: Hyperemesis*.)

Some caregivers recommend pyridoxine (vitamin B_6) as a reasonable first-line pharmacologic treatment for nausea and vomiting of pregnancy. It has a good safety profile and minimal side effects. It can be administered alone or with doxylamine succinate, an antihistamine that improves efficacy. Typical dosing is pyroxidine 10 to 25 mg orally three times daily and one 25-mg over-the-counter tablet of doxylamine (sold as Unisom Sleep Tabs) at bedtime (O'Donnell et al., 2016). Diclegis (a combination of doxylamine succinate and pyridoxine hydrochloride [vitamin B_6]) is often used. It is administered daily on an empty stomach. The starting dose is two tablets taken at bedtime and may be increased to four tablets daily by adding one tablet in the morning and one midafternoon (ACOG, 2018b). If this is not effective, other pharmacologic options include promethazine (Phenergan), metoclopramide (Reglan), and ondansetron (Zofran).

If the woman with intractable nausea and vomiting does not respond to frequent, small meals of simple carbohydrates and the occasional use of antiemetics, she may require IV fluids on an outpatient basis. If the woman's symptoms do not improve, hospitalization and total parenteral nutrition may be necessary.

The initial workup should include an ultrasound to exclude the possibility of molar pregnancy. Initially, the woman is given nothing by mouth; IV fluids are administered to correct dehydration. Potassium chloride is typically added to the IV infusion to prevent hypokalemia. Replacement of thiamine (vitamin B_1) and pyroxidine (vitamin B_6) is important to correct deficiencies of these vitamins and prevent peripheral neuropathy and Wernicke encephalopathy (WE) (confusion, loss of memory, gait ataxia, oculomotor dysfunction).

If the woman does not respond to this management, total parenteral nutrition may be used to meet the caloric and nutritional needs of the woman and her fetus. When the woman's condition has improved, oral feedings are started. Six small dry feedings followed by clear liquids is one suggested treatment. Another method is 1 ounce of water offered each hour, followed as tolerated by clear, then nourishing liquids, progressing on succeeding days to low-fat, soft, and regular diets.

Complementary Health Approaches

Hyperemesis

Complementary and alternative therapies that have been tried to treat hyperemesis include:

- Ginger, which has beneficial effects on motion sickness and nausea (raw ginger is discouraged)
- Acupuncture or acupressure, which may lead to a reduction in the severity of symptoms (ACOG, 2018b)
- Hypnosis, which has been helpful in some women.

●○● NURSING MANAGEMENT

For the Woman with Hyperemesis Gravidarum

Nursing Assessment and Diagnosis

When a woman is hospitalized for control of vomiting, she must be regularly assessed for the amount and character of further emesis, intake and output, fetal heart rate, maternal vital signs, initial and daily weights, evidence of jaundice or bleeding, and her emotional state.

Nursing diagnoses that may apply to the woman with hyperemesis gravidarum include:

- ***Nutrition, Imbalanced: Less Than Body Requirements,*** related to persistent vomiting secondary to hyperemesis
- ***Fluid Volume: Deficient,*** related to severe dehydration secondary to persistent vomiting

(NANDA-I © 2017)

Nursing Plan and Implementation

Community-Based Nursing Care

The initial evaluation of the woman is designed to distinguish between nausea and vomiting of pregnancy (NVP), also called *morning sickness*, which is amenable to self-care, and hyperemesis gravidarum, which presents a real malnutrition risk. Take this opportunity to evaluate possible family and lifestyle stressors. It is wise to include both the woman and her family in the discussion of strategies to reduce nausea and vomiting that she can try at home, including such tactics as small carbohydrate meals, high-protein snacks, total avoidance of fatty foods, resting with her feet up and head elevated, or slowly sipping carbonated beverages when nauseated. Herbal teas, such as spearmint, peppermint, raspberry, chamomile, or ginger root, may be helpful. Known noxious odors, very hot or cold liquids, ice, and straws should be avoided. If the nausea and vomiting progress to a point where oral intake is not tolerated and dehydration is evident, medical intervention is required.

Hospital-Based Nursing Care

Nursing care should be supportive and directed at maintaining a relaxed, quiet environment away from food odors or offensive smells. Once oral feedings are started, food should be attractively served. Oral hygiene is important because the mouth is dry and may be irritated from vomitus. Weight gain or loss should be monitored regularly. Because emotional factors have been found to play a major role in this condition, psychotherapy may be recommended. With proper treatment, the prognosis is favorable.

As part of patient teaching, review actions the woman can take to prevent or decrease nausea. These are discussed further in Chapter 13. See *Case Study: Azia Askari.*

Evaluation

Expected outcomes of nursing care include:

- The woman is able to explain hyperemesis gravidarum, its therapy, and its possible effects on her pregnancy.
- The woman's condition is corrected, and possible complications are avoided.

●○●

Care of the Woman with a Hypertensive Disorder

Hypertensive disorders of pregnancy affect 10% of women and are one of the most common medical disorders that increase maternal and perinatal morbidity and mortality (Sibai, 2017). Preeclampsia alone is responsible for 75,000 deaths per year worldwide (Markham & Funai, 2014).There is only one cure for hypertensive disorders during pregnancy and that is delivery of the placenta.

The classification of hypertension (HTN) in pregnancy is as follows (Safe Motherhood Initiative, 2017):

- Preeclampsia-eclampsia
- Chronic hypertension
- Chronic hypertension with superimposed preeclampsia
- Gestational hypertension.

Table 18–3 describes the defining features of each hypertensive disorder in pregnancy. The pathophysiology and collaborative care of women with these disorders are quite different.

Preeclampsia and Eclampsia Syndrome

Preeclampsia is exclusively a disease of pregnancy. It is characterized by new-onset hypertension and proteinuria, usually after 20 weeks' gestation (Markham & Funai, 2014). It affects about 5 to 10% of all pregnancies in the United States (Sibai, 2017).

Preeclampsia, a syndrome of systemic vasospasm that affects both mother and fetus, is clinically defined as an increase

CASE STUDY: Azia Askari

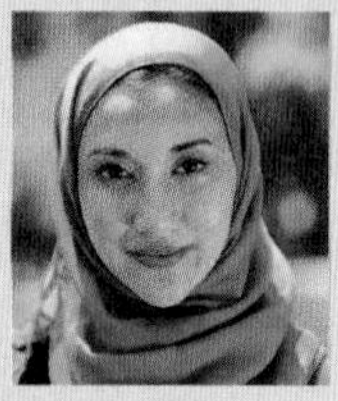

SOURCE: HONGQI ZHANG/123RF.

Azia is now 13 weeks pregnant and reports that she still has daily nausea and vomiting. The nurse notes that her urine is positive for protein and ketones and is extremely concentrated. She has lost 5.5 pounds and has a -7 lb weight gain since her new patient appointment. She states she cannot keep down any solids and despite eating saltine crackers in the morning, she still vomits each day. The doctor diagnoses her with hyperemesis gravidarum and orders laboratory studies, a urine culture, and urinalysis. Azia's blood pressure is 104/70 and pulse is 102. She is being sent over to the maternity unit for intravenous fluids and is to follow-up with the nutritionist.

Question to Ponder

What patient education would you provide Azia with today?

TABLE 18–3 Hypertensive Disorders in Pregnancy

	PREECLAMPSIA	PREECLAMPSIA WITH SEVERE FEATURES	GESTATIONAL HTN	CHRONIC HTN	HELLP SYNDROME
Pathophysiology	End organ dysfunction due to vasospasm	End organ dysfunction due to vasospasm		Can progress to superimposed preeclampsia	Severe consequence of preeclampsia
Definition	New-onset HTN (gestational hypertension) and proteinuria greater than 20 weeks (usually in third trimester)	New-onset HTN greater than 20 weeks; features more severe than preeclampsia; proteinuria not necessary	New-onset HTN that does not meet preeclampsia criteria greater than 20 weeks and that resolves by day 42 postpartum	HTN before 20 weeks	Hemolysis, elevated liver enzymes, low platelets
Symptoms/signs	Mild to severe	Severe	Absent or mild	Mild to severe	Severe
Blood pressure (BP): Twice 4–6 hours apart, not more than 7 days apart	Greater than 140 systolic OR Greater than 90 diastolic 2 × 4–6 hrs. apart AND protein as follows	Greater than 160 systolic OR Greater than 110 diastolic 2 × 4 hrs. apart	Greater than 140 systolic OR Greater than 90 diastolic 2 × 4–6 hrs. apart	140/90 prior to pregnancy with HTN greater than or equal to 12 weeks postpartum	Variable BP
Proteinuria	Protein greater than 0.3g/24 hrs. OR Protein/creatinine ratio greater than 0.3	No specific amount protein necessary	Proteinuria less than 300 mg per 24-hr collection	No proteinuria unless superimposed pre-eclampsia develops	No specific amount of protein necessary
Platelets	Greater than 100,000	Less than 100,000			Less than 100,000
Hepatic changes	Alanine aminotransferase (ALT)/ aspartate aminotransferase (AST): ALT/AST 2 × normal	Severe RUQ epigastric pain ALT/AST greater than or equal to 2 × normal • LDH greater than 600 • Bilirubin greater than1.2 (Lambert, Brichant, Hartstein, et al., 2014)			ALT/AST greater than 2 × normal
CNS changes	May or may not have headache with visual changes (scotomata)	30% will experience: Visual changes Severe headache Altered mentation			
Pulmonary changes		Pulmonary edema			

SOURCES: Choubey & Witter, 2015; Safe Motherhood Initiative, 2017; Sibai, 2017.

in blood pressure after 20 weeks' gestation accompanied by proteinuria in a previously normotensive woman (Markham & Funai, 2014). Historically, edema (extracellular fluid accumulation) was included in the diagnostic triad; however, it is too nonspecific to be utilized as diagnostic criteria, as many women without preeclampsia develop edema toward the end of pregnancy. Some women with preeclampsia will not present with proteinuria. In the latter case, evidence of thrombocytopenia, renal insufficiency, liver involvement, cerebral symptoms, or pulmonary edema with hypertension can help make the diagnosis (Cunningham et al., 2018). Preeclampsia is further classified as preeclampsia with severe features. (The term *mild preeclampsia* is no longer used [Sibai, 2017].) Table 18–3 helps to differentiate the hypertensive disorders of pregnancy.

SAFETY ALERT!

Sudden onset of severe edema warrants close evaluation to rule out preeclampsia or other pathologic processes such as renal disease. It is important to remember that severe preeclampsia can occur without edema.

Eclampsia is the occurrence of a seizure or coma in a woman with preeclampsia who has no other cause for seizure. Eclamptic seizures may occur during the antepartum, intrapartum, or postpartum periods.

PATHOPHYSIOLOGY OF PREECLAMPSIA-ECLAMPSIA SYNDROME

The etiology of preeclampsia is still unknown (Sibai, 2017). The mechanisms behind the pathogenesis of preeclampsia remain unclear, but include (Sibai, 2017):

- Impaired trophoblastic invasion and/or poor implantation
- Abnormal immunologic response to paternal antigens
- Imbalance in angiogenesis; an exaggerated systemic inflammatory response
- Increased oxidative stress
- Vascular endothelial dysfunction and coagulation abnormalities
- Genetic propensity for the development of preeclampsia.

Key features of preeclampsia involve (Sibai, 2017):

- Failure of the uterine spiral arteries to transform from thick-walled muscular vessels to saclike flaccid vessels, leading to an exaggerated inflammatory response and eventual inappropriate endothelial cell activation and dysfunction.
- Loss of normal vasodilatation of uterine arterioles resulting in decreased placental perfusion (Figure 18–4), and potentially leading to intrauterine fetal growth restriction (IUGR) and chronic hypoxia or distress.
- Systemic maternal vasospasm resulting in decreased perfusion to virtually all organs, including the placenta (Figure 18–5).
- Decrease in plasma volume, activation of the coagulation cascade, and alterations in glomerular capillary endothelium.
- Increased sensitivity to pressor agents (substances that increase blood pressure) rather than less sensitivity to them, as in a normal pregnancy.
- Imbalance between prostacyclin and thromboxane may play a role. Prostacyclin, a vasodilator produced by endothelial cells, decreases blood pressure, prevents platelet aggregation, and promotes uterine blood flow. Thromboxane, produced by platelets, causes vessels to constrict and platelets to clump together. Prostacyclin is decreased in preeclampsia, allowing the potent vasoconstrictor and platelet-aggregating effects of thromboxane to dominate.
- Decreased production of nitric oxide (NO), which is a potent vasodilator and important regulator of maternal blood pressure. Additionally, NO inhibits platelet aggregation and adhesion to vascular endothelium (Markham & Funai, 2014).

The role of prostacyclin-thromboxane imbalance in preeclampsia has prompted several randomized trials designed to evaluate the effect of low-dose aspirin (50–150 mg/day), which suppresses thromboxane, to prevent preeclampsia. The incidence of severe preeclampsia, eclampsia, IUGR, and preterm birth are reduced in women identified to be at risk for preeclampsia, especially if the low-dose regimen commences after 12 weeks' gestation (Sibai, 2017).

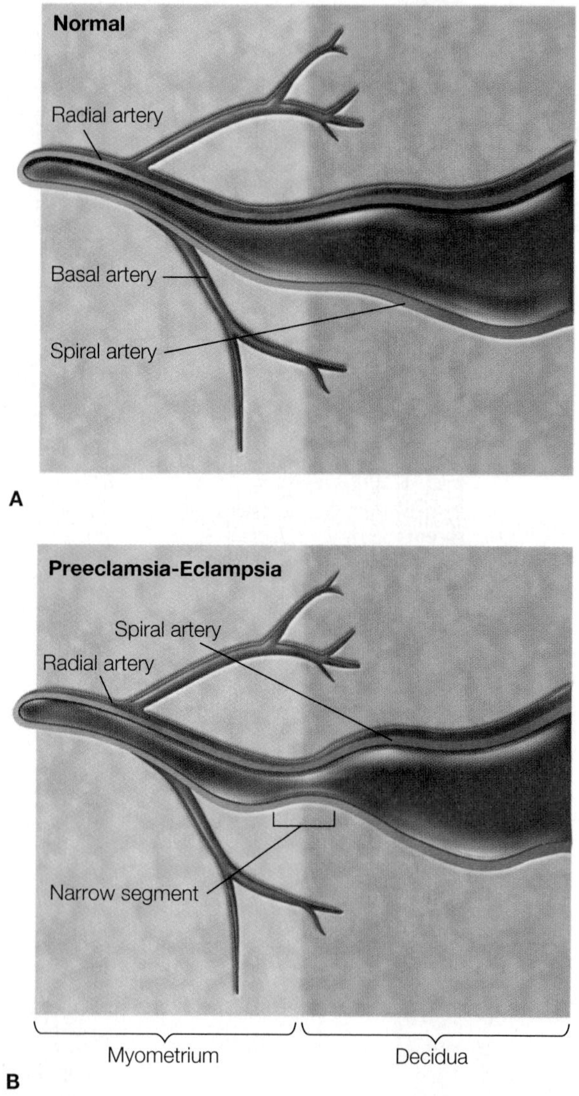

Figure 18–4 A. In a normal pregnancy, the passive quality of the spiral arteries permits increased blood flow to the placenta. B. In preeclampsia, vasoconstriction of the myometrial segment of the spiral arteries occurs.

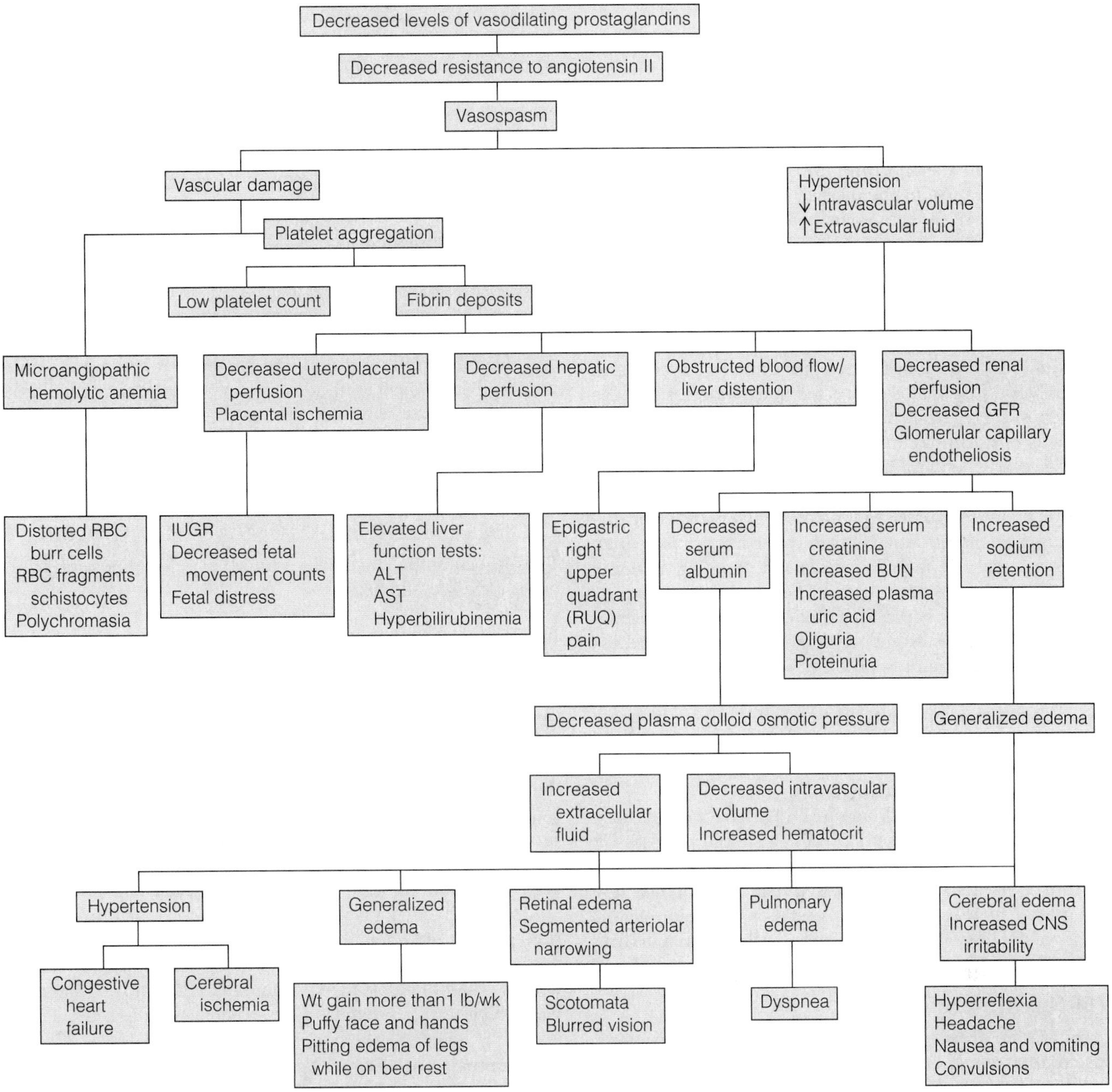

Figure 18–5 Clinical manifestations and possible pathophysiology of preeclampsia-eclampsia.

First pregnancies, adolescent pregnancies, out-of-wedlock pregnancies, and conception with a new partner increase the risk of preeclampsia. Paternal contribution to the risk of development of preeclampsia is suggested by the observation that men who have previously fathered a child with a woman who developed preeclampsia are more likely to father a subsequent preeclamptic birth with a new partner (Katsi et al., 2015).

Decreased renal perfusion is associated with preeclampsia. With a reduction in glomerular filtration rate (GFR), serum levels of creatinine, blood urea nitrogen (BUN), and uric acid begin to rise from normal pregnant levels, whereas urine output diminishes. For each 50% decrease in GFR, serum creatinine and BUN plasma levels double, whereas sodium is retained in increased amounts. Sodium retention results in increased extracellular volume and increased sensitivity to angiotensin II. The typical kidney lesion of preeclampsia involves swollen glomerular capillary endothelial cells containing fibrin deposits. Stretching of the capillary walls allows the large protein molecules, primarily albumin, to escape into the urine, decreasing serum albumin.

Edema is usually more profound in preeclampsia than in normal pregnancy, although some of the most severe forms of the disease may occur without edema. The pathologic basis of edema is twofold:

1. The higher salt retention draws out intravascular fluid.
2. Plasma colloid osmotic pressure decreases because of serum albumin loss through edematous renal glomeruli and damaged vascular endothelium. This causes fluid movement to extracellular spaces, also known as *third spacing*. Some edema may be so great as to have leaking through the skin pores that mimics sweating. This is called *anasarca*.

The decreased intravascular volume causes increased viscosity of the blood and a corresponding rise in hematocrit.

HELLP SYNDROME

HELLP syndrome (**h**emolysis, **e**levated **l**iver enzymes, and **l**ow **p**latelet count) is thought to be a variant of preeclampsia, as it does not always develop with hypertension or proteinuria (Markham & Funai, 2014). It complicates 0.5 to 0.9% of pregnancies and usually manifests between 27 and 37 weeks' gestation (Dusse, Alpoim, Silva, et al., 2015). Most cases occur in White women. As progression of the disease is insidious, the nurse must be attuned to vague symptoms such as malaise.

The hemolysis that occurs is termed *microangiopathic hemolytic anemia*. It is thought that red blood cells are distorted or fragmented during passage through small, damaged blood vessels. Vascular damage is associated with vasospasm, and platelets aggregate at sites of damage, resulting in *thrombocytopenia* (a low platelet count less than 150,000/mm^3). Elevated liver enzymes occur from blood flow that is obstructed in hepatocytes because of fibrin deposits. Hyperbilirubinemia and jaundice may be seen.

Deposits of fibrin-like material found in the hepatic sinusoids cause obstruction and hepatocellular injury. This necrosis is the classic hepatic lesion associated with HELLP. Increase in intrahepatic pressure causes swelling of the liver, and liver distention causes epigastric pain. Ultimately, the liver capsule may rupture. Symptoms can include nausea and vomiting, malaise, flulike symptoms, or epigastric pain. This can lead to misdiagnoses of gastroenteritis, hepatitis, gallbladder disease, pyelonephritis, renal disease, or thrombocytopenia purpura. Regardless of blood pressure or the presence or absence of protein in the urine, a woman presenting with the preceding symptoms should have a CBC with platelet count and a complete metabolic panel (CMP) with liver enzymes drawn. Perinatal morbidity and mortality with HELLP syndrome are high; therefore, the possibility of HELLP should be considered carefully.

Women with HELLP syndrome are best cared for in a tertiary care center. Initially, the mother's condition should be assessed and stabilized, especially if her platelets are very low (less than 50,000/mm^3). The fetus is also assessed using a nonstress test (NST; if greater than 26 to 28 weeks' gestation) and biophysical profile (if greater than 36 weeks' gestation). All women with true HELLP syndrome should give birth regardless of gestational age.

MATERNAL RISKS

Preeclampsia syndrome impacts end organ systems, causing serious complications. Central nervous system (CNS) changes include hyperreflexia, headache, and eclamptic seizure. The underlying cause of the seizures is not known. Once thought to be from cerebral edema, there is some controversy as to whether cerebral edema is a feature of eclampsia or a postmortem phenomenon.

Acute tubular necrosis may result from underperfusion of the kidneys. This is associated with hypovolemia and renal vasoconstriction. One of the more common problems related to preeclampsia is pulmonary edema due to increased capillary permeability.

Thrombocytopenia is the most common hematologic complication of severe preeclampsia (Sibai, 2017). The exact mechanism is not fully understood, but platelet consumption is believed to be related to endothelial damage as described previously and activation of thrombin. Abruptio placentae is a risk associated with preeclampsia and may cause release of procoagulants, such as thromboplastin, which can result in acute DIC.

Subcapsular hematoma of the liver is a rare but important occurrence in women with preeclampsia and HELLP syndrome. Rupture of a subcapsular hematoma is a life-threatening event. The woman may complain of right shoulder pain or severe epigastric pain persisting for several hours before circulatory collapse is evident. This is a surgical emergency requiring a multidisciplinary approach to management. Maternal and fetal mortality is over 50%, and women who survive are at risk for adult respiratory distress syndrome (ARDS), pulmonary edema, and acute renal failure in the postoperative period (Markham & Funai, 2014).

FETAL-NEONATAL RISKS

Newborns of women with preeclampsia during pregnancy tend to be small for gestational age (SGA) because of intrauterine growth restriction (IUGR). The cause is related specifically to maternal vasospasm and hypovolemia, which result in uteroplacental insufficiency (UPI), fetal hypoxia, and malnutrition. Placental abruption secondary to hypertension may result in profound fetal hypoxia and even death. In addition, the newborn may be premature because the treatment for the disorder may require early childbirth.

At birth, the newborn may be oversedated because of medications administered to the woman. The newborn may also have hypermagnesemia caused by treatment of the woman with large doses of magnesium sulfate.

CLINICAL MANIFESTATIONS AND DIAGNOSIS

The most commonly occurring clinical manifestations and diagnoses are discussed here.

Preeclampsia. Preeclampsia is the presence of gestational hypertension plus proteinuria. See Table 18–3. With preeclampsia, proteinuria is generally between 300 mg/L (1+ dipstick) and 1 g/L (2+ dipstick). This is measured in a midstream clean-catch or catheter-derived urine specimen.

The gold standard for the measurement of proteinuria is the 24-hour urine. Excretion of more than 300 mg of protein in a 24-hour period is considered abnormal. Alternatively, a spot protein-to-creatinine ratio can be collected and analyzed. This entails collection of one random urine sample. A result greater than 0.30 would indicate an abnormality (Sibai, 2017).

Although edema is no longer considered a diagnostic criterion, generalized edema, seen as puffy face, hands, and dependent areas such as the ankles and lower legs, may be present. Edema is identified by a weight gain of more than 4 pounds in 1 week (Sibai, 2017). Edema is assessed on a 1+ to 4+ scale.

Preeclampsia with Severe Features. Preeclampsia with severe features may develop suddenly. The following clinical signs and symptoms are often present (ACOG, 2013; Sibai, 2017):

- Blood pressure of 160/110 mmHg or higher on two occasions at least 4 to 6 hours apart while the woman is on bedrest
- Oliguria: Urine output less than or equal to 500 mL in 24 hours
- Cerebral or visual disturbances
- Pulmonary edema or cyanosis
- Epigastric or right upper quadrant pain
- Impaired liver function (elevated hepatic enzymes–alanine aminotransferase [ALT] or aspartate aminotransferase [AST] at least twice normal)
- Thrombocytopenia (less than 100,000 platelets per cubic millimeter)
- Intrauterine fetal growth restriction.

Other signs or symptoms that may be present include severe headache or one that persists despite analgesic therapy, blurred vision or scotomata (visual distortions before the eyes), narrowed segments on the retinal arterioles when examined with an ophthalmoscope, retinal edema (retinas appear wet and glistening) on funduscopy, dyspnea due to pulmonary edema, moist breath sounds on auscultation, pitting edema of lower extremities while on bedrest, epigastric pain, hyperreflexia, nausea and vomiting, irritability, and emotional tension. Proteinuria is no longer necessary as part of the diagnosis (Sibai, 2017).

Eclampsia. Eclampsia, characterized by convulsion or coma, may occur before the onset of labor, during labor, or early in the postpartum period. Late postpartum eclampsia (convulsions occurring more than 48 hours following birth) rarely occurs but has been documented. Some women experience only one convulsion, especially if it occurs late in labor or during the postpartum period, while others may have from 2 to 20 or more. Unless they occur extremely frequently the woman often regains consciousness between convulsions.

CLINICAL THERAPY

The goals of medical management for the woman include prevention of cerebral hemorrhage, convulsion, hematologic complications, and renal and hepatic diseases. Medical management aims to birth an uncompromised newborn as close to term as possible, although preterm delivery may be necessary for worsening maternal or fetal disease (e.g., fetal growth restriction). There are two goals in accomplishing a good outcome for mother and newborn: (1) reduction of elevated blood pressure and (2) prevention of seizures.

Antepartum Management. The only definitive treatment for preeclampsia-eclampsia syndrome is the delivery of the placenta (Sibai, 2017).

Home Care of Gestational Hypertension and Preeclampsia. In general, women with proteinuric preeclampsia should be admitted to the hospital. However, with changes in healthcare, more attention has been given to decreasing inpatient hospital days for women whose symptoms allow. Close maternal monitoring is essential to establish the severity and progression of the disease. The woman must be able to comply with frequent maternal and fetal evaluations and have ready access to medical care.

A woman should be considered for outpatient management in her home if she meets the following criteria: Blood pressure less than or equal to 150/100 mmHg, proteinuria less than 1 gram/24 hours or 3+ dipstick, platelet count greater than 120,000 mm^3, and normal fetal growth on serial ultrasounds. She must have a basic understanding of her condition, be able to recognize the signs and symptoms of worsening preeclampsia (Table 18–4), be able to accurately count fetal movements, be cooperative, and know when to call the doctor. She must be willing to come for twice-weekly fetal surveillance with NSTs or biophysical profiles, in addition to a weekly obstetric visit for blood pressure assessments and weekly bloodwork that includes a CBC and CMP. Although decreased activity is generally recommended, she is not restricted to bedrest but is encouraged to rest frequently, especially in the left lateral position.

The woman monitors her blood pressure and weight daily. Weight gain of 1.4 kg (3 lb) in 24 hours or 1.8 kg (4 lb) in a 7-day period is generally cause for concern. Nursing contact varies from daily to weekly, depending on clinician request. Laboratory testing regularly evaluates platelet counts, creatinine and BUN, liver enzymes, and 24-hour urine specimens for creatinine clearance and total protein, or a spot protein-to-creatinine ratio. Use of uric acid and lactic dehydrogenase to determine severity of preeclampsia is variable (Markham & Funai, 2014). Estimates of fetal growth and amniotic fluid volume should be made at the time preeclampsia is diagnosed and repeated every 2 to 4 weeks if normal. Any woman with worsening symptoms or severe preeclampsia should be hospitalized.

Hospital Care of Preeclampsia. The woman is placed on bedrest, primarily in the left lateral recumbent position, to decrease pressure on the vena cava and aorta, thereby increasing venous return, circulatory volume, and placental and renal perfusion. Improved renal blood flow helps decrease angiotensin II levels, promotes diuresis, and lowers blood pressure.

Her diet should be well balanced and nutritious. Excessively salty foods should be avoided, but strict sodium restriction and diuretics are not necessary when treating preeclampsia (Markham & Funai, 2017).

Tests to evaluate fetal status are done more frequently as a pregnant woman's preeclampsia progresses. These tests are described in detail in Chapter 16. Monitoring fetal well-being is essential to achieving a safe outcome for the fetus. The following tests are used:

- Fetal movement record or fetal kick counts
- Nonstress test: Reactive is normal
- Amniotic fluid index: Normal is greater than 5 centimeters
- Ultrasonography at least every 2 to 4 weeks for serial determination of growth: Normal is intrauterine growth greater than the 10th percentile
- Biophysical profile weekly, if not daily in some institutions
- Amniocentesis to determine fetal lung maturity in the event early birth is necessary
- Doppler velocimetry beginning at 30 to 32 weeks to screen for uteroplacental insufficiency and fetal compromise.

Maternal well-being is monitored by:

- Blood pressure four times daily
- Daily weight and daily evaluation for worsening edema, persistent headache, visual changes, or epigastric pain
- Daily urine dipstick for protein (variable)
- Periodic assessment of laboratory values to include: CBC with platelet count; CMP that includes liver function tests (AST, ALT), serum creatinine, and blood urea nitrogen; lactic dehydrogenase (LDH); uric acid; bilirubin; and 24-hour urine for protein and creatinine clearance or spot protein-to-creatinine ratio.

TABLE 18–4 Signs and Symptoms of Worsening Preeclampsia

- Increasing edema, especially of hands and face (if on bedrest, observe for sacral edema)
- Worsening headache
- Epigastric pain
- Visual disturbances
- Decreasing urinary output
- Nausea and vomiting
- Bleeding gums
- Disorientation
- Generalized complaints of not feeling well

Hospital Care of Preeclampsia with Severe Features. Any woman with severe preeclampsia is hospitalized immediately. It is widely accepted that childbirth should be considered in all pregnant women who develop preeclampsia after 34 weeks' gestation because the risks of prolonging the pregnancy are severe for the mother and the fetus. Expectant management may be used in selected women who are less than 34 weeks because the approach significantly improves neonatal outcomes. Fetal well-being is assessed daily, and birth is indicated regardless of gestational age if maternal or fetal condition worsens (Sibai, 2017). Other medical therapies for severe preeclampsia include:

- ***Bedrest.*** Bedrest must be complete. Stimuli that may bring on seizure activity should be reduced.
- ***Diet.*** A high-protein diet is given as long as the woman is alert and has no nausea or indication of impending seizure. Sodium restriction is no longer recommended (Markham & Funai, 2014).
- ***Anticonvulsants.*** Magnesium sulfate is the treatment of choice for seizure prophylaxis in severe preeclampsia and treatment of eclamptic convulsions and has been used for more than 60 years because of its CNS-depressant action (Sibai, 2017). Blood levels of magnesium sulfate should be maintained at therapeutic levels (levels vary according to laboratory). Excessive blood levels may produce respiratory paralysis or cardiac arrest. Anticonvulsant therapy may prevent seizures, but does not prevent the ultimate progression of the disease. The antidote for magnesium sulfate toxicity is 10% calcium gluconate in 10 milliliters (1 gram) intravenous push.
- ***Corticosteroids.*** A series of betamethasone or dexamethasone is often administered to the woman whose fetus has an immature lung profile to promote fetal lung maturation.
- ***Fluid and electrolyte replacement.*** The goal of fluid intake is to achieve a balance between correcting hypovolemia and preventing circulatory overload. Fluid intake may be oral or supplemented with IV therapy. IV fluids may be started "to keep lines open" in case they are needed for drug therapy, even when oral intake is adequate. Criteria vary for determining appropriate fluid intake. Electrolytes are replaced as indicated by daily serum electrolyte levels as noted on the CMP. Women with preeclampsia are at risk for hyponatremia (low blood sodium), which is indicative of low serum osmolality. A rapid decrease in serum osmolality can cause seizures as a result of cerebral dysfunction. It is imperative that serum sodium levels be evaluated to assess the need for fluid restriction and the switch to IV administration of isotonic sodium chloride.
- ***Antihypertensives.*** The major indication for antihypertensive therapy is the prevention of stroke. "The goal is not to normalize BP, but to achieve a range of 140–150/90–100 mm Hg in order to prevent repeated, prolonged exposure to severe systolic hypertension, with subsequent loss of cerebral vasculature autoregulation" (ACOG, 2017a, p. e91). In general, antihypertensive therapy is given for sustained systolic blood pressure of at least 160 mmHg or diastolic blood pressures of 105 to 110 mmHg or above for at least 15 minutes, which constitutes a hypertensive emergency (Sibai, 2017).

The therapeutic goal is to maintain the diastolic blood pressure between 90 and 100 mmHg. Decreasing the diastolic below 90 mmHg may decrease uterine blood flow, causing fetal compromise. Methyldopa is often used for long-term control of mild to moderate hypertension in pregnancy because it is effective and has a well-documented fetal and maternal safety record. However, its slow onset of action does not make it an option for treatment of elevated blood pressure in severe preeclampsia. Labetalol and hydralazine are considered first-line medications for the treatment of acute hypertension in pregnancy and are generally administered by IV boluses; oral rapid-acting nifedipine may be added to achieve desired blood pressure (ACOG, 2013, 2017a). Parenteral labetalol should be avoided in women with moderate to severe asthma, bradycardia, or congestive heart failure (Sibai, 2017). For women with severe preeclampsia undergoing expectant management remote from term, oral labetalol and nifedipine are acceptable choices (Sibai, 2017). Some guidelines recommend against using any calcium channel blocker with magnesium sulfate because of a potential drug interaction resulting in a neuromuscular blockade and hypotension; however, magnesium sulfate and nifedipine may be used together safely and effectively.

Hospital Care of Eclampsia. Eclampsia is defined as the occurrence of either seizure or coma associated with pregnancy and not caused by other neurologic disease. Seizures may be focal, multifocal, or generalized. The possible etiology of the seizure is likely related to cerebral vasospasm, edema, hemorrhage, ischemia, or loss of autoregulation of cerebral blood flow due to high systemic pressure (hypertensive encephalopathy), but no mechanism has been proven conclusively. Many women experience an increase in deep tendon reflexes (DTRs) before seizure, but seizures may also occur without hyperreflexia. The woman with preeclampsia should be monitored for signs and symptoms of impending eclampsia: Scotomata, which can appear as dark spots or flashing lights in the field of vision; blurred vision; epigastric pain; vomiting; persistent or severe headache, generally frontal in location; neurologic hyperactivity or confusion; pulmonary edema; and cyanosis. Eclamptic seizures are almost always self-limiting, although there may be more than one, and generally last no more than 3 to 4 minutes.

If a seizure occurs, nursing assessment should include time of onset and duration, body involvement, presence of incontinence, status of the fetus, and signs of placental abruption. The airway should be maintained, oxygen administered during the seizure, and a pulse oximeter applied. The woman is positioned on her side to avoid aspiration. Suctioning may be necessary to keep the airway clear; a tongue blade should not be inserted into the back of the throat because it may stimulate the gag reflex. To prevent injury, side rails should be up and padded, but the woman should not be restrained.

Magnesium sulfate has long been used in the treatment of preeclampsia. A bolus (or loading dose) of 4 to 6 g magnesium sulfate is administered intravenously in 100 mL of IV fluid over 15 to 20 minutes followed by a maintenance infusion of 2 g/hour IV infusion (Cunningham et al., 2018). In 10% of cases, an eclamptic woman will experience a second seizure. An additional bolus of 2 g of magnesium sulfate can be administered intravenously over 3 to 5 minutes (Sibai, 2017). If convulsions continue, lorazepam (Ativan) 2 mg over 3 to 5 minutes may be administered intravenously.

Side effects with the magnesium sulfate loading dose may include flushing, a feeling of warmth, headache, nystagmus, nausea, dry mouth, dysphoria, and dizziness. Other side effects include lethargy and sluggishness and a risk of pulmonary edema if the woman has predisposing conditions such as multiple gestation or infection, has had excessive IV fluid administration, or has concurrent β-sympathomimetic therapy. Fetal side effects may include hypotonia and lethargy that persist for 1 or

2 days following birth, hypoglycemia, and hypocalcemia. Anticonvulsant therapy is used to prevent or control seizure activity. Antihypertensive agents are used to prevent stroke by keeping the diastolic blood pressure between 90 and 100 mmHg, while avoiding a potential reduction in uteroplacental blood flow or cerebral perfusion.

Clinical Tip

When caring for a woman with severe preeclampsia who is receiving IV magnesium sulfate, it is imperative to follow protocols for monitoring blood levels of magnesium but even more vital to provide close surveillance with astute nursing assessments. You are probably already aware of the common signs of increasing magnesium levels, such as diminished reflexes, decreased respiratory rate, and depressed level of consciousness. However, there are some subtle clues you can also watch for that may suggest either the therapeutic or toxic range. When a woman's magnesium level is in the therapeutic range, she usually has some slurring of speech, awkwardness of movement, and decreased appetite. If the woman is slow to arouse, has slow/shallow respirations, or begins to have difficulty swallowing and begins to drool, she may be approaching the toxic range.

During a seizure, fetal bradycardia, transient late decelerations, and decreased variability occur. Following the seizure, compensatory tachycardia may occur. Stabilizing the mother can help the fetus recover in utero. If the fetal heart tracing remains nonreassuring for more than 10 to 15 minutes despite intrauterine resuscitative efforts (positioning the woman in the left lateral recumbent position, administering oxygen, and maintaining IV access), emergency birth should be considered. An eclamptic seizure increases uterine irritability and may cause a precipitous birth. Therefore, a minimum ratio of one nurse to one woman is imperative to assess fetal and maternal status continuously. Although she may still be unconscious, the woman should be observed for onset of labor. The woman is also observed for signs of placental separation (see Chapter 23). She should be checked every 15 minutes for vaginal bleeding, which may or may not be present with abruptio placentae, and the abdomen palpated for uterine rigidity. Fetal monitoring with a tocotransducer and tocodynamometer should be continuous.

Following a seizure, frequent auscultation of maternal lungs is required to assess for complications from aspiration and to rule out pulmonary edema, which, while not common in women who have experienced eclampsia, can be associated with increased morbidity and mortality (Markham & Funai, 2014). The woman is watched for circulatory and renal failure and for signs of cerebral hemorrhage. Furosemide (Lasix) may be given in low doses for pulmonary edema; digitalis may be given for circulatory failure. An indwelling Foley catheter is often inserted, and intake and output are monitored hourly.

A woman may have a single convulsion or many convulsions, usually followed by a period of unresponsiveness. She may be combative and confused as she awakens, but having a family member at her side helps to reduce her agitation. Also, it is important to avoid bright light, loud noises, and frequent disturbances. The most serious complication, cerebral hemorrhage, arises from uncontrolled hypertension. Loss of vision, which is usually temporary, is a sign of impending hemorrhage. IV options for the treatment of hypertension are hydralazine, labetalol, or immediate-release oral nifedipine. In an extreme emergency when the aforementioned does not control the hypertension, nitroprusside may be used for the shortest amount of time possible. Concerns about cyanide and thiocyanate toxicity in the woman and fetus or newborn are real, including increased intracranial pressure with potential worsening of cerebral edema in the woman (ACOG, 2017a).

Intrapartum Management of Preeclampsia. Labor may be induced by IV oxytocin when there is evidence of fetal lung maturity and cervical readiness. In very severe cases, cesarean birth may be necessary regardless of fetal maturity.

The woman may receive both IV oxytocin and magnesium sulfate simultaneously. Because magnesium sulfate has a depressant action on smooth muscle, uterine contractions may diminish, and labor may be augmented with oxytocin. Equipment and IV lines for both fluids must be checked frequently to ensure that they are being administered at the proper rate. Infusion pumps should be used to guarantee accuracy. IV bags and tubing must be labeled carefully.

Narcotics may be given via IV judiciously, especially if administered with a coexisting infusion of magnesium sulfate, for pain relief in labor. An epidural, spinal, or combined spinal-epidural can be safely administered to the woman with preeclampsia in the absence of thrombocytopenia (platelets less than 70,000/mm^3 or per anesthesia protocol). Hypotension is a major side effect of neuraxial analgesia and can be avoided by attention to technique during placement and activation of the epidural and careful volume expansion. The woman with preeclampsia is in total body fluid overload but has a depleted intravascular volume, making her prone to hypotension when the vascular bed dilates in response to epidural/spinal administration.

Childbirth in the Sims position should be considered. If the lithotomy position is used, a wedge should be placed under the right buttock to displace the uterus off the great vessels lying underneath to maximize placental perfusion and return of blood to the heart. The wedge should also be used if birth is by cesarean. Oxygen is administered to the woman during labor if the need is indicated by fetal response to the contractions.

Intrapartum Management of Eclampsia. In recent years, the usefulness of invasive hemodynamic monitoring using either a central venous pressure (CVP) or a pulmonary artery catheter (PAC) has been called into question. Nonetheless, many experts consider hemodynamic monitoring essential for the critically ill pregnant woman (Markham & Funai, 2014). Both these procedures carry risk to the woman, and the decision to use them should be made judiciously. Invasive hemodynamic monitoring may be indicated for the woman with the following:

- Oliguria
- Severe cardiac disease
- Severe renal disease
- Pulmonary edema resulting in impaired maternal oxygenation
- Refractory hypertension with administration of a vasoactive drug, such as nitroprusside or dopamine.

When the woman's vital signs have stabilized, urinary output is good, and the maternal and fetal hypoxic and acidotic states are alleviated, birth of the fetus should be considered. Birth of the placenta is the only known cure for preeclampsia-eclampsia syndrome. If the newborn will be preterm, it may be necessary to transfer the woman to a tertiary center where there is a NICU. The woman and her partner deserve careful explanation about treatment regarding her status and that of the fetus. Plans for childbirth and further treatment must be discussed with them.

A neonatal provider must be available to care for the newborn at birth. This caregiver must be aware of all medications the woman has received during labor, including the amounts and times of administration, to anticipate any adverse side effects on the newborn.

Postpartum Management. Immediately postpartum, a woman who required magnesium sulfate in the antepartum period will continue to receive the infusion for about 24 hours. While blood pressure improves dramatically within 48 hours postpartum, it can rise again 3 to 6 days postpartum. Therefore, nurses should be acutely aware that there is the possibility of worsening disease after the mother has been discharged from the hospital that includes HELLP syndrome, liver rupture, hypertensive crisis, or seizures. Antihypertensive medication may be required for 4 to 6 weeks postpartum to control persistent blood pressures of 160 mmHg systolic or 100 mmHg diastolic.

Some women may develop late-postpartum eclampsia (seizures occurring more than 48 hours but less than 4 weeks postpartum). As all women remain at risk for preeclampsia-eclampsia syndrome for 4 weeks postpartum, it is important for the nurse to educate about the warning signs and symptoms of preeclampsia-eclampsia (headache, scotomata, right upper quadrant pain) prior to discharge and to strongly advise women to call their providers or present to the emergency department if symptoms appear. Hypertension remaining past the 84th day postpartum is classified as chronic hypertension (Markham & Funai, 2014).

The recurrence rate of preeclampsia is substantially higher in women with new partners or sperm donors, multiple gestations, early-onset or severe previous preeclampsia-eclampsia syndrome, previous HELLP syndrome, preexisting hypertension, renal disease, or underlying vascular disease (Markham & Funai, 2014).

●○● NURSING MANAGEMENT

For the Woman with Preeclampsia

See *Nursing Care Plan: The Woman with Preeclampsia* for information on nursing care.

Nursing Assessment and Diagnosis

An essential part of nursing assessment is to obtain a baseline blood pressure early in pregnancy. Arterial blood pressure varies with position and is highest when the woman is sitting, intermediate when she is supine, and lowest when she is in the left lateral recumbent position. Therefore, it is important that the woman be in the same position when the blood pressure is measured at each visit, that is, in the sitting position with legs uncrossed.

Blood pressure is taken and recorded at each antepartum visit. If the blood pressure rises or if the normal slight decrease in blood pressure expected between 8 and 28 weeks of pregnancy does not occur, the woman should be followed closely.

Blood pressure elevations should be based on at least two determinations at least 4 to 6 hours apart and not more than 7 days apart. To minimize errors in blood pressure measurements and improve reproducibility, the following precautions should be taken when measuring blood pressure:

- Take blood pressure measurements while the woman is seated, with feet supported and her arm at the level of the heart.
- Use Korotkoff phase V (sound disappearance) to measure the diastolic pressure.
- Calibrate the mercury sphygmomanometer and use the nearest 2 mm measurement.
- If using an electronic device, use one that has been validated for pregnancy.

When blood pressure and other signs indicate that the preeclampsia is worsening, hospitalization is necessary to monitor the woman's condition closely. At that time the following should be assessed:

- ***Blood pressure.*** Determine blood pressure every 1 to 4 hours, more frequently if indicated by medication or other changes in the woman's status.
- ***Temperature.*** Determine temperature every 4 hours, every 2 hours if elevated or if premature rupture of the membranes (PROM) has occurred.
- ***Pulse and respirations.*** Determine pulse rate and respirations along with blood pressure.
- ***Fetal heart rate (FHR).*** Determine the FHR with the blood pressure or monitor continuously with the electronic fetal monitor.
- ***Urinary output.*** Measure every voiding. If the woman has preeclampsia with severe features, she will have an indwelling catheter. In this case, hourly urine output can be assessed. Output should be 700 mL or greater in 24 hours, or at least 30 mL per hour.
- ***Urine protein.*** Determine urinary protein hourly if an indwelling catheter is in place, or with each voiding. Readings of 3+ or 4+ indicate loss of 5 g or more protein in 24 hours.
- ***Urine specific gravity.*** Determine specific gravity of the urine hourly or with each voiding. Readings over 1.040 correlate with oliguria and proteinuria.
- ***Edema.*** Inspect and palpate for edema: Face (especially eyelids and cheekbone area), fingers, hands, arms (ulnar surface and wrist), legs (tibial surface), ankles, feet, and sacral area. The degree of pitting is determined by pressing over bony areas.
- ***Weight.*** Weigh the woman daily at the same time, wearing the same robe or gown and slippers. Weighing may be omitted if the woman is to maintain strict bedrest or a bed scale may be used.
- ***Pulmonary edema.*** Observe the woman for coughing, shortness of breath, or difficult breathing. The lungs are auscultated for moist respirations.

Professionalism in Practice **Measuring Blood Pressure**

Common errors in measuring blood pressure (BP) include:

- Incorrect cuff size—a cuff that is too small results in a falsely elevated BP, whereas one that is too large falsely lowers BP.
- Korotkoff phase—when BP is checked during pregnancy, the disappearance of the sound (phase V) is the preferred indicator rather than the muffling of the sound (phase IV).
- The BP should be checked with the woman in the sitting position in the clinic and in the semi-reclining position in the hospital setting, not in the left lateral recumbent position, as this falsely lowers the true BP (Sibai, 2017).
- Anxiety, exercise, and smoking can elevate BP. Allow 10 minutes for the woman to rest before checking the BP.

- ***Deep tendon reflexes.*** Assess the woman for evidence of hyperreflexia in the brachial, wrist, patellar, or Achilles tendons (Table 18–5). The patellar reflex is the easiest to assess (Figure 18–6).
- ***Clonus.*** Assess clonus bilaterally by vigorously dorsiflexing the woman's foot while her knee is held in a flexed position. Normally no clonus is present. If it is present, it is measured as one to four beats, or sustained (the nurse must stop the tapping of the foot), and is recorded as such.
- ***Placental separation.*** Assess the woman hourly for vaginal bleeding and/or uterine rigidity.

TABLE 18–5 Deep Tendon Reflex Rating Scale

RATING	ASSESSMENT
4+	Hyperactive; very brisk, jerky, or clonic response; abnormal
3+	Brisker than average; may not be abnormal
2+	Average response; normal
1+	Diminished response; low normal
0	No response; abnormal

Nursing Care Plan: The Woman with Preeclampsia

1. Nursing Diagnosis: *Fluid Volume: Imbalanced, Risk for,* related to fluid shift from intravascular to extravascular space secondary to vasospasm (NANDA-I © 2017)

Goal: Patient is restored to normal fluid volume levels.

INTERVENTION	RATIONALE
• Encourage woman to lie in the left lateral recumbent position.	• The left lateral recumbent position decreases pressure on the vena cava and aorta, thereby increasing venous return, circulatory volume, and placental and renal perfusion. Angiotensin II levels are decreased when there is improved renal blood flow, which helps to promote diuresis and lower blood pressure.
• Assess blood pressure every 1 to 4 hours as necessary.	• Frequent monitoring will assess for progression of the disorder and allow for early intervention to ensure maternal and fetal health and well-being.
• Monitor urine for volume and proteinuria every shift or every hour per agency protocol.	• Monitoring provides information to assess renal perfusion. Proteinuria is the last cardinal sign of preeclampsia to appear. As the disorder worsens, the capillary walls of the glomerular endothelial cells stretch, allowing protein molecules to pass into the urine. Normally urine does not contain protein. Readings of 3+ and 4+ indicate loss of 5 g or more protein in 24 hours. Urinary output decreases when there is a reduction of the glomerular filtration rate. Urinary output that falls below 30 mL per hour or less than 700 mL in a 24-hour period should be reported.
• Assess deep tendon reflexes and clonus.	• Hyperreflexia may occur as preeclampsia worsens. Eliciting deep tendon reflexes provides information about CNS status and is also used to assess for magnesium sulfate toxicity. Reflexes are graded on a scale of 0 to 4+ using the Deep Tendon Reflex Rating Scale. A rating of 4+ is abnormal and indicates hyperreflexia. A rating of 0 or no response is also abnormal and is seen with high maternal serum magnesium levels. Clonus, an abnormal finding, is present if the foot "jerks" or taps the examiner's hand, at which time the examiner counts the number of taps or beats. The presence of clonus indicates a more pronounced hyperreflexia and is indicative of CNS irritability.
• Assess for edema.	• Edema develops as fluid shifts from the intravascular to the extravascular spaces. Edema is assessed either by weight gain (more than 4 pounds in 1 week) or by assessing for pitting edema (assessed by using finger pressure to a swollen area, usually the lower extremities, and grading on a scale of 1+ to 4+).
• Administer magnesium sulfate per infusion pump as ordered.	• As preeclampsia worsens, the risk of an eclamptic seizure increases. Magnesium sulfate is the treatment of choice for seizures because of its CNS depressant action. As a secondary effect, magnesium sulfate relaxes smooth muscles and may therefore transiently decrease the blood pressure. Magnesium sulfate is contraindicated in women with myasthenia gravis.
• Assess for magnesium sulfate toxicity.	• Side effects of magnesium sulfate are dose related. Therapeutic levels are in the range of 4.8–8.4 mg/dL. As maternal serum magnesium levels increase, toxicity may occur. Signs of toxicity include decreased or absent DTRs, urine output below 30 mL/hr, respirations below 12, confusion, and ultimately respiratory arrest. Have 10% calcium gluconate 10 mL available as an antidote.
• Provide a balanced diet that includes 80–100 g/day or 1.5 g/kg/day of protein.	• A diet rich in protein is necessary to replace protein that is excreted in the urine.

EXPECTED OUTCOME: The signs and symptoms of preeclampsia will diminish as evidenced by decreased blood pressure, urine protein levels of zero, and a return of the deep tendon reflexes to normal.

(continued)

Nursing Care Plan: The Woman with Preeclampsia (*continued*)

2. Nursing Diagnosis: ***Injury, Risk for,*** **to the fetus, related to uteroplacental insufficiency secondary to vasospasm (NANDA-I © 2017)**

Goal: The fetus avoids complications related to uteroplacental insufficiency.

INTERVENTION	RATIONALE
• Instruct patient to count fetal movements three times a day for 20 to 30 minutes.	• Fetal activity provides reassurance of fetal well-being. Decrease in fetal movement or cessation of movement may indicate fetal compromise.
• Encourage patient to rest in the left lateral recumbent position.	• Lying in the left lateral recumbent position decreases pressure on the vena cava, which increases venous return, circulatory volume, and placental and renal perfusion. Blood flow to the fetus is increased, thereby reducing the risk of fetal hypoxia and malnutrition.
• **Collaborative:** Assist with serial ultrasounds	• Maternal vasospasm and hypovolemia result from preeclampsia, which may lead to intrauterine growth restriction and oligohydramnios. Ultrasound provides assessment of fetal growth and fluid levels.
• Perform NST as ordered.	• A nonstress test is performed to assess the fetal heart rate in response to fetal movement. Accelerations of fetal heart rate with fetal movement may indicate the fetus has adequate oxygenation and an intact central nervous system. (Refer to Chapter 16 for interpretation of NST results.)
• Describe for the woman the purposes of a biophysical profile (BPP).	• Preeclampsia or eclampsia places the woman at risk for uteroplacental insufficiency due to the loss of normal vasodilation of uterine arterioles and maternal vasospasm. This results in decreased uteroplacental perfusion, which may lead to fetal hypoxia. A BPP is one assessment tool used to evaluate fetal well-being. Providing explanation of the diagnostic test helps relieve anxiety and ensures the woman understands what the test evaluates and what the results mean.
• Assist with amniocentesis to determine fetal lung maturity if early birth is indicated.	• Women with preeclampsia may give birth before term. Amniotic fluid may be analyzed to determine the maturity of the fetal lungs. An L/S (lecithin/sphingomyelin) ratio of 2:1 or greater in a woman without diabetes indicates fetal lung maturity and is usually achieved by 35–36 weeks' gestation. The presence of phosphatidylglycerol (PG) also indicates lung maturity. In addition, a lamellar body count (LBC) of the amniotic fluid greater than 50,000/mcL indicates lung maturity.
• Explain the purpose of Doppler flow studies.	• Doppler flow studies (umbilical velocimetry) help to assess placental function and sufficiency. Uteroplacental insufficiency is a risk for a woman with preeclampsia. If fetal growth restriction is present (less than 10th percentile), Doppler velocimetry of the umbilical artery is useful for fetal surveillance. An abnormal value would be greater than 3.

EXPECTED OUTCOME: The fetus will have an adequate supply of oxygen and nutrients as evidenced by absence of signs of nonreassuring fetal status and fetal diagnostic test results within normal limits.

3. Nursing Diagnosis: ***Health Maintenance, Ineffective,*** **related to deficient knowledge about new diagnosis (preeclampsia) (NANDA-I © 2017)**

Goal: The woman will describe the condition and treatment regimen.

INTERVENTION	RATIONALE
• Assess the woman and the family's understanding of preeclampsia and its implications for pregnancy.	• This assessment provides information about the woman's cognitive level and her understanding of her diagnosis. Behavior changes occur when teaching strategies are appropriate for the woman and family's cognitive level.
• Provide information about the disease process, impact on maternal well-being, risks of progression, implications for the fetus, and dangers of eclampsia.	• Basic understanding of the condition and its implications is necessary for the woman to understand the treatment plan. A woman who shows signs of early preeclampsia often feels well and may have difficulty accepting the need to rest.
• Emphasize the importance of self-monitoring for signs that her condition is worsening and the importance of regular prenatal care for the purpose of maternal and fetal surveillance.	• The woman should be able to identify signs of disease progression, including evidence of increasing edema, decreased urine output, signs of cerebral disturbance (frontal headache, blurred vision, scotomata), epigastric or right upper quadrant pain, nausea and vomiting, and increased irritability.

EXPECTED OUTCOME: Woman will demonstrate understanding of preeclampsia and its implications as evidenced by verbalization of basic condition, signs and symptoms of progression, importance of sufficient rest in side-lying position, and need to follow prescribed diet.

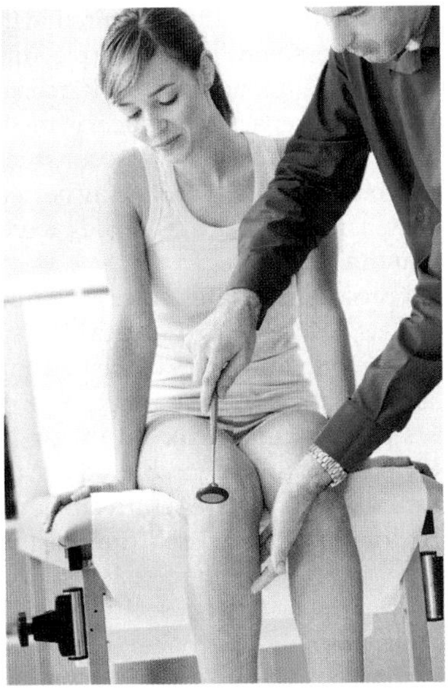

Figure 18–6 Correct position for eliciting patellar reflex: Sitting.

SOURCE: B. Boissonnet/BSIP SA/Alamy Stock Photo.

- *Headache.* Question the woman about the existence and location of any headache and its response to acetaminophen.
- *Visual disturbance.* Question the woman about any visual blurring or changes, including scotomata. Record the results of the daily funduscopic exam on the chart.
- *Epigastric pain.* Ask the woman about any epigastric pain. It is important to differentiate it from simple heartburn, which tends to be familiar and less intense. Nausea and vomiting or right upper quadrant pain, occasionally radiating to the back, are also of concern.
- *Laboratory blood tests.* Daily tests of hematocrit to measure hemoconcentration; BUN, creatinine, and uric acid levels to assess kidney function; clotting studies for any indication of thrombocytopenia (platelet count) or DIC; liver enzymes; and electrolyte levels for deficiencies are all indicated.
- *Level of consciousness.* Observe the woman for alertness, mood changes, and any signs of impending convulsion or coma.
- *Emotional response and level of understanding.* Assess the woman's emotional response carefully so that support and teaching can be planned accordingly.

In addition, continue to assess the effects of any medications administered. Because the administration of prescribed medications is an important aspect of care, you will, of course, be familiar with the more commonly used medications, their purpose, implications, and associated untoward or toxic effects.

Examples of nursing diagnoses that may apply for the pregnant woman with preeclampsia-eclampsia include:

- *Fluid Volume: Risk for Imbalanced,* related to fluid shift from the intravascular to extravascular space secondary to vasospasm and endothelial injury
- *Injury, Risk for,* related to convulsion secondary to cerebral edema
- *Maternal/Fetal Dyad, Risk for Disturbed,* related to lack of opportunities for interaction due to maternal medical needs.

(NANDA-I © 2017)

Nursing Plan and Implementation

Community-Based Nursing Care

A woman with preeclampsia may have fears about her health and that of the fetus. If she is on bedrest at home, she may have to deal with boredom and concerns about how her family is coping. Her partner may be stressed and/or blame the woman for his or her additional responsibilities, while also worrying about the woman's health and that of the fetus.

Identify and discuss each of these areas with the woman and her partner. It is necessary to explain to them the reasons for bedrest. A woman with mild preeclampsia may feel very well and be unable to see the need for resting even a few hours a day. Refer the couple to community resources, such as homemaking services, a support group for the partner, or a hotline. Arrangements may be made for the partner to attend childbirth classes alone if the mother is not able to, or someone may be found to teach the classes privately. In addition, childbirth classes can be accessed over the internet, thereby enabling the couple to participate together even if the woman is limited to bedrest at home.

Health Promotion

- Ensure that the woman knows which symptoms are significant and should be reported at once.
- Emphasize that although she is usually seen once or twice a week, she may need to come in earlier if symptoms indicate the condition is progressing.
- Describe in detail and be sure that she understands her diet plan, which must match her culture, finances, and lifestyle.

Hospital-Based Nursing Care

The development of worsening preeclampsia is a cause for increased concern to the woman and her family. The most immediate concerns of the woman and her partner are usually about the prognosis for herself and the fetus. She may also worry about separation from her partner and children and the impact on those relationships. There may be concerns about finances and how to provide for the children at home. Offer honest, hopeful information. Explain the plan of therapy and the reasons for procedures to the extent that the woman or her partner is interested. Keep the couple informed of the fetal status and take the time to discuss other concerns the couple may express. Provide as much information as possible and seek other sources of information or aid for the family as needed. Offer to contact a member of the clergy or counselor for additional support if the couple so chooses. In addition, you can provide educational videos that help address the couple's educational needs and access other support services including social services, a nutritionist, and even a lactation consultant if the woman is hospitalized for an extended period of time.

Maintain a quiet, low-stimulus environment for the woman, such as a private room in a quiet location where she can be watched closely. Limit visitors to close family or main support persons. The woman should maintain the left lateral recumbent position most of the time, with side rails up for her protection. Unlimited phone calls are avoided because the phone ringing unexpectedly may be too jarring. To avoid a sense of isolation, however, some women find it preferable to limit calls to a certain time of the day rather than refusing all calls.

For the woman on strict bedrest, venous thromboembolism prophylaxis should be initiated. Compression stockings, a sequential compression device, and low-molecular-weight heparin may all be ordered.

Nursing Management of Eclampsia

The occurrence of a convulsion is frightening to any family member who may be present, although the woman will not be able to recall it when she becomes conscious. Therefore, offering explanations to family members, and to the woman herself later, is essential.

When the tonic phase of the convulsion begins, turn the woman to her side (if she is not already in that position) to aid circulation to the placenta. Turn her head face down to allow saliva to drain from her mouth. Attempting to insert a padded tongue blade has been questioned, and in many facilities it is no longer advocated. In others, it is used if it can be done without force because it may prevent injury to the woman's mouth and tongue. The side rails should be padded or a pillow put between the woman and each side rail. After 15 to 20 seconds, the clonic phase starts. In approximately 30 to 90 seconds, when the thrashing subsides, intensive monitoring and therapy begin. An oral airway may be inserted, the woman's nasopharynx is suctioned, and oxygen administration is begun by nasal catheter. A pulse oximeter is placed and IV access established (if not already done). Notify the attending healthcare provider and anesthesiologist immediately. Monitor fetal heart tones continuously and monitor maternal vital signs every 5 minutes until they are stable, then every 15 minutes.

Nursing Management During Labor and Birth

The plan of care for the woman with preeclampsia in labor depends on both maternal and fetal condition. The woman may have mild or severe preeclampsia, may become eclamptic during labor, or may have been eclamptic before the onset of labor. Therefore, careful monitoring of blood pressure and checking for edema and proteinuria are necessary for all women in labor. Obtain the prenatal record so that current blood pressure readings may be compared with the baseline reading from early in her pregnancy.

During labor, keep the woman with preeclampsia positioned on her side as much as possible. Monitor both woman and fetus carefully throughout labor. Note signs of progressing labor. In addition, be alert for indications of worsening preeclampsia, placental separation, pulmonary edema, circulatory or renal failure, and nonreassuring fetal status.

During the second stage of labor encourage the woman to push while lying on her side or with a wedge under her hip. If she is unable to do so comfortably or effectively, help her to a semi-sitting position for pushing and resume the lateral position between each contraction. Birth is in the side-lying position, if possible. If the lithotomy position is used, place a wedge under the woman's hip.

Encourage a family member to stay with the woman as long as possible throughout labor and childbirth. This is especially needed if the woman has been transferred to a high-risk center from another facility. Orient the woman in labor and the family member or support person to the new surroundings and keep them informed of progress and the plan of care. When possible, the same nurses should care for the woman throughout her hospital stay.

Nursing Management During the Postpartum Period

Carefully note the amount of postpartum vaginal bleeding. Because the woman with preeclampsia is hypovolemic, even normal blood loss can be serious. Rising pulse rate and falling urine output are late indications of excessive blood loss. Palpate the uterus frequently and massage the fundus when needed to keep it contracted. If magnesium sulfate is required in the postpartum period, meticulous assessment of uterine bleeding is required, as the medication, being a smooth muscle relaxant, can cause uterine atony. No ergot preparations, such as methylergonovine (Methergine), are given because their vasoconstrictive action has a hypertensive effect. Other uterotonics may be necessary to control bleeding, such as misoprostol (Cytotec), oxytocin (Pitocin), and/or prostaglandin $F_{2\alpha}$.

Check blood pressure and pulse every 4 hours for 48 hours. Hematocrit, platelets, uric acid, AST, and ALT may be measured daily. Instruct the woman to report any headache, visual disturbance, or epigastric pain. Continue intake and output recordings for 48 hours postpartum. Increased urinary output within 48 hours after birth is a highly favorable sign. With the diuresis, edema recedes and blood pressure returns to normal.

Postpartum depression or postpartum posttraumatic stress disorder can develop after the long ordeal of a difficult pregnancy. Urge family members to visit and allow as much mother–newborn contact as possible. There may be fears about a future pregnancy. The couple needs information about the chance of preeclampsia occurring again. Also give family-planning information. Combined oral contraceptives (COCs) may be used if the woman's blood pressure has returned to normal by the time they are prescribed (usually 4 to 6 weeks postpartum). Any progestin-only method of contraception (progesterone-only pills, Depo-Provera, Nexplanon) may be prescribed regardless of hypertension and may be a good alternative for a woman with chronic hypertension or if breastfeeding. An intrauterine contraceptive device is an excellent option.

Evaluation

Expected outcomes of nursing care include:

- The woman is able to explain preeclampsia, its implications for her pregnancy, the treatment regimen, and possible complications.
- The woman suffers no eclamptic seizures.
- The woman and her caregivers detect signs of increasing severity of the preeclampsia or possible complications early so that appropriate treatment measures can be instituted.
- The woman gives birth to a healthy newborn.

Chronic Hypertension

Chronic hypertension is defined as hypertension present prior to pregnancy or before the 20th week of pregnancy or hypertension that persists for more than 3 months following childbirth (Sibai, 2017). For the majority of women with chronic hypertension, the disease is mild. One of the challenges the healthcare team faces is differentiating chronic hypertension from preeclampsia. This is even more difficult if a woman arrives for her first prenatal visit during the second trimester when blood pressure is generally lower and preexisting hypertension is more difficult to recognize. If the diastolic blood pressure is greater than 80 mmHg during the second trimester, chronic hypertension should be suspected.

Early prenatal care is important to determine accurately the gestational age and the severity of hypertension. Adverse maternal and neonatal outcomes are increased in women with chronic hypertension, even if they do not develop superimposed preeclampsia. These risks include fetal growth restriction, preterm birth, and cesarean birth, as well as the associated economic burden of longer maternal hospitalization and neonatal intensive care admission.

At the time of the first visit, the woman should be counseled on several aspects of her pregnancy:

- ***Nutrition.*** Women should be advised about recommended weight gain according to the Institute of Medicine (IOM) guidelines and encouraged to make healthy food choices. There is no evidence to limit sodium intake.
- ***Bed rest.*** Frequent rest periods are not necessary if blood pressure is stable.
- ***Medication.*** Studies have shown that women with mild chronic hypertension have outcomes similar to the general maternity population if BP remains equal to or less than 160/105 and there is no end organ damage. Therefore, the ACOG Task Force (2013) recommends initiating antihypertensive medications when the systolic BP is equal to or greater than 160 mmHg or the diastolic BP is equal to or greater than 105 mmHg. The goal is to maintain BP between 120 and 160 mmHg systolic and 80 and 105 mmHg diastolic. Methyldopa (Aldomet) or labetalol (Coreg) is generally the first choice for use in pregnancy when medication is required. Angiotensin-converting enzyme (ACE) inhibitors are contraindicated during the second and third trimesters due to fetal risks of renal failure, IUGR, and death (ACOG, 2013). For women with end organ damage, the goal for BP is maintenance of 140/90.
- ***Prenatal visits.*** Counseling regarding the importance of frequent prenatal visits and antenatal fetal surveillance (NSTs, BPPs) to reduce the incidence of adverse outcomes for mother or fetus is stressed.
- ***Blood pressure monitoring.*** The woman and her partner can be taught how to monitor blood pressure at home and maintain a record to be brought to each prenatal visit. Home monitoring is often more accurate because the woman is in a familiar environment and relaxed.
- ***Fetal surveillance.*** Starting at about 24 weeks, the woman should begin to keep fetal movement records (discussed in Chapter 16) and notify her care provider of any significant decrease in fetal movement. Serial ultrasounds every 2 to 4 weeks to assess fetal growth and amniotic fluid volume is indicated. Antepartum fetal testing may begin as early as 26 weeks. Nonstress tests can be reactive after 28 weeks and biophysical profiles are indicated after 36 weeks. Twice weekly testing (NST and BPP) is a standard and usually begins at 32 weeks, unless earlier testing is indicated.

During the first prenatal visit, the woman should have a thorough physical examination, which includes a funduscopic examination, blood pressure and pulses in all four extremities, and auscultation of heart and lungs. Laboratory work includes routine prenatal labs (blood type, Rh factor, antibody screen, Rubella immunity, etc.); a urinalysis and 24-hour urine collection for total protein; urine for culture and sensitivity; complete metabolic panel (serum electrolytes, LFTs, BUN/creatinine); and a glucose tolerance test. An ultrasound to confirm gestational age is done. Preexisting chronic hypertension is the most likely explanation for hypertension in early pregnancy, although a thorough evaluation can rule out causes of secondary hypertension such as diabetes, kidney disease, pheochromocytoma, or coarctation of the aorta.

A woman with chronic hypertension generally has more frequent prenatal visits. She should be seen every 2 to 3 weeks in the first two trimesters and then more frequently in the third trimester, depending on how she and the fetus are progressing. Twenty-four-hour urine collections, serum creatinine, uric acid, hematocrit, platelets, and ultrasound examinations are repeated at least once in the second and third trimesters if the blood pressure remains stable. See *Case Study: Benita Cartier*.

Chronic Hypertension with Superimposed Preeclampsia

Preeclampsia develops in approximately 25% of women previously found to have chronic hypertension (Markham & Funai, 2014). The development of superimposed preeclampsia can be difficult to diagnose. After 20 weeks' gestation the onset of proteinuria and worsening hypertension is suggestive of superimposed preeclampsia (Sibai, 2017). If the woman has underlying renal disease it may be very difficult to confirm the diagnosis of superimposed preeclampsia. A rise in serum uric acid, when compared to a baseline value, is helpful in identifying preeclampsia, which frequently occurs late in the second trimester or early in the third.

Gestational Hypertension

Gestational hypertension exists when transient elevations of blood pressure occur for the first time after midpregnancy without proteinuria or other signs of preeclampsia. The final determination that the woman has gestational hypertension is made retrospectively in the postpartum period. If preeclampsia does not develop and blood pressure returns to normal by 12 weeks postpartum, the diagnosis of gestational hypertension may be assigned. If the blood pressure elevation persists after 12 weeks postpartum, the woman is diagnosed with chronic hypertension.

CASE STUDY: Benita Cartier

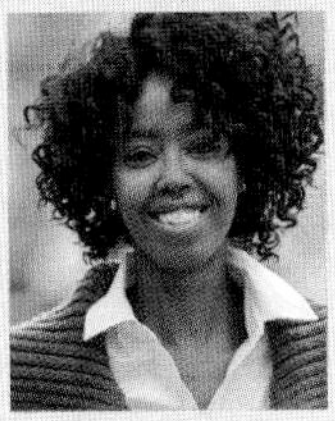

SOURCE: blvdone/Shutterstock.

Benita calls the labor and delivery unit nursing line this morning and reports blurred vision and a headache that has not responded to Tylenol. She is 32 weeks pregnant and tells the nurse she has a history of chronic hypertension. The nurse advises Benita that she should secure child care for her daughter and come in immediately for a blood pressure check, laboratory studies, and fetal monitoring.

Upon admission and testing, the nurse calls Benita's nurse-midwife and reports that the FHR monitoring is reassuring, labs are pending, but Benita's blood pressure is 162/90.

Questions to Ponder

What nursing interventions are needed at this time? What laboratory findings are important to review and why? What additional physical assessment data should the nurse on the labor and delivery unit obtain?

Care of the Woman with a Perinatal Infection Affecting the Fetus

Fetal infection can develop at any time during pregnancy. In general, perinatal infections are most likely to cause catastrophic harm when the embryo is exposed during first-trimester organ development. Infections later in the second and especially third trimesters of pregnancy create various concerns such as growth restriction, nonimmune hydrops, and neurologic sequelae. (The acronym **TORCH**—**t**oxoplasmosis, **o**ther (HIV, parvovirus, listeria, Zika), **r**ubella, **c**ytomegalovirus, and **h**erpes—is occasionally used to identify the most common of these perinatal infections.) This section addresses the most commonly occurring viral and parasitic infections that may have an impact on the fetus if acquired during pregnancy.

Toxoplasmosis

Toxoplasmosis is caused by the protozoan *Toxoplasma gondii*. The pregnant woman may contract the organism by eating raw or undercooked meat, by drinking unpasteurized goat's milk, or by contact with the feces of infected cats, either through the cat litter box or by gardening in areas frequented by cats. Half of all adults in the United States have IgG antibody to toxoplasmosis, and generally it is a barely noticeable infection that mimics mononucleosis. However, when contracted in pregnancy, it can profoundly and adversely affect the fetus, creating long-term catastrophic neurologic sequelae, such as microcephaly. The greatest risk of perinatal transmission is in the third trimester, and if the mother has been acutely infected, there is a 40% chance the newborn will have evidence of congenital infection (Duff & Birsner, 2017).

FETAL-NEONATAL RISKS

Maternal infection during the first trimester is associated with the lowest incidence of congenital infection but the most fetal damage, and the pregnancy often ends in a spontaneous abortion. The highest rate of congenital infection (60%) occurs when the mother contracts the infection in the third trimester (ACOG, 2015a). Congenital clinical manifestations include chorioretinitis (inflammation of the retina and choroid layer of the eye), disseminated purpuric rash, hepatosplenomegaly, ascites, fever, seizures, periventricular calcifications, microcephaly, and ventriculomegaly. Survivors are often blind, deaf, and severely neurodevelopmentally impaired.

CLINICAL THERAPY

Diagnosis can be made by serologic testing using IgM and IgG antibody titer tests. IgM is the first antibody to respond to an infection, so a negative IgM test would exclude recent or current infection, unless the incubation period is not yet over. IgG is the antibody that confers immunity and indicates a previous infection (ACOG, 2015). However, with toxoplasmosis, both IgM and IgG antibody titers can remain elevated for years. Therefore, any positive IgM result or high IgG titer must be followed by confirmatory testing by an amniocentesis to rule out congenital infection. A polymerase chain reaction (PCR) for *T. gondii* DNA in amniotic fluid should be completed and is the best way to diagnose fetal infection. Ultrasound can then be used to reveal findings suggestive of severe fetal infection such as ascites, ventriculomegaly, microcephaly, and intrauterine growth restriction (Duff & Birsner, 2017).

Maternal infection with toxoplasmosis should be treated with sulfadiazine and pyrimethamine to minimize the risk of congenital infection. Pyrimethamine (Daraprim) is teratogenic and should be added after the first trimester. Alternatively, a macrolide, spiramycin, can reduce transplacental transfer and the risk of congenital infection. Spiramycin is not commercially available in the United States, but can be obtained for treatment through the CDC. Newborns with congenital infection are treated with pyrimethamine, sulfadiazine, and leucovorin for 1 year (ACOG, 2015; Duff & Birsner, 2017).

●○● NURSING MANAGEMENT

For the Pregnant Woman with Toxoplasmosis

Nursing Assessment and Diagnosis

The incubation period for the disease is 10 days. The woman with acute toxoplasmosis may be asymptomatic, or she may develop myalgia, malaise, rash, splenomegaly, fever, headache, and enlarged posterior cervical lymph nodes. Symptoms usually disappear in a few days or weeks.

Nursing diagnoses that might apply to the pregnant woman with toxoplasmosis include:

- ***Knowledge, Readiness for Enhanced***, related to a desire to understand the ways in which a pregnant woman can contract toxoplasmosis
- ***Grieving*** related to potential effects on baby of maternal toxoplasmosis

(NANDA-I © 2017)

Nursing Plan and Implementation

When caring for women during the antepartum period, you have the primary opportunity to discuss methods of prevention of toxoplasmosis with the childbearing woman. The woman must understand the importance of avoiding poorly cooked or raw meat, whether game or commercial meats, especially pork, beef, lamb, and, in the arctic region, caribou. Fruits and vegetables should be washed. If she has a cat, she should avoid contact with the cat litter box by having someone else clean it. In addition, because it takes approximately 48 hours for a cat's feces to become infectious, the litter should be cleaned frequently. Discuss the importance of wearing gloves when gardening and avoiding garden areas frequented by cats.

Evaluation

Expected outcomes of nursing care include:

- The woman is able to discuss toxoplasmosis, its method of transmission, the implications for her fetus, and measures she can take to avoid contracting it.
- The woman implements health measures to avoid contracting toxoplasmosis.
- The woman gives birth to a healthy newborn.

Rubella

Rubella is a mild illness in children and adults, of which 20 to 50% of cases are asymptomatic. Congenital rubella syndrome (CRS) in the fetus can have overwhelming consequences. In the United States, large epidemics of rubella are rare because of immunization. Still, there are pockets of unvaccinated people and cases continue to occur among babies born to women who emigrate from countries without rubella vaccination programs (Bernstein, 2017). Prepubertal girls and nonpregnant women of childbearing age who do not have antirubella antibodies (IgG antibodies) should be immunized with the live, attenuated rubella vaccine. Although no fetal infection has resulted from immunization of a pregnant woman, pregnancy should be avoided for 1 month after immunization (CDC, 2016b). Be aware of the importance of postpartum immunization of the nonimmune woman to decrease unnecessary perinatal transmission.

FETAL-NEONATAL RISKS

The period of greatest risk for the teratogenic effects of rubella on the fetus is during the first trimester, when maternal–fetal transmission occurs in up to 80% of cases of maternal rubella infection (Bernstein, 2017). Defects are rare when infection develops after 20 weeks' gestation (Cunningham et al., 2018). The most common clinical signs of CRS are cataracts, sensorineural deafness, and congenital heart defects (particularly patent ductus arteriosus). Other abnormalities, such as intellectual disability or cerebral palsy, may become evident in infancy. Diagnosis in the newborn can be conclusively made in the presence of these conditions and with an elevated rubella IgM antibody titer at birth.

Newborns with CRS are infectious and should be isolated. Their care should be provided by people who are immune to rubella. These babies may continue to shed the virus for up to 12 months and should be considered contagious (Bernstein, 2017).

CLINICAL THERAPY

The best therapy for rubella is prevention. Live, attenuated vaccine is available and should be given to all children. Women of childbearing age should be tested for immunity and vaccinated if susceptible, after it is established that they are not pregnant. Health counseling in high school and during routine health visits in the clinic should stress the importance of screening before planning a pregnancy. As part of the prenatal laboratory screen, the woman is evaluated for rubella using hemagglutination inhibition (HAI), a serology test. The presence of an IgG titer is evidence of immunity. At what value the titer confers immunity will be based on the laboratory findings. It is incumbent upon the nurse to know what titer value confers immunity when interpreting laboratory results. When in doubt, the nurse should call microbiology.

Because the vaccine is made with attenuated virus, pregnant women are not vaccinated. However, it is considered safe for newly vaccinated children to have contact with pregnant women. Children should be given a single dose of the rubella vaccine at 1 year of age or at 15 months as part of the measles, mumps, and rubella (MMR) vaccine. All rubella-susceptible women (titer nonimmune) should receive the MMR vaccine in the postpartum period.

If a woman who is pregnant becomes infected with rubella during the first trimester, therapeutic abortion may be an alternative.

●○● NURSING CARE MANAGEMENT

For the Pregnant Woman with Rubella

Nursing Assessment and Diagnosis

A woman who develops rubella during pregnancy may be asymptomatic or may show signs of a mild infection, including a maculopapular rash, lymphadenopathy, muscular achiness, and joint pain. The presence of IgM antirubella antibody is diagnostic of a recent infection. These titers remain elevated for approximately 1 month following infection.

Nursing diagnoses that may apply to the woman who develops rubella early in her pregnancy include:

- ***Coping, Ineffective***, related to an inability to accept the possibility of fetal anomalies secondary to maternal rubella exposure
- ***Health Maintenance, Ineffective***, related to lack of knowledge about the importance of rubella immunization before becoming pregnant

(NANDA-I © 2017)

Nursing Plan and Implementation

Nursing support and understanding are vital for the couple contemplating abortion because of a diagnosis of rubella infection. Such a decision may initiate a crisis for the couple who have planned their pregnancy. They need objective data to understand the possible adverse effects of CRS on their fetus and the prognosis for their offspring.

Evaluation

Expected outcomes of nursing care include:

- The woman is able to describe the implications of rubella exposure during the first trimester of pregnancy.
- If exposure occurs in a woman who is not immune, she is able to identify her options and make a decision about continuing her pregnancy that is acceptable to her and her partner.
- The nonimmune woman receives the rubella vaccine during the early postpartum period.
- The woman gives birth to a healthy baby.

Cytomegalovirus

Cytomegalovirus (CMV) belongs to the herpes simplex virus group and causes both congenital and acquired disorders. The virus has subtypes, placing an infected individual at risk for reinfection. A primary infection in the pregnant woman can be catastrophic to the fetus, while reinfections may have less severe consequences. Most infected pregnant women are asymptomatic, yet the virus can be transmitted to the fetus across the placenta or by exposure to cervical secretions during birth. It is the most common congenital infection and responsible for sensorineural hearing loss (ACOG, 2015).

The virus can be found in urine, saliva, cervical mucus, semen, and breast milk. It can be passed between humans by any close contact such as kissing, breastfeeding, and sexual intercourse. Asymptomatic CMV infection is particularly common in children and gravid women. Transmission is common in daycare centers, especially among children between the ages of 1 and 3 years. It is a chronic, persistent infection and the infected individual may shed the virus continually over many years. Although the virus is usually innocuous in adults and children, it may be fatal to the fetus. Currently there is no treatment.

Accurate diagnosis in the pregnant woman is best documented by seroconversion (positive IgM antibodies and negative IgG antibodies initially, changing to negative IgM antibodies and positive IgG antibodies). Shedding of the virus in urine and saliva can be intermittent and does not distinguish primary infection from recurrent infection. Identification of the virus in amniotic fluid by PCR or viral culture is the most sensitive and specific way of diagnosing congenital infection (ACOG, 2015; Bernstein, 2017). Ultrasound findings may include fetal hydrops, growth restriction, hydramnios, cardiomegaly, and fetal ascites.

FETAL-NEONATAL RISKS

CMV is the most common viral cause of infection in the human fetus. Subclinical infections in the newborn can produce intellectual disability and hearing loss, sometimes not recognized for several months, or learning disabilities not seen until childhood. In children, congenital CMV is the leading cause of hearing loss (Bernstein, 2017).

For the fetus/newborn, serious long-term complications most often follow a primary maternal infection in the first half of pregnancy (Bernstein, 2017). For the fetus, this infection can result in extensive intrauterine tissue damage that leads to fetal death; to survival with microcephaly, hydrocephaly, cerebral palsy, or intellectual disability; or to survival with no damage at all. The infected newborn is often SGA.

At present, no treatment exists for maternal CMV or for the congenital disease in the newborn (Bernstein, 2017). Thus, prevention is important. The pregnant woman should be advised to avoid areas with high concentrations of young children such as daycare centers, if possible, and to practice good hand hygiene techniques.

Herpes Simplex Virus

It has been estimated that one in six people between the ages of 14 and 49 (16.2%) are infected with genital herpes in the United States (ACOG, 2016b). *Herpes simplex virus (HSV-I or HSV-II)* infection can cause painful lesions in the genital area. Lesions may also develop on the cervix. This condition and its implications for nonpregnant women are discussed in Chapter 5. However, because the presence of herpes lesions in the genital tract may profoundly affect the fetus, herpes infection, as it relates to a pregnant woman, is discussed here.

FETAL-NEONATAL RISKS

A primary herpes simplex infection can increase the risk of spontaneous abortion when infection occurs in the first trimester. Preterm labor (PTL), IUGR, and neonatal infection are greater risks if the primary infection occurs late in the second trimester or early in the third trimester and maternal viremia develops or placental transfer occurs. Recurrent infections during pregnancy do not appear to increase the risk for abortion or low-birth-weight newborns.

The risk of transmission to the newborn by direct contact during birth will vary by the route of birth (vaginal versus cesarean birth), whether a lesion is present at the time, and whether it is a primary or recurrent lesion. If HSV-1 or HSV-2 is acquired close to the time of labor (primary outbreak), the risk of transmission to the fetus is 30 to 50% during a vaginal birth. Exposure to a recurrent/secondary lesion drops the risk of transmission to the newborn to between 2 and 5% (ACOG, 2016b). For a woman with either a primary or a secondary outbreak of genital herpes during labor, or with symptoms that may indicate an impending outbreak (called *aura*), the preferred method of childbirth is cesarean birth. Although fetal transmission with recurrent outbreaks is low, a cesarean birth is warranted because of the serious nature of the disease in the newborn. Vaginal birth is appropriate for women with a history of HSV but no evidence of active genital disease or aura at the time of childbirth (ACOG, 2016b).

The infected newborn is often asymptomatic at birth, but symptoms can occur any time after birth and up to 4 weeks of age. Symptoms include vesicular skin lesions, respiratory distress, fever (or hypothermia), seizures, and poor feeding. Newborns with disseminated disease present the earliest, usually within the first week after birth. CNS symptoms generally occur during the second or third week. All newborns with neonatal herpes should be evaluated promptly and treated with acyclovir. Care of infected newborns is addressed in Chapter 31.

CLINICAL THERAPY

A woman planning a pregnancy who has no history of HSV, but who has had a partner with genital HSV, should have type-specific serology testing to determine her risk of acquiring HSV. If she is already pregnant, this should be done as early in pregnancy as possible. Type-specific serology for HSV-1 and HSV-2 will confirm a "yes" or a "no" for past infection, but will not detail where the infection might be (mouth, anus, vagina). For this reason, couples should take precautions to decrease the chance of transmission.

Antiviral therapy is recommended after 36 weeks' gestation for women who experience recurrent outbreaks during pregnancy (ACOG, 2016b). Oral antiviral therapies are available, including acyclovir, famciclovir, and valacyclovir. Famciclovir and valacyclovir have the advantage of better absorption and a longer half-life than acyclovir. Currently, there is no evidence that there are any adverse fetal effects related to exposure to these antiviral drugs during any trimester.

●○● NURSING MANAGEMENT

For the Pregnant Woman with Herpes Simplex Virus

Nursing Assessment and Diagnosis

During the initial prenatal visit, it is important to learn whether the woman or her partner have had previous herpes infections. If so, ongoing assessment is indicated as pregnancy progresses.

Nursing diagnoses that may apply to the pregnant woman with HSV include:

- ***Pain, Acute***, related to the presence of lesions secondary to herpes infection
- ***Coping, Ineffective***, related to depression secondary to the risk to the fetus if herpes lesions are present at birth

(NANDA-I © 2017)

Nursing Plan and Implementation

Nurses need to be particularly concerned with patient education about this fast-spreading disease. Inform women about what herpes is, how it is spread, and preventive measures. Condoms do not afford complete protection (approximately 50% effective); therefore, advise couples to abstain from sexual contact while prodromal symptoms or lesions are present on the infected partner (ACOG, 2016b). Provide women with information about the association of genital herpes with spontaneous abortion, attendant neonatal mortality and morbidity, and the possibility of cesarean birth. A woman who has a history of HSV infection needs to inform her future healthcare providers.

Adolescents who acquired HSV may become concerned about the possible risks of HSV infection as they mature and become young adults who want to have families. Counsel these women in a manner that allows expression of the anger, shame, and depression so often experienced by women with herpes. Literature may be helpful and is available from many public health agencies.

Evaluation

Expected outcomes of nursing care include:

- The woman is able to describe her infection with regard to its method of transmission, expected medical therapy, comfort measures, implications for her pregnancy, and long-term implications.
- The woman has appropriate laboratory testing (serology, viral cultures) as recommended throughout her pregnancy.
- The woman gives birth to a healthy baby.

Group B Streptococcus Infection

Group B streptococcus (GBS) infection is a bacterial infection found in the lower GI or urogenital tract. Women may transmit GBS to their fetus in utero or during childbirth. GBS is a leading cause of infectious neonatal sepsis and mortality. Fortunately, improved recognition and rapid treatment of infected newborns have reduced morbidity and mortality rates considerably.

An estimated 10 to 40% of pregnant women are carriers of GBS (ACOG, 2016c). The reservoir for GBS is thought to be the GI tract. Most women are asymptomatic and considered to be *carriers*. In symptomatic women, GBS is responsible for considerable maternal morbidity from infections such as pyelonephritis, chorioamnionitis, postpartum endometritis, sepsis, wound infections, and, in rare instances, meningitis.

FETAL-NEONATAL RISKS

Newborns become infected either by vertical transmission from the mother when passing through the birth canal, resulting in early-onset GBS in the first week of life, or from horizontal transmission from colonized nursery personnel or babies in the nursery, which may result in late-onset GBS (after the first week of life). GBS can also result in unexpected intrapartum stillbirths (Cunningham et al., 2018). Although most newborns who are born to colonized mothers will be born healthy, the transmission rate is influenced by how heavily the mother is colonized, whether or not she is persistently culture positive, the site of colonization (rectal vs. vaginal), and other risk factors.

Risk factors for GBS neonatal sepsis include:

- Prematurity
- Maternal intrapartum fever
- Membranes ruptured for longer than 18 hours
- A previously infected baby with GBS disease
- GBS bacteriuria in the current pregnancy
- Young maternal age
- African American or Hispanic race.

GBS causes severe, invasive disease in affected newborns. The majority of cases occur within the first week of life and are thus designated as early-onset disease. Late-onset disease occurs 1 week or more after birth. Early-onset GBS is often characterized by signs of serious illness including respiratory distress or pneumonia, apnea, and shock. Newborns with late-onset GBS often develop meningitis. Long-term neurologic complications are common in survivors of both types of GBS.

CLINICAL THERAPY

Guidelines for the detection of carriers and preventive treatment of newborns at risk include (CDC, 2016a):

- All pregnant women should be screened for both vaginal and rectal GBS colonization at 35 to 37 weeks' gestation. This is known as *universal GBS screening*. Treatment should be based on these results, even if cultures were done earlier in pregnancy.
- Women with a positive GBS screen between 35 and 37 weeks should receive intrapartum antibiotic prophylaxis (IAP) at the onset of labor or the rupture of membranes.
- Women with GBS in their urine at any time during the pregnancy should receive IAP because they typically have heavy colonization with GBS and thus have an increased risk of giving birth to a newborn with early-onset disease. These women do not need vaginal and rectal cultures at 35 to 37 weeks because therapy is already indicated.
- Women who have already given birth to a newborn with invasive GBS disease should receive IAP. Culture-based universal screening is not necessary.
- If the results of GBS screening are not known when labor begins, IAP is indicated for women with any of the following risk factors: Gestation less than 37 weeks, membranes ruptured equal to or longer than 18 hours, or a temperature greater than 100.4°F (38°C).

IAP is not indicated in the following circumstances:

- Regardless of GBS status, women who undergo a cesarean birth, have not been in labor, and have intact membranes
- Positive GBS culture in a previous pregnancy with a negative culture result in the current pregnancy
- Negative vaginal and rectal GBS screening results done at the appropriate gestational age regardless of intrapartum risk factors.

Figure 18–7 provides an algorithm for assessing the need for intrapartum antibiotic prophylaxis.

Intrapartum antibiotic prophylaxis for GBS (IAP-GBS) is recommended as follows: Initial dose of penicillin G 5 million units IV followed by 2.5 to 3.0 million units IV every 4 hours until childbirth. Alternately, ampicillin may be used. Women at high risk for an anaphylactic reaction to penicillin because of marked allergy may be treated with clindamycin; if the GBS strain is resistant to clindamycin, vancomycin may be given (CDC, 2016a).

Human B19 Parvovirus

Human B19 parvovirus causes erythema infectiosum (EI), or *fifth disease*. It produces a characteristic "slapped cheek" rash on the face and is one of the usual childhood diseases along with mumps, measles, rubella, and chickenpox (the other four diseases). It is transmitted via hand-to-hand contact or respiratory droplets. Symptoms in adults include myalgia, arthralgia, and coryza (inflammation of the nasal membranes with profuse nasal discharge), as well as headache, fever, and nausea, which coincides with contagiousness. More than 50% of pregnant women will be immune to parvovirus B19 as evidenced by a positive IgG titer (ACOG, 2015). Nonimmune women (negative IgG titer) with school-age children are more likely to acquire parvovirus B19 and should have serologic evaluation of IgM titer if exposed.

Although there is a low risk of fetal morbidity, transplacental (vertical) transmission is reported to be as high as 33%. Severe effects occur most frequently if maternal infection occurred before 20 weeks' gestation. Fetal infection is associated with spontaneous abortion, fetal hydrops, and stillbirth (Bernstein, 2017). The major concern for the fetus is nonimmune hydrops fetalis and fetal anemia, which, if left untreated, may result in death. If maternal infection is confirmed, weekly measurements of peak systolic velocity of the MCA (middle cerebral artery) are indicated to detect signs of fetal anemia. If fetal anemia and hydrops are diagnosed, intrauterine fetal transfusion may reduce the mortality. Fetal death may occur at 4 to 12 weeks postinfection; therefore, fetal surveillance should be maintained for 8 to 12 weeks. The risk of fetal death remains several months post maternal infection, even when fetal hydrops is not evident. In fetuses who survive the infection, long-term development appears to be normal.

Zika Virus

Zika is relatively new on the scene and information is being updated so rapidly there remains a paucity of well-designed studies.

Vaginal and rectal GBS screening cultures at 35–37 weeks' gestation for ALL pregnant women (unless client had GBS bacteriuria during the current pregnancy or a previous infant with invasive GBS disease)

Intrapartum prophylaxis indicated
- Previous infant with invasive GBS disease
- GBS bacteriuria during current pregnancy
- Positive GBS screening culture during current pregnancy (unless a planned cesarean birth, in the absence of labor or amniotic membrane rupture, is performed)
- Unknown GBS status (culture not done, incomplete, or results unknown) and any of the following:
    - Birth at less than 37 weeks' gestation*
    - Amniotic membrane rupture longer than or equal to 18 hours†
    - Intrapartum temperature greater than or equal to 100.4F (less than or equal to 38C) †

Intrapartum prophylaxis not indicated
- Previous pregnancy with a positive GBS screening culture (unless a culture was also positive during the current pregnancy)
- Planned cesarean birth performed in the absence of labor or membrane rupture (regardless of maternal GBS culture status)
- Negative vaginal and rectal GBS screening culture in late gestation during the current pregnancy, regardless of intrapartum risk factors

* If onset of labor or rupture of amniotic membrane occurs at less than 37 weeks' gestation and there is a significant risk for preterm birth (as assessed by the clinician).
† If amnionitis is suspected, broad-spectrum antibiotic therapy that includes an agent known to be active against GBS should replace GBS prophylaxis.

Figure 18–7 Indications for intrapartum antibiotic prophylaxis to prevent perinatal GBS disease under a universal prenatal screening strategy based on combined vaginal and rectal cultures collected at 35 to 37 weeks' gestation from all pregnant women.

SOURCE: Centers for Disease Control and Prevention (CDC).

Zika is a viral infection caused by a bite from the *Aedes* species of mosquito (Figure 18–8). To become infected, the mosquito must bite and feed from an infected host. The Zika virus can also be transmitted by infected individuals via blood, sex, handling of specimens in the laboratory, and perinatal transmission. There is no vaccine, and there is no cure. Anyone who has been to a known Zika-infested area and develops acute-onset fever, rash, joint pain, or conjunctivitis should be tested according to the latest CDC and state health department guidelines.

The virus is responsible for *congenital Zika syndrome (CZS)*, which can cause microcephaly in one out of 10 fetuses whose mothers are infected (Figure 18–9). It also can cause decreased brain tissue with a specific pattern of brain damage; damage to the back of the eye; joints with limited range of motion, such as clubfoot; and too much muscle tone, restricting body movement soon after birth. Women planning a pregnancy should follow the current CDC (2017a) guidelines if they have been infected

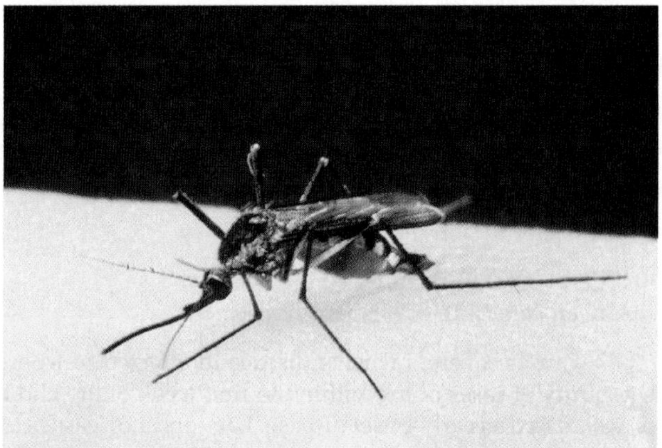

Figure 18–8 The *Aedes* species of mosquito, which is responsible for transmitting the Zika virus.

SOURCE: Centers for Disease Control and Prevention (CDC)/Robert S. Craig.

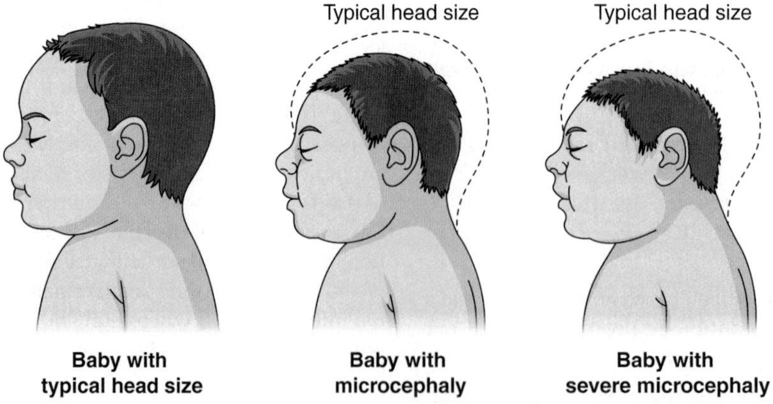

Figure 18–9 One of the most devastating outcomes of Zika infection during pregnancy is microcephaly. This figure compares a baby with a typical head size to babies with microcephaly and a severe version of microcephaly.

SOURCE: Centers for Disease Control and Prevention (CDC).

with Zika per laboratory confirmation: Delay conception at least 2 months from onset of symptoms; and men should delay conception for 6 months from onset of symptoms.

Women of reproductive age who are planning a pregnancy in the upcoming year, or who are already pregnant, should absolutely avoid Zika-infested areas. The mosquito lives indoors and outdoors in swampy areas and bites day and night. Should any woman need to travel to a high-risk area, she should wear DEET-covered clothing or apply DEET liberally to prevent a bite from an infected mosquito. Should she develop symptoms of a Zika infection, she should call her healthcare provider immediately. If her male partner becomes infected, or if they are both infected, they should use condoms to prevent transmission of the virus for 6 months.

According to the CDC (2017b), the test that is offered to pregnant women depends on the timing of exposure to the Zika virus and the subsequent development of symptoms:

- Up to 2 weeks after symptom onset or last possible exposure, urine or serum RNA nucleic acid testing; a positive test confirms the diagnosis of recent maternal Zika virus infection.
- From 2 to 12 weeks after symptom onset or last date of possible exposure, serologic assays can be offered to detect Zika virus–specific IgM antibodies.

Once infection has been confirmed, referral to maternal-fetal medicine is essential for determining evidence of fetal infection and possible catastrophic neurologic sequelae. The nurse can help the mother and family to verbalize their feelings and facilitate appropriate counseling.

Other Infections in Pregnancy

Table 18–6 summarizes other urinary tract, vaginal, and sexually transmitted infections that put pregnancy at risk. (Infections in the nonpregnant woman are described in detail in Chapter 5.) Spontaneous abortion is frequently the result of a severe maternal infection, and research links infection with prematurity. In addition, if the pregnancy is carried to term in the presence of infection, the risk of maternal and fetal morbidity and mortality increases. Thus, it is essential to maternal and fetal health that infection be diagnosed and treated promptly.

TABLE 18–6 Infections That Put Pregnancy at Risk

CONDITION AND CAUSATIVE ORGANISM	SIGNS AND SYMPTOMS	TREATMENT	IMPLICATIONS FOR PREGNANCY
Urinary Tract Infections (UTIs)			
Asymptomatic bacteriuria (ASB): *Escherichia coli*, *Klebsiella*, *Proteus* most common	Bacteria present in urine and on culture with no accompanying symptoms.	Cephalosporins and ampicillin in early and late pregnancy; sulfonamides or nitrofurantoin in middle pregnancy. Organism sensitivity to antibiotics will guide the selection of an appropriate antibiotic.	Women with ASB in early pregnancy may go on to develop cystitis or acute pyelonephritis by third trimester if not treated. Oral sulfonamides taken in the last few weeks of pregnancy may lead to neonatal hyperbilirubinemia and kernicterus.
Cystitis (lower UTI): Causative organisms same as for ASB	Dysuria, urgency, frequency, low-grade fever, and hematuria may occur. Urine culture (clean catch) shows presence of leukocytes. Presence of 10^5 (100,000) or more colonies bacteria/mL urine.	Same	If not treated, infection may ascend and lead to acute pyelonephritis.
Acute pyelonephritis: Causative organisms same as for ASB	Sudden onset. Chills, high fever, flank pain, nausea and vomiting, malaise. May have decreased urine output, severe colicky pain, dehydration. Marked bacteriuria in urine culture, pyuria, WBC casts. Presence of 10^5 (100,000) or more colonies bacteria/mL urine.	Hospitalization; IV antibiotic therapy. Broad-spectrum antibiotics may be required until the urine culture is ready. Catheterization if urine output is low or absent. Supportive therapy or pain medication for comfort. Follow-up urine cultures are necessary.	Increased risk of premature birth and IUGR. Risk of Gram-negative septicemia.
Vaginal Infections			
Vulvovaginal candidiasis (yeast infections): *Candida albicans*	Often thick, white, curdy discharge, severe itching, dysuria, dyspareunia. Diagnosis based on presence of hyphae and spores in a wet-mount preparation of vaginal secretions.	Topical agents only are recommended during pregnancy. This includes intravaginal insertion of miconazole butoconazole, or clotrimazole, or other topical azole preparations (CDC, 2015).	If the infection is present at birth and the fetus is born vaginally, the fetus may contract thrush.
Bacterial vaginosis: *Gardnerella vaginalis*	White, homogenous vaginal discharge with a foul odor often described as "fishy." Wet-mount preparation with normal saline reveals "clue cells." Application of potassium hydroxide (KOH) to a specimen of vaginal secretions produces a pronounced fishy odor, known as a "positive whiff test."	Metronidazole 500 mg PO BID × 7 days or metronidazole 250 mg PO TID × 7 days or clindamycin 300 mg PO BID × 7 days (CDC, 2015).	Multiple studies have failed to demonstrate a teratogenic effect from metronidazole. BV during pregnancy is associated with PROM, PTL, intra-amniotic infection, and endometritis postpartum in high-risk pregnancies (CDC, 2015).

(continued)

TABLE 18–6 Infections That Put Pregnancy at Risk *(continued)*

CONDITION AND CAUSATIVE ORGANISM	SIGNS AND SYMPTOMS	TREATMENT	IMPLICATIONS FOR PREGNANCY
Vaginal Infections *(continued)*			
Trichomoniasis: *Trichomonas vaginalis*	Occasionally asymptomatic. May have frothy greenish-gray vaginal discharge, pruritus, and urinary symptoms. Strawberry patches may be visible on vaginal walls or cervix. Wet-mount preparation of vaginal secretions shows motile flagellated trichomonads.	Single 2-g dose of metronidazole orally or single 2-g dose of tinidazole orally (CDC, 2015).	Increased risk for PROM, preterm birth, and low birth weight.
Sexually Transmitted Infections			
Chlamydial infection: *Chlamydia trachomatis*	Majority of women asymptomatic, but symptoms include thin or purulent discharge, urinary burning and frequency, and/or lower abdominal pain. Often diagnosed during routine prenatal cervical DNA swab or urine DNA (the Aptima Combo).	Doxycycline, ofloxacin, and levofloxacin are contraindicated during pregnancy. Thus, pregnant women are treated with azithromycin or amoxicillin followed by repeat culture in 3 weeks (CDC, 2015).	Neonate of woman with untreated chlamydial infection may develop newborn conjunctivitis, which can be treated with erythromycin eye ointment (but not silver nitrate). Newborn may also develop chlamydial pneumonia. May be responsible for premature labor and fetal death.
Syphilis: *Treponema pallidum*, a spirochete	Primary stage: Chancre, slight fever, malaise. Chancre lasts about 4 weeks, then disappears. Secondary stage occurs 6 weeks to 6 months after infection. Skin eruptions (condyloma lata), also symptoms of acute arthritis, liver enlargement, iritis, chronic sore throat with hoarseness. Diagnosed by blood tests such as RPR, Treponemal IgG, FTA-ABS.	Treatment for pregnant women follows the regimen recommended for the general population and is based on the stage of syphilis. For early latent syphilis (less than 1-year duration), 2.4 million units benzathine penicillin G IM. For late latent syphilis (more than 1-year duration) or latent syphilis of unknown duration, 2.4 million units benzathine penicillin G IM once a week for 3 weeks. Pregnant women who are allergic to penicillin should be desensitized and then treated with penicillin. Sexual partners should also be screened and treated. If one dose is missed, the series of three must be implemented again (CDC, 2015).	Syphilis can be passed transplacentally to the fetus. If untreated, one of the following can occur: Second-trimester abortion, stillborn at term, congenitally infected, or uninfected live newborn.
Gonorrhea: *Neisseria gonorrhoeae* (Gram-negative anaerobe)	Majority of women asymptomatic, but symptoms include purulent vaginal discharge, dysuria, urinary frequency, inflammation, swelling of the vulva and the appearance of erosion in the cervix. Often diagnosed during routine prenatal cervical DNA swab or urine DNA (the Aptima Combo).	Pregnant women are treated with a cephalosporin (ceftriaxone, cefixime). Spectinomycin is not available in the United States; thus azithromycin 2 g PO may be used if the woman cannot tolerate a cephalosporin. The woman is also treated for chlamydia using azithromycin or amoxicillin (CDC, 2015). All sexual partners are also treated.	Infection at time of birth may cause ophthalmia neonatorum in the newborn.
Condylomata acuminata: Caused by human papillomavirus (HPV)	Soft, grayish-pink lesions on the vulva, vagina, cervix, or anus	Podophyllin, podofilox, and imiquimod are contraindicated during pregnancy. Some caregivers recommend removing warts by surgical methods, cryotherapy, or laser because the warts can proliferate and become friable (bleed easily) during pregnancy.	Possible teratogenic effect of podophyllin. Large doses have been associated with fetal death. Cesarean birth is only indicated for women with warts that obstruct the pelvic outlet or if vaginal birth would result in significant bleeding (CDC, 2015).

Care of the Woman Requiring Surgery During Pregnancy

Although elective surgery should be delayed until the postpartum period, essential surgery should be undertaken at any gestational period during pregnancy. The most common essential surgeries include appendectomy, cholecystectomy, and ovarian torsion. The early second trimester is the best time to operate because there is less risk of spontaneous abortion or early labor and the uterus is not so large as to impinge on the abdominal field (ACOG, 2017b).

General preoperative and postoperative care is similar for pregnant and nonpregnant women; however, special considerations must be kept in mind whenever the surgical patient is pregnant. If a chest x-ray is done, the fetus should be shielded from radiation. The decreased intestinal motility and delayed gastric emptying that occur in pregnancy increase the risk of vomiting when anesthetics are given and during the postoperative period. Thus, a nasogastric tube may be recommended before major surgery. An indwelling urinary catheter prevents bladder distention, decreases risk of injury to the bladder, and permits monitoring of output. FHR must be monitored electronically before, during, and after surgery.

Pregnancy causes increased secretions of the respiratory tract and engorgement of the nasal mucous membrane, often making breathing through the nose difficult. Because of this, pregnant women often need an endotracheal tube for respiratory support during surgery. Caregivers must guard against maternal hypoxia during surgery because uterine circulation will be decreased and fetal oxygenation can decline very quickly. During surgery and the recovery period, the woman is positioned to allow optimal uteroplacental–fetal circulation. A wedge is placed under her hip to tip the uterus and thereby avoid pressure by the gravid uterus on the maternal vena cava and aorta.

Spinal or epidural anesthesia is preferred because neuraxial anesthetics are not associated with birth defects. Caution must be exercised because this type of anesthesia may produce hypotension and respiratory apnea in the pregnant woman. The frequency and degree of the hypotension increase with higher anesthetic levels.

Blood loss during surgery is monitored carefully. Because of the normal increased blood volume of pregnancy, uterine blood flow may be reduced significantly before the maternal blood pressure begins to fall. Fluid replacement should be done with balanced electrolyte solution and, if needed, with whole blood.

●○● NURSING MANAGEMENT

For the Pregnant Woman Requiring Surgery

Nursing Assessment and Diagnosis

During the preoperative period, assess the pregnant woman's health status in the same way that any preoperative patient is assessed. Is there any sign of respiratory infection, fever, urinary tract infection, or anemia? Are laboratory values all within normal limits for surgery (except in the case of emergency surgery, which may, of necessity, be done even with abnormal laboratory values)? Do the woman and her family understand the surgical procedure? Do they know what to expect postoperatively? Do they have any questions or concerns?

Pre/intra/postoperatively, fetal heart rate should be assessed, if at all possible. If the gestation is viable, continuous fetal monitoring is recommended. Postoperatively, complete all necessary assessments as would be done for any patient.

Nursing diagnoses that might apply to the pregnant woman who requires surgery include:

- ***Anxiety*** related to lack of knowledge of preoperative and postoperative procedures
- ***Fear*** related to the possible effect of surgery on fetal outcome

(NANDA-I © 2017)

Nursing Plan and Implementation

Much of the nurse's care during the preoperative period is directed toward the educational needs of the woman and her family. Plan time to review the procedure and answer any questions the family may have. Recognize that the need for surgery during pregnancy is probably very distressing for the woman and her family. Help decrease their anxiety by providing information and emotional support.

Pre/intra/postoperatively, you are caring for two patients: The mother and her unborn child. In addition to monitoring the status of both, you must consider how to provide trimester-appropriate care. If surgery is done in the first trimester, be aware of the potential teratogenic effect of any medications prescribed and discuss the implications with the surgeon and obstetrician. After 20 weeks' gestation, recognize the potential for vena cava syndrome if the woman lies flat on her back and help her to maintain a side-lying position. To avoid inadequate oxygenation, encourage the woman to turn, breathe deeply, and cough regularly and also to use any ventilation therapy, such as incentive spirometry, to avoid developing pneumonia. The pregnant woman is also at increased risk for thrombophlebitis, so apply sequential compression devices (SCDs) and antiembolism stockings; encourage leg exercises while the woman is confined to bed; administer low-molecular-weight heparin as thromboembolic prophylaxis, if ordered; and begin ambulation as soon as possible. In addition, encourage the woman to maintain or resume an adequate diet as soon as possible. If cultural factors influence the woman's dietary practices, work together with the dietician to meet the woman's needs.

Discharge teaching is especially important. The woman and her family should have a clear understanding of what to expect regarding activity level, discomfort, diet, medications, and any other special considerations. In addition, they ought to know any warning signs that they should report to their physician immediately.

Evaluation

Expected outcomes of nursing care include:

- The woman is able to explain the surgical procedure, its risks and benefits, and its implications for her pregnancy.
- Caregivers maintain adequate maternal oxygenation throughout surgery and postoperatively.
- Potential complications are avoided or detected early and treated successfully.
- The woman is able to describe any necessary postdischarge activities, limitations, and follow-up and agrees to cooperate with the recommended regimen.
- The woman maintains her pregnancy successfully.

Care of the Woman Suffering Major Trauma

Trauma complicates from 6 to 7% of pregnancies, and trauma from motor vehicle crashes and falls is the leading cause of fetal and maternal death (Robbins, Martin, & Wilson, 2014). Violence that includes domestic violence and assault, fractures, and suicide attempts are the next most common causes of injury.

In early pregnancy, physiologic changes from progesterone can lead to fatigue, syncopal episodes (fainting spells) from vasodilation, and hyperventilation that increase the potential for injury. Later in pregnancy, the woman has less balance and coordination and may fall. Her protruding abdomen is vulnerable to a variety of minor injuries. The fetus is usually well protected by the amniotic fluid, which distributes the force of a blow equally in all directions, by the muscle layers of the uterus and abdominal wall, and by the maternal adipose layer, which acts as a cushion. In early pregnancy, while the uterus is still in the pelvis, it is shielded from blows by the surrounding pelvic organs, muscles, and bony structures.

The normal physiologic changes of pregnancy have clinical implications for victims of trauma. Generally, the pregnant woman has a greater volume of blood loss compared with a nonpregnant woman before evidence of shock is seen. The pregnant woman with significant volume loss is able to maintain hemodynamic stability temporarily by decreasing uteroplacental perfusion, thereby compromising fetal status. In the second and third trimesters, supine positioning can decrease blood return to the heart and cause overt hypotension and even loss of consciousness. During pregnancy, minute ventilation and oxygen consumption increase (Robbins et al., 2014). This makes the gravid woman more susceptible to hypoxemia with apnea. Clotting factors normally increase in pregnancy, making it a hypercoagulable state. Thus, the risk of thrombosis after injury is increased. DIC occurs commonly with severe trauma.

Trauma that causes concern includes blunt trauma, penetrating abdominal injuries, and the complications of maternal shock, premature labor, and spontaneous abortion. Maternal mortality most often occurs from head trauma or hemorrhage. Uterine rupture is a rare but life-threatening complication of trauma. It may result from strong deceleration forces in a motor vehicle crash, with or without seat belts. Traumatic separation of the placenta can occur (abruptio), which causes a high rate of fetal mortality. Premature labor, often following rupture of membranes during a motor vehicle crash, is another serious hazard to the fetus. Premature labor can begin even if the woman is not injured. To help prevent trauma from motor vehicle crashes, all pregnant women should wear both lap seat belts (i.e., not across the abdomen) and shoulder harnesses.

Fractures of the pelvis can result in significant retroperitoneal hemorrhage. If there is an unstable or dislocated fracture of the pelvis, cesarean birth will probably be necessary, but with a slightly displaced pelvic fracture, vaginal birth may be attempted. Hematuria or difficulty placing a urinary catheter may be associated with injuries to the bladder or urethra.

Penetrating trauma includes gunshot wounds and stab wounds. The mother generally fares better than the fetus if the penetrating trauma involves the abdomen, as the enlarged uterus is likely to protect the mother's bowel from injury. Blood flow is shunted away from the uterus to provide for the mother, which can be at the expense of the fetus.

Clinical Therapy

The goals of clinical therapy are to stabilize the injury and promote well-being for both mother and fetus. Thus, clinical therapy initially focuses on ensuring airway adequacy, maintaining ventilation and adequate circulatory volume, controlling acute bleeding, and splinting fractures to prevent vascular or tissue injury. The Glasgow Coma Scale is useful in evaluating for neurologic deficit. Once the mother is stabilized, fetal status is assessed.

Care must be taken at the scene of the injury to avoid the development of supine hypotensive syndrome, which can result in a reduction of blood return to the heart and a decrease in cardiac output, especially when the woman is supine, which is the preferred position for CPR in the nonpregnant population. Placing a wedge under the woman's right hip to 30 degrees displaces the uterus to the left and is critical in restoring cardiac output. A neck brace is used if a neck injury is suspected, or the woman is placed on a backboard and the entire board is tilted to displace the uterus. Prompt treatment of maternal hypotension or hypovolemia also averts poor fetal oxygenation. Obstetric consultation is necessary to ensure that the needs of both mother and fetus are met.

In cases of noncatastrophic trauma, that is, where the mother's life is not directly threatened, monitoring of the mother and fetus for 4 to 24 hours (if greater than 20 weeks' gestation, although some sources would say greater than 23 weeks' gestation to account for the lowest limit of viability) is recommended to observe for vaginal bleeding, uterine tenderness, contractions, or amniotic fluid leakage (Brown, 2017). In many facilities this may be called the *obstetric trauma protocol*. A baseline CBC is drawn and compared to a follow-up 4 hours later. If the hematocrit has dropped, it may indicate internal bleeding. A Kleihauer-Betke test to examine the number of fetal red blood cells (RBCs) in the maternal system is ordered. A large number may indicate a maternal–fetal hemorrhage. An ultrasound to examine for a retroplacental clot is performed. All Rh-negative women are given Rh immune globulin. If there are not four contractions per hour, if there is no vaginal bleeding, and all labwork and diagnostic imaging is within normal limits, the woman is discharged home in 4 hours.

Abruptio placentae may occur following a blow to the abdomen as the flexible myometrium of the uterus sustains a contour-changing impact that the relatively inelastic placenta cannot match. The increased intrauterine pressure during the blow further shears the placenta from the underlying decidua basalis. Increased uterine irritability in the first few hours following trauma helps identify women who may be at high risk for this potentially catastrophic complication.

Fetomaternal hemorrhage may occur and is more likely in women whose placenta is located on the anterior wall of the uterus. Fetal jeopardy from significant fetal hemorrhage is generally accompanied by fetal tachycardia, loss of variability, or a sinusoidal fetal heart rate pattern.

Perimortem cesarean birth is advocated if CPR on the mother is unsuccessful in the first 5 minutes. Chest compressions are less effective in the third trimester because of compression of the inferior vena cava by the gravid uterus. Cesarean birth alleviates this compression and improves resuscitation efforts in both the fetus and the mother.

●○● NURSING MANAGEMENT

For the Woman Suffering Major Trauma

Nursing Assessment and Diagnosis

Each woman must be assessed individually according to the type and extent of her injuries. As with all trauma victims, initial assessments focus on adequacy of the airway, evidence of breathing, existence of cardiovascular stability, extent of injury, and a brief neurologic assessment. When an injured woman is pregnant, it is also necessary to assess fetal status to avoid fetal hypoxia. Frequent maternal blood gas determinations are indicated if respiratory function is compromised. If the fetus is viable, continuous electronic fetal monitoring may be indicated.

Ongoing assessments include evaluation of uterine tone, contractions and tenderness, fundal height, fetal heart rate and variability, intake and output and other indicators of shock, postoperative evaluation in those women requiring surgery, determination of neurologic status, and assessment of mental outlook and anxiety level.

Nursing diagnoses that might apply to the pregnant woman suffering trauma include:

- ***Pain, Acute,*** related to the effects of the trauma experienced
- ***Constipation*** related to immobility secondary to the effects of the trauma
- ***Fear*** related to the effects of the trauma on fetal well-being

(NANDA-I © 2017)

Nursing Plan and Implementation

As a member of the healthcare team, you are actively involved in the ongoing assessment of the status of the woman and fetus. A primary responsibility is to assess the childbearing woman's emotional state. The trauma victim must be oriented to her situation and receive explanation and reinforcement as necessary to help her understand any interventions. Family members should be involved as appropriate. Give the pregnant woman an opportunity to discuss her feelings and concerns. See *Case Study: Melissa Bond-James*.

Evaluation

Expected outcomes of nursing care include:

- The woman and her family are able to understand the effects of the trauma on her and on her unborn child.
- Adequate maternal oxygenation is maintained to ensure fetal well-being.
- The woman's pain is adequately relieved, and her trauma is treated.
- Potential complications are quickly identified, and appropriate interventions are instituted.
- The woman gives birth to a healthy newborn.
- If the trauma results in fetal demise, the woman is able to verbalize her feelings and begin working through the grief process.

Care of the Pregnant Woman Experiencing Intimate Partner Violence

The true extent of intimate partner violence (IPV) during pregnancy is difficult to determine, but estimates suggest 6 to 22% of women are victimized (Brown, 2017) (Figure 18–10).

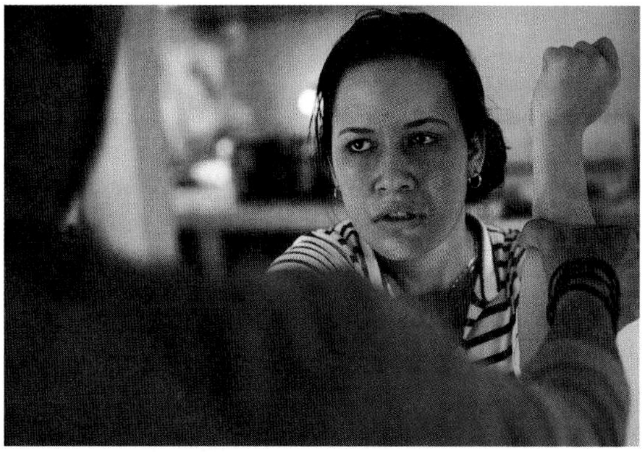

Figure 18–10 **Intimate partner violence may begin or escalate during pregnancy.**

SOURCE: Diego Cervo/Shutterstock.

Violence may escalate during pregnancy, and homicide by an intimate partner is a significant cause of maternal mortality (Brown, 2017). Being the victim of physical, sexual, or psychologic abuse is one of the strongest predictors that an individual will become either a perpetrator or a victim of IPV. Other known risk factors include low socioeconomic status, unemployment/family financial difficulties, heavy alcohol or drug use, antisocial personality traits, belief in strict gender roles (e.g., male dominance and aggression in relationships), negative or volatile family dynamics, low social support, and weak community sanctions against IPV (CDC, 2017b).

Battering may result in psychologic distress, loss of pregnancy, preterm labor, low-birth-weight babies, injury to the fetus, and fetal death. Complications such as poor maternal weight gain, infection, anemia, and second- and third-trimester bleeding are also seen more frequently among pregnant women who are abused. Women who are battered may also experience sexual abuse and are at increased risk of contracting sexually transmitted infections from their partners. This pattern of violence may escalate during pregnancy and may occur even more frequently in the postpartum period when there is a new baby in the home that requires frequent attention. In some instances, abuse may decrease during pregnancy, and the woman feels safe while she is pregnant, only to have the abuse resume shortly after childbirth. These women may repeatedly become pregnant to escape abuse. Chronic psychosomatic symptoms can be an indicator of abuse. The woman may have nonspecific or vague complaints. It is important to assess old scars around the head, chest, arms, abdomen, and genitalia. Any bruising or evidence of pain is also evaluated. The nurse should be especially alert for signs of bruising or injury to the woman's breasts, abdomen, or genitals because these areas are common targets of violence during pregnancy. Other indicators include a decrease in eye contact, silence

CASE STUDY: Melissa Bond-James

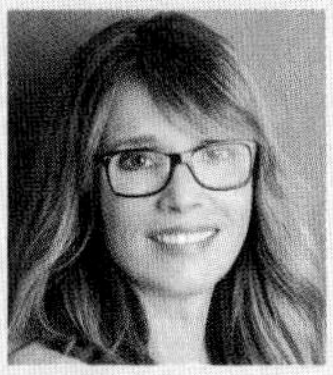

SOURCE: Kinga/Shutterstock.

Melissa calls the nurse and reports that she was involved in a motor vehicle accident (MVA) and was hit from the back by another car. She states she is fine, but has some mild cramping and may have hurt her abdomen. She reports the seat belt tightened around her lower abdomen when the car was struck. She is 31 weeks' gestation and denies bleeding. The baby seems to be sleeping but she has felt some movement since the accident.

Question to Ponder

What advice would you give Melissa?

when the partner is in the room, and a history of nervousness, insomnia, drug overdose, or alcohol problems. Frequent visits to the emergency department and a history of accidents or injuries without understandable causes are possible indicators of abuse.

The goals of treatment are to identify the woman at risk, increase her decision-making abilities to decrease the potential for further abuse, and provide a safe environment for her and her unborn child. Screening must be done in a private setting and by using direct questions. All women should be screened for intimate partner violence at the first prenatal visit, at least once per trimester, and at the postpartum visit. See Chapter 8 for discussion of specific screening questions.

Once domestic violence is identified, the next step is to determine the immediate safety of the woman. She needs to be aware of community resources available to her, such as emergency shelters; police, legal, and social services; and counseling. It is important to establish an exit plan in situations of ongoing violence. Pocket cards and resource materials can be handed to women or left in restrooms for them to pick up. Nurses need to recognize that, ultimately, it is the woman's decision either to seek assistance or to return to old patterns, and understand that even women with money and means find it difficult to leave an abusive situation. Lack of finances, needs of the other children, ongoing threats of physical harm, and extended family member denial all play a part in the woman staying with the abuser. For further information, see Chapter 8.

Care of the Woman at Risk for Rh Alloimmunization

Red blood cells contain antigens. One that has caused enormous obstetric morbidity and mortality is the Rh blood group (RhD antigen), which is present on the surface of erythrocytes of most of the population. When it is present, a person is said to be Rh positive. Those without the RhD antigen are Rh negative. The incidence varies by race and ethnicity. While approximately 15% of Caucasian Americans are Rh negative, that percentage drops to 5 to 8% of African Americans and 1 to 2% of Asian Americans and Native Americans (ACOG, 2018a).

If an Rh-negative person is exposed to Rh-positive blood (RhD), an antigen–antibody response occurs, antibodies are formed, and the person is said to become *alloimmunized/sensitized/isoimmunized*. Subsequent exposure to more Rh-positive blood can cause a robust production of antibodies that leads to destruction of RhD antigen or hemolysis of RBCs. RhD alloimmunization can occur when an Rh-negative woman carries an Rh-positive fetus to term, or to termination by miscarriage or induced abortion, or as an ectopic pregnancy. Also, during pregnancy Rh-positive fetal blood can enter the maternal circulation of an Rh-negative woman subsequent to trauma or interventional procedures such as a chorionic villus sample, amniocentesis, or external cephalic version. Rh-positive blood can also enter the bloodstream of an Rh-negative nonpregnant woman if she receives an Rh-positive blood transfusion.

Routine prenatal labwork ordered at the first obstetrical visit includes blood type, Rh status (factor present or absent), and an antibody screen. The latter can determine if alloimmunization of an Rh-negative mother has occurred by identifying the production of antibodies against the Rh-positive blood group. These are called anti-D antibodies. The use of **Rh immune globulin (RhIg)**, such as RhoGAM or RhoPhylac, has resulted in a marked decrease in the prevalence of alloimmunization in pregnancy. However, because there are over 400 atypical antigens on RBCs capable of causing an antigen–antibody reaction, it is prudent for the nurse to know that there are more antibodies than anti-D that can cause fetal hemolysis. No prophylaxis, such as RhIg, is available to prevent the formation of antibodies to other red cell antigens such as Duffy (produces anti-Duffy antibodies), Kell (produces anti-K1 antibodies), and others.

Pathophysiology of RhD Alloimmunization

During a normal pregnancy, small amounts of fetal blood cross the placenta. If this did not occur as a normal part of the pregnancy, we would not be able to perform noninvasive prenatal testing (NIPT) using cell-free DNA (cfDNA). An Rh-negative mother may develop anti-D antibodies in response to this exposure if she has a fetus who is Rh positive with the RhD antigen. During delivery of the placenta or as a result of trauma, larger quantities of fetal blood can enter the maternal circulation. After exposure to the Rh-positive antigen, the primary immune response is development of immunoglobulin M (IgM) antibodies. This primary response develops slowly over several weeks or months, with a detectable titer developing 5 to 16 weeks after the sensitizing event. IgM antibodies are large and do not cross the placenta. Because this transfer of RBCs usually occurs at birth, and because IgM antibodies/immunoglobulins are the first to respond and do not cross the placenta, the first child is usually not affected. Prevention is essential, as once an Rh-negative woman develops anti-D antibodies, she is "alloimmunized" for life.

Following the primary response, the body forms IgG immunoglobin (IgG) for lifetime immunity. Unfortunately, a subsequent exposure to the RhD antigen (such as during a subsequent pregnancy) may result in a rapid production of anti-D IgG immunoglobulins, or anti-D antibodies. Depending on the woman's immune system, these antibodies may develop days after exposure. IgG is capable of crossing the placenta, coating the fetal RhD-positive RBCs and causing hemolysis.

The secondary response produces a response that is stronger than the primary response (Figure 18–11). Thus, although hemolysis is not generally a problem for the fetus during a first pregnancy, it may create serious problems during subsequent pregnancies. The destruction of fetal RBCs causes anemia in the fetus that can lead to death. The earlier in the pregnancy the fetal hemolysis begins, the worse the prognosis. To prevent alloimmunization after exposure to Rh-positive blood by an Rh-negative woman, RhIg is administered.

Fetal-Neonatal Risks

Although RhD alloimmunzation can now be prevented by administration of RhIg, its incidence has increased in recent years due to the migration to more developed countries of Rh-negative alloimmunized women from countries with lower healthcare standards or limited resources to RhIg (Moise, 2017).

If the woman is alloimmunized, the hemolysis caused by the maternal IgG antibodies that cross the placenta to the fetus creates fetal anemia. The fetus responds by increasing RBC production of immature cells that still have a nucleus. The presence of nucleated RBCs (erythroblasts) is why the term **erythroblastosis fetalis** was coined for this severe *hemolytic disease of the fetus and newborn (HDFN)*. This anemia can also cause marked fetal edema, called **hydrops fetalis**. Congestive heart failure may result. RBC destruction also leads to hyperbilirubinemia and jaundice (called *icterus gravis*), which can lead to neurologic damage (*kernicterus*). Fetal death can be from severe anemia or hypoxia and cardiac arrest. See Chapter 31 for further discussion of kernicterus and of treatment of the newborn affected by Rh alloimmunization.

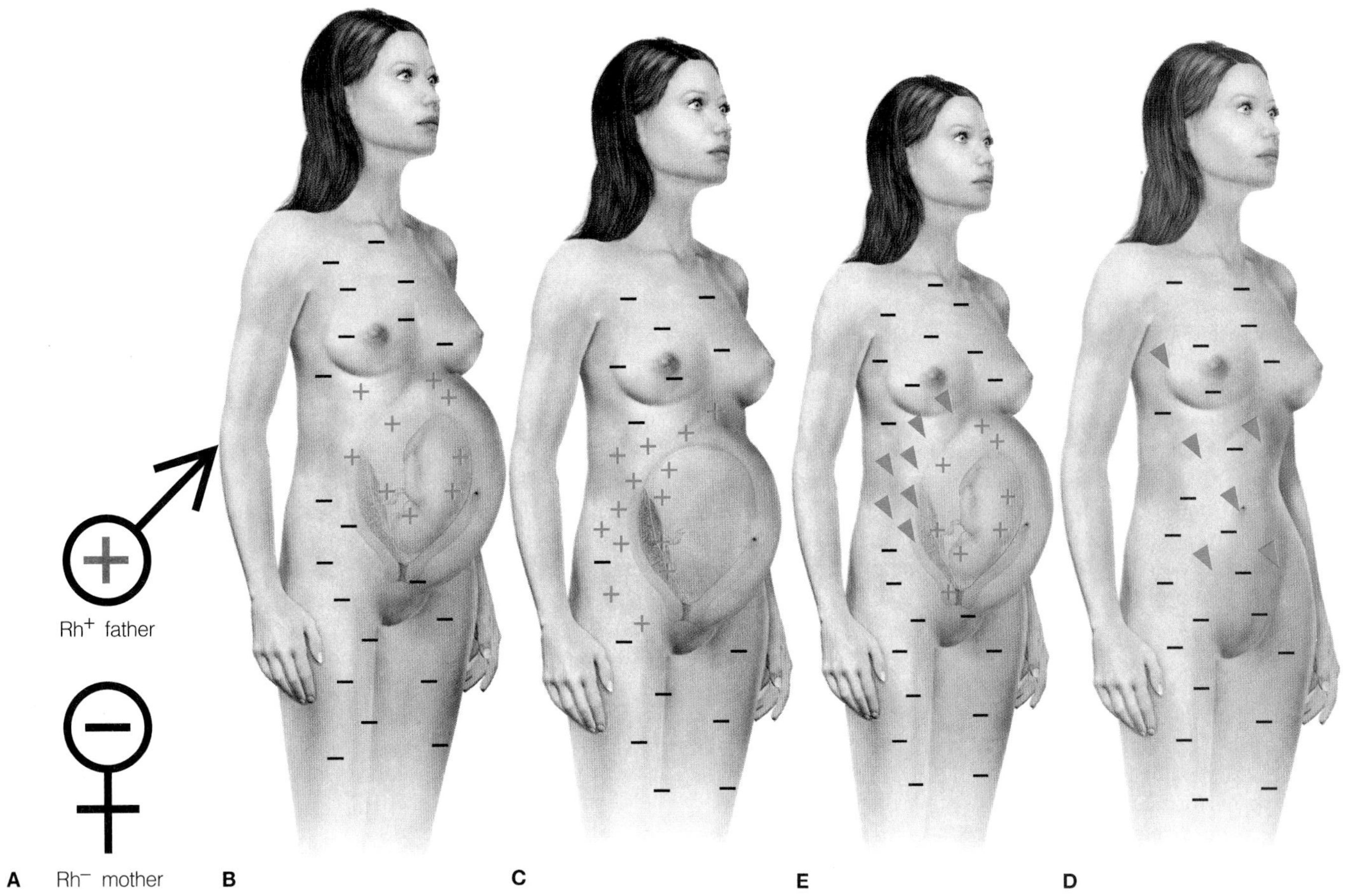

Figure 18–11 Rh alloimmunization sequence. A. Rh-positive father and Rh-negative mother. B. Pregnancy with Rh-positive fetus. Some Rh-positive blood enters the mother's blood. C. As the placenta separates, the mother is further exposed to the Rh-positive blood. D. The mother is sensitized to the Rh-positive blood; anti-Rh-positive antibodies (triangles) are formed. E. In subsequent pregnancies with an Rh-positive fetus, Rh-positive red blood cells are attacked by the anti-Rh-positive maternal antibodies, causing hemolysis of red blood cells in the fetus.

SCREENING FOR RH INCOMPATIBILITY AND ALLOIMMUNIZATION

At the first prenatal visit, healthcare providers should:

1. Take a history of past pregnancies, previous alloimmunization, abortions, blood transfusions, or children who developed jaundice or anemia during the newborn period.
2. Determine maternal blood type (ABO) and Rh factor and do a routine antibody screen.
3. Identify other medical complications such as diabetes, infections, or hypertension.

An antibody screen (*indirect Coombs test*) is done to determine whether an Rh-negative woman has become alloimmunized (developed anti-D antibodies) to the Rh-positive antigen. The test measures the number of antibodies in the maternal blood. If the pregnant woman is not alloimmunized, RhIg (RhoGAM, RhoPhylac) is administered prophylactically at 28 weeks' gestation and then after delivery of an Rh-positive fetus. If the woman has a positive antibody screen, follow-up will depend on the amount of anti-D antibody in her serum, as determined by a titer. A woman with an elevated antibody titer beyond 1:1 or 1:2 should be considered as suspicious for alloimmunization and her pregnancy should be managed closely. Each laboratory determines the titer at which HDNF is likely, usually a titer between 1:8 and 1:32. It is imperative that any positive titer and subsequent titers be run at the same lab due to the difference in reagents between labs. Once a titer doubles, or reaches 1:8, the woman is highly alloimmunized and should be seen by maternal-fetal medicine for an individualized and specialized plan of care.

If the Rh-negative woman is not alloimmunized, 300 mcg of Rh immune globulin is administered IM prophylactically at 28 weeks' gestation. RhIg is also administered after any trauma, any procedure (CVS, ECV, amniocentesis), and within 72 hours of birth of an Rh-positive newborn.

Clinical Therapy

The goal of medical management is the prevention of Rh alloimmunization or, if alloimmunization has occurred, birth of a mature fetus that has not developed severe hemolysis in utero. This requires early identification and treatment of maternal conditions that predispose the baby to hemolytic disease and coordinated care and treatment by maternal-fetal medicine, obstetrics, and neonatology.

ANTEPARTUM MANAGEMENT OF THE NONALLOIMMUNIZED PREGNANT WOMAN

Four RhIg products are available: RhoGAM (the first approved for clinical use) and HyperRHO, which are administered intramuscularly, and Rhophlac and WinRho-SDF, which can be administered intramuscularly or intravenously. When the woman is Rh negative and not alloimmunized and the father is Rh positive or unknown, RhIg is given prophylactically at 28 weeks' gestation. It is also given after each spontaneous or induced abortion, ectopic pregnancy, chorionic villus sampling, multifetal pregnancy reduction, partial molar pregnancy, amniocentesis, percutaneous umbilical blood sampling (PUBS), antepartum hemorrhage, fetal death in the second or third trimester, blunt trauma to the maternal abdomen, or external cephalic version.

Whether alloimmunization is the result of a blood transfusion or fetal–maternal hemorrhage for any reason, a Kleihauer-Betke or rosette test can be performed to determine the amount of Rh-positive blood present in the maternal circulation and to calculate the amount of RhIg needed. The standard dose of RhIg (300 mcg) can prevent alloimmunization after exposure of up to 30 mL of Rh-positive fetal whole blood or 15 mL of packed red cells. Up to five doses of Rh immune globulin can be administered in a 24-hour period if there was a large maternal–fetal hemorrhage such as after a motor vehicle crash. Should a large dose be required, it may be preferable to use one of the intravenous forms to avoid multiple injections.

ANTEPARTUM MANAGEMENT OF THE ALLOIMMUNIZED PREGNANT WOMAN

A woman who is Rh negative is homozygous for the lack of the antigen (dd). If the father's Rh status is unknown, he is asked to come to the healthcare provider's office to be checked. If he is homozygous for Rh positive (DD), all of his offspring will be Rh positive. If he is heterozygous (Dd), 50% of his offspring will be Rh negative and 50% heterozygous for Rh positive. If the father is Rh negative, all their children will be Rh negative, and no Rh incompatibility with the mother will occur. If the father is Rh positive or the mother is known to have previously carried an Rh-positive fetus, further testing and careful management are needed. RhD genotyping of the fetus can be determined by cfDNA testing (Moezzi et al., 2016).

If the father is heterozygous or if paternity is questionable or unknown, fetal DNA testing should be done to determine the fetal Rh status (Moezzi et al., 2016). If the father is Rh negative, or if the fetus is Rh negative, no further intervention is needed.

In women who are alloimmunized for the first time, ultrasound should be done in the first trimester to best determine gestational age (ACOG, 2016d). Follow-up ultrasounds can also be used to detect ascites and subcutaneous edema, which are signs of severe fetal hemolysis. Other indicators of the fetal condition include an increase in fetal heart size and hydramnios.

Maternal anti-D antibody titers should be determined monthly until 24 weeks' gestation and then every 2 weeks thereafter. Negative antibody titers can consistently identify the fetus not at risk. However, the titers cannot reliably point out the fetus in danger because the level of the titer does not correlate with the severity of the disease. If titers remain below critical levels, birth at term is planned (Moise, 2017).

If the titers are higher than critical levels (this will be lab dependent, but usually a two-fold increase or greater than 1:32), Doppler ultrasound to measure peak systolic velocity in the middle cerebral artery (MCA-PSV) of the fetus is used to detect fetal anemia beginning at 24 weeks. The decreasing fetal red cell mass and concurrent decrease in blood viscosity result in an increase in fetal cardiac output and an increase in the velocity of blood flow through the middle cerebral artery, which is demonstrated by an increase in the peak systolic velocities. MCA-PSV correlates well over time with increasing levels of bilirubin from hemolysis in the amniotic fluid. If serial MCA Doppler scans indicate a peak velocity of 1.5 multiples of the median (MoM) or more, PUBS is done to determine fetal hematocrit. If the hematocrit is 30% or less, intrauterine transfusion is indicated. If the fetal hematocrit is greater than 30%, the PUBS is repeated in 1 to 2 weeks. After 35 weeks' gestation, the false-positive rate for the prediction of anemia with the use of MCA-PSV increases (Moise, 2017).

Intrauterine transfusion is done to correct the anemia produced by fetal RBC hemolysis from maternal anti-D antibody attack and thereby improve fetal oxygenation. This may be done either intravascularly through PUBS or intraperitoneally as early as 18 weeks. Intravascular transfusion has greatly improved the outcome for severely affected fetuses. Under ultrasound visualization, the umbilical vein is entered and the fetus is temporarily paralyzed with 0.01 mg/kg estimated fetal weight of vecuronium. A fetal hematocrit is obtained, then leukocyte-poor Rh-negative packed red blood cells (PRBCs) are transfused. The volume of PRBCs is determined by a formula based on estimated normal blood volume, the pretransfusion hematocrit, the hematocrit of the blood to be transfused, and the desired hematocrit. Repeat transfusions can be scheduled as necessary until the fetus is of a viable age and sufficiently mature to tolerate extrauterine life. If access to the umbilical vein is problematic, intrauterine transfusions can be performed by introducing the needle into the fetal abdomen and peritoneal cavity. Blood is transfused through a catheter into the peritoneal cavity, where diaphragmatic lymphatics absorb the RBCs into fetal circulation (Moise, 2017).

Most transfused fetuses survive. However, the procedure poses risks for the fetus. Complications include nonreassuring fetal status, umbilical vein hematoma, fetal-maternal hemorrhage, fetal death, and chorioamnionitis. Birth is delayed until at least 32 weeks' gestation, if possible. Premature newborns are generally more susceptible to damage from hemolytic disease. They often require exchange transfusion in the nursery and intensive care.

Historically, management of Rh disease was done with delta optical density (ΔOD_{450}) analysis, a test that determines the amount of bilirubin pigment found in the amniotic fluid via spectrography. Because the amount of bilirubin found in the amniotic fluid correlates roughly with the extent of the hemolysis, the ΔOD_{450} analysis serves as an indirect predictor of the severity of the fetal anemia after 35 weeks' gestation, if necessary, as MCA-PSV screening sensitivity falls off after this (Moise, 2017).

POSTPARTUM MANAGEMENT

The goals of postpartum care are to prevent alloimmunization in the as-yet-unsensitized woman and to treat the hemolytic disease in the newborn of a sensitized woman.

The Rh-negative mother who has not developed anti-D antibodies as evidenced by a negative titer or who is indirect Coombs negative, and who has given birth to an Rh-positive fetus (direct Coombs negative), is given an intramuscular injection of 300 mcg Rh immune globulin within 72 hours. This protocol reduces the incidence of antenatal alloimmunization dramatically. Although not completely understood, it is possible the RhD immunoglobulins work to destroy the fetal cells in the maternal circulation before alloimmunization occurs, thereby blocking maternal antibody production. It is possible circulating exogenous anti-D immunoglobulins also fool the woman's immune system into believing she has already produced them. This provides a type of temporary passive immunity for the mother, which prevents the development of permanent active immunity (antibody formation). The normal dose of Rh immune globulin should suppress the immune response to approximately 30 mL Rh-positive whole blood or 15 mL of PRBCs. As discussed previously, if a larger fetal–maternal hemorrhage might have occurred, a qualitative test, the rosette test, can be performed. If this is positive, the quantitative Kleihauer-Betke test can then be performed to obtain an estimate of the extent of the bleed and the dose of Rh immune globulin (RhIg or anti-D antibody) can be calculated.

Rh immune globulin is not given to the newborn or the father. It is not effective and should not be given to a previously alloimmunized woman. However, sometimes after childbirth or an abortion, the results of the blood test do not clearly show whether the mother is already alloimmunized to the Rh-positive antigen. In such cases, Rh immune globulin should be given because it will cause no harm.

●○● NURSING MANAGEMENT

For the Woman with Alloimmunization

Nursing Assessment and Diagnosis

As part of the initial prenatal history, ask the mother whether she knows her blood type and Rh factor. Many women are aware that they are Rh negative and that this status has implications for pregnancy. If the woman knows she is Rh negative, her knowledge of what that means should be assessed. Also ask the woman whether she ever received Rh immune globulin, whether she has had any previous pregnancies and their outcomes, and whether she knows her partner's Rh factor. Should the partner be Rh negative, there is no risk to the fetus, which will also be Rh negative. Uncertain paternity is an awkward situation; nevertheless, it is essential for the healthcare provider to have this information. Nurses often have a more intimate relationship with pregnant women, allowing them to obtain sensitive information that is vital in the management of pregnancy. When paternity is uncertain or the father is unavailable for testing, the fetus is assumed to be RhD positive until proven otherwise because its prevalence in the general population is so much higher than Rh negativity.

Ethics In Action!

How would you respond to an Rh-negative pregnant woman who asks you what to do when she learns that her husband, who is also Rh negative, is not the father of her Rh-positive child?

If the woman does not know what her Rh factor status is, intervention cannot begin until the initial laboratory data are obtained. If the woman is Rh negative, it is imperative to obtain the father's Rh factor status and, if he is Rh positive, whether he is hetero- or homozygous (DD or Dd). Once that is complete, you can plan intervention based on the findings.

If the woman becomes sensitized during her pregnancy, nursing assessment focuses on the knowledge level and coping skills of the woman and her family. Provide ongoing assessment during procedures, such as ultrasound and amniocentesis, to evaluate fetal well-being.

Postpartum, review data about the Rh status of the fetus. If the fetus is Rh positive, the mother is Rh negative, and no alloimmunization has occurred, nursing assessment reveals the need to administer RhIg within 72 hours of birth. If inadvertently the dose of RhIgG is not given within the 72-hour window, some protection has been documented with administration within 13 days. The recommendation is to administer the dose up to 28 days after birth.

Nursing diagnoses that might apply to the pregnant woman at risk for Rh sensitization include:

- ***Knowledge, Readiness for Enhanced***, related to an expressed desire to understand the treatment of Rh incompatibility and the purpose of Rh immune globulin (RhIg)
- ***Coping, Ineffective***, related to stress and concerns for fetal well-being

(NANDA-I © 2017)

Nursing Plan and Implementation

During the antepartum period, explain the mechanisms involved in alloimmunization and answer any questions the woman and her partner may have. It is imperative that the woman understand the importance of receiving Rh immune globulin after every spontaneous or therapeutic abortion or ectopic pregnancy if she is not already alloimmunized. Also explain the purpose of prophylactic RhIg administered at 28 weeks and after the birth of an Rh-positive newborn if not alloimmunized.

> "As a nurse for many years, I remember when RhoGAM first started to be used—what a difference it made in the lives of so many women and their unborn babies. Today, young women who are Rh negative will hopefully never know the pain and tragedy that this blood incompatibility caused. RhoGAM was nothing short of miraculous!"

If the woman is alloimmunized to the Rh factor, it poses a threat to any Rh-positive fetus she carries. Provide emotional support to the family to help them deal with their grief and any feelings of guilt about the condition of the fetus or newborn. Should an intrauterine transfusion become necessary, continue to provide emotional support while also assuming responsibilities as part of the healthcare team.

During labor, when caring for an Rh-negative woman who has not been sensitized, ensure that the woman's blood is assessed for any antibodies and has also been cross-matched for Rh immune globulin. On the postpartum unit, the nurse is generally responsible for administering the RhIg (see *Clinical Skill 18–1: Administration of Rh Immune Globulin [RhoGAM, WinRho-SDF, HyperRho S/D, Rhophlac]*). See *Key Facts to Remember: Rh Alloimmunization* for a summary of the major considerations in caring for an Rh-negative woman. Treatment of hemolytic disease of the fetus and newborn is discussed in detail in Chapter 31.

Evaluation

Expected outcomes of nursing care include:

- The woman is able to explain the process of Rh alloimmunization and its implications for her unborn fetus or newborn and for subsequent pregnancies.
- If the woman has not been alloimmunized, she is able to explain the importance of receiving Rh immune globulin when necessary and cooperates with the recommended dosage schedule.
- The woman gives birth to a healthy newborn.
- If complications develop for the fetus (or newborn), they are detected quickly, and therapy is instituted.

Clinical Skill 18–1

Intramuscular Administration of Rh Immune Globulin (RhoGAM, WinRho-SDF, HyperRho S/D, Rhophlac)

NURSING ACTION

Preparation

- Confirm that Rh immune globulin (RhIg) is indicated by checking the woman's blood type, Rh factor, and antibody screen (indirect Coombs) from prenatal and intrapartum records. Verify from the most current lab results that she is Rh negative and no alloimmunization has occurred (maternal indirect Coombs negative or anti-D antibody screen negative). Confirm that the newborn is Rh positive (usually from a cord blood sample) and that there is no active hemolysis of newborn RBCs (a negative direct Coombs test). RhIg is *not* indicated if the newborn is also Rh negative.

Rationale: *RhIg is only indicated for Rh-negative, nonalloimmunized women with an Rh-positive newborn.*

- Confirm that the woman does not have a history of allergies to immune globulin preparations by checking entries on medication allergies in her chart and by asking her whether she has ever had any allergic reactions to medications, globulins, or blood products.

Rationale: *RhIg is made from the plasma portion of blood. Allergic reactions are possible.*

- Explain purpose and procedure. Have consent form signed if required by agency policy.

Rationale: *Many agencies require separate consent for the administration of RhIg because it is a blood product. The woman should clearly understand the purpose of RhIg, its rationale, the administration procedure, and any related risks. Generally, the primary side effects are redness and tenderness at the injection site and allergic responses.*

Equipment and Supplies

- RhIg is obtained from the blood bank or pharmacy according to agency protocol. Lot numbers for the drug and the cross-match should be the same.
- Syringe and IM needle

Procedure

1. Confirm the woman's identity and administer one or more vial(s) of 300 mcg Rh immune globulin IM in the deltoid muscle.

Rationale: *The normal 300-mcg dose provides passive immunity following exposure to 15 mL of transfused RBCs or 30 mL of fetal whole blood.*

2. An immune globulin microdose (50 mcg) is used after miscarriage, elective abortion, ectopic pregnancy, or molar pregnancy that occurs before 13 0/7 weeks' gestation. Antepartum, RhIg is generally given within 3 hours but not longer than 72 hours of the event.
3. If a larger bleed is suspected at birth (as in cases of severe abruptio placentae), additional doses may be administered at one time using multiple sites at regular intervals as long as all doses are given within 72 hours of childbirth.
4. Provide opportunities for the woman to ask questions and express concerns.

Rationale: *Many women, especially primigravidas, are not aware of the risks for an Rh-positive fetus of an alloimmunized Rh-negative mother. They need to understand the importance of receiving RhIg for each pregnancy to ensure continued protection.*

5. Chart according to agency policy. Most agencies chart lot number, route, dose, and patient education.

Key Facts To Remember

Rh Alloimmunization

When trying to work through Rh alloimmunization problems, the nurse should remember the following:

- A potential problem exists when an Rh-negative mother and an Rh-positive father conceive a fetus who is Rh positive.
- In this situation, the mother may become alloimmunized by producing antibodies against her fetus's Rh-positive blood.

The following tests are used to detect sensitization:

- Antibody screen—antibodies developed against the Rh-positive antigen are known as anti-D antibodies.
- Indirect Coombs tests—done on the mother's blood to measure the number of anti-D antibodies.
- Direct Coombs test—done on the newborn's cord blood to detect the presence of Rh-positive RBCs coated by maternal anti-D antibody.

Based on the results of these tests, the following may be done:

- If the mother's indirect Coombs test is negative and the newborn's direct Coombs test is negative (confirming that alloimmunization has not occurred), the mother is given Rh immune globulin within 72 hours of birth.
- If the mother's indirect Coombs test is positive (she has anti-D antibodies and a high titer) and her Rh-positive newborn has a positive direct Coombs test, RhIg is *not* given; in this case, the newborn is carefully monitored for HDFN.
- It is recommended that RhIg be given at 28 weeks antenatally to decrease possible transplacental bleeding concerns.
- RhIg is also administered after each abortion (spontaneous or therapeutic), antepartum hemorrhage mismatched blood transfusion, ectopic pregnancy, amniocentesis, chorionic villus sampling (CVS), percutaneous umbilical blood sampling (PUBS), external cephalic version, or maternal trauma.

Clinical Tip

In most cases, Rh immune globulin is administered in the deltoid muscle. However, in an extremely thin woman, or in the cases of a larger-than-normal dose, consider administering the medication in the ventrogluteal or posterior gluteal site. You may also divide the dose into multiple injections. Both Rhophlac and WinRho-SFD may be administered intravenously.

Care of the Woman at Risk Due to ABO Incompatibility

Tests ordered on blood include blood type, Rh factor, and antibody screen. The tests determine the blood group (A, B, AB, or O), the presence or absence of the Rhesus factor (RhD positive or negative), and the presence or absence and identification of antibodies in the serum (such as anti-D).

Many antibodies in the serum are developed in response to antigens in the environment, such as foods eaten, and this includes anti-A and anti-B antibodies. Unlike HDFN caused by RhD incompatibility, newborns with ABO incompatibility rarely have serious life-threatening scenarios because the antigen/antibody response is not as robust. ABO incompatibility of the newborn is fairly common and, in most cases, is limited to type O mothers with a type A or B fetus. It is almost exclusively seen after birth of the newborn, as the larger anti-A and anti-B antibodies do not readily cross the placenta, plus they attach to organs throughout the maternal body rather than just targeting fetal RBCs. This allows for a less severe antigen–antibody reaction. The group B fetus/newborn of a group A mother, and the group A fetus/newborn of a group B mother, are only occasionally affected. Group O newborns, because they have no antigenic sites on the RBCs, are never affected regardless of the mother's blood type. The incompatibility occurs as a result of the maternal antibodies present in her serum and interaction between the antigen sites on the newborn RBCs.

Anti-A and anti-B antibodies are naturally occurring; that is, women are naturally exposed to the A and B antigens through the foods they eat and through exposure to infection by Gram-negative bacteria. As a result, some women have high serum anti-A and anti-B titers before they become pregnant. Once the woman becomes pregnant, the maternal serum anti-A and anti-B antibodies cross the placenta and produce hemolysis of the fetal RBCs. With ABO incompatibility, the first baby can be affected but typically hemolysis of fetal RBCs occurs after birth. No relationship exists between the appearance of the disease and repeated sensitization from one pregnancy to the next.

Unlike the case of Rh incompatibility, treatment is never warranted antepartum. As part of the initial assessment, however, the nurse should note whether the potential for an ABO incompatibility exists. This alerts caregivers so that following birth, the newborn can be assessed carefully for the development of hyperbilirubinemia (see Chapter 31). Affected neonates usually have only mild anemia, and the severity of the disease demonstrated with the first-born baby is generally similar in all subsequent pregnancies.

Focus Your Study

- Several health problems associated with bleeding arise from the pregnancy itself, such as spontaneous abortion, ectopic pregnancy, and gestational trophoblastic disease. The nurse needs to be alert to early signs of these situations, to guard the woman against heavy bleeding and shock, to facilitate the medical treatment, and to provide educational and emotional support.
- Hyperemesis gravidarum, excessive vomiting during pregnancy, may cause fluid and electrolyte imbalance, dehydration, signs of starvation in the mother, and, if severe enough, death of the fetus. Treatment is aimed at controlling the vomiting, correcting fluid and electrolyte imbalance, correcting dehydration, and improving nutritional status.
- Hypertension may exist before pregnancy or, more often, may develop during pregnancy. Preeclampsia can lead to intrauterine growth restriction of the fetus. If untreated, it may lead to convulsions (eclampsia) and even death for the mother and fetus. Antihypertensive or anticonvulsive drugs may be part of the therapy. There is no evidence to support maintaining periods of bedrest in the left lateral position to prevent preeclampsia.
- Toxoplasmosis, rubella, cytomegalovirus (CMV), parvovirus B19, herpes, group B streptococcus (GBS) infection, and other perinatal infections all pose a grave threat to the fetus. Prevention is the best therapy. There is no known treatment for rubella, parvovirus B19, or Zika, but antimicrobial drugs are available for toxoplasmosis, herpes, and GBS. A vaccine for CMV may be available in the near future.
- Universal vagino-rectal screening for GBS is now recommended for all pregnant women at 35 to 37 weeks' gestation.
- The impact of surgery or trauma on the pregnant woman and her fetus is related to timing in the pregnancy, seriousness of the situation, and other influencing factors. In addition to the critical state of the mother, whether or not the fetus has met the age of viability will determine management.
- Physical violence often begins or continues during pregnancy. The nurse needs to be alert for signs of abuse, including bruising or injury to the breasts, abdomen, and genitals. The nurse should provide the woman information about the cycle of violence and community resources available to assist her.
- Rh incompatibility can exist when an Rh-negative woman and an Rh-positive partner conceive a fetus that is Rh positive. The use of Rh immune globulin has greatly decreased the incidence of severe sequelae due to Rh incompatibility, however, the exact mechanism of action is still unknown.
- ABO incompatibility of the newborn is far more common than Rh incompatibility and, in most cases, is limited to type O mothers with a type A or B fetus. Antepartum treatment is never indicated and the newborn generally does well.

In order to make safe and effective judgments using NANDA-I © 2017 nursing diagnoses, it is essential that nurses refer to the definitions and defining characteristics of the diagnoses used in this text, which can be found in Appendix C.

References

American College of Obstetricians and Gynecologists (ACOG). (2013). *Hypertension in pregnancy* (ACOG Task Force and Work Group Report). Washington, DC: Author.

American College of Obstetricians and Gynecologists (ACOG). (2015). *Cytomegalovirus, parvovirus B19, varicella zoster, and toxoplasmosis in pregnancy* (ACOG Practice Bulletin No. 151). Washington, DC: Author.

American College of Obstetricians and Gynecologists (ACOG). (2016a). *Diagnosis and treatment of gestational trophoblastic disease* (ACOG Practice Bulletin No. 53). Washington, DC: Author.

American College of Obstetricians and Gynecologists (ACOG). (2016b). *Management of herpes in pregnancy* (ACOG Practice Bulletin No. 82). Washington, DC: Author.

American College of Obstetricians and Gynecologists (ACOG). (2016c). *Prevention of early-onset Group B streptococcal disease in newborns* (ACOG Committee Opinion No. 485). Washington, DC: Author.

American College of Obstetricians and Gynecologists (ACOG). (2016d). *Ultrasound in pregnancy* (ACOG Practice Bulletin No. 175). Washington, DC: Author.

American College of Obstetricians and Gynecologists (ACOG). (2017a). *Emergent therapy for acute-onset, severe hypertension during pregnancy and the postpartum period* (ACOG Committee Opinion No. 692). Washington, DC: Author.

American College of Obstetricians and Gynecologists (ACOG). (2017b). *Nonobstetric surgery during pregnancy* (ACOG Committee Opinion No. 696). Washington, DC: Author.

American College of Obstetricians and Gynecologists (ACOG). (2018a). *Management of alloimmunization during pregnancy* (ACOG Practice Bulletin No. 192). Washington, DC: Author.

American College of Obstetricians and Gynecologists (ACOG). (2018b). *Nausea and vomiting of pregnancy* (ACOG Practice Bulletin No. 189). Washington, DC: Author.

American College of Obstetricians and Gynecologists (ACOG). (2018c). *Tubal ectopic pregnancy. Interim update* (ACOG Practice Bulletin No. 193). Washington, DC: Author.

Bernstein, H. B. (2017). Maternal and perinatal infection. In S. G. Gabbe, J. R. Niebyl, J. L. Simpson, M. B. Landon, H. L. Galan, E. R. M. Jauniaux, . . . & W.A. Grobman (Eds.), *Obstetrics: Normal and problem pregnancies* (7th ed., pp.1099–1129). Philadelphia, PA: Elsevier.

Brown, H. L. (2017). Trauma and related surgery in pregnancy. In S. G. Gabbe, J. R. Niebyl, J. L. Simpson, M. B. Landon, H. L. Galan, E. R. M. Jauniaux, . . . & W.A. Grobman (Eds.), *Obstetrics: Normal and problem pregnancies* (7th ed., pp.565–577). Philadelphia, PA: Elsevier.

Centers for Disease Control and Prevention (CDC). (2015). *2015 sexually transmitted diseases treatment guidelines.* Retrieved from https://www.cdc.gov/std/tg2015

Centers for Disease Control and Prevention (CDC). (2016a). *Group B Strep (GBS)—Obstetric providers.* Retrieved from https://www.cdc.gov/groupbstrep/clinicians/obstetric-providers.html

Centers for Disease Control and Prevention (CDC). (2016b). *Maternal vaccines: Part of a healthy pregnancy.* Retrieved from https://www.cdc.gov/vaccines/pregnancy/pregnant-women/index.html

Centers for Disease Control and Prevention (CDC). (2017a). *Intimate partner violence: Risk and protection factors.* Retrieved from https://www.cdc.gov/violenceprevention/intimatepartnerviolence/riskprotectivefactors.html

Centers for Disease Control and Prevention (CDC). (2017b). *Zika virus.* Retrieved from https://www.cdc.gov/zika/pregnancy/index.html

Choubey, V., & Witter, F. R. (2015). Hypertensive disorders of pregnancy. In C. T. Johnson, J. L. Hallock, J. L. Bienstock, H. E. Fox, & E. E. Wallach (Eds.), *The Johns Hopkins manual of gynecology and obstetrics* (5th ed., pp.198–207). Philadelphia, PA: Wolters Kluwer.

Cunningham, F. G., Leveno, K. J., Bloom, S. L., Dashe, J. S., Hoffman, B. L., Casey, B. M., & Spong, C. Y. (2018). *Williams obstetrics* (25th ed.). New York, NY: McGraw-Hill.

Duff, P., & Birsner, M. (2017). Maternal and perinatal infection in pregnancy: Bacterial. In S. G. Gabbe, J. R. Niebyl, J. L. Simpson, M. B. Landon, H. L. Galan, E. R. M. Jauniaux, . . . W. A. Grobman (Eds.), *Obstetrics: Normal and problem pregnancies* (7th ed., pp. 1130–1146). Philadelphia, PA: Elsevier.

Dusse, L. M., Alpoim, P. N., Silva, J. T., Rios, D. R., Brandão, A. H., & Cabral, A. C. (2015). Revisiting HELLP syndrome. *Clinica Chimica Acta, 451*(Pt. B), 117–120. DOI: 10.1016/j.cca.2015.10.024

Fields, L., & Hathaway, A. (2016.) Key Concepts in pregnancy of unknown location: Identifying ectopic pregnancy and providing patient-centered care. *Journal of Midwifery and Women's Health, 62*(2), 172–179. DOI: 10.1111/jmwh.12526.

Katsi, V., Felekos, I., Siristatidis, C., Kasioni, S., Drakontaidis, A., Farmakides, G., . . . & Kallikazaros, I. (2015). Preeclampsia: What does the father have to do with it? *Current Hypertension Reports, 17*(8), 60. DOI: 10.1007/s11906-015-0576-7

Lambert, G. Brichant, J. F., Hartstein, G., Bonhomme, V., & Dewandre, P. Y. (2014). Preeclampsia: An update. *Acta Anaesthesiolgica Belgica, 65,* 137–149.

Markham, K. B., & Funai, E. F. (2014). Pregnancy-related hypertension. In R. K. Creasy, R. Resnik, J. D. Iams, C. J. Lockwood, T. R. Moore, & M. F. Greene (Eds.), *Creasy & Resnik's maternal-fetal medicine principles and practice* (7th ed., pp. 871–899). Philadelphia, PA: Elsevier Saunders.

Mensah, V., & Yates, M. (2015). Ectopic pregnancy. In C. T. Johnson, J. L. Hallock, J. L. Bienstock, H. E. Fox, & E. E. Wallach (Eds.). *The Johns Hopkins manual of gynecology and obstetrics* (5th ed., pp. 379–388). Philadelphia, PA: Wolters Kluwer.

Moezzi, L., Keshavarz, Z., Ranjbaran, R., Aboualizadey, F., Behzad-Behbahani, A., Abudullahi, M., Ramezani, A., . . . Sharifzadeh, S. (2016). Fetal RHD genotyping using real-time polymerase chain reaction analysis of cell-free fetal DNA in pregnancy of RhD negative women in south of Iran. *International Journal of Fertility and Sterility, 10*(1), 62–70.

Moise, K. J. (2017). Red cell alloimmunization. In S. G. Gabbe, J. R. Niebyl, J. L. Simpson, M. B. Landon, H. L. Galan, E. R. M. Jauniaux, . . . W. A. Grobman (Eds.), *Obstetrics: Normal and problem pregnancies* (7th ed., pp. 770–785). Philadelphia, PA: Elsevier.

Ngan, H. Y. S., Seckl, M. J., Berkowitz, R. S., Xiang, Y., Golfier, F., Sekharan, P. K., & Lurain, J. R. (2015). FIGO CANCER REPORT 2015, Update on the diagnosis and management of gestational trophoblastic disease. *International Journal of Gynecology and Obstetrics, 131,* S123–S126.

Niemeijer, M. N., Grooten, I. J, Voss, N., Bais, J. M. J., van der Post, J. A., Mol, B. W., . . . Leeflang, M. G. (2014). Diagnostic markers for hyperemesis gravidarum: A systematic review and metaanalysis. *American Journal of Obstetrics and Gynecology, 211*(2), 150.e1–150.e15.

O'Donnell, A., McParlin, C., Robson, S. C., Beyer, F., Moloney, E., Bryant, A., . . . & Vale, L. (2016). Treatments for hyperemesis gravidarum and nausea and vomiting in pregnancy: A systematic review and economic assessment. *Health Technology Assessment, 20*(74), 1–268.

Robbins, K. S., Martin, S. R., & Wilson, W. C. (2014). Intensive care considerations for the critically ill parturient. In R. K. Creasy, R. Resnik, J. D. Iams, C. J. Lockwood, T. R. Moore, & M. F. Greene (Eds.), *Creasy & Resnik's maternal-fetal medicine: Principles and practice* (7th ed., pp. 1180–1192). Philadelphia, PA: Elsevier Saunders.

Safe Motherhood Initiative. (2017). *Maternal safety bundle for severe hypertension in pregnancy.* Retrieved from https://www.acog.org/-/media/Districts/District-II/Public/SMI/v2/HTNSlideSetJuly2017.pdf?dmc=1&ts=20180313T1543532026

Salani, R., & Copeland, L. J. (2017). Malignant diseases and pregnancy. In S. G. Gabbe, J. R. Niebyl, J. L. Simpson, M. B. Landon, H. L. Galan, E. R. M. Jauniaux, . . . W. A. Grobman (Eds.), *Obstetrics: Normal and problem pregnancies* (7th ed., pp. 1057–1074). Philadelphia, PA: Elsevier.

Sibai, B. M. (2017). Preeclampsia and hypertensive disorders. In S. G. Gabbe, J. R. Niebyl, J. L. Simpson, M. B. Landon, H. L. Galan, E. R. M. Jauniaux, . . . W. A. Grobman (Eds.), *Obstetrics: Normal and problem pregnancies* (7th ed., pp. 661–705). Philadelphia, PA: Elsevier.

Simpson, J. L., & Jauniaux, E. R. M. (2017). Early pregnancy loss and stillbirth. In S. G. Gabbe, J. R. Niebyl, J. L. Simpson, M. B. Landon, H. L. Galan, E. R. M. Jauniaux, . . . W. A. Grobman (Eds.), *Obstetrics: Normal and problem pregnancies* (7th ed., pp. 578–594). Philadelphia, PA: Elsevier.

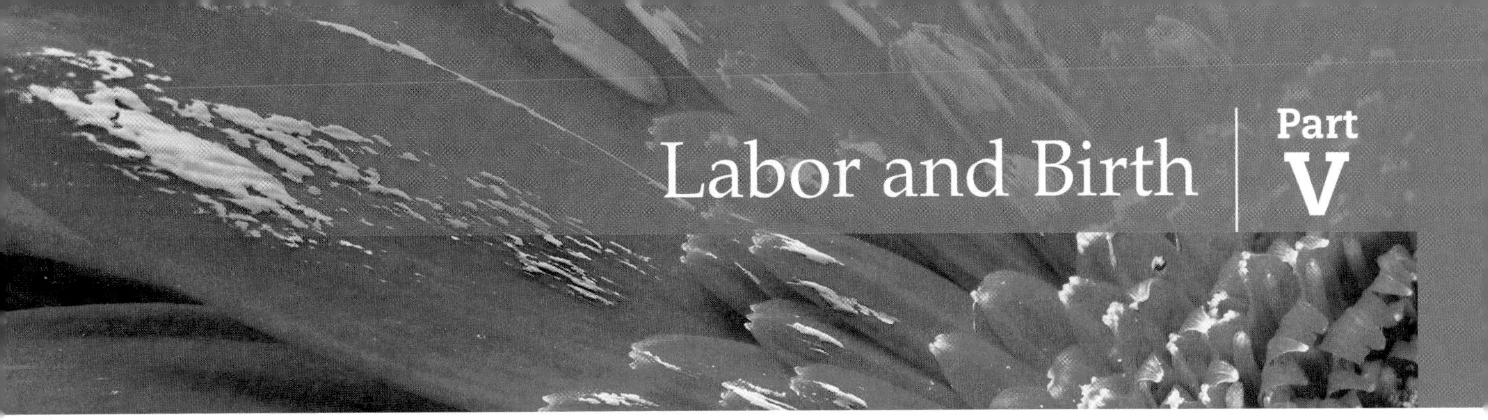

Labor and Birth | Part V

Chapter 19

Processes and Stages of Labor and Birth

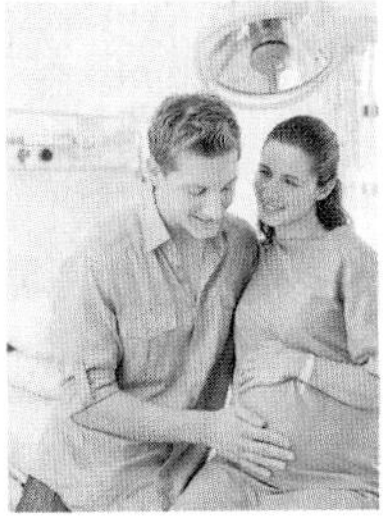

SOURCE: OJO Images/
Exactostock - 1775/Superstock.

Just as a woman's heart knows how and when to pump, her lungs to inhale, and her hand to pull back from fire, so she knows when and how to give birth. —Virginia

Learning Outcomes

19.1 Compare methods of childbirth preparation.

19.2 Examine the five critical factors that affect the labor process.

19.3 Describe the physiology of labor.

19.4 Discuss premonitory signs of labor.

19.5 Differentiate between false and true labor.

19.6 Describe the characteristics of the four stages of labor and their accompanying phases.

19.7 Describe the physiologic and psychosocial changes that are indicative of the maternal progress during each of the stages of labor.

19.8 Summarize maternal systemic responses to labor.

19.9 Describe fetal adaptations to labor.

Healthy People 2020

(MICH-10) Increase the proportion of pregnant women who receive early and adequate prenatal care

(MICH-12) (Developmental) Increase the proportion of pregnant women who attend a series of prepared childbirth classes

(MICH-16) Increase the proportion of women delivering a live birth who received preconception care services and practiced key recommended preconception health behaviors

During the weeks of pregnancy, both mother and baby prepare for birth. The fetus develops and grows in readiness for life outside the womb. The expectant woman undergoes various physiologic and psychosocial changes that gradually prepare her for childbirth and for the role of mother. With good prenatal care, she is educated about the experience of childbirth and learns methods of preparing for and undergoing labor and birth, such as relaxation and coping techniques and breathing exercises to use during labor.

The onset of labor begins a remarkable change in the relationship between the woman and her baby. During labor, particularly at the end, a woman instinctively knows she is engaging in one of the most important tasks she will ever do. A precious life is about to emerge. In those hours and moments, the birth process may seem to carry all the power in the universe. The mother-to-be and her partner may be stretched beyond all of their normal limits of concentration, purpose, endurance, and pain. The dynamic nature of this experience is what makes the birth of a baby both a physiologic and a psychosocial transition into parenthood.

Methods of Childbirth Preparation

Various types of childbirth preparation are taught in North America. Childbirth preparation classes are usually taught by certified childbirth educators. Vital to each method is the educational component, which helps alleviate fear. The classes vary in coverage of subjects related to the maternity cycle, but all teach relaxation and coping techniques, as well as what to expect during labor and birth. Most classes also feature exercises to relax and condition muscles and breathing exercises for use in labor. The greatest differences among the methods lie in the theories of why they work and in the specific comfort techniques and breathing patterns they teach.

Childbirth preparation offers several advantages. It helps a pregnant woman and her support person understand the choices in the birth setting, promotes awareness of available options, and provides tools for them to use during labor and birth. Another advantage is the satisfaction of the parents, for whom childbirth becomes a shared and profound emotional experience. In addition, each method has been shown to shorten labor. All nurses should know how these techniques differ, so that they can support each birth experience effectively. A Cochrane Review and ongoing research has found that women who receive continuous support during labor require less analgesia, have fewer cesarean and instrument births, and experience a shorter period of labor (Hodnett, Gates, Hofmeyr, et al., 2011; Tharp, Farley, & Jordan, 2016). This provides additional evidenced-based practice guidance regarding the need to provide ongoing support of the woman's partner/support person during the labor and birth process.

Programs for Preparation

Some antepartum classes, specifically oriented to preparation for labor and birth, have a name associated with a theory of pain reduction in childbirth. In modern pregnancy preparation, it is less common to select a specific method for childbirth education (CBE). Most women who receive CBE with alternative resources select methods with specific techniques that are taught in a private setting, usually outside of the hospital setting. See Box 19–1 for commonly used childbirth education methods.

One of the most important components of childbirth education is instilling confidence in a woman's ability to give birth (Tharp et al., 2016). Many childbirth education specialists and educators embrace contemporary models that focus on the interconnectedness of the body and spirit. After that connection is established and understood by pregnant women, coping strategies, stress reduction, and relaxation techniques can be taught.

BOX 19-1

Most Commonly Used Childbirth Education Methods in the United States

METHOD NAME	DESCRIPTION OF CBE TECHNIQUE
Lamaze (psychoprophylactic)	Dissociative relaxation, controlled muscle relaxation, and specified breathing patterns are used to promote birth as a normal process.
Bradley (partner-assisted)	Consists of a 12-week session in which the woman works on controlled breathing and deep abdominopelvic breathing with a focus on achieving natural childbirth.
Hypnobirthing	Breathing and relaxation techniques help prepare the body to work in neuromuscular harmony to make the birth process easier, safer, and more comfortable.

SAFETY ALERT!

Explain to women who are using internet childbirth education resources that some sites may not use health professionals or experts in the childbirth field and may be written by individuals who lack formal education and training. Advise women to look for resources that are supported by licensed professionals or well-known, credible organizations.

Another prominent organization that provides educational resources and certification for educators is the International Childbirth Education Association (ICEA). This organization does not advocate a particular method of childbirth preparation but rather promotes a philosophy of "freedom of choice based on knowledge of alternatives" (ICEA, 2017). Many expectant parents find this approach consistent with their own desires to experience birth as informed healthcare consumers. ICEA educators often teach a combination of techniques designed to meet individual needs.

Body-Conditioning Exercises

Some body-conditioning exercises, such as the pelvic tilt, pelvic rock, and Kegel exercises, are taught in childbirth preparation classes. Other exercises strengthen the abdominal muscles for the expulsive phase of labor. (See Chapter 13 for a description of some recommended exercises.) Exercises aimed at adducting the legs into an extended *McRoberts position*, which is performed by flexing the mother's thighs toward her shoulders while she is lying on her back, help enable the woman to stretch her hamstring muscles, a task usually required during the second stage of labor (Arulkumaran, 2016). Many childbirth methods utilize body conditioning as a portion of their education program. With the encouragement of daily exercise in pregnancy, women can incorporate exercises into their daily programs that will help build endurance and strength for the labor and birth process.

Relaxation Exercises

Relaxation during labor allows the woman to conserve energy and the uterine muscles to work more efficiently. Most childbirth education methods use a form of relaxation exercise as part of their philosophical basis. Without practice, it is difficult to relax the whole body in the midst of intense uterine contractions. Progressive relaxation exercises such as those taught to induce sleep can be helpful during labor.

The *touch relaxation technique* is often used as a pain relief measure in which the partner's touch enhances the woman's ability to relax or release tense muscles. During labor, the partner's touch can include light touching, stroking, or massaging as a nonverbal cue to relax. The method often combines patterned abdominal breathing with focused touch relaxation. The laboring woman learns to release tension in the specific areas or in a generalized manner when her partner touches her. The partner observes and becomes attuned to the woman's tense, tightened muscles or verbal cues that indicate discomfort. Box 19–2 provides information on the technique of the touch relaxation method.

An additional exercise is *disassociation relaxation*. The woman is taught to become familiar with the sensation of contracting and relaxing the voluntary muscle groups throughout her body. She then learns to contract a specific muscle group and relax the rest of her body. The exercise conditions the woman to relax uninvolved muscles while the uterus contracts, creating an active relaxation pattern.

Other strategies to induce relaxation include visualization, imagery, and meditation. See Box 19–3.

BOX 19-2
Touch Relaxation Technique

- The partner initially touches the woman's brow.
- The woman is encouraged to begin abdominal breathing, in which she breathes in through her nose, allowing her abdomen to rise as much as possible. The woman then breathes out through her mouth while simultaneously allowing her abdomen to fall. The partner reminds her to focus on muscle relaxation as the breath is released and to attempt to completely relax her body as she exhales.
- The partner continues gently touching the woman's brow while providing encouragement, telling her "You are doing fine, you are releasing the tension in your forehead." After five or more breaths, the partner touches the woman's shoulders and the pattern described above is repeated.
- The partner then systematically focuses on the arms, chest, abdomen, thighs, and calves. The last instruction is for the woman to breathe in deeply and relax her entire body. The partner is advised to encourage this complete relaxation strategy at the end of each contraction to allow the woman to rest and reserve her energy between labor contractions.
- The couple should be encouraged to practice this technique prior to labor. Some couples may verbalize understanding of the technique, but actual practice should be encouraged prior to labor. This enables the woman to identify specific touch techniques that she personally finds helpful.
- Couples should be encouraged to practice the technique simulating a true labor pattern to become accustomed to the frequency needed to maintain the actual length of time and duration that will occur when the woman is in true labor. Women who regularly practice with their partners often become cued by touch alone and can begin the relaxation technique as soon as the partner touches her brow. Couples often individualize the technique to their own comfort levels and should be encouraged to make modifications that feel natural to them.

SOURCES: Data from Perez & Hutchins, 2014; Simpkin & Ancheta, 2011.

BOX 19-3
Visualization, Imagery, and Meditation

Visualization and imagery	During pregnancy, visualization and imagery are used to induce a state of relaxation. The woman is advised to focus on a calming and relaxing image. Some women may envision a special peaceful place, while others may envision holding their baby or another pleasant event. Images can be suggested by the partner or practitioner or may be chosen by the woman herself. The partner or practitioner describes a tranquil image, such as a sparkling brook with sunshine peeking through the trees and birds singing gently in the background. During labor, this technique assists the woman with muscle relaxation and provides a positive distraction from uterine contractions, which helps conserve energy and fight fatigue.
Meditation	Meditation is a practice in which the woman remains upright in an alert position and focuses on stilling or emptying her mind. The woman focuses and repeats a particular word or sound, called a mantra, while attempting to reach a state of dissociation. In this state, she is detached from interacting with the environment and becomes an observer of her surroundings rather than an active participant. Mindfulness is a type of meditation that focuses on the present moment. The participant is aware of her environment and observes her thoughts and feelings without judgment. In mindfulness, the woman is encouraged to embrace the labor experience.

Breathing Techniques

Breathing techniques are a key element of most childbirth preparation programs. Breathing techniques increase the woman's pain threshold, encourage relaxation, provide distraction, enhance the ability to cope with uterine contractions, and allow the uterus to function more efficiently. In addition, they help keep the mother and her unborn baby adequately oxygenated. Breathing techniques are best taught during the final trimester of pregnancy. The nurse then supports the mother's use of breathing techniques during labor.

Patterned-paced breathing, which is commonly used in the *Lamaze method*, has three levels. The woman tends to begin with the first level and then proceed to the next when she feels the need. Regardless of the level of breathing used, a cleansing breath begins and ends each pattern. A cleansing breath involves only the chest. It consists of inhaling through the nose and exhaling through pursed lips (as if blowing on a spoonful of hot food).

Other childbirth education models encourage different types of breathing exercises. Abdominal breathing, which is commonly used in the *Bradley method*, encourages the woman to move the abdominal wall upward as she inhales and downward as she exhales. This method tends to lift the abdominal wall off the contracting uterus and thus may provide some pain relief. The breathing is deep and rhythmic. A less commonly used technique, known as the *Kitzinger method*, utilizes chest breathing in collaboration with abdominal relaxation. *Hypnobirthing* utilizes deep, slow breathing as a center component of its philosophy. If the woman has not been trained in a particular technique, she can be taught during labor the "quick method," which uses a pant–pant–blow breathing pattern; this may help her from breathing too rapidly. See *Case Study: Angelina Newman*.

Preparation for Childbirth That Supports Individuality

Childbirth educators stress the value of individuality when providing information to expectant parents. The goal is to encourage women to incorporate their own natural responses into coping with the pain of labor and birth. Self-care activities that may be used include vocalization or "sounding" to relieve tension in pregnancy and labor, massage (light touch) to facilitate relaxation, use of warm water for showers or bathing during labor,

CASE STUDY: Angelina Newman

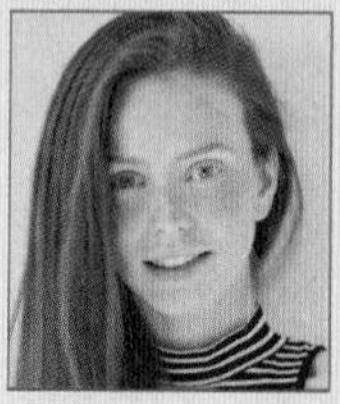

SOURCE: WAYHOME studio/Shutterstock

Angelina is extremely apprehensive about her upcoming labor and birth. She is reluctant to go to childbirth classes because she is afraid that the married couples there will judge her for being pregnant so young. She says she does not see the benefit in attending and is already overwhelmed by her classes in school. She states she does not have time to study more subjects and learn additional "worthless information."

Questions to Ponder

How you would encourage Angelina to attend classes? Discuss how you would explain that they differ from school-based learning. What are the benefits to the pregnant woman, of any age, of attending childbirth education classes?

visualization (imagery), relaxing music, subdued lighting, and the use of a birthing ball (see Figure 21–1).

Additional ways in which the nurse can help the couple during labor and birth include:

- Identify the methods of childbirth preparation commonly used in your area and learn the basics of their approaches to relaxation and breathing; practice these methods so that you can support a laboring couple more effectively.
- Encourage expectant mothers and couples to make the birth a personal experience.
- Suggest the couple bring items from home that help create a more personal birthing space, such as warm socks, extra pillows or a favorite blanket, bath powder, lotion, or meaningful photos.
- Encourage the couple to listen to soothing music on their cell phone or MP3 player or watch favorite DVDs to increase personalization of the childbearing experience.

Educational content in prenatal preparation classes should include techniques and strategies to provide adequate coping mechanisms. Expectant couples should be taught the physiological changes that occur during labor so they can gain an understanding of the physical process that is associated with certain symptoms. The critical factors in labor, physiological changes that occur in pregnancy, premonitory signs of labor, differences between true and false labor, the stages of labor, and the physiological and psychological maternal and fetal responses that occur during labor are essential concepts that the woman and her partner should be familiar with. It is often helpful to utilize instructional materials, videos, online visual technology, and pelvic models to aid in childbirth education.

Critical Factors in Labor

Five factors are important in the process of labor and birth: (1) the birth passage (birth canal), (2) the fetus (passenger), (3) the relationship between the passage and the fetus, (4) the physiologic forces of labor, and (5) the woman's psychosocial considerations (Table 19–1). The progress of labor is critically dependent on the complementary relationship of these five factors. Abnormalities that affect any component of these critical forces can alter the outcome of labor and jeopardize both the expectant woman and her baby. Complications during labor and birth are discussed in Chapter 24.

TABLE 19–1 Critical Factors in Labor

CRITICAL FACTOR	COMPONENTS
1. Birth passage	• Size of the maternal pelvis (diameters of the pelvic inlet, midpelvis, and outlet) • Type of maternal pelvis (gynecoid, android, anthropoid, platypelloid, or a combination) • Ability of the cervix to dilate and efface and ability of the vaginal canal and the external opening of the vagina (the introitus) to distend
2. Fetus	• Fetal head (size and presence of molding) • Fetal attitude (flexion or extension of the fetal body and extremities) • Fetal lie • Fetal presentation (the body part of the fetus entering the pelvis in a single or multiple pregnancy)
3. The relationship between the passage and the fetus	• Engagement of the fetal presenting part • Station (location of fetal presenting part in the maternal pelvis) • Fetal position (relationship of the presenting part to one of the four quadrants of the maternal pelvis)
4. Physiologic forces of labor	• Frequency, duration, and intensity of uterine contractions as the fetus moves through the passage • Effectiveness of the maternal pushing effort
5. Psychosocial considerations	• Mental and physical preparation for childbirth • Sociocultural values and beliefs • Previous childbirth experience • Support from significant others • Emotional status

Genetic Facts Predicting the Baby's Size

The size of a couple's baby is partially related to genetic tendencies. The birth size of the mother and the baby's father can be predictive of their own baby; however, due to other variables, it is not a precise prediction, but can be one of the factors to consider when estimating fetal/neonatal size.

Birth Passageway

The true pelvis and soft tissues of the cervix, vagina, and the pelvic floor form the birth passageway. The true pelvis is the critical factor of the passageway because the fetus must progress through this bony canal during the vaginal birth process. The true pelvis is divided into three sections: The inlet, the pelvic cavity (midpelvis), and the outlet (see Figure 12–4).

PELVIC TYPES

The Caldwell-Moloy classification of pelvises is sometimes used to differentiate types of bony pelvises (Caldwell & Moloy, 1933). *Gynecoid*, *android*, *anthropoid*, and *platypelloid* are the four basic types (see Figure 19–1). Each type of pelvis has a characteristic shape, and each shape has implications for labor and birth. However, variations in the female pelvis are great and pelvic shapes often occur that differ from these categories.

Implications of each approximate type of pelvis for childbirth are described in Table 19–2. The ability of the cervix to dilate and efface and the ability of the vaginal canal and the external opening of the vagina (the introitus) to distend are additional

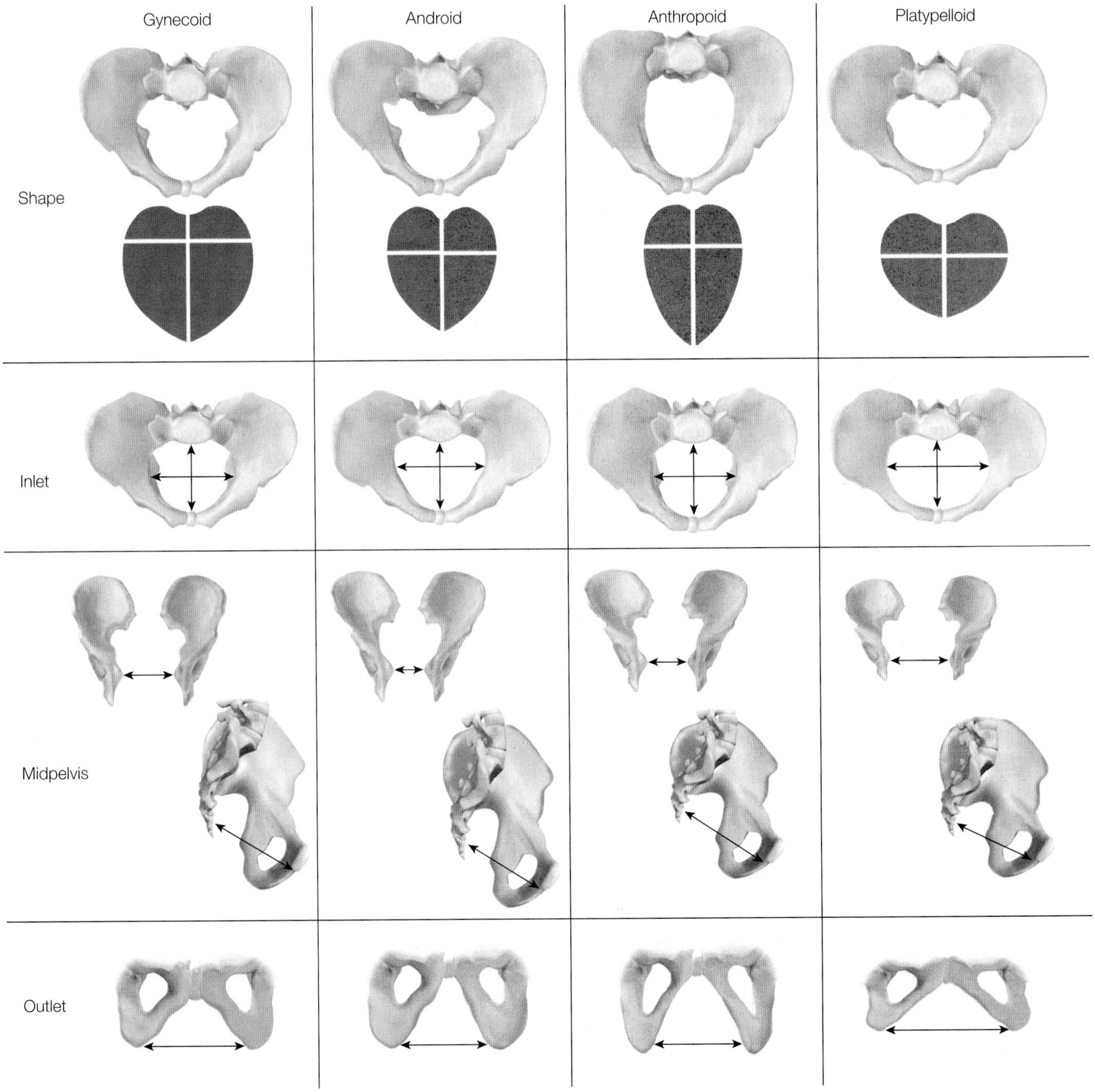

Figure 19–1 **Comparison of the four basic pelvic types.**

TABLE 19–2 Implications of Pelvic Type for Labor and Birth

PELVIC TYPE	PERTINENT CHARACTERISTICS	IMPLICATIONS FOR BIRTH
Gynecoid	Inlet rounded with all inlet diameters adequate	Favorable for vaginal birth
	Midpelvis diameters adequate with parallel side walls	
	Outlet adequate	
Android	Inlet heart-shaped with short posterior sagittal diameter	Not favorable for vaginal birth
	Midpelvis diameters reduced	Descent into pelvis is slow
	Outlet capacity reduced	Fetal head enters pelvis in transverse or posterior position with arrest of labor frequent
Anthropoid	Inlet oval in shape, with long anteroposterior diameter	Favorable for vaginal birth
	Midpelvis diameters adequate	
	Outlet adequate	
Platypelloid	Inlet oval in shape, with long transverse diameters	Not favorable for vaginal birth
	Midpelvis diameters reduced	Fetal head engages in transverse position
	Outlet capacity inadequate	Difficult descent through midpelvis
		Frequent delay of progress at outlet of pelvis

NOTE: Description of pelvic shape is exaggerated for easier comprehension.

factors of the birth passageway. See Chapter 12 for techniques to assess the size and shape of the pelvis.

Birth Passenger (Fetus)

Several aspects of the fetus's body and the way the fetus moves through the mother's birth canal are considered critical factors of the passenger that affect the outcome of labor. These interacting factors are the fetal head, fetal attitude, fetal lie, fetal presentation, and fetal position. The placenta must also pass through the birth canal but rarely impedes the labor process, except in cases of placenta previa (see Chapter 23 for placental complications).

FETAL HEAD

The fetal head is composed of bony parts, which can either hinder childbirth or make it easier. Once the head (the least compressible and largest part of the fetus) has been born, the birth of the rest of the body is rarely delayed.

The fetal skull has three major parts: The face, the base of the skull (cranium), and the vault of the cranium (roof). The bones of the face and cranial base are well fused and essentially fixed. The base of the cranium is composed of the two temporal bones, each with a sphenoid bone and an ethmoid bone. The bones composing the vault are the two frontal bones, the two parietal bones, and the occipital bone (Figure 19–2). These bones are not fused, allowing this portion of the head to adjust as it passes through the narrow portions of the maternal pelvis. The cranial bones overlap under pressure of the powers of labor and the demands of the unyielding pelvis. This overlapping is called **molding**.

The **sutures** of the fetal skull are membranous joints that unite the cranial bones; they allow for molding of the fetal head and help the clinician identify the position of the fetal head during vaginal examination. The important sutures of the cranial vault are (see Figure 19–2):

- ***Frontal suture.*** Located between the two frontal bones; becomes the anterior continuation of the sagittal suture
- ***Sagittal suture.*** Located between the parietal bones; divides the skull into left and right halves; runs anteroposteriorly, connecting the two fontanelles

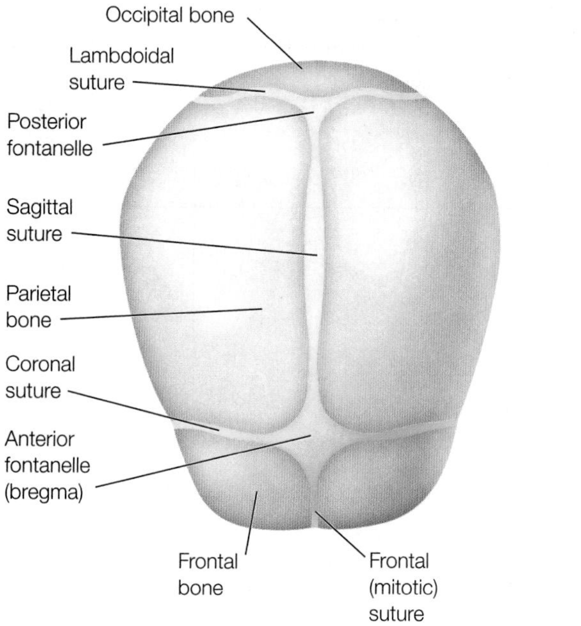

Figure 19–2 **Superior view of the fetal skull.**

- ***Coronal sutures.*** Located between the frontal and parietal bones; extend transversely left and right from the anterior fontanelle (bregma)
- ***Lambdoidal suture.*** Located between the two parietal bones and the occipital bone; extends transversely left and right from the posterior fontanelle.

The intersection of several cranial sutures forms an irregular space that is enclosed by a membrane and is called a **fontanelle**. The anterior and posterior fontanelles are clinically useful in identifying the position of the fetal head in the pelvis and in assessing the status of the newborn after birth. The greater, or anterior, fontanelle (bregma) is diamond shaped, measures 2 to 3 cm, and is situated at the junction of the sagittal, coronal, and frontal sutures. It permits growth of the brain by remaining

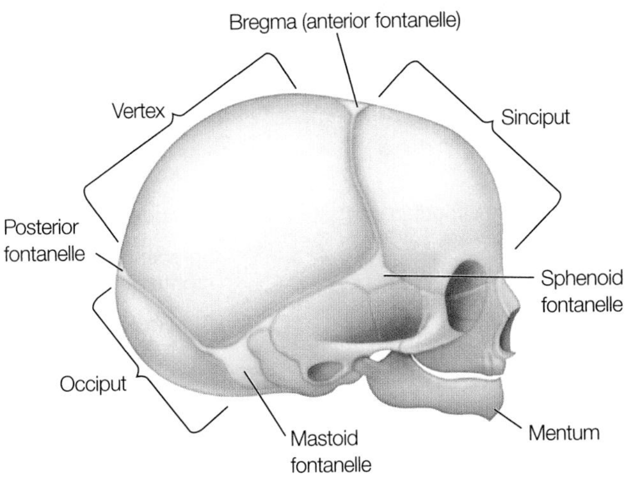

Figure 19–3 **Lateral view of the fetal skull identifying the landmarks that have significance during birth.**

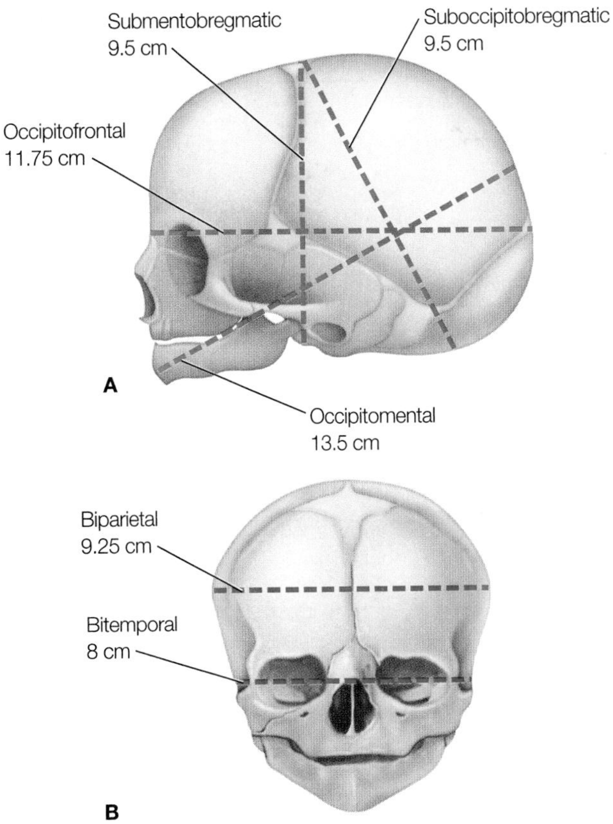

Figure 19–4 **A. Anteroposterior diameters of the fetal skull. When the vertex of the fetus presents and the fetal head is flexed with the chin on the chest, the smallest anteroposterior diameter (suboccipitobregmatic) enters the birth canal. B. Transverse diameters of the fetal skull.**

unossified for as long as 18 months. The lesser, or posterior, fontanelle is shaped like a small triangle, measures about 1 to 2 cm, and is situated at the intersection of the sagittal and lambdoidal sutures. It closes within 2 to 3 months after birth.

Following are several other important landmarks of the fetal skull (Figure 19–3):

- ***Mentum.*** The fetal chin
- ***Sinciput.*** The anterior area known as the brow
- ***Vertex.*** The area between the anterior and posterior fontanelles
- ***Occiput.*** The area of the fetal skull occupied by the occipital bone, beneath the posterior fontanelle.

The diameters of the fetal skull vary considerably within normal limits. Some diameters shorten and others lengthen as the head is molded during labor. Fetal head diameters are measured between the various landmarks on the skull (Figure 19–4A). For example, the suboccipitobregmatic diameter is the distance from the undersurface of the occiput to the center of the bregma (anterior fontanelle). The biparietal diameter is the largest part of the fetal head (Figure 19–4B).

Fetal Attitude

Fetal attitude refers to the relation of the fetal body parts to one another and describes the posture the fetus assumes as it conforms to the shape of the uterine cavity. The normal attitude of the fetus is termed *general flexion*, where the head is flexed so that the chin is on the chest with the arms crossed over the chest and the legs flexed at the knees with the thighs on the abdomen (Figure 19–5).

Changes in fetal attitude, particularly in the position of the head, cause the fetus to present larger diameters of the fetal head to the maternal pelvis. These deviations from a normal fetal attitude often contribute to a longer, more difficult labor.

FETAL LIE

Fetal lie refers to the relationship of the long, or cephalocaudal, axis (spinal column) of the fetus to the long, or cephalocaudal, axis of the mother. The fetus may assume either a longitudinal (vertical) or a transverse (horizontal) lie. A *longitudinal lie* occurs when the cephalocaudal axis of the fetus is parallel to the woman's spine. A *transverse lie* occurs when the cephalocaudal axis of the fetal spine is at a right angle to the woman's spine (see Figure 24–11). A transverse lie is associated with a shoulder presentation and can lead to complications in the later stages of labor; this is discussed in detail in Chapter 24. Table 19–3 identifies the characteristics associated with a longitudinal versus a transverse fetal lie.

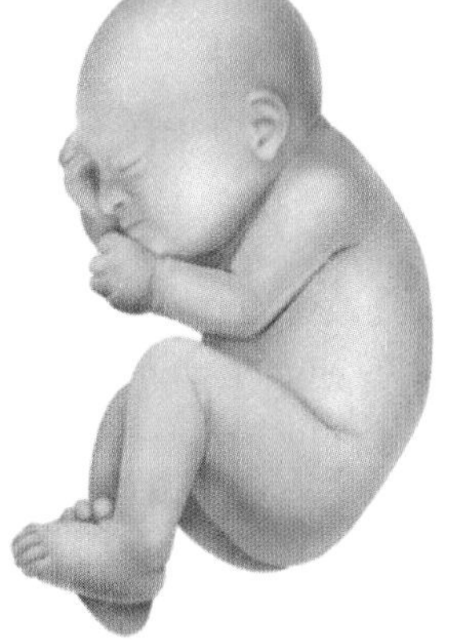

Figure 19–5 **Fetal attitude. The attitude (or relationship of body parts) of this fetus is normal. The head is flexed forward with the chin almost resting on the chest. The arms and legs are flexed.**

TABLE 19–3 Characteristics Associated with Longitudinal versus Transverse Fetal Lie

FETAL LIE	ATTITUDE	PRESENTING PART	LANDMARK
Longitudinal Lie (99.5%)			
Cephalic presentation (96–97%)	Flexion of fetal head onto chest	Vertex (posterior part—occiput)	Occiput (O)
	Military (no flexion, no extension)	Vertex (median part)	Occiput (O)
	Partial extension	Brow	Forehead (frontum) (Fr)
	Complete extension of the head	Face	Chin (mentum) (M)
Breech Presentation (Approximately 3%)			
Complete breech	Flexed hips and knees	Buttocks	Sacrum (S)
Frank breech	Flexed hips, extended knees with legs against abdomen and chest	Buttocks	Sacrum (S)
Footling breech: Single, double	Extended hips and at least one knee extended with foot in cervical canal	Feet (one or two)	Sacrum (S)
Kneeling breech: Single, double	Extended hips, flexed knees	Knees	Sacrum (S)
Transverse or Oblique Lie (Approximately 0.5%)			
Shoulder presentation	Variable	Shoulder, arm	Scapula (Sc or A)

FETAL PRESENTATION

Fetal presentation is determined by fetal lie and refers to the body part of the fetus that enters the maternal pelvis first and leads through the birth canal during labor. The **presenting part**, or the portion of the fetus that is felt through the cervix on vaginal examination, determines the presentation. Fetal presentation may be *cephalic* (head first), *breech* (buttocks or feet first), or *shoulder*.

The most common presentation is cephalic. When this presentation occurs, labor and birth are more likely to proceed normally. Breech and shoulder presentations are associated with difficulties during labor and do not proceed as normal; therefore, they are called **malpresentations**. (See Chapter 24 for nursing management of malpresentations.)

Cephalic Presentation. The fetal head presents to the birth passage in approximately 97% of term births. The cephalic presentation can be further classified into vertex, sinciput, brow, or face presentation according to the degree of flexion or extension of the fetal head (attitude).

Vertex Presentation.

- When the presenting part is the occiput, the presentation is noted as vertex.
- Vertex is the most common type of presentation.
- The fetal head is completely flexed onto the chest.
- The smallest diameter of the fetal head (suboccipitobregmatic) presents to the maternal pelvis (Figure 19–6A).

Sinciput Presentation.

- The fetal head is partially flexed.
- The occipitofrontal diameter presents to the maternal pelvis.
- The top of the head is the presenting part (Figure 19–6B).

Brow Presentation.

- The fetal head is partially extended.
- The occipitomental diameter, the largest anteroposterior diameter, is presented to the maternal pelvis (Figure 19–6C).

Face Presentation.

- The fetal head is hyperextended (complete extension).
- The submentobregmatic diameter presents to the maternal pelvis (Figure 19–6D).

Breech Presentation. A breech presentation indicates that the presenting part is the lower extremities or buttocks. Breech presentations occur in approximately 3% of all term births (Cunningham et al., 2016). These presentations are classified according to the attitude of the fetus's hips and knees. In all variations of the breech presentation (complete, frank, or footling breech), the sacrum (the bone on the buttocks that is felt when palpating) is the landmark.

Complete Breech.

- The fetal knees and hips are both flexed, the thighs are on the abdomen, and the calves are on the posterior aspect of the thighs.
- The buttocks and feet of the fetus present to the maternal pelvis.

Frank Breech.

- The fetal hips are flexed, and the knees are extended.
- The buttocks of the fetus present to the maternal pelvis.

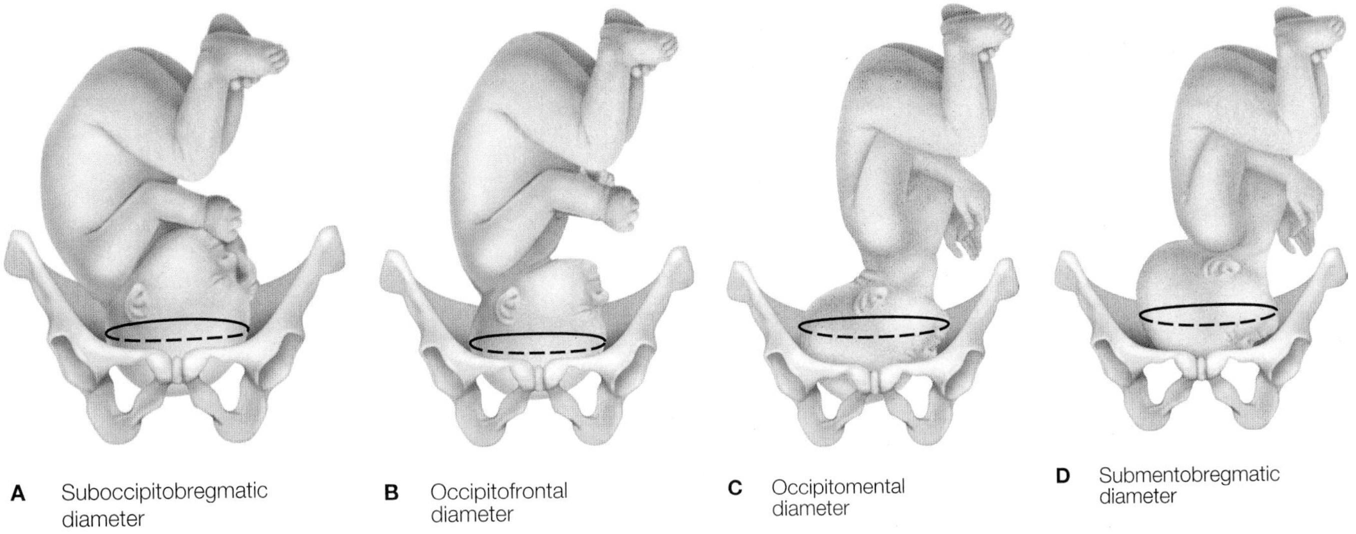

Figure 19–6 Cephalic presentation. A. Vertex presentation. Complete flexion of the head allows the suboccipitobregmatic diameter to present to the pelvis. B. Sinciput (median vertex) presentation (also called *military presentation*) with no flexion or extension. The occipitofrontal diameter presents to the pelvis. C. Brow presentation. The fetal head is in partial (halfway) extension. The occipitomental diameter, which is the largest diameter of the fetal head, presents to the pelvis. D. Face presentation. The fetal head is in complete extension, and the submentobregmatic diameter presents to the pelvis.

Footling Breech.

- The fetal hips and legs are extended.
- The feet of the fetus present to the maternal pelvis.
- In a single footling one foot presents; in a double footling both feet present.

Shoulder Presentation. When the fetal shoulder is the presenting part, the fetus is in a transverse lie and the acromion process of the scapula is the landmark. This type of presentation occurs less than 1% of the time (Cunningham et al., 2016).

Relationship of Maternal Pelvis and Presenting Part

The third critical factor, in addition to the birth passage and fetus, is the relationship between these two factors. When assessing the relationship of the maternal pelvis and the presenting part of the fetal body, the nurse considers engagement, station, and fetal position.

ENGAGEMENT

Engagement of the presenting part occurs when the largest diameter of the presenting part reaches or passes through the pelvic inlet (Figure 19–7A). When the fetal head is flexed, the biparietal diameter is the largest dimension of the fetal skull to pass through the pelvic inlet in a cephalic presentation. The intertrochanteric diameter (transverse diameter between the right and left trochanter) is the largest to pass through the inlet in a breech presentation.

Engagement can be determined by vaginal examination. In primigravidas, engagement usually occurs 2 weeks before term. Multiparas, however, may experience engagement several weeks before the onset of labor or during the process of labor.

The presenting part is said to be *floating* (or *ballottable*) when it is freely movable above the inlet (see Figure 19–7B). The fetus will continue to descend into the inlet of the pelvis as labor continues (see Figure 19–7C). Once the presenting part reaches the level of the inlet, engagement is said to have occurred.

STATION

Station refers to the relationship of the presenting part to an imaginary line drawn between the ischial spines of the maternal pelvis. In a normal pelvis, the ischial spines mark the narrowest diameter through which the fetus must pass. These spines are not sharp protrusions but rather blunted prominences at the midpelvis. The ischial spines as a landmark have been designated as zero station (Figure 19–8). If the presenting part is higher than the ischial spines, a negative number is assigned, noting centimeters above zero station. Station –5 is at the inlet, and station +4 is at the outlet. If the presenting part can be seen at the woman's perineum, birth will occur momentarily. During labor the presenting part should move progressively from the negative stations to the midpelvis at zero station and into the positive stations. Failure of the presenting part to descend in the presence of strong contractions may be due to disproportion between the maternal pelvis and fetal presenting part.

FETAL POSITION

Fetal position refers to the relationship of the landmark on the presenting fetal part to the anterior, posterior, or sides (right or left) of the maternal pelvis. The landmark on the fetal presenting part is related to four imaginary quadrants of the maternal pelvis: Left anterior, right anterior, left posterior, and right posterior. These quadrants designate where the presenting part is directed. If the landmark is directed toward the center of the side of the pelvis, fetal position is designated as transverse, rather than anterior or posterior.

The landmark chosen for vertex presentations is the occiput, and the landmark for face presentations is the mentum. In breech presentations the sacrum is the designated landmark, and the acromion process on the scapula is the landmark in shoulder presentations.

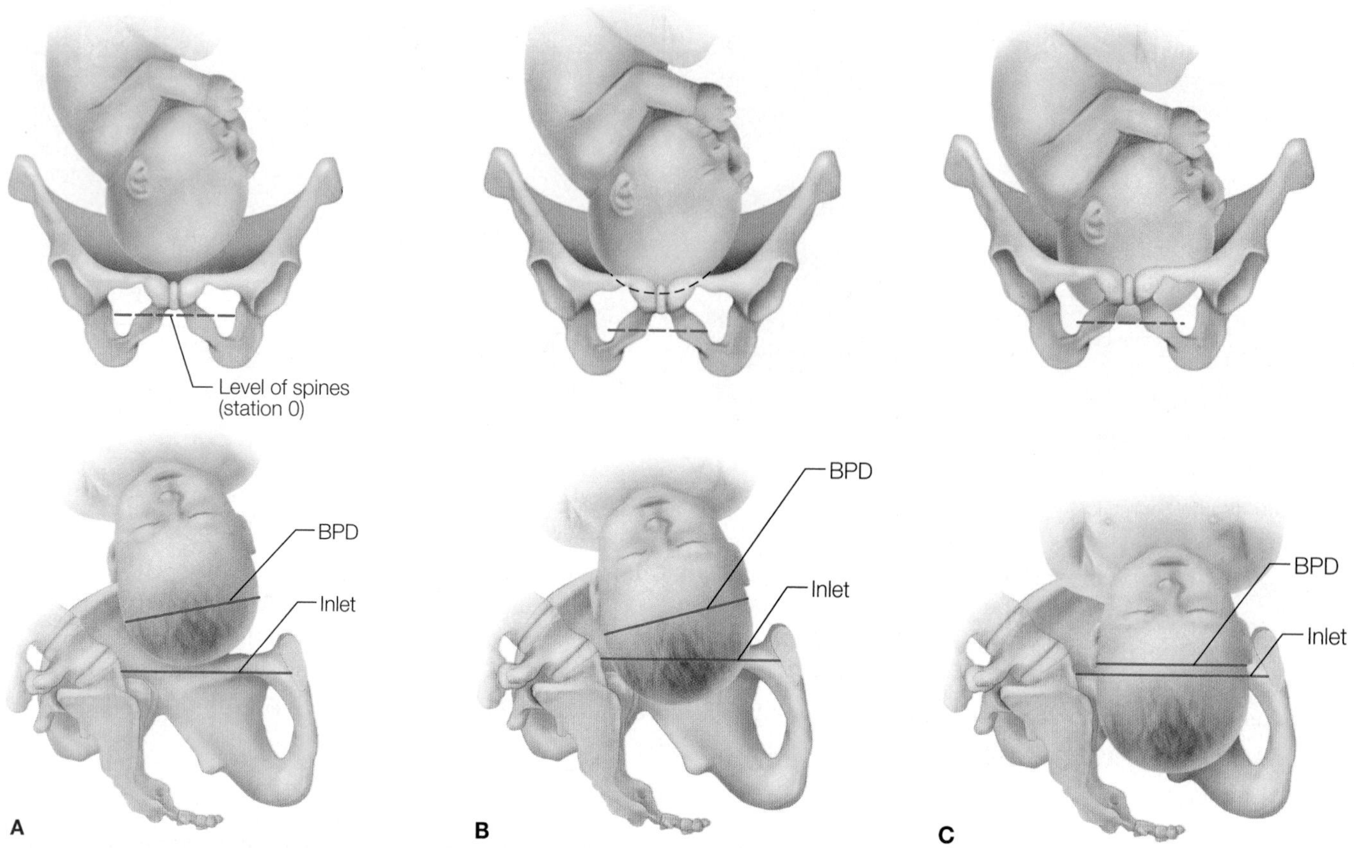

Figure 19–7 **Process of engagement in cephalic presentation. A. Engaged. The biparietal diameter (BPD) of the fetal head is in the inlet of the pelvis. In most instances, the presenting part (occiput) will be at the level of the ischial spines (0 station). B. Floating. The fetal head is directed down toward the pelvis but can still easily move away from the inlet. C. Descending. The fetal head descends into the inlet but can be moved away by exerting pressure on the fetus.**

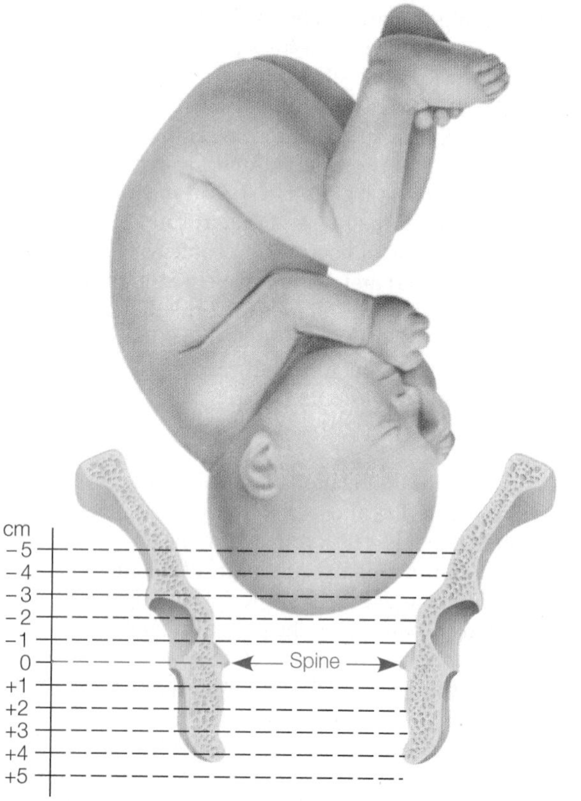

Figure 19–8 **Measuring the station of the fetal head while it is descending. In this view the station is –2.**

In summary, three notations are used to describe the fetal position:

- ***Right (R)*** or ***left (L)*** side of the maternal pelvis
- The landmark of the fetal presenting part: ***Occiput (O)***, ***mentum (M)***, ***sacrum (S)***, or ***acromion (scapula [Sc]) process (A)***
- ***Anterior (A)***, ***posterior (P)***, or ***transverse (T)***, depending on whether the landmark is in the front, back, or side of the pelvis.

The abbreviations of these notations help the healthcare team communicate the fetal position. Thus, when the fetal occiput is directed toward the back and to the left of the passage, the abbreviation used is LOP (left-occiput-posterior). Table 19–4 lists positions and abbreviations used for various fetal presentations, some of which are illustrated in Figure 19–9.

The fetal position influences labor and birth. For example, the fetal head presents a larger diameter in a posterior position than in an anterior position. A posterior position increases the pressure on the maternal sacral nerves, causing the laboring woman to experience backache and pelvic pressure. As a result, the woman may bear down or feel the urge to push earlier than needed. In addition, the second stage of labor may be prolonged when the fetal head remains in a posterior position.

The most common fetal position is occiput anterior. When this position occurs, the labor and birth are more likely to proceed normally. Positions other than occiput anterior are more frequently associated with problems during labor; therefore, they are called *malpositions*. (See Chapter 24 for discussion of malpositions and their management.)

TABLE 19–4 Abbreviations Used for Fetal Position

POSITIONS IN VERTEX PRESENTATION	POSITIONS IN FACE PRESENTATION
ROA: Right-occiput-anterior	RMA: Right-mentum-anterior
ROT: Right-occiput-transverse	RMT: Right-mentum-transverse
ROP: Right-occiput-posterior	RMP: Right-mentum-posterior
LOA: Left-occiput-anterior	LMA: Left-mentum-anterior
LOT: Left-occiput-transverse	LMT: Left-mentum-transverse
LOP: Left-occiput-posterior	LMP: Left-mentum-posterior
POSITIONS IN BREECH PRESENTATION	**POSITIONS IN SHOULDER PRESENTATION***
RSA: Right-sacrum-anterior	RADA: Right-acromion-dorsal-anterior
RST: Right-sacrum-transverse	RADP: Right-acromion-dorsal-posterior
RSP: Right-sacrum-posterior	LADA: Left-acromion-dorsal-anterior
LSA: Left-sacrum-anterior	LADP: Left-acromion-dorsal-posterior
LST: Left-sacrum-transverse	
LSP: Left-sacrum-posterior	

* The term *dorsal (D)* is added when denoting the fetal position in a shoulder presentation; it refers to the fetal back. Thus, the abbreviation *RADA* indicates that the acromion process of the scapula is directed toward the woman's right and the fetus's back is anterior.

Assessment techniques to determine fetal position include inspection and palpation of the maternal abdomen and vaginal examination. (See Chapter 20 for discussion of assessment of fetal position.)

Physiologic Forces of Labor

Primary and secondary forces work together to deliver the fetus, the fetal membranes, and the placenta from the uterus into the external environment. The *primary force* is uterine muscular contractions, which cause the changes of the first stage of labor—complete effacement and dilatation of the cervix. The *secondary force* is the use of abdominal muscles to push during the second stage of labor. The pushing adds to the primary power after full dilatation.

CONTRACTIONS

A uterine **contraction** is the rhythmic tightening and shortening of the uterine muscles during labor. Each contraction has three phases:

1. ***Increment:*** The "building-up" of the contraction (the longest phase)
2. ***Acme:*** The peak of the contraction
3. ***Decrement:*** The "letting-up" of the contraction.

Between contractions is a period of relaxation. This period of relaxation allows uterine muscles to rest and provides respite for the laboring woman. It also restores uteroplacental circulation, which is important to fetal oxygenation and adequate circulation in the uterine blood vessels.

When describing uterine contractions during labor, caregivers use the terms *frequency*, *duration*, and *intensity*.

Frequency refers to the time between the beginning of one contraction and the beginning of the next contraction. The **duration** of each contraction is measured from the beginning of the contraction to the completion of the contraction (Figure 19–10). In beginning labor, the duration is 30 to 40 seconds. As labor continues, duration increases to 30 to 90 seconds.

Intensity refers to the strength of the uterine contraction during acme. In most instances the intensity is estimated by palpating the contraction, but it may be measured directly with an intrauterine catheter attached to an electronic fetal monitor. Intensity of uterine contractions cannot be accurately measured by external monitoring with an electronic fetal monitor because several variables affect the external monitor, including maternal weight, specifically the amount of adipose tissue, and positioning of the monitor on the maternal abdomen. When estimating intensity by palpation, the nurse determines whether it is mild, moderate, or strong by judging the amount of indentability of the uterine wall during the acme of a contraction. If the uterine wall can be indented easily, the contraction is considered mild. Strong intensity exists when the uterine wall cannot be indented. Moderate intensity falls between these two ranges. When intensity is measured with an intrauterine catheter, the normal resting tonus (between contractions) is about 10 to 12 mmHg of pressure. During acme the intensity ranges from 25 to 40 mmHg in early labor, 50 to 70 mmHg in active labor, 80 to 100 mmHg during transition, and greater than 100 mmHg while the woman is pushing in the second stage (Cunningham et al., 2016). (See Chapter 20 for further discussion of assessment techniques.)

At the beginning of labor the contractions are usually mild, of short duration, and relatively infrequent. As labor progresses, duration and intensity increase and the frequency is every 2 to 3 minutes. Because the contractions are involuntary, the laboring woman cannot control their duration, frequency, or intensity.

BEARING DOWN

After the cervix is completely dilated, the maternal abdominal musculature contracts as the woman pushes. This pushing is called *bearing down*. The pushing aids in the expulsion of the fetus and the placenta. If the cervix is not completely dilated, bearing down can cause cervical edema (which retards dilatation), possible tearing and bruising of the cervix, and maternal exhaustion. The combined involuntary pressure of the uterine contractions and the voluntary muscle contractions of the abdomen force the fetus toward the outlet so birth can occur.

Psychosocial Considerations

Thus far, the discussion has focused on physical influences on labor outcomes. But the final critical factor is the parents' psychosocial readiness, including their fears, anxieties, birth fantasies, and level of social support. Similar psychosocial factors affect

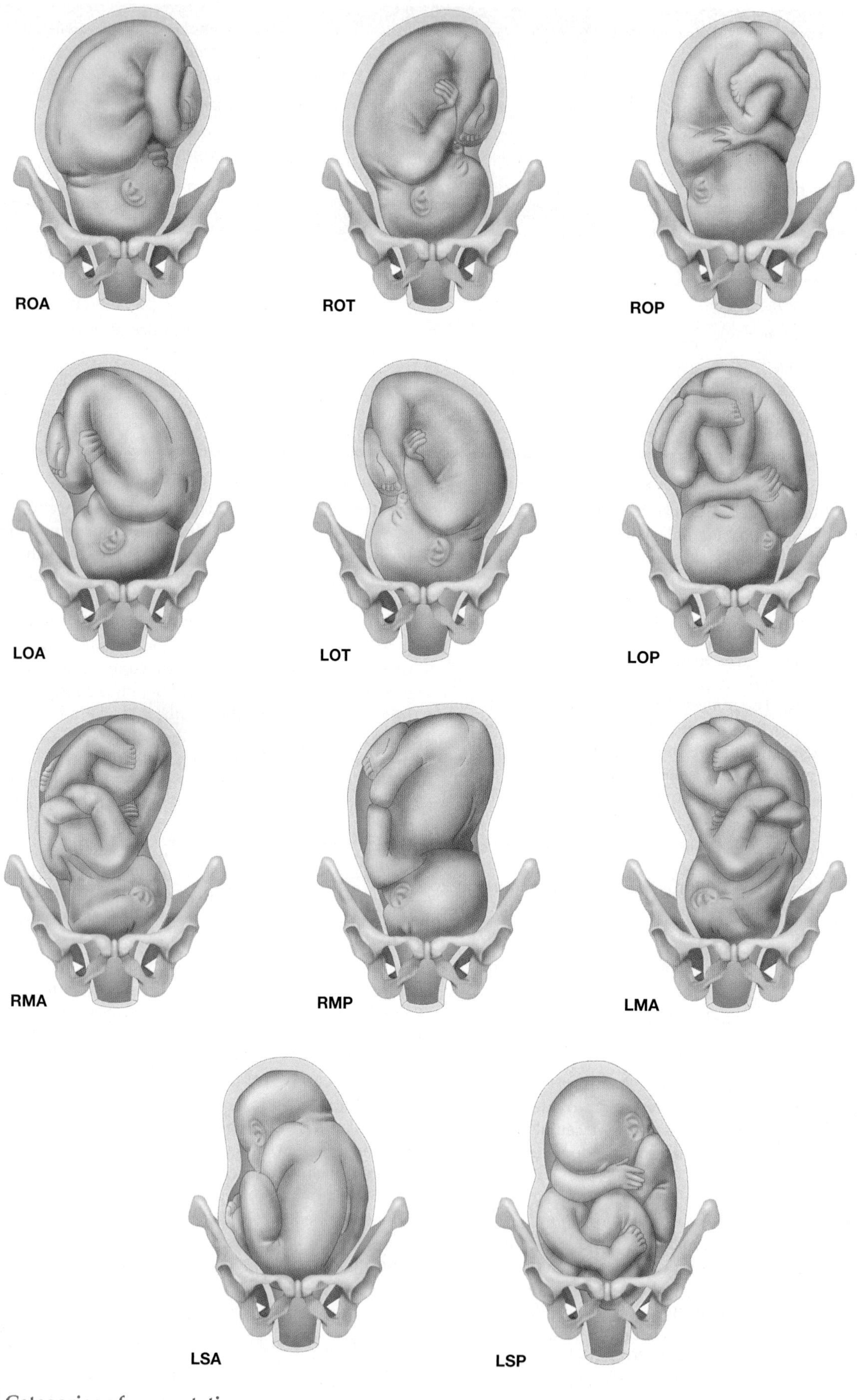

Figure 19–9 Categories of presentation.

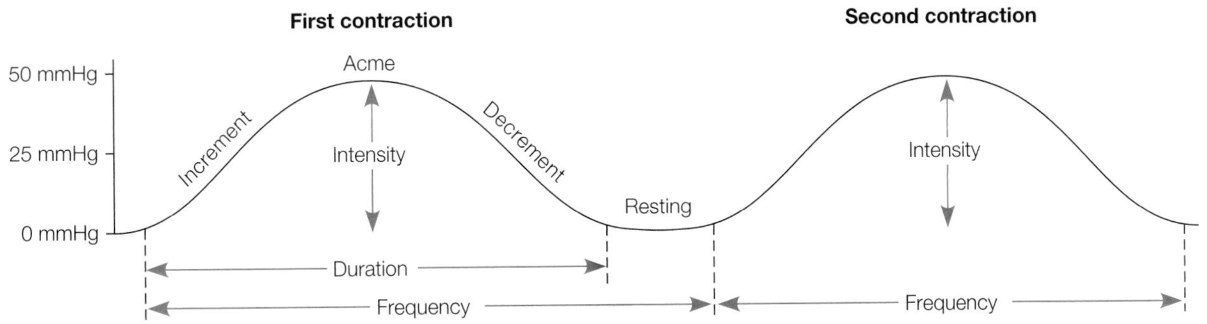

Figure 19–10 Characteristics of uterine contractions.

both parents. Both are making a transition into a new role and both have expectations of themselves and their partner during the labor and birth experience. Although many prospective parents attend childbirth preparation classes, they still tend to be concerned about what labor will be like. Concerns include whether they will each be able to perform the way they expect, whether the discomfort and pain will be more than the mother expects or is able to cope with, whether the father or partner can provide helpful support, and whether they can maintain a sense of control and be advocates for themselves. In addition, both partners face an irrevocable event—the birth of a new family member—and, consequently, disruption of lifestyle, relationships, and self-image.

Many women have preconceived ideas about what birth should be like and some fear "losing control" of their body functions, emotions, or ability to handle the pain associated with labor. Women whose birth experiences do not meet their preconceived ideas may feel loss and disappointment. They may also feel that they have failed to live up to the expectations of friends, family, and peers.

Various factors influence a woman's reaction to labor and contribute to a positive birth experience (Table 19–5). Her accomplishment of the tasks of pregnancy, usual coping mechanisms in response to stressful life events, previous experiences, support system, preparation for childbirth, and cultural influences are all significant factors.

Many women have dreams about their birthing experience, their baby, and their early parenting experiences. Dreaming and fantasizing about the unborn baby are a developmental process of pregnancy. The nurse can encourage the woman to share her dreams and fantasies and use them as a tool to examine the woman's expectations, fears, and coping mechanisms. This can assist the woman in forming a maternal role and facilitate bonding with her fetus.

When a woman is facing labor, especially for the first time, she may worry about her ability to withstand the pain of contractions. Some women may place great emphasis on withstanding the pain of childbirth stoically—without medication, crying, moaning, or making other sounds. The nurse's role is to help childbearing families explore options and identify interventions to help each woman cope with the discomfort of labor in a way that is acceptable to her.

The laboring woman's support system may also influence the course of labor and birth. Although some women may prefer not to have a support person or family member with them, for many women the presence of her partner and other significant persons (especially the nurse) tends to have a positive effect. A labor partner's presence at the bedside provides a means to enhance communication and to demonstrate feelings of love. Communication needs may include talking and the use of affectionate and understanding words from the partner. Showing love may take the form of holding hands, hugging, or touching.

How the woman views the birth experience in hindsight may have implications for mothering behaviors. A significant relationship exists between the birth experience and mothering behaviors (MacKinnon et al., 2017). It appears that any activities by the expectant woman or by healthcare providers that enhance the birth experience will be beneficial to the mother-baby connection. The father's experience of childbirth and his opportunities for bonding may have important implications for fathering as well.

TABLE 19–5 Factors Associated with a Positive Birth Experience

- Motivation for the pregnancy
- Attendance at childbirth education classes
- A sense of competence or mastery
- Self-confidence and self-esteem
- Positive relationship with partner
- Maintaining control during labor
- Support from partner or other person during labor
- Not being left alone in labor
- Trust in the medical/nursing staff
- Having personal control of breathing patterns, comfort measures
- Choosing a physician/certified nurse-midwife who has a similar philosophy of care
- Receiving clear information regarding procedures

Physiology of Labor

In addition to considering the five critical factors affecting the progress of labor and birth, it is essential to explore the physiology of the normal labor experience.

Possible Causes of Labor Onset

Labor usually begins between the 38th and the 42nd week of gestation, when the fetus is mature and ready for birth. Despite medical advances, there is still no full understanding of the biochemical substances and interactions that stimulate labor and birth. Some important aspects have been identified. For example, estrogen is known to stimulate uterine muscle contractions to permit softening, stretching, and eventual thinning of the cervix. Collagen fibers in the cervix are broken down by the action of enzymes such as collagenase and elastase. As the collagen fibers change, their ability to bind is decreased because of increasing amounts of hyaluronic acid (which loosely binds collagen fibrils) and decreasing amounts of dermatan sulfate (which tightly binds collagen fibrils). There is also an increase in the water content of the cervix. All these changes result in a weakening and softening of the cervix, which facilitates cervical stretching and effacement.

Hypotheses have also been formed about the roles of progesterone withdrawal, of prostaglandin, and of corticotropin-releasing hormone.

PROGESTERONE WITHDRAWAL HYPOTHESIS

Progesterone produced by the placenta relaxes uterine smooth muscle by interfering with conduction of impulses from one cell to the next. For this reason, the uterus is usually without coordinated contractions during pregnancy. Biochemical changes toward the end of gestation result in decreased availability of progesterone to myometrial cells. The decrease in availability may be associated with a yet-unknown antiprogestin that inhibits the relaxant effect on the uterus but allows other progesterone actions such as lactogenesis (Cunningham et al., 2016).

PROSTAGLANDIN HYPOTHESIS

Although the exact relationship between prostaglandin and the onset of labor is not yet established, the effect is clinically demonstrated by the successful induction of labor after vaginal application of prostaglandin E. In addition, preterm labor may be stopped by using an inhibitor of prostaglandin synthesis such as indomethacin (Cunningham et al., 2016).

The amnion and decidua are the focus of research on the source of prostaglandins. Once prostaglandin is produced, stimuli for its synthesis may include rising levels of estrogen, decreased availability of progesterone, increased levels of oxytocin or response to oxytocin, platelet-activating factor, and endothelin-1 (Cunningham et al., 2016).

CORTICOTROPIN-RELEASING HORMONE HYPOTHESIS

Corticotropin-releasing hormone (CRH) is also a focus for researchers. Its possible role in onset of labor is suggested by the fact that CRH concentration increases throughout pregnancy, with a sharp increase at term. Also, CRH may play a role in increased risk for preterm birth, and CRH levels are elevated in multiple gestations. Finally, CRH is known to stimulate the synthesis of prostaglandin F and prostaglandin E by amnion cells (Cunningham et al., 2016).

Myometrial Activity

In true labor the uterus divides into two portions. This division is known as the *physiologic retraction ring*. The upper portion, which is the contractile segment, becomes progressively thicker as labor advances. The lower portion, which includes the lower uterine segment and cervix, is passive. As labor continues, the lower uterine segment expands and thins out.

With each contraction, the muscles of the upper uterine segment shorten and exert a longitudinal traction on the cervix, causing effacement. **Effacement** is the taking-up (or drawing-up) of the internal os and the cervical canal into the uterine side walls. The cervix changes progressively from a long, thick structure to a structure that is tissue-paper thin (Figure 19–11). In primigravidas effacement usually precedes dilatation. The uterine muscle remains shorter and thicker and does not return to its original length. This phenomenon is known as *brachystasis*. The space in the uterine cavity decreases as a result of brachystasis, and this places downward pressure on the fetus (Groll, 2015).

The uterus shortens with each contraction, which in turn pulls the lower uterine segment upward. This shortening causes flexion of the fetal body, which thrusts the presenting part down toward the lower uterine segment and the cervix. The pressure exerted by the fetus is called *fetal axis pressure*. As the uterus shortens, the longitudinal muscle fibers elongate, and the lower uterine segment is more distensible and removes resistance on the presenting part as the uterus is pulled upward. This action and the hydrostatic pressure of the fetal membranes cause **cervical dilatation**, which is when the cervical os and cervical canal widen from less than 1 cm to approximately 10 cm, allowing birth of the fetus. When the cervix is completely dilated and retracted up into the lower uterine segment, it can no longer be palpated.

The round ligament pulls the fundus forward, aligning the fetus with the bony pelvis. This facilitates engagement of the presenting part. Pressure exerted on the cervix by the presenting part aids in both effacement and cervical dilatation (Cunningham et al., 2016).

Musculature Changes in the Pelvic Floor

The levator ani muscle and fascia of the pelvic floor draw the rectum and vagina upward and forward with each contraction, along the curve of the pelvic floor. As the fetal head descends to the pelvic floor, the pressure of the presenting part causes the perineal structure, which was once 5 cm in thickness, to change to a structure less than 1 cm thick. A normal physiologic anesthesia is produced as a result of the decreased blood supply to the area. The anus everts, exposing the interior rectal wall as the fetal head descends forward (Cunningham et al., 2016).

Premonitory Signs of Labor

Most primigravidas and many multiparas experience one or more of the following signs and symptoms of impending labor.

LIGHTENING

Lightening describes the effects that occur when the fetus begins to settle into the pelvic inlet (engagement). With fetal descent, the uterus moves downward, and the fundus no longer presses on the diaphragm, which eases breathing.

However, with increased downward pressure of the presenting part, the woman may notice the following (Cunningham et al., 2016):

- Leg cramps or pains due to pressure on the nerves that course through the obturator foramen in the pelvis
- Increased pelvic pressure
- Increased venous stasis, leading to edema in the lower extremities
- Increased urinary frequency
- Increased vaginal secretions resulting from congestion of the vaginal mucous membranes.

BRAXTON HICKS CONTRACTIONS

Before the onset of labor, *Braxton Hicks contractions*—the irregular, intermittent contractions that have been occurring throughout the pregnancy—may become uncomfortable. The pain seems to be in the abdomen and groin but may feel like the "drawing" sensations experienced by some women with dysmenorrhea. When these contractions are strong enough for the woman to believe she is in labor, she is said to be in false labor.

CERVICAL CHANGES

Considerable change occurs in the cervix during the prenatal and intrapartum period. At the beginning of pregnancy the cervix

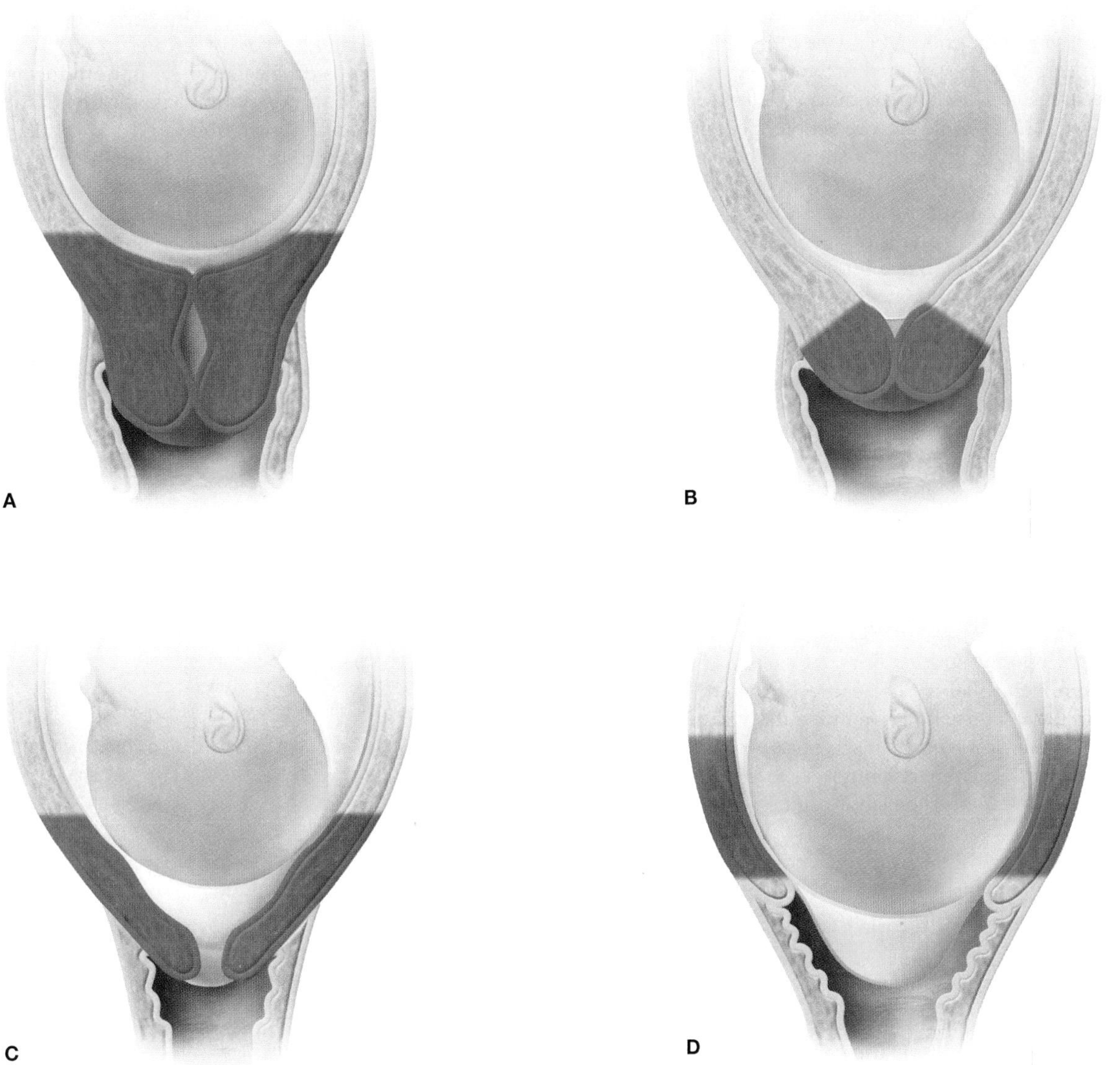

Figure 19–11 **Effacement of the cervix in the primigravida. A. At the beginning of labor, there is no cervical effacement or dilatation. The fetal head is cushioned by amniotic fluid. B. Beginning cervical effacement. As the cervix begins to efface, more amniotic fluid collects below the fetal head. C. Cervix is about one-half (50%) effaced and slightly dilated. The increasing amount of amniotic fluid below the fetal head exerts hydrostatic pressure on the cervix. D. Complete effacement and dilatation.**

is rigid and firm, and it must soften so that it can stretch and dilate to allow fetal passage. This softening of the cervix, called *ripening*, is under the influence of hormonal factors, which are discussed shortly.

BLOODY SHOW

During pregnancy, cervical secretions accumulate in the cervical canal to form a barrier called a *mucous plug*. With softening and effacement of the cervix, the mucous plug is often expelled, resulting in a small amount of blood loss from the exposed cervical capillaries. The resulting pink-tinged secretions are called **bloody show**.

Bloody show is considered a sign of impending labor, usually within 24 to 48 hours. Vaginal examination that includes manipulation of the cervix may also result in a blood-tinged discharge, which is sometimes confused with bloody show. However, this discharge is typically brownish in color and is not accompanied by the mucous plug.

RUPTURE OF MEMBRANES

In approximately 12% of women, the amniotic membranes rupture before the onset of labor. This breaking-open of the amniotic membranes is called **rupture of membranes (ROM)**. After membranes rupture, 80% of women will experience spontaneous labor within 24 hours. If membranes rupture and labor does not begin spontaneously within 12 to 24 hours, labor may be induced to avoid infection (once the membranes have ruptured there is an open pathway into the uterine cavity). An induction of labor is done only if the pregnancy is near term.

At the beginning of labor, the amniotic membranes bulge through the cervix in the shape of a cone. When the membranes rupture, the amniotic fluid may be expelled in large amounts. *Spontaneous rupture of membranes (SROM)* generally occurs at the height of an intense contraction with a gush of the fluid out of the vagina. If engagement has not occurred, the danger exists that the umbilical cord may be expelled with the fluid (prolapsed cord). Because of these potential problems, the woman is advised to notify her certified nurse-midwife (CNM) or physician and proceed to the hospital or birthing center. In some instances the fluid is expelled in small amounts and may be confused with episodes of urinary incontinence associated with urinary urgency, coughing, or sneezing. The discharge should be checked to ascertain its source and to determine further action. (See Chapter 20 for assessment techniques.) In some instances, the membranes are ruptured by the physician/CNM, using an instrument called an amniohook. This procedure is called *amniotomy* or *artificial rupture of membranes (AROM)* and is discussed in Chapter 25.

Spontaneous rupture of membranes and leakage of amniotic fluid before the onset of labor at any gestational age is known as *premature rupture of membranes (PROM)*. When the membranes rupture and leakage of amniotic fluid from the vagina occurs before 37 weeks of gestation, the term *preterm premature rupture of membranes (PPROM)* is used. PPROM occurs in up to 25% of all cases of preterm labors, complicates more than 3% of pregnancies each year, and is associated with more than one-third of preterm births (Cunningham et al., 2016). Infection often precedes PPROM. When PPROM is suspected, strict sterile technique should be used in any vaginal examination. (For a complete discussion of PROM and PPROM, see Chapter 23.)

SUDDEN BURST OF ENERGY

Some women report a sudden burst of energy approximately 24 to 48 hours before labor. The cause of the energy spurt is unknown. In prenatal teaching the nurse should warn prospective mothers not to overexert themselves and to eat small, nutritious meals during this energy burst so that they will not be excessively tired or weak when labor begins.

OTHER SIGNS

Other premonitory signs include:

- Weight loss of 2.2 to 6.6 kg (1 to 3 lb) resulting from fluid loss and electrolyte shifts produced by changes in estrogen and progesterone levels
- Increased backache and sacroiliac pressure from the influence of relaxin hormone on the pelvic joints
- Diarrhea, indigestion, or nausea and vomiting just before the onset of labor (the causes of these signs are unknown).

Differences Between True Labor and False Labor

The contractions of true labor produce progressive dilatation and effacement of the cervix. They occur regularly and increase in frequency, duration, and intensity. The discomfort of true labor contractions usually starts in the back and radiates around to the abdomen. The pain is not relieved by ambulation (in fact, walking may intensify the pain) or by resting.

The contractions of false labor do not produce progressive cervical effacement and dilatation. Classically, they are irregular and do not increase in frequency, duration, and intensity. The contractions may be perceived as a hardening or "balling-up" without discomfort or discomfort may occur mainly in the lower abdomen and groin. The discomfort may be relieved by ambulation, changes of position, resting, or a hot bath or shower (Groll, 2017). See *Key Facts to Remember: Comparison of True Labor and False Labor*.

Key Facts to Remember

Comparison of True Labor and False Labor

True Labor	False Labor
Contractions are at regular intervals.	Contractions are irregular.
Intervals between contractions gradually shorten.	Usually no change.
Contractions increase in duration and intensity.	Usually no change.
Discomfort begins in back and radiates around to abdomen.	Discomfort is usually in abdomen.
Intensity usually increases with walking.	Walking has no effect on or lessens contractions.
Cervical dilatation and effacement are progressive.	No change.
Contractions do not decrease with rest or warm tub bath.	Rest and warm tub baths lessen contractions.

NURSE'S RESPONSE TO FALSE LABOR

During the third trimester, the woman will find it helpful to learn the characteristics of true labor contractions as well as the premonitory signs of ensuing labor. The nurse informs the woman that false labor is common and many times cannot be distinguished from true labor except by vaginal examination. The woman must feel free to come in for accurate assessment of labor and should be counseled not to feel foolish if the labor is false. See *Case Study: Angelina Newman*.

In addition, false labor can last for several hours and can be exhausting. The nurse can suggest interventions to decrease the anxiety and physical discomforts associated with false labor such as walking, changing position, or a warm tub bath.

CASE STUDY: Angelina Newman

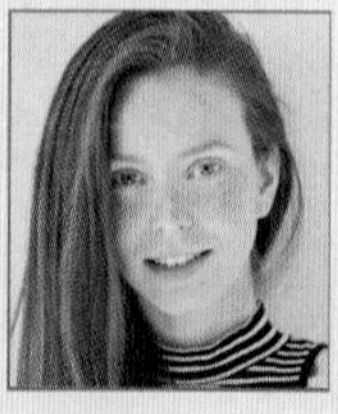

SOURCE: WAYHOME studio/Shutterstock

Angelina comes to the hospital with concerns she is in labor at 37 1/7 weeks gestation. She began having contractions 2 hours ago, notes good fetal movement, and denies her water broke or any vaginal bleeding. The nurse performs a vaginal exam and tells her that her cervix is soft, 1 centimeter dilated, 50% effaced, and in a posterior position, with the baby's station being –2. The nurse palpates mild contractions, and the fetal monitor shows contractions are occurring irregularly and lasting 25 to 35 seconds. After Angelina walks for 1.5 hours, the nurse reexamines her and finds no cervical change. Her contractions have spaced out and are rare now. Angelina asks if she can just stay and have the baby.

Question to Ponder

How would you educate Angelina on the reasons why reaching 39 weeks of gestation is desirable?

Stages of Labor and Birth

To assist caregivers, common terms have been developed as benchmarks to subdivide the process of labor into *stages* and *phases* of labor. It is important to note, however, that these represent theoretic separations in the process. A laboring woman will not usually experience distinct differences from one to the other. The first stage begins with the beginning of true labor and ends when the cervix is completely dilated at 10 cm. The second stage begins with complete dilatation and ends with the birth of the neonate. The third stage begins with the birth of the neonate and ends with the expulsion of the placenta.

Some clinicians identify a fourth stage of labor. During this stage, which lasts 1 to 4 hours after expulsion of the placenta, the uterus effectively contracts to control bleeding at the placental site (Groll, 2017). Nursing care of the laboring woman is discussed in Chapter 21.

The following discussion characterizes the four stages and their accompanying phases.

First Stage

The first stage of labor is divided into the latent or early, active, and transition phases. Each phase of labor is characterized by physical and psychologic changes.

LATENT OR EARLY PHASE

The *latent* or *early phase* begins with the onset of regular contractions. As the cervix begins to dilate it also effaces, although little or no fetal descent is evident. For a woman in her first labor (nullipara), the latent or early phase averages 7.3 to 8.6 hours, with 95% of women completing this stage by 17 to 21 hours. This early phase in multiparas averages 4.1 to 5.3 hours, with 95% of women completing this stage within 12 to 14 hours (Gabbe et al., 2015). Table 19–6 presents labor characteristics by stage of labor.

Uterine contractions become established during the latent phase and increase in frequency, duration, and intensity. They may start as mild contractions lasting 20 to 40 seconds with a frequency of 10 to 30 minutes. They average 25 to 40 mmHg by intrauterine pressure catheter at acme (Gabbe et al., 2015).

In the early or latent phase of the first stage of labor, contractions are usually mild. The woman feels able to cope with the discomfort. She may be relieved that labor has finally started. Although she may be anxious, she is able to recognize and express those feelings of anxiety. The woman is often talkative and smiling and is eager to talk about herself and answer questions. Excitement is high, and her partner or other support person is often as elated as she is.

ACTIVE PHASE

When the woman enters the early *active phase*, her anxiety tends to increase as she senses the intensification of contractions and pain. She begins to fear a loss of control and may use a variety of coping mechanisms. Some women exhibit a decreased ability to cope and a sense of helplessness. Women who have support persons and family available may experience greater satisfaction and less anxiety than those without support. During this phase the cervix dilates from about 4 to 7 cm. Fetal descent is progressive. The cervical dilatation mean time varies with the specific dilatation of the cervix and the woman's parity status. Multiparous women show more rapid dilatation prior to 6 cm compared to nulliparous women. Prior to 4 cm, the nulliparous women averages 1.8 cm per hour; however, cervical progression between 4 and 5 cm is basically the same, regardless of parity (1.3 to 1.4 cm/hr). After a woman reaches 6 cm, the progression

TABLE 19–6 Characteristics of Labor

	LATENT/EARLY PHASE	FIRST STAGE (ACTIVE/TRANSITION)	SECOND STAGE	SECOND STAGE, WITH EPIDURAL
Nullipara	7.3–8.6 hr mean with 95% between 17–21 hours	6–13.3 hrs mean with 95% between 16.6–30 hours	36–57 minutes mean with 95% between 122–197 minutes	79 minutes mean with 95% by 336 minutes
Multipara	4.1–5.3 hr mean with 95% between 12–14 hours	5.7–7.5 hours with 95% between 12.5–13.7 hours	17–19 minutes mean with 95% between 57–81 minutes	45 minutes mean with 95% by 255 minutes
Cervical dilatation	0–3 cm	Active labor 4–7 cm Transition 8–10 cm		
Contractions				
Frequency	Every 10–30 min	Active labor every 2–3 min Transition every 1.5–2 minutes	Every 1.5–2 min	Every 1.5–2 min
Duration	20–40 sec	Active labor 40–60 sec Transition 60–90 sec	60–90 sec	60–90 sec
Intensity	Begin as mild and progress to moderate; 25–40 mmHg by intrauterine pressure catheter (IUPC)	Begin as moderate and progress to strong, 50–70 mmHg by IUPC Strong by palpation; 70–90 mmHg by IUPC	Strong by palpation; 70–100 mmHg by IUPC	Strong by palpation; 70–100 mmHg by IUPC

SOURCE: Data from Gabbe et al., 2015.

of dilatation accelerates and is not vastly different between the nullipara and multipara, although multiparous women do dilate a bit more quickly overall than their nulliparous peers (Gabbe et al., 2015).

TRANSITION PHASE

The *transition phase* is the last part of the first stage. When the woman enters the transition phase, she may demonstrate significant anxiety. She becomes acutely aware of the increasing force and intensity of the contractions. She may become restless, frequently changing position. By the time the woman enters the transition phase, she is often inner directed and tired. She may fear being left alone at the same time that the support person may be feeling the need for a break. The nurse should reassure the woman that she will not be left alone. It is crucial that the nurse be available as a relief support at this time and keep the woman informed about where her labor support people are, if they leave the room.

Cervical dilatation during transition averages 0.5 cm/hr for nulliparous women and 0.3 cm/hr for multiparous women. During this phase, the rate of fetal descent increases. For 95% of women, the transition phase is completed within 4.6 hours for nulliparas; 3.2 hours for women with one previous birth; and 2.9 hours for women who have given birth two or more times previously (Gabbe et al., 2015). The total duration of the first stage may be increased if epidural anesthesia is used.

During the active and transition phases, contractions become more frequent, are longer in duration, and increase in intensity. At the beginning of the active phase, the contractions have a frequency of 2 to 5 minutes, a duration of 40 to 60 seconds, and are moderate to strong in intensity. During transition, contractions have a frequency of 1.5 to 2 minutes, a duration of 60 to 90 seconds, and are strong in intensity (Gabbe et al., 2015).

As dilatation approaches 10 cm, there may be increased rectal pressure and an uncontrollable urge to bear down, an increase in bloody show, and ROM (if this has not already occurred). The woman may also fear that she will be "torn open" or "split apart" by the force of the contractions. The woman may experience a sensation of pressure so great with the peak of a contraction that it seems to her that her abdomen will burst open. The woman should be informed that this is a normal sensation and reassured that such bursting will not happen.

During transition the woman will most likely withdraw into herself. Increasingly she may doubt her ability to cope with labor. The woman may become apprehensive and irritable. Although she may be terrified of being left alone, she may not want anyone to talk to her or touch her. However, with the next contraction she may ask for verbal and physical support. She may need help regaining focus. Other characteristics that may accompany this phase include:

- Hyperventilation, as the woman increases her breathing rate
- Restlessness
- Difficulty understanding directions
- A sense of bewilderment and anger at the contractions
- Generalized discomfort, including low back pain, shaking, and cramping in the legs
- Increased sensitivity to touch
- Increased need for partner's and/or nurse's presence or support
- Increased apprehension and irritability
- Statements that she "can't take it anymore"
- Requests for medication
- Hiccupping, belching or nausea and vomiting
- Beads of perspiration on the upper lip
- Increasing rectal pressure
- Curling of her toes
- Loss of control
- Crying or yelling.

The woman in this phase is anxious to "get it over with." She may be amnesic and sleep between her now-frequent contractions. Her support persons may start to feel helpless and may turn to the nurse for increased participation as their efforts to alleviate her discomfort seem less effective.

Second Stage

The second stage of labor begins when the cervix is completely dilated (10 cm) and ends with the birth of the neonate. Contractions continue with a frequency of 1.5 to 2 minutes, a duration of 60 to 90 seconds, and strong intensity. Descent of the fetal presenting part continues until it reaches the perineal floor (Gabbe et al., 2015). Refer to Table 19–6.

Some women will feel an unbearable urge to immediately begin pushing, whereas others may not. It is important to remember that women without this urge to push should be encouraged to relax and let the baby "labor down." As the fetus continues to descend with the contractions, the sensation to push will increase as the fetus descends and creates the feeling of rectal pressure. For women with epidural anesthesia who have little sensation, it is sometimes necessary to reduce the rate of the epidural medication so some return of feeling can occur and her instinct to push as a result of rectal pressure can be restored. As the fetal head descends, the woman has the urge to push because of pressure of the fetal head on the sacral and obturator nerves. As she pushes, intra-abdominal pressure is exerted from contraction of the maternal abdominal muscles.

Women should be instructed to push naturally with an open glottis. Screaming, grunting, or other sounds may be voiced during the pushing stage. Open glottis pushing typically results in 5 seconds of sustained pushing for three to five times per contraction.

As the fetal head continues its descent, the perineum begins to bulge, flatten, and move anteriorly. The amount of bloody show may increase. The labia begin to part with each contraction. Between contractions, the fetal head appears to recede. With succeeding contractions and maternal pushing effort, the fetal head descends farther. **Crowning** occurs when the fetal head is encircled by the external opening of the vagina (introitus) and means birth is imminent. Some women feel acute, increasingly severe pain and a burning sensation as the perineum distends. The woman may continue to fear that she will tear apart. The nurse needs to instruct the woman to "push through the pain and burning."

Usually, a childbirth-prepared woman feels relieved that the acute pain she felt during the transition phase is over. She also may be relieved that the birth is near and she can now push. Some women feel a sense of control now that they can be actively involved. Others, particularly those without childbirth preparation, may become frightened. They tend to fight each contraction and any attempt of others to persuade them to push with contractions. The woman may feel she has lost control and become embarrassed and apologetic, or she may demonstrate extreme irritability toward the staff or her supporters in an attempt to regain control over external forces against which she feels helpless. Such behavior may be frightening and disconcerting to her support persons. The nurse needs to provide reassurance to the support person(s) that this is a common reaction.

Developing Cultural Competence **Fathers in the Birthing Room**

The presence of the father during labor and at birth, although now common in countries such as the United States, Canada, and Australia, is not a universal norm. Rather, it is strongly influenced by cultural practices. The father is not present at the birth in many countries, including Algeria, Brazil, China, Ethiopia, and Korea. Similarly, Orthodox Judaism does not allow men to attend the labor and birth (McFarland & Wehbe-Alamah, 2014).

In many Middle Eastern countries, it is uncommon for men to be present in the birthing room. The rationale for excluding the father is vague and has been cited as concerns for future sexual relations from seeing the birth itself, increasing stress on the laboring woman, or fear of the father fainting. Other rationales are based on staff preferences because the presence of a man at a birth would result in female care providers having to wear hijab in the work setting, and that and the presence of husbands would interfere with their work preferences (Benoit, 2017).

Note: It is unwise to attribute specific attitudes or beliefs to all members of a cultural group. The information in the Developing Cultural Competence boxes offers possible insights into caring for women from different cultural groups.

SPONTANEOUS BIRTH (VERTEX PRESENTATION)

As the head distends the vulva with each contraction, the perineum becomes extremely thin, and the anus stretches and protrudes. As extension occurs under the symphysis pubis, the head is born. When the anterior shoulder meets the underside of the symphysis pubis, a gentle push by the mother aids in birth of the shoulders. The body then follows. Figure 19–12 shows a birth sequence.

POSITIONAL CHANGES OF THE FETUS

For the fetus to pass through the birth canal, the fetal head and body must adjust to the maternal pelvis by certain positional changes. These changes, called **cardinal movements** or *mechanisms of labor*, are described in the order in which they occur (Figure 19–13).

Descent. Descent is thought to occur because of four forces: (1) pressure of the amniotic fluid, (2) direct pressure of the fundus of the uterus on the breech of the fetus, (3) contraction of the abdominal muscles, and (4) extension and straightening of the fetal body. The head enters the inlet in the occiput transverse or oblique position because the pelvic inlet is widest from side to side. The sagittal suture is an equal distance from the maternal symphysis pubis and sacral promontory.

Flexion. Flexion occurs as the fetal head descends and meets resistance from the soft tissues of the pelvis, the musculature of the pelvic floor, and the cervix. As a result of the resistance, the fetal chin flexes downward onto the chest.

Internal Rotation. The fetal head must rotate to fit the diameter of the pelvic cavity, which is widest in the anteroposterior diameter. As the occiput of the fetal head meets resistance from the levator ani muscles and their fascia, the occiput rotates from left to right, and the sagittal suture aligns in the anteroposterior pelvic diameter.

Extension. The resistance of the pelvic floor and the mechanical movement of the vulva opening anteriorly and forward assist with extension of the fetal head as it passes under the symphysis pubis. With this positional change the occiput, then brow and face, emerge from the vagina.

Restitution. The shoulders of the fetus enter the pelvis obliquely and remain oblique when the head rotates to the anteroposterior diameter through internal rotation. Because of this rotation the neck becomes twisted. Once the head emerges and is free of pelvic resistance, the neck untwists, turning the head to one side (restitution), and aligns with the position of the back in the birth canal.

External Rotation. As the shoulders rotate to the anteroposterior position in the pelvis, the head is turned farther to one side (external rotation).

Expulsion. After the external rotation and through expulsive efforts of the laboring woman, the anterior shoulder meets the undersurface of the symphysis pubis and slips under it. As lateral flexion of the shoulder and head occurs, the anterior shoulder is born before the posterior shoulder. The body follows quickly.

Third Stage

The third stage of labor is defined as the period of time from the birth of the baby until the completed delivery of the placenta.

PLACENTAL SEPARATION

After the baby is born, the uterus contracts firmly, diminishing its capacity and the surface area of placental attachment. The placenta begins to separate because of this decrease in surface area. This separation is accompanied by bleeding, leading to the formation of a hematoma between the placental tissue and the remaining decidua. This hematoma accelerates the separation process. The membranes are the last to separate. They are peeled off the uterine wall as the placenta descends into the vagina.

Signs of placental separation usually appear around 5 minutes after the birth of the baby, but can take up to 30 minutes to manifest. These signs are (1) a globular-shaped uterus, (2) a rise of the fundus in the abdomen, (3) a sudden gush or trickle of blood, and (4) further protrusion of the umbilical cord out of the vagina.

PLACENTAL DELIVERY

When the signs of placental separation appear, the woman may bear down to aid in placental expulsion. If this fails and the physician/CNM has ascertained that the fundus is firm, gentle traction may be applied to the cord while pressure is exerted on the fundus. The weight of the placenta as it is guided into the placental pan (a basin that holds the placenta once it is expelled) aids in the removal of the membranes from the uterine wall. A placenta is considered to be *retained* if more than 30 minutes have elapsed from completion of the second stage of labor.

If the placenta separates from the inside to the outer margins, it is expelled with the fetal (shiny) side presenting

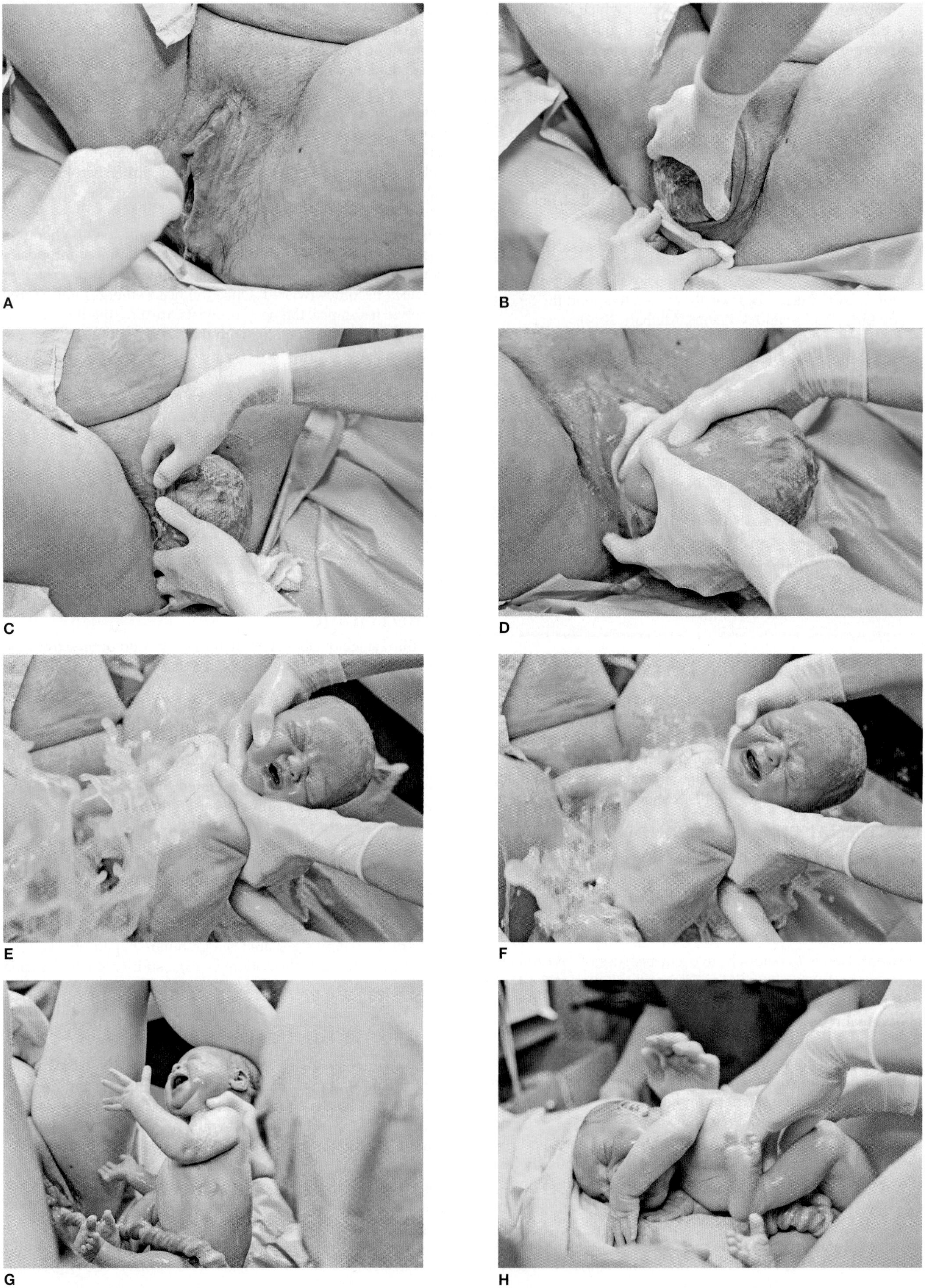

A B C D E F G H

Figure 19–12 **The birth sequence.** SOURCE: Michele Davidson.

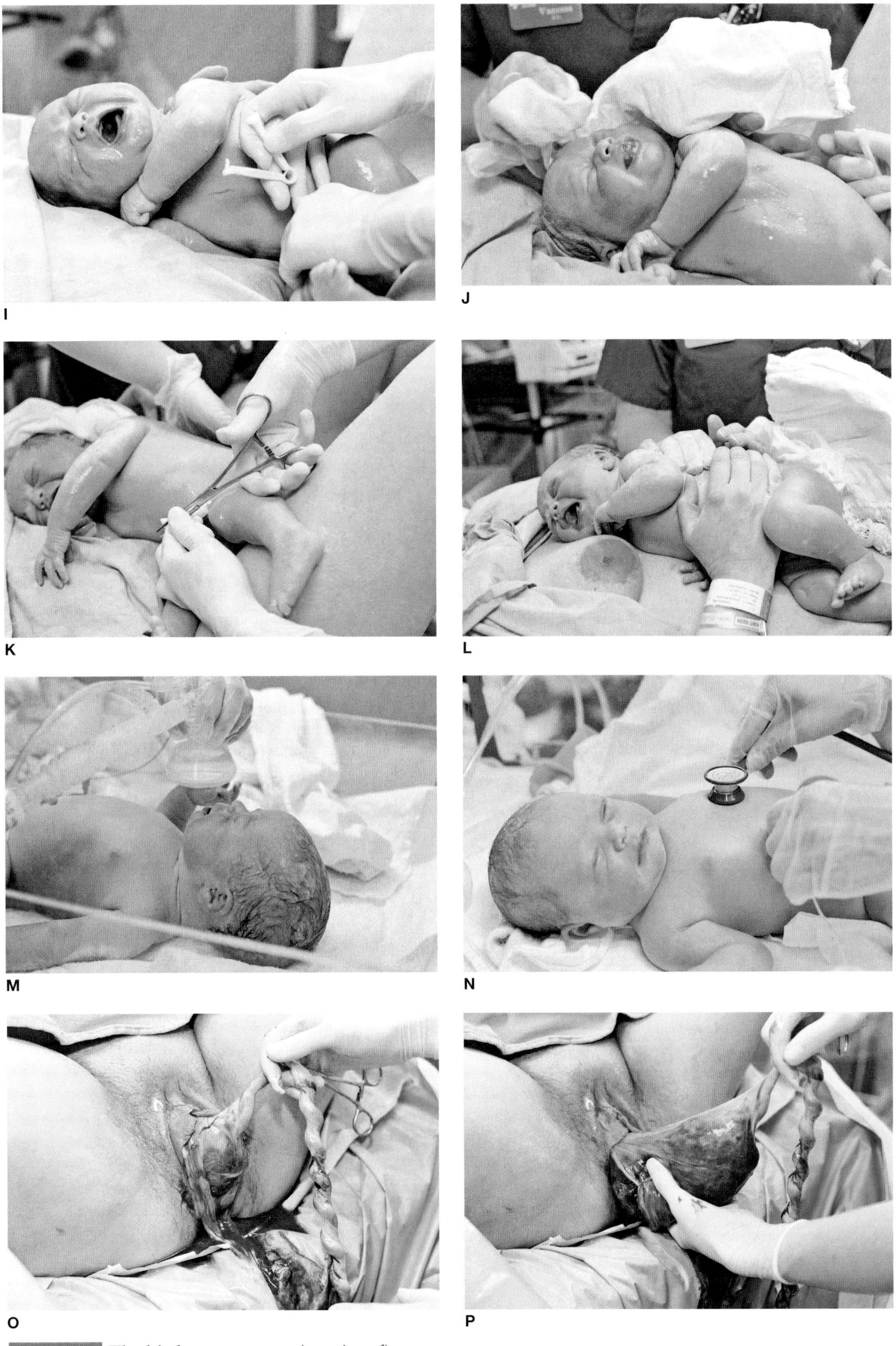

Figure 19–12 **The birth sequence.** *(continued)* **SOURCE:** Michele Davidson.

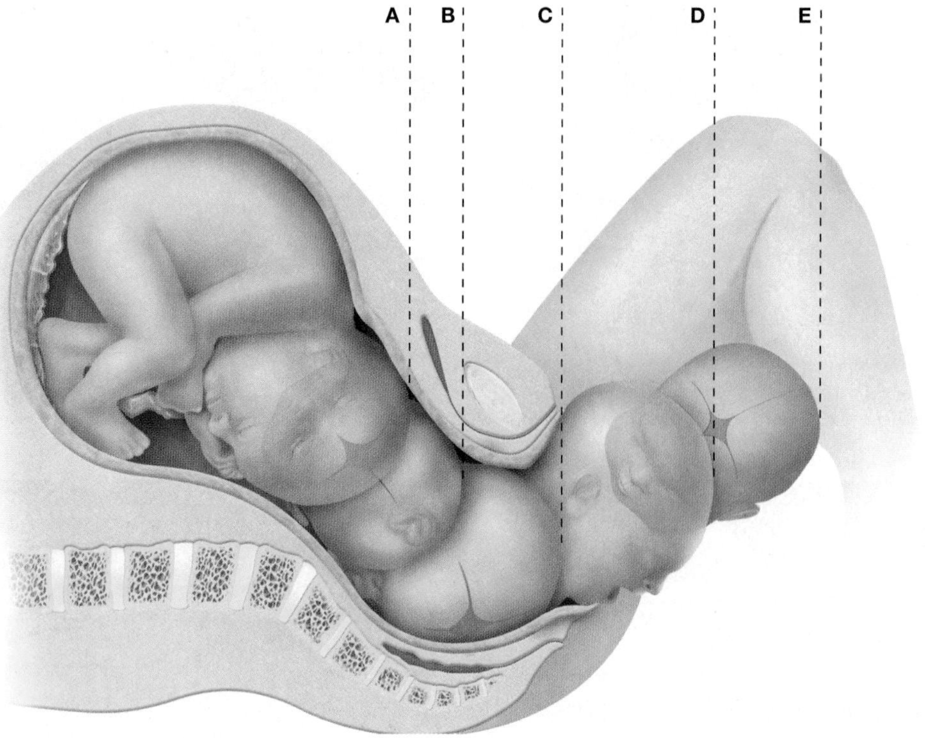

Figure 19–13 **Cardinal movements (mechanisms of labor). A. and B. Descent. C. Internal rotation. D. Extension. E. External rotation.**

(Figure 19–14A). This is known as the *Schultze mechanism* of placental delivery or, more commonly, *Shiny Schultze.* If the placenta separates from the outer margins inward, it will roll up and present sideways with the maternal surface delivering first. This is known as the *Duncan mechanism* of placental delivery and is commonly called *Dirty Duncan* because the placental surface is rough (Figure 19–14B). Also see Figure 9–23 and Figure 9–24.Nursing and medical interventions during the third stage of labor are discussed in Chapter 21.

Fourth Stage

The fourth stage of labor is the time from 1 to 4 hours after birth in which physiologic readjustment of the mother's body begins. With the birth, hemodynamic changes occur. Blood loss at birth

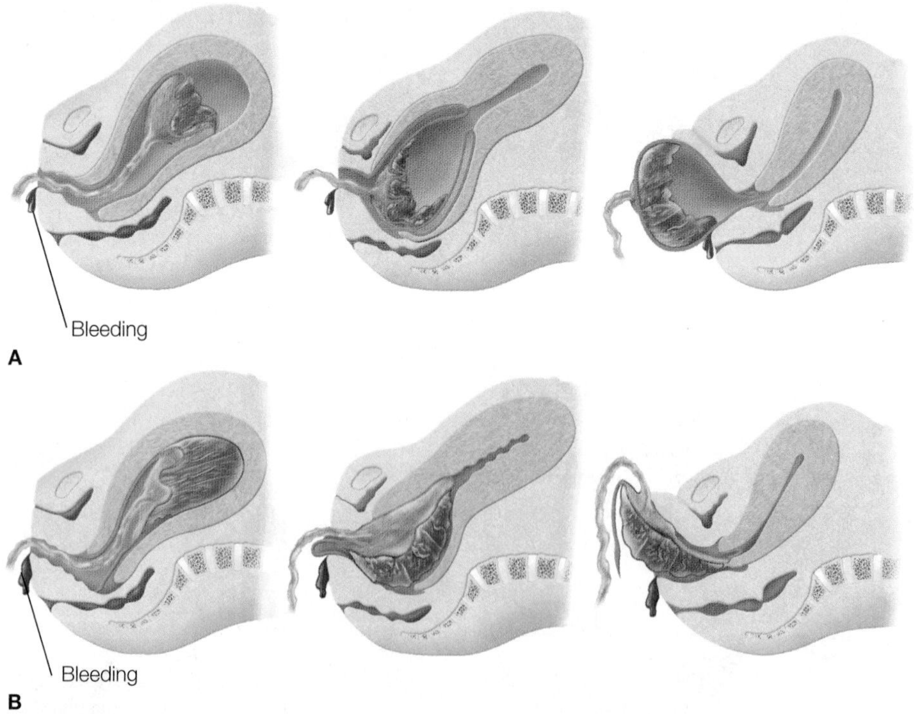

Figure 19–14 **Placental separation and expulsion. A. Schultze mechanism. B. Duncan mechanism.**

ranges from 250 to 500 mL. With this blood loss and the easing of pressure exerted by the pregnant uterus on the surrounding vessels, blood is redistributed into venous beds. This results in a moderate drop in both systolic and diastolic blood pressure, increased pulse pressure, and moderate tachycardia (Cunningham et al., 2016).

The uterus remains contracted and is in the midline of the abdomen. The fundus is usually midway between the symphysis pubis and umbilicus. Its contracted state constricts the vessels at the site of placental implantation. Immediately after birth of the placenta, the cervix is widely spread and thick.

Nausea and vomiting experienced during transition usually cease. The woman may be thirsty and hungry. She may experience a shaking chill, which is thought to be associated with the ending of the physical exertion of labor. The bladder is often hypotonic due to trauma during the second stage and/or the administration of anesthetics that may decrease sensations. Hypotonic bladder leads to urinary retention. Nursing care during this stage is discussed in Chapter 21.

> “I have had the privilege of practicing nursing in the birthing area for many years. In my head I know all the factors that must work together to bring this new life into the world. But it is in my heart and in working with and watching the laboring woman (and her partner if she has one) that I truly believe each labor and birth is a miracle. I, along with these parents, get to participate in a moment of time that will never occur again for any of us. I will never tire of this and will never get enough.”

Maternal Systemic Response to Labor

The labor process affects nearly every major body system. Each system adapts to these changes through various compensation mechanisms.

Cardiovascular System

The woman's cardiovascular system is stressed both by the uterine contractions and by the pain, anxiety, and apprehension the woman experiences. In pregnancy, the resting pulse rate increases by 10 to 18 beats per minute (Gabbe et al., 2016). During labor there is a significant increase in cardiac output. Each strong contraction greatly decreases or completely stops the blood flow in the branches of the uterine artery that supply the intervillous space (in the placenta). This leads to a redistribution of about 300 to 500 mL of blood into the peripheral circulation and an increase in peripheral resistance, resulting in increased systolic and diastolic blood pressure, an increasing pulse rate and an increase of about 30% in cardiac output (Gabbe et al., 2016).

Maternal position also affects cardiac output, blood pressure, and pulse. When the laboring woman turns to a side-lying position, cardiac output increases by about 22%, the pulse rate decreases by about 6 beats per minute, and stroke volume increases by 27%. When the woman is supine, cardiac output increases 25%, stroke volume increases 33%, pulse pressure increases more than 26%, blood pressure rises significantly, and transient tachycardia occurs (Gabbe et al., 2016).

There is an additional effect on hemodynamics during the bearing-down efforts in the second stage. When the laboring woman holds her breath and pushes against a closed glottis (Valsalva maneuver), intrathoracic pressure rises. As intrathoracic pressure increases, the venous return is interrupted, increasing venous pressure. In addition, the blood in the lungs is forced into the left atrium, which leads to a transient increase in cardiac output, blood pressure, and pulse pressure and causes bradycardia. As venous return to the lungs continues to be diminished while the breath is held, a decrease in blood pressure, pulse pressure, and cardiac output occurs.

When the next breath is taken (Valsalva maneuver is interrupted), the intrathoracic pressure is decreased. Venous return increases, refilling the pulmonary bed and resulting in recovery of the cardiac output and stroke volume. This process is repeated with each pushing effort.

Immediately after birth, cardiac output peaks with an 80% increase over prelabor values. Then in the first 10 minutes it decreases 20 to 25%. Cardiac output further decreases in the first hour after the birth. However, these decreases still leave the woman with an elevated cardiac output for at least 24 hours after the birth (Gabbe et al., 2016).

Blood Pressure

As a result of increased cardiac output, systolic blood pressure rises during uterine contractions. In the first stage, systolic pressure may increase by 35 mmHg, and there may be further increases in the second stage during pushing efforts. Diastolic pressure also increases by about 25 mmHg in the first stage and 65 mmHg in the second stage. These increases begin just before the uterine contraction, with a return to baseline as soon as the contraction ends. Blood pressure may also rise as a result of fear, apprehension, and pain (Gabbe et al., 2016).

Blood pressure may drop precipitously when the woman lies in a supine position and experiences aortocaval compression. In addition to hypotension, there is an increase in the pulse rate, diaphoresis, nausea, weakness, and air hunger. These changes are attributed to the decreased cardiac output and a subsequent drop in stroke volume.

Women with hydramnios, women with multiple gestation, and obese women have the highest risk of developing aortocaval compression. Other predisposing factors include hypovolemia, dehydration, hemorrhage, metabolic acidosis, administration of narcotics (which results in vasodilation and inhibits compensatory mechanisms), and administration of epidural anesthesia, which results in *sympathetic blockade* (blocking of the sympathetic nervous system, leading to vasodilation and hypotension).

Fluid and Electrolyte Balance

Profuse perspiration (diaphoresis) occurs during labor. Hyperventilation also occurs, altering electrolyte and fluid balance from insensible water loss. The muscle activity elevates the body temperature, which increases sweating and evaporation from the skin. As the woman responds to the work of labor, the rise in the respiratory rate increases the evaporative water volume because each breath of air must be warmed to the body temperature and humidified. With the increased evaporative water volume, maintaining adequate oral fluids/hydration is important. Parenteral intravenous fluids may be used to maintain fluid and electrolyte balance.

Respiratory System

Oxygen demand and consumption increase at the onset of labor because of the presence of uterine contractions. Approximately 50% of the increased oxygen is used by the placenta, the uterus, and the fetus (Gabbe et al., 2016). As anxiety and pain from uterine contractions increase, hyperventilation frequently occurs. With hyperventilation there is a fall in $PaCO_2$, and respiratory alkalosis results (Cunningham et al., 2016).

As labor progresses and contractions become more frequent, stronger, and prolonged, the workload, tension, and anxiety of the woman continue to change. A mild increase in the respiratory rate is normal in labor and is related to the increase in metabolism (Gabbe et al., 2016).

By the end of the first stage most women have developed a mild metabolic acidosis compensated by respiratory alkalosis. As she pushes in the second stage of labor, the woman's $PaCO_2$ levels may rise along with blood lactate levels (due to muscular activity), and mild respiratory acidosis occurs. By the time the baby is born (end of second stage), there is metabolic acidosis uncompensated by respiratory alkalosis (Cunningham et al., 2016).

The changes in acid–base status that occur in labor are quickly reversed in the fourth stage because of changes in the woman's respiratory rate. Acid–base levels return to pregnancy levels by 24 hours after birth, and nonpregnant values are attained a few weeks after birth.

Renal System

During labor there is an increase in maternal renin, plasma renin activity, and angiotensinogen. This elevation is thought to be important in the control of uteroplacental blood flow during birth and the early postpartum period (Cunningham et al., 2016).

Polyuria is common during labor. This results from the increase in cardiac output, which causes an increase in the glomerular filtration rate and renal plasma flow. Slight proteinuria occurs in one-third to one-half of women in labor (Gabbe et al., 2016).

Structurally, the base of the bladder is pushed forward and upward when engagement occurs. The pressure from the presenting part may impair blood and lymph drainage from the base of the bladder, leading to edema of the tissues (Cunningham et al., 2016). Hematuria may be present as a result of trauma to the lower urinary tract.

Gastrointestinal System

During labor, gastric motility and absorption of solid food are reduced. Gastric emptying time is prolonged, and gastric volume (amount of contents that remain in the stomach) remains over 25 mL, regardless of the time the last meal was taken. This is even more marked in women who have received analgesia agents (Cunningham et al., 2016). These women may be at risk for aspiration should general anesthesia be necessary. During labor, anaerobic and aerobic carbohydrate metabolism rises due to an increase in skeletal muscle activity and maternal anxiety (Gabbe et al., 2016).

The fluid requirements of women in labor have not been clearly established. In some instances oral hydration is the primary goal. In other situations a saline lock may be inserted so that intravenous access is available, if needed. If intravenous fluids are used, it is important to remember that when hypertonic glucose infusions are used, there is an increase in maternal blood glucose; this can lead to fetal hyperglycemia and hyperinsulinemia and to hypoglycemia in the newborn.

Immune System and Other Blood Values

The white blood cell (WBC) count increases to $25{,}000/mm^3$ to $30{,}000/mm^3$ during labor and early postpartum (Groll, 2017). The change in WBC count is due mostly to increased neutrophils resulting from a physiologic response to stress. The increased WBC count makes it difficult to identify the presence of an infectious process.

Maternal blood glucose levels decrease because glucose is used as an energy source during uterine contractions. The decreased blood glucose levels lead to a decrease in insulin requirements (Groll, 2017). Glucose levels can drop significantly during a prolonged or difficult labor.

Pain

Pain during labor comes from a complexity of physical causes. Each woman will experience and cope with pain differently. Multiple factors affect a woman's reaction to labor pain.

PAIN DURING LABOR

The pain associated with the first stage of labor is unique in that it accompanies a normal physiologic process. Even though perception of the pain is determined to some extent by cultural patterning, there is unquestionably a physiologic basis for pain during labor. Pain during the first stage of labor arises from (1) dilatation of the cervix, (2) hypoxia of the uterine muscle cells during contraction, (3) stretching of the lower uterine segment, and (4) pressure on adjacent structures. The primary source of pain is dilatation or stretching of the cervix. Nerve impulses travel through the uterine plexus, to the pelvis through hypogastric plexuses, and then into the lumbar sympathetic chain (Figure 19–15). They enter the spinal cord through the posterior roots of the 10th through 12th thoracic and 1st lumbar nerves.

As with other visceral pain, pain from the uterus is also directly referred to the dermatomes supplied by the 10th through 12th thoracic nerves. The areas of referred pain include the lower

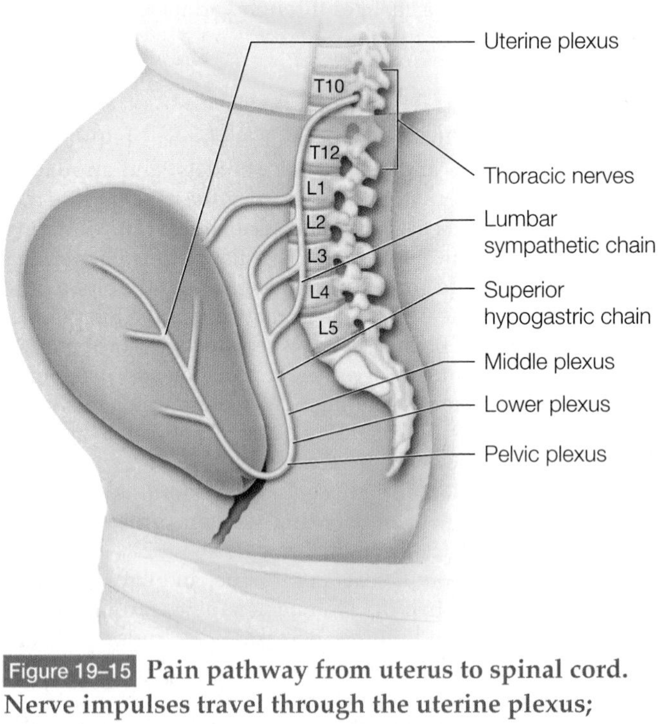

Figure 19–15 Pain pathway from uterus to spinal cord. Nerve impulses travel through the uterine plexus; pelvic plexus; lower, middle, and superior hypogastric plexuses; and lumbar sympathetic chain. They enter the neuroaxis through the 10th, 11th, and 12th thoracic and 1st lumbar spinal segments.

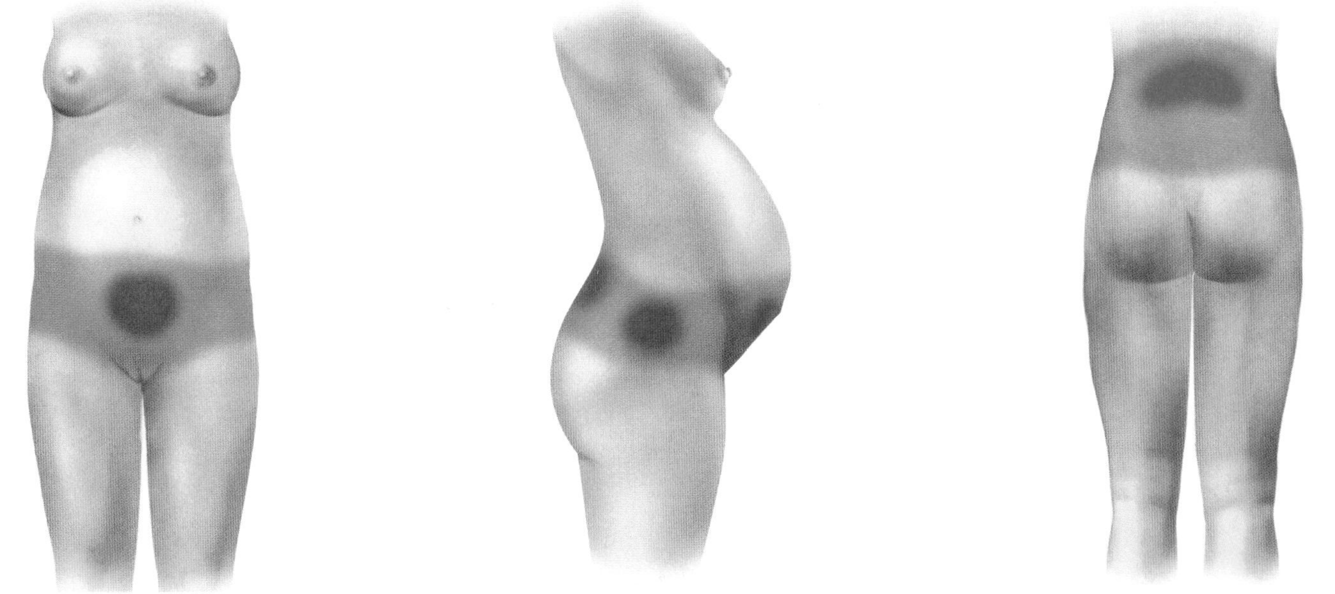

Figure 19–16 Area of reference of labor pain during the first stage. Pain is most intense in the darker colored areas.

abdominal wall and the areas over the lower lumbar region and the upper sacrum (Figure 19–16).

During the second stage of labor, pain is due to (1) hypoxia of the contracting uterine muscle cells, (2) distention of the vagina and perineum, and (3) pressure on adjacent structures including the lower back, buttocks, and thighs. The nerve impulses from the vagina and perineum are transmitted by way of the pudendal nerve plexus and enter the spinal cord through the posterior roots of the 2nd through 4th sacral nerves. The area of pain increases as shown in Figure 19–17.

Pain during the third stage results from uterine contractions and cervical dilatation as the placenta is expelled. Sensations of pain are felt above the symphysis pubis bone in the perineal area and in the lower back (Figure 19–18). The mechanism for the transmission of nerve impulses is the same as for the first stage of labor. The third stage of labor is short, and after this phase anesthesia is needed primarily for episiotomy repair.

FACTORS AFFECTING RESPONSE TO PAIN

Many factors affect the individual's perception of pain impulses. Some psychologic and environmental influences particularly appropriate to labor are discussed here.

Preparation for childbirth (previously discussed) has been shown to reduce the need for analgesia during labor. Preparing

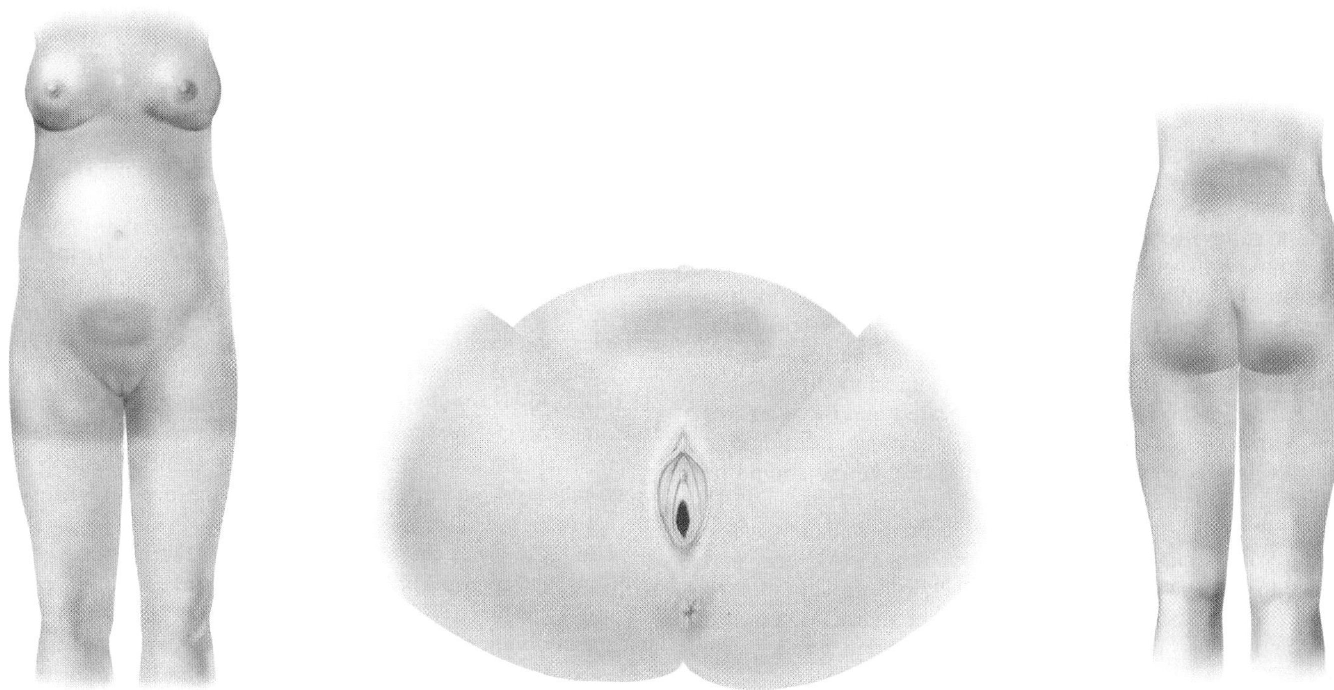

Figure 19–17 Distribution of labor pain during the later phase of the first stage and early phase of the second stage. The darkest colored areas indicate the location of the most intense pain; moderate color, moderate pain; and light color, mild pain. The uterine contractions, which at this stage are very strong, produce intense pain.

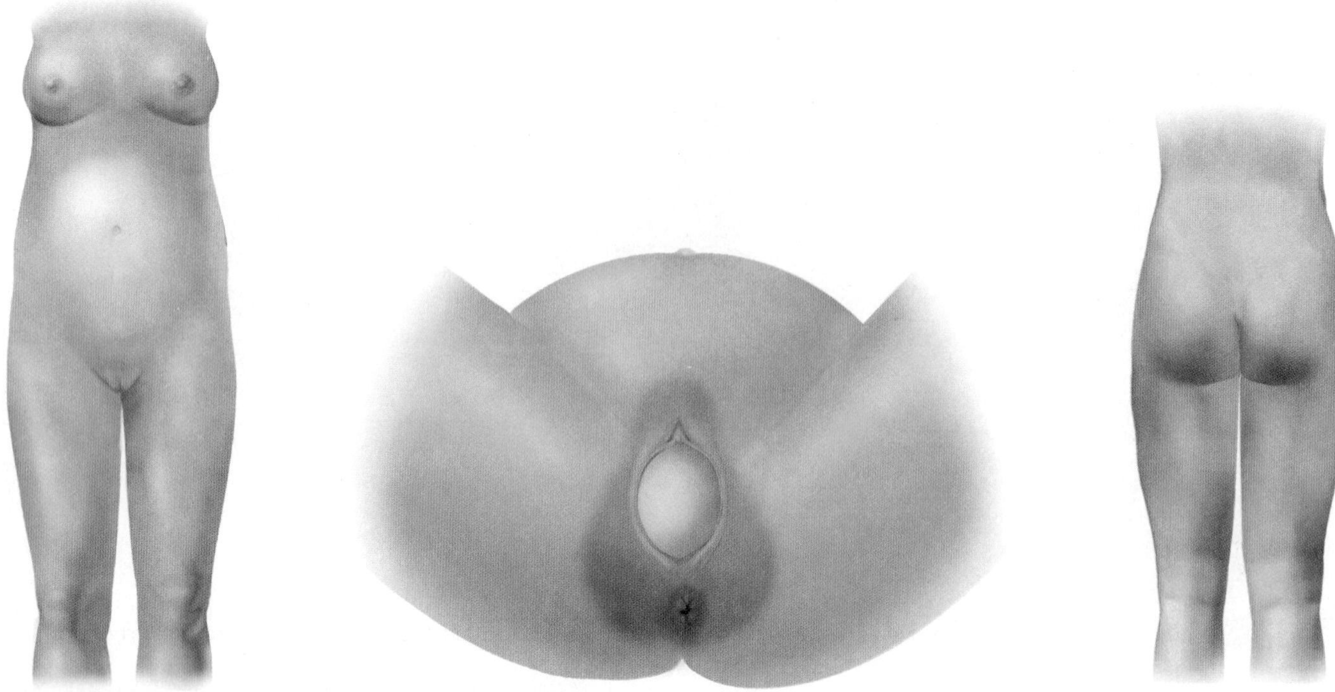

Figure 19–18 **Distribution of labor pain during the later phase of the second stage and actual birth. The perineal component is the primary cause of discomfort. Uterine contractions contribute much less.**

for labor and birth through reading, talking with others, or attending a childbirth preparation class frequently have positive effects for the laboring woman and her partner. The woman who knows what to expect and what techniques she may use to increase comfort tends to be less anxious during the labor. A tour of the birthing center and an opportunity to see and feel the environment also help reduce anxiety because during admission (especially with the first child) many new things are happening and they seem to occur all at once. The more the woman and her partner learn during classes and through their own efforts, the more likely their anxiety will lessen.

Individuals tend to respond to painful stimuli in the way that is acceptable in their culture. In some cultures, it is natural to communicate pain, no matter how mild, whereas members of other cultures stoically accept pain out of fear or because it is expected. Nurses need to be aware of cultural norms and demonstrate culturally sensitive care to women and their families in the intrapartum setting (Spector, 2017).

Families will react to the healthcare system based on their own cultural beliefs. Nurses need to identify specific cultural norms with each individual family so appropriate care can be provided. Whenever possible, requests that include the family's cultural preferences should be incorporated into the woman's care. Nurses should avoid making generalizations about specific cultures. Instead, individual preferences and beliefs should be explored.

Another factor that may influence response to pain is *fatigue* and *sleep deprivation*. The fatigued woman has less energy and ability to use such strategies as distraction or imagination to deal with pain. As a result, she may lose her ability to cope with labor and choose analgesics or other medications to relieve the discomfort.

The woman's *previous experience with pain* also affects her ability to manage current and future pain. Those who have had experience with pain seem more sensitive to painful stimuli than those who have not.

Anxiety can affect a woman's response to pain. Unfamiliar surroundings and events can increase anxiety, as does separation from family and loved ones. The woman's anticipation of discomfort and concerns about whether she can cope with the contractions may also increase her anxiety level. It is not uncommon for laboring women to worry about their partners or other family members. Reassurance from family members that things are being "taken care of at home" can help.

Both attention and distraction have an influence on the perception of pain. When pain sensation is the focus of attention, the perceived intensity is greater. A sensory stimulus such as a backrub can be a distraction that focuses the woman's attention on the stimulus rather than the pain. The nurse can offer suggestions to support persons on interventions to initiate physical distractions for the laboring woman.

As part of the culture of healthcare, nursing and medical professionals have their own (collective and individual) expectations of the woman in labor and those who support her. In one setting, the woman may be expected to use a breathing technique and relaxation methods, whereas in another, most women receive an epidural block. Some nurses may believe that the woman and her support persons should take care of themselves and ask for assistance only if really necessary; other nurses may believe that frequent interaction and support are essential as long as the woman and her support persons are comfortable with the interaction.

The healthcare professional is most likely to interpret pain according to the norms of the healthcare culture, although various other cultures have different ways of responding to pain. The absence of crying and moaning does not necessarily mean that pain is absent, nor does the presence of crying and moaning necessarily mean that pain relief is desired at that moment. It is very important for the nurse to accept and respect the fact that the pain is whatever the woman says it is and to assist her in coping with it. Chapter 22 focuses on pharmacologic pain management.

Fetal Response to Labor

When the fetus is normal, the mechanical and hemodynamic changes of normal labor have no adverse effects.

Heart Rate Changes

Fetal heart rate decelerations can occur with intracranial pressures of 40 to 55 mmHg. The currently accepted explanation of this early deceleration is hypoxic depression of the central nervous system, which is under vagal control. The absence of these head compression decelerations (early decelerations) in some fetuses during labor is explained by the existence of a threshold that is reached more gradually in the presence of intact membranes and lack of maternal resistance. Early decelerations are harmless in the normal fetus.

Acid–Base Status in Labor

The blood flow to the fetus is slowed during the acme of the contraction, which leads to a slow decrease in the fetal pH. During the second stage, as uterine contractions become stronger and last longer and the woman pushes with each contraction, there is a more rapid decrease in fetal pH. There is also an increase in fetal base deficit and in $PaCO_2$ and a drop in fetal oxygen saturation. Persistent acid–base imbalance can lead to multiorgan dysfunction in the newborn, including neurologic impairment.

Hemodynamic Changes

The adequate exchange of nutrients and gases in the fetal capillaries and intervillous spaces depends in part on the fetal blood pressure. Fetal blood pressure is a protective mechanism for the normal fetus during the anoxic periods caused by the contracting uterus during labor. The fetal and placental reserve is enough to see the fetus through these anoxic periods unharmed.

Behavioral States

The human fetus develops behavioral states between 36 and 38 weeks of gestation. The behavioral states seem to continue during labor even in the presence of uterine contractions. Two sleep states (quiet and active) are most prevalent, although quiet and active awake states are occasionally observed. A decrease in fetal heart rate variability accompanies the quiet sleep state, and there is also a decrease in fetal breathing movements and other general body activity. The quiet sleep state generally lasts less than 40 minutes.

Fetal Sensation

Beginning at about 37 or 38 weeks' gestation (full term), the fetus is able to experience sensations of light, sound, and touch. Fetal hearing begins to develop at 23 to 24 weeks but is not considered reliable until 28 weeks (Polin & Abman, 2016). Even in utero, the fetus is sensitive to light and will move away from a bright light source. Additionally, the term baby is aware of pressure sensations during labor such as the touch of the caregiver during a vaginal exam or pressure on the head as a contraction occurs. Although the fetus may not be able to process this input, as the woman labors the fetus is experiencing the labor as well.

Focus Your Study

- Most childbirth classes include information on body-conditioning exercises, relaxation techniques, and breathing methods.
- Five factors that continually interact during labor and birth are the birth passage, the birth passenger (fetus), the relationship between the birth passage and the fetus, the physiologic forces of labor, and factors associated with the woman's psychosocial status.
- Four types of pelvises have been identified, and each has a different effect on labor. The diameters of gynecoid and anthropoid pelvises are usually large enough for labor and birth to progress normally. In the android and platypelloid types, the pelvic diameters are diminished (smaller than in gynecoid and anthropoid). Labor is more likely to be difficult (longer) and a cesarean birth is more likely.
- Important dimensions of the maternal pelvis include the diameters of the pelvic inlet, pelvic cavity, and pelvic outlet.
- The fetal head contains bones in the top portion (cranial vault) that are not fused. This allows them to overlap somewhat in response to the pressures on the fetal head during labor. The pressure and overlapping of the sutures, which are membranous spaces between the cranial bones, result in a change in the shape of the head called molding.
- Fetal attitude refers to the relation of the fetal parts to one another. The head is usually held in midline and not to one side or the other, and the extremities are usually flexed and held close to the body because there is little extra room within the uterine cavity.
- Fetal lie refers to the relationship of the cephalocaudal (head to sacral area) axis of the fetus to the maternal spine. The fetal lie is either longitudinal (both the maternal and fetal spines are vertical) or transverse (the fetal spine is at a right angle to the maternal spine).
- Fetal presentation is determined by the body part lying closest to the inlet of the maternal pelvis. In a longitudinal lie the fetal presentation is usually cephalic (head first) but may also be breech (buttocks or one or both feet first). In a transverse lie the fetal shoulder is usually closest to the pelvic inlet.
- Engagement of the presenting part occurs when the largest diameter of the fetal presenting part reaches or passes through the pelvic inlet.
- Station refers to the relationship of the presenting part to an imaginary line drawn between the maternal ischial spines, which are in the midpoint of the pelvic cavity. The fetal presenting part enters the pelvic inlet at what is termed about a –5 and descends

toward the ischial spines, where it is called a 0 (zero) station. Further descent from 0 to +4 occurs as the presenting part descends below the ischial spines toward the vaginal opening.

- Fetal position is the relationship of a specified landmark on the presenting fetal part to the sides, front, or back of the maternal pelvis. Once the position is known, the positions of the fetal head and back can be determined.
- Each uterine contraction has an increment, acme, and decrement.
- Contraction frequency is the time from the beginning of one contraction to the beginning of the next contraction.
- Duration of contractions refers to the period of time from the beginning to the end of one contraction.
- Intensity of contractions refers to the strength of the contraction during acme. Intensity of contractions is termed mild, moderate, or strong.
- Labor stresses the coping skills of women. Women with prenatal education about childbirth usually report more positive responses to labor.
- Women with support persons tend to use their coping skills more effectively than those who lack support.
- Premonitory signs of labor include lightening, Braxton Hicks contractions, cervical softening and effacement, bloody show, sudden burst of energy, weight loss, and, sometimes, rupture of membranes.
- True labor contractions occur regularly with an increase in frequency, duration, and intensity. The contractions usually start in the back and radiate around the abdomen. The discomfort is not relieved by ambulation, rest, or warm tub baths. False labor contractions do not produce progressive cervical effacement and dilatation. They are irregular and do not increase in intensity. The discomfort may be relieved by ambulation, rest, or warm tub baths.
- Possible causes of labor onset include the progesterone withdrawal hypothesis, the prostaglandin hypothesis, and the corticotropin-releasing hormone hypothesis.
- There are four stages of labor and birth. The first stage is from beginning of true labor to complete dilatation of the cervix. The second stage is from complete dilatation of the cervix to birth. The third stage is from birth to expulsion of the placenta. The fourth stage is from expulsion of the placenta to a period of 1 to 4 hours after.
- The fetus accommodates to the maternal pelvis in a series of movements called the cardinal movements of labor, which include descent, flexion, internal rotation, extension, restitution, external rotation, and expulsion.
- Placental separation is indicated by lengthening of the umbilical cord, a small spurt of blood, change in uterine shape, and a rise of the fundus in the abdomen.
- The placenta is expelled by the Schultze or Duncan mechanism. This is determined by the way it separates from the uterine wall.
- Maternal systemic responses to labor involve the cardiovascular, respiratory, renal, gastrointestinal, and immune systems. Cardiac output and blood pressure increase, as do oxygen demand and consumption. Polyuria is common, and gastric motility and absorption are reduced. The white blood cell count increases, and blood glucose levels decrease.
- Factors that affect the response to labor pain include education, cultural beliefs, fatigue and sleep deprivation, personal significance of pain, previous experience, anxiety, and the availability of coping techniques.
- The fetus is usually able to tolerate the labor process with no untoward changes.

References

Arulkumaran, S. (Ed.). (2016). *Best practice in labor and delivery* (2nd ed.). Cambridge, UK: Cambridge University Press.

Benoit, B. (2017). *About Islam: Should husbands attend their wives labors?* Retrieved from http://aboutislam.net/family-society/husbands-wives/should-husbands-attend-their-wives-labor/

Caldwell, W. E., & Moloy, H. C. (1933). Anatomical variations in the female pelvis and their effect on labor with a suggested classification [Historical article]. *American Journal of Obstetrics and Gynecology, 26*, 479–505.

Cunningham, F. G., Leveno, K. J., Bloom, S. L., Spong, C., Dashe, J. S., Hoffman, B. L., Casey, B. M., & Sheffield, J. S. (2016). *Williams obstetrics* (25th ed.). New York, NY: McGraw-Hill.

Gabbe, S. G., Niebyl, J. R., Galan, H. L., Jauniaux, E. R. M., Landon, M. B., Simpson, J. L., & Driscoll, D. A. (2015). *Obstetric essentials: Normal and problem pregnancies.* St. Louis, MO: Saunders.

Gabbe, S. G., Niebyl, J. R., Galan, H. L., Jauniaux, E. R. M., Landon, M. B., Simpson, J. L., & Driscoll, D. A. (2016). *Obstetrics: Normal and problem pregnancies, expert consult* (6th ed.). Philadelphia, PA: Elsevier.

Groll, C. G. (2015). *Fast facts for the L&D nurse.* New York, NY: Springer.

Hodnett, E. D., Gates, S., Hofmeyr, G. J., Sakala, C., & Weston, J. (2011). Continuous support for women during childbirth. *Cochrane Database of Systematic Reviews,* Issue 2. Article No. CD003766. DOI: 10.1002/14651858.CD003766.pub3

International Childbirth Education Association (ICEA). (2017). *ICEA philosophy statement.* Retrieved from http://icea.org/about

MacKinnon, A. L., Yang, L., Feeley, N., Gold, I., Hayton, B., & Zelkowitz, P. (2017). Birth setting, labour experience, and postpartum psychological distress. *Midwifery, 50*, 110–116. DOI: http://dx.doi.org/10.1016/j.midw.2017.03.023

McFarland, M. R., & Wehbe-Alamah, H. B. (2014). *Leininger's culture care diversity and universality: A worldwide nursing theory* (3rd ed.). New York, NY: Jones & Bartlett.

Perez, P., & Hutchins, C. (2014). *The nurturing touch at birth: A labor support handbook* (3rd ed.). Johnson, VT: Cutting Edge Press.

Polin, R. A., & Abman, S. H. (2016). *Fetal and neonatal physiology* (5th ed.). Philadelphia, PA: Elsevier.

Simpkin, P., & Ancheta, R. (2011). *The labor progress handbook* (3rd ed.). New York, NY: Wiley-Blackwell

Spector, R. E. (2017). *Cultural diversity in health and illness* (8th ed.). Hoboken, NJ: Pearson.

Tharpe, N. L., Farley, C. L., & Jordan, R. G. (2016). *Clinical practice guidelines for midwifery and women's health* (5th ed.). Burlington, MA: Jones & Bartlett Learning.

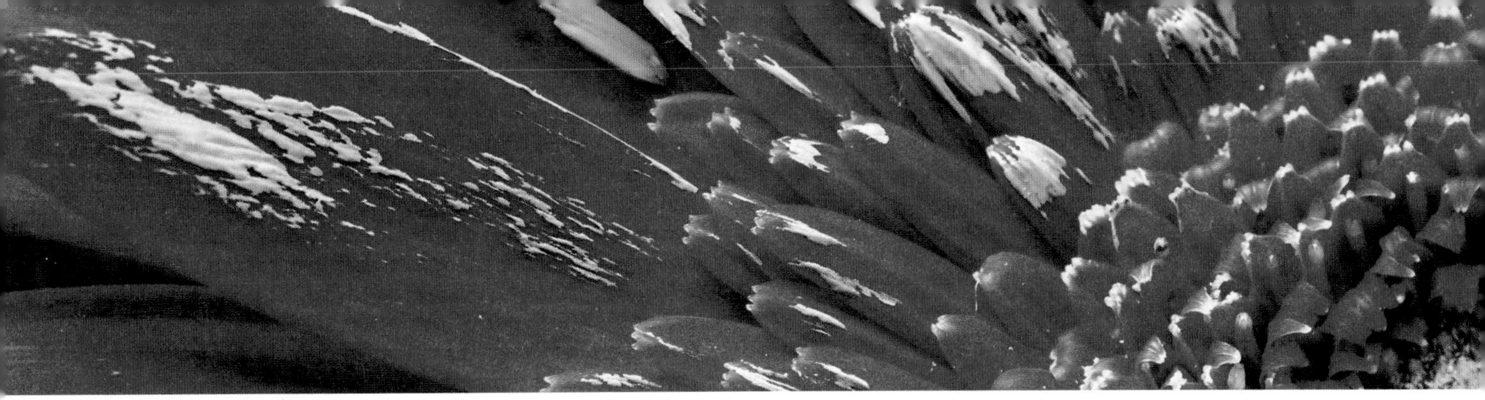

Chapter 20
Intrapartum Nursing Assessment

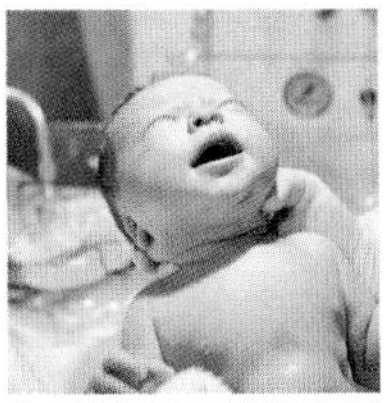

SOURCE: Tetra Images/SuperStock.

Birth is the sudden opening of a window, through which you look out upon a stupendous prospect. For what has happened? A miracle. You have exchanged nothing for the possibility of everything.
—William MacNeile Dixon

Learning Outcomes

20.1 Describe the intrapartum physical, psychosocial, and cultural assessments necessary for optimum maternal-fetal outcome.

20.2 Discuss the outer limits of normal progress of each of the phases and stages of labor.

20.3 Compare the various methods of monitoring fetal heart rate and contractions, giving advantages and disadvantages of each.

20.4 Describe the procedure for performing Leopold maneuvers and the information they provide.

20.5 Differentiate between baseline and periodic changes in the fetal heart rate.

20.6 Examine the differences between fetal tachycardia and fetal bradycardia.

20.7 Discuss fetal heart rates and patterns using National Institute of Child Health and Human Development (NICHD) terminology.

20.8 Explain the steps to be performed in the systematic evaluation of fetal heart rate tracings.

20.9 Evaluate abnormal findings on a fetal heart rate tracing.

20.10 Explain the interventions that are indicated when a nonreassuring fetal heart rate pattern is identified.

20.11 Describe the steps used to perform fetal scalp stimulation.

Healthy People 2020

(MICH-10) Increase the proportion of pregnant women who receive early and adequate prenatal care

(MICH-6) Reduce maternal illness and complications due to pregnancy (complications during hospitalized labor and delivery)

(MICH-7) Reduce cesarean births among low-risk (full-term, singleton, vertex presentation) women

The labor process is a period of increased physiologic stress for the pregnant woman and her fetus. The physiologic events that occur during the intrapartum period require many changes and rapid adaptations. Accurate and frequent assessment by the nurse is crucial to ensure the health and well-being of both the woman and her baby. The primary purpose of the intrapartum assessment is to collect the essential data used to individualize care, to evaluate the response of the mother or fetus, and to monitor the well-being of the maternal-fetal unit throughout labor. The nurse in the birth setting uses a wide variety of assessment skills, including observation, palpation, and auscultation to provide care for two primary patients, the mother and her fetus. The expectant mother's support person—who may be a spouse, a partner, a family member, or a friend—is also an important member of the birthing team, and assessments of their coping, interactions, and teamwork are integral to the nurse's knowledge base. The nurse's physical presence with the laboring woman provides the best opportunity for ongoing assessment, even as the nurse quietly provides comfort measures and gently assists the woman's support person to help her throughout the labor experience.

In current practice, hands-on techniques can be augmented by the use of technology. For example, the nurse or clinician can use a fetoscope, Doppler ultrasound (US), or an electronic fetal monitor to listen to or obtain the fetal heart rate (FHR). Palpation can be performed by the nurse to manually feel uterine contractions or electronic fetal monitoring (EMF) can be used to record contractions. No matter what technology is used, it is important for the nurse to remember that a machine or any tool used for assessment provides information, but it does not replace the human interaction and support that are provided by the nurse. In the birth setting that utilizes "high-touch" nursing care, the use of "low-tech" or "high-tech" assessments are easily integrated to provide comprehensive, high-quality care.

This chapter discusses the assessments that are an important part of nursing care in maternity settings such as a birthing center or hospital. Home birth would also involve many of the same assessments, but the equipment available would be limited.

Maternal Assessment

The goal of a maternal assessment is to create an accurate database of information from which healthcare providers are able to formulate an optimal plan of care for a patient given her current clinical situation. Assessment of the intrapartum woman begins with a patient history and screening for intrapartum risk factors. Data collection includes a variety of data assessment methods: The prenatal record, admission interviews of the patient and family members to obtain historical data, a psychologic assessment, and the initial and ongoing assessments of the mother and fetus throughout labor.

Assessment and evaluation of the woman presenting as a potential intrapartum patient may vary from patient to patient depending on the woman's current labor and medical status, risk factors, membrane status, and stage of labor. Evidence-based practice standards have shown that many labor and birth interventions do not result in approved maternal or newborn outcomes, but may increase the risk of surgical intervention and decrease the woman's level of satisfaction (American College of Obstetricians and Gynecologists [ACOG], 2017a). ACOG (2016) states that pregnant women who present to the acute care setting should be evaluated in a timely manner. Women may often need to be triaged upon presentation to the hospital obstetrical unit or birth center; thus, nursing staff may be required to perform intrapartum assessments in various phases of labor in order to facilitate prompt and efficient care for patients. For example, the initial evaluation of a laboring woman may only include assessment of her vital signs, FHR, status of uterine contractions, and any abnormal symptoms or signs of potential problems such as vaginal bleeding, acute abdominal pain, temperature above 100.4°F, premature labor, preterm premature rupture of membranes (PPROM), term premature rupture of membranes (PROM) indicating that the amniotic sac ruptures prior to the onset of labor, hypertension, or nonreassuring fetal patterns (Gabbe, Niebyl, Simpson, et al., 2017).

If the initial assessment reveals any complications or high-risk conditions, such as preterm labor, PROM or PPROM, preeclampsia, FHR abnormalities, or vaginal bleeding, or if the woman presents with ruptured membranes, the nurse should promptly continue the assessment of the mother and fetus and initiate appropriate treatment. If a woman is in early labor or complications are not identified, the nurse may defer the complete physical assessment and admission of the mother once fetal well-being has been determined. Assessment and evaluation may be limited to determine if there is any change from the most recently documented prenatal care visit or other evaluation and to determine any ongoing or newly developed risk factors that could impact medical decision making during the present admission. On the other hand, a woman who has received no prenatal care may require a complete assessment including history and physical, obstetrical evaluation, laboratory tests, ultrasound, and other indicated procedures as her condition warrants (ACOG, 2016). Regardless of status, the well-being of the mother and fetus are of primary concern, and it is the responsibility of the nursing and medical staff to obtain accurate and appropriate data regarding the patient and to provide appropriate services as needed. See *Case Study: Melissa Bond-James*.

CASE STUDY: Melissa Bond-James

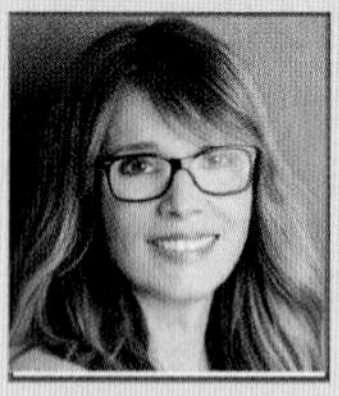

SOURCE: Kinga/Shutterstock

Melissa and her wife, Nancy, present to the labor and delivery unit at 29 weeks' gestation after being advised to go to the hospital by the nurse at her obstetrician's office. Melissa has continued running throughout her pregnancy and after her 3-mile run that morning she began to experience contractions. She states she sometimes has uterine irritability during her runs, but after drinking two or three glasses of water and resting, it goes away completely. Today, she drank four glasses of water and rested, but the contractions are getting more frequent, occurring every 10 minutes at regular intervals. Nancy, who has been timing them, states they seem longer and are stronger in the last 45 minutes. The couple is quite concerned and afraid the baby is at risk to be born prematurely.

Questions to Ponder

What baseline data should the labor and delivery nurse obtain? Nancy asks you what tests they are likely to order and what the tests will tell them. Outline their probable plan of care and what tests will be needed to determine if the contractions are a result of preterm labor. If preterm labor has been diagnosed, what medications are likely to be ordered for Melissa? Review the possible medications, their indications, and desired outcomes.

Prenatal Record

When a pregnant woman approaches approximately 36 weeks' gestation, a copy of the prenatal record should be available at the facility where she will give birth so that the medical record is accessible to members of the healthcare delivery team. If the prenatal record is available, it can provide the foundation for the intrapartum assessment. Health conditions, risk factors, abnormal test results, and ongoing assessments are necessary in determining patient care needs. Information should be verified, if possible, to avoid conflicts during subsequent patient interviews.

Historical Data

During assessment interviews, the pregnant patient is likely to be the primary source of information. Her spouse, partner, or another family member may be present and capable of providing information in the event that the mother cannot concentrate or participate in the interview because of her physical state or stage of labor. The patient's privacy should be safeguarded and confidentiality maintained.

The historical or background data are the foundation for the intrapartum assessment and includes the patient's demographic and socioeconomic information; medical, surgical, family, obstetrical, and gynecologic histories; psychosociocultural assessments; and physical examination. See Box 20–1.

Intrapartum High-Risk Screening

Screening for intrapartum high-risk factors is an integral part of assessment of the normal laboring woman. While obtaining the history, the nurse notes the presence of any factors that may be associated with a high-risk condition. The Association of Women's

Box 20-1
Historical Data for the Intrapartum Assessment

Demographic Information

- Name and age
- Attending obstetrician or certified nurse-midwife (CNM)
- Pediatrician/family physician

Socioeconomic Factors

- Housing, transportation
- Ability to provide for the new baby
- Support system

Psychosocial Assessment

- Cultural factors
- Resources and support systems
- Domestic violence screening
- Substance abuse/exposure, including tobacco and marijuana use
- History of mental health illness, including family history of mental illness, especially postpartum mood and anxiety disorders

Medical and Surgical Histories

- History of previous illness, such as tuberculosis, heart disease, diabetes, convulsive disorders, immune system abnormalities, hematologic disorders, thyroid disorders, gastrointestinal abnormalities, asthma, sickle cell disease, Tay-Sachs disease, and other inherited disorders
- Environmental exposures (mercury, pesticides, asbestos, solvents, metals, chemicals, radiation, smoking)
- Surgeries

Family History

- Genetic disorders, medical conditions, psychiatric conditions
- Family violence history, intimate partner violence (IPV)

Obstetric History

- Past pregnancies
- Complications during pregnancy (e.g., preeclampsia/eclampsia, gestational diabetes, anemia, hyperemesis, hydramnios or oligohydramnios, placenta previa)
- Labor complications (e.g., dystocia [malpresentation, cephalopelvic disproportion (CPD), macrosomia, failure to progress], precipitous or prolonged labor, prolonged pushing, hemorrhage, placenta abruption or accreta, cord prolapse, embolism, mechanical delivery [forceps or vacuum], pain management [epidural or medications], episiotomy/laceration)
- Postpartum complications (e.g., hemorrhage, infection, thrombus, postpartum depression, difficulty breastfeeding)
- High-risk factors
- Previous abortions, term and preterm newborns, number of living children, neonatal deaths
- Mode of birth
- Current pregnancy
- Gravidity, parity
- High-risk factors
- Blood type; Rh factor; results of serology testing; complete blood count (CBC); glucose testing; screens for STIs and group beta strep; quadruple screen; and results of any genetic diagnostic tests (nuchal translucency testing, chorionic villus sampling, amniocentesis) and specialized tests (Tay-Sachs, cystic fibrosis, sickle cell disease)
- Allergies to medications, foods, or substances
- Drug and alcohol consumption and smoking during pregnancy
- Elevated blood pressure, bleeding problems, recurrent urinary tract infection
- Medications used during the pregnancy, including prescription medication, over-the-counter medications, and herbal supplements
- Method chosen for newborn/infant feeding
- Type of prenatal education (childbirth preparation classes)
- Birth plan with the woman's preferences regarding labor and birth, such as no episiotomy, no analgesics or anesthetics, or the presence/participation of the father/partner or others at the birth
- Gestational age assessment
- Fetal activity

(continued)

Box 20-1 *(continued)*

- Leopold maneuvers
- Fetal positioning

Clinical Assessment

- Maternal vital signs
- Maternal weight, height, and weight gain this pregnancy
- Nutritional status
- Uterine activity
- Contraction assessment
- Onset, duration, frequency of uterine contractions
- Fetal response to uterine contractions
- Membrane status
- Status of membranes, color of amniotic fluid
- Date and time of rupture
- Vaginal examination
- Vaginal bleeding and discharge
- Cervical exam

Biochemical Examinations During Pregnancy

- Laboratory studies
- CBC, blood type, and Rh and antibody screen
- Toxicology screening (if ordered)
- Blood glucose screening
- Urine for protein and sugar
- Infectious disease evaluation
- Chlamydia, gonorrhea, group beta strep, hepatitis B, rubella, syphilis
- Optional infectious disease evaluation: Cytomegalovirus, tuberculosis, trichomonas, HIV, human papillomavirus (HPV), hepatitis A and C, herpes simplex virus

Fetal Assessment

- Gestational age assessment
- Last menstrual period (LMP)
- Fetal movement
- Ultrasound exams for dating
- Fetal activity
- Fetal movement by maternal report
- Fetal movement by palpation
- Antenatal assessments
- Nonstress tests (NSTs)
- Contraction stress tests (CSTs)
- Biophysical profiles
- Ultrasounds
- Amniotic fluid index (AFI)
- Method of monitoring
- Auscultation
- External
- Tocodynamometer
- Internal
- Fetal spiral electrode
- Intrauterine pressure catheter

SOURCE: Data from Gabbe et al., 2017.

Health, Obstetric, and Neonatal Nurses (AWHONN) has also created the Maternal Fetal Triage Index (MFTI), a five-level standardized method for assigning an acuity score to pregnant women presenting to the hospital for care (ACOG, 2016; Killion, 2016). For example, the woman who reports a physical symptom such as term gestation with heavy vaginal bleeding needs immediate assessment to rule out abruptio placentae or placenta previa before the admission process continues. This scenario would be considered a level "1-stat" MFTI requiring immediate lifesaving intervention for a woman and/or her fetus. In addition to identifying the presence of a high-risk condition, the nurse must recognize the implications of the condition for the laboring woman and her fetus. For example, in the case of an abnormal fetal presentation, the nurse understands that the labor may be prolonged, prolapse of the umbilical cord may be more likely, and there is a greater possibility of a cesarean birth.

Although physical conditions are frequently listed as the major factors that increase risk in the intrapartum period, psychosocial and cultural variables such as poverty, nutrition, the amount of prenatal care, and cultural beliefs regarding pregnancy can also precipitate a high-risk situation in the intrapartum period. It is important for the nurse to begin gathering data about these psychosocial and cultural factors as the woman enters the birthing area. In a recent systematic review of the literature, researchers found that intimate partner violence (IPV) was directly related to significantly higher adverse birth outcomes such as preterm birth, low birthweight, and small for gestational age (Donovan, Spracklen, Schweizer, et al., 2016; Hill, Pallitto, McCleary-Sills, et al., 2016). A woman's mental health condition plays a role in predicting postpartum mental health and, sometimes, traumatic birth or adverse birth outcomes and bonding problems. Furthermore, a traumatic experience such as giving birth to a high-risk neonate is an additional predictor of postpartum posttraumatic stress disorder and postpartum depression (ACOG, 2015).

Communication problems can also affect the course of labor, as well as the nurse's ability to provide support and education. Thus, the nurse observes the communication pattern between the woman and her support person(s) and their responses to admission questions and initial teaching. If the nurse or other birthing room staff does not speak the primary language of the woman and her support person(s) or if the woman is hearing impaired, an appropriate interpreter should be obtained so that the patient can make informed decisions. Communication may also be affected by cultural standards regarding when it is acceptable to speak, who should ask questions, or whether it is acceptable for the woman to let others know if she is experiencing discomfort (National Institutes of Health, 2016).

An IPV assessment should be performed on all women throughout the pregnancy and at admission to the intrapartum unit. Victims of IPV are more likely to experience an unintended pregnancy and to abuse substances during pregnancy and are at risk for depression and postpartum depression (Alhusen, Ray, Sharps, et al., 2015).

A partial list of intrapartum risk factors appears in Table 20–1. The factors precede the Intrapartum Assessment Guide because they must be kept in mind during the assessment.

TABLE 20–1 Intrapartum High-Risk Factors

FACTOR	MATERNAL IMPLICATION	FETAL-NEONATAL IMPLICATION
Abnormal presentation	↑ Incidence of cesarean birth ↑ Incidence of prolonged labor ↑ Incidence of fibroids	↑ Incidence of placenta previa Prematurity ↑ Risk of congenital abnormality Neonatal physical trauma ↑ Risk of intrauterine growth restriction (IUGR)
Multiple gestation	↑ Uterine distention → ↑ risk of postpartum hemorrhage ↑ Risk of cesarean birth ↑ Risk of preterm labor	Low birth weight Prematurity ↑ Risk of congenital anomalies Feto-fetal transfusion
Hydramnios	↑ Discomfort ↑ Dyspnea ↑ Risk of preterm labor Edema of lower extremities/varicosities	↑ Risk of esophageal or other high alimentary tract atresias ↑ Risk of central nervous system (CNS) anomalies (myelocele) ↑ Risk of TORCH (toxoplasmosis, rubella, cytomegalovirus, herpes virus hominis type 2) infections ↑ Risk of prolapse cord
Oligohydramnios	Maternal fear of "dry birth"	↑ Incidence of congenital anomalies ↑ Incidence of renal lesions ↑ Risk of IUGR ↑ Risk of fetal acidosis ↑ Risk of cord compression Postmaturity
Meconium staining of amniotic fluid	↑ Psychologic stress due to fear for baby	↑ Risk of fetal asphyxia ↑ Risk of meconium aspiration ↑ Risk of pneumonia due to aspiration of meconium
Premature rupture of membranes	↑ Risk of infection (chorioamnionitis) ↑ Risk of preterm labor ↑ Anxiety/fear for the baby Prolonged hospitalization ↑ Incidence of tocolytic therapy	↑ Perinatal morbidity Prematurity ↓ Birth weight ↑ Risk of respiratory distress syndrome (RDS) Prolonged hospitalization
Induction of labor	↑ Risk of uterine rupture ↑ Length of labor if cervix not ready ↑ Anxiety	Prematurity if gestational age not assessed correctly ↑ Risk of hypoxia
Abruptio placentae/placenta previa	Hemorrhage Uterine atony ↑ Incidence of cesarean birth ↑ Maternal morbidity	Fetal hypoxia/acidosis Fetal exsanguination ↑ Perinatal mortality
Failure to progress in labor	Maternal exhaustion ↑ Incidence of augmentation of labor ↑ Incidence of cesarean birth	Fetal hypoxia/acidosis Intracranial birth injury
Precipitous labor (less than 3 hours)	Perineal, vaginal, cervical lacerations ↑ Risk of postpartum hemorrhage	Neonatal tentorial (brain) tears Trauma—neural or tissue, cephalohematoma
Prolapse of umbilical cord	↑ Fear for baby Cesarean birth ↑ emergent	Acute fetal hypoxia/acidosis
Fetal heart decelerations	↑ Fear for baby ↑ Risk of cesarean birth, forceps, vacuum Continuous electronic monitoring and intervention in labor	Tachycardia, chronic asphyxic insult, bradycardia Acute asphyxic insult Chronic hypoxia Congenital heart block
Uterine rupture	Hemorrhage Cesarean birth/hysterectomy ↑ Risk of morbidity/mortality	Fetal anoxia Fetal hemorrhage ↑ Neonatal morbidity and mortality

(continued)

TABLE 20–1 Intrapartum High-Risk Factors *(continued)*

FACTOR	MATERNAL IMPLICATION	FETAL-NEONATAL IMPLICATION
Postdates (greater than 42 weeks)	↑ Anxiety ↑ Incidence of induction of labor ↑ Incidence of cesarean birth ↑ Use of technology to monitor fetus ↑ Risk of shoulder dystocia	Postmaturity syndrome ↑ Risk of fetal-neonatal mortality and morbidity ↑ Risk of antepartum fetal death ↑ Incidence/risk of large baby ↑ Hypoglycemia
Diabetes	↑ Risk of hydramnios ↑ Risk of hypoglycemia or hyperglycemia ↑ Risk of preeclampsia	↑ Risk of malpresentation ↑ Risk of macrosomia ↑ Risk of IUGR ↑ Risk of RDS ↑ Hypoglycemia, polycythemia ↑ Birth trauma ↑ Risk of congenital anomalies
Preeclampsia	↑ Abruptio placentae ↑ Risk of seizures ↑ Risk of stroke ↑ Risk of HELLP	↑ Risk of small-for-gestational-age (SGA) baby ↑ Risk of preterm birth ↑ Risk of mortality
AIDS/STIs	↑ Risk of additional infections	↑ Risk of transplacental transmission

Intrapartum Physical and Psychosociocultural Assessment

A physical examination is part of the admission procedure and part of the ongoing care of the patient. Although the intrapartum physical assessment is not as complete and thorough as the initial prenatal physical examination (see Chapter 12), it does involve assessment of some body systems and the actual labor process.

The physical assessment includes assessments performed immediately on admission as well as ongoing assessments. When labor is progressing very quickly, the nurse may not have time for a complete assessment. In this case, the critical physical assessments would include maternal vital signs, labor status, fetal status, and laboratory findings. Psychologic disorders can also affect the intrapartum course. For example, the woman suffering from clinical depression may exhibit fear or a feeling of hopelessness, apathy, weariness or lack of energy, trouble concentrating, increased inflammatory activity and impaired immune function, and impaired quality of mother–baby interaction (Gabbe et al., 2017). Women diagnosed with depression are significantly more likely to have preterm labor and birth, low-birth-weight babies, and decreased rates of breastfeeding initiation compared with women without depression.

The woman with a panic disorder may have short-lived, unpredictable episodes of intense anxiety, whereas the woman with a generalized anxiety disorder may experience continual and excessive anxiety or worrying. The woman with obsessive–compulsive disorder may have irrational impulses that are relieved only with performing a ritualistic behavior, such as repetitive hand washing. Psychosis is one of the most disabling psychiatric disorders, and the woman may experience hallucinations and delusions. Women with acute psychosis typically require inpatient hospitalization.

Pregnancy further complicates psychiatric disorders because of fear that the medications used to treat the symptoms may be contraindicated in pregnancy. It is essential that women with psychiatric disorders or those that appear to have psychiatric symptoms be collaboratively managed by a psychiatrist or psychiatric mental health nurse practitioner who is knowledgeable in psychopharmacology. For these reasons, the woman with a psychologic disorder may require additional support from the nurse. The nurse plays a key role in maintaining the collaborative management plan for the woman and her healthcare team.

Assessment of psychosocial history is a critical component of intrapartum nursing assessment. Because of the prevalence of physical and sexual assault against women in our society (see Chapter 8), the nurse needs to consider the possibility that the woman may have experienced violence at some point in her life. If this is the case, she may be anxious about the labor process or anxiety may arise during labor. Therefore, it is essential to review the woman's prenatal record and any other available records for information that may indicate abuse.

A transcultural nursing assessment provides a starting point for a plan that honors the values and beliefs of the laboring woman. Nurses are entrusted with the care of patients from various cultural backgrounds, with differing values from their own, and must deliver care that is culturally sensitive and free of biases based on gender, race, or religious affiliation (Giger, 2017). Frequently, however, the nurse feels uncertain about what to ask or consider, perhaps because there has been no personal opportunity to become aware of varying cultural values and beliefs. It is important to remember that despite one's cultural background, variations in different individuals and families can be dramatic. Some individuals may not embrace cultural beliefs that are inherent in their culture. The cultural assessment section of the assessment guide helps to encourage cultural sensitivity in the nurse (Giger, 2017).

The final section of the guide addresses psychosocial factors. The laboring woman's psychosocial status is an important part of the total assessment. The woman has previous ideas, knowledge, and fears about childbearing. The adequacy of resources, such as housing, transportation, utilities, and access to social services, should also be assessed. By assessing her psychosocial status, the nurse can meet the woman's needs for information and support. The nurse can then support the woman and her partner or family member; in the absence of a partner/family member, the nurse may become the support person. *Assessment Guide: Intrapartum—First Stage of Labor* provides a framework that the maternity nurse can use when examining the laboring woman.

ASSESSMENT GUIDE | Intrapartum—First Stage of Labor

Physical Assessment/Normal Findings	Alterations and Possible Causes*	Nursing Responses to Data†
Vital Signs		
Blood Pressure (BP): Less than or equal to 120/80 mmHg	High blood pressure (essential hypertension, gestational hypertension, preeclampsia, renal disease, apprehension, anxiety or pain) Low blood pressure (supine hypotension) Hemorrhage/hypovolemia Shock Drugs *Maternal Early Warning Criteria* (Mhyre et al., 2014): Systolic BP <90 or >160 Diastolic BP >100 *Severe range* (ACOG, 2013a): Systolic BP >160 Diastolic BP >110 or higher	Evaluate history of preexisting disorders and check for presence of other signs of preeclampsia. Do not assess during contractions; implement measures to decrease anxiety and reassess. Turn woman on her side and recheck BP. Provide quiet environment. Have oxygen (O_2) available. Notify physician/CNM.
Pulse: 60–100 beats/min; rate may increase 10 beats/min during pregnancy or more during labor and birth	Decreased pulse rate may indicate a deterioration in maternal condition Increased pulse rate (excitement or anxiety, cardiac disorders, early shock, drug use); decreased pulse rate ($MgSO_4$ toxicity, maternal hemorrhage) *Maternal Early Warning Criteria* (Mhyre et al., 2014): <50 or >120 beats/min	Evaluate cause, reassess to see if rate continues; report to physician/CNM.
Respirations: 12–20 breaths/min (or pulse rate divided by 4)	Marked tachypnea (respiratory disease), hyperventilation in transition phase Decreased respirations (narcotics) Hyperventilation (anxiety/pain) *Maternal Early Warning Criteria* (Mhyre et al., 2014): <10 or >30 breaths/min	Assess between contractions; if marked tachypnea continues, assess for signs of respiratory disease or respiratory distress. Encourage slow breaths if woman is hyperventilating.
Pulse oximetry 95% or greater; women living in high altitudes can have reduction down to 92%	Less than 90%: Hypoxia, hypotension, hemorrhage, pulmonary embolism, or cardiac concern	Apply O_2; notify physician/CNM.
Temperature: 36.2–37.6°C (98–99.6°F)	Elevated temperature (infection, dehydration, prolonged ROM, epidural regional block)	Assess for other signs of infection or dehydration.
Recommended Weight Gain		
If prepregnant BMI is less than 18.5, a 28–40 lb gain is recommended; if BMI is 18.5–24.9, a 25–35 lb gain is recommended; if BMI is 25–29.9, a 15–25 lb gain is recommended; if BMI is 30 or greater, an 11–20 lb gain is recommended (ACOG, 2013b).	Weight gain greater than recommendations may indicate fluid retention, obesity, large fetus, diabetes mellitus, preeclampsia; weight gain less than 15 lb may indicate SGA fetus, substance abuse, psychosocial problems	Assess for signs of edema. Evaluate dietary patterns. Assess for substance abuse and eating disorders.
Lungs		
Normal breath sounds, clear and equal	Rales, rhonchi, friction rub (infection), pulmonary edema, asthma	Reassess; refer to physician/CNM.

(continued)

Assessment Guide | Intrapartum—First Stage of Labor (continued)

Physical Assessment/Normal Findings	Alterations and Possible Causes*	Nursing Responses to Data†
Fundus		
At 40 weeks' gestation located just below xiphoid process	Uterine size not within 2–3 cm below expected size for a singleton pregnancy may indicate SGA fetus, fetal malposition, or oligohydramnios. Fundal height greater than 2–3 cm of expected size may indicate large for gestational age (LGA) fetus, molar pregnancy, polyhydramnios, full bladder, incorrectly calculated gestational age, BMI > 40, multiple pregnancy, placental/fetal anomalies, malpresentation), IUGR	Reevaluate history regarding pregnancy dating. Refer to physician/CNM for additional assessment.
Edema		
Slight amount of dependent edema	Pitting edema of face, hands, legs, abdomen, sacral area (preeclampsia vs. dependent edema)	Check deep tendon reflexes for hyperactivity; check for clonus; refer to physician/CNM.
Hydration		
Normal skin turgor, elastic	Poor skin turgor (dehydration)	Assess skin turgor; refer to physician for deviations. Provide fluids per physician/CNM orders.
Perineum		
Tissues smooth, pink color (see *Assessment Guide: Initial Prenatal Assessment* in Chapter 12)	Varicose veins of vulva, herpes lesions/genital warts	Note on patient record need for follow-up in postpartum period; reassess after birth; refer to physician/CNM.
Clear mucus; may be blood-tinged with earthy or human odor	Profuse, purulent, foul-smelling drainage	Suspected gonorrhea or chorioamnionitis; report to physician/CNM; initiate care to newborn's eyes; notify neonatal nursing staff and pediatrician.
Presence of small amount of bloody show that gradually increases with further cervical dilatation	Hemorrhage, placental abruption	Assess BP and pulse, pallor, diaphoresis; report any marked changes. Use standard precautions. For increased bright red bleeding, report to physician/CNM.
Labor Status		
Uterine Contractions (UC): Regular pattern	Failure to establish a regular pattern, prolonged latent phase	Evaluate whether woman is in true labor; ambulate if in early labor.
	Active phase	Evaluate patient status and contractile pattern per birth setting policy.
	Hypertonicity systole	Provide oxygen, stop Pitocin, and administer terbutaline.
	Hypotonicity	Obtain a 30-minute electronic fetal monitoring (EFM) strip.
	Dehydration	Notify physician/CNM. Provide hydration.
Cervical Dilatation: Progressive cervical dilatation from size of fingertip to 10 cm (see Table 20–2 and *Clinical Skill 20–1: Performing an Intrapartum Vaginal Examination*)	Rigidity of cervix (frequent cervical infections, scar tissue, failure of presenting part to descend)	Evaluate contractions, fetal engagement, position, and cervical dilatation. Inform patient of progress.
Cervical Effacement: Progressive thinning of cervix (see *Clinical Skill 20–1*)	Failure to efface (rigidity of cervix, failure of presenting part to engage); cervical edema (pushing effort by woman before cervix is fully dilated and effaced, trapped cervix)	Evaluate contractions, fetal engagement and position. Notify physician/CNM if cervix is becoming edematous; work with woman to prevent pushing until cervix is completely dilated. Keep vaginal exams to a minimum.

Physical Assessment/Normal Findings	Alterations and Possible Causes*	Nursing Responses to Data†
Fetal Descent: Progressive descent of fetal presenting part from station −5 to +4 (see Figure 20–1 in *Clinical Skill 20–1*)	Failure of descent (abnormal fetal position or presentation, macrosomic fetus, inadequate pelvic measurements)	Evaluate fetal position, presentation, and size.
Membranes: May rupture before or during labor	Rupture of membranes more than 12–24 hours before initiation of labor	Assess for ruptured membranes using Nitrazine test tape before doing vaginal exam. Follow standard precautions. Instruct woman with ruptured membranes to remain on bedrest if presenting part is not engaged and firmly down against the cervix. Keep vaginal exams to a minimum to prevent infection. When membranes rupture in the birth setting, *immediately assess FHR* to detect changes associated with prolapse of umbilical cord (FHR slows).
Findings on Nitrazine Test Tape Membranes probably intact: Yellow — pH 5.0 Olive — pH 5.5 Olive green — pH 6.0	False-positive results may be obtained if large amount of bloody show is present, previous vaginal examination has been done using lubricant, infection is present, or tape is touched by nurse's fingers.	Assess fluid for consistency, amount, odor; assess FHR frequently. Assess fluid at regular intervals for presence of meconium staining. Follow standard precautions while assessing amniotic fluid.
Membranes probably ruptured: Blue-green — pH 6.5 Blue-gray — pH 7.0 Deep blue — pH 7.5		Teach woman that amniotic fluid is continually produced (to allay fear of "dry birth"). Teach woman that she may feel amniotic fluid trickle or gush with contractions. Change Chux pads often.
Amniotic fluid clear, with earthy or human odor, no foul-smelling odor	Greenish amniotic fluid (nonreassuring fetal status) Bloody fluid (vasa previa, abruptio placentae)	Assess FHR; do vaginal exam to evaluate for prolapsed cord; apply fetal monitor for continuous data; report to physician/CNM.
	Strong or foul odor (amnionitis)	Take woman's temperature and report to physician/CNM.
Fetal Status		
FHR: 110–160 beats/min Tachycardia Bradycardia	Less than 110 or greater than 160 beats/min (nonreassuring fetal status); abnormal patterns on fetal monitor: Decreased variability, late decelerations, variable decelerations, absence of accelerations with fetal movement	Initiate interventions based on particular FHR pattern.
Presentation: Cephalic, 97% Breech, <3% Shoulder, <1%	Face, brow, breech, or shoulder presentation	Report to physician/CNM; after presentation is confirmed as face, brow, breech, or shoulder, woman may be prepared for cesarean birth.
Position: Left-occiput-anterior (LOA) most common	Persistent occipital-posterior (OP) position; transverse arrest	Carefully monitor maternal and fetal status. Reposition mother side-lying or on hands and knees to promote rotation of fetal head.

(continued)

Assessment Guide | Intrapartum—First Stage of Labor (continued)

Physical Assessment/Normal Findings	Alterations and Possible Causes*	Nursing Responses to Data†
Activity: Fetal movement	Uterine tachysystole (more than five contractions in 10 minutes) (may precede fetal hypoxia) Complete lack of movement (nonreassuring fetal status or fetal demise)	Carefully evaluate FHR; apply fetal monitor. Report to physician/CNM.
Laboratory Evaluation		
Hematologic Tests *Hemoglobin:* 12–16 g/dL	Less than 11 g/dL (anemia, hemorrhage, sickle cell disorders, pernicious anemia)	Evaluate woman for problems due to decreased oxygen-carrying capacity caused by lowered hemoglobin.
CBC: *Hematocrit:* 38%–47% *RBC:* 4.2–5.4 million/mm^3 *WBC:* 4500–11,000/mm^3, although leukocytosis to 20,000/mm^3 is not unusual *Platelets* 150,000–400,000/mm^3	Presence of infection or blood dyscrasias, loss of blood (hemorrhage, disseminated intravascular coagulation [DIC])	Evaluate for other signs of infection or for petechiae, bruising, or unusual bleeding.
Serologic Testing: Serologic test for syphilis (STS), Venereal Disease Research Laboratory (VDRL) test, or rapid plasma reagent (RPR) test: Nonreactive Rh Rh negative	Positive reaction (see *Assessment Guide: Initial Prenatal Assessment* in Chapter 12) Rh-positive fetus in Rh-negative woman or O+ woman	For reactive test, notify newborn nursery and pediatrician. Assess prenatal record for titer levels during pregnancy. Obtain cord blood for direct Coombs at birth.
Hepatitis B	Presence of infection	Assess mother to see if active infection. Monitor liver functions. Notify nursery and pediatrician and administer hepatitis B vaccination to newborn immediately following birth.
Human immunodeficiency virus (HIV)	Presence of infection	Obtain immune status functioning. Notify nursery and pediatrician upon admission. Refer to infectious disease specialist to begin antiretroviral therapy. Give maternal intravenous antivirals during labor. Begin antivirals on newborn immediately following birth.
Urinalysis: Glucose: Negative	Glycosuria (low renal threshold for glucose, diabetes mellitus)	Assess blood glucose; test urine for ketones; ketonuria and glycosuria require further assessment of blood sugars. (Glycosuria should not be discounted and its presence necessitates follow-up.)
Ketones: Negative	Ketonuria (starvation ketosis)	Assess nutritional status.
Proteins: Negative	Proteinuria (urine specimen contaminated with vaginal secretions, fever, infection, kidney disease); proteinuria of 2+ or greater found in uncontaminated urine may be a sign of ensuing preeclampsia	Instruct woman in collection technique; incidence of contamination from vaginal discharge is common. Report any increase in proteinuria to physician/CNM.
Red blood cells: Negative	Blood in urine (calculi, cystitis, glomerulonephritis, neoplasm)	Assess collection technique (may be bloody show).

Physical Assessment/Normal Findings	Alterations and Possible Causes*	Nursing Responses to Data†
White blood cells: Negative	Presence of white blood cells (infection in genitourinary tract)	Assess for signs of urinary tract infection.
Casts: None	Presence of casts (nephrotic syndrome)	
Nitrites	Infection	Assess for signs of urinary tract infection.
Sexually transmitted infections (STIs):		
Chlamydia Gonorrhea	Presence of infection	Antibiotic treatment for mother and partner with test of cure culture in 2 weeks following completion of treatment. Stress importance of condom use. Rescreen at 36 weeks prior to onset of labor. Observe newborn for conjunctivitis.
Human papillomavirus (HPV)	Presence of infection	Explain need for regular Pap smear testing. Document on maternal obstetrical record. Observe for any external warts. If abnormal Pap, colposcopy may be warranted.
Cultural Assessment§	***Variations to Consider**	**Nursing Responses to Data†**
Cultural influences determine customs and practices regarding intrapartum care.	Individual preferences may vary.	
Ask these questions: Who would you like to remain with you during your labor and birth?	She may prefer only her support person to remain or may also want family or friends.	Provide support for her wishes by encouraging desired people to stay. Provide information to others (with the woman's permission) who are not in the room.
What would you like to wear during labor?	She may be more comfortable in her own clothes.	Offer supportive materials such as Chux, if needed, to protect her own clothing. Avoid subtle signals to the woman that she should not have chosen to remain in her own clothes. Have other clothing available if the woman desires. If her clothing becomes contaminated, it will be simple to place it in a plastic bag.
What activity would you like during labor?	She may want to ambulate most of the time, stand in the shower, sit in the whirlpool bath, sit on a chair/stool/birthing ball, remain on the bed, and so forth.	Support the woman's wishes; provide encouragement and complete assessments in a manner so her activity and positional wishes are disturbed as little as possible.

(*continued*)

Assessment Guide | Intrapartum—First Stage of Labor (continued)

Cultural Assessment§	*Variations to Consider	Nursing Responses to Data†
What position would you like for the birth?	She may feel more comfortable in lithotomy with stirrups and her upper body elevated; side-lying or sitting in birthing bed; standing; squatting; or on hands and knees.	Collect any supplies and equipment needed to support her in her chosen birthing position. Provide information to the coach regarding any changes that may be needed based on the chosen position.
Is there anything special you would like?	She may want the room darkened or to have curtains and windows open, music playing, a Leboyer birth, her support person to cut the umbilical cord, to save a portion of the umbilical cord, to save the placenta, to videotape the birth, and so forth.	Support requests, and communicate requests to any other nursing or medical personnel (so requests can continue to be supported and not questioned). If another nurse or physician does not honor the request, act as advocate for the woman by continuing to support her unless her desire is truly unsafe.
Ask the woman if she would like fluids, and ask what temperature she prefers.	She may prefer clear fluids other than water (tea, clear juice). She may prefer iced, room-temperature, or warmed fluids. Oral intake in labor is preferable unless a cesarean birth is anticipated or if risk factors for cesarean are present.	If the woman has a low-risk pregnancy, the nurse may provide PO fluids and solid food as desired. However, this should also be done in accordance with the birth setting policy and risk factors for labor and birth and risk for possible cesarean birth (American College of Nurse-Midwives [ACNM], 2016; Sperling, Dahlke, & Sibai, 2016).
Observe the woman's response when privacy is difficult to maintain and her body is exposed.	Some women do not seem to mind being exposed during an exam or procedure; others feel acute discomfort.	Maintain privacy and respect the woman's sense of privacy. If the woman is unable to provide specific information, the nurse may draw from general information regarding cultural variation. For example, Southeast Asian women may not want any family member in the room during exam or procedures. Her partner may not be involved with coaching activities during labor or birth. Muslim women may need to remain covered during the labor and birth and avoid exposure of any body part. The support person may need to be in the room but remain behind a curtain or screen.
The newborn should be placed on the chest of the mother as soon as possible after birth so that skin-to-skin contact can be initiated.	Some women may request the newborn to be cleaned off prior to skin-to-skin contact. If skin-to-skin contact with the mother is not an option, skin-to-skin contact with the father, partner, or other support person should be offered.	
If the woman is to breastfeed, ask if she would like to feed her baby immediately after birth.	She may want to feed her baby right away or she may want to wait a little while.	

Psychosocial Assessment	Variations to Consider	Nursing Responses to Data†
Preparation for Childbirth		
Woman has some information regarding process of normal labor and birth.	Some women do not have any information regarding childbirth.	Add to present information base.
Woman has breathing or relaxation techniques to use during labor.	Some women do not have any method of relaxation or breathing to use, and some do not desire them.	Support breathing and relaxation techniques that patient is using; provide information, if needed.

Psychosocial Assessment	Variations to Consider	Nursing Responses to Data†
Woman and support person have done extensive preparation for childbirth (examples include Bradley or Lamaze classes or hypnobirthing).	Some women have strong opinions regarding labor and birth preparation.	Support woman's wishes to participate in her birth experience; support birth plan.
Response to Labor		
Early or Latent Phase (0–3 cm): Relaxed, excited, anxious for labor to be well established	May cope well or feel unable to cope with contractions because of fear, anxiety, or lack of information.	Provide support and encouragement; establish trusting relationship.
Active Phase (4–7 cm): Becomes more intense, begins to tire	May remain quiet and without any sign of discomfort or anxiety; may insist that she is unable to continue with the birthing process.	Provide support and coaching, if needed.
Transitional Phase (8–10 cm): Feels tired, may feel unable to cope, needs frequent coaching to maintain breathing patterns		
Coping Mechanisms: Ability to cope with labor through use of support system, breathing, relaxation techniques, and comfort measures including frequent position changes in labor, warm water immersion, and massage	May feel marked anxiety and apprehension, may not have coping mechanisms that can be brought into this experience or may be unable to use them at this time.	Support coping mechanisms if they are working for the woman; provide information and support if she exhibits anxiety or needs alternative to present coping methods.
	Survivors of sexual abuse may demonstrate fear of IVs or needles, may recoil when touched, may insist on a female caregiver, may be very sensitive to body fluids and cleanliness, and may be unable to labor lying down. May show extreme distress with vaginal examinations.	Encourage participation of partner or other support person such as a doula or family member if a supportive relationship seems apparent. Establish rapport and a trusting relationship. Provide information that is true and offer your presence.
Anxiety		
Some anxiety and apprehension is within normal limits.	May show anxiety through rapid breathing, nervous tremors, frowning, grimacing, clenching of teeth, thrashing movements, crying, increased pulse and blood pressure.	Provide support, encouragement, and information. Teach relaxation techniques; support controlled breathing efforts. May need to provide a paper bag to breathe into if woman says her lips are tingling. Note FHR.
Sounds During Labor		
	Some women are very quiet; others moan or make a variety of noises.	Provide a supportive environment. Encourage woman to do what feels right for her.
Support System		
Physical intimacy between mother and father/partner (or mother and support person/doula): Caretaking activities such as soothing conversation, touching	Some women would prefer no contact; others may show clinging behaviors.	Encourage caretaking activities that appear to comfort the woman; encourage support for the woman; if support is limited, the nurse may take a more active role.
Support person stays in close proximity	Limited interaction may come from a desire for quiet.	Encourage support person to stay close (if this seems appropriate).

(continued)

Assessment Guide | Intrapartum—First Stage of Labor (continued)

Psychosocial Assessment	Variations to Consider	Nursing Responses to Data†
Relationship between mother and father/partner (or support person): Involved interaction	The support person may seem to be detached and maintain little support, attention, or conversation.	Support interactions; if interaction is limited, the nurse may provide more information and support. Ensure that coach/significant other has short breaks, especially prior to transition.

§These are only a few suggestions. We do not mean to imply that this is a comprehensive cultural assessment; rather, it is a tool to encourage cultural sensitivity.

*Possible causes of alterations or variations are identified in parentheses.

†This column provides guidelines for further assessment and initial nursing intervention.

TABLE 20–2 Duration of Centimeter Change in Cervical Dilatation by Parity in Spontaneous Labor*

CERVICAL DILATATION	NULLIPAROUS	MULTIPAROUS
4–5 cm	6 hr	7 hr
5–6 cm	3 hr	3 hr
6–7 cm	2 hr	2 hr
7–8 cm	1.5 hr	1 hr
8–9 cm	1.5 hr	1 hr
9–10 cm	2 hr	1 hr
Second stage with epidural	≥4 hr	≥3 hr
Second stage without epidural	≥3 hr	≥2 hr

*All values represent the normal parameters for the 95th percentile of laboring women.

SOURCES: Data from Ehsanipoor & Satin, 2017;Milton, 2017.

Evaluating Labor Progress

Intrapartum nursing care requires competent assessment, clinical skills, and a comprehensive knowledge of maternal-fetal anatomy and the physiology of the labor process. An ongoing, accurate assessment of both the mother and fetus and their responses to labor is necessary to provide the data required to make sound clinical judgments and provide appropriate care. Labor can be monitored in a number of ways, each having its own benefits and limitations. If a "low-technology" approach is desired, a nurse can monitor uterine contractions and the FHR intermittently using techniques such as palpation and auscultation. However, if the clinical situation demands, as in the case of a high-risk pregnancy, the laboring woman may be monitored electronically, which is called **electronic fetal monitoring (EFM)**. External devices (tocodynamometer and ultrasound) or internal devices (intrauterine pressure catheter and fetal scalp electrode) may be used when a continuous graphic data record is needed to evaluate the mother and fetus during labor.

"Trying to figure out if I was in labor was quite a task. Here I was, a birthing room nurse, and I couldn't decide if my contractions were the real thing. I timed them, and about the time I decided this was it, they would slow down. How exasperating not to know! It was so hard on me. But now I see that all women are in this spot. They want so much to be right, and we often treat them as if they should be able to sense when it is the real thing. I'd like the birthing room nurses to remember this."

The method of monitoring during labor may vary, depending on the presence of risk factors at admission, the preferences of the woman and healthcare provider, and the institution's policies (ACOG, 2017a). In a recent ACOG Committee Opinion (2017a), the lowest level of intervention that can safely assess and monitor the maternal-fetal patient should be used, as interventions are not associated with improved outcomes and may in fact set the woman up for additional testing procedures that are not indicated and may be perceived as intrusive and uncomfortable. When intermittent monitoring, which is recommended for low-risk women, is used, the nurse must perform a hands-on assessment, including auscultation of fetal heart tones (FHT) and palpation of uterine contractions (UC). If continuous EFM is needed and is used, the amount of physical, hands-on care may vary depending on whether an internal or external mode of monitoring is used. EFM provides a continuous tracing of the FHR.

Professional associations, such as the American College of Obstetricians and Gynecologists (ACOG), American College of Nurse-Midwives (ACNM), and Association of Women's Health, Obstetric and Neonatal Nurses (AWHONN), and individual healthcare institutions generally set the guidelines for the level of intrapartum monitoring. Nurses will need to be aware of the policy for the individual birth settings in which they are caring for laboring women. The frequency of the maternal-fetal assessment and documentation depends on the mother's stage of labor and the presence of risk factors. When EFM is used, ACOG recommends that the nurse or physician/CNM review EFM data at least every 30 minutes. According to ACOG (2017a), low-risk pregnancies with Category I (normal) tracings do not need EFM but may be monitored with intermittent auscultation. FHR should be assessed every 30 minutes in the first stage of labor and every 15 minutes in the second stage of labor. Women with Category II (indeterminate) or Category III (abnormal) tracings or women with risk factors should be assessed and tracings evaluated every 15 minutes in first-stage labor and every 5 minutes in second-stage labor. Periodic documentation should accompany each review of the FHR tracing. See Table 20–3 for the frequency of recommended assessments and documentations.

The recommended frequency of FHR tracing assessment and documentation is only a guideline for practice. At times, the nurse may find it necessary to monitor the FHR more frequently. There may be times when a woman with low-risk factors may be placed on EFM, but if the patterns reveal a Category I tracing and she remains free of risk factors, a return to intermittent monitoring is preferred. The placement of a temporary EFM may be warranted with certain clinical events such as vaginal exams; rupture of membranes; abnormal uterine activity patterns; administration of medications; procedures such as epidurals, amniocentesis, and external versions; and other adverse events that have the potential to affect the FHR tracing. It is beneficial to assess the FHR tracing before and after such events or any time a nonreassuring FHR tracing is detected (Holley, 2017).

In 2002, approximately 85% of all live births were monitored electronically, making EFM the most prevalent assessment procedure in maternal-fetal health care (Gabbe et al., 2017). As research and evidence-based practice trends continue to evolve, the use of intermittent monitoring in low-risk women with Category I tracings is now the preferred assessment technique. When oxytocin is initially started, risk factors become known, or a change in the heart rate occurs, EFM may be indicated. Intermittent auscultation for low-risk women receiving oxytocin should be every 15 minutes and occur after an oxytocin increase. In addition, one-on-one nurse–patient support is associated with improved maternal satisfaction and improved pain perception (ACOG, 2017c).

UTERINE ACTIVITY ASSESSMENT

Monitoring uterine activity throughout labor is essential and provides data regarding the labor progress and fetal well-being. Numerous internal and external factors affect maternal and fetal well-being. UCs interrupt the flow of blood to the placenta and reduce the amount of oxygen immediately available to the fetus. Decreased oxygen and blood flow directly affect the FHR. The pattern and intensity of contractions have a direct effect on the duration and progress of labor and the ability of the fetus to adapt to the intrapartum process.

UCs occur in wavelike patterns. Adequate labor is generally defined as three to five contractions in 10 minutes, or a contraction every 2 to 3 minutes in active labor. A uterine contraction begins at the fundus (top or apex of the uterus), progresses downward through the lower segments of the uterus, and is followed by a similar wave of relaxation. The contraction of the upper uterine segment increases intrauterine pressure and leads to cervical dilatation and effacement and the descent of the fetus. During and between UCs, the fundus changes shape and firmness, reflecting the intensity of the UC. By monitoring the changes in the fundus, the nurse can determine the frequency, duration, and relative strength of the UC, as well as the resting tone of the uterus between contractions (Miller, Miller, & Cypher, 2017). The intensity and frequency of the UC vary from woman to woman and labor to labor. Three methods of monitoring UCs are currently used: Palpation, electronic monitoring with an external tocodynamometer, and electronic monitoring with an internal intrauterine pressure catheter. Each method is discussed in the following sections.

Palpation. **Palpation** is the technique of assessing a uterine contraction by touch. To assess UCs, the nurse places the fingertips of one hand on the top of the uterus. Hand placement is usually on the fundus, but the location may vary based on maternal or fetal position, uterine size and shape, and maternal body composition. Gentle pressure is applied to the abdomen until the firmness of the underlying uterine wall is felt.

The *frequency* of the contractions is measured from the beginning of one contraction to the beginning of the next. The length

TABLE 20–3 Frequency of Maternal-Fetal Assessment and Documentation

PREGNANCY RISK STATUS	ACTIVE LABOR: FIRST STAGE	ACTIVE LABOR: SECOND STAGE	ORGANIZATION
Low risk without oxytocin	Every 30 min	Every 15 min	AWHONN[a]
With oxytocin or risk factors	Every 15 min	Every 5 min	
Low risk	Every 30 min	Every 15 min	ACOG[b]
High risk	Every 15 min	Every 5 min	
Low risk	Every 15–30 min	Every 5 min	ACNM[c]
Documentation	Objective and factual information Ongoing assessments of both mother and fetus Ongoing FHR and uterine activity assessments Interventions and evaluation of responses Communication with patient, support people, providers as indicated[a]		

SOURCES: Data from

[a]AWHONN, 2015.

[b]ACOG, 2017c.

[c]ACNM, 2015.

of the contraction, referred to as the *duration*, is measured from the beginning of the contraction, when the muscle begins to tense, to the end of the same contraction, when the muscle is completely relaxed. Uterine resting tone is determined between UCs, when optimum uterine relaxation is achieved (Gabbe et al., 2017; Kilpatrick & Garrison, 2017).

During the acme (peak) of the contraction, intensity can be evaluated subjectively by estimating the firmness of the fundus. It can be useful to compare the contraction to the firmness of a nose, chin, or forehead. A tense fundus that is easily indented (tip of the nose) is considered mild intensity. When the fundus becomes firm and difficult to indent with the fingertips (chin), the strength of the UC is considered moderate. The fundus that is hard and cannot be indented (forehead) is classified as strong. The nurse should assess successive contractions to provide reliable data. Direct uterine palpation is used with intermittent auscultation of the fetal heart or in conjunction with continuous EFM. The frequency of palpation depends on the risk status of the mother and fetus and the stage of labor along with the quality of contraction tracing from an internal or external monitor (AWHONN, 2015; Gabbe et al., 2017).

Palpation has its capabilities, benefits, and limitations. Palpation allows the nurse to assess relative frequency, duration, and subjective strength of the contraction and uterine resting tone. UC assessment by palpation is beneficial over electronic monitoring because it (1) is noninvasive and does not increase the risk for infection or patient injury; (2) is readily accessible, requiring no equipment; (3) increases the "hands-on" care of the patient, which can be reassuring to her; and (4) allows the mother freedom from restricting and sometimes uncomfortable abdominal belts, thus permitting her to move freely and ambulate if her condition permits. Palpation is limited because it does not provide actual quantitative measure of uterine pressure; thus, subjective differences between nurses and nurse-to-patient interpretations may exist. Palpation offers no permanent record, which can hinder interpretation by others. Maternal size and increased adipose tissue from obesity and maternal positioning may prevent direct palpation of the fundus. The limitations of palpation may outweigh the benefits in some clinical situations, and electronic monitoring may be a more appropriate choice for uterine assessment (Gabbe et al., 2017).

Electronic Monitoring with External Tocodynamometer. Electronic monitoring of uterine contractions can be done externally by using a tocodynamometer or tocotransducer (toco). A *toco* is a pressure-monitoring device that is placed on the maternal abdomen at or near the fundus (the area of greatest contractility) and held in place with an elastic belt, belly band, or other adhesive material. By placing the toco over a fetal part in the fundus rather than a pocket of amniotic fluid, a better contraction tracing can be obtained (Gabbe et al., 2017). As the uterus contracts, pressure exerted against the toco is amplified and transmitted to the EFM and recorded on graph paper.

The procedure for applying the tocotransducer begins with palpation of the uterus to locate the fundus. The toco monitors uterine activity transabdominally by detecting changes in the abdominal wall and converting the fundal movement into electronic impulses. The toco can be used to assess UCs for *frequency* (timing) and *duration* (length). However, it cannot determine UC intensity (strength). The displayed numbers and graph tracing for UC intensity are arbitrary and are influenced by how tightly the belt is applied around the maternal abdomen or the maternal position. Palpation must be used to assess UC intensity when the external toco monitor is used. When the belt is tight enough, the nurse should be able to note the beginning of contractions on the monitor just before or at the same time the woman begins to feel them (Gabbe et al., 2017).

A beltless tocodynamometer system featuring remote telemetry is available. This system consists of an adhesive transducer that is applied to the most prominent part of the woman's abdomen with a double-sided adhesive film. The nonbelted tocodynamometer tends to be preferred by the laboring woman because it allows more freedom of movement, is easily applied, needs readjustment infrequently, and is generally more convenient. It enables upright positions, which promote fetal descent by gravity, as well as ambulation, which can shorten the labor course and increase comfort for the laboring woman (Gabbe et al., 2017).

The advantages to using a toco for assessing uterine contractions are that it is noninvasive, is easy to place, and may be used both before and following rupture of membranes. Because it is noninvasive, it can be used intermittently to allow the woman to ambulate, shower, or use a whirlpool bath. The toco also provides a permanent, continuous recording of the duration and frequency of contractions for future evaluation. Placement of the tocotransducer influences the accuracy of the uterine graphic tracing. As with any type of technology, no toco is flawless, and the monitor cannot fill the role of the nurse. The nurse should routinely palpate the intensity of the contractions and the relaxation of the uterus between contractions and compare the assessment with data recorded by the monitor. Another disadvantage is that sometimes the belt may become uncomfortable because it must be worn snugly to monitor UCs accurately. The belt may require frequent readjustment as the mother changes position. The mother may also feel inhibited to move or as though she needs to remain in one position so as not to disturb the belt.

Electronic Monitoring by Internal Pressure Catheter. Electronic monitoring of UCs can be done internally by using an **intrauterine pressure catheter (IUPC)**. The IUPC is a catheter that is inserted into the uterine cavity through the cervical os. With correct placement in the uterus, usually in the area of the fetal small parts (arms or legs), the catheter reflects the pressure inside the uterine cavity. As the pressure changes in the uterus, the changes are relayed through a transducer to the fetal monitor, producing a tracing on graph paper. The IUPC can measure the resting tone of the uterus between contractions and the actual amount of intrauterine pressure during contractions, referred to as UC intensity (Gabbe et al., 2017).

IUPCs can be one of two types: Fluid-filled catheters and solid-tipped catheters. Fluid-filled catheters are a single-lumen catheter connected to a pressure-sensitive diaphragm outside the uterus. As intrauterine pressure changes, the column of fluid in the catheter fluctuates and exerts pressure on the diaphragm, sending signals to the transducer and fetal monitor. The solid-tipped catheter uses more recent technology in that the catheter contains a solid-state micropressure transducer (electronic sensor) at its tip, and the catheter is inserted directly into the uterine cavity through the cervical os. The catheter is then connected by a cable to the EFM. The catheter also incorporates a second lumen, permitting amnioinfusion while simultaneously providing accurate monitoring of intrauterine pressure (Gabbe et al., 2017). Regardless of the type of catheter, fluid filled or solid tipped, the IUPC can be used only after membranes are ruptured and the patient has adequate cervical dilation, usually 2 to 3 cm or more (Gabbe et al., 2017).

The IUPC has several benefits over an external tocotransducer or palpation. Because the IUPC is inserted directly into the uterus, it provides near-exact pressure measurements for contraction intensity and uterine resting tone. The increased sensitivity of the IUPC allows for very accurate timing of UCs, thus making it extremely useful in cases when the provider needs closer uterine monitoring; additionally, it is less affected by increased maternal BMI than other methods. The IUPC may be the preferred method of monitoring when it is particularly important to avoid tachysystole and possible uterine rupture in a woman with a previous history of cesarean birth who is attempting a vaginal birth after cesarean (VBAC) and is receiving oxytocin. If the woman's labor is prolonged, internal monitoring can be used to accurately assess the frequency and strength of contractions. If a nonreassuring FHR tracing is present, internal monitoring with IUPC and fetal scalp electrode may be essential to correlate UC timing and FHR pattern response. IUPCs are also placed when meconium-stained amniotic fluid is present (Raghuraman, & Cahill, 2017).The IUPC provides a permanent record of the uterine activity for future analysis and documentation, making it useful in patient care decision making.

With all of its benefits, however, the IUPC has its limitations and risks. Use of IUPCs is limited by the clinical situation. Membranes must be ruptured and adequate cervical dilatation must be achieved for insertion. The procedure is invasive and increases the risk of uterine infection or uterine perforation or trauma (Harper, Shanks, Tuuli, et al., 2013). When an intrauterine catheter is used, there is a slight risk of infection, but this seems to depend on the duration of ruptured membranes and length of labor (Euliano et al., 2016; Gabbe et al., 2017). Invasive equipment like the IUPC is contraindicated in cases when active infections can be transmitted vertically through the cervix into the uterus to the fetus. Insertion of an IUPC with a low-lying placenta can result in placenta puncture, which can cause hemorrhage and nonreassuring fetal status (Gabbe et al., 2017). IUPCs also require proper insertion and zeroing procedures; thus, competency in insertion technique and equipment maintenance and troubleshooting is essential.

CERVICAL ASSESSMENT

Cervical dilatation (see Table 20–2) and effacement are evaluated directly by vaginal examination (see *Clinical Skill 20–1: Performing an Intrapartum Vaginal Examination*). The vaginal examination can also provide information regarding fetal position, station of the presenting part, and membrane status (intact or ruptured). To assist in evaluating membrane status, the nurse assesses for the presence of amniotic fluid (see *Clinical Skill 20–2: Assessing for Amniotic Fluid*).

Clinical Skill 20-1

Performing an Intrapartum Vaginal Examination

NURSING ACTION

Preparation

- Explain the procedure, the indications for the exam, what the exam may feel like, and that it may cause discomfort.
- Assess for latex allergies.
- Position the woman with her thighs flexed and abducted. Instruct her to put the heels of her feet together. Drape the woman with a sheet, leaving a flap to access the perineum.

Rationale: *This position provides access to the woman's perineum. The drape ensures privacy.*

- Encourage the woman to relax her muscles and legs.
- Inform the woman before touching her. Be gentle.

Rationale: *Relaxation decreases muscle tension and increases comfort.*

Equipment and Supplies

Clean disposable gloves if membranes not ruptured

Sterile gloves if membranes ruptured

Lubricant

Nitrazine test tape

Slide

Sterile cotton-tipped swab (Q-tip)

Before the Procedure: Test for Fluid Leakage

If fluid leakage has been reported or noted, use Nitrazine test tape and Q-tip with slide for fern test before performing the exam (see *Clinical Skill 20–2*).

Procedure

Clean gloves (sterile if membranes ruptured)

CLINICAL TIP

Digital examination may be deferred if the woman has ruptured membranes but is not in active labor (Simkin, Hanson, & Ancheta, 2017).

1. Pull glove onto dominant hand.

Rationale: *Single glove is worn when membranes are intact. If a sterile exam is needed, both hands will be gloved with sterile gloves.*

2. Using your gloved hand, position the hand with the wrist straight and the elbow tilted downward. Insert your well-lubricated second and index fingers of the gloved hand gently into the vagina until they touch the cervix. Use care when positioning your hand.

Rationale: *This position allows the fingertips to point toward the umbilicus and find the cervix.*

3. If the woman verbalizes discomfort, acknowledge it and apologize. Pause for a moment and allow her to relax before progressing.

Rationale: *This validates the woman's discomfort and helps her feel more in control.*

(continued)

Clinical Skill 20-1 *(continued)*

4. To determine the status of labor progress, perform the vaginal examination during and between contractions.

Rationale: *Cervical effacement, dilatation, and fetal station are affected by the presence of a contraction.*

5. Palpate for the opening, or a depression, in the cervix. Estimate the diameter of the depression to identify the amount of dilatation (Figure 20–1).

Rationale: *Allows determination of effacement and dilatation.*

6. Determine the status of the fetal membranes by observing for leakage of amniotic fluid. If fluid is expressed, test for amniotic fluid and note any foul odor or discoloration.
7. Palpate the presenting part (Figure 20–2).

Rationale: *Determining the presenting part is necessary to assess the position of the fetus and to evaluate fetal descent.*

8. Assess the fetal descent (Figure 20–3) and station by identifying the position of the posterior fontanelle in relation to the ischial spines.
9. Record findings on woman's chart/EMR.

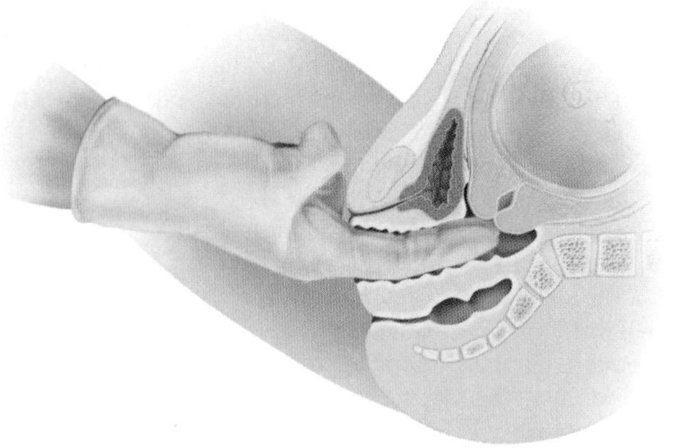

Figure 20–1 **To gauge cervical dilatation, the nurse places the index and middle fingers against the cervix and determines the size of the opening. Before labor begins, the cervix is long (approximately 2–5 cm), the sides feel thick, and the cervical canal is closed, so an examining finger cannot be inserted. During labor, the cervix begins to dilate, and the size of the opening progresses from 1 cm to 10 cm in diameter.**

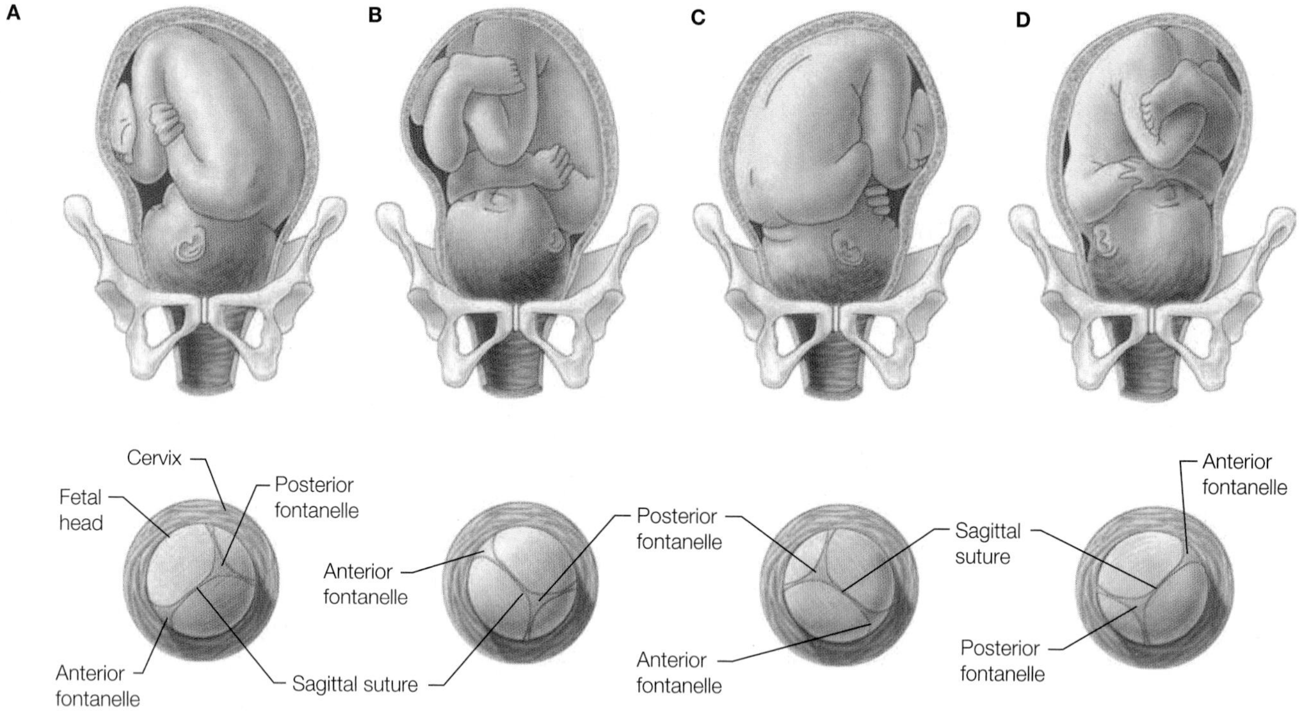

Figure 20–2 **Palpation of the presenting part (the portion of the fetus that enters the pelvis first). A. Left occiput anterior (LOA). The occiput (area over the occipital bone on the posterior part of the fetal head) is in the left anterior quadrant of the woman's pelvis. When the fetus is in LOA, the posterior fontanelles (located just above the occipital bone and triangular in shape) are in the upper left quadrant of the maternal pelvis. B. Left occiput posterior (LOP). The posterior fontanelle is in the lower left quadrant of the maternal pelvis. C. Right occiput anterior (ROA). The posterior fontanelle is in the upper right quadrant of the maternal pelvis. D. Right occiput posterior (ROP). The posterior fontanelle is in the lower right quadrant of the maternal pelvis.**

NOTE: The anterior fontanelle is diamond shaped. Because of the roundness of the fetal head, only a portion of the anterior fontanelle can be seen in each of the views, so it appears to be triangular in shape.

10. Document that the procedure was explained to the patient and that the woman verbalized understanding and provided consent before the vaginal examination. The woman's reaction and how the procedure was tolerated should be documented. The findings of the examination should be clearly documented using a facility-appropriate documentation form.

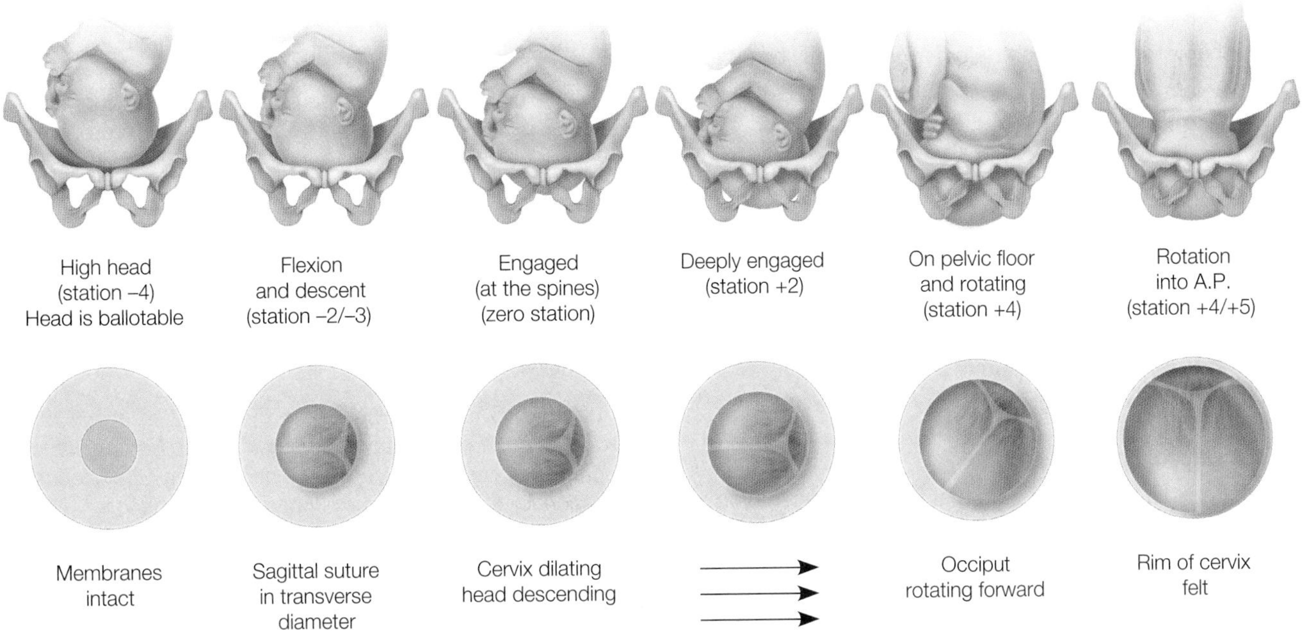

Figure 20–3 Descent of the fetus through the maternal pelvis can be assessed by determining station (the relationship of the presenting part to an imaginary line between the maternal ischial spines). As the fetus moves downward, cardinal movements occur. The nurse assesses the station and identifies the cardinal movements by determining the position of the posterior fontanelle. The upper panels depict the fetal head progressing downward through the pelvis. From left to right, the first four views depict descent and flexion of the fetal chin onto the fetal chest. In the last two views, internal rotation occurs. Each view also depicts downward movement of the fetal head through the maternal pelvis as measured by the change in station. The lower panels depict the cervix, which is still rather thick (little effacement has occurred). The amniotic membranes are still intact over the fetal head. When the fetus is at –4 station, the fetal head is ballotable (when it is touched by the examining nurse's finger, the head floats upward and resettles downward). In the second view, note the thinner cervix (which indicates that more effacement has occurred). The sagittal suture and posterior fontanelle can be palpated. The next two views depict further effacement and descent of the fetal head from 0 station to +2. The last two views depict continuing effacement and position that would be felt on vaginal examination of the presenting part while the fetal head is completing internal rotation.

Fetal Assessment

A complete intrapartum fetal assessment requires determination of the fetal position and presentation and evaluation of the fetal status.

Determination of Fetal Position and Presentation

Fetal position is determined in several ways, including:

- Inspection of the woman's abdomen
- Palpation of the woman's abdomen (Leopold maneuvers)
- Vaginal examination to determine the presenting part
- Ultrasound.

INSPECTION

The nurse should observe the woman's abdomen for size and shape. The lie of the fetus should be assessed by noting whether the uterus projects up and down (longitudinal lie) or left to right (transverse lie) (Gabbe et al, 2017; Holley, 2017).

PALPATION: LEOPOLD MANEUVERS

Leopold maneuvers are a systematic way to evaluate the maternal abdomen (Figure 20–4). Frequent practice increases the examiner's skill in determining fetal position by palpation. Leopold maneuvers may be difficult to perform on an obese woman or on a woman who has excessive amniotic fluid (hydramnios).

Care should be taken to ensure the woman's comfort during Leopold maneuvers. The woman should have recently emptied her bladder and should lie on her back with her abdomen

Clinical Skill 20-2

Assessing for Amniotic Fluid

NURSING ACTION

Preparation

- Explain the procedure, indications for the procedure, what the woman will feel, and information that may be obtained.
- Determine whether she has noted the escape of any fluid from her vagina.

Equipment and Supplies

Nitrazine test tape
Sterile speculum
A glass slide and a sterile cotton-tipped swab (Q-tip)
Sterile syringe
Microscope

Procedure: Sterile Gloves

1. Complete this test before doing an examination that requires the use of lubricant.

2. Put on sterile gloves. With one gloved hand, spread the labia, and with the other gloved hand place a small section of Nitrazine tape (approximately 2 in. long) against the vaginal opening. Take care not to touch the tape with bare fingers before the test.

Rationale: *Contamination of the Nitrazine test tape with lubricant can make the test unreliable. Enough fluid needs to be placed on the test tape to make it wet.*

3. Compare the color on the test tape to the guide on the back of the Nitrazine test tape container to determine test results.

Rationale: *Amniotic fluid is alkaline, and an alkaline fluid turns the Nitrazine test tape a dark blue. If the test tape remains a beige color, the test is negative for amniotic fluid. The normal vaginal pH is 3.8 to 4.5, whereas amniotic fluid has a pH of 7.1 to 7.3.*

4. Amniotic fluid may also be obtained by speculum exam. This is indicated in preterm premature rupture of membranes. If fluid is present in sufficient amount to draw some into a syringe, a small amount should be collected, or the pool of fluid in the posterior vagina can be obtained with a sterile cotton swab. A small amount of fluid is placed on a glass slide, allowed to dry, and then examined under a microscope or sent to the lab. A ferning pattern confirms the presence of amniotic fluid. See Figure 4–1B for an example of ferning.

Rationale: *Obtaining a specimen by speculum examination reduces the contamination of the fluid with other substances such as blood and cervical mucus and reduces the chance of infection for the woman who is not actively laboring.*

5. Record the findings on the labor record. Documentation of the status of membranes should include whether they are intact or ruptured. Other characteristics, such as color, odor, and amount of fluid present, should also be recorded, along with the time of rupture.

uncovered. To aid in relaxation of the abdominal wall, the shoulders should be raised slightly on a pillow and the knees drawn up a little. The procedure should be completed between contractions. The examiner's hands should be warm. The order in which Leopold maneuvers are performed may vary from one clinician to another.

While inspecting and palpating the maternal abdomen, the nurse should consider these questions:

- Is the fetal lie longitudinal or transverse?
- What is in the fundus? Am I feeling buttocks or head?
- Where is the fetal back?
- Where are the small parts or extremities?
- What is in the inlet? Does it confirm what I found in the fundus?
- Is the presenting part engaged, floating, or descending into the inlet? (See Figure 19–8 in Chapter 19.)
- Is there fetal movement?
- How large is the fetus (appropriate, large, or small for gestational age)?
- Is there one fetus or more than one?
- Is fundal height proportionate to the estimated gestational age?

First Maneuver. While facing the woman, the nurse palpates the upper abdomen with both hands (see Figure 20–4A). The nurse determines the shape, size, consistency, and mobility of the form that is found. The fetal head is firm, hard, and round and moves independently of the trunk. The breech feels softer and symmetric and has small bony prominences; it moves with the trunk.

Second Maneuver. After ascertaining whether the head or the buttocks occupies the fundus, the nurse tries to determine the location of the fetal back and notes whether it is on the right or left side of the maternal abdomen. Still facing the woman, the nurse palpates the abdomen with deep but gentle pressure, using the palms (see Figure 20–4B). The right hand should be steady while the left hand explores the right side of the uterus. The nurse then repeats the maneuver, probing with the right hand and steadying the uterus with the left hand. The fetal back should feel firm and smooth and should connect what was found in the fundus with a mass in the inlet. Once the back is located, the nurse validates the finding by palpating the fetal extremities (small irregularities and protrusions) on the opposite side of the abdomen.

Third Maneuver. Next, the nurse should determine what fetal part is lying above the inlet by gently grasping the lower portion of the abdomen just above the symphysis pubis with the thumb

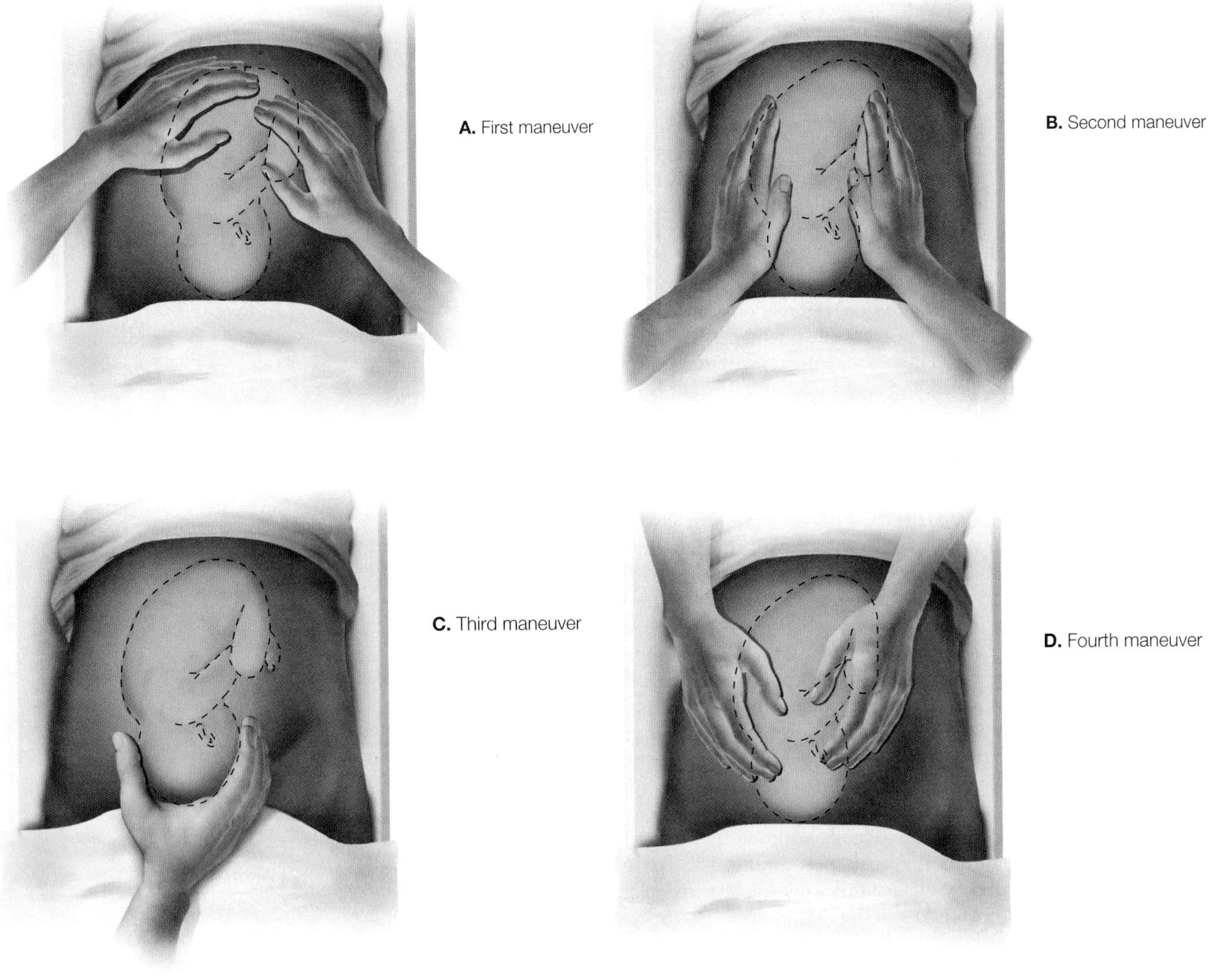

Figure 20–4 **Leopold maneuvers for determining fetal head position, presentation, and lie.**

NOTE: Some practitioners may perform the sequence differently. Many nurses do the fourth maneuver first to identify the part of the fetus in the pelvic inlet.

and fingers of the right hand (see Figure 20–4C). This maneuver yields the opposite information from what was found in the fundus and validates the presenting part. If the head is presenting and is not engaged, it may be gently pushed back and forth.

Fourth Maneuver. For this portion of the examination, the nurse faces the woman's feet and attempts to locate the cephalic prominence or brow. Location of this landmark assists in assessing the descent of the presenting part into the pelvis. The fingers of both hands are moved gently down the sides of the uterus toward the pubis (see Figure 20–4D). The cephalic prominence (brow) is located on the side where there is greatest resistance to the descent of the fingers toward the pubis. It is located on the opposite side from the fetal back if the head is well flexed. However, when the fetal head is extended, the occiput is the first cephalic prominence felt, and it is located on the same side as the back. Therefore, when completing the fourth maneuver, if the nurse finds that the first cephalic prominence palpated is on the same side as the back, the head is not flexed. If the first prominence found is opposite the back, the head is well flexed (Gabbe et al., 2017; Miller et al., 2017).

VAGINAL EXAMINATION

The vaginal examination reveals information regarding the fetus such as presentation, position, station, degree of flexion of the fetal head, and any swelling that may be present on the fetal scalp (caput succedaneum).

Clinical Tip

If you are having difficulty reaching the posterior cervix, ask the woman to place her fists under her buttocks or use a bedpan to facilitate a pelvic tilt, which will make the cervix more accessible.

ULTRASOUND

Real-time ultrasound (US) is frequently available in the birth setting. It may be used to assess fetal lie, presentation, and position; obtain measurements of biparietal diameter to estimate gestational age; assess for anomalies when a vaginal examination reveals suspicious findings; and assess placement of the placenta. Ultrasound is often helpful to pinpoint the fetal heart location when the nurse is having difficulty finding it, such as in cases where there are multiple fetuses. It can also be used to diagnose a fetal demise. (See Chapter 16 for further discussion of the use of ultrasound for fetal assessment.)

Auscultation of Fetal Heart Rate

Auscultation is the direct auditory monitoring and interpretation of the fetal heart in utero. The number of fetal heartbeats per minute (beats/min) is referred to as the fetal heart rate (FHR). Auscultation uses a handheld instrument, such as a fetoscope or ultrasound Doppler, to listen to and count the FHR. Each instrument uses slightly different technology. The fetoscope is an older assessment tool; however, some clinicians and women prefer it because it is "natural" and does not rely on ultrasound. Fetoscopes magnify actual fetal heart sounds, whereas Dopplers use ultrasound to convert fetal myocardial movement into sound waves that are then amplified and sent through a speaker from which the heart rate can be counted. Some Dopplers display a digital readout in addition to the audible sound produced.

Before listening to the FHR the first time, the nurse may choose to perform Leopold maneuvers to determine the probable location to best hear the FHR. The FHR is heard most clearly at the fetal back (Gabbe et al., 2017) (Figure 20–5). Thus, in a cephalic presentation, the FHR is best heard in the lower quadrant of the maternal abdomen. In a breech presentation it is heard at or above the level of the maternal umbilicus. In a transverse lie the FHR may be heard best just above or just below the umbilicus. As the presenting part descends and rotates through the maternal pelvis during labor, the FHR tends to descend and move toward the midline. In some instances, the monitor may track the maternal heart rate instead of the FHR. However, the nurse can avoid the error by comparing the maternal pulse with the FHR.

After the FHR is located, it is usually counted for 30 to 60 seconds to obtain the number of beats per minute. The nurse should listen before, during, and just after a contraction to detect any abnormal heart rate, especially if the FHR is over 160 (tachycardia), if it is under 110 (bradycardia), or if irregular beats (such as a deceleration) are heard. Listening through a contraction may be difficult because of maternal movement or a muffling of the FHR sounds. It is especially important to listen during and after the contraction to detect any deceleration that might occur. It is also important to listen immediately after each contraction when the woman is pushing during the second stage because fetal bradycardia frequently occurs as pressure is exerted on the fetal head during descent. See *Clinical Skill 20–3: Auscultation of Fetal Heart Rate* and Table 20–4 for guidelines regarding how often to auscultate FHR.

Auscultation has been used for many years and remains a very valuable assessment technique even though it uses less technology than EFM. Research and standards have shown that intermittent auscultation is equally effective for monitoring the FHR as EFM when a 1:1 nurse-to-patient ratio is maintained and the pregnant patient remains low risk. There are several other advantages as well; for example, it is less expensive, it allows the laboring woman to have freedom of movement, it is more comfortable than wearing the bands required for EFM, and it allows easier assessment of the FHR during hydrotherapy or in positions other than supine in bed (Miller et al., 2017).

Use of auscultation to assess the FHR does have some limitations for the nurse to consider. It may be hard to hear the FHR when the maternal conditions include obesity or polyhydramnios. There is no visual or permanent recording of the FHR as there is with the use of the electronic fetal monitor. There is no way to assess FHR variability or to hear or see the changes in fetal heart rate patterns, especially when there is only intermittent assessment of the FHR, thus making it recommended only for use in low-risk pregnancies (Miller et al., 2017). Low-risk status has been defined as a pregnancy with no pregnancy risk factors, clear amniotic fluid with no evidence of meconium, and normal labor patterns. Women receiving Pitocin augmentation or induction that meet this criteria are also considered low risk and can be monitored intermittently as long as the labor pattern and FHR are within the normal range. Outside these parameters, intermittent auscultation may not be appropriate and should not be used to assess high-risk pregnancies (Gabbe et al., 2017). Figure 20–6 shows the use of a Doppler to auscultate the FHR.

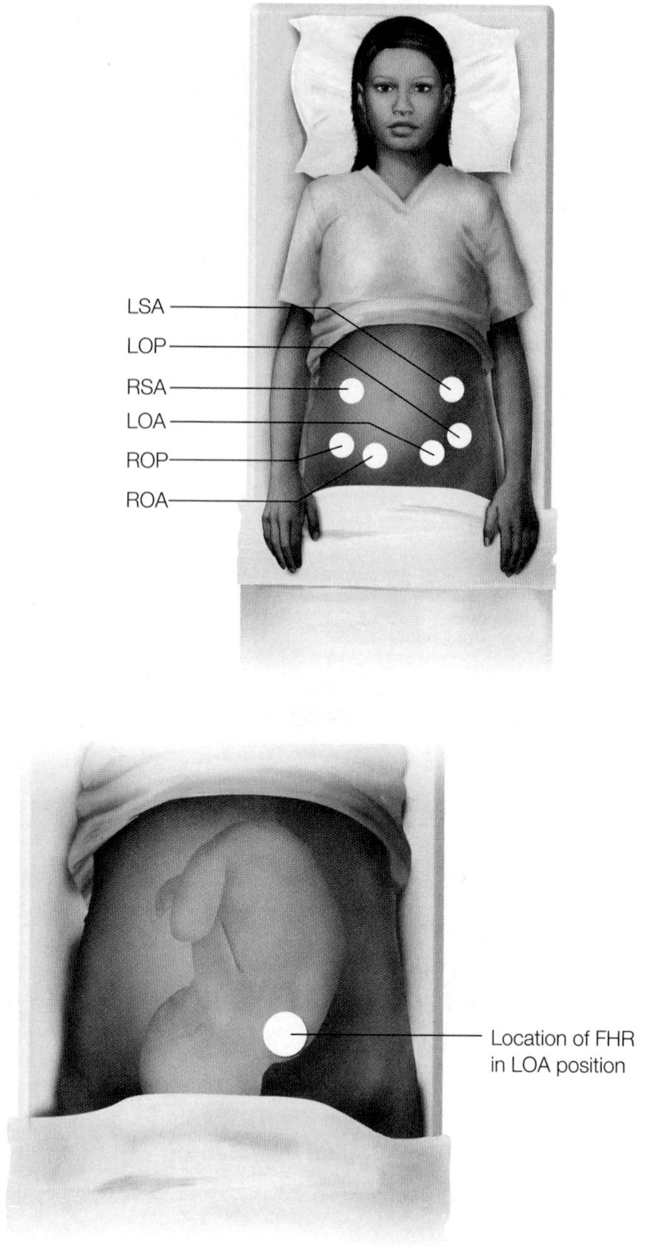

Figure 20–5 **Location of FHR in relation to the more commonly seen fetal positions. The FHR is heard more clearly over the fetal back.**

Auscultation is a learned skill and requires practice and knowledge of its benefits and limitations as an assessment tool. Identifying patterns and nonreassuring FHR is difficult and requires training. Auscultation must be practiced to ensure accurate interpretation of data.

Clinical Skill 20-3

Auscultation of Fetal Heart Rate

NURSING ACTION

Preparation

- Explain the procedure, the indications for it, and the information that will be obtained.
- Uncover the woman's abdomen.

Equipment and Supplies

Handheld Doppler device or fetoscope

Ultrasonic gel if using a Doppler device

CLINICAL TIP

The fetal heart rate is heard most clearly through the fetal back. Locate the fetal back using Leopold maneuvers.

Procedure

1. Listening for the fetal heart rate using the Doppler:
   - Place ultrasonic gel on the diaphragm of the Doppler. Gel is used to maintain contact with the maternal abdomen and enhances conduction of sound.
   - The diaphragm should be warmed prior to using the Doppler.
   - Place the Doppler diaphragm on the woman's abdomen halfway between the umbilicus and symphysis and in the midline. You are most likely to hear the FHR in this area. Listen carefully for the sound of the fetal heartbeat.
2. Check the woman's pulse against the fetal sounds you hear. If the rates are the same, reposition the Doppler and try again.

Rationale: *If the rates are the same, you are probably hearing the maternal pulse and not the FHR.*

3. If the rates are not similar, count the FHR for 1 full minute. Note that the FHR has a double rhythm and only one sound is counted.
4. If you do not locate the FHR, move the Doppler laterally.
5. Auscultate the FHR between, during, and for 30 seconds following a uterine contraction.
6. Frequency recommendations:
   - Low-risk women: Every 30 minutes during the first stage and every 15 minutes in the second stage.
   - High-risk women: Every 15 minutes during the first stage and every 5 minutes in the second stage.

Rationale: *This evaluation provides the opportunity to assess the fetal status and response to labor.*

7. Document that the procedure was explained to the woman and that she verbalized understanding. The location of the FHR, FHR baseline, changes in FHR that occur with contractions, and presence of accelerations or decelerations should be included. Other characteristics should include variability, maternal position, type of device used, uterine activity, maternal pulse, and nursing interventions that were performed.

Auscultation with the Fetoscope

The fetoscope is an older assessment tool; however, some clinicians prefer it because it is "natural" and does not rely on ultrasound. Some women seeking prenatal care outside of a traditional care environment may request the use of a fetoscope.

TABLE 20–4 Frequency of Auscultation: Assessment and Documentation

ASSESS FHR BEFORE:
Initiation of labor-enhancing procedures (e.g., artificial rupture of membranes)
Periods of ambulation
Administration of medications
Administration or initiation of analgesia/anesthesia
ASSESS FHR FOLLOWING:
Rupture of membranes
Recognition of abnormal uterine activity patterns, such as increased basal tone or tachysystole
Evaluation of oxytocin (maintenance, increase, or decrease of dosage)
Administration of medications (at time of peak action)
Expulsion of enema
Urinary catheterization
Vaginal examination
Periods of ambulation
Evaluation of analgesia and/or anesthesia (maintenance, increase, or decrease of dosage)

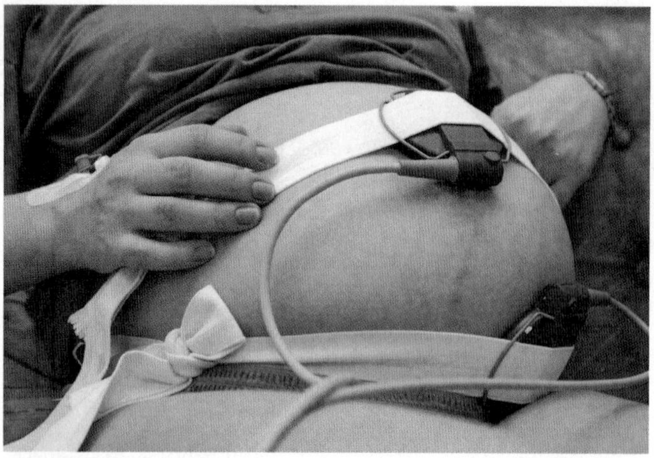

Figure 20–6 **The nurse uses a Doppler to assess the fetal heart rate. Doppler monitors can be used for intermittent labor monitoring or in the outpatient or community setting.**

SOURCE: Artur Steinhagen/Fotolia.

Identifying UCs and the FHR simultaneously is necessary to determine patterns in the FHR and the relationship between the FHR and the UC. Auscultation does not allow for the detection of small changes in the FHR and cannot determine baseline variability. It may also be limited by maternal obesity and movement by the mother and fetus (Simkin et al., 2017). In such instances, it may be essential to monitor using electronic means, regardless of the patient's risk status.

Electronic Fetal Monitoring

Electronic fetal monitoring provides a continuous tracing of the fetal heart rate, allowing characteristics of the FHR to be observed and evaluated (see Figure 20–7 and *Clinical Skill 20–4: Electronic Fetal Monitoring*). EFM requires advanced assessment and clinical judgment skills, regardless of the setting in which it is used. Therefore, licensed, experienced healthcare professionals should perform each aspect of fetal heart monitoring (FHM), consistent with their state or provincial scope of practice. AWHONN maintains that fetal heart monitoring includes (1) application of fetal monitoring components, (2) intermittent auscultation, (3) ongoing monitoring and interpretation of FHR data, (4) initial assessment of the laboring woman and fetus, and (5) ongoing clinical interventions and evaluations of the woman and fetus (Simkin et al., 2017).

Initiation of monitoring and ongoing clinical evaluation should only be performed by healthcare professionals who have education and skills validation in FHM and in the care of the laboring woman. AWHONN regards these healthcare professionals with expertise in fetal monitoring as (1) registered nurses; (2) certified nurse midwives (CNMs), certified midwives (CMs), and registered midwives (RMs [Canada]); (3) other advanced practice nurses such as nurse practitioners and clinical nurse specialists; (4) physicians; and (5) physician assistants (PAs).

In an effort to resolve controversy surrounding the benefits and interpretations of EFM and interventions for nonreassuring tracings, the National Institute of Child Health and Human Development (NICHD) Research Planning Workshop was held in the late 1990s. As a result, standardized, unambiguous definitions for FHR tracings were proposed (Simkin et al., 2017). In 2004, the Joint Commission on Accreditation of Healthcare

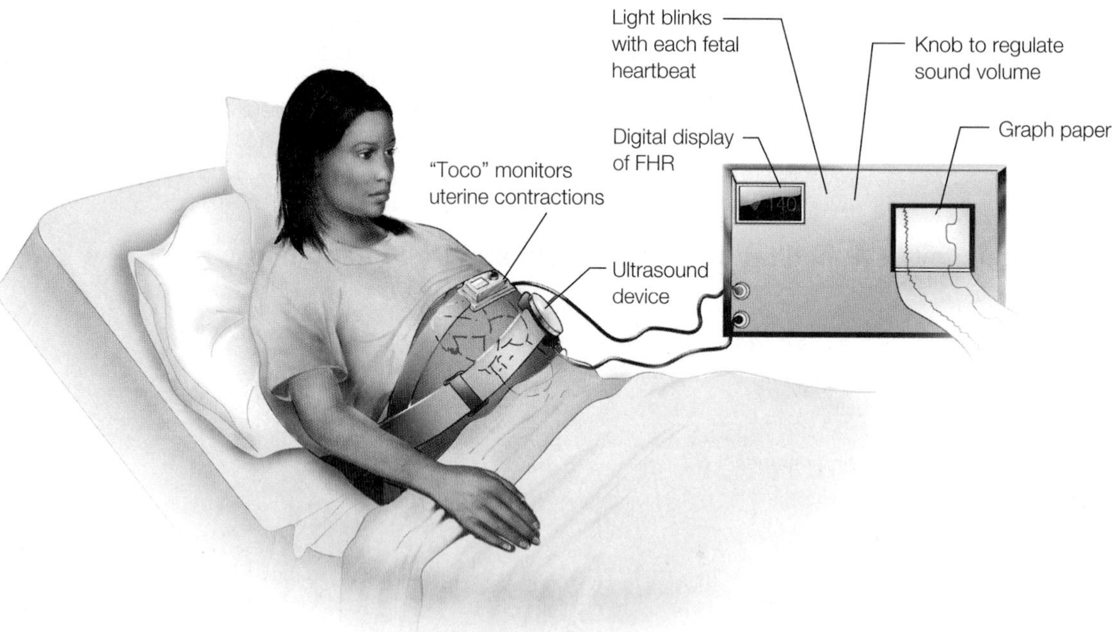

Figure 20–7 **Electronic monitoring by external technique. The ultrasound device is placed over the area of the fetal back and transmits information about the FHR. The tocodynamometer (toco) is placed over the uterine fundus to provide information used to monitor uterine contractions. Information from both devices is transmitted to the electronic fetal monitor. The FHR is shown in a digital display (as a blinking light), on the special monitor paper, and audibly (by adjusting a knob on the monitor). The uterine contractions are displayed on the special monitor paper as well.**

Clinical Skill 20–4

Electronic Fetal Monitoring

NURSING ACTION

Preparation

- Explain the procedure, the indications for it, and the information that will be obtained.

Equipment and Supplies

Monitor
Two elastic monitor belts
Tocodynamometer (toco)
Ultrasound transducer
Ultrasound gel

CLINICAL TIP

Evaluating the FHR tracing provides information about fetal status and response to the stress of labor. The presence of reassuring characteristics is associated with good fetal outcomes. Rapid identification of nonreassuring characteristics allows prompt interventions and the opportunity to determine the fetal response to the interventions.

Procedure

1. Turn on the monitor.
2. Place the two elastic belts around the woman's abdomen.
3. Place the toco over the uterine fundus off the midline on the area palpated to be firmest during contractions. Secure it with one of the elastic belts.

Rationale: *The uterine fundus is the area of greatest contractility.*

4. Note the UC tracing. The resting tone tracing (i.e., without a UC) should be recording on the 10 or 15 mmHg pressure line. Adjust the line to reflect that reading.

Rationale: *If the resting tone is set on the zero line, there is often a constant grinding noise.*

5. Apply the ultrasonic gel to the diaphragm of the ultrasound transducer.

Rationale: *Ultrasonic gel is used to maintain contact with the maternal abdomen. The ultrasonic beam is directed toward the fetal heart.*

6. Place the diaphragm on the maternal abdomen in the midline between the umbilicus and the symphysis pubis.
7. Listen for the FHR, which will have a whiplike or galloping sound. Move the diaphragm laterally, if necessary, to obtain a stronger sound (refer to Figure 20–5).
8. When the FHR is located, attach the second elastic belt snugly to the transducer.

Rationale: *Firm contact is necessary to maintain a steady tracing.*

9. Place the following information on the beginning of the fetal monitor paper: Date, time, woman's name, gravida, para, membrane status, and name of healthcare provider.
10. Ongoing documentation should provide information about FHR including baseline rate in beats per minute (beats/min), variability, response to uterine contractions (accelerations or decelerations), procedures performed, changes in position, and the like, as well as any therapy initiated. The maternal pulse should be assessed and documented to ensure the tracing is not detecting the maternal heartbeat. Tracing should be categorized using the three-tier system (see later discussion).

Note: Each birthing unit may have specific guidelines about additional information to include. A full description of fetal monitoring analysis is beyond the scope of this text.

Organizations (JCAHO) recommended standardized and consistent use of fetal monitoring terminology among all healthcare professionals and the development of clear guidelines for fetal monitoring of potential high-risk patients.

In 2008, ACOG, NICHD, and the Society for Maternal-Fetal Medicine sponsored a workshop updating the EFM nomenclature. A three-tiered intrapartum categorization system was recommended, with nomenclature and interpretation for management of fetal heart rate patterns. In November 2010, ACOG issued a Practice Bulletin on intrapartum FHR tracings that provides a framework for evaluation and management of intrapartum EFM patterns based on the three-tiered categorization system (ACOG, 2017c). This chapter reflects the most recent guidelines at the time of this book's publication instituted by ACOG, AWHONN, and NICHD for FHR tracings.

INDICATIONS FOR ELECTRONIC FETAL MONITORING

AAP and ACOG state that the method of FHR monitoring used during labor should be based on risk assessment at admission, patient and obstetric staff preference, and departmental policy. Although there is no standardized list, Table 20–5 identifies some common indications for EFM. Low-risk women should be monitored with intermittent auscultation.

EXTERNAL MONITORING

Electronic monitoring of the FHR can be done externally by using an ultrasound transducer. The US transducer is a Doppler device with computerized logic to interpret and count the Doppler signals (Simkin et al., 2017). The US transducer is placed on the maternal abdomen over the fetal back (as determined by Leopold

TABLE 20–5 Possible Indications for Electronic Fetal Monitoring

Fetal Factors
Decreased fetal movement
Abnormal auscultatory FHR
Meconium passage
Abnormal presentations/positions
IUGR or SGA fetus
Postdates (greater than 41 weeks)
Multiple gestation
Maternal Factors
Fever
Infections
Preeclampsia
Disease conditions (e.g., hypertension, diabetes)
Anemia
Obesity
Rh alloimmunization
Previous perinatal death
Grand multiparity
Previous cesarean birth
Borderline/contracted pelvis
Uterine Factors
Dysfunctional labor
Failure to progress in labor
Oxytocin induction/augmentation
Uterine anomalies
Complications of Pregnancy
Prolonged rupture of membranes
Premature rupture of membranes
Preterm labor
Marginal abruptio placentae
Partial placenta previa
Occult/frank prolapse of cord
Amnionitis
Regional Anesthesia
Elective Monitoring

maneuvers), where the FHR is usually the loudest, and is held in place with an elastic belt. A water-soluble gel is applied to the underside of the transducer to aid in conduction of the fetal heart sounds. The US transducer then emits ultrasonic beams that reflect off the moving fetal myocardium and return to the transducer. The transducer receives the signal and interprets it before amplifying it in the fetal monitor and recording it on graph paper (refer to Figure 20–7). The US image can be influenced by other moving structures in the maternal abdomen, such as maternal arterial blood flow and maternal or fetal movement. Interference is generally filtered out; however, on occasion the maternal heart rate is detected by the US transducer and must be distinguished from the FHR by comparing the signal with the maternal pulse.

The external US transducer can be more beneficial than auscultating the FHR because it produces a continuous graphic recording. The US transducer can show the baseline (BL), baseline variability (BL VAR), and changes in the FHR. It is noninvasive and does not require rupture of membranes or minimal cervical dilation. FHR monitoring by US transducer is limited because it is susceptible to interference from maternal and fetal movement, as discussed earlier, and may produce a weak signal (King et al., 2014; Simkin et al., 2017). The tracing may become sketchy and difficult to interpret. Repeating the procedure for US placement usually remedies the weak signal and tracing.

INTERNAL MONITORING

Internal fetal monitoring is accomplished with a fetal scalp electrode (FSE), a fine surgical spiral wire attached to the fetal scalp. The FSE is the most precise method of monitoring because it is a direct electrocardiogram (ECG) of the FHR and produces the most accurate FHR tracing. The FSE is attached to the fetus during a vaginal exam. Once in place, the electrode is connected to the fetal monitor. The monitor determines the time between fetal "R" waves in the "QRS" complex and calculates the findings into a FHR. The FHR is then recorded on graph paper.

For the spiral electrode to be inserted, the cervix must be dilated at least 2 cm, the presenting fetal part must be accessible by vaginal examination, and the membranes must be ruptured. Even though it is not possible to apply the electrode and catheter under strict sterile conditions, the procedure should be performed as aseptically as possible. After determining fetal position by vaginal examination, the examiner (physician, midwife, or nurse) inserts the electrode, which is encased in a plastic guide, to the level of the internal cervical os and attaches it to the presenting part, being careful not to apply it to the face, suture lines, fontanelles, cervix, or perineum if the fetus is in a breech presentation (Gabbe et al., 2017; King et al., 2014). The electrode is rotated clockwise until it is attached to the presenting part and is then disengaged from the guide tube (Figure 20–8). The guide tube is removed, and the end wires are connected to a leg plate that is attached to the woman's thigh. The cable from the leg plate is connected to the monitor. Infections and injuries from internal electrodes and catheters are a small but actual risk.

Because the risk of transmission to the fetus is increased by the small puncture in the fetal scalp, the use of a FSE should be avoided if at all possible in the presence of intact fetal membranes; any contraindication to cervical exams, such as active vaginal bleeding from an unknown source or placenta previa or known maternal infections such as HIV, herpes simplex virus (HSV), or hepatitis. The Centers for Disease Control and Prevention (CDC, 2016) states that there is insufficient data at this time to determine if use of a FSE is associated with an increased risk for early-onset group B streptococcus (GBS) in the neonate; therefore, a decision to use it should be based on risks versus benefits for laboring women who test GBS positive. Fetal scalp monitors are also avoided in preterm babies because of the increased risk of ventricular hemorrhage (Gabbe et al., 2017; Simkin et al., 2017). The fetal scalp electrode is removed prior to birth.

The FHR tracing at the top of Figure 20–9 was obtained by internal monitoring, and the uterine contraction tracing at the bottom was obtained by external monitoring. A comparison shows that the spiral electrode provides an instantaneous and continuous recording of FHR that is clearer than the data provided by external monitoring. Notice that the FHR shows variability (the tracing moves up and down instead of in a straight line), ranging between about 140 and 155 beats/min.

TELEMETRY

As discussed previously, FHR and uterine activity may also be monitored by a telemetry system. Equipment consists of US along with external uterine pressure transducers connected to a small battery-operated transmitter. Signals are transmitted to a

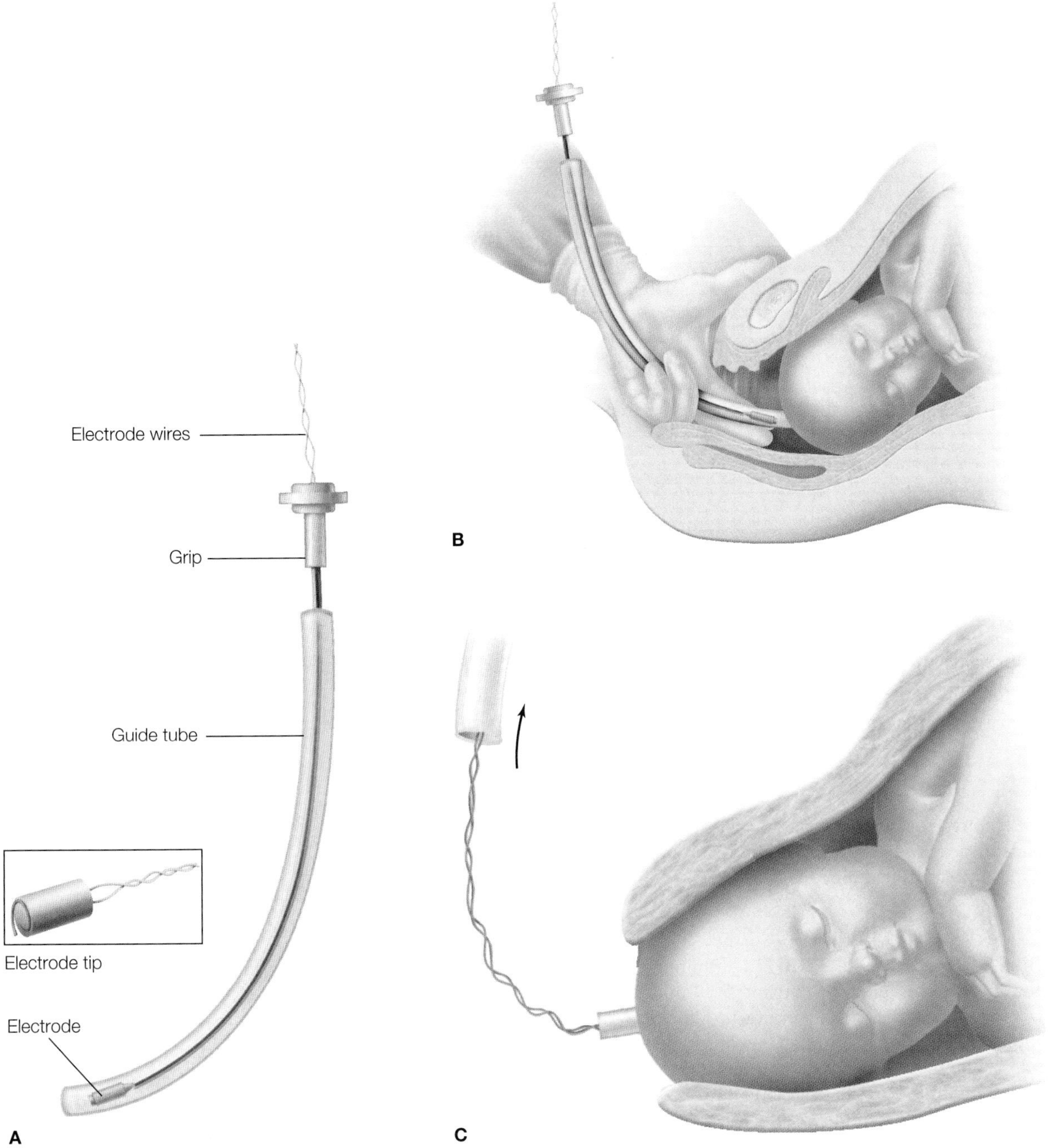

Figure 20–8 **Techniques for internal, direct fetal monitoring. A. Spiral electrode. B. Attaching the spiral electrode to the scalp. C. Attached spiral electrode with guide tube removed.**

receiver connected to a monitor that displays FHR and uterine activity data. A printout provides documentation. This system, which can be worn on a shoulder strap, allows the woman to ambulate, helping her to feel more comfortable and less confined during labor, yet provides for continuous monitoring. Telemetry provides for direct as well as indirect monitoring of FHR, indirect monitoring of uterine pressure, and dual FHR monitoring of twins.

Fetal Heart Rate Patterns

When the FHR is monitored electronically, the interval between two successive fetal heartbeats is continually measured. The rate is displayed as if the beats occurred at the same interval for 60 seconds. For example, if the interval between beats is 0.5 second per 60 seconds, then divide the interval time into the time frame. The rate for the full minute would then be 60 seconds/0.5 = 120 beats/min.

Fetal heart rate patterns are described by baseline rate, variability, accelerations, and decelerations and are categorized using a three-tier system (Simkin et al., 2017). *Periodic patterns* are those associated with uterine contractions, and *episodic patterns* are those not associated with uterine contractions. The definitions for FHR pattern categorization—jointly developed in 2008 by NICHD, ACOG, and SMFM—have a three-tier classification for interpretation (shown in Table 20–7 later in the chapter) (Gabbe et al, 2017). Standardized terminology minimizes variation among care providers, allows for accurate documentation of fetal status

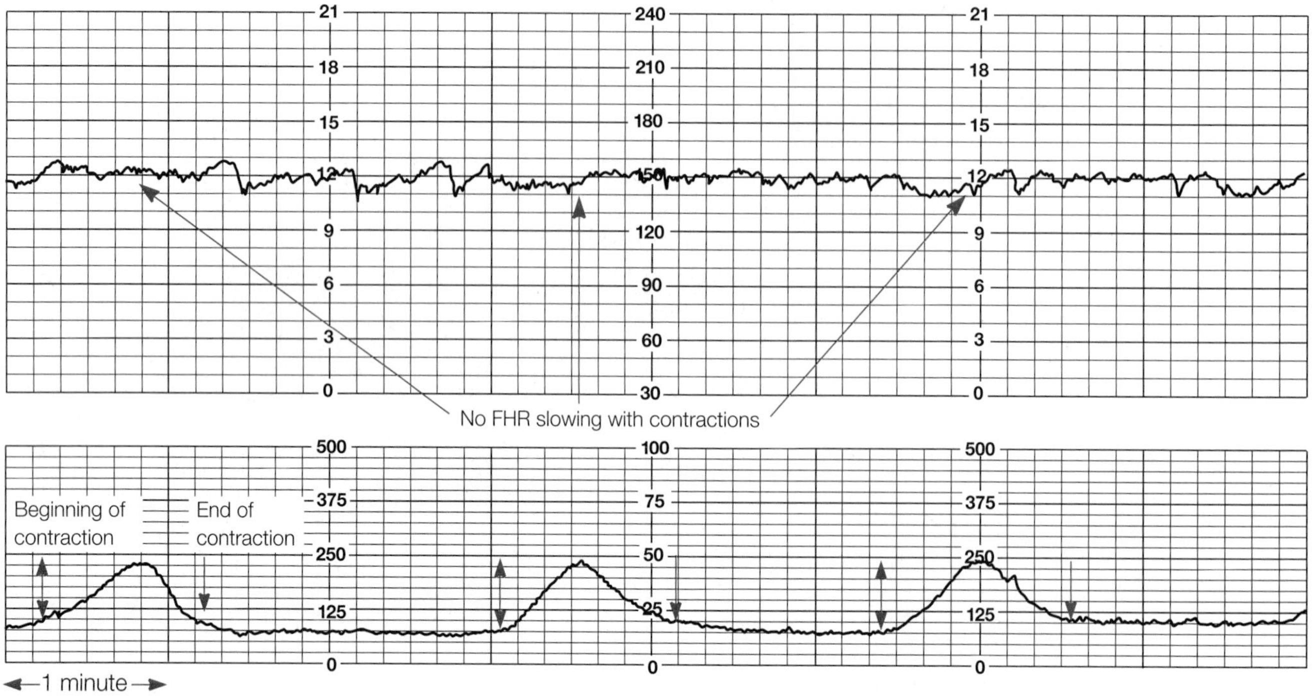

Figure 20–9 *Top:* **An FHR tracing obtained by internal monitoring. Normal FHR range is 110 to 160 beats/min. This tracing indicates an FHR range of 140 to 155 beats/min.** *Bottom:* **A uterine contraction tracing obtained by external monitoring. Each dark vertical line marks 1 minute, and each small rectangle represents 10 seconds. The contraction frequency is about every 3 minutes, and the duration of the contractions is 50 to 60 seconds.**

in medical records, serves as a basis for better communication between healthcare providers, and should result in more timely interventions and improved outcomes.

Baseline Fetal Heart Rate

The **baseline fetal heart rate (BL FHR)** is determined by approximating the mean (average) FHR during a 10-minute period, rounded to increments of 5 beats/min (e.g., 125, 130, 135, 140). Accelerations, decelerations, and periods of marked FHR variability (>25 beats/min) are excluded. There must be at least 2 minutes of identifiable baseline segments (not necessarily contiguous) in any 10-minute window, or the baseline for that period is indeterminate, and the preceding 10-minute window must be used to determine the baseline. For example, if the FHR over a period of 10 minutes fluctuates between 142 beats/min and 156 beats/min, the BL FHR would be documented as 150 beats/min with moderate variability.

The normal BL rate ranges from 110 to 160 beats/min, depending on gestational age. As the gestational age of the fetus increases, the FHR decreases. The FHR decreases an average of 16 beats/min between 16 weeks' gestation and term. The slowing of the FHR occurs as the parasympathetic nervous system (PNS) matures and exerts control over the fetal heart activity (Gabbe et al., 2017).

TACHYCARDIA

Fetal tachycardia is a BL FHR greater than 160 beats/min for at least a 10-minute period. The possible causes of tachycardia may be idiopathic, maternal, fetal, or a combination of maternal and fetal. However, it should be kept in mind that tachycardia in the presence of good variability is not a sign of fetal distress. Some of the most common causes are (Gabbe et al., 2017):

Maternal

- Fever (metabolism of the fetus accelerates because of increased maternal temperature)
- Dehydration
- Anxiety
- Betasympathomimetic or sympathetic drugs, such as ritodrine, terbutaline, atropine, and isoxsuprine (these drugs have a cardiac stimulant effect)
- Maternal hyperthyroidism (thyroid-stimulating hormones may cross the placenta and stimulate the FHR)
- Supraventricular tachycardia

Fetal

- Early fetal hypoxia (leads to stimulation of the sympathetic nervous system [SNS] as the fetus compensates for reduced blood flow)
- Asphyxia
- Fetal anemia (heart rate increases as a compensatory mechanism to improve tissue perfusion)
- Infection
- Prematurity
- Prolonged fetal stimulation
- Fetal heart failure.

Tachycardia is considered a nonreassuring sign if it is accompanied by other FHR patterns such as late decelerations, severe variable decelerations, or decreased or absent variability. If tachycardia is associated with maternal fever, treatment may consist of antipyretics, cooling measures, and antibiotics. Fetal arrhythmia or dysrhythmia needs to be ruled out. The pediatrician should be notified because tachycardia may cause heart failure in the newborn.

Intervention for tachycardia usually requires treatment of the underlying cause. Additional testing and monitoring may be used to further determine fetal well-being.

BRADYCARDIA

Fetal bradycardia is by definition an FHR baseline less than 110 beats/min for at least a 10-minute period. The lower limits of the FHR have been debated in the past. An FHR as low as 90 beats/min with good variability has been classified as benign and reassuring. When bradycardia is accompanied by decreased variability, late decelerations, or both, it is considered ominous and a sign of advanced fetal compromise (Gabbe et al., 2017). The possible causes of bradycardia include (Gabbe et al., 2017):

Maternal

- Drugs that stimulate PNS or block the SNS (anesthesia and regional analgesia)
- Maternal hypotension (results in decreased blood flow to the fetus)
- Accidental monitoring of maternal pulse

Fetal

- Stimulation of the vagus nerve (prolonged head compression as in early decelerations, application of the forceps or vacuum extractor, or prolonged scalp stimulation)
- Prolonged umbilical cord compression (fetal baroreceptors are activated by cord compression, which produces vagal stimulation, and in turn decreases FHR)
- Fetal dysrhythmia (associated with complete heart block in the fetus)
- Hypoxemia or late fetal asphyxia (depression of myocardial activity)
- Occiput posterior or transverse position.

WANDERING BASELINE

A *wandering baseline* is a smooth, meandering, unsteady BL that fluctuates in the normal BL range without variability (Gabbe et al., 2017). The possible causes of this type of BL may be a congenital defect or metabolic acidosis. Immediate interventions should be taken to enhance fetal oxygenation, and birth should be anticipated (Gabbe et al., 2017).

SINUSOIDAL FETAL HEART RATE PATTERN

A *sinusoidal FHR pattern* is defined as having a visually apparent, smooth, wavelike, undulating sine pattern in FHR baseline (Miller et al., 2017). The pattern has a series of cycles that are extremely smooth and regular (not necessarily identical) in amplitude and duration. It resembles a perfect letter "S" lying on its side. The FHR undulates in a sine pattern between 120 and 160 beats/min with variability amplitude of 5 to 15 beats/min. The pattern has a cycle frequency of 3 to 5/minute that persists for 20 minutes or more. Accelerations do not occur spontaneously, nor can they be induced (Figure 20–10).

Sinusoidal patterns may be benign (pseudosinusoidal) or pathologic (true sinusoidal) patterns. Pathologic sinusoidal patterns are indicative of nonreassuring fetal status and require immediate attention (Gabbe et al., 2017). The possible causes of a true sinusoidal pattern include (Gabbe et al., 2017):

- Fetal anemia
- Chronic fetal bleeding
- Fetal isoimmunization
- Twin-to-twin transfusion
- Umbilical cord occlusion
- CNS malformations.

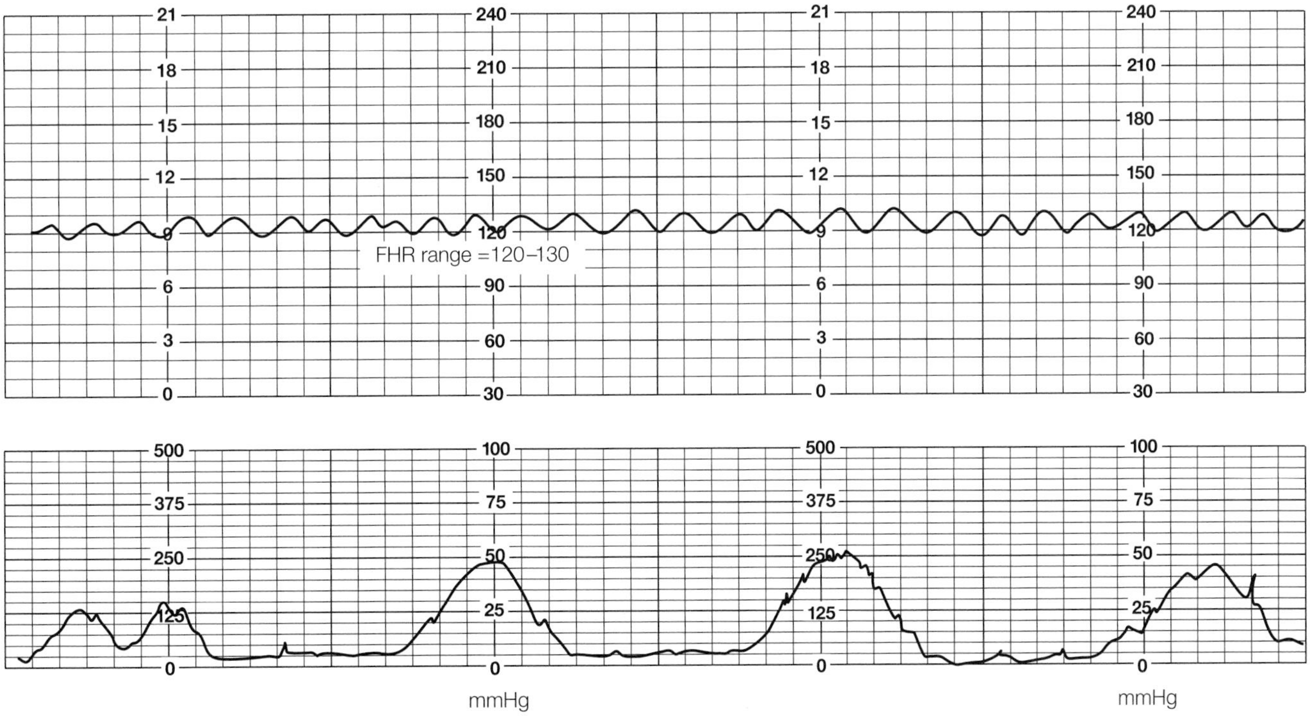

Figure 20–10 **Sinusoidal pattern. Note the undulating waveform evenly distributed between the 120 and 130 beats/min baseline. There is minimal variability.**

If the sinusoidal pattern is uncorrectable, interventions include immediate notification of the healthcare provider and expeditious birth of the baby.

ARRHYTHMIAS AND DYSRHYTHMIAS

Arrhythmias, a term often used interchangeably with *dysrhythmias*, are disturbances in the FHR pattern that are not associated with abnormal electrical impulse formation or conduction in the fetal cardiac tissue. Fetal arrhythmias can be divided into three categories: Irregular rhythms, sustained tachycardia, and sustained bradycardia. The majority of fetal arrhythmias are irregular rhythms (Miller et al., 2017). An arrhythmic pattern demonstrates a normal P wave and QRS complexes (Miller et al., 2017). However, dysrhythmic FHR patterns may exhibit abnormal electrical impulse formation and/or conduction in the fetal cardiac tissues, resulting in abnormal P waves, QRS complexes, or both. Arrhythmic and dysrhythmic patterns get their names from the origin of the pattern, for example, sinus node variants, atrial node patterns, or ventricular patterns (Miller et al., 2017).

FHR dysrhythmias are estimated to occur in 2 to 14% of all pregnancies. Whereas 90% of dysrhythmias are benign, 10% can be life-threatening and require the consultation of a neonatal or pediatric cardiology expert (Miller et al., 2017). For this reason, it is important to accurately diagnose abnormal FHR patterns and distinguish fetal arrhythmias from artifact and electrical interference. Fetal dysrhythmias can be difficult to diagnose because detection of the fetal cardiac electrical activity is best accomplished by invasive or advanced monitoring techniques such as fetal scalp electrode, real-time ultrasound, Doppler velocimetry, fetal echocardiogram, and echocardiogram monitoring (e.g., M-mode echocardiography and pulsed Doppler echocardiography) (Miller et al., 2017). With the exception of the fetal scalp electrode, more advanced and expensive diagnostic testing may not be readily available. The most common causes of FHR dysrhythmias are discussed in Table 20–6.

Baseline Variability

Baseline variability (BL VAR) is a reliable indicator of fetal cardiac and neurologic function and well-being. The opposing "push–pull" balancing between the sympathetic nervous system and the parasympathetic nervous system directly affects the FHR. ACOG, AWHONN, and NICHD define baseline variability as BL fluctuations in the baseline FHR that are irregular in amplitude and with a frequency of over two cycles per minute. The fluctuations are visually quantified as the amplitude range of the peak-to-trough of the FHR fluctuations and measured in beats/min (Miller et al., 2017) (Figure 20–11). Variability is classified by ACOG (2017c) and AWHONN (2015) as follows:

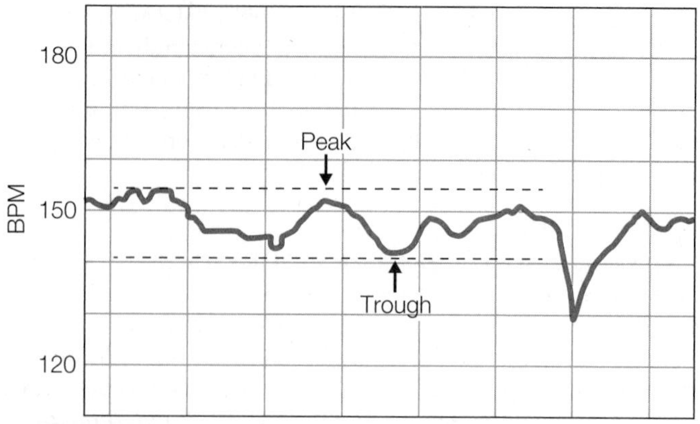

Figure 20–11 **This tracing shows an amplitude range of ~10 beats/min (moderate variability).**

- Absent FHR variability—amplitude range undetected
- Minimal FHR variability—amplitude range detectable but 5 beats/min or less
- Moderate FHR variability (normal)—amplitude range of 6 to 25 beats/min
- Marked FHR variability—amplitude range greater than 25 beats/min

Figure 20–12 and Figure 20–13 illustrate examples of each of these categories.

Fetal Heart Rate Changes

In addition to changes in the average BL FHR range, the FHR may also exhibit intermittent or transient deviations or changes from the BL that are commonly referred to as accelerations and decelerations. These transient deviations or changes in BL are categorized as *episodic* or *periodic*. Episodic changes (formerly referred to as nonperiodic changes) are not associated with UCs. Periodic changes occur with UCs. If a periodic change occurs with 50% or more of UCs in a 20-minute period, it is further categorized as a recurrent change or pattern.

The nurse must remember that it is very important to examine all changes in FHR in relation to the surrounding BL and uterine activity. A comprehensive evaluation of maternal–fetal interaction facilitates effective and efficient treatment and fetal well-being.

TABLE 20–6 Common Causes of Various Types of Fetal Dysrhythmias

SINUS NODE VARIANTS	ATRIAL DYSRHYTHMIAS	VENTRICULAR DYSRHYTHMIAS
• Bradycardia • Tachycardia • Marked sinus arrhythmia • Infections • CNS disturbances	• Parasympathetic response to fetal hypoxemia • Maternal ingestion of stimulants (e.g., caffeine, tobacco, alcohol, cocaine) • Abnormal reentry conduction • Cardiomyopathy • Fetal–maternal placental hemorrhage • Nonimmune hydrops fetalis • Wolf-Parkinson White syndrome • Cardiac structural abnormalities (e.g., atrial septal defect [ASD], ventricular septal defect [VSD], valve malformation)	• Beta-blocker drugs • Complete heart blocks (AV malformation) • Congenital heart disease • Autoimmune disease (AV malformation) • Maternal collagen disorders (AV malformation)

SOURCES: Data from Anderson & Stone, 2013; Gabbe et al., 2017; Miller et al., 2017.

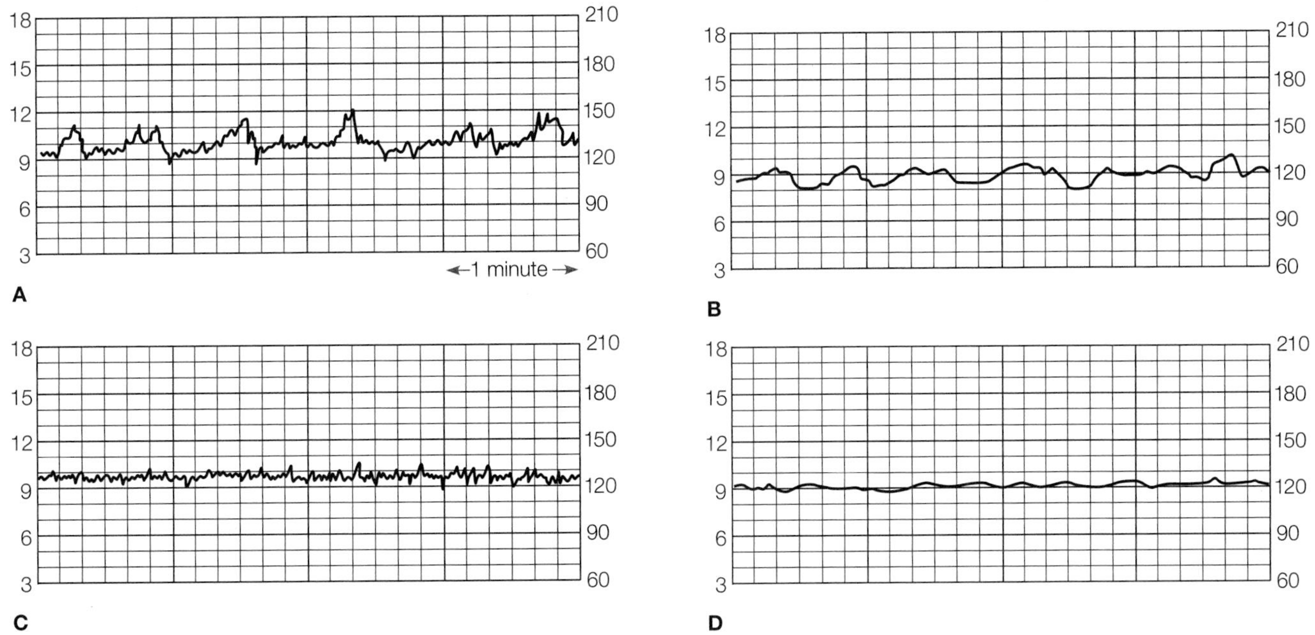

Figure 20–12 **A. and B. Moderate variability. C. Minimal variability. D. Absent variability.**

ACCELERATIONS

An **acceleration**, also called an *accel*, is described as a visually apparent, abrupt increase in the BL FHR, with an onset-to-peak of less than 30 seconds and lasting less than 2 minutes overall, beginning at the most recently calculated BL. To be called an acceleration, the peak must be 15 beats/min or more and the acceleration must last 15 seconds or more from the onset to the return to BL when the fetus is equal to or greater than 32 weeks of gestational age. The duration of the acceleration is defined as the time from the initial change in FHR from the BL to the return of the FHR to the BL. At gestations of less than 32 weeks, accelerations are defined as having a peak of 10 beats/min or more and a duration of 10 seconds or more. A *prolonged acceleration* is any acceleration that lasts 2 minutes or more but less than 10 minutes in duration. Prolonged accelerations that last more than 10 minutes are defined as a baseline change (Miller et al., 2017).

As discussed earlier in this chapter, accelerations can be either episodic or periodic. *Episodic accelerations* are not associated with contractions and tend to be more peaked and abrupt. They are often associated with fetal movement, stimulation, or an environmental stimulus. Episodic accelerations are reassuring FHR patterns, whether or not they are accompanied by fetal movement. *Periodic accelerations* are associated with uterine

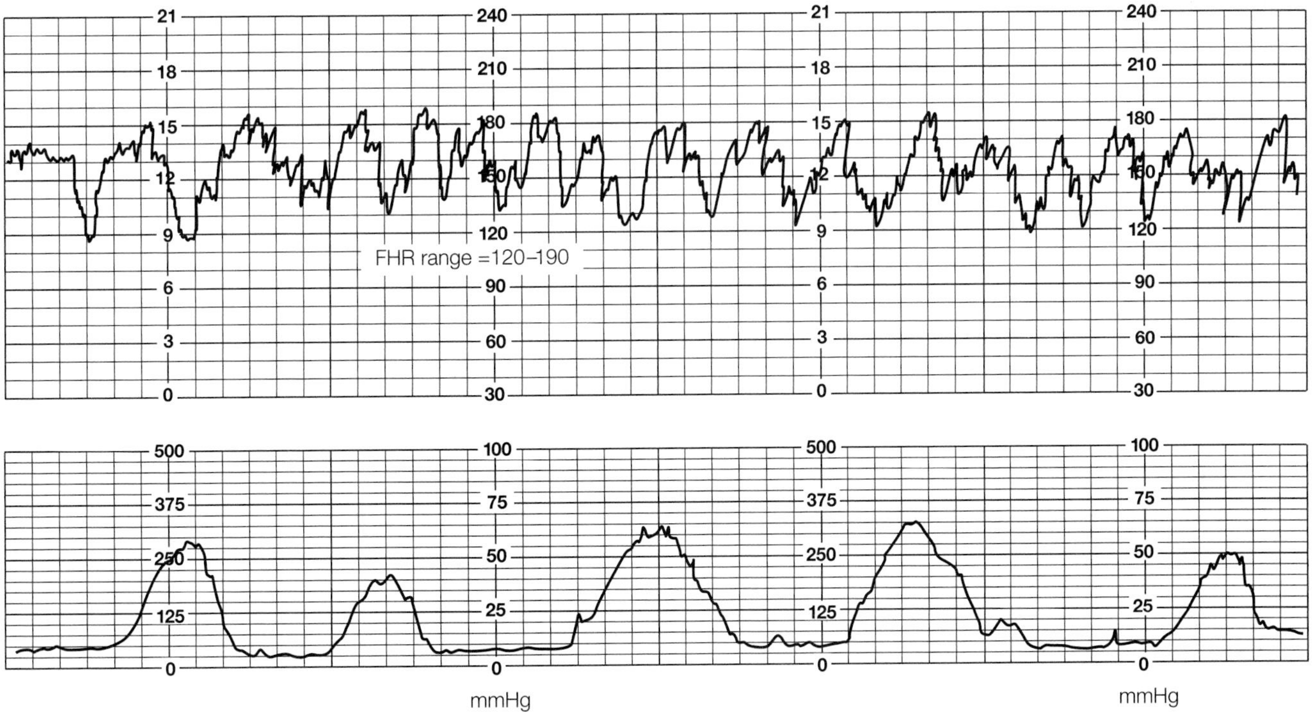

Figure 20–13 **Marked variability. FHR varies markedly between 120 and 190 beats/min. With this type of pattern, it is not possible to determine average baseline FHR because of the wide, marked variations.**

contractions. When they occur on a repetitive basis, they may be smooth in configuration, multiphasic, and may precede variable decelerations. Various types of accelerations are shown in Figure 20–14.

Accelerations can occur during labor without any apparent stimulus but are generally associated with the stimulation of the autonomic nervous system (ANS), specifically the SNS, which increases the FHR. If the heart rate increases with CNS stimulation, it usually indicates an intact fetal nervous system and fetal well-being. FHR accelerations can be associated with fetal movement, vaginal exams, application of a fetal scalp electrode, occiput posterior presentation and uterine contractions, fundal pressure, abdominal palpation, vibroacoustic stimulation (VAS), scalp stimulation, and other environmental stimuli (Miller et al., 2017). Fetuses of extreme prematurity are less likely to accelerate because of their immature PNS. In fetuses of less than 32 gestational weeks, an acceleration of at least 10 beats/min for 10 seconds is reassuring (Miller et al., 2017). Fetuses suffering from IUGR experience fewer accelerations than normal, healthy, well-oxygenated fetuses. Medications administered to the mother may inhibit accelerations because of their effect on the SNS. Some of the drugs seen to affect fetuses are beta blockers and CNS depressants. Hypoxia is also a large contributing factor to lack of accelerations and may be the first sign of a nonreassuring FHR tracing.

Accelerations are generally benign because they are associated with an intact fetal nervous system, lack of fetal hypoxia, and acidosis. The patterns are considered reassuring, thus no intervention is required.

DECELERATIONS

Decelerations, often referred to as *decels*, are generally defined as decreases in the FHR below the BL. Each deceleration has its own unique characteristics, etiology, and significance. Each deceleration consists of several components:

- ***Onset:*** Point at which the deceleration leaves the BL FHR
- ***Descent:*** Time from onset to nadir
- ***Nadir:*** Lowest point of the deceleration
- ***Depth:*** Level (in beats per minute) a deceleration reaches at its nadir
- ***Recovery:*** Time from nadir to return to BL
- ***Duration:*** Total length of time from onset to return to BL.

Decelerations in the FHR are categorized as early, late, variable, or prolonged and are based on specific characteristics of their shape, appearance, rate of decent, and timing in relation to uterine contractions (Figure 20–15). Decelerations are measured by depth in beats per minute below the baseline and duration in minutes and seconds (Miller et al., 2017).

Variable decelerations may be accompanied by other characteristics, the clinical significance of which requires further research investigation. Miller et al. (2017) provide some examples of these characteristics and explain the physiologic mechanism of variable decelerations, including a slow return of the FHR after the end of the contraction, biphasic decelerations, tachycardia after variable deceleration(s), accelerations preceding or following a deceleration (sometimes called "shoulders" or "overshoots"), and fluctuations in the FHR in the trough of the deceleration. See Figure 20–16.

Miller et al. (2017) describe characteristics of decelerations according to the 2008 *NICHD Workshop Report on Electronic Fetal Monitoring: Update on Definitions, Interpretation, and Research Guidelines* as follows:

Early Deceleration

- Visually apparent, usually symmetrical, gradual decrease and return of the FHR associated with a uterine contraction.
- A gradual FHR decrease is defined as one from the onset to the FHR nadir of 30 seconds or more.
- The decrease in FHR is calculated from the onset to the nadir of the deceleration.
- The nadir of the deceleration occurs at the same time as the peak of the contraction.

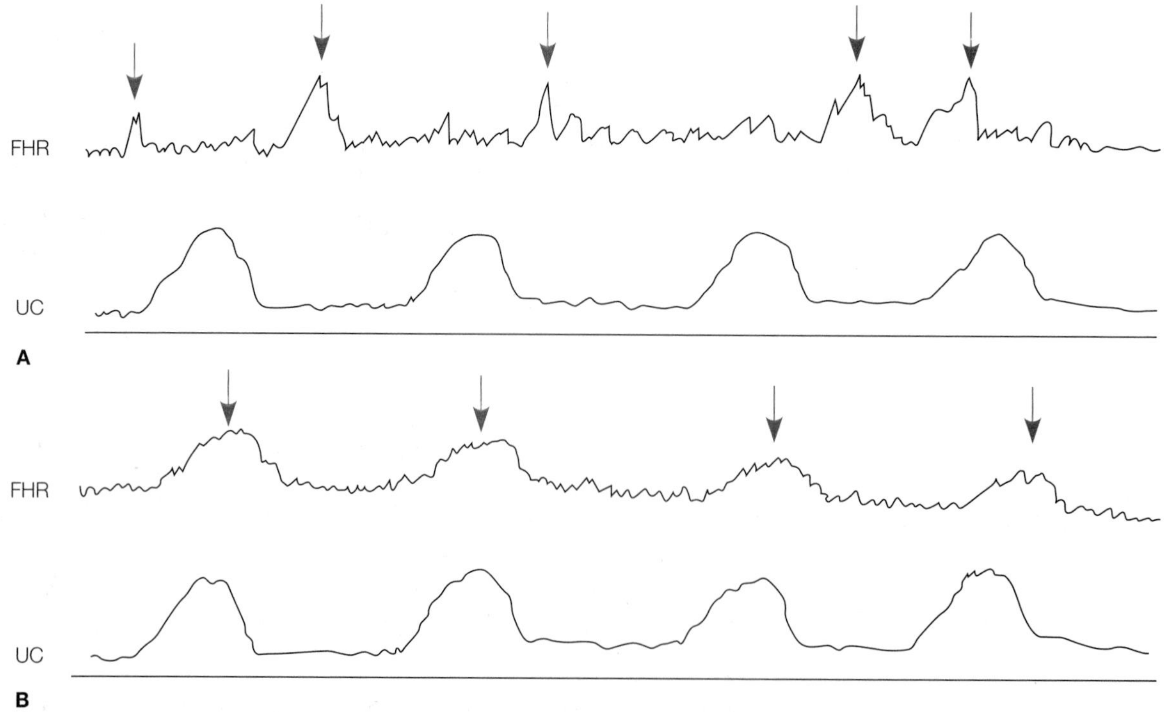

Figure 20–14 **Types of accelerations. A. Episodic accelerations. B. Periodic accelerations.**

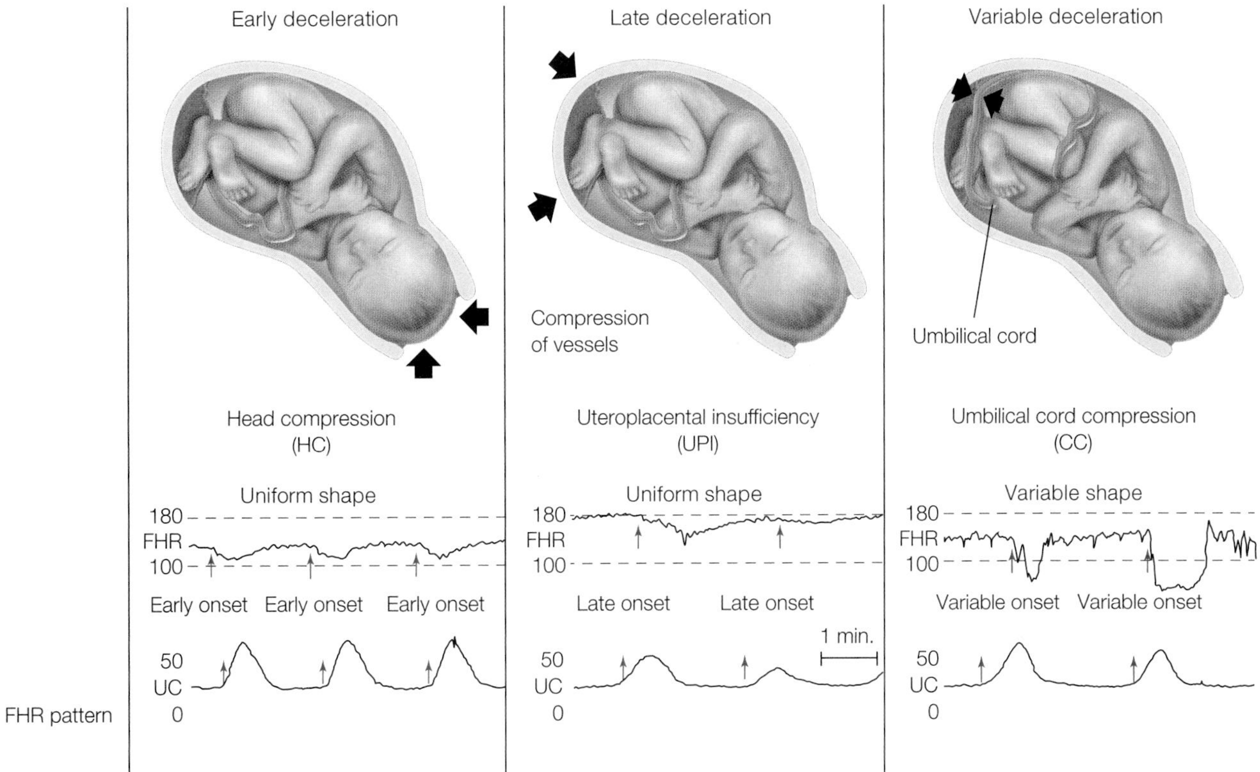

	Early deceleration	Late deceleration	Variable deceleration
Shape	Waveform consistently uniform; inversely mirrors contraction	Waveform uniform; shape reflects contraction	Waveform variable; generally sharp drops and returns
Onset	Just prior to or early in contraction	Late in contraction	Abrupt with fetal insult; not related to contraction
Lowest level	Consistently at or before midpoint of contraction	Consistently after the midpoint of the contraction	Variable around midpoint
Range	Usually within normal range of 120–160 beats/min	Usually within normal range of 120–130 beats/min	Not usually within normal range
Ensemble	Can be single or repetitive	Occasional, consistent, gradual increase—repetitive	Variable—single or repetitive

Figure 20–15 **Types and characteristics of early, late, and variable decelerations.**

- In most cases the onset, nadir, and recovery of the deceleration are coincident with the beginning, peak, and ending of the contraction, respectively.

Late Deceleration

- Visually apparent, usually symmetrical, a gradual decrease and return of the FHR to BL, associated with a uterine contraction.
- A gradual FHR decrease is defined as from the onset to the FHR nadir of 30 seconds or more.
- The decrease in FHR is calculated from the onset to the nadir of the deceleration.
- The deceleration is delayed in timing, with the nadir of the deceleration occurring after the peak of the contraction.
- In most cases, the onset, nadir, and recovery of the deceleration occur after the beginning, peak, and ending of the contraction, respectively.

Variable Deceleration

- Visually apparent abrupt decrease in FHR. (An abrupt FHR decrease is defined as from the onset of the deceleration to the beginning of the FHR nadir of 30 seconds or less. The decrease in FHR is calculated from the onset to the nadir of the deceleration.)
- The decrease in FHR is 15 beats/min or more, lasting 15 seconds or more but less than 2 minutes in duration.
- When variable decelerations are associated with uterine contractions, their onset, depth, and duration commonly vary with successive uterine contractions.

Early decelerations are a result of vagal nerve stimulation caused by fetal head compression that occurs during UCs (Figure 20–17). They are usually uniform in shape and mirror the shape of the UC. The depth of the deceleration is rarely more than 30 to 40 beats/min (Figure 20–18). Early decels are not associated with loss of variability, tachycardia, or other FHR changes that

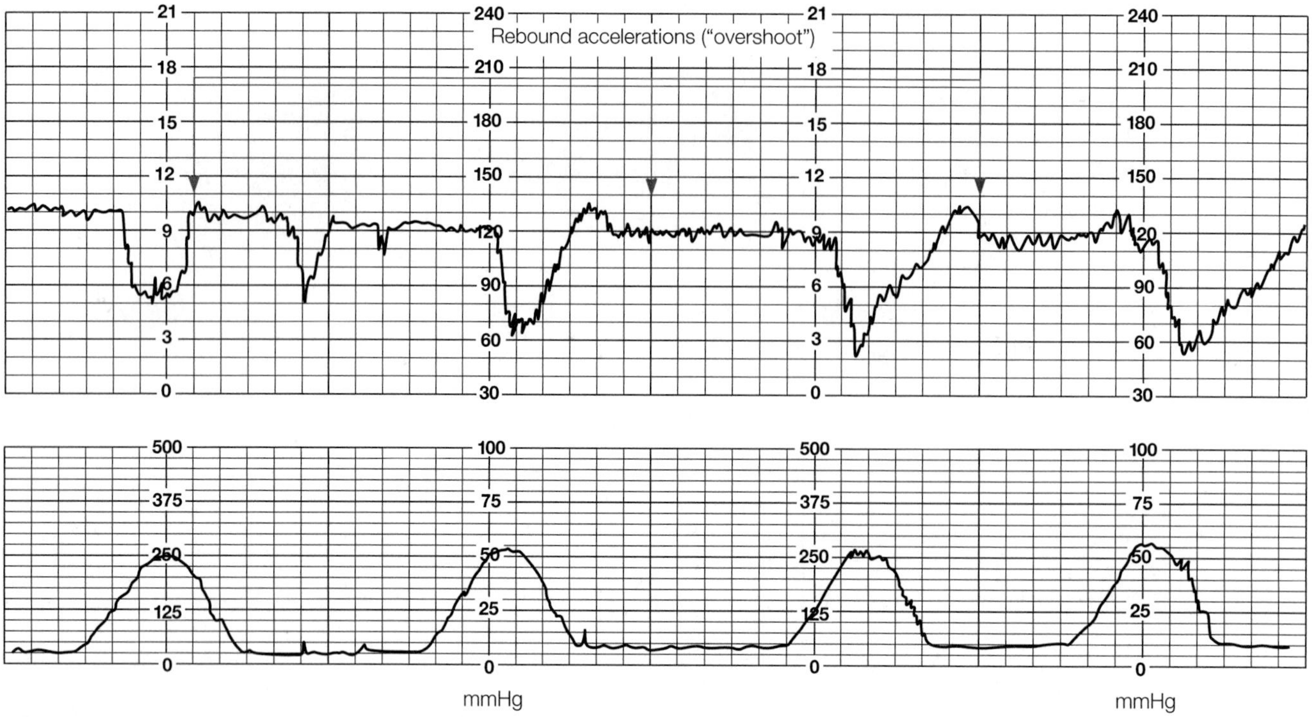

Figure 20–16 Variable decelerations with overshoot. The timing of the decelerations is variable, and most have a sharp decline. A rebound acceleration (overshoot) occurs after most of the decelerations. Baseline FHR is 115 to 130 beats/min. Nadir of decelerations is 55 to 80 beats/min. Variability is minimal.

are associated with fetal hypoxia, acidosis, or low Apgar scores. They are viewed as reassuring unless they are seen with the lack of descent of the fetal head into the pelvis (Gabbe et al., 2017).

Late decelerations, often referred to as *lates* or *late decels*, are due to uteroplacental insufficiency and are a result of decreased blood flow or oxygen transfer to the fetus through the intervillous space during contractions. Late decels may be one of two types: Reflexive or myocardial. The pathophysiology of late decels is complicated and is not always understood.

When uteroplacental reserve is adequate, the fetus normally tolerates the transient stress of repetitive contractions. If a decrease in uteroplacental blood flow (for example, from maternal hypotension or excessive uterine activity) lowers the oxygen level in the intervillous space to a level lower than the oxygen level in the fetus, fetal chemoreceptors are stimulated

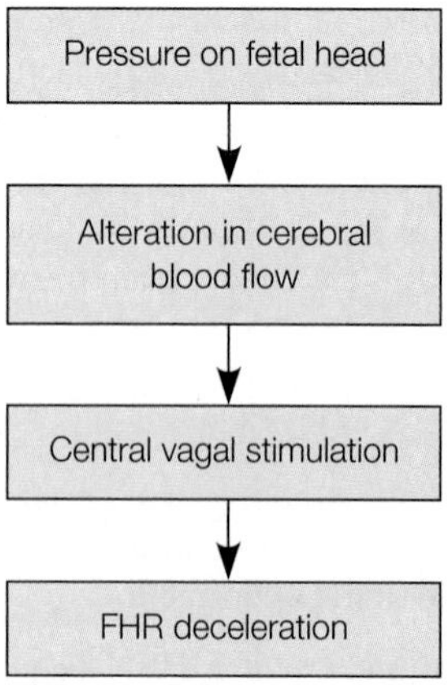

Figure 20–17 Mechanism of early deceleration (head compression).

SOURCE: Adapted from Freeman, R. K., & Garite, T. J. (1981). The physiologic basis of fetal monitoring. In *Fetal heart rate monitoring* (p. 13). 1981 Lippincott, Williams & Wilkins.

and FHR decreases. This response to the lowered oxygen level is reflexive because it is a normal physiologic chemical response to low oxygen levels in the blood. The delay in the FHR deceleration is due to the time it takes for the normal physiologic response of the neurologic system to respond to the lowered oxygen environment. This type of late decel is generally considered nonacidemic and is associated with moderate BL VAR. The BL VAR is the key to determining an intact fetal CNS and should always be considered when evaluating late decelerations and the level of intervention required (Gabbe et al., 2017).

In some cases, repetitive or chronic episodes of decreased oxygen in the intervillous space exist and the fetus experiences a chronic state of hypoxia that leads to metabolic acidosis. The fetal CNS is affected by the metabolic acidosis and progresses to myocardial depression. Late decelerations are produced by the myocardial depression (Miller et al., 2017) (Figure 20–19).

The decrease in heart rate resulting from late decelerations is usually shallow, typically 10 to 20 beats/min; however, it may approach 30 to 40 beats/min below the BL (Gabbe et al., 2017) (Figure 20–20). The depth of the late deceleration is usually proportional to the strength of the UC; late decelerations are considered a nonreassuring sign. When they are repetitive and uncorrectable and associated with minimal or absent BL VAR or BL rate changes, they indicate fetal hypoxia and acidemia and require prompt attention and intervention. The objective of intervention is to improve fetal oxygenation and uteroplacental perfusion while assessing and eliminating the stressor as reflected by the deceleration (Miller et al, 2017). If this is not possible, immediate birth may be indicated.

Sometimes late or variable decelerations are due to the supine position of the laboring woman. In this case, the decrease in uterine blood flow to the fetus may be alleviated by raising the woman's upper trunk or turning her to the side to displace pressure of the gravid uterus on the inferior vena cava. If the

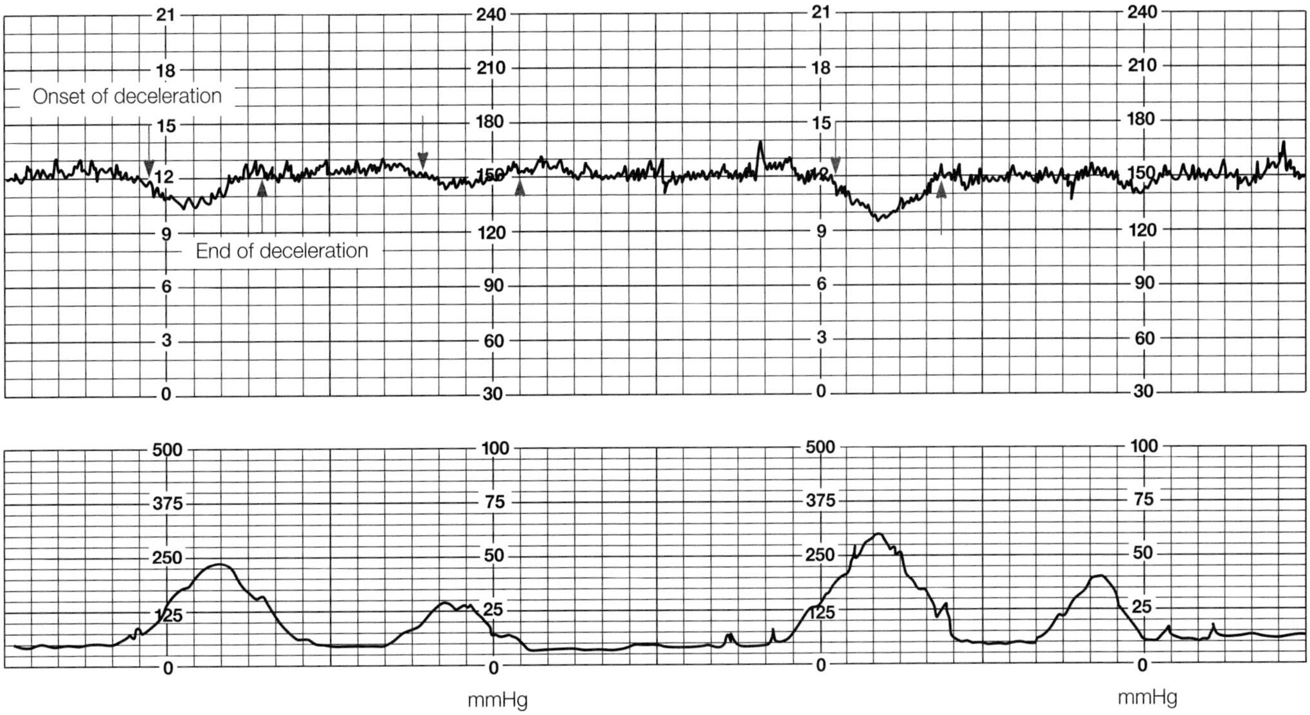

Figure 20–18 **Early decelerations. Baseline FHR is 150 to 155 beats/min. Nadir (lowest point) of decelerations is 130 to 145 beats/min.**

woman remains flat on her back, the fetus will continue to have decelerations because of oxygen compromise. Immediate nursing interventions include changing the maternal position and increasing the administration of intravenous fluids. Oxygen should be provided to the mother via face mask if hypoxia is suspected, such as when there is absent or minimal variability. If oxytocin (Pitocin) is being administered, the infusion should be stopped immediately until the FHR recovers or the physician/CNM has instructed that the infusion be resumed. The physician/CNM should be notified immediately in the event that late decelerations occur.

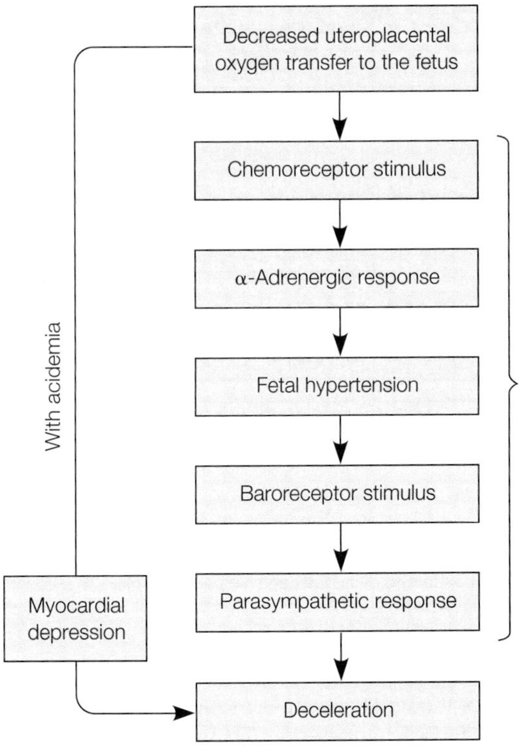

Figure 20–19 **Mechanism of late deceleration.**

SOURCE: Reprinted from Freeman, R. K., & Garite, T. J. (1981). The physiologic basis of fetal monitoring. In *Fetal heart rate monitoring* (p. 15). Copyright © 1981 Lippincott, Williams & Wilkins.

Late decelerations normally occur within the normal heart range (110 to 160 beats/min) and may be quite obvious or very subtle and almost indistinguishable. Some fetuses at highest risk demonstrate a flat BL FHR with late decelerations that are barely noticeable (Miller et al., 2017).

Episodic or Periodic Decelerations. Decelerations can be episodic or periodic. As discussed earlier in this chapter, episodic decelerations imply that the deceleration occurred without relationship to UCs. Episodic decelerations may occur without or between contractions and usually are the result of environmental stimuli, such as vaginal exams, rupture of membranes, the administration of regional anesthesia or medications, or other events (Gabbe et al., 2017). Also discussed earlier, periodic refers to decelerations that occur in direct association with UCs. Episodic or periodic decelerations are considered *repetitive* if they occur with 50% or more of UCs (Miller et al., 2017).

Early or Late Decelerations. Periodic decelerations associated with UCs are also classified by their timing with respect to them. The etiology and clinical significance of each type of deceleration are unique. Clinical interventions and treatments are based on the systematic assessment of the FHR tracing and the overall evaluation of the mother, the fetus, and labor status. Deceleration characteristics and the discussion of their clinical significance and interventions are included in the following sections.

Prolonged Decelerations. Prolonged decelerations are visually apparent decreases in the FHR of 15 beats/min or more below the

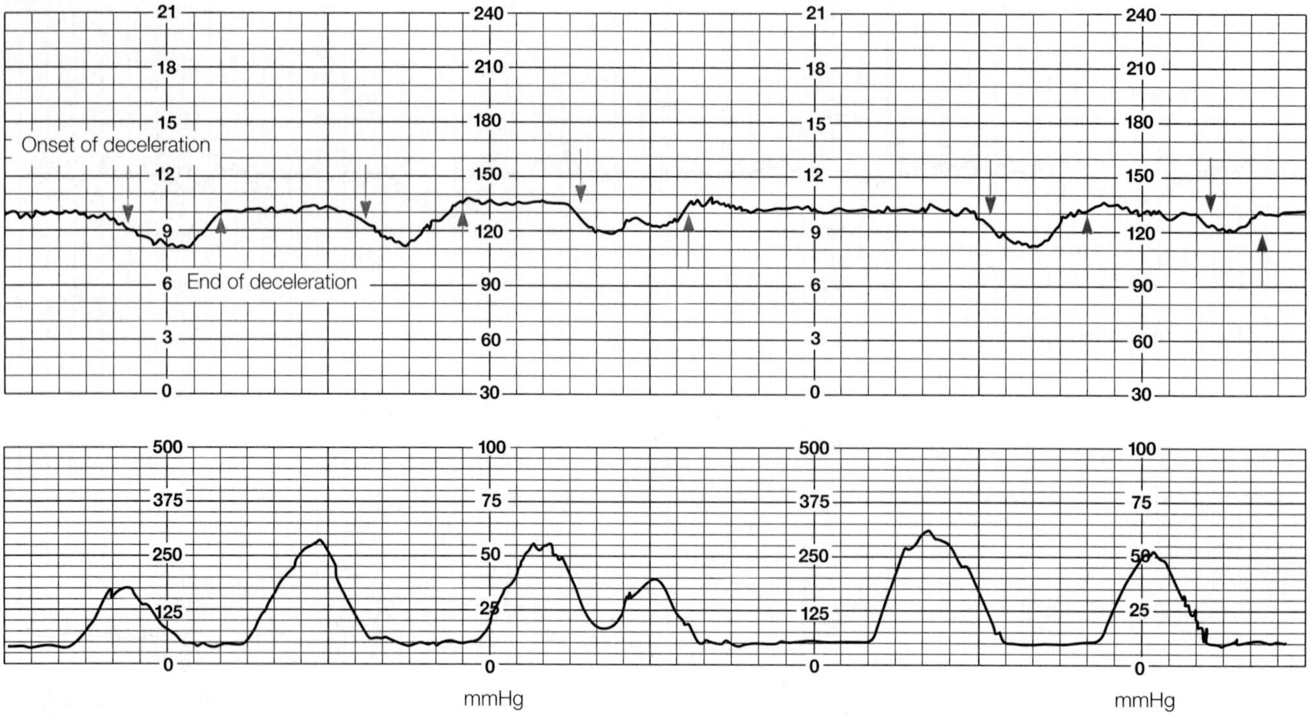

Figure 20–20 **Late decelerations. Baseline FHR is 130 to 148 beats/min. Nadir (lowest point) of decelerations is 110 to 120 beats/min. Absent variability.**

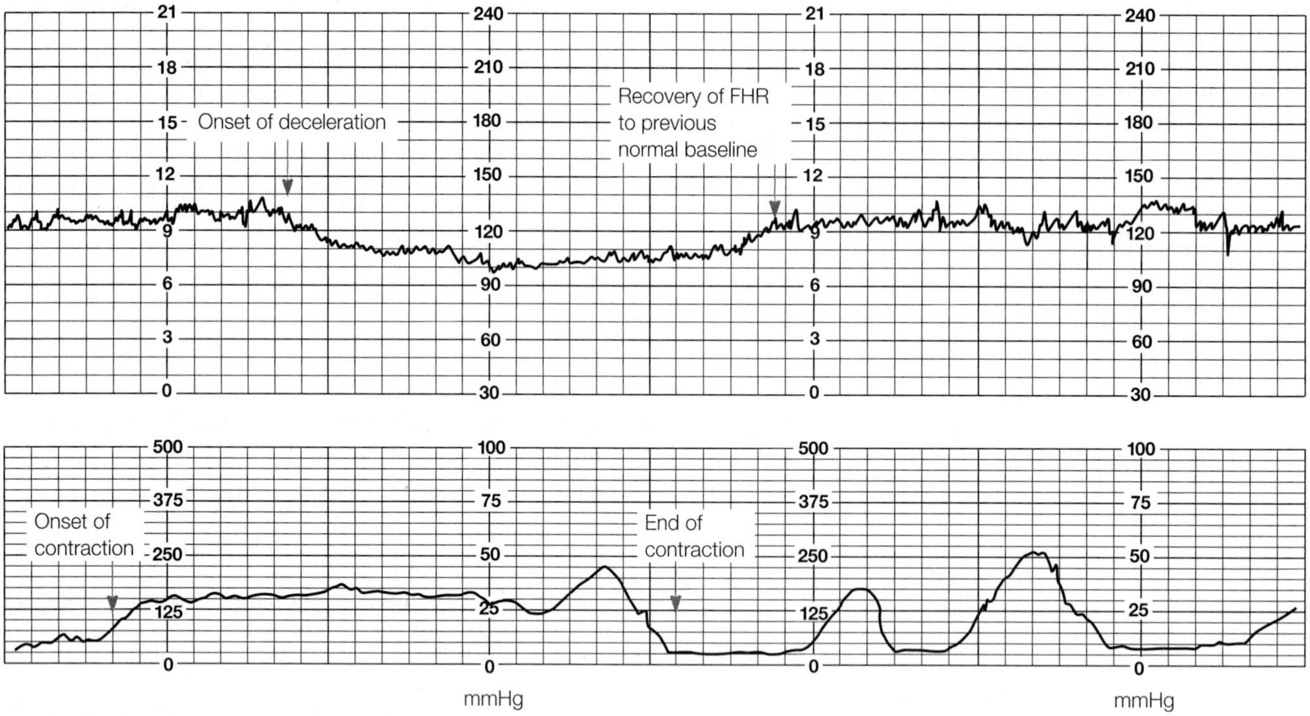

Figure 20–21 **The prolonged deceleration depicted lasts approximately 160 seconds.**

NOTE: The prolonged contraction is 120 seconds. The deceleration begins after 80 seconds of uterine contraction. Note the beginning return of FHR 30 seconds after uterine tone returns to normal resting tone (contraction ends). Minimal variability is present despite the deceleration.

BL that last more than 2 minutes and less than 10 minutes from onset to return to BL (Figure 20–21).

Variable Decelerations. Variable decelerations are those that have a U or V shape and are typically associated with cord compression. They may vary somewhat in shape but have an abrupt onset and return to normal abruptly as well. They vary in intensity and duration and usually correlate to uterine contractions. They are thought to result from vagus nerve firing resulting from umbilical cord compression. They are usually not concerning unless the deceleration is less than 70 beats/min and lasts more than 60 seconds. In addition, if the variable is slow to return to baseline, it could be an indication of hypoxia and warrants intervention (Miller et al., 2017) (Figure 20–22 and Figure 20–23).

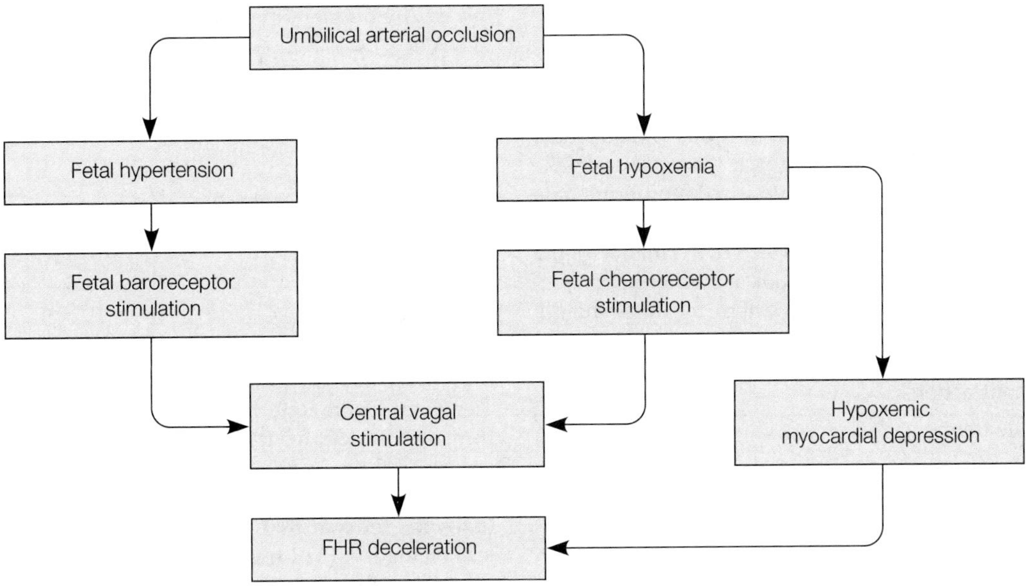

Figure 20–22 Mechanism of variable deceleration.

SOURCE: Adapted with permission from Freeman, R. K., & Garite, T. J. (1981). The physiologic basis of fetal monitoring. In *Fetal heart rate monitoring* (p. 13). Copyright © 1981 Lippincott, Williams & Wilkins.

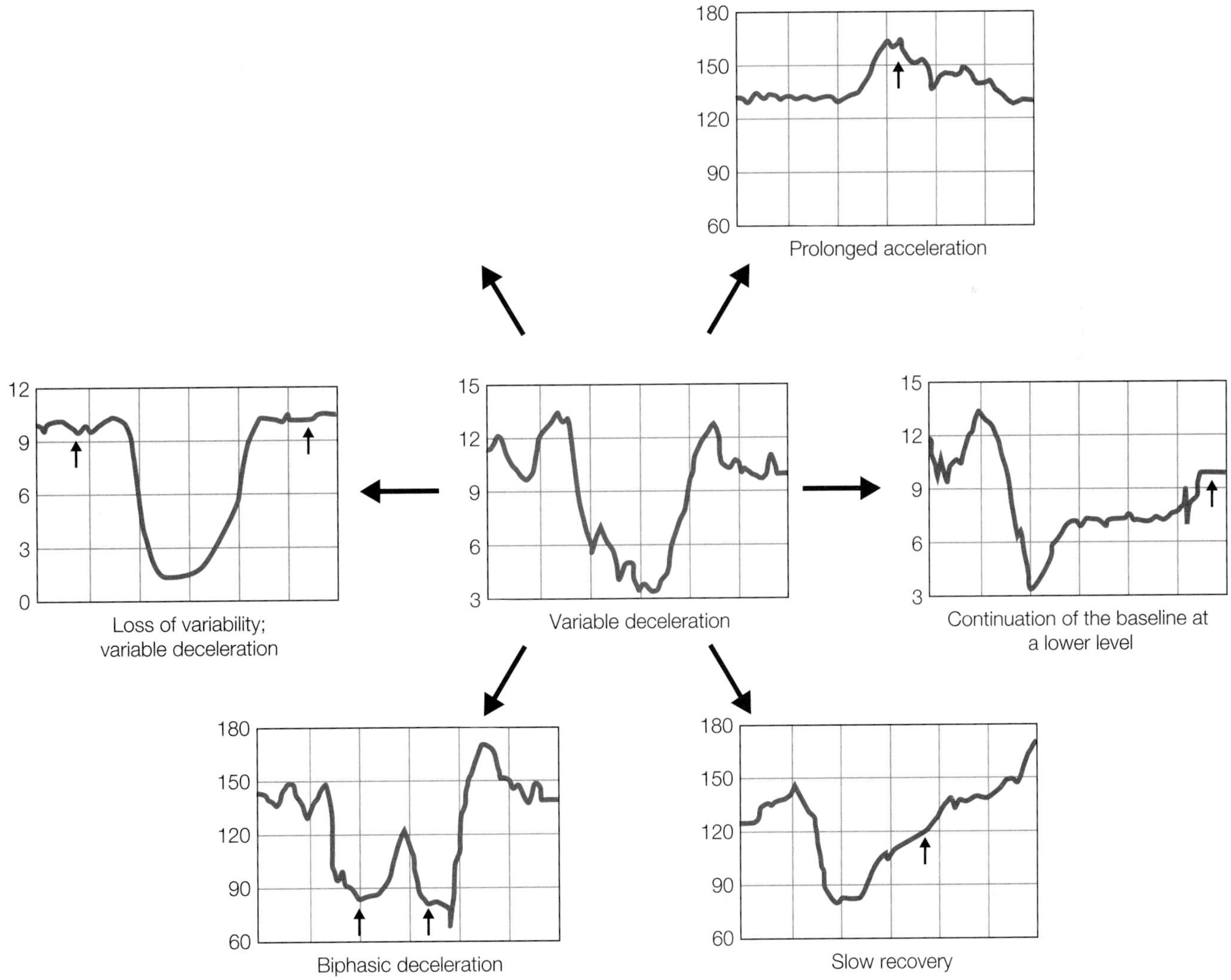

Figure 20–23 Atypical variable decelerations. The presence of any of these types of variable decelerations strongly suggests fetal hypoxia, especially when variability is decreased.

Interpretation of Fetal Heart Rate Patterns

The effective nurse uses a systematic approach in evaluating FHR tracings to avoid interpreting findings on the basis of inadequate or erroneous data. With a systematic approach, the nurse can make a more accurate and rapid assessment; easily communicate data to the woman, physician/CNM, and staff; and have a universal language for documenting the woman's record. Evaluation of the electronic monitor tracing begins with a look at the uterine contraction pattern. To evaluate the contraction pattern, the nurse should:

1. Determine the uterine resting tone.
2. Assess the contractions:
   a. What is the frequency?
   b. What is the duration?
   c. What is the intensity (if internal monitoring)?

The next step is to evaluate the FHR tracing.

1. Determine the baseline:
   a. Is the baseline within normal range?
   b. Is there evidence of tachycardia?
   c. Is there evidence of bradycardia?
2. Determine FHR variability:
   a. Is variability absent, minimal, or moderate? Is variability minimal or marked?
3. Determine whether a sinusoidal pattern is present.
4. Determine whether there are periodic changes.
   a. Are accelerations present?
   b. Is there a reassuring tracing or FHR pattern?
   c. Are decelerations present?
   d. Are they uniform in shape? If so, determine if they are early or late decelerations.
   e. Are they nonuniform in shape? If so, determine if they are variable decelerations.
5. Determine the category.
   a. Category I
   b. Category II
   c. Category III

After evaluating the FHR tracing for the factors listed, the nurse may categorize the tracing according to the Three-Tier Fetal Heart Rate Interpretation System (Table 20–7). The three-tier system for the categorization of FHR patterns is recommended by ACOG, AWHONN, and NICHD (Gabbe et al., 2017; Miller et al., 2017). Categorization of the FHR tracing evaluates the fetus at that point in time; tracing patterns can and will change. A FHR tracing may move back and forth between categories depending on the clinical situation and management strategies employed.

Category I FHR tracings are normal. They are strongly predictive of normal fetal acid–base status at the time of observation. The FHR tracings may be followed in a routine manner, and no specific action is required.

Category II FHR tracings are indeterminate. They are not predictive of abnormal fetal acid–base status, yet there is not enough adequate evidence at present to classify these as Category I or Category III. Category II tracings require evaluation and continued surveillance and reevaluation, taking into account the entire associated clinical circumstances.

TABLE 20–7 Three-Tier Fetal Heart Rate Interpretation System

CATEGORY I REASSURING FETAL HEART RATE TRACINGS	CATEGORY II PATTERNS WARRANTING CONTINUAL ASSESSMENT	CATEGORY III PATTERNS OF NONREASSURING FETAL STATUS THAT WARRANT IMMEDIATE INTERVENTION
• Normal range FHR 110–160 beats/min • Moderate FHR variability • Absence of variable, late, or prolonged decelerations • Accelerations may be present or may be absent • Early decelerations may be present or may be absent; they do not represent a nonreassuring status	• Includes all FHR tracings that do not meet criteria to be placed in Category I or III Examples include: • Baselines that include bradycardia with continued variability or tachycardia • Baseline changes in variability that include minimal variability, absent variability without decelerations, or marked baseline variability • Lack of accelerations with fetal acoustic or scalp stimulation • Episodic decelerations that include recurrent variable decelerations with minimal or moderate variability, prolonged decelerations lasting >2 minutes but <10 minutes in duration, or recurrent late decelerations that maintain moderate variability • Variable deceleration patterns that include overshoots, shoulders, or slow return to baseline status	• Absent variability in baseline FHR with recurrent late decelerations, recurrent variable decelerations, or bradycardia for at least 10 minutes • Sinusoidal FHR patterns for at least 20 minutes

SOURCES: Data from ACOG, 2009, 2017; Macones, Hankins, Spong, et al., 2008; Miller et al., 2017.

Category III FHR tracings are abnormal. They are predictive of abnormal fetal acid–base status at the time of observation if they continue. They require prompt evaluation. Depending on the clinical situation, efforts to expeditiously resolve the abnormal FHR pattern may include, but are not limited to, provision of maternal oxygen, change in maternal position, discontinuation of labor stimulation, and treatment of maternal hypotension. If they are not immediately corrected, acidemia will occur; therefore, birth is required via the fastest route possible.

Professionalism in Practice FHR and Legal Responsibilities

Nurses caring for women during childbirth are legally responsible for correctly interpreting FHR patterns, initiating appropriate nursing interventions based on those patterns, and documenting the outcomes of those interventions.

PROVISION OF EMOTIONAL SUPPORT

It is important to provide information to the laboring woman regarding the FHR pattern and the interventions that will help her fetus. Sharing information with the laboring woman reassures her that a potential or actual problem has been identified and that she is an active participant in the interventions. Occasionally, a problem arises that requires immediate intervention. In that case, the nurse can say something like, "It is important for you to turn on your side right now because the baby is having a little difficulty. I'll explain what is happening in just a few moments." This type of response lets the woman know that although an action needs to be accomplished rapidly, information will soon be provided. In the haste to act quickly, the nurse must not forget that it is the woman's body and her baby. See *Case Study: Melissa Bond-James*.

Labor and birth nurses must be skilled and competent in evaluating electronic FHR patterns and responding appropriately (see *Key Facts to Remember: Guidelines for Management of Variable, Late, and Prolonged Deceleration Patterns*). Competence can be maintained through frequent in-services, formal courses, and continuing education programs.

Indirect Methods of Fetal Assessment

When there is a question regarding fetal status, indirect methods such as **scalp stimulation** (pressing on the fetal scalp with the examining fingers during a vaginal exam to elicit an acceleration of FHR), *acoustic stimulation* (using a sound device placed against the maternal abdomen to elicit an acceleration in FHR), or stimulation by maternal abdominal palpation (patting or shaking the abdomen) can be used to assess the fetus. Ongoing scalp stimulation is not recommended and should not be used by nurses (Miller et al., 2017). When one of the indirect methods is used, the fetus who is not in any stress responds with an acceleration of the FHR, described as a reactive response (acceleration of 15 beats per minute (beats/min) amplitude with a duration of 15 seconds). Whereas reactivity is associated with fetal well-being, the absence of acceleration does not diagnose acidemia or predict fetal compromise (Miller et al., 2017). Further observation and assessment measures are indicated.

Cord Blood Analysis at Birth

In cases in which significant abnormal FHR patterns have been noted before birth, amniotic fluid is meconium stained, or the newborn is depressed at birth, umbilical cord blood may be analyzed immediately after birth to assess the baby's respiratory status. The cord is usually clamped before the neonate takes his or her first breath to provide an evaluation of blood gas status before the baby interacts with the extrauterine environment because values can change after only a few seconds of neonatal breathing.

An 8- to 10-inch segment of the umbilical cord is double-clamped and cut, and a small amount of blood is aspirated from one of the umbilical arteries (arterial blood seems to provide the most reliable indication of blood gas status and fetal tissue pH). Blood is collected in a heparinized syringe unless it is to be analyzed immediately; it should not be allowed to remain in the segment of cord longer than 30 minutes. Some clinicians may collect a segment of cord and send blood samples only if the Apgar score is below 7 at 5 minutes, as recommended by ACOG (2017b). In this instance, values might be used to clarify the cause of a low Apgar score while minimizing any medical-legal exposure and expense. Determination of pH and base deficit values can differentiate whether fetal acidemia is due to hypoperfusion of the placenta or to cord compression.

CASE STUDY: Melissa Bond-James

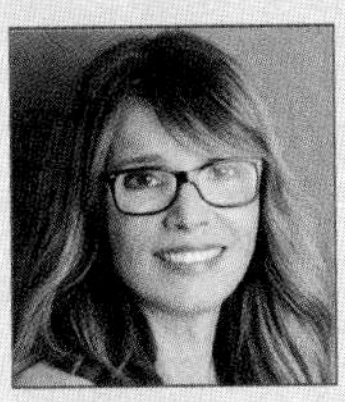

SOURCE: Kinga/ Shutterstock

Melissa once again presents to the labor and delivery unit after having contractions while she was out to dinner with Nancy and some friends. One of the friends is a nurse who urged her to come to the hospital to be assessed because the contractions were becoming more frequent, more painful, and closer together. After placing her on the fetal monitor, the nurse notes Melissa is having mild variable decelerations. Nancy asks if this means Melissa will have to have a cesarean birth. She states her sister had decelerations and she was rushed to the operating room for a cesarean birth when she had her baby 2 months ago.

Questions to Ponder

As a nurse, you know there are three different types of decelerations. Explain the different types of decelerations and which ones are considered normal and which ones would be cause for concern. What are variable decelerations often related to?

Key Facts to Remember

Guidelines for Management of Variable, Late, and Prolonged Deceleration Patterns

Pattern	Nursing Interventions to Consider
Variable decelerations	Report findings to physician/CNM and document in chart.
Isolated or occasional	Provide explanation to woman and partner.
Moderate	Change maternal position to one in which FHR pattern is most improved.
	Discontinue oxytocin if it is being administered and other interventions are unsuccessful.
	Perform vaginal examination to assess for prolapsed cord or change in labor progress.
	Monitor FHR continuously to assess current status and for further changes in FHR pattern.
	Give oxygen, if indicated.
	Assess visually for possible rupture of membranes or vaginal bleeding.
Variable decelerations	Give oxygen via face mask at 7–10 L/min.
Severe and uncorrectable decelerations	Change maternal position to one in which FHR pattern is most improved, typically the left.
	Increase IV fluids to maintain volume and hydration (normal saline or lactated Ringers).
Late decelerations	Discontinue oxytocin if it is being administered and late decelerations persist despite other interventions.
Late decelerations with tachycardia or variability decreasing	Provide explanation to woman and partner while performing the initial interventions.
	Report findings to physician/CNM and document in chart.
	Prepare for probable cesarean birth.
	Vaginal birth may be possible if woman has reached the second stage and it is anticipated to be short; otherwise, prepare for possible operative vaginal birth if pushing is not yielding fetal descent or cesarean section if slow or no progress.
	Monitor for further FHR changes.
	Maintain maternal position on appropriate side.
	Maintain good hydration with intravenous (IV) fluids (normal saline or lactated Ringers).
	Monitor maternal blood pressure and pulse for signs of hypotension; possibly increase flow rate of IV fluids to treat hypotension.
	Follow physician's orders for treatment for hypotension, if present.
Prolonged decelerations	Perform vaginal examination to rule out prolapsed cord or to determine progress in labor status.
	Administer oxygen via face mask at 7–10 L/min.
	Change maternal position as needed to try to alleviate decelerations.
	Discontinue oxytocin if it is being administered.
	Notify physician/CNM of findings/initial interventions and document in chart.
	Provide explanation to woman and partner.
	Increase IV fluids (normal saline or lactated Ringers).
	Administer tocolytic if hypertonus noted and ordered by physician/CNM.
	Anticipate normal FHR recovery following deceleration if FHR previously normal.
	Anticipate intervention if FHR previously abnormal or deceleration lasts greater than 3 minutes.

Focus your study

- Intrapartum assessment includes attention to both physical and psychosociocultural parameters of the laboring woman, assessment of the fetus, and ongoing assessment for conditions that place the woman and her fetus at an increased risk.
- Birthing room nurses have responsibilities for recognizing and interrupting fetal monitoring patterns, notifying the physician/CNM of problems, and initiating corrective and supportive measures when needed.
- Uterine contractions (UCs) may be assessed externally through palpation or by an electronic monitor. An intrauterine pressure catheter can be placed internally to measure uterine activity more accurately.
- A vaginal examination determines the status of cervical dilatation, effacement, and fetal presentation, position, and station.
- Fetal presentation can also be assessed by inspection, vaginal examination, or ultrasound (US).

- Leopold maneuvers provide a systematic evaluation of fetal presentation and position.
- Intermittent auscultation is the preferred method of fetal assessment in low-risk women in spontaneous labor with Category I tracings.
- Indications for electronic fetal monitoring (EFM) include fetal, maternal, and uterine factors; presence of pregnancy complications; regional anesthesia; and elective monitoring.
- The fetal heart rate (FHR) may be assessed by auscultation or electronic fetal monitoring.
- Electronic fetal monitoring (EFM) is accomplished by indirect ultrasound or by direct methods that require the placement of a spiral electrode on the fetal presenting part.
- Variability refers to baseline (BL) fluctuations of two cycles per minute or greater in the FHR, and it is classified by the visually quantified amplitude of peak-to-trough in beats per minute.
- The normal range of FHR is 110 to 160 beats per minute.
- Baseline changes in the FHR include tachycardia, bradycardia, and variability.
- Tachycardia is defined as a rate of 160 beats per minute or more for at least a 10-minute segment of time.
- Bradycardia is defined as a rate of 110 beats per minute or less for at least a 10-minute segment of time.
- Baseline variability is an important parameter of fetal well-being.
- Periodic changes in the FHR from baseline include decelerations and accelerations. Accelerations are normally caused by fetal movement.
- Decelerations are categorized as early, late, or variable according to NICHD categories.
- Early decelerations are due to compression of the fetal head during contractions and are generally considered benign when they occur with ongoing fetal descent. They typically do not require intervention.
- Late decelerations are associated with uteroplacental insufficiency.
- Variable decelerations are associated with compression of the umbilical cord.
- Sinusoidal patterns are characterized by an undulant sine wave.

References

Alhusen, J. L., Ray, E., Sharps, P., & Bullock, L. (2015). Intimate partner violence during pregnancy: Maternal and neonatal outcomes. *Journal of Women's Health, 24*(1), 100–106. DOI: 10.1089/jwh.2014.4872

American College of Nurse-Midwives (ACNM). (2015). Intermittent auscultation for intrapartum fetal heart rate surveillance. *Journal of Midwifery & Women's Health, 61*(1), 134. DOI: 10.1111/jmwh.12372

American College of Nurse-Midwives (ACNM). (2016). Clinical bulletin: Providing oral nutrition to women in labor. *Journal of Midwifery & Women's Health, 61*(4), 528–534. DOI: 10.1111/jmwh.12515

American College of Obstetricians and Gynecologists (ACOG). (2009). *Intrapartum fetal heart rate monitoring: Nomenclature, interpretation, and general management principles* (ACOG Practice Bulletin No. 106). *Obstetrics & Gynecology, 114*(1), 192–202. DOI: 10.1097/AOG.0b013e3181aef106

American College of Obstetricians and Gynecologists (ACOG). (2010). *Management of fetal heart rate tracings* (ACOG Practice Bulletin No.116). *Obstetrics & Gynecology, 116*(5), 1232–1240.

American College of Obstetricians and Gynecologists (ACOG). (2013a). *Hypertension in pregnancy* (ACOG Task Force Report). Washington, DC: Author.

American College of Obstetricians and Gynecologists (ACOG). (2013b). *Weight gain during pregnancy* (ACOG Committee Opinion No.548). Washington, DC: Author.

American College of Obstetricians and Gynecologists (ACOG). (2015). *Screening for perinatal depression* (ACOG Committee Opinion No. 630). Washington, DC: Author. Retrieved from https://www.acog.org/Resources-And-Publications/Committee-Opinions/Committee-on-Obstetric-Practice/Screening-for-Perinatal-Depression

American College of Obstetricians and Gynecologists (ACOG). (2016). *Hospital-based triage of obstetric patients* (ACOG Committee Opinion No. 667). Washington, DC: Author. Retrieved from https://www.acog.org/Resources-And-Publications/Committee-Opinions/Committee-on-Obstetric-Practice/Hospital-Based-Triage-of-Obstetric-Patients

American College of Obstetricians and Gynecologists (ACOG). (2017a). *Approaches to limit intervention during labor and birth* (ACOG Committee Opinion No. 687). Washington, DC: Author. Retrieved from https://www.acog.org/Resources-And-Publications/Committee-Opinions/Committee-on-Obstetric-Practice/Approaches-to-Limit-Intervention-During-Labor-and-Birth

American College of Obstetricians and Gynecologists (ACOG). (2017b). *Delayed umbilical cord clamping after birth* (ACOG Committee Opinion No. 684). Washington, DC: Author.

American College of Obstetricians and Gynecologists (ACOG). (2017c). *Management of intrapartum fetal heart rate tracings* (ACOG Practice Bulletin No. 116). ACOG: Washington, D.C.

Anderson, B. A., & Stone, S. (2013). *Best practices in midwifery: Using the evidence to implement change.* New York, NY: Springer.

Association of Women's Health, Obstetric and Neonatal Nursing (AWHONN). (2015). Fetal heart rate monitoring. *Journal of Obstetric, Gynecologic, & Neonatal Nursing, 44*(5), 683–686. DOI: 10.1111/1552-6909.12743

Centers for Disease Control and Prevention (CDC). (2016). *Questions & answers about implementing the 2010 guidelines for obstetric providers.* Retrieved from https://www.cdc.gov/groupbstrep/clinicians/QAs-obstetric.html

Donovan, B. M., Spracklen, C. N., Schweizer, M. L., Ryckman, K. K., & Saftlas, A. F. (2016). Intimate partner violence during pregnancy and the risk for adverse infant outcomes: A systematic review and meta-analysis. *British Journal of Obstetrics and Gynaecology, 123*(8), 1289–1299. DOI: 10.1111/1471-0528.13928

Ehsanipoor, R. M., & Satin, A. J. (2017). *Normal and abnormal labor progression.* UpToDate. Retrieved from https://www.uptodate.com/contents/normal-and-abnormal-labor-progression

Euliano, T. Y., Nguyen, M. T., Darmanjian, S., Busowski, J. D., Euliano, N., & Gregg, A. R. (2016). Monitoring uterine activity during labor: Clinician interpretation of electrohysterography versus intrauterine pressure catheter and tocodynamometry. *American Journal of Perinatology, 33*(9), 831–838. DOI: 10.1055/s-0036-1572425

Gabbe, S. A., Niebyl, J. R., Galan, H. L., & Jauniaux, E. R. M. (2017). *Obstetrics: Normal and problem pregnancies: Expert consult.* St. Louis, MO: Saunders.

Giger, J. N. (2017). Introduction to transcultural nursing. In J. N. Giger (Ed.), *Transcultural nursing* (pp. 2–18). St. Louis, MO: Elsevier.

Harper, L. M., Shanks, A. L., Tuuli, M. G., Roehl, K. A., & Cahill, A. G. (2013). The risks and benefits of internal monitors in laboring patients. *American Journal of Obstetrics and Gynecology, 209*(1), 38.e1–38.e6.

Hill, A., Pallitto, C., McCleary-Sills, J., & Garcia-Moreno, C. (2016). A systematic review and meta-analysis of intimate partner violence during pregnancy and selected birth outcomes. *International Journal of Gynaecology and Obstetrics, 133*(3), 269–276. DOI: 10.1016/j.ijgo.2015.10.023

Holley, S. L. (2017). Admission assessment of the fetus. In B. B. Kennedy, S. B. McMurtry, & E. J. Martin (Eds.), *Intrapartum management modules* (5th ed., pp. 69–89). Philadelphia, PA: Wolters Kluwer Health.

Killion, M. M. (2016). The maternal fetal triage index: a standardized approach to OB triage. *MCN: The American Journal of Maternal/Child Nursing, 41*(6), 372.

Kilpatrick, S., & Garrison, E. (2017). Normal labor and delivery. In S. G. Gabbe, J. R. Niebyl, J. L. Simpson, M. B. Landon, H. L. Galan, E. R. M., Jauniaux, D. A., . . . W. A. Grobman, (Eds.), *Obstetrics: Normal and problem pregnancies* (7th ed., pp. 246–270). Philadelphia, PA: Elsevier.

King, T. L., Brucker, M. C., Kriebs, J. M., Fahey, J. O., Gegor, C. L., & Varney, H. (2014). *Varney's midwifery* (5th ed.). Burlington, MA: Jones & Bartlett Learning.

Macones, G. A., Hankins, G. D., Spong, C. Y., Hauth, J., & Moore, T. (2008). The 2008 National Institute of Child Health and Human Development workshop report on electronic monitoring: Update on definitions, interpretation, and research guidelines. *Obstetrics & Gynecology, 112*(3), 661–666.

Miller, L. A., Miller, D. A., & Cypher, R. L. (2017). Methods and instrumentation. *Mosby's pocket guide to fetal monitoring: A multidisciplinary approach* (8th ed., pp. 30–32). St. Louis, MO: Elsevier.

Milton, S. H. (2017). *Normal labor and delivery.* Medscape. Retrieved from https://emedicine.medscape.com/article/260036-overview

Mhyre, J. M., D'Oria, R. Hameed, A. B., Lappen, J. R, Holley, S. L., Hunter, S. K., . . . D'Alton. M. E. (2014). The maternal early warning criteria: A proposal from the national partnership for maternal safety. *Obstetrics & Gynecology, 124*(4), 782–786. DOI: 10.1097/AOG.0000000000000480

National Institutes of Health. (2016). *Clear communication: Cultural respect.* Retrieved from https://www.nih.gov/institutes-nih/nih-office-director/office-communications-public-liaison/clear-communication/cultural-respect

Raghuraman, N., & Cahill, A. G. (2017). Update on fetal monitoring: Overview of approaches and management of category II tracings. *Obstetrics and Gynecology Clinics, 44*(4), 615–624. DOI: 10.1016/j.ogc.2017.08.007

Simkin, P., Hanson, L., & Ancheta, R. (2017). *The labor progress handbook: early interventions to prevent and treat dystocia.* Boston, MA: Wiley.

Sperling, J. D., Dahlke, J. D., & Sibai, B. M. (2016). Restriction of oral intake during labor: Whither are we bound? *American Journal of Obstetrics & Gynecology, 214*(5), 592–596. DOI: 10.1016/j.ajog.2016.01.166

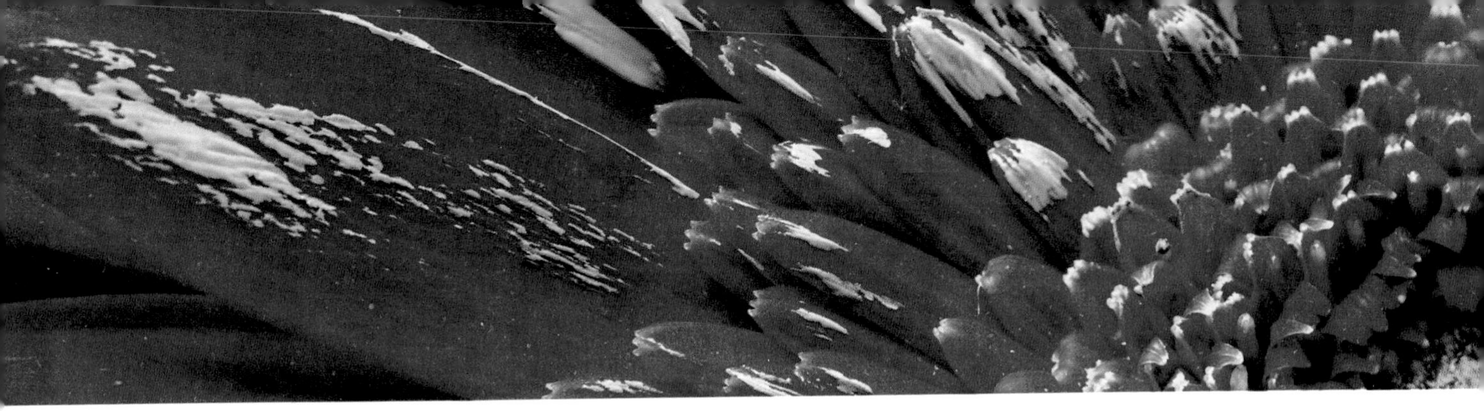

Chapter 21
The Family in Childbirth: Needs and Care

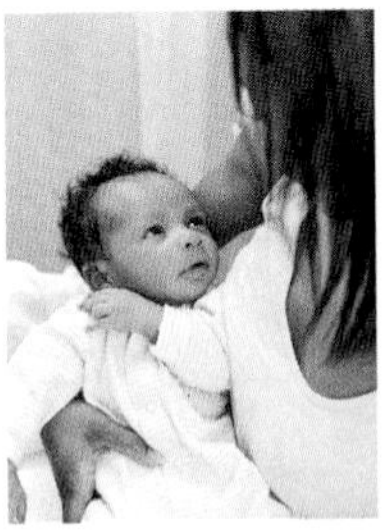

SOURCE: RubberBall/SuperStock.

The moment our daughter was born, time seemed to stand still. We couldn't keep our eyes off of her. I remember vividly the first time I touched her tiny finger and stroked her cheek. Those moments together as a family are forever engraved in my memory.

Learning Outcomes

21.1 Identify nursing diagnoses specific to the first, second, third, and fourth stages of labor.

21.2 Describe factors that are assessed in the laboring woman during the admission process.

21.3 Discuss the components of a social history and its function in caring for the laboring woman.

21.4 Summarize the importance of incorporating family expectations and cultural beliefs into the nursing care plan.

21.5 Discuss nursing interventions to meet the care needs of the laboring woman and her partner during each stage of labor.

21.6 Describe nursing interventions for promoting the woman's comfort during each stage of labor.

21.7 Summarize immediate nursing care of the newborn following birth.

21.8 Discuss the components of care for the woman during the third stage of labor.

21.9 Discuss initial measures to help the woman and family integrate the newborn into family life.

21.10 Explore the nurse's role in providing sensitive, developmentally responsive care to adolescent parents.

21.11 Delineate management of a nurse-managed precipitous labor and birth.

Healthy People 2020

(MICH-1) Reduce the rate of fetal and infant deaths

(MICH-6) Reduce maternal illness and complications due to pregnancy (complications during hospitalized labor and delivery)

(MICH-7) Reduce cesarean births among low-risk (full-term, singleton, vertex presentation) women

It is time for a child to be born. The waiting is over; labor has begun. The dreams and wishes of the past months fade as the expectant family faces the reality of the tasks of childbearing and childrearing that are ahead.

The woman and her husband, partner, or support person are about to undergo one of the most meaningful and stressful events in life together. Physical and psychologic resources, coping mechanisms, and support systems will all be challenged.

Despite avid planning, childbirth education classes, internet research, and reading childbirth materials, the woman may question her ability to cope with labor. The support person may doubt his or her ability to perform in the expected role.

Some childbearing families may fear they will be denied adequate care during labor due to lack of medical insurance or immigration status. In 1986, the Emergency Medical Treatment and Labor Act (EMTLA) was passed by Congress to ensure that patients requiring emergency medical services, including women in labor, had access to medical services regardless of their ability to pay for services or their immigration status (American College of Emergency Physicians [ACEP], 2016).

Many childbearing families look to the nurse for support and guidance. For some women, the nurse may be their only support. It is essential that the nurse provides holistic care that addresses the patient's or couple's physiologic, psychologic, and comfort needs throughout the process of labor and birth.

The previous two chapters present information that lays the foundation for this chapter. Chapter 19 presents a database of information regarding physiologic and psychologic changes during labor and birth, and Chapter 20 discusses intrapartum assessment. This chapter discusses nursing care during labor and birth.

Nursing Diagnoses During Labor and Birth

In devising a plan of care for the intrapartum period, the nurse can develop a comprehensive plan that includes the time from the onset of labor to the fourth stage, or a plan for each stage of labor and birth can be developed. The nurse's plan of care should be based on current nursing and medical research. By providing evidence-based guided care, the nurse ensures that the woman and her family are appropriately cared for during their labor and birth. An overall plan presents an overview of the whole process, but it is usually general in nature. A plan of care that identifies nursing diagnoses for (at least) each stage provides an opportunity to identify more specific nursing interventions.

In the first stage of labor, nursing diagnoses that may apply include:

- ***Anxiety*** related to discomfort of labor and unknown labor outcome
- ***Knowledge, Readiness for Enhanced,*** regarding information about the fetal monitor related to an expressed desire to understand equipment used
- ***Coping: Family, Compromised,*** related to the labor process
- ***Pain, Acute,*** related to uterine contractions, cervical dilatation, and fetal descent
- ***Knowledge, Deficient,*** related to lack of information about the normal labor process and comfort measures
- ***Fear*** related to unknown birth outcome and anticipated discomfort

(NANDA-I © 2017)

Nursing diagnoses for the second and third stages may include:

- ***Pain, Acute,*** related to uterine contractions, birth process, and/or perineal trauma from birth
- ***Knowledge, Deficient,*** related to lack of information about pushing methods
- ***Coping, Ineffective,*** related to the birth process
- ***Fear*** related to outcome of the birth process

(NANDA-I © 2017)

In the fourth stage, possible nursing diagnoses include:

- ***Pain, Acute,*** related to perineal trauma
- ***Knowledge, Deficient,*** related to lack of information about the involutional process and self-care needs
- ***Family Processes, Readiness for Enhanced,*** related to incorporation of the newborn into the family

(NANDA-I © 2017)

Women with Special Needs **Mental Disabilities**

Women with mental disabilities, such as PTSD, may experience flashbacks and excessive fear during labor. Supportive care with one nurse is preferred so that a personal relationship and trust can be established. Labor often triggers painful flashbacks in women who have been sexually abused or sexually assaulted.

Nursing Care During Admission

Many families worry that they will not reach the birthing center in time for the birth or that cues indicating the onset of labor will be missed. Sometimes labor occurs so rapidly that birth is imminent upon admission, but this is rare, especially in nulliparous women. Usually, the family is advised to arrive at the birth setting at the beginning of the active phase of labor or when the following occur:

- Rupture of membranes (ROM)
- Decreased fetal movement
- Regular, frequent uterine contractions (UCs) (nulliparas, about 5 minutes apart for 1 hour; multiparas, 6 to 8 minutes apart for 1 hour)
- Any vaginal bleeding.

If time permits and the family is not familiar with what will occur during labor, the nurse can provide information on admission. (See *Teaching Highlights: What to Expect During Labor.*) The family may be facing a number of unfamiliar procedures. It is important to remember that each woman has the right to determine what happens to her body. Informed consent should be obtained before any procedure that involves touching the body.

Establishing a Positive Relationship

The initial interaction with the nurse and how it is perceived by the woman and her partner greatly influences the course of her hospital stay. Sometimes, the hospital environment can appear

TEACHING HIGHLIGHTS What to Expect During Labor

- Describe aspects of the admission process
  - Abbreviated history
  - Physical assessment (maternal vital signs, fetal heart rate, contraction status, status of membranes)
  - Assessment of uterine contractions (frequency, duration, intensity)
  - Orientation to surroundings and staff introductions
  - Determine couple's expectations of the nurse.
- Advise of ongoing care time frame parameters (such as frequency of maternal vital signs, fetal heart rate, and contraction assessments).
- Explain type of monitoring to be used with rationale for use and what to expect from the equipment.
- Explain what "normal" data look like and what characteristics are being watched for.
- Advise that assessment frequency increases as labor progresses.
- Explain the vaginal examination and the information obtained.
- Review comfort techniques and ascertain what the woman thinks will promote comfort.
- Review breathing techniques; if the woman is unfamiliar with techniques, review them in simple-to-understand language and encourage her to practice.
- Review comfort and support measures such as positioning, back rub, touch, distraction techniques, and ambulation.
- If the woman is in early labor, offer her a tour of the birthing area.
- Have printed materials available for reference in the woman's native language.
- If time permits, videos showing coping skills and what to expect during labor may be helpful.

cold, impersonal, and technical, resulting in anxiety and stress. If the family is greeted by the nurse in a brusque, harried manner, they are less likely to look to the nurse for support. A calm, pleasant manner, in contrast, indicates to the family that they are important and can instill a sense of confidence in the staff's ability to provide quality care and ensure safety.

It is important to establish rapport and to create a supportive environment for the family in which they feel free to ask questions. Before performing an assessment, explain the procedure and allow time for questions. The support and encouragement of the nurse begins with the initial encounter and should continue throughout the woman's stay. Continuous rather than intermittent support during the labor process has been validated as having positive outcomes in terms of fewer cesarean and operative deliveries and fewer requests for pain medications. In addition, newborns were found to have higher 5-minute Apgar scores (MacKinnon et al., 2017).

During the admission, the woman is asked to sign informed consent for treatment and is often given information on arranging advance directives. An identification and allergy bracelet should be double-checked with the woman and then applied to her wrist.

Another important aspect of the initial contact is communicating in the woman and family's primary language. Interpreters should be available for patients who do not speak English fluently and for women or family members who are deaf.

Women with Special Needs Hearing Loss

It is estimated that 15% of adults have some form of hearing loss, with the majority being adults over the age of 60 (National Institute on Deafness and Other Communication Disorders, 2016). Pregnant women who are deaf often do not have access to interpreters, which can impact newborn outcomes. Women who are deaf are at an increased risk for low birth weight and preterm birth (Mitra, Akobirshoev, McKee, et al., 2016).

Culture plays a major role in how a woman and her family view the labor and birth process. Trends in American culture are moving toward a shared partnership model between the woman and her partner in which the partner is actively involved in the birth process and often stays with the mother throughout the labor and birth. In contrast, some Iranian and Turkish women may be less likely to have their partner with them in the labor and birth setting and may prefer to have female family members or friends with them (Spector, 2016). The nurse should never assume a patient's preferences based on race, ethnicity, or geographic background because most families embrace various customs and traditions unique to their own family unit. See *Developing Cultural Competence: Home Births in Amish Communities*.

Developing Cultural Competence Home Births in Amish Communities

Approximately 40 to 80% of Amish women give birth at home or in an Amish-run birthing center. The factors for these choices are often driven by costs (the Amish have no commercial health insurance), geographic distance, and preference to be cared for in the home setting. Amish women in the United States, many of whom have eight or more children, are cared for by CNMs, lay midwives, and, in rare cases, physicians who attend home births. Because the Amish do not utilize electricity, caregivers must bring specialized equipment for the birth. At most Amish births, the husband is the only family member in attendance. Many Amish families decline medical interventions, such as vitamin K injections, eye ointment, hepatitis B vaccines, or circumcision. Once an Amish woman gives birth, a young single Amish girl is typically employed as a maid in the home for 4 to 6 weeks to perform household chores for the family (Wente, 2015).

Note: It is unwise to attribute specific attitudes or beliefs to all members of a cultural group. The information in the Developing Cultural Competence boxes offers possible insights into caring for women from different cultural groups.

Labor Assessment

Following the initial greeting, the woman may either be taken into a labor assessment area (sometimes called a *triage area*) for evaluation or admitted directly into a birthing room. Ideally, the nurse should ask the woman if she prefers to complete the assessment process alone or have her partner or family members present. During the admission history, the nurse can initiate any immediate interventions needed and establish individualized priorities. The nurse is then able to make effective nursing decisions regarding intrapartum care:

- Is the woman in labor, or is she a candidate to be sent home with a clear understanding of when to return?
- Are there factors that put the laboring woman or the fetus at risk?
- Should ambulation or bedrest be encouraged?
- Is more frequent monitoring needed?
- What are the woman's wishes and special requests for the labor and birth?
- Who will be with the laboring woman for social support?

The woman is assisted into a comfortable position. If she wants to rest in bed, a sidelying or semi-Fowler position rather than a supine position is most comfortable and avoids supine hypotensive syndrome (vena cava syndrome).

After obtaining the essential information from the woman and her prenatal records from her physician/CNM, the nurse begins the intrapartum assessment. (Chapter 20 discusses intrapartum assessment in depth.)

As the assessments begin, the nurse auscultates the fetal heart rate (FHR) (detailed information on monitoring FHR is presented in Chapter 16), vital signs, contraction status (frequency, duration, and intensity), cervical dilatation and effacement, and fetal presentation and station. A determination of whether the woman is admitted or sent home is then made. Some women may be advised to ambulate to determine if labor is progressing and admission is warranted. Women who are admitted in the latent phase are more likely to have a longer duration of labor, increased use of epidural analgesia for pain, and increased use of oxytocin to augment labor than women who are clearly in the active phase at admission.

A vaginal examination is performed to assess for advanced labor (frequent contractions, advanced cervical dilatation, and/or an urge to bear down). If the labor is progressing rapidly or if the woman is in advanced labor, the physician/CNM is notified immediately while preparations for the birth are made. If there are signs of excessive bleeding upon admission or if the woman reports episodes of painless bleeding in the last trimester, placenta previa may be present; in such cases, vaginal examination is not performed because it may stimulate copious bleeding.

Results of the comprehensive assessment determine if the admission is routine or if urgency is needed. Indicators of normal labor are included in Table 21–1.

If high-risk or emergency data are identified, the nurse immediately reports the findings to the physician/CNM; otherwise, all assessment data should be gathered before initiating contact with the healthcare provider. The report should include this information:

- Cervical dilatation and effacement
- Station
- Presenting part
- Status of the membranes
- Contraction pattern
- Fetal heart rate
- Vital signs that are not in the normal range
- Response to labor by the woman and her wishes for the birth and desire for analgesia/anesthesia.

Collecting Laboratory Data

After admission data are obtained, multiple laboratory tests are performed to provide more extensive physiologic data that are used to determine appropriate care for the woman and her fetus. A clean-voided midstream urine specimen is tested for the presence of protein, ketones, glucose, and leukocytes by using a dipstick before sending the sample to the laboratory. This procedure is especially important if nondependent edema or elevated blood pressure is noted on admission. Proteinuria of +1 or more may be a sign of preeclampsia. Glycosuria is found frequently in pregnant women because of the increased glomerular filtration rate in the proximal tubules and the inability of these tubules to increase glucose reabsorption. However, it may also be associated with gestational diabetes

TABLE 21–1 Indicators of Normal Labor Process on Admission

INDICATOR	NORMAL CHARACTERISTICS
Uterine contractions	Frequency of not less than 2 minutes
	Duration of less than 75 seconds
	Uterine relaxation between contractions
	Most intense discomfort only with contractions (Some women, especially those with occiput posterior position, complain of less intense lower abdominal and/or back pain between contractions.)
Fetal heart rate	Rate 110–160 with average variability
	Absence of late decelerations
Maternal vital signs	BP at or less than 120/80 or less than a 30 systolic or 15 diastolic increase above prepregnancy readings
	Pulse 60–100
	Temperature between 36.5°C and 37.5°C (97.8°F and 99.6°F)
If membranes ruptured	Fluid clear without odor

and should not be discounted. Leukocytes can be found in the urine when bacteria are present. The presence of a urinary tract infection can contribute to uterine irritability, pelvic pressure, and back pain, all symptoms that can be mistaken for labor.

Laboratory tests are performed in the outpatient setting; however, some labs are also done upon admission. Hemoglobin and hematocrit values help determine the oxygen-carrying capacity of the circulatory system and the ability of the woman to withstand blood loss at birth. Elevation of the hematocrit indicates hemoconcentration of blood, which occurs with edema or dehydration. A low hemoglobin, in the absence of other evidence of bleeding, suggests anemia. Blood is typed and cross-matched on most women admitted to the labor unit. A serology test for syphilis is obtained. The Centers for Disease Control and Prevention (CDC), American Congress of Obstetricians and Gynecologists (ACOG), Association of Women's Health, Obstetric, and Neonatal Nurses (AWHONN), and the U.S. Preventative Services Task Force recommend that all women undergo voluntary screening for HIV during pregnancy. Women who have not been screened during the pregnancy should be screened for HIV in the intrapartum setting once consent has been obtained (CDC, 2015).

Social Assessment

Once initial physical assessments are performed, the nurse can then take a detailed social history that provides a comprehensive view of both the woman's social habits and psychologic factors that may affect her birth experience. The presence of certain risk factors—including family violence or sexual assault (see Chapter 8); use of drugs, alcohol, or tobacco; and presence of sexually transmitted infections—can influence a woman's labor, birth, and future childrearing choices. It is imperative to ask the woman about domestic violence and to assess any degree of psychologic or physical harm, either potential or real. Because many women find questions about psychosocial risk factors embarrassing, the nurse should always ask such questions when the woman is alone and should use a straightforward, nonjudgmental approach. For example, a question such as "How many times per week do you drink alcohol?" prompts the woman to be specific in her answer. If the woman reports that she does drink alcohol on a daily basis, the nurse then asks about the amount. Drug use can be assessed in a similar manner.

A social assessment should also include data about the woman's current living situation, availability of resources, preparedness for the newborn, community resources, and the woman's social support network. This dialogue provides an opportunity for the nurse to continue to build support, to provide information when requested, and to be direct yet supportive. Referrals to social services, the Special Supplemental Nutrition Program for Women, Infants, and Children (WIC), and new parent support programs can be initiated. It is important to begin this dialogue early in the admission process so that adequate resources can be obtained for the family.

Documentation of Admission

A nursing admission note is entered into the computer or the charting system and should include the reason for admission; the date, time, and method of the woman's arrival; notification of the physician/CNM; the condition of the woman; labor and membrane status; current level of pain; presence of support system; and pertinent social assessment information.

Nursing Care During the First Stage of Labor

After completing the nursing assessment and diagnosis steps, the nurse creates a plan of care. During the first stage of labor, the nurse is concerned about the physical safety of the woman and fetus, along with the woman and her partner's emotional well-being. The nurse continually assesses the effects and pattern of the UCs, FHR, and fetal well-being, maternal vital signs (VS), cervical changes, and intake and output. Additionally, the nurse monitors the responses to labor of the woman, her support person, and family.

Labor support is a primary role for nurses during the first stage of labor. The woman and her family look to their nurse for information about labor progress, pain management, procedures, and examinations and for assistance with pain management techniques such as breathing and relaxation. Reassurance that labor is progressing well and explanations about deviations from normal are needed. The couple will also benefit from positive encouragement and praise. For most families, the nurse's presence in the room is reassuring and desired; however, the nurse should assess the woman's individual preferences, because some women may prefer privacy. Clinical research has established that laboring women have fewer complications and shorter labors when they perceive support from their nurse, doula, and/or friends and family members (Simkin, Hanson, & Ancheta, 2017).

Integration of Family Expectations

Laboring families have certain expectations of the experience, of themselves, of the nurse, and of the physician/CNM. In some cases, expectations may not be realistic. Unrealistic expectations can increase anxiety levels for the woman and her partner. The labor nurse should assess the family's expectations to integrate them into the labor plan and/or assist the family in reestablishing expectations that are realistic. Some families may present to the facility with a birth plan (see Chapter 13). The plan should be reviewed and requests should be incorporated into the woman's nursing care plan whenever possible. Requests that cannot be met should be discussed and a clear rationale should be provided.

With the variety of expectations patients have of nurses, it becomes a challenge to provide individualized care. The nurse needs to assess and respond to the woman's needs and desires. To determine preferences, the nurse can look for cues. When the woman and her support person are admitted, do they seem to take control and know what is going to happen? Do they have a birth plan that they have already worked out, or do they seem hesitant and unsure of the process?

Although these two ends of the spectrum are obvious, they are a starting point. The nurse can also gain more information by asking questions such as, "Other than the assessments that I will be making, what kind of involvement would you like from me? Would you like to call me when you need something or have me come in now and then, or would you be more comfortable if I stay in the room most of the time?" This gives them an opportunity to make their wishes known. This approach also provides them with the opportunity to ask questions and seek advice as needed. It is also important that the woman knows that the nurse understands that her wishes may change during labor and that the nurse will be available for her throughout the process.

During the labor process, the nurse also serves as an advocate for the woman and her support person. The support person may need support, guidance, or an opportunity for rest periods. The nurse models behavior to family members who may feel uncomfortable or uneasy in the labor and birth setting (Groll, 2017).

Integration of Cultural Beliefs

Values, customs, and practices of different cultures are as important during labor as they are in the prenatal period. Research indicates that an individual's experiences in labor are highly dependent upon social and cultural norms. Without this knowledge, a nurse is less likely to understand a family's behavior and may impose personal values and beliefs upon them. As cultural sensitivity increases, so does the likelihood of providing high-quality care (Spector, 2016).

The following sections briefly present a few possible cultural responses to labor. Additional information on culturally sensitive care is provided in Chapter 2. It is difficult to present such a limited discussion without appearing to advance stereotypes. No statement of a specific behavior can accurately reflect the preference of all people in a group. Within every culture, each person develops his or her own beliefs and value system. Nurses must regard general information about any culture or belief system as background information to help them determine the person's own needs and desires.

MODESTY

Modesty is an important consideration for women, regardless of the culture to which they belong. However, some women may be more uncomfortable than others with the degree of exposure needed for some procedures. Some women may be particularly uncomfortable when men are present and feel more comfortable with women; others may be uncomfortable with exposure of personal body parts regardless of the gender of the examiner or person who assists them. The nurse needs to be observant of the woman's responses to examinations and procedures and to provide appropriate draping and privacy (Spector, 2016). It is more prudent to assume that embarrassment will occur with exposure and take measures to provide privacy than to assume that it will not matter to the woman.

Clinical Tip

It is best not to assume that women of any culture have the information they desire about birth, self-care, and newborn care, regardless of the number of children they have had. An important aspect of nursing is to teach, so always offer culturally sensitive information. Be sensitive, and ask what is important to the mother. For example, is there special clothing she wants the newborn to wear, or does she have any preference about how she wants the umbilical stump cared for? Remain aware that the information you learned in class or a text primarily reflects the nursing culture and the Western, chiefly European, culture. To believe that the health-care practices of these two cultures are relevant to all people is an example of ethnocentrism. Strive to increase your understanding of other cultures as your clinical practice base grows.

For example, some Hispanic women may fear loss of privacy, so they labor at home as long as possible. Some Asian women are not accustomed to male physicians and attendants, and some Muslims forbid any male (other than the husband) to see a woman who is uncovered. The nurse should be aware that in traditional Muslim cultures, the man is the primary source of information. It may be necessary to speak to the man before interacting with the woman. This communicates respect and shows cultural sensitivity. The nurse should ensure coverage of the woman whenever possible, even during vaginal exams and the second stage (Spector, 2016).

“I am in an area with a very small Muslim population, and one of the nursing students with me had the opportunity to work with a Muslim couple during labor, birth, and then in the postpartum area the following day. During labor, the woman's sister remained at her side, and her husband sat on the other side of a drawn curtain inside the labor room and close to the door. He requested that a sign be placed on the door indicating that no males were to enter the room. We took care to ensure that we asked for a female lab tech for blood drawing, and a female physician attended the birth. The labor and birth went smoothly, and the woman did not utter any sound, even during pushing. After the birth, the father was shown the child before his wife held the newborn boy. The father was very pleased and talked quietly to his son, with his head down beside the newborn's ear. The next day, the student was once again assigned to this family. The sign remained on the door, and at all times that day, the sister and father remained in the room, the father always sitting away from the bed, close to the door. This was the woman's fifth child, so at first the student thought that she would not want much self-care, newborn, or breastfeeding information. But she began to talk to the woman, with her husband interpreting all questions and giving answers, and as each topic was brought up, the mother indicated that she wanted more information. Building on the trust that they had established the previous day in labor, the father told the student to "give the instruction," and he left the room. The mother and sister were full of questions about their health and their bodies—questions they had had for years! The student was proud that she did not make assumptions and was able to share so much information with them. It was an experience that the student and I will always remember with great joy.”

PAIN EXPRESSION

Women's reactions to the discomfort of labor vary greatly. Some turn inward and remain very quiet during the whole process, whereas others may be very vocal, with behaviors such as counting out loud, moaning quietly or loudly, crying, or cursing. They may also turn from side to side or change positions frequently. The nurse supports a woman's individual expression of pain, whatever it may be, to enhance the birthing experience for mother, baby, and family.

In the Korean culture, for example, it used to be important for the laboring woman to be silent so she would not bring shame on her family. However, today women are encouraged to be less passive. Vocalization is more common, although older family members may discourage shouting or outcries as aggressive behavior. Some Hmong women may be quiet during labor, although behavior varies from one individual to the next. European Americans demonstrate a wide variety of behaviors in response to pain. Especially in the transitional phase, some women want to squeeze their partner's (or the nurse's) hand, and some may be tempted to bite during the most intense part of the contraction. Some Latina women use less pain medication and often avoid epidural anesthesia due to cultural-based beliefs that women should endure labor without medication (Spector, 2016).

In working with women from another culture, the nurse needs an awareness of the individual couple's beliefs, values, and practices to understand their needs. The maternity nurse would do well to make it a priority to become acquainted with the beliefs and practices of the various cultures in the community while keeping in mind that stereotyping should be avoided. Instead, an open conversation with the couple to learn about their various practices and wishes for the birth is far more important. In the birthing situation, the nurse supports the family's cultural practices as long as it is safe to do so.

CASE STUDY: Azia Askari

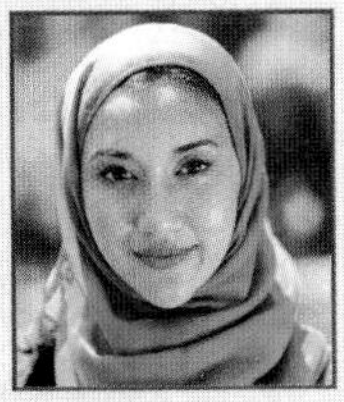

SOURCE: HONGQI ZHANG/123RF.

Azia presents to the local hospital with reports of beginning contractions yesterday after walking with her daughters outdoors to a nearby playground. Her sister-in-law has brought her to the hospital and is translating for the nurse. The hospital has an interpreter who speaks Farsi who is en route to the hospital to translate. Her sister-in-law reports that the contractions have increased in frequency, duration, and strength and they are now occurring every 3 to 5 minutes, lasting 45 to 60 seconds, and they are getting stronger. She stresses that the family has a firm preference for female-only care providers based on their cultural beliefs and Muslim religion.

Question to Ponder

What steps would you take to support Azia's cultural beliefs in this situation?

Provision of Care in the First Stage

Throughout the first stage, the nurse needs to evaluate physical parameters of the woman and her fetus. Maternal temperature is monitored every 4 hours unless the temperature is over 37.5°C (99.6°F); in such cases, it must be taken every hour. Once the amniotic fluid has ruptured, temperature should be monitored every 2 hours.

The nurse monitors blood pressure, pulse, and respirations every hour. If the woman's blood pressure is greater than a 30 systolic or 15 diastolic increase above prepregnancy readings or her pulse is more than 100, the physician/CNM must be notified. The blood pressure and pulse are then reevaluated more frequently. The nurse palpates uterine contractions for frequency, intensity, and duration.

Intrapartum vaginal exams are done to assess cervical changes, status of membranes, fetal position, and station. However, frequent vaginal exams increase the risk of infection and should be performed only when needed. Some providers advocate performing vaginal examinations only when a change of management will occur, such as before an epidural or to provide scalp stimulation.

The fetal heart rate (FHR) is auscultated every 30 minutes as long as it remains between 110 and 160 beats per minute (beats/min) without the presence of decelerations (AWHONN, 2016). The FHR should be auscultated throughout one contraction and for about 15 seconds after the contraction to ensure that there are no decelerations. If the FHR is not in the 110 to 160 range and/or decelerations are heard, continuous electronic monitoring is recommended. The nurse documents labor progress, status of fetus, and interventions in the woman's chart. See *Key Facts to Remember: Nursing Assessments in the First Stage of Labor.*

Clinical Tip

If the monitor is no longer recording the fetal heart tracing, check that there is adequate gel under the transducer and reposition it before you assume there is a problem with the baby.

Key Facts to Remember

Nursing Assessments in the First Stage of Labor

Phase	Mother	Fetus
Latent	Blood pressure, respirations each hour if in normal range Temperature every 4 hours unless over 37.5°C (99.6°F) or membranes ruptured, then every hour Uterine contractions every 15–30 minutes	FHR every 30 minutes for low-risk women and every 15 minutes for high-risk women if normal characteristics present (presence of variability, baseline [BL] in the 110–160 beats/min range, without late decelerations) Note fetal activity If electronic fetal monitor in place, assess for reactive nonstress test (NST)
Active	Blood pressure, pulse, respirations every hour if in normal range Uterine contractions palpated every 15–30 minutes	FHR every 30 minutes for low-risk women and every 15 minutes for high-risk women if normal characteristics are present (AWHONN, 2016)
Transition	Blood pressure, pulse, respirations every 15–30 minutes Contractions palpated at least every 15–30 minutes	FHR every 15–30 minutes if normal characteristics are present

LATENT PHASE

If the laboring woman has not had childbirth education classes, the latent phase is a time when the nurse can give anticipatory guidance. Most women are eager to know what to expect. Most women are not too uncomfortable during contractions in this phase and are responsive to learning breathing and other coping techniques. The unprepared woman may hesitate to ask questions but can benefit from anticipatory guidance offered by the nurse.

As long as there are no contraindications (such as vaginal bleeding or rupture of membranes with the fetus unengaged), the woman may be encouraged to ambulate to encourage fetal head descent. A tour of the birthing facility decreases anxiety and can provide a distraction. Many women feel more comfortable walking and changing position and prefer not to remain in bed. Some may be unaware that ambulation is an option and should be advised that ambulation aids in fetal descent, increases the frequency and intensity of contractions, and allows the woman to make her own choices for positioning when contractions occur (Figure 21–1).

The nurse should offer fluids and light snacks as desired for women with low-risk pregnancies. Women with high-risk pregnancies may have clear liquids throughout labor, however, if a cesarean birth is anticipated or scheduled, oral hydration should be stopped due to the reduced gastric emptying time and risk of aspiration with surgical birth. A recent meta-analysis and systematic review showed that oral intake during labor does not result in adverse maternal or fetal outcomes and actually reduces the duration of labor (Ciardulli, Saccone, Anastasio, et al., 2017). Vomiting during labor does sometimes occur during the transition phase and is related to decreased gastric emptying time. The nurse should reassure the woman and provide oral care.

ACTIVE PHASE

During the active phase, the contractions have a frequency of 2 to 3 minutes, a duration of 50 to 60 seconds, and moderate intensity. Contractions need to be palpated every 15 to 30 minutes. As the contractions become more frequent and intense, intrapartum vaginal examination may be performed to assess cervical dilatation and effacement and fetal station and position. During the active phase, the cervix dilates from 4 to 7 cm, and vaginal discharge and bloody show increase. The woman should be encouraged to void because a full bladder can interfere with fetal descent. If the woman is unable to void, catheterization may be necessary. Maternal vital signs, including blood pressure, pulse, and respirations, should be assessed every hour for low-risk women (unless previously elevated) and every 30 minutes for high-risk women. The FHR is auscultated every 30 minutes for women without complications and more frequently (every 15 minutes) for women with complications (ACOG, 2017b).

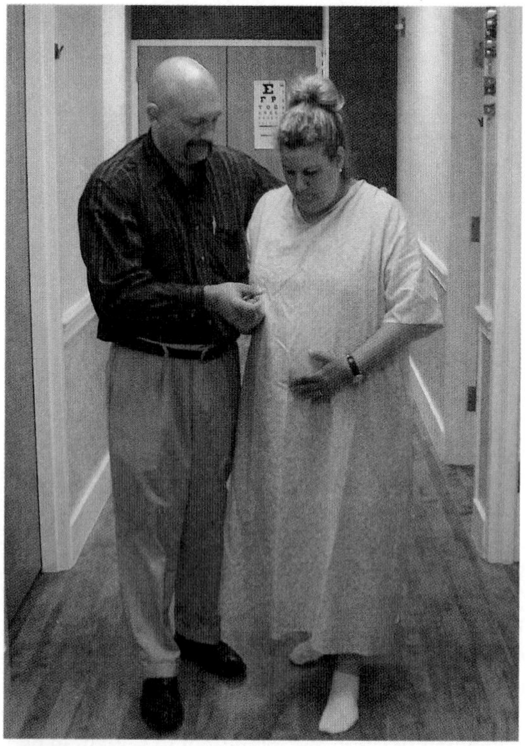

Figure 21–1 Woman and her partner walking in the hospital during labor.

SOURCE: Michele Davidson.

For the woman experiencing slow progress of labor or the inability to tolerate fluids, an intravenous (IV) electrolyte solution may be started to provide energy and prevent dehydration. If an IV is started, it becomes even more important to encourage voiding every 1 to 2 hours to prevent bladder distention.

If the amniotic membranes have not ruptured previously, the physician/CNM may do so when the first stage of labor is near completion. Routine amniotomy is not indicated if the labor is progressing normally and the fetal status is stable. Amniotomy may be performed if additional monitoring is warranted (ACOG, 2017b). When the membranes rupture, the nurse notes the color and odor of the amniotic fluid and the time of rupture and immediately auscultates the FHR. The fluid should be clear with no odor.

Meconium-stained amniotic fluid may be a sign of a compromised fetus or may be present when the fetus is in a breech presentation. In the case of a breech fetus, meconium staining may not indicate a compromised fetus. In a cephalic presentation, however, meconium staining may indicate a compromised fetal state. When the fetus is compromised, the intestines and anal sphincter relax, leading to the release of meconium into the amniotic fluid. Meconium turns the fluid greenish brown. Whenever the nurse notes meconium-stained fluid, an electronic monitor is applied to continuously assess the FHR (ACOG, 2017b). The time of rupture is noted because the incidence of amnionitis increases with rupture over 24 hours.

Clinical Tip

Catheterizing a woman during a contraction is uncomfortable for her and difficult to do because of the increased downward pressure. To avoid these problems, pass the catheter between contractions. If the baby's head is low in the pelvis, you will have to change the direction of the catheter. Visualize passing it up and over the baby's head rather than straight into the urethra.

An additional concern is prolapse of the umbilical cord, which occurs when membranes rupture and the fetus is not engaged. The concern is that the amniotic fluid coming through the cervix will propel the umbilical cord through the cervix (prolapsed cord). Prolapsed cord is assessed by monitoring for signs of nonreassuring fetal status and performing a vaginal examination with a sterile glove. The FHR is auscultated because a drop in the rate might indicate an undetected prolapsed cord. Immediate intervention is necessary to remove pressure on a prolapsed umbilical cord until a cesarean birth can be performed (see Chapter 25). See Table 21–2 for additional deviations from normal. See *Promotion of Comfort in the First Stage* later in the chapter for comfort management for the patient.

TRANSITION PHASE

During transition, the contraction frequency is every 1.5 to 2 minutes, duration is 60 to 90 seconds, and intensity is strong. Cervical dilatation increases from 8 to 10 cm, effacement is complete (100%), and a heavy amount of bloody show is usually present. Some multiparous women may not completely efface prior to the birth. Nulliparous women should completely efface prior to the birth of the baby. Contractions are palpated at least every 15 minutes. Sterile vaginal examination can be done during this stage of labor to assess rapid changes in status. Maternal blood pressure, pulse, and respirations are taken at least every 30 minutes, and FHR is auscultated every 30 minutes for low-risk women and every 15 minutes for high-risk women (ACOG, 2017b).

TABLE 21–2 Deviations from Normal Labor Process Requiring Immediate Intervention

PROBLEM	IMMEDIATE ACTION
Women admitted with vaginal bleeding or history of painless vaginal bleeding	• Do not perform vaginal examination. • Assess FHR. • Evaluate amount of blood loss. • Evaluate labor pattern. • Notify physician/CNM immediately.
Presence of greenish or brownish amniotic fluid	• Continuously monitor FHR. • Evaluate dilatation of cervix and determine if umbilical cord is prolapsed. • Evaluate presentation (vertex or breech). • Maintain woman on complete bedrest on left side. • Notify physician/CNM immediately. • Have suction equipment and laryngoscope at the bedside to provide immediate suctioning upon delivery.
Decrease in FHR below 110 beats/min	• Perform vaginal examination to assess for prolapsed cord. • Turn woman to a sidelying or hands-and-knees position. • Administer oxygen by face mask. • Discontinue pitocin. • Call the physician/CNM. • Continue continuous external monitoring or place internal fetal monitor if hospital protocol allows and rupture of membranes (ROM) has occurred. • Provide fetal scalp stimulation.
Absence of FHR and fetal movement	• Notify physician/CNM. • Provide truthful information and emotional support to laboring couple. • Remain with the couple.
Prolapse of umbilical cord	• Relieve pressure on cord manually. • Continuously monitor FHR; watch for changes in FHR pattern. • Notify physician/CNM. • Assist woman into knee-chest position or place in Trendelenburg position. • Administer oxygen.

Woman admitted in advanced labor; birth imminent	• Prepare for immediate birth.
	• Obtain critical information:
	  • Estimated date of birth (EDB)
	  • History of bleeding problems
	  • History of medical or obstetric problems
	  • Past and/or present use/abuse of prescription/OTC/illicit drugs
	  • Problems with this pregnancy
	  • FHR and maternal vital signs
	  • Whether membranes are ruptured and how long since rupture
	  • Blood type and Rh
	• Direct another person to contact physician/CNM.
	• Do not leave woman alone.
	• Provide support to couple.
	• Put on gloves.

Throughout labor the woman's center of focus gradually turns inward. She becomes less aware of what is going on around her and intensely aware of her uterine contractions. She experiences body boundary diffusion, which hampers her ability to know where her body ends and her external environment begins. Women during this time will reach out to others but may be uncomfortable with others touching them.

The woman's ability to speak in coherent sentences can be impaired during the transitional phase. This makes it difficult for the woman to communicate her needs to healthcare providers and her support team. The support person(s) and nurse need to follow the woman's cues and change interventions as needed.

The nurse should encourage the woman to rest between contractions by instructing the woman at the end of her contraction to take a deep breath and to let it out slowly while she relaxes her muscles. Helping to maintain a quiet room between contractions can also enhance the woman's ability to rest. The woman during this phase is present focused; thus, providing instruction between contractions should be kept to a minimum.

Some women have difficulty coping with the intensity of labor during this time and need assistance in performing breathing techniques. Either the support person or the nurse can breathe along with the woman during each contraction to help her maintain her pattern. It is helpful to encourage her and assure her that she is doing a good job. The woman will begin to feel increased rectal pressure as the fetal presenting part moves down the birth canal and sometimes a burning sensation as the tissues begin to stretch. The nurse encourages the woman to refrain from pushing until the cervix is completely dilated. For the woman who is unmedicated, the urge to push may seem unbearable. Specific instructions, such as encouraging the woman to "blow in short breaths like you are blowing out a candle" or "pant like a puppy," can help prevent the woman from involuntarily pushing. This measure also helps prevent cervical edema or lacerations.

The end of transition and beginning of the second stage may be indicated by involuntary passage of flatus or stool and the movement of the fetus from the side of the maternal abdomen to the midline. Other indications include a change in the woman's voice or the sounds she is making. As the fetus moves down and she feels increased pressure and a bearing-down sensation, her voice tends to deepen. A moan during a contraction takes on a more guttural quality. Labor nurses recognize this sound as a sign that the woman may have entered the second stage.

Promotion of Comfort in the First Stage

The first step in planning care for the laboring woman is to talk with the woman and her partner or support person to identify their goals. Usually the main concern is discomfort, so it is important to identify factors that may contribute to discomfort. These factors include uncomfortable positions, diaphoresis, continual leaking of amniotic fluid, a full bladder, dry mouth, anxiety, and fear. Nursing interventions can minimize the effects of these factors. See Personal Comfort Measures later in this section.

In labor, the more common pain reactions—such as increased pulse and respiratory rates, dilated pupils, increased blood pressure, and muscle tension—are transitory because the pain is intermittent. However, increased muscle tension may impede the progress of labor; therefore, the nurse encourages the woman to relax her skeletal muscles and avoid holding her breath.

Sounds are an important part of the labor and birthing process. Some women naturally make sounds such as moans and grunts and feel that it helps them cope and do the work of labor; they are responding to what their body tells them to do. Others begin to make loud sounds (screams) only as they lose their ability to cope and feel they do not have any other options.

Some women may want physical contact during contractions. They may provide verbal and nonverbal signs, such as crying, moaning, and beseeching the coach or nurse to hold their hand or rub their back. They may look at the support person or reach out for help to indicate their anxiety. Touch may be used to convey support and enhance comfort for the woman. She may be soothed by a neck or back rub or by holding the hand of her partner or the nurse. A woman generally wants touching and physical contact during the first part of labor, but when she moves into the transition phase, she may rebuff all efforts and pull away. Other women do not want to be touched at all, regardless of the phase of labor. Speaking in a low, calm voice conveys support and shows that the nurse and others are present.

A decrease in the intensity of discomfort is one of the goals of nursing support during labor. Nursing measures to decrease pain include:

- Encouraging position changes
- Assisting with personal comfort measures
- Decreasing anxiety
- Providing information
- Using specific supportive relaxation techniques
- Encouraging paced breathing
- Administering pharmacologic agents as desired by the woman.

POSITION CHANGES

The maternal position for birth varies based on maternal preference to standard protocols. It can vary from remaining ambulatory to the standard lithotomy position to sidelying or kneeling.

The woman is encouraged to ambulate if the fetal head is engaged and the intermittent fetal monitoring has shown a reassuring FHR pattern. However, to avoid the risk of umbilical cord prolapse, the woman is generally instructed to remain in bed if membranes are ruptured and the presenting part is not engaged.

Even if the woman prefers not to walk around, upright positions such as sitting in a rocker or leaning against a wall or bed can enhance comfort. Women can also utilize birthing balls for comfort during labor (Figure 21–2). If she stays in bed, the woman is encouraged to assume any position that she finds comfortable. Some women may wish to stand at the bedside leaning on the bedside tray for support. An upright position assists with fetal descent.

A side-lying position is generally the most advantageous for the laboring woman. Care should be taken that all body parts are supported, with the joints slightly flexed. Pillows may be placed against her chest and under the uppermost arm. A pillow or folded bath blanket is placed between her knees to support the uppermost leg and relieve tension or muscle strain. A pillow (or warmed rolled blanket) placed at the woman's midback also helps provide support. If the woman is more comfortable on her back, the head of the bed should be elevated to relieve the pressure of the uterus on the vena cava, and the uterus should be tilted by placing a towel or blanket under the woman's back. Pillows may be placed under each arm and under the knees to provide support. Because a pregnant woman is at increased risk for thrombophlebitis, excessive pressure behind the knee and calf should be avoided, and frequent assessment of pressure points needs to be made.

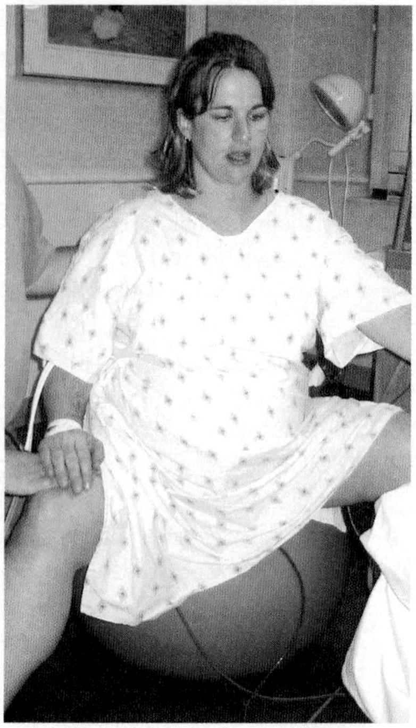

Figure 21–2 **The laboring woman is encouraged to choose a position of comfort. While often promoting maternal comfort during labor, the birthing ball also facilitates fetal descent and rotation and helps increase the diameter of the pelvis.**

SOURCE: Olly/Fotolia.

Clinical Tip

When assisting with position changes, provide the woman with a sheet to provide continued coverage and assist with modesty and maintaining dignity throughout labor.

Frequent position changes (at least every hour) seem to achieve more efficient contractions and contribute to comfort and relaxation. It is also helpful for the woman to sit up in a rocking chair or other comfortable chair, or in the shower.

PERSONAL COMFORT MEASURES

Because vaginal discharge increases, the nurse needs to change the underpads frequently. Washing the perineum with soap and warm water removes secretions and increases comfort. The nurse needs to use standard precautions to avoid exposure to vaginal secretions.

Diaphoresis and the constant leaking of amniotic fluid can dampen the woman's gown and bed linens. Fresh, smooth, dry bed linens promote comfort. To avoid having to change the bottom sheet following rupture of membranes (ROM), the nurse may replace the underpads at frequent intervals (standard precautions need to be followed). The perineal area should be kept as clean and dry as possible to promote comfort. The woman may also find comfort in applying a cool washcloth to her forehead or behind the back of her neck.

A full bladder adds to the discomfort during a contraction and may prolong labor by interfering with the descent of the fetus. Even though the woman is voiding, urine may be retained because of the pressure of the fetal presenting part. A full bladder can be detected by palpation directly over the symphysis pubis. Some of the procedures for regional analgesia during labor contribute to the inability to void, and catheterization may be necessary. The woman should be encouraged to empty her bladder about every 1 to 2 hours. The nurse should offer the woman a bedpan before catheterization because some women are able to void despite anesthesia, and spontaneous voiding decreases the risk of infection that is associated with repeated catheterizations.

The woman may experience dryness of her mouth because her breathing is more rapid. The woman can be instructed to breathe in through her nose and out through her mouth. Clear fluids and light snacks along with ice chips are usually offered unless a complication exists that makes cesarean birth a possibility. The nurse can also apply A & D ointment or a lip emollient to the dry lips. Some prepared childbirth programs advise the woman to bring lollipops to suck on to help combat the dryness that occurs with some of the breathing patterns. If the woman vomits, the nurse should wipe her mouth and offer water to rinse her mouth.

Some women feel discomfort from cold feet. Wearing socks or slippers may increase their comfort. Some women may wish to wear their own nightgown, although they need to know that the gown will most likely be soiled and may be more difficult to move around in.

Birthing balls—large, heavy plastic balls that accommodate an adult's weight—are used by some laboring women to increase comfort (see Figure 21–2). The woman sits on the ball and can roll it back and forth gently. The slow rock is thought to widen the pelvis and enhance fetal descent, while leaning forward on the knees with the head, arms, and chest over the ball simulates a hands-and-knees position and may facilitate rotation of an occiput-posterior. When a birthing ball is used, the nurse should remain close by the woman to help provide balance. Many balls come with aluminum frames to prevent falls.

Some family members or support persons can assist the woman with comfort measures. They may help with position changes, provide ice chips, walk with the laboring woman, and give back rubs (Figure 21–3). If the family is not already involved in providing comfort measures and seems to want to be, the nurse can act as a role model while providing comfort measures and then invite the support person(s) to join in if they like.

Family members also need to be encouraged to maintain their own comfort. As their attention is directed toward the laboring woman, they may forget their own needs. The nurse may have to encourage them to take breaks, maintain food and fluid intake, and rest.

REDUCING ANXIETY

The anxiety experienced by women entering labor is related to a combination of factors inherent to the process. A moderate amount of anxiety enhances the ability to deal with the pain. But an excessive degree of anxiety decreases the woman's ability to cope with the pain.

To decrease anxiety that is not related to pain, the nurse can give information (which eases fear of the unknown), establish rapport with the couple (which helps them preserve their personal integrity), express confidence in the couple's ability to work with the labor process, and assist with breathing and relaxation techniques. In addition to being a good listener, the nurse needs to demonstrate genuine concern for the laboring woman. Remaining with the woman as much as possible conveys a caring attitude and dispels fear of abandonment. Praise for correct breathing, relaxation efforts, and pushing efforts not only encourages repetition of the behavior but also decreases anxiety about the ability to cope with labor.

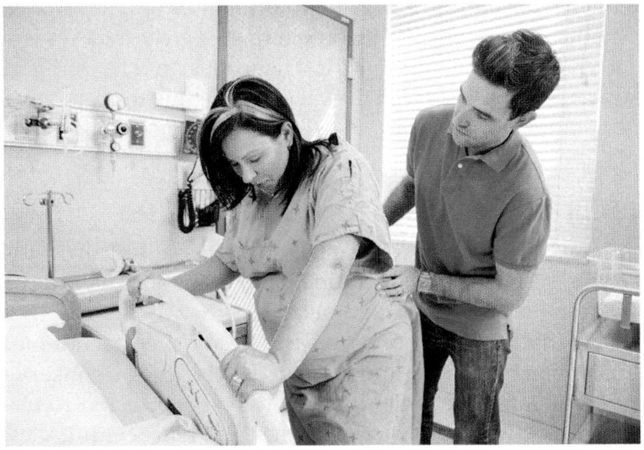

Figure 21–3 **The woman's partner provides support and encouragement during labor.**

SOURCE: Tyler Olson/Shutterstock.

The woman's support person and other members of her family may also experience increasing anxiety as the woman advances through labor. Their anxiety may be reduced or kept at a minimum by keeping them informed about the progress of labor, reassuring them that the sounds and behaviors of the woman in labor are normal, explaining procedures and the use of equipment, and praising them for their assistance in supporting the woman through labor.

Labor and childbirth may be a time of increased anxiety for the woman with a history of sexual abuse or rape. All women entering the healthcare arena need to be assessed for a history of sexual abuse or rape. It is not uncommon for women to deny sexual abuse or rape because this information is difficult to share with a stranger. It is important to be alert for nonverbal cues, such as unexplained anxiety, unrelenting pain, or intense fear during vaginal examinations. The nurse should offer support, provide information, and introduce relaxation techniques to aid the woman in coping to offset her anxiety.

PROVIDING INFORMATION

Providing information about the nature of the discomfort that will occur during labor is important and is best achieved in the early portion of labor. Stressing the intermittent nature and maximum duration of the contractions can be most helpful. The woman can cope with pain better when she knows how far she has progressed and that a period of relief will follow. Describing the type of discomfort and specific sensations that will occur as labor progresses helps the woman recognize these sensations as normal and expected when she does experience them.

A thorough explanation of surroundings, procedures, and equipment being used also decreases anxiety, thereby reducing pain. For some patients, changing from intermittent monitoring to continuous monitoring can create distress and concern. If continuous monitoring is warranted during labor, the nurse should explain the purpose of the monitor and the monitor strip and show the woman and her support persons how the monitor can help them use controlled breathing techniques to relieve pain. The monitor may indicate the beginning of a contraction just seconds before the woman feels it. The woman and her support person can learn how to read the tracing to identify the beginning of the contraction.

SUPPORTIVE RELAXATION TECHNIQUES

Tense muscles increase resistance to the descent of the fetus and contribute to maternal fatigue and anxiety. This fatigue increases pain perception and decreases the woman's ability to cope with the pain. Comfort measures, massage, techniques for decreasing anxiety, and patient teaching can conserve energy. The laboring woman needs to be encouraged to use the periods between contractions to rest and relax her muscles.

Distraction is a method of increasing relaxation and coping with discomfort. During early labor, conversation or activities such as light reading, cards, or other games serve as distractions.

Touch is another type of distraction. See *Box 19–2: Touch Relaxation Techniques*. Nurses can make themselves available to the woman who desires touch. The nurse can place a hand on the side of the bed within the woman's reach. The person who needs touch will reach out for contact, and the nurse can pick up and follow through with this behavioral cue.

Back pain associated with labor may be relieved more effectively by firm pressure on the lower back or sacral area. To apply firm pressure, the nurse or a support person places a hand or a rolled, warmed towel or blanket in the small of the woman's back. Warm compresses can also provide relief.

Visualization techniques also enhance relaxation. See *Box 19–3: Visualization, Imagery, and Meditation*.

In addition to these measures, the nurse can enhance the woman's relaxation by providing encouragement and support for controlled breathing techniques. See Chapter 19 for more information about breathing techniques.

In utilizing breathing techniques over a prolonged period of time, **hyperventilation** may occur. Hyperventilation is the result of an imbalance of oxygen and carbon dioxide (i.e., too much carbon dioxide is exhaled, and too much oxygen remains in the body). The signs and symptoms of hyperventilation are tingling or numbness in the tip of the nose, lips, fingers, or toes; dizziness; spots before the eyes; or spasms of the hands or feet (carpal-pedal spasms). If hyperventilation occurs, the woman should be encouraged to slow her breathing rate and to take shallow breaths. If the signs and symptoms continue or become more severe (that is, if they progress from numbness to spasms), the woman can breathe into a paper surgical mask or into her cupped hands, which causes rebreathing of carbon dioxide, until symptoms abate.

Many women utilize alternative relaxation and breathing exercises during labor to reduce pain, anxiety, and reduce the stress of labor. Another alternative practice in labor is hydrotherapy, either showering or soaking in a tub or whirlpool bath. Yoga is also a common practice in pregnancy and labor. Aromatherapy, massage, music therapy, use of heat to the back or abdomen with heating pad, and acupuncture are all alternative strategies that can result in reduced need for medications and shorter births.

EVIDENCE-BASED PRACTICE | Relaxation Therapies During Labor

Clinical Question

For women who would like to avoid pharmacologic or invasive methods of pain management in labor, what relaxation therapies may be effective pain relief alternatives?

The Evidence

Some women would like to experience childbirth without pharmacologic or invasive pain management techniques. Yet the pain in childbirth can be intense, and alternative therapies are often used. This Cochrane Review evaluated whether mind–body techniques for relaxation could reduce women's pain and improve their overall experience of childbirth. The authors of this systematic review, experts in the field, reviewed 15 studies involving more than 1700 women to determine if breathing techniques, visualization, yoga, or music helped reduce pain. Studies represented an international sample of women. This type of review, published in the Cochrane database, comprises the gold standard for evidence for practice.

Mind–body techniques for relaxation and pain management are widely accessible to women regardless of socioeconomic status. Many of these techniques help the mother cope with pain, reduce stress, and enhance the birth experience (Smith et al., 2018).

Relaxation techniques, yoga, and music therapy all demonstrated a role in reducing pain and increasing overall satisfaction with pain relief. While these effects were demonstrated across multiple studies, the actual difference in pain relief was small. There was an associated perception of a greater sense of control over the birth experience among the women using these techniques. There was no indication that any of these techniques is unsafe for mother or baby. There was a great deal of variation in how these techniques were applied, and the evidence provides little guidance in actual implementation (Smith et al., 2018).

Best Practice

The use of relaxation therapies, yoga, or music may be helpful in reducing the level of pain during childbirth and enhancing a mother's overall satisfaction with the birth experience. Women may feel more control over the experience, enhancing their well-being. More research is needed as to the specific ways these techniques should be used. The nurse can feel confident counseling women who choose alternative therapies for relaxation that they may be helpful and will not be harmful (Smith et al., 2018).

Clinical Reasoning

How could these therapies be standardized to better assess their effectiveness? What assessments might tell the nurse that a mother would be a candidate for relaxation therapies during labor?

In some instances, analgesic agents or regional anesthetic blocks may be used to enhance comfort and relaxation during labor. See Chapter 22 for a discussion of pharmacologic pain management.

Table 21–3 summarizes labor progress, possible responses of the laboring woman, and nursing care during the first and second stages of labor.

Nursing Care During the Second Stage of Labor

Nursing care in the second stage entails both physical and psychologic support, continual encouragement, and appropriate patient teaching to facilitate birth.

TABLE 21–3 Normal Progress, Psychologic Characteristics, and Nursing Support During First and Second Stages of Labor

PHASE	CERVICAL DILATATION	UTERINE CONTRACTIONS	WOMAN'S RESPONSE	SUPPORT MEASURES
Stage 1				
Latent phase	1–3 cm	Every 10–20 minutes, 15–20 seconds' duration Mild intensity progressing to every 5–7 minutes, 30–40 seconds' duration Moderate intensity	Usually happy, talkative, and eager to be in labor Exhibits need for independence by taking care of own bodily needs and seeking information	Establish rapport on admission and continue to build during care. Assess information base and learning needs. Be available to consult regarding breathing technique, if needed; teach breathing technique, if needed and in early labor. Orient family to room, equipment, monitors, and procedures. Encourage woman and partner to participate in care as desired. Provide needed information. Assist woman into position of comfort; encourage frequent change of position; encourage ambulation during early labor. Offer fluids/light snacks/ice chips. Keep couple informed of progress. Encourage woman to void every 1 to 2 hours. Assess need for an interest in using visualization to enhance relaxation and teach, if appropriate.
Active phase	4–7 cm	Every 2–3 minutes, 50–60 seconds' duration Moderate to strong intensity	May experience feelings of helplessness Exhibits increased fatigue and may begin to feel restless and anxious as contractions become stronger Expresses fear of abandonment Becomes more dependent as she is less able to meet her needs	Encourage woman to maintain breathing patterns. Provide quiet environment to reduce external stimuli. Provide reassurance, encouragement, support; keep couple informed of progress. Promote comfort by giving back rubs, sacral pressure, cool cloth on forehead, assistance with position changes, support with pillows. Provide ice chips/clear liquids, if requested, and ointment for dry mouth and lips. Encourage to void every 1 to 2 hours. Offer shower/whirlpool/warm bath, if available.
Transition phase	8–10 cm	Every 1.5–2 minutes, 60–90 seconds' duration Strong intensity	Tires and may exhibit increased restlessness and irritability May feel she cannot keep up with labor process and is out of control Physical discomforts Fear of being left alone May fear tearing open or splitting apart with contractions	Encourage woman to rest between contractions. If she sleeps between contractions, wake her at beginning of contraction so she can begin breathing pattern (increases feeling of control). Provide support, encouragement, and praise for efforts. Keep couple informed of progress; encourage continued participation of support persons. Promote comfort as listed previously but recognize many women do not want to be touched when in transition. Provide privacy. Provide ice chips, ointment for lips. Encourage to void every 1 to 2 hours.
Stage 2				
	Complete	Every 1.5–2 minutes	May feel out of control, helpless, or panicky or may be happy that she can take a more active role in pushing	Assist woman in pushing efforts. Encourage woman to assume position of comfort. Provide encouragement and praise for efforts. Keep couple informed of progress. Provide ice chips. Maintain privacy as woman desires.

Provision of Care in the Second Stage

The second stage begins when the cervix is completely dilated (10 cm). The uterine contractions continue as in the transition phase. Sterile vaginal examinations are performed to assess fetal descent. Maternal pulse, blood pressure, and fetal heart rate (FHR) are assessed every 5 to 15 minutes (depending on risk factors); some protocols recommend assessment after each contraction (Gabbe et al., 2016). See *Key Facts to Remember: Nursing Assessments in the Second Stage of Labor*.

Key Facts to Remember
Nursing Assessments in the Second Stage of Labor

Mother	Fetus
Blood pressure, pulse, respiration every 5–15 minutes (depending on risk factors)	FHR every 5–15 minutes (depending on risk factors)
Uterine contractions palpated continuously	

As the woman pushes during the second stage, she may make a variety of sounds. At times, nurses and physicians may feel the need to help her or encourage her to be more quiet. Other nurses feel more comfortable with maternal sounds and use them as cues. For example, if the woman begins to feel she is losing control, her sound may change to a high-pitched cry or whimper, or she may even shriek in pain. The nurse stays sensitive to changes in the sounds for clues that the woman needs help coping with her pain. The nurse needs to be aware that maternal sounds may be a coping mechanism for some women and may assist in their pain management.

The research focusing on pushing during the second stage recommends that the woman be allowed to rest for up to 90 minutes at the beginning of the second stage and to begin pushing when she feels the natural urge to bear down. Some studies have shown that this has been associated with reduction of maternal fatigue and increased fetal oxygenation with fewer decelerations noted when women delay pushing until they feel the urge to push (Huang, 2018). Other studies have shown an increased risk of cesarean birth and postpartum hemorrhage (Yee et al., 2016). Close monitoring during the second stage is warranted to determine continual maternal and fetal assessment.

When the woman reports feeling an uncontrollable urge to push (bear down), the nurse can help her greatly by letting her know that these new sensations are normal. This is because some women interpret the increased rectal pressure as a need to move her bowels. The instinctive response is to tighten muscles rather than bear down. The woman may also report that she fears she is "splitting apart" or that she feels a "ring of fire." The woman who expects these sensations and understands that bearing down contributes to progress at this stage is more likely to do so.

> "When I tried to push with the contractions, I felt as if I would tear apart. It hurt so badly that I was shaking. I knew it was time to push and my body was telling me to, but it hurt so much. The nurse kept saying, 'Just push and you will feel better.' I wanted to scream at her. She had no idea what was happening to me."

When the contraction begins, the nurse tells the woman to take two short breaths, then to take a third breath and hold it while pulling back on her knees and pushing down with her abdominal muscles (Figure 21–4). Positioning is an important component of safe and effective pushing. An upright position or lateral position is preferred over supine positioning because it has fewer negative maternal hemodynamic changes (Cunningham et al., 2016). The nurse should encourage the woman to choose a position of comfort and to change positions frequently, which aids in fetal descent. Forcing women's legs back against their abdomen during pushing should be avoided because this can result in extensive perineal stretching that can increase the risk of perineal lacerations (Dresang & Yonke, 2015). Some women prefer to exhale slightly (exhale breathing) while pushing to avoid the physiologic effects of the Valsalva maneuver. With this method the woman takes several deep breaths and then holds her breath for 5 to 6 seconds. Then, through slightly pursed lips, she exhales slowly every 5 to 6 seconds while continuing to hold her breath. The woman takes another breath and continues exhale breathing and pushing during the contraction.

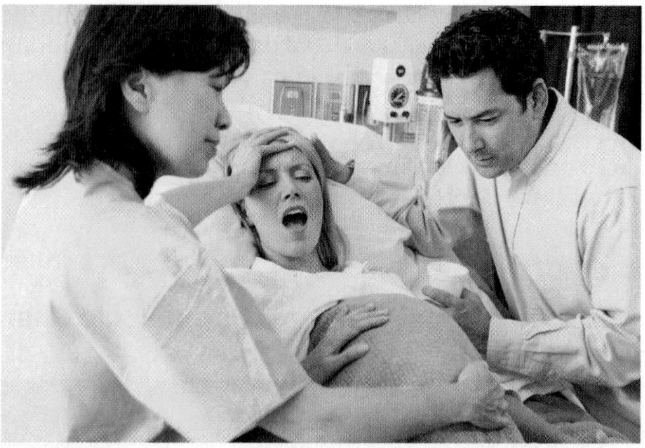

Figure 21–4 The nurse provides encouragement and support during pushing efforts.
SOURCE: Monkey Business Images/Shutterstock.

> "I knew when I was completely dilated. I knew when to push and I did it without tearing. My body told me to listen. I knew what to do. When I began pushing, I felt in control because I could do something . . . I could push the baby out. I knew he was ready to be born."
>
> —Harriette Hartigan, *Women in Birth*

The woman is encouraged to rest between contractions. Although the laboring woman may appear exhausted at this time, most experience relief at being able to push with contractions. Perspiration increases with the pushing efforts, and a cold washcloth for the forehead and face is most soothing. Some women may wish to bring a small fan with them and use it during the second stage. The birthing woman may also appreciate sips of fluid or ice chips at this time.

The nurse and/or support person can assist the woman into a comfortable position for pushing. Maternal positions—such as standing, squatting while leaning back on a partner or leaning forward on a birthing bar, lying in a lateral or Sims position, or crouching on hands and knees—may increase comfort and effectiveness of pushing. Some women feel that sitting on a toilet seat is a comfortable position that assists their pushing efforts. This position may cause anxiety in the caregivers, however, for fear that the birth may occur quickly in this most inopportune place. Some women benefit from gripping the hands of the support person or nurse. This technique increases intra-abdominal pressure, which aids in the expulsion effort. Another variation of this technique, which can be quite effective, is to have the woman grip a towel while the support person or nurse pulls the towel in the opposite direction. Care should be taken that the nurse or support person does not suffer a back injury. Pushing efforts should be maximized by having the woman place her chin to her chest and avoid hyperextension of the neck by having her "curl around the baby" to facilitate descent into the pelvis.

If anticipated progress is not made or the laboring woman wants to try other positions for pushing, the nurse should support her. Some nurses have their own preferences and may be more comfortable directing the laboring woman to use these preferred positions; however, it is important to remember that the nurse is there to support the birth, and that frequent changes in position may assist in the descent of the baby.

If the maternal pushing effort diminishes because of frustration or fatigue, many women benefit from short rest periods. Rest periods are appropriate if maternal and fetal assessments are stable. In addition, the physician/CNM should be informed of the actual time that has been spent pushing and not the time that has elapsed since the beginning of the second stage. If the maternal vital signs are stable and the FHR is reassuring, rest periods can be used to prevent maternal exhaustion (Groll, 2017).

Throughout the second stage, it remains important to provide information regarding progress and what is happening in the labor. It is also imperative to address the woman's questions honestly, to acknowledge her concerns, and to continue to provide support.

A nullipara is usually prepared for birth when the perineum begins to bulge. A multipara usually progresses much more quickly, so she may be prepared for the birth when the cervix is dilated 7 to 8 cm.

The woman's blood pressure and the FHR are monitored between contractions, and the contractions are palpated until the birth. The nurse continues to assist the woman in her pushing efforts. Both the woman and the support person are kept informed of procedures and of progress, and both are supported throughout the birth.

In addition to assisting the woman and her partner, the nurse assists the physician/CNM in preparing for the birth. The physician/CNM usually dons a sterile gown and gloves and may place sterile drapes over the woman's abdomen and legs. Some providers may perform a sterile preparation before birth; others may not do so as part of their normal routine. Although some physicians/CNMs may place the woman in stirrups for birth, others may opt to drop the foot of the bed lower than the upper portion and let the woman rest her feet on the bed to facilitate maternal comfort. An episiotomy should only be performed if there is a medical indication for one and, when needed, should be performed just before birth. See the discussion of episiotomy in Chapter 25.

Promotion of Comfort in the Second Stage

Most of the comfort measures that have been used during the first stage remain appropriate at this time. Cool cloths to the face and forehead may help provide cooling as the woman is involved in the intense physical exertion of pushing. If she has been diaphoretic, a dry gown may be comforting. The woman may feel hot and want to remove some of the covering. Care still needs to be taken to provide privacy even though covers are removed. Some women may want to remove all of their clothing. Healthcare providers should allow the woman to give birth in a way that will promote her comfort.

Additional comfort measures may be used during this stage. Warm perineal, abdominal, and back compresses may be used to increase muscle relaxation. Perineal massage and stretching with a lubricant may be performed, although evidence does not show that it reduces perineal lacerations (Ommolbanin, Hajar, & Mahbobeh, 2014) and the use of perineal massage before imminent crowning can result in considerable perineal edema. For this reason, some institutions may limit perineal massage to physicians/CNMs. When used, perineal massage should be limited.

The woman can be encouraged to rest and "let all muscles go" during the period between contractions. The nurse and support person(s) can assist the woman into a pushing position with each contraction to further conserve energy. Sips of fluid or ice chips may be used to provide moisture and relieve dryness of the mouth. Constant reassurance is imperative.

Visualization techniques may be helpful. The woman can be encouraged to envision the baby descending the birth canal and the vagina opening up. Phrases such as "Open to your baby" and "Let the baby come; don't try to hold back" can be useful and calming. Many women benefit from visualizing the descent of the fetus in a mirror. The nurse should ask the woman if she would like to watch in the mirror.

Assisting the Woman and Physician/CNM During Birth

Shortly before the birth, the birthing room or delivery room is prepared with equipment and materials that may be needed. Family members do not need to change into other clothing if the birth occurs in a birthing room; they don a disposable scrub suit if the birth is to occur in a delivery room or surgery suite. Meticulous hand hygiene is required of the nurses and physician/CNM. Nurses who will be in direct contact with the mother at the time of birth need to wear protective clothing, such as an apron or gown with a splash apron, disposable gloves, and eye covering. The physician/CNM will also need to wear a gown with a splash apron or a plastic apron, eye covering, and sterile gloves.

Most facilities now use one room for labor, delivery, and recovery (LDR) rooms. Use of a separate birthing room is rare. If the laboring woman is to give birth in a separate birthing room, she will be moved shortly before birth on her bed or a cart. It is important to preserve her privacy during the transfer, and safety must be provided by raising the side rails into a locked position. In the birthing room, the labor bed or transfer cart must be carefully supported against the delivery table; this ensures the woman's safety during the transfer.

If the woman is to be moved from one bed to another, it should be done between contractions. During the contraction, the woman feels increased discomfort and may be involved in pushing efforts. Perineal bulging may be occurring, which adds to the discomfort and difficulty in moving. All of these factors make moving the woman very uncomfortable. If birth seems imminent (within the next minute), it is safer for the woman to give birth in her labor bed or on the cart. Transfer to the delivery table is then delayed until after the baby is born and the cord has been clamped and cut.

Even though there are differences in the birthing room setting, the family can still be together during the birth. It is important to provide encouragement for family members to participate because the delivery room environment may be unfamiliar and seem less relaxed. The support person may be hesitant to continue to provide support for fear of interfering or being in the way. The nurse can ensure that family members are included throughout the birthing process by giving them simple directions about how they can assist and be involved in the process.

MATERNAL BIRTHING POSITIONS

The woman is usually positioned for birth on a bed, birthing chair, or delivery table. In some instances, she may give birth standing at the side of the bed or on her hands and knees on the floor. The position the woman assumes is determined not only by her individual wishes but also by the physician/CNM.

If stirrups are used, they should be padded to alleviate pressure, and both legs should be lifted simultaneously to avoid strain on abdominal, back, and perineal muscles. The stirrups should be adjusted to fit the woman's legs. The feet are supported in the stirrup holders. The height and angle of the stirrups are adjusted so there is no pressure on the back of the knees or the calf, which might cause discomfort and postpartum vascular problems. This is particularly true of women with epidural anesthesia. The birthing bed is elevated 30 to 60 degrees to help the woman bear down, and handles are provided so she may pull back on them.

The upright posture for birth was considered normal in most societies until modern times. Alternatively, women selected squatting, kneeling, standing, and sitting for birth. Only within the last 200 years has the recumbent position become the norm in the Western world. Its use in this century has been reinforced because of the convenience it offers in applying new technology, and it has thus become the conventional manner in which North American women give birth in hospitals. In searching for alternative positions, consumers and professionals alike continue to refocus on the comfort of the laboring woman and the advantages of alternative positions rather than on the convenience of the physician/CNM (Table 21–4).

Recumbent Position. The recumbent (lithotomy) position for birth is sometimes used to enhance the maintenance of asepsis, assessment of FHR, and performance of episiotomy and repair. This position may not be ideal as the uterine axis is directed toward the symphysis pubis instead of the pelvic inlet, thus interfering with fetal alignment. Additionally, this position is working directly against gravity. These disadvantages may be lessened slightly if the woman has her back elevated 30 to 40 degrees.

Lateral Sims Position. A common position favored by some women and birth attendants is the lateral Sims or sidelying position. In assuming this position for birth, for example, the woman lies on her left side with her left leg extended and her right knee drawn against her abdomen or flexed by her side or with both legs bent at the knees. Although the frequency of contractions may decrease in this position, the intensity increases, yielding greater uterine efficiency. Those who favor this position find that it increases overall comfort, does not compromise venous return from the lower extremities, puts less stress and pressure on the maternal neck, and diminishes the chances of aspiration should vomiting occur. Women also perceive the lateral Sims as a more natural and comfortable position and less intrusive with no stirrups or overhead lights required (Figure 21–5). Many providers recommend laying on the left side to facilitate blood flow to the heart, but women in labor often alternate from side to side to aid in fetal descent. Birth attendants have found that the position has a positive effect on the management of fetal shoulder dystocias. Sidelying positions are also helpful in labors in which the fetus is in a posterior position because this position allows the uterine weight and the fetus to tip away from the maternal back. Fewer episiotomies are required in this position because the perineum tends to be more relaxed.

Squatting Position. Squatting is favored by some women primarily for the positive use it makes of gravity, which allows the abdominal wall to relax. Squatting is thought to facilitate the entrance of the presenting part into the pelvic inlet, thus hastening engagement. This engagement facilitates pressure being applied to the cervix, which aids in dilatation and effacement. This in turn can stimulate the myometrium to produce more intense uterine contractions and shorten the length of labor. A squatting bar (birthing bar) may be used across a bed or on the floor to increase the woman's balance and provide some support. During the second stage of labor, squatting increases the size of the pelvic outlet by 6 to 8 mm providing more space for fetal descent (Desseauve, Fradet, Lacouture, et al., 2017), allows the pressure from the thighs to compress the uterus to further aid in fetal descent, and facilitates a favorable fetal position. This position can have drawbacks for the birth attendants because it makes the perineum somewhat inaccessible, making it more difficult to control the birth process. It can also make it difficult to administer perineal or pudendal analgesia, use instruments, and monitor fetal status. Because perineal edema can also occur from prolonged squatting, the intermittent application of ice should be used to decrease edema. Women with epidural anesthesia may be unable to assume this position because of the heaviness in their lower extremities.

Semi-Fowler Position. Some care providers advocate a semi-Fowler position as an appropriate middle ground between the recumbent and upright positions. This position has been associated with shorter first and second stages of labor because it enhances the effectiveness of the abdominal muscle efforts while the woman is pushing. Raising and supporting the torso helps the woman view the birth process. At the same time the birth attendant has access to the perineum.

Sitting Position. The sitting position is becoming an option for more women with the increased availability of birthing chairs. Birthing chairs or stools have been used for centuries and are sometimes used during the second stage of labor. A supported sitting position may also be achieved in a birthing bed.

The upright sitting position offers advantages similar to squatting, including stronger, more effective uterine contractions that result from the fetus's weight, creating additional force to aid descent into the birth canal. Some practitioners will utilize the birthing chair or a supported sitting position prior to an operative assisted birth. This position may also be preferred for women with severe back pain as it enables the woman to curl forward and grasp her knees and ankles during pushing efforts, allowing her to visualize the birth without mirrors. Use of this position can result in additional maternal blood loss, so close monitoring is warranted.

Hands-And-Knees Position. The hands-and-knees position is more comfortable for a woman experiencing back labor as there is less pressure on the maternal back from the fetus, and the fetus may be able to rotate more easily from the posterior position. The mother can be well supported by dropping the foot of the birthing bed and supplying extra pillows upon which she can rest her forearms. Because there is less pressure on the perineum,

TABLE 21–4 Comparison of Birthing Positions

POSITION	ADVANTAGES	DISADVANTAGES	NURSING ACTIONS
Recumbent	Enhances ability to maintain sterile field. May be easier to monitor FHR. Easier to perform episiotomy or laceration repair.	May decrease blood pressure. It is difficult for the woman to breathe due to pressure on the diaphragm. There is an increased risk of aspiration. May increase perineal pressure, making laceration more likely. May interfere with uterine contractions.	Ensure that stirrups do not cause excess pressure on the legs. Assess legs for adequate circulation and support.
Left lateral Sims	Does not compromise venous return from lower extremities. Increases perineal relaxation and decreases need for episiotomy. Appears to prevent rapid descent.	It is difficult for the woman to see the birth.	Adjust position so that the upper leg lies on the bed (scissor fashion) or is supported by the partner or on pillows.
Squatting	Size of pelvic outlet is increased. Gravity aids descent and expulsion of newborn. Second stage may be shortened (Gabbe et al., 2016).	It may be difficult to maintain balance while squatting.	Help woman maintain balance. Use a birthing bar, if available.
Semi-Fowler	Does not compromise venous return from lower extremities. Women can view birth process.	If legs are positioned wide apart, relaxation of perineal tissues is decreased.	Assess that upper torso is evenly supported. Increase support of body by changing position of bed or using pillows as props.
Sitting in birthing bed	Gravity aids descent and expulsion of the fetus. Does not compromise venous return from lower extremities. Woman can view the birth process. Leg position may be changed at will.		Ensure that legs and feet have adequate support.
Sitting on birthing stool	Gravity aids descent and expulsion of baby. Does not compromise venous return from lower extremities. Woman can view birth process.	It is difficult to provide support for the woman's back.	Encourage woman to sit in a position that increases her comfort.
Hands and knees	Increases perineal relaxation and decreases need for episiotomy. Increases placental and umbilical blood flow and decreases nonreassuring fetal status. Improves fetal rotation. Better able to assess perineum. Better access to fetal nose and mouth for suctioning at birth. Facilitates birth of baby with shoulder dystocia.	Woman cannot view birth. There is decreased contact with birth attendant. Caregivers cannot use instruments. There may be increased maternal fatigue.	Adjust birthing bed by dropping the foot down. Supply extra pillows for increased support.

there is less need for an episiotomy; in addition, the incidence of lacerations is lessened. The birth attendant has better access to the perineum for stretching and for suctioning of the fetal nose and mouth at the time of birth. This position may also increase placental and umbilical blood flow during episodes of nonreassuring fetal status, while increasing the intensity of contractions. This position may increase the pelvic diameter and facilitate a less traumatic birth of a baby with shoulder dystocia. Disadvantages of this position include decreased eye contact between the mother and birth attendant, the inability to use instruments, maternal fatigue, and the need to reposition the mother if perineal repair is needed.

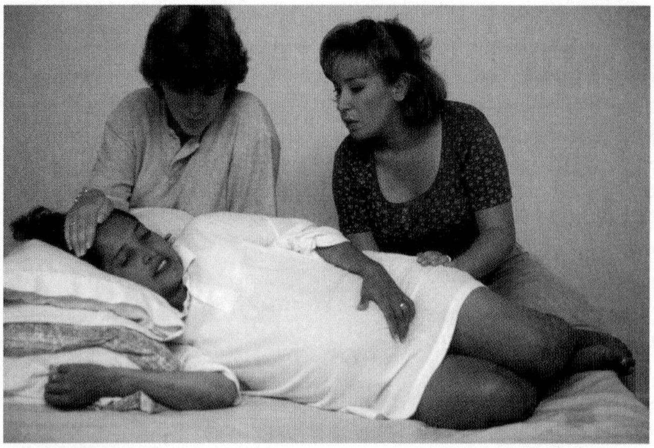

Figure 21–5 **Sidelying laboring or birthing position.**

SOURCE: Angela Hampton Picture Library/Alamy Stock Photo.

CLEANSING THE PERINEUM

If a perineal prep is to be performed, the woman is positioned for the birth, and her vulvar and perineal area is cleansed to increase her comfort and to remove the bloody discharge that is present before the actual birth. An aseptic technique such as the one that follows is recommended.

After thorough handwashing, the nurse opens the sterile prep tray, dons sterile gloves, and cleans the vulva and perineum with the cleansing solution. Beginning with the mons pubis, the area is cleansed up to the lower abdomen. A second sponge is used to clean the inner groin and thigh of one leg, and a third is used to clean the other leg, moving outward to avoid carrying material from surrounding areas to the vaginal outlet. The last three sponges are used to clean the labia and vestibule with one downward sweep each. The used sponges are discarded and should not be placed on the delivery table. Once the cleansing is completed, the woman returns to the desired birthing position. Not all birthing facilities use such formalized cleansing procedures. Some facilities use a spray bottle with povidone-iodine (Betadine) or other cleansing agent and simply spray the perineal area. Because birth is not truly a "sterile procedure," some providers do not perform perineal cleansing techniques.

SUPPORT DURING THE SECOND STAGE

The nurse assesses the woman's support person(s) for comfort and knowledge and assists them in supporting the woman during the second stage. Some support persons will want to take an active role, whereas others will prefer simply to be observers. The nurse provides calm reassurance while assessing the roles the members of the support team desire and offers suggestions and support, keeps the support team informed of the woman's progress, provides explanations of the process, and praises them for their supportive activities, all of which are associated with a positive experience.

ASSISTING WITH THE BIRTH OF THE BABY

When the fetal head has distended the perineum, the clinician may perform a hand maneuver, such as supporting the perineum between the thumb and four fingers, which is believed to prevent undue trauma to the fetal head and maternal soft tissues. The woman may be asked to breathe rapidly, pant, or blow to avoid too-rapid birth of the fetal head. The woman may also be instructed to push and take a breath intermittently to avoid rapid expulsion.

After the baby's head is born, the clinician palpates the neck for the presence of a cord, which can be slipped over the fetal head if it is loose. If the cord is tight, it is double-clamped and cut.

Restitution and external rotation occur after the head is born. The only assistance needed during this time is support of the maternal perineum. While awaiting completion of external rotation, the clinician suctions the newborn's nose and mouth to remove mucus. When the newborn's shoulder appears at the symphysis pubis, the clinician may use both hands to grasp the newborn's head gently and pull downward for release of the anterior shoulder. Gentle upward traction facilitates release of the posterior shoulder.

Birth of the newborn's body may be controlled by grasping the posterior shoulder with one hand, palm turned toward the perineum. The left hand may be used for this if the newborn is left occiput anterior (LOA). The right hand then follows along the baby's back, and the feet are grasped as they are expelled. The newborn's head is kept down and to the side as the feet, legs, and body are tucked under the clinician's left arm in a football hold. The clinician's right hand is then free for further care of the newborn, and the newborn is securely held. CNMs often place the newborn directly on the mother's abdomen. The nose and mouth are suctioned with a bulb syringe, and respiratory passages are cleared. Figure 19–3 depicts an entire birthing experience.

ASSISTING WITH CLAMPING THE UMBILICAL CORD

Delayed umbilical cord clamping is now recommended for all healthy term neonates. If the newborn is held at or below the vagina as cord clamping is delayed, as much as 50 to 100 mL of blood may be shifted from the placenta to the newborn. The extra amount of blood may reduce the frequency of iron deficiency anemia, which can occur later in infancy. There is a small increase in hyperbilirubinemia (excessive amount of bilirubin in the blood), however, the benefits appear to outweigh this small risk (ACOG, 2017a). Chapter 26 discusses delayed umbilical cord clamping in depth.

Some parents may specify a preference in their birth plan regarding exactly when the umbilical cord is to be cut. Delayed cord clamping for greater than 30 seconds in preterm neonates is associated with fewer transfusions, a decreased incidence of anemia, lower rates of intraventricular hemorrhage, decreased need for transfusions, and a lower incidence of sepsis. When immediate cord clamping is required in preterm newborns needing resuscitation, some practitioners use a cord milking technique wherein they push the blood in the cord toward the baby to increase the volume of blood, even though delayed clamping cannot be performed.

The umbilical cord is usually clamped with two Kelly clamps and cut between them. The father, partner, other support person, or the mother may wish to cut the cord after it has been clamped by the physician/CNM.

The physician/CNM may double-clamp the cord so that a section can be made available for the collection of cord blood gases. After the cord has been cut, cord blood is collected and sent to the lab as needed. If cord blood banking is being performed, the physician/CNM begins collection procedures at this time. If cord blood banking is desired, immediate clamping will increase the amount of cells collected and may be performed in these circumstances (ACOG, 2017a).

If the physician/CNM has not placed a cord clamp on the newborn's umbilical stump, it is the responsibility of the nurse to do so. Before applying the cord clamp, the nurse examines the cut end for the presence of two arteries and one vein. The umbilical vein is the largest vessel, and the arteries are smaller vessels.

The presence of only one artery in the umbilical cord is associated with genitourinary abnormalities. The number of vessels is recorded on the birth and newborn records.

The cord is clamped approximately 0.5 to 1 inch from the abdomen to allow room between the abdomen and clamp as the cord dries (Figure 21–6). Abdominal skin must not be clamped because this will cause necrosis of the tissue. The clamp is removed in the newborn nursery approximately 24 hours after birth if the cord has dried.

CORD BLOOD COLLECTION FOR BANKING

Growing numbers of parents are arranging for cord blood banking either for their own storage or for donation. Immediately after the newborn's umbilical cord is clamped and cut and before the placenta is expelled, the physician/CNM withdraws blood from the umbilical cord. The blood is placed in a special container that parents receive from the Cord Blood Registry and bring with them for the birth. The parents will have any special directions that are required for storage and care of the container. Although current recommendations for cord blood banking include a family history of an illness that can be treated with fetal cells and children whose parents are from a nontraditional lineage, such as mixed-race backgrounds or other ethnic combinations that are uncommon, many families are choosing to bank their neonates' cord blood.

Stem cell transplants are now used to treat many different types of diseases. The future of stem cell transplantation is promising, with rapid expansion of uses. Because cord blood, like bone marrow, contains hematopoietic stem cells, it can be used to treat numerous cancers, genetic and blood disorders, cerebral palsy, and immune disorders. Cord blood has advantages over bone marrow. It is a no-risk procedure, causes no discomfort to the newborn or mother, and is less likely to trigger a potentially fatal rejection response. Cord blood can also work with a less than perfect match and is more readily available than bone marrow. Although cord blood banks have been established in the United States, universal cord blood collection does not exist. While some facilities collect volunteer donations, the majority of hospitals do not. Most of the banking performed in the United States is done by for-profit agencies where the parents pay a set fee to collect the blood and have it processed, followed by an annual storage fee. The main drawback of cord blood banking is the cost.

Cord blood transfusions can be utilized to treat a growing number of disorders. It is estimated that over 35,000 transfusions had been performed as of 2015 (National Cord Blood Registry, 2015). Both ACOG and the American Academy of Pediatrics support the process of cord blood banking; therefore, the advantages and disadvantages should be discussed with parents. While universal cord blood banking is not routinely recommended, parents who have an older child who may benefit from a cord blood transfusion or unusual genetic inherited disorders should consider cord blood banking. Recent recommendations have also been made that women at risk of giving birth prematurely should consider cord blood banking because these babies are more at risk for cerebral palsy and other neurologic injuries (National Cord Blood Registry, 2015).

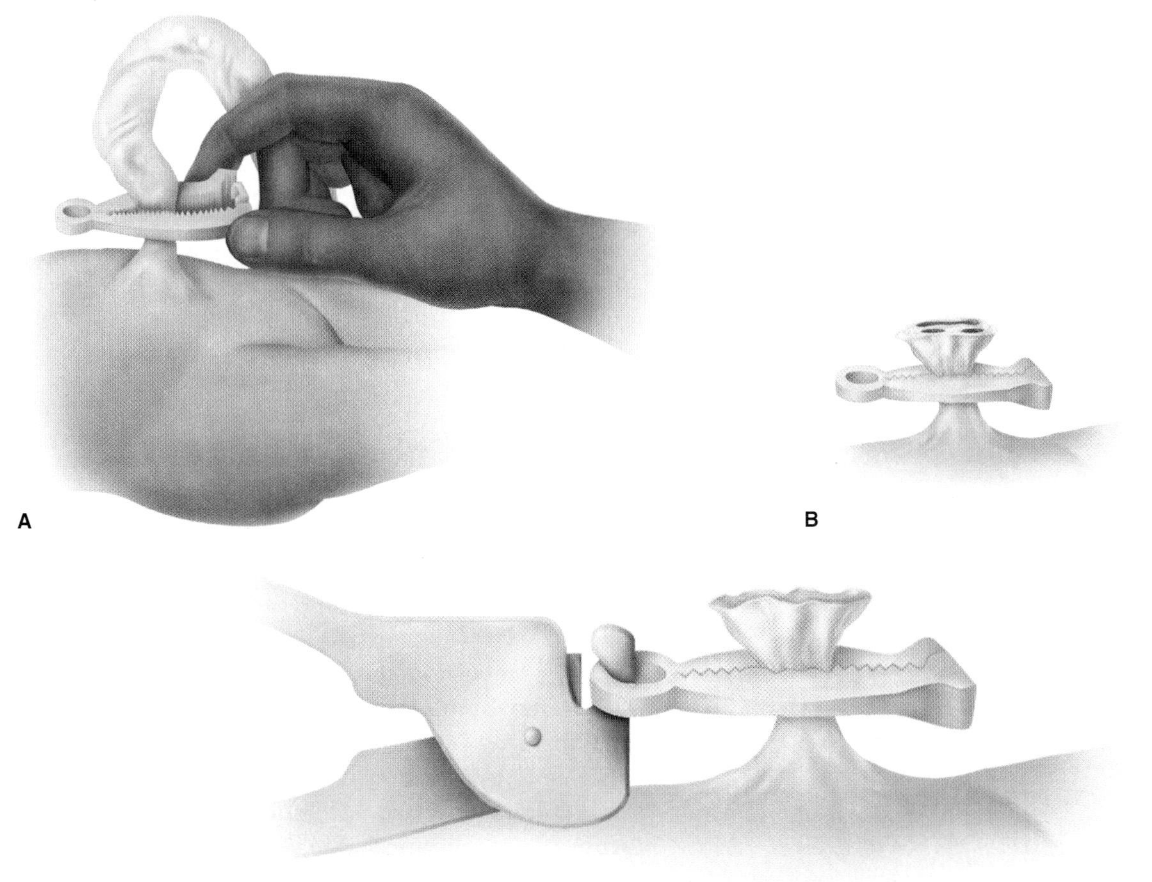

Figure 21–6 Hollister cord clamp. A. Clamp is positioned 0.5 to 1 inch from the abdomen and then secured. B. Cut cord. The one vein and two arteries can be seen. C. Plastic device for removing clamp after cord has dried. After the cord has dried, the nurse grasps the Hollister clamp on either side of the cut area and gently separates it.

Once collected, the blood is tested for infectious and genetic disorders before it is frozen. Abnormal blood results are communicated to the parents. Written consent is required for both collection and storage of cord blood.

Nursing Care During the Third Stage of Labor

Nursing care in the third stage focuses on providing initial newborn care and assisting with birth of the placenta.

Provision of Initial Newborn Care

The physician/CNM places the newborn on the mother's abdomen or chest so skin-to-skin contact can be initiated. Skin-to-skin contact provides optimal warmth for the newborn, facilitates bonding, and fosters early breastfeeding. If the newborn needs additional supportive care or suctioning, a radiant-heated unit can be used and positioned as close to the bed as possible, although the standard of care is to provide skin-to-skin contact immediately upon birth.

Because the first priority is to maintain respirations, the newborn is placed in a modified Trendelenburg position to aid drainage of mucus from the nasopharynx and trachea. The newborn is also suctioned with a bulb syringe or DeLee mucus trap as needed. Suctioning with a DeLee mucus trap is typically only utilized when meconium is present (Sawyer, 2015). See *Clinical Skill 21–1: Performing Nasal Pharyngeal Suctioning*.

The second priority is to provide and maintain warmth, so the newborn is dried immediately with warmed, soft baby blankets with the immediate removal of wet blankets because

CLINICAL SKILL 21–1

Performing Nasal Pharyngeal Suctioning

NURSING ACTION

Preparation

- Suction equipment is always available in the birthing area to clear secretions from the newborn's nose or oropharynx if respirations are depressed or if amniotic fluid was meconium stained.
- Tighten the lid on the DeLee mucus trap or other suction device collection bottle.

Rationale: *This avoids spillage of secretions and prevents air from leaking out of the lid.*

- Connect one end of the DeLee tubing to low suction.

Equipment and Supplies

DeLee mucus trap or other suction device

Procedure: Clean Gloves

1. Don gloves.
2. Without applying suction, insert the free end of the DeLee tubing 3 to 5 inches into the newborn's nose or mouth (Figure 21–7).

Rationale: *Applying suction while passing the tube would interfere with smooth passage of the tube.*

3. Place your thumb over the suction control and begin to apply suction. Continue to suction as you slowly remove the tube, rotating it slightly.

Rationale: *Suctioning during withdrawal removes fluid and avoids redepositing secretions in the newborn's nasopharynx.*

4. Continue to reinsert the tube and provide suction for as long as fluid is aspirated.

Note: Excessive suctioning can cause vagal stimulation, which decreases the heart rate.

5. If it is necessary to pass the tube into the newborn's stomach to remove meconium secretions that the newborn swallowed before birth, insert the tube through the newborn's mouth into the stomach. Apply suction and continue to suction as you withdraw the tube.

Rationale: *Because the newborn's nares are small and delicate, it is easier and faster to pass the suction tube through the mouth.*

6. Document the completion of the procedure and the amount and type of secretions.

Rationale: *This documentation provides a record of the intervention and the status of the neonate at birth.*

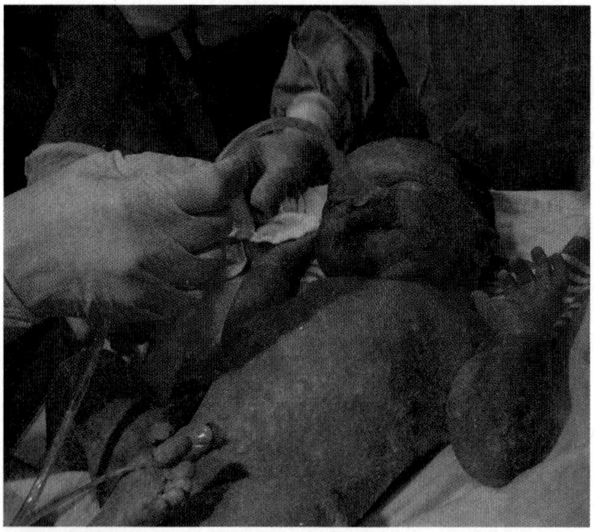

Figure 21–7 **DeLee mucus trap being used to suction a newborn's mouth to remove excess secretions. One end of the suction tubing is connected to low suction, and the other end of the tubing is inserted 3 to 5 inches into the newborn's nose or mouth. Suction is applied as the tubing is pulled out. The process is repeated for as long as fluid is aspirated.**

SOURCE: Wilson Garcia.

contact with wet blankets can result in heat loss. The newborn's head is dried first to minimize heat loss. Once the newborn in placed skin-to-skin on the mother, warmed blankets are placed over both of them to maintain warmth. If the newborn must be placed in a radiant-heated unit, he or she is dried, laid on a dry blanket, and left uncovered under the radiant heat. Because radiant heat warms the outer surface of objects, a newborn wrapped in blankets will receive no benefit. A stocking cap is commonly placed on the newborn's head to conserve heat. See Chapter 26 and Chapter 28 for more information on neonatal heat loss and keeping newborns warm.

APGAR SCORING SYSTEM

The Apgar scoring system (Table 21–5) was designed in 1952 by Dr. Virginia Apgar, an anesthesiologist. The purpose of the **Apgar score** is to evaluate the physical condition of the newborn at birth. The newborn is rated 1 minute after birth and again at 5 minutes and receives a total score ranging from 0 to 10 based on this criteria:

1. The heart rate is auscultated or palpated at the junction of the umbilical cord and skin. This is the most important assessment. A newborn heart rate of less than 100 beats/min indicates the need for immediate resuscitation.
2. The respiratory effort is the second most important Apgar assessment. Complete absence of respirations is termed *apnea*. A vigorous cry indicates good respirations.
3. The muscle tone is determined by evaluating the degree of flexion and resistance to straightening of the extremities. A normal term newborn's elbows and hips are flexed, with the knees positioned up toward the abdomen.
4. The reflex irritability is evaluated as the newborn is dried or by lightly rubbing the soles of the feet. A cry is a score of 2. A grimace is 1 point, and no response is 0.
5. The skin color is inspected for cyanosis and pallor. Newborns generally have blue extremities, and the rest of the body is pink, which merits a score of 1. This condition, termed *acrocyanosis*, is present in 85% of normal newborns at 1 minute after birth. A completely pink newborn scores a 2, and a totally cyanotic, pale baby is scored 0. Newborns with darker skin pigmentation will not be pink. Their skin color is assessed for pallor and acrocyanosis, and a score is selected based on the assessment.

A score of 7 to 10 indicates a newborn in good condition and requires only nasopharyngeal suctioning. An Apgar score between 4 and 7 indicates the need for stimulation; a score under 4 indicates the need for resuscitation (Groll, 2017).

TABLE 21–5 The Apgar Scoring System

SCORE SIGN	0	1	2
Heart rate	Absent	Slow; less than 100 beats/min	Greater than 100 beats/min
Respiration	Absent	Slow; irregular	Good breathing with crying
Muscle tone	Flaccid	Some flexion of extremities	Active movement of extremities
Reflex response	Absent	Grimace; noticeable facial movement	Vigorous cry; coughs; sneezes; pulls away when touched
Skin color	Pale or blue	Pink body, blue extremities	Pink body and extremities

SOURCE: Data from Apgar, V. (1966).

NEWBORN PHYSICAL ASSESSMENT BY THE NURSE

An abbreviated systematic physical assessment is performed by the nurse in the birthing area immediately after birth to detect any abnormalities (Table 21–6). First, the nurse notes the size of the newborn and the contour and size of the head in relationship to the rest of the body. The newborn's posture and movements indicate tone and neurologic functioning. The appearance of the head is noted along with palpation of the fontanelles. The face should be inspected along with the ears and neck.

The skin is inspected for discoloration, presence of vernix caseosa and lanugo, and evidence of trauma and desquamation (peeling of skin). *Vernix caseosa* is a white, cheesy substance normally found on newborns that is absorbed within 24 hours after birth. Vernix is abundant on preterm newborns and absent on postterm newborns. A large quantity of fine hair (*lanugo*) is more common on preterm newborns, whereas desquamation of the skin is often seen in postterm newborns.

The nares are observed for flaring, the palate is assessed to determine if a cleft palate is present. The presence of mucus is documented and is removed with the bulb syringe. The chest is inspected for respiratory rate (30–60 breaths/min), retractions, grunting, or stridor. The lungs are auscultated bilaterally for breath sounds. Absence of breath sounds on one side may indicate pneumothorax. Rales may be heard immediately after birth because a small amount of fluid may remain in the lungs; this fluid will be absorbed. Rhonchi indicates aspiration of oral secretions. The abdomen is inspected and palpated for masses. The heart is assessed for heart rate (110–170 beats/min), rhythm, and the presence of any murmurs. The umbilical cord is inspected, and the number of vessels is recorded.

The genital area, buttocks, and anus are inspected. The spine is inspected to ensure it is intact. The elimination of urine or meconium is recorded. The extremities are inspected and compared for symmetry. Reflexes are assessed to determine central nervous system maturity. A complete and detailed newborn assessment can be found in Chapter 27.

NEWBORN IDENTIFICATION

To ensure correct identification and for security purposes, the mother and newborn have identification bands with identical codes attached in the birthing or delivery room. The mother receives a bracelet on her wrist and typically has the option of giving the second adult band to the father/partner or a support person. Two bracelets are snugly placed on the newborn to prevent loss—one on the wrist and one on the ankle.

SAFETY ALERT!

Newborns should never be removed from the birthing or delivery room until identification bands have been placed. The bands should remain in place until the mother and baby are discharged home.

TABLE 21–6 Initial Newborn Evaluation

ASSESS	NORMAL FINDINGS
Respirations	Rate 30–60 irregular No retractions, no grunting
Apical pulse	Rate 110–170 and somewhat irregular
Temperature	Skin temp above 36.5°C (97.8°F)
Skin color	Body pink with bluish extremities
Umbilical cord	Two arteries and one vein
Gestational age	Preterm, near term, and term newborns may remain with parents for extended time as long as baby is stable (Stanford Medicine, 2017).
Sole creases	Sole creases that involve the heel
In general, expect scant amount of vernix on upper back, axilla, groin, lanugo only on upper back; ears with incurving of upper two-thirds of pinnae and thin cartilage that springs back from folding; male genitals—testes palpated in upper or lower scrotum; female genitals—labia majora larger; clitoris nearly covered.	
In the following situations, newborns should generally be stabilized rather than remaining with parents in the birth area for an extended period of time. • Apgar less than 8 at 1 minute and less than 9 at 5 minutes or baby requires resuscitation measures (other than whiffs of oxygen) • Respirations below 30 or above 60, with retractions and/or grunting • Apical pulse below 110 or above 170 with marked irregularities • Skin temperature below 36.5°C (97.8°F) • Skin color pale blue or circumoral pallor • Baby less than 38 or more than 42 weeks' gestation • Baby very small or very large for gestational age • Congenital anomalies involving open areas in the skin (meningomyelocele)	

Most healthcare facilities use newborn alarm safety devices to prevent abduction and ensure the safety of newborns in hospital settings. Umbilical cord alarms are one type of security device that are placed at the time the cord clamp is applied. The cord clamp and alarm are left in place until the mother and baby are discharged home. An alarm system that is attached to either the wrist or ankle by a band is another newborn safety device that may be utilized by some facilities (Figure 21–8). A newer option, a skin-sensing tag alarm, is placed on the wrist or ankle and senses if the tag has been removed by monitoring changes in temperature that would occur if the tag were to be removed or become dislodged from the newborn. All three devices sound an alarm if the baby is removed from the hospital unit or if the device is cut or disengaged. The need for proper disinfection techniques for devices that are reused in clinical practice is imperative.

Additional security measures are now commonplace in many maternity settings. Staff must wear appropriate identification; parents receive education to not allow individuals without proper identification to remove their baby from the room under any circumstances, to keep the newborn on the side of the bed farthest from the door, and to return the baby to the nursery if the mother plans to nap or shower if no other family member is present.

While hospital abductions are rare, they are catastrophic to the family, hospital, and community. Because many abductors pose as medical personnel to gain access to the baby, parents should not only check for proper identification, but should be advised that if family feels uneasy with anyone, they should immediately alert the nurse and refuse to provide access to the baby until additional verification can be performed. If a woman is reluctant to allow a student nurse to transport her baby, the staff nurse should be asked to assist the student.

Footprinting was once considered a security procedure but is now only performed to provide a souvenir for parents. To prepare the newborn for footprinting, the nurse wipes the soles of both the newborn's feet to remove any vernix caseosa. The footprint can be placed on a card or in the parents' baby book.

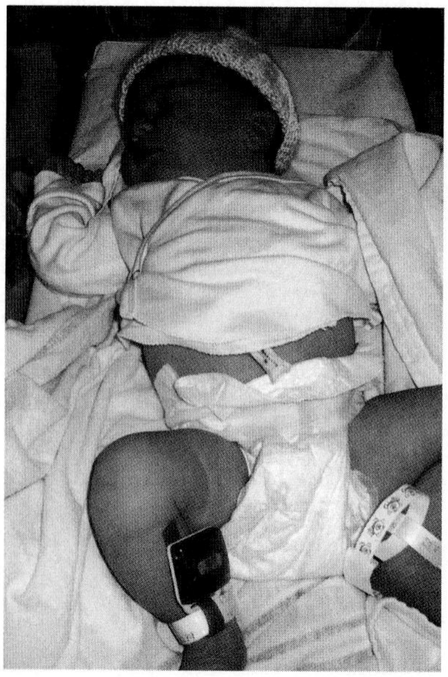

Figure 21–8 A newborn with a security device in place on one ankle.

SOURCE: Anne Garcia.

INITIATION OF ATTACHMENT

The birth of the baby is usually an emotionally charged time for all members of the family. The sight of the new baby and the sounds of the first cry may fill the parents with utter amazement. As the baby is placed on the mother's abdomen or chest, she frequently reaches out to touch and stroke her baby. When the newborn is placed in this position, the father or partner also has a very clear, close view and can also reach out to touch the baby.

When the parents feel comfortable in the environment, they may talk to the newborn, and some mothers talk to their babies in a high-pitched voice, which seems to soothe newborns. Some couples verbally express amazement and pride when they see they have produced a beautiful, healthy baby. Their verbalization enhances feelings of accomplishment and profound happiness.

Dimming the lights in the birthing area often encourages the newborn to open his or her eyes wide and gaze at the surroundings. In this first hour after birth, the newborn is usually quiet and continues to gaze. This is a wonderful opportunity for eye contact with the parents, and many parents are content to gaze quietly at their newborn.

The nurse completes assessments and interventions such as footprinting, obtaining vital signs, and applying identification bracelets while the baby is on the mother's chest and can assist the mother to a more comfortable position for holding the newborn. Breastfeeding can be encouraged if the mother and baby desire. When the baby is held close to the breast, the baby will seek out the nipple. Even if the newborn does not actively nurse, the baby can lick, taste, and smell the mother's skin. This activity stimulates the maternal release of prolactin, which promotes the onset of lactation.

The initial parental–newborn attachment period can be enhanced by minimizing assessments, delaying the instillation of ophthalmic antibiotic for the first hour, keeping the room slightly darkened, avoiding loud noises, talking in quiet tones, and providing privacy. Both parents need to be encouraged to do whatever they feel most comfortable doing. Some may desire immediate and unlimited time, while others may prefer to wait until all birth-related activities are completed (the placenta is expelled and episiotomy repair is completed); other parents may prefer limited contact immediately after birth and quiet time later. Although immediate contact may be important for attachment and initiation of breastfeeding, the parents' wishes need to be supported.

Parents can be encouraged to delay phone calls and visits from friends until after the first hour of birth because the baby is the most alert at that time. Most facilities have policies in place where the newborn is taken to the nursery for assessment and bathing after the initial time spent with parents. This is an excellent time for phone calls and visits with family and friends.

> "I was hungry for the baby as he was born. I wanted to see, hold him. It was hours before I realized or even thought love in relation to him."
>
> —Harriette Hartigan, *Women in Birth*

Delivery of the Placenta

After the cord has been clamped and cut, the physician/CNM observes for these signs of placental separation:

1. The uterus rises upward in the abdomen because the placenta settles downward into the lower uterine segment.
2. As the placenta proceeds downward, the umbilical cord lengthens.
3. A sudden trickle or spurt of blood appears.
4. The uterus changes from a discoid to a globular shape.

While waiting for these signs, the nurse gently palpates the uterus to check for ballooning caused by uterine relaxation and subsequent bleeding into the uterine cavity.

After the placenta has separated, it may be expelled by various techniques such as maternal bearing-down effort, controlled cord traction, and fundal pressure. Maternal effort allows the placenta to be expelled spontaneously and is best accomplished in an upright position. When the mother is in a dorsal recumbent or lithotomy position, she or the nurse can help the process by splinting or supporting her abdominal muscles. The mother or nurse can place her palms over the lower abdomen, or the mother can flex her thighs over her abdomen. The mother then bears down to expel the placenta.

To help the woman expel her placenta, the physician/CNM first ensures that separation has occurred and then places one hand above the symphysis pubis with the palm against the anterior surface of the uterus. The uterus is displaced upward and backward as the mother is asked to relax her abdominal muscles and breathe through an open mouth. The elevation of the uterus straightens out the birth canal and facilitates expulsion of the placenta, as well as protecting the uterus from inversion. Gentle traction is exerted on the umbilical cord. Excessive pulling may increase the risk of uterine inversion, snapping-off of the cord, and subsequent hemorrhage. During this procedure, the nurse encourages the mother to continue breathing through an open mouth and to relax her abdominal muscles.

Fundal pressure is not a method of choice because it is very uncomfortable for the mother, may damage uterine supports, and may invert the uterus. If this method is needed, the mother is asked to relax her abdominal muscles, and then the hand of the physician/CNM is placed behind the uterus with the fingers directed downward toward the maternal spine. With a quick "scooping" motion, the contracted uterus is pressed downward in an arc. This motion is different from direct downward pressure, which folds the uterus over the lower segment and does not enhance movement of the placenta. During the procedure, the nurse provides continued encouragement to maintain abdominal relaxation. This is very difficult because of the discomfort of the procedure.

After expulsion of the placenta, the physician/CNM inspects the placental membranes to make sure they are intact and that all cotyledons are present. This inspection is especially important with placentas expelled via the Duncan mechanism (the chance of tearing off a portion of a cotyledon [lobe] is greatest with this mechanism of placental separation). If there is a defect or a part missing from the placenta, a digital uterine examination is done. The time and mechanism (Schultze or Duncan) of expulsion of the placenta are noted on the birth record (see Chapter 9 and Figure 9–23 and Figure 9–24). See *Case Study: Melissa Bond-James.* The vagina and cervix are inspected for lacerations, and any necessary repairs are made. An episiotomy or laceration may be repaired now if it has not been done previously. (See further discussion of episiotomy in Chapter 25.) The fundus of the uterus is palpated; normal position is at the midline and below the umbilicus. If the fundus is displaced, it may be because of a full bladder or a collection of blood in the uterus.

Clinical Tip

When the woman's bladder is full after birth and spontaneous voiding cannot be achieved, urinary cauterization is needed to empty the bladder and prevent postpartum hemorrhage.

CASE STUDY: Melissa Bond-James

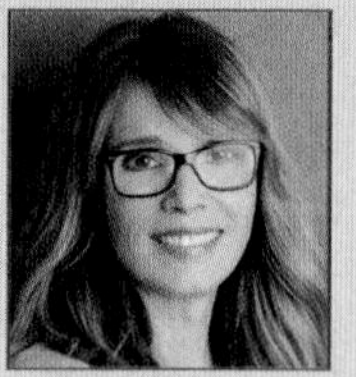
SOURCE: Kinga/ Shutterstock.

Melissa and her wife, Nancy, present to the hospital at 38 weeks and 2 days. Melissa was treated for preterm labor on two occasions, but is now term with no additional complications of pregnancy. She tells the nurse she would like to keep the afterbirth and is planning on having placenta encapsulation performed. Placenta encapsulation involves having the placenta steamed, dehydrated, ground, and placed into capsules. The practice of placenta consumption, or *placentophagy*, has its roots in Chinese medicine. Few studies have examined its therapeutic effects, but anecdotal reports include improved mood, increased energy, improved lactation, and decreased postpartum bleeding (Young, Gryder, Zava, et al., 2016). Other women have used the capsules and reported improvement in menstrual and menopausal symptoms. Melissa indicates that she hopes it will decrease her risk for postpartum depression because her sister had it after both of her children were born.

Question to Ponder

What steps should the labor nurse take to ensure hospital policies for proper disposal of the placenta are met and the proper protocol is followed before giving the placenta to Nancy to take home?

Use of Oxytocics

Some physicians/CNMs advocate the use of an oxytocic drug (Pitocin) to stimulate uterine contractions after birth and reduce the incidence of third-stage hemorrhage.

The physician/CNM may request that 10 units of oxytocin be given intramuscularly either when the baby is crowning or at the time of placenta expulsion as a means to prevent uterine atony and excessive bleeding. Other practitioners prefer to add 10 to 20 units of oxytocin to IV fluids administered over a period of hours. Methylergonovine maleate (Methergine) 0.2 mg can be administered intramuscularly when heavy bleeding occurs but should never be given if preeclampsia is present. Carboprost tromethamine (Hemabate) 250 mcg/mL can also be administered intramuscularly for postpartum hemorrhage. See *Drug Guide: Carboprost Tromethamine (Hemabate)*. Although the use of misoprostol (Cytotec) in treating postpartum hemorrhage is an off-label use, it is used in some settings with favorable results; however, it does have undesirable side effects including shivering, pyrexia, and diarrhea (Wilson, Shannon, & Shields, 2017).

Drug Guide
Carboprost Tromethamine (Hemabate)

PREGNANCY RISK CATEGORY: D

OVERVIEW OF ACTION

Carboprost tromethamine (Hemabate) is used to reduce blood loss secondary to uterine atony. It stimulates myometrial contractions to control postpartum hemorrhaging that is unresponsive to usual techniques. Carboprost tromethamine can also be used to induce labor in women desiring an elective termination of a pregnancy. The drug is also used to induce labor in cases of intrauterine fetal death and hydatidiform mole (Wilson et al., 2017).

ROUTE, DOSAGE, FREQUENCY

In cases of immediate postpartum hemorrhage, when other measures have failed, the usual intramuscular dose is 250 mcg (1 mL), which can be repeated every 1.5 to 3.5 hours if uterine atony persists. In severe bleeding, an initial dose of 400 mcg may be considered. The dosage can be increased to 500 mcg (2 mL) if uterine contractility is inadequate after several doses of 250 mcg. The total dosage should not exceed 12 mg. The maximum duration of use is 48 hours (Wilson et al., 2017).

CONTRAINDICATIONS

The drug is contraindicated in women with active cardiac, pulmonary, hepatic, or renal disease. It should not be administered during pregnancy or in women with acute pelvic inflammatory disease (Wilson et al., 2017).

SIDE EFFECTS

The most common side effects are nausea and vomiting and diarrhea. Fever, chills, and flushing can occur. Headache and muscle, joint, abdominal, or eye pain can also occur (Wilson et al., 2017).

NURSING CONSIDERATIONS

1. Pretreatment or concurrent administration of antiemetic and antidiarrheal drugs may be given to decrease nausea and vomiting and diarrhea.
2. The injection should be given in a large muscle with a tuberculin syringe. Aspiration should be performed to avoid injection into a blood vessel, which can result in bronchospasm, tetanic contractions, and shock.
3. After administration, monitor uterine status and bleeding carefully.
4. Report excess bleeding to the physician/CNM.
5. Check vital signs routinely, observing for an increase in temperature, elevated pulse, and decreased blood pressure.
6. Breastfeeding should be delayed for 24 hours after administration (Wilson et al., 2017).

Nursing Care During the Fourth Stage of Labor

The period immediately following expulsion of the placenta is referred to as the fourth stage of labor and birth. The label is misleading, however, because labor and birth are completed with delivery of the placenta, and the next few hours are actually the immediate recovery phase. The fourth stage is usually defined as lasting from 1 to 4 hours after the birth or until vital signs are stable. Nursing care in this phase involves the basics of postpartum nursing care.

Immediately after the placenta is expelled, the episiotomy or vaginal lacerations are repaired. The uterus is palpated at frequent intervals, usually every 15 minutes for an hour until bleeding is within normal limits, to ensure that it remains firmly contracted. Although labor is completed, the uterus is sensitive to touch. Palpation of the uterine fundus will be uncomfortable for the woman. If the mother has not held her baby, immediate newborn care should be completed at her side and within her reach so that she can touch her baby during this time. As soon as immediate care is completed, the new mother is usually eager to cuddle and explore her baby. If she plans to breastfeed and the baby is interested, she should be encouraged and helped to do so right after birth while the baby is awake and alert. Care should be taken not to try to force an uninterested baby to breastfeed because it will just lead to frustration for both mother and baby.

Behavioral characteristics of the mother vary, according to such factors as the length of labor, level of fatigue, extent of interruption in normal sleep patterns, and cultural norms. After the initial excitement of becoming acquainted with their new baby and notifying others of the birth, many new mothers are very tired and want to rest. Others are wide awake, eager to talk about their labor, and satisfy basic body needs, such as hunger and thirst.

Provision of Care in the Fourth Stage

As soon as the physician/CNM completes the repair of any perineal lacerations or an episiotomy, drapes (if used) are removed. If the mother is to remain in the birthing bed, the nurse places clean absorbent pads beneath her and applies maternity pads. A cold pack may be placed directly on the perineum if perineal edema is present or an episiotomy has been done. If a mother prefers to shower immediately after birth, the nurse can assist her as needed and change the bed linens while the mother is up.

If stirrups were used, her perineum is cleansed and maternity pads applied before her legs are removed from the stirrups. To avoid muscle strain, both legs are removed from the stirrups at the same time. The legs may be held together and gently pushed toward the woman's abdomen, back to a neutral position, and then gently lowered toward her right side and then the left side to promote circulation return. If the woman has given birth on a delivery table, she is transferred to a recovery room bed. If the mother has not had a chance to hold her baby, she may do so before she is transferred from the birthing room. The nurse ensures that the mother and father/partner and newborn are given time to begin the attachment process.

In addition to encouraging family celebration of the birth, the immediate recovery period involves assessing both maternal bleeding and newborn stabilization. The most significant source of bleeding is from the site where the placenta was implanted and where uterine vessels previously provided pooling of maternal blood to nourish the fetus. It is therefore critical that the fundus stay well contracted to clamp off these uterine vessels and prevent hemorrhage. It is the nurse's responsibility to assess the mother's blood pressure, pulse, firmness and position of fundus, and amount and character of vaginal blood flow every 15 minutes for the first 1 or 2 hours. Deviations from the normal ranges require more frequent checking.

Blood pressure should return to the prelabor level, and pulse rate should be slightly lower than it was in labor. The maternal blood pressure should be monitored at 5- to 15-minute intervals. The return of the blood pressure is due to an increased volume of blood returning to the maternal circulation from the uteroplacental shunt. Baroreceptors cause a vagal response, which slows the pulse. The physiologic slowing may be offset by excitement, increased temperature, or dehydration. A rise in the blood pressure may be a response to oxytocic drugs or may be caused by preeclampsia. Blood loss may be reflected by a lowered blood pressure and a rising pulse rate. See *Key Facts to Remember: Maternal Adaptations Following Birth.*

Key Facts to Remember
Maternal Adaptations Following Birth

Characteristic	Normal Finding
Blood pressure	Returns to prelabor level
Pulse	Slightly lower than in labor
Uterine fundus	In the midline at the umbilicus or 1–2 fingerbreadths below the umbilicus
Lochia	Red (rubra), small to moderate amount (from spotting on pads to 25–50% of pad covered in 15 minutes) Doesn't exceed saturation of one pad in first hour
Bladder	Nonpalpable
Perineum	Smooth, pink, without bruising or edema
Emotional state	Wide variation, including excited, exhilarated, smiling, crying, fatigued, verbal, quiet, pensive, and sleepy

The fundus should be firm at the umbilicus or lower and in the midline. The uterus should be palpated but not massaged unless boggy (atonic). See *Clinical Skill 21–2: Assessing the Uterine Fundus Following Vaginal Birth.* When the uterus becomes boggy, pooling of blood occurs within it, resulting in the formation of clots. Anything left in the uterus prevents it from contracting effectively. Thus, if it becomes boggy or appears to rise in the abdomen, the fundus should be massaged until firm. The uterus at this time is very tender, and palpation and massage cause discomfort. All palpation and massage should be done as gently as possible.

A boggy uterus feels very soft instead of firm and hard. The uterus may have relaxed so much that it cannot be found when the nurse attempts to palpate it. In this case the nurse places a hand in the midline of the abdomen at the level of the umbilicus and begins to make kneading motions. This motion stimulates the uterine fundus to contract, and the nurse will feel the fundus tighten to a firm, hard object.

Clinical Tip

Teach the woman to gently massage her own uterus by feeling for the uterus at the level of the umbilicus. Describe the uterus as a commonly known identifiable object, such as a grapefruit or a softball, to provide a visual cue for the woman. Once she identifies her uterus, she can massage gently it to increase uterine contractions.

CLINICAL SKILL 21–2

Assessing the Uterine Fundus Following Vaginal Birth

NURSING ACTION

Preparation

- Explain the procedure, the information it provides, and what it might feel like.
- Ask the woman to void.

Rationale: *A full bladder can cause uterine atony.*

- Have the woman lie flat in bed with her head on a pillow. If the procedure is uncomfortable, she may find that it helps to flex her legs.

Rationale: *The supine position prevents falsely high assessment of fundal height. Flexing the legs relaxes the abdominal muscles.*

Equipment and Supplies

A clean perineal pad

Procedure

1. Gently place one hand on the lower segment of the uterus. Using the side of the other hand, palpate the abdomen until you locate the top of the fundus.

Rationale: *One hand stabilizes the uterus while the other hand locates the top of the fundus.*

2. Determine whether the fundus is firm. If it is, it will feel like a hard, round object in the abdomen. If it is not firm, massage the abdomen lightly until the fundus is firm.

Rationale: *A firm fundus indicates that the uterine muscles are contracted and bleeding will not occur.*

3. Measure the top of the fundus in fingerbreadths above, below, or at the fundus. See Figure 21–9.

Rationale: *Fundal height gives information about the progress of involution.*

4. Determine the position of the fundus in relation to the midline of the body. If it is not in the midline, locate it and then evaluate the bladder for distention.

Rationale: *The fundus may deviate from the midline when the bladder is full because the enlarged bladder pushes the uterus aside.*

5. If the bladder is distended, use nursing measures to help the woman void. If she is not able to void after a specified period of time, catheterization may be necessary.

6. Measure urine output for the next few hours until normal elimination is established.

Rationale: *During the postpartum as diuresis occurs, the bladder may fill far more rapidly than normal, putting the woman at risk for uterine atony and hemorrhage.*

7. Assess the lochia.

CLINICAL TIP

Gloves may be put on before assessing the abdomen and fundus or when you are ready to assess the perineum and lochia.

8. Document the position (midline, deviated to the left or right), fundal height in relation to the umbilicus (F @ U or F @ U ↑ 1 or F @ U ↓ 1), and consistency (firm, boggy). The bladder status should also be recorded (distended, appears empty), along with the time of the last void.

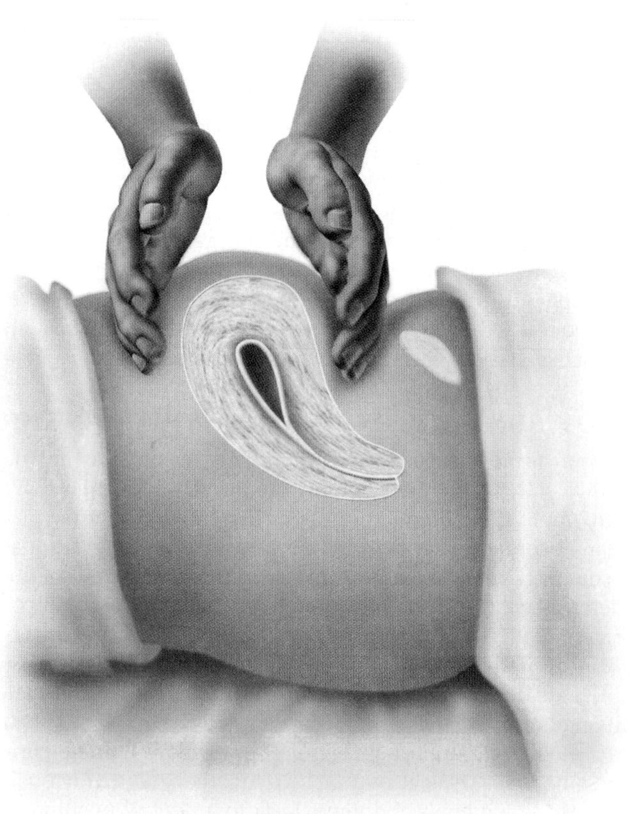

Figure 21–9 **Suggested method of palpating the fundus of the uterus during the fourth stage. The left hand is placed just above the symphysis pubis, and gentle downward pressure is exerted. The right hand is cupped around the uterine fundus.**

The nurse inspects the bloody vaginal discharge, called *lochia*, for amount and charts it as minimal, moderate, or heavy (see Chapter 32). It should be bright red. Because different brands of maternity pads absorb varying amounts of blood, it may be necessary to weigh the maternity pad to determine actual blood loss. A gram scale is used, and 1 g is equivalent to approximately 1 mL of blood. If the perineal pad becomes soaked in a 15-minute period or if blood pools under the buttocks, continuous observation is necessary. As long as the woman remains in bed during the first hour, bleeding should not exceed saturation of one pad. Laceration of the vagina, cervix, or an unligated vessel in the episiotomy may be indicated by a continuous trickle of blood even though the fundus remains firm. (See *Clinical Skill 32–2: Evaluating Lochia.*)

If the fundus rises and displaces to the right, the nurse palpates the bladder to determine whether it is distended. All measures should be taken to enable the mother to void. If she is unable to void, catheterization is necessary. Postpartum women have decreased sensations to void as a result of the decreased tone of the bladder caused by the trauma imposed on the bladder and urethra during childbirth. The bladder fills rapidly as the body attempts to rid itself of the extra fluid volume returned from the uteroplacental circulation and of IV fluid that may have been received during labor and birth. If the mother is unable to void, a warm towel placed across the lower abdomen, warm water poured over the perineum, or spirits of peppermint poured into a bedpan may help the urinary sphincter relax and thus facilitate voiding. A distended bladder can cause uterine atony, thus increasing postpartum bleeding.

The perineum is inspected for edema and hematoma formation. With an episiotomy or laceration, an ice pack often reduces swelling and alleviates discomfort. To fully visualize the episiotomy or laceration site, the nurse has the woman lie on her side and lifts her anterior buttock to visualize the suture line. The site should be well approximated and may appear swollen or bruised. No active bleeding at the site should be observed.

These conditions should be reported to the physician/CNM:

- Hypotension
- Tachycardia
- Uterine atony
- Excessive bleeding
- Temperature over 100.4°F (or as per agency's guidelines).

The nurse should be aware that the blood pressure may not fall rapidly in the presence of dangerous bleeding in postpartum mothers because of the extra systemic volume. However, an increasing pulse rate may be noted before a decrease in blood pressure is detected. A normal blood pressure with the mother in the Fowler position is a good confirmation of a normotensive woman.

Promotion of Comfort in the Fourth Stage

Women frequently have tremors in the immediate postpartum period. It has been proposed that this shivering response is caused by exhaustion or a difference in internal and external body temperatures (higher temperature inside the body than on the outside). Another theory is that the woman is reacting to the fetal cells that have entered the maternal circulation at the placental site. A heated bath blanket placed next to the woman and perhaps a warm drink tend to alleviate the problem.

The couple may be tired, hungry, and thirsty. Some hospitals serve them a meal. The tired mother may initially have a period of excitement but may then drift off into a welcome sleep because of exhaustion from the energy that was exerted during labor. The father/partner or support person should also be encouraged to rest because the supporting role is physically and mentally tiring. The mother is usually transferred from the birthing unit to the postpartum unit after 2 hours or more, depending on agency policy and whether these criteria are met: Stable vital signs, stable lochia, nondistended bladder, firm fundus, and sensations fully recovered from any anesthetic agent received during childbirth.

Nursing Care of the Adolescent

Adolescent patients need ongoing support and developmental responsiveness throughout labor and the birth process. Each adolescent in labor is different. The nurse must assess what each patient brings to the experience by asking these questions:

- Has the young woman received prenatal care?
- What are her attitudes and feelings about the pregnancy?
- How does her developmental stage influence her behavior, and how are her specific needs different?
- Who will support her during the birth, and what is the person's relationship to her?
- What preparation has she had for the experience?
- What are her expectations and fears regarding labor and birth?
- How has her culture influenced her?
- What are her usual coping mechanisms?
- Does she have adequate social support?
- Does she plan to keep the newborn? If so, does she need to learn parenting skills?
- Will the father of the baby be involved in the labor and birth experience?

Adolescents are at highest risk for pregnancy and labor complications and must be assessed carefully. Any adolescent who has not had prenatal care requires especially close observation during labor. The status of the fetus is monitored to ensure its well-being. The young woman's prenatal record is carefully reviewed for risks. The adolescent is more likely to have poor nutritional intake, preeclampsia, cephalopelvic disproportion (CPD), anemia, prematurity, drugs ingested during pregnancy, sexually transmitted infections, fetal death, and size–date discrepancies (gestation appears to be less than dates indicate because of minimal weight gain) (March of Dimes, 2017). Babies born to teenage mothers are more likely to have lower birth weights. They are also more likely to be exposed to alcohol, drugs, and tobacco in utero and in early childhood (CDC, 2017).

The nurse's support role depends on the young woman's support system during labor. When the patient is not accompanied by someone who will stay with her during childbirth, it is even more important for the nurse to establish a trusting relationship with her. In this way, the nurse can help her cope with labor and understand what is happening to her. Establishing rapport without recrimination will provide emotional support and encouragement. The adolescent who is given positive reinforcement for "work well done" will leave the experience with increased self-esteem, despite the emotional stress and difficulty of giving birth at a young age.

The adolescent who has taken childbirth education classes is generally better prepared than the adolescent who has had no preparation. The nurse must keep in mind, however, that the younger the adolescent, the less she may be able to participate actively in the process.

Age-Related Responses to Labor and Birth

The very young adolescent (under age 14) has fewer coping mechanisms and less experience to draw on than her older counterparts have. Because her cognitive development is incomplete, the younger adolescent may have fewer problem-solving capabilities. Her ego integrity may be more threatened by the experience, and she may be more vulnerable to stress and discomfort.

The very young woman needs someone to rely on at all times during labor. She may be more childlike and dependent than older teens. The nurse must be sure that instructions and explanations are simple and concrete. During the transition phase, the young teenager may become withdrawn and unable to express her need to be nurtured. Touch, soothing encouragement, and measures to promote her comfort help her maintain control and meet her needs for dependence. During the second stage of labor, the young adolescent may feel as if she is losing control and may reach out to those around her. By remaining calm and giving directions, the nurse helps her control feelings of helplessness.

“One of the most memorable expectant mothers I cared for during my nursing course was Cara, a 13-year-old. I met her each week as she came into the OB clinic at our hospital and stayed with her as she waited for her appointment and was then seen by the medical student. I noticed that with each passing visit, she became more and more anxious. I did my best to determine the source of her anxiety, provide general teaching, and try to answer all of her questions. I consulted with my professor, and she sat in with me during some visits. But Cara became more and more anxious. Near term, she began asking if she could just have the baby cut out. Finally, in the 38th week, after 2½ months of building trust, she told me she was afraid because her baby had gotten too big, and it would never be able to come out through her belly button. I was speechless for a moment. For 2½ months, I had answered questions and felt so proud of my support and teaching, and for all this time, she had not been able to ask the most important question of all—the question that paralyzed her with fear. I was finally able to provide specific information, made drawings on a paper towel, had the medical student talk with her, and best of all, was able to be on call and be with her in labor and during birth. The beautiful smile on her face as her baby daughter was born was unbelievable. Cara wasn't afraid! It's been 39 years since then, and I still remember her.”

The middle adolescent (ages 14 to 16 years) often attempts to remain calm and unflinching during labor. If unable to break through the teenager's stoic barrier, the nurse needs to rise above frustration and realize that a caring attitude will still positively affect the young woman.

Many older adolescents (ages 16 to 19 years) feel that they "know it all," but they may be no more prepared for childbirth than their younger counterparts. The nurse's reinforcement and nonjudgmental manner will help them save face. If the adolescent has not taken classes, she may require preparation and explanations. The older teenager's response to the stresses of labor is similar to that of the adult woman.

The Adolescent Father

Consideration of the adolescent father is a very important aspect of labor and birthing care. In modern society, the role of the father has undergone tremendous transformation. Nurses need to be aware that this is a stressful time for the young father. Interventions that are inclusive, foster the new father's role, and support paternal attachment are imperative at this time of family development (Sriyasak, Sridawruang, Almqvist, et al., 2018). There are some specific interventions that increase comfort, enhance education, and perhaps decrease stress. In the early part of labor, the nurse can talk with the father about his expectations for parenting the newborn and what resources are available in the community. Many adolescents are reluctant to ask questions, but an accepting attitude may help in establishing rapport and gaining trust.

The teen father may need encouragement to provide supportive care and to know what actions are acceptable in the birthing area. He may be encouraged to hold the mother's hand, to sit on the bed beside her, to give a back massage, or to stroke her forehead. He may need assistance in how to give a shoulder rub or back rub; he can watch the nurse first and then perform the action himself with the encouragement of the nurse. He may need more encouragement than the older father to share a Jacuzzi or shower or to support the mother in changing positions and ambulating. It is important for the nurse to speak in lay terms and to anticipate questions, to answer all vocalized questions honestly, and to provide opportunities for the parents to ask for further information.

Other Members of the Support Team

In addition to the adolescent's partner, the mother may want her parents or friends with her as members of her support team. Some teens may want their mothers as their primary support person, whereas others may strive to prove their independence and "do this on their own." Still other young women may look to friends for advice and support. The nurse includes parents and friends of the adolescent mother in the patient teaching and other aspects of the mother's care. It is important to respect the young woman's privacy and honor her wishes regarding whom she wants in the room for the birth. The nurse may have to advocate for the young woman in certain circumstances.

Teaching the Adolescent Mother

During the latent phase of labor, the nurse can explain to the young woman what changes in body sensations and emotional reactions she might anticipate as labor and birth progress. The adolescent also needs teaching about what possible medical procedures, such as electronic fetal monitoring (EFM), might be used, as well as what nursing care measures are available. Some adolescents might not realize that they can request the nurse's presence, touch, or advice, unless the nurse specifically informs them that these options are available.

Adolescents are oriented to the present time and may not adequately predict future needs for themselves or their baby. The nurse should assess to make sure adequate resources are available, including baby and postpartum supplies, transportation to and from follow-up visits, and child care, if the adolescent mother is planning on returning to school or work.

Young mothers may need more information on newborn/infant care and feeding choices than older women. Some adolescents may be reluctant to breastfeed because of embarrassment

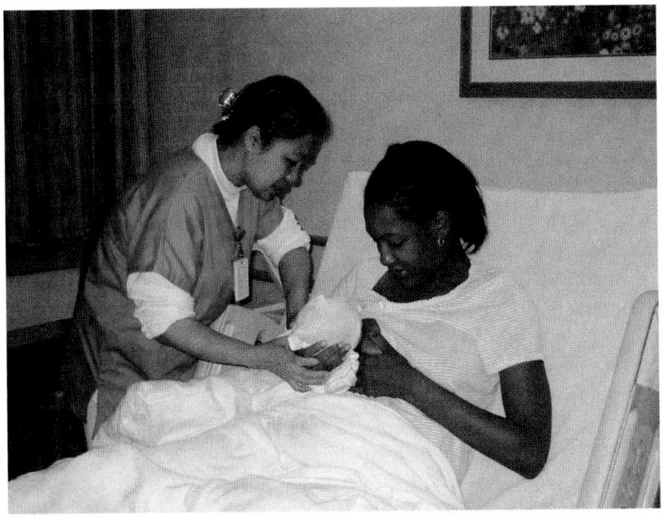

Figure 21–10 **An adolescent mother receives breastfeeding assistance in the immediate postpartum period.**

SOURCE: Michele Davidson.

or lack of information. The nurse can assist the young woman to explore her feelings related to breastfeeding and provide information (Figure 21–10). The nurse should provide encouragement and support the young mother's decision. Sometimes, young women feel "pressured" to breastfeed their babies when they truly do not feel comfortable with this feeding choice. The nurse should give the young mother permission to make her own decision. Young women who choose to use formula should be given clear instructions on the importance of mixing the formula per the manufacturer's directions because overdiluting or underdiluting can cause adverse side effects for the baby.

Although rarer than in previous decades, some adolescents may choose to relinquish their newborns. In these situations, the nurse informs the adolescent that seeing the baby can facilitate the grieving process but lets her know that seeing the newborn is her choice. (See Chapter 33 for further discussion of the relinquishing mother and the adolescent parent.)

Nursing Care During Precipitous Labor and Birth

Occasionally labor progresses so rapidly that the maternity nurse is faced with the task of managing the actual birth of the baby. The terms **precipitous labor** and **precipitous birth** are used when the labor and birth occur in 3 hours or less. The attending nurse has the primary responsibility for providing a physically and psychologically safe experience for the woman and her baby.

A woman whose physician/CNM is not present may feel disappointed, frightened, cheated, and abandoned, especially if she is not prepared through childbirth education. The nurse can support the woman by keeping her informed about the labor progress and assuring her that the nurse will stay with her. If birth is imminent, the nurse must not leave the mother alone. Auxiliary personnel can be directed to contact the attending physician/CNM or other physicians/CNMs that are in the facility. The auxiliary personnel should also retrieve the emergency pack (*precip pack*), which should be readily accessible to the birthing/labor rooms. A typical pack contains these items:

- Small drape that can be placed under the woman's buttocks to provide a sterile field
- Bulb syringe to clear mucus from the newborn's mouth
- Two sterile clamps (Kelly or Rochester) to clamp the umbilical cord before applying a cord clamp
- Sterile scissors to cut the umbilical cord
- Sterile umbilical cord clamp, either Hesseltine or Hollister
- Baby blanket to wrap the newborn in after birth
- Package of sterile gloves

Clinical Tip

When birth is imminent and a physician/CNM is not present, do not take the bed apart (or "break the bed") because this increases the risk that the newborn could be dropped at the time of birth. Lower the foot of the bed slightly to create space beneath the buttocks so you are able to adequately deliver the head without the risk of a newborn fall.

As the materials are being gathered, the nurse must remain calm. The woman is reassured by the nurse's composure and feels that the nurse is competent. The primary goal of nursing care is the safe birth of the baby.

Birth of the Baby

The nurse manages precipitous birth in the hospital by encouraging the woman to assume a comfortable position. If time permits, the nurse scrubs both hands with soap and water and puts on sterile gloves. Sterile drapes are placed under the woman's buttocks.

At all times during the birth, the nurse gives clear instructions to the woman, supports her efforts, and provides reassurance. The nurse needs to remain calm and proceed in a slow, confident manner.

Most neonates will be born in vertex presentation. When the baby's head crowns, the nurse instructs the woman to either blow or pant, which decreases her urge to push. The nurse checks whether the amniotic sac is intact. If it is, the nurse tears the sac with a clamp so that the newborn will not breathe in amniotic fluid with the first breath.

The nurse may place an index finger inside the lower portion of the vagina and the thumb on the outer portion of the perineum and gently massage the area to aid in stretching of perineal tissues and to help prevent perineal lacerations. This is called *ironing the perineum*.

With one hand, the nurse applies gentle pressure against the fetal head to maintain flexion and prevent it from popping out rapidly. The nurse does not hold the head back forcibly. Rapid birth of the head may tear the woman's perineal tissues. The rapid change in pressure within the fetal head may cause subdural or dural tears. The nurse supports the perineum with the other hand and allows the head to be delivered between contractions.

As the woman continues to blow or pant, the nurse inserts one or two fingers along the back of the fetal head to check for the umbilical cord. If the cord is around the neck, the nurse bends her fingers like a fish hook, grasps the cord, and pulls it over the baby's head, loosens it, or slips it down over the shoulders. It is important to check that the cord is not wrapped around more than one time. If the cord is tightly looped and cannot be slipped over the baby's head, the nurse places two clamps on the cord, cuts it between the clamps, and unwinds the cord. Because this ceases oxygenation to the baby, all efforts should be made to reduce (remove) the cord over the head whenever possible. The head typically rotates (restitutes) to the left or right. The nurse needs to let the head rotate (restitute) to the side before attempting delivery of the head.

Immediately after birth of the head, the nurse suctions first the mouth, throat, and then the nasal passages. The nurse places a hand on each side of the head and instructs the woman to push gently so that the rest of the body can be expelled quickly. The newborn must be supported as it emerges.

Breech vaginal births are quite rare. Because the incidence of breech presentations is only 3%, most breech presentations are scheduled for cesarean births, and women are advised to come to the hospital immediately if labor does begin spontaneously. Because the primary concern in a breech birth is to prevent the entrapment of the head in the cervix, intervention is avoided until the buttocks are born. The nurse then pulls down a loop of cord (to avoid stress on its point of insertion) and supports the breech in both hands. The baby's body is lifted slightly upward for birth of the posterior shoulder and arm. The newborn may then be lowered, and the anterior shoulder and arm will pass under the symphysis pubis. Suprapubic pressure should be applied to maintain the normal flexion of the baby's head and should be continued until the baby is born. The nape of the neck pivots under the symphysis, and the rest of the head is born over the perineum by a movement of flexion.

Regardless of the presentation at birth, the newborn is held at the level of the uterus to facilitate blood flow through the umbilical cord immediately after birth. The combination of amniotic fluid and vernix makes the newborn very slippery, so the nurse must be careful to avoid dropping the baby. Placing the woman in stirrups is not recommended for this reason; instead, the foot of the bed can be lowered. The nurse suctions the nose and mouth of the newborn again, using a bulb syringe. The nurse then dries the newborn quickly to prevent heat loss. Wet blankets should be removed and replaced with warmed, dry blankets.

As soon as the nurse determines that the newborn's respirations are adequate, the baby can be placed on the mother's abdomen. The newborn's head should be slightly lower than the body to aid drainage of fluid and mucus. The weight of the newborn on the mother's abdomen stimulates uterine contractions, which aid in placental separation. The umbilical cord should not be pulled. The Apgar score is assessed at 1 and 5 minutes.

The nurse is alert for signs of placental separation. When these signs are present, the nurse places one hand just above the symphysis pubis to guard the uterus and uses the other hand to maintain gentle downward traction on the cord while instructing the mother to push so that the placenta can be expelled. In some instances the mother can squat, and this usually helps expel the placenta. The nurse inspects the placenta to determine whether it is intact. Because the physician/CNM is usually en route, delivery of the placenta can be delayed until the practitioner arrives. Traction should not be applied because this can result in hemorrhage or detaching the umbilical cord from the placenta.

The nurse checks the firmness of the uterus. Palpation of the uterus should not be performed before separation of the placenta. The fundus may be gently massaged to stimulate contractions and decrease bleeding. Putting the newborn to breast also stimulates uterine contractions through release of oxytocin from the pituitary gland.

The umbilical cord may now be cut. Two sterile clamps are placed approximately 2 to 4 inches from the newborn's abdomen. The cord is cut between them with sterile scissors. A sterile cord clamp (Hollister or Hesseltine) can be placed adjacent to the clamp on the newborn's cord, between the clamp and the newborn's abdomen. The clamp must not be placed snugly against the abdomen because the cord will dry and shrink.

The area under the mother's buttocks is cleaned, and her perineum is inspected for lacerations. Bleeding from lacerations may be controlled by pressing a clean perineal pad against the perineum and instructing the woman to keep her thighs together. Further evaluation by the physician/CNM will be needed to determine if lacerations are present that need to be repaired.

If the arrival of the physician/CNM is delayed or if the newborn is having respiratory distress, the newborn should be transported immediately to the nursery. The newborn must be properly identified before leaving the birthing area.

Record Keeping

The nurse notes and places on the record this information:

1. Position of fetus at birth
2. Presence of cord around neck or shoulder (nuchal cord)
3. Time of birth
4. Apgar scores at 1 and 5 minutes after birth
5. Gender of newborn
6. Time of expulsion of placenta
7. Method of placental expulsion
8. Appearance and intactness of placenta
9. Mother's condition
10. Any medications that were given to mother or newborn (per agency protocol).

Clinical Tip

Since time is typically very limited and rushed in a precipitous birth, the nurse can write interventions and birth outcomes on the FHR monitoring strip so that times and details are more precise and exact.

Postbirth Interventions

Postbirth interventions are the same as those discussed in the *Nursing Care During the Third Stage of Labor* section.

Evaluation

Evaluation provides an opportunity to determine the effectiveness of nursing care. As a result of comprehensive nursing care during the intrapartum period, these outcomes may be anticipated:

- The mother's physical needs and the psychologic well-being of the family have been maintained and supported.
- The baby's physical and psychologic well-being has been protected and supported.
- The family has had input into the birth process, and members have participated as much as they desired.
- The birth was safe and promoted family cohesiveness.

Focus Your Study

- Admission to the birth setting involves assessment of many physiologic, psychologic, and social factors. The information gained helps the nurse establish priorities of care.
- Before initiating care, the nurse explains what will be done, the reasons, potential benefits and risks, and possible alternatives, if appropriate. This helps the woman determine what happens to her body and is a critical element in the process of obtaining informed consent.
- Behavioral responses to labor vary with the phase of labor, the woman's preparation and previous experience, cultural beliefs, and developmental level.
- Each woman's cultural beliefs affect her need for privacy, her expression of discomfort, her expectations for the birth, and the role she wishes the father/partner/support person to play in the birth event.
- The laboring woman's comfort may be increased by general comfort measures, supportive relaxation techniques, methods of handling anxiety, controlled breathing, and support by a caring person.
- The laboring woman fears being alone during labor. Even though there is a support person available, the woman's anxiety may be decreased when the nurse remains with her.
- Maternal birthing positions include a wide variety of possibilities, such as recumbent, sidelying, sitting, squatting, and crouching on hands and knees.
- Immediate assessments of the newborn include evaluation of the Apgar score and an abbreviated physical assessment. These early assessments help determine whether there is a need for resuscitation and whether the newborn's adaptation to extrauterine life is progressing normally. The newborn that is not experiencing problems may remain with the parents for an extended period of time following birth.
- Immediate care of the newborn following birth also includes maintaining respirations, promoting warmth, preventing infection, and providing accurate identification.
- The new parents and their baby are given time together as soon as possible after birth.
- Nursing assessments continue after the birth and are important to ensure that normal physiologic adaptations are taking place.
- The adolescent has special needs in the birth setting. Her developmental needs require specialized nursing care.
- Nurse-assisted births are sometimes performed in the absence of the physician/CNM or when birth is imminent.

In order to make safe and effective judgments using NANDA-I © 2017 nursing diagnoses, it is essential that nurses refer to the definitions and defining characteristics of the diagnoses used in this text, which can be found in Appendix C.

References

American College of Emergency Physicians (ACEP). (2016). *Emergency Medical Treatment and Labor Act (EMTALA)*. Retrieved from https://www.acep.org/Liability-Reform-HR-836/#sm.0000yuhqa9dqud8ftos294ozebgci

American College of Obstetricians and Gynecologists (ACOG). (2017a). *Delayed cord clamping after birth* (ACOG Committee Opinion No. 684). Washington, DC: Author.

American College of Obstetricians and Gynecologists (ACOG). (2017b). *Intrapartum fetal heart rate monitoring: Nomenclature, interpretation, and general management principles* (ACOG Practice Bulletin No. 106). Washington, DC: Author.

Apgar, V. (1966). *The newborn (Apgar) scoring system, reflections and advice*. Retrieved from http://profiles.nlm.nih.gov/ps/access/CPBBJY.pdf

Association of Women's Health, Obstetric, and Neonatal Nurses (AWHONN). (2017). *AWHONN's high risk and critical care obstetrics*. Washington, DC: Author.

Centers for Disease Control and Prevention (CDC). (2015). *2015 Sexually transmitted diseases treatment guidelines. HIV infection: Detection, counseling, and referral*. Retrieved from https://www.cdc.gov/std/tg2015/hiv.htm

Centers for Disease Control and Prevention (CDC). (2017). *About teen pregnancy*. Retrieved from https://www.cdc.gov/teenpregnancy/aboutteenpreg.htm

Ciardulli, A., Saccone, G., Anastasio, H., & Berghella, V. (2017). Less-restrictive food intake during labor in low-risk singleton pregnancies: A systematic review and meta-analysis. *Obstetrics & Gynecology, 129*(3), 473–480.

Cunningham, F. G., Leveno, K. J., Bloom, S. L., Spong, C., Dashe, J.S., Hoffman, B.L., . . . Sheffield, J. S. (2016). *Williams obstetrics* (25th ed.). New York, NY: McGraw-Hill.

Desseauve, D., Fradet, L., Lacouture, P., & Pierce, F. (2017). Position for labor and birth: State of knowledge and biomechanical perspectives. *European Journal of Obstetrics and Gynecology and Reproductive Biology, 208*, 46–54. DOI: http://dx.doi.org/10.1016/j.ejogrb.2016.11.006

Dresang, L. T., & Yonke, N. (2015). Management of spontaneous vaginal delivery. *American Family Physician, 92*(3), 202–208.

Gabbe, S. G., Niebyl, J. R., Simpson, J. L., Galan, H. L., & Jauniaux, E. R. M., Driscoll, D. A., . . . Grobman, W. A. (2016). *Obstetrics: Normal and problem pregnancies, expert consult.* (6th ed.). St. Louis, MO: Saunders.

Groll, C. G. (2017). *Fast facts for the labor and delivery nurse*. New York, NY: Springer.

Huang, Y. C. (2018). Correlations between pushing skills and pushing perceptions, second-stage labor duration, postpartum fatigue, and birth satisfaction. *World Academy of Science, Engineering and Technology, International Journal of Nursing and Health Sciences, 5*(2).

MacKinnon, A. L., Yang, L., Feeley, N., Gold, I., Hayton, B., & Zelkowitz, P. (2017). Birth setting, labour experience, and postpartum psychological distress. *Midwifery, 50*, 110–116.

March of Dimes (MOD). (2017). *Quick reference: Fact sheets: Teenage pregnancy.* Retrieved from https://www.marchofdimes.com/professionals/14332_1159.asp

Mitra, M., Akobirshoev, I., McKee, M. M., & Iezzoni, L. I. (2016). Birth outcomes among US women with hearing loss. *American Journal of Preventive Medicine, 51*(6), 865–873. Retrieved from https://doi.org/10.1016/j.amepre.2016.08.001

National Cord Blood Registry. (2015). *Cord blood can save lives.* Retrieved from https://www.nationalcordbloodprogram.org

National Institute on Deafness and Other Communication Disorders. (2016). *Quick statistics about hearing.* Retrieved from https://www.nidcd.nih.gov/health/statistics/quick-statistics-hearing

Ommolbanin, Z., Hajar, P., & Mahbobeh, F. (2014). Effect of perineal massage on the incidence of episiotomy and perineal laceration. *Health, 6*(1), 10–14. DOI: 10.4236/health.2014.61003

Sawyer, T. L. (2015). *Intubation and tracheal suctioning for meconium aspiration.* Retrieved from https://emedicine.medscape.com/article/1413467-overview#a2

Simkin, P., Hanson, L., & Ancheta, R. (2017). *The labor progress handbook: Early interventions to prevent and treat dystocia* (4th ed.). Hoboken, NJ: Wiley.

Smith, C., Levett, K., Collins, C., Armour, M., Dahlen, H., & Suganuma, M. (2018). Relaxation techniques for pain management in labour. *Cochrane Database of Systematic Reviews 2018*, Issue 3. Article No.: CD009514. Retrieved from https://www.cochrane.org/CD009514/PREG_relaxation-techniques-pain-management-labour

Spector, R. E. (2016). *Cultural diversity in health and illness* (9th ed.). Boston, MA: Pearson.

Sriyasak, A., Sridawruang, C., Almqvist, A. L., & Häggström-Nordin, E. (2018). Parents' experiences of their teenage children's parenthood: An interview study. *Nursing and Health Sciences, 20*(1), 39–45. DOI: 10.1111/nhs.12378

Standford Medicine. (2017). *Infants born <38 weeks gestation or <6 lbs.* Retrieved from https://med.stanford.edu/newborns/professional-education/breastfeeding/babies-at-risk/infants---38-weeks-or-less-than-6-pounds.html

Wente, S. (2015). An Amish homebirth. *Spectrum Health: Health Beat.* Retrieved from https://healthbeat.spectrumhealth.org/amish-homebirth/

Wilson, B. A., Shannon, M. T., & Shields, K. A. (2017). *Pearson nurse's drug guide: 2018.* Hoboken, NJ: Pearson.

Yee, L. M., Sandoval, G., Bailit, J., Reddy, U. M., Wapner, R. J., Varner, M. V. V., . . . & Eunice Kennedy Shriver National Institute of Child Health and Human Development (NICHD) Maternal-Fetal Medicine Units (MFMU) Network. (2016). Maternal and neonatal outcomes with early compared with delayed pushing among nulliparous women. *Obstetrics & Gynecology, 128*(5), 1039–1047.

Young, S. M., Gryder, L. K., Zava, D., Kimball, D. W., & Benyshek, D. C. (2016). Presence and concentration of 17 hormones in human placenta processed for encapsulation and consumption. *Placenta, 43*, 86–89. DOI: 10.1016/j.nutres.2016.04.005

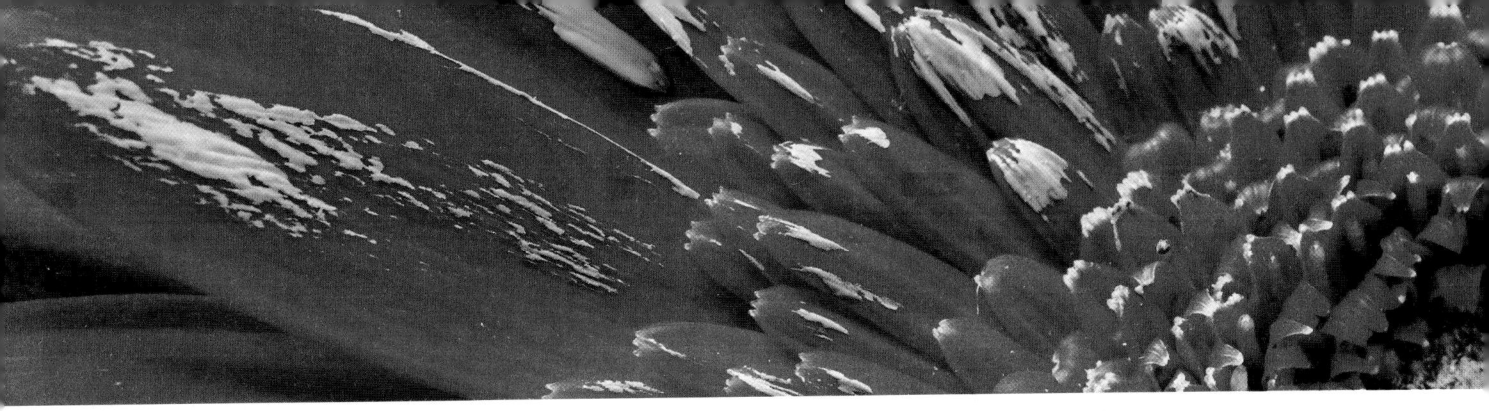

Chapter 22
Pharmacologic Pain Management

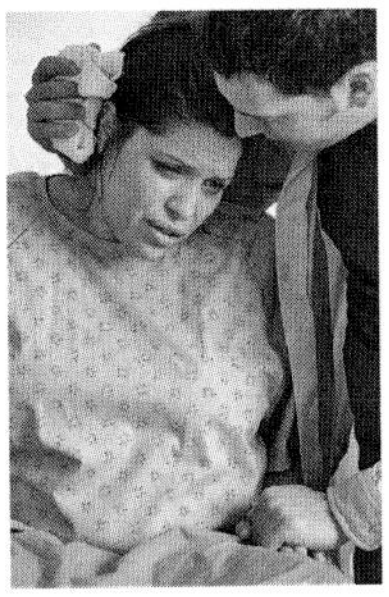

We had attended childbirth classes and practiced through the last few weeks, and I had hoped to go through all of labor and birth without medication. But when the contractions really came on strong, I just wasn't ready for the amount and the kind of pain that I felt. I've always been able to tolerate pain well, but this was different. My husband and I talked about it, and he reassured me that, if I felt I needed something, it was okay with him. My nurse was also very supportive. She helped me feel I was making a good decision and wasn't failing somehow.

SOURCE: Radius/SuperStock.

Learning Outcomes

22.1 Discuss the nurse's role in supporting pharmaceutical pain relief measures in labor.

22.2 Identify how opioid abuse, dependence, and addiction affects women's options for pharmacologic pain relief in labor and birth.

22.3 Describe the use of systemic analgesics to promote pain relief during labor.

22.4 Compare the major types of regional analgesia and anesthesia, including the area affected, advantages, disadvantages, techniques, and nursing implications.

22.5 Summarize possible complications of regional anesthesia.

22.6 Describe the indication for the use of general anesthesia in labor and birth.

22.7 Describe the nurse's role in caring for a woman experiencing major complications of general anesthesia.

22.8 Identify contraindications to specific types of analgesia and anesthesia for high-risk mothers.

When a childbearing woman experiences discomfort during labor and birth, the nurse can assist her to have a positive birth experience by providing effective comfort measures while continuing to assess her and her baby's well-being. Nursing interventions directed toward pain relief begin with the nonpharmacologic measures described in Chapter 21, such as providing information, encouragement, back rubs, and clean linens; suggesting positional changes; and assisting with relaxation and breathing techniques. Many women need no further interventions.

For other women, the progression of labor brings increasing levels of pain that interfere with their ability to cope effectively. For these women, pharmacologic agents may be used to decrease discomfort, increase relaxation, and reestablish the ability to participate more actively in the labor and birth experience. Options include systemic analgesics, regional nerve blocks (epidural, spinal, and combined spinal–epidural), and local anesthetic blocks (pudendal and perineal). These methods are not mutually exclusive and may be used in combination with nonpharmacologic comfort measures.

Medicated Birth

Nurses need to recognize that the decision to have an unmedicated or a medicated birth involves many factors and reflects a great deal of thought and planning for most women and their families. Some of these factors include patient and caregiver preferences, availability of anesthesia and analgesia, fear of risks and complications, past life experiences, previous experiences with pain, and cultural influences. Other factors, such as the amount of sleep the woman has had or the length of labor, can also influence the need or desire for pharmacologic pain relief measures. The woman should be supported regardless of her decision even if it changes during the course of labor.

Each year in the United States, close to 4 million babies are born. Approximately two-thirds of women in the United States who give birth have regional anesthesia, most commonly some form of epidural (Martin, Hamilton, Osterman, et al., 2017).

Many women and couples who participate in childbirth education approach their birth experiences confident that the techniques they have learned will enable them to cope with the pain of labor. Nurses should respect their choices and provide support to help them meet their goals. Analgesics and anesthetics affect the fetus and can result in maternal side effects. Following an unmedicated birth, many women report a quicker postpartum recovery and are often able to ambulate, urinate, shower, and eat within an hour of giving birth. Additionally, many women feel an enormous sense of empowerment after successfully having an unmedicated birth.

For the woman who has advised the nursing staff that she wants no pharmacologic remedies, the nurse should offer alternative comfort measures. All nurses in the intrapartum setting need to be familiar with various nonpharmacologic techniques available to help women cope with the pain they may experience (see Chapter 21). The nurse should not offer pharmacologic options to women who have stated they want an unmedicated birth unless the woman specifically asks about them. When women do request pharmacologic options, nurses should discuss them with the woman between contractions when she is most comfortable.

On the other hand, many women are simply unprepared for the intense pain of active labor and may request medication. They may begin labor undecided about whether to use medication, and then request pain relief as contractions intensify. Frequently, feelings of inadequacy and guilt accompany such decisions. The nurse plays a special role in assisting the woman and her partner/support person to explore options for pain relief realistically. The nurse can explain that, although pharmacologic agents do affect the fetus, so do the pain and stress experienced by the laboring mother. Physiologic and emotional responses to labor include:

- Increased respiratory rate
- Increased oxygen consumption
- Metabolic acidosis
- Release of catecholamines, leading to constriction of maternal blood vessels
- Fear and anxiety
- Feeling of being out of control
- Stalled labor progression.

The nurse, as a trusted member of the birth team, plays a significant role in shaping the woman's perception of her birth experience by helping the woman understand that the empowering aspect of birth is not in meeting someone else's expectations, but in being an active participant in her own plan of care, choosing which interventions she wants, and being present for the birth of her baby.

"I felt really prepared for labor! We went through all of the classes and had envisioned the 'perfect birth.' After 16 hours of labor and no progress, I was exhausted and frustrated; sobbing, I totally broke down. I felt like a failure for getting an epidural. My nurse, Madison, was great! She comforted me and reinforced that I was not a failure. She reassured me that in the end the most important thing would be holding my daughter in my arms. She was right—my despair was forgotten when I was able to enjoy the rest of labor and get some much needed sleep before Katherine was born. As I gazed at my newborn daughter, I learned what was really important that day and in my life!"

Systemic Analgesia

The goal of systemic analgesia during labor is to provide maximal pain relief with minimal risk for the woman and fetus. **Systemic analgesia** is pain medication given intravenously, intramuscularly, or via inhalation that does not result in complete loss of sensation or a reduction of motor functioning. While systemic analgesics do lessen the pain sensations, they typically do not eliminate pain completely.

Multiple factors must be considered in the use of analgesic agents:

- Effects on the woman
- Effects on the fetus
- Effects on the labor contractions
- Medical status of the woman
- History of substance abuse; current use of substances, including alcohol
- Progress of labor.

The effects on the mother are of primary importance because the well-being of the fetus depends on adequate functioning of the maternal cardiopulmonary system. Any alteration of function that disturbs the woman's homeostatic mechanism affects the fetal environment. Maintaining the maternal respiratory rate and blood pressure within normal range is thus of prime importance. The use of electronic fetal monitoring (EFM) (discussed in Chapter 20) provides a means of accurately assessing the effects of pharmacologic agents on fetal well-being and uterine contractions.

All systemic analgesics can cross the placental barrier by simple diffusion, with some agents crossing more readily than others. Drug action in the body depends on the rate at which the substance is metabolized by liver enzymes and excreted by the kidneys. The fetal liver enzymes and renal systems are inadequate to metabolize analgesic agents, so high doses remain active in fetal circulation for a prolonged period of time. The percentage of blood volume flowing to the fetal brain increases during intrauterine stress, so the hypoxic fetus receives an even larger amount of a depressant drug. The blood–brain barrier is more permeable at the time of birth, a factor that also increases the amount of drug carried to the central nervous system (Baysinger, Bucklin, & Gambling, 2016).

As with other healthcare issues, the use of systemic analgesics in labor has been affected by the opioid abuse crisis in the United States (see Chapter 17 for a discussion of the pregnant woman affected by substance abuse). Because of a lack of research and evidenced-based practice on pain management during labor for women with opioid dependencies, in practice most physicians do not offer analgesic options during labor and direct the woman to have an epidural. Due to long-term opioid use, a woman may experience greater-than-average levels of pain. Early epidural placement may be beneficial in ensuring the woman receives effective analgesia (Pan & Zakowski, 2017). Epidurals have not been shown to be any less effective for women with opioid dependence or addiction, so they are considered a safe as well as effective option. Nurses in the intrapartum setting should be aware of factors that may impact pharmacologic decision making related to the abuse of opioids in laboring women and the need for a plan of care for pain management during recovery and on discharge.

Clinical Tip

Preexisting opioid addiction can impact pharmacologic options in labor. A comprehensive review of substance abuse discussed with the woman in a nonjudgmental manner is more likely to yield truthful information.

Administration of Analgesic Agents

The optimal time for administering analgesia is determined after a complete assessment of many factors. In the past, there was a debate on the ideal timing of medication administration; however, both the American College of Obstetricians and Gynecologists (ACOG) and the American Society of Anesthesiologists (ASA) agree that a woman's request for pain medications is ample reason to administer them (ACOG, 2017b). A laboring woman should receive pain medication when she requests it in response to discomfort or pain. Most analgesic agents are best used to alleviate discomfort of early labor; to give relief and rest to a woman in false or prolonged prodromal labor; or to assist a woman, who does not want an epidural, to get through early active labor and into transition. Most analgesia that is given too late is of no value to the woman and may cause neonatal respiratory depression. In many institutions, the nurse decides when to give the analgesic agent prescribed by the physician, certified nurse-midwife (CNM), or certified registered nurse anesthetist (CRNA).

The exception to timing of analgesia is with use of nitrous oxide inhalation, which can be administered at any point in labor including during second stage and even during perineal repair. Nitrous oxide requires an order from a physician, CNM, or CRNA; however, the nurse prepares, implements, and manages the administration of nitrous oxide to the laboring woman, making it a viable option for women at facilities without an available anesthesiologist. Nitrous oxide has a rapid offset and has not been shown to cause neonatal respiratory depression (Zanardo et al., 2017).

The nurse observes the woman for cues that indicate she would benefit from the administration of analgesics. The nurse performs needed assessments of both the mother and fetus and then notifies the physician/CNM. The decision to administer pain medication is based on a complete assessment of the woman, her fetus, and the progress of labor. The physician/CNM may evaluate the woman at the bedside or may rely on the nurse's assessment and provide an order for the nurse to administer the medications. In most institutions, the CRNA is available to monitor analgesia-related complications and provide ongoing monitoring for women who later receive an epidural. The American Society for Anesthesiologists practice guidelines mandate that all women undergo a history and physical examination prior to the initiation of anesthesia (Baysinger et al., 2016). Facilities may have anesthesiologists (physicians who specialize in administering anesthesia) or CRNAs provide these services.

Before administering the medication, the nurse once again ascertains whether the woman has a history of any drug reactions or allergies and provides information regarding the medication (see Box 22–1). After giving the medication, the nurse documents the drug name, dose, route, site, and the woman's blood pressure and pulse (before and after) on the institution's charting system. The nurse also assesses the fetal heart rate (FHR) for possible side effects. A common expected side effect is a decrease in variability due to neonatal sedation. With some analgesics, the FHR pattern takes on an even, undulating pattern, called a *pseudosinusoidal pattern*, an expected pattern that does not warrant any intervention. Any other nonreassuring factors, however, must be addressed.

SAFETY ALERT!

Before administering analgesic medication, the nurse should review fall prevention procedures with the woman, which may include raising bed rails and calling for assistance for toileting, depending on the hospital's policies.

Box 22–1
What Women Need to Know About Pain Relief Medications

Before receiving medications, the woman should understand:

- Type of medication administered
- Route of administration
- Expected effects of medication
- Implications for fetus/newborn
- Safety measures needed (e.g., remain in bed with side rails up)
- Side effects/complications.

MATERNAL ASSESSMENT

These maternal assessments are critical before administering systemic analgesics:

- The woman is willing to receive medication after being advised about it (Box 22–1).
- Vital signs are stable.
- Contraindications (such as drug allergies, respiratory compromise, and current or past drug dependence) are not present.
- Knowledge of other medications being administered, such as magnesium sulfate or tocolytics.

FETAL ASSESSMENT

These assessments of the fetus are also required:

- FHR is between 110 and 160 beats per minute.
- Moderate variability is present.
- Late decelerations or recurrent variable decelerations are absent.

ASSESSMENT OF LABOR

These assessment parameters must also be evaluated:

- Contraction pattern
- Cervical dilatation
- Cervical effacement
- Fetal presenting part
- Station of the fetal presenting part.

If normal parameters are not present relative to maternal or fetal factors, the nurse may need to complete further assessments with the physician/CNM. In addition, no complications that would preclude administering an analgesic agent should be present, such as drug allergies or drug-specific contraindications.

ROUTES OF ADMINISTRATION

Oral analgesics are not used because they are poorly absorbed and gastric emptying time is prolonged during labor. The intramuscular (IM), intravenous (IV), or subcutaneous (SC) routes, as well as inhalation, are used instead. For IM administration, the needle must be of sufficient length to penetrate the muscle and the subcutaneous fat. The IV route is preferred over IM because it results in prompt, smooth, and more predictable action with a smaller total dose required. When an agent is given intravenously, it is suggested that the injection be given with the onset of a contraction, when the blood flow to the uterus and the fetus is normally decreased (Baysinger et al., 2016).

When an analgesic medication is administered by IM or SC route, it takes a few minutes for the effect to be felt. The nurse can continue with other supportive measures to enhance comfort until the effect of the medication is perceived. When the medication begins to take effect, the woman may be able to sleep between contractions. This short period of rest can restore her energy. With an IV administration, however, the woman feels the effect of the drug faster, so if any change of position is necessary or if the woman needs to void, the nurse may suggest that these activities be completed before the drug is administered (Gabbe et al., 2016). Sometimes analgesics are administered via IV and IM routes simultaneously. The benefit of this technique is that the woman receives a rapid onset from the IV route as well as the longer duration of pain control that is achieved with the IM route (Baysinger et al., 2016).

Nitrous oxide, as an inhaled analgesic, is self-administered by the woman. Nitrous oxide inhalation has a rapid onset of 30 seconds and leaves the body quickly through exhalation—within 1 to 2 minutes (Collins, 2017). Because it is self-administered, many women report high rates of satisfaction with their analgesia when nitrous oxide is used (Richardson, Lopez, Baysinger, et al., 2017).

Clinical Tip

The anesthesiologist or CRNA should be notified of any complications or unexpected outcomes that occur as the result of medication administration.

Sedatives

In current labor and birth practice, sedatives are used primarily in the early latent phase of labor, when the cervix is long, closed, and thick, and when rest is prescribed for the expectant woman. Sedatives promote relaxation and allow the woman to sleep for a few hours. Upon the woman's awakening, contractions have either ceased (i.e., the woman was in false labor) or contractions return and take on a regular pattern that promotes changes in cervical dilatation and effacement.

Sedatives have minimal analgesic properties and can actually increase the reaction to painful stimuli. They should be administered only to decrease anxiety and promote sleep because they cross the placenta and can cause depression in the newborn (Berghella, 2016). Sedatives should not be given when a woman is in active labor because they can cause respiratory depression in the newborn should birth occur sooner than expected.

BENZODIAZEPINES

Benzodiazepines, such as lorazepam (Ativan) or midazolam (Versed), are no longer used for pain management in labor. They may be used to treat severe anxiety only after the baby is born. Their primary role in the intrapartum setting is as an anticonvulsant and are given after magnesium sulfate for seizures in the presence of preeclampsia. Flumazenil, the drug used to reverse benzodiazepine sedative effects, should be kept on hand in case of accidental overdose.

H_1-RECEPTOR ANTAGONISTS

H_1-receptor antagonists block the action of histamines at the receptor sites. These drugs cross the blood–brain barrier and inhibit N-methyltransferase, which is a by-product of histamine. It is this mechanism that leads to the sedative effects of this class of drugs. In addition, these drugs also have anti-Parkinson and antiemetic effects. There are seven subtypes of H_1-receptor antagonists. These drugs cause drowsiness and may be used in early labor to promote sleep and decrease anxiety. The degree of drowsiness experienced depends on which drug is administered. Common H_1-receptor antagonists used in early or false labor are promethazine (Phenergan) and diphenhydramine (Benadryl).

Promethazine (Phenergan), which is a phenothiazine, results in marked sedation and is often combined with opiates because it potentiates their effect. It also has strong antiemetic effects and can be given with opiates to relieve nausea and vomiting, which can be a side effect of certain opiates. All phenothiazines cross the placental barrier and can result in decreased variability in the FHR. Promethazine has not, however, resulted in lower Apgar scores. Phenothiazines can also bind to bilirubin binding sites in newborns whose mothers are exposed to the drug at term. This can result in an increased incidence of neonatal hyperbilirubinemia and jaundice (Wilson, Shannon, & Shields, 2017). The combination of promethazine with fentanyl results in sedation so the mother can rest. Women in false labor are able to rest and frequently will awaken to find that their uterine contractions have dissipated. Alternatively, women who receive this combination in early or prodromal labor are able to rest and may wake to find themselves in active labor.

Diphenhydramine (Benadryl) is an ethanolamine subtype of the H_1 antagonists. Most commonly, this over-the-counter medication is used to treat allergic rhinitis and urticaria; however, it also possesses sedative and antiemetic properties that can be used to treat women in early labor. The drug has a relatively short half-life (1 to 4 hours) and can last up to 6 to 8 hours (Wilson et al., 2017). Sometimes healthcare providers advise women to use this drug at home if medically indicated because it is readily available. It should be noted that this drug causes agitation in some women. If this side effect occurs, women should discontinue the medication (Wilson et al., 2017).

Nursing Care. Carefully assess the woman before administration of analgesic agents. Because they are not indicated for women in active labor, assess and determine the stage of labor based on frequency, duration, and intensity of her contractions (Simpson & Creehan, 2014). Perform a vaginal exam to determine if cervical change has occurred. Fetal well-being is established by obtaining electronic fetal monitoring and ensuring a Category I fetal heart rate tracing (see Chapter 20 and Table 20–7 for a discussion of fetal heart rate tracing categories). Explain to the woman the desired effects of the medication and possible side effects. Review safety precautions such as staying in bed and obtaining assistance with toileting. Most institutions require continuous or intermittent fetal monitoring for a period of time after medication administration.

Clinical Tip

Some women experience extreme anxiety as the intensity of labor increases. Provide interventions to decrease anxiety, such as speaking in a calm voice, providing explanations on the physiologic changes the woman is experiencing, offering distractions, and using breathing and stress-reduction techniques to decrease anxiety levels. Reassuring the woman that what she is experiencing is normal labor progression can alleviate much anxiety.

Narcotic Analgesics

Narcotic analgesic agents that are injected into the circulation have their primary action at sites in the brain. Specifically, a narcotic that diffuses out of cerebral capillaries and reaches the periventricular/periaqueductal gray matter of the brain activates the neurons that descend to the spinal cord and inhibits the transmission of pain impulses in the substantia gelatinosa. Nausea and vomiting are produced by stimulation of the medullary chemoreceptor trigger zone.

A brief discussion of some selected narcotic analgesic agents follows. Both narcotic and nonnarcotic analgesic drugs are summarized in Table 22–1.

FENTANYL (SUBLIMAZE)

Fentanyl (Sublimaze) is a short-acting synthetic opioid with moderate analgesia and mild sedation properties. The main advantages of fentanyl are a rapid onset and short half-life. In addition, the drug has limited placental transfer and thus has a lower incidence of reduced fetal heart rate variability. Because of its short half-life, women who receive fentanyl are less likely to give birth to a baby experiencing respiratory depression, however, repeated doses are required. The usual dosage is 50 to 100 mcg every 1 hour (Wilson et al., 2017). Fentanyl is a very useful choice for the woman who presents in active labor, is 5 cm dilated, and needs something to help her over the hump to transition and second stage.

Nursing Care. Prior to administration, confirm that the woman does not have any opioid dependency or addiction. Naloxone (Narcan) is used to reverse respiratory depression; however,

TABLE 22–1 Analgesics Used in Labor

DRUG/CLASS	DOSAGE, ROUTE, FREQUENCY	COMMON SIDE EFFECTS	LIFE-THREATENING REACTIONS	CONTRAINDICATIONS
Nitrous oxide	Inhaled with contractions or during procedures	Sedation, nausea, dizziness		Vitamin B_{12} deficiency
Nubain (nalbuphine hydrochloride): CNS agent, analgesic, narcotic agonist, antagonist	10–20 mg every 3–6 hours PRN SC/IM/IV	Sedation; sweaty, clammy skin; nausea and vomiting	Respiratory depression	Hypersensitivity to drug
Morphine (morphine sulfate): CNS agent, analgesic, narcotic agonist	IV 2.5–15 mg every 4 hours IM/SC 5–20 mg every 4 hours	Pruritus (itching), constipation, nausea	Anaphylactic reaction, respiratory depression; overdose; respiratory arrest, cardiac arrest	Hypersensitivity to opiates, increased intracranial pressure, convulsive disorders, acute alcoholism, acute asthma, chronic pulmonary diseases, decreased respirations, pulmonary edema, biliary tract surgery, anastomosis, pancreatitis, acute ulcerative colitis, liver/renal insufficiency, Addison disease, hypothyroidism
Phenergan (promethazine hydrochloride): Gastrointestinal (GI) agent, antiemetic, antivertigo agent, phenothiazine	23–50 mg every 3–4 hours po/pr/IM/IV	Sedation, drowsiness, dry mouth, blurred vision	Respiratory depression, agranulocytosis	Hypersensitivity to phenothiazines, glaucoma, peptic ulcer, pyloroduodenal obstruction, bladder neck obstruction, epilepsy, bone marrow depression, breastfeeding
Benadryl (diphenhydramine hydrochloride): Antihistamine, antiemetic, antivertigo, antitussive, sedative-hypnotic	23–50 mg every 6 hours po/IM/IV	Drowsiness, sedation, dry mouth, hypotension, nausea and vomiting, GI symptoms	Anaphylaxis, seizures, coma, respiratory depression	Hypersensitivity to drug. Can be used during an acute asthma attack. Use with caution in glaucoma, bladder obstruction, hypertension, hypothyroidism, and renal disease.

giving naloxone to a woman with an unknown addiction may put her into immediate withdrawal, which will adversely affect her and her baby. Administering fentanyl with other central nervous system depressants, such as sedatives, phenothiazides, other tranquilizers, hypnotic agents, and general anesthetics, can exacerbate respiratory depression and cause other effects. For this reason, evaluate the woman's respiratory and cardiac status by careful observation of vital signs and pulse oximetry; also check the woman's level of consciousness frequently.

Continuous electronic monitoring of the FHR pattern is recommended. Respiratory depression in the mother or fetus/newborn can be improved by the administration of naloxone, which is a specific antagonist for this agent, particularly when birth occurs sooner than expected. Ensure that naloxone is readily available when administering opiates to a laboring woman.

NALBUPHINE HYDROCHLORIDE (NUBAIN)

Nalbuphine hydrochloride (Nubain) is a synthetic agonist–antagonist narcotic analgesic and may precipitate drug withdrawal if the woman is physically dependent on narcotics (Gabbe et al, 2016). Nalbuphine crosses the placenta to the fetus and can cause nonreassuring fetal status and neonatal respiratory depression (Wilson et al., 2017). Nalbuphine may be given by the IV, IM, or SC route. It is most frequently given by the IV route in the birth setting or by combined IV and IM for longer duration. The usual dose for adults is 10 mg/70 kg. If given intravenously, onset of action occurs in 2 to 3 minutes, peak of action occurs in 15 to 20 minutes, and duration is 3 to 6 hours. When given by the IM or SC route, the onset of action occurs in less than 15 minutes, peak of action occurs in 30 to 60 minutes, and duration is 3 to 6 hours. When given by the IV route, nalbuphine may be given directly into the tubing of a running IV infusion; 10 mg should be administered over 3 to 5 minutes (Wilson et al., 2017). Adverse maternal effects include respiratory depression, drowsiness, dizziness, crying, blurred vision, nausea, diaphoresis, and urinary urgency (Wilson et al., 2017). Another use of nalbuphine is to offset severe pruritis after spinal anesthesia for cesarean delivery; however, as an agonist–antagonist drug, doing so can also reduce the analgesic effect of the spinal. Because of this side effect, diphenhydramine may be a better choice to relieve intense itching.

Nursing Care. Assess the woman's history to identify contraindications to use of nalbuphine, such as the possibility of current narcotic drug dependence, sensitivity to sulfites, and history of asthma (Wilson et al., 2017). If no contraindications exist, the IV route is frequently used during labor. The woman's respiratory rate, quality of respirations, and characteristics of the FHR must be carefully assessed. A Category I pattern is preferred prior to the administration of nalbuphine, as it can result in decreased variability, including presenting as a pseudosinusoidal pattern. Because the woman may experience dizziness and sedation, use of a bedpan may be necessary. The nurse should also be prepared for a precipitous birth after nalbuphine administration by having naloxone (Narcan) nearby due to the increased risk of neonatal resuscitation.

OPIATE ANTAGONIST: NALOXONE (NARCAN)

Because naloxone (Narcan) is an antagonist with little or no agonistic effect, it exhibits little pharmacologic activity in the absence of narcotic agents. Naloxone can be used to reverse the mild respiratory depression, sedation, and hypotension following small doses of opiates (Gabbe et al., 2016). Naloxone exerts its effect by competing for opiate receptors and taking the place of the opiate on the receptor. In this manner, it blocks or reverses the action of the narcotic analgesic (Gabbe et al., 2016). The drug is useful for respiratory depression caused by nalbuphine (Nubain) and fentanyl (Sublimaze) (Gabbe et al., 2016). Naloxone is the drug of choice when the depressant is unknown because it will cause no further depression. Its duration of action is less than that of most narcotic analgesics; however, respiratory depression may return as the antagonistic effect of naloxone wears off. Accordingly, careful ongoing assessment of the mother and newborn is necessary after naloxone administration.

Clinical Tip

Ongoing evaluation of the patient's progress in labor relative to analgesic administration allows the nurse to be prepared by pulling naloxone (Narcan) from the medication cabinet when delivery is imminent and notifying appropriate staff of the increased risk for neonatal resuscitation.

Nursing Care. When naloxone is administered to the laboring mother or to the newborn just after birth, resuscitative measures and trained personnel should be readily available in the event that additional respiratory support is needed. When administered to the laboring mother, naloxone may be injected undiluted at a rate of 0.4 mg over 15 seconds into the tubing of a running IV infusion. Titrated doses of naloxone are more likely to be used in a postoperative setting when epidural analgesia has been given with a cesarean birth. After the direct IV administration, obtain maternal vital signs at 5-minute intervals until the respiratory rate has been stabilized and then every 30 minutes. Neonatal administration can be administered via IV, IM, or endotracheal (ET) routes. The standard neonatal dosage is 0.01 mg/kg (American Academy of Pediatrics [AAP] & American Heart Association [AHA], 2016). The duration of naloxone is shorter (minutes to hours) than the analgesic drug it is acting as an antagonist for, so be alert for the return of respiratory depression and the need for repeated doses.

SAFETY ALERT!

Withdrawal symptoms may occur when naloxone (Narcan) is given to a woman or a newborn who is physically dependent on narcotics. A careful assessment that includes opiate drug use is imperative.

NITROUS OXIDE

Nitrous oxide is making a comeback in obstetrics in the United States, partly due to the availability of new Food and Drug Administration–approved devices for administration as well as the approval of its administration and management by nurses. A safe, effective, and inexpensive option for pain relief in labor, nitrous oxide has been used in Canada, Europe, and Australia for more than a hundred years. It has not been shown to have an impact on the rate of spontaneous vaginal births, uterine activity, or the risk of complications (Collins, 2015; Pinyan, Curlee, Keever, et al., 2017). As a nurse-driven option, nitrous oxide inhalation is a low-cost solution for an institution, which means it is a viable, effective option for women in hospitals without in-house anesthesiologists.

For obstetric purposes, nitrous oxide is mixed in a concentration of 50% nitrous oxide and 50% oxygen, compared to a 70/30 ratio found in the dental setting, where many people are already familiar with its use. Rather than a continuous flow of gas, the apparatus uses a demand valve that releases the mixture only when the woman has a tight seal on the mask or mouthpiece and inhales. The woman exhales back into the apparatus as well, using a scavenging system that prevents gas from being released into the environment, thus reducing the risk of exposure to healthcare staff.

Nitrous oxide inhalation is the only analgesia that is completely controlled by the woman. The woman holds the mask and decides when to inhale the medication and when to stop. Women report high satisfaction with nitrous oxide, even when it was not considered to be fully effective in pain management (Richardson et al., 2017). The aspect of self-administration of the analgesia may contribute to this finding. Women who used nitrous oxide solely as their method of pain management report they would do so again in subsequent births (Collins, 2015). The use of nitrous oxide does not prevent the woman from choosing to move to other forms of analgesia, including an epidural regional block, though some institutions may have policies regarding administration of other systemic analgesics while using nitrous oxide.

In addition to analgesia, nitrous oxide has anxiolytic properties. Stress and anxiety interfere with effective coping with labor as well as labor progression, so nitrous oxide may help a woman feel less overwhelmed by labor and more empowered to manage it without additional analgesia or regional blocks such as epidurals. The anxiolytic effect can benefit women who begin labor with significant anxiety or fear, as well as women who, in active labor, enter transition and experience self-doubt (Collins, 2015).

Nitrous oxide is a safe option for analgesia. If the woman is too sedated, she will not be able to bring the mask to her face to inhale more of the medication, preventing overdose. Nitrous oxide has a rapid onset and offset. If the woman does not tolerate the medication, its effect wears off within 1 to 2 minutes, versus an analgesic administered intravenously that may last for 4 to 6 hours. Nitrous oxide will cross the placenta, but does not affect the fetal heart rate pattern or result in neonatal depression. Moreover, should the woman deliver while on nitrous oxide, the newborn will blow off whatever medication is left within the first few breaths. Use of nitrous oxide has not been shown to have an impact on Apgar scores or the ability to breastfeed (Pinyan et al., 2017).

Nitrous oxide inhalation is a versatile option for pain management because there is no "window" for its use as there are with other systemic analgesics. The effects on the mother and the newborn are the same with either short- or long-term use. It can be used in early labor, active labor, and even second stage. It can also be used during obstetric procedures such as cervical Foley bulb placement, external cephalic version, manual removal of the placenta, and perineal repair (Collins, 2015). Nitrous oxide use has been associated with increased patient satisfaction scores related to the birth experience and increased breastfeeding rates at 7 days and 3 months postpartum (Zanardo et al., 2017).

There are few contraindications for nitrous oxide. Because it inactivates vitamin B_{12}, it is contraindicated in women with vitamin B_{12} deficiency and related disorders such as Crohn disease, celiac disease, pernicious anemia, alcoholism, and anorexia. Nitrous oxide is also contraindicated in women who have had recent bariatric surgery or who have a potential space that could be filled such as pneumothorax or obstructed bowel; however, these rarely appear in laboring women. Other contraindications include inability of the woman to hold her own mask or inability to tolerate potential side effects such as dizziness or nausea.

Nursing Care. Assess the woman and the fetus for well-being prior to the administration of any systemic analgesic. Consents and an order for the medication must be performed by the physician/CNM. Once an order is made, manage the implementation of nitrous oxide, assessing its use by the woman and its effectiveness.

Provide education and support as the woman learns how to use the apparatus. This can be challenging if she is in active labor during education. Ensure that the woman is able to place the mask or mouthpiece to make a tight seal. Instruct the woman to begin breathing 30 seconds prior to the onset of the contraction in order to allow for a therapeutic level to be achieved before its peak. Help the woman develop her own rhythm of inhalation.

Encourage family-centered care by including the woman's partner/support person in the labor process, teaching that person how to play an active role in supporting the woman, such as cueing her when the contraction is about to start either using a timer or tocodynamometer, as well as continuing to provide other nonpharmacologic methods of support.

Educate the partner/support person and any other persons present about patient-controlled analgesia, stressing that no one else should help the woman hold the mask or mouthpiece. For her safety, only the woman can hold the mask or mouthpiece. Moreover, no other person in the room may experiment by inhaling nitrous oxide themselves. Unauthorized use of nitrous oxide could result in the person being removed from the birth room or, perhaps worse, the analgesia being removed as a pain relief option for the laboring woman.

The woman is a fall risk. However, since the medication leaves the body so quickly, women using nitrous oxide can generally walk around between contractions or use the restroom freely. Assess the woman's response to the medication for signs of dizziness or difficulty ambulating. The woman is not to be left alone while using nitrous oxide. Institutional policy may dictate the nurse must stay; however, other institutions may allow a support person to serve this purpose.

Continue to assess the woman's vital signs and fetal heart rate pattern per institution policy. There is no evidence that nitrous oxide affects the cardiovascular system, respiratory system, or fetal heart rate, so a change in blood pressure, respiratory rate, or fetal status would need to be investigated further rather than being attributed to the use of nitrous oxide. Document the woman's use, tolerance, and effectiveness or satisfaction with the analgesia per institutional policy. See *Case Study: Azia Askari*.

CASE STUDY: Azia Askari

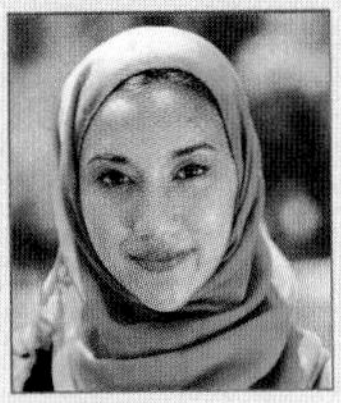

SOURCE: HONGQI ZHANG/123RF.

Azia is experiencing severe pain with her contractions, even though she has been ambulating and changing positions frequently. Although she has had unmedicated births in the past, she and her husband have decided she would like to have something for pain since this labor is longer and more painful. She describes how her sister, Asal, recently gave birth in Iran and used gas to ease the pain. While nitrous oxide is not widely used in Iran or the United States, the medical facility has just begun using it. Azia is fearful of needles and feels this would be the best option for her.

Questions to Ponder

What safety considerations are warranted for Azia if she should begin using nitrous oxide? What education is necessary prior to obtaining an order for its use in labor?

Regional Anesthesia and Analgesia

Regional anesthesia is the temporary and reversible loss of sensation produced by injecting an anesthetic agent (called a *local anesthetic*) into an area that will bring the agent into direct contact with nervous tissue. Loss of sensation occurs because the local agents stabilize the cell membrane, which prevents initiation and transmission of nerve impulses. The regional anesthetic blocks most commonly used in childbearing include epidural, spinal, or combined spinal–epidural. Epidural blocks may be used for analgesia during labor and vaginal birth and for anesthesia for an unplanned cesarean birth. Spinal blocks are used for planned cesarean births. A combined spinal–epidural block may be used to provide the fast onset of pain relief provided by the spinal and ongoing anesthesia for the labor and birth provided by the epidural, though this is a less common option as epidurals have become more effective.

An epidural relieves pain associated with the first stage of labor by blocking the sensory nerves supplying the uterus. Pain associated with the second stage of labor and with birth can be alleviated with epidural, combined spinal–epidural, and pudendal blocks (Figure 22–1 and Table 22–2).

Regional anesthesia carries considerably less risk than general anesthesia. Risk of maternal death with general anesthesia during a cesarean birth is primarily related to intubation difficulties, respiratory failure, and drug reactions (Baysinger et al., 2016).

Clinical Tip

If the laboring woman has voiced a plan to have epidural anesthesia, advise her to make the request ahead of the time when she might want it so the anesthesiologist has ample time to arrive before the woman's pain level becomes too intense.

Until recently, the same anesthetic agents used for regional epidural anesthesia were also used to produce regional analgesia during labor. **Regional analgesia** is the temporary and reversible loss of pain sensation produced by injecting an analgesic agent into the nervous tissue supplying a region of the body. This approach was somewhat problematic because anesthetic agents alter the transmission of impulses to the bladder, making voiding difficult. The agents also interfere with the woman's ability to maintain her blood pressure and move her lower extremities. In addition, the descent of the fetus may be slowed because the agents also decrease the woman's ability to push effectively during the second stage of labor (Gabbe et al., 2016). To address these problems, regional analgesia is now obtained by injecting a narcotic agent such as fentanyl along with only a small amount of a local anesthetic agent. This approach yields effective pain relief without the troubling side effects of epidural anesthesia. The woman's pain is relieved, her blood pressure remains stable, and, because there is no motor blockage, she may be able to adjust her position more easily. Urinary retention can still occur, but it can be treated with the placement of an indwelling Foley catheter or an intermittent in-and-out catheter (Gabbe et al., 2016). Urinary retention is usually a short-term complication that resolves on its own after the anesthesia has completely worn off.

The intrathecal (or spinal) injection of narcotics results in another type of regional analgesia. In this case, the narcotic is injected into the subarachnoid (spinal) space. Fentanyl citrate and preservative-free morphine are the most frequently used narcotic agents. The woman's pain is usually relieved; however, she may experience urinary retention. Delayed respiratory depression may also occur and seems to be more frequent with the use of morphine (Wilson et al., 2017).

It is important for the laboring woman to have information about the regional analgesia or anesthesia that is to be administered. As with other procedures, the woman needs to know how the block is given, the expected effect on her and the fetus, advantages and disadvantages, and possible risks. Many women discuss possible analgesic and anesthetic blocks with their physician/CNM during the pregnancy. Some women, in their desire throughout their pregnancy to have an unmedicated birth, arrive in labor with no prior information about these options. They should still have an opportunity to ask questions and obtain

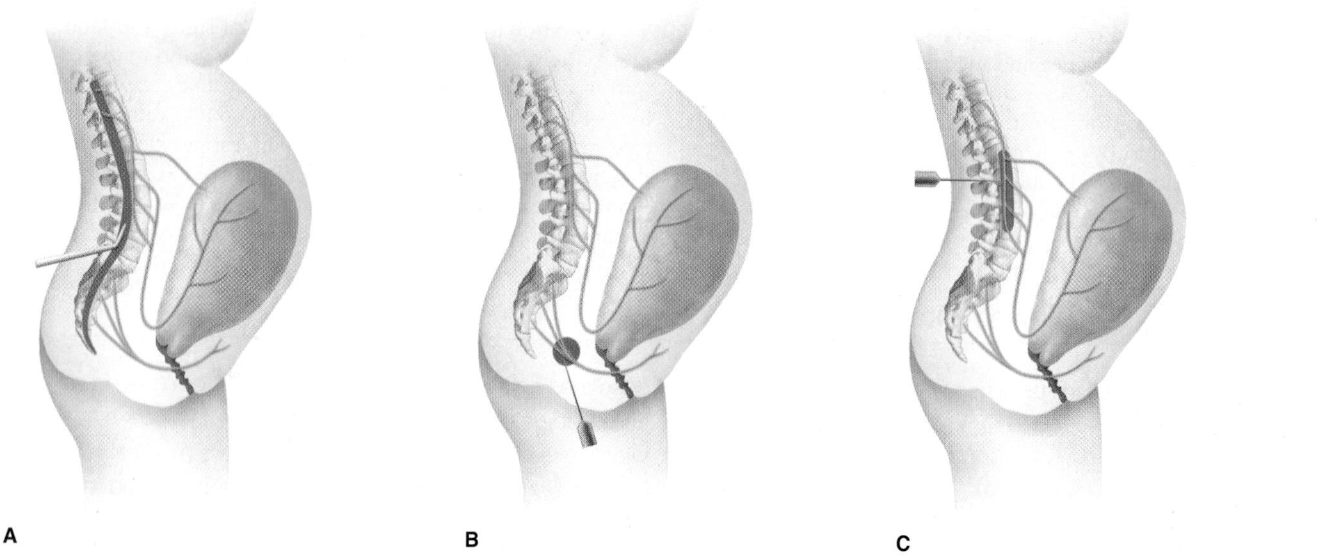

Figure 22–1 Schematic diagram showing pain pathways and sites of interruption. A. Lumbar sympathetic (spinal) block: Relief of uterine pain only. B. Pudendal block: Relief of perineal pain. C. Lumbar epidural block: Dark area demonstrates peridural (epidural) space and nerves affected, and the gray tube represents a continuous plastic catheter.

TABLE 22–2 Summary of Commonly Used Regional Blocks

TYPE OF BLOCK	AREAS AFFECTED	USE DURING LABOR AND BIRTH	NURSING ACTIONS
Lumbar epidural	Uterus, cervix, vagina, and perineum	Given in first stage and second stage of labor.	Assess woman's knowledge regarding the block. Act as advocate to help her obtain further information, if needed. Monitor maternal blood pressure to detect the major side effect, which is hypotension. Provide support and comfort. See *Nursing Care Plan: For Epidural Anesthesia* for further nursing actions.
Combined spinal-epidural	Uterus, cervix, vagina, and perineum	Spinal analgesia may be given in late active labor for pain relief. Epidural is placed at the same time for ongoing anesthesia.	Assess woman's knowledge regarding the block. Monitor maternal vital signs and FHR status. Provide comfort measures.
Pudendal	Perineum and lower vagina	Given in the second stage just before birth to provide anesthesia for episiotomy or for low forceps birth.	Assess woman's knowledge regarding the block. Act as advocate to help her obtain further information, if needed.
Local infiltration	Perineum	Administered just before birth to provide anesthesia for episiotomy or after birth for repair of a laceration.	Assess woman's knowledge regarding the block. Provide information as needed. Provide comfort and support. Observe perineum for bruising or other discoloration in the recovery period.
Spinal	Uterus, cervix, vagina, and perineum	Given for cesarean birth. Provides immediate onset of anesthesia.	Assess woman's knowledge regarding the block. Monitor maternal vital signs and FHR status.

information before receiving any regional analgesia or anesthesia while in labor. The nurse should answer questions and address concerns in early labor before the onset of acute pain. This ensures that the woman fully understands the information and can make an informed choice. Informed consent is obtained in writing before the procedure begins.

Action and Absorption of Anesthetic Agents

Local anesthetic agents block nerve conduction by impairing propagation of the action potential in axons along with impairing the transmission of nerve impulses by stabilizing the cell membrane. The agents interact directly with specific receptors on the sodium channel, inhibiting sodium ion influx and thus the continuation of the action potential (Wilson et al., 2017). The types of nerve fibers are differentially sensitive to the various anesthetic agents. In general, the smaller the fiber, the more sensitive it is to local agents. For example, it is possible to block the small C and A delta fibers, which transmit pain, touch, and temperature, without blocking the larger A alpha, A beta, and A gamma fibers, which continue to maintain a sense of pressure, muscle tone, position sense, and motor function (Wilson et al., 2017).

Absorption of local anesthetic agents depends primarily on the vascularity of the area of injection. The agents cause vasodilation, increasing blood flow (Baysinger et al., 2016). Higher concentrations cause greater vasodilatation. Good maternal physical condition or a high metabolic rate aids absorption. Malnutrition, dehydration, electrolyte imbalance, and cardiovascular and pulmonary problems increase the potential for toxic effects. The pH of tissues affects the rate of absorption, which has implications for fetal complications such as acidosis (Baysinger et al., 2016). The addition of vasoconstrictors, such as epinephrine, delays absorption and prolongs the anesthetic effect. Epinephrine decreases uteroplacental blood flow, making it an undesirable additive in many situations. The breakdown of local anesthetics in the body is accomplished by the liver and plasma esterase, and the resulting substance is eliminated by the kidneys. It is important to use the weakest concentration and the smallest amount necessary to produce the desired results (Baysinger et al., 2016).

Types of Local Anesthetic Agents

Three types of local anesthetic agents are currently available:

- *Ester types:* Include chloroprocaine hydrochloride (Nesacaine) and tetracaine hydrochloride (Pontocaine)
- *Amide types:* Include bupivacaine hydrochloride (Marcaine), mepivacaine hydrochloride (Carbocaine), ropivacaine hydrochloride (Naropin), levobupivacaine (Chirocaine), and lidocaine hydrochloride (Xylocaine)
- *Opiate types:* Include morphine (Duromorph) and fentanyl (Sublimaze)

Esters are rapidly metabolized; therefore, toxic maternal levels are not as likely to be reached, and placental transfer to the fetus is prevented.

Amide types are more powerful and longer-acting agents than ester types. They readily cross the placenta, can be measured in the fetal circulation, and affect the fetus for a prolonged period. Newer amide types of local anesthetic agents, such as ropivacaine (Naropin) and levobupivacaine (Chirocaine), are becoming more commonly used because they have a long action but fewer toxic effects (Baysinger et al., 2016).

Opioids are used with epidural blocks to produce analgesia for labor. When only opioids are used epidurally, the amount of pain relief is not as great as when a combination of opioids and a low dose of a local anesthetic agent is used to achieve better pain control with reduced motor impairment (Baysinger et al., 2016). There does appear to be a higher incidence of pruritus when this combination method is used. While the use of opiates has been associated with undesirable side effects, such as nausea and vomiting, hypotension, respiratory depression, and sedation, the incidence appears to be low. These agents are commonly used, especially in women undergoing a cesarean birth, because of their high effectiveness rates in controlling postpartum pain (Baysinger et al., 2016).

Women who receive fentanyl can experience interference with early breastfeeding, with higher dosages having more negative impact than lower dosages (Baysinger et al., 2016). Other evidence supports the use of fentanyl in labor. There are no differences in cesarean and operative birth rates between women who received epidural opiates and those who received systemic analgesia. In fact, women who receive epidural opiates sometimes have a shorter first stage than those who receive systemic analgesic agents (Baysinger et al., 2016).

A variety of anesthetic agents and a wide range of doses have been used for epidural anesthesia with varying results. The most commonly used agents are lidocaine 2% with epinephrine 1:200,000, bupivacaine 0.23%, and 2-chloroprocaine 3%. Each agent provides adequate anesthesia with 15 to 20 mL of the solution, but each has been associated with side effects. The pharmacology of each drug must be understood before it is used.

Adverse Maternal Reactions to Anesthetic Agents

Reactions to local anesthetic agents range from mild symptoms to cardiovascular collapse. Mild reactions include palpitations, vertigo, tinnitus, apprehension, confusion, headache, and a metallic taste in the mouth. Common side effects include pruritus, vertigo, dizziness, and urinary retention (Baysinger et al., 2016). Moderate reactions include more severe degrees of the mild symptoms plus nausea and vomiting, hypotension, and muscle twitching, which may progress to convulsions and loss of consciousness. Severe reactions are sudden loss of consciousness, coma, severe hypotension, bradycardia, respiratory depression, and cardiac arrest (Baysinger et al., 2016). High concentrations of the agents may also cause local toxic effects on tissues. It is important to remember that when the mother experiences an adverse reaction, the fetus is also affected.

Systemic toxic reactions most commonly occur with an excessive dose—either too great a concentration or too large a volume. Pregnant women in labor generally require less medication because of hormonal factors, uterine compression, an increase in cardiac output, and an increased sensitivity of the neural axons (Baysinger et al., 2016). Accidental intravenous (IV) injection that suddenly increases the amount of the drug in maternal circulation results in depression of vasomotor, respiratory, and other medullary centers of the brain (Baysinger et al., 2016). It also depresses the heart and peripheral vascular bed. A massive intravascular dose can result in sudden circulatory collapse within 1 minute. Reactions to subcutaneous and extradural injection occur in 5 to 40 minutes. The short-acting agent procaine can produce toxic reactions in 10 to 15 minutes, and the long-acting agent mepivacaine in 20 to 40 minutes (Baysinger et al., 2016). It is imperative that the woman is under close supervision by knowledgeable personnel throughout the time that an agent is being used and that a patent, large-bore IV line is in place prior to any procedure.

If epinephrine has been added to the anesthetic agent to prolong the anesthesia, it is necessary to differentiate between reaction to the anesthetic agent and to the epinephrine. Reaction to epinephrine is characterized by pallor, perspiration, dyspnea, and a greater increase in blood pressure and pulse than occurs with reactions to anesthetic agents.

Psychogenic reactions such as severe anxiety, hallucinations, inability to move or speak, or catatonic appearance can also occur, with symptoms similar to those occurring with systemic toxic reactions (Baysinger et al., 2016). This phenomenon may occur as the procedure is begun and before the injection of the anesthetic agent. Regardless of the cause, the symptoms must be treated.

Allergic reactions to anesthetic agents may also occur. The manifestations of the antigen–antibody reaction include urticaria, laryngeal edema, joint pain, swelling of the tongue, and bronchospasm.

TREATMENT OF SYSTEMIC TOXICITY

Preferred treatment of mild toxicity involves the administration of oxygen by mask and IV injection of a short-acting barbiturate to decrease anxiety (Wilson et al., 2017). The clinician should anticipate the possibility of convulsions or cardiovascular collapse and make appropriate preparations to treat them.

TREATMENT OF CONVULSIONS

The best treatment for convulsions is to establish the airway and administer 100% oxygen. Benzodiazepines or propofol may be administered to stop convulsions (Wilson et al., 2017). Small doses are adequate and help avoid cardiorespiratory depression.

TREATMENT OF SUDDEN CARDIOVASCULAR COLLAPSE

In sudden cardiovascular collapse, the nurse's first priority is to begin cardiopulmonary resuscitation, as per the American Heart Association (2016) basic life support algorithm. For the pregnant woman, a manual displacement of the uterus is necessary to maximize venous return to the heart. If CPR is warranted, the woman should be placed on her back to allow optimal positioning for chest compressions and the insertion of an advance airway (Cobb & Lipman, 2017). Monitoring of the fetus at this point is not necessary and could delay or inhibit maternal resuscitation efforts.

After 4 minutes of resuscitative measures, a bedside cesarean birth must be started in order for delivery of the baby within 5 minutes. Unfortunately, despite national guidelines recommending a perimortem cesarean delivery (PMCD), one study showed that one-third of the women who died in pregnancy remained undelivered (Cobb & Lipman, 2017). Birth of the baby often makes resuscitative efforts easier and more successful in obtaining a return of spontaneous circulation. It is believed that this is mostly due to the sudden relief of aortocaval compression.

Institutions should have an emergency code to alert all team members to a maternal cardiac arrest to ensure the presence of experts in obstetrics, anesthesiology, and neonatology at the bedside as soon as possible after a cardiac arrest has been identified.

Lumbar Epidural Block

A lumbar **epidural block** involves injection of a local anesthetic agent into the epidural space, which is accessed through the lumbar area. The epidural space is a potential space between the dura mater and the ligamentum flavum, extending from the base of the skull to the end of the sacral canal (Figure 22–2). It contains areolar and adipose tissues, lymphatic vessels, and the internal vertebral venous plexus (Baysinger et al., 2016). The epidural, used as a continuous block, provides analgesia and anesthesia from active labor through the birth and episiotomy repair. Complete pain relief is achieved for 85% of women; 12% experience partial relief; and only 3% of women report no relief at all (Gabbe et al., 2016).

Lumbar epidural block has become fairly common during labor and birth given that it generally provides adequate pain relief, does not pass through the placenta to affect the fetus, and

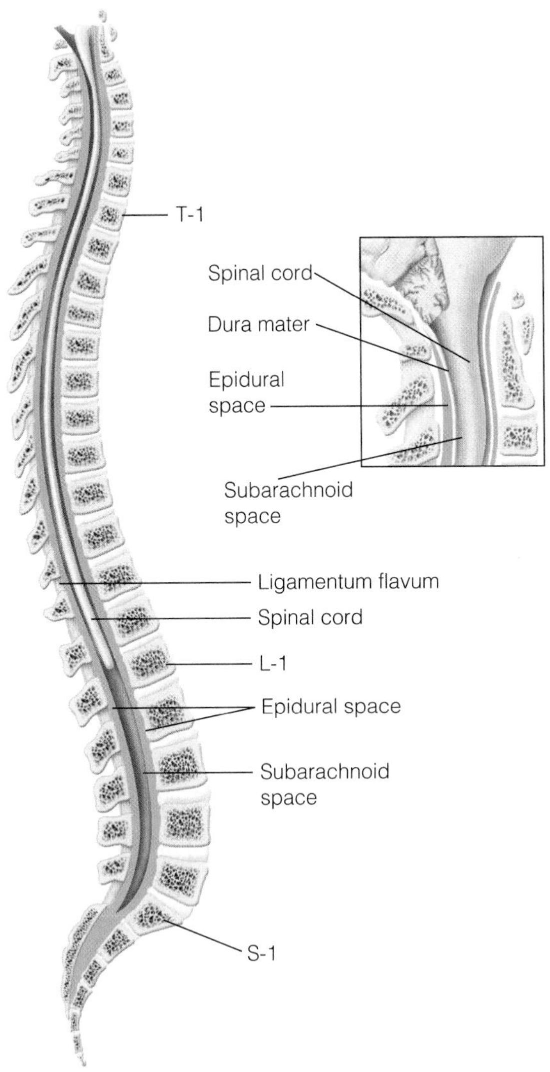

Figure 22–2 **The epidural space lies between the dura mater and the ligamentum flavum, extending from the base of the skull to the end of the sacral canal.**

allows the woman some sensation to feel pressure and push. Epidural anesthesia has become the preferred method of pain relief for laboring women.

Ethics in Action!

How do you respond to a woman whose partner does not want her to get an epidural for pain relief during labor?

Epidural blocks can be administered in a number of ways. To provide analgesia and anesthesia during labor, the block can be administered as a single dose with an epidural needle, as a single dose through an epidural catheter with additional doses (called *top-ups* or *top-offs*) given as needed, or as a continuous epidural. The most commonly used epidural technique for laboring women is the continuous epidural infusion via a pump that allows the woman to get a predetermined amount of medication on a continual basis. If the woman becomes uncomfortable, a bolus of additional medication can be given to achieve comfort. Some institutions use patient-controlled pumps that allow the woman to administer her own bolus under controlled conditions.

Many women equate the quality of their labor experience directly with their satisfaction with the anesthesia they receive while in labor. Although many women desire the pain relief from regional anesthesia, many do not like its side effects, such as inability to void, decreased motor sensation in the lower extremities, and the need to stay in bed.

The American Society of Anesthesiologists (ASA) states that epidural placement should be performed when the woman experiences pain and asks for an epidural (Sng & Sia, 2017). One study showed that women who received epidurals on request experienced fewer side effects and had less operative-assisted births (Sng & Sia, 2017). The woman should be educated that epidurals do increase the risk for complications, including:

- Urinary catheterization
- Pitocin augmentation of labor
- Intrauterine pressure catheter use
- Fetal malpresentation associated with decreased maternal movement during labor
- Increased rates of assisted vaginal deliveries (forceps or vacuum assistance)
- Spinal headaches.

These complications may increase maternal risks for infection and long-term residual morbidities such as dyspareunia (painful intercourse), urinary complications, back pain at insertion sites, and residual headaches.

Regional anesthesia may affect labor progression. In a study comparing regional anesthesia to systemic analgesics, the first stage of labor was shorter in women with epidurals (ACOG, 2017b). Women with an epidural, however, may have a longer second stage (ACOG, 2017b). Adequate time should therefore be given for allowing fetal descent to occur after complete dilatation (called "laboring down") for up to 2 hours (ACOG, 2017a). These recommendations have extended the time for pushing before declaring failure to progress or arrest of descent, allowing up to 3 hours of effective pushing efforts for the primiparous woman to provide the best opportunity for a vaginal delivery.

ADVANTAGES

The lumbar epidural block produces good analgesia that alters maternal physiologic responses to pain. The woman is fully awake during labor and birth. The continuous technique allows different blocking for each stage of labor so that internal rotation of the fetus can be accomplished. In many cases, the dose of anesthetic agent can be adjusted to preserve the woman's reflex urge to bear down. Once the pump is stopped, the effects of the epidural wear off within the first 2 hours. Most importantly, compared to sedatives, epidurals do not enter the vascular system and are not passed on to the fetus through the placenta. Consequently, precipitous delivery after epidural placement will not require neonatal resuscitation secondary to the anesthesia used. Another advantage is that should a woman's labor not progress as expected, or should the fetus show signs of not tolerating labor, the epidural catheter can be used to provide anesthesia for a cesarean birth, avoiding the use of general anesthesia. It is important to note that the use of an epidural has not been shown to increase the risk for cesarean birth (ACOG, 2017b).

DISADVANTAGES

The most common complication of an epidural block is maternal hypotension secondary to peripheral vasodilatation. This is increased by the blockade of the sympathetic nerve supply to the adrenal glands, which prevents the release of catecholamines (Baysinger et al., 2016). Maternal hypotension is generally prevented by preloading with a rapid infusion of IV fluids, then providing IV fluids continuously until birth. Although hypotension can occur, the incidence of hypotension requiring ephedrine is relatively low, less than 2% (Gabbe et al., 2016). Variability of the FHR may decrease, and late decelerations can occur if maternal hypotension develops. Other serious complications, although rare, have been reported, including postdural puncture seizures, meningitis, cardiorespiratory arrest, and vertigo (vestibulocochlear dysfunction) (Baysinger et al., 2016).

Another disadvantage of an epidural block is that the onset of analgesia may not occur for up to 30 minutes. Some women with epidurals may have decreased sensation and movement, or they may have essentially no control over movement in the anesthetized region. Some studies have demonstrated that epidural use contributes to the need to augment labors with oxytocin. On the other hand, other clinical studies, along with healthcare providers, assert that epidural analgesia may shorten the active and transition phases because of the pain relief. A meta-analysis showed that women who had received continuous infusion epidural anesthesia had a longer second stage compared to women who received parenteral opioids (ACOG, 2017b). Nevertheless, women with epidurals experienced greater pain relief than those who received opioids by intramuscular or intravenous routes (Sng & Sia, 2017).

In addition, an epidural block requires skilled personnel for administration and close observation of the woman and her fetus. The anesthesia provider must be careful while administering the block to avoid perforating the dura mater, which would place the needle in the subarachnoid space; if the error is not recognized, the anesthetic agent would be injected into the spinal canal. Skilled nurses are also required to maintain close observation of the laboring woman and her fetus. Finally, epidural anesthesia is more costly than systemic agents, which may be a crucial factor for women and families without insurance who are paying out of pocket for their birthing costs.

CONTRAINDICATIONS

Absolute contraindications for epidural block are (ACOG, 2017b):

- Maternal refusal
- Local or systemic infection
- Uncorrected hypovolemia
- Coagulation disorders
- Actual or anticipated maternal hemorrhage
- Increased intracranial pressure
- Allergy to a specific class of local anesthetic agents.

Relative contraindications include:

- Platelet count less than 100,000/mm^3
- Severe anatomic abnormalities of the spine
- Uncooperative patient
- Sepsis
- Hypertension.

Patients with previous back surgery, suspicion of neurologic disease, long-term use of aspirin or anti-inflammatory agents, abruptio placentae, or acute infection at the epidural site, as well as a lack of trained staff at the facility, are also causes for concern that need to be evaluated on an individual basis.

Epidurals can be used in women with heart failure or aortic stenosis, although invasive monitoring may be needed to evaluate blood pressure variations (Arendt, 2017). A cesarean birth may be indicated to prevent the stress associated with the second stage and maternal pushing efforts; however, preventing cardiac stress can also be accomplished by laboring down and having an operative birth, which is always preferable to surgery (Arendt, 2017).

TECHNIQUE FOR CONTINUOUS LUMBAR EPIDURAL BLOCK

In administering a continuous lumbar epidural block, the following actions are taken (Baysinger et al., 2016):

1. Maternal and fetal status and labor progress are assessed. Because maternal blood pressure and pulse will be taken frequently, an automatic blood pressure device, such as a continuous pulse oximeter, may be useful. FHR is continuously monitored by EFM and assessed by the nurse.
2. Oxygen and resuscitative equipment are readied. The nurse ensures that all equipment is in the room and properly functioning.
3. An IV infusion is begun, and a preload of 500 to1000 mL of IV fluid (e.g., 0.45% normal saline or lactated Ringer solution) is given over approximately 15 to 30 minutes by the nurse.
4. With the assistance of the nurse, the woman may be positioned on her left or right side at the edge of the bed (the mattress is firmer and provides more support) with her legs slightly flexed, or she may be asked to sit on the edge of the bed. She is advised to drop her shoulders, round out the small of her back, and place her chin on her chest. It may be helpful to advise the woman to push out her lower back "like an angry cat" to achieve the proper position. This is especially effective for positioning obese women. The spinal column is not kept convex because the convex position reduces the peridural space to a greater degree and stretches the dura mater, making it more susceptible to puncture. The epidural space is decreased during pregnancy because of venous engorgement. It is also smaller in obese and short individuals (Gabbe et al., 2016). A small pillow may be placed under the woman's head and in front of her chest to provide support for her arms. The nurse typically stands beside the woman, offering support and assisting her in maintaining this position. The nurse assists the woman with breathing techniques and alerts the anesthesia provider when a contraction occurs. See Figure 22–3 for incorrect (A, B) and correct (C, D, E) positions for a lumbar epidural block.
5. The skin is prepared with an antiseptic agent by the anesthesia provider.
6. A skin wheal of a small amount of local anesthesia is given intradermally by the anesthesia provider to anesthetize the supraspinous and interspinous ligaments.
7. The anesthesia provider then inserts a short, beveled 16- to 18-gauge needle with stylet that is passed to the ligamentum flavum in the widest interspace below the second lumbar vertebra (usually in the third or fourth lumbar interspace) (Figure 22–4). The ligamentum flavum is identified by its resistance to injection of saline or air (called *loss of resistance technique*). Resistance disappears as the epidural space is entered.

8. The anesthesia provider then injects 5 mL of preservative-free saline in order to pass the catheter into the epidural space more easily.
9. The catheter is inserted approximately 1 to 2 cm into the epidural space by the anesthesia provider. The needle is removed. Aspiration for blood (indicating that a vessel has been inadvertently entered) or cerebrospinal fluid (indicating the dura mater has been punctured) is attempted.
10. If aspiration tests are negative, a test dose of local anesthetic agent containing 1.5% lidocaine with 1:200,000 concentration of epinephrine or 3 mL of 0.23% bupivacaine with 1:200,000 concentration of epinephrine is injected. The anesthesiologist usually injects the medication after aspiration and after a uterine contraction to minimize the risk of tachycardia that can occur if the drug is directly injected into a vessel (Gabbe et al., 2016). If the subarachnoid space has been entered, sensory and motor changes occur in the woman's extremities. If there are no untoward effects, additional anesthetic agent is injected. The catheter is securely taped so that its placement will not be disturbed. Pain relief should occur within 15 to 20 minutes after administration (Gabbe et al., 2016).
11. The nurse then assists the woman into a semireclining position with a lateral tilt of her uterus for 10 minutes to allow for distribution of the block. This also prevents aortocaval compression (see Chapter 11).
12. The anesthesia provider and the nurse then monitor the maternal blood pressure every 5 minutes for the first 15 minutes past the injection and then every 15 minutes until the block wears off. Maternal vital signs are evaluated by either the nurse or the anesthesia provider against baseline readings obtained just before the beginning of the procedure. The nurse is responsible for documentation of assessment data that are obtained throughout the procedure.
13. The woman must be attended by a nurse, nurse anesthetist, or an anesthesiologist at the bedside for the first 20 minutes following the initial dose and after administration of any additional dose.

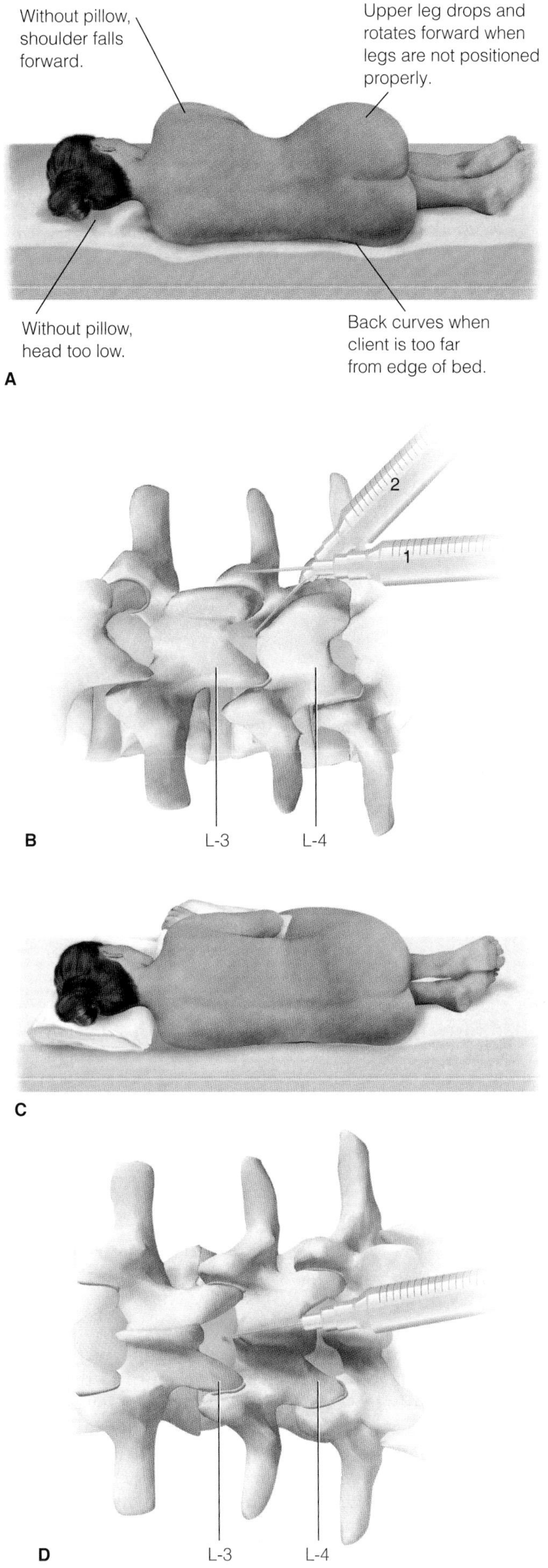

Figure 22–3 Positioning woman for epidural anesthesia block. A. Incorrect maternal positioning for placing subarachnoid or epidural block. The upper shoulder has fallen forward, upper leg has rotated forward, and the patient is positioned on the center of the bed so that there is no support from the edge and the back can curve. B. Vertebral position with patient in incorrect position. The vertebrae rotate forward and, if the needle is inserted in the usual way (needle 1), the apophyseal joints are encountered. Needle 2 shows the proper insertion of the needle entering the epidural space. C. Correct maternal positioning. The back is straight and vertical, the shoulders are square, and the upper leg is prevented from rolling forward. D. Vertebral position with the woman correctly positioned.

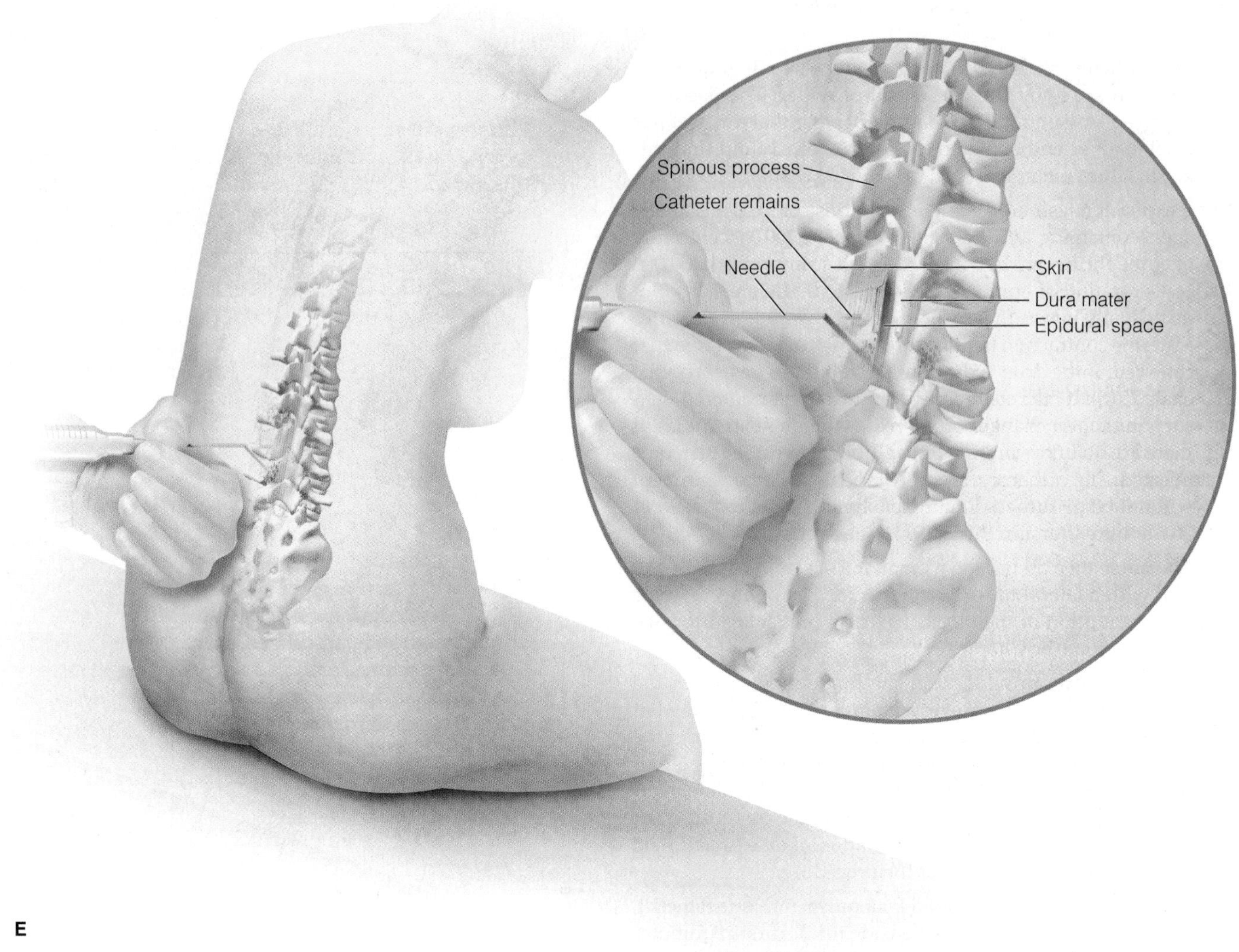

Figure 22–3 *(continued)* **Positioning woman for epidural anesthesia block. E. Sitting position with the shoulders rolled forward and back exposed for needle insertion.**

14. The maternal blood pressure and pulse and the FHR continue to be monitored by the nurse throughout infusion until the birth.
15. If the epidural is not being administered by continuous pump, the anesthesiologist aspirates the catheter each time before administering subsequent doses.

PROBLEMS AND ADVERSE EFFECTS

The major adverse effect of epidural anesthesia is maternal hypotension caused by a spinal blockade, which lowers peripheral resistance, decreases venous return to the heart, and subsequently lessens cardiac output and lowers blood pressure. Maternal hypotension will cause uteroplacental insufficiency in the fetus, which appears as late decelerations on the fetal monitoring strip. The risk of hypotension can be minimized by hydrating the vascular system with 500 to 1000 mL of IV solution (Baysinger et al., 2016) before the procedure, changing the woman's position to a sidelying one, and/or increasing the IV rate afterward. If maternal hypotension occurs, the nurse must initiate intrauterine resuscitation measures—one way to remember these interventions is to think of *flip*, *flush*, and *O*. The first intervention is to reposition the woman fully on her side. If she is on her side, reposition (*flip*) her to the opposite side. The goal is to maximize blood flow back to the heart and to the uterus. The second intervention is to increase fluids per the institution's policy in order to increase blood volume and increase perfusion of the placenta (*flush*). Finally, the nurse can administer 10 L oxygen by non-rebreather face mask. By providing additional oxygenation (*O*), the nurse is adding oxygen that is not bound to maternal hemoglobin and is easier for fetal hemoglobin to pick up in the chorionic villus. Should these initial interventions not improve maternal blood pressure, the nurse may also administer 5 to 15 mg ephedrine per orders by the anesthesiologist to reverse vasodilation caused by the epidural. Usually, these inventions are sufficient to restore normal maternal blood pressure and normal fetal heart rate patterns. If these interventions do not

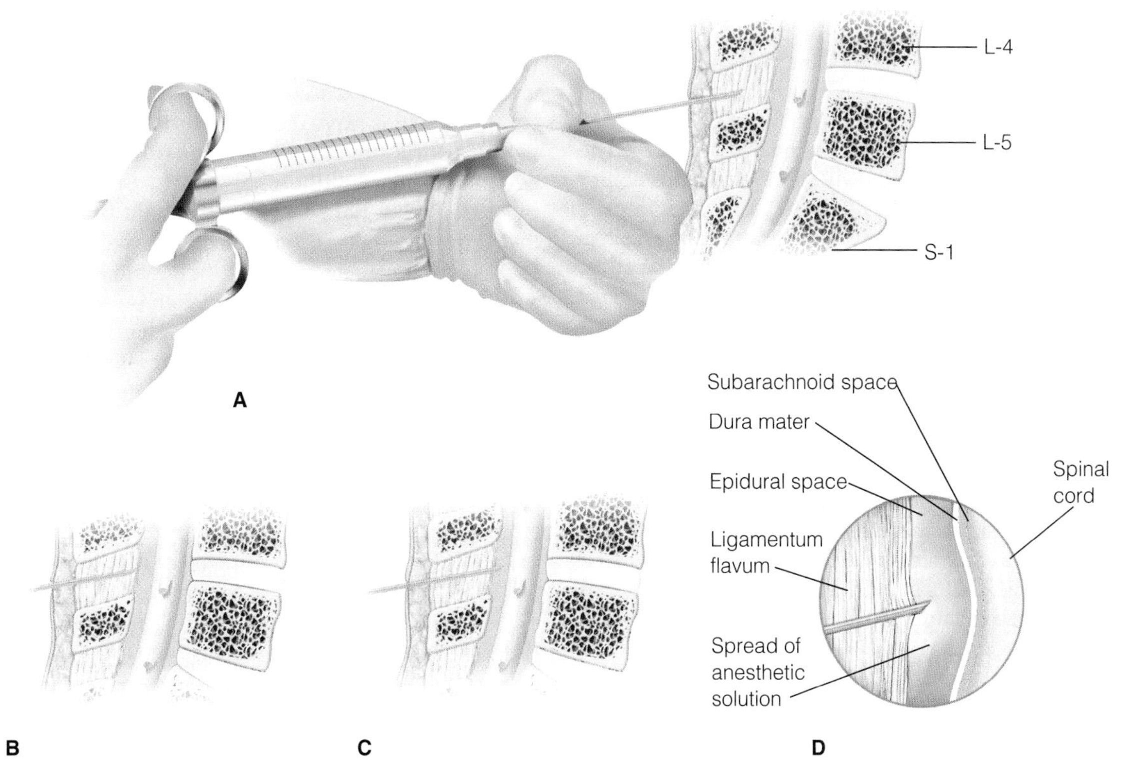

Figure 22–4 **Technique for lumbar epidural block. A. Proper position of insertion. B. Needle in the ligamentum flavum. C. Tip of needle in epidural space. D. Force of injection pushing dura away from tip of needle.**

resolve late decelerations, the nurse must begin to consider other causes of placental insufficiency.

Throughout the rest of her labor, the woman must maintain a lateral tilt or sidelying position to maximize venous return to the heart, minimize the risk of maternal hypotension, and maintain adequate perfusion of the placenta. The nurse should help reposition the woman, alternating sides, which also helps with the descent of the fetus and the even distribution of the anesthetic agents through the epidural. If the woman needs to be in a supine position for vaginal exams, the nurse maintains a lateral tilt during the procedure as much as possible and then repositions her on her side after the procedure is complete.

A potentially distressing maternal problem is an inadequate block, unilateral block, or block failure. Epidural anesthesia has a higher failure rate than spinal anesthesia because the catheter must be properly placed to produce adequate anesthesia (Baysinger et al., 2016). A one-sided block is fairly common and can be overcome by having the woman lie on the unanesthetized side and injecting more of the local anesthetic agent. If the woman has a continuous epidural block, she should turn from side to side every hour to avoid a one-sided block. A block may be effective except for a "spot" or "window" of pain in the inguinal or suprapubic area. Breakthrough pain may occur at any time during the epidural infusion. It usually occurs when the continuous infusion rate of the anesthetic agent is below the recommended rate for a therapeutic dose. Breakthrough pain can also occur when the woman has a full bladder, when there is a rapid dilatation or fetal descent, or when the cervix is completely dilated. The nurse assesses the woman carefully before calling the anesthesia provider for additional medication administration. Breakthrough pain may also occur when the infusion pump rate is altered or the integrity of the epidural line is broken.

Pruritus may occur at any time during the epidural infusion and is estimated to occur in 50 to 100% of women who receive epidural anesthesia. It typically begins on the face, neck, or torso and is generally the result of the agent used in the epidural infusion. Traditionally, Benadryl, an antihistamine, has been administered with some relief noted (Gabbe et al., 2016). One study examined the use of prophylactic pentazocine, which showed a 69% reduction in itching in women who received a single 15-mg dose of IV pentazocine after delivery (Hirabayashi, Doi, Imamachi, et al., 2017).

Maternal temperature may be elevated to 37.8°C (100.4°F) or higher with the use of epidural anesthesia. Sympathetic blockade may decrease sweat production and, in turn, diminish heat loss. It has also been suggested that heat loss may result from a failure of the central nervous system to regulate temperature. Headaches, migraine headaches, neck aches, and tingling of the hands and fingers have also been reported (Gabbe et al., 2016).

Short-term localized tenderness at the needle puncture site occurs in about 40% of women during the first week after birth. Backache is fairly common and thought to result from maternal positions under anesthesia that inadvertently cause muscle strain. In repositioning the woman, the nurse must assess for apparent unnatural positions and avoid prolonged positioning. Long-term back pain is uncommon. Other problems or adverse effects include urinary retention, shivering, and nausea and vomiting.

COMPLICATIONS

One of the most serious complications of regional anesthesia, systemic toxic reaction, was discussed previously in the section "Adverse Maternal Reactions to Anesthetic Agents." Toxic reactions following a lumbar epidural block may be caused by unintentional placement of the drug in the arachnoid or subarachnoid space, excessive amount of the drug in the epidural space (massive epidural), or accidental intravascular injection (Baysinger et al., 2016). Because large quantities of anesthetic agent are used for epidural block, the likelihood of toxic reactions is higher than with some of the other regional procedures. The incidence of drug reactions is relatively low, but the possibility is always present.

Pain during cesarean birth with epidural anesthesia has been reported by a growing number of women. In light of this, some anesthesiologists use both temperature and pinprick tests to assess sensory loss. Dermatomes from T_4 to S_3 should be tested for sensory loss before beginning a cesarean birth (Baysinger et al., 2016). The method of assessment and the results should be documented in the anesthesia record.

Spinal headaches can also be a complication that occurs with epidural anesthesia. Spinal headaches occur when the dura is accidently punctured during epidural placement (Baysinger et al., 2016). Spinal headaches may heal on their own, or they may require the placement of a blood patch, a procedure in which a small amount of the woman's blood is injected into the epidural space to clot and close the area that is leaking. See *Case Study: Azia Askari*.

Nursing Care. Assess the maternal vital signs and the FHR for baseline information and to ensure that both maternal and fetal vital signs are within normal limits. (*Note:* All information regarding assessments, procedures, and other activities is recorded on the woman's chart. Some facilities may use checklists or electronic charting systems.)

Explain the procedure and expected results, and answer the woman's questions. Act as an advocate for the woman and arrange for consultation with the anesthesiologist if questions arise. The husband/partner/support person should be included to promote a family-centered approach. Informed consent for the epidural should be obtained by the anesthesiologist. The earlier you initiate these discussions, the less likely the woman will be in too much pain to fully process information and respond appropriately.

Many women are concerned about the timing of the epidural placement. Your ability to educate the woman and set expectations for pain management with an epidural will have a large influence on the woman's later perception of her birth experience. Explain that the total time from request, to placement, to medication administration, to pain relief can take 30 to 45 minutes. Encourage her to request an epidural when she is managing her contractions but beginning to get tired, not when she has no coping ability left.

Provide physical and emotional support throughout the procedure, identifying the steps as they occur in order to provide reassurance that the process is progressing normally. Ensure family members are safe and not at risk of breaking the sterile field. It is a good idea to have only the father/partner sitting near the woman to minimize the risk of passing out and to have all other support persons leave the room during the procedure.

If during the course of labor, additional local anesthetic agents are injected, the regimen of assessing maternal blood pressure and initial surveillance should be repeated each time the epidural catheter is reinjected. If the woman's legs have been in stirrups during a vaginal birth, her blood pressure should be assessed as soon as her legs are taken out of the stirrups. While the legs were elevated, circulating blood volume in the trunk increased. Restoring circulation to the legs decreases the overall blood volume and may precipitate hypotension. See *Nursing Care Plan: For Epidural Anesthesia* for more information about maternal hypotension associated with epidural anesthesia.

Shivering may be caused by heat loss from increased peripheral blood flow or alteration of thermal input to the central nervous system when warm but not cold sensations have been suppressed. Changes in core body temperature may be responsible for shivering that is associated with epidural anesthesia. One study examined the administration of an intraoperative dexmedetomidine infusion, which resulted in cessation of shivering and further stabilized hemodynamic effects (Hu, Zhu, Cao, et al., 2017). Although warming intravenous fluids, applying warm blankets, providing a forced-air warming device, and providing reassurance can make the woman feel more at ease, it does not aid in reducing or stopping the shivering.

SAFETY ALERT!

Nursing care following an epidural block includes frequent assessment of the bladder to avoid bladder distention. Catheterization may be necessary because most women are unable to void; however, the nurse should first offer the woman a bedpan because catheterization increases the risk of urinary tract infections.

Assess the woman's level of pain relief. Assess the equal distribution of the anesthetic agent by assessing the temperature of the woman's feet. If one foot warms more quickly than the other, the woman should be positioned with the cooler side dependent. It is important for the woman to turn from side to side every hour to promote equal distribution of the anesthetic agent. In the presence of break-through pain or inadequate relief, assess for advanced cervical dilatation and bladder distention. If positioning changes and emptying the bladder do not help and the woman has inadequate pain relief, notify the anesthesia provider. During a continuous epidural block, the

CASE STUDY: Azia Askari

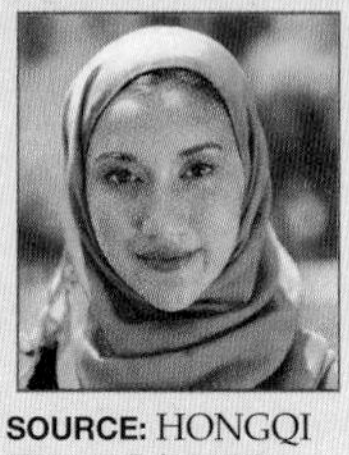

SOURCE: HONGQI ZHANG/123RF.

Azia is in the labor and delivery unit and is 4 centimeters dilated. She is accompanied by her sister-in-law and her husband. Azia tells her sister-in-law that she is fearful because things seem to be going much faster this time and she is experiencing more pain with this labor. She asks about the use of nitrous oxide but is afraid it won't be effective for her pain. Azia asks you if getting an epidural will make her "pushing part" last longer.

Question to Ponder

How do you counsel Azia on how the epidural may affect the labor progression?

Nursing Care Plan For Epidural Anesthesia

1. NURSING DIAGNOSIS: *Injury, Risk for*, related to maternal hypotension associated with epidural anesthesia secondary to vasodilation and venous pooling (NANDA-I © 2017)

Goal: Maternal and fetal effects associated with hypotension will be minimized.

INTERVENTION	RATIONALE
• Obtain baseline maternal vital signs and fetal heart rate.	• Normal ranges during labor include temperature 36.6°C to 37.5°C (98°F to 99.6°F), pulse 60 to 100, respirations 12 to 20/min, blood pressure 90–140 (60–90), fetal heart rate 110 to 160 beats/min.
• Insert IV with large-gauge catheter.	• Allows for IV fluid to be administered quickly if hypotension occurs.
• Provide hydration with 500 to 1000 mL of intravenous solution (e.g., lactated Ringer solution) 15 to 30 min before procedure. Dextrose-free solution is recommended.	• Increases intravascular volume and maintains cardiac output by preloading the patient before epidural anesthesia. Rapid infusion of dextrose solution can cause fetal hyperglycemia and rebound neonatal hypoglycemia.
• Educate the patient about treatment measures to expect if unwanted side effects from the epidural occur.	• Advance preparation will decrease anxiety and the patient will be more compliant. Treatment measures include oxygen administration, increase of IV fluids, possible administration of a vasopressor such as ephedrine, and repositioning the patient.
• Assist the patient into position following the procedure.	• Place patient in a lateral tilt position for 15 min following administration of block to allow medication to diffuse bilaterally. Once complete pain relief is achieved, position patient on side.
• Monitor blood pressure every 5 min for the first 15 min and then every 15 min until the block wears off.	• Close monitoring will allow for quick assessment and treatment of any changes from baseline blood pressure before the procedure.
• Monitor fetal heart rate pattern, noting the baseline, variability, presence of accelerations, and presence or absence of decelerations.	• Maternal hypotension may present first in the fetal heart rate. Variability and the absence of late decelerations indicate normal placental perfusion.

EXPECTED OUTCOMES: A baseline of maternal blood pressure and fetal heart rate pattern is established, and the woman is prepared should treatment be needed.

• Observe, record, and report symptoms of hypotension, including nausea and vomiting, apprehension, restlessness, dizziness, tinnitus, and headache, or the development of late decelerations on the fetal heart rate tracing.	• These signs, immediately following epidural placement, are related to hypotension and must be treated even in the absence of a significant drop in the systolic blood pressure.

EXPECTED OUTCOMES: Hypotension is quickly identified and treatment measures started.

• Initiate treatment measures to reverse hypotension.	• Treatment measures include: Place woman in left lateral position, increase IV rate, administer oxygen by face mask at 7 to 10 L/min as needed. (Remember, "Flip, Flush, and O.") If necessary, administer vasopressors as ordered (usually ephedrine 5 to 10 mg IV). Notify analgesia provider or certified nurse anesthetist.

EXPECTED OUTCOMES: Hypotension is treated successfully. Blood pressure returns to normal limits, increasing blood flow to the fetus. Fetal heart rate returns to a Category I tracing.

anesthesiologist should titrate the infusion to maintain a sensory level of T_{10}, and the presence of motor block and height of sensory block should be documented at least hourly (Baysinger et al., 2016).

Respiratory rate and quality of the respirations should be assessed at least every 15 to 30 minutes. Notify the anesthetist of any significant decreases in respiratory rate or respiratory pattern changes. If the respiratory rate falls below 14 respirations per minute, naloxone (Narcan) may be given to remove the effect of the anesthetic agent; respirations will then return to a normal rate (Baysinger et al., 2016).

Ask the woman if she is experiencing pruritus and be alert for signs of scratching, especially on the face, neck, and torso. If present, pruritus is usually treated with diphenhydramine (Benadryl), 25 mg administered IV or 50 mg IM per physician's or CNM's order (Gabbe et al., 2016).

During the second stage of labor, the woman may require assistance with pushing because she may not feel her contractions or experience the urge to push. If the woman does not feel the urge to push, you may collaborate with the anesthesia provider so that the block can be turned down or temporarily turned off until the urge to push returns. The woman may also need assistance holding or controlling her legs in order to push, often provided by you and the father/partner or other support person. When supporting the woman's legs, do not place pressure to force them back, which can cause ligament or nerve damage in the leg. Have the woman pull her own legs back as she will naturally apply the appropriate amount of force.

After birth, return of complete sensation and the ability to control the legs are essential before ambulation is attempted. This may take several hours, depending on the agent and the total dose. The woman must also be able to maintain blood pressure in a sitting and then standing position.

Spinal Block

In a **spinal block**, a local anesthetic agent is injected directly into the spinal fluid in the subarachnoid space to provide anesthesia for cesarean birth. The subarachnoid space is the fluid-filled area between the dura mater and the spinal cord. During pregnancy, the space decreases because of the distention of the epidural veins. Thus, a specific dose of anesthetic produces a much higher level of anesthesia in the pregnant woman than in the nonpregnant woman. When a spinal block is properly administered, failure rate is low. Unlike epidural anesthesia, spinal blocks allow the anesthesia to mix directly with the cerebrospinal fluid, which eliminates "windows" where anesthesia coverage is not obtained (Baysinger et al., 2016). Cesarean birth requires anesthetic blockade to the T_4 dermatome (Figure 22–5).

ADVANTAGES

The advantages of spinal block are immediate onset of anesthesia, relative ease of administration, a smaller drug volume, and maternal compartmentalization of the drug. Spinal anesthesia is frequently the regional block of choice in acute obstetric emergencies because it is the safest and fastest anesthesia technique (Baysinger et al., 2016).

DISADVANTAGES

The primary disadvantage of spinal block is intense blockade of sympathetic fibers, resulting in a high incidence of hypotension. This leads to a greater potential for fetal hypoxia. In addition, uterine tone is maintained, which makes intrauterine manipulation difficult. Spinal anesthesia is traditionally short acting, and it is difficult to maintain adequate anesthesia coverage for prolonged procedures (Baysinger et al., 2016).

CONTRAINDICATIONS

Spinal anesthesia is contraindicated for women with severe hypovolemia, regardless of cause; central nervous system disease; infection over the site of puncture; maternal coagulation problems; and allergy to local anesthetic agents (Baysinger et al., 2016). Sepsis and active genital herpes may be considered relative rather than absolute contraindications. Spinal block is also contraindicated for women who do not wish to have spinal procedures or are unable to appropriately consent (Gabbe et al., 2016).

TECHNIQUE

These steps are followed in administering a subarachnoid block (Baysinger et al., 2016):

1. The nurse assists the woman into a sitting or left lateral position.
2. Intravenous infusion is checked for patency.
3. The nurse helps the woman into the same position as for a lumbar epidural block.
4. The anesthesiologist/nurse anesthetist prepares the skin carefully, maintaining sterility before initiating the procedure.
5. A skin wheal is made over L_3 or L_4.
6. An 18- or 19-gauge needle is introduced through the skin and into the interspinous ligament. Then, a 24- to 27-gauge pencil-point needle is introduced inside the larger needle and inserted into the ligamentum flavum, the epidural space through the dura mater, and into the subarachnoid space (Figure 22–6).
7. The appropriate amount of anesthetic agent is injected slowly and then both needles are removed.
8. Upon removal, a drop of cerebrospinal fluid can be seen in the hub of the needle if the subarachnoid space has been entered.
9. With hyperbaric solutions, the woman remains sitting up for 45 seconds.
10. The nurse assists the woman onto her back with a pillow under her head and a wedge under her right side. Position changes can alter the dermatome level if done within 3 to 5 minutes. After 10 minutes, a position change will not affect the level of anesthesia.
11. The nurse monitors blood pressure, pulse, and respirations every 1 to 2 minutes for the first 10 minutes, then every 5 to 10 minutes.

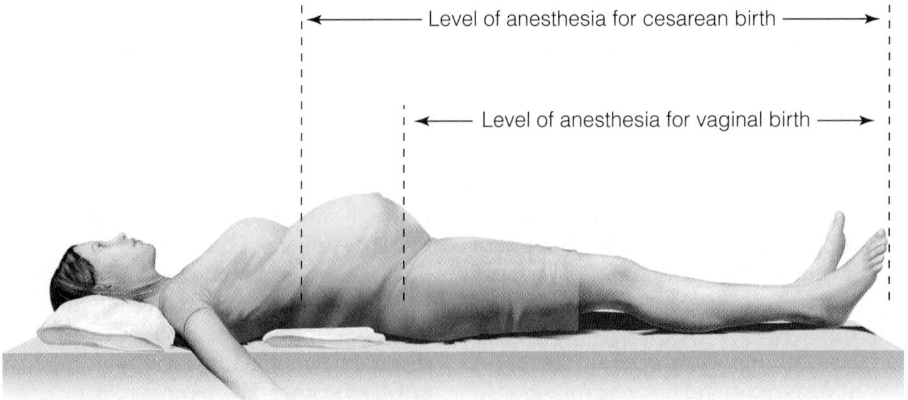

Figure 22–5 **Levels of anesthesia for vaginal and cesarean births.**

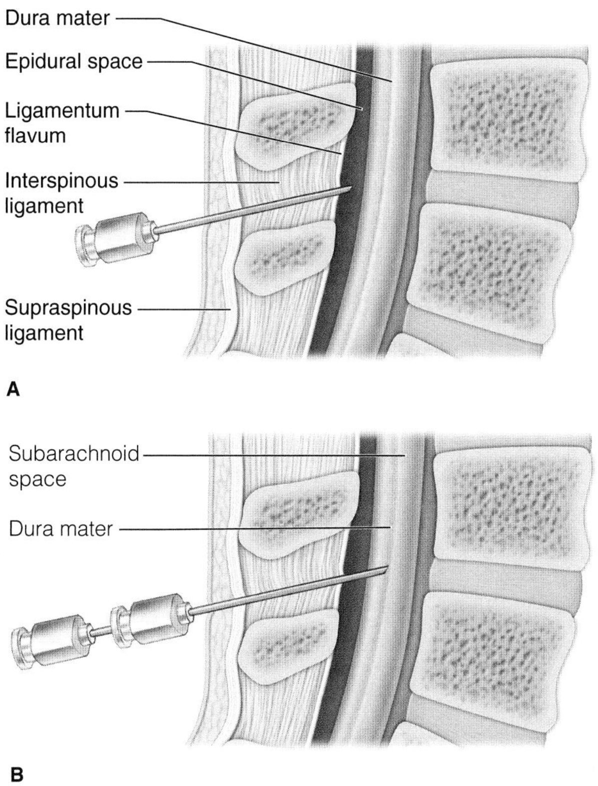

Figure 22–6 **Double-needle technique for spinal injection. A. Large needle in epidural space. B. A 23-gauge needle in a larger needle entering the subarachnoid space.**

In the absence of maternal hypotension or toxic reaction, a spinal block exerts no direct effect on the fetus. The amount of anesthetic used is too small to reach fetal circulation in a quantity that might cause fetal depression. Spinal anesthesia has been shown to be well tolerated by a healthy fetus when a maternal IV fluid preload in excess of 500 to 1000 mL precedes the administration of the spinal.

COMPLICATIONS

The complications of spinal anesthesia include hypotension, drug reaction, total spinal neurologic sequelae, and spinal headache. The side effects include nausea, shivering, and urinary retention.

Hypotension can be minimized by prehydrating with 500 to 1000 mL of non–dextrose-containing fluids and displacing the uterus to a lateral position. The practice of placing an already hypotensive woman in a sitting position following injection to prevent upward spread of the anesthetic solution is dangerous because it will cause venous pooling in the lower extremities, further decreasing the maternal blood pressure (Baysinger et al., 2016). The normal curve of the thoracic spine prevents cranial spread of an intrathecal agent. A pillow is placed under the woman's head to exaggerate the curve.

Treatment of hypotension is the same as with an epidural block: Positioning the woman in a lateral and head-down position and rapidly infusing IV fluids. Preventing cardiovascular collapse requires early detection, supplemental oxygen, assisted ventilation, and measures to maintain the blood pressure. The extent to which the fetus is affected relates to the degree of maternal hypotension. When maternal hypotension has been reversed, it is best to delay the birth for 4 to 5 minutes to allow the fetus to recover. If hypotension does not resolve in a short period of time, ephedrine can be administered IV. Resuscitative equipment and trained personnel must be available to treat the mother and baby.

Complications that involve anesthesia can occur in the phrenic nerve (C_3–C_5) or higher (Baysinger et al., 2016). In a *high-level* block, respiratory function becomes impaired, requiring mechanical ventilation to maintain adequate respiratory functioning until the block recedes. Another extremely rare complication is the *complete spinal* in which respiratory assistance is needed and loss of consciousness also occurs. A *total spinal* block occurs when there is paralysis of the respiratory muscles. It is a relatively rare but critical event. The symptoms include apnea, dilation of pupils, loss of consciousness, and absence of blood pressure. The onset of symptoms usually occurs within minutes of the injection but can occur in a span of time ranging from 30 seconds to 45 minutes. Resuscitative treatment, airway control, and support of blood pressure must begin immediately. If this complication occurs, it is important to remember that the woman is not asleep; although she may be paralyzed, she may be aware of everything going on around her. She requires assurance that her respiratory status will be maintained until she can breathe on her own again (Baysinger et al., 2016).

Conversely, a spinal block can render inadequate anesthesia coverage (in which the anesthesia does not reach the T_4 level) and discomfort can occur, sometimes presenting in the middle of surgery. Such cases may warrant the need for general anesthesia (Baysinger et al., 2016).

Neurologic complications may occur coincidentally with spinal anesthesia, for example, with preexisting disease or faulty positioning of the woman. Hypotension and apnea can occur, decreasing oxygen to the brain. The woman should be positioned with a left tilt, and fluids should be administered to treat hypotension (Gabbe et al., 2016). Genuine neurologic sequelae, such as paralysis, are extremely rare.

Although much less serious than other complications, headache may be an unpleasant aftermath of spinal anesthesia. It is the most frequent complication, with an incidence of about 1 to 3% (Gabbe et al., 2016). Leakage of spinal fluid at the site of dural puncture is thought to be the cause. Several techniques have been suggested to decrease the possibility of headache. The use of a narrow-gauge pencil-point anesthesia needle (24 to 27 gauge) reduces the incidence of spinal headache. Conservative treatments, such as hyperhydration and keeping the woman flat in bed after birth, have been used with minimal success. An abdominal binder may provide some relief. Postdural headaches can last up to 7 days and not only are painful but can also interfere with maternal–newborn interactions and breastfeeding success. In severe cases, a blood patch can be performed. A small amount of the woman's blood is drawn and, before coagulation occurs, injected into the epidural space at the site of the puncture, which generally results in immediate pain relief.

Nursing Care. Assist in positioning the woman, provide oxygen via nasal cannula or mask, assess and record baseline vital signs of the mother and fetus. A bolus of fluid should be given before initiation of the block whenever possible (Baysinger et al., 2016). The anesthesiologist is responsible for assessing and recording the level of the spinal block.

Position the woman as described earlier and support her in this position. Palpate the woman's uterus to detect the beginning of a contraction. Intrathecal agents are not administered during a contraction because the increased pressure could cause a higher level of anesthesia than desired. After the agent has been administered, assist the woman to the supine position with a wedge under her right hip to displace the uterus, and place a pillow under her head. After the block is instilled, continue to monitor maternal blood pressure, pulse, and respiration until the anesthesiologist takes over. In the surgical setting, a safety belt is placed across the woman's thighs to prevent injury. Sequential compression devices can be used to prevent the development of blood clots due to immobility. The woman should be kept informed of everything that is going on in the birthing area, particularly if she is receiving mask oxygen.

If hypotension should occur, the IV fluids should be increased and the uterus displaced manually to the left (Baysinger et al., 2016). If the woman reports that she is having difficulty breathing, she needs to be assessed very carefully. Some women recognize the loss of sensation of the normal rise and fall of the chest with respirations and become anxious that they are not breathing. Provide reassurance that the feeling is a normal side effect. Although rare, total spinal block can occur, therefore the possibility must always be kept in mind. Observe the woman for apnea, unconsciousness, pupil dilation, and unobtainable blood pressure. Prompt treatment, which may include the use of a vasopressor (such as ephedrine), may avert maternal or fetal death. It is essential to establish an airway and give oxygen with positive pressure until the woman can be intubated and other emergency measures instituted.

Combined Spinal–Epidural Block

Spinal anesthesia may be combined with an epidural block. The combined spinal–epidural (CSE) can be used for labor analgesia and for cesarean birth. The anesthetic and analgesic agents used differ according to the purpose of the CSE. A CSE is accomplished by inserting an epidural needle into the epidural space. A narrow-gauge pencil-point anesthesia needle (24 to 27 gauge) is inserted through the epidural needle, through the dura, and into the cerebrospinal fluid. A small amount of local anesthetic agent, opioid, or both is injected, and the needle is withdrawn. An epidural catheter is then threaded through the epidural needle into the epidural space. The epidural needle is removed, and the epidural catheter is securely placed against the woman with tape.

An advantage of CSE is that the spinal agent will have a faster onset than medications that are injected into the epidural space. Nevertheless, as the spinal can cause uterine hypertonicity, it can result in additional interventions for intrauterine resuscitation. Given that epidural blocks have become more effective, CSEs are not as commonly used.

Pudendal Block

The **pudendal block** technique is performed by the obstetrician and provides perineal anesthesia for the second stage of labor, birth, and episiotomy repair. An anesthetic agent is injected below the pudendal plexus, as shown in Figure 22–1B. The pudendal plexus arises from the anterior division of the second and third sacral nerves and the entire fourth sacral nerve. Below the plexus, the branches converge into the pudendal nerve, which crosses the sacrosciatic notch and passes the tip of the ischial spine, where it divides into the perineal, dorsal, and inferior hemorrhoidal nerves of the pudendal plexus. The perineal nerve, which is the largest branch of the pudendal plexus, supplies the skin of the vulvar area, the perineal muscles, and the urethral sphincter. The dorsal nerve supplies the clitoris, and the inferior hemorrhoidal nerve supplies the skin and muscles of the perineal region as well as the internal anal sphincter. Pudendal block provides relief of pain from perineal distention but does not relieve pain of uterine contractions (Figure 22–7).

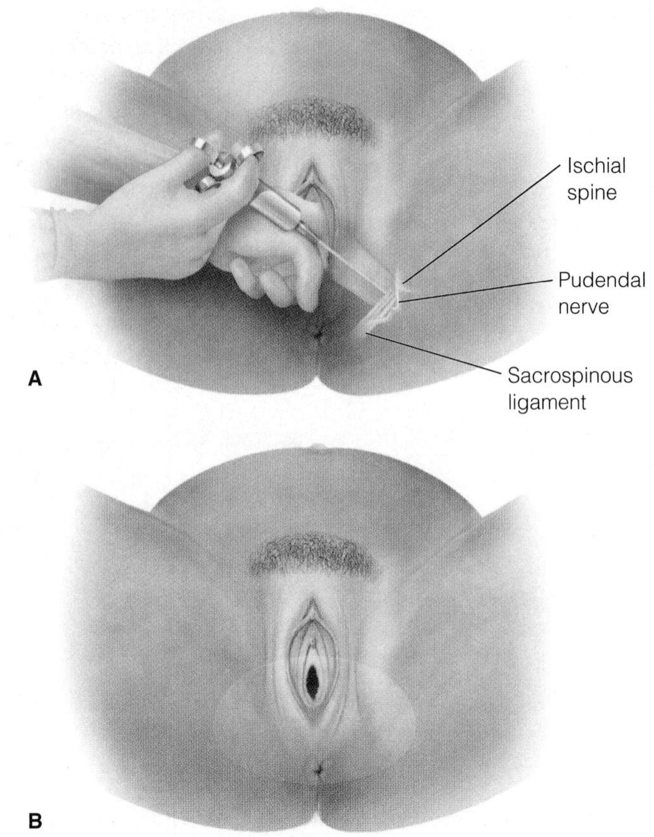

Figure 22–7 A. Pudendal block by the transvaginal approach. B. Area of perineum affected by pudendal block.

ADVANTAGES

The advantages of pudendal block are ease of administration and absence of maternal hypotension. It also allows the use of low forceps or vacuum extraction for birth. A moderate dose of anesthetic agent (10 mL per side) has minimal ill effects on the woman and the course of labor.

DISADVANTAGES

The urge to bear down during the second stage of labor may be decreased, but the woman is able to do so with appropriate coaching. There is usually little effect on the uncompromised fetus unless overly rapid or intravascular injection occurs. The block may be done by a transvaginal or transperineal approach. The woman may experience a burning sensation when the block is administered. Transvaginal injection is simpler, safer, and more direct, making it the procedure of choice.

COMPLICATIONS

A systemic toxic reaction can occur from accidental vascular injection. Other possible maternal complications specific to pudendal block include broad ligament hematoma, perforation of the rectum, and trauma to the sciatic nerve.

Nursing Care. Explain the procedure and the expected effect and answer any questions. Pudendal block does not alter maternal vital signs or FHR, so assessments in addition to the expected ones are not necessary.

Local Infiltration Anesthesia

Local anesthesia is accomplished by injecting an anesthetic agent into the intracutaneous, subcutaneous, and intramuscular areas

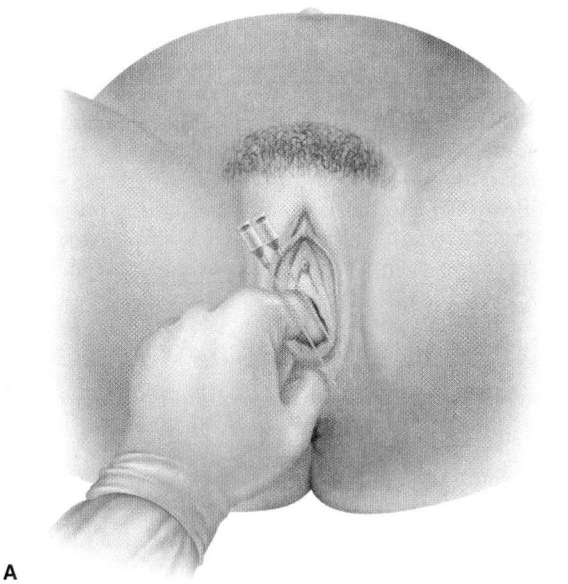

A

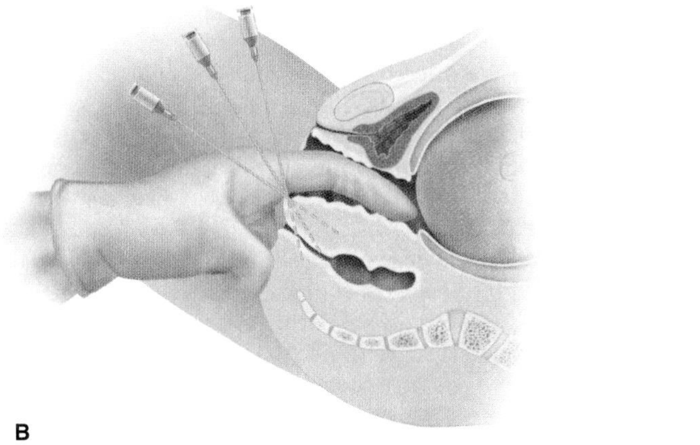

B

Figure 22–8 Local infiltration anesthesia. A. Technique of local infiltration for episiotomy and repair. B. Technique of local infiltration showing fan pattern for the fascial planes.

of the perineum (Figure 22–8). It is generally used at the time of birth for episiotomy and repair or after birth if a laceration has occurred; it is especially useful for women giving birth without previous pharmacologic interventions. The procedure is essentially free from complications. The woman may experience a burning sensation at the time of administration.

ADVANTAGES

The major advantage of the local block is that it involves the use of the least amount of anesthetic agent. It can be done if an episiotomy is needed just before the birth. It can also be used when a laceration has occurred and a repair is needed.

DISADVANTAGES

The major disadvantage is that large amounts of solution must be used. Although any local anesthetic may be used, chloroprocaine (Nesacaine), lidocaine (Xylocaine), and mepivacaine (Carbocaine) are the agents of choice in local infiltration because of their capacity for diffusion. A burning sensation at the time of injection is common. See *Case Study: Melissa Bond-James*.

Nursing Care. Explain the procedure and the expected effect and answer any questions. Local anesthetic agents have no effect on maternal vital signs or FHR, so additional assessments are unnecessary.

Transversus Abdominis Plane Block

The **transversus abdominis plane (TAP) block** is growing in use for postoperative pain management after cesarean birth. Guided by ultrasound, an anesthesiologist injects local anesthetic bilaterally into the space between the transverse abdominus and the internal oblique muscles, filling the connective tissue and providing pain relief to the abdominal area (Baysinger et al., 2016). A TAP block is therefore sometimes referred to as a *fill block* instead of a regional block. The block targets the peripheral sensory nerves innervating the anterior abdominal wall, which makes it particularly useful for managing pain secondary to cesarean births with a vertical or Pfannensteil incision. It does not affect motor function. TAP blocks are administered at the end of surgery while the patient is still under the influence of general anesthesia or a spinal or epidural regional block, eliminating discomfort during the procedure.

ADVANTAGES

TAP blocks can provide up to 12 hours of postoperative analgesia without the need for additional opioids, reducing or even eliminating the need for intravenous opioids for women who required general anesthesia for surgery. TAP blocks are a useful pain relief option for women who cannot or should not use opioids after surgery. They reduce opioid-related side effects such as sedation, nausea and vomiting, and decreased bowel motility. TAP blocks have been shown to reduce the use of opioids postoperatively, improve a woman's satisfaction with her pain management postoperatively, and improve mobility after surgery compared to using oral or IV pain medication (Champaneria, Shah, Wilson, et al., 2016).

CASE STUDY: Melissa Bond-James

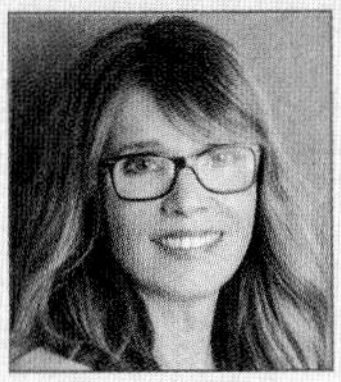

SOURCE: Kinga/Shutterstock.

Melissa is in active labor and is breathing through her contractions. She advises the nurse and the clinical technician that she would like to have a natural birth and does not want to be asked about pain medications. She completed childbirth classes and appears to have good control using breathing techniques to help her cope with contractions. Her wife, Nancy, asks if there is anything Melissa can be given after the birth if she has a tear. Melissa reinforces she does not want an episiotomy.

Question to Ponder

What will you tell Melissa and Nancy about pain medication approaches that can be used for Melissa if she needs a repair and sutures for a perineal laceration after birth?

There are no known reported disadvantages because it is a low-risk procedure that involves two injections into the fascia of the abdominal wall. Throughout the procedure, the anesthesiologist will draw back on the syringe to ensure medication is not being injected into the vascular system.

CONTRAINDICATIONS

The only contraindications for the procedure are infection at the injection site, refusal or inability to consent by the woman, or allergies to local anesthetics.

General Anesthesia

General anesthesia (induced unconsciousness) may be needed for cesarean birth and surgical intervention with some obstetric complications. The method used to achieve general anesthesia is a combination of intravenous analgesics and inhaled agents. The use of general anesthesia in the obstetric setting continues to decline because of adverse fetal effects and the increase in maternal risks. In order to decrease the length of fetal exposure and teratogenic effects, it is recommended that the woman be fully prepped and the obstetrician be fully prepared to make the initial incision prior to the administration of anesthesia.

The most common indications for general anesthesia include perceived lack of time for regional anesthesia, contraindications to regional anesthesia, failure of regional anesthesia, and patient refusal of regional anesthesia (Baysinger et al., 2016). The risk of general anesthesia, in the obstetric setting, must always be weighed against the well-being of the mother and fetus. In the case of abruption, for example, general anesthesia allows for the most rapid birth of the compromised fetus and for the initiation of resuscitative measures for the woman.

Intravenous Anesthetics

Propofol (Diprivan) is a short-acting sedative, which means that it exerts its effect rapidly and has a brief duration of action. Propofol produces sedation within 30 seconds after IV administration and is frequently used for initiating unconsciousness prior to intubation. Ketamine (Ketalar) is an intermediate-acting barbiturate that may be used for anesthesia induction. The effects typically last 20 to 60 minutes. The drug is contraindicated in women with preeclampsia or chronic hypertension. Ketamine may also be used to supplement an epidural or spinal block that becomes less effective during surgery. Ketamine has known hallucinogenic effects; accordingly, it is often given with midazolam (Versed), which produces an amnesic effect.

Inhaled Anesthesia Agents

The most commonly used inhaled anesthesia agent is nitrous oxide due to its analgesic and anxiolytic properties. Nitrous oxide does not produce significant uterine relaxation. Although it crosses the placenta immediately after administration, fetal tissue uptake occurs 20 minutes after administration, which results in a lower fetal arterial concentration and less neonatal depression. Nitrous oxide is commonly mixed with oxygen at a 1:1 ratio; this combination is known as Entonox (Alaj, 2017). When using nitrous oxide, the woman holds the face mask to her nose and mouth and breaths deeply. Once the pain ceases, she removes it from her face until it is needed again (Alaj, 2017).

Halogenated agents, such as isoflurane, sevoflurane, and desflurane, are also used, often in combination with nitrous oxide. The use of sevoflurane has been associated with uterine relaxation when administered in high dosages, suggesting that the lowest dose possible should be used (Baysinger et al., 2016). Many times, halogenated agents are used in combination with nitrous oxide in order to reduce this side effect.

Inhaled anesthetic agents have also been used in combination with spinal or epidural techniques when the epidural anesthesia was ineffective or severe maternal anxiety was present. Inhaled agents may also be used for women with aortic stenosis instead of regional anesthesia if advised by the cardiologist. Inhaled anesthetic agents have been associated with cardiovascular stability throughout surgery without adverse fetal outcomes (Gabbe et al., 2016).

Complications of General Anesthesia

A primary danger of general anesthesia is fetal respiratory depression secondary to maternal respiratory depression or medication administration. The woman is hyperoxygenated by face mask prior to intubation to ensure the fetus gets as much oxygen as possible. Most general anesthetic agents reach the fetus in about 2 minutes. The respiratory depression of the fetus is directly proportional to the depth and duration of the anesthesia. The long-term significance of fetal respiratory depression in a normal birth has not been determined. The poor fetal metabolism of general anesthetic agents is similar to that of analgesic agents administered during labor. General anesthesia is not advocated when the fetus is considered to be at high risk, particularly in preterm birth.

Most general anesthetic agents cause some degree of uterine relaxation, although the inhalation agents affect uterine relaxation to a lesser degree than the IV agents. They may also cause vomiting and aspiration.

Pregnancy results in decreased gastric motility, and the onset of labor halts the process almost entirely. Food eaten hours earlier may remain undigested in the stomach. Even when food and fluids have been withheld, the gastric juice produced during fasting is highly acidic and can produce chemical pneumonitis if aspirated. This pneumonitis is known as Mendelson syndrome. The signs and symptoms are chest pain, respiratory distress, cyanosis, fever, and tachycardia. Women undergoing emergency cesarean births appear to be at considerable risk for adverse events. The leading cause of maternal deaths in women who have had general anesthesia is the failure to establish a patent airway (Baysinger et al., 2016).

Care During General Anesthesia

Prophylactic antacid therapy is given to reduce the acidic content of the stomach before general anesthesia. Administration of a nonparticulate antacid (such as Bicitra) may be used; Reglan or Pepcid may also be used (Gabbe et al., 2016).

Before the induction to anesthesia, the woman should have a wedge placed under her hip to displace the uterus and avoid vena caval compression in the supine position. She should also be preoxygenated with 3 to 5 minutes of 100% oxygen. IV fluids should be started so that access to the intravascular space is immediately available.

Before surgery, the nurse assists the anesthesiologist in applying cardiac monitors, blood pressure cuff, and oxygen saturation device. The nurse can also hold the face mask for oxygenating the woman while the anesthesiologist draws up needed medication. The nurse also provides emotional support to the woman given that support persons may not attend cesarean birth performed under general anesthesia.

During the process of rapid induction of anesthesia, the nurse applies cricoid pressure, as the pregnant woman is more susceptible to aspiration. Cricoid pressure is accomplished by depressing the cricoid cartilage 2 to 3 cm posteriorly so that the

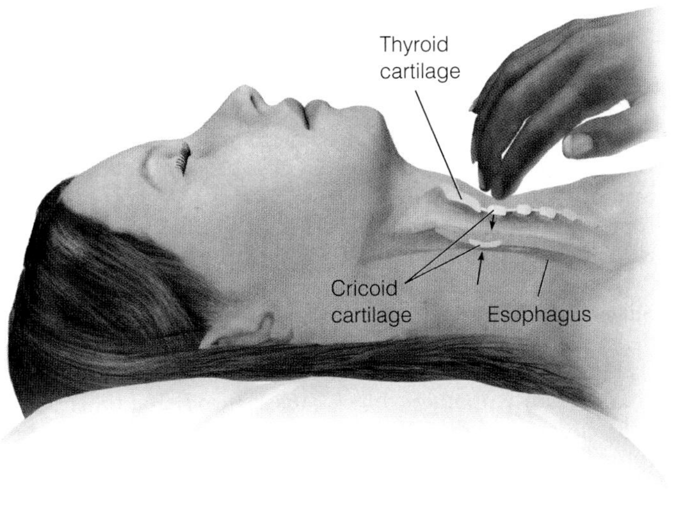

Figure 22–9 **Proper position for fingers in applying cricoid pressure until a cuffed endotracheal tube is placed by the anesthesiologist or certified nurse anesthetist. The cricoid cartilage is depressed 2 to 3 cm so that the esophagus is occluded.**

esophagus is occluded. Pressure is continued until the anesthesiologist has placed the cuffed endotracheal tube and indicates that the pressure can be released. Figure 22–9 shows the appropriate technique. The woman's neck can be supported by the nurse's other hand.

Clinical Tip

Women who receive general anesthesia are slower to initiate breastfeeding in the immediate postpartum period, which could have long-term effects on breastfeeding success. Women who receive general anesthesia and undergo a cesarean birth may need more assistance with breastfeeding than women who deliver vaginally. Encourage the woman to breastfeed as soon as she is alert enough to hold the baby.

Neonatal Neurobehavioral Effects of Anesthesia and Analgesia

Studies have focused on the neurobehavioral effects on the newborn of pharmacologic agents used during labor and birth. Although analgesic and anesthetic agents may alter the behavioral and adaptive function of the newborn, physiologic factors such as hunger, degree of hydration, time within the sleep–wake cycle, gestational age, and birth weight may also exert an influence (Berghella, 2016).

Analgesic and Anesthetic Considerations for the High-Risk Mother and Fetus

Up to this point the discussion of obstetric analgesia and anesthesia has dealt with the healthy woman and healthy fetus. Pain relief for high-risk women during labor and birth requires skill in decision making, close observation, and awareness of potential threats to the woman and fetus. Safety for all involved requires the close cooperation of the obstetrician, anesthesiologist, pediatrician or neonatologist, and labor nurse. The pathophysiologic changes that accompany maternal disorders have a direct influence on the choice of agent or technique. It is difficult to separate maternal and fetal complications because whatever alters the woman's response will also affect the fetus. The effects on the woman cannot be considered without the potential effects on the fetus.

Preterm Labor

The preterm fetus has special risks and requirements. An immature fetus is more susceptible to depressant drugs because he or she has less protein available for binding; has a poorly developed blood–brain barrier, which increases the likelihood that pharmacologic agents will attain a higher concentration in the central nervous system; and has a decreased ability to metabolize and excrete drugs after birth (Baysinger et al., 2016). Analgesia during labor should be avoided whenever possible. If it becomes necessary, the smallest dose that will provide relief should be administered. General anesthesia should be avoided in premature gestations (Berghella, 2016). Emotional support will be very valuable to the woman in this situation.

Preeclampsia

Pregnancies complicated by preeclampsia are high-risk situations, as discussed in Chapter 18. The potential for chronic placental insufficiency or preterm birth is also present. The woman with mild preeclampsia usually may have the analgesia or anesthesia of choice, although the incidence of hypotension with epidural anesthesia is increased (Baysinger et al., 2016). If hypotension occurs with the epidural block, it provides further stress on an already compromised cardiovascular system. Hypotension can usually be managed with judicious fluid increase and positioning. The nurse must realize that any drop in blood pressure for a hypertensive woman, even a drop to normal limits, may actually compromise her and the fetus.

The woman with severe preeclampsia poses a real challenge. Regional anesthesia seems to be the preferred method as long as hypotension can be avoided. Raising the central venous pressure by 3 to 4 cm H_2O with IV fluids helps avoid hypotension, but it must be remembered that this woman is already threatened with heart failure (Berghella, 2016). The effect of fluid intake can be monitored with a pulmonary artery occlusion pressure monitoring catheter. Pulmonary artery catheterization is used to correct volume deficits and appears more accurate than central pressure catheters in monitoring left- and right-side cardiac filling pressures, cardiac output, and systemic vascular resistance (Berghella, 2016). Although invasive monitoring is indicated, it is not associated with better maternal or neonatal outcomes (Gabbe et al., 2016). It is important to monitor and record the fluid intake and output. Some physicians use vasopressors; others avoid them because of the possible decrease in uterine blood flow to an already compromised fetus and the threat of a maternal cerebral vascular accident (Berghella, 2016). Spinal anesthesia is rarely used because of the greater potential for hypotension.

The use of general anesthesia poses a risk of aggravating maternal hypertension. In general, the safest method for general anesthesia is intubation, but because it may cause a hypertensive episode, it is avoided if possible. Another important consideration is that women with preeclampsia are more prone to have mucosal edema in the oral cavity and glottis, making intubation more difficult (Berghella, 2016).

Diabetes Mellitus

The fetus of a mother with diabetes mellitus may have a reduction in placental blood flow. Hypotension, which can result during regional anesthesia, can deplete this blood flow even further. If the fetus is tolerating labor well without an indication of fetal compromise, the continuous epidural technique may be undertaken. If a change in fetal status occurs, cesarean birth may be necessary, making a previously placed epidural useful in preventing the need for general anesthesia.

Anesthesia for cesarean birth requires special consideration in this case. The woman with diabetes is more likely to experience cardiovascular depression during a regional block because of higher sympathetic blockade (Baysinger et al., 2016). If a regional block is selected, it is recommended that acute hydration (preload) be provided by administering dextrose-free solution. In addition, left uterine displacement is initiated before the administration of the block and maintained throughout the surgery. Hypotension is treated promptly.

Cardiac Disease

Pregnancy imposes significant risks for the woman with cardiac disease. With mild mitral stenosis, the preferred anesthetic is continual epidural anesthesia with low forceps birth. This method avoids the cardiovascular changes associated with contractions and the Valsalva maneuver during bearing down in the second stage of labor. Hypotension can be avoided with carefully controlled IV fluids and by measuring central venous pressure to avoid overload. Epidural block or general anesthesia may be used in cesarean birth. Ketamine should be avoided because it produces tachycardia (Baysinger et al., 2016). Women at risk for congestive heart failure require invasive pulmonary artery occlusion pressure monitoring (Berghella, 2016).

Bleeding Complications

The current trend in treating bleeding complications during labor is to schedule cesarean birth when possible. When the maternal cardiovascular system is stable and there is no evidence of fetal compromise, an epidural may be given for birth. However, when either of these conditions results in active bleeding, the threat of hypovolemia must be treated immediately. Maternal hypovolemia and shock produce fetal hypoxia, acidosis, and possible fetal death (Berghella, 2016).

Regional blocks are contraindicated during active bleeding because the sympathetic block causes vasodilatation and further reduction of the vascular volume. Women with thrombocytopenia should also avoid regional blocks. Platelet status is an important consideration when choosing the best approach for anesthesia; when at all possible, hematologic conditions should be corrected before initiating birth (Berghella, 2016). General anesthesia is recommended for these cases. Following birth of the baby and placenta, oxytocin should *not* be given as an intravenous (IV) bolus to contract the uterus because it causes vasodilatation, which in turn causes a decrease in blood pressure and in total peripheral resistance. Oxytocin should be given as a dilute infusion to gain an oxytocic effect to treat uterine atony (relaxation) and to control postpartum bleeding. Resources that should be on hand to handle hemorrhagic emergencies include large-bore IV catheters, a fluid warmer, a forced-air body warmer, the woman's specific blood type or O negative blood, trained personnel, and equipment to infuse blood products rapidly (Baysinger et al., 2016).

Focus Your Study

- Pain relief during labor may be enhanced by nonpharmacologic methods and administration of analgesic agents and regional anesthesia blocks. The nurse can offer alternative comfort measures, avoid offering pain medication to women who do not desire pain medication, provide the woman who does desire pain medication with the opportunity to explore available options, and provide education and reassurance to the expectant woman and her support person.
- The goal of pharmacologic analgesia during labor is to provide maximal pain relief with minimal risk for the woman and fetus.
- The optimal time for administering analgesia is determined after a complete assessment of vital factors, including maternal, fetal, and labor assessments, and the woman's perception of her pain level and her need and desire for pain medication.
- Two common analgesic agents are nalbuphine (Nubain) and nitrous oxide.
- Opiate antagonists, such as naloxone (Narcan), counteract the respiratory depressant effect of the opiate narcotics by acting at specific receptor sites in the central nervous system.
- Sedatives, including barbiturates, benzodiazepines, and H_1-receptor antagonists, are primarily used in latent or early labor to promote rest and allow the woman to sleep.
- Regional anesthesia is achieved by injecting local anesthetic agents into an area that will bring the agent into direct contact with nerve tissue. Methods most commonly used in childbearing include lumbar epidural, spinal block, combined spinal–epidural block, pudendal block, local infiltration, and TAP blocks.
- Three types of local anesthetic agents used in regional blocks are esters, amides, and opiates. The esters are metabolized more rapidly and have only limited placental transfer. The amides are absorbed quickly and can be found in maternal blood within minutes after administration. Opiates act on specific opiate receptors in the spinal cord and have a greater analgesic effect when combined with a low dose of local anesthetic.
- Possible maternal complications of regional anesthesia, although rare, include systemic toxicity, convulsions, and sudden cardiovascular collapse.
- Agents in use for epidural and spinal routes include the opioids morphine and fentanyl. Adverse reactions of the woman to local anesthetic agents range from mild symptoms, such as

palpitations, to cardiovascular collapse. The newer amides, including ropivacaine and levobupivacaine, are longer acting and have fewer side effects.

- Pudendal blocks provide perineal anesthesia during the second stage of labor, birth, episiotomies, or laceration repair.
- General anesthesia can be achieved by a combination of intravenous injection and inhalation of anesthetic agents.
- The goal of general anesthesia is to provide maximal pain relief with minimal side effects to the woman and her fetus.
- Complications of general anesthesia include fetal depression, uterine relaxation, vomiting, and aspiration.
- The choice of analgesia and anesthesia for the high-risk woman and fetus requires careful evaluation.

In order to make safe and effective judgments using NANDA-I © 2017 nursing diagnoses, it is essential that nurses refer to the definitions and defining characteristics of the diagnoses used in this text, which can be found in Appendix C.

References

Alaj, A. N. (2017). *Nitrous oxide administration.* Retrieved from https://emedicine.medscape.com/article/1413427-overview#a4

American Academy of Pediatrics (AAP) & American Heart Association (AHA). (2016). *Textbook of neonatal resuscitation (7th ed.).* Elk Grove Village, IL: American Academy of Pediatrics.

American College of Obstetricians and Gynecologists (ACOG). (2017a). *Approaches to limit intervention during labor and birth.* (ACOG Committee Opinion No. 687). Washington, DC: Author.

American College of Obstetricians and Gynecologists (ACOG). (2017b). *Obstetric analgesia and anesthesia.* (ACOG Practice Bulletin No. 177). Washington, DC: Author.

American Heart Association (AHA). (2016). *Advanced cardiovascular life support (ACLS) provider manual 2015 guidelines.* Dallas, TX: Author.

Arendt, K.W. (2017). *Anesthesia for labor and delivery in high-risk heart disease: General considerations.* Retrieved from https://www.uptodate.com/contents/anesthesia-for-labor-and-delivery-in-high-risk-heart-disease-general-considerations?search=anesthesia-for-labor-and-delivery-in-high-risk-heartdisease-general-considerations&source=search_result&selectedTitle=2~150&usage_type=default&display_rank=2

Baysinger, C. L., Bucklin, B. A., & Gambling, D. (2016). *A practical approach to obstetric anesthesia* (2nd ed.). New York, NY: Wolters Kluwer.

Berghella, V. (2016). *Maternal-fetal evidence-based guidelines* (3rd ed.). Boca Raton, FL: CRC Press.

Champaneria, R., Shah, L., Wilson, M. J., & Daniels, J. P. (2016). Clinical effectiveness of transversus abdominis plane (TAP) blocks for pain relief after caesarean section: A meta-analysis. *International Journal of Obstetric Anesthesia, 28,* 45–60. DOI: 10.1016/j.ijoa.2016.07.009

Cobb, B., & Lipman, S. (2017). Cardiac arrest: Obstetric CPR/ACLS. *Clinical Obstetrics and Gynecology, 60*(2), 425–430.

Collins, M. (2015). A case report on the anxiolytic properties of nitrous oxide during labor. *Journal of Obstetric, Gynecologic, & Neonatal Nursing, 44*(1), 87–92. DOI: 10.1111/1552-6909.12522

Collins, M. (2017). Nitrous oxide utility in labor and birth: A multipurpose modality. *The Journal of Perinatal & Neonatal Nursing, 31*(2), 137–144. DOI: 10.1097/JPN.0000000000000248

Gabbe, S. G., Niebyl, J. R., Simpson, L., Landon, M. B., Galan, H. L., Jauniaux, E. R. M., . . . Grobman, W. A. (2016). *Obstetrics: Normal and problem pregnancies* (7th ed.). Philadelphia, PA: Elsevier.

Hirabayashi, M., Doi, K., Imamachi, N., Kishimoto, T., & Saito, Y. (2017). Prophylactic pentazocine reduces the incidence of pruritus after cesarean delivery under spinal anesthesia with opioids: A prospective randomized clinical trial. *Anesthesia & Analgesia, 124*(6), 1930–1934. DOI: 10.1213/ANE.0000000000002060

Hu, J., Zhu, M., Cao, L., Chen, J., & Lu, Y. (2016). Dexmedetomidine reduces shivering during epidural anesthesia. *International Journal of Clinical and Experimental Medicine, 9*(6), 11355–11360.

Martin, J. A., Hamilton, B. E., Osterman, M. J., Driscoll, A. K., & Mathews, T. J. (2017). Births: Final data for 2015. *National Vital Statistics Report, 66*(1), 1.

Pan, A., & Zakowski, M. (2017). Peripartum anesthetic management of the opioid-tolerant or buprenorphine/suboxone-dependent patient. *Clinical Obstetrics and Gynecology, 60*(2), 447–458. DOI: 10.1097/GRF.0000000000000288

Pinyan, T., Curlee, K., Keever, M., & Baldwin, K. M. (2017). A nurse-directed model for nitrous oxide use during labor. *MCN: The American Journal of Maternal Child Nursing, 42*(3), 160–165. DOI: 10.1097/NMC.0000000000000336

Richardson, M. G., Lopez, B. M., Baysinger, C. L., Shotwell, M. S., & Chestnut, D. H. (2017). Nitrous oxide during labor: Maternal satisfaction does not depend exclusively on analgesic effectiveness. *Anesthesia and Analgesia, 124*(2), 548–553. DOI: 10.1213/ANE.0000000000001680

Simpson, K. R., & Creehan, P. A. (2014). *AWHONN's perinatal nursing* (4th ed). Washington, DC: Association of Women's Health, Obstetric, and Neonatal Nurses.

Sng, B. L., & Sia, A. T. H. (2017). Maintenance of epidural labor analgesia: The old, the new and the future. *Best Practice & Research Clinical Anaesthesiology, 31*(1), 15–22. DOI: 10.1016/j.bpa.2017.01.002

Wilson, B. A., Shannon, M. T., & Shields, K. (2017). *Pearson nurse's drug guide: 2018.* Hoboken, NJ: Pearson.

Zanardo, V., Volpe, F., Parotto, M., Gilbert, L., Selman, A., & Straface, G. (2017). Nitrous oxide labor analgesia and pain relief memory in breastfeeding women. *Journal of Maternal Fetal Neonatal Medicine,* pp. 1–6. DOI: 10.1080/14767058.2017.1368077

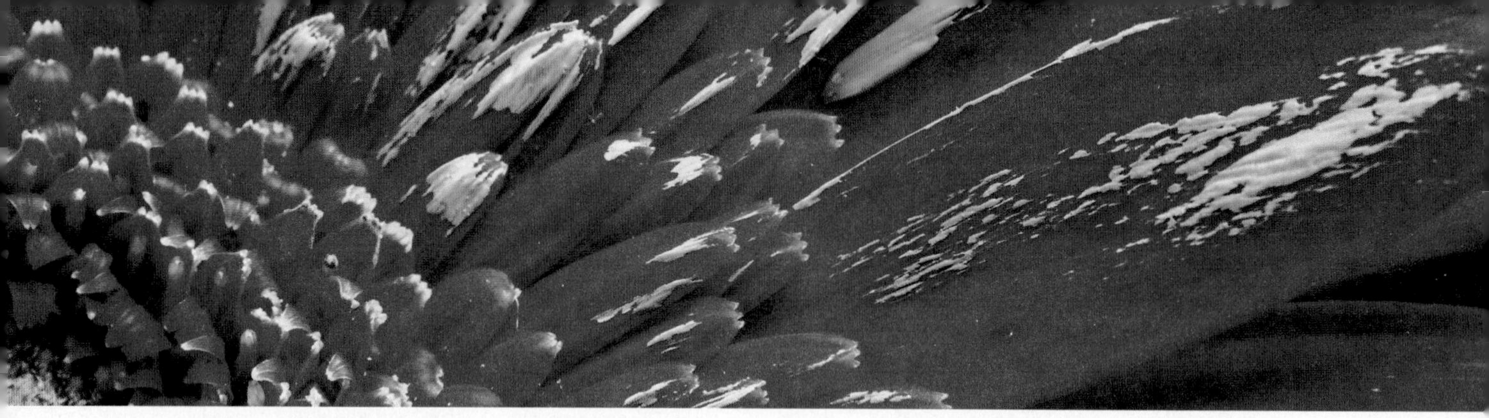

Chapter 23

Childbirth at Risk: Prelabor Onset Complications

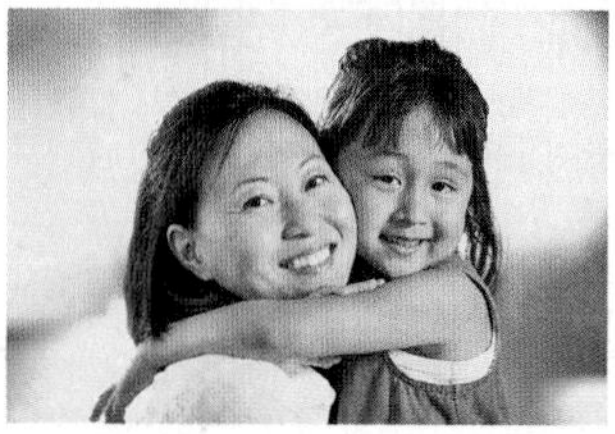

As a fourth-time mother, I was unprepared to deal with the hardship of 6 months of bedrest after having three uncomplicated pregnancies. Each day brought me closer to a safe delivery, but the stress and strain of three active young children and the worry of the condition of my unborn baby made each day a struggle.

SOURCE: Greer & Associates, Inc./Purestock/SuperStock.

Learning Outcomes

23.1 Analyze the implications and maternal and fetal risks of preterm labor.

23.2 Identify the causes and risk factors for premature rupture of membranes.

23.3 Describe the clinical therapy for premature rupture of membranes and preterm labor in determining hospital-based and community-based nursing management of the woman and her fetus-newborn.

23.4 Compare placenta previa and abruptio placentae, including implications for the mother and fetus and their nursing care.

23.5 Discuss the differences between developmental and degenerative placental problems.

23.6 Identify the causes and risk factors of cervical insufficiency.

23.7 Describe the clinical therapies and appropriate nursing interventions for the mother with cervical insufficiency and her unborn fetus.

23.8 Analyze the maternal and fetal-newborn implications and clinical therapy in determining community-based and hospital-based nursing care of the woman with a multiple gestation.

23.9 Describe the identification of the woman with hydramnios and the maternal and fetal-neonatal implications.

23.10 Describe the identification of the woman with oligohydramnios and the maternal and fetal-neonatal implications.

23.11 Compare the clinical therapy and nursing management of the woman with hydramnios and the woman with oligohydramnios.

Healthy People 2020

(MICH-1.2) Reduce the rate of fetal and infant deaths during perinatal period (28 weeks of gestation to less than 7 days after birth)

(MICH-8.1) Reduce low birth weight (LBW)

(MICH-8.2) Reduce very low birth weight (VLBW)

(MICH-9) Reduce preterm births

(MICH-16) Increase the proportion of women delivering a live birth who received preconception care services and practiced key recommended preconception health behaviors

After the first trimester, the majority of pregnancies progress smoothly to term. In some cases, however, complications can occur before the onset of labor that significantly impact the outcome of pregnancy. This chapter presents information related to the most common of these conditions. Labor-related complications are discussed in Chapter 24.

Care of the Woman at Risk Due to Preterm Labor

In 2013, the American College of Obstetricians and Gynecologists (ACOG) introduced new definitions for pregnancy duration. Pregnancy is based on the premise that pregnancies last 40 weeks. ACOG has defined *early-term birth* as birth occurring between 37 weeks and 38 weeks 6 days; *full-term birth* as birth occurring between 39 weeks and 40 weeks 6 days; and *late-term birth* as birth occurring after the 41st week. *Postterm birth* is defined as birth occurring after 42 weeks (ACOG, 2015). **Preterm labor (PTL)** is defined as labor that occurs after 20 and before 37 completed weeks of pregnancy. Prematurity continues to be the number one cause of neonatal mortality and long-term neurologic disabilities in the United States. Preterm birth is the second leading cause of neonatal death after congenital and chromosomal abnormalities, and the economic implications of preterm birth exceed $26 billion per year in healthcare and societal costs (Centers for Disease Control and Prevention [CDC], 2017).

In the United States, preterm births were at a decade low in 2012, but rates have risen slightly. In the United States, 17.7% of African American women give birth prematurely; a little more than 10% of Native American/Alaskan Native populations and a little less than 10% of Caucasian American and Asian American women have premature births (March of Dimes, 2018). It is unclear why racial background plays a role in premature births. In addition, women younger than 17 and older than 35 have increased risk for premature birth (March of Dimes, 2018). Table 23–1 presents a list of risk factors for spontaneous preterm labor.

Maternal Risks

The most significant risk factor for preterm birth is a previous preterm birth. Screening for risk factors prior to pregnancy is one approach to identify women at risk and to reduce or eliminate modifiable risk factors, such as smoking, substance abuse, stress, alcohol use, and other behavioral factors. Screening can be done at regular well-woman visits for women planning pregnancies within the next 1 to 2 years or those who are at risk for an unintended pregnancy. Women should undergo preconception counseling that includes optimal timing of pregnancy and birth, optimal weight and weight gain recommendations, prepregnancy screening for infectious disease, and optimal control of preexisting conditions that increase the risk of preterm labor or increase the risks of needing to undergo an early birth due to maternal medical conditions.

Prenatal teaching aimed at helping women recognize the early signs and symptoms are imperative for early identification of preterm labor. If symptoms do occur, prompt assessment is warranted to confirm or rule out preterm labor. It is important to identify the causal factor so treatment can be initiated; however, there are times when the causal factor is unclear. High-risk women warrant more frequent prenatal visits to monitor for pregnancy complications and for preexisting medical conditions that can result in poor labor outcomes when early birth is indicated. Once an etiological factor is identified, the provider should conduct the proper assessment to initiate appropriate treatments as soon as possible. For women in geographically isolated areas, this may include transfer to a more appropriate medical setting (Davidson, Armstrong, & Sampson, 2016).

Fetal-Neonatal Risks

Mortality increases for newborns born before 37 weeks' gestation. Babies born prior to 32 gestational weeks are nine times more likely to die in the neonatal period (first 4 weeks of life) compared to newborns born at 39 to 40 weeks (Matthews, MacDorman, & Thoma, 2016). In fact, preterm birth accounts for 25% of neonatal deaths and 36% of infant deaths (deaths occurring within the first

TABLE 23–1 Risk Factors for Spontaneous Preterm Labor

Abdominal surgery during the second or third trimester	Foreign body (intrauterine device [IUD])	Native American/Alaskan Native ancestry
Abdominal trauma	History of cervical procedures	Periodontal disease
African ancestry	History of pyelonephritis or other maternal infection	Previous preterm birth
Antepartum hemorrhage	Hypertension	Previous preterm labor with term birth
Age (less than 18 or more than 35)	Intimate partner violence	Prolonged standing or lifting
Anemia	In vitro fertilization (singleton or multiple gestation)	Previous second-trimester abortion
Asymptomatic bacteriuria	Inadequate prenatal care	Sexually transmitted infection (STI) (trichomoniasis, chlamydia)
Bacterial vaginosis, *E. coli* (ascending intrauterine infection)	Insulin-dependent diabetes	Shortened cervical length
Cervical insufficiency; cerclage in place	Lack of social support	Sickle cell disease
Cervix dilated more than 1 cm at 32 weeks	Less than 6-month interval between pregnancies	Stress
Chorioamnionitis	Low maternal weight; poor weight gain	Substance use: Alcohol, drugs, tobacco
Elevated maternal serum alphafetoprotein level	Low socioeconomic status	Urinary tract infections
Exposure to certain environmental toxins	Maternal coagulation disorders	Uterine anomaly; fibroids
Febrile illness	Maternal obesity	Uterine irritability
Fetal abnormality	More than two first-trimester abortions	Uteroplacental ischemia
	Multiple gestation	Vaginal bleeding

SOURCES: Robinson & Norwitz, 2017; Ross, 2017.

12 months of life) (March of Dimes, 2016). Although the preterm baby is faced with many maturational deficiencies (fat storage, heat regulation, immaturity of organ systems), the most critical factor is the lack of development of the respiratory system—to the extent that life cannot be supported.

Periviable birth refers to birth that occurs between 20 0/7 weeks and 25 6/7 weeks of gestation. Babies who are born in this gestational period account for the majority of neonatal deaths and 40% of infant deaths (ACOG, 2016c). **Extremely preterm births** are those that occur prior to 28 gestational weeks and account for 0.5% of all births. While recent research has shown some gains in survivability in extremely premature neonates, despite survival, most extremely premature babies who survive do so with significant neurodevelopmental impairment. For example, of babies born between 22 0/7 and 22 6/7 weeks, only 1% survive and do not have any neurodevelopmental impairment (ACOG & SMFM, 2016). In general, as the gestational age decreases at the time of birth, the level of long-term respiratory, neurocognitive, and visual and auditory deficits increases. These statistics warrant open and honest discussions with expectant parents on the management that they would like to pursue if a periviable birth cannot be prevented. Some may request palliative care measures for the neonate, whereas other parents may request every available resuscitation effort be made (Perinatal Hospice & Palliative Care, 2017). Realistic expectations on the neonate's prognosis, long-term medical complications, and risks of neurodevelopmental complications should be discussed. It is important to remember that it is the parents' decision to make, and healthcare providers should support and guide them through the process. Healthcare providers need to understand that these discussions are associated with significant grief reactions. (Chapter 36 discusses grief and loss in the childbearing family.) It is recommended that the physician meet with the family on more than one occasion to discuss options and clarify information (Perinatal Hospice & Palliative Care, 2017).

In some instances, such as severe maternal diabetes or serious isoimmunization, continuation of the pregnancy may be more life-threatening to the fetus than the hazards of prematurity. See Chapter 30 for in-depth consideration of the preterm newborn. See *Genetic Facts: Genetic Patterns and the Risk of Preterm Birth.*

Genetic Facts Genetic Patterns and the Risk of Preterm Birth

Clinicians have hypothesized for generations that familial patterns can directly impact the risk of preterm birth and the duration of gestations. Genetic studies have now identified gene variants to support these beliefs. Specifically, variants at the *EBF1, EEFSEC, AGTR2, WNT4, ADCY5,* and *RAP2C* loci are associated with gestational duration and variants at the *EBF1, EEFSEC,* and *AGTR2* loci are associated with preterm birth. These genes have also been associated with factors related to uterine development, maternal nutrition, and vascular control (Zhang et al., 2017).

CLINICAL THERAPY

The prevention and treatment of PTL have been widely studied. Current practice supports short-term tocolytic medications used to delay birth by 48 to 72 hours so the maximum benefit of corticosteroids can be administered to reduce the risks of respiratory distress syndrome (RDS). The most commonly used tocolytic agent is nifedipine (Procardia), which has been associated with a reduction in RDS, necrotizing enterocolitis, intraventricular hemorrhage, neonatal jaundice, and admission to the neonatal intensive care unit (NICU) when given prior to 34 weeks' gestation (Ross, 2017).

Survival of newborns prior to 26 gestational weeks is much lower than those born after 27 weeks. Survival outcomes are associated primarily with gestational age, but are also significantly impacted by gestational weight, sex, plurality, and the administration of corticosteroids prior to birth (Ehrenkranz & Mercurio, 2017). Table 23–2 provides an overview of recommended interventions based on periviable fetal gestational age. All women and their families facing a periviable birth should receive supportive nursing care and family-centered teaching on the implications of periviable birth and should be managed by a perinatologist in a Level III medical facility that can provide neonatal intensive care services. For women in rural settings, a transfer to a more appropriate facility should be facilitated as soon as maternal stability has been established.

Diagnosis. The signs and symptoms of PTL are listed in *Key Facts to Remember: Signs and Symptoms of Preterm Labor*. It is important to diagnose PTL as quickly as possible so interventions can be implemented to avoid a preterm birth. Table 23–3 summarizes common criteria for diagnosing PTL.

Key Facts To Remember
Signs and Symptoms of Preterm Labor

- Uterine contractions that occur every 10 minutes or less, with or without pain
- Mild menstrual-like cramps felt low in the abdomen
- Constant or intermittent feelings of pelvic pressure that may feel like the baby pressing down
- Rupture of membranes
- Low, dull backache, which may be constant or intermittent
- A change in vaginal discharge (an increase in amount, a change to more clear and watery, or a pinkish tinge)
- Urinary frequency, urgency, hesitancy, or hematuria
- Abdominal cramping with or without diarrhea

No attempt is made to stop labor if any of the following conditions exists:

- Fetal demise
- Lethal fetal anomaly
- Severe preeclampsia/eclampsia
- Hemorrhage/abruptio placentae
- Chorioamnionitis
- Severe fetal growth restriction
- Fetal maturity
- Category III fetal heart rate tracing
- Gestational age less than 24 weeks
- Oligohydramnios (less than normal amount of amniotic fluid)
- Absent or reversed diastolic flow upon Doppler examination of umbilical blood flow
- Repetitive severe variable decelerations
- Significant vaginal bleeding consistent with abruption, unless patient is stable and fetal well-being is established.

TABLE 23–2 Selected Interventions for Periviable Fetus in Preterm Labor

GESTATIONAL AGE	SUGGESTED INTERVENTIONS
20 0/7 – 21 6/7 weeks	• May consider antenatal antibiotics if preterm premature rupture of membranes (PPROM) without imminent birth and no evidence of chorioamnioitis is present.[1]
22 0/7 – 22 6/7 weeks	• May consider antenatal antibiotics if PPROM without imminent birth and no evidence of chorioamnioitis is present.[1]
23 0/7 – 23 6/7 weeks	• Decision to initiate life-saving measures determined by parental request and clinical assessment. • If interventions desired, ensure facility has NICU and neonatologists available. • May consider tocolytic administration for up to 48 hours.[1] • May consider administration of corticosteroids to facilitate fetal lung maturity if birth is expected within 7 days.[1] • May consider antenatal antibiotics if PPROM without imminent birth and no evidence of chorioamnioitis is present.[1] • May consider a 7-day course of therapy of intravenous ampicillin and erythromycin.[2] • May consider group beta streptococcus (GBS) intrapartum antibiotic treatment regimen.[1] • May consider magnesium sulfate for fetal neuroprotective benefits. • Neonatal consult for consideration of resuscitation of newborn upon birth.[1] • In some cases, a cesarean birth may be considered based on maternal and fetal risk factors.[1]
24 0/7 – 24 6/7 weeks	• Perform comprehensive clinical assessment. • Ensure facility has NICU and neonatologists available; if transfer warranted, transfer as soon as maternal stability is established. • Begin tocolytic administration for up to 48 hours.[2] • Administer corticosteroids to facilitate fetal lung maturity.[2] • If PPROM has occurred, administer a 7-day course of therapy of intravenous ampicillin and erythromycin.[2] • Based on GBS status, intrapartum antibiotic treatment regimen should be initiated.[2] • Administer magnesium sulfate for fetal neuroprotective benefits.[2] • Neonatal consult for resuscitation of newborn upon birth.[1] • In some cases, a cesarean birth may be considered based on maternal and fetal risk factors.[1]
25 0/7 – 25 6/7 weeks	• Perform comprehensive clinical assessment. • Ensure facility has NICU and neonatologists available; if transfer warranted, transfer as soon as maternal stability is established. • Begin tocolytic administration for up to 48 hours.[2] • Administer corticosteroids to facilitate fetal lung maturity.[2] • If PPROM has occurred, administer a 7-day course of therapy of intravenous ampicillin and erythromycin.[2] • Based on GBS status, intrapartum antibiotic treatment regimen should be initiated.[2] • Administer magnesium sulfate for fetal neuroprotective benefits.[2] • Neonatal consult for resuscitation of newborn upon birth.[1] • A cesarean birth may be considered based on maternal and fetal risk factors.[1]

SOURCES: ACOG, 2018; ACOG & SMFM, 2016; Ehrenkranz & Mercurio, 2017.
[1] Little empirical evidence to support recommendations, but may be offered for parents who demand interventions.
[2] Weak empirical evidence exists, but moderate evidence supports recommendation.

TABLE 23–3 Criteria for Diagnosis of Preterm Labor in Gestations of 20 to 36 6/7 Weeks

Uterine contractions every 5 minutes for 20 minutes
or
8 contractions in a 60-minute period
and
Documented cervical change or cervical effacement of 80% or more
or
Cervical dilation greater than 1 cm

Some women have frequent contractions without changes in the cervix. *Fetal fibronectin (fFN)*, an extracellular matrix protein that is an adhesive "glue" produced by the fetal membranes that binds the membranes and placenta to the decidua, may be detected between 22 and 34 weeks in women prior to a preterm birth. Based on this physiological knowledge, fFN testing has been used in preterm gestations as a screening tool to determine if a woman was at risk for preterm birth in the next 7 days.

The presence of fFN in the cervicovaginal fluid is normal in the first half of pregnancy as the gestational sac attaches to the inside of the uterus. After 20 weeks' gestation, its presence is abnormal and can signal inflammatory or mechanical disruption of the fused membranes. fFN is also found in the amniotic fluid, and a positive test can indicate ruptured membranes. Near term, it is normal for fFN to once again appear in vaginal secretions. Negative results are highly predictive in 96.1% of women, meaning that less than 4% of women with a negative fFN test delivered within 7 days (Esplin, Elovitz, & Iams, 2017); however, false positives are more common. There has been some research that has shown that fFN testing using quantitative values (producing a numerical value) rather than qualitative values (positive/negative) may produce more accurate findings (Esplin et al., 2017).

False-positive testing results can be associated with recent sexual intercourse, vaginal examination, bacterial vaginosis, and vaginal bleeding. As the body of evidence continues to evolve, the predictive value of true positive testing has become a source of debate because fFN does not provide a good indication of those women who will give birth in the next 14 days. ACOG (2016c) does not recommend routine screening, although some clinicians continue to utilize fFN testing as a tool among other factors to guide clinical decision making.

Contraction frequency alone is not enough to establish a diagnosis of preterm labor. A woman suspected of being in PTL should have a digital cervical examination once rupture of the membranes has been ruled out. If fFN testing is planned, this should be performed before a digital or endovaginal ultrasound exam. Electronic fetal monitoring should take place for a minimum of 1 to 2 hours to detect uterine contractions.

Assessing cervical length by endovaginal ultrasonography is another diagnostic tool that has been used to identify a preterm birth. Demonstrated cervical change or presumed prior cervical change (transvaginal cervical length less than 20 mm, cervical effacement greater than 50%, or cervical dilation greater than or equal to 2 cm) has been the criteria used for diagnosis of preterm birth when contractions are present. In addition, cervical length of at least 30 mm (3 cm) is good evidence that the woman is not in PTL. However, some women have shorter cervical lengths and do not give birth prematurely; hence, cervical length should be part of a more extensive clinical assessment and not the only identifiable diagnostic factor. A cervical length of less than 20 mm in the presence of regular contractions, or a digital exam that identifies the cervix to be 3 cm or more dilated or 80% or more effaced in the presence of regular contractions, establishes the diagnosis of PTL (ACOG, 2016c).

Interventions. Intervention to reduce preterm birth can be divided into primary prevention and secondary prevention. Primary prevention includes diagnosis and treatment of infections, progesterone administration, and cervical cerclage.

Primary Prevention Strategies. Maternal bacterial infection has been implicated as a causative factor of PTL, with microbial invasion of the amniotic cavity present in approximately 10% of women with PTL (Gabbe et al., 2016). The microbial colonization may even precede conception and ascend from the cervix and vagina into the uterus. A woman who is diagnosed with a sexually transmitted infection (STI) has a 25% risk of becoming reinfected within the next 12 months (CDC, 2015). Lower genital tract infections that are associated with preterm birth include bacterial vaginosis (BV), trichomoniasis, chlamydia, urinary group B streptococcus (GBS), mycoplasmas, gonorrhea, high concentration of anaerobes, and aerobic Gram-negative rods. It is hypothesized that there may be an association with the ability of a species of bacteria to stimulate prostaglandin production.

BV is the most common lower genital tract infection among women of reproductive age and has consistently been associated with increased risks of PTL, preterm premature rupture of membranes (PPROM), spontaneous abortion, chorioamnionitis, endometritis, and cesarean section wound infections. In spite of this, it remains unclear whether screening and treatment of BV will reduce the frequency of these complications (CDC, 2015). Treatment of BV in low-risk populations has not been shown to improve obstetric outcomes, but some studies have shown that women with a history of preterm birth who received oral treatment with metronidazole or clindamycin had a reduction in preterm birth or premature rupture of membranes (PROM).

An estimated 20 to 30% of all women are GBS carriers. Neonatal infection from GBS is a potentially severe consequence of maternal GBS infection; nevertheless, there is no association of preterm birth and vaginal GBS colonization. Women with preterm labor should be screened for GBS, and if birth is possible, positive women should be treated with an antibiotic therapy regimen. Women at risk for birth with unknown GBS status should also be treated to prevent neonatal infection. GBS is discussed more fully in Chapter 18.

PTL is also associated with urinary tract infections (UTIs), so it is prudent to obtain a clean-catch or catheterized urine specimen to identify and treat the infection. If untreated, asymptomatic bacteriuria is associated with increased risks of pyelonephritis later in pregnancy and a significant increase in preterm birth (Impey & Child, 2017). Even asymptomatic bacteriuria alone increases the risk of preterm birth; therefore, screening and treatment of all pregnant women at the first prenatal visit are important components of care. Women with a positive culture should be retested following therapy to ensure that the infection is resolved. Because asymptomatic bacteriuria is common during pregnancy, women with frequent UTIs can be given low-dose suppression therapy with daily antibiotics.

Women with risk factors for bacteriuria or urinary tract infections should be screened at more frequent intervals. A urine dip at each visit can be used to assess for leukocytes and proteinuria. Women living in poverty have a five-fold increased incidence of bacteriuria. Women with sickle cell trait have double the risk of bacteriuria. Other risk factors for bacteriuria include diabetes mellitus, neurogenic bladder retention, history of vesicoureteral reflux (treated or untreated), previous renal transplantation, and a history of previous UTIs (Brusch, 2017).

A link has been identified between preterm, low-birth-weight newborns and gum disease, and it suggests that periodontal treatment during pregnancy reduces preterm birth (Puertas et al., 2017).

Progesterone supplementation (hydroxyprogesterone) is recommended for the prevention of recurrent preterm birth for women with a singleton pregnancy and a prior spontaneous preterm birth due to spontaneous preterm labor or premature rupture of membranes. Hydroxyprogesterone should be initiated in at-risk women at 16 to 21 weeks' gestation. Vaginal progesterone 100 mg twice per day is the usual dosage and route. Intramuscular progesterone 250 mg (1mL) is also effective, but is associated with injection site pain and may be associated with additional healthcare costs (nurse's visit, injection fees, etc.). Progesterone is normally produced by the corpus luteum in early pregnancy and is maintained through placental production after 12 weeks. Progesterone promotes uterine relaxation, suppresses contractions, and prevents gestational immune tolerance (Impey & Child, 2017). If the efficacy of progesterone is a result of immune suppression, this may explain why progestogens can be effective if given prophylactically but not once labor has started. Progesterone supplementation is not typically used in multiple gestations.

Cervical cerclage is a surgical intervention used as a primary preventive strategy and involves the placement of a suture to prevent dilatation and effacement of the cervix. This is done to prevent cervical insufficiency in women with a previous history of painless cervical dilatation that has resulted in a second-trimester birth or a fetal loss that occurred in a previous pregnancy. (Cervical insufficiency and cerclage is discussed in detail later in the chapter.)

Secondary Prevention Strategies. Secondary prevention strategies include antibiotic treatment, emergency cervical cerclage placement, and tocolysis.

Antibiotics are used to treat infection that may occur during pregnancy, most commonly, vaginal or urinary infections. The antibiotic selected is based on culture results and what is most effective for that organism. Drug allergies should be reviewed and updated in the electronic medical record (EMR) prior to prescribing new medications. The nurse reinforces the need to take all of the medication, regardless if symptoms have resolved. Once the woman has completed the antibiotic regimen, a follow-up culture is done to confirm the infection is no longer present. If the infection is one that is sexually transmitted, the woman should be advised not to have sexual relations and should ensure her partner is treated as well. Both partners should have a test of culture. Condoms are an effective way to reduce reinfection between partners and should be recommended as a means of reducing the woman's risk of contracting the infection again.

Women who experience painless premature dilatation are at a significant risk for fetal loss or extremely preterm birth. If a shortened cervix is identified on a routine second-trimester exam, an *emergency* or *rescue* cerclage may be placed. Cerclage placement can be performed if the cervix has not completely effaced and if the membranes have not ruptured.

Tocolysis is the use of medications in an attempt to stop labor. These medications may delay birth for 24 to 48 hours (ACOG, 2016c). Although the delay of childbirth in itself may not improve neonatal outcome, it may permit the administration of betamethasone for fetal surfactant induction or allow for the transport of the mother to a tertiary care facility where equipment, services, and specialized and appropriately trained staff are present. If labor cannot be arrested, the priority becomes successful preterm birth and management of its psychologic effect on the woman and her partner.

The selection of a short-term tocolytic should be made based on maternal history and risk factors. There are several different drugs currently used for tocolysis including beta-adrenergic agonists (also called β-mimetics or β-agonists) (terbutaline), magnesium sulfate, calcium channel blockers (nifedipine), and prostaglandin synthetase inhibitors (celecoxib, sulindac, indomethacin, ketorolac). Terbutaline was once used extensively for preterm labor, but in 2011, a black box warning was issued; evidence indicates that prolonged terbutaline use is associated with maternal cardiac arrhythmias; therefore, the use of terbutaline should not exceed 48 to 72 hours (Cunningham et al., 2016).

There is no clear choice for a tocolytic; instead, a pharmacologic agent is chosen on an individual basis based on the presentation of labor and maternal history. The use of β-mimetics does pose a significant risk to the mother in PTL. β-mimetics, which may be administered intravenously, intramuscularly, subcutaneously, or orally, can significantly affect maternal cardiovascular and metabolic physiology. The most serious effects include hypotension, cardiac arrhythmia, tachycardia, palpitations, myocardial ischemia, pulmonary edema, and maternal hyperglycemia.

Magnesium sulfate is often selected as the tocolytic of choice in preterm labor due to its effectiveness in short-term reduction in labor contractions and its neuroprotective fetal effects. Magnesium sulfate should not be used in conjunction with select medications, such as calcium channel blockers, or when myasthenia gravis or neuromuscular disorders exist (ACOG, 2016c). The usual recommended loading dose is 4 to 6 g intravenously in 100 mL of intravenous (IV) fluid over 20 minutes. The maintenance dose is then 2 to 4 g/hr titrated to deep tendon reflexes and serum magnesium levels. The therapy is maintained for 12 to 24 hours at the lowest rate to significantly diminish contractions (Wilson, Shannon, & Shields, 2017). The infusion is typically continued so that two doses of corticosteroids can be administered to promote fetal lung maturation. The maternal serum level that is usually necessary for tocolysis seems to be 5.5 to 7.5 mg/dL.

Side effects with the loading dose may include flushing, a feeling of warmth, headache, nystagmus, nausea, dry mouth, and dizziness. Other side effects include lethargy and sluggishness and a risk of pulmonary edema if the woman has predisposing conditions such as multiple gestation or infection; has had excessive IV fluid administration; or has concurrent β-sympathomimetic therapy (ACOG, 2016c). Fetal side effects may include hypotonia and lethargy that persist for 1 or 2 days following birth, hypoglycemia, and hypocalcemia.

Of the calcium channel blockers approved for use in the United States, nifedipine is the most frequently used as a tocolytic. Nifedipine acts by reducing the flow of extracellular calcium ions into the intracellular space of the myometrial smooth muscle cells, thereby inhibiting contractile activity. Nifedipine is well absorbed either orally or sublingually, has fewer side effects than comparative agents, and is just as effective (ACOG, 2016c). The most common side effects are related to arterial vasodilation, that is, hypotension, tachycardia, facial flushing, and headache. Because the mechanism of action of nifedipine is different from the beta-adrenergic drugs, coadministration of nifedipine and terbutaline or ritodrine may prove beneficial in the treatment of PTL. Because both magnesium sulfate and nifedipine block calcium, however, coadministration of them has been implicated in serious maternal side effects related to low calcium levels and has resulted in maternal cardiovascular collapse. Nifedipine is contraindicated in women with heart disease, cardiovascular compromise, intrauterine infection, multiple pregnancy, and maternal hypertension (ACOG, 2016c).

Prostaglandins enhance the formation of myometrial gap junctions and stimulate the influx of intracellular calcium ions needed for muscle contraction. Prostaglandin synthetase inhibitors, therefore, are a logical choice for tocolysis. Indomethacin, sulindac, or celecoxib are the prostaglandin synthetase inhibitors most often used to suppress labor. Maternal side effects are few. Dyspepsia, nausea and vomiting, depression, and dizzy spells may occur. On rare occasions, psychosis or renal failure may result. These drugs are best administered with an antacid or taken with meals to reduce the chance of gastrointestinal (GI) upset. Prostaglandin synthetase inhibitors are generally not used in women with drug-induced asthma, coagulation disorders, hepatic or renal insufficiency, or peptic ulcer disease.

Indomethacin crosses the placenta readily, and oligohydramnios and premature closure of the fetal ductus arteriosus may occur with long-term use. Consequently the drug, which is no longer widely used, is not recommended after 34 weeks' gestation or for a course of therapy longer than 48 hours. Indomethacin has been associated with necrotizing enterocolitis in the newborn with long-term use. Indomethacin may be considered for longer use in very preterm laboring women when the risks of extreme prematurity outweigh potential complications (Dutta, Behnia, Harirah, et al., 2016).

The National Institute of Child Health and Human Development (NICHD) recommends that corticosteroids (typically betamethasone or dexamethasone) be administered antenatally to women at risk of preterm birth because of their beneficial effect on fetal lung maturation. Any women who are candidates for tocolysis are candidates for antenatal corticosteroids, regardless of fetal gender, race, or availability of surfactant therapy for the newborn, especially between 24 and 34 weeks' gestation.

●○● NURSING MANAGEMENT

For the Woman at Risk for Preterm Labor

Nursing Assessment and Diagnosis

During the antepartum period, identify the woman at risk for PTL by noting the presence of predisposing factors. The primary areas for ongoing assessment are change in risk status for PTL, educational needs of the woman and her partner/family members, and the woman's responses to medical and nursing interventions.

Nursing diagnoses that may apply to the woman with PTL include:

- ***Knowledge, Readiness for Enhanced,*** related to an expressed desire to understand the causes, identification, and treatment of PTL and its implications
- ***Fear*** related to early labor and birth
- ***Coping, Ineffective,*** related to need for constant attention to pregnancy
- ***Anxiety*** related to the possibility of a preterm birth (PTB)

(NANDA-I © 2017)

Nursing Plan and Implementation

Community-Based Nursing Care

Once uterine activity stops, the woman is sometimes placed on continued pharmacologic therapy. Some insurance companies provide care management by nurses who provide risk assessment over the phone and opportunities for questions and support as a means of preventing preterm births and reducing costs associated with preterm births.

Home Care

Outpatient management of a woman at risk for preterm birth includes frequent office visits to assess symptoms and cervical length and in-depth patient education about the signs and symptoms of PTL.

> **Women with Special Needs** **Uterine Monitoring**
>
> For women with mobility disabilities, such as paralysis or neuromuscular conditions, that cause an inability to feel uterine contractions, home uterine monitoring may be considered.

The woman's ability to care for herself, the impact of the changes in relationships that will occur, and care of any young children in the home are among the issues that affect the woman's ability to cope effectively with this situation. Be alert to any signs that the woman is failing to achieve the emotional and developmental tasks of pregnancy, such as lack of maternal attachment. An individualized nursing management plan helps focus on each woman's specific needs.

Health Promotion

Once the woman at risk for PTL has been identified, teach her about the importance of recognizing the onset of labor. Increasing the woman's awareness of the subtle symptoms of PTL is one of your most important teaching objectives (see *Teaching Highlights: Preterm Labor*).

Teach her also to evaluate contraction activity once or twice a day. The woman does so by lying down tilted to one side with a pillow behind her back for support. She places her fingertips on the fundus of the uterus (which is above the umbilicus after 20 weeks' gestation). She checks for contractions (hardening or tightening in the uterus) for about 1 hour. It is important for the pregnant woman to know that uterine contractions occur occasionally throughout the pregnancy. If they occur every 10 minutes for 1 hour, however, the cervix could begin to dilate, and labor could continue.

Ensure that the woman knows when to report signs and symptoms. If contractions occur every 10 minutes (or less) for 1 hour, if any of the other signs and symptoms is present for 1 hour, or if clear fluid begins leaking from the vagina, she should telephone her physician/CNM, clinic, or hospital birthing unit and make arrangements to be checked for ongoing labor. If the woman experiences any PTL symptoms for more than 15 minutes while physically active, instruct her to:

- Empty her bladder
- Lie down tilted toward her side
- Drink 3 to 4 (8 oz) cups of fluid
- Palpate for uterine contractions, and if contractions occur 10 minutes apart or less for 1 hour, notify the healthcare provider
- Soak in a warm tub bath
- Rest for 30 minutes after the symptoms have subsided and gradually resume activity
- Call her healthcare provider if symptoms persist, even if uterine contractions are not palpable.

Caregivers need to be aware that the woman is knowledgeable and attuned to changes in her body and to take her call seriously. When a woman is at risk for PTL, she may have many episodes of contractions and other signs or symptoms. If she is treated positively, she will feel freer to report problems as they arise. Other preventive measures the woman might follow are presented in Table 23–4.

> **TEACHING HIGHLIGHTS** | Preterm Labor
>
> - Describe the dangers of preterm labor, especially the risk of prematurity in the baby, and all the potential problems.
> - Explain that many of the early symptoms of labor, such as backache and increased bloody show, may be subtle initially.
> - Describe the signs and symptoms of preterm labor (refer to *Key Facts to Remember: Signs and Symptoms of Preterm Labor*).
> - Summarize self-care measures (see Table 23–4) the woman can take to prevent preterm labor.
> - Teach the woman how to palpate for uterine contractions. Demonstrate and ask for a return demonstration.

TABLE 23–4 Self-Care Measures to Prevent Preterm Labor

- Rest two or three times a day, lying on your left side.
- Drink 2 to 3 quarts of water or liquids each day. Avoid caffeine drinks. Filling a quart container and drinking from it will eliminate the need to keep track of numerous glasses of fluid.
- Empty your bladder at least every 2 hours during waking hours.
- Avoid lifting heavy objects. If small children are in the home, work out alternatives for picking them up, such as sitting on a chair and having them climb on your lap.
- Pace necessary activities to avoid overexertion.
- Sexual activity may need to be curtailed or eliminated.
- Find pleasurable ways to help compensate for limitations of activities and boost the spirits.
- Try to focus on 1 day or 1 week at a time rather than on longer periods of time.

SOURCE: Prepared in consultation with the Prematurity Prevention Program at the University of Washington Medical Center.

Hospital-Based Nursing Care

Providing supportive nursing care to the woman in PTL is important during hospitalization. This care consists of promoting rest, monitoring vital signs, measuring intake and output, and continuously monitoring fetal heart rate (FHR) and uterine contractions. Activities that increase uterine contractions should be avoided. Placing the woman on her left side facilitates maternal-fetal circulation. Vaginal examinations are kept to a minimum. If tocolytic agents are being administered, the mother and fetus are monitored closely for any adverse effects.

Whether PTL is arrested or proceeds, the woman and her family experience intense psychologic stress. Decreasing the anxiety associated with the unknown and the risk of a preterm newborn is one of your primary aims. Recognize the stress of prolonged bedrest and lack of sexual contact with her husband or partner and help the couple find satisfactory ways of dealing with these stresses. With empathetic communication, facilitate the couple's expression of their feelings, which commonly include guilt and anxiety, thereby helping the couple identify and implement coping mechanisms. Keep the couple informed about the labor progress, the treatment regimen, and the status of the fetus so that their full cooperation can be elicited. In the event of imminent vaginal or cesarean birth, offer the couple brief but ongoing explanations to prepare them for the actual birth process and the events following the birth. You may also offer to arrange consultations for the woman and her support person with the neonatologist, social worker, or hospital chaplain, if requested. See *Case Study: Benita Cartier*.

Evaluation

Expected outcomes of nursing care include:

- The woman can discuss the cause, diagnosis, and treatment of PTL.
- The woman affirms that her fears about early labor are decreased.
- The woman states that she feels comfortable in her ability to cope with her situation and has resources to call on, if needed.
- The woman can identify signs and symptoms of PTL that need to be reported to her caregiver.
- The woman can describe appropriate self-care measures to initiate in the event that she experiences any symptoms of PTL.
- The woman successfully gives birth to a healthy baby.

Care of the Woman with Premature Rupture of Membranes

Spontaneous rupture of the membranes before the onset of labor is known as **premature rupture of membranes (PROM)**. Some authorities define PROM as the rupture of the bag of waters any time after 37 completed weeks but before the onset of labor; some have further defined PROM as a specific period elapsed without labor, generally between 1 and 12 hours. PROM occurs in 8% of all pregnancies, with 95% of women giving birth within 28 hours (ACOG, 2016c). **Preterm PROM (PPROM)** is described as rupture of the membranes before 37 weeks' gestation and is associated with more adverse outcomes, specifically related to prematurity. **Prolonged rupture of the membranes** is rupture more than 24 hours before birth.

In the United States, PPROM complicates approximately 3% of pregnancies each year and is associated with more than 50% of preterm births (ACOG, 2016c). Pregnancies complicated with PPROM are associated with intra-amniotic infection (15 to 25%), postpartum infection (15 to 20%), and abruptio placentae (2 to 5%).

CASE STUDY: Benita Cartier

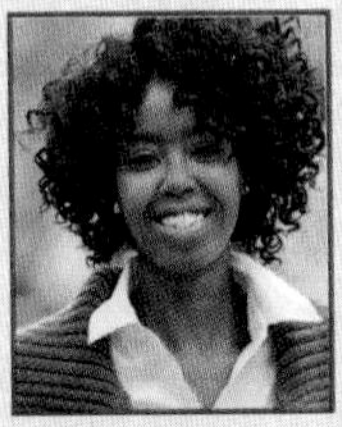

SOURCE: blvdone/Shutterstock.

Benita has been caring for her 25-month-old daughter while her husband, who is a pilot, has a series of flights out of the country. They have been walking down to the playground throughout the summer months. Benita notes achiness in her lower pelvis and cramping. When questioned further, she notes a semiregular pattern and feels they could be contractions. She is concerned because she has several risk factors including chronic hypertension, a previous history of preeclampsia, sickle cell trait, and a history of urinary tract infections. Based on her medical history and risk factors, she is advised to come in for evaluation. When she arrives, Benita asks you what tests will likely be performed.

Question to Ponder

What types of assessments and laboratory testing do you anticipate will be ordered?

Infection rates increase with the degree of prematurity, with younger gestational ages being more likely to develop infection. When cases of PPROM occur prior to 24 weeks' gestation, it is associated with a 95% mortality rate (Linehan et al., 2016).

Whereas preterm labor tends to be the cause of preterm birth in more educated and affluent women, PPROM is seen more frequently in women with lower socioeconomic status (CDC, 2017). Although the cause of PPROM is unknown, it is thought that PPROM occurs because of multiple, interrelated factors. One of the most significant risk factors for PPROM are previous preterm birth and previous PPROM; hence, cervical insufficiency may be the cause of second-trimester PPROM. Other risks factors include:

- Cervicitis
- Urinary tract infection
- Gonorrhea infection
- Asymptomatic bacteriuria
- Amniocentesis
- Placenta previa
- Abruptio placentae
- Hydramnios
- History of laser conization or loop electrosurgical excision procedure (LEEP)
- Multiple pregnancy
- Maternal genital tract anomalies
- Smoking
- Substance abuse
- Connective tissue disorders
- Fetal anomalies.

Once membranes have ruptured, the majority of women proceed to active labor and deliver soon after PPROM. With appropriate therapy and conservative management, approximately 50% of all pregnancies deliver within a week after the membranes have ruptured. Resealing of membranes is uncommon and occurs in less than 10% of pregnancies, mostly subsequent to amniocentesis (Jazayeri, 2017). See *Evidence-Based Practice: Initial Management of Preterm Premature Rupture of Membranes.*

EVIDENCE-BASED PRACTICE | Initial Management of Preterm Premature Rupture of Membranes

Clinical Question

What is best practice for initial management of preterm premature rupture of membranes?

The Evidence

Preterm premature rupture of membranes (PPROM), also referred to as *preterm prelabor rupture of membranes*, affects approximately 3% of all pregnancies in the United States. PROM is defined as rupture of the membranes before 37 weeks of gestation and before the onset of labor. It is a major cause of the 12% of births that are preterm and it carries significant risks of neonatal morbidity and mortality. Management of PPROM is influenced by complicating factors (e.g., clinical infection) and gestational age of the fetus. Accurate gestational estimation and assessment of maternal and fetal risks will necessarily drive the approach to treating PPROM.

The American College of Obstetricians and Gynecologists (ACOG, 2018) issued a Practice Bulletin updating the optimal method of initial management of a mother with PPROM. This was based on a systematic review of evidence and expert knowledge and forms the strongest level of evidence for practice.

In all women who present with PPROM, gestational age, fetal presentation, and fetal well-being should be determined. The initial assessment should evaluate for signs of infection, placental issues, and fetal compromise. Most women with PPROM will deliver within 96 hours. The most significant complication for the mother is intrauterine infection; for the baby, prematurity causes the most mortality and morbidity (ACOG, 2018).

Initial management of PPROM generally falls into two categories: Expectant management, involving hospital-based monitoring and watchful waiting, or induction using an oxytocin infusion. Expectant management is appropriate when the fetus is less than 34 weeks' gestation and no fetal or maternal contraindications exist. In these cases, mothers should be given antenatal corticosteroids and antibiotics to attempt to gain fetal maturation to viability. The mother should be carefully counseled about the potential complications of ongoing pregnancy without intact membranes (ACOG, 2018).

For fetuses at 34 weeks' or greater gestation, the meta-analysis reported in this guideline found that induction of labor reduced the time from rupture of membrane to birth, and as a result, rates of intrauterine infection were lower. The largest trial also concluded that women found induction of labor less stressful than watchful waiting and viewed their labor more positively than women who were managed expectantly. There was no evidence to support the use of prophylactic antibiotics to reduce infection rates in the absence of a confirming culture of group B streptococci (ACOG, 2018).

Best Practice

Expectant management is appropriate for women who experience PPROM before 34 weeks' gestation. Medical treatment and monitoring are essential to gain further fetal maturation. Outpatient management has not been sufficiently studied to establish safety and is not recommended. Women who experience PPROM after 34 weeks' gestation will benefit from labor induction if natural labor does not immediately commence. This approach is recommended for all women with ruptured membranes after 34 weeks' gestation. However, expectant management may be acceptable for these mothers who do not desire induction if there are no maternal complications and fetal conditions are monitored and reassuring. These women should be counseled about the risks of prolonged PPROM without delivery (ACOG, 2018).

Clinical Reasoning

Develop a counseling plan for a woman with preterm premature rupture of the membranes. What are the most important risks and benefits to discuss with the mother? What assessments should be carried out during the monitoring period?

Maternal Risks

Maternal risk is related to infection, specifically *chorioamnionitis* (intra-amniotic infection resulting from bacterial invasion and inflammation of the membranes before birth) and *endometritis* (postpartum infection of the endometrium that may be related to chorioamnionitis or may occur independently).

Chorioamnionitis is more common in women with a history of premature birth, preterm labor, and premature rupture of membranes. The incidence of chorioamnionitis rises with earlier gestations. Infection is the primary causative factor in 40 to 60% of all preterm births (Sherman, 2017). Collection of amniotic fluid by amniocentesis permits analysis of the fluid for subclinical chorioamnionitis. Gram stain, white cell count, glucose concentration, and culture of the fluid are useful in determining treatment; however, the results of the amniotic fluid culture could take as long as 48 hours. Placenta cultures are also used to assess for chorioamnioitis. Placental inflammation is present in 42% of preterm births of extreme low-birth-weight neonates. Blood cultures are another means of assessing for neonatal infection, although the screening is typically limited to newborns who are febrile or symptomatic. In addition, fluid gathered either by amniocentesis or from fluid that has pooled in the vagina can be analyzed for fetal lung maturity. The lecithin/surfactant ratio is the biochemical marker associated with fetal lung maturity. A ratio greater than 2:0 is associated with fetal lung maturity. When the fetal lungs are mature, the risk of serious pulmonary complication in newborns is minimal, and labor is allowed to progress naturally.

Abruptio placentae occurs more frequently in women with PPROM. It is not clear whether infection causes inflammation of the decidua, which facilitates premature separation, or whether the bleeding episode contributes to a weakening of the membranes, which eventually leads to rupture. Childbirth may be complicated by malpresentation and reduced amniotic fluid volume (Gabbe et al., 2016).

Fetal-Neonatal Risks

The most significant cause of neonatal morbidity and mortality is prematurity and its associated complications such as respiratory distress syndrome, necrotizing enterocolitis, and intraventricular hemorrhage (see Chapter 31). Neonatal infection (sepsis) occurs in 2 to 4% of newborns, but the preterm newborn is much more likely to develop sepsis and die than a baby born at term. Fetal hypoxia may occur from cord prolapse or cord compression. In cases of early, prolonged PPROM, the oligohydramnios that occurs may result in fetal pulmonary hypoplasia, facial anomalies, limb position defects, and fetal growth restriction (Sherman, 2017).

CLINICAL THERAPY

Any time a pregnant woman complains of watery vaginal discharge or a sudden gush of fluid, rupture of the membranes must be considered. The woman should be questioned about the time of initial loss of fluid; if continuous leaking is occurring; the color, consistency, and amount of the fluid; and any odor noted. These questions not only help to determine whether there is blood, meconium, or vernix present but also may help to differentiate PROM/PPROM from increased vaginal secretions associated with infection or preterm labor, urinary incontinence, normal leukorrhea of pregnancy, or the passage of the mucous plug.

During the initial physical inspection, any fluid leaking from the vaginal introitus can be checked with nitrazine paper or nitrazine swabs. This test relies on the fact that amniotic fluid is more alkaline (pH 7 to 7.5) than normal vaginal secretions (pH 4.5 to 5.5). A color change in the paper to blue-green or blue is highly suggestive of ruptured membranes. Factors that can yield a false-positive result are contamination of the fluid with semen, urine, 50% or more blood in the specimen, or antiseptic cleansers and soap. The elevated pH associated with bacterial vaginosis can also lead to misleading results. If there is copious fluid leaking from the vaginal introitus, the diagnosis of PROM/PPROM is considered to be confirmed.

If further evaluation is required, a sterile speculum exam is done. Unless the woman is in active labor, direct digital exam of the cervix or vagina is avoided until PPROM is ruled out or a management plan has been determined. Speculum exam relies on gross pooling of amniotic fluid in the vaginal vault. The woman can be asked to "bear down," performing a Valsalva maneuver, if fluid is not visualized in the vagina. The woman may also remain in a supine position for several hours to allow collection of fluid to occur; the exam is then repeated.

In addition to performing a nitrazine test on the fluid, a fern test can be performed by applying a thin sample of secretions onto a clean slide and looking for microscopic evidence of a fernlike pattern (see Figure 4–1B). Rapid bedside immunoassay tests can be used to detect amniotic fluid proteins in cervicovaginal fluids and confirm or rule out rupture of membranes. The Amnisure ROM and the ROM Plus are two commercially available tests that can be utilized when PROM/PPROM cannot be confirmed by other methods or when obstetric providers are not available in a practice setting; however, it is reserved for these circumstances because the test is costly (Igbinosa, Moore, Johnson, et al., 2017). Traditional methods of confirmation, such as patient history, positive nitrazine testing, and positive ferning, have high degrees of accuracy. Vaginal cultures for group B streptococcus, chlamydia, and gonorrhea may be obtained at this time. Ultrasound can be used in conjunction with other tests to look for reduced amniotic fluid.

Concurrently, fetal well-being should be assessed through a fetal heart rate tracing or biophysical profile. In addition, the gestational age of the fetus must be calculated to decide on a management plan (Table 23–5). At greater than 36 weeks' gestation, labor will begin in 50% of women within 12 hours. Labor induction may be delayed for 12 to 24 hours unless a situation exists that would preclude expectant management. In fetuses of less than 32 weeks' gestation, antenatal magnesium sulfate has been shown to reduce the incidence of cerebral palsy (ACOG, 2016c).

Management of PPROM in the absence of infection and gestation of less than 37 weeks is usually conservative. Amniocentesis may be done to evaluate for intra-amniotic infection. Fetal lung maturity studies will also be done if the fetus is nearing 34 weeks' gestation. The woman is hospitalized on bedrest. Upon admission, a complete blood count (CBC) and urinalysis are obtained. Nonstress tests (NSTs) or biophysical profiles are used to monitor fetal well-being. Typically, NSTs are performed every shift (8–12 hours per institution policy) or the frequency is determined by physician/CNM order. Biophysical profiles should be performed every 24 hours (Gabbe et al., 2016). Maternal blood pressure, pulse, and temperature are assessed every 4 hours. Regular laboratory evaluations should be performed to detect maternal infection.

If PPROM occurs and a cerclage is already in place, management is based on the gestational age. In pregnancies less than 23 weeks, the cerclage should be removed (AGOG, 2016a). Cerclages that are left in place require close monitoring to ensure they are intact and not strained, pulling, or in danger of tearing from uterine contractility. (Cervical insufficiency and the cerclage procedure are discussed later in the chapter.)

When a woman chooses conservative treatment, she is advised to continue bedrest (with bathroom privileges); monitor her temperature four times a day; keep a fetal movement record; and avoid intercourse, douches, or insertion of any object into the

TABLE 23–5 Currently Used Plans for Women with Premature Rupture of Membranes

Preterm

- Expectant management (observation); birth when labor or clinical infection develops
- Fetal pulmonary status determined by amniotic fluid testing; birth if fetus is mature
- Risk of infection determined by amniotic fluid Gram stain; white cell count, glucose, and culture; maternal white cell count and assessment for maternal fever or uterine tenderness; assessment for fetal well-being through electronic fetal monitoring or ultrasound for biophysical profile scoring; birth if infection develops
- Penicillin G or ampicillin for treatment of group B streptococcus (GBS), or antibiotic prophylaxis if GBS status unknown in gestations above 24 weeks
- Adjunctive antibiotic therapy with erythromycin or azithromycin for 7 days to increase latency period from PPROM to birth if the fetus is more than 24 gestational weeks
- Administration of corticosteroids, with or without birth in 48 hours after first dose; tocolytics as needed to delay birth for 48 hours to promote fetal lung maturity in fetuses greater than 24 weeks
- Birth after an arbitrary latent period (e.g., 16–72 hours)
- Assess for GBS, chlamydia, or *Neisseria gonorrhoeae*; treatment indicated if positive
- Combinations of the above

Term

- Induction if spontaneous labor does not begin in approximately 12 hours, if cervix is ripe, or if there are other complications (e.g., preeclampsia)
- Expectant management for women with uncomplicated pregnancies and cervix unfavorable for induction

vagina ("pelvic rest"). The woman is advised to contact her provider and return to the hospital if she has fever (100.4°F or higher), uterine tenderness or contractions, increased leakage of fluid, decreased fetal movement, or a foul vaginal discharge. During this time, twice-weekly NSTs and CBCs and weekly ultrasound and cervical visualization may be completed. Research indicates no significant difference in latency periods, gestational age at birth, infection, or perinatal outcomes between home care and hospitalization when this regimen is followed (Gabbe et al., 2016).

Authorities disagree regarding the ideal management of PPROM. Prophylactic antibiotics are administered to any woman with an unknown GBS status or a history of a positive culture during the present pregnancy (Gabbe et al., 2016). The goal of antibiotic use for PPROM is to treat or prevent ascending infection to prolong the interval from rupture of membranes to childbirth. Antibiotic use may also allow sufficient time for corticosteroids used to enhance fetal lung maturity to take effect. In addition, the neonatal mortality rate is significantly lower in newborns whose mothers received antibiotics (ACOG, 2016c). If vaginal cultures are positive, antibiotics will be continued for at least 7 days. If amniotic fluid studies indicate a low glucose level, high white blood cell (WBC) count, a positive Gram stain, or organisms in the fluid, immediate birth is indicated.

Betamethasone, a corticosteroid, decreases the likelihood of neonatal respiratory distress syndrome, necrotizing enterocolitis, intraventricular hemorrhage, and perinatal death in neonates who are born prematurely. Administration of single-course betamethasone (12 mg intramuscularly [IM] with a second dose in 24 hours or dexamethasone 6 mg IM every 12 hours for two doses) is the current recommendation to increase fetal lung maturity (ACOG, 2016c). Respiratory status is a significant indicator of death rates, long-term survival, and presence of long-term neurodevelopmental impairments. The National Institutes of Health (NIH), ACOG, and the Royal College of Medicine (RCP) all recommend corticosteroid administration for any fetus between 24 0/7 weeks and 33 6/7 weeks. Fetuses between 34 0/7 and 36 6/7 weeks' gestation who are at risk of birth within 7 days and have not already received corticosteroids should be given a single dose as well (ACOG, 2017). Corticosteroid administration is associated with improved neonatal reductions in intraventricular hemorrhage and necrotizing enterocolitis (ACOG, 2017; Wilson et al., 2017).

Use of tocolytics may be indicated in the woman who has ruptured membranes to allow a course of steroids to be given to improve fetal lung maturity and reduce neonatal complications; however, if a maternal fever is present, delay of the birth is not recommended (ACOG, 2017).

Families with PPROM with gestational ages below 24 weeks should be counseled on grave outcomes associated with very preterm birth. The vast majority of births that occur prior to 24 weeks' gestation result in neonatal death or severe neurodevelopmental disabilities (ACOG, 2016c). Women with a fetus less than 24 weeks can be offered an induction of labor since the fetal respiratory system is unable to develop without the presence of amniotic fluid, which is needed for spontaneous respiratory breathing to occur. Women with gestational ages of 23 to 24 weeks can either be observed in the acute care setting or return home with careful observation measures in place. Early gestations that are maintained and result in live births are at significant risk to have long-term adverse outcomes and are the major cause of disabilities in children.

●○● NURSING MANAGEMENT

For the Woman with PROM or PPROM

Nursing Assessment and Diagnosis

Determining the time, amount, color, odor, and duration of the rupture of membranes is a significant component of the antepartum assessment. Ask the woman when her membranes ruptured and when contractions began because the risk of infection may be directly related to the time involved. The color and odor are important variables that can indicate possible infection or meconium passage. Gestational age is determined to prepare for the possibility of a preterm birth. Observe the mother for signs and symptoms of infection, especially by reviewing her WBC count, temperature, and pulse rate and the character of her amniotic fluid. If the mother has a fever, check hydration status. Fetal heart rate tracings should be watched for tachycardia, loss of variability, or decelerations. When a preterm or cesarean birth is anticipated, evaluate the childbirth preparation and coping abilities of the woman and her partner.

Nursing diagnoses that may be used for the woman with PPROM include:

- *Infection, Risk for,* related to premature preterm rupture of membranes
- *Gas Exchange, Impaired,* of the fetus, related to compression of the umbilical cord secondary to prolapse of the cord
- *Coping, Ineffective,* related to unknown outcome of the pregnancy

(NANDA-I © 2017)

Nursing Plan and Implementation

Nursing actions should focus on the woman, her partner, and the fetus. Uterine activity and fetal response to the labor are evaluated, but vaginal exams are not done unless absolutely necessary. Encourage the woman to rest on her right or left side to promote optimal uteroplacental perfusion. Comfort measures may help promote rest and relaxation. Ensure that hydration is maintained, particularly if the woman's temperature is elevated.

Education is another important aspect of nursing care. The couple needs to understand the implications of PROM/PPROM and all treatment methods. It is important to address side effects and alternative treatments. The couple needs to know that although the membranes are ruptured, amniotic fluid continues to be produced. Accurate information about neonatal outcomes for the given gestational age will help the woman and those she looks to for support have a more realistic view of the situation. This is often done by a healthcare provider experienced in the care of high-risk newborns such as a neonatologist or a neonatal nurse practitioner. Providing psychologic support for the couple is critical. Reduce anxiety by listening empathetically, relaying accurate information, and providing explanations of procedures. It may be necessary to prepare the couple for a cesarean birth, a preterm newborn, and the possibility of fetal or neonatal demise.

Evaluation

Expected outcomes of nursing care include:

- The woman's risk of infection and cord prolapse is decreased.
- The couple is able to discuss the implications of PROM/PPROM and all treatment options.
- The pregnancy is maintained without trauma to the mother or fetus.

TABLE 23–6 Causes and Sources of Hemorrhage

CAUSES AND SOURCES	SIGNS AND SYMPTOMS
Antepartum Period	
Abortion	Vaginal bleeding Intermittent uterine contractions Rupture of membranes
Placenta previa	Painless vaginal bleeding after seventh month
Abruptio placentae	
Partial	Vaginal bleeding: No increase in uterine pain
Severe	Vaginal bleeding may or may not be present Extreme tenderness of abdominal area Rigid, boardlike abdomen Increase in size of abdomen
Intrapartum Period	
Placenta previa	Bright red vaginal bleeding
Abruptio placentae	Same signs and symptoms listed above
Uterine atony in Stage III	Bright red vaginal bleeding Ineffectual contractility
Postpartum Period	
Uterine atony	Boggy uterus Dark vaginal bleeding Presence of clots
Retained placental fragments	Boggy uterus Dark vaginal bleeding Presence of clots
Lacerations of cervix or vagina	Firm uterus Bright red blood

Care of the Woman and Fetus at Risk Because of Placental Problems

Maintaining placental function is paramount to ensuring fetal well-being and continuation of the pregnancy. Because the placenta is highly vascular, problems that develop are usually associated with maternal and possibly fetal hemorrhage. Causes and sources of hemorrhage are reviewed in Table 23–6. Other placental problems are discussed in Chapter 24.

Abruptio Placentae

Abruptio placentae is the premature separation of a normally implanted placenta from the uterine wall. The incidence of abruptio placentae requiring delivery is 1% of all pregnancies, but it accounts for 15% of perinatal mortality (Ananth & Kinzler, 2017). It is more frequent in pregnancies complicated by smoking, premature rupture of membranes, multiple gestation, advanced maternal age, cocaine use, chorioamnionitis, and hypertension (Ananth & Kinzler, 2017). The risk of recurrence is 10 times higher if a previous abruption has occurred (Ananth & Kinzler, 2017).

The cause of abruptio placentae is largely unknown. Theories have been proposed relating its occurrence to decreased blood flow to the placenta through the sinuses during the last trimester. It is estimated that maternal hypertension is the most common cause (44%), with maternal trauma accounting for 2 to 10% of the cases (Ananth & Kinzler, 2017). Domestic violence, abdominal trauma, presence of fibroids, uterine overdistention, fetal growth restriction, alcohol consumption, a short umbilical cord, and high parity also contribute (Ananth & Kinzler, 2017). Abruptions also appear to be more common in certain ethnic groups. Caucasian American and African American women have higher incidences of abruptions than Asian American and Latin American women. Classification of abruption is based on the extent of separation (Table 23–7). The most commonly occurring abruption is class 1 (Gabbe et al., 2016).

TABLE 23–7 Classification of Abruption

CLASS	AMOUNT OF BLEEDING	UTERINE TETANY	NONREASSURING FETAL STATUS	MATERNAL SHOCK	FREQUENCY OF OCCURRENCE
0	None	None	None	None	Diagnosed after birth
1	Scant/mild	May or may not be present	Usually none	May or may not be present	48%
2	Moderate	May or may not be present	May or may not be present	May or may not be present	27%
3	Severe	Severe	Usually severe; fetal death may occur	Present with possible coagulopathy; risk of maternal death	24%

SOURCES: Gaufberg, 2008; Han, Schatz, & Lockwood, 2011.

PATHOPHYSIOLOGY

Premature separation of the placenta may be divided into four types:

1. ***Marginal:*** The blood passes between the fetal membranes and the uterine wall and escapes vaginally. Separation begins at the periphery of the placenta; this marginal sinus rupture may or may not become more severe. (Figure 23–1A)
2. ***Central:*** The placenta separates centrally, and the blood is trapped between the placenta and the uterine wall. Entrapment of the blood results in concealed bleeding. (Figure 23–1B)
3. ***Partial.*** Separation occurs but is not complete. May be minimal or moderate. Partial separation can progress to complete separation.
4. ***Complete:*** Massive vaginal bleeding is seen in the presence of almost total separation. (Figure 23–1C)

Different authors may classify abruptions using alternative terminology. *Revealed* or *external* indicates that bright red or dark and clotted blood is being expelled from the vagina. *Concealed* or *internal* notes absence of vaginal bleeding or very scant bleeding and is typically associated with a blood accumulation behind the placenta that is not being expelled from the vagina. *Mixed* or *combined* indicates the bleeding is a combination of the two and vaginal bleeding is present with additional accumulation of internal blood behind the placenta.

Abruptio placentae may also be graded according to the severity of clinical and laboratory findings as follows (Deering, 2015):

- ***Grade 1 (Mild).*** Mild separation with slight vaginal bleeding. FHR pattern and maternal blood pressure unaffected. Accounts for 48% of abruptions.
- ***Grade 2 (Moderate).*** Partial abruption with moderate bleeding. Significant uterine irritability is present. Maternal pulse may be elevated, although blood pressure is stable. Signs of fetal compromise evident in FHR. Accounts for 27% of abruptions.
- ***Grade 3 (Severe).*** Large or complete separation with moderate to severe bleeding. Maternal shock and painful uterine contractions present. Fetal death common. Accounts for about 24% of abruptions.

In severe cases of central abruptio placentae, a blood clot forms behind the placenta. With no place to escape, the blood

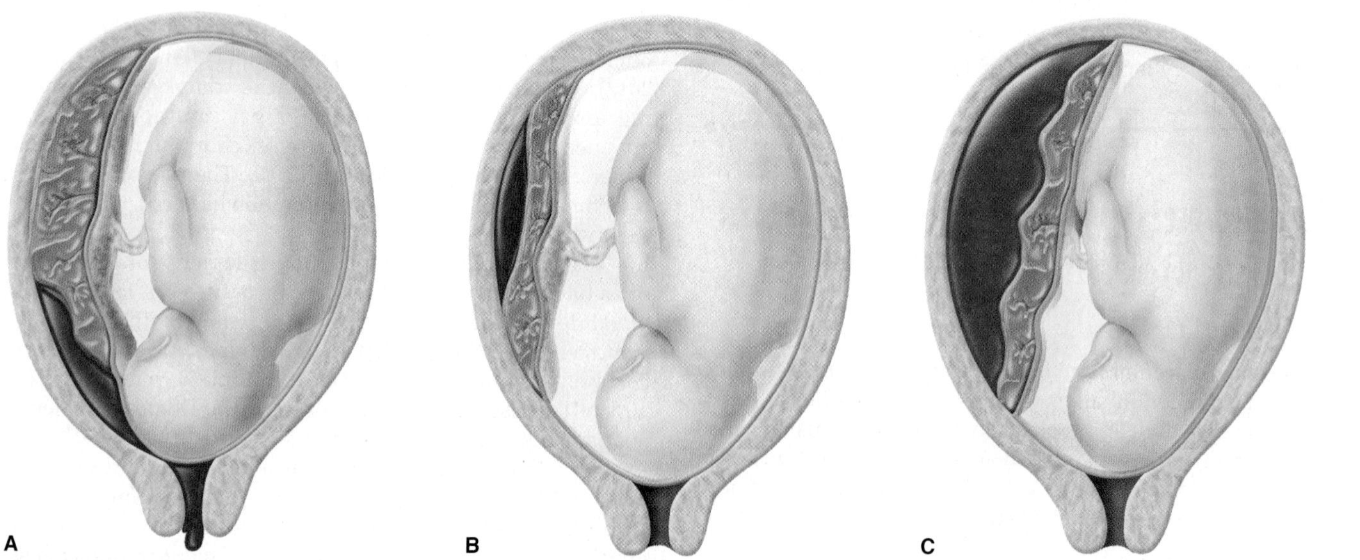

Figure 23–1 Abruptio placentae. A. Marginal abruption with external hemorrhage. B. Central abruption with concealed hemorrhage. C. Complete separation.

invades the myometrial tissues between the muscle fibers. This occurrence accounts for the uterine irritability that is a significant sign of premature separation of the placenta. If hemorrhage continues, eventually the uterus turns entirely blue in color. After the baby is born, the uterus has difficulty contracting. This syndrome is known as a *Couvelaire uterus* and frequently necessitates hysterectomy.

As a result of the damage to the uterine wall and the retroplacental clotting with covert abruption, large amounts of thromboplastin are released into the maternal blood supply, which in turn triggers the development of *disseminated intravascular coagulation (DIC)* (a rare, life-threatening condition in which small blood clots develop throughout the bloodstream, blocking small blood vessels and potentially causing hemorrhage) and the resultant hypofibrinogenemia. Fibrinogen levels, which are ordinarily elevated in pregnancy, may drop to incoagulable amounts within a matter of minutes as a result of rapidly developing premature separation of the placenta. Additional information on DIC may be found in a medical-surgical nursing textbook.

MATERNAL RISKS

Although maternal mortality has dramatically decreased in the last 100 years, maternal morbidity is still common. Problems following the birth depend in large part on the severity of the intrapartum bleeding coagulation defects such as DIC, hypofibrinogenemia, and length of time between separation and the birth. Moderate to severe hemorrhage results in hemorrhagic shock, which ultimately may prove fatal to the mother if not reversed. In the postpartum period, women who have suffered this disorder are at risk for hemorrhage and renal failure due to shock, vascular spasm, intravascular clotting, or a combination of the three. Another cause of renal failure is incompatible emergency blood transfusion. Failure is directly proportional to the number of units transfused. In some cases, hysterectomy is performed if bleeding cannot be controlled.

FETAL-NEONATAL RISKS

Perinatal mortality associated with abruptio placentae is approximately 25% (Gabbe et al., 2017). In severe cases in which separation occurs to approximately 50% of the placenta, newborn mortality is 100%. In less severe separation, fetal outcome depends on the level of maturity. The most serious complications in the newborn arise from preterm labor, anemia, and hypoxia. If fetal hypoxia progresses unchecked, irreversible brain damage or fetal demise may result. Neurologic defects within the first year of life occur in approximately 14% of babies who survive (Gabbe et al., 2016). With thorough assessment and prompt action on the part of the healthcare team, fetal and maternal outcome can be optimized.

CLINICAL THERAPY

Because of the risk of DIC, evaluating the results of coagulation tests is imperative. DIC occurs as a complication secondary to a major medical complication. In DIC, fibrinogen levels and platelet counts are usually decreased; prothrombin times (PT) and partial thromboplastin times (PTT) are normal to prolonged (Polin, Abman, Rowitch, et al., 2016). If the values are not markedly abnormal, serial testing may be helpful in establishing an abnormal trend that is indicative of coagulopathy. Another very sensitive test determines fibrin degradation products; these levels rise with DIC. See Table 23–8.

After the diagnosis is established, emphasis is placed on maintaining the cardiovascular status of the mother and developing a plan for achieving the birth of the fetus. Intravenous access with a large-gauge cannula is warranted along with continuous electronic fetal monitoring (EFM). Which birth method is selected depends on the condition of the woman and fetus; in many circumstances cesarean birth may be the safest option.

TABLE 23–8 Abnormal Clotting Factors Indicative of Abruptio Placentae

- PT longer than 15 seconds
- PTT longer than 60 seconds
- Fibrinogen levels less than 150 mg/dL
- Platelet count less than 100,000/mm^3
- Fibrinogen degradation products greater than 100 mg/Ml

If the separation is mild and gestation is near term, labor may be induced, and the fetus may be born vaginally with as little trauma as possible. If rupture of membranes and oxytocin infusion by pump do not initiate labor within a short time, a cesarean birth is usually done. A longer delay would increase the risk of hemorrhage, with resulting hypofibrinogenemia. Supportive treatment to decrease risk of DIC includes typing and cross-matching for blood transfusions (at least three units), clotting mechanism evaluation, and intravenous fluids (Polin & Abman, 2016).

In cases of moderate to severe placental separation, a cesarean birth is done after hypofibrinogenemia has been treated by intravenous infusion of cryoprecipitate or fresh frozen plasma (FFP). Vaginal birth is impossible in the event of a Couvelaire uterus because it could not contract properly in labor. Cesarean birth is necessary in the face of severe hemorrhage to allow an immediate hysterectomy to save both woman and fetus.

The hypovolemia that accompanies severe abruptio placentae is life-threatening and must be combated with whole blood. If the fetus is alive but experiencing stress, emergency cesarean birth is the method of choice. With a stillborn fetus, vaginal birth is preferable unless shock from hemorrhage is uncontrollable. Intravenous fluids of a balanced salt solution such as lactated Ringer solution are given through a 16- or 18-gauge cannula (Gabbe et al., 2016). Central venous pressure (CVP) monitoring may be needed to evaluate intravenous fluid replacement. Hemodynamic monitoring is an essential aspect of nursing care for the woman with abruption. If there is any evidence of hypovolemia, two venous lines should be started. Urine output should be monitored with an indwelling catheter. If the output drops below 30 mL per hour with adequate fluid replacement, CVP should be used to assess for hypovolemia. CVP will be the guide to fluid replacement. An absolute level is not as significant as the response to fluid replacement. Pulmonary artery catheter measurement, such as with a Swan-Ganz catheter, may be necessary to manage the hemodynamic changes. However, a significant abruption may preclude placing a catheter in the jugular or subclavian vein because the DIC is causing bleeding from multiple sites. The CVP is evaluated hourly, and results are communicated to the physician. Elevations of CVP may indicate fluid overload and pulmonary edema. The hematocrit is maintained at 30% through the administration of packed red cells or whole blood or both (Gabbe et al., 2016).

Laboratory testing is ordered to provide ongoing data regarding hemoglobin, hematocrit, and coagulation status. A clot observation test may be done at the bedside to evaluate coagulation status (see Table 23–8). A red-topped glass tube containing 5 mL of maternal blood is inverted four to five times. If a clot fails to form in 6 minutes, a fibrinogen level of less than 150 mg/dL is suspected. If a clot is not formed in 30 minutes, the fibrinogen level may well be less than 100 mg/dL. A clot observation test may be completed by a physician or a nurse.

Measures are taken to stimulate labor to effect vaginal birth as indicated by the condition of the mother and fetus. The birth may be hastened by performing an amniotomy (discussed in Chapter 25) and by oxytocin stimulation. Previously, birth within 6 hours of the diagnosis of severe placental abruption was recommended to reduce maternal mortality and morbidity. Currently, changing medical practice directed to ensuring adequate fluid replacement, especially blood, appears to accomplish the same outcome (Gabbe et al., 2016). These interventions should be started immediately, as birth is to be facilitated without delay.

A Kleihauer-Betke test is also needed to determine the amount of fetal-maternal hemorrhage in Rh-negative women. The appropriate amount of Rh D immunoglobulin is calculated based on the test results and number of units of blood that is given (Polin & Abman, 2016).

●○● NURSING MANAGEMENT

For the Woman with Abruptio Placentae

Nursing Assessment and Diagnosis

Electronic monitoring of the uterine contractions and resting tone between contractions provides information regarding the labor pattern and effectiveness of the oxytocin induction. Because uterine resting tone is frequently increased with abruptio placentae, it must be evaluated frequently for further increase. Abdominal girth measurements may be ordered hourly and are obtained by placing a tape measure around the maternal abdomen at the level of the umbilicus. Another method of evaluating uterine size, which increases as more bleeding occurs at the site of abruption, is to place a mark at the top of the uterine fundus. The distance from the symphysis pubis to the mark may be evaluated hourly.

Nursing diagnoses that may apply to the woman with abruptio placentae include:

- ***Fluid Volume: Risk for Deficient,*** related to hypovolemia secondary to excessive blood loss
- ***Tissue Perfusion: Peripheral, Ineffective,*** related to blood loss secondary to uterine atony following birth
- ***Anxiety*** related to concern for personal status and the baby's safety
- ***Gas Exchange, Impaired,*** of the fetus, related to decreased blood volume and hypotension

(NANDA-I © 2017)

Nursing Plan and Implementation

The psychologic aspects of nursing care are very important. Maternal apprehension increases as the clinical picture changes. Factual reassurance and an explanation of the procedures and what is happening are essential for the emotional well-being of the expectant mother. Reinforce positive aspects of the woman's condition, such as normal FHR, normal vital signs, and decreased evidence of bleeding.

Other nursing care measures are addressed in *Nursing Care Plan: Hemorrhage in the Third Trimester,* which appears at the end of this section.

Evaluation

Expected outcomes of nursing care include:

- The woman and her baby have a safe labor and birth without further complications for the mother or child.
- The woman and family verbalize understanding of reasons for medical therapy and risks.

●○●

Ethics in Action!

How do you provide compassionate nursing care to a young woman who has just experienced a fetal demise secondary to placental abruption due to cocaine use?

Placenta Previa

In **placenta previa**, the placenta is improperly implanted in the lower uterine segment. This implantation may be on a portion of the lower segment or over the internal os (Figure 23–2). As the lower uterine segment contracts and dilates in the later weeks of pregnancy, the placental villi are torn from the uterine wall, thus exposing the uterine sinuses at the placental site. Bleeding begins, but because the amount depends on the number of sinuses exposed, it may initially be either scanty or profuse.

In the past, placenta previa terminology was sometimes considered vague and nonspecific. In response to the use of subjective terminology, the American College of Radiology (ACR) (2015) created the American College of Radiology Appropriateness Criteria, which recommends a grading system that includes four grades that provide a quantifiable description of the relationship between the cervical os and the placenta, as shown in Table 23–9. The descriptions in parentheses are the formerly used terms.

The cause of placenta previa is unknown. Statistically, it occurs in about 1 in 200 pregnancies (Gabbe et al., 2016). Factors associated with placenta previa are previous placenta previa, multiparity, increasing age, placenta accreta (discussed in a following section), defective development of blood vessels in the decidua, prior cesarean birth or other uterine surgery, cocaine use, smoking, a recent spontaneous or induced abortion, and a large placenta (Gabbe et al., 2016).

Another condition, **vasa previa**, occurs when the fetal vessels course through the amniotic membranes and are present at the cervical os. Vasa previa occurs in 1 in 2500 pregnancies. Although this is a rare cause of antepartum bleeding, it is associated with a high rate of fetal death (Gabbe et al., 2016).

CLINICAL THERAPY

Women who present with vaginal bleeding should be questioned regarding any history of abnormal placenta placement that was diagnosed during the pregnancy. When possible, prenatal records should be reviewed. Women who have not had a routine ultrasound examination and have no history of bleeding during the pregnancy may have an undiagnosed placenta previa. The goal of medical care is to identify the cause of bleeding and to provide treatment that will ensure birth of a mature newborn. It must be determined whether the cause of the bleeding is placenta previa or advanced labor with copious bloody show (which is normal). Indirect diagnosis is made by localizing the placenta via tests that require no vaginal examination. The

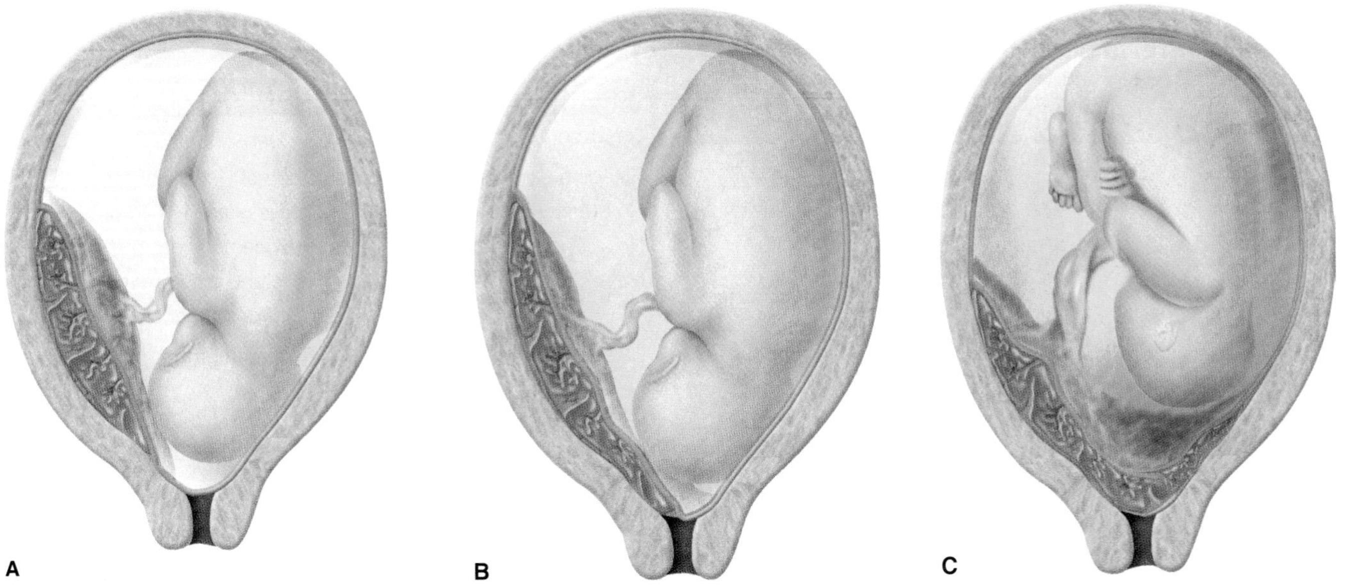

Figure 23–2 Grades of placenta previa. A. Grade 1, low-lying placental implantation. B. Grade 3, partial placenta previa. C. Grade 4, complete placenta previa.

TABLE 23–9 Grades of Placenta Previa

GRADE	DESCRIPTION
Grade 1	Placenta lies in lower uterine segment but its lower edge does not abut the internal cervical os (i.e., lower edge 0.5–5.0 cm from internal os) (Figure 23–2A) (Low-lying placenta)
Grade 2	Placental tissue reaches the margin of the internal cervical os, but does not cover it (Marginal placenta previa)
Grade 3	Placenta partially covers the internal cervical os (Figure 23–2B) (Partial placenta previa)
Grade 4	Placenta completely covers the internal cervical os (Figure 23–2C) (Total placenta previa)

most commonly employed diagnostic test is the transabdominal ultrasound scan. Abdominal or transvaginal sonography is used to identify the presence of placenta previa. If placenta previa is ruled out, a vaginal examination can be performed with a speculum to determine the cause of bleeding (such as cervical lesions or polyps).

Direct diagnosis of placenta previa can be made only by feeling the placenta inside the cervical os. However, such an examination may cause profuse bleeding due to tearing of tissue in the cotyledons of the placenta. Because of the danger of bleeding, a vaginal examination is generally contraindicated and is performed only if ultrasound is not available, the pregnancy is near term, and there is already profuse vaginal bleeding. The examination is done by a physician using a double setup procedure; that is, the delivery room is set up for the vaginal examination and a normal vaginal birth and also for a cesarean birth should placenta previa be present and the examination precipitate brisk bleeding. Adequate personnel must be present to respond to treatment decisions.

Clinical Tip

When assessing a woman for vaginal bleeding, make sure to have the woman lift her bottom completely off the bed so you can observe for blood loss beneath the buttocks.

The differential diagnosis of placental or cervical bleeding takes careful consideration. Table 23–10 provides a comparison of the signs and symptoms of placenta previa and abruptio placentae. Partial separation of the placenta may also present with painless bleeding, and a true placenta previa may not demonstrate overt bleeding until labor begins, thus confusing the diagnosis. In fact, the causes of slight to moderate antepartum bleeding episodes in 20 to 25% of women are never accurately diagnosed.

Care of the woman with painless late gestational bleeding depends on (1) the week of gestation during which the first bleeding episode occurs and (2) the amount of bleeding (Table 23–11). If the pregnancy is less than 37 weeks' gestation, expectant management is employed to delay birth until about 37 weeks' gestation to allow the fetus to mature. Expectant management involves stringent compliance with:

- Bedrest with bathroom privileges only as long as the woman is not bleeding
- No vaginal examinations
- Monitoring of blood loss, pain, and uterine contractility
- Evaluation of FHR with external monitor
- Monitoring of maternal vital signs
- Complete laboratory evaluation: Hemoglobin, hematocrit, Rh factor, and urinalysis

TABLE 23–10 Differential Signs and Symptoms of Placenta Previa and Abruptio Placentae

SIGNS/ SYMPTOMS	PLACENTA PREVIA	ABRUPTIO PLACENTAE
Onset	Slow	Immediate
Bleeding	External	External or internal
Color of blood	Bright red	Dark in color, if present
Drop in hemoglobin	= Blood loss	Greater than apparent blood loss
Shock	= Blood loss	Greater than apparent blood loss
Preeclampsia	Absent	May be present
Pain	With labor	Severe and constant
Uterine tenderness	Absent	Painful to touch
Uterine tone	Soft and palpable	Firm and hard
Uterine contour	Normal	May change shape with uterine enlargement
Fetal heart tones	Usually present	Present or absent
Engagement	Absent	May be present
Presentation	May be abnormal	No relationship
Maternal drug screen	Usually negative	May be positive
Abdominal trauma	Usually not present	May have occurred

TABLE 23–11 Assessment and Management of Placenta Previa

ASSESSMENT	MANAGEMENT/ACTION
Gestation Less Than 37 Weeks	
Bleeding stopped No uterine contractions No abdominal pain NST reactive	Bedrest Vital signs every 4 hours Provide IV fluids Type and cross-match blood Monitor patient closely
Bleeding begins again *or* Labor has begun *or* Maternal vital signs decline *or* Fetal status is nonreassuring	Cesarean birth
Complete previa	Cesarean birth
Gestation More Than 37 Weeks	
Bleeding minimal or stopped Reassuring fetal status	Induction of labor possible if: Low-lying or marginal previa Cervix is ripe Cephalic presentation Fetal head down in pelvis
Bleeding continues *or* Complete previa	Cesarean birth

SOURCE: Data from Lockwood & Stieglitz, 2017.

- Administration of intravenous fluid (lactated Ringer solution) with drip rate monitored
- Availability of two units of cross-matched blood for possible transfusion
- Administration of betamethasone to facilitate fetal lung maturity
- Administration of RhD immunoglobulin in RhD-negative women

If frequent, recurrent, or profuse bleeding persists or if fetal well-being appears threatened, a cesarean birth needs to be performed.

●○● NURSING MANAGEMENT

For the Woman with Placenta Previa

Nursing Assessment and Diagnosis

Assessment of the woman with placenta previa must be ongoing to prevent or treat complications that are potentially lethal to the mother and fetus. Painless, bright red vaginal bleeding is the best diagnostic sign of placenta previa. If this sign should develop during the last 3 months of a pregnancy, placenta previa should always be considered until ruled out by ultrasound examination. The first bleeding episode is generally scanty; however, each subsequent hemorrhage is more profuse. No vaginal examinations should be performed unless the placenta location has been established via ultrasound.

The uterus remains soft, and if labor begins, it relaxes fully between contractions. The FHR usually remains stable unless profuse hemorrhage and maternal shock occur. As a result of the placement of the placenta, the fetal presenting part is often unengaged, and transverse lie is common.

Appraise and quantify blood loss, pain, and uterine contractility from both subjective and objective perspectives (Association of Women's Health, Obstetric, & Neonatal Nurses [AWHONN], 2015b). Maternal vital signs and the results of blood and urine tests will provide additional data about the woman's condition. FHR is evaluated with an external fetal monitor. Another nursing responsibility is observing and verifying the family's ability to cope with the anxiety associated with an unknown outcome.

Nursing diagnoses that may apply to the woman experiencing placenta previa are:

- ***Fluid Volume, Deficient,*** related to hypovolemia secondary to excessive blood loss
- ***Tissue Perfusion: Peripheral, Ineffective,*** related to blood loss secondary to uterine atony following birth
- ***Anxiety*** related to concern for own personal status and the baby's safety
- ***Gas Exchange, Impaired,*** related to decreased blood volume and hypotension
- ***Fear*** related to concern for safety of the baby

(NANDA-I © 2017)

Nursing Plan and Implementation

Continue to monitor the woman and her fetus to determine the status of the bleeding and to determine the mother's and baby's responses. Evaluate the electronic monitor tracing to determine the fetal status. Maternal vital signs, intake and output, and other pertinent assessments must be made frequently. AWHONN has advocated for Obstetric Vital Sign Alert programs to improve obstetrical outcomes for high-risk women. Several tools have been proposed that are implemented in the EMR system to alert care providers when women meet certain thresholds of risk. The frequency of monitoring vital signs has been a factor that has been examined in these programs, designed to reduce maternal morbidity and mortality. When antepartum bleeding occurs, the frequency of vital signs can range from every 5 minutes, 15 minutes, or 30 minutes depending on the degree of bleeding, range of vital sign findings, and other maternal and fetal factors (AWHONN, 2015a).

CLINICAL TIP

When faced with an emergent situation, tell the woman she needs to follow your instructions quickly and that you will explain what is happening as soon as possible once you take the necessary measures to ensure that she and the baby are safely cared for.

Emotional support for the family is an important nursing care goal. When active bleeding is occurring, the assessments and management must be directed toward physical support. However, emotional aspects need to be addressed simultaneously. Explain to the woman and family the assessments being completed and the treatment measures that need to be done. Provide time for questions and act as an advocate in obtaining information for the family. Offer emotional support by staying with the family and by the use of touch.

The newborn's hemoglobin, cell volume, and erythrocyte count should be checked immediately after birth and then monitored closely. The newborn may require oxygen and administration of blood and admission into a neonatal intensive care unit.

Additional information regarding nursing care is addressed in *Nursing Care Plan: Hemorrhage in the Third Trimester*.

Evaluation

Expected outcomes of nursing care include:

- The cause of hemorrhage is recognized promptly, and corrective measures are taken.
- The woman's vital signs remain in the normal range.
- The woman and her baby have a safe labor and birth.
- The family understands what has happened and the implications and associated problems of placenta previa.

Nursing Care Plan: Hemorrhage in the Third Trimester

1. Nursing Diagnosis: *Fluid Volume: Risk for Deficient*, related to excessive vascular loss during pregnancy (NANDA-I © 2017)

Goal: Woman will not experience significant fluid volume deficit during the third trimester of pregnancy.

INTERVENTION	RATIONALE
• Monitor vital signs (i.e., temperature—normal range is 96.8°–100.4°F, pulse—normal is 60–100, respirations—normal is 12–20, blood pressure—normal is 120/80, central venous pressure—normal range is 5–10 mm H_2O). Compare present blood pressure with woman's baseline blood pressure. Note pulse pressure.	• Any deviations in a woman's baseline vital signs could indicate intravascular fluctuations.
• Weigh pads and chux. If the woman has bathroom privileges, instruct her on initiating pad counts. Teach the woman how to weigh pads and chux, with each gram equal to approximately 1 mL of blood loss.	• The combination of weighing and counting pads and chux assists medical personnel in determining the woman's blood loss.
• Report amount of blood loss within a specific period (e.g., 50 mL of bright-red blood on pad in 20 minutes).	
• Monitor urinary output hourly and measure urine specific gravity (normal: 1.010–1.025).	• A decrease in urinary output (less than 30 mL/hr) and an increase in specific gravity suggest dehydration and a need for an increase in fluid intake.
• Palpate bilateral peripheral pulses (normal: Equal and strong) and note capillary refill (normal: Less than 3 seconds). Also, assess skin color and temperature (normal: Pink, warm, dry, and intact).	• Helps determine signs of circulatory loss or hypovolemic shock, which include weak pulses, capillary refill greater than 3 seconds, skin color that is cyanotic or pallor, and skin temperature that is cool and clammy.
• Assess mental status at frequent intervals.	• Excessive blood loss can lead to changes in mentation.
• Assess the woman for signs and symptoms of disseminated intravascular coagulation.	• Provides vital information on maternal status.

(continued)

Nursing Care Plan: Hemorrhage in the Third Trimester (*continued*)

INTERVENTION	RATIONALE
• Instruct the woman on the importance of strict bedrest and avoidance of any sexual activity that involves nipple stimulation or that might lead to orgasm.	• Bleeding may cease with limited activity. Pressure on the abdomen and orgasms can stimulate uterine activity, thereby causing bleeding. Nipple stimulation may result in uterine contractions, as can orgasm.
• Monitor fetal status and uterine activity by continuous fetal monitoring.	• May determine the origin of bleeding and fetal well-being.
• **Collaborative:** Collect and review blood work as ordered: Complete blood count (CBC), type and cross-match, Rh titer, fibrinogen levels, platelet count, activated partial thromboplastin time (APTT), prothrombin time (PT), and human chorionic gonadotropin (hCG) levels.	• Determines blood loss and need for intervention if bloodwork is abnormal.
• Administer appropriate isotonic IV solutions and blood products (e.g., plasma expanders, whole blood, serum albumin, or packed red blood cells) as ordered by the physician.	• Reverses shock symptoms by increasing blood volume.
• Insert Foley catheter.	• Close monitoring of urinary output will aid in determining adequate renal perfusion.

EXPECTED OUTCOME: The woman will show signs of adequate fluid volume during pregnancy as evidenced by vital signs within normal limits, capillary refill in less than 3 seconds, adequate sensorium, and urine output greater than 30 mL/hr.

2. Nursing Diagnosis: *Tissue Perfusion: Peripheral, Ineffective* (uteroplacental), related to hypovolemia secondary to excessive maternal blood loss (NANDA-I ©2017)

Goal: The fetus will have no evidence of hypoxia during pregnancy.

INTERVENTION	RATIONALE
• Assess maternal vital signs.	• Closely monitoring maternal physiologic status and circulatory status will assist in determining if an episode of bleeding has occurred and allow for interventions to protect maternal and fetal well-being.
• Monitor fetal heart tones continuously, assessing for variability, accelerations, and decelerations, and record.	• Continuous electronic fetal monitoring will aid in detecting signs of fetal hypoxia and allow time for appropriate intervention.
• Assess fundal height.	• Determines an approximate gestational age.
• Assess labor progression by determining cervical dilatation and effacement if contractions are present.	• Provides information on maternal labor status.
• **Collaborative:** Perform scalp stimulation to assess fetal accelerations.	• FHR acceleration is considered 15 beats above the baseline lasting for 15 seconds and is indicative of fetal well-being.
• Assess amniotic fluid for meconium.	• Impaired gas exchange relaxes fetal intestinal motility, causing expulsion of meconium into amniotic fluid.
• Assist the physician during ultrasonography and amniocentesis for lecithin/sphingomyelin (L/S) ratio sample.	• Determines viability and alerts appropriate medical personnel of fetal age if birth is imminent.

EXPECTED OUTCOME: Fetus will demonstrate adequate tissue perfusion as evidenced by fetal heart tones that remain within 110–160 beats/min, long-term variability and short-term variability present, positive periodic changes (no variable or late decelerations), and fetal scalp blood pH greater than 7.25 (if indicated).

3. Nursing Diagnosis: *Fear/Anxiety* related to personal and fetal well-being secondary to third-trimester hemorrhage (NANDA-I © 2017)

Goal: The woman will verbalize a decrease in fear and anxiety.

INTERVENTION	RATIONALE
• Maintain frequent contact with the woman and family members.	• Establishes trust with the woman and her family members, so the patient will not feel alone or abandoned.

Nursing Care Plan: Hemorrhage in the Third Trimester (*continued*)

INTERVENTION	RATIONALE
• Provide the woman with accurate, reliable information concerning diagnosis and prognosis.	• Fear and anxiety will lessen when the woman is informed of health status and is allowed to make decisions based on present situation.
EXPECTED OUTCOME: The woman will actively seek information about diagnosis and prognosis.	
• Allow the woman and family members to verbalize the origin of fears.	• Recognizing the origin of fears gives the woman and her family the appropriate tool to begin the process of developing coping strategies for dealing with the fears.
• Explain all procedures in an easy-to-understand, non-threatening manner, and allow the woman and family members to ask questions.	• Accurate information prepares the woman and family members for the impending procedures, thereby reducing fear of the unknown.
EXPECTED OUTCOME: The woman and her family members develop appropriate coping strategies that decrease anxiety.	

Care of the Woman with Cervical Insufficiency

Many questions remain unanswered about cervical insufficiency. The classic definition presents **cervical insufficiency** as painless dilatation of the cervix without contractions because of a structural or functional defect of the cervix. The woman is usually unaware of contractions and presents with advanced effacement and dilatation and, possibly, bulging membranes. It is difficult to determine the incidence because of the inconsistency in definition and lack of clear diagnostic criteria.

The origin of cervical insufficiency is multifactorial; the etiology may be either congenital or acquired. Factors that may contribute to the tendency for the cervix to dilate prematurely can be divided into three categories: Congenital factors, acquired factors, and biochemical (hormonal) factors. Congenitally insufficient cervix may be found in women exposed to diethylstilbestrol (DES) or those with a bicornuate uterus. Acquired cervical insufficiency may be related to inflammation, infection, subclinical uterine activity, cervical trauma, cone biopsy, late second-trimester elective abortions, or increased uterine volume (as with a multiple gestation). Loop electrosurgical excision procedure (LEEP) of the cervix has been found to significantly increase the risk of preterm births in both singleton and twin gestations (ACOG, 2016b). The hormone relaxin may be an endocrine cause of cervical insufficiency.

A woman's obstetric history may give her healthcare provider an indication of increased risk for cervical insufficiency. Factors include multiple gestations, repetitive second-trimester losses, previous preterm birth, progressively earlier births with each subsequent pregnancy, short labors, previous elective abortion or cervical manipulation, DES exposure, or other uterine anomaly. These women will benefit from close surveillance of cervical length with transvaginal ultrasound beginning between 16 and 24 weeks' gestation. Cervical effacement occurs from the internal os out and can be seen on ultrasound as "funneling." Alteration is apparent in transvaginal scan when fundal pressure is applied or the woman assumes a standing position. In addition, women at risk for cervical insufficiency need to be informed early in pregnancy of warning signs of impending birth, such as lower back pain, pelvic pressure, and changes in vaginal discharge.

A number of contemporary studies have concluded that endovaginal ultrasound measurements of cervical length between 15 and 28 weeks' gestation identify groups at risk for preterm birth. However, the placement of a cervical cerclage (see the following discussion) does not substantially reduce the risk of prematurity (ACOG, 2016a). This has led to a reconsideration of both medical and surgical treatment options for women with a history of midtrimester losses. Medical therapies used are serial cervical ultrasound assessments, progesterone supplementation, antibiotics, and anti-inflammatory drugs (ACOG, 2016a).

Cerclage Procedures

A **cerclage** is a surgical procedure in which a stitch is placed in the cervix to prevent a spontaneous abortion or premature birth. (See Figure 23–3.) Surgical options include the various types of cerclage procedures. An elective cervical cerclage may be placed

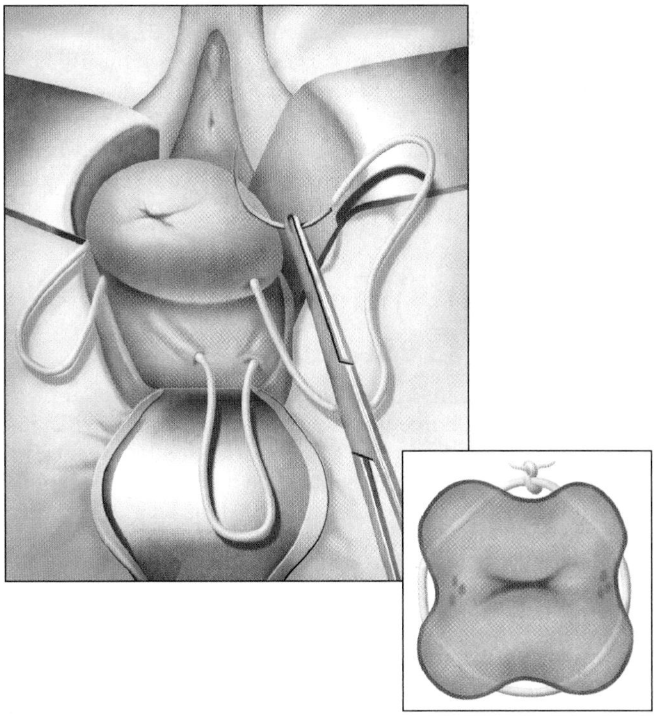

Figure 23–3 A cerclage or purse-string suture is inserted in the cervix to prevent preterm cervical dilatation and pregnancy loss. After placement, the string is tightened and secured anteriorly.

late in the first trimester or early in the second trimester with a 93% success rate in preventing fetal loss, with a mean age of 35 gestational weeks at the time of birth. An emergency cerclage is associated with a 92% success rate in preventing fetal loss with a mean gestational age of 32 weeks at the time of birth (ACOG, 2016a).

An emergency or rescue cerclage is one that is placed for emergent reasons, when dilatation and effacement have already occurred. It carries far graver outcomes, resulting in PPROM in one-third of cases, a 64% neonatal death rate, and an average age of 26 gestational weeks at the time of birth. Additionally, the chance of cerclage failure is increased when compared with an elective placement of a cerclage. When preforming a rescue cerclage, decompression of a bulging amniotic sac must be accomplished immediately before the cerclage placement. In this situation, a preoperative evaluation for infection, ruptured membranes, and uterine activity may be prudent. Tocolytics (drugs that stop labor), broad-spectrum antibiotics, and anti-inflammatory agents are given perioperatively and for ongoing treatment.

An abdominal cerclage approach may be required for women with a congenitally short or amputated cervix, cervical defects, a cervix previously scarred, or unhealed lacerations or subacute cervicitis. Laparoscopic abdominal cerclage placement is replacing the traditional open laparotomy approach (Gunasheela, Nayak, Roy, et al., 2016). Figure 23–4A–B compare a cervix of normal length with one indicative of cervical shortening. Figure 23–4C shows a cerclage in place.

An uncomplicated elective cerclage may be done on an outpatient basis and the woman is typically discharged home once she is able to ambulate and void. An emergency (or rescue) cerclage, however, usually requires hospitalization. Once the cerclage is placed, the woman is monitored for infection by monitoring vital signs, uterine contractions, and fetal heart rate and assessed for ruptured membranes. A CBC is typically done the next day to assess the WBC level and then as needed based on clinical indicators. Most women are advised to avoid heavy lifting and to refrain from coitus until at least 32 to 34 weeks (Jazayeri, 2015). Women with cervical cerclages typically have serial ultrasound measurements of the cervix either weekly or biweekly. After 36 to 37 completed weeks' gestation, the suture may be cut and vaginal birth permitted, or the suture may be left in place and a cesarean birth performed to avoid repeating the procedure in subsequent pregnancies.

Care of the Woman with a Multiple Gestation

The incidence of twins in the United States accounts for approximately 33 per 1000 live births. Higher numbers of twins and multiple fetal gestations are directly correlated to advances in reproductive technologies. It is estimated that triplets and higher-order multiples occur in 103.6 of 100,000 births in the United States (Martin, Hamilton, Osterman, et al., 2017). The incidence of these higher-order births is declining because of recent recommendations from the American College of Obstetricians and Gynecologists to reduce the number of fetuses transferred during in vitro fertilization procedures. Because twin birth is by far the most common multiple birth, the discussion focuses on this type and also identifies specific variations for triplets and higher-order multiple gestations as appropriate. The embryology of multiple gestations is discussed in Chapter 9.

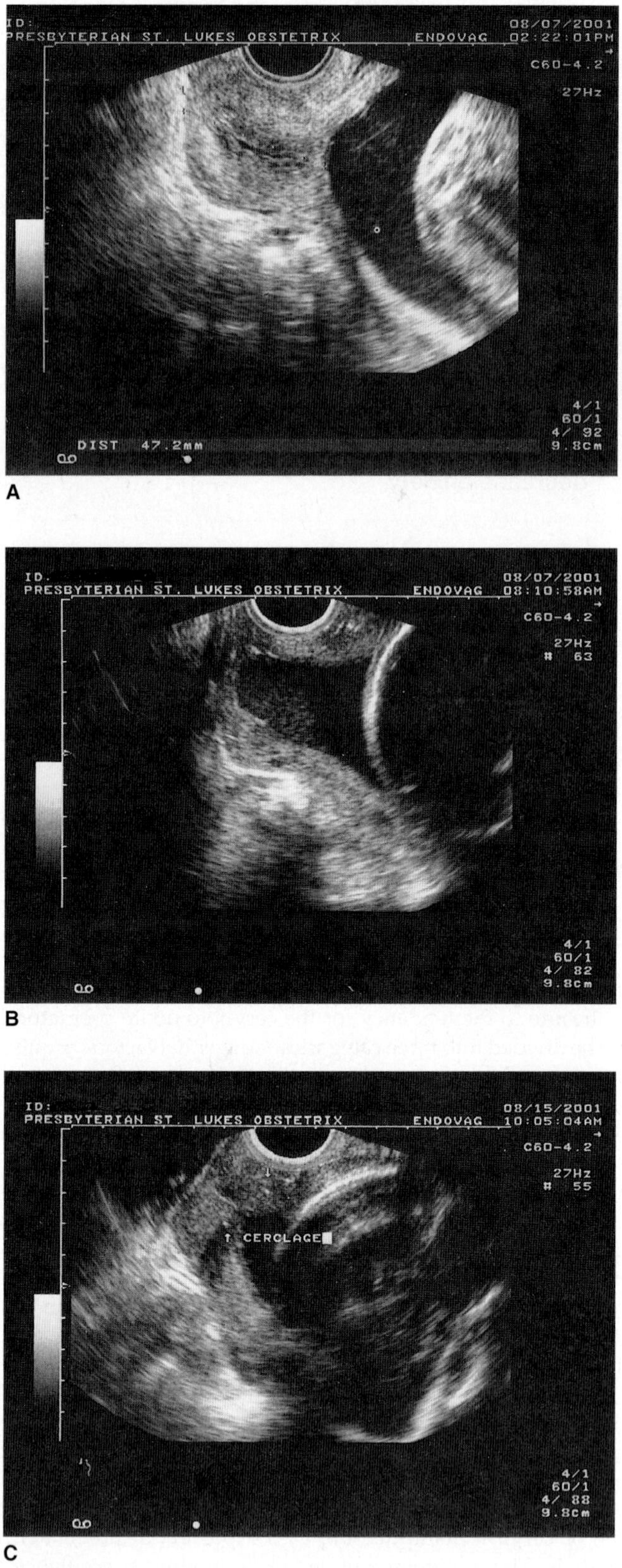

Figure 23–4 **Endocervical ultrasound of the cervix. A. Normal cervix measuring 47.2 mm. B. Woman at 24 weeks' gestation with chorioamnionitis and preterm labor. Cervix is fully effaced and dilated 2 cm. C. Arrow indicates stitch placement of cerclage. Cervix is 18.5 mm in length.**

SOURCE: A.–C. Debbie McGee, MSN, PNNP, RDMS.

Pregnancy Loss in Multiple Gestation

The development of sensitive human chorionic gonadotropin (hCG) assays and increasingly sensitive ultrasound techniques has made it possible to determine more accurately the early pregnancy loss rate of twins, including both complete pregnancy loss and spontaneous resorption of one twin (called the "vanishing twin" phenomenon). Of all twin pregnancies, approximately 25% are lost before the end of the first trimester (Polin & Abman, 2016). Causative factors in the loss of both twins in the first trimester include environmental factors, infectious organisms, trophoblast dysfunction, poor embryo quality, or a lower concentration of placentally produced substances. Although loss of one twin can occur at any time during the pregnancy, it more commonly occurs in the first trimester. Marginal and velamentous cord insertions (discussed in Chapter 24) are more likely to be present when there is a vanishing twin, and the presence of a monochorionic placenta is more likely to result in either a singleton gestation (because of a vanishing twin) or complete pregnancy loss (Polin & Abman, 2016).

Pregnancy loss of twins in the second trimester is associated with congenital anomalies, growth restriction, chromosomal abnormalities, and cervical insufficiency. Congenital anomalies are twice as likely to occur in twin gestations (Kore, 2016). In a monochorionic placenta, there may be a vascular anastomosis that leads to twin-to-twin transfusion syndrome. When this syndrome is present, blood is chronically drained from one fetus to the other. The donor fetus becomes growth restricted, and oligohydramnios develops. The recipient fetus becomes polycythemic and hydropic, and hydramnios develops. If the fetuses become severely affected during the second trimester, untreated mortality may be 100% (Gabbe et al., 2016).

The incidence of preterm birth is also higher in multiple gestations. Preterm birth occurs in 58.8% of twins, 94.4% of triplets, and 98.3% of quadruplets (Kore, 2016). New guidelines have been introduced that recommend optimal delivery for multiple gestations (Table 23–12). If spontaneous labor has not occurred in a multiple gestation by the recommended gestational age, induction or birth via cesarean is initiated.

POTENTIAL COMPLICATIONS

A woman with a multiple gestation is more likely to develop complications, which include (Kore, 2016):

- Spontaneous abortions are more common.
- Gestational diabetes; 3 to 6% of twin pregnancies and 22 to 39% of triplet pregnancies are complicated by gestational diabetes.
- Hypertension is the major maternal complication. The risk of developing severe hypertension or preeclampsia is 2.6 times higher in twins and significantly higher in triplets.
- HELLP (hemolytic anemia, elevated liver enzymes, and low platelet count) syndrome, a complication resulting from eclampsia or preeclampsia (discussed in Chapter 18), is more common.
- Acute fatty liver, which is manifested by severe coagulopathy, hypoglycemia, and hyperammonemia, which can lead to maternal and fetal death, is more common.
- Pulmonary embolism is six times more likely to develop during pregnancy with multiple gestations.
- Maternal anemia occurs because of demands of the multiple gestation. The hemoglobin averages 10 g/dL from the 20th week on. Anemia is indicated by hemoglobin levels below 11 g/dL in the first or third trimester or below 10.5 g/dL in the second trimester. When decreased hemoglobin is accompanied by serum ferritin concentration of less than 12 mg/dL, iron deficiency anemia is diagnosed.

TABLE 23–12 Guidelines for Timing of Birth in Multiple-Gestation Pregnancies

TYPE OF AMNIOTIC SAC OR COMPLICATIONS PRESENT	RECOMMENDED INTERVAL FOR BIRTH
Uncomplicated twin pregnancy with separate placentas and amniotic sacs	38 weeks' gestation
Uncomplicated twin pregnancy with single placenta but two separate amniotic sacs	34–37 6/7 weeks' gestation
Twins with single placenta and single amniotic sac	32–34 weeks' gestation
Fetal growth restriction in one twin with two separate placentas and amniotic sacs	36–37 weeks' gestation
Fetal growth restriction in one twin with single placenta and two separate amniotic sacs	32–34 weeks' gestation
Twin gestation with intrauterine growth restriction in one twin with additional risk factors, such as abnormal Doppler studies, oligohydramnios, hydramnios, preeclampsia, gestational diabetes, etc.	32–34 weeks' gestation
Twin gestation with fetal death of one twin	If greater than 34 weeks' gestation, consider birth; if less than 34 weeks' gestation, laboratory and fetal monitoring warranted
Twin gestation with single placenta and single amniotic sac	32–34 weeks' gestation if reassuring fetal status
Triplet or quadruplet	35 weeks' gestation

SOURCES: Data from ACOG, 2016b; Kore, 2016).

- Hydramnios may be due to increased renal perfusion from cross-vessel anastomosis of monozygotic twins.
- Premature rupture of membranes, cervical insufficiency, and intrauterine growth restriction occur more commonly.
- Twin-to-twin transfusion, conjoined (Siamese) twins, and *acardia* (twin reversed arterial perfusion sequence) are rare complications associated with twins.
- Preterm labor, uterine dysfunction due to an overstretched myometrium, abnormal fetal presentations, instrumental or cesarean birth, and postpartum hemorrhage may be labor complications.
- Pulmonary edema is more common in multiple gestations due to cardiovascular changes.
- Dermatologic complications, such as pruritic urticarial papules and plagues of pregnancy (PUPP), occur in 2.9% of twin and 14% of triplet pregnancies.
- Multiple births account for 21% of low-birth-weight newborns, 19 to 24% of very low-birth-weight newborns, 20% of neonatal intensive care unit (NICU) admissions, and 26% of neonatal deaths.

The woman with a multiple gestation may experience more physical discomfort during her pregnancy, such as shortness of breath, dyspnea on exertion, backaches, round ligament pain, heartburn, pelvic or suprapubic pressure, and pedal edema because of the oversized uterus.

CLINICAL THERAPY

The goals of medical care are to promote normal fetal development, to prevent maternal complications, to prevent preterm birth, and to diminish fetal trauma during labor.

Ultrasound examinations play a crucial role in the care and treatment of multiple gestations. Ultrasound assists with identifying the presence of more than one fetus early in the pregnancy, providing accurate dating of the pregnancy, and detecting fetal anomalies. Because the incidence of perinatal mortality and morbidity is increased in twins, use of ultrasound in the first and second trimesters can be particularly helpful. Evidence supports the use of ultrasound for accurately determining chorionicity and amnionicity in multiple pregnancies (Kore, 2016).

Knowledge of chorionicity is essential in differentiating twin-to-twin transfusion from fetal growth restriction secondary to abnormal placental blood flow. Knowledge of chorionicity is also important in determining the management of a multiple pregnancy in which one twin is sonographically abnormal. If the twins are dichorionic/diamniotic (DC/DA) (see Chapter 9), then selective termination could be considered.

Determination of amnionicity is based on ultrasound visualization or the lack of visualization of an intertwin membrane. Visualization of this membrane becomes more difficult as the gestation advances because of progressive thinning of the intertwin membrane, fetal crowding, and an increasing incidence of oligohydramnios. Knowledge regarding the presence of one amnion is crucial because management of monochorionic/monoamniotic (MC/MA) twins (see Chapter 9) requires more intensive surveillance and earlier birth, usually by cesarean (Kore, 2016). Women with MC/MA twins are frequently cared for by perinatologists in a facility that has high-risk services available.

Preventing preterm labor is a major goal. Prenatal care should begin early, and more frequent visits are usually scheduled. Many practitioners perform vaginal examinations at each visit after 28 weeks to identify cervical changes, such as cervical shortening, effacement, or dilatation, or the beginning of bulging membranes. Assessing cervical length via ultrasound has been predictive in identifying women at risk for preterm birth (PTB). A cervical length of less than 25 mm between 14 and 20 weeks is associated with PTB prior to 32 weeks. Cervical length less than 25 mm for triplets between 15 and 20 weeks is associated with a 100% delivery rate by 28 weeks (Kore, 2016). Digital examinations are often helpful as well, but to be accurate they should be performed by the same examiner at each prenatal visit (Kore, 2016). Fetal fibronectin (fFN) as a predictor of preterm labor has been well established in singleton pregnancies. A study of 147 twin gestations revealed that a negative fFN test is associated with a less than 3% risk of PTB in the following 2-week period. This test can be beneficial because women with multiple gestations are often asymptomatic. Further research is needed to determine if this test results in fewer PTBs.

The administration of corticosteroids is now recommended for multiple pregnancies between 24 and 34 weeks if a risk to deliver within the next 7 days is suspected. Based on a family's desire for aggressive management, women as early as 23 0/7 weeks can be given this option as well. A single repeat dose of corticosteroids can be given to women less than 34 weeks who have received previous steroids at least 14 days prior. Repeated dosages beyond this are not recommended (ACOG, 2016b). Fetuses at risk for preterm birth prior to 32 weeks should be administered magnesium sulfate as a neuroprotection to reduce the incidence and severity of cerebral palsy (ACOG, 2016c).

Interventions such as routine cervical cerclage placement, reduced activity and work, home uterine monitoring, prophylactic bedrest, or routine hospitalization for unidentified medical indications have not been found to reduce preterm birth and are not recommended for routine care (ACOG, 2016b).

Some areas offer twin clinics, which provide many advantages for the woman with a multiple gestation. These advantages include consistent evaluation, intensive prenatal education, counseling, and support from the same healthcare providers.

Intrapartum management and assessment require careful attention to maternal and fetal status. The mother should have an intravenous infusion in place with a large-bore needle. Anesthesia and cross-matched blood should be readily available. The twins are monitored by dual EFM. The labor may progress very slowly or very quickly.

The decision about method of birth may not be made until labor occurs, and the method depends on a variety of factors. The presence of maternal complications such as placenta previa, abruptio placentae, or severe preeclampsia usually indicates the need for cesarean birth. Fetal factors such as severe intrauterine growth restriction (IUGR), preterm birth, fetal anomalies, nonreassuring fetal status, or unfavorable fetal position or presentation also require cesarean birth. Typically, a cesarean birth is performed if the presenting twin is in a presenting position other than vertex and cannot be turned to a vertex presentation.

Birth of three or more fetuses is best accomplished by cesarean because of the risk of fetal insult due to decreased placental perfusion and hemorrhage from the separating placenta during the intrapartum period (Gabbe et al., 2016). Complicated obstetric maneuvers such as breech extraction and podalic version, the risk of prolapse of the cord, and an increase in fetal collision provide additional reasons for cesarean birth.

Any combination of presentations and positions can occur with twins (Figure 23–5). Approximately 40% of twins present in a vertex/vertex presentation. Diamniotic twin gestations with the first twin in vertex presentation can undergo a trial of labor and attempt a vaginal birth. Women with one previous low

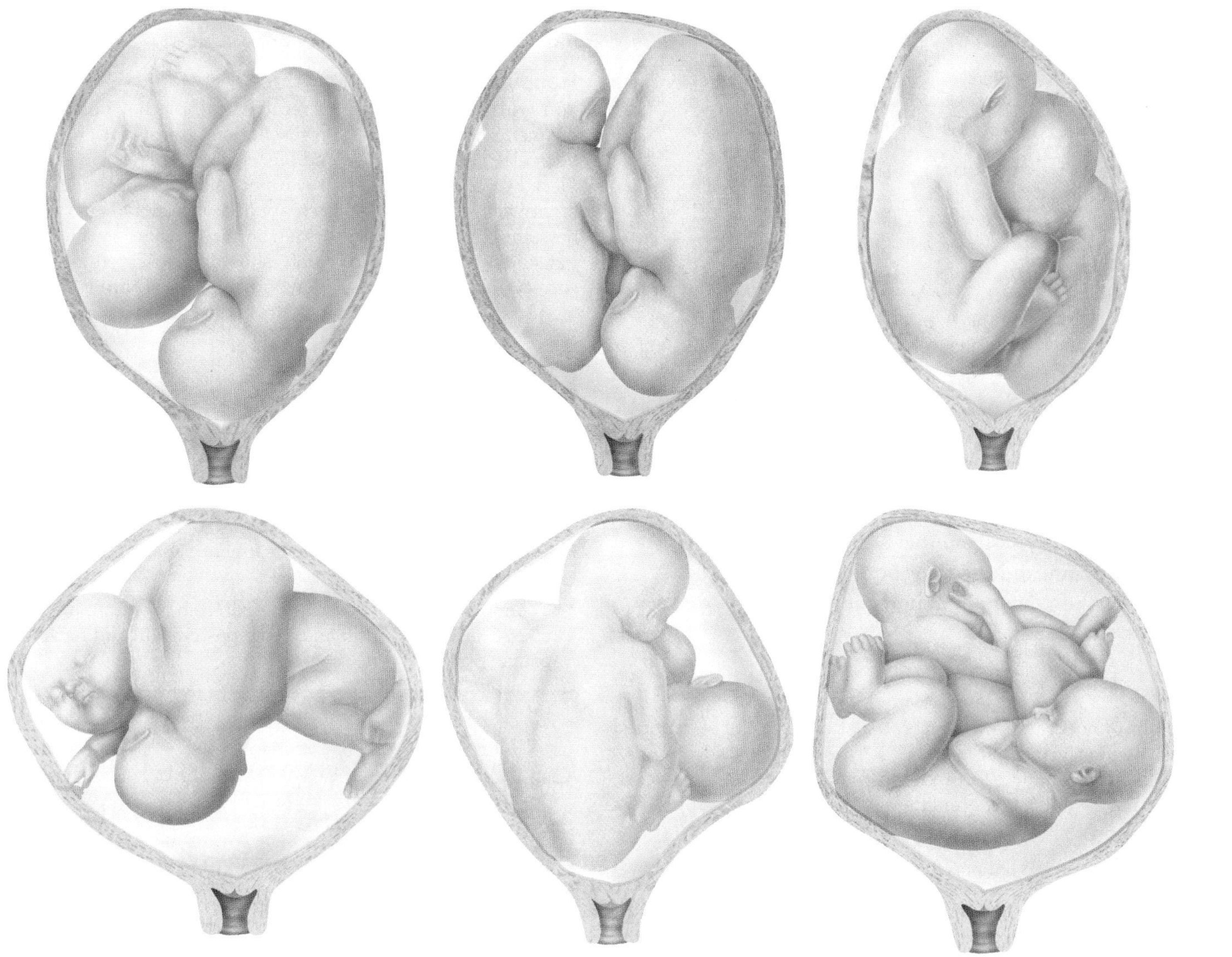

Figure 23–5 Twins may be in any of these presentations in utero.

transverse cesarean can also undergo a trial of labor (ACOG, 2016b). Vaginal birth is a viable option when the presenting twin is in vertex position, although practitioner experience with podalic version and breech vaginal birth is becoming less and less common and contributes to increases in the cesarean birth rates in twin gestations.

The placentas are examined after the birth. If the twins are of the same sex, the placentas are sent to the pathology laboratory for examination to determine whether they are monozygotic or dizygotic twins.

●○● NURSING MANAGEMENT

For the Woman with Multiple Gestation

Nursing Assessment and Diagnosis

When obtaining a maternal history at the beginning of antenatal care, identify any family history of twinning. Equally important is a history of medication taken to enhance fertility or artificial reproductive technology that may have been used to conceive. Note these facts on the antepartum record.

At each antepartum clinic visit, measure the fundal height. During the prenatal period, a fundal height greater than expected for the weeks of gestation and auscultation of two heartbeats that differ by at least 10 beats per minute are the most likely clues of twin pregnancy. Some women experience severe nausea and vomiting and develop severe anemia despite the intake of multiple-vitamin therapy.

Any growth, fetal movement, or heart tone auscultation out of proportion to gestational age by dates is indicative of twins. During palpation, you may feel many small parts on all sides of the abdomen (Figure 23–6). If twins are suspected, attempt to auscultate two separate heartbeats in different quadrants of the maternal abdomen. Use of the Doppler device may be helpful. Conclusive evidence of twins is found on sonography.

Determine the family's level of preparation for integrating more than one new member during the prenatal visits. Although the thought of having twins can be very exciting, the reality of attaching to two babies and adapting to the parental role may be trying.

During labor it is important to monitor each fetus. In the case of twins, an external electronic monitor can be applied to both, or if conditions permit, the internal monitor can be applied to twin A and the external monitor to twin B. The heart rates may be auscultated on different quadrants of the maternal abdomen, but continuous monitoring is more beneficial.

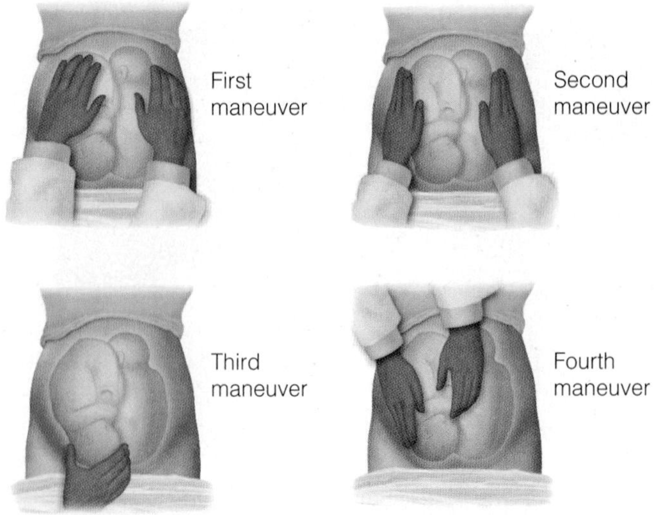

Figure 23–6 **Leopold maneuvers in twin pregnancy for determining fetal head positions, presentations, and lie. The fetus on the mother's right side is in cephalic presentation, and the fetus on the left is in breech presentation. Leopold maneuvers may be done in a different sequence.**

Signs of nonreassuring heart rate patterns should be reported to the physician/CNM.

After a multiple birth, closely monitor the mother for postpartum hemorrhage. Nursing diagnoses that may apply to a woman with a multiple gestation include:

- *Fear* related to unknown outcome of the birth process
- *Coping, Ineffective,* related to uncertainty about the labor and birth plan
- *Knowledge, Deficient,* related to lack of information about the problems associated with multiple gestation
- *Gas Exchange, Impaired,* (fetuses) related to decreased oxygenation secondary to cord compression

(NANDA-I © 2017)

Nursing Plan and Implementation

Community-Based Nursing Care

Antepartum, the woman may need counseling about diet and daily activities. Help her plan meals to meet her increased needs. A daily intake of 4000 kcal (minimum) and 135 g of protein are recommended for optimal weight gain and fetal growth. A prenatal vitamin and 1 mg of folic acid and iron should also be taken daily. A weight gain of 35 to 45 lb is recommended.

Maternal hypertension is treated with bedrest in the lateral position to increase uterine and kidney perfusion. Back discomfort can be alleviated by pelvic rocking, good posture, and good body mechanics. Help the woman schedule frequent periods of rest during the day. Family members or friends may be willing to care for the woman's other children periodically to allow her time to get rest. Community support systems, such as neighbors or church members, may be available to assist the family with meals, grocery shopping, and household chores. Many communities now have support groups specifically designed for mothers of multiples. Members provide invaluable peer support throughout pregnancy and the postpartum period. Teaching regarding prevention and recognition of preterm labor is very important.

Hospital-Based Nursing Care

You will need to prepare to receive multiple newborns. This means a multiplication of resuscitation equipment and newborn identification papers and bracelets. The newborns may be placed in individual radiant warmers or in the same one once identification bands have been applied. Additional staff members should be available for newborn resuscitation, monitoring, and care. Special precautions should be observed to ensure correct identification of the newborns. The first born is usually tagged Baby A; the second, Baby B; and so on.

Evaluation

Expected outcomes of nursing care include:

- The woman is able to discuss the implications and problems associated with a multiple gestation.
- The woman feels she is able to cope with the pregnancy and birth.
- The woman understands the treatment plan and how to gain further information.
- The mother, father/partner, and babies have a safe prenatal course, labor, and birth and a safe postpartum and newborn course.

Care of the Woman and Fetus at Risk Because of Amniotic Fluid-Related Complications

Complications related to amniotic fluid include hydramnios and oligohydramnios.

Hydramnios

Hydramnios (also called *polyhydramnios*) occurs when there is over 2000 mL of amniotic fluid. It typically occurs in 1% of all pregnancies (Gabbe et al., 2016). The exact cause of hydramnios is unknown; however, it often occurs in cases of major congenital anomalies. It is postulated that a major source of amniotic fluid is found in special amnion cells that lie over the placenta (Gabbe et al., 2016). In cases of hydramnios, no pathology has been found in this amniotic epithelium. However, during the second half of the pregnancy, the fetus normally begins to swallow and inspire amniotic fluid and to urinate, which contributes to the amount present. Fetal malformations that affect this swallowing mechanism—as well as neurologic disorders in which the fetal meninges are exposed in the amniotic cavity—can result in hydramnios (Gabbe et al., 2016).

This condition is also found in cases of anencephaly in which the fetus is thought to urinate excessively because of overstimulation of the cerebrospinal centers. When a monozygotic twin manifests hydramnios, it is possible that the twin with the increased blood volume urinates excessively. The weight of the placenta has been found to be increased in some cases of hydramnios, indicating that increased functioning of the placental tissue may contribute to the problem.

There are two types of hydramnios: Chronic and acute. The chronic type, in which the fluid volume gradually increases, is a problem of the third trimester. Most cases are of this variety. In acute cases, the volume increases rapidly over a period of a few days. The acute type is usually diagnosed between 20 and 24 weeks' gestation.

When the amount of amniotic fluid is over 3000 mL, the woman experiences shortness of breath and edema in the lower extremities from compression of the vena cava. If hydramnios is severe enough, she can experience intense pain. The acute form of hydramnios tends to be more severe. Milder forms of hydramnios occur more frequently and are associated with minimal symptoms. Hydramnios is associated with such maternal disorders as diabetes and Rh sensitization. It can also occur as a result of infections such as syphilis, toxoplasmosis, cytomegalovirus, herpes, and rubella (Gabbe et al., 2016).

Fetal malformations and preterm birth are common with hydramnios; thus, there is a fairly high rate of perinatal mortality. Prolapsed umbilical cord can occur when the membranes rupture, which adds a further complication for the fetus. The incidence of malpresentations is also increased (Gabbe et al., 2016).

CLINICAL THERAPY

Hydramnios is managed with supportive treatment unless the intensity of the woman's distress and symptoms dictate otherwise.

If the accumulation of amniotic fluid is severe enough to cause maternal dyspnea and pain, hospitalization and removal of the excessive fluid are required. This can be done vaginally by artificial rupture of membranes (AROM) or by amniocentesis. If the infant is preterm, an abdominal approach may be indicated, but the need for fluid removal is uncommon. In term or near-term gestations, the dangers of performing AROM vaginally are prolapsed cord and the inability to remove the fluid slowly. A *needle amniotomy* (discussed in Chapter 25) may be preferred because this releases the fluid at a slower rate and allows the presenting part to descend gradually.

A needle amniotomy is performed by the physician/CNM. A needle or a fetal scalp electrode is used to make a small puncture in the amniotic sac. There is a risk that the force of the fluid could make a larger hole in the amniotic sac, thus increasing the risk of a prolapsed cord. If amniocentesis is performed, it should be done with the aid of sonography to prevent inadvertent damage to the fetus and placenta. Women with excess amniotic fluid should undergo a vaginal examination after an amniotomy to ensure the presenting part is well applied to the cervix before they ambulate. If the fetal part is not well applied, bedrest is then indicated to reduce the risk of a prolapsed umbilical cord.

A prostaglandin synthesis inhibitor (indomethacin) may be used to treat hydramnios if the amount of amniotic fluid is creating respiratory distress for the mother. The medication works by reducing the fetal urine production. Indomethacin has been shown to decrease amniotic fluid volume by 90 to 100% within the first week of administration, except in cases where hydrocephalus or a fetal neuromuscular disorder is present. The woman then undergoes weekly ultrasounds to determine the amount of amniotic fluid and if additional administration of a prostaglandin synthesis inhibitor is warranted (Carter, 2017).

●○● NURSING MANAGEMENT

For the Woman with Hydramnios

Nursing Assessment and Diagnosis

Hydramnios should be suspected when the fundal height increases out of proportion to the gestational age.

With increased fluid, you may have difficulty palpating the fetus and auscultating the FHR. In more severe cases the maternal abdomen appears extremely tense and tight on inspection. On sonography large spaces can be identified between the fetus and the uterine wall.

Nursing diagnoses that may apply for a woman with hydramnios include:

- ***Gas Exchange, Impaired,*** related to pressure on the diaphragm secondary to hydramnios
- ***Fear*** related to unknown outcome of the pregnancy
- ***Pain, Acute,*** related to abdominal pressure secondary to hydramnios

(NANDA-I © 2017)

Nursing Plan and Implementation

When amniocentesis is performed, sterile technique is used to prevent infection. Offer support to the couple by explaining the procedure to them. After the procedure is completed, uterine and fetal monitoring should be continued for 1 to 2 hours to ensure fetal well-being and that uterine contractions have not been stimulated. While the mother may report some pain at the needle insertion site and mild cramping, vaginal bleeding, regular uterine contractions, or loss of amniotic fluid are complications and need to be reported immediately. Light activity the day of the procedure is recommended, and intercourse should be avoided for 2 days (Ghidini, 2017).

If the fetus has been diagnosed with a congenital defect in utero or is born with the defect, psychologic support is needed to assist the family. Collaborate with social services to offer the family this additional help. Offer to contact chaplain services at the family's request.

Evaluation

Expected outcomes of nursing care include:

- The woman and her partner can discuss the procedure, implications, risks, and characteristics that need to be reported to the caregiver.

Oligohydramnios

Oligohydramnios is defined as a less than normal amount of amniotic fluid (approximately 500 mL is considered normal). Although no exact amount of fluid has been definitively identified as diagnostic of this condition, oligohydramnios is diagnosed when the largest vertical pocket of amniotic fluid visible on ultrasound examination reveals a 5 cm or less pocket of amniotic fluid (Gabbe et al., 2016). The exact cause of oligohydramnios is unknown. It is found in cases of postmaturity, with intrauterine growth restriction (IUGR) secondary to placental insufficiency, and in fetal conditions associated with major renal malformations, including renal aplasia with dysplastic kidneys and obstructive lesions of the lower urinary tract. If oligohydramnios occurs in the first part of pregnancy, there is a danger of fetal adhesions (one part of the fetus may adhere to another part).

During the gestational period, fetal skin and skeletal abnormalities may occur because fetal movement is impaired as a result of inadequate amniotic fluid volume. Because there is less fluid available for the fetus to use during fetal breathing movements, pulmonary hypoplasia may develop. During the labor and birth, the lessened amounts of fluid reduce the cushioning effect for the umbilical cord, and cord compression is more likely to occur.

CLINICAL THERAPY

During the antepartum period, oligohydramnios may be suspected when the uterus does not increase in size in accordance with established gestational dating, the fetus is easily palpated and outlined by the examiner, and the fetus is not ballottable. The fetus can be assessed by biophysical profile (BPP), nonstress tests (NSTs), and serial ultrasounds. During labor the fetus will be monitored by continuous EFM to detect cord compression, which will be indicated by nonperiodic decelerations. Amnioinfusion can replace some fluid volume and remove pressure on the umbilical cord (see Chapter 25).

●○● NURSING MANAGEMENT

For the Woman with Oligohydramnios

Nursing Assessment and Diagnosis

Oligohydramnios should be suspected when the fundal height is less than the gestational age and the fetal parts are easily palpated through the fundal wall. Continuous EFM is an important part of assessment during the labor and birth. Evaluate the EFM tracing for the presence of nonperiodic decelerations or other nonreassuring signs (such as increasing or decreasing baseline, decreased variability, or presence of periodic decelerations). If nonperiodic decelerations are noted, change the woman's position (to relieve pressure on the umbilical cord) and then notify the physician/CNM. If position changes are insufficient to relieve the pattern, an amnioinfusion may be performed. After the birth, the newborn is evaluated for signs of congenital anomalies, pulmonary hypoplasia, or postmaturity.

On sonography there is a lack of amniotic fluid. An amniotic fluid index is typically performed to determine the amount of amniotic fluid. Less than 5 cm of amniotic fluid is considered low, and the diagnosis of oligohydramnios is made (Simpson & Creehan, 2014).

Nursing diagnoses that may apply for a woman with hydramnios include:

- ***Gas Exchange, Impaired,*** related to cord compression secondary to oligohydramnios
- ***Fear*** related to unknown outcome of the pregnancy

(NANDA-I © 2017)

Nursing Plan and Implementation

The fetus is continually monitored during labor and birth. An amnioinfusion (discussed in Chapter 25) is often performed to increase the amount of fluid surrounding the fetus and to decrease the incidence of variable decelerations. In the event that the fetal heart rate tracing is nonreassuring, late decelerations occur, and birth is not imminent, a cesarean birth may be performed. See *Case Study: Melissa Bond-James.*

Evaluation

Expected outcomes of nursing care include:

- The woman and her partner can discuss the diagnosis, implications, and risks to the caregiver.
- The fetus remains uncompromised during labor and birth.

CASE STUDY: Melissa Bond-James

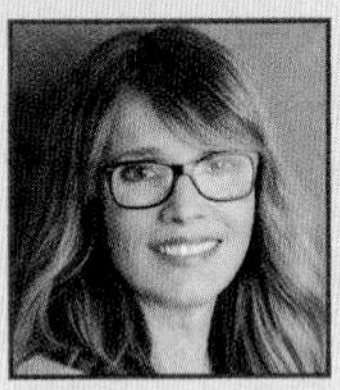

SOURCE: Kinga/Shutterstock.

When Melissa presented to one of her regular prenatal visits she appeared to be measuring smaller than expected based on her gestational age. She noted that she had been feeling regular fetal movement and felt fine. The healthcare provider recommended an ultrasound and arranged for her to go to the hospital immediately following the appointment. At that time, Melissa was 37 weeks 5 days and was due soon but was not experiencing contractions. The ultrasound revealed that Melissa's amniotic fluid index was 4.5 cm.

Questions to Ponder

What was the main purpose of the ultrasound that was ordered due to Melissa's measurements being smaller than expected? When the ultrasound revealed that her amniotic fluid index was 4.5 cm, what would be a likely plan of care for Melissa?

Focus Your Study

- Preterm labor is often treated with tocolytics, which can be effective in stopping labor; however, they do have side effects.
- Both premature rupture of membranes (PROM) and preterm labor place the fetus at risk. Women with preterm premature rupture of membranes (PPROM) and no signs of infection are managed conservatively with bedrest and careful monitoring of fetal well-being.
- Abruptio placentae is the separation of the placenta from the uterine wall before the birth of the baby that often results in painful vaginal bleeding. Abruptio placentae may be central, marginal, or complete.
- Placenta previa occurs when the placenta implants low in the uterus or over the cervix. A low-lying or marginal placenta is one that lies near the cervix. In a partial placenta previa, part

of the placenta lies over the cervix. In a complete placenta previa, the entire placenta covers the cervix. Bleeding associated with placenta previa is typically painless.

- Placental problems can be either developmental or degenerative.
- Cervical insufficiency, the premature dilatation of the cervix, is the most common cause of second-trimester abortion. It is treated surgically with a cerclage, which involves placing a suture in the cervix to keep it from opening.
- Multiple gestation is associated with both maternal and fetal/neonatal complications.
- Hydramnios, also known as polyhydramnios, occurs when there is more than 2000 mL of amniotic fluid contained within the amniotic membranes.
- Oligohydramnios occurs when there is a severely reduced volume of amniotic fluid. Oligohydramnios is associated with intrauterine growth restriction (IUGR), postmaturity, and fetal renal and urinary malformations. The fetus is more likely to experience variable decelerations because the amniotic fluid is insufficient to keep pressure off the umbilical cord.

In order to make safe and effective judgments using NANDA-I © 2017 nursing diagnoses, it is essential that nurses refer to the definitions and defining characteristics of the diagnoses used in this text, which can be found in Appendix C.

References

American College of Obstetricians and Gynecologists (ACOG). (2015). *Definition of term pregnancy* (ACOG Committee Opinion No. 579). Washington, DC: Author.

American College of Obstetricians and Gynecologists (ACOG). (2016a). *Cervical cerclage for cervical insufficiency* (ACOG Practice Bulletin No. 142). Washington, DC: Author.

American College of Obstetricians and Gynecologists (ACOG). (2016b). *Multifetal gestations: Twin, triplet, and higher-order multifetal pregnancies* (ACOG Practice Bulletin No. 169). Washington, DC: Author.

American College of Obstetricians and Gynecologists (ACOG). (2016c). *Prediction and prevention of preterm birth* (ACOG Practice Bulletin No. 130). Washington, DC: Author.

American College of Obstetricians and Gynecologists (ACOG). (2017). *Antenatal corticosteroid therapy for fetal lung maturation* (ACOG Committee Opinion No. 713). Washington, DC: Author.

American College of Obstetricians and Gynecologists (ACOG). (2018). *Prelabor rupture of membranes* (ACOG Practice Bulletin No. 188). *Obstetrics & Gynecology, 131*(1), e1–14.

American College of Obstetricians and Gynecologists (ACOG) & Society of Maternal-Fetal Medicine (SMFM). (2016). *Periviable birth* (Obstetric Care Consensus, No. 4). Washington, DC: ACOG.

American College of Radiology (ACR). (2015). *American College of Radiology appropriateness criteria.* Retrieved from https://acsearch.acr.org/list

Ananth, C. V., & Kinzler, W. L. (2017). *Placental abruption: Clinical features and diagnosis.* UpToDate. Retrieved from https://www.uptodate.com/contents/placental-abruption-clinical-features-and-diagnosis

Association of Women's Health, Obstetric, and Neonatal Nurses (AWHONN). (2015a). Development of an obstetric vital sign alert to improve outcomes in acute care obstetrics. *Nursing for Women's Health, 19*(2), 128–141. DOI: http://dx.doi.org/10.1111/1751-486X.12185

Association of Women's Health, Obstetric, and Neonatal Nurses. (AWHONN). (2015b). *Quantification of blood loss* (AWHONN Practice Brief No. 1). Washington, DC: Author.

Brusch, J. L. (2017). *Urinary tract infection (UTI) and cystitis (bladder infection) in females treatment and management.* Medscape. Retrieved from https://emedicine.medscape.com/article/233101-treatment

Carter, B. S. (2017). *Polyhydramnios and oligohydramnios.* Medscape. Retrieved from https://reference.medscape.com/article/975821-overview#a5

Centers for Disease Control and Prevention (CDC). (2015). *Chlamydial infections.* Retrieved from https://www.cdc.gov/std/tg2015/chlamydia.htm

Centers for Disease Control and Prevention (CDC). (2017). *Preterm birth.* Retrieved from https://www.cdc.gov/reproductivehealth/maternalinfanthealth/pretermbirth.htm

Cunningham, F. G., Leveno, K. J., Bloom, S. L., Spong, C., Dashe, J.S., Hoffman, B.L., . . . Sheffield, J. S. (2016). *Williams obstetrics* (25th ed.). New York, NY: McGraw-Hill.

Davidson, M. R., Armstrong, S., & Sampson, M. (2016). Childbearing in geographically isolated communities: The Smith Island experience. *Journal of Women's Health Care & Social Issues, 6*(1). DOI: 10.4172/2325-9795.1000262

Deering, S. H. (2015). *Abruptio placentae.* eMedicine. Retrieved from http://emedicine.medscape.com/article/252810-overview#a0101

Dutta, E. H., Behnia, F., Harirah, H., Costantine, M., & Saade, G. (2016). Perinatal outcomes after short versus prolonged indomethacin for tocolysis in women with preterm labor. *American Journal of Perinatology, 33*(09), 844–848.

Ehrenkranz, R. A., & Mercurio, M. R. (2017). *Periviable birth (limit of viability).* UpToDate. Retrieved from https://www.uptodate.com/contents/periviable-birth-limit-of-viability

Esplin, M. S., Elovitz, M. A., & Iams, J. A. (2017). Predictive accuracy of serial transvaginal cervical lengths and quantitative vaginal fetal fibronectin levels for spontaneous preterm birth among nulliparous women. *Journal of the American Medical Association, 317*(10), 1047–1056. DOI: 10.1001/jama.2017.1373

Gabbe, S., Niebyl, J., Simpson, J. L., Landon, M. B., Galan, H. L., . . . & Grobman, W. A. (2016). *Normal and problem pregnancies* (7th ed.). Philadelphia, PA: Elsevier.

Gaufberg, S. A. (2008). Abruptio placenta. *eMedicine Journal.* Retrieved from https://www.emedicine.com/emerg/topic12.htm

Ghidini, A. (2017). *Patient education: Amniocentesis (beyond the basics).* UpToDate. Retrieved from https://www.uptodate.com/contents/amniocentesis-beyond-the-basics

Gunasheela, D., Nayak, R., Roy, P., Kumar, V., & Menon, J. (2016). Interval laparoscopic abdominal cerclage for recurrent pregnancy loss. *Journal of Reproductive Biotechnology and Fertility, 5,* 1–4. DOI: 10.1177/2058915816633522

Han, C. S., Schatz, F., & Lockwood, C. J. (2011). Abruption-associated prematurity. *Clinics in Perinatology, 38*(3), 407–421. DOI: http://doi.org/10.1016/j.clp.2011.06.001

Igbinosa, I., Moore, F. A., Johnson, C., & Block, J. E. (2017). Comparison of rapid immunoassays for rupture of fetal membranes. *BMC Pregnancy & Childbirth, 17,* 128. DOI: 10.1186/s12884-017-1311-y

Impey, L., & Child, T. (2017). *Obstetrics and gynecology* (5th ed). New York, NY: Wiley-Blackwell.

Jazayeri, A. (2015). *Cervical cerclage.* Medscape. Retrieved from https://emedicine.medscape.com/article/1848163-overview

Jazayeri, A. (2017). *Premature rupture of membranes.* Medscape. Retrieved from https://emedicine.medscape.com/article/261137-overview

Kore, S. (2016). *Multiple gestations: Basics and beyond.* New Delhi: Jaypee Brothers Medical Publishing.

Linehan, L. A., Walsh, J., Morris, A., Kenny, L., O'Donoghue, K., Dempsey, E., & Russell, N. (2016). Neonatal and maternal outcomes following midtrimester preterm premature rupture of the membranes: A retrospective cohort study. *BMC Pregnancy and Childbirth, 16*(25). DOI: 10.1186/s12884-016-0813-3

Lockwood, C. J., & Stieglitz, K. R. (2017). *Placenta previa: Management.* UpToDate. Retrieved from https://www.uptodate.com/contents/placenta-previa-management

March of Dimes. (2016). *Premature babies.* Retrieved from https://www.marchofdimes.org/complications/premature-babies.aspx

March of Dimes. (2018). *Preterm labor and premature birth: Are you at risk?* Retrieved from https://www.marchofdimes.org/complications/preterm-labor-and-premature-birth-are-you-at-risk.aspx

Martin, J. A., Hamilton, B. E., Osterman, M. J., Driscoll, A. K., & Mathews, T. J. (2017). Births: Final data for 2015. *National Vital Statistics Report, 66*(1), 1.

Matthews, T. J., MacDorman, M. F., & Thoma, M. E. (2015). Infant mortality statistics from the 2013 period linked birth/infant death data set. *National Vital Statistics Report, 64*(9), 1–29.

Perinatal Hospice and Palliative Care. (2017). *Continuing your pregnancy when your baby's life is expected to be brief.* Retrieved from https://www.perinatalhospice.org/

Polin, R. A., Abman, S. H., Rowitch, D., & Benitz, W. E. (2016). *Fetal and neonatal physiology* (5th ed.). Atlanta, GA: Elsevier.

Puertas, A., Magan-Fernandez, A., Blanc, V., Revelles, L., O'Valle, F., Pozo, E., . . . & Mesa, F. (2017). Association of periodontitis with preterm birth and low birth weight: A comprehensive review. *Journal of Maternal Fetal Neonatal Medicine, 31*(5), 1–6. DOI: 10.1080/14767058.2017.1293023

Robinson, J. N., & Norwitz, E. R. (2017). *Preterm birth: Risk factors and interventions for risk reduction.* Retrieved from https://www.uptodate.com/contents/preterm-birth-risk-factors-and-interventions-for-risk-reduction

Ross, M. G. (2017). *Preterm labor.* Medscape. Retrieved from https://emedicine.medscape.com/article/260998-overview

Sherman, M. P. (2017). *Chorioamnioitis.* Medscape. Retrieved from https://emedicine.medscape.com/article/973237-overview#a6

Simpson, K. R., & Creehan, P. A. (2014). *AWHONN perinatal nursing* (4th ed.). Philadelphia, PA: Lippincott, Williams & Wilkins.

Wilson, B. A., Shannon, M. T., & Shields, K. (2017). *Pearson nurse's drug guide 2018.* Hoboken, NJ: Pearson.

Zhang, G., Feenstra, B., Bacelis, J., Liu, X., Muglia, L. M., Juodakis, J., . . . & Muglia, L. J. (2017). Genetic associations with gestational duration and spontaneous preterm birth. *New England Journal of Medicine, 377*, 1156–1167. DOI: 10.1056/NEJMoa1612665

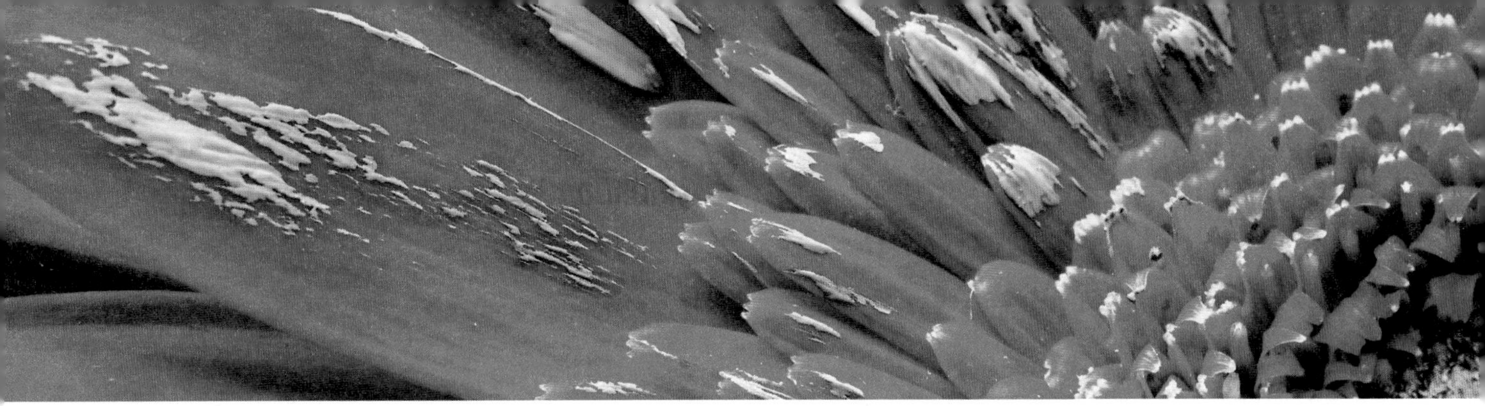

Chapter 24
Childbirth at Risk: Labor-Related Complications

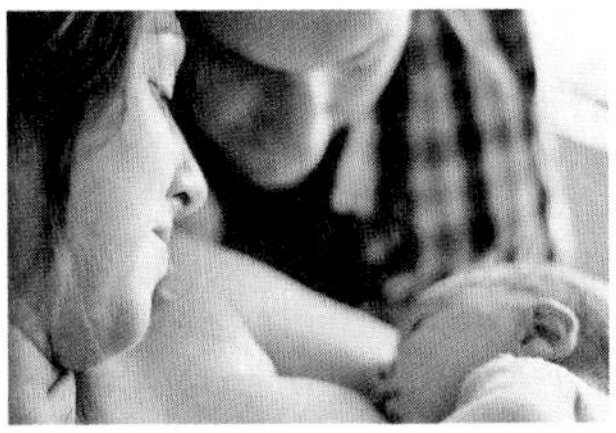

SOURCE: Fancy Collection/SuperStock.

I couldn't wait to begin labor. I wasn't afraid. We had wonderful plans for our labor and birth. My nurse helped me with my breathing as I entered transition. Everything was going so well. Suddenly, the baby began having decelerations. The nurse assisted me onto my side and called for assistance. Time seemed to stand still as the once rapidly beating heart suddenly sounded so slow. It seemed like it took forever to return to its previous rapid pace. For an instant, I was terrified, but after that one episode, there were no further problems.

Learning Outcomes

24.1 Discuss dysfunctional labor patterns.

24.2 Describe the impact of postterm pregnancy on the childbearing family.

24.3 Summarize various types of fetal malposition and malpresentation and possible associated problems.

24.4 Discuss the implications of macrosomia and hydrocephalus on the woman and the fetus.

24.5 Analyze the implications of abnormal placenta and umbilical cord variations.

24.6 Discuss the interventions needed in caring for a woman with a prolapsed umbilical cord.

24.7 Discuss the identification, management, and nursing care of women with anaphylactoid syndrome of pregnancy.

24.8 Identify the signs and symptoms associated with a uterine rupture.

24.9 Delineate the effects of pelvic contractures on labor and birth.

24.10 Identify complications related to uterine rupture.

24.11 Discuss complications of the third and fourth stages of labor.

Healthy People 2020

(MICH-1.2) Reduce the rate of fetal and infant deaths during perinatal period (28 weeks of gestation to less than 7 days after birth)

(MICH-6) Reduce maternal illness and complications due to pregnancy (complications during hospitalized labor and delivery)

(MICH-16) Increase the proportion of women delivering a live birth who received preconception care services and practiced key recommended preconception health behaviors

The successful completion of the 40-week gestational period requires the harmonious functioning of the critical factors we discussed in Chapter 19: The birth passage, the fetus, the relationship between the passage and fetus, and the forces of labor. Disruptions in any of these components may result in dystocia (at-risk or difficult labor). Some of the most common at-risk conditions during labor are discussed in this chapter.

Care of the Woman Experiencing Dystocia Related to Dysfunctional Uterine Contractions

Dystocia is an abnormal labor pattern in which abnormalities occur with the *power* (uterine contractions or maternal expulsion forces), the *passenger* (fetal size, position, or presentation), or the *passage* (soft tissues or pelvis). Dystocia is defined as a rate of cervical dilatation of less than 0.5 cm per hour over 4 hours during the active stage of labor or less than 1 cm per hour of fetal descent during the second stage of labor (Senger, 2015). Dystocia encompasses many problems in labor, the most common of which is dysfunctional (or uncoordinated) uterine contractions that result in a prolongation of labor. Figure 24–1 depicts normal, tachysystole, and hypotonic uterine contraction patterns. Risk factors for labor dystocia include:

- Advanced maternal age
- Maternal obesity
- Nulliparity
- Short maternal height
- Pregnancy complications
- Labor induction
- Premature rupture of membranes
- Prolonged latent phase
- Epidural anesthesia
- Chorioamnionitis
- Postterm gestation
- Large-for-gestational-age (LGA) fetus
- Malposition
- Malpresentation.

Tachysystole Labor Patterns

Tachysystole is defined as uterine contraction frequency of more than five contractions in a 10-minute period with less than 60 seconds of relaxation between contractions or contractions lasting greater than 2 minutes. Risk factors for uterine tachysystole include:

- High-dose oxytocin titration regimens
- Oxytocin incremental intervals less than 30 minutes
- Cocaine use
- Uterine rupture
- Placental abruption.

Fetal-neonatal risks include:

- Nonreassuring fetal status because contractions and increased resting tone interfere with the uteroplacental exchange

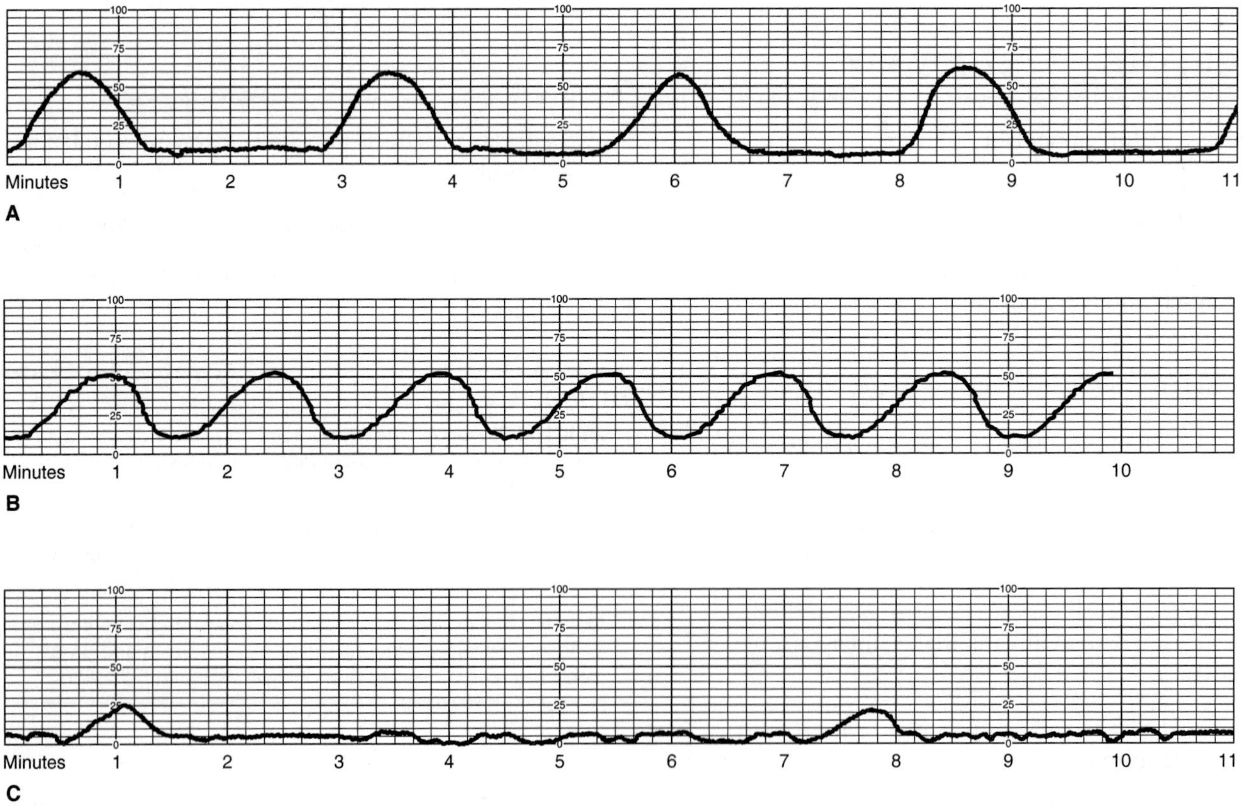

Figure 24–1 **Comparison of labor patterns. A. Normal uterine contraction pattern. Note that the contraction is every 3 minutes; duration is 60 seconds. The baseline resting tone is below 10 mmHg. B. Tachysystole uterine contraction pattern. Note that the contraction frequency is every 1.5 minutes, with a duration of 90 seconds. The baseline resting tone is 10 mmHg. C. Hypotonic uterine contraction pattern. Note in this example that the contraction frequency is every 7 minutes with some uterine activity between contractions, duration is 50 seconds, and intensity increases approximately 25 mmHg during contractions.**

- Category II and III fetal tracings (discussed later in the chapter)
- Prolonged pressure on the fetal head, which may result in cephalohematoma, caput succedaneum, or excessive molding.

CLINICAL THERAPY

Continuous fetal monitoring is warranted for the woman with a tachysystole labor pattern. If the woman is receiving oxytocin (Pitocin), the infusion should be stopped immediately. If contractions normalize to a desirable pattern with normal fetal heart rate tracings, a tocolytic agent should be administered.

NURSING MANAGEMENT

For the Woman Experiencing Tachysystole Labor

Nursing Assessment and Diagnosis

As part of the labor assessment, monitor the frequency, duration, and intensity of labor contractions. Contractions should not occur more frequently than every 2 minutes and should have a period of 60 seconds of relaxation between contractions. Uterine contractions should last less than 2 minutes in length. Contractions outside of these parameters in frequency or duration are considered tachysystole and warrant immediate intervention.

Nursing diagnoses that may apply to the woman in tachysystole labor include:

- ***Pain, Acute,*** related to the woman's inability to relax secondary to tachysystole uterine contractions
- ***Coping, Ineffective,*** related to ineffectiveness of breathing techniques to relieve discomfort
- ***Anxiety*** related to frequency of contractions and lack of an adequate uterine relaxation period

(NANDA-I © 2017)

Nursing Plan and Implementation

A key nursing responsibility is to provide comfort and support to the laboring woman and her partner. The woman experiencing a tachysystole labor pattern will probably be very uncomfortable because of the increased force of contractions. Her anxiety level and that of her partner may be high. It is important to do all you can to reduce the woman's discomfort and promote a more effective labor pattern.

Suggest supportive measures such as a change of position: Left lateral side-lying, high Fowler, rocking in a rocking chair, or sitting up (Cunningham et al., 2016). Continuous fetal monitoring is essential. Institute comfort measures such as maintaining a quiet environment, back rub, therapeutic touch, visualization, effleurage, and relaxation exercises. The oxytocin infusion (if one is being used), should be stopped immediately. Any breast stimulation that may be used to stimulate contractions should also be stopped. If the contraction pattern continues, an order for a tocolytic agent is obtained and immediately administered. The physician/CNM should be advised of the patient's status and the contraction pattern. Although extremely rare, tachysystole can be associated with placenta abruption or uterine rupture, both of which are life-threatening complications. Nonreassuring fetal status often occurs with a tachysystole contraction pattern, so intrauterine resuscitation measures may become warranted and can include the following:

- Position the woman on her left side.
- Apply oxygen via face mask.
- Increase intravenous fluids by at least 500 mL bolus.
- Call for anesthesia provider for support.
- Call the physician/CNM to the bedside.

The labor partner may also need assistance in understanding the situation and helping the woman cope. Maintain a calm, understanding approach; this will provide the woman and her partner further support. It is important to offer information about the cause of the tachysystole labor pattern and assure the woman that she is not overreacting to the situation. Families with English as a second language may have difficulty understanding the explanation so an interpreter should be brought in to adequately explain the circumstances as soon as possible.

Patient education is key for the woman experiencing tachysystole labor. She needs information about the dysfunctional labor pattern and the possible implications for herself and her baby. Information will help relieve anxiety and decrease fear about the interventions that may rapidly be occurring. Explain the purpose of the treatment and offer opportunities to ask questions.

Evaluation

Anticipated outcomes of nursing care include:

- The woman's labor pattern normalizes with contractions of normal frequency, duration, and intensity.
- The woman and her partner are able to cope with the abnormal labor pattern and interventions.
- The woman's level of pain becomes more tolerable.

Hypotonic Labor Patterns

Hypotonic uterine contractions are a common cause of dystocia in the first stage and typically occur in nulliparous women. When cervical dilatation and effacement are not occurring, other factors should be ruled out, including cephalopelvic disproportion, malposition, malpresentation, and macrosomia. Other factors that increase the risk of hypotonic labor include induced labor with an unripe cervix, false labor, early amniotomy, and premature rupture of membranes.

Clinical Tip

Normal cervical dilatation in a first-time mother—commonly known as a "primip"—is just over 1 cm per hour, and dilatation in a "multip" is about 1.5 cm per hour. If your assessments reveal that this expected pattern is not occurring, consider that a problem may be developing. The most likely causes of the problem are related either to the contractions or to fetal position or size.

CLINICAL THERAPY

When uterine contractions are irregular and of low amplitude and there is commonly less than 1 cm cervical dilatation per hour (called *prolonged labor*) or there has been no change of cervical dilatation for 2 hours (*arrest of progress*), the physician/CNM evaluates for contraindications to oxytocin (Pitocin), the size of the maternal pelvis, the position and presentation of the fetus, and fetal weight. Cephalopelvic disproportion (CPD) must be excluded. Station is a key component when evaluating for CPD. If the presenting part is not engaged ("out of the pelvis"), especially in a nulliparous woman, it is possible that CPD is present.

If CPD exists, oxytocin (Pitocin) augmentation should not be used and a cesarean birth is indicated.

When CPD is ruled out, an amniotomy (artificial rupture of membranes [AROM]) can be performed if membranes are intact.

Amniotomy is associated with a reduction in the length of labor and reduced cesarean birth rates and should be performed under the following circumstances:

- Active labor has been established.
- The presenting part is well applied to the cervix.
- Hypotonic labor patterns are present.
- Hypercontractibility is present.

Clinical Tip

Amniotomy should not be performed if the presenting part is not well applied to the cervix because this increases the risk of cord prolapse.

Oxytocin is the drug of choice for labor augmentation or labor induction. Oxytocin should be used with caution since it is a drug that appears on the high-alert list due to its ability to cause uterine tachysystole. (See *Drug Guide: Oxytocin [Pitocin]* in Chapter 25.)

The American College of Obstetricians and Gynecologists has outlined two regimens of oxytocin administration: A low-dose regimen and a high-dose regimen (see complete discussion in Chapter 25). Low-dose regimens are associated with less uterine tachysystole, although fetal outcomes have not differed between the two groups. High-dose regimens are associated with a shorter length of labor, decreased second stage, reduced chorioamnionitis and neonatal sepsis, and reduced incidence of cesarean births related to dystocia; however, they are associated with increased rates of uterine tachysystole with adverse fetal heart rate (FHR) changes (Cunningham et al., 2016). Continuous electronic fetal monitoring (EFM) is required for any woman receiving oxytocin. With augmentation of labor, the contraction pattern and progressive cervical dilatation pattern should improve, and fetal descent (measured by station) should occur. If there is no improvement in these areas, cesarean birth may be necessary.

●○● NURSING MANAGEMENT

For the Woman Experiencing Hypotonic Labor

Nursing Assessment and Diagnosis

Assessing maternal vital signs, contractions, cervical dilatation, fetal descent, and FHR characteristics provides the data you will use to evaluate maternal-fetal status. Be sure also to assess for signs and symptoms of infection and dehydration. During the vaginal examination, assess the fetal presenting part (usually vertex) for the development of a caput. If the fetal vertex presses down on the cervix during contractions without further descent, a *caput succedaneum* may occur. As hypotonic labor continues, the caput increases in size; it seems that the head is descending, but it is not (Figure 24–2).

Because labor progress is slow, assess the woman's stress and coping, noting whether anxiety is having a deleterious effect on labor progress. Evidence of increasing frustration and discouragement on the part of the mother and her partner may become apparent as labor continues.

The laboring woman should maintain adequate fluid and nourishment throughout labor. Oral fluid intake or intravenous fluids can be provided. Women can eat light snacks in early labor as well. Ensure that adequate urinary output is occurring.

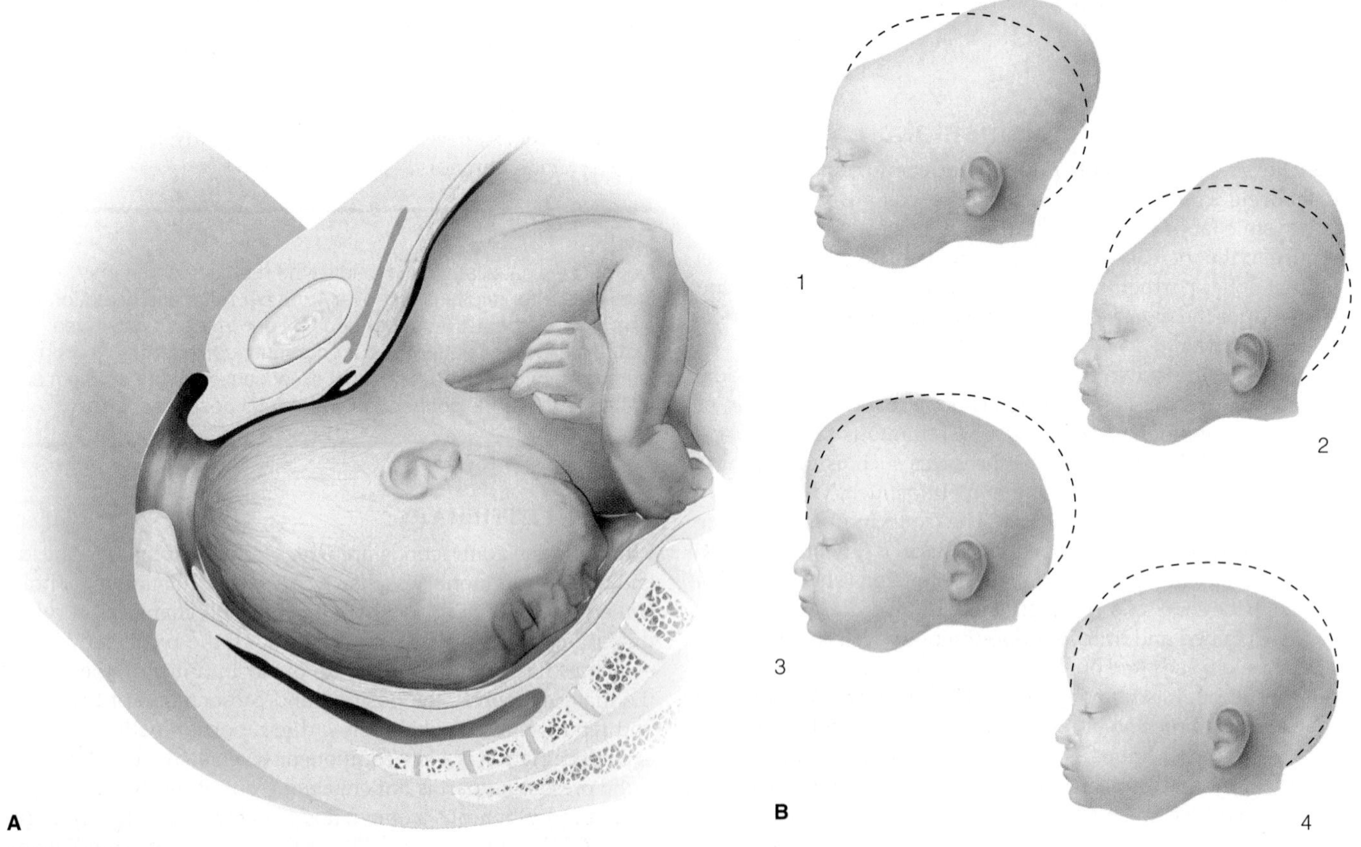

Figure 24–2 Effects of labor on the fetal head. A. Caput succedaneum formation. The presenting portion of the scalp area is encircled by the cervix during labor, causing swelling of the soft tissue. B. Molding of the fetal head in cephalic presentations: (1) occiput anterior, (2) occiput posterior, (3) brow, (4) face.

Nursing diagnoses that may apply to the woman experiencing dysfunctional labor include:

- ***Pain, Acute***, related to rapid increase in frequency and intensity of uterine contractions
- ***Coping, Ineffective***, related to ineffectiveness of breathing techniques to relieve discomfort
- ***Anxiety*** related to slow labor progress

(NANDA-I © 2017)

Nursing Plan and Implementation

Nursing measures are aimed at promoting maternal and fetal well-being. Frequently monitor maternal vital signs; note the frequency, duration, and strength of contractions; and assess the FHR. Once the amniotic membranes are ruptured, assess the amount of fluid and the presence of blood or meconium (dark green, light green, yellowish, or black stool present in the large intestine of the fetus). Because meconium can be associated with a compromised fetus, ongoing observation of the amniotic fluid is critical. Once meconium-stained fluid is identified, continuous fetal monitoring is warranted.

Maternal hydration status can be monitored by recording intake and output. Assess the bladder every 2 hours for distention; an in-and-out catheterization can be performed for women unable to void on their own. Alternatively, a Foley catheter may be inserted during the first stage of labor to reduce the need for multiple in-and-out catheterizations, which can increase the risk of urinary tract infections. The catheter should be removed before maternal pushing.

Ongoing evaluation for symptoms of infection should be performed, especially for prolonged labors. These symptoms include fever, chills, foul-smelling amniotic fluid, and fetal tachycardia. Vaginal examinations should be kept to a minimum to reduce the incidence of infection.

The laboring woman needs information about the hypotonic labor pattern and the possible implications for herself and her baby. You will need to:

- Address the woman's and her partner's concerns and questions.
- Provide clear, accurate information.
- Keep the woman and her partner informed of labor progress.
- Advise the woman and her partner of possible treatment measures.
- Discuss disadvantages and treatment alternatives.

Evaluation

Expected outcomes of nursing care include:

- The woman and her partner understand the labor pattern and its possible implications.
- The woman and her partner are able to cope with the labor.
- The woman's comfort increases and her anxiety decreases.
- The woman experiences a more effective labor pattern.

Care of the Woman with Postterm Pregnancy

Postterm pregnancy is one that extends more than 294 days or 42 completed weeks past the first day of the last menstrual period. It is important to understand that 42 completed weeks refers to the completion of 42 weeks, meaning that the seventh day has elapsed. The incidence of postterm pregnancy is approximately 7% of all pregnancies in the United States (Norwitz, 2017). Postterm pregnancy has been associated with primiparity, previous postterm pregnancy, placental sulfatase deficiency, fetal anencephaly, male fetus, maternal obesity, and genetic predisposition (Norwitz, 2017).

Many times postterm pregnancies are related to inaccurate pregnancy dating. A frequent cause of inaccurate pregnancy dating is error in determining the time of ovulation and conception according to the first day of the last menstrual period. This error can be corrected by performing a first-trimester scan, which is the most accurate ultrasonic gestational age assessment. During the first trimester, the crown-rump length (CRL) is used. In a second-trimester ultrasound, which is less accurate, the biparietal diameter of the fetal head is measured and then compared with conventional dating tables. First-trimester dating reduces the number of estimated postterm pregnancies and decreases unnecessary interventions (Norwitz, 2017).

Maternal Risks

Although postterm pregnancy does not pose any significant risk to the woman during the pregnancy, the labor and birth process may be affected. Maternal symptoms and complications may include:

- Increased discomforts of pregnancy
- Maternal anxiety
- Insomnia
- Cesarean birth
- Operative vaginal birth (forceps or vacuum extractor)
- Perineal trauma and damage
- Maternal hemorrhage.

"When I went over my due date, I felt so anxious and overwhelmed. I was mentally prepared to carry my baby until a certain date, but once that date was reached, I felt unable to deal with all of the discomforts of pregnancy. I couldn't sleep well. I was uncomfortable eating, walking, even putting on my shoes. Well-wishing friends and family would call and say, 'Haven't you had that baby yet?' The calls just made it worse. I can't tell you how relieved I was when labor started, and I knew I would soon meet my new baby."

Fetal-Neonatal Risks

True postterm pregnancies are frequently associated with placental changes that cause a decrease in the uterine–placental–fetal circulation. The perinatal mortality rate after 42 weeks is twice that of term fetuses and increases sixfold during the 43rd gestational week (Norwitz, 2017). Complications related to alternations in placenta functioning include:

- Reduced placental blood supply
- Decreased fetal oxygenation
- Reduced nutritional supply.

Other fetal-newborn complications may include:

- Oligohydramnios
- Risk of umbilical cord compression

- Small for gestational age (SGA)
- Large for gestational age (LGA)
- Macrosomia
- Higher incidence of birth trauma
- Risk of shoulder dystocia
- Cephalopelvic disproportion (CPD)
- Meconium, which can be associated with nonreassuring fetal status and meconium aspiration at birth
- Low umbilical artery pH
- Low 5-minute Apgar scores
- Nonreassuring fetal status
- Increased category II and III FHR tracings
- Hypoglycemia
- Seizures
- Respiratory distress.

Approximately 20% of all postterm fetuses experience *dysmaturity syndrome*, which is associated with uteroplacental insufficiency (resembling intrauterine growth restriction), meconium aspiration, and short-term neonatal complications (Norwitz, 2017).

Ethics in Action!

How would you respond if a woman with an unfavorable cervix is pressuring you to schedule an induction so that her mother can be present for the birth before leaving on a trip?

CLINICAL THERAPY

When the 40th week of gestation is completed and birth has not occurred, most practitioners begin using the nonstress test (NST), biophysical profile (BPP), or a modified BPP (ultrasound measurement of the amniotic fluid volume plus an NST) as assessment tools. While there is no consensus on the frequency of antenatal surveillance, many practitioners use twice-weekly testing providing the amniotic fluid level is normal. Any time that tests indicate fetal problems or there is decreased amniotic fluid volume, induction of labor is recommended (Norwitz, 2017). Most practitioners consider induction at 41 gestational weeks to reduce maternal and fetal-newborn risks associated with postterm pregnancy (Norwitz, 2017).

●○● NURSING MANAGEMENT

For the Woman with Postterm Pregnancy

Nursing Assessment and Diagnosis

When the woman is admitted into the birthing area, it is important to establish the estimated date of birth (EDB) and ascertain the type of antenatal testing that has been completed. During labor, ongoing assessments of the FHR by continuous EFM are important to identify reassuring characteristics (lack of decelerations, accelerations with fetal movement) and to determine the presence of variable decelerations or late decelerations so that corrective actions may be taken. When amniotic membranes rupture, assess the fluid for the presence of meconium. Ongoing assessments of labor progress (contractions, progressive cervical dilatation and effacement, and fetal descent) may provide clues to the presence of a macrosomic fetus because labor may be lengthened and fetal descent may not occur. See *Case Study: Angelina Newman*.

Possible nursing diagnoses for the woman with postterm pregnancy include:

- ***Fear*** related to the unknown outcome for the baby
- ***Coping: Family, Compromised,*** related to concern regarding the status of the baby
- ***Injury, Risk for,*** to the fetus related to the birth of a macrosomic baby
- ***Injury, Risk for,*** to the mother related to perineal trauma
- ***Pain, Acute,*** related to the birthing process

(NANDA-I © 2017)

Nursing Plan and Implementation

Community-Based Nursing Care

If the woman has not been assessing fetal activity every day, teach her how to do it so that she can identify inadequate fetal movement and contact her healthcare provider (see Chapter 16 for discussion of techniques to detect fetal movement). Explain antenatal testing procedures and the rationale for the need for testing, and stress the importance of antenatal fetal testing. It is important to provide education on implications, potential fetal risks, and possible treatment options. You will perform most antenatal testing, and you must be knowledgeable regarding the testing procedures, interpretation of results, and collaboration with the physician/CNM. Always provide an opportunity for the woman and her partner to ask questions and clarify information.

CASE STUDY: Angelina Newman

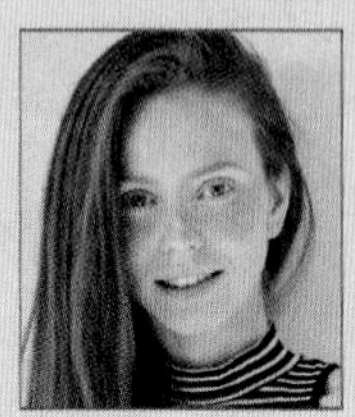

SOURCE: WAYHOME studio/Shutterstock.

Angelina was due to have her baby 8 days ago. She was advised to watch for signs of preterm labor when she was 32 weeks because of contractions. She is now more than a week overdue and is distraught, exhausted, and growing frustrated. She is having difficulty arranging transportation to the additional medical appointments and does not understand why she can't just have a cesarean birth since the baby "will not come out." The midwife advised her that she will be scheduled to be induced on Wednesday if she does not go into labor before that time. The midwife plans to admit her for cervical ripening and then a Pitocin induction.

Question to Ponder

How would you explain to Angelina why it is necessary for her to first have cervical ripening agents prior to the induction?

Hospital-Based Nursing Care

In the birth setting, the response of the fetus during labor is assessed carefully; thus continuous electronic monitoring is warranted. If variable decelerations are present, change the laboring woman's position to attempt to take pressure off the umbilical cord and reevaluate the FHR. When an amnioinfusion is performed to increase the volume of fluid or to dilute meconium-stained fluid, assist with the procedure and monitor the infusion and the response of the FHR. (See Chapter 25 for further discussion.) See *Case Study: Melissa Bond-James*.

Evaluation

Expected outcomes of nursing care include:

- The woman is able to explain the implications of the postterm pregnancy.
- The woman and her partner and family feel supported and able to cope with the labor and birth.
- Fetal problems are identified quickly.

Care of the Woman and Fetus at Risk Because of Fetal Malposition

Persistent occiput posterior (OP) position of the fetus is the most common fetal malposition and occurs when the head remains in the direct OP position throughout labor. In early labor approximately 15% of fetuses are in OP position, although only 5% remain in that position at the time of birth (Gabbe et al., 2016). This position may be normal in some races, particularly those in which women tend to have small pelvises or in women with anthropoid pelvises. The position is related to transverse narrowing of the midpelvis. For a fetus in an OP position to rotate to an occiput anterior (OA) position, it must rotate 135 degrees (right-occiput-posterior [ROP] to right-occiput-transverse [ROT] to right-occiput-anterior [ROA] to OA) (see Figure 19–9) and, in most cases, this rotation is accomplished. In others, however, it is not. Labor progress may cease, or the fetus may be born in a posterior position. Occiput posterior positions are associated with a higher incidence of vacuum-assisted births.

Maternal-Fetal-Neonatal Risks

The woman usually experiences intense pain in the small of her back throughout the labor, unless the baby rotates. At birth, if the fetus remains in a posterior position, the woman may suffer a third- or fourth-degree perineal laceration or extension of a midline episiotomy. There is no increased risk of fetal mortality because of the OP position unless labor is protracted or an operative birth is performed. There is a higher incidence of operative vaginal deliveries in fetuses who fail to rotate from the OP position. Maternal risks of OP malposition include (Simkin & Ancheta, 2017):

- Higher rates of cesarean birth
- Prolonged first and second stage of labor
- Oxytocin augmentation
- Anal sphincter injury
- Severe perineal lacerations
- Episiotomy
- Blood loss greater than 500 mL
- Postpartum infection
- Accidental lacerations of the lower uterine segment during cesarean
- Instrument delivery.

CLINICAL THERAPY

Medical treatment focuses on close monitoring of both maternal and fetal status and labor progress to determine whether vaginal or cesarean birth is the safer method. Prenatally, use of a hands-and-knees position twice daily has been helpful in correcting the persistent OP position if it is diagnosed prenatally (Simkin & Ancheta, 2017). Vaginal birth is possible via the following methods:

1. Spontaneous birth
2. Forceps-assisted birth with the occiput directly posterior
3. Forceps rotation of the occiput to the anterior position and birth (Scanzoni maneuver) (Figure 24–3)
4. Manual rotation to the anterior position followed by spontaneous or forceps-assisted birth (Figure 24–4).

If the pelvis has larger diameters and the perineal muscles are relaxed, as found in grand multiparity (a woman who has had five or more children), the fetus may have no particular problem emerging spontaneously in the OP position. If, however, the perineum is rigid, the second stage of labor may be prolonged. A prolonged second stage is one that lasts over an hour in multiparas and 2 hours or more in nulliparas.

In the event of a prolonged second stage with arrest of descent due to the OP position, a forceps or manual rotation may be done if no cephalopelvic disproportion (CPD) is present; however, many obstetricians opt to perform a cesarean birth. If CPD is suspected, cesarean birth is warranted.

CASE STUDY: Melissa Bond-James

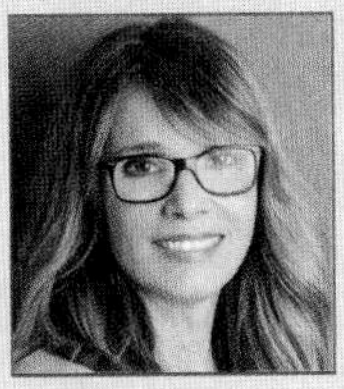

SOURCE: Kinga/Shutterstock.

The nurse enters the labor room and notes that Melissa is having some decelerations with contractions. Upon further assessment, the nurse notes that the fetal heart rate begins to decrease after the contraction ceases. The pattern is repetitive and occurs with each contraction. The nurse informs Melissa she will call the nurse midwife and share these findings but before she leaves, she must perform certain interventions.

Question to Ponder

What interventions do you expect will be performed as a result of seeing late decelerations on the fetal monitoring strip?

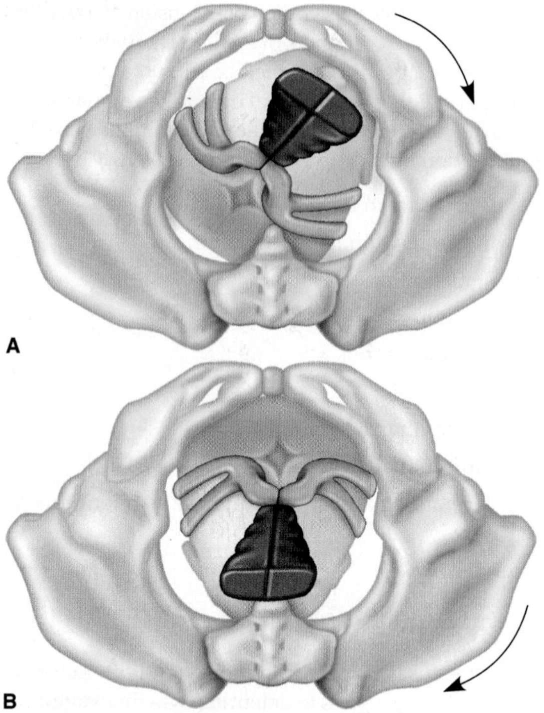

Figure 24–3 **Scanzoni maneuver, anterior rotation. A. Forceps are applied to the fetal head, which is in ROP position. Fetal head is then rotated 45 degrees to ROT, then another 45 degrees to ROA, then a final 45 degrees to OA. B. The fetal position has now changed from ROP to OA for a total rotation of 135 degrees. The forceps are now upside-down, so they are removed and reapplied to provide the traction necessary for a forceps-assisted birth.**

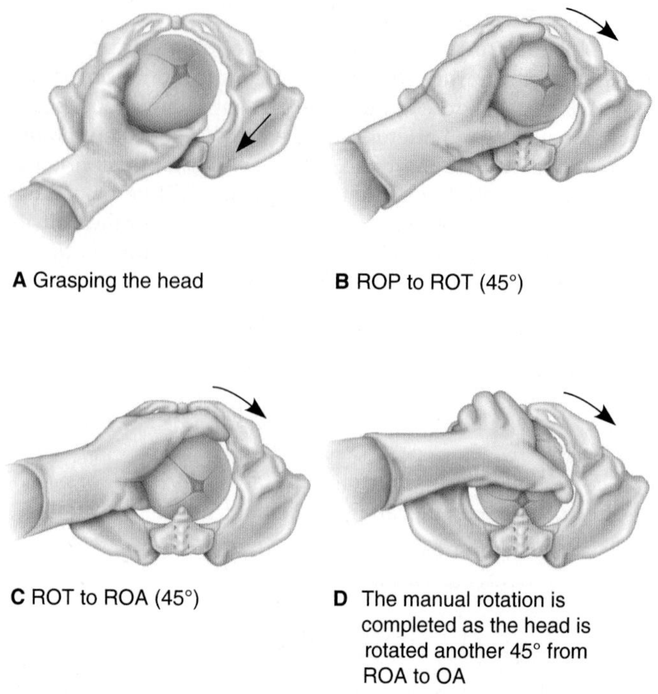

Figure 24–4 **Manual rotation of ROP to OA. A. The physician's left hand is inserted into the vagina and the back of the fetal head is grasped. B. The head is flexed and then rotated 45 degrees to ROT. C. The head is rotated another 45 degrees to ROA. D. The manual rotation is completed as the head is rotated another 45 degrees from ROA to OA. During the manual rotation, the physician's other hand is placed on the maternal abdomen, and the body is turned in the same direction as the head by applying pressure to the fetal breech or shoulders.**

Women with Special Needs Autonomic Dysreflexia

Autonomic dysreflexia is a rare complication that can occur in women with a spinal cord injury. It is caused by overstimulation of the nerve pathways and is characterized by paroxysmal hypertension, intense throbbing headaches, profuse perspiration, nasal stuffiness, anxiety, and skin flushing. Cognitive impairment may also occur. The condition is life-threatening and requires prompt intervention and immediate evaluation from the obstetrician and anesthesiologist.

●○● NURSING MANAGEMENT

For the Laboring Woman with a Fetus in Occiput Posterior Position

Nursing Assessment and Diagnosis

The first sign of OP position is intense back pain in the first stage of labor. The back pain is caused by the fetal occiput compressing the sacral nerves. Other signs and symptoms may include:

- Dysfunctional labor pattern
- Prolonged active phase
- Secondary arrest of dilatation
- Arrest of descent
- Depression in the maternal abdomen above the symphysis pubis
- FHR auscultated far laterally on the maternal abdomen
- A wide diamond-shaped anterior fontanelle in the anterior portion of the pelvis is felt upon vaginal examination.

Leopold maneuvers should be performed to detect positional changes (see Chapter 20 and Figure 20–4). Intrapartum ultrasound is another effective tool for detecting fetal malposition.

Nursing diagnoses that may apply to women with persistent OP position include:

- ***Pain, Acute,*** related to back discomfort secondary to occiput posterior position
- ***Coping, Ineffective,*** related to persistent back pain

(NANDA-I © 2017)

Nursing Plan and Implementation

Labor management interventions for the woman include:

- Forward leaning, hands and knees, straddling, kneeling, or side-lying positioning
- Pelvic rocking
- Whirlpool or shower
- Adequate fluid and hydration during labor
- Judicious use of anesthesia as needed
- Oxytocin infusion

- Amniotomy
- Anticipate possible need for vacuum or forceps
- Birthing ball use (see Figure 21–2).

Evaluation

Expected outcomes of nursing care include:

- The woman's discomfort is decreased.
- The woman and her partner apply comfort measures and position changes that assist her.
- The woman's coping abilities are strengthened.
- The woman and her partner state that they feel supported and encouraged.

Care of the Woman and Fetus at Risk Because of Fetal Malpresentation

In a normal cephalic presentation, the occiput is the presenting part, and the head is flexed with the chin on the chest (Figure 24–5A). Three cephalic malpresentations are possible: *Sinciput* (also called *military*), *brow*, and *face* (Figure 24–5B–D). The fetal body straightens out in these malpresentations from the classic fetal position to an S-shaped position. Of these, the military presentation is probably the least difficult for the woman and fetus. In most cases, as soon as the head reaches the pelvic floor, flexion occurs and a vaginal birth results. Thus, of the cephalic malpresentations, only brow and face are discussed here.

In addition to the cephalic malpresentations, the breech, shoulder (transverse lie), and compound presentations can cause significant difficulty during labor. These malpresentations are also discussed in this chapter.

Brow Presentation

Brow presentations are the least common of all presentations, with an incidence of 1 in 500 births to 1 in 1400 births (Lin, 2016). In a brow presentation, the forehead of the fetus becomes the presenting part and the head is slightly extended instead of flexed, which results in the head entering the birth canal with the widest diameter of the head (occipitomental) foremost (see Figure 24–5C). Proposed causes include:

- High parity
- Placenta previa
- Uterine anomaly
- Hydramnios
- Fetal anomaly
- Low birth weight
- Cephalopelvic disproportion
- Large-for-gestational-age fetus.

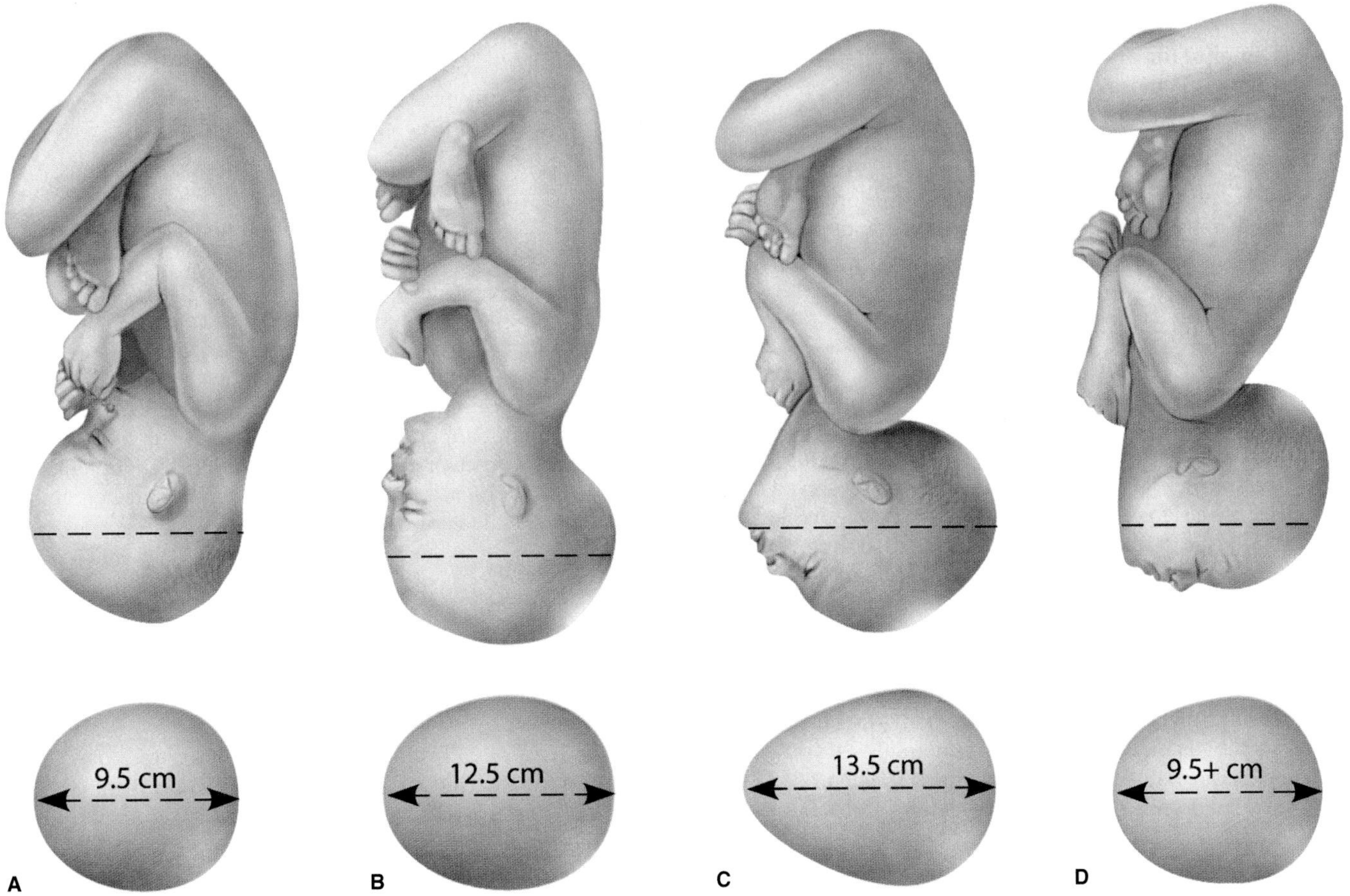

Figure 24–5 Types of cephalic presentations. A. The occiput is the presenting part because the head is flexed and the fetal chin is against the chest. The largest anteroposterior (AP) diameter that presents and passes through the pelvis is approximately 9.5 cm. B. Military (sinciput) presentation. The head is neither flexed nor extended. The presenting AP diameter is approximately 12.5 cm. C. Brow presentation. The largest diameter of the fetal head (approximately 13.5 cm) presents in this situation. D. Face presentation. The AP diameter is 9.5 cm.

In labors in which a brow presentation exists, 33 to 50% will result in a prolonged labor or a secondary arrest of labor (Lin, 2016). In the presence of CPD, failure to convert to a vertex presentation or face presentation indicates that a cesarean birth may be necessary. If a vaginal birth is attempted, the woman will probably need an episiotomy and may require extension of the episiotomy at the moment of birth.

Fetal mortality is increased because of injuries received during the birth. Trauma during the birth process can include cerebral and neck compression and damage to the trachea and larynx.

CLINICAL THERAPY

Active medical intervention is not necessary as long as cervical dilatation and fetal descent are occurring. If labor progress is slow, clinical pelvimetry findings and ultrasound to determine the presence of fetal anomalies are important. Brow presentations should be managed expectantly because a cesarean birth is most frequently warranted (Lin, 2016). Oxytocin may be used with caution to correct an inadequate labor pattern. Use of forceps or manual conversion is contraindicated. If problems occur, cesarean birth is indicated.

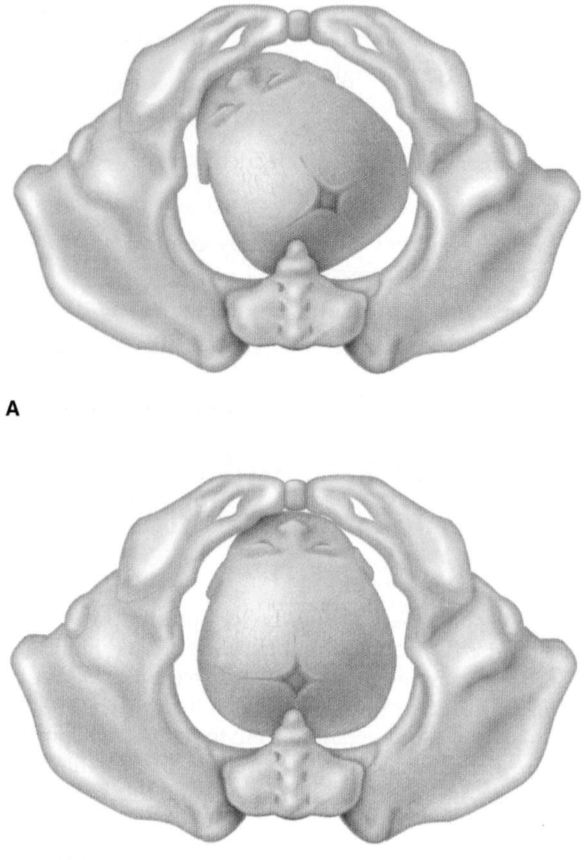
A

B

Figure 24–6 **Brow presentation. A. Descent. B. Internal rotation in the pelvic cavity.**

●○● NURSING MANAGEMENT

For the Laboring Woman with the Fetus in Brow Presentation

Nursing Assessment and Diagnosis

Leopold maneuvers suggest a brow presentation when both the chin and occiput are palpable. A brow presentation may be detected on vaginal examination by palpation of the diamond-shaped anterior fontanelle and orbital ridges (Figure 24–6).

Nursing diagnoses that may apply to brow presentation include:

- ***Anxiety*** or ***Fear*** related to outcome for fetus
- ***Knowledge, Deficient,*** related to lack of information about possible maternal-fetal effects of brow presentation
- ***Injury, Risk for,*** to the fetus related to pressure on fetal structures secondary to brow presentation

(NANDA-I © 2017)

Nursing Plan and Implementation

Nursing management of the brow presentation includes close observation of the woman for labor aberrations and of the fetus for signs of nonreassuring fetal status. The fetus should be observed closely during labor for signs of hypoxia as evidenced by late decelerations.

Explain the position of the fetus to the laboring couple or interpret what the physician/CNM has told them. Stay close at hand to reassure the couple, inform them of any changes, and assist them with labor-coping techniques.

In both brow and face presentations, the appearance of the newborn may be affected. The couple may need help in beginning the attachment process because of the newborn's facial appearance. After the baby is inspected for gross abnormalities, you and the pediatrician can assure the couple that the facial edema and excessive molding are only temporary and will subside in a few days.

Evaluation

Expected outcomes of nursing care include:

- The woman and her partner understand the implications and associated problems of brow presentation.
- The mother and her baby have a safe labor and birth.
- The woman and her baby initiate the bonding process.

●○●

Face Presentation

In a face presentation (Figure 24–5D), the face of the fetus is the presenting part. The fetal head is hyperextended even more than in the brow presentation. Face presentations occur in 1 in 600 to 800 births and occur most commonly in women with a contracted pelvis (Cunningham et al., 2016). They also occur frequently in multiparous women or women with a pendulous abdomen. Most face presentations occur during labor when the face enters the pelvic inlet. Fetal factors include:

- Macrosomia
- Nuchal cord
- Anencephaly
- Fetal malformations, such as thyroid goiter or soft tissue tumors of the fetal neck.

The risks of CPD and prolonged labor are increased with face presentation. As with any prolonged labor, the chance of infection is increased. The fetus may develop edema, making vaginal examination for placement of heart rate electrodes difficult. If a fetal scalp electrode is applied, it should be placed on the mentum. After birth, the edema gives the newborn an unusual appearance. As with the brow presentation, the neck and internal structures may swell as a result of trauma received during descent. Petechiae, swelling, and facial bruising are often seen in the superficial layers of the facial skin because of birth trauma. The perinatal mortality rate is 2 to 3% not including nonviable malformations and extreme prematurity (Lin, 2016).

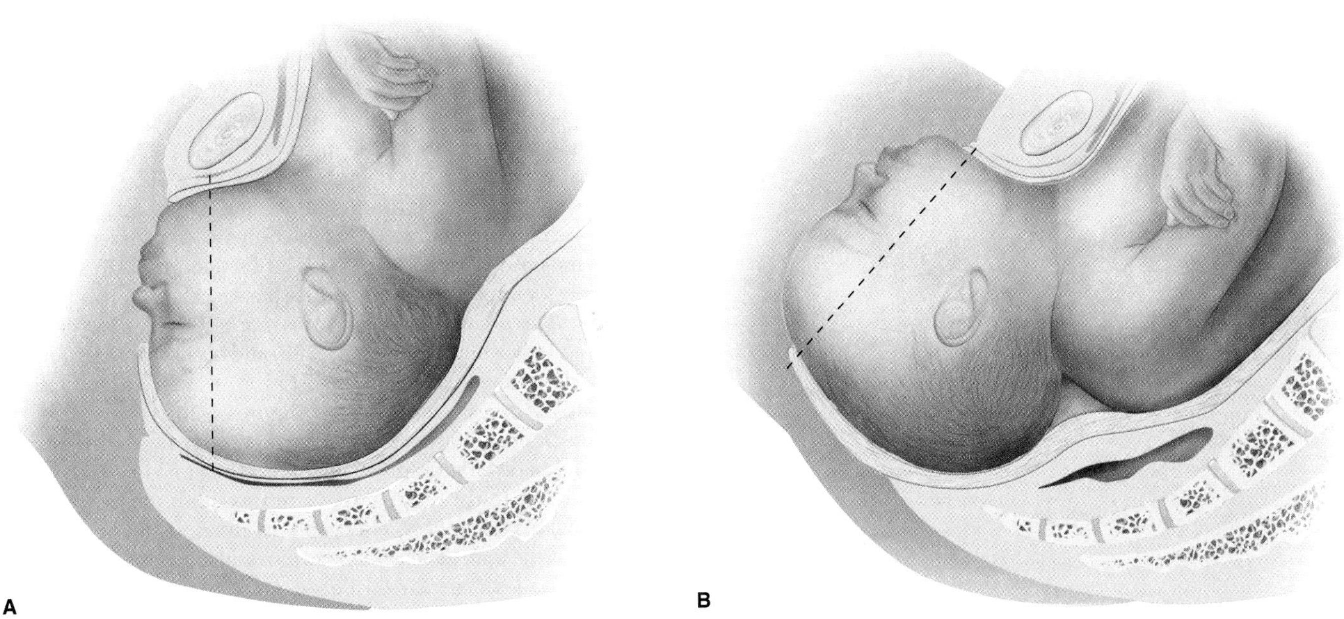

Figure 24–7 **Face presentation. Mechanism of birth in mentoanterior position. A. The submentobregmatic diameter at the outlet. B. The fetal head is born by movement of flexion.**

CLINICAL THERAPY

If no CPD is present, the mentum (chin) is anterior, and the labor pattern is effective, the objective of medical treatment is a vaginal birth (Figure 24–7). The success rate of vaginal delivery is 70 to 80%. Oxytocin may be administered as needed for hypotonic labor patterns. Attempts at manual rotation should not be made because this increases perinatal mortality and maternal morbidity (Lin, 2016). Mentum posteriors can become wedged on the anterior surface of the sacrum (Figure 24–8). In this case as well as in the presence of CPD, cesarean is the preferred method of birth.

●○● NURSING MANAGEMENT

For the Laboring Woman with the Fetus in Face Presentation

Nursing Assessment and Diagnosis

When performing Leopold maneuvers, you may find that the back of the fetus is difficult to outline, and a deep furrow can be palpated between the hard occiput and the fetal back (Figure 24–9A). Fetal heart tones can be heard on the side where the fetal feet are palpated. It may be difficult to determine by vaginal examination whether a breech or a face is presenting, especially if facial edema is already present. During the vaginal examination, palpation of the saddle of the nose and the gums should be attempted (Figure 24–9B). When assessing engagement, remember that the face has to be deep within the pelvis before the biparietal diameter has entered the inlet. The majority of face presentations are diagnosed via vaginal exam later in labor, and some are not diagnosed until the time of birth (Lin, 2016).

Nursing diagnoses that may apply to the woman with a fetus in face presentation include:

- ***Fear*** related to unknown outcome of the labor and appearance of the baby
- ***Injury, Risk for,*** to the newborn's face related to edema secondary to the birth process

(NANDA-I © 2017)

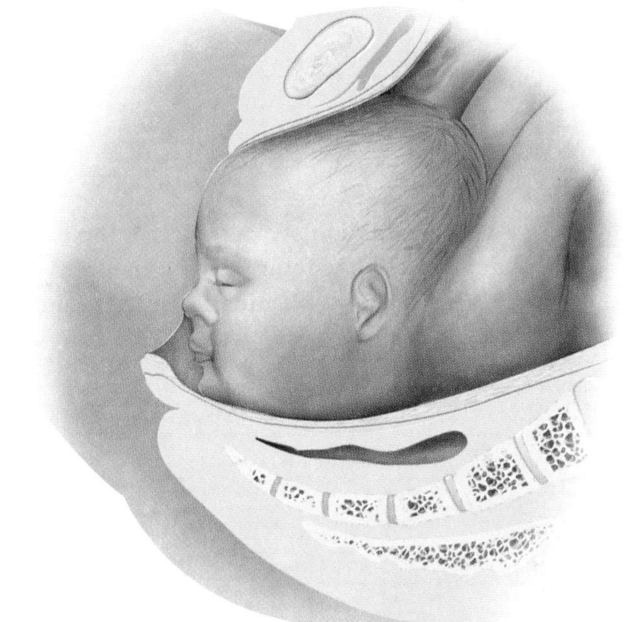

Figure 24–8 **Face presentation. Mechanism of birth in mentoposterior position. Fetal head is unable to extend farther. The face becomes impacted.**

Nursing Plan and Implementation

Nursing interventions are the same as for the brow presentation.

Evaluation

Expected outcomes of nursing care include:

- The woman and her partner understand the implications and problems of face presentation.
- The mother and her baby have a safe labor and birth.
- The woman and her baby initiate the bonding process.

●○●

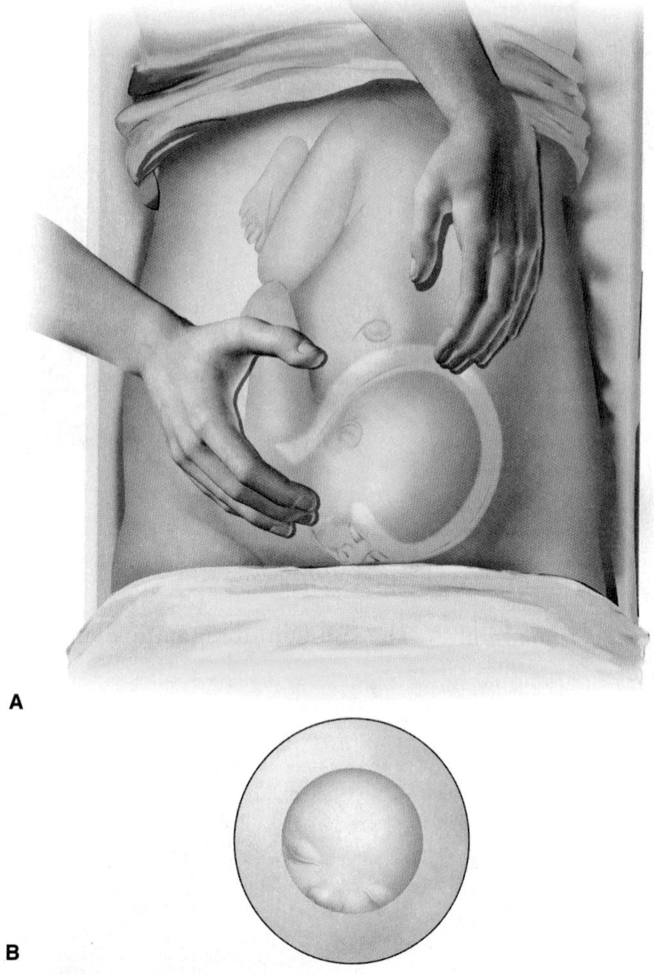

Figure 24–9 Face presentation. A. Palpation of the maternal abdomen with the fetus in right mentum posterior (RMP). B. Vaginal examination may permit palpation of facial features of the fetus.

Breech Presentation

Breech presentation is the most common malpresentation, with an overall incidence of approximately 4% of births. The incidence of breech presentation is directly related to gestational age: At 25 to 26 weeks' gestation, the incidence is about 25%, but by 32 weeks, the incidence has decreased to 7% (Lin, 2016).

Frank breech is the most common type of breech (especially at term) and is characterized by flexed hips and extended knees. It occurs in about 50 to 70% of breech births (Figure 24–10A). Single or double footling breech (incomplete breech), characterized by one or both hips extended and a foot presenting, accounts for about 10 to 30% of breech births (Figure 24–10B) and occurs more frequently in preterm fetuses. The remaining 5 to 10% of breech presentations are complete breech presentations (Figure 24–10C) (Lin, 2016).

Breech presentation is most frequently associated with placenta previa, implantation of the placenta in one of two cornual regions close to the uterus, hydramnios, high parity, oligohydramnios, hydrocephaly, anencephaly, previous breech presentation, uterine anomalies, pelvic tumors, multiple gestation, and fetal anomalies (Lin, 2016). Because the presenting part does not completely fill the space in the lower uterine segment, once membranes rupture, cord prolapse is more likely. The incidence of cord prolapse is more likely in a breech presentation than in other presentations. Babies born after breech presentation have higher newborn/infant mortality and neonatal complications. Factors associated with breech presentation include a decreased muscle tone in the fetus and an abnormal fetal motor ability. Breech fetuses are more likely to have neuromuscular disorders. Children who presented in breech presentation scored lower on motor functioning during the first 5 years of life than children who had presented in cephalic presentation (Lin, 2016). These birth defects can be associated with factors that caused the breech presentation (birth defects or intrauterine growth restriction) or with damage that occurred during birth (Lin, 2016).

Head trauma during vaginal birth is more likely in breech presentation because it does not allow for the slow molding that occurs in a cephalic presentation as the fetal head moves through the birth canal. The head is the largest and least resilient part of the fetal body. It is the last to come through the maternal pelvis in breech presentations; thus, molding does not occur. In the case

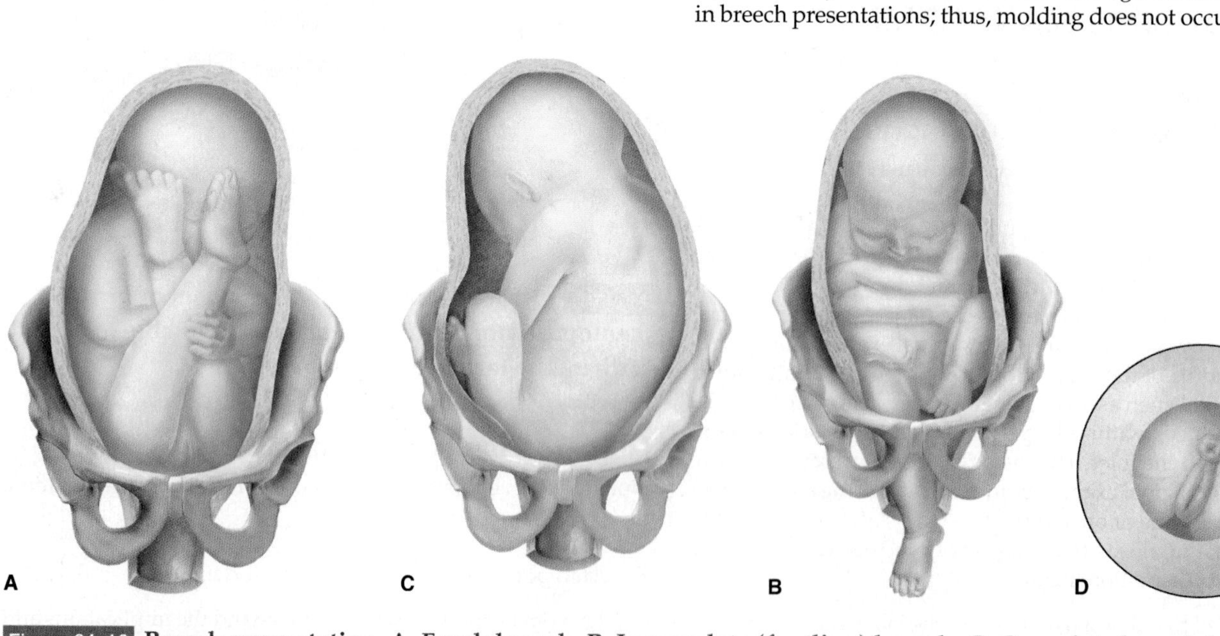

Figure 24–10 Breech presentation. A. Frank breech. B. Incomplete (footling) breech. C. Complete breech in left sacral anterior (LSA) position. D. On vaginal examination, the nurse may feel the anal sphincter. The tissue of the fetal buttocks feels soft.

of a preterm breech, a single or double footling and the torso may emerge through a cervix that is not completely dilated, leaving the larger head entrapped by the cervix. Entrapment may also occur with cesarean birth if the incision is inadequate or uterine relaxation is less than optimal. Vaginal breech birth also carries higher risks of meconium aspiration and fetal asphyxia (Sloman, Wanat, Burns, et al., 2016).

Studies have demonstrated that planned cesarean births of breech fetuses had a lower risk of perinatal morbidity and mortality than planned vaginal births (Sloman et al., 2016). It is now recommended that the mode of birth for a single fetus should be based on the healthcare provider's experience and expertise; there is a decrease of expertise in this area of obstetrics. The mother should be informed that there are more complications associated with planned vaginal breech delivery than with planned cesarean birth in these fetuses (Sloman et al., 2016).

CLINICAL THERAPY

An external cephalic version (ECV) is usually attempted at 37 to 38 weeks' gestation. The ECV, which is discussed in detail in Chapter 25, can reduce breech presentation by 50% (Sloman et al., 2016).

Maternal positioning exercises can also be utilized to facilitate the rotation of the fetus. The mother should be advised to assume a position where her hips are higher than her torso, which can give the fetus ample room to move into a cephalic presentation. The mother should be encouraged to perform these exercises two or three times daily. Once she feels a large movement, however, she should be advised to discontinue the exercises until a healthcare provider has determined if the desirable position has been achieved. See *Case Study: Azia Askari.*

If the version is unsuccessful or the fetus spontaneously turns back into a breech presentation, the physician will evaluate the possibility of a vaginal birth or plan a cesarean birth. Many physicians recommend a cesarean birth when a breech presentation is detected, especially if the woman is nulliparous, because breech births have higher mortality and morbidity rates as well as an increased incidence of cord prolapse, birth trauma, and fetal cervical spinal cord injuries due to hyperextension of the head (Senger, 2015). Contraindications for labor and vaginal birth include:

- Fetal weight less than 1500 g or more than 3800 g
- Hyperextension of the fetal neck of more than 90 degrees
- Extension of the fetal arms over the head
- Anomalies, such as hydrocephalus
- Diminished maternal pelvic measurements.

If a vaginal birth is being attempted, narcotic agents or an epidural block may be used for pain relief. Epidural anesthesia may be advantageous during the latter portion of labor because it will help prevent the pushing sensation the woman may feel before complete dilatation. If the woman pushes before cervical dilatation is complete, the fetal body may be expelled and the head entrapped. At the time of birth the physician may have an assistant available in case forceps are needed. Once the fetal body is born, an assistant supports the fetal body as the physician applies Piper forceps to assist in birth of the fetal head (called the *aftercoming head*) (Skinner, Davies-Tuck, Wallace, et al., 2017). See *Complementary Health Approaches: Moxibustion to Promote Version in Breech Presentation.*

Complementary Health Approaches

Moxibustion to Promote Version in Breech Presentation

Moxibustion is a traditional Chinese medicine (TCM) technique in which certain herbs are burned close to the skin near a particular acupressure or acupuncture point, thus stimulating the point and allowing energy to flow through it. To promote version in breech presentations, mugwort is burned close to acupoint BL67, located beside the outer corner of the fifth toenail. The heat and pungency of the burning mugwort stimulate the pressure point, much like acupressure or acupuncture does, and energy is released. It is believed that the effect of moxibustion increases fetal activity. Moxibustion has been shown to decrease the need for ECV and reduce the use of oxytocin before and during labor (Gabbe et al., 2016).

NURSING MANAGEMENT

For the Laboring Woman with the Fetus in Breech Presentation

Nursing Assessment and Diagnosis

At times, the nurse is the first person to recognize a breech presentation. On palpation using Leopold maneuvers, you may feel the hard vertex in the fundus and can perform ballottement of the head independently of the fetal body. The wider sacrum is palpated in the lower part of the abdomen. If the sacrum has not descended, on ballottement the entire fetal body will move. Furthermore, fetal heart tones (FHTs) are usually auscultated above the umbilicus. Passage of meconium from compression of the fetus's intestinal tract during descent may occur.

CASE STUDY: Azia Askari

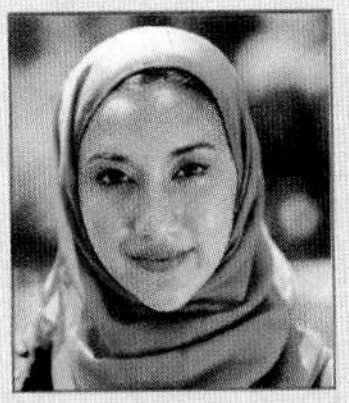

SOURCE: HONGQI ZHANG/123RF.

Azia has previously had two term uncomplicated pregnancies in Iran. This pregnancy has been uneventful, so Azia is surprised and concerned when the nurse practitioner reveals that her baby is in a breech position. Azia really wants to have a normal birth and is adamant she wants to do everything to avoid a cesarean birth. She is almost 39 weeks, with early prenatal care that confirms her dates. The NP discusses options with her including an external cephalic version or an elective cesarean birth.

Questions to Ponder

What educational information should be reviewed with Azia when discussing the option of an external cephalic version? Is it likely to be more successful or less successful in a multiparous woman?

Be particularly alert for a prolapsed umbilical cord, especially in single or double footling breeches, because there is space between the cervix and presenting part through which the cord can slip. If the fetus is small and the membranes rupture, the danger is even greater. This is one reason why any woman admitted to the birthing area with a history of ruptured membranes should not ambulate until a full assessment, including vaginal examination, is performed.

Nursing diagnoses that may apply to breech presentation include:

- ***Health Management, Readiness for Enhanced,*** related to an expressed desire to understand the implications of the procedure
- ***Injury, Risk for,*** to the fetus due to head entrapment from a planned vaginal breech birth

(NANDA-I © 2017)

Nursing Plan and Implementation

During labor, the fetus is at increased risk for prolapse of the cord. Some agency protocols may therefore call for continuous EFM even though there are no current research studies to support its use. Because women with a breech presentation are at an increased risk for a prolapsed umbilical cord, maternal ambulation is usually not recommended until the presenting part is well engaged. Ongoing assessments of contractions, cervical dilatation, effacement, and fetal descent are also important to monitor labor progress. Emotional support and sharing of information are critical to the childbearing woman and her support person. They need to be kept apprised of the labor's current status as well as the possible treatment plans so they can continue to make informed choices.

During a vaginal birth, continue to assess the FHR and to provide encouragement and support for the couple. Piper forceps need to be readily available to the physician; you may be expected to assist the physician if forceps are needed for the birth.

Evaluation

Expected outcomes of nursing care include:

- The woman and her partner can describe the implications and associated problems with breech presentation.
- The mother and baby have a safe labor and birth.
- Major complications are recognized early, and corrective measures are instituted.

Transverse Lie (Shoulder Presentation) of a Single Fetus

In *transverse lie* the fetus's long axis lies across the woman's abdomen, and on inspection the contour of the maternal abdomen appears widest from side to side (Figure 24–11). It is not uncommon in multiple gestations for one or more of the fetuses to be in a transverse lie. An incidence of transverse lie of a single fetus is approximately 1 in 300 term births (Skinner et al., 2017).

Maternal conditions associated with a transverse lie are grand multiparity with lax uterine musculature (the most common cause); obstructions such as bony dystocia, placenta previa, neoplasms, and fetal anomalies; hydramnios; and preterm fetus.

Vaginal birth is impossible with a transverse lie. Labor should not be allowed to continue, and a cesarean birth is done quickly. Frequently a vertical incision is made in the uterus because the fetal head and fetal feet lie in the upper portion of the uterus; a low transverse incision may lead to difficulties in extracting the fetus (Skinner et al., 2017).

If labor is allowed to continue, the fetal shoulder will be forced down into the pelvis and the fetus will become impacted. With no relief, uterine rupture may occur.

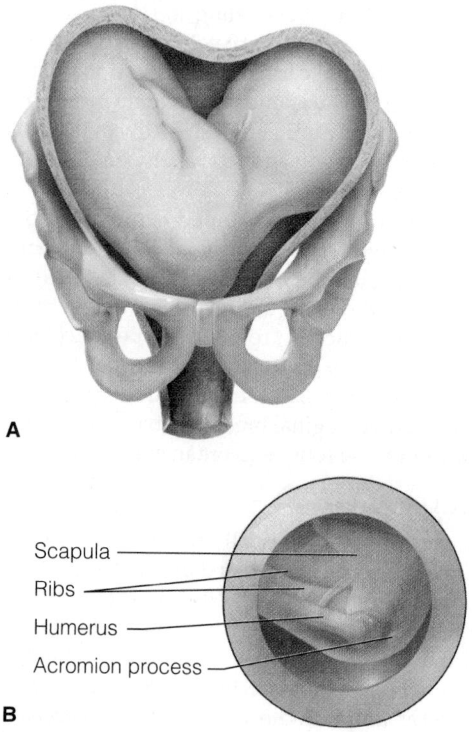

Figure 24–11 Transverse lie. A. Shoulder presentation. B. On vaginal examination, the nurse may feel the acromion process as the fetal presenting part.

CLINICAL THERAPY

Transverse lie may be diagnosed using Leopold maneuvers and can then be confirmed by ultrasound. At the time of the ultrasound examination, it is important to confirm fetal position, fetal biparietal diameters (to confirm gestational age), and location of the placenta and to carry out an examination for the presence of fetal anomalies and structural abnormalities of the uterus such as leiomyoma (fibroid tumor) or adnexal tumors.

Management varies, depending on the length of gestation, because many transverse lies convert to either cephalic or breech presentation by full term (39 weeks). If the fetus is still in a transverse lie at term, an ECV (see Chapter 25) may be done if (1) there is no contraindication to vaginal birth (e.g., a fetal anomaly, complete placenta previa, or a structural problem in the uterus) and (2) fetal pulmonary lung maturity is confirmed either by ultrasound measurements or by amniocentesis for assessment of phospholipids (2:1 lecithin/sphingomyelin [L/S] ratio and the presence of phosphatidylglycerol). An ECV is most likely to be successful close to term. Spontaneous version will likely occur if performed before 37 weeks. The use of tocolytics for the procedure may be helpful for nulliparas. The fetus is assessed with a nonstress test (NST) or biophysical profile (BPP) before the procedure. If the version is successful, the woman may be induced if she is at term and her cervix is favorable. However, scientific studies do not support immediate induction as a routine to minimize the chance the fetus will return to the original position (Skinner et al., 2017).

NURSING MANAGEMENT

For the Laboring Woman with the Fetus in Transverse Lie

Nursing Assessment and Diagnosis

A transverse lie can be identified by inspection and palpation of the abdomen, by auscultation of FHTs in the midline of the abdomen (not conclusive), and by vaginal examination.

On palpation, no fetal part is felt in the fundal portion of the uterus or above the symphysis pubis. The head may be palpated on one side and the breech on the other. FHTs are usually auscultated just below the midline of the umbilicus. On vaginal examination, if a presenting part is palpated, it is the ridged thorax or possibly an arm that is compressed against the chest. Women with a transverse lie may report less shortness of breath, pelvic pressure, and urinary frequency than other women because pressure is not exerted on the diaphragm and the bladder.

Nursing diagnoses that may apply when transverse lie is present include:

- ***Gas Exchange, Impaired,*** related to decrease in blood flow secondary to cord compression associated with prolapsed cord
- ***Powerlessness, Risk for,*** related to unknown outcome
- ***Fear*** related to unknown outcome of birth

(NANDA-I © 2017)

Nursing Plan and Implementation

The primary nursing actions are to help evaluate the fetal presentation and to provide information and support to the couple. If an ECV has been accomplished and an induction is started, complete all interventions related to the induction (see the discussion in Chapter 25). If transverse lie is discovered when the woman is admitted to the birthing unit in labor, provide information regarding the need for either an ECV or a cesarean birth and assist with preparation for the birth. If an ECV is not performed or is unsuccessful, a cesarean birth will be performed. Before the cesarean, watch for rupture of membranes and the possibility of prolapse of the umbilical cord. (See Chapter 25 for further information regarding cesarean birth.)

Evaluation

Expected outcomes of nursing care include:

- The transverse lie is recognized promptly, and crucial assessments are completed.
- Measures to perform an ECV or a cesarean birth are completed.
- The mother and baby have a safe birth.
- The couple can describe the implications and associated problems of transverse lie.

Compound Presentation

A compound presentation is one in which there are two presenting parts. It can occur when the pelvic inlet is not totally occluded by the primary presenting part. If the prolapsed part is a hand, the birth is generally not difficult. Sometimes the hand slips back, and occasionally it is born alongside the head. This may increase the chance of laceration. Cesarean birth is indicated in the presence of uterine dysfunction or nonreassuring fetal status and is more common in obese women (Kaplan, 2017).

Care of the Woman and Fetus at Risk Because of Macrosomia

Fetal **macrosomia** is defined as weight of more than 4000 g. It is important to remember that the mean birth weight varies throughout the world. The definition of macrosomia will thus differ according to the ethnic group being discussed.

A woman who is obese is twice as likely to have a macrosomic fetus (Phillips, Skelly, King, et al., 2018). Obesity has been defined in a number of ways. For a complete discussion on maternal obesity, see Chapter 14. There is also an association between macrosomia and both pregestational and gestational diabetes. Increased maternal glucose levels have also been shown to increase fetal weight. Other risk factors include postterm pregnancy, multiparity, grand multiparity, previous macrosomic newborn, previous shoulder dystocia, male sex, and maternal birth weight.

A woman's pelvis that is adequate for an average-sized fetus may be disproportionately small for an oversized fetus. Distention of the uterus causes overstretching of the myometrial fibers, which may lead to dysfunctional labor and an increased incidence of postpartum hemorrhage. If the oversized fetus is not able to descend, the chance of uterine rupture during labor increases. Vaginal birth poses an increased risk of perineal lacerations and extensions of an episiotomy. The mother is also at risk for postpartum hemorrhage and puerperal infection. The incidence of vacuum and forceps birth increases with fetal size.

The most significant complication in macrosomia is *shoulder dystocia*, which is an obstetric emergency. However, shoulder dystocia may occur with fetuses weighing less than 4000 g, and risk factors are not reliable predictors. Following birth of the head, the anterior shoulder of the macrosomic fetus may not emerge either spontaneously or with gentle traction (Phillips et al., 2018). If shoulder dystocia is not managed correctly, permanent injury to the baby may result. **Brachial plexus injury** is an injury due to improper or excessive traction applied to the fetal head during birth that results in damage to the network of nerves that sends signals from the spine to the shoulder, arm, and hand.

Other injuries that may occur include fractured clavicles, meconium aspiration, asphyxia, hypoglycemia, polycythemia, and hyperbilirubinemia. Other neurologic damage to the fetus can also occur.

In addition, macrosomic neonates are more likely to become obese in childhood and adolescence. These children are also at risk to develop diabetes later in life (Phillips et al., 2018).

CLINICAL THERAPY

The occurrence of the maternal and fetal problems associated with macrosomic fetuses may be somewhat lessened by identifying macrosomia before the onset of labor. The diagnosis is not precise. There is good evidence to show that estimating fetal size with ultrasound is no more accurate than a clinical estimate from Leopold maneuvers (Ray & Alhusen, 2016). However, ultrasound is usually employed as an assessment measure in diagnosing macrosomia. If a large fetus is suspected, the maternal pelvis should be evaluated carefully. An estimation of fetal size can be made by palpating the crown–rump length (CRL) of the fetus in utero, but the greatest errors in estimation occur on both ends of the spectrum–the macrosomic fetus and the very small fetus. Whenever the uterus appears excessively large, hydramnios, an oversized fetus, or a multiple pregnancy must be considered.

Labor and vaginal birth for a fetus greater than 4500 g may warrant a cesarean birth to reduce the risks associated with vaginal births. The best method of birth for a fetus weighing 4000 to 4500 g is debated. If a vaginal birth is attempted and difficulty extracting the shoulders occurs during the birth, the physician/CNM may direct the woman to sharply flex her thighs up against her abdomen (McRoberts maneuver). This position is thought to change the maternal pelvic angle and therefore reduce the force needed to extract the shoulders, thereby decreasing the incidence of brachial plexus stretching and clavicular fracture (Figure 24–12A–C). The maternal head should be lowered, and the nurse applies suprapubic pressure directly over the symphysis pubis to aid release of the anterior shoulder. Fundal pressure (pressure exerted at the top of the maternal fundus) should not be performed because this can further wedge the shoulder against the suprapubic bone. See *Evidence-Based Practice: Managing Shoulder Dystocia.*

In addition, the physician/CNM may incorporate other interventions, such as checking the placement of the shoulder, performing an episiotomy, and using the Woods screw maneuver (which consists of rotating the anterior shoulder 180 degrees to the posterior position). In cases where these interventions fail, the physician/CNM may electively break the clavicle to facilitate extraction of the shoulders.

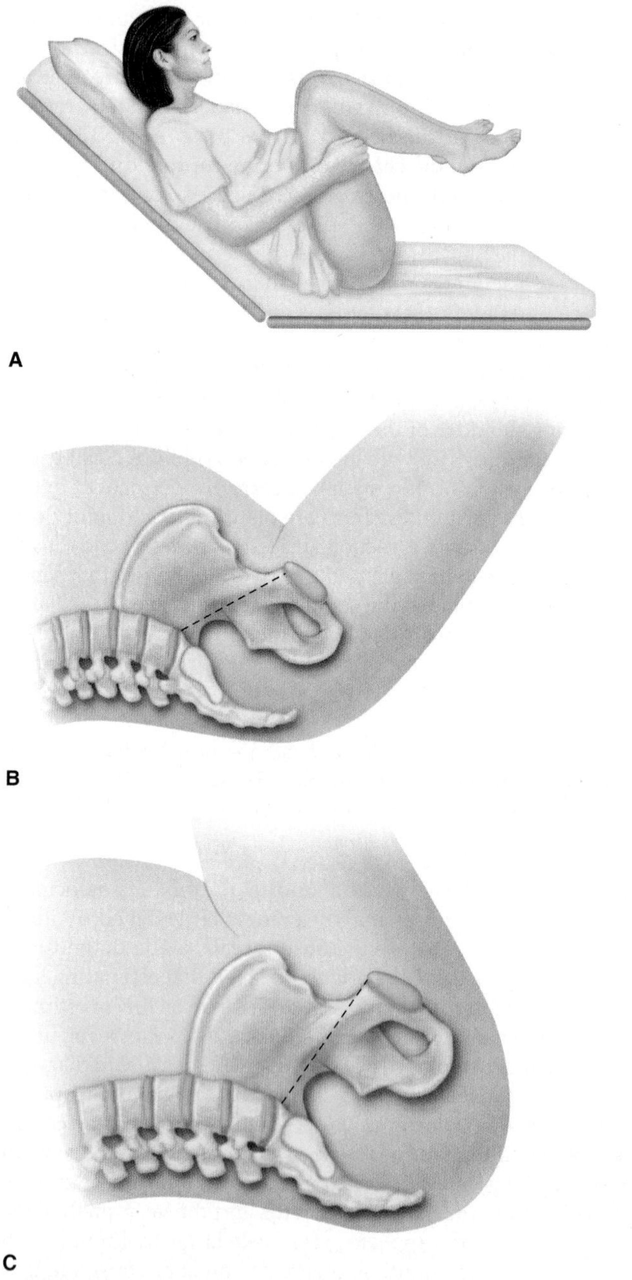

Figure 24–12 McRoberts maneuver. A. The woman flexes her thighs up onto her abdomen. B. The angle of the maternal pelvis before McRoberts maneuver. C. The angle of the pelvis with McRoberts maneuver.

●○● NURSING MANAGEMENT

For the Laboring Woman and the Fetus at Risk for Macrosomia

Nursing Assessment and Diagnosis

Assist in identifying factors associated with macrosomic fetuses. During the intrapartum period, the risk factors include slow descent of the fetus and prolonged second stage. Because women with these risk factors are prime candidates for dystocia and its complications, frequently assess the FHR for nonreassuring heart rate patterns, which may indicate fetal stress; evaluate the rate of cervical dilatation; and assess fetal descent.

Nursing diagnoses that may apply to the woman with a macrosomic fetus include:

- ***Injury, Risk for,*** to the fetus related to trauma during the birth process
- ***Infection, Risk for,*** related to traumatized tissue secondary to maternal tissue damage during birth
- ***Injury, Risk for,*** to the mother related to perineal trauma associated with macrosomic birth

(NANDA-I © 2017)

Nursing Plan and Implementation

Monitor labor closely for a dysfunctional pattern, assessing FHR and reporting any sign of labor dysfunction or nonreassuring heart rate patterns to the physician/CNM. Note any arrest of descent, excessive molding of the fetal head, or the presence of caput succedaneum, which can also indicate a large fetus or CPD.

Provide support for the laboring woman and her partner and information regarding the implications and possible associated problems. Give the couple directions for proper positioning at the time of birth to facilitate extraction of the shoulders. If you anticipate a possible shoulder dystocia, notify additional staff and inform appropriate support personnel for the newborn. During the birth, continue to provide support and encouragement to the couple. Informing the woman that possible suprapubic pressure may be needed may help reduce anxiety for the couple.

After the birth, inspect the newborn for cephalohematoma, Erb palsy (caused by overstretching of the brachial plexus and damage to C_5, C_6, C_7), and fractured clavicles (exhibited by nonmovement of one arm or palpation of the clavicle to detect an irregularity of the bone structure) and inform the admission nursery of any problems. The newborn will need to be observed closely for cerebral and neurologic damage.

Postpartum, check the uterus for potential atony and the maternal vital signs for deviations suggesting hypovolemic shock. Frequent fundal checks should be performed to evaluate the woman for postpartum bleeding. If postpartum hemorrhage occurs, intravenous (IV) or intramuscular (IM) oxytocin (Pitocin) should be administered to stimulate contraction of the uterus.

Evaluation

Expected outcomes of nursing care include:

- The woman and her partner can describe the implications of macrosomia and possible associated problems.
- The mother and baby have a safe labor and birth.

EVIDENCE-BASED PRACTICE | Managing Shoulder Dystocia

Clinical Question

What is best practice in managing deliveries at risk of or complicated by shoulder dystocia?

The Evidence

Shoulder dystocia occurs when the anterior shoulder of the fetus cannot descend because it is obstructed by the symphysis pubis or the sacral promontory. It occurs during delivery and is diagnosed when gentle downward pressure on the fetal head is not followed by the shoulder. The condition usually requires additional obstetric maneuvers to achieve delivery. Shoulder dystocia is associated with an increased risk of postpartum hemorrhage, in part due to higher risk of perineal injury. Most of these cases are managed without injury to the fetus, although nerve and bone injuries can occur. This practice guideline, sponsored by the American College of Obstetricians and Gynecologists (ACOG, 2017) and carried out by a team of clinical experts, is the strongest level of evidence for practice.

There are few predictors of shoulder dystocia, and so it is rarely diagnosed until it occurs. There is no pattern of prolonged or precipitous labor that reliably leads to shoulder dystocia. About 10% of women whose births occur with shoulder dystocia will have the condition in a subsequent birth. Induction of labor had no effect on the occurrence of the condition, and cesarean birth does not appear to reduce the rate of injury to mother and baby. While no single maneuver works in all situations, the McRoberts maneuver should be attempted first because it is a simple and effective technique. This maneuver is carried out by two assistants, each of whom grasps one of the mother's legs and sharply flexes the thigh against the abdomen. The maneuver causes rotation of the symphysis pubis that can free the shoulder of the fetus. Suprapubic pressure may be used simultaneously to abduct and rotate the shoulder free from the pubis.

Practitioners who receive simulation experiences and shoulder dystocia protocols can reduce the incidence of morbidity associated with shoulder dystocia (ACOG, 2017).

Best Practice

There are no predictors for shoulder dystocia, and so the nurse should be prepared to assist in maneuvers to free the fetus's shoulder from the mother's symphysis pubis. This may involve the McRoberts maneuver or suprapubic pressure or both. Facilitating delivery is desirable to minimize perineal damage for the mother and potential nerve or bone damage for the baby.

Clinical Reasoning

Describe the anatomical processes during birth that would allow the McRoberts maneuver to be effective. What role might the nurse play in assisting with the delivery of a fetus with shoulder dystocia?

Care of the Woman and Fetus in the Presence of Nonreassuring Fetal Status

When the oxygen supply is insufficient to meet the physiologic demands of the fetus, a nonreassuring fetal status may result. *Nonreassuring fetal status* is the term used to identify data describing the fetal status. Previously, the term fetal distress was used; however, its use implied an ill fetus despite the fact that the condition is often transient, not chronic.

A variety of factors may contribute to a nonreassuring fetal status. The most common are related to cord compression and uteroplacental insufficiency associated with placental abnormalities and preexisting maternal or fetal disease. If the resultant hypoxia persists and metabolic acidosis follows, the situation can be life-threatening to the fetus.

The most common initial signs of nonreassuring fetal status are meconium-stained amniotic fluid (in a vertex presentation) and changes in the FHR. The presence of ominous FHR patterns—such as late or severe variable decelerations, decrease in or lack of variability, and progressive acceleration in the FHR baseline—are indicative of hypoxia (see Chapter 20).

CLINICAL THERAPY

When there is evidence of possible nonreassuring fetal status, treatment centers on relieving the hypoxia and minimizing the effects of anoxia on the fetus. Initial interventions include changing the mother's position, increasing infusion rates of intravenous fluids, and administering oxygen by mask at 6 to 10 L per minute. If EFM has not yet been used, it is usually instituted at this time. If oxytocin is in use, it should be discontinued. If EFM is ineffective, the physician/CNM may utilize internal monitoring devices to more accurately assess FHR changes. Table 24–1 summarizes intrapartum management of nonreassuring fetal status heart rate patterns.

TABLE 24–1 Management of Nonreassuring Fetal Status

- Recognize pattern changes that are indicative of nonreassuring fetal status such as:
  - Deep, repetitive variable decelerations
  - Prolonged decelerations
  - Ongoing late decelerations
- Begin intrauterine resuscitation measures:
  - Change maternal position.
  - Correct maternal hypotension.
  - Discontinue Pitocin.
  - Administer medications, such as terbutaline, to decrease uterine activity.
  - Increase intravenous fluid rate or begin IV immediately if not already established.
  - Assess for prolapsed cord via vaginal examination.
- If abnormal patterns resolve, continue with continuous electronic fetal monitoring.
- If abnormal patterns do not resolve and vaginal birth is imminent, proceed with vaginal birth as quickly as possible.
- If birth is not imminent and bradycardia persists, or if a scalp pH level is less than 7.20, a cesarean birth is indicated.
- If these tests are reassuring, cautious assessments can continue every 15 minutes until birth occurs.
- If testing becomes nonreassuring, a cesarean should be performed.

NURSING MANAGEMENT

For the Laboring Woman and Fetus in the Presence of Nonreassuring Fetal Status

Nursing Assessment and Diagnosis

Review the woman's prenatal history to anticipate the possibility of nonreassuring fetal status. When the membranes rupture, it is important to assess FHR and to observe for meconium staining. A sterile vaginal examination should be performed to rule out cord prolapse. As labor progresses, be particularly alert for even subtle changes in the FHR pattern and the fetal scalp pH, if available. Reports by the mother of increased or greatly decreased fetal activity may also be associated with nonreassuring fetal status. For further discussion of FHR patterns and characteristics and evaluation of fetal status during labor, see Chapter 20.

Nursing diagnoses that may apply in the presence of nonreassuring fetal status include:

- ***Cardiac Output, Decreased***, of the fetus related to decreased uteroplacental perfusion secondary to maternal hypotension, decreased blood volume, or vasoconstriction with preeclampsia
- ***Anxiety*** related to knowledge of nonreassuring fetal status

(NANDA-I © 2017)

Nursing Plan and Implementation

Staff members may become so involved in assessing fetal status and initiating corrective measures that they fail to give explanations and emotional support to the woman, her partner, and other family members. It is imperative to provide both full explanations of the problem and comfort to the couple. In many instances, if birth is not imminent, the woman must undergo cesarean birth. Anticipation of this surgery may cause fear and frustration for the couple, especially if they were committed to a shared, prepared birth experience.

Evaluation

Expected outcomes of nursing care include:

- The woman and her family become less anxious and more able to cope with their situation.
- The FHR remains in normal range, or, alternatively, supportive measures maintain the FHR as normal as possible.

Care of the Woman Experiencing Placental and Umbilical Cord Problems

Placental Problems

Problems of the placenta can be divided into those that are developmental and those that are degenerative. Developmental problems of the placenta include placental lesions, succenturiate placenta, circumvallate placenta, and battledore placenta (Table 24–2). Degenerative changes include infarcts and placental calcification.

SUCCENTURIATE PLACENTA

In *succenturiate placenta*, one or more accessory lobes of fetal villi have developed on the placenta, with vascular connections of fetal origin (see Table 24–2). Vessels from the major to the minor lobe(s) are supported only by the membranes, thus increasing the risk of the minor lobe's being retained during the third stage of labor.

The gravest maternal danger is postpartum hemorrhage if this minor lobe is severed from the placenta and remains in the uterus. All placentas should be examined closely for intactness. If vessels appear to be severed at the margin of the placenta, the uterus should be explored for retained placental tissue. This condition is not usually diagnosed until after the birth of the placenta.

Fetal/newborn implications can be life-threatening if the vascular connections rupture between the placenta lobes because a fatal fetal hemorrhage can result. Examination of the fetal membrane following birth may reveal a small hole with vessels running toward it. This is another indication of a retained lobe (Endler, Saltvedt, & Papadogiannakis, 2016). At birth, the baby should be inspected for pallor, cyanosis, retractions, tachypnea, tachycardia, and feeble pulse. The newborn's cry will be weak and the muscle tone flaccid.

CIRCUMVALLATE PLACENTA

In *circumvallate placenta*, the fetal surface of the placenta is exposed through a ring opening around the umbilical cord (see Table 24–2). The vessels descend from the cord and end at the margin of the ring instead of coursing through the entire surface area of the placenta. The ring is composed of a double fold of amnion and chorion with some degenerative decidua and fibrin between. The cause of this condition is unknown. Maternal-fetal problems include an increased incidence of late abortion or fetal death, antepartum hemorrhage, prematurity, and abnormal maternal bleeding during or following the third stage of labor, resulting from improper placental separation or shearing of membranes from the placenta.

BATTLEDORE PLACENTA

In *battledore placenta*, the umbilical cord is inserted at or near the placental margin (see Table 24–2). As a result, all fetal vessels transverse the placental surface in the same direction. The chances of preterm labor are high because of interference with fetal circulation and nutrition. Nonreassuring fetal status or bleeding during labor is also likely because of cord compression or vessel rupture.

PLACENTAL INFARCTS AND CALCIFICATIONS

As the placenta grade matures (previously discussed in Chapter 23), the placenta may develop infarcts and calcifications. They become significant if they cover a large enough area to interfere with the uterine–placental–fetal exchange. Altered exchange can also occur with certain maternal disease processes, such as hypertension. Infarcts are most often seen in cases of severe preeclampsia and in women who smoke.

Umbilical Cord Abnormalities

Umbilical cord abnormalities include congenital absence of an umbilical artery, insertion variations, cord length variations, and knots and loops of the cord. Insertion variations include velamentous insertion and vasa previa, and cord length problems include long and short cords.

CONGENITAL ABSENCE OF UMBILICAL ARTERY

Absence of an umbilical artery may have serious fetal implications. Newborns with two vessel cords have increased anomalies and pregnancy complications. Approximately 15% of fetuses experience intrauterine growth restriction. If anomalies are

TABLE 24–2 Placental and Umbilical Cord Variations

PLACENTAL VARIATION	MATERNAL IMPLICATIONS	FETAL-NEONATAL IMPLICAIONS	
SUCCENTURIATE PLACENTA			
One or more accessory lobes of fetal villi will develop on the placenta.	Postpartum hemorrhage from retained lobe	None, as long as all parts of the placenta remain attached until after birth of the fetus	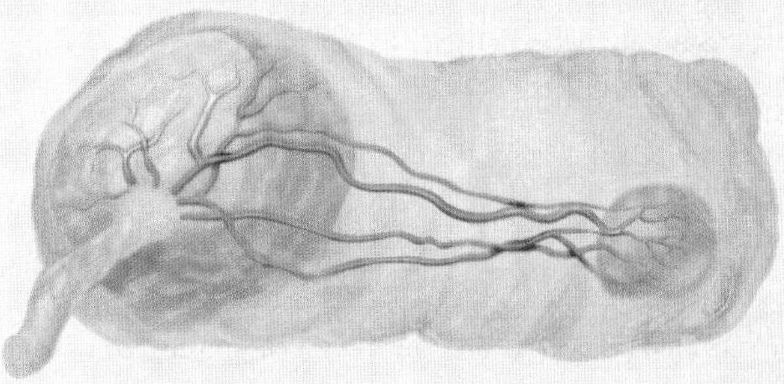
CIRCUMVALLATE PLACENTA			
A double fold of chorion and amnion form a ring around the umbilical cord, on the fetal side of the placenta.	Increased incidence of late abortion, antepartum hemorrhage, and preterm labor	Intrauterine growth restriction, prematurity, fetal death	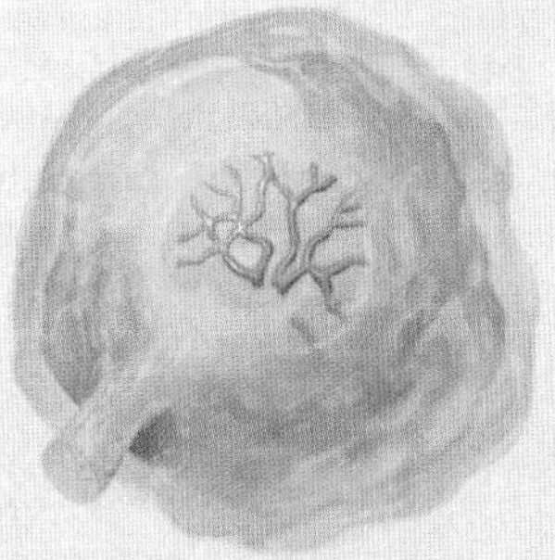
BATTLEDORE PLACENTA			
The umbilical cord is inserted at or near the placental margin.	Increased incidence of preterm labor and bleeding	Prematurity, fetal stress	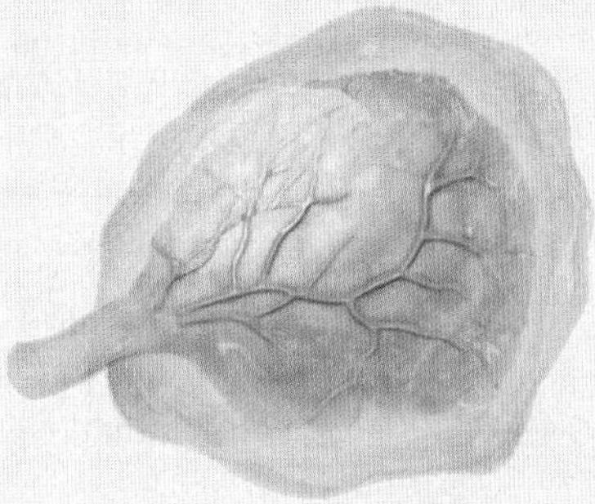
VELAMENTOUS INSERTION OF THE UMBILICAL CORD			
The vessels of the umbilical cord divide some distance from the placenta in the placental membranes.	Hemorrhage if one of the vessels is torn	Fetal stress, hemorrhage	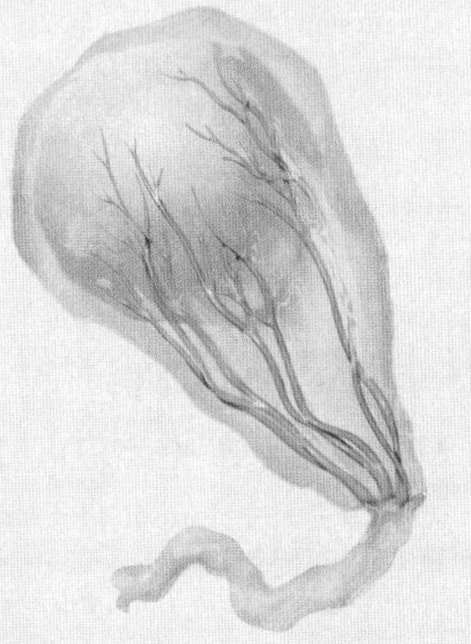

SOURCE: Data from Creasy, Resnik, Iams, et al., 2014.

present, there is a 50% risk of aneuploidy, although it is not associated with trisomy 21 (Elghazaly, Ali, & Babikir, 2016).

Immediately after the umbilical cord is cut, it should be inspected to determine whether the correct number of vessels is present. If an artery is absent, the nurse should examine the newborn closely for anomalies and gestational-age problems and alert the attending pediatrician.

INSERTION VARIATIONS

In a *velamentous insertion*, the vessels of the umbilical cord divide some distance from the placenta in the placental membranes (see Table 24–2). Velamentous insertions occur more frequently in multiple gestations than in singletons. Other placental anomalies, such as succenturiate placenta, often accompany this condition. The velamentous insertion is more easily compressed or kinked during pregnancy or labor because of the lack of Wharton jelly to protect it. If the vessels become torn during labor, fetal hemorrhage can occur, and blood can escape from the vagina. When fetal hemorrhage occurs, it results in FHR abnormalities.

When the vessels of a velamentous insertion transverse the internal os and appear in front of the fetus, a vasa previa has occurred. Fetal hemorrhage with asphyxia is likely to result because as the fetal blood escapes out of the vagina the hemorrhage will probably be diagnosed as maternal.

CORD LENGTH VARIATIONS

The average length of the umbilical cord is 55 cm. Although short cords rarely cause complications directly, they have been associated with umbilical hernias in the fetus, abruptio placentae, and cord rupture. Long cords tend to twist and tangle around the fetus, causing transient variable decelerations. A long cord rarely causes fetal death, however, because it is generally not pulled tight until descent at the time of birth. With a long cord and an active fetus, one or more true knots can result. Again, these knots are usually not pulled tight enough to cause fetal stress until the baby has been born, and the cord can then be clamped and cut.

CLINICAL THERAPY

The goals of medical treatment are to prevent serious fetal complications and to examine the newborn for anomalies that coexist with umbilical cord abnormalities.

Any vaginal bleeding during labor warrants continuous monitoring of the fetus, preferably with an external electronic monitor. Any signs of nonreassuring heart rate patterns should be reported immediately. In the presence of bleeding, laboratory tests may be used to differentiate fetal from maternal red blood cells. Fetal hemorrhage is resolved by terminating the pregnancy vaginally or through cesarean birth and by correcting neonatal anemia. Expediting the birth, whether vaginally or surgically, is paramount when a severe nonreassuring heart rate pattern is apparent. Following the birth, the pediatric team identifies and treats any neonatal complications or anomalies.

●○● NURSING MANAGEMENT

For the Laboring Woman and the Fetus with Umbilical Abnormalities

Nursing Assessment and Diagnosis

Umbilical abnormalities may not become evident until the birth of the fetus. During labor, observe for signs of nonreassuring fetal status and excessive bleeding (with velamentous insertion and vasa previa).

Nursing diagnoses that may apply include:

- *Gas Exchange, Impaired,* of the fetus related to decreased blood flow secondary to placental abnormalities
- *Knowledge, Deficient,* regarding information about placental abnormalities related to an expressed desire to understand the implications of the finding

(NANDA-I © 2017)

Nursing Plan and Implementation

Be alert for an unusual amount of bleeding during the labor and birth. Following the birth, inspect the placenta for abnormalities. Examination of the placenta by a pathologist may be indicated.

Often any mild or moderate variable deceleration can be successfully managed by the nurse. Repositioning of the woman often alleviates pressure on the cord if this is the reason for the deceleration.

Evaluation

Expected outcomes of nursing care include:

- The mother and baby have a safe labor and birth.
- The woman's bleeding is assessed quickly, and corrective measures are taken.
- The family is able to cope successfully with fetal or neonatal anomalies, if they exist.

Care of the Woman and Fetus with a Prolapsed Umbilical Cord

An umbilical cord that precedes the fetal presenting part is known as a **prolapsed umbilical cord**. It occurs when the cord falls or is washed down through the cervix into the vagina and becomes trapped between the presenting part and the maternal pelvis. The incidence of cord prolapse is 3% of vertex presentations and 3.7% of all breech presentations. It can also occur in compound presentations. Because of this entrapment, the vessels carrying blood to and from the fetus are compressed. In rare circumstances a prolapsed cord may be visible at the lower edge of the vagina. In other cases, the umbilical cord lies beside or just ahead of the fetal head; this is called *occult cord prolapse.*

Any time that the pelvic inlet is not completely filled by the fetus or the presenting part is not firmly against the cervix and the membranes rupture, the umbilical cord can be washed down into the birth canal in front of the presenting part (Figure 24–13). The incidence of prolapse of the cord is 20 times greater with abnormal axis lie (Fazil, Zafar, Asifa, et al., 2016)—especially footling breech and shoulder presentations—low birth weight, a multipara with more than five previous births, multiple gestation, polyhydramnios, unengaged presenting part, obstetric manipulation (amniotomy), and the presence of a long cord (longer than 80 cm). Approximately 50% of cord prolapses occur in the second stage of labor. Many cord prolapses occur as a result of some obstetric intervention, such as amniotomy, application of fetal scalp electrode, intrapressure catheter, or external cephalic version (Cunningham et al., 2016).

Maternal-Fetal-Neonatal Risks

Although a prolapsed cord does not directly precipitate physical alterations in the woman, her immediate concern for the baby creates enormous stress. The woman may need to deal with some

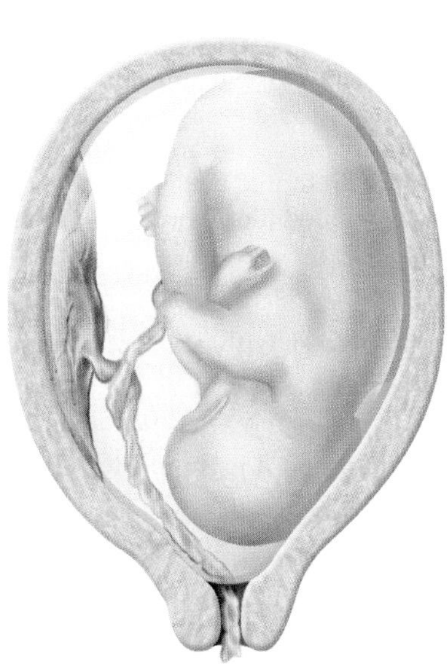

Figure 24–13 **Prolapse of the umbilical cord.**

unusual interventions, a cesarean birth, and, in some circumstances, death of the fetus.

The fetus is affected because compression of the umbilical cord occludes blood flow through the umbilical vessels. Bradycardia (baseline fetal heart rate [BL FHR]) below 110 beats per minute) and persistent variable decelerations may develop. If labor is occurring, the cord is compressed further with each contraction. If the pressure on the cord is not relieved, the fetus will die.

CLINICAL THERAPY

Preventing the occurrence of cord prolapse is the preferred medical approach. For all laboring women with a history of ruptured membranes, bedrest is usually indicated until engagement with no cord prolapse has been documented. When prolapse does occur, it is usually discovered by the nurse, and relieving the compression of the cord by pushing back the presenting part (discussed shortly) is critical for the fetus. It is also effective to place the woman in a knee-to-chest position to relieve pressure on the cord (Figure 24–14). The method of birth will most likely be cesarean unless a vaginal birth is imminent.

●○● NURSING MANAGEMENT

For the Laboring Woman and the Fetus with a Prolapsed Umbilical Cord

Nursing Assessment and Diagnosis

In the intrapartum area, review the nursing history and ascertain whether the woman is likely to be at risk for prolapse of the cord. Be sure to observe the perineum and assess the FHR for

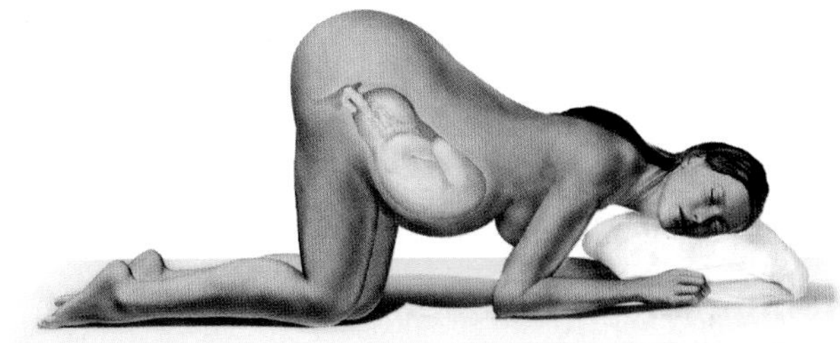

Figure 24–14 **Knee-chest position is used to relieve cord compression during cord prolapse emergency.**

bradycardia and severe, recurrent, variable decelerations, particularly when the presenting part is not engaged and spontaneous or artificial rupture of the membranes occurs. In addition, the pulsing cord could also be the presenting part, even in cases where dilatation and effacement have not yet occurred.

Nursing diagnoses that may apply to the woman with a prolapsed cord include:

- ***Gas Exchange, Impaired,*** of the fetus related to decreased blood flow secondary to compression of the umbilical cord
- ***Fear*** related to unknown outcome

(NANDA-I © 2017)

Nursing Plan and Implementation

Because there are few outward signs of cord prolapse, every pregnant woman is advised to call her physician/CNM when the membranes rupture and to go immediately to the office, clinic, or birthing facility. A sterile vaginal examination determines whether there is danger of cord prolapse. If the presenting part is well engaged, the risk is minimal and ambulation may be encouraged. If the presenting part is not well engaged, bedrest is recommended to prevent cord prolapse. Maintaining bedrest after rupture of membranes can lead to conflict if the laboring woman and her partner wish to utilize ambulation. You can ease this situation by helping communication between the physician/CNM and the couple.

If membranes have not yet ruptured when the woman arrives at the facility, at the time of spontaneous rupture or amniotomy the FHR should be monitored by EFM or auscultated for at least a full minute and again at the end of a contraction and after a few contractions. In the presence of cord prolapse, EFM tracings show baseline bradycardia or severe, moderate, or prolonged nonperiodic decelerations. If these patterns are found, perform a vaginal examination.

If a loop of cord is discovered, leave your gloved fingers in the vagina and push the presenting part upward to lift the fetal part off the cord and relieve cord compression until the physician/CNM arrives. This is a lifesaving measure. Oxygen is administered, and FHR is monitored by EFM to see if the cord compression is adequately relieved (baseline will rise above 110 beats per minute, and variable decelerations are lessened or relieved). You may also feel pulsation in the cord; however, in some instances a pulsation cannot be felt, and FHR can be detected only by EFM. A large-gauge intravenous cannula is inserted and intravenous fluids should be initiated. Anesthesia and neonatology services should be notified of impending birth.

In some cases, another nurse may insert an indwelling bladder catheter while the other nurse is still supporting the presenting part. The indwelling bladder catheter is inserted using a sterile asepto syringe or infusion device, and the bladder is filled with approximately 500 mL of warmed, sterile normal saline. The filled bladder lifts the fetal head upward and relieves pressure on the umbilical cord. Filling the woman's bladder and maintaining her in a side-lying position may be all that is needed to relieve the pressure on the cord. If the bladder is not filled, the force of gravity can be incorporated. In this instance, maintain pressure on the presenting part and instruct the woman to assume the knee-chest position or have the other nurse adjust the bed to the Trendelenburg position. Maintain pressure on the presenting part while the woman is transported to the birthing or operating room in this position. Maintain this position until the fetus is born via cesarean birth.

Evaluation

Expected outcomes of nursing care include:

- The FHR remains in normal range with supportive measures.

- The fetus is born safely.
- The woman and her partner feel supported.
- The woman and her partner understand the problem and the corrective measures that are undertaken.

Care of the Woman and Fetus at Risk Because of Anaphylactoid Syndrome of Pregnancy

Anaphylactoid syndrome of pregnancy, which is also called *amniotic fluid embolism*, occurs when a bolus of amniotic fluid, fetal cells, hair, or other debris enters the maternal circulation and then the maternal lungs. The cause of this obstetric emergency is unknown. A meta-analysis based on 13 population studies and 36 case studies consisting of two or more women found a mortality rate of 20.3% (Benson, 2017). Because amniotic fluid embolism is a rare complication, a national registry was initiated in 1988 to collect retrospective data for analysis.

CLINICAL THERAPY

When an amniotic fluid embolism is suspected, intravenous access is obtained as quickly as possible. The crash cart is accessed and on hand so supplies are readily available if a code is indicated. The mother is stabilized and an emergency cesarean birth is warranted. Symptoms generally occur rapidly, so a quick response is imperative. Diagnosis is made by symptomology by the physician. Symptoms include shortness of breath, hypoxia, cyanosis, and cardiovascular and respiratory collapse (Benson, 2017). Supportive nursing measures include preparations for an emergency birth and transfer of the mother to the intensive care unit after surgery is completed.

NURSING MANAGEMENT

For the Woman and Fetus at Risk Because of Anaphylactoid Syndrome of Pregnancy

Nursing Assessment and Diagnosis

Nursing diagnoses that may apply to the woman with anaphylactoid syndrome of pregnancy include:

- ***Gas Exchange, Impaired***, of the fetus related to decreased blood flow secondary to maternal hypoxia
- ***Gas Exchange, Impaired***, of the mother related to decreased blood flow secondary to amniotic fluid embolism
- ***Fear*** related to unknown outcome

(NANDA-I © 2017)

Nursing Plan and Implementation

In the absence of the physician/CNM, administer oxygen under positive pressure until medical help arrives. An intravenous line is quickly established. If respiratory and cardiac arrest occurs, cardiopulmonary resuscitation (CPR) is initiated immediately. The obstetrician and anesthesiologist should be called immediately. If a perinatologist and/or hospital intensivist is on staff, they should also be called.

Prepare the equipment necessary for blood transfusion and for the insertion of a central venous pressure (CVP) line. As the blood volume is replaced, using fresh whole blood to provide clotting factors, the CVP is monitored frequently. In the presence of *cor pulmonale* (abnormal enlargement of the right side of the heart as a result of disease of the lungs or the pulmonary blood vessels), fluid overload could easily occur. The fetus is continually monitored. In women who are unresponsive to CPR, an emergent cesarean birth should be performed in an effort to save the fetus. CPR is continued throughout the cesarean procedure.

Evaluation

- The mother is treated with appropriate interventions to achieve stabilization.
- The fetus is delivered safely via cesarean birth.
- The family is informed and supported during emergency procedures.

Care of the Woman with a Uterine Rupture

Uterine rupture is a nonsurgical disruption of the uterine cavity. The incidence of uterine rupture is approximately 1 in 2000 births (Gabbe et al., 2016). A *complete rupture* is one in which the endometrium, myometrium, and serosa have separated. An *incomplete* or *partial rupture* is one in which not all layers, but some, have been disrupted. The extent of maternal and fetal distress is proportional to the degree of rupture. Rupture preceding labor is rare. It is most commonly associated with a previous uterine incision that ruptures during the labor process. It can also be caused from uterine manipulation (such as a version), an operative vaginal delivery, abdominal trauma, interval of birth between deliveries less than 18 months, postpartum fever during a previous cesarean birth, or a one-layer closure performed with a previous cesarean birth (Gabbe et al., 2016).

CLINICAL THERAPY

Uterine rupture can only be diagnosed via a surgical incision, but suspected uterine rupture is based on maternal and fetal symptomology. If the rupture is accompanied by vaginal bleeding, the nurse initiates a pad count to keep track of bleeding. Preparations are made for an emergency birth, and neonatology services are obtained, if available in the practice setting. Neonatal resuscitation should be anticipated.

NURSING MANAGEMENT

For the Woman with a Uterine Rupture

Nursing Assessment and Diagnosis

A nonreassuring fetal heart rate is commonly the earliest warning sign of a possible uterine rupture. It is sometimes associated with variable or late decelerations, followed by bradycardia (Gabbe et al., 2016). Upon palpation, there may be loss of a fetal station since the presenting part is no longer being held in place by the uterine wall. Maternal symptoms include constant abdominal pain, uterine tenderness, change in uterine shape, cessation of contractions, hematuria, and signs of shock. Uterine rupture can be suspected clinically but is confirmed surgically.

Nursing Plan and Implementation

When a nonreassuring fetal pattern is identified, immediately contact the physician/CNM. Risk factors for uterine rupture should be reviewed. Women with a previous history of cesarean birth or uterine surgery are at risk for uterine rupture. Maternal signs and symptoms should be assessed, including pain, bleeding, and hematuria. Leopold maneuvers and maternal vital signs should be performed. Birth via cesarean is warranted. Prepare the woman for an emergency cesarean birth. The anesthesiologist should be called immediately. Blood should be typed and matched for possible transfusion. An additional intravenous line using an 18-gauge or larger cannula is placed. During the cesarean birth, the degree of rupture is assessed. If the uterus is unable to be repaired or if the mother is hemodynamically unstable, a hysterectomy is performed.

Nursing diagnoses for women experiencing a uterine rupture include:

- *Gas Exchange, Impaired,* of the fetus related to decreased blood flow secondary to uterine rupture
- *Gas Exchange, Impaired,* of the mother related to decreased blood flow secondary to uterine rupture
- *Fear* related to unknown outcome
- *Anxiety* related to emergency procedures and unknown fetal outcome
- *Coping, Ineffective,* due to emergent situation secondary to uterine rupture

(NANDA-I © 2017)

Evaluation

- The mother remains hemodynamically stable throughout emergency cesarean birth.
- The fetus retains optimal oxygenation until a safe birth is achieved.

Care of the Woman with Cephalopelvic Disproportion

The birth passage includes the maternal bony pelvis, beginning at the pelvic inlet and ending at the pelvic outlet, and the maternal soft tissues within these anatomic areas. A contracture (narrowing) in any of the described areas can result in **cephalopelvic disproportion (CPD)**. Abnormal fetal presentations and positions occur in CPD as the fetus moves to accommodate passage through the maternal pelvis.

The gynecoid and anthropoid pelvic types are usually adequate for vertex birth, but the android and platypelloid types predispose to CPD. Certain combinations of types can also result in pelvic diameters inadequate for vertex birth. (See Chapter 19 for a description of the types of pelvises and their implications for childbirth.) Clues that may lead to suspicion of contractures of the maternal pelvis are presented in Table 24–3. Women with a history of pelvic fractures may also be at risk for CPD (Gabbe et al., 2016).

TABLE 24–3 Clues Suggesting Contractures of Maternal Pelvis

- Diagonal conjugate less than 11.5 cm (contracture of inlet); outlet less than 8 cm (contracture of outlet)
- Unengaged fetal head in early labor in primigravidas (consider contracture of inlet, malpresentation, or malposition)
- Hypotonic uterine contraction pattern (consider contracted pelvis)
- Deflexion of fetal head (fetal head not flexed on fetal chest; may be associated with occiput posterior)
- Uncontrollable pushing before complete dilatation of cervix (may be associated with occiput posterior)
- Failure of fetal descent (consider contracture of inlet, midpelvis, or outlet)
- Edema of anterior portion (lip) of cervix (consider obstructed labor at the inlet)

Types of Contractures

There are two types of contractures: *Contractures of the inlet* and *contractures of the outlet*.

CONTRACTURES OF THE INLET

The pelvic inlet is contracted if the shortest anterior–posterior diameter is less than 10 cm or the greatest transverse diameter is less than 12 cm. The anterior–posterior diameter may be approximated by measuring the diagonal conjugate, which in the contracted inlet is less than 11.5 cm. Clinical and x-ray pelvimetry are used to determine the smallest anterior–posterior diameter through which the fetal head must pass.

The treatment goal is to allow the natural forces of labor to push the biparietal diameter of the fetal head beyond the potential interspinous obstruction. Although forceps may be used, they cause difficulty because pulling on the head destroys flexion and because they further diminish the available space. A bulging perineum and crowning indicate that the obstruction has been passed.

CONTRACTURES OF THE OUTLET

An interischial tuberous diameter of less than 8 cm constitutes an outlet contracture. Outlet and midpelvic contractures frequently occur simultaneously. Whether vaginal birth can occur depends on the woman's interischial tuberous diameters and the fetal posterosagittal diameter.

Implications of Pelvic Contractures

Labor is prolonged and protracted in the presence of CPD, and premature rupture of the membranes (PROM) can result from the force of the unequally distributed contractions being exerted on the fetal membranes. In obstructed labor (the fetus is not able to pass through the birth canal), uterine rupture can also occur. With delayed descent, necrosis of maternal soft tissues can result from pressure exerted by the fetal head. Eventually, necrosis can cause fistulas from the vagina to other nearby structures. Difficult forceps-assisted births can also result in damage to maternal soft tissue.

If the membranes rupture and the fetal head has not entered the inlet, there is a danger of cord prolapse. Extreme molding of the fetal head can result. Traumatic forceps-assisted births can damage the fetal skull and CNS.

CLINICAL THERAPY

Fetopelvic relationships can be assessed by comparing the estimated weight of the fetus as obtained by ultrasound measurements to pelvic measurements obtained by a manual examination before labor and by computed tomography (CT). Occasionally, in high-risk centers magnetic resonance imaging (MRI) is used to identify adequacy of pelvic diameters.

When the pelvic diameters are borderline or questionable, a *trial of labor (TOL)* may be advised. In this process the woman continues to labor, and careful assessments of uterine contractions, cervical dilatation, and fetal descent are made by the physician/CNM and nurse. As long as there is continued progress, the TOL continues. If progress ceases, the decision for a cesarean birth is made.

●○● NURSING MANAGEMENT

For the Woman with Cephalopelvic Disproportion

Nursing Assessment and Diagnosis

The adequacy of the maternal pelvis for a vaginal birth should be assessed intrapartum as well as antepartum. During the intrapartum assessment, the size of the fetus and its presentation, position, and lie must also be considered. (See Chapter 20 for intrapartum assessment techniques.)

Suspect CPD when labor is prolonged, cervical dilatation and effacement are slow, and engagement of the presenting part is delayed or lack of fetal descent occurs.

Nursing diagnoses that may apply include:

- ***Knowledge, Deficient***, related to lack of information about implications of CPD
- ***Fear*** related to unknown outcome of labor

(NANDA-I © 2017)

Nursing Plan and Implementation

Nursing actions during the TOL are similar to care during any labor, with the exception that the assessments of cervical dilatation and fetal descent are done more frequently. Monitor contractions and chart labor progress. Monitor the fetus frequently. Report any signs of fetal stress to the physician/CNM immediately.

The woman may be positioned in a variety of ways to increase the pelvic diameters. Sitting or squatting increases the outer diameters and may be effective in instances where there is failure of or slow fetal descent. Changing from one side to the other or maintaining a hands-and-knees position may assist the fetus in occiput posterior (OP) position to change to an occiput anterior (OA) position. The woman may instinctively want to assume one of these positions. If not, you may encourage a change of position. Standing with support can facilitate fetal decent by using gravity as an aid. Women with an epidural may use position changes with adequate support.

The woman and her partner may need help in coping with the stresses of complicated labor. Keep the couple informed of what is happening and explain the procedures that are being used. This should reassure the couple that measures are being taken to resolve the problem.

Evaluation

Expected outcomes of nursing care include:

- The woman's fear is lessened.
- The woman has additional knowledge regarding the problems, implications, and treatment plans.

Care of the Woman at Risk Because of Complications of Third and Fourth Stages of Labor

Common complications of the third and fourth stages of labor include retained placenta, lacerations, and placenta accrete.

Retained Placenta

Retention of the placenta beyond 30 minutes after birth is termed **retained placenta**. It occurs in 2 to 3% of all vaginal births. Bleeding as a result of a retained placenta can be excessive. If placenta expulsion does not occur, a manual removal of the placenta by the physician/CNM is attempted. In women who do not have an epidural in place, intravenous sedation may be required because of the discomfort caused by the procedure. Retained placenta may be a symptom of an accreta, increta, or percreta (to be discussed shortly). Failure to retrieve the placenta via manual removal usually necessitates surgical removal by curettage. If the woman does not have an epidural in place, the procedure can be performed under general anesthesia.

Lacerations

Lacerations of the cervix or vagina may be present when bright red vaginal bleeding persists in the presence of a well-contracted uterus. The incidence of lacerations is higher among childbearing women who are young, are nulliparous, have an epidural block, undergo forceps-assisted or vacuum-assisted birth, or undergo an episiotomy. Vaginal and perineal lacerations are often categorized in terms of degree:

- ***First-degree laceration***: Limited to the fourchette, perineal skin, and vaginal mucous membrane
- ***Second-degree laceration***: Involves the perineal skin, vaginal mucous membrane, underlying fascia, and muscles of the perineal body; it may extend upward on one or both sides of the vagina
- ***Third-degree laceration***: Extends through the perineal skin, vaginal mucous membranes, and perineal body and involves the anal sphincter; it may extend up the anterior wall of the rectum
- ***Fourth-degree laceration***: Similar to the third degree but extends through the rectal mucosa to the lumen of the rectum; it may be called a third-degree laceration with a rectal wall extension

Placenta Accreta

In **placenta accreta**, the chorionic villi attach directly to the myometrium of the uterus. Two other types of placental adherence are **placenta increta**, in which the myometrium is invaded, and **placenta percreta**, in which the myometrium is penetrated. These placenta-adherent disorders can be life-threatening. The adherence itself may be total, partial, or focal, depending on the amount of placental involvement. The incidence of placenta accreta is 1 in 2000 births (Gabbe et al., 2016). Placenta accreta is the most common type of adherent placenta. Previous cesarean births increase the risk of placenta accreta. This is of concern with the rapidly rising cesarean section rate within the United States.

The primary complication of placenta accreta is maternal hemorrhage and failure of the placenta to separate following birth of the baby. An abdominal hysterectomy may be the necessary treatment, depending on the amount and depth of involvement. Chapter 35 discusses hemorrhage following birth.

The at-risk conditions during labor discussed in this chapter can, in some cases, lead to fetal demise. See Chapter 36 for an in-depth discussion of caring for the family experiencing perinatal loss.

Focus Your Study

- Hypotonic labor patterns begin normally and then progress to infrequent, less intense contractions. If there are no contraindications, oxytocin is administered intravenously as treatment.
- Postterm pregnancy is one that extends more than 294 days, or 42 weeks, past the first day of the last menstrual period.
- The occiput posterior position of the fetus prolongs the labor process, causes severe back discomfort in the laboring woman, and predisposes her to vaginal and perineal trauma and lacerations during birth.
- The types of fetal malpresentations include face, brow, breech, and shoulder.
- A fetus or newborn weighing more than 4000 g is termed *macrosomic*. Macrosomia may lead to problems during labor and birth and in the early neonatal period.
- Prolapsed umbilical cord results when the umbilical cord precedes the fetal presenting part. When this occurs, pressure is placed on the umbilical cord, and blood flow to the fetus is diminished.
- Anaphylactoid syndrome of pregnancy, or amniotic fluid embolism, occurs when a bolus of amniotic fluid enters the maternal circulation and then enters the maternal lungs. Maternal mortality is very high with this complication.
- Uterine rupture occurs when the layers of the uterine cavity are separated by a nonsurgical event and requires an emergency cesarean birth to be performed immediately.
- Cephalopelvic disproportion occurs when there is a narrowed diameter in the maternal pelvis. The narrowed diameter is called a contracture, and it may occur in the pelvic inlet, midpelvis, or outlet. If pelvic measurements are borderline, a trial of labor may be attempted. Failure of cervical dilatation or fetal descent would then necessitate a cesarean birth.
- Third- and fourth-stage complications usually involve a hemorrhage. Causes of hemorrhage include lacerations of the birth canal or cervix, retained placenta, and placenta accreta.
- Nonreassuring fetal status is indicated by persistent late decelerations, persistent severe variable decelerations, and prolonged decelerations. If fetal stress is recognized and treated appropriately, the fetus may be spared any permanent damage.

In order to make safe and effective judgments using NANDA-I © 2017 nursing diagnoses, it is essential that nurses refer to the definitions and defining characteristics of the diagnoses used in this text, which can be found in Appendix C.

References

American College of Obstetricians and Gynecologists (ACOG). 2017. *Shoulder dystocia* (ACOG Practice Bulletin No. 178). *Obstetrics & Gynecology, 129*(5), e123–e133.

Benson, M. D. (2017). Amniotic fluid embolism mortality rate. *Journal of Obstetrics and Gynaecology Research, 43*(11), 1714–1718. DOI: 10.1111/jog.13445

Creasy, R. K., Resnik, R., Iams, J. D., & Lockwood, C. J. (2014). *Creasy & Resnik's maternal-fetal medicine: Principles and practice* (7th ed.). Philadelphia, PA: Saunders Elsevier.

Cunningham, F. G., Leveno, K. J., Bloom, S. L., Spong, C., Dashe, J.S., Hoffman, B.L., . . . Sheffield, J. S. (2016). *Williams obstetrics* (25th ed.). New York, NY: McGraw-Hill.

Elghazaly, E. A., Ali, Q. M., & Babikir, H. H. (2016). Umbilical cord abnormalities. *Sudan Medical Monitor, 11*(1), 1. DOI: 10.4103/1858-5000.178489

Endler, M., Saltvedt, S., & Papadogiannakis, N. (2016). Macroscopic and histological characteristics of retained placenta: A prospectively collected case-control study. *Placenta, 41*, 39–44. DOI: 10.1016/j.placenta.2016.02.013

Fazil, A., Zafar, F., Asifa, A., Akmal, N., & Karim, A. (2016). Prevalence and perinatal mortality of cord prolapse and presentation. *Annals of King Edward Medical University, 11*(3). DOI: 10.21649/akemu.v11i3.1026

Gabbe, S. G., Niebyl, J. R., Simpson, J. L., Landon, M. B., Galan, H. L., Jauniaux, E. R. M., . . . Grobman, W. A. (Eds.). (2016). *Obstetrics: Normal and problem pregnancies* (7th ed.). Philadelphia, PA: Elsevier.

Kaplan, A. I. (2017). Compound presentation, obese mother, bad outcome: This shoulder dystocia case presented several hurdles tor the defense. *Contemporary OB/GYN, 62*(4), 65–68.

Lin, S. L. (2016). Malpresentation and abnormal lie. In K. Singh (Ed.), *Integrated approach to obstetrics and gynaecology* (p. 423). Singapore: World Scientific Publishing.

Norwitz, E. (2017). Patient education: Postterm pregnancy (Beyond the basics). *Up-to-Date.* Retrieved from https://www.uptodate.com/contents/postterm-pregnancy-beyond-the-basics

Phillips, J. K., Skelly, J. M., King, S. E., Bernstein, I. M., & Higgins, S. T. (2018). Associations of maternal obesity and smoking status with perinatal outcomes. *Journal of Maternal-Fetal & Neonatal Medicine, 31*(12), 1620–1626. DOI: https://www.tandfonline.com/doi/full/10.1080/14767058.2017.1322950

Ray, E. M., & Alhusen, J. L. (2016). The suspected macrosomic fetus at term: A clinical dilemma. *Journal of Midwifery & Women's Health, 61*(2), 263–269.

Senger, P. L. (2015). *Pathways to pregnancy and parturition* (3rd ed.). Redmond, OR: Current Conceptions.

Simkin, P., & Ancheta, R. (2017). Prolonged prelabor and latent first stage. *The labor progress handbook: Early interventions to prevent and treat dystocia* (4th ed., pp. 95–121). Hoboken, NJ: Wiley.

Skinner, S., Davies-Tuck, M., Wallace, E., & Hodges, R. (2017). Perinatal and maternal outcomes after training residents in forceps before vacuum instrumental birth. *Obstetrics & Gynecology, 130*(1), 151–158. DOI: 10.1097/AOG.0000000000002097

Sloman, R., Wanat, M., Burns, E., & Smith, L. (2016). Midwives' views, experiences and feelings of confidence surrounding vaginal breech birth: A qualitative study. *Midwifery, 41*, 61–67.

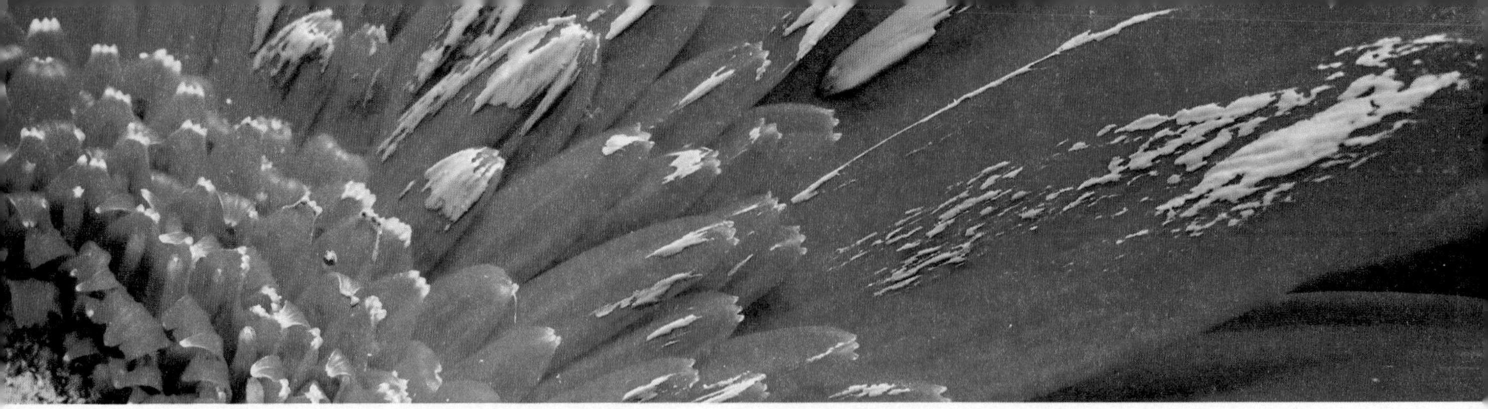

Chapter 25
Birth-Related Procedures

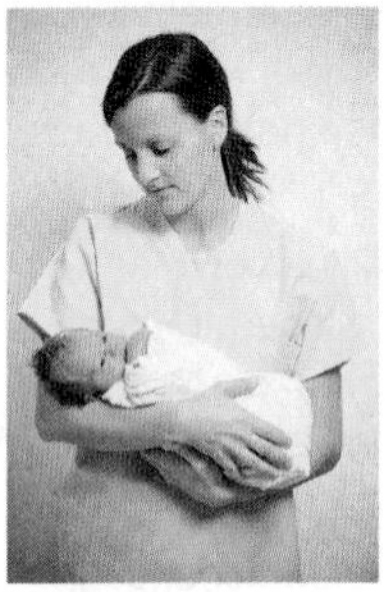

With our first baby, I suddenly had to have a cesarean. Everything happened so fast, but our son was OK, and that's all that mattered. With our second baby, I wanted to try for a vaginal birth, but nevertheless I was afraid. I don't know what I would have done without my nurse. She stayed with me the whole time I labored and kept giving me support. She explained everything, so I knew what was happening. I felt safe. I had a beautiful baby girl after 8 hours of labor. Everything went well postpartum, and I am so glad I was able to avoid another cesarean. We don't plan to have another baby, but if we did, I wouldn't be so afraid.

SOURCE: RubberBall/SuperStock.

Learning Outcomes

25.1 Describe the impact of an unanticipated obstetric procedure on the childbearing woman and her partner.

25.2 Contrast the methods of external cephalic version and internal version and the related nursing management.

25.3 Discuss the use of amniotomy in current maternal-newborn care.

25.4 Compare methods for inducing labor, explaining their advantages and disadvantages.

25.5 Discuss the use of transcervical intrapartum amnioinfusion.

25.6 Describe the types of episiotomies performed, the rationale for each, and the associated nursing interventions.

25.7 Summarize the indications for forceps-assisted birth, types of forceps that may be used, complications, and related interventions.

25.8 Discuss the use of vacuum extraction, including indications, procedure, complications, and related nursing management.

25.9 Explain the indications for cesarean birth, impact on the family unit, preparation and teaching needs, and associated nursing management.

25.10 Examine the risks, guidelines, and nursing care of the woman undergoing vaginal birth after cesarean birth (VBAC) or a trial of labor after cesarean birth (TOLAC).

Healthy People 2020

(MICH-6) Reduce maternal illness and complications due to pregnancy (complications during hospitalized labor and delivery)

(MICH-7.1) Reduce cesarean births among low-risk (full-term, singleton, and vertex presentation) women

(MICH-7.2) Reduce cesarean birth among low-risk women giving birth with a prior cesarean birth

Most births occur without the need for operative obstetric intervention. In some instances, however, obstetric procedures are necessary to maintain the safety of the woman and the fetus. The most common obstetric procedures are electronic fetal monitoring (discussed in Chapter 20), version, amniotomy, induction of labor, episiotomy, cesarean birth, and vaginal birth following a previous cesarean birth.

Generally, women are aware of the possible need for an obstetric procedure during their labor and birth, and many women accept whatever procedure is recommended based on the belief that the healthcare provider knows what is needed and that it is in the baby's best interest. However, some women expect to have a "natural" birth experience and do not desire or anticipate any medical intervention. These women may feel disappointed or even guilty when an unanticipated obstetric procedure is needed. The nurse can provide information regarding the procedure to enhance the understanding of the woman and her partner of what is proposed, the anticipated benefits and possible risks, and any possible alternative treatments.

The nurse must provide emotional support to the woman and her family to assist them in accepting the unanticipated procedure. Although the physical responses to interventions are constantly monitored and documented, it is especially important for nurses to continually assess and document the family's emotional responses to interventions. Most times it is the nurse who plays a key role in emotional support and teaching. The importance of this role is just as imperative to any physical care that the nurse performs for the laboring woman and her family.

Care of the Woman During Version

Version, or turning the fetus, is a procedure used to change the fetal presentation by abdominal or intrauterine manipulation. The most common type of version is **external cephalic version (ECV)**, in which the fetus is changed from a breech, transverse, or oblique lie to a cephalic presentation by external manipulation of the maternal abdomen (Figure 25–1). The success rates for version are the highest for transverse presentations. Overall, success rates for version average 60% (Cunningham et al., 2014). Successful ECVs decrease the chances of nonvertex and cesarean births.

The other type of version, called a **podalic version** (also called an *internal version*), is used only with the second twin during a vaginal birth. In a podalic version, the physician places a hand inside the uterus, grabs the fetus's feet, and then turns the fetus from a transverse or noncephalic presentation to a breech presentation (Figure 25–2). The fetus is then born in a breech presentation. This maneuver is used only when the second twin is not in a cephalic position. It is considered superior to an external cephalic version because it causes fewer decelerations (Cunningham et al., 2014). Some physicians may elect to have the second twin be born by cesarean if the twin is not in a cephalic presentation.

External Cephalic Version

If breech or shoulder presentation (transverse lie) is detected in the later weeks of pregnancy, ECV may be attempted. The version is usually done after 36 to 37 weeks' gestation because most fetuses still in breech presentation at this time will not spontaneously change back to a vertex presentation. This provides time for the fetus to assume a vertex position spontaneously. In addition, if complications arise from the procedure, the risk of prematurity is eliminated. Even when ECV is successful, there is some evidence that the stress of the procedure may increase the rate of intrapartum cesarean births. Breech fetuses have been shown to have smaller head circumferences, lower birth weight, and lower fetoplacental ratios. Fetuses that were previously breech tend to have higher rates of nonreassuring fetal status and dystocia. These mothers may also have a smaller pelvis, which may be the cause of the breech presentation in the first place (Simpson & Creehan, 2014). Factors associated with higher success rates include higher parity, adequate amniotic fluid, lack of fetal engagement, transverse lie, a palpable fetal head, and a relaxed uterus. Factors associated with higher failure rates include nulliparity, advanced dilatation, fetal weight less than 2500 g, anterior placenta, a low station, maternal obesity, decreased amniotic fluid volume, and anterior or posterior positioning of the fetal spine (Cunningham et al., 2014).

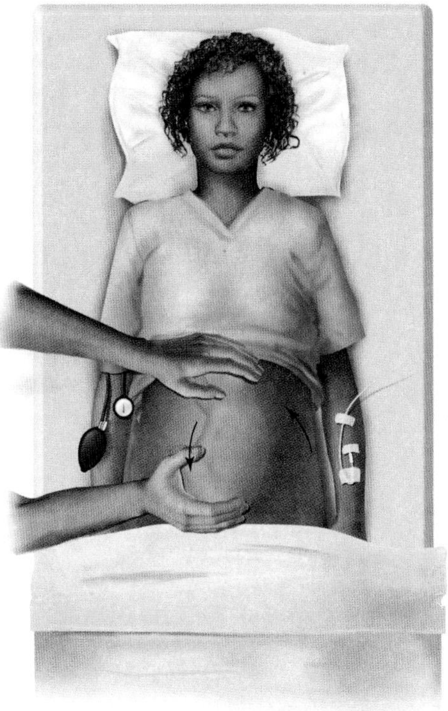

Figure 25–1 **External (or cephalic) version of the fetus. The technique involves applying pressure to the fetal head and buttocks so that the fetus completes a "backward flip" or "forward roll."**

CRITERIA FOR EXTERNAL CEPHALIC VERSION

The following criteria should be met before performing ECV (Simpson & Creehan, 2014):

- A single fetus (also called a *singleton*) must be present. If a multiple gestation exists, a variety of concerns preclude an external version. For example, a cesarean rather than vaginal birth may need to be considered, and the fetuses might become entangled during a version.
- The fetal breech is not engaged. Once the presenting part is engaged, it is difficult, if not impossible, to do a version.
- An adequate amount of amniotic fluid must exist. The amniotic fluid helps ease movement of the fetus and provides adequate room for the umbilical cord to float without being compressed.
- A reactive nonstress test (NST) should be obtained immediately before performing the version. A reactive NST indicates fetal well-being.
- The fetus must be 36 to 37 or more weeks' gestation. A version may be accompanied by complications that require immediate birth by cesarean. If gestation is less than 37 weeks, a preterm birth would result.

(*Note:* Occasionally, a physician may do an external version while the woman is in early labor before the presenting part has become engaged.)

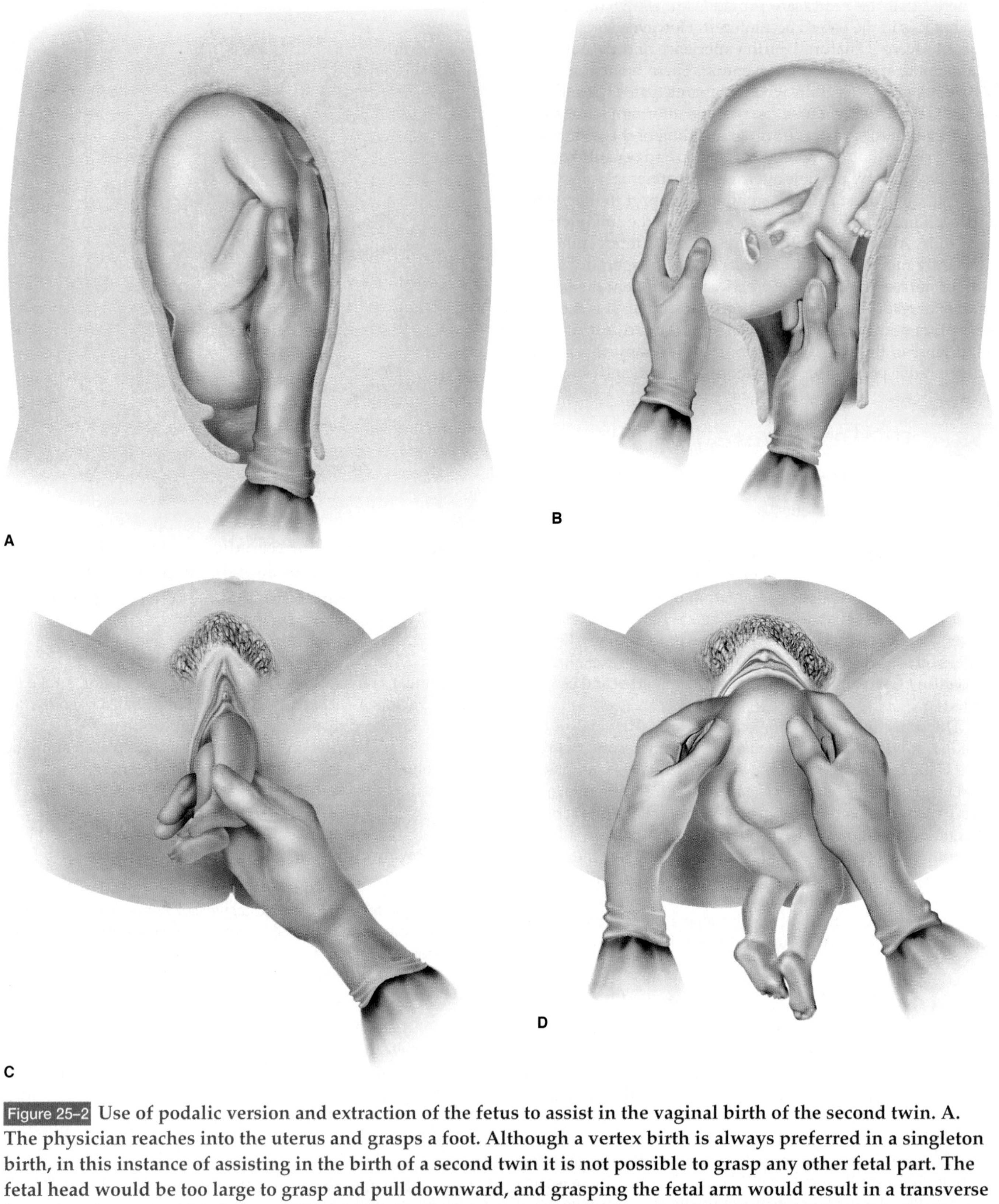

Figure 25–2 Use of podalic version and extraction of the fetus to assist in the vaginal birth of the second twin. A. The physician reaches into the uterus and grasps a foot. Although a vertex birth is always preferred in a singleton birth, in this instance of assisting in the birth of a second twin it is not possible to grasp any other fetal part. The fetal head would be too large to grasp and pull downward, and grasping the fetal arm would result in a transverse lie and make vaginal birth impossible. B. While applying pressure on the outside of the abdomen to push the baby's head up toward the top of the uterus with one hand, the physician pulls the baby's foot down toward the cervix. C. Both feet have been pulled through the cervix and vagina. D. The physician now grasps the baby's trunk and continues to pull downward on the baby to assist the birth.

CONTRAINDICATIONS FOR EXTERNAL CEPHALIC VERSION

Absolute contraindications to ECV include (Cunningham et al., 2014):

- ***Suspected intrauterine growth restriction.*** The fetus has been stressed and amniotic fluid may be decreased.
- ***Fetal anomalies.*** This category includes major abnormalities.
- ***Presence of an abnormal fetal heart rate (FHR) tracing.*** A nonreassuring FHR pattern might indicate that the fetus is already stressed and other action needs to be taken.
- ***Rupture of the membranes.*** Rupture of the membranes would result in an inadequate amount of amniotic fluid.
- ***Planned cesarean birth.*** ECV should not be attempted if there is a contraindication to vaginal delivery.
- ***Maternal problems.*** Maternal problems include gestational diabetes that has required insulin, uncontrolled chronic hypertension, preeclampsia, or maternal cardiac disease.
- ***Amniotic fluid abnormalities.*** Oligohydramnios (amniotic fluid index less than 5 cm) makes the fetus difficult to maneuver and increases risk of umbilical cord compression. Hydramnios (amniotic fluid index greater than 25 cm) stretches the uterine walls, increasing pressure and decreasing the chance the fetus will remain in a cephalic presentation.

Relative contraindications to ECV include:

- ***Previous lower uterine segment cesarean birth.*** Prior scarring of the uterus may increase the risk of uterine tearing or uterine rupture.
- ***Nuchal cord.*** A nuchal cord may tighten around the fetal neck and decrease circulation to the fetus.
- ***Multiple gestation.***
- ***Evidence of uteroplacental insufficiency.***
- ***Significant third-trimester bleeding.***
- ***Uterine malformation.***

EXTERNAL CEPHALIC VERSION PROCEDURE

The high rate of cesarean section for breech presentations suggests that ECV is not performed routinely even for suitable candidates. Women who are appropriate candidates should be informed that 50% of external versions are successful. Even though fetal risks associated with external version are reported at 1 to 2%, some women may opt for a cesarean section (Sharoni, Lyell, & Weiniger, 2015). Over 90% of fetuses in breech presentation are delivered by elective cesarean section, with approximately 12% of cesarean deliveries in the United States performed for breech presentation. The percentage is higher when deliveries for repeat cesarean sections secondary to a history of a prior cesarean indicated for breech presentation are included (Ehrenberg-Buchner & Smith, 2015).

The external version is accomplished in a birthing unit, rather than an outpatient setting, in case further intervention (such as emergency cesarean birth) is necessary. The physician/CNM uses ultrasound to confirm the presence of a single fetus, the amount of amniotic fluid, the location of the placenta, the position of the umbilical cord, and that a breech presentation still exists. Maternal vital signs are assessed, and continuous electronic fetal monitoring (EFM) is done to evaluate the FHR, to obtain a reactive NST, and to evaluate the presence of uterine activity. Blood work may be done, including a complete blood count (CBC) and a blood type and antibody screen (if not already available). The physician explains the procedure, and the patient signs a consent form.

An intravenous line is established for medication administration and in case of difficulties. A beta-mimetic agent (a subcutaneous dose of terbutaline) or intravenous infusion of magnesium sulfate (if a beta-mimetic agent is contraindicated because of a medical condition) is administered to achieve uterine relaxation. Several studies have explored the use of various tocolytics, but terbutaline was shown to be most successful when given 5 to 20 minutes prior to ECV (Ehrenberg-Buchner & Smith, 2015). The use of regional analgesia has shown mixed results in randomized trials, indicating that further research is needed (American College of Obstetricians and Gynecologists [ACOG], 2016a).

The woman is placed in a supine or slight Trendelenburg position. Once uterine relaxation is achieved, the maternal abdomen is copiously covered with warmed ultrasound gel to decrease excessive manipulation and friction, and the physician grasps the fetal breech between the index finger and the thumb. First the presenting part is gently pushed upward or lifted out of the maternal pelvis by exerting pressure over the skin on the maternal abdomen. If the fetal breech can be lifted out, then the breech and head are rotated or moved out in opposite directions. In most cases, a direction similar to a forward roll is attempted initially. If that is not successful, a roll in the opposite direction is attempted. The procedure should be concluded when any of the following occur: The fetal head is moved to a head-down position; repeated failures have occurred; the woman has indicated that the procedure has become too painful or stressful; or signs of maternal or fetal problems occur, including a nonreassuring FHR pattern (ACOG, 2016a). Intermittent monitoring with ultrasound throughout the procedure can be used to assess the FHR and the fetal position and determine if progress has occurred (ACOG, 2016a). The tocolytic agent is discontinued, and frequently the fetus is held in the new presentation by either the physician or the nurse until the uterus regains tone.

In the event of a failed version, a repeat attempt can be made within a week if the procedure was well tolerated by the woman and her fetus. The risk of maternal-fetal hemorrhage is 2.4% (Simpson & Creehan, 2014). (See Chapter 18.) Ultrasound is performed to confirm the fetal position. A vaginal examination may be performed to evaluate cervical dilatation and fetal descent. Spontaneous reversion is rare and occurs in 3% of women, but the risk is decreased with term gestations compared with earlier gestations.

Clinical Tip

Spontaneous version after a failed ECV may also occur, so it is imperative to check for the fetal position prior to a scheduled cesarean birth. When the fetus is at a high station and not engaged, or if maternal obesity or hydramnios are present, it may be difficult to identify the position. Position should be confirmed via ultrasound if uncertainty with the physical examination occurs. It is important to confirm the presenting part and to palpate the fundal part using Leopold maneuvers to ensure accuracy.

NURSING MANAGEMENT

For the Expectant Woman During External Cephalic Version

Ensure that the woman understands the procedure, knows that the procedure may be uncomfortable or very painful, and realizes that she can tell the physician/CNM to stop if the pain is too great.

The possibility of failure of the ECV and the slight risk of a cesarean birth if the fetus exhibits a nonreassuring fetal status should also be discussed. Before the version, explain the procedure and possible outcomes, and then complete initial maternal and fetal assessments, provide ongoing evaluation of FHR, and perform the NST. Place an intravenous line. Obtain bloodwork and alert the obstetrical team regarding the procedure in the rare event that a cesarean birth should be necessary. Check to ensure that the woman has signed the consent form with the physician and has had all questions answered prior to the beginning of the procedure. Provide psychologic support through reassurance and continuous explanations throughout the procedure.

Continue to monitor maternal blood pressure and pulse about every 2 minutes throughout the period of time the betamimetic agent is used and for about 30 minutes after. Monitor the FHR for at least 30 minutes or longer if clinically indicated following the ECV (ACOG, 2016a). Assess the maternal-fetal response to the tocolytic agent. Continue to provide information by reiterating aftercare instructions, such as monitoring for uterine contractions, being aware of fetal movement (fetal kick counts), and recognizing signs of reversion (excessive movement or a sensation described as the fetus "turning around").

Care of the Woman During Cervical Ripening

Each year four million women in the United States give birth and over 20% of them undergo induction of labor (Levine et al., 2016). Induction of labor may be necessary or beneficial in certain clinical situations. When the cervix is unfavorable, the use of cervical ripening agents increases the likelihood of a successful induction of labor (see Table 25–3 later in the chapter). Misoprostol (Cytotec) and formulations of prostaglandin E_2 (PGE_2) for **cervical ripening** (softening and effacing the cervix) are drugs that may be used for the pregnant woman at or near term when there is a medical or obstetric indication for induction of labor. Mechanical methods designed to ripen the cervix employ the use of balloon catheters to encourage mechanical dilatation. Current research is revealing the advantage of the combined use of mechanical (balloon catheter) and pharmacologic (misoprostol [Cytotec]) methods, resulting in a shortened time to delivery (Levine et al., 2016).

Contraindications to cervical ripening include, but are not limited to (Goldberg & Smith, 2015):

- Prematurity
- Active herpes
- Fetal malpresentation
- Nonreassuring fetal surveillance
- History of prior traumatic delivery
- Regular contractions
- Unexplained vaginal bleeding
- Placenta previa
- Vasa previa
- Prior uterine myomectomy involving the endometrial cavity or classic cesarean delivery.

Use of Misoprostol (Cytotec)

Misoprostol (Cytotec) is a synthetic PGE_1 analog that can be used to soften and ripen the cervix and to induce labor. It is available as a tablet that is inserted into the vagina, or it can be taken orally or sublingually.

Misoprostol (Cytotec) has been found to be more effective than oxytocin or prostaglandin agents and is less costly. Women who receive misoprostol to induce labor typically deliver within 24 hours of administration. The use of the drug is also associated with lower cesarean birth rates. Most adverse maternal and fetal outcomes associated with misoprostol have been associated with doses beyond the recommended 25 mcg. Misoprostol intravaginally has been found to be as efficacious or superior to dinoprostone gel (Cunningham et al., 2014). Guidelines for misoprostol induction include (Goldberg & Smith, 2015):

- Initial dosage of 25 mcg
- Recurrent administration not to exceed dosing intervals of more than 3 to 6 hours
- Oxytocin (Pitocin) not administered less than 4 hours after the last misoprostol (Cytotec) dose
- Misoprostol to be administered only when uterine activity and FHR can be monitored continuously for an initial observation period.

Contraindications for misoprostol include:

- Nonreassuring FHR tracing
- Frequent uterine contractions of moderate intensity
- Previous cesarean birth
- Previous uterine surgery/scar
- Placenta previa
- Undiagnosed vaginal bleeding.

Use of Prostaglandin Agents (Cervidil, Prepidil)

The two most commonly used types of prostaglandins are Prepidil and Cervidil. Prepidil gel contains 0.5 mg dinoprostone (a form of prostaglandin E_2) and is placed intracervically. Cervidil is packaged in an intravaginal insert that resembles a 2-cm square piece of cardboard-like material. It is placed in the posterior vagina and is left in place to provide a slow release of 10 mg dinoprostone at a rate of 0.3 mg/hr over 12 hours (Cunningham et al., 2014). See *Drug Guide: Dinoprostone (Cervidil) Vaginal Insert* and *Drug Guide: Dinoprostone (Prepidil).*

Drug Guide

Dinoprostone (Cervidil) Vaginal Insert
Pregnancy Risk Category: C

OVERVIEW OF MATERNAL-FETAL ACTION

Dinoprostone is a naturally occurring form of prostaglandin E_2. Dinoprostone can be used at term to ripen the cervix and can stimulate the smooth muscle of the uterus to enhance uterine contractions. A single vaginal insert may be used to ripen the cervix, and then oxytocin can be administered 30 minutes later (Ferring Pharmaceuticals, 2016).

ROUTE, DOSAGE, AND FREQUENCY

The vaginal insert contains 10 mg of dinoprostone. The insert is placed transversely in the posterior fornix of the vagina, and the patient is kept supine for 2 hours but then may ambulate. The dinoprostone is released at approximately 0.3 mg/hr over a 12-hour period. The vaginal insert should be removed by pulling on the retrieval string upon onset of uterine contractions or after 12 hours (Ferring Pharmaceuticals, 2016).

CONTRAINDICATIONS

- Patient with known sensitivity to prostaglandins
- Presence of nonreassuring fetal status
- Unexplained bleeding during pregnancy
- Strong suspicion of cephalopelvic disproportion
- Patient already receiving oxytocin
- Patient with six or more previous term pregnancies
- Patient who is not anticipated to be able to give birth vaginally.

Dinoprostone vaginal insert should be used with *caution* in patients with ruptured membranes, a fetus in breech presentation, presence of glaucoma, or history of asthma (Ferring Pharmaceuticals, 2016).

MATERNAL SIDE EFFECTS

Uterine hyperstimulation with or without nonreassuring fetal status has occurred in a very small number (2.8 to 4.7%) of patients. Less than 1% of patients have experienced fever, nausea and vomiting, diarrhea, or abdominal pain (Ferring Pharmaceuticals, 2016).

EFFECTS ON FETUS/NEWBORN

Nonreassuring FHR patterns.

NURSING CONSIDERATIONS

- Assess for presence of contraindications.
- Monitor maternal vital signs, cervical dilatation, and effacement carefully.
- Monitor fetal status for presence of reassuring FHR pattern (baseline 110–160 beats/min, average variability, presence of accelerations with fetal movement, absence of late or variable decelerations).
- Remove vaginal insert if uterine hyperstimulation, sustained uterine contractions, nonreassuring fetal status, spontaneous rupture of membranes, or any other maternal adverse actions occur.

Source: Ferring Pharmaceuticals, 2016.

Drug Guide

Dinoprostone (Prepidil)
Pregnancy Risk Category: C

OVERVIEW OF MATERNAL-FETAL ACTION

Dinoprostone cervical gel is a synthetically prepared form of prostaglandin E_2. Dinoprostone can be given at term and acts directly on the myometrial fibers to stimulate uterine contractility. Dinoprostone directly softens the cervix, relaxing smooth muscle in the cervix itself, and assists the uterus in producing coordinated contractions with lower doses of pitocin (Wilson, Shannon, & Shields, 2018).

ROUTE, DOSAGE, AND FREQUENCY

Prepidil is packaged as a single-dose syringe that contains 0.5 mg of dinoprostone in a 2.5-mL viscous gel. The package contains two soft plastic catheters that are used for intracervical administration. The plastic catheter is introduced into the external cervical os for placement. The catheters come in two different lengths and have a shield to prevent instillation of the medication into the internal os. The medication can be placed directly during a digital examination or a speculum can be used to visualize the cervix. The woman is placed in a reclining position and bedrest is maintained to prevent the medication from leaking from the vagina. The woman should be monitored using EFM for at least 30 minutes and up to 2 hours after placement to assess the contraction pattern and the fetal status. Prepidil may be repeated every 6 hours up to three doses. Pitocin should not be administered for at least 6 to 12 hours because the effects of dinoprostone can be heightened when oxytocin is administered (Wilson et al., 2018).

CONTRAINDICATIONS

- Known sensitivity to prostaglandins
- Presence of nonreassuring fetal status
- Unexplained vaginal bleeding during pregnancy
- Current use of oxytocin
- Grandmultiparous women with more than six previous term vaginal births
- Known contraindications for vaginal birth
- Suspected cephalopelvic disproportion
- Previous surgical scar on uterus.

Dinoprostone should be used with caution in women with a history of asthma; ruptured membranes; or renal, hepatic, or cardiovascular disease (Wilson et al., 2018).

MATERNAL SIDE EFFECTS

Uterine hyperstimulation can occur, resulting in a nonreassuring FHR pattern. Rarely, fever, nausea and vomiting, and diarrhea have also been noted to occur. In the past, women who have had a previous cesarean birth and have been given dinoprostone have had a uterine rupture as a result.

EFFECTS ON FETUS/NEWBORN

Nonreassuring FHR patterns.

NURSING CONSIDERATIONS

- Assess fetal status before administration.
- Assess for contractions.

(continued)

Drug Guide

Dinoprostone (Prepidil)
Pregnancy Risk Category: C *(continued)*

- Monitor vital signs, cervical changes, and potential side effects.
- Monitor for reassuring fetal status (FHR of 110–160, presence of variability, accelerations with fetal movement, absence of late or variable decelerations).
- Report uterine hyperstimulation, sustained uterine contractions, nonreassuring fetal status, spontaneous ruptured membranes. or adverse maternal reactions to physician or certified nurse-midwife (CNM) immediately.
- Use caution in handling this product to prevent contact with skin. Wash hands thoroughly with soap and water after administration.

Source: Pharmacia & Upjohn. Division of Pfizer, Inc., New York, NY, 2014.

ADVANTAGES AND DISADVANTAGES OF PROSTAGLANDIN ADMINISTRATION

An advantage of Cervidil is that it can be removed easily if uterine hyperstimulation occurs (Ferring Pharmaceuticals, 2016). Both Prepidil and Cervidil have been demonstrated to cause cervical ripening, shorter labor, and lower requirements for oxytocin during labor induction. Vaginal birth is achieved within 24 hours for most women. The incidence of cesarean birth is reduced when prostaglandin agents are used before labor induction (Cunningham et al., 2014).

The most frequent complication of prostaglandin administration is uterine over activity. Hyperstimulation (tachysystole or hypertonus associated with abnormalities in FHR), tachysystole (persistent pattern of five or more contractions in 10 minutes), and hypertonus (a single contraction lasting longer than 2 minutes) are all forms of uterine over activity (ACOG, 2016b).

Contraindications to labor induction are found in Table 25–1. Women with a previous uterine incision should not receive prostaglandin agents, as the risk of uterine rupture is greatly increased (Simpson & Creehan, 2014). Prostaglandin should be used with caution in women with compromised cardiovascular, hepatic, or renal function and in women with asthma or glaucoma (Ferring Pharmaceuticals, 2016).

PROSTAGLANDIN AGENT INSERTION PROCEDURE

It is recommended that prostaglandin gel be used only in a hospital birthing unit and that a physician be readily available in case an emergency cesarean birth is needed. The use of prostaglandin E (PGE) in outpatient settings and birth centers is currently under study. When Prepidil is used, it is introduced by means of a prefilled syringe with a catheter attached to the hub. The catheter is inserted through the vagina and into the endocervix, where the gel is injected. The catheter has a small shield at the top so that the gel cannot be deposited above the internal os. Prepidil is available as a gel that may be placed in a diaphragm and applied to the cervix and as a suppository that is placed in the posterior fornix of the vagina.

When Cervidil is used, the vaginal insert is placed in the posterior vagina. The woman should be instructed to call the nurse if it becomes dislodged so it can be reinserted. The woman is then monitored so her contractions and the fetus can be assessed. If hyperstimulation does occur, the insert can be removed. If active labor is established, the insert should also be removed. Women who receive Cytotec typically remain in the acute care setting, and oxytocin is started to facilitate birth.

TABLE 25–1 Contraindications to Labor Induction or Augmentation

- Vasa previa or complete placenta previa
- Transverse fetal lie
- Umbilical cord prolapse
- Previous classical cesarean delivery
- Active genital herpes infection
- Previous myomectomy entering the endometrial cavity

SOURCE: Data from ACOG, 2016b.

Mechanical Methods of Cervical Ripening and Labor Induction

Mechanical methods to ripen the cervix or induce labor, such as balloon catheters and extra-amniotic saline infusion (EASI), can be used as an alternative or in conjunction with other agents. Advantages of mechanical agents for cervical ripening are similar in efficacy when compared to hormonal agents, are less costly, have a lower incidence of systemic side effects, and have less incidence of uterine hyperstimulation (Cunningham et al., 2014).

Balloon catheters have been used for cervical ripening for many years to promote mechanical dilatation. A Foley catheter with a 30-mL to 50-mL balloon is passed through the undilated cervix and then inflated. The weighted balloon applies pressure on the internal os of the cervix and acts to ripen the cervix. This technique can be used alone or in conjunction with other induction methods, such as vaginal misoprostol (Cytotec), intravenous oxytocin (Pitocin), or extra-amniotic saline infusion where additional saline is inserted into the Foley bulb, which is pulled snugly against the cervical os (Goldberg & Smith,2015).

Use of Nitric Oxide Donor Agents

Nitric oxide (NO) donor agents are being studied for their ripening of the cervix without producing contractions and therefore may be of use in the outpatient setting. Such NO donor agents include isosorbide mononitrate, isosorbide dinitrate, nitroglycerin, and sodium nitroprusside. The use of NO donor agents leads to little or no difference in the labor process and delivery outcomes when compared to intracervical catheters, intracervical prostaglandins, or vaginal misoprostol (Cytotec), but may be associated with dizziness or nausea (ACOG, 2017a).

●○● NURSING MANAGEMENT

For the Expectant Woman During Cervical Ripening

Physicians/CNMs and labor and delivery nurses who have had special education and training may administer agents for cervical ripening. Maternal vital signs are assessed for a baseline, and an electronic fetal monitor is applied for at least 30 minutes to obtain an external tracing of uterine activity, FHR pattern, and a reactive NST. If a nonreactive test is obtained, consultation with the physician/CNM is required. After the gel, intravaginal insert, or tablet is inserted, instruct the woman to remain lying down with a rolled blanket or hip wedge under her right hip to tip the uterus slightly to the left for the first 30 to 60 minutes to maintain the placement of the cervical ripening agent. Gel may leak from the endocervix. Monitor the woman for uterine tachysystole (hyperstimulation of the uterus) and FHR abnormalities (changes in baseline rate, variability, and presence of decelerations) for 30 minutes to 2 hours if a prostaglandin gel agent is used (Goldberg & Smith, 2015). If tachysystole of the uterus greater than five contractions in 10 minutes occurs, position the woman on her left side and administer oxygen if nonreassuring fetal status develops. The administration of a tocolytic agent (such as a subcutaneous injection of 0.25 mg terbutaline) should be considered if the uterine tachysystole pattern continues. The gel may be removed if uterine tachysystole, severe nausea and vomiting, or cardiac tachysystole develops (Wilson et al., 2018). Treatment with antiemetics, antipyretics, and antidiarrheal agents is usually not indicated. Women who receive Cervidil or Cytotec tend to remain in the acute care setting so the contraction pattern and fetal status can be monitored continuously for an initial observation period (Goldberg & Smith, 2015).

Women undergoing induction via balloon catheters do not need continuous fetal monitoring. Perform intermittent monitoring along with the maternal vital signs. Assess the location of the catheter to ensure the catheter has not become displaced. This can be achieved by marking the catheter tubing at the introitus and noting whether movement has occurred. After the catheter is inserted, the woman should remain in a recumbent position. Vaginal examinations should not be performed. A bedpan should be used, as ambulation should be avoided.

Care of the Woman During Induction or Augmentation of Labor

The American College of Obstetricians and Gynecologists (American College of Obstetricians and Gynecologists, 2015) defines labor induction as the stimulation of uterine contractions before the spontaneous onset of labor, with or without ruptured fetal membranes, for the purpose of accomplishing birth. In the United States over 22% of pregnant women undergo induction of labor (ACOG, 2016b). **Labor augmentation** refers to the artificial stimulation of uterine contractions when spontaneous contractions have failed to result in progressive cervical dilation or the descent of the fetus (Cunningham et al., 2014).

Induction or augmentation may be indicated in the presence of the following:

- Maternal medical conditions (diabetes mellitus, hypertensive disorders, renal disease, chronic pulmonary disease, antiphospholipid syndrome)
- Preeclampsia, eclampsia
- Premature rupture of membranes (PROM)
- Chorioamnionitis
- Fetal demise
- Postterm pregnancy
- Fetal compromise (severe fetal growth restriction, isoimmunization, oligohydramnios, and nonreassuring antepartum testing, such as a poor biophysical profile score)
- Risk of rapid labor or extensive distance from the hospital setting
- Mild abruptio placentae
- Nonreassuring FHR.

Contraindications to Labor Induction or Augmentation

All contraindications to spontaneous labor and vaginal birth are contraindications to the induction or augmentation of labor (see Table 25–1).

Before induction is attempted, appropriate assessment must indicate that both the woman and fetus are ready for the onset of labor. Assessment of the individual patient and the clinical situation should be considered. This includes evaluation of fetal maturity and cervical readiness. In order to reduce the likelihood of delivery of a late-preterm neonate, confirmation of a gestational age of at least 39 weeks should be ascertained. Inductions should not be performed prior to 39 weeks without an absolute medical indication (ACOG, 2016b).

The gestational age of the fetus is best evaluated by accurate menstrual dating and ultrasound visualization of the gestational sac between 5 and 6 weeks' gestation. When needed, amniotic fluid studies for lecithin/sphingomyelin (L/S) ratio and phosphatidylglycerol are also beneficial in assessing fetal lung maturity (see Chapter 16). See Table 25–2 for confirmation of gestational age to ensure a term newborn.

BISHOP SCORE

The findings on vaginal examination will help determine whether cervical changes favorable for induction have occurred. Bishop (Bishop, 1964) developed a prelabor scoring system that is still helpful in predicting the inducibility of women (Table 25–3). Components evaluated are cervical dilatation, effacement, consistency, and position, as well as the station of the fetal presenting part. A score of 0, 1, 2, or 3 is given to each assessed characteristic. The higher the total score for all the criteria, the more likely that labor will occur. The lower the total score, the higher the failure rate. A favorable cervix is the most important criterion for a successful induction (Cunningham et al., 2014). The presence of a cervix that is anterior, soft, 50% effaced, and dilated at least 2 cm, with the fetal head at +1 station or lower (Bishop score of 9), is favorable for successful induction (Bishop, 1964). Low Bishop scores have been correlated with prolonged labors and a higher incidence of cesarean births (Cunningham et al., 2014).

TABLE 25–2 Confirmation of Gestational Age

- Ultrasound measurement obtained prior to 20 weeks that demonstrates gestational age of at least 39 weeks.
- Presence of fetal heart tones via Doppler or ultrasound present for at least 30 gestational weeks.
- Documented positive serum or urine human chorionic gonadotropin pregnancy test result indicating at least 36 weeks have passed since initial test results.

SOURCE: Data from ACOG, 2016b

TABLE 25–3 Prelabor Status Evaluation Scoring System

	ASSIGNED VALUE: BISHOP SCORE			
FACTOR	0	1	2	3
Cervical dilatation	Closed	1–2 cm	3–4 cm	5 cm or more
Cervical effacement	0 to 30%	40 to 50%	60 to 70%	80% or more
Fetal station	–3	–2	–1, 0	+1, or lower
Cervical consistency	Firm	Moderate	Soft	
Cervical position	Posterior	Midposition	Anterior	

SOURCE: Data from Bishop, 1964.

Methods of Inducing or Augmenting Labor

When the cervix is favorable, the most frequently used methods of induction or augmentation are stripping the amniotic membranes, amniotomy, intravenous oxytocin (Pitocin) infusion, and complementary methods.

STRIPPING THE MEMBRANES

A nonpharmacologic method of induction or augmentation frequently used by physicians/CNMs is called *stripping* (or *sweeping*) *the amniotic membranes*. The physician/CNM inserts a gloved finger as far as possible into the internal cervical os and rotates the finger 360 degrees, twice. This motion separates the amniotic membranes that are lying against the lower uterine segment and internal os from the distal part of the lower uterine segment. The stripping or sweeping is thought to release prostaglandin $F_{2\alpha}$ ($PGF_{2\alpha}$) from the amniotic membranes or prostaglandin E_2 (PGE_2) from the cervix. Membrane sweeping has been associated with a reduced risk of postterm pregnancy and a reduction in labor inductions (Ugwu, Obi, Iferikigwe, et al., 2014). Women should be advised that this procedure can cause significant discomfort. In addition, uterine contractions, cramping, scant bleeding, and a bloody discharge can occur after the procedure is performed. Although the procedure is not 100% effective as a labor induction method, if labor is initiated, it typically begins within 24 to 48 hours. As an augmentation method, stripping of the membranes can be performed in the birthing room in an attempt to strengthen contractions without the need for oxytocin administration. If contractions fail to become adequate, however, oxytocin may need to be considered.

OXYTOCIN INFUSION

Intravenous administration of oxytocin is an effective method of initiating uterine contractions. Contraction frequency is only a partial assessment of uterine activity; the duration and intensity of contractions are also important measures of the quality of a contraction. The goal is to achieve an adequate uterine contraction pattern without producing tachysystole. Normal contraction activity is described as five contractions or less in 10 minutes, averaged over a 30-minute window. More than five contractions in 10 minutes (averaged over a 30-minute window) constitutes tachysystole.

When augmentation is needed because of an arrest of labor or failure of the presenting part to descend, oxytocin is given intravenously to achieve a desirable labor pattern with strong contractions that will result in cervical dilatation and fetal descent. Typically, augmentation is warranted if there are fewer than three contractions in a 10-minute period or if the intensity is less than 25 mmHg as indicated by an internal uterine pressure catheter during the active phase of labor. An assessment of the maternal pelvis, fetal station, and fetal position is performed before starting the oxytocin infusion. In addition, cephalopelvic disproportion should be ruled out because it is a contraindication. The other contraindications for labor augmentation are the same as for labor induction.

A primary bag of intravenous fluid is prepared and used to start and maintain the infusion. This avoids the risk of infusing a large dose of oxytocin as the line is begun and provides additional fluids while the oxytocin solution is being kept at a low infusion rate. After the infusion is started, the oxytocin solution is piggybacked into the primary tubing port closest to the catheter insertion. This allows only a small amount of oxytocin to back flow into the tubing and ensures greater dosage accuracy. The oxytocin should be administered with a device that permits precise control of the flow rate. Oxytocin for induction of labor should not be administered intramuscularly or without the aid of an intravenous electric pump. Over the past few years, differences in opinion regarding oxytocin dosage have surfaced.

Clinical Tip

Attach the IVPB oxytocin (Pitocin) to the medication port closest to the insertion site. If the Pitocin needs to be turned off quickly, there will be little left to infuse through the primary IV line.

Ten to 20 units of oxytocin (Pitocin) are added to 1 liter of a secondary line of isotonic intravenous fluid (usually 5% dextrose in balanced saline solution—for example, 5% dextrose in lactated Ringer solution). The resulting mixture will contain 10 or 20 milliunits of oxytocin per milliliter (1 mU/min/6 mL/hr or 2 mU/min/12 mL/hr), and the prescribed dose can be calculated easily. Some facilities are now using 30 units of oxytocin per 500 mL of intravenous fluid to reduce the risk of pulmonary edema in the postpartum period. Other dilutions can also be used. Other dosage concentrations are presented in the *Drug Guide: Oxytocin (Pitocin)*. It is imperative that the nurse be familiar with the specific dosage used within the institution to avoid medication errors. See *Professionalism in Practice: Recommended Medical Practice Guidelines.*

Drug Guide

Oxytocin (Pitocin)

OVERVIEW OF OBSTETRIC ACTION

Oxytocin (Pitocin) exerts a selective stimulatory effect on the smooth muscle of the uterus and blood vessels. Oxytocin affects the myometrial cells of the uterus by increasing the excitability of the muscle cell, increasing the strength of the muscle contraction, and supporting propagation of the contraction (movement of the contraction from one myometrial cell to the next). Its effect on the uterine contraction depends on the dosage used and on the excitability of the myometrial cells. During the first half of gestation, there is little excitability of the myometrium, and the uterus is fairly resistant to the effects of oxytocin. However, from midgestation on, the uterus responds increasingly to exogenous intravenous oxytocin. Cautious use of diluted oxytocin administered intravenously at term results in a slow rise of uterine activity.

The circulatory half-life of oxytocin is 3 to 5 minutes. It takes approximately 40 minutes for a particular dose of oxytocin to reach a steady-state plasma concentration (Wilson et al., 2018).

The effects of oxytocin on the cardiovascular system can be pronounced. Blood pressure may initially decrease but after prolonged administration increase by 30% above the baseline. Cardiac output and stroke volume increase. With doses of 20 milliunits/min or above, oxytocin exerts an antidiuretic effect, decreasing free water exchange in the kidney and markedly decreasing urine output.

Oxytocin is used to induce labor at term and to augment uterine contractions in the first and second stages of labor. Oxytocin may also be used immediately after birth to stimulate uterine contraction and thereby control uterine atony.

ROUTE, DOSAGE, AND FREQUENCY

For induction of labor: Add 10 units of Pitocin (1 mL) to 1000 mL of intravenous solution. (The resulting concentration is 10 mU oxytocin per 1 mL of intravenous fluid.) Using an infusion pump, administer IV, starting at 0.5–1 milliunit/min and increase by 1–2 milliunits/min every 40–60 minutes. Alternatively, start at 1–2 milliunits/min and increase by 1 milliunit/min every 15 minutes until a good contraction pattern (every 2–3 minutes and lasting 40–60 seconds) is achieved.

MATERNAL CONTRAINDICATIONS

- Severe preeclampsia, eclampsia
- Predisposition to uterine rupture (in nullipara over 35 years of age, multigravida 4 or more, over distention of the uterus, previous major surgery of the cervix or uterus)
- Cephalopelvic disproportion
- Malpresentation or malposition of the fetus, cord prolapse
- Preterm fetus
- Rigid, unripe cervix; total placenta previa
- Presence of nonreassuring fetal status.

MATERNAL SIDE EFFECTS

Hyperstimulation of the uterus results in hypercontractility, which in turn may cause the following:

- Abruptio placentae
- Impaired uterine blood flow, leading to fetal hypoxia
- Rapid labor, leading to cervical lacerations
- Rapid labor and birth, leading to lacerations of the cervix, vagina, or perineum; uterine atony; fetal trauma
- Uterine rupture
- Water intoxication (nausea and vomiting, hypotension, tachycardia, cardiac arrhythmia) if oxytocin is given in electrolyte-free solution or at a rate exceeding 20 milliunits/min; hypotension with rapid IV bolus administration postpartum.

EFFECT ON FETUS-NEWBORN

- Fetal effects are primarily associated with the presence of hypercontractility of the maternal uterus. Hypercontractility decreases the oxygen supply to the fetus, which is reflected by irregularities or decrease in FHR.
- Hyperbilirubinemia (Wilson et al., 2018) when administered for augmentation of labor
- Trauma from rapid birth.

NURSING CONSIDERATIONS

- Explain induction or augmentation procedure to patient.
- Apply fetal monitor and obtain 15- to 20-minute tracing and NST to assess FHR before starting IV oxytocin.
- For induction or augmentation of labor, start with primary IV and piggyback secondary IV with oxytocin and infusion pump.
- Ensure continuous monitoring of the fetus and uterine contractions.
- The maximum rate is 40 milliunits/min (Wilson et al., 2018). Not all protocols recommend a maximum dose, and the safest maximum dose has not been established. When indicated, the maximum dose is generally between 16 and 40 milliunits/min (Wilson et al., 2018).Decrease oxytocin by similar increments once labor has progressed to 5–6 cm dilatation. Protocols may vary from one agency to another.

  0.5 milliunit/min = 3 mL/hr
  1.0 milliunit/min = 6 mL/hr
  1.5 milliunits/min = 9 mL/hr
  2 milliunits/min = 12 mL/hr
  4 milliunits/min = 24 mL/hr
  6 milliunits/min = 36 mL/hr
  8 milliunits/min = 48 mL/hr
  10 milliunits/min = 60 mL/hr
  12 milliunits/min = 72 mL/hr
  15 milliunits/min = 90 mL/hr
  18 milliunits/min = 108 mL/hr
  20 milliunits/min = 120 mL/hr

- Assess FHR, maternal blood pressure, pulse, frequency and duration of uterine contractions, and uterine resting tone before each increase in the oxytocin infusion rate.
- Record all assessments and IV rate within the electronic medical record (EMR).
- Record oxytocin infusion rate in milliunits/min and mL/hr (e.g., 0.5 milliunit/min [3 mL/hr]).
- Document all patient activities (such as change of position, vomiting), procedures done (amniotomy, sterile vaginal examination), and administration of analgesic agents to allow for interpretation and evaluation of tracing.
- Assess cervical dilatation as needed.
- Apply nursing comfort measures.
- Discontinue IV oxytocin infusion and infuse primary solution when (1) nonreassuring fetal status is noted (bradycardia, late or variable decelerations); (2) uterine contractions are more frequent than every 2 minutes;

(continued)

Drug Guide

Oxytocin (Pitocin) *(continued)*

(3) duration of contractions exceeds more than 60 seconds; or (4) insufficient relaxation of the uterus between contractions or a steady increase in resting tone is noted (Wilson et al., 2018). In addition to discontinuing IV oxytocin infusion, turn patient to side, and if nonreassuring fetal status is present, administer oxygen by tight face mask at 7–10 L/min; notify physician.

- Maintain intake and output record.

FOR AUGMENTATION OF LABOR

Prepare and administer IV Pitocin as for labor induction. Increase rate until labor contractions are of good quality. The flow rate is gradually increased at no less than every 30 minutes to a maximum of 10 milliunits/min (Wilson et al., 2018). In some settings or in a situation when limited fluids may be administered, a more concentrated solution may be used. When 10 units of Pitocin are added to 500 mL IV solution, the resulting concentration is 1 milliunit/min = 3 mL/hr. If 10 units Pitocin are added to 250 mL IV solution, the concentration is 1 milliunit/min = 1.5 mL/hr.

FOR ADMINISTRATION AFTER EXPULSION OF PLACENTA

- One dose of 10 units of Pitocin (1 mL) is given intramuscularly or 10 to 20 units are added to IV fluids for continuous infusion.
- Assess maternal vital signs.
- Record all assessments and IV rate on patient's chart. Record oxytocin infusion rate in milliunits/min and mL/hr (e.g., 0.5 milliunit/min [3 mL/hr]).
- Apply nursing comfort measures or pharmacologic agents for afterbirth pain associated with Pitocin administration.
- Maintain intake and output record.

Professionalism in Practice Recommended Medical Practice Guidelines

In some cases during augmentation of labor, a provider may order more than 40 milliunits/min of oxytocin. Because this contradicts ACOG guidelines and the manufacturer's recommended maximum dosage, the nurse can politely advise the ordering provider that they cannot advance the dosage above this rate. Institutional guidelines should be in place to protect nurses from being asked to override recommended medical practice guidelines.

Practitioners use both low-dose and high-dose regimens. The low-dose regimen uses a starting dose of 0.5 to 2 milliunits/min with increases of 1 to 2 milliunits/min every 15 to 40 minutes until an adequate labor pattern is established. The high-dose regimen has a starting dose of up to 6 milliunits/min with incremental increases of 3 to 6 milliunits/min every 20 to 40 minutes. If tachysystole arises with the high-dose regimen, the incremental dose is reduced to3 milliunits/min; if tachysystole is recurrent, the incremental dose is reduced to 1 milliunit/min. Higher-dose regimens have been associated with a shorter labor, less incidence of dystocia, lower cesarean birth rates, and a lower incidence of chorioamnionitis, but have a higher incidence of tachysystole, which can cause nonreassuring fetal status (Simpson & Creehan, 2014).

Oxytocin induction is not without some associated risks; however, most side effects are dose-related. The most common side effect of oxytocin administration is tachysystole of the uterus (with or without FHR changes), resulting in uterine contractions that are too frequent (more often than every 2 minutes), uterine contractions that are too intense, or an increased uterine resting tone. Category 2 or 3 FHR tracing changes have been associated with tachysystole. Other risks include uterine rupture and water intoxication.

COMPLEMENTARY HEALTH APPROACHES

In addition to the allopathic cervical ripening and induction methods previously discussed, there are a variety of more "natural" and noninvasive methods that CNMs tend to suggest or administer either in the home setting or in tertiary care centers. These methods include sexual intercourse/lovemaking; self or partner stimulation of the woman's nipples and breasts; the use of herbs, such as blue/black cohosh, evening primrose oil, and red raspberry leaves; the use of homeopathic solutions, such as caulophyllum or pulsatilla; castor oil; enemas; and acupressure/acupuncture.

Although not widely described in nursing and medical textbooks, the use of complementary health approaches has risen dramatically. It is estimated that 30% of adults and 12% of children use such methods regularly (National Center for Complementary and Integrative Health [NCCIH], 2016). Natural methods can be very effective and are frequently the preferred choice of many CNMs and their patients. It is important for nursing students, nurses, and consumers to be aware of all aspects of pregnancy care.

Sexual intercourse has been suggested as a logical method of stimulating cervical ripening and uterine contractions. Female orgasm stimulates uterine contractions and the male ejaculate contains a rich source of natural prostaglandins, but there is no definitive evidence that reflects successful induction of labor. However, breast and nipple stimulation, which are a frequent part of lovemaking, stimulates the release of endogenous oxytocin, which in turn stimulates the uterus to contract. Nipple stimulation for cervical ripening may be done at term or to augment labor. It also has been found to initiate spontaneous labor (Cunningham et al., 2014). There are multiple suggested methods, including manual manipulation and use of the electric breast pump. A recent systematic review of clinical trials comparing breast stimulation for third-trimester cervical ripening or induction of labor to other or no interventions found that breast stimulation increased the likelihood that women would go into labor. Breast stimulation is therefore not recommended in high-risk women, and care should be taken to monitor uterine contractility because hyperstimulation can occur.

Plant-based homeopathic solutions—such as caulophyllum, pulsatilla, and others—are used for cervical ripening and induction of labor. Herbal preparations including black and blue cohosh and evening primrose oil have been used; however, evidence to support their safety and use in pregnancy is inadequate; therefore, nurses should not encourage women to use these remedies. A recent systematic review that evaluated outcomes of herbal remedies during labor found that that the use of black cohosh has been associated with increased meconium-stained amniotic fluid and cesarean births (Boltman-Binkowski, 2016). There are no current guidelines for their use in augmenting labor. The physician/CNM must have thorough personal knowledge of homeopathic remedies or ongoing consultation with a homeopathic physician.

Castor oil has been used for many years but has not been studied frequently as a method of labor induction and augmentation. The method by which castor oil stimulates uterine contractions is not understood, but is thought to be a result of the release of prostaglandin E_2 as a consequence of increased peristalsis and diarrhea after ingestion of the drug. Safe use of this method is unproven (NCCIH, 2016).

Acupressure and acupuncture are not as accepted in the United States as in other countries. However, the rising interest in and use of holistic practices and alternative medicine are prompting a closer look at acupuncture as a method of inducing and augmenting labor and relieving labor pain. In acupuncture, sterile needles are inserted into the body at specific predetermined sites to elicit a desired response, such as initiation of contractions or relief of pain. Although acupuncture requires extensive education and training, some CNMs can work with an acupressurist/acupuncturist to learn manual massage of acupuncture and acupressure points, shiatsu, and other touch techniques.

●○● NURSING MANAGEMENT

For the Expectant Woman During Labor Induction

No matter which induction or augmentation method is used, close observation and accurate assessments are mandatory to provide safe, optimal care for both woman and fetus. Obtain maternal vital signs (temperature, pulse, respirations, and blood pressure) before beginning an oxytocin infusion. Induction protocols also recommend obtaining a 20- to 30-minute electronic fetal monitor recording demonstrating a reassuring FHR and a reactive NST and contraction status before the infusion is started. Patient teaching includes the purpose and procedure for the induction, as well as a review of the care that will be provided, including assessments and comfort measures. See *Nursing Care Plan: For Induction of Labor*.

During the oxytocin infusion, a physician should be readily accessible to manage any complication that occurs. A fetal monitor is used to provide continuous data. Women may ambulate if a portable or walking monitor is available.

Nursing Care Plan: For Induction of Labor

1. Nursing Diagnosis: ***Injury, Risk for*, related to hyperstimulation of uterus caused by induction of labor (NANDA-I © 2017)**

Goal: Progression of labor without difficulty or complications

INTERVENTION	RATIONALE
• Obtain a baseline for maternal blood pressure, pulse, respirations, temperature, and pain level.	• Oxytocin (Pitocin) induction can affect the cardiovascular system. Blood pressure may initially be decreased. If the induction is prolonged the blood pressure may increase by 30%. Respirations can become elevated because of pain sensation, anxiety, or physiologic causes. Temperature is obtained to monitor for infection. The pain level is assessed continuously to determine if pain medication is warranted or changes in vital signs are caused by maternal discomfort.
• Place patient on external fetal monitor for 20 minutes to obtain a baseline for fetal heart rate (FHR) and variability.	• Assesses for fetal well-being. Normal FHR ranges from 110 to 160 beats/min. Variability measuring three to five fluctuations in 1 minute is documented as average. Continuous electronic fetal monitoring (EFM) is performed during an oxytocin induction.
• Perform nonstress test.	• A nonstress test is performed to assess the FHR in response to fetal movement. Accelerations of FHR with fetal movement may indicate the fetus has adequate oxygenation and an intact central nervous system. A reactive nonstress test indicates there were at least two accelerations of 15 beats/min above baseline, lasting 15 seconds in a 20-minute period.
• Insert IV line and begin primary infusion with 1000 mL of electrolyte solution.	• An electrolyte solution such as lactated Ringer solution is used for the primary solution. A primary IV allows continuous intravenous access and fluid infusion in the event the oxytocin drip needs to be discontinued.
• Piggyback oxytocin solution into primary IV tubing, via pump, in the port closest to the IV insertion site.	• Oxytocin is mixed in 1000 mL of an electrolyte solution (usually 5% dextrose in lactated Ringer solution) and piggybacked to main IV line. A pump is used to ensure dosage accuracy.
• Begin oxytocin infusion per agency protocol.	• The rate to be used is determined by physician/CNM orders or agency protocol.
• Monitor infusion pump and connections.	• This ensures adequate dosing. Early identification of problems with the infusion site, the piggyback connection, or flow rate will minimize effects on uterine contractions and FHR. If a problem is found, correct and restart infusion at the beginning dose.
• Monitor and evaluate maternal blood pressure and pulse before each increase in the oxytocin infusion rate.	• Prolonged inductions may increase the blood pressure by 30%. The oxytocin infusion rate should not be advanced if maternal hypertension or hypotension is present or if there are any radical changes in pulse rate.

(continued)

Nursing Care Plan: For Induction of Labor (*continued*)

• Evaluate urine output.	• There is an antidiuretic effect with dosages of oxytocin above 20 milliunits/min. This level decreases free water exchange in the kidneys, therefore markedly decreasing urine output.
• Evaluate and document FHR before each increase in oxytocin infusion rate.	• During oxytocin infusion, FHR should range between 110 and 160 beats/min. Hypercontractility of the maternal uterus may cause nonreassuring fetal status. Fetal bradycardia may occur along with a decrease in variability, leading to fetal hypoxia. Fetal tachycardia may also occur. If persistent fetal bradycardia or fetal tachycardia occurs, the oxytocin is discontinued.
• Evaluate and document contraction pattern before each increase of the oxytocin infusion rate.	• Contractions every 2 to 3 minutes, lasting 40 to 60 seconds with moderate intensity, are considered adequate. Cervical dilatation progresses an average of 1.2 cm/hr to 1.5 cm/hr (0.5 in./hr to 0.6 in./hr) during the active phase of labor.
• Increase oxytocin infusion dosage until adequate contractions are achieved or the maximum dose per agency protocol is reached.	• Oxytocin may be increased every 30 to 60 minutes until an adequate contraction pattern is achieved.
• Evaluate contraction frequency, duration, and intensity before increasing the infusion rate. Discontinue oxytocin infusion and infuse primary solution if signs of hyperstimulation of the uterus are detected.	• Signs of hyperstimulation include contraction frequency less than 2 minutes, duration exceeding 60 seconds, and increased resting tone. Hyperstimulation of the uterus puts the patient at risk for abruptio placentae and uterine rupture.
• Initiate treatment measures to reverse the effects of oxytocin infusion if fetal tachycardia or bradycardia occurs.	• When the FHR falls outside the normal range (110 to 160 beats/min), treatment measures should be initiated. To reverse the effects of oxytocin, immediately discontinue, infuse primary solution, administer oxygen by tight face mask at 7 to 10 L/min, place patient in side-lying position, and notify physician/CNM.

EXPECTED OUTCOME: Contractions will increase in frequency, duration, and intensity. An increase in cervical dilatation, effacement, and intensity will be achieved. The uterus will remain soft between contractions.

Women who are undergoing alternative methods of induction also need continuous assessment and nursing support. For women who have entered labor after stripping of the amniotic membranes, a normal labor pattern should ensue. Intermittent external fetal monitoring can be used if the fetus is reactive and the maternal vital signs are within normal parameters. Women should be advised that they may continue to have a blood-tinged discharge from the procedure. Women who have their membranes stripped are less likely to go past their due dates. Continue to assess the contraction pattern, including the frequency, intensity, and duration of the contractions.

Women who choose to use nipple stimulation as a means of inducing labor should be continuously monitored with the external fetal monitor while the electric breast pump is in use. Release of oxytocin stimulated by breast pumping can result in surges of oxytocin release, which can lead to nonreassuring fetal status. Some fetuses who are unable to tolerate the release of oxytocin from breast pumping may react without stress to intravenous oxytocin administration, as this results in a small amount of oxytocin being released in a controlled manner.

In cases where homeopathic or herbal remedies have been used to induce labor, normal intermittent monitoring and assessment of maternal vital signs can be performed. If oxytocin is to be administered, inform the physician/CNM of what has been given, the dose, the last time administered, and the immediate effects that were achieved. An assessment is performed before administration of pharmacologic substances.

Expected outcomes of nursing care include:

- The woman and family are fully informed; understand the induction process; are able to relate the advantages, disadvantages, risks, and possible outcomes; and have had an opportunity to have their questions answered.
- The woman's labor is successfully induced.
- The labor progresses at a normal rate and maternal vital signs remain in normal range.
- The fetal status remains reassuring throughout the labor period.

Care of the Woman During an Amniotomy

Amniotomy is the *artificial rupture of the amniotic membranes (AROM)* and has been one of the most common procedures performed in obstetrics. Because the amniotomy requires that an instrument be inserted through the cervix, at least 2 cm of cervical dilatation must be present. The amniotomy may be performed as a method of induction of labor (to stimulate the beginning of labor). Recent guidelines suggest that routine amniotomy should not be performed if labor is progressing normally because it could increase the risk of infection (ACOG, 2017a). Amniotomy is indicated during labor to allow access to the fetus in order to apply an internal fetal heart monitoring electrode to the scalp or to insert an intrauterine pressure catheter (ACOG, 2017a).

Advantages and Disadvantages of Amniotomy

Amniotomy as a method of labor induction has these advantages:

- Contractions can be elicited for women who wish not to receive or who refuse pharmacologic interventions, but have a medical indication to induce labor.
- There is usually no risk of hypertonus or rupture of the uterus, as with intravenous oxytocin induction.
- The woman does not require the same intensive monitoring as with intravenous oxytocin induction.
- EFM is facilitated because, once the membranes are ruptured, a fetal scalp electrode may be applied and an intrauterine catheter may be inserted to assist in evaluating an FHR pattern.
- The color and composition of amniotic fluid can be evaluated.
- Amniotomy is a less costly procedure compared to other methods of induction.

The disadvantages of amniotomy are:

- Once an amniotomy is done, the risk for infection begins to rise if labor proceeds beyond 24 hours because microorganisms can now invade the intrauterine cavity and cause amnionitis.
- The danger of a prolapsed cord is increased once the membranes have ruptured, especially if the fetal presenting part is not firmly pressed down against the cervix.
- Compression and molding of the fetal head are increased because of loss of the cushioning effect of the amniotic fluid for the fetal head during uterine contractions.
- Fetal injury can occur if the amniohook causes a laceration on the presenting part.
- Bleeding can occur if an undiagnosed vasa previa is present.
- Severe variable decelerations can occur, which increases the likelihood of a cesarean birth.
- The intervention can cause an increase in pain, making labor more difficult to manage.

Amniotomy Procedure

Before an amniotomy is performed, the fetus is assessed for presentation, position, station, and FHR. Unless the fetal head is well engaged in the pelvis, practitioners do not advocate an amniotomy because of the danger of prolapsed cord (refer to Chapter 24 for discussion of prolapsed cord). Other risks are abruptio placentae (because of rapid decompression of the uterus with the rapid loss of amniotic fluid), infection (because of the introduction of organisms into the cervix and intrauterine cavity), and amniotic fluid embolus (because of rapid decompression of the uterus and small amounts of fluid entering the maternal vascular system from under the edge of the placenta). These complications may also be associated with spontaneous rupture of membranes (SROM).

While performing a sterile vaginal examination, the physician/CNM introduces an amnihook (or other rupturing device) into the vagina, through the cervix, and against the amniotic membrane, which is in front of the fetal presenting part. A small tear is made in the amniotic membrane. Following rupture of the membrane, amniotic fluid is allowed to escape slowly.

NURSING MANAGEMENT

For the Woman Undergoing Artificial Rupture of the Amniotic Membranes

First, explain the procedure to the woman. Assess the fetal presentation, position, and station because amniotomy should be delayed until engagement has occurred (to decrease the risk of a prolapsed cord when the fluid is expelled). Position the woman in a semireclining position and drape her to provide privacy. Place disposable underpads and/or towels under the woman's buttocks to absorb the amniotic fluid. The FHR is assessed just before and immediately after the amniotomy, and the two FHR assessments are compared. If there are marked changes, check for prolapse of the cord. Inspect the amniotic fluid for amount, color, odor, and the presence of meconium or blood. While wearing disposable gloves, cleanse and dry the perineal area and change the disposable underpads. Advise the woman that fluid will continue to be expelled from her vagina. Frequent pericare and pad changes should be done to increase patient comfort. Because there is now an open pathway for organisms to ascend into the uterus, strict sterile technique must be observed during vaginal examinations. In addition, the number of vaginal examinations must be kept to a minimum to reduce the chance of introducing an infection, and the woman's temperature should be monitored every 2 hours. As long as the presenting part is well applied to the cervix, the woman can ambulate and change positions. Bedrest is only required when the presenting part is not engaged or is not firmly applied to the cervix because this increases the risk of a prolapsed cord. Provide information about the amniotomy and the expected effects. Some women may worry that all the amniotic fluid will be gone and that they will experience a "dry birth." It is important for them to know that amniotic fluid is constantly produced.

Care of the Woman During Amnioinfusion

Amnioinfusion (AI) is a technique by which a volume of warmed, sterile, normal saline or Ringer lactate solution is introduced into the uterus through the use of an intrauterine pressure catheter (IUPC). AI can be used during the intrapartum period to increase the volume of fluid when oligohydramnios is present and the physician wants either to prevent the possibility of variable decelerations by increasing the volume of amniotic fluid or to treat nonperiodic decelerations that are already occurring. The AI increases the volume of fluid, relieving pressure on the umbilical cord and promoting increased perfusion to the fetus. The use of AI has been determined to be effective in reducing fetal decelerations, improving neonatal outcomes, and reducing delivery by cesarean section (Cunningham et al., 2014).

Contraindications to AI include patients with a contraindication to vaginal delivery, amnionitis, hydramnios, uterine hypertonus, multiple gestation, known fetal anomaly, uterine anomaly, nonreassuring fetal status requiring immediate birth, nonvertex presentation, scalp pH below 7.2, placenta previa, vasa previa, or abruptio placentae (Cunningham et al., 2014). AI can also be associated with rare serious risk factors, including umbilical cord prolapse, amniotic fluid embolism, and uterine rupture (Cunningham et al., 2014).

There are several different amnioinfusion protocols, however, most procedures involve infusing a bolus of 500 to 800 mL of warmed normal saline through an intrauterine catheter using a continuous infusion of approximately 3 mL per minute (Cunningham et al., 2014).

NURSING MANAGEMENT

For the Woman Undergoing Amnioinfusion

The nurse is frequently the first person to detect changes in FHR associated with cord compression or FHR changes. When cord compression is suspected, the immediate intervention is to assist the laboring woman to another position in an effort to relieve the compression and to apply O_2 via face mask (see Chapter 24 for further discussion). If this intervention is not successful, an amnioinfusion may be considered. Assist with the AI and monitor the woman's vital signs (blood pressure, pulse, and respiration) and contraction status (frequency, duration, intensity, resting tone, and associated maternal discomfort). FHR is monitored by continuous EFM. Provide ongoing information to the laboring woman and her partner and answer questions as they arise. Comfort measures and positioning are very important because AI requires the woman to be on bedrest.

The AI should not cause pain or discomfort for the laboring woman other than the need for bedrest. Ensure that the fluid infused is being expelled from the woman's vagina. This is achieved with frequent examination of the woman's sanitary pad or an absorbent pad that is placed beneath her buttocks. Advise the woman that fluid will leak from her vagina. Change absorbent pads and provide pericare on a regular basis.

Care of the Woman During an Episiotomy

An **episiotomy** is a surgical incision of the perineal body. In the past, some providers performed episiotomies with the belief that an episiotomy would prevent damage to the periurethra, perineum, anal sphincter, and rectum from lacerations during the birth; prevent damage to the posterior wall of the vagina; prevent jagged tears from lacerations; reduce mechanical and metabolic risk to the fetus/newborn; protect the maternal bladder; and prevent future perineal relaxation.

Although the incidence of episiotomies in the United States has continued to decline since evidenced-based practice guidelines advised against the use of routine episiotomies, some practitioners continue routine episiotomy due to local professional norms, education provided during previous training, and individual practitioner preference rather than the consideration of the needs of the individual woman at the time of delivery. Routine episiotomy (performed without a medical indication) has no maternal benefits and is associated with a number of maternal complications. In the United States, less than 10% of women receive routine episiotomies (Simpson & Creehan, 2014). Typically, CNMs tend to perform fewer episiotomies than physicians. See *Developing Cultural Competence: Birth-Related Procedures*.

Developing Cultural Competence Birth-Related Procedures

Although many women from Western cultures feel comfortable advocating for themselves, women in some cultures may be less verbal or feel uncomfortable discussing birth-related procedures or letting practitioners know of their own personal preferences. Nurses should discuss possible birth procedures with all women and provide modeling by bringing these topics up to the healthcare provider when care is being provided.

Current evidence supports the prevention of lacerations by protecting the perineum manually by holding the perineum between the thumb and the fingers, whereas the performance of an episiotomy makes it more likely that the woman will have deep perineal tears. It has also been suggested that perineal lacerations heal more quickly in the absence of episiotomy (Simpson & Creehan, 2014). Major perineal trauma (extension to or through the anal sphincter) is *more* likely to occur if a midline episiotomy is performed. Women who are allowed to tear spontaneously have less sexual dysfunction than women who have undergone episiotomies (Simpson & Creehan, 2014). See *Case Study: Melissa Bond-James*.

Additional complications associated with an episiotomy are blood loss, infection, pain, and perineal discomfort that may continue for days or weeks past birth, including dyspareunia (painful intercourse). Flatal incontinence (uncontrollable passage of gas) has also been reported (Cunningham et al., 2014). There are no scientific data to support the beliefs that episiotomies yield a shorter second stage, improved Apgar scores, or a decrease in perinatal asphyxia (Cunningham et al., 2014). In light of the debate over the value of episiotomy, it is now suggested that the procedure be used selectively to facilitate birth if shoulder dystocia, breech delivery, operative vaginal delivery (use of forceps or vacuum), macrocosmic fetuses, or persistent occiput posterior positions are anticipated, or in the occurrence of maternal or fetal distress (Cunningham et al., 2014).

Although practices of episiotomies differ, when instruments such as forceps are used, most practitioners perform the episiotomy after the application of the blades (Cunningham et al., 2014).

CASE STUDY: Melissa Bond-James

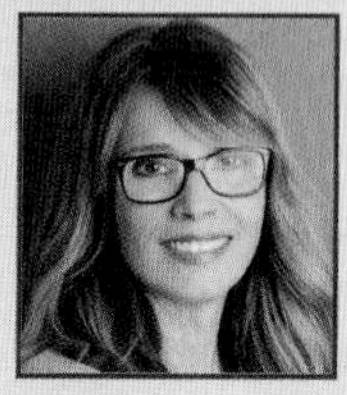

SOURCE: Kinga/Shutterstock.

Melissa has begun pushing in second stage and the nurse notes the baby is moving down very well. After 25 minutes of pushing, the physician arrives and preps Melissa's perineum for birth. As the baby is expelled, Melissa has a laceration occur. After the placenta is delivered and Melissa is breastfeeding her baby, the physician tells her she will do a repair under local anesthesia.

Questions to Ponder

What comfort measures should be provided upon completion of the repair? What education should be provided to Melissa to ensure proper hygiene is performed that will promote healing?

Risk Factors That Predispose Women to Episiotomy

Overall factors that place a woman at increased risk for an episiotomy are:

- Primigravid status
- Large or macrosomic fetus
- Occiput-posterior position
- Use of forceps or vacuum extractor
- Shoulder dystocia
- White race
- Physician provider
- Private practice physician
- Nocturnal birth times.

Other factors that predispose a woman to episiotomy may be mitigated by nurses and physicians/CNMs. These include:

- Use of lithotomy position or other recumbent position (causes excessive perineal stretching)
- Encouraging or requiring sustained breath holding during second-stage pushing (causes excessive perineal stretching, can adversely affect blood flow in the mother and fetus, and encourages the woman to be responsive to caregiver directions rather than to her own urges to push spontaneously)
- Arbitrary time limit placed by the physician/CNM on the length of the second stage.

See *Professionalism in Practice: Decreasing Episiotomy Rates.*

Clinical Tip

Women can be encouraged to wait to begin pushing once they are completely dilated and effaced until they feel a strong urge to push. This allows the contractions to continue to push the fetus into the birth canal. Once the fetus reaches the pelvic floor, the woman will feel an uncontrollable urge to push. This can reduce the length of second stage and prevent maternal fatigue and exhaustion.

Professionalism in Practice Decreasing Episiotomy Rates

Nursing advocacy is needed to promote selective rather than routine episiotomies. The nurse can begin by encouraging pregnant women to read about prenatal perineal preparation and to talk with their physicians/CNMs about their personal beliefs and the incidence of episiotomy in their practices. Nurses can share current research with nursing colleagues through staff meetings and explore and strongly encourage nursing care interventions that avoid the lithotomy position. The woman should be encouraged to respond to her body's urges to push during the second stage. Just as patients ask physicians/CNMs about their episiotomy philosophy and incidence, patients may ask labor and birthing nurses to provide information about their actions to help decrease episiotomy rates. It is imperative that nurses continue to stay current about new information and research in order to maintain current practice standards.

Episiotomy Procedure

The episiotomy is performed with a sharp scissors that has rounded points, just before birth, when approximately 3 to 4 cm of the fetal head is visible during a contraction (Cunningham et al., 2014). There are two types of episiotomy: Midline and mediolateral (Figure 25–3).The midline episiotomy is a vertical incision that begins at the vaginal opening and extends downward toward the rectum. The mediolateral incision begins in the middle of the vaginal opening and extends down toward the buttocks at a 45-degree angle. Analgesia may be enhanced with the existing labor epidural, or with the use of bilateral pudendal nerve blockade or by a 1% lidocaine infiltration. The episiotomy is usually performed during a contraction when the head is crowning, but may be performed without anesthesia in case of an emergency delivery (Cunningham et al., 2014).

The midline episiotomy is preferred over the mediolateral episiotomy because it heals easier, is associated with less blood loss, and is generally less painful than a mediolateral episiotomy, although the midline is associated with an increased risk of third- and fourth-degree lacerations (Cunningham et al., 2014). Repair of the episiotomy (episiorrhaphy) and any lacerations is usually performed after expulsion of the placenta, although some providers may perform a repair between the birth of the baby and the placenta. Many providers wait until after expulsion of the placenta in case a manual removal of the placenta or a uterine exploration is indicated (Cunningham et al., 2014).

●○● NURSING MANAGEMENT

For the Woman Undergoing an Episiotomy

Support the woman during the episiotomy and the repair because she may feel some pressure sensations. It is not uncommon for her to feel a "pulling" or "tugging" sensation. In the absence of adequate anesthesia, she may feel pain. Place a hand on her shoulder and talk with her to provide comfort and distraction from the repair process. If the woman is having more discomfort than she can comfortably handle, act as an advocate in communicating the woman's needs to the physician/CNM. At all times, the woman needs to be the one who decides whether the amount of discomfort is tolerable, and her perception of pain should never be minimized. She is the person experiencing the discomfort, and her evaluation needs to be respected. If there are just a few (three to five) stitches left, she may choose to forgo more local anesthesia, but she should be given the choice. For women with severe pain or anxiety, intravenous medication such as Fentanyl or Nubain can be administered for both pain and anxiety control.

Note the type of episiotomy on the birth record. This information should also be included in a report to the postpartum nurse so that adequate assessments can be made and relief measures can be instituted, if necessary.

Pain relief measures may begin immediately after birth with application of an ice pack to the perineum. For optimal effect, the ice pack should be applied for 20 to 30 minutes and removed for at least 20 minutes before being reapplied. This is advisable because the ice causes vasoconstriction; however, if the ice pack is left in place more than 30 minutes, vasodilation and subsequent edema may occur. The perineal tissues should be assessed frequently to prevent injury from the ice pack. Inspect the episiotomy site every 15 minutes during the first hour after the birth for redness, swelling, tenderness, and hematomas. As a part of postpartum care, give the mother instruction in perineal hygiene

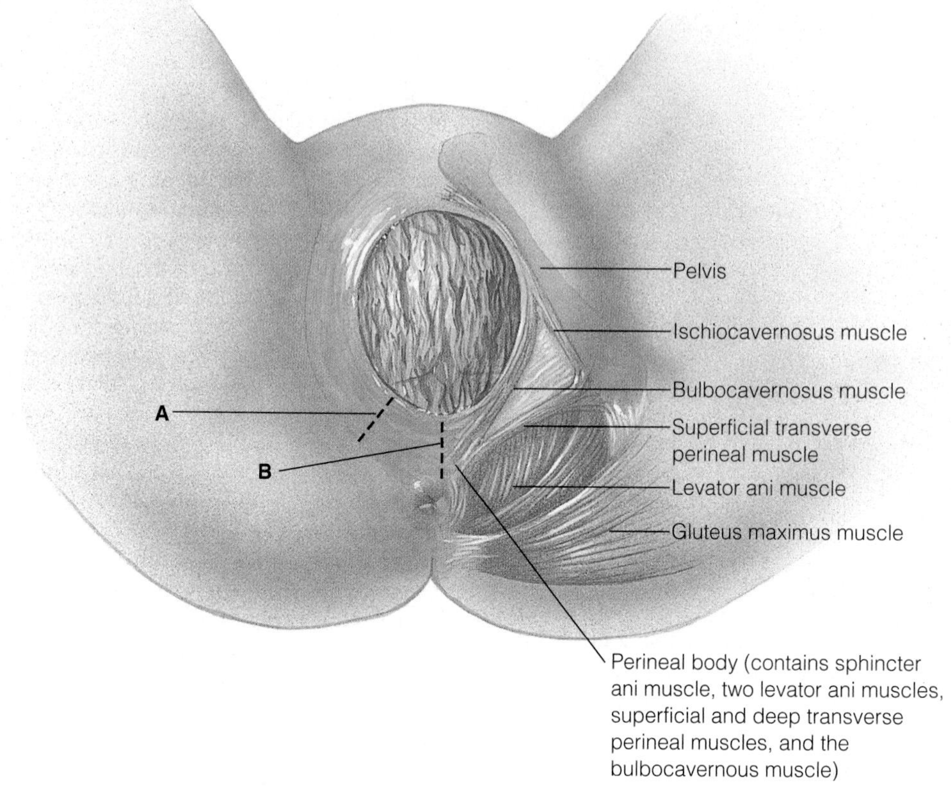

Figure 25–3 The two most common types of episiotomies are midline and mediolateral. A. Right mediolateral. B. Midline.

care and comfort measures. (See Chapter 33 for additional discussion of relief measures for the immediate postpartum period.)

It is important to recognize that perineal pain continues for a period of time. Women who experience prolonged pain tend to have other problems, such as breastfeeding difficulties and depression, and are more reluctant to reestablish sexual activity. Risk factors for subsequent lacerations include use of repeat episiotomy and instrument-assisted births.

Care of the Woman During Forceps-Assisted Birth

Forceps are designed to assist the birth of a fetus by providing traction or by providing the means to rotate the fetal head to an occiput-anterior position. In medical literature and practice, **forceps-assisted birth** is also known as *instrumental delivery*, *operative delivery*, or *operative vaginal delivery*. There are many different types of forceps, each with special functions. For example, Piper forceps are designed to be used with a breech presentation (buttocks as presenting part); they are applied after the birth of the body, when the fetal head is still in the birth canal and assistance is needed. In conversational language, Piper forceps are said to be applied to the after coming head. All other forceps are used in situations when the fetus is in a cephalic (head down) presentation. In such situations, the forceps are applied to the sides of the head. The type of forceps used is determined by the physician assisting with the birth.

Criteria for Forceps Application

ACOG has classified the definitions of forceps applications into three categories: Outlet, low, and midforceps. Criteria for *outlet forceps* application are as follows (Cunningham et al., 2014):

1. Forceps are applied when the fetal skull has reached the pelvic floor and is at or on the perineum. (There is bulging of the perineum.)
2. The scalp is visible between contractions without separating the labia. (Earlier in labor, as the woman pushes during the contraction, the fetal scalp may be visible, but when the pushing effort ceases, the scalp recedes and is no longer visible. This criterion indicates that the scalp remains visible even when the woman is not pushing.)
3. The sagittal suture is not more than 45 degrees from the midline. The sagittal suture is the anterior–posterior suture on the top of the fetal head. At this point in a spontaneous birth, extension has almost been completed, external rotation is beginning, and the sagittal suture is between the midline and 45 degrees from the midline. (For example, think of a clock face. If 12:00 is the maternal symphysis pubis and the fetus is in left occiput anterior [LOA], the sagittal suture and the occiput are between 12:00 and 1:30.) (See Chapter 19.) The important aspect of this criterion is that with outlet forceps, the fetal head is moving naturally from extension to external rotation, and the forceps are being used to guide or lift the head out.

The criterion for *low forceps* application is that the leading edge (presenting part) of the fetal skull must be at a station of plus 2 (+2) or below (e.g., +3) but not on the pelvic floor. The rotation (internal rotation, which is part of the cardinal movements) of the fetal head is less than 45 degrees (right or left occiput anterior to occiput anterior, or right or left occiput posterior to occiput posterior) (Cunningham et al., 2014).

The criterion for *midforceps* application is that the fetal head must be engaged (largest diameter of the head reaches or passes through the pelvic inlet), but the leading edge (presenting part) of the fetal skull is above a plus 2 (+2) station (e.g., +1, 0, −1, −2). When midforceps are used, the goal is to apply traction and, frequently, to rotate the head and facilitate the vaginal birth.

High forceps are not indicated in current obstetric practice. A woman whose fetus is at a station of −3 or is above the pelvic inlet should give birth by cesarean. Types of forceps are depicted in Figure 25–4.

Indications for Use of Forceps

Indications for the use of forceps include the presence of any condition that threatens the mother or fetus and that can be relieved by birth. Conditions that put the woman at risk include heart disease, acute pulmonary edema or pulmonary compromise, certain neurologic conditions, intrapartum infection, prolonged second stage, or exhaustion. Fetal conditions include premature

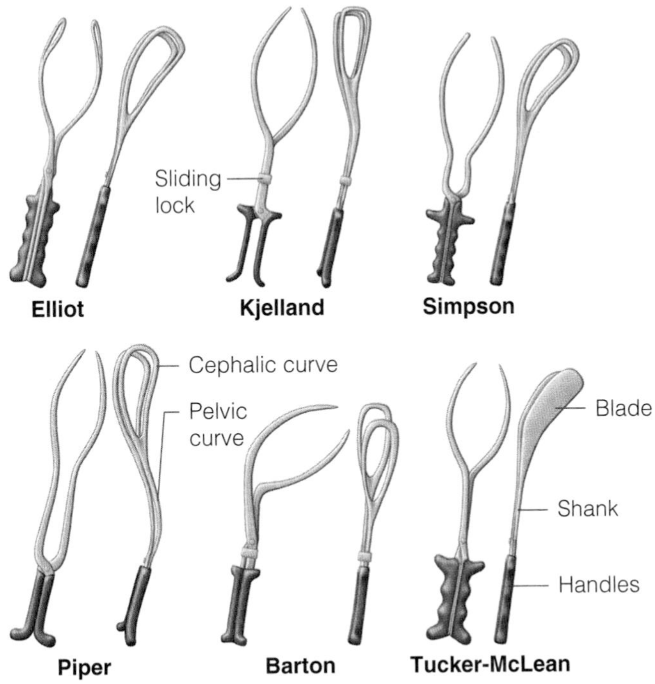

Figure 25–4 Forceps are composed of a blade, shank, and handle and may have a cephalic and pelvic curve. (Note labels on Piper and Tucker-McLean forceps.) The blades may be fenestrated (open) or solid. The front and lateral views of these forceps illustrate differences in blades, open and closed shanks, and cephalic and pelvic curves. Elliot, Simpson, and Tucker-McLean forceps are used as outlet forceps. Kielland and Barton forceps are used for midforceps rotations. Piper forceps are used to provide traction and flexion of the after coming head (the head comes after the body) of a fetus in breech presentation.

placental separation, prolapsed umbilical cord, and nonreassuring fetal status. Forceps may be used electively to shorten the second stage of labor and spare the woman's pushing effort (when exhaustion or heart disease is present) or when regional anesthesia has affected the woman's motor innervation, and she cannot push effectively. In the past, outlet forceps have been used to protect the head of a preterm fetus during birth; however, the advantages of this practice are now being questioned (Cunningham et al., 2014).

Risk factors for a forceps- or vacuum-assisted birth (discussion to follow) are (Cunningham et al., 2014):

- Nulliparity
- Maternal age (35 and over)
- Maternal height of less than 150 cm (4 ft 11 in.)
- Pregnancy weight gain of more than 15 kg (33 lb)
- Postdate gestation (41 weeks or more)
- Epidural anesthesia
- Fetal presentation other than occipitoanterior
- Presence of dystocia
- Presence of a midline episiotomy
- Abnormal FHR tracing.

Neonatal and Maternal Risks

Complications of a forceps-assisted birth for the newborn may include (Cunningham et al., 2014):

- Ecchymosis
- Edema
- Forceps marks
- Caput succedaneum
- Cephalohematoma
- Hyperbilirubinemia
- Transient facial paralysis
- Low Apgar scores
- Corneal abrasions, retinal hemorrhage, Descemet membrane tear, or other ocular trauma
- Erb palsy
- Fractured clavicle
- Elevated neonatal bilirubin levels
- Prolonged newborn hospital stay.

Maternal risks of a forceps-assisted birth may include (Cunningham et al., 2014):

- Third- or fourth-degree lacerations of the birth canal, urethra, or cervix
- Extensions of a median episiotomy into the anus
- Increased bleeding and bruising
- Hematomas
- Pelvic floor injuries
- Increased perineal pain
- Sexual dysfunction in the postpartum period
- Postpartum infections, including metritis
- Prolonged hospital stays
- Urinary and rectal incontinence; anal sphincter injury; fistulas.

Prerequisites for Forceps Application and Birth

It is very important that all of the prerequisites be met before the forceps procedure is attempted. The prerequisites are (Cunningham et al., 2014):

- The physician must be knowledgeable about the advantages and disadvantages of different types of forceps and their use.
- The cervix must be completely dilated.
- The fetal head must be engaged and the station, presentation, and exact position of the head must be known. The fetus should be in a vertex or a face presentation with the chin anterior.
- Amniotic membranes must be ruptured to allow a firm grasp on the fetal head.
- The type of pelvis should be identified because certain pelvic types do not permit rotation. In addition, there must be no disproportion between the fetal head and the maternal pelvis.
- Maternal bladder should be empty.
- There must be no obstructions to the birth below the fetal head, such as an incurving coccyx that will not allow the fetus to pass or a disproportion between the size of the head and the outlet or the midpelvis.
- Adequate anesthesia must be given for the type of forceps procedure that is anticipated. For instance, low forceps may be done with a pudendal block; however, midforceps or a rotation of more than 45 degrees requires an epidural, spinal-epidural, or general anesthesia.

Trial or Failed Forceps Procedure

The use of forceps or vacuum may be considered when the clinician believes a successful outcome can occur. In a trial forceps procedure, the physician attempts to use forceps with the knowledge that there could be a degree of cephalopelvic disproportion. A complete setup for immediate cesarean birth needs to be available before the forceps are applied. If a good application cannot be obtained or if no descent occurs with the application, a vacuum technique can be attempted. If this yields no descent, then a cesarean birth is the method of choice. See *Case Study: Azia Askari.*

NURSING MANAGEMENT

For the Woman Undergoing a Forceps-Assisted Birth

Direct nursing care measures toward the variable(s) that may be positively affected by specific nursing interventions. For instance, dystocia may be corrected by changing maternal position, ambulation, rocking, frequent bladder emptying, and so on. FHR abnormalities may be affected by utero–placental–fetal circulation, so ambulation should be considered (if not contraindicated), in addition to frequent position changes, intake of adequate fluids, and monitoring to detect early FHR changes.

If a forceps-assisted birth is required, explain the procedure briefly to the woman and her partner. With adequate regional anesthesia, the woman should feel some pressure but no pain. Encourage her to avoid pushing during application of the forceps (Figure 25–5 depicts the application). Monitor contractions and advise the physician/CNM when one is present because traction is applied only with a contraction. During the contraction, as the forceps are applied, advise the woman to avoid pushing. With each contraction, *after the forceps are in place*, the physician/CNM provides traction on the forceps as the woman pushes. It is not uncommon to observe mild fetal bradycardia as traction is applied to the forceps. This bradycardia results from head compression and is transient.

Following birth, the newborn is assessed for facial edema, bruising, caput succedaneum, cephalohematoma, corneal abrasion, and any sign of cerebral edema. In the fourth stage, assess the woman for perineal swelling, bruising, hematoma, excessive bleeding, and hemorrhage. In the postpartum period it is important to assess for signs of infection if lacerations occurred during the procedure.

Answer questions and reiterate explanations provided, review nursing assessments of the woman and her newborn, and provide opportunities for the woman and partner to ask further questions. Some women may feel a sense of loss or failure as a result of needing forceps for birth. Provide reassurance to the woman and her partner.

Care of the Woman During Vacuum Extraction

Vacuum extraction is an obstetric procedure used by physicians/CNMs to assist the birth of a fetus by applying suction to the fetal head. The vacuum extractor accounts for 68% of all operative

CASE STUDY: Azia Askari

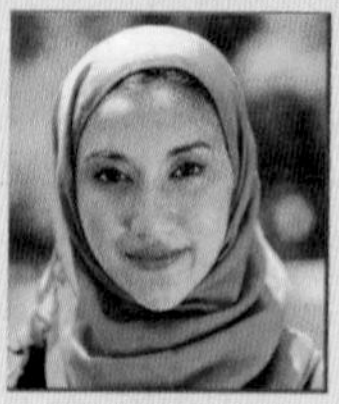

SOURCE: HONGQI ZHANG/123RF.

Azia has been admitted to the hospital for the last 9.5 hours. Her mother, sister-in-law, and husband are with her. Azia started second stage 1.5 hours ago and has been pushing since that time. There is little fetal descent and the midwife reports that the baby is presenting posteriorly but feels the obstetrician may be able to use forceps to turn the baby's head slightly and facilitate a vaginal birth. Her husband is growing very frustrated and states he does not want her to have a cesarean birth because her recovery will be too long. The midwife informs the couple the only experienced obstetrician that is available to do the procedure is a male.

Questions to Ponder

How would you explain the benefits of the procedure while still supporting the family's cultural beliefs? How can you support Azia's and her husband's individual choices in this situation?

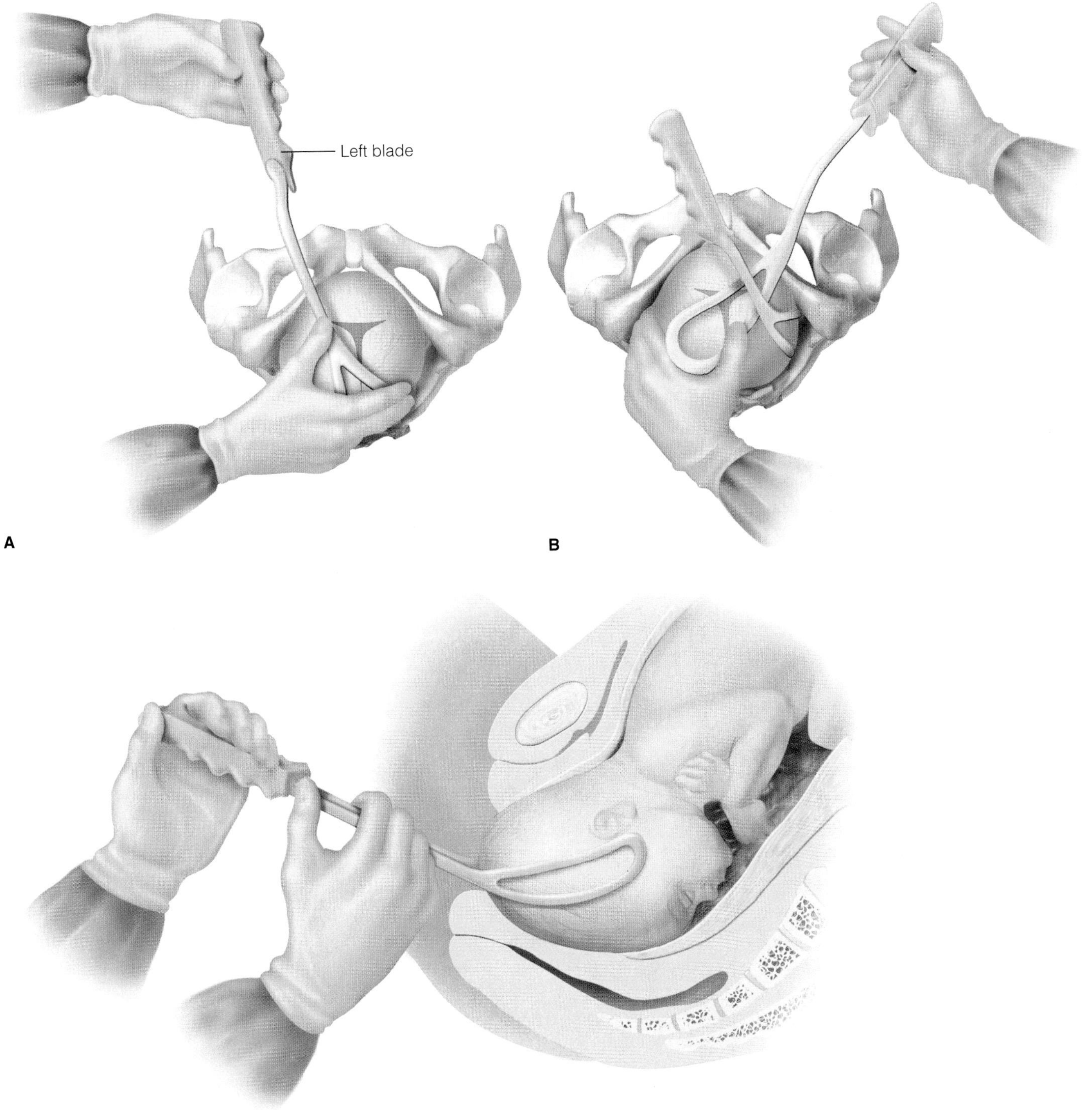

Figure 25–5 Application of forceps in occiput-anterior (OA) position. A. The left blade is inserted along the left side wall of the pelvis over the parietal bone. B. The right blade is inserted along the right side wall of the pelvis over the parietal bone. C. With correct placement of the blades, the handles lock easily. During uterine contractions, traction is applied to the forceps in a downward and outward direction to follow the birth canal.

vaginal births. Its use has increased by 41% since 1990 and continues to rise (Cunningham et al., 2014). The vacuum extractor is composed of a soft suction cup attached to a suction bottle (pump) by tubing. The suction cup, which comes in various sizes, is placed against the occiput of the fetal head. Care must be taken to ensure that no cervical or vaginal tissue is trapped under the cup. The pump is used to create negative pressure (suction) of approximately 50 to 60 mmHg in a stepwise sequence or rapid application. An artificial caput ("chignon") is formed as the fetal scalp is pulled into the cup. The physician/CNM then applies traction in coordination with uterine contractions. The fetal head should descend with each contraction until it emerges from the vagina (Figure 25–6).

Research indicates that negative suction applied for more than 10 minutes is associated with a greater incidence of scalp injury. The longer the duration of suction, the more likely the newborn will have scalp injury. Although there are no data on the duration of use, ACOG advises a 30-minute time limit (Simpson & Creehan, 2014). Many practitioners limit the time to 20 minutes. Although there are no specifications on the number of attempts, failure to descend with multiple attempts is an indicator that a cesarean birth may be needed. In addition, if more than three "pop-offs" occur (the suction cup pops off the fetal head), the procedure should be discontinued. The most common indication for the use of the vacuum extractor is a prolonged second stage of labor or nonreassuring heart rate pattern. Vacuum extraction is also used to relieve the woman of pushing effort, when analgesia or fatigue interferes with her ability to push effectively, or in cases of nonreassuring fetal status when prompt birth is indicated. The vacuum extractor is preferred to forceps in cases of borderline cephalopelvic

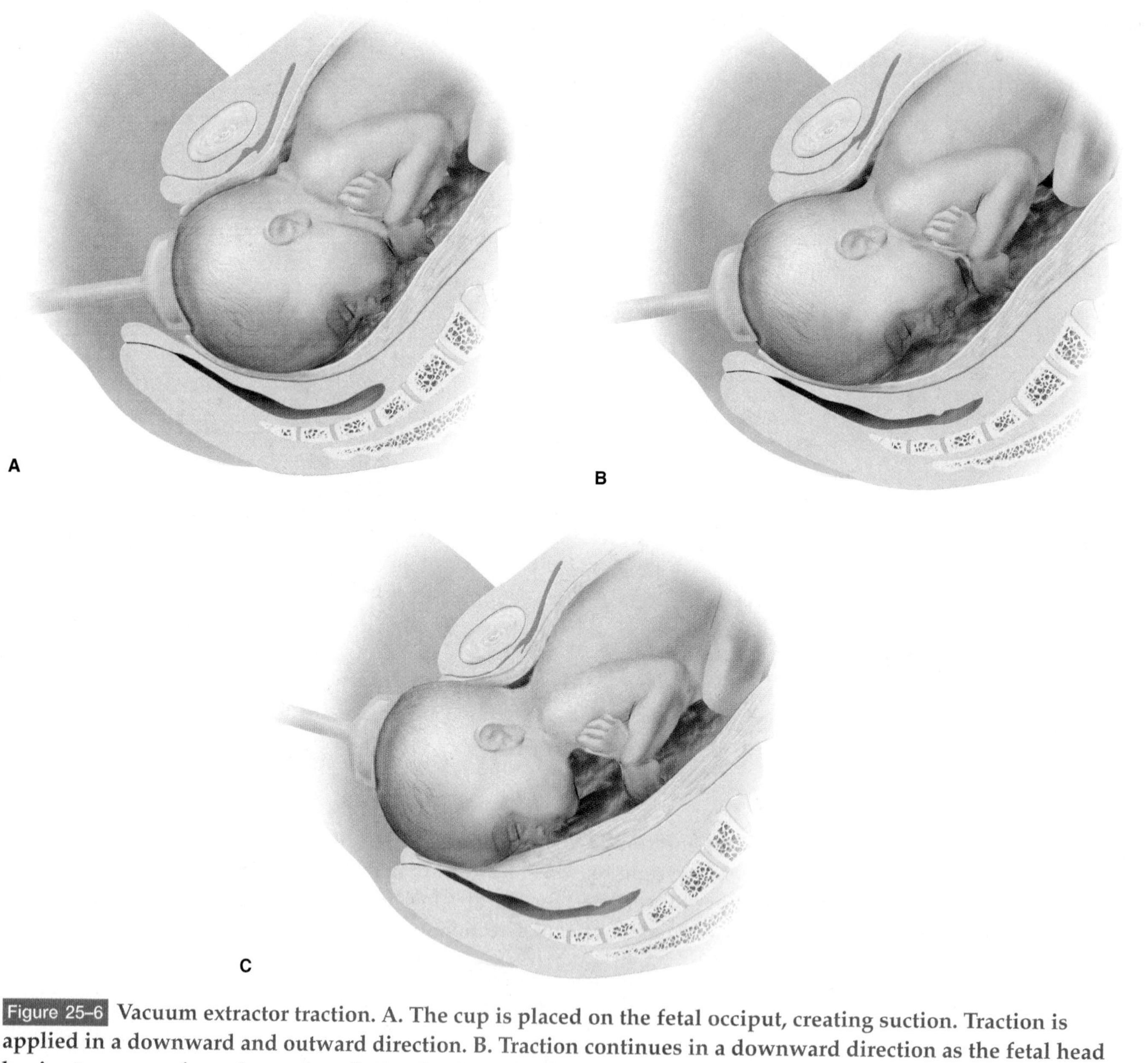

Figure 25–6 Vacuum extractor traction. A. The cup is placed on the fetal occiput, creating suction. Traction is applied in a downward and outward direction. B. Traction continues in a downward direction as the fetal head begins to emerge from the vagina. C. Traction is maintained to lift the fetal head out of the vagina.

disproportion (CPD), when successful passage of the fetal head requires all potential space inside the vaginal canal. True CPD is an absolute contraindication to vacuum extraction. Other contraindications include nonvertex presentations, maternal or suspected fetal coagulation defects, known or suspected hydrocephalus, and fetal scalp trauma (Cunningham et al., 2014). Relative contraindications include suspected fetal macrosomia, high fetal station, face or breech presentation, gestation less than 34 weeks, incompletely dilated cervix, and previous fetal scalp blood sampling (Cunningham et al., 2014).

Neonatal complications include scalp lacerations, bruising, subgaleal hematomas, cephalohematomas, intracranial hemorrhages, subconjunctival hemorrhages, neonatal jaundice, fractured clavicle, Erb palsy, damage to the sixth and seventh cranial nerves, ocular injuries, retinal hemorrhage, and fetal death. In addition, there is an increased incidence of shoulder dystocia (Cunningham et al., 2014). There appear to be more neonatal complications and injuries with use of a metal suction cup device than with soft cup devices. In the presence of a preterm gestation, risk of periventricular-intraventricular hemorrhage (PV-IVH) has been a concern, and some studies provide conflicting recommendations. Maternal complications include perineal trauma, edema, third- and fourth-degree lacerations, postpartum pain, and infection (Simpson & Creehan, 2014). Women who give birth with the aid of a vacuum extractor report more sexual difficulties in the postpartum period. Maternal genital tract and anal sphincter injuries occur less frequently with the vacuum extractor than with forceps.

In 1998, the U.S. Food and Drug Administration (FDA) released a health advisory statement that vacuum extraction can cause serious or fatal complications. Twelve deaths and nine serious injuries occurred between 1994 and 1998. The FDA recommended caution in using rocking movements when using the device. They also recommended that pediatricians be alerted when a vacuum-assisted birth occurred so the newborn can be closely monitored for related injuries. In addition, the following guidelines are recommended when a birth is facilitated by a vacuum extractor (Cunningham et al., 2014):

- The criteria used to evaluate the appropriateness of a forceps birth should also be used to determine the appropriateness of a vacuum birth (station).
- The same indications and contraindications should be used for both forceps and vacuum births.
- The presenting part must be vertex and must be at 0 station or below.
- Vacuum-assisted births should be performed only by an experienced practitioner.
- The procedure should be terminated immediately if descent does not occur or if the vacuum device pops off more than three times.

●○● NURSING MANAGEMENT

For the Woman Undergoing a Vacuum-Assisted Birth

There are different types of vacuum extractors. Be familiar with the types used within the birthing setting and learn the pressure limits of each type.

Inform the woman about what is happening during the procedure. If adequate regional anesthesia has been administered, the woman feels only pressure during the procedure. Pump the vacuum to the appropriate level to provide suction by the physician/CNM. The FHR is auscultated at least every 5 minutes or assessed by continuous EFM. The parents need to be informed that the caput (chignon) on the baby's head will disappear within 2 to 3 days. Continue to assess the newborn for complications such as bruising, newborn jaundice, cephalohematomas, intracranial hemorrhage, and retinal hemorrhages.

Care of the Family During Cesarean Birth

Cesarean birth is the birth of the baby through an abdominal and uterine incision. This method of delivery is one of the oldest surgical procedures known. Until the 20th century, cesareans were primarily equated with an attempt to save the fetus of a dying woman. As the maternal and perinatal morbidity and mortality rates associated with cesarean birth steadily decreased throughout the 20th century, the rate of cesarean births increased.

The rate of cesarean birth in the United States in 2015 was 32% (CDC, 2017). Sweden and the Netherlands have maintained cesarean birth rates of 10% for decades. Many Latin American countries also have low rates, including Peru, with a cesarean birth rate below 10%, and Honduras, with a rate of 12%. England and Canada have rates below 20%. However, some countries, such as Chile, have rates as high as 40% (Cunningham et al., 2014). The rising international cesarean rate is concerning given that the World Health Organization has proposed that a rate greater than 10 to 15% is not justifiable in any region of the world (Cunningham et al., 2014).

Many factors affect the cesarean birth rate, and they need to be considered in discussions about decreasing the current rate in the United States. These factors include a rising number of nulliparous women, who are at an increased risk for cesareans, giving birth; a rise in the maternal age, which is associated with a higher incidence of cesarean birth; changing philosophies regarding the best method of birth with a breech presentation; interpretations of EFM tracings; a decrease in the use of forceps and vacuum extractors to facilitate a vaginal birth; and a dramatic rise in obesity, another risk factor for cesarean birth. Other risks include changing practice related to vaginal birth after cesarean birth, increased use of epidural anesthesia, physician convenience, and type of provider (Cunningham et al., 2014). Interestingly, some women are now requesting a primary cesarean birth because of fear of labor, convenience, and concern about pelvic floor damage that could result in long-term medical complications. See *Women with Special Needs: Dwarfism in Childbearing Women*.

Women with Special Needs Dwarfism in Childbearing Women

There are over 200 types of dwarfism that may impact childbearing women. Women with dwarfism are at risk for alterations in ambulation as the center of gravity changes. In addition, due to their pelvic bone anatomy, these women are unable to have a vaginal birth. Women with dwarfism should be scheduled for an elective cesarean birth at 39 gestational weeks. Should spontaneous labor occur prior to the surgery date, they should be advised to proceed directly to the birthing facility for a cesarean birth.

One of the most significant healthcare factors dominating the 21st century is the concern related to medical malpractice litigation. Failure to perform a cesarean birth is one of the most common malpractice claims in obstetrical practice. Although there is no association between performing a cesarean birth and a reduction in childhood neurologic problems, including a decline in neonatal seizures or cerebral palsy, fear of litigation remains a driving force in obstetrical practice. The malpractice crisis has become so grave that some physicians/CNMs are abandoning obstetrical practice because of fear of litigation and high malpractice premiums. See *Genetic Facts: Labor and Its Effect on Gene Expression*.

Genetic Facts Labor and Its Effect on Gene Expression

An emerging theory that warrants further study is that labor is a critical physiologic life event that has influential environmental and immunological effects affecting gene expression (Merideth & Hugill, 2016). One study demonstrated that variations in genes involved in oxytocin receptor (OXTR) signaling correlate to the duration of labor and the risk of cesarean birth in women undergoing near-term induction (Jacobson, 2017).

Indications

Cesarean births are performed in the presence of a variety of maternal and fetal conditions. Events such as cord prolapse and placenta previa are instances in which delivery by cesarean is unconditional and can be lifesaving (Ye et al., 2016). Commonly accepted indications also include CPD, placental abruption, active genital herpes, umbilical cord prolapse, failure to progress in labor, proven nonreassuring fetal status, and benign and malignant tumors that obstruct the birth canal. Indications that are more controversial include breech presentation, previous cesarean birth, major congenital anomalies, cervical cerclage, severe Rh isoimmunization, and maternal preference for cesarean birth. The majority of cesarean births performed in the United States are done because of a previous cesarean birth and dystocia (Cunningham et al., 2014).

Maternal Mortality and Morbidity

Cesarean births have a higher maternal mortality rate than vaginal births. In the United States, women undergoing a cesarean birth have a fourfold risk of death when compared with women who give birth vaginally (Cunningham et al., 2014). In England, emergency cesarean birth has a ninefold risk of death when compared with vaginal delivery, and elective cesarean births have a threefold risk (Cunningham et al., 2014).

There also exists a higher rate of acute and long-term morbidities associated with delivery by cesarean section. These include wound infection, excessive blood loss, injury to internal organs, increased hospital stay, more negative emotions, lower Apgar scores, and greater incidence of neonatal respiratory problems (Molina et al., 2015).

Education of the woman about her informed choice regarding a cesarean birth is an important discussion that must occur between the woman and her healthcare provider. Although there is not enough data to determine recommendations, there is a consensus that cesarean birth should not be performed based solely on maternal request prior to 39 weeks' gestation unless there is proven fetal lung maturity.

Surgical Techniques

Cesarean birth requires both a skin and a uterine incision, which are not necessarily the same type of incision.

SKIN INCISIONS

The skin incision for a cesarean birth is either transverse (Pfannenstiel) or vertical (midline incision) and is not indicative of the type of incision made into the uterus. The type of skin incision is determined by time factor, patient preference, cosmetic reasons, or physician preference.

The transverse incision (Figure 25–7) is made across the lowest and narrowest part of the abdomen. Because the incision is made just below the pubic hair line, it is almost invisible after healing. Other advantages of this type of incision include less bleeding and better healing. The limitations of this type of skin incision are that it does not allow for extension of the incision if needed. Because it usually requires more time, this incision is used when time is not of the essence (e.g., with failure to progress and no fetal or maternal stress). This type of incision may result in suboptimal visualization, especially in obese women. This type of incision may also develop more scar tissue if subsequent surgeries, such as repeat cesarean, are performed (Cunningham et al., 2014).

The vertical (infraumbilical midline) incision is made between the navel and the symphysis pubis. This incision is quicker and is therefore preferred in cases of nonreassuring fetal status when rapid birth is indicated, with preterm or macrosomic fetuses, or when the woman is obese (Cunningham et al., 2014).

UTERINE INCISIONS

The type of uterine incision depends on the need for the cesarean. The choice of incision affects the woman's opportunity for a subsequent vaginal birth and her risks of a ruptured uterine scar with a subsequent pregnancy. See *Developing Cultural Competence: Translating Operative Reports*.

Developing Cultural Competence Translating Operative Reports

Women from other countries who have had a previous cesarean birth typically have a vertical skin incision; however, the skin incision does not provide data on the type of uterine incision that was performed. Obtain an operative report, if possible. Operative reports in other languages need to be translated by personnel familiar with medical terminology. If an operative report cannot be obtained, which is common, provide the woman with a thorough explanation regarding the need for a repeat cesarean.

The two major locations of uterine incisions are the lower uterine segment and the upper segment of the uterine corpus (Figure 25–8). The most common lower uterine segment incision is a transverse incision (Figure 25–8A). A vertical incision can be made in the lower uterine segment in certain circumstances (Figure 25–8B). Another incision, the classic vertical incision (Figure 25–8C), which is made into the upper uterine segment, was the method of choice for many years but is nearly never performed in modern obstetrics. More blood loss results, and it is more difficult to repair. Most important, it carries an increased risk of uterine rupture with subsequent pregnancy, labor, and birth because the upper uterine segment is the most contractile portion of the uterus. See Table 25–4 for the advantages and disadvantages of the three types of uterine incisions.

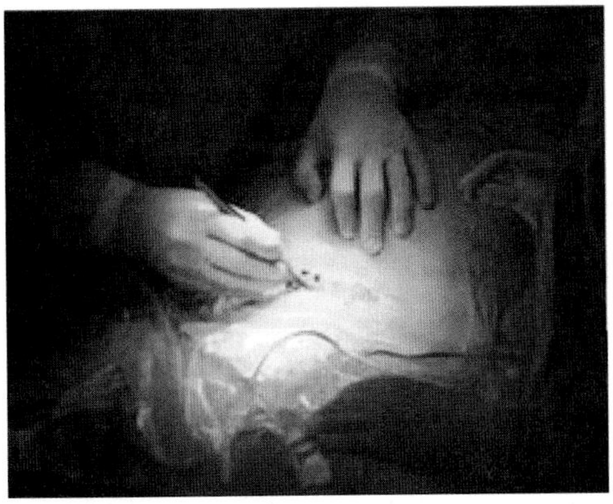

Figure 25–7 **Transverse skin incision for a cesarean birth.**

SOURCE: Wilson Garcia.

Analgesia and Anesthesia

There is no perfect anesthesia for cesarean birth. Each has its advantages, disadvantages, possible risks, and side effects. Goals for analgesia and anesthesia administration include safety, comfort, and emotional satisfaction for the patient. See Chapter 22 for more information.

●○● NURSING MANAGEMENT

For the Woman Undergoing a Cesarean Birth

Preparation for Cesarean Birth

Preparing the woman and her family for the possibility of cesarean birth is an integral part of prenatal education (American Academy of Family Physicians [AAFP], 2015). Some circumstances that are typically a part of vaginal delivery may require modification if a cesarean birth occurs. Encourage all pregnant women and their partners to discuss with their physician/CNM

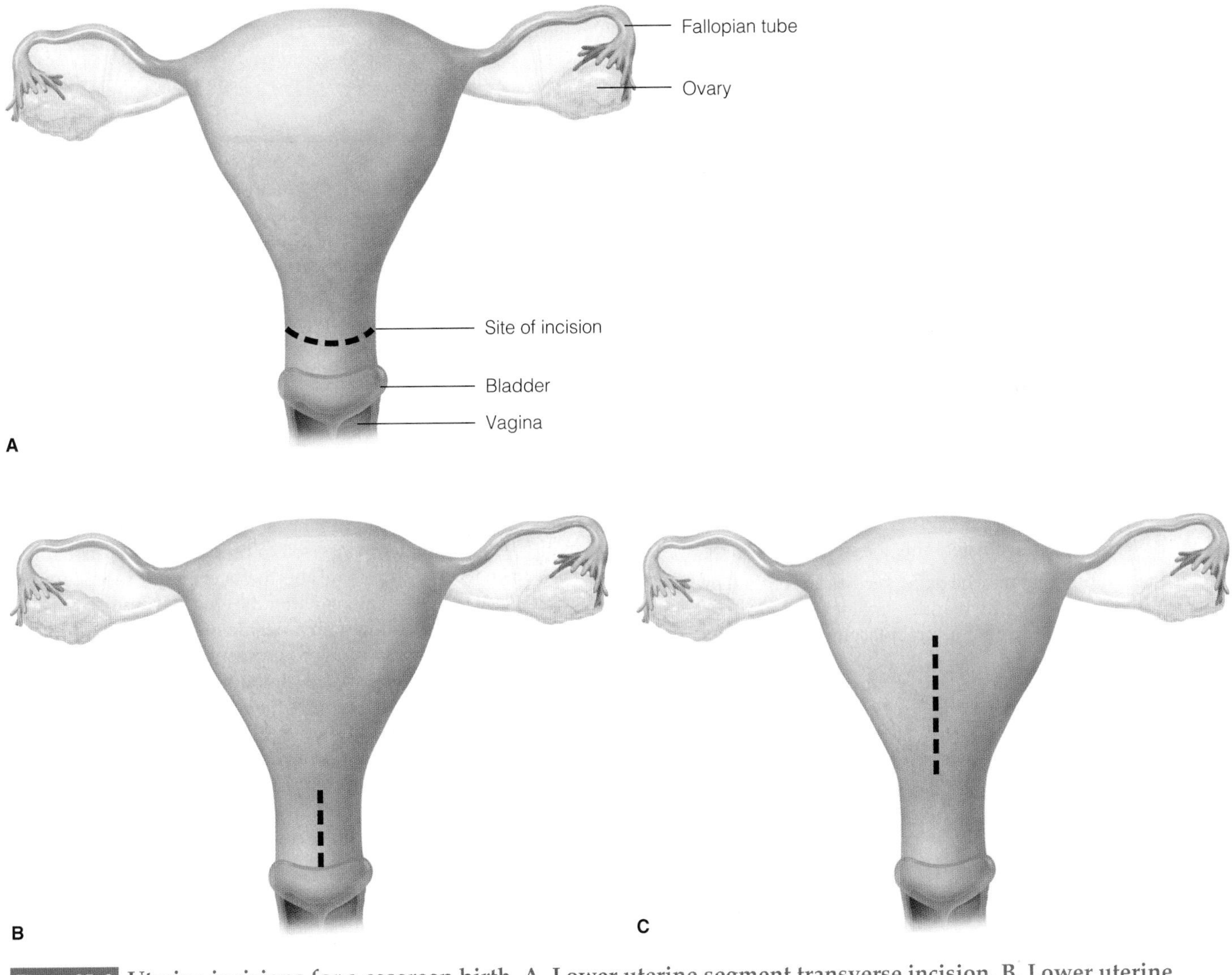

Figure 25–8 **Uterine incisions for a cesarean birth. A. Lower uterine segment transverse incision. B. Lower uterine segment vertical incision. C. This view illustrates the classical uterine incision that is done in the body (corpus) of the uterus. The classical incision was commonly done in the past and is associated with increased risk of uterine rupture in subsequent pregnancies and labor.**

TABLE 25–4 Types of Uterine Incisions for Cesarean Birth

ADVANTAGES	DISADVANTAGES
LOWER UTERINE SEGMENT TRANSVERSE INCISION (MOST COMMONLY USED)	
Less blood loss because it is the thinnest part of the uterus Easier to repair Requires minimal dissection of the bladder from underlying myometrium Less chance of adherence of bowel or omentum to the incision line Area is less likely to rupture during subsequent pregnancies	Takes longer to make a transverse incision and complete the repair Size of incision is limited because of the presence of major vessels on either side of the uterus Can extend laterally into the uterine vessels Incision may stretch and become a thin sheath, causing problems in subsequent labors
LOWER UTERINE SEGMENT VERTICAL INCISION (NOT COMMONLY USED)	
Preferred for: Multiple gestation Placenta previa Nonreassuring fetal status Abnormal presentation Preterm and macrosomic fetuses	Incision may extend into the cervix Extensive dissection of the bladder Controlling bleeding and closure can be difficult Carries a high risk of rupture with subsequent labor Future births need to be cesarean
UPPER UTERINE SEGMENT VERTICAL INCISION (CLASSICAL)	
None; no longer in use	Heavy blood loss Difficult to repair Increased risk of uterine rupture with subsequent pregnancy

SOURCE: Data from Cunningham et al., 2014.

what approach would be taken in the event of a cesarean. They can also discuss their needs and desires as a couple under those circumstances. Their preferences may include:

- Participating in the choice of anesthetic
- Presence of the father/partner during the procedures in the recovery or postpartum room
- Audio or video recording and/or photographing of the birth
- Delayed instillation of eye drops to promote eye contact between parent and newborn in the first hour after birth
- Physical contact or holding the newborn while on the operating room table or in the recovery room (If the mother cannot hold the newborn, the father/partner can hold the baby for her.)
- Breastfeeding immediately after the surgery has been completed
- Preparation that may be done, such as abdominal prep, insertion of an indwelling bladder catheter, and starting an intravenous infusion and epidural placement
- Description or viewing of the operating room
- Types of anesthesia for birth and analgesia available postpartum
- Sensations that may be experienced
- Role of father/partner
- Interaction with the newborn
- Immediate recovery phase
- Postpartum phase.

Preparing the woman for surgery involves more than the procedures of establishing intravenous lines and a urinary indwelling catheter or doing an abdominal prep. As discussed previously, good communication skills are essential in assisting the couple. Therapeutic use of touch and eye contact (if culturally acceptable and possible) do much to maintain reality orientation and control. These measures reduce anxiety for the woman during the stressful preparatory period.

If the cesarean birth is scheduled and not an emergency, you have ample time for preoperative teaching. The woman needs to practice her turning, coughing, and deep breathing. It is helpful if she is taught to splint her abdominal muscles when she coughs. Have the mother sign an informed consent form once a thorough discussion about the procedure has occurred. To prepare the woman for the surgery, give her nothing by mouth. To reduce the likelihood of serious pulmonary damage should aspiration of gastric contents occur, antacids may be administered within 30 minutes of surgery. If epidural anesthesia is used, you may assist with the procedure, monitor the woman's blood pressure and response, and continue EFM. An abdominal and perineal prep is done, and an indwelling catheter is inserted to prevent bladder distention. For women receiving epidural anesthesia, it may be more comfortable to place the Foley catheter after the epidural has been placed. Start an intravenous line with a needle of adequate size to permit blood administration and order preoperative medication. The pediatrician, neonatologist, and/or the staff of the neonatal intensive care unit (NICU) should be notified and adequate preparation made to receive the newborn. Be sure that the warmer is functional and that appropriate resuscitation equipment is available.

Assist in positioning the woman on the operating table. Ascertain FHR before surgery and during preparation because fetal hypoxia can result from aortocaval compression. The operating table may be adjusted so it slants slightly to one side, or a wedge (folded blanket or towels) may be placed under the right hip. The uterus should be displaced about 15 degrees from the midline. This helps relieve the pressure of the heavy uterus on the vena cava and lessens the incidence of vena cava compression and supine maternal hypotension. The woman is strapped onto the table to prevent falls or injuries from occurring during the surgery. If a cauterization device is being used, the grounding source is secured on the woman's leg after the device has been checked to make sure it is in working order. The suction should be in working order, and the urine collection bag should be positioned under the operating table to ensure visibility and proper urinary drainage. Auscultation or electronic monitoring of the FHR should be continued until immediately before the surgery. A last-minute check is done to ensure that the fetal scalp electrode has been removed if the fetus was internally monitored. Continue to provide reassurance and describe the various procedures being performed, along with a rationale, to ease anxiety and give the woman a sense of control.

To facilitate the safety of the patient, a "time-out" is indicated prior to the start of the procedure (The Joint Commission, 2015). The concept of a time-out was introduced by The Joint Commission in 2003 to prevent surgical interventions from being performed on the wrong patient, wrong procedure, or the wrong site. A time-out is called prior to the procedure so an instrument count can be performed. Another pause, or time out, is performed after the procedure and before closure of the incision that includes a count of all instruments that were used during the operative procedure, including the use of fluid-absorbing sterile "tapes" that may have been introduced into the abdominal cavity during the procedure. Typically, this count is repeated three times throughout the operation to ensure that no instruments are left in the woman's abdomen. The nurse or scrub technician is responsible for ensuring that the instrument and tape count is correct. In the event the count is not correct or if a count was not done initially because of emergency circumstances, a portable x-ray screening is performed to ensure that no instruments or tapes remain in the maternal abdomen. Time-out procedures have been implemented to reduce errors in the hospital setting.

Preparation for Repeat Cesarean Birth

When a couple is anticipating a repeat cesarean birth, they have time to reflect on their past experiences, analyze and synthesize the new information they are given, and prepare for the experience. Couples who have had previous negative experiences need an opportunity to describe what they felt contributed to these events. Encourage them to identify what they would like to have altered and to list interventions that would make the experience more positive. Those who have had positive experiences need reassurance that their needs and desires will be met in the same manner. In addition, provide an opportunity for the couple to discuss any fears or anxieties. Some women who undergo an elective repeat cesarean birth may continue to grieve the loss of the ideal birth experience or continue to exhibit mixed emotions regarding their choices for the birth. These women need reassurance and support throughout the birth process.

Preparation for Emergency Cesarean Birth

The period preceding surgery must be used to its greatest advantage. If possible, the couple needs some time for privacy to assimilate the information given to them and to ask for additional information. It is imperative that caregivers use their most effective communication skills. You must address what the couple may anticipate during the next few hours. Asking the couple, "What questions do you have about the decision?" gives them an opportunity for further clarification. You can prepare the woman in stages, giving her information and the rationale for each procedure before commencing. Before carrying out a procedure, it is essential to tell the woman (1) what is going to happen, (2) why it is being done, and (3) what sensations she may experience. This allows the woman to be informed and to consent to the procedure. The woman experiences a sense of control and therefore feels less helpless and powerless.

Supporting the Father/Partner

Every effort should be made to include the father/partner/support person in the cesarean birth experience. When the father/partner/support person attends the cesarean birth, he or she must wear a surgical gown and mask as do others in the operating suite. The individual can sit on a stool placed beside the woman's head to provide physical touch, visual contact, and verbal reassurance to the mother.

Many support persons worry about their own reactions to the operative procedure. A sterile drape is placed between the woman's head and the sterile field. Advise the support person that this can be used as a partition if he or she does not wish to view the procedure itself. Encourage support persons to eat before the surgery, if possible. Most support persons who fear "fainting" or "feeling queasy" do not have difficulties in the operating room and frequently forget these fears as they are swept away in the excitement of the birth.

Other measures, such as the following, can be taken to promote the participation of the father/partner who chooses not to be present in the delivery room:

- Allow the father/partner to be in a place near the operating room, where the newborn's first cry can be heard
- Encourage the father/partner to carry or accompany the newborn to the nursery for the initial assessment
- Involve the father/partner in postpartum care in the recovery room.

In the event that the father/partner/support person cannot be with the woman during the cesarean birth, such as in situations involving emergencies, you may obtain consent from the woman before the surgery and then provide updates to the person to alleviate undue fear and anxiety.

Immediate Postpartum Recovery Period

After birth, assess the Apgar score and complete the initial assessment and identification procedures as after a vaginal birth. Every effort must be made to assist the parents in bonding with the newborn. If the mother is awake, free one of her arms to enable her to touch and stroke the baby. Give the newborn to the father/partner to hold until the baby is taken to the nursery.

Check the woman's vital signs every 5 minutes until they are stable, and then every 15 minutes for an hour, and every 30 minutes until she is discharged to the postpartum unit. Remain with the woman until she is stable.

Check the dressing and perineal pad every 15 minutes for at least an hour, and gently palpate the fundus to determine whether it is remaining firm. Place your hand to support the incision when palpating the fundus. Intravenous oxytocin is usually administered to promote the contractility of the uterine musculature. If the woman has had general anesthesia, position her on her side to facilitate drainage of secretions, turn her, and assist her with coughing and deep breathing every 2 hours for at least 24 hours. If she has received a spinal or epidural anesthetic, check the level of anesthesia every 15 minutes. It is important to monitor intake and output and to observe the urine for bloody tinge, which could mean surgical trauma to the bladder. If the physician prescribes medication to relieve the mother's pain and nausea, administer it as needed. Some physicians use a single dose of epidural morphine (5 to 7.5 mg) for postsurgical pain relief. Facilitation of parent–newborn interaction following birth and postpartum care is discussed in Chapter 33.

Care of the Woman Undergoing Trial of Labor After Cesarean and Vaginal Birth After Cesarean

In the late 1980s there was an increasing trend to have a **trial of labor after cesarean (TOLAC)**,which is a planned attempt to labor by a woman who has previously undergone a cesarean delivery and desires a subsequent vaginal delivery, and attempt **vaginal birth after cesarean (VBAC)** in cases of nonrecurring indications for a cesarean (e.g., twins, umbilical cord prolapse, placenta previa, nonreassuring fetal status). This trend was influenced by consumer demand and studies that support VBAC as a viable and safe alternative.

Women's interest in a VBAC has increased, as more evidence has shown the incidence of uterine rupture and infant mortality and morbidity is less than previously suspected (Hehir, Mackey, & Robson, 2017). Women should be made aware of the risks associated with VBAC compared to repeat cesarean and how these are related to personal beliefs and desires associated with childbirth (Merideth & Hugill, 2016). Although the absolute risks of VBAC are small, there is a 0.1 to 0.7% risk of uterine rupture when women attempt a trial of labor after previously undergoing a cesarean birth (Cunningham et al., 2014). According to 2013 data, among women who had one previous cesarean birth, only one in five attempted a trial of labor even though 70% of mothers who did were successful (CDC, 2015). For some women, the mode of delivery is an attempt to control a situation that may seem unpredictable by determining the date and planning ahead (Tolmacheva, 2015).

ACOG guidelines state that the following aspects should be met when identifying candidates for TOLAC and VBAC (Cunningham et al., 2014):

- One previous cesarean birth and a low transverse uterine incision
- An adequate pelvis
- No other uterine scars or previous uterine rupture
- A physician who is able to do a cesarean is available throughout active labor
- In-house anesthesia personnel are available for emergency cesarean births, if warranted.

TOLAC does carry some risks, although they are rare and isolated in actual numbers. Repeat cesarean births are associated with greater risks, including increased incidence of abnormal placentation in subsequent pregnancies and the increased risk of mortality secondary to surgery. The incidence of abnormal placentation increases in chance with each additional pregnancy.

TABLE 25–5 Risks Associated with Repeat Cesarean Delivery

- Blood loss
- Abnormal placentation
- Surgical injury to bowel or bladder
- Adhesions
- Postsurgical complications
- Longer hospitalization
- Increased cost
- Hysterectomy

Examples of abnormal placentations include placenta previa, placenta accreta, and placenta abruption. Additional risks for repeat cesarean delivery are included in Table 25–5.

With recent recommendations for TOLAC as the standard of care, success rates for VBAC have been encouraging. Women whose previous cesarean was performed for breech presentation had the highest success rates for VBAC (91%). Women who had a previous cesarean birth for nonreassuring fetal status had an 84% success rate, whereas a woman diagnosed with previous dystocia had a 67% success rate. Women who were previously diagnosed with dystocia before 5-cm dilatation had a 67% success rate, whereas women who had previously progressed to 6 to 9 cm had a 73% success rate. Women who had been labeled as having dystocia in the second stage had a 75% success rate (Cunningham et al., 2014). See *Evidence-Based Practice: Risks and Benefits of TOLAC*. See *Concept Map: Failure to Progress in Labor; Trial of Labor After Cesarean (TOLAC)*.

●○● NURSING MANAGEMENT

For the Woman Undergoing Trial of Labor after Cesarean

The nursing care of a woman undergoing TOLAC varies according to institutional protocols. Generally, if the woman is at very low risk (has had one previous cesarean with a lower uterine segment incision), her blood count, type, and screen are obtained on admission; a saline lock is inserted for intravenous access, if needed; continuous EFM is used; and clear fluids may be taken. If the woman is at higher risk, NPO status should be maintained and, in addition to the care listed, an intrauterine catheter may be inserted to monitor intrauterine pressures during labor.

Supportive and comfort measures are very important. The woman may be excited about this opportunity to experience labor and vaginal birth, or she may be hesitant and frightened about the possibility of complications. Provide information and encouragement for the laboring woman and her partner.

EVIDENCE-BASED PRACTICE | Risks and Benefits of TOLAC

Clinical Question

What are the risks and benefits of a trial of labor after cesarean (TOLAC) for mothers who desire a vaginal birth? What factors increase the likelihood of a failed trial of labor after a previous cesarean birth?

The Evidence

The rate of cesarean births increased dramatically between 1970 and 2016 in the United States. That number fluctuated recently as more mothers opted to try for a vaginal birth after a surgical one. Although cesarean rates dropped, they rebounded after some women experienced serious complications from TOLAC, with subsequent liability claims.

In 2010, the National Institutes for Health (NIH) brought together a conference of experts to determine the safety and efficacy of TOLAC and vaginal birth after cesarean (VBAC). They believed that TOLAC was a safe option for many women who desired the experience of a vaginal birth. The NIH charged the panel to identify the characteristics of women who could successfully attempt VBAC and to provide practice guidelines for counseling these patients. This type of practice guideline, developed by content experts, supported by the NIH and the American College of Obstetricians and Gynecologists (ACOG), is the strongest level of evidence for practice.

VBAC is associated with several health advantages for women. Mothers who successfully labor and deliver vaginally avoid major abdominal surgery and have lower rates of serious complications, such as thromboembolism and infection. They have a shorter recovery period than mothers with surgical births. Long-term outcomes are also advantageous, as multiple cesarean births are associated with a higher lifetime risk of hysterectomy, bowel issues, or bladder injuries. The success rate is high; the published vaginal delivery rate after TOLAC is between 60 and 80% (ACOG, 2017c).

TOLAC also carries risk; most maternal mortality and morbidity is associated with an emergency cesarean birth after a trial of labor. The conclusion: VBAC is associated with fewer complications than elective repeat cesarean delivery, but a failed TOLAC is associated with more maternal morbidity and mortality (ACOG, 2017c). It is critical, then, to determine the characteristics of mothers most likely to have a successful VBAC after laboring.

Women whose first cesarean birth was due to a nonrecurring problem (e.g., breech presentation) are more likely to be successful then women whose surgical birth was due to a labor disorder. Women who require labor induction or augmentation are also less likely to achieve VBAC. Other negative influences include increased maternal age, high body mass index, large birth weight, and gestation beyond 40 weeks. The most successful mothers are those with a healthy pregnancy (e.g., no preeclampsia) who have previously had at least one vaginal birth. The data are not definitive on the risks associated with attempted VBAC after more than one cesarean birth. There is no risk difference between vertical and horizontal cesarean incisions that are in the lower uterine segment; however, classical incisions that are typically in the mid- to upper uterus and T-incisions, are associated with higher uterine dehiscence and uterine rupture rates (ACOG, 2017c). There does not appear to be a difference between twin and singleton gestations. There is no evidence to support epidural analgesia as a factor in VBAC success, and regional anesthesia has not been demonstrated to mask signs of uterine rupture, as this condition is recognized from fetal heart tracing abnormalities. Women attempting TOLAC have labor patterns similar (in both intensity and length) to those with no prior cesarean delivery (ACOG, 2017c).

Best Practice

Women who express interest in a vaginal delivery after a previous cesarean birth should be counseled about the potential risks and benefits of both TOLAC and elective repeat cesarean delivery. The mother's specific risk factors should be a part of this discussion, as well as the potential outcomes for mother and baby if an emergency cesarean delivery is required after TOLAC. This discussion should happen early in the woman's prenatal period, to allow the most time for her to consider options, since many of the risk factors for failed VBAC are identifiable early in pregnancy.

Clinical Reasoning

What might a nursing assessment include prior to counseling about TOLAC and VBAC? What assessments during labor can indicate that an emergency cesarean birth may be required?

Concept Map

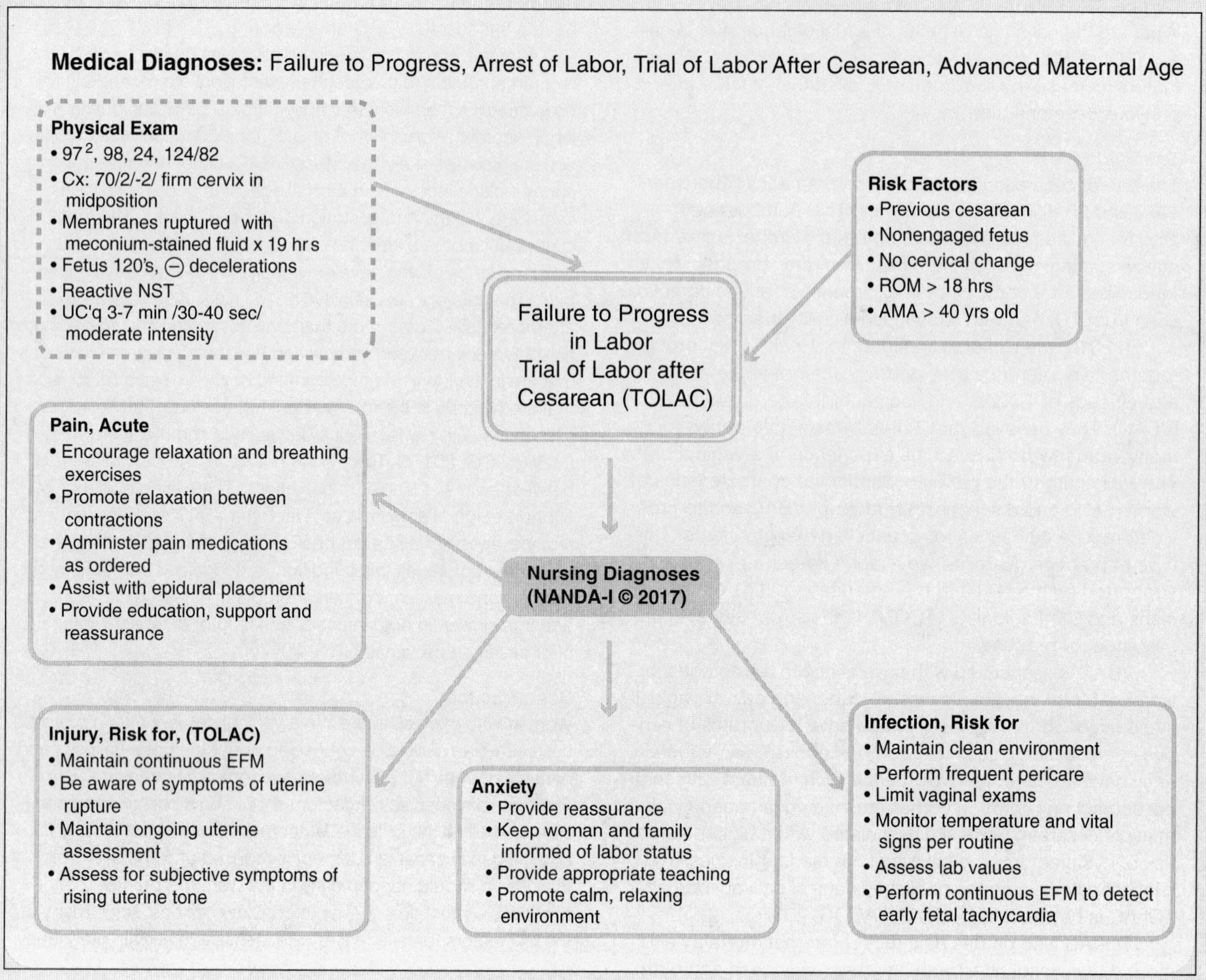

Focus Your Study

- An external (or cephalic) version may be done after 37 weeks' gestation to change a breech presentation to a cephalic presentation, thereby making a lower-risk vaginal birth more possible.
- The version is accomplished with the use of tocolytic agents to relax the uterus. An internal (podalic) version is used only when needed during the vaginal birth of a second twin.
- Amniotomy (AROM) is performed to hasten labor. The risks are prolapse of the umbilical cord and infection.
- Prostaglandin E_2 may be used before an induction of labor to soften the cervix (called cervical ripening). These agents are inserted into the vagina to make the cervix more favorable for induction.
- Labor is induced for many reasons. The methods include amniotomy, stripping of the membranes, intravenous oxytocin infusion, and alternative and complementary methods. Nursing responsibilities are heightened during an induced labor.
- Amnioinfusions are used in cases of oligohydramnios or nonperiodic decelerations to increase the volume of amniotic fluid, which relieves cord compression and promotes perfusion to the fetus.
- An episiotomy may be performed just before birth of the fetus.Current evidence shows a limited number of indications for its use.

- Forceps-assisted birth can be accomplished using outlet forceps, low forceps, or midforceps. Outlet forceps are the most common and are associated with few maternal-fetal complications. Midforceps are associated with more complications but, when needed, are an important aid to birth.
- A vacuum extractor is a soft, pliable cup attached to suction that can be applied to the fetal head and used in much the same way as forceps.
- Approximately one in three births is accomplished by cesarean. The nurse has a vital role in providing information, support, and encouragement to the couple participating in a cesarean birth.
- Vaginal birth after cesarean (VBAC) or trial of labor after cesarean (TOLAC) carries a low risk of uterine rupture; however, many physicians perform repeat cesarean births out of fear of malpractice issues. Overcoming the old fears of uterine rupture is a high priority for both the parents and the medical and nursing community.

In order to make safe and effective judgments using NANDA-I © 2017 nursing diagnoses, it is essential that nurses refer to the definitions and defining characteristics of the diagnoses used in this text, which can be found in Appendix C.

References

American Academy of Family Physicians (AAFP). (2015). Planning for labor and vaginal birth after cesarean delivery: Guidelines from the AAFP. *American Family Physician, 91*(3), 197–198.

American College of Obstetricians and Gynecologists (ACOG). (2016a). *External cephalic version* (ACOG Practice Bulletin No. 161). Washington, DC: Author.

American College of Obstetricians and Gynecologists (ACOG). (2009, reaffirmed 2016b). *Induction of labor* (ACOG Practice Bulletin No. 107). Washington, DC: Author.

American College of Obstetricians and Gynecologists. (2017a). *Approaches to limit intervention during labor and birth* (ACOG Committee Opinion No. 687). Washington, DC: Author.

American College of Obstetricians and Gynecologists. (2017b). *Medications for pain relief in labor and delivery* (ACOG Frequently Asked Questions No. FAQ86). Washington, DC: Author.

American College of Obstetricians and Gynecologists (ACOG). (2017c). *Vaginal birth after cesarean delivery* (ACOG Practice Bulletin No. 184). *Obstetrics & Gynecology, 130*(5), e217–233.

Bishop, E. H. (1964). Pelvic scoring for elective induction. *Obstetrics and Gynecology, 24*(2), 266.

Boltman-Binkowski, H. (2016). A systematic review: Are herbal and homeopathic remedies used during pregnancy safe? *Curationis, 39*(1), 1–8. Retrieved from https://dx.doi.org/10.4102/curationis.v39i1.1514

Centers for Disease Control and Prevention (CDC). (2015). Maternal morbidity for vaginal and cesarean deliveries, according to previous cesarean history: New data from the birth certificate, 2013. *National Vital Statistics, 64*(4), 1–13.

Centers for Disease Control and Prevention (CDC). (2017). *National Center for Health Statistics: Births—Method of delivery.* Retrieved from https://www.cdc.gov/nchs/fastats/delivery.htm

Cunningham, F. G., Leveno, K. J., Bloom, S. L., Spong, C. Y., Dashe, J., Hoffman, B. L., . . . Sheffield, J. S. (2014). *Williams obstetrics* (24th ed.). New York,NY: McGraw-Hill.

Eherenberg-Buchner, S., & Smith, C. V. (2015). *External cephalic version.* Retrieved from http://emedicine.medscape.com/article/1848353-overview#a01

Ferring Pharmaceuticals. (2016). *Cervidil manufacture's drug information.* Retrieved from https://www.cervidil.com/hcp?gclid=CL7biJfKmtECFVe2wAodTi0JzQ

Goldberg, A. E., & Smith, C.V. (2015). *Cervical ripening.* Retrieved from https://emedicine.medscape.com/article/263311-overview#aw2aab6b7

Hehir, M. P., Mackie, A., & Robson, M. S. (2017). Simplified and standardized intrapartum management can yield high rates of successful VBAC in spontaneous labor. *Journal of Maternal-Fetal & Neonatal Medicine, 30*(12), 1504–1508. DOI:10.1080/14767058.2016.1220522

Jacobson, A. (2017). Oxytocin-related gene expression predicts outcomes in induced near-term labor. *Clinical Practice Today.* Retrieved from http://www.clinicalpracticetoday.com/oxytocin-related-gene-expression-predicts-outcomes-in-induced-near-term-labor/

The Joint Commission (TJC). (2015). *The importance of a safe and effective time out.* Retrieved from https://www.jointcommission.org/search/?Keywords=time+out&sitename=Joint+Commission&guid=15f03a20f69a4b90bf03481043d0051f&f=sitename%252ckeyword&keyword=Time+Out

Levine, L. D., Downes, K. L., Elovitz, M. A., Parry, S., Sammel, M. D., & Srinivas, S. K. (2016). Mechanical and pharmacologic methods of labor induction. *Obstetrics & Gynecology, 128*(6), 1357–1364.

Merideth, D., & Hugill, K. (2016). Once a caesarean, always a caesarean?: Challenging perceptions around vaginal birth after caesarean. *British Journal of Midwifery, 24*(9), 616–623.

Molina, G., Weiser, T. G., Lipsitz, S. R., Esquivel, M. M., Uribe-Leitz, T., Azad, T., . . . Haynes, A. B. (2015). Relationship between cesarean delivery rate and maternal and neonatal mortality. *Journal of the American Medical Association, 314*(21), 2263–2270.

National Center for Complementary and Integrative Health (NCCIH). (2016). *Herbs at a glance.* Retrieved from https://nccih.nih.gov/health/herbsataglance.htm

Sharoni, L., Lyell, D. J., & Weiniger, C. F. (2015). Too late to back out?: Options for breech presentation management. *Epidemiology Community Health, 69*(12), 1135–1137.

Simpson, K. R., & Creehan, P. A. (2014). *AWHONN's perinatal nursing* (4th ed.). Washington, DC: AWHONN.

Tolmacheva, L. (2015). Vaginal birth after caesarean or elective caesarean—What factors influence women's decisions? *British Journal of Midwifery, 23*(7), 470–475.

Ugwu, E. O., Obi, S. N., Iferikigwe, E. S., Dim, C. C., & Ezugwu, F. O. (2014). Membrane stripping to prevent post-term pregnancy in Enugu, Nigeria: A randomized controlled trial. *Archives of Gynecology and Obstetrics, 289*(1), 29–34.

Wilson, B. A., Shannon, M. T., & Shields, K. M. (2018). *Pearson nurse's drug guide 2019.* Hoboken, NJ: Pearson.

Ye, J., Zhang, J., Mikolojczyk, R., Torloni, M. R., Gülmerzoglu, A. M., & Betran, A. P. (2016). Association between rates of caesarean section and maternal and neonatal mortality in the 21st century: A worldwide population-based ecological study with longitudinal data. *British Journal of Obstetrics Gynecology, 123*(5), 745–753.

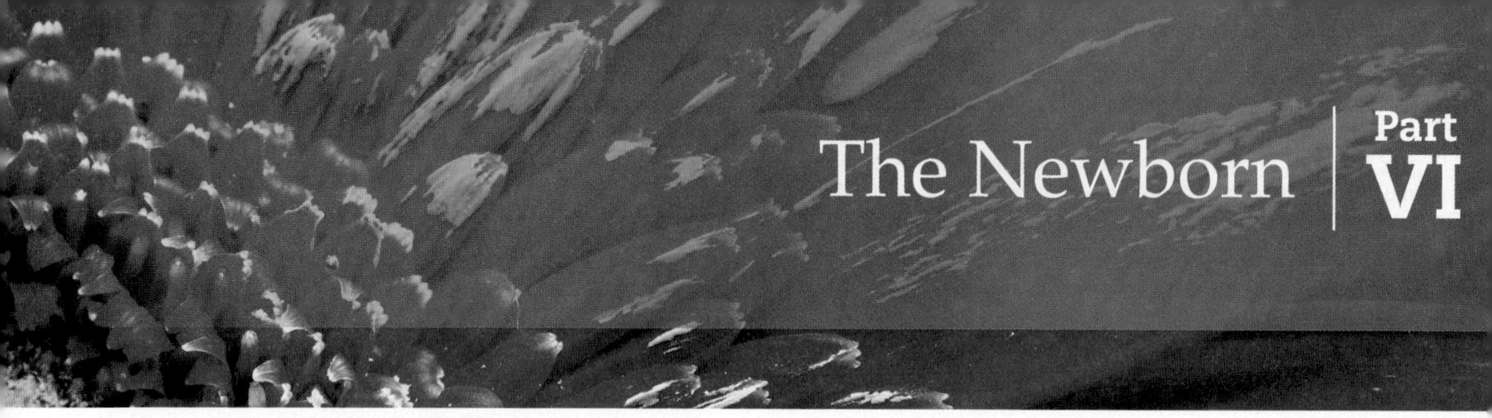

The Newborn | Part VI

Chapter 26

Physiologic Responses of the Newborn to Birth

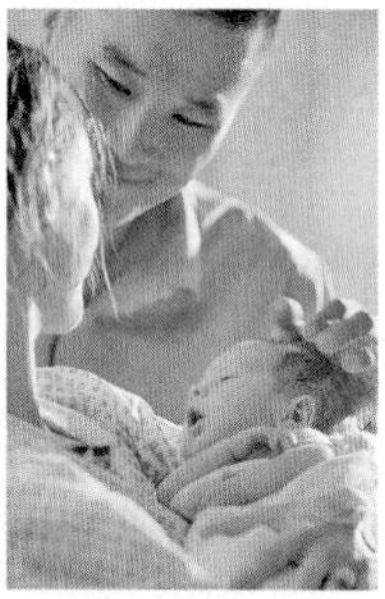

SOURCE: Photodisc/ Exactostock/Superstock.

The incredible attributes of the newborn have a major purpose. They prepare the baby for interaction with the family and for life in the world.

—Marshall H. Klaus & Phyllis H. Klaus,

The Amazing Newborn

Learning Outcomes

26.1 Review the significant developments of the fetal respiratory system.

26.2 Summarize the cardiopulmonary changes that must occur for the newborn to successfully transition to extrauterine life.

26.3 Explain the differences in fetal and adult hemoglobin and why this is important in transition to extrauterine life.

26.4 Relate the process of thermogenesis and the major mechanisms of heat loss to the challenge of maintaining newborn thermal stability.

26.5 Discuss the reasons a newborn may develop hyperbilirubinemia and the nursing interventions that can decrease the probability of jaundice.

26.6 Delineate the functional abilities of the newborn's gastrointestinal tract and liver.

26.7 Relate the development of the newborn kidney to the newborn's ability to maintain adequate fluid and electrolyte balance.

26.8 Describe basic newborn immunologic responses.

26.9 Explain the physiologic and behavioral characteristics of newborn neurologic functioning, patterns of behavior during the periods of reactivity and possible nursing interventions.

26.10 Describe the normal sensory/perceptual abilities and behavioral states present in the newborn period and the associated nursing care.

Healthy People 2020

(NWS-21) Reduce iron deficiency among young children and females of childbearing age

(MICH-21) Increase the proportion of newborns who are breastfed

(ENT-VSL-1) Increase the proportion of newborns who are screened for hearing loss by no later than age 1 month, have audiologic evaluation by age 3 months, and are enrolled in appropriate intervention services no later than age 6 months

The newborn period is the time from birth through the 28th day of life. The first 6 hours of life, in which the newborn stabilizes respiratory and circulatory functions, is called **transition**. With the first breath and the clamping of the umbilical cord, the newborn begins the transition from intrauterine to extrauterine life. This transition from fetus to newborn is the most complex physiologic adaptation that occurs in the human experience and involves virtually every organ system of the body. The nurse needs to be knowledgeable about a newborn's normal physiologic and behavioral adaptations and be able to recognize alterations from normal transition.

Fetal Respiratory System

Fetal Lung Development

The respiratory system is in a continuous state of development during fetal life, and lung development continues into early childhood. During the first 20 weeks of gestation, lung development is limited to the differentiation of pulmonary, vascular, and lymphatic structures. At 20 to 24 weeks, alveolar ducts begin to appear, followed by primitive alveoli at 24 to 28 weeks. During this time, the alveolar epithelial cells begin to differentiate into type I cells (structures necessary for gas exchange) and type II cells (structures that provide for the synthesis and storage of surfactant). **Surfactant** is composed of surface-active phospholipids (lecithin and sphingomyelin), which are critical for alveolar expansion and stability.

At 28 to 32 weeks of gestation, the number of type II cells increases, and surfactant is produced within them. Surfactant production peaks at about 35 weeks of gestation and remains high until term, paralleling late fetal lung development. At this time, the lungs are structurally developed enough to maintain good lung expansion and adequate exchange of gases at birth.

During intrauterine development, the lungs are filled with fetal lung fluid produced by the pulmonary epithelium, which stretches the lung tissue and stimulates growth of alveoli. Production and maintenance of a normal volume of fetal lung fluid are essential for normal lung growth (Blackburn, 2018). Through intermittent fetal breathing movements, the fetus practices respiration, develops the chest wall muscles and the diaphragm, and regulates lung fluid volume. Figure 26–1 depicts the changes in fetal lung fluid with the first and subsequent breaths.

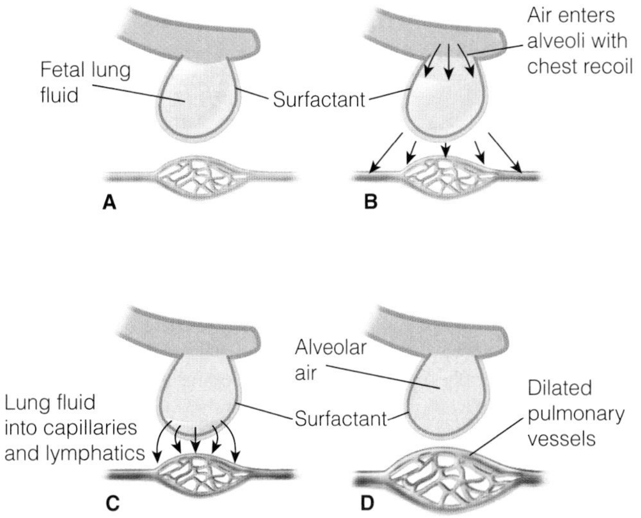

Figure 26–1 Process of absorption of fetal lung fluid during breathing after birth. A. Fetal alveoli filled to functional residual capacity with fetal lung fluid. Fetal lung fluid is produced by the alveoli, fills the airways, and eventually enters the amniotic fluid. B. After fetal chest compression, one-third of the fetal lung fluid is squeezed out, allowing air to enter passively as the chest recoils. C. With each subsequent breath, the lungs expand, facilitating the movement of the remaining fetal lung fluid into the capillaries and lymphatic system. Pulmonary blood flow is increasing. D. Normal alveoli after removal of fetal lung fluid and dilatation of pulmonary arteries. Surfactant has lined the inside of the alveoli to prevent collapse.

Fetal Circulation

In utero, the placenta is the organ of gas exchange. The low vascular resistance of the placenta and the high vascular resistance of the fluid-filled lungs result in shunts characteristic of fetal circulation. From the placenta, highly oxygenated blood (oxygen saturation of 65 to 70%) flows through the umbilical vein. A small amount of blood perfuses the liver, with the majority of blood volume flowing through the inferior vena cava and to the right atrium. Due to intracardiac streaming, blood is preferentially directed from the right atrium across the **foramen ovale (FO)** (an opening in the septum between the atria) into the left atrium, the left ventricle, and the ascending aorta. This results in better oxygenated fetal blood directed to the myocardium and fetal brain.

A smaller volume of blood enters the right ventricle and is pumped through the pulmonary artery. Because pulmonary vascular resistance is very high due to the fluid-filled fetal lungs, more than 60% of right-ventricular output bypasses the lung and flows through the **ductus arteriosus (DA)** (a tubular connection between the pulmonary artery and descending aorta) into the descending aorta (Blackburn, 2018). This mixing of well-oxygenated and poorly oxygenated blood results in an oxygen saturation of 45% in the blood that perfuses the lower part of the body. Vascular resistance of the placenta is low; approximately 30 to 50% of the combined ventricular cardiac output flows through the umbilical arteries to the placenta, where it releases carbon dioxide and waste products and collects oxygen and nutrients (Blackburn, 2018). Therefore, in fetal circulation the right and left ventricles function together, in parallel, rather than sequentially (one after the other), to perfuse the fetal body and the placenta. See *Key Facts to Remember: Fetal and Newborn Circulation*.

Cardiopulmonary Adaptation

Marked changes occur in the cardiopulmonary system at birth. During late gestation, lung fluid secretion decreases. The onset of labor stimulates the production of catecholamines and other hormones, causing fetal pulmonary epithelial cells to begin reabsorption of fluid from the alveolar spaces (Blackburn, 2018). With birth, the change in the sensory environment from the warm, dark womb to the brightly lighted, cold delivery room is an important stimulus for the initiation of breathing. The cold stimulates skin sensory receptors, and the newborn responds with rhythmic respirations. A number of physical and sensory influences help to sustain respiration after birth. They include the numerous tactile, auditory, visual, and painful stimuli of birth and the normal handling after delivery. Joint movement

Key Facts To Remember
Fetal and Newborn Circulation

System	Fetal	Newborn
Pulmonary blood vessels	Constricted with very little blood flow (high pulmonary vascular resistance); lungs not expanded and fluid-filled	Vasodilatation and increased blood flow (decreasing pulmonary vascular resistance); lungs expanded; increased PaO_2 stimulates vasodilation.
Systemic blood vessels	Dilated with low peripheral vascular resistance; blood mostly in placenta	Arterial pressure rises due to cord clamping with loss of placental reservoir; increased systemic blood volume causes increased peripheral vascular resistance.
Ductus arteriosus	Large with no tone; blood flow from pulmonary artery to aorta (right to left shunting)	Reversal of blood flow. Now from aorta to pulmonary artery (left to right shunting) because of increased left-atrial pressure and increased systemic vascular pressures. Ductus is sensitive to increased PaO_2 and a decline in circulating prostaglandins and begins to constrict.
Foramen ovale	Patent with large blood flow from right atrium to left atrium	Increased pressure in left atrium attempts to reverse blood flow and shuts one-way valve.

results in enhanced proprioceptor stimulation to the respiratory center. Thoroughly drying the newborn and placing him or her in skin-to-skin contact with the mother provides stimulation in a comforting way, as well as decreases heat loss.

The newborn's first breaths of air initiate a sequence of events that empties the airways of fluid, establishes volume and function of the newborn's lungs, and causes fetal circulation to convert to newborn circulation. The initial first breaths generate a high negative pressure, driving fluid from the lungs and filling the alveoli with air. As the lungs expand and are exposed to high concentrations of oxygen (room air), pulmonary vascular resistance falls, causing pulmonary vasodilation and increased blood flow to the lungs. Figure 26–2 summarizes the initiation of respiration.

When the umbilical cord is clamped, the low-resistance placenta is excluded from circulation; cessation of blood flow through the umbilical vein facilitates collapse of the *ductus venosus (DV)*, and the systemic vascular resistance increases. Thus, the fetal pulmonary to systemic pressure relationships are reversed, and systemic pressure becomes greater than pulmonary pressure. These pressure changes cause the foramen ovale to close. As pressure in the pulmonary artery decreases and pressure in the aorta increases, the shunt across the ductus arteriosus reverses to left to right and constricts, leading to closure in the first few days of life. This closure of fetal shunts establishes the serial arterial–venous circulation indicative of newborn circulation. See Figure 26–3.

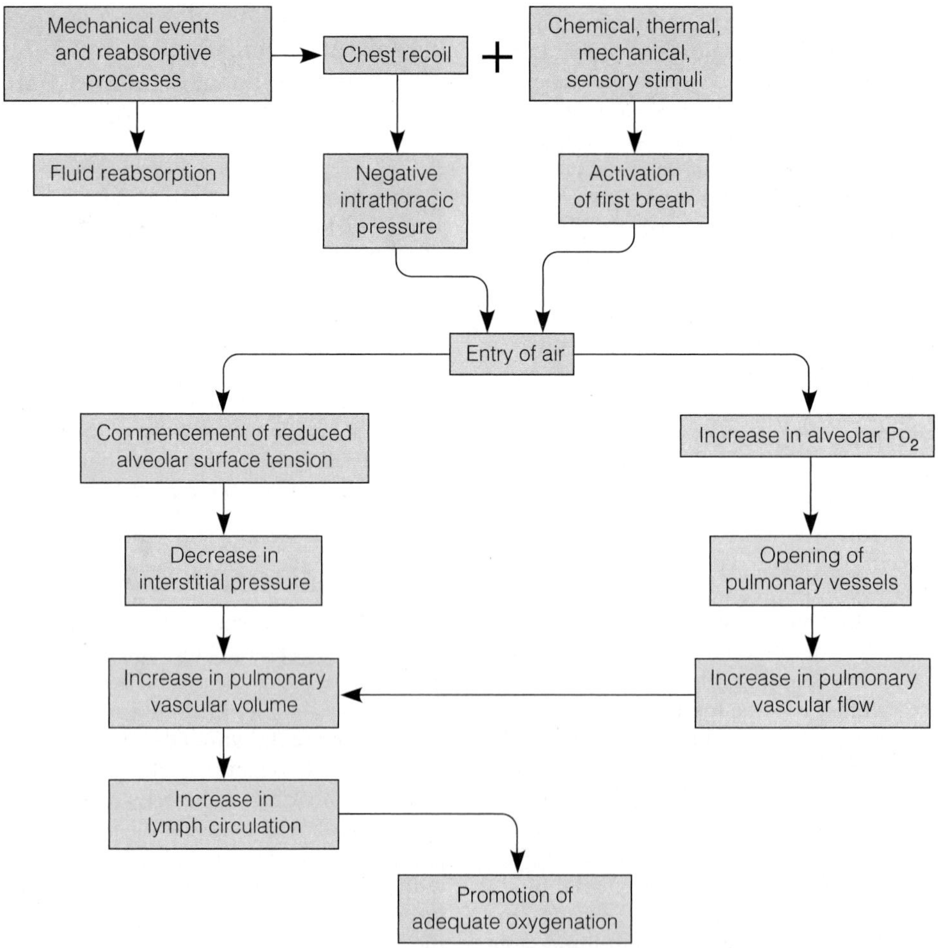

Figure 26–2 **Initiation of respiration in the newborn.**

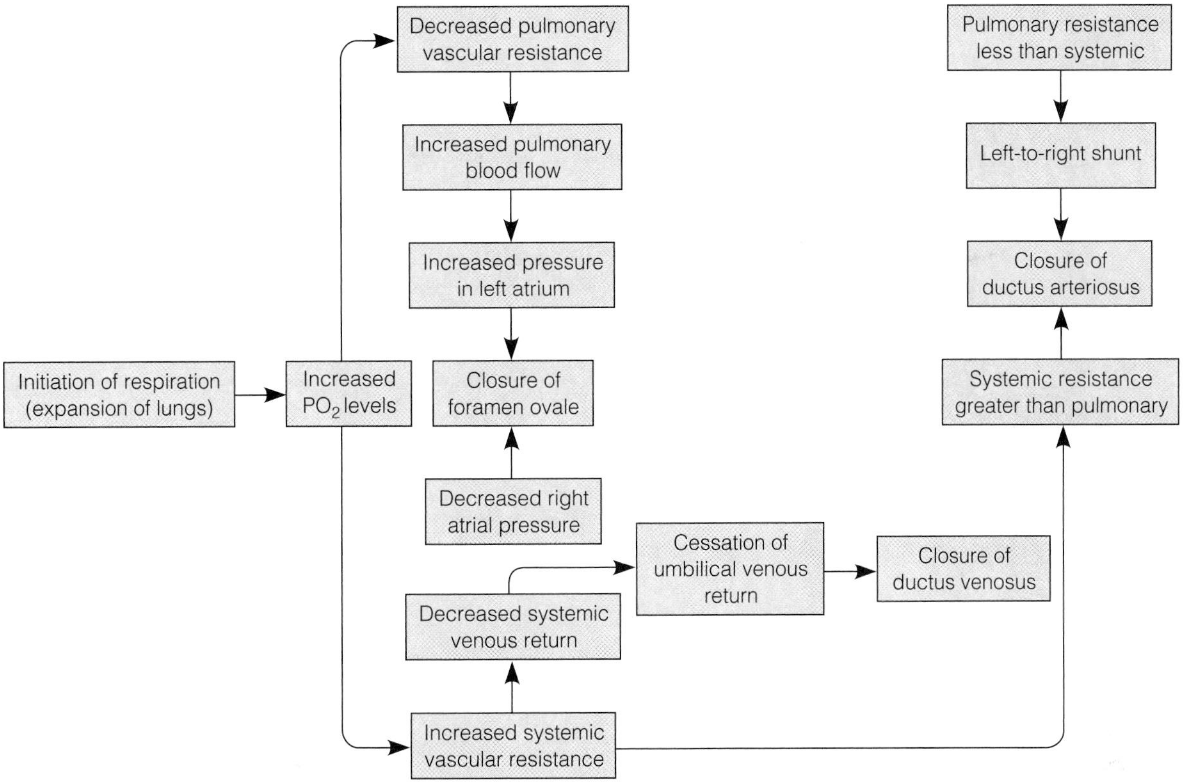

Figure 26–3 **Transitional circulation: Conversion from fetal to newborn circulation.**

In summary, the four major cardiopulmonary changes (Figure 26–4) are:

1. ***Increased systemic vascular resistance and decreased pulmonary vascular resistance.*** With the loss of the low-resistance placenta, systemic vascular resistance increases, resulting in greater systemic pressure. At the same time, lung expansion and exposure to high oxygen concentrations increase pulmonary blood flow and dilate pulmonary blood vessels. The combination of vasodilation and increased pulmonary blood flow decreases pulmonary vascular resistance. As the pulmonary vascular beds open, the systemic vascular pressure increases, enhancing perfusion of the other body systems.
2. ***Closure of the foramen ovale.*** Closure of the foramen ovale is a function of changing arterial pressures. In utero, pressure is greater in the right atrium, and the foramen ovale is open after birth, shunting blood from the right atrium to the left. The decreased pulmonary vascular resistance and the decreased umbilical venous return to the right atrium also cause a decrease in right-atrial pressure. The pressure gradients across the atria are now reversed, with left-atrial pressure greater; this causes the foramen ovale to functionally close 1 to 2 hours after birth or, in some newborns, not until several days later. Anatomic closure of the foramen ovale occurs within 30 months (Blackburn, 2018).
3. ***Closure of the ductus arteriosus.*** Initial elevation of the systemic vascular pressure above the pulmonary vascular pressure increases pulmonary blood flow by reversing the flow through the ductus arteriosus. Blood now flows from the aorta into the pulmonary artery. An increase in blood PO_2 triggers the ductus arteriosus to constrict. In utero, the placenta produces prostaglandin E_2 (PGE_2), which causes ductus vasodilation. With the loss of the placenta and increased pulmonary blood flow, PGE_2 levels drop, leaving the active constriction by PO_2 unopposed. Functional closure of the ductus arteriosus in the well newborn starts within 18 hours after birth; fibrosis or anatomic closure occurs within 2 to 3 months after birth (Blackburn, 2018).
4. ***Closure of the ductus venosus.*** Closure of the ductus venosus is related to mechanical pressure changes that result from severing the cord, redistribution of blood, and cardiac output. Closure of the ductus venosus forces perfusion of the liver. Fibrosis or anatomic closure of the ductus venosus occurs within 2 weeks, at which time it becomes known as the ligamentum venosum (Blackburn, 2018). See Figure 26–5.

Clinical Tip

Gentle physical contact by thoroughly drying the newborn and placing the baby in skin-to-skin contact with the mother's chest and abdomen will provide ample external stimulation for the first breaths in a comforting way. These actions will also decrease heat loss and promote mother–newborn bonding.

Maintaining Respiratory Function

The ability of the lung to maintain oxygenation and ventilation (the exchange of oxygen and carbon dioxide) is influenced by such factors as **lung compliance** and airway resistance. Lung compliance is influenced by the elastic recoil of the lung tissue and by anatomic differences in the newborn. The newborn has a relatively large heart and mediastinal structures that reduce available lung space. Also, the newborn chest is equipped with weak intercostal muscles, a rigid rib cage with horizontal ribs, and a high diaphragm that restricts the space available for lung expansion. The large abdomen further encroaches on the diaphragm to decrease lung space. Another factor that limits ventilation is airway resistance, which depends on the radius length and number of airways. Airway resistance is increased in the newborn when compared with adults.

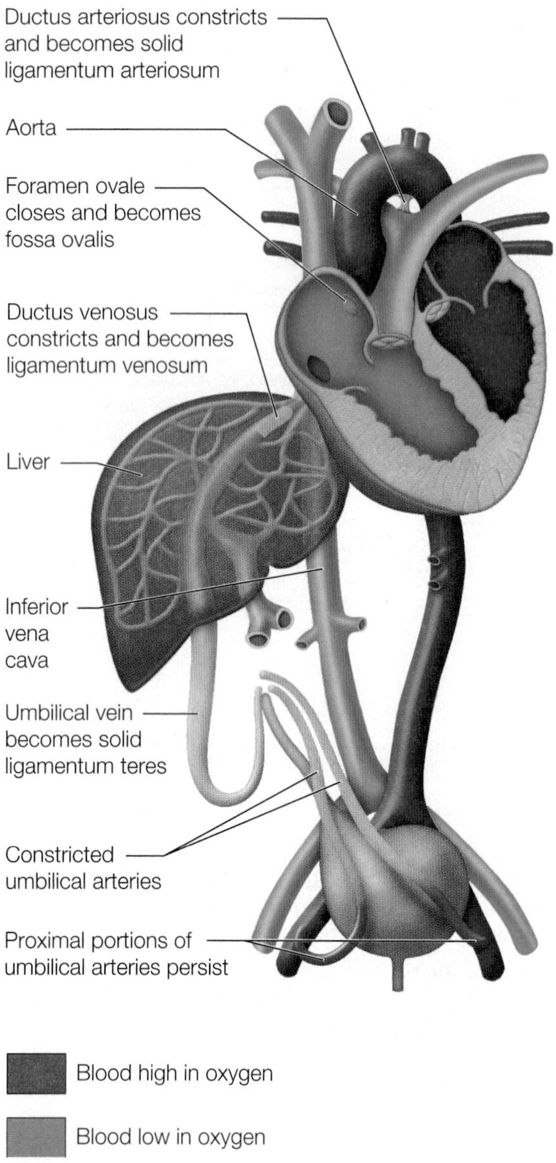

Figure 26–4 Major changes that occur in the newborn's circulatory system.

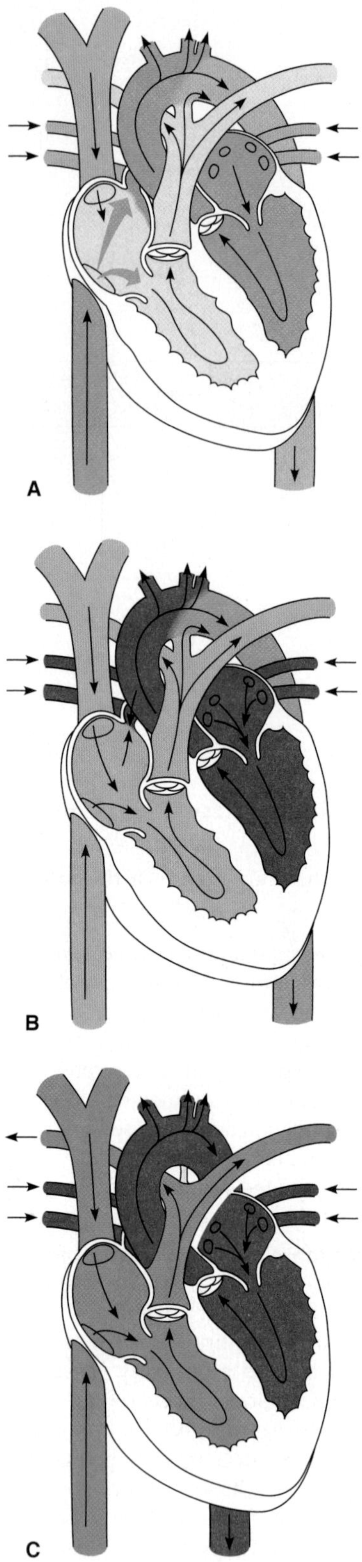

Figure 26–5 Fetal-newborn circulation. A. Pattern of blood flow and oxygenation in fetal circulation. B. Pattern of blood flow and oxygenation in transitional circulation of the newborn. C. Pattern of blood flow and oxygenation in newborn circulation.

Characteristics of Newborn Respiration

The normal newborn respiratory rate is 30 to 60 breaths per minute (America Academy of Pediatrics [AAP] & American College of Obstetricians and Gynecologists [ACOG], 2017). Initial respirations may be largely diaphragmatic, shallow, and irregular in depth and rhythm. The abdomen's movements are synchronous with chest movements. Breathing patterns in newborns can be irregular and variable. Periodic breathing is common in preterm newborns, but can also be seen in term newborns. **Periodic breathing** is defined as "vigorous respiration followed by up to a 20 seconds pause" (Fraser, 2019, p. 82). Periodic breathing is rarely associated with changes in skin color or heart rate, and it has no prognostic significance. Tactile or other senses stimulate the respiratory center and convert periodic breathing patterns to normal breathing patterns during newborn transition. With deep sleep, the pattern is reasonably regular. Periodic breathing occurs with rapid eye movement (REM) sleep, and grossly irregular breathing is evident with motor activity, sucking, and crying. Cessation of breathing lasting more than 20 seconds is defined as *apnea* and is abnormal in term newborns. Apnea may or may not be associated with changes in skin color or heart rate (a drop below 100 beats per minute [beats/min]). Apnea always needs to be further evaluated.

Newborns are obligatory nose breathers because the nasal route is the primary means of air entry. This is because of the high position of the epiglottis and the position of the soft palate (Blackburn, 2018). Although many term newborns can breathe orally when nasally occluded, nasal obstructions can cause respiratory distress. Any obstruction will cause some degree of respiratory distress, so it is important to keep the throat and nose clear.

Immediately after birth and for approximately the next 2 hours, respiratory rates of 60 to 70 breaths per minute (breaths/min) are normal. Acrocyanosis is normal for the first 24 hours. If respirations drop below 30 or exceed 60 per minute when the baby is at rest, or if retractions, central cyanosis, nasal flaring, or expiratory grunting occur, the primary care provider should be notified. Any increased use of the intercostal muscles (retractions) may indicate respiratory distress. (See Chapter 31 and Table 31–2 for signs of respiratory distress.) Institutions may perform pulse oximetry, which should be greater than 95% in term newborns; however, it takes about 10 minutes on average for pulse oxygen saturations to rise above 90% (Eichenwald, Hansen, Martin, et al., 2017). See agency protocol.

Characteristics of Cardiac Function

HEART RATE

Shortly after the first cry and the start of changes in cardiopulmonary circulation, the newborn heart rate can accelerate to 180 beats/min. The average resting heart rate in the first week of life is 110 to 160 beats/min in a healthy full-term newborn but may vary significantly during deep sleep or active awake states. In full-term newborns, the heart rate may drop to a low of 70 to 90 beats/min during deep sleep (Vargo, 2019).

Apical pulse rates should be obtained by auscultation (Figure 26–6) for a full minute, preferably when the newborn is asleep. The heart rate should be evaluated for abnormal rhythms or beats. Peripheral pulses of all extremities should also be evaluated to detect any inequalities or unusual characteristics. While radial pulses are usually readily found, pedal pulses may be difficult to palpate in the newborn. Additionally, brachial and femoral pulses are usually easily palpated in the well newborn.

BLOOD PRESSURE

The blood pressure tends to be highest immediately after birth, and then it descends to its lowest level at about 3 hours of age.

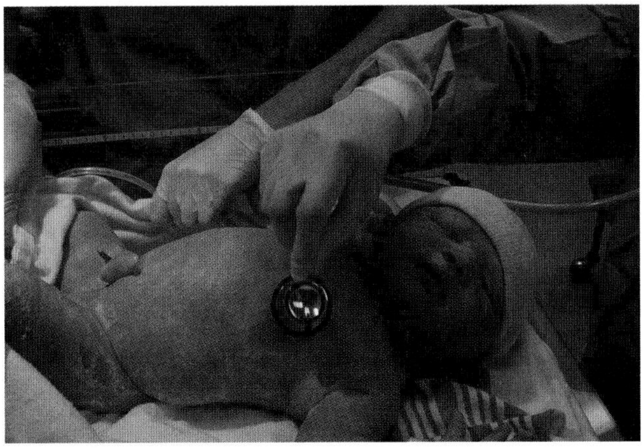

Figure 26–6 **Apical pulse rates should be obtained by auscultation for a full minute, preferably when the newborn is asleep.**

SOURCE: Wilson Garcia.

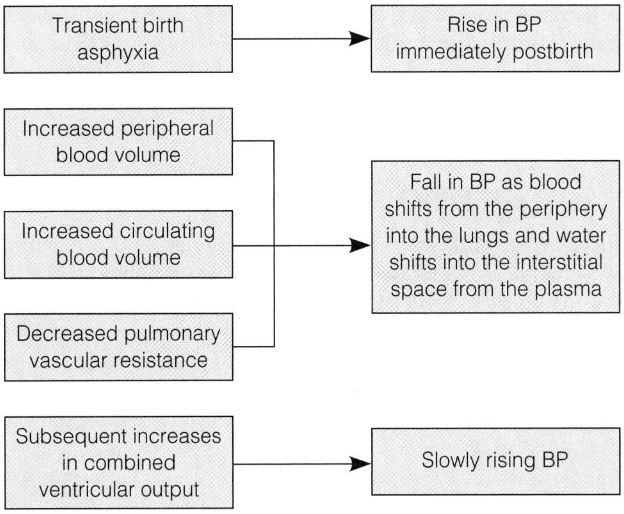

Figure 26–7 **Response of blood pressure to changes in newborn blood volume.**

By 4 to 6 days of life, the blood pressure rises and plateaus at a level approximately the same as the initial level. Blood pressure is sensitive to the changes in blood volume that occur in the transition to newborn circulation. Figure 26–7 diagrams this response. Peripheral perfusion pressure is a particularly sensitive indicator of the newborn's ability to compensate for alterations in blood volume before changes in blood pressure. Capillary refill should be less than 3 seconds when the skin is blanched.

Blood pressure values during the first 12 hours of life vary with the birth weight and gestational age. The average mean blood pressure is 50 to 55 mmHg in full-term resting newborns over 3 kg during the first 12 hours of life (Gardner & Hernandez, 2016). In the preterm newborn, the average mean blood pressure varies according to weight and degree of illness. Crying may cause an elevation in both the systolic and diastolic blood pressure; thus, accuracy is more likely in the quiet newborn. Blood pressure in the lower extremities is usually higher than that in the upper extremities.

CARDIAC MURMURS

Murmurs are produced by turbulent blood flow. In newborns, 90% of all murmurs are transient and *not associated with anomalies.*

Cardiac murmurs are often present in the initial newborn period as transition from fetal to newborn circulation occurs. These murmurs heard in the transition period (the first 48 hours of life) should be followed up (Vargo, 2019). Such murmurs usually involve incomplete closure of the ductus arteriosus or foramen ovale. Soft murmurs may be heard as the pulmonary branch arteries increase their blood flow from 7 to 50% of the combined ventricular output during transition, causing a physiologic peripheral pulmonary stenosis. Clicks may normally be heard at the lower left sternal border as the great vessels dilate to accommodate systolic blood flow in the first few hours of life. Because of the current practice of early discharge, murmurs associated with ventricular septal defect and patent ductus arteriosus are often not picked up until the first well-baby checkup at 4 to 6 weeks of age. Thus, newborns with serious cardiac anomalies may not be identified until weeks after discharge from the birthing facility.

CARDIAC WORKLOAD

Before birth, the right ventricle does approximately two-thirds of the cardiac work, resulting in increased size and thickness of the right ventricle at birth. After birth, the left ventricle must assume a larger share of the cardiac workload, and it progressively increases in size and thickness. This may explain why right-sided heart defects are better tolerated than left-sided ones and why left-sided defects rapidly become symptomatic after birth.

Hematopoietic Adaptations

Birth brings dramatic changes in circulation and oxygenation, which affect hematopoiesis. The mean hemoglobin level in cord blood at term is 17 g/dL (Eichenwald et al., 2017). Normally the hemoglobin and hematocrit values rise in the first several hours after birth because of the movement of plasma from the intravascular to the extravascular space. By 3 to 5 days after birth, nucleated red blood cells (RBCs) are normally no longer found in the blood of term or preterm newborns, but may be present in marked elevated numbers in the presence of hemolysis or hypoxic stress (Blackburn, 2018).

Oxygen Transport

The transportation of oxygen to the peripheral tissues depends on the type of hemoglobin in the RBCs. In the fetus and newborn, a variety of hemoglobin types exist, with the most significant being fetal hemoglobin (HbF) and adult hemoglobin (HbA). Approximately 70 to 90% of hemoglobin in the fetus and newborn is HbF. The greatest difference between HbF and HbA relates to the transport of oxygen and release of it to tissues.

Because HbF has a greater affinity for oxygen than does HbA, the oxygen saturation in the newborn's blood is greater than in the adult's, but the amount of oxygen available to the tissues is less. This situation is beneficial prenatally because the fetus must maintain adequate oxygen uptake in the presence of very low oxygen tension (umbilical venous PO_2 cannot exceed the uterine venous PO_2). Because of this high concentration of oxygen in the blood, hypoxia in the newborn is particularly difficult to recognize. Clinical manifestations of cyanosis do not appear until low blood levels of oxygen are present.

In addition, alkalosis (increased pH) and hypothermia can result in less oxygen being available to the body tissues, whereas acidosis, hypercarbia, and hyperthermia can result in less oxygen being bound to hemoglobin and more oxygen being released to the body tissues.

In the first days of life, hemoglobin may rise 1 to 2 g/dL above fetal levels as a result of placental transfusion, low oral fluid intake, and diminished extracellular fluid volume. The fetal hemoglobin concentration in blood decreases after birth by approximately 3% per week and is less than 5 to 8% of total hemoglobin by 6 months of age. The hemoglobin level declines progressively during the first 2 months of life (Blackburn, 2018). This initial decline in hemoglobin creates a phenomenon known as **physiologic anemia of the newborn**. The lowest hemoglobin level is reached at about 3 months of age and is called the *physiologic nadir*. The newborn usually tolerates this physiologic state without any clinical difficulties. Hemoglobin values fall mainly from a decrease in red cell mass rather than from the diluting effect of increasing plasma volume. The fact that red cell survival is lower in newborns than in adults, and that red cell production is less, also contributes to this anemia. Neonatal RBCs have a lifespan of 60 to 70 days, approximately two-thirds the lifespan of adult RBCs (Blackburn, 2018). Erythropoiesis resumes normally when levels of erythropoietin rise in response to low hemoglobin levels and tissue oxygen needs (Blackburn, 2018). Once erythropoiesis resumes, iron stores will be used to produce new RBCs. Most newborns require supplemental iron to maintain adequate iron stores.

By 3 to 5 days after birth, nucleated red blood cells are normally no longer found in the blood of term or preterm newborns, but may be present in markedly elevated numbers in the presence of hemolysis or hypoxic stress. The absolute number of neutrophils in the blood of the newborn is greater than that found in older children, while the absolute number of lymphocytes is equivalent to that in older children. The platelet count of the newborn is comparable to adult values. A number of maternally administered pharmacologic agents have been implicated in hematologic abnormalities of the fetus or newborn. Therefore, obtaining an accurate maternal history, including medications, is important.

Blood volume is approximately 80 mL/kg of body weight for a term newborn (Eichenwald et al., 2017). For example, a 3.6-kg (8-lb) newborn has a blood volume of 288 mL. Blood volume varies based on the amount of placental transfusion received during the delivery of the placenta, as well as other factors, including:

- ***Gestational age.*** There appears to be a positive association among gestational age, RBC numbers, and hemoglobin concentration.
- ***Prenatal and/or perinatal hemorrhage.*** Significant prenatal or perinatal bleeding decreases the hematocrit level and causes hypovolemia.
- ***Site of the blood sample.*** Hemoglobin and hematocrit levels are significantly higher in capillary blood than in venous blood. Sluggish peripheral blood flow creates RBC stasis, thereby increasing RBC concentration in the capillaries. Consequently, blood samples taken from venous blood sites are more accurate than those from capillary sites.

Delayed Cord Clamping

In utero, the fetus's blood flows through the umbilical cord to and from the fetus and the placenta, bringing oxygen and nutrition to the fetus from the mother's blood. If the umbilical cord is left unclamped for a short period of time after birth, some of the blood from the placenta passes to the newborn (this is called *placental transfusion*) to increase the neonate's blood volume and improve blood flow to the baby's organs (ACOG, 2017). For many years, the standard of care has included immediate clamping of the umbilical cord at birth. The World Health Organization was the first to recommend delayed cord clamping as a standard for all newborns at birth. Although many randomized controlled trials of term and preterm newborns have evaluated the benefits and risks of immediate umbilical cord clamping versus delayed umbilical cord clamping (generally defined as umbilical cord clamping performed 30 to 60 seconds after birth), delayed cord clamping is recommended (ACOG, 2017).

Physiologic studies in term newborns have demonstrated that placental blood is rapidly transferred into the newborn via the uninterrupted umbilical cord in a stepwise fashion during the initial seconds after birth. Approximately 80 mL of blood is transferred by 1 minute after birth, reaching approximately 100 mL at 3 minutes after birth (ACOG, 2017). Providing babies with additional blood through delayed umbilical cord clamping may facilitate transition from fetal to neonatal circulation (ACOG, 2017). Reviews of multiple clinical trials found that delayed umbilical cord clamping had both positive and negative effects on neonatal outcomes. Newborns in the delayed umbilical cord clamping group had significantly higher levels of hemoglobin compared with newborns in the immediate umbilical cord clamping group. Newborns in the delayed umbilical cord clamping group also had higher ferritin levels until 6 months of age and fewer suffered from iron deficiency anemia. However, a slight increase was noted in the need for phototherapy for jaundice in the delayed umbilical cord clamping group.

The benefits of delayed umbilical cord clamping for the preterm newborn are much more compelling. Clinical trials in preterm newborns found that delaying umbilical cord clamping was associated with fewer babies who required blood transfusion for anemia and/or low blood pressure. Also, a significant reduction in the incidence of intraventricular hemorrhage and less risk of necrotizing enterocolitis (a severe infection in the bowel) were found in neonates in the delayed umbilical cord clamping group (ACOG, 2017; Katheria et al., 2015). These effects may be related to an improvement in the circulating neonatal blood volume and better control of blood pressure following placental transfusion. However, there are some legitimate arguments for clamping the umbilical cord soon after birth in cases of placenta previa or placental abruption. In general, delayed cord clamping does not increase postpartum hemorrhage (ACOG, 2017). The concern that delayed umbilical cord clamping could hinder the timely initiation of resuscitation is not valid because the placenta still performs gas exchange after delivery and sick and preterm neonates can benefit from the additional blood volume (ACOG, 2017).

The concentration of serum electrolytes in the blood indicates the fluid and electrolyte status of the newborn. See Table 26–1 for normal term newborn serum electrolytes and blood gas values.

TABLE 26–1 Normal Term Newborn Cord Blood and Cord Blood Gas Values

LABORATORY DATA	NORMAL RANGE
Cord Blood Values	
Hemoglobin	14–20 g/dL
Hematocrit	43–63%
WBC	10,000–30,000/mm^3
WBC differential	
Neutrophils	40–80%
Lymphocytes	20–40%
Monocytes	3–10%
Platelets	150,000–350,000/mm^3
Reticulocytes	3–7%
Sodium	127–144 mEq/L
Potassium	3.4–9.9 mEq/L
Chloride	103–111 mEq/L
Bicarbonate	18–23 mEq/L
Carbon dioxide	13–27 mmol/L
Calcium	8.2–111 mg/dL
Glucose	45–96 mg/dL
Total protein	4.8–7.3 g/dL
Cord Blood Gas Values	
Venous Blood Gas	
pH	7.25–7.35
PO_2	2–32 mmHg
PCO_2	40–50 mmHg
Base excess	± 0–5
HCO_3	22
Arterial Blood Gas	
pH	7.14–7.4
PO_2	16–20 mmHg
PCO_2	32–68 mmHg
Base excess	± 0–10
HCO_3	15–26.8

SOURCE: Data from Fanaroff & Martin, 2015.

Coagulation

The platelet count of the newborn is comparable to adult values; however, the newborn may have transient diminished platelet function. Transient neonatal thrombocytopenia may occur in newborns born to mothers with severe hypertension or HELLP syndrome (hemolysis, elevated liver enzymes, and low platelet count) (see Chapter 18 for a discussion of HELLP syndrome) and in newborns born to mothers who have idiopathic isoimmune thrombocytopenia. Coagulation factors II, VII, IX, and X (synthesized in the liver) require vitamin K for the final steps of synthesis. The absence of intestinal flora needed to synthesize vitamin K in the newborn gut results in a quick decrease of these clotting factors after birth. These clotting factors then slowly increase, but do not approach adult levels for several weeks or later (Blackburn, 2018). This decrease may be lessened by administration of vitamin K, effectively preventing early-occurring hemorrhagic disease of the newborn. Although newborn bleeding problems are rare, an injection of vitamin K (AquaMEPHYTON) is given prophylactically shortly after birth (AAP & ACOG, 2017). (Hemorrhagic disease of the newborn is discussed in more depth in Chapter 30.)

Thermoregulation

Temperature regulation is the maintenance of thermal balance by the loss of heat to the environment at a rate equal to heat production. Newborns are *homeothermic*; they attempt to stabilize their internal (core) body temperatures within a narrow range in spite of significant temperature variations in their environment.

Thermoregulation in the newborn is closely related to the rate of metabolism and oxygen consumption. The **neutral thermal environment (NTE)** is the temperature range in which heat production is at the minimum needed to maintain normal body temperature. The normal newborn requires higher environmental temperatures than adults do to maintain a neutral thermal environment.

Several newborn characteristics affect establishment of thermal stability:

- Heat transfer from newborn organs to skin surface is increased compared to adults due to the newborn's decreased subcutaneous fat and large body surface-to-weight ratio.
- Newborns rely on nonshivering thermogenesis for heat production via metabolism of brown adipose tissue.
- Blood vessels in the newborn are closer to the skin than those of an adult. Therefore the circulating blood is influenced by changes in environmental temperature and in turn influences the hypothalamic temperature-regulating center.
- The flexed posture of the term newborn decreases the surface area exposed to the environment, thereby reducing heat loss.

There are tables listing neutral thermal environmental temperatures that give a recommended temperature range depending on the weight and age of the newborn. Generally speaking, the smaller babies in each weight group will require a temperature in the higher temperature range and the younger the baby, the higher the temperature required. For example, the preterm or small-for-gestational-age (SGA) newborn has less adipose tissue and is hypoflexed, and therefore requires higher environmental temperatures to achieve a thermal neutral environment. Larger, well-insulated, full-term newborns may be able to cope with lower environmental temperatures. If the environmental temperature falls below the lower limits of the NTE, the newborn responds with increased oxygen consumption and increased metabolism, which results in greater heat production and decreased weight gain and growth. Prolonged exposure to the cold may result in depleted glycogen stores and acidosis. Oxygen consumption also increases if the environmental temperature is above the NTE.

Heat Loss

A newborn is at a distinct disadvantage in maintaining a normal temperature. With a large body surface in relation to mass and a limited amount of insulating subcutaneous fat, the full-term newborn loses about four times as much heat as an adult does. The newborn's poor thermal stability is due primarily to excessive heat loss rather than to impaired heat production. Because of the risk of hypothermia and possible cold stress, minimizing heat loss in the newborn after birth is essential. Two major routes of heat loss are from the internal core of the body to the body surface and from the external surface to the environment. Usually the core temperature is higher than the skin temperature, resulting in continuous transfer or conduction of heat to the surface. The greater the difference in temperature between core and skin, the more rapidly heat transfers. The transfer is accomplished through an increase in oxygen consumption, depletion of glycogen stores, and metabolization of brown fat. Heat loss from the body surface to the environment takes place in four ways—by convection, radiation, evaporation, and conduction (Figure 26–8).

- **Convection** is the loss of heat from the warm body surface to the cooler air currents. Air-conditioned rooms, air currents with a temperature below the newborn's skin temperature, unwarmed oxygen by mask, and removal of the newborn from an incubator for procedures increase convective heat loss of the newborn. The amount of heat transferred depends on the velocity of the moving air, the temperature difference between the air and the baby's skin, and the proportion of body surface area exposed.
- **Radiation** losses occur when body heat is transferred to cooler surfaces and objects not in direct contact with the body. The walls of a room or of an incubator are potential causes of heat loss by radiation, even if the ambient temperature of the incubator is within the neutral thermal range for the newborn. Placing cold objects (such as ice for blood gases) onto the incubator or near the newborn in the radiant warmer will increase radiant heat losses.
- **Evaporation** is the loss of heat incurred when water is converted to a vapor. The newborn is particularly prone to heat loss by evaporation immediately after birth (when the baby is wet with amniotic fluid) and during baths; thus, drying the newborn is critical. Evaporation also occurs from expired air from the respiratory tract. Radiant warming beds and phototherapy lights also accentuate evaporative loss.

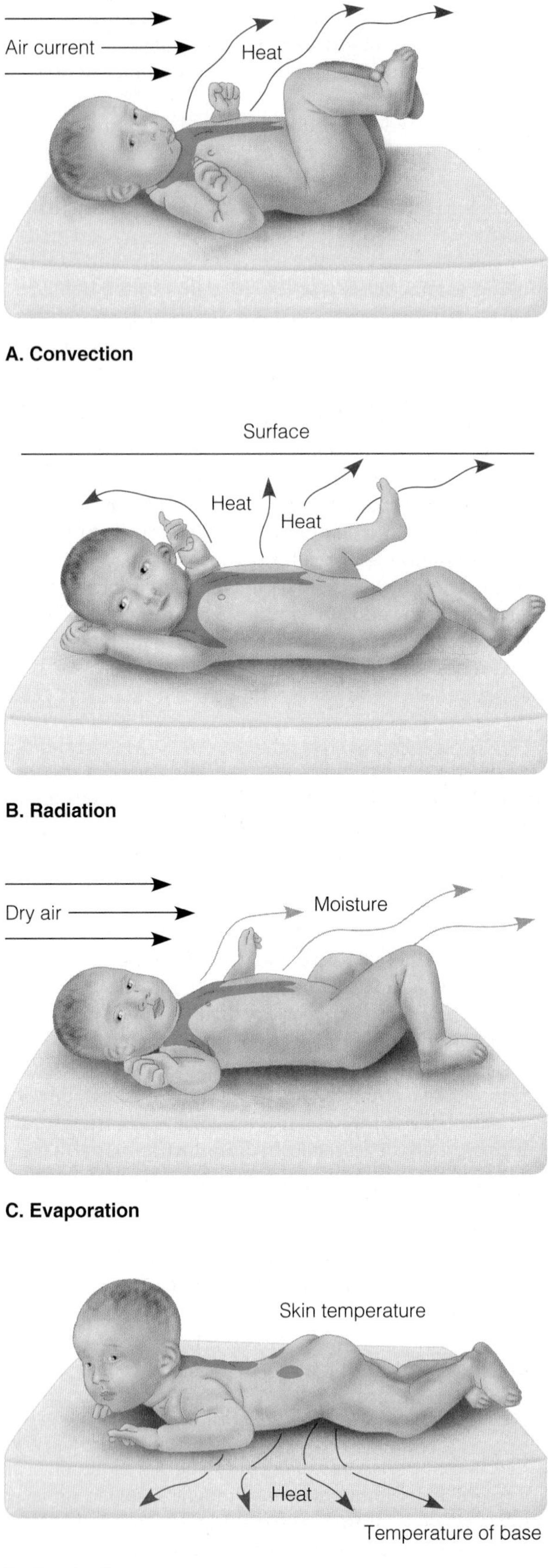

Figure 26–8 **Methods of heat loss. A. Convection. B. Radiation. C. Evaporation. D. Conduction. The shaded areas of the baby's body in images A–D denote the presence of brown adipose tissue.**

- **Conduction** is the loss of heat to a cooler surface by direct skin contact. Chilled hands, cool scales, cold examination tables, and cold stethoscopes can cause heat loss by conduction.

The newborn can respond to the cooler environment with peripheral vasoconstriction and increased muscular activity, but this is not always effective due to the minimal amount of fat insulation present, the large body surface area, and ongoing thermal conduction. Because of these factors, minimizing the baby's heat losses and preventing hypothermia are imperative. Nursing measures for preventing hypothermia are described in Chapter 28, and Chapter 31 discusses care of the newborn with cold stress.

Clinical Tip

Bath time is when many newborns experience cold stress. To minimize the risk, always bathe newborns in a warm room, gather all supplies prior to beginning the bath, and prewarm soaps or shampoos. Dry newborns with warmed blankets and dress immediately. The newborn's head accounts for a large portion of body surface area and has great capacity for heat loss, so placing a hat on the baby is an effective way to minimize heat loss. Placing newborns skin to skin with mother after bathing is a good way to help them rewarm and maintain body temperature.

Once the baby has been dried after birth, the highest losses of heat generally result from radiation and convection. Most hospitalized newborns are weighed daily. Placing unclothed newborns on a cold scale can induce heat loss. Therefore the undressed newborn should be examined in a warm environment with an external heat source such as a radiant warmer.

Developing Cultural Competence Newborn Baths in Jordan

In Jordan, the birth of a male baby is a much celebrated event. The newborn is bathed daily during the first week of life. During the final bath, salt is added to the water to help the newborn's skin adjust to the external environment and protect it from changes in the weather.

Heat Production (Thermogenesis)

When exposed to a cool environment, the newborn requires additional heat. The newborn has several physiologic mechanisms that increase heat production, or **thermogenesis**. These include increased metabolic rate, muscular activity, and nonshivering thermogenesis.

Nonshivering thermogenesis (NST), an important mechanism of heat production unique to the newborn, is the major mechanism through which heat is produced. It occurs when skin receptors perceive a drop in environmental temperature and, in response, transmit sensations to stimulate the sympathetic nervous system. NST uses the newborn's stores of **brown adipose tissue (BAT)** (also called *brown fat*) to provide heat. BAT first appears in the fetus at 26 to 30 weeks' gestation and continues to increase until the early weeks after the birth of a term newborn, unless it is depleted by cold stress (Blackburn, 2018). Brown fat is deposited in the midscapular area, around the neck, and in the axillae, with deeper placement around the trachea, esophagus, abdominal aorta, kidneys, and adrenal glands (see the shaded areas in the baby's body in Figure 26–8). BAT receives its name from the tissue's dark color, which is caused by its enriched blood supply, dense cellular content, and abundant nerve endings. These characteristics promote rapid metabolism, heat generation, and heat transfer to the peripheral circulation. The large numbers of brown fat cells increase the speed with which triglycerides are metabolized to produce heat but cause increased oxygen consumption and caloric output in the already compromised newborn.

Shivering, a form of muscular activity common in the cold adult, is rarely seen in the newborn. NST from BAT is the primary source of heat in the hypothermic newborn. If a newborn is SGA, intrauterine growth restricted (IUGR), or premature, his or her brown fat stores will be inadequate to produce sufficient heat. Brown fat stores cannot be replenished once they are used.

An increase in metabolism as a result of hypothermia results in an increase in oxygen and glucose consumption. A decrease in the environmental temperature of 2°C, from 33°C to 31°C (91.4°F to 87.8°F), is a drop sufficient to double the oxygen consumption of a term newborn and can cause the newborn to show signs of respiratory distress.

When exposed to cold, the preterm newborn may be unable to increase ventilation to the necessary level of oxygen consumption. (See Chapter 31 for a discussion of cold stress.) Because oxidation of fatty acids depends on the availability of oxygen and glucose, the newborn's ability to generate heat can be altered by pathologic events such as hypoxia, acidosis, and hypoglycemia or by medications that block the release of norepinephrine. Newborn hypothermia prolongs as well as potentiates the effects of many analgesic and anesthetic drugs in the newborn.

Hepatic Adaptations

The liver performs many essential functions, including the production of bile, regulation of plasma proteins and glucose, and the biotransformation of drugs and toxins. The newborn has less than 20% of the hepatocytes that are present in the adult liver, and liver growth continues after birth until it reaches its mature size.

Iron Storage

Iron is an essential micronutrient that plays a significant role in critical cellular functions in all organ systems. The serum iron level in umbilical cord blood is elevated compared to maternal levels (Blackburn, 2018). As RBCs are destroyed after birth, their iron content is stored in the liver until needed for new RBC production. Newborn iron stores are determined by total body hemoglobin content and length of gestation. The term newborn has about 270 mg of iron at birth, and about 140 to 170 mg of this amount is in the hemoglobin. If the mother's iron intake has been adequate, enough iron will be stored to last until 5 months of age.

Glucose Homeostasis

Glucose not used for immediate energy needs is converted to glycogen and stored in the liver, heart, and skeletal muscles as glycogen. During fasting, glycogen is broken down to reform glucose and is released by the liver. Fetal glucose levels are approximately 80% of the mother's glucose level. Glycogen storage for postnatal energy needs begins early in gestation, with most glycogen stores accumulating during the third trimester.

After umbilical cord clamping, the newborn's blood glucose level falls, reaching a nadir at about 1 to 2 hours of age. In these first hours after birth, the neonatal brain metabolizes the newborn's abundant stores of lactate, so that even though the glucose concentration may be low, the baby's brain is not energy deficient. By secreting glucagon and suppressing insulin release, the newborn gradually mobilizes glucose to meet his or her energy needs. Thus, even if a healthy term newborn is not fed soon after birth, blood glucose levels rise at 3 to 4 hours of age. However, hepatic glycogen is rapidly depleted if feeding is not established early. The nurse may assess the glucose level on admission if risk factors are present or per agency protocol (see Chapter 31).

Conjugation of Bilirubin

Bilirubin is primarily the metabolic end product of erythrocyte (RBC) breakdown. *Conjugation*, or the changing of bilirubin into an excretable form, is the conversion of the yellow lipid-soluble pigment (unconjugated, indirect) into water-soluble pigment (excretable, direct). Unconjugated bilirubin is fat soluble, has a propensity for fatty tissues, is not in an excretable form, and is a potential toxin. **Total bilirubin** is the sum of conjugated (direct) and unconjugated (indirect) bilirubin.

Fetal unconjugated bilirubin crosses the placenta to be excreted, so the fetus does not need to conjugate bilirubin. Total bilirubin at birth is less than 3 mg/dL unless an abnormal hemolytic process has occurred in utero. After birth, the newborn's liver must begin to conjugate bilirubin. This produces a rise in serum bilirubin in the first few days of life. The unconjugated bilirubin formed, after RBCs are destroyed, is transported in the blood bound to albumin. The bilirubin is transferred into the hepatocytes and bound to intracellular proteins. These proteins determine the amount of bilirubin that is held in the liver cells for processing and consequently determine the amount of bilirubin uptake into the liver. The activity of uridine diphosphoglucuronosyl transferase (UDPGT) enzyme results in the attachment of unconjugated bilirubin to glucuronic acid (a product of liver glycogen), producing bilirubin glucuronides (conjugated, direct bilirubin). Direct (water-soluble) bilirubin is excreted into the bile ducts and duodenum. The (direct) conjugated bilirubin then progresses down the intestines, where bacteria transform it into urobilinogen (urine bilirubin) and stercobilinogen. Stercobilinogen is not reabsorbed but is excreted as a yellow-brown pigment in the stools.

Even after the bilirubin has been conjugated and bound, it can be changed back to unconjugated bilirubin via the enterohepatic circulation. In the intestines, β-D-glucuronidase enzyme acts to split off (deconjugate) the bilirubin from bilirubin glucuronides if it is not first acted upon by gut bacteria to produce urobilinogen; the free bilirubin is reabsorbed through the intestinal wall and brought back to the liver via portal vein circulation. The longer the direct bilirubin remains in the newborn's gut, the greater chance it has of becoming deconjugated. Because of this, newborns who establish gut motility and active stooling through early and frequent feedings are less likely to develop physiologic jaundice. Conjugation of bilirubin in newborns is depicted in Figure 26–9.

The newborn liver has relatively less metabolic and enzymatic activity at birth and in the first few weeks of life than an adult liver. This reduction in hepatic activity, along with a relatively large bilirubin load, decreases the liver's ability to conjugate bilirubin and increases susceptibility to jaundice. *Jaundice (icterus)* is the yellowish coloration of the skin and sclera caused by the presence of bilirubin in elevated concentrations. *Hyperbilirubinemia* is an elevated total serum bilirubin level. Abnormal values differ by gestational age, days of life, and presence of risk factors.

Physiologic Jaundice

Physiologic jaundice (nonpathologic unconjugated hyperbilirubinemia) develops in more than 60% of term newborns and 80% of preterm newborns and is visible when the serum bilirubin concentration is greater than 4 to 6 mg/dL (Hardy, D'Agata, & McGrath, 2016). Usually bilirubin levels increase soon after birth due to increased bilirubin production and/or delayed bilirubin elimination, as well as by a unique neonatal phenomenon of enterohepatic recirculation of bilirubin. However, by the end of the first week of life the bilirubin levels decline. Peak bilirubin levels are reached between days 3 and 4 in the full-term newborn and between days 5 and 6 in the preterm newborn (Hardy et al., 2016). This condition does not have a pathologic basis, but rather is a normal biologic response of the newborn. Note that these values are established for Caucasian European and American newborns. Chinese, Japanese, Korean, and Native American newborns have considerably higher bilirubin levels that are not as apparent and that persist for longer periods with no apparent ill effects. See *Genetic Facts: Jaundice in East Asian or Mediterranean Families*.

Genetic Facts Jaundice in East Asian or Mediterranean Families

A baby born to a family of East Asian or Mediterranean heritage is at a higher risk of becoming jaundiced. Also, some families inherit conditions (such as G6PD deficiency), and their babies are more likely to get jaundice (Centers for Disease Control and Prevention [CDC], 2016).

Because of the shorter lifespan of fetal RBCs, newborns have a two to three times greater production or breakdown of bilirubin. Bruising from the delivery process can also increase the amount of bilirubin to be handled by the liver. The low volume and inadequate caloric intake of the newborn's initial feedings increase reabsorption of bilirubin and are further aggravated by decreased gastrointestinal activity characteristic of the early postnatal period (Bhutani, Vilms, & Hamerman-Johnson, 2010). Enterohepatic recirculation of bilirubin is the deconjugation and reabsorption of bilirubin that occurs in the bowel. The signs of physiologic jaundice appear *after* the first 24 hours postnatally. This differentiates physiologic jaundice from pathologic jaundice, which is clinically seen at birth or within the first 24 hours of postnatal life (see Care of the Newborn with Jaundice in Chapter 31).

In some newborns the rise of bilirubin continues or accelerates. Thus, unmonitored and untreated severe hyperbilirubinemia may progress to excessive levels that are associated with bilirubin neurotoxicity. All newborns should be routinely monitored for the development of jaundice, and nurseries should have protocols for the assessment of jaundice. Jaundice can be detected by blanching the skin with digital pressure on the forehead, mid sternum, or knee to reveal the underlying color of the skin (Bhutani et al., 2010). The newborn develops jaundice in cephalocaudal progression, meaning that jaundice is first seen in the face and then travels down the trunk.

Several newborn care procedures will decrease the probability of high bilirubin levels:

- Maintain the newborn's skin temperature at 36.5°C (97.8°F) or above; cold stress results in acidosis. Acidosis decreases

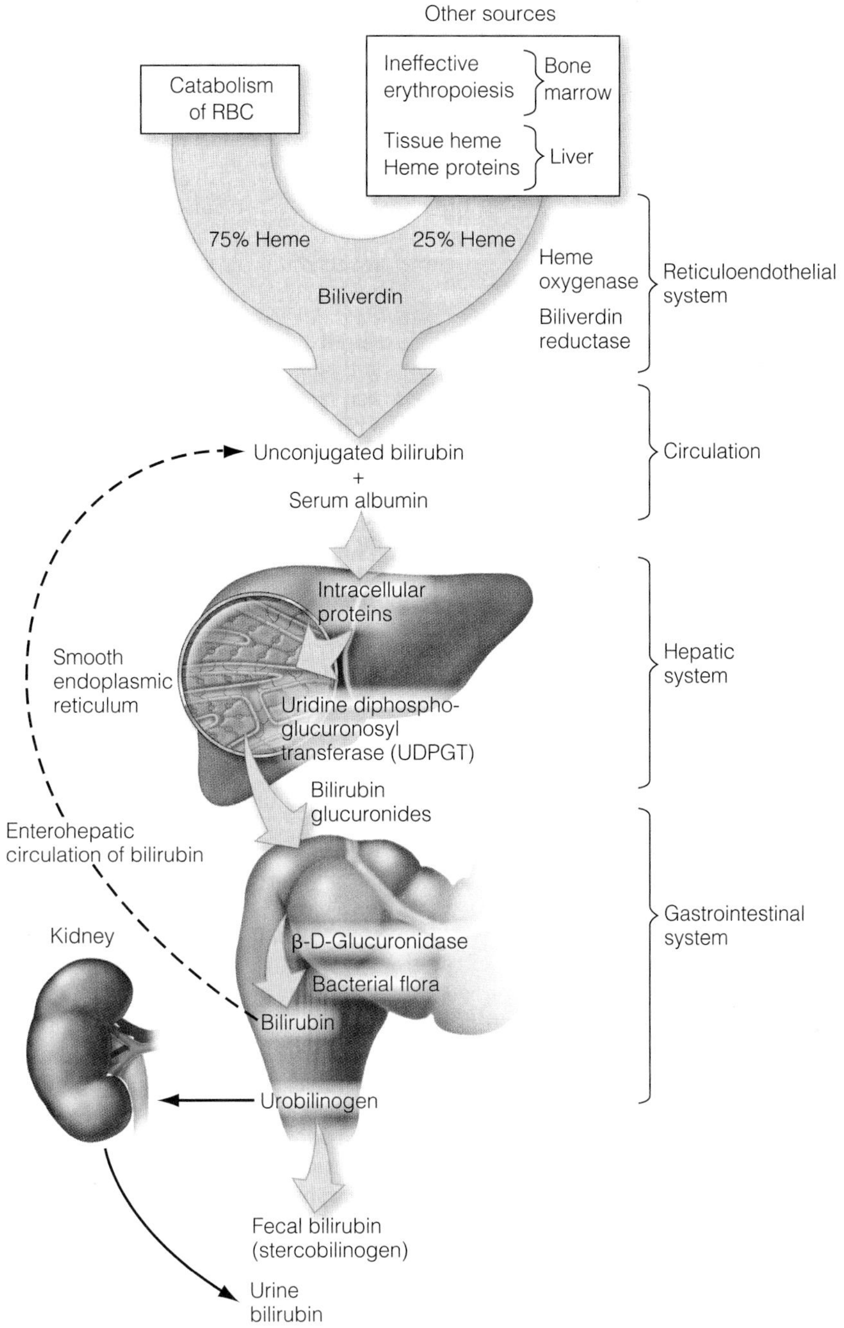

Figure 26–9 Conjugation of bilirubin in newborns.

available serum albumin-binding sites, weakens albumin-binding powers, and causes elevated unconjugated bilirubin levels.

- Monitor stool for amount and characteristics. Bilirubin is eliminated in the feces; inadequate stooling may result in reabsorption and recycling of bilirubin. Early breastfeeding should be encouraged because the laxative effect of colostrum increases excretion of meconium and transitional stool.
- Encourage early feedings to promote intestinal elimination and bacterial colonization and provide caloric intake necessary for hepatic binding proteins to form.

SAFETY ALERT!

Universal screening for hyperbilirubinemia, not visual inspection alone, is necessary to identify elevated bilirubin levels in newborns (AWHONN, 2017).

Absence of jaundice, however, is not an indication of absence of hyperbilirubinemia. Therefore, screening using hour-specific bilirubin measurement and clinical risk factors can identify newborns who are likely to develop severe hyperbilirubinemia. Predischarge bilirubin screening identifies newborns with bilirubin levels higher than the 75th percentile for age in hours. Clinical risk factors for severe hyperbilirubinemia include exclusive and insufficient breast milk feedings, family history of neonatal jaundice, bruising, assisted delivery with vacuum or forceps, cephalohematoma, Asian ethnicity, maternal age (>25 years), male gender, and gestational age.

If jaundice becomes apparent, nursing care is directed toward keeping the newborn well hydrated and promoting intestinal elimination. For specific nursing management and therapies, see *Nursing Care Plan: For the Newborn with Hyperbilirubinemia* in Chapter 31.

Physiologic jaundice may be very upsetting to parents; they require emotional support and thorough explanation of the condition. If the baby is placed under phototherapy, a few additional days of hospitalization may be required, which may also be disturbing to parents. The nurse should encourage parents to provide for the emotional needs of their newborn by continuing to feed, hold, and caress the baby. If the mother is discharged, the parents are encouraged to return for feedings and to telephone or visit whenever they wish. In many instances, the mother, especially if she is breastfeeding, may elect to remain hospitalized with her newborn; the nurse should support this decision. If insurance limitations make this unrealistic, it may be possible to find an empty room for the discharged mother and her family to use while visiting the newborn. As an alternative to continued hospitalization, the newborn may be treated with home phototherapy. (See the Phototherapy section in Chapter 31 for more information.)

Breastfeeding Jaundice

Breastfeeding is implicated in jaundice in some newborns. *Breastfeeding jaundice* occurs in the first days of life in breastfeeding newborns and is related to inadequate fluid intake with some element of dehydration and not with any abnormality in milk composition (Hardy et al., 2016). Prevention and treatment of early breastfeeding jaundice includes encouraging frequent (every 2 to 3 hours) breastfeeding, avoiding supplementation in nondehydrated newborns, and accessing maternal lactation counseling. Breastfeeding jaundice is self-limiting; it peaks around day 3 as enteral intake increases, then resolves. See *Developing Cultural Competence: Interpreting Illness Through Cultural Beliefs*.

Developing Cultural Competence Interpreting Illness Through Cultural Beliefs

Cultural beliefs lead mothers to interpret illness within their cultural framework, especially when left without clear and understood explanations (Lauderdale, 2016). For example, some Latina women believe that showing strong maternal emotions during pregnancy and during breastfeeding can be detrimental. They may blame jaundice in their newborn on "bili" associated with anger. Such maternal reactions can be lessened by careful explanations to the mother about the diagnosis, prognosis, duration, and management options for jaundice and possibility for recurrence.

NOTE: *It is unwise to attribute specific attitudes or beliefs to all members of a cultural group. The information in the Developing Cultural Competence boxes offers possible insights into caring for women from different cultural groups.*

Breast Milk Jaundice

Breast milk jaundice occurs in less than 1 in 200 term newborns with an onset after 3 to 5 days of life and peaking by 2 weeks of life (Blackburn, 2018). The exact mechanism of true breast milk jaundice is unknown, but it is thought to be due to unidentified factors in breast milk interfering with bilirubin metabolism, causing an exaggerated physiologic jaundice (Eichenwald et al., 2017). In contrast to breastfeeding jaundice, breast milk jaundice is related to milk composition promoting increased bilirubin reabsorption from the intestine. For example, some women's breast milk may contain several times the normal concentration of certain free fatty acids. These free fatty acids may compete with bilirubin for binding sites on albumin and inhibit the conjugation of bilirubin or increase lipase activity, which disrupts the RBC membrane. Increased lipase activity enhances absorption of bile across the gastrointestinal tract membrane, thereby increasing the enterohepatic circulation of bilirubin.

Clinical Tip

Breastfeeding mothers need encouragement and support in their desire to breastfeed their newborns, assistance and instruction about pumping and expressing milk during the interrupted breastfeeding period, and reassurance that nothing is wrong with their milk or mothering abilities.

Newborns with breast milk jaundice appear well, and *kernicterus* (toxic levels of bilirubin in the brain) with this type of jaundice has not been documented. Temporary cessation of breastfeeding may be advised if bilirubin reaches presumed toxic levels of approximately 20 mg/dL or if the interruption is necessary to establish the cause of the hyperbilirubinemia. Total serum bilirubin levels may reach 12 to 20 mg/dL and persist up to 2 months. In cases of breast milk jaundice, within 24 to 36 hours after breastfeeding is discontinued, the newborn's serum bilirubin levels begin to fall dramatically. With resumption of breastfeeding, the bilirubin concentration may show a slight rise of 2 to 3 mg/dL with a subsequent decline. See *Key Facts to Remember: Factors in Physiologic, Breast Milk, and Breastfeeding Jaundice*.

Key Facts To Remember
Factors in Physiologic, Breast Milk, and Breastfeeding Jaundice

Physiologic Jaundice

- Physiologic jaundice occurs after the first 24 hours of life.
- During the first week of life, bilirubin should not exceed 13 mg/dL. Some pediatricians allow levels up to 15 mg/dL.
- Bilirubin levels peak at 3 to 5 days in term newborns.

Breast Milk Jaundice

- Bilirubin levels begin to rise after the first week of life when mature breast milk comes in.
- A peak of 5 to 10 mg/dL is reached at 2 to 3 weeks of age.
- It may be necessary to interrupt breastfeeding for a short period when bilirubin reaches 20 mg/dL.

Breastfeeding Jaundice

- Bilirubin levels rise after the first 24 hours of age.
- Levels peak on the third or fourth day of life and decline through the first month to normal levels.
- The incidence can be decreased by increasing the number of breastfeeding episodes to 8 to 12 in 24 hours.

Gastrointestinal Adaptations

During pregnancy, the fetus receives a continuous supply of energy substrates (glucose, fats, and carbohydrates), oxygen, vitamins, and water across the placenta that provide for its metabolism and growth needs. The central roles of the gastrointestinal tract are to act as a barrier between the outer environment and the body, to digest food, and to absorb nutrients. In utero, fetal swallowing is accompanied by gastric emptying and peristalsis of the fetal intestinal tract. By the end of gestation, peristalsis becomes much more active in preparation for extrauterine life. Fetal peristalsis is also stimulated by anoxia, causing the expulsion of meconium into the amniotic fluid in more mature or stressed fetuses. By 36 to 38 weeks of fetal life, the gastrointestinal tract is adequately mature, with the presence of enzymatic activity and the ability to transport nutrients.

Digestion and Absorption

Birth represents a dramatic change of nutrition from a fetal diet rich in carbohydrates and poor in fat to a neonatal diet rich in fat and poor in carbohydrates. As soon as lactation is initiated, the newborn receives a high-fat, low-carbohydrate diet, since colostrum and the initial milk are rich in fat and poor in lactose.

The full-term newborn has adequate intestinal and pancreatic enzymes to digest most simple carbohydrates, fats, and proteins. The carbohydrates requiring digestion in the newborn are usually disaccharides (lactose, maltose, sucrose), which are split into monosaccharides (galactose, fructose, and glucose) by the enzymes of the intestinal mucosa. Lactose is the primary carbohydrate in the breastfeeding newborn and is generally easily digested and well absorbed. The only enzyme lacking at birth is pancreatic amylase, which remains relatively deficient during the first few months of life. Newborns have trouble digesting starches (changing more complex carbohydrates into maltose), so they should not eat them until after the first 6 months of life.

Although proteins require more digestion than carbohydrates, they are well digested and absorbed from the newborn intestine. The newborn digests and absorbs fats less efficiently because of the minimal activity of the pancreatic enzyme lipase. The newborn excretes 10 to 20% of the dietary fat intake, compared with 10% for the adult. The fat in breast milk is absorbed more completely by the newborn than is the fat in cow's milk because it consists of more medium-chain triglycerides and contains lipase. (See Chapter 29 for a more detailed discussion of newborn/infant nutrition.) Following intestinal absorption, nutrients are delivered to the liver by the portal blood and directly delivered to the peripheral tissues.

The fetal gastrointestinal tract is sterile. Microbes begin to establish as soon as the newborn's oral mucosa is exposed to the environment. The gastrointestinal microbiota is important in the development of immune tolerance to allergens. The mode of delivery sets the pattern of gastrointestinal tract colonization. Newborns born by vaginal delivery become colonized by microbes present in the birth canal and mother's gastrointestinal tract, whereas newborns born by cesarean section are initially colonized by skin flora (Blackburn, 2018; Mueller, Bakacs, Combellick, et al., 2015). The establishment and type of feeding are major factors influencing the composition of gastrointestinal-tract microbes. Formula-fed newborns have elevated levels of *Clostridia* and *Bacteroides*, while the microbiota of the breastfed newborn has abundant *Bifidobacteria* due to natural prebiotics in human breast milk (Mueller et al., 2015). Breast milk confers significant anti-infective benefits.

By birth, the newborn has experienced swallowing, gastric emptying, and intestinal propulsion. Air enters the stomach immediately after birth. The small intestine is air filled within 2 to 12 hours, and the large bowel within 24 hours. The salivary glands are immature at birth, and little saliva is manufactured until the baby is about 3 months old. The newborn's stomach can hold 50 to 60 mL. It empties intermittently, starting within a few minutes of the beginning of a feeding and ending between 2 and 4 hours after feeding. Bowel sounds are present within the first 30 to 60 minutes of birth, and the newborn can successfully feed during this time. The newborn's gastric pH becomes less acidic about a week after birth and remains less acidic than that of adults for the next 2 to 3 months.

The cardiac sphincter is immature, as is neural control of the stomach, so some regurgitation may be noted in the newborn period. Continuous vomiting or regurgitation should be monitored closely and reported promptly, as it may be indicative of a more serious problem. Bilious vomiting is abnormal and must be evaluated thoroughly because it might represent a condition that warrants prompt surgical intervention.

Adequate digestion and absorption are essential for newborn growth and development. If optimal nutritional support is available, postnatal growth ideally should parallel intrauterine growth. After 30 weeks of gestation the fetus gains 30 g (1.06 oz) per day and adds 1.2 cm (0.5 in.) to body length weekly. To gain weight at the intrauterine rate, the term newborn requires 120 kcal/kg/day. Following birth, caloric intake is often insufficient for weight gain until the newborn is 5 to 10 days old. During this time there may be a weight loss of 5 to 10% in term newborns. A shift of intracellular water to extracellular space and insensible water loss account for the 5 to 10% weight loss. Thus, failure to lose weight when caloric intake is inadequate may indicate fluid retention.

Elimination

Term newborns normally pass meconium within 24 hours of life–and almost always within 48 hours. **Meconium** is formed in utero from the amniotic fluid and its constituents, with intestinal secretions and shed mucosal cells. It is recognized by its thick, tarry, black (or dark green) appearance. Transitional (thin brown to green) stools consisting of part meconium and part fecal material are passed for the next day or two, after which the stools become entirely fecal. Generally, the stools of a breastfed newborn are pale yellow (but may be pasty green); they are more liquid and more frequent than those of formula-fed newborns, whose stools are paler and often the consistency of peanut butter. Frequency of bowel movement varies but initially ranges from one every 2 to 3 days to as many as 10 daily. Mothers should be counseled that there is no constipation as long as the bowel movement remains soft. See Figure 29–15 in Chapter 29 for progression of stools in the breastfed newborn. See *Key Facts to Remember: Physiologic Adaptations to Extrauterine Life*.

Urinary Adaptations

Kidney Development and Function

In utero the placenta is the organ responsible for fluid and electrolyte homeostasis. After birth the kidney assumes the role of regulation. The kidney is structurally developed with a full complement of functioning nephrons by 34 to 36 weeks of gestation.

Glomerular filtration occurs as blood passes through the capillaries and plasma is filtered through the glomerular capillary walls. Filtrate is collected in the Bowman space and the tubules, where composition is modified until it is excreted as urine. Glomerular filtration rate (GFR) doubles in the first few days of life in term newborns to 15 to 60 mL/kg/day (Blackburn, 2018). The newborn's

Key Facts To Remember
Physiologic Adaptations to Extrauterine Life

- Periodic breathing may be present.
- Desired skin temperature 36°C–36.5°C (96.8°F–97.7°F); stabilizes 4 to 6 hours after birth.
- Desired blood glucose level reaches 60–70 mg/dL by third postnatal day.
- Progression of stool:
  - Meconium (thick, tarry, black; meconium plug may be expelled)
  - Transitional stools (thin, brown to green)
  - Breastfed newborns (yellow gold, soft, or mushy)
  - Formula-fed newborns (pale yellow, formed, and pasty)

ability to dilute urine is fully developed, but concentrating ability is limited. A major function of the kidneys is to maintain osmolality of extracellular fluid within the narrow range compatible with optimal cellular function. The ability to concentrate urine fully is attained by 3 months of age. Feeding practices may affect the osmolarity of the urine but have limited effect on concentration of the urine.

Characteristics of Newborn Urinary Function

Many newborns void immediately after birth, and the voiding frequently goes unnoticed. Among normal newborns, 90% void by 24 hours after birth, and 99% void by 48 hours after birth (Eichenwald et al., 2017). A newborn who has not voided by 48 hours should be assessed for adequacy of fluid intake, bladder distention, restlessness, and symptoms of pain. The appropriate healthcare providers should be notified, if indicated.

The initial bladder volume is 6 to 44 mL of urine. The first 2 days postnatal, the newborn may void two to six times daily, with a urine output of 15 mL/kg/day. The newborn subsequently voids five to 25 times every 24 hours, with a volume of 25 mL/kg/day. Observation and documentation of adequate urinary output are a component of transitional care.

Following the first voiding, the newborn's urine frequently appears cloudy (because of mucus content) and has a high specific gravity, which decreases as fluid intake increases. Occasionally pink stains ("brick dust spots") appear on the diaper. These are caused by urates and are innocuous. Blood may occasionally be observed on the diapers of female newborns. This *pseudomenstruation* is related to the withdrawal of maternal hormones. Males may have bloody spotting from a circumcision, if performed. In the absence of apparent causes for bleeding, the healthcare provider should be notified. During early infancy, normal urine is straw-colored and almost odorless, although odor occurs when there is a metabolic disorder or when infection is present. Table 26–2 summarizes urinalysis values of the normal newborn.

TABLE 26–2 Newborn Urinalysis Values

- Protein less than 5–10 mg/dL
- WBC less than 2–3/hpf
- RBC 0
- Casts 0
- Bacteria 0
- Color pale yellow

Immunologic Adaptations

Neonatal defense against infections in utero or after delivery is dependent on maternal immunity because newborns lack immunologic memory (exposure to infectious agens) and often have slower capacities to develop immune responses (Blackburn, 2018). Maternal-fetal infection transmission (transplacental, perinatal, postnatal) is a major cause of morbidity and mortality in newborns. The immune responses in newborns are usually functionally impaired when compared with adults. The differences in the neonatal immune response put the newborn at risk for development of bacterial and viral infections, resulting in increased mortality.

The general purposes of the newborn immune system are those of defense (fighting microorganisms), homeostasis (disposition of worn-out cells), and surveillance (recognition and destruction of foreign or aberrant cells).

Components of the immune system include both nonspecific mechanisms and specific immune responses. Nonspecific immune mechanisms include phagocytosis, inflammatory response, complement, and coagulation.

- *Phagocytosis* is a major mechanism to remove pathogens and cell debris.
- *Inflammatory response* is the complex biologic response of vascular tissues to harmful stimuli such as pathogens, damaged cells, or irritants.
- *Complement* helps or "complements" the ability of antibodies and phagocytic cells to clear pathogens from an organism.
- *Coagulation* is the process by which blood forms a clot.

These nonspecific immune mechanisms function without prior exposure, can be identified early in gestation, and reach functional development at 32 to 33 weeks' gestation.

Humoral Immunity

The specific immune responses consist of cell-mediated (T cell) and humoral (B cell) systems. The maturation of specific immune responses begins in utero at about 7 to 12 weeks' gestation. The newborn's immune system has a decreased ability to develop effective antibody responses. Humoral immunity is a specific antibody-mediated response that functions most effectively if there has been recent exposure.

The pregnant woman forms antibodies in response to illness or immunization. This process is called **active acquired immunity**. When antibodies are transferred to the fetus in utero, **passive acquired immunity** results because the fetus does not produce the antibodies itself.

Of the major types of immunoglobins involved in immunity—IgG, IgM, IgA, and IgE—immunoglobulin G (IgG) is the major immunoglobulin of serum and interstitial fluid and provides immunity against bacterial and viral pathogens. IgG is transferred via active or passive placental transfer, with the majority passed in the third trimester. IgM does not cross the placental barrier. However, synthesis begins early in gestation, with detectable levels at approximately 30 weeks' gestation, and rapidly increases after birth. IgA is the most common immunoglobulin in the gastrointestinal and respiratory tract; it does not cross the placenta, but is secreted in human colostrum and human milk. IgA does not increase to detectable levels until 2 to 3 weeks of age. IgE is present in very small amounts in serum and secretions and plays a major role in allergic reactions.

Cellular Immunity

Specific cellular immunity is mediated by T lymphocytes, which enhance the efficiency of the phagocytic response. T lymphocytes are activated by antigens to which they have become sensitized. There are three types of activated T cells:

- *Cytotoxic:* Kills foreign or virus-infected cells
- *Helper:* Enables T or B cells to respond to antigens
- *Suppressor:* Represses responses to specific B or T lymphocytes to antigens

T lymphocytes modify the behavior of phagocytic cells and increase their antimicrobial activity. Because of the enhanced susceptibility of newborns to infection, recognition of the signs and symptoms of infection is a priority during the transition period.

Neurologic Adaptation

The human brain is an intricate, fragile organ that begins development in the first 4 weeks of gestation. Two major developmental events begin in utero, but do not complete until years postnatal:

- **Neuronal organization** provides the basis for brain function and its complex circuitry by achieving stabilization of cell connections. This includes cell differentiation, programmed cell death, synaptic development, neurotransmitters, and myelination. Neuronal organization peaks at about 20 weeks' gestation and continues for several years after birth (Blackburn, 2018).
- **Myelination** involves myelin deposition around axons, which enhances intracellular communication. Myelin is a fatty covering that insulates the brain circuitry, prevents leakage of current, and enables rapid, efficient transmission of nerve impulses. Myelination begins in the second trimester of pregnancy and continues into adult life (Blackburn, 2018).

Unlike the cardiovascular or respiratory systems, which undergo tremendous changes at birth, the nervous system is minimally influenced by the actual birth process.

Intrauterine Environmental Influence on Newborn Behavior

Newborns respond to and interact with the environment in a predictable pattern of behavior that is shaped somewhat by their intrauterine experience. This intrauterine experience is affected by intrinsic factors such as maternal nutrition and drug exposure and external factors such as the mother's physical environment. Depending on the newborn's intrauterine experience and individual temperament, newborn behavioral responses to different stresses vary. Some newborns react quietly to stimulation, others become overreactive and tense, and some may exhibit a combination of the two.

Factors such as exposure to intense auditory stimuli in utero can eventually be manifested in the behavior of the newborn. For example, the fetal heart rate (FHR) initially increases when the pregnant woman is exposed to auditory stimuli, but repetition of the stimuli leads to decreased FHR. Thus, the newborn who was exposed to intense noise during fetal life is significantly less reactive to loud sounds postnatal.

Characteristics of Newborn Neurologic Function

Perinatal factors will affect how the newborn interacts with the environment. Type of labor and delivery, drugs given to the mother during labor, overall neonatal health, and of course gestational age of the newborn are all matters that affect neonatal behavior. The environment itself also plays into newborn response. A quiet, dim, warm, calming environment will elicit different newborn behavior than a noisy, bright, or cold surrounding will.

Normal newborns are usually in a position of partially flexed extremities with the legs near the abdomen. When awake, the newborn may exhibit purposeless, uncoordinated bilateral movements of the extremities. The organization and intensity of the newborn's motor activity are influenced by a number of factors, including (Brazelton & Nugent, 2011):

- Sleep–wake states
- Presence of environmental stimuli, such as heat, light, cold, and noise
- Conditions causing a chemical imbalance, such as hypoglycemia
- Hydration status
- State of health
- Recovery from the stress of labor and birth.

The newborn's body grows in a cephalocaudal (head-to-toe), proximal–distal fashion. Muscle tone should be symmetric. Diminished muscle tone and flaccidity may indicate neurologic dysfunction.

Reflexes—including the Moro, grasping, rooting, and sucking reflexes—are characteristics of neurologic integrity. (For further discussion of reflexes, see Chapter 27.) Complex behavioral patterns reflect the newborn's neurologic maturation and integration. Newborns who can bring a hand to the mouth are demonstrating motor coordination as well as a self-quieting technique, thus increasing the complexity of the behavioral response. **Self-quieting ability** is the ability of newborns to use their own resources to quiet and comfort themselves.

Habituation is the newborn's ability to process and respond to complex stimulation. For example, when a bright light is flashed into the newborn's eyes, the initial response is blinking, constriction of the pupil, and perhaps a slight startle reaction. However, with repeated stimulation, the newborn's responses gradually diminish and disappear. The capacity to ignore repetitious disturbing stimuli is a defense mechanism that allows the newborn to shut out overwhelming and disturbing stimuli. Sensory abilities include visual, auditory, olfactory, taste, and tactile capacities.

Periods of Reactivity

The newborn usually shows a predictable pattern of behavior during the first several hours after birth, characterized by two **periods of reactivity** separated by a sleep phase. In a classic description of periods of reactivity that is still used today, Desmond, Rudolph, and Phitaksphraiwan (1966) organized these changes into three periods: The first period of reactivity, the period of inactivity to sleep phase, and the second period of reactivity.

FIRST PERIOD OF REACTIVITY

The first period of reactivity lasts approximately 30 minutes after birth. During this period the newborn is awake and active and may appear hungry and have a strong sucking reflex. This is

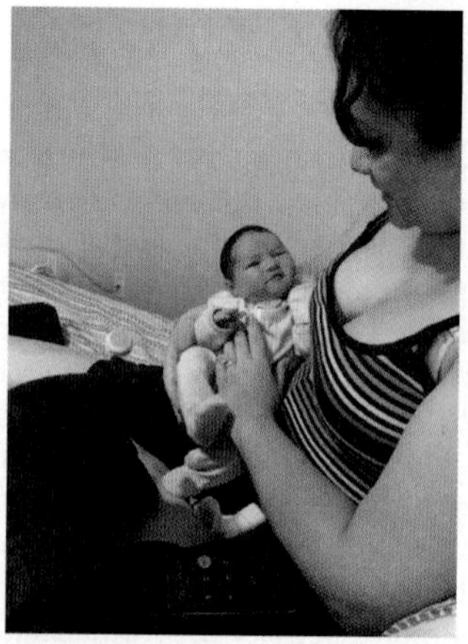

Figure 26–10 **Mother and baby gaze at each other. This quiet alert state is the optimal state for interaction.**

SOURCE: Craig London.

the natural and best opportunity to initiate breastfeeding if the mother has chosen to breastfeed (Figure 26–10). Bursts of random, diffuse movements alternating with relative immobility may occur. Respirations are rapid and there may be retraction of the chest, transient flaring of the nares, and grunting. The heart rate is rapid, and the rhythm may be irregular. Bowel sounds are usually absent.

PERIOD OF INACTIVITY TO SLEEP PHASE

After approximately half an hour the newborn's activity gradually diminishes, and the heart rate and respirations decrease as the newborn enters the sleep phase. The sleep phase may last from a few minutes to 2 to 4 hours. During this period, the newborn will be difficult to awaken and will show no interest in sucking. Bowel sounds become audible, and cardiac and respiratory rates return to baseline values.

SECOND PERIOD OF REACTIVITY

During the second period of reactivity, the newborn is again awake and alert. This period lasts 4 to 6 hours in the normal newborn. Physiologic responses are variable during this stage. The heart and respiratory rates increase; however, the nurse must be alert for apneic periods, which may cause a drop in the heart rate and oxygen level (desaturation). The newborn is stimulated to continue breathing during such times. The newborn may develop rapid color changes and become mildly cyanotic or mottled during these fluctuations. Production of respiratory and gastric mucus increases, and the baby responds by gagging, choking, and regurgitating.

Continued close observation and intervention may be required to maintain a clear airway during this period of reactivity. The gastrointestinal tract becomes more active. The newborn often passes the first meconium stool and may also have an initial voiding. The newborn will indicate readiness for feeding by such behaviors as sucking, rooting, and swallowing. If feeding was not initiated in the first period of reactivity, it is done at this time. (See Chapter 28 for further discussion of this first feeding.)

SAFETY ALERT!

Because newborns are often unable to handle oral secretions effectively enough to protect their airway, parents must be instructed in the proper use of the bulb syringe. The bulb syringe used correctly creates mild suction for removal of oral and nasal secretions. Overuse or vigorous use of the bulb syringe causes unnecessary trauma and inflammation of the small nasal airways, resulting in swelling and partial airway obstruction. See *Clinical Skill 21–1: Performing Nasal Pharyngeal Suctioning* in Chapter 21.

Behavioral States of the Newborn

The behavior of the newborn can be divided into two categories: Sleep states and alert states (Vittner & McGrath, 2019). These postnatal behavioral states are similar to those that have been identified during pregnancy. Subcategories are identified under each major category.

SLEEP STATES

The sleep states are:

1. ***Deep or quiet sleep.*** Deep or quiet sleep is characterized by closed eyes with no eye movements; regular, even breathing; and jerky motions or startles at regular intervals. Behavioral responses to external stimuli are likely to be delayed. Startles are rapidly suppressed, and changes in state are not likely to occur. Heart rate may range from 100 to 120 beats per minute when startled.
2. ***Active or light sleep (REM sleep).*** The baby has irregular respirations; eyes closed, with REM; irregular sucking motions; minimal activity; and irregular but smooth movement of the extremities. Environmental and internal stimuli may initiate a startle reaction and a change of state.

Newborn sleep cycles have been recognized and defined according to duration. The length of the sleep cycle depends on the age of the newborn. At term, REM active sleep and quiet sleep occur in intervals of 50 to 60 minutes (Gardner, Goldson, & Hernandez, 2016). About 45 to 50% of the newborn's total sleep is active/light sleep, 35 to 45% is deep/quiet sleep, and 10% is transitional between these two periods. Growth hormone secretion depends on regular sleep patterns. Any disturbance of the sleep–wake cycle can result in irregular spikes of growth hormone. REM sleep stimulates the highest peaks of growth hormone and the growth of the neural system. Over time, the newborn's sleep–wake patterns become diurnal; that is, the newborn sleeps at night and stays awake during the day. (See Chapter 27 for a short discussion of Brazelton's assessment of newborn states.)

ALERT STATES

In the first 30 to 60 minutes after birth, many newborns display a quiet alert state, characteristic of the first period of reactivity. Nurses should use these alert states to encourage bonding and breastfeeding. These periods of alertness tend to be short the first 2 days after birth to allow the baby to recover from the birth process. Subsequent alert states are of choice or of necessity. Increasing choice of wakefulness by the newborn indicates a maturing capacity to achieve and maintain consciousness. Heat, cold, and hunger are but a few of the stimuli that can cause wakefulness by necessity. Once the disturbing stimuli are removed, the newborn tends to fall back asleep.

The following are subcategories of the alert state (Vittner & McGrath, 2019).

1. ***Drowsy or semidozing.*** The behaviors common to the drowsy state are open or closed eyes, fluttering eyelids, semidozing appearance, and slow, regular movements of the extremities. Mild startles may be noted from time to time. Although the reaction to a sensory stimulus is delayed, a change of state often results.

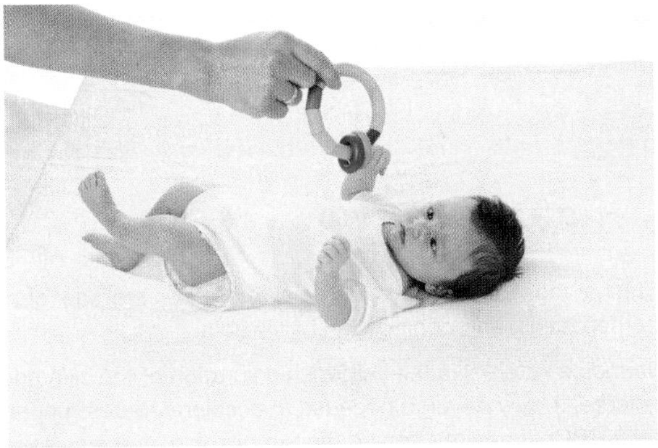

Figure 26–11 Newborn in active alert state turning his head to follow an object.

2. *Quiet alert.* In the wide-awake state, the newborn is alert and follows and fixates on attractive objects, faces, or auditory stimuli. Motor activity is minimal, and the response to external stimuli is delayed.
3. *Active alert.* In the active alert awake state, the newborn's eyes are open and motor activity is quite intense, with thrusting movements of the extremities. Environmental stimuli increase startles or motor activity, but individual reactions are difficult to distinguish because of the generally high activity level (Figure 26–11).
4. *Crying.* Intense crying is accompanied by jerky motor movements. Crying serves several purposes for the newborn. It may be a distraction from disturbing stimuli such as hunger and pain. Fussiness often allows the newborn to discharge energy and reorganize behavior. Most important, crying elicits an appropriate response of help from the parents.

Clinical Tip

While the mother/newborn couplet is in the hospital, the nurse has a perfect opportunity to teach parents techniques to deal with newborn crying and fussiness. Most importantly, it is necessary for parents and caregivers to know that for the first several months crying is the only means of communication available to the newborn and usually signifies unmet needs.

Sensory/Perceptual Capacities of the Newborn

VISUAL CAPACITY

Orientation is the newborn's ability to be alert to, to follow, and to fixate on complex visual stimuli that have a particular appeal and attraction. The newborn prefers the human face and eyes and bright shiny objects. As the face or object is brought into the line of vision, the newborn responds with bright, wide eyes, still limbs, and fixed staring. This intense visual involvement may last several minutes, during which time the newborn is able to follow the stimulus from side to side. Figure 26–11 illustrates this response. The newborn uses this sensory capacity to become familiar with family, friends, and surroundings.

AUDITORY CAPACITY

The newborn responds to auditory stimulation with a definite, organized behavior repertoire. During all interactions, care providers should observe the newborn's response to sound. The stimulus used to assess auditory response should be selected to match the state of the newborn. A rattle is appropriate for light sleep, a voice for an awake state, and a clap for deep sleep. As the newborn hears the sound, the cardiac rate rises, and a minimal startle reflex may be seen. If the sound is appealing, the newborn will become alert and search for the site of the auditory stimulus. Newborns prefer the sound of the human voice to nonhuman sounds. The newborn's hearing should be evaluated prior to discharge. (See Chapter 27 for a discussion of newborn hearing screening tests.)

OLFACTORY CAPACITY

Newborns develop the sense of smell rapidly and can differentiate their mother by smell within the first week of life (Cheffer & Rannali, 2016). Newborns are able to distinguish their mother's breast pads from those of other mothers at just 1 week postnatal and will turn preferentially toward the mother's smell (Cheffer & Rannali, 2016).

TASTE AND SUCKING

Newborns respond differently to varying tastes. They can distinguish between sweet and sour at 3 days of age (Cheffer & Rannali, 2016). Sugar, for example, increases sucking, and newborns tend to have a preference for sweet tastes. When breastfeeding, the newborn sucks in bursts with frequent regular pauses. The bottle-fed newborn tends to suck at a regular rate with infrequent pauses.

When awake and hungry, the newborn displays rapid searching motions in response to the rooting reflex. Once feeding begins, the newborn establishes a sucking pattern according to the method of feeding. Finger sucking happens not only postnatal, but also in utero. The newborn frequently uses nonnutritive sucking as a self-quieting activity, which assists in the development of self-regulation.

TACTILE CAPACITY

The newborn is very sensitive to being touched, cuddled, and held; thus, touch may be the most important of all of the senses for the newborn. Often a mother's first response to an upset or crying newborn is touching or holding. Swaddling, placing a hand on the abdomen, or holding the arms to prevent a startle reflex are other ways to soothe the baby. The settled newborn is then able to attend to and interact with the environment. Touch is also used to rouse a drowsy newborn, making the baby more alert for feeding.

Focus Your Study

- The newborn period is the time from birth through the 28th day of life.
- The production of surfactant is crucial to keeping the lungs expanded during expiration by reducing alveolar surface tension.
- Onset of respirations stimulates cardiovascular changes: Air enters the lungs; oxygen content rises in alveoli and stimulates relaxation of pulmonary arteries. This leads to a decrease in pulmonary vascular resistance, which allows complete vascular flow to the lungs. With increased oxygenated pulmonary blood flow and loss of the placenta, systemic blood flow increases and the foramen ovale and ductus arteriosus begin to close.
- The newborn is an obligatory nose breather. Respirations move from being primarily shallow, irregular, and diaphragmatic to synchronous abdominal and chest breathing.
- Normal respiratory rate is 30 to 60 breaths/min.
- The status of the cardiopulmonary system may be measured by evaluating the heart rate, blood pressure, and presence or absence of murmurs. The normal heart rate is 80 to 160 beats/min.
- Oxygen transport in the newborn is significantly affected by the presence of greater amounts of HbF (fetal hemoglobin) than HbA (adult hemoglobin). HbF holds oxygen more efficiently but releases it to the body tissues only at low PO_2 levels.
- Newborn blood values are affected by gestational age, prenatal and/or perinatal hemorrhage, site of the blood drawing, and timing of the clamping of the umbilical cord.
- Thermoregulation in the newborn is closely related to the rate of metabolism and oxygen consumption.
- Evaporation is the primary heat loss mechanism in newborns who are wet from amniotic fluid or a bath. In addition, excessive heat loss occurs from radiation and convection because of the newborn's larger surface area compared with weight and from thermal conduction because of the marked difference between core temperature and skin temperature.
- The primary source for heat production in the cold-stressed newborn is brown adipose tissue (BAT).
- By secreting glucagon and suppressing insulin release, the newborn gradually mobilizes glucose to meet his or her energy needs.
- The newborn's liver plays a crucial role in iron storage, glucose homeostasis, and conjugation of bilirubin.
- Jaundice (icterus) is the yellowish coloration of the skin and sclerae. It may develop because of accelerated destruction of fetal RBCs, impaired conjugation of bilirubin, and increased bilirubin reabsorption from the intestinal tract.
- The newborn possesses the ability to digest and absorb nutrients necessary for newborn growth and development but has trouble digesting starches.
- The newborn's stools change from meconium (thick, tarry, black) to transitional stools (thinner, brown to green) and then to the distinct forms for either breastfed newborns (yellow-gold, soft, or mushy) or formula-fed newborns (pale yellow, formed, and pasty). Most newborns pass their first stool within 24 to 48 hours of birth.
- The newborn's kidneys are characterized by a decreased rate of glomerular flow, limited tubular reabsorption, limited excretion of solutes, and limited ability to concentrate urine. Most newborns void within 24 hours of birth.
- The immune system in the newborn is not fully activated until it begins to produce its own immunity at about 4 weeks of age. The newborn does possess some immunologic abilities and has passive immunity from the mother, lasting from 4 weeks to 8 months.
- Neurologic and sensory perceptual functioning in the newborn is evident from the newborn's interaction with the environment, presence of synchronized motor activity, and well-developed sensory capacities.
- The first period of reactivity lasts for 30 minutes after birth. The newborn is alert and hungry at this time, making this a natural opportunity to promote attachment.
- The second period of reactivity requires close monitoring by the nurse because apnea, decreased heart rate, gagging, choking, and regurgitation are likely to occur and require nursing intervention.
- Behavioral states in the newborn can be divided into sleep states and alert states.
- Some of the behavioral capabilities of the newborn that assist in adaptation to extrauterine life include self-quieting ability and habitation.

References

American College of Obstetricians and Gynecologists (ACOG). (2017). Delayed umbilical cord clamping after birth (ACOG Committee Opinion No. 684). *Obstetrics & Gynecology, 129*(1), e5–10.

Association of Women's Health, Obstetric and Neonatal Nurses (AWHONN). (2009, reaffirmed 2017). *Clinical position statement: Universal screening for hyperbilirubinemia.* Washington, DC: Author.

American Academy of Pediatrics (AAP) Committee on Fetus and Newborn & American College of Obstetricians and Gynecologists (ACOG) Committee on Obstetrics. (2017). *Guidelines for perinatal care* (8th ed.). Evanston, IL: Author.

Bhutani, V. K., Vilms, R. J., & Hamerman-Johnson, L. (2010). Universal bilirubin screening for severe neonatal hyperbilirubinemia. *Journal of Perinatology, 30,* S6–S15.

Blackburn, S. T. (2018). Maternal, fetal, neonatal physiology: A clinical perspective (5th ed.). St. Louis, MO: Elsevier.

Brazelton, T. B., & Nugent, J. K. (2011). *The neonatal behavioral assessment scale* (4th ed.). London, UK: MacKeith.

Centers for Disease Control and Prevention (CDC). (2016). *Facts about jaundice and kernicterus.* Retrieved from https://www.cdc.gov/ncbddd/jaundice/facts.html

Cheffer, N. D., & Rannali, D. A. (2016). Transitional care of the newborn. In S. Mattson & J. E. Smith (Eds.), *Core curriculum for maternal-newborn nursing* (5th ed., pp. 345–362). St. Louis, MO: Saunders.

Desmond, M. M., Rudolph, A. J., & Phitaksphraiwan, P. (1966). The transitional care nursery. A mechanism for preventive medicine in the newborn. *Pediatric Clinics of North America, 13*(3), 651–668.

Eichenwald, E. C., Hansen, A. R., Martin, C. R., & Stark, A. R. (2017). *Cloherty and Stark's manual of neonatal care* (8th ed.). Philadelphia, PA: Lippincott Williams & Wilkins.

Fanaroff, A. A., & Martin, R. J. (Eds.). (2015). *Neonatal-perinatal medicine* (10th ed.). St. Louis, MO: Mosby.

Fraser, D. (2019). Chest and lung assessment. In E. P. Tappero & M. E. Honeyfield (Eds.), *Physical assessment of the newborn* (6th ed., pp. 79–91). Petaluma, CA: NICU INK.

Gardner, S. L., Goldson, E., & Hernandez, J. A. (2016). The neonate and the environment: Impact on development. In S. L. Gardner, B. S. Carter, M. Enzman-Hines, & J. A. Hernandez (Eds.), *Merenstein & Gardner's handbook of neonatal intensive care* (7th ed., pp. 270–331). St. Louis, MO: Mosby.

Gardner, S. L., & Hernandez, J.A. (2016). Initial nursery care. In S. L. Gardner, B. S. Carter, M. Enzman-Hines, & J. A. Hernandez (Eds.), *Merenstein & Gardner's handbook of neonatal intensive care* (7th ed., pp. 71–104). St. Louis, MO: Mosby.

Hardy, W., D'Agata, A., & McGrath, J. M. (2016). The infant at risk. In S. Mattson & J. E. Smith (Eds.), *Core curriculum for maternal-newborn nursing* (5th ed., pp. 363–416). St. Louis, MO: Saunders.

Katheria, A. C., Truong, G., Cousins, L., Oshiro, B., & Finer, N. N. (2015). Umbilical cord milking versus delayed cord clamping in preterm. *Pediatrics 136*(1), 61–69. DOI: 10.1542/peds.2015-0368

Lauderdale, J. (2016). Transcultural perspectives in childbearing. In M. M. Andrews & J. S. Boyle (Eds.), *Transcultural concepts in nursing care* (7th ed., pp. 120–152). Philadelphia, PA: Lippincott.

Mueller, N. T., Bakacs, E., Combellick, J., Grigoryan, Z., & Domingquez-Bello, M. G. (2015). Infant microbiome development: Mom matters. *Trends in Molecular Medicine, 21*(2), 109–117. DOI: 10.1016/j.molmed.2014.12.002

Vargo, L. (2019). Cardiovascular assessment. In E. P. Tappero & M. E. Honeyfield (Eds.), *Physical assessment of the newborn* (6th ed., pp. 93–111). Petaluma, CA: NICU INK.

Vittner, D., & McGrath, J. M. (2019). Behavioral assessment. In E. P. Tappero & M. E. Honeyfield (Eds.), *Physical assessment of the newborn* (6th ed., pp. 193–218). Petaluma, CA: NICU INK.

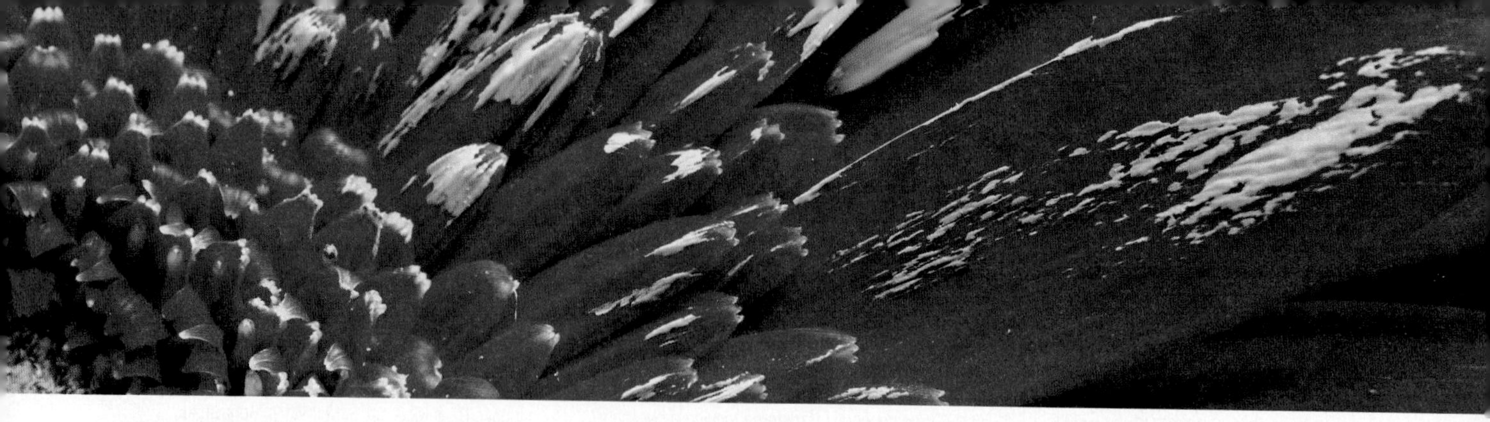

Chapter 27
Nursing Assessment of the Newborn

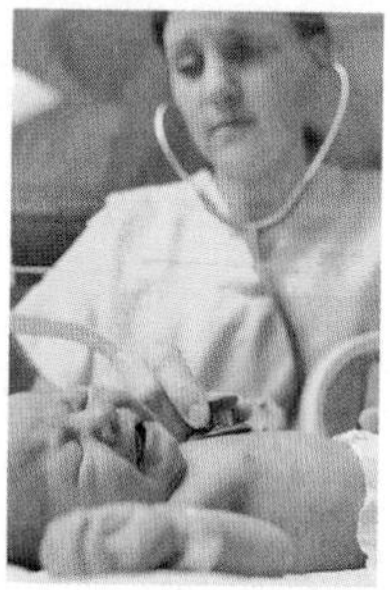

Something very special occurs within the first hour after birth. If the environment is quiet, the birthing without complications, the lights lowered, the handling diminished, newborn infants—aside from all the physiological adaptations they must make—begin in a uniquely human way to adapt to the new experience of being in the world.

—Marshall H. Klaus & Phyllis H. Klaus, *The Amazing Newborn*

SOURCE: RubberBall/SuperStock.

Learning Outcomes

27.1 Identify the major assessment time periods for the newborn.

27.2 Describe the physical and neuromuscular maturity characteristics assessed to determine the gestational age of the newborn.

27.3 Summarize the components of a systematic physical newborn assessment and the significance of normal variations and abnormal findings.

27.4 Describe the components of a newborn neurologic assessment and the neurologic/neuromuscular characteristics of the newborn.

27.5 Identify the newborn reflexes that are present at birth.

27.6 Correlate normal behavioral characteristics of the newborn with variations that may be present.

27.7 Describe how to use the assessment procedure and results of the newborn physical, neurologic, and behavioral assessments to teach and involve the parents in their baby's care and to allay their concerns.

Healthy People 2020

(MICH-8) Reduce low birth weight (LBW) and very low birth weight (VLBW)

(MICH-1.8) Reduce the rate of infant deaths from sudden infant death syndrome (SIDS)

Unlike adults, newborns communicate their needs primarily by their behavior. Because nurses are the most consistent professional observer of the newborn, they can translate this behavior into information about the newborn's condition and respond with appropriate nursing interventions. This chapter focuses on the assessment of the newborn and interpretation of findings.

Timing of Newborn Assessments

During the first 24 hours of life, the newborn makes the critical transition from intrauterine to extrauterine life. The risk of mortality and morbidity is statistically high during this period. Assessment of the newborn is essential to ensure that the transition is proceeding successfully.

There are three major time frames for assessing newborns while they are in the birth facility.

1. ***Delivery room disposition.*** The first assessment is done in the birthing area immediately after birth to determine the need for resuscitation or other interventions. The stable newborn should stay with the family after birth to initiate early attachment. The newborn with complications is usually taken to the special nursery for further evaluation and intervention.
2. ***Nursery or couplet care admission examination.*** A second assessment may be done by the nursery nurse as part of

routine admission procedures. During this assessment, the nurse carries out a brief physical examination to estimate gestational age and evaluate the newborn's adaptation to extrauterine life. No later than 2 hours after birth, the admitting nursery nurse should evaluate the newborn's status and any problems that place the newborn at risk.

3. ***Before discharge examination.*** A certified nurse-midwife (CNM), physician, or nurse practitioner will carry out an exam similar to the well-baby admission exam and a behavioral assessment and review additional information from the baby's stay in the birthing unit to assess if the newborn is ready for routine care at home. A complete physical examination is done to detect any emerging or potential problems. When the birthing center stay is short, a combination admission-discharge exam is appropriate.

See *Key Facts to Remember: Timing and Types of Newborn Assessments* for an at-a-glance summary of newborn assessment.

Assessment of the newborn is a continuous process used to evaluate development and adjustments to extrauterine life. In the birthing area, Apgar scoring and careful observation of the newborn form the basis of the assessment and are correlated with information such as:

- Maternal prenatal care history
- Birthing history
- Maternal analgesia and anesthesia
- Complications of labor or birth
- Treatment instituted immediately after birth, in conjunction with determination of clinical gestational age
- Consideration of the newborn's classification by weight and gestational age and by neonatal mortality risk
- Physical examination of the newborn.

The nurse incorporates data from these sources with the assessment findings during the first 1 to 4 hours after birth to formulate a plan for nursing intervention. See *Evidence-Based Practice: Sickness Severity Scores.*

The various newborn assessments and the data obtained from them are only valuable to the degree to which they are shared with the parents. The parents must be included in the assessment process from the moment of their child's birth. The *Apgar score* and its meaning should be explained immediately to the family (see further discussion in Chapter 21). As soon as possible, the parents should take part in the physical and behavioral assessments as well.

The nurse encourages the parents to identify the unique behavioral characteristics of their newborn and to learn nurturing activities. Attachment is promoted when parents have the opportunity to explore their newborn in private, identifying individual physical and behavioral characteristics. The nurse's supportive responses to the parents' questions and observations are essential throughout the assessment process. The newborn physical examination is the beginning of newborn health surveillance and health education for the newborn's family that continues into the community setting. See *Case Study: Melissa Bond-James.*

Ethics in Action!

How would you respond to a parent who immediately after her child's birth observes a birth defect not noted on the prenatal ultrasound?

Estimation of Gestational Age

It is essential to establish the newborn's gestational age in the first 4 hours after birth so that careful attention can be given to age-related problems. Traditionally, a newborn's gestational age was determined from the date of the pregnant woman's last menstrual period. This method was accurate only 75 to 85% of the time. Because of the problems that develop with the newborn who is preterm or whose weight is inappropriate for gestational age, a more accurate system was developed to evaluate the newborn. Once learned, the procedure can be done in a few minutes.

SAFETY ALERT!

It is essential that the nurse wear gloves when assessing the newborn in these early hours after birth and before the first bath until amniotic fluid, vaginal secretions, and blood on the skin are removed.

Clinical **gestational age assessment tools** have two components: External physical characteristics and neurologic or

Key Facts To Remember

Timing and Types of Newborn Assessments

Delivery Room Disposition	Nursery or Couplet Care Admission Examination	Before Discharge Examination
• Need for resuscitation • Whether newborn is stable and can be placed with parents to initiate early attachment/bonding	• Progress of newborn's adaptation to extrauterine life • Determination of gestational age • Ongoing assessment for high-risk problems	• Complete physical examination (Depending on agency protocol, the nurse may complete some components independently with the certified nurse-midwife/physician/nurse practitioner completing the exam before discharge.) • Nutritional status and ability to formula-feed or breastfeed satisfactorily • Behavioral state organization abilities

EVIDENCE-BASED PRACTICE | Sickness Severity Scores

Clinical Question

Which assessment tools most accurately reflect the severity of sickness in neonates admitted to the neonatal intensive care unit (NICU)?

The Evidence

Sickness severity scores are often used to estimate the intensity of illness among neonates admitted to the NICU. These scores help determine appropriate treatments, predict the likely course of illness, assess the risk of mortality, and estimate long-term outcomes. Hospitals may use these scores as an indicator of quality of care. Garg, Sharma, and Farahbakhsh (2018) conducted an extensive literature search to determine the reliability and validity of the most commonly used neonatal sickness severity scores and the relative quality of each. This type of review of nearly 50 publications representing thousands of neonates is the strongest level of evidence for practice.

The commonly used Clinical Risk Index for Babies (CRIB) and the updated version CRIB II score were strong predictors of neonatal sickness. The Score for Neonatal Acute Physiology (SNAP) and its extensions, SNAP-PE and SNAP-II, also performed well. All these scores rely heavily on birthweight and gestational age to predict morbidity and mortality, but additional measures are used. The CRIB scores were considered simple to use and did not require sophisticated equipment. This may be helpful in less-developed healthcare settings. The SNAP and its derivatives were also excellent predictors of mortality and morbidity, but their major drawback was their complexity. The SNAP requires more than 25 physiologic measures, many requiring a professional laboratory to complete. One scoring instrument—the National Therapeutics Interventions Scoring System (NTISS)—was highly predictive of mortality, but only in neonates less than 1500 grams in weight. In each of these cases, the overall scoring system was a better predictor than birth weight and gestational age alone (Garg et al., 2018).

Best Practice

Scoring systems for severity of sickness in neonates admitted to NICUs can help predict neonatal mortality and morbidity reliably and with a moderate level of certainty. The CRIB scores are useful when simplicity is valued and technology is limited. The SNAP scores are useful when professional laboratory values are available and multiple measurements can be conducted. The NTISS is an effective predictor for neonates weighing less than 1500 grams at birth. All these systems are more effective than using gestational age and birth weight alone (Garg et al., 2018).

Clinical Reasoning

How can the neonatal nurse use severity of sickness scores efficiently in the NICU? How can these scores be used in counseling parents about the baby's prognosis?

neuromuscular development evaluations. Physical characteristics generally include:

- Sole creases
- Amount of breast tissue
- Amount of lanugo
- Cartilaginous development of the ear
- Testicular descent and scrotal rugae in the male
- Labial development in the female.

These objective clinical criteria are not influenced by labor and birth and do not change significantly within the first 12 hours after birth.

Neurologic examination facilitates assessment of functional or physiologic maturation in addition to physical development. However, the newborn's nervous system is unstable during the first 24 hours of life; neurologic evaluation findings based on reflexes or assessments dependent on the higher brain centers may not be reliable. If the neurologic findings drastically deviate from the gestational age derived by evaluation of the external characteristics, a second assessment is done in 24 hours. The neurologic assessment components (excluding reflexes) are especially helpful in assessing the gestational age of newborns less than 34 weeks' gestation. Between 26 and 34 weeks, neurologic changes are significant, whereas significant physical changes are less evident.

Ballard et al. (1991) developed the *estimation of gestational age by maturity rating*, a simplified version of the well-researched *Dubowitz tool*. The Ballard tool omits some of the neuromuscular tone assessments, such as head lag, ventral suspension (which is difficult to assess in very ill newborns or those on respirators), and leg recoil. In Ballard's tool, each physical and neuromuscular finding is given a point value, and the total score is matched to a gestational age. The maximum score on the Ballard tool is 50, which corresponds to a gestational age of 44 weeks.

For example, on completing a gestational assessment of a 1-hour-old newborn, the nurse gives a score of 3 to all the physical characteristics, for a total of 18, and gives a score of 3 to all the neuromuscular assessments, for a total neurologic score of 18.

CASE STUDY: Melissa Bond-James

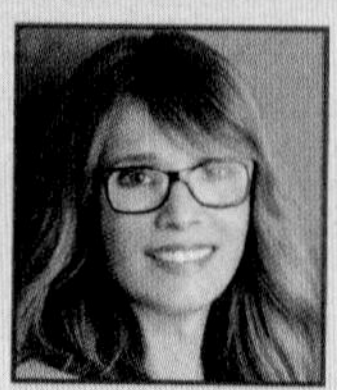

SOURCE: Kinga/ Shutterstock.

Upon admission to the labor and delivery unit, Melissa had presented an extensive birth plan that specifically said that she did not want the baby taken out of her arms for at least 1 hour after birth.

Questions to Ponder

As the nurse who will likely be present for the birth, how would you explain what complications or circumstances would warrant removal of the baby before this time? Can you describe how you would perform an assessment and still maintain the mother's wishes within the birth plan?

The physical characteristics score of 18 is added to the neurologic score of 18 for a total score of 36, which correlates with 38 or more weeks' gestation. Because all newborns vary slightly in the development of physical characteristics and maturation of neurologic function, scores will usually vary instead of all being 3, as in this example.

Postnatal gestational age assessment tools can overestimate preterm gestational age and underestimate postterm gestational age. The tools have been shown to lose accuracy when newborns of less than 28 weeks' or more than 43 weeks' gestation are assessed. In the **New Ballard Score (NBS)**, Ballard et al. (1991) added criteria for more accurate assessment of the gestational age of newborns between 20 and 28 weeks' gestation and less than 1500 g. They suggest that the assessment be made within 12 hours of birth to optimize accuracy, especially in newborns of less than 26 weeks' gestational age. Also, the Ballard assessment may be overstimulating to babies of less than 27 weeks' gestation (Cavaliere & Sansoucie, 2014).

Some maternal conditions such as preeclampsia, diabetes, and maternal analgesia and anesthesia may affect certain gestational assessment components and warrant further evaluation (see Chapter 16 and Chapter 22). Maternal diabetes, while it appears to accelerate fetal physical growth, seems to decelerate maturation. Maternal hypertension states, which slow fetal physical growth, seem to speed maturation.

Newborns of women with preeclampsia have a poor correlation with the criteria involving active muscle tone and edema. Maternal analgesia and anesthesia may cause the baby to have respiratory depression. Babies with respiratory distress syndrome (RDS) tend to be flaccid and edematous and to assume a "froglike" posture (see Chapter 31). These characteristics affect the scoring of the neuromuscular components of the assessment tool used. The NBS gestational age assessment tool is used throughout this chapter to demonstrate the assessment of the physical and neuromuscular criteria associated with gestational age.

Assessment of Physical Maturity Characteristics

The nurse first evaluates observable characteristics without disturbing the baby. Selected physical characteristics common to the Dubowitz and Ballard gestational assessment tools are presented here in the order in which they might be most effectively evaluated:

1. *Resting posture*, although a neuromuscular component, should be assessed as the baby lies undisturbed on a flat surface (Figure 27–1).
2. *Skin* in the preterm newborn appears thin and transparent, with veins prominent over the abdomen early in gestation. As the newborn approaches term, the skin appears opaque because of increased subcutaneous tissue. Disappearance of the protective vernix caseosa promotes skin desquamation, and this is commonly seen in postmature newborns (babies greater than 42 weeks' gestational age and those showing signs of placental insufficiency; see Chapter 30 for a discussion of postmature newborns).
3. **Lanugo**, a fine hair covering, decreases as gestational age increases. The amount of lanugo is greatest at 28 to 30 weeks. It is most abundant over the back (particularly between the scapulae), although it will be noted over the face, legs, and arms. Lanugo disappears first from the face and then from the trunk and extremities (Figure 27–2).
4. *Sole (plantar) creases* are reliable indicators of gestational age in the first 12 hours of life. Later, the skin of the foot begins drying, and superficial creases appear. Development of sole creases begins at the top (anterior) portion of the sole and, as gestation progresses, proceeds to the heel (Figure 27–3). Peeling may also occur. Plantar creases vary with race. In newborns of African descent, sole creases may be less developed at term.

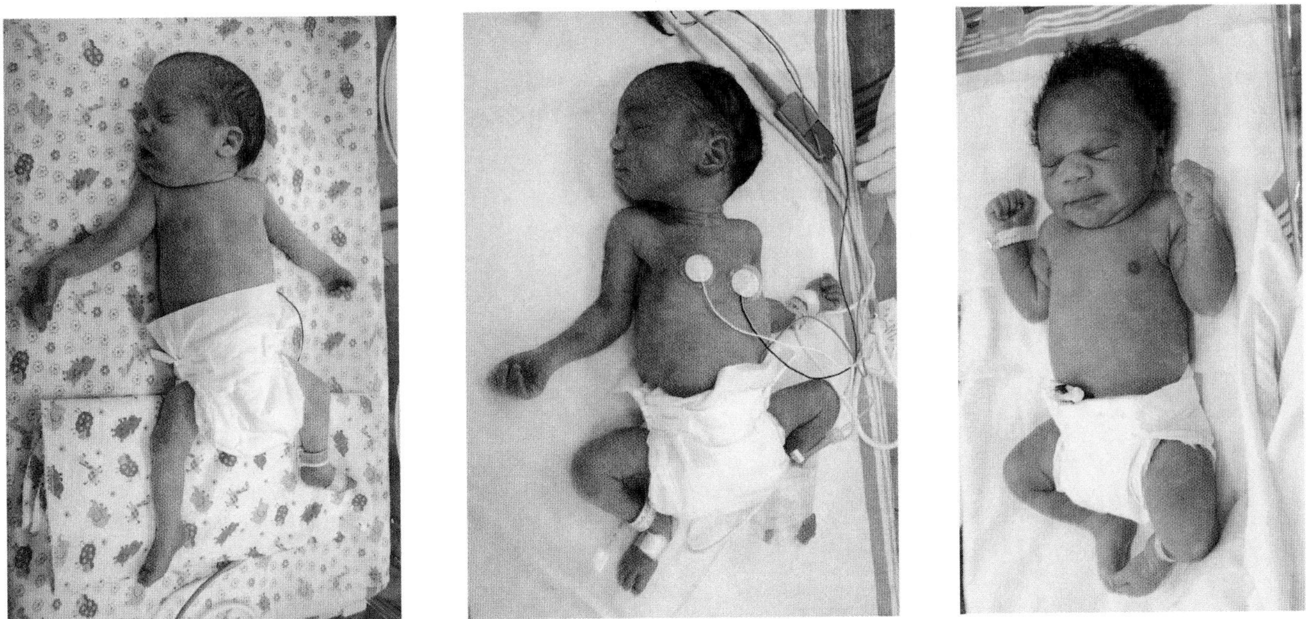
A B C

Figure 27–1 Resting posture. A. Newborn exhibits beginning of flexion of the thigh. The gestational age is approximately 31 weeks. Note the extension of the upper extremities. Score 1 or 2. B. Newborn exhibits stronger flexion of the arms, hips, and thighs. The gestational age is approximately 35 weeks. Score 3. C. The full-term newborn exhibits hypertonic flexion of all extremities. Score 4.

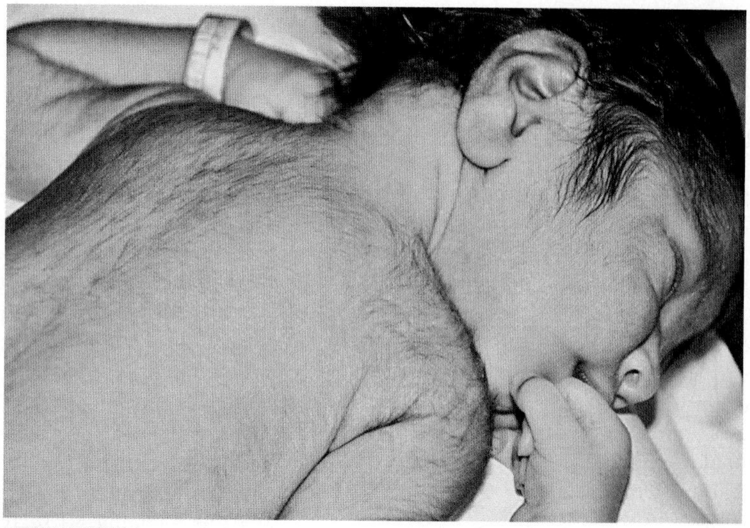

Figure 27–2 **Lanugo.**

SOURCE: Vanessa Howell RN, MSN, NNP-BC.

5. The nurse inspects the *areola* and gently palpates the breast bud tissue by applying the forefinger and middle finger to the breast area and measuring the tissue between them in centimeters or millimeters (Figure 27–4). At term gestation, the tissue will measure between 0.5 and 1 cm (5 and 10 mm). During the assessment, the nipple should not be grasped firmly because skin and subcutaneous tissue will prevent accurate estimation of size. The nurse must perform this procedure gently to avoid causing trauma to the breast tissue.

   As gestation progresses, the breast bud and areola enlarge. However, a large breast tissue mass can occur as a result of conditions other than advanced gestational age or the effects of maternal hormones on the baby. In the large-for-gestational-age (LGA) newborn of a mother with diabetes, accelerated development of breast tissue is a reflection of subcutaneous fat deposits. Asymmetrical (head sparing), small-for-gestational-age (SGA), term, or postterm newborns may have used subcutaneous fat (which would have been deposited as breast tissue) to survive in utero; as a result, their lack of breast tissue may indicate a gestational age of 34 to 35 weeks, even though other factors indicate a term or postterm newborn (Eichenwald, Hansen, Martin, et al., 2017).

6. *Ear form and cartilage distribution* develop with gestational age. The cartilage gives the ear its shape and substance (Figure 27–5). In a newborn of less than 34 weeks' gestation, the ear is relatively shapeless and flat; it has little cartilage, so the ear folds over on itself and remains folded. By approximately 36 weeks' gestation, some cartilage and slight incurving of the upper pinna are present, and the pinna springs back slowly when folded. (The nurse tests this response by holding the top and bottom of the pinna together with the forefinger and thumb and then releasing it, or by folding the pinna of the ear forward against the side of

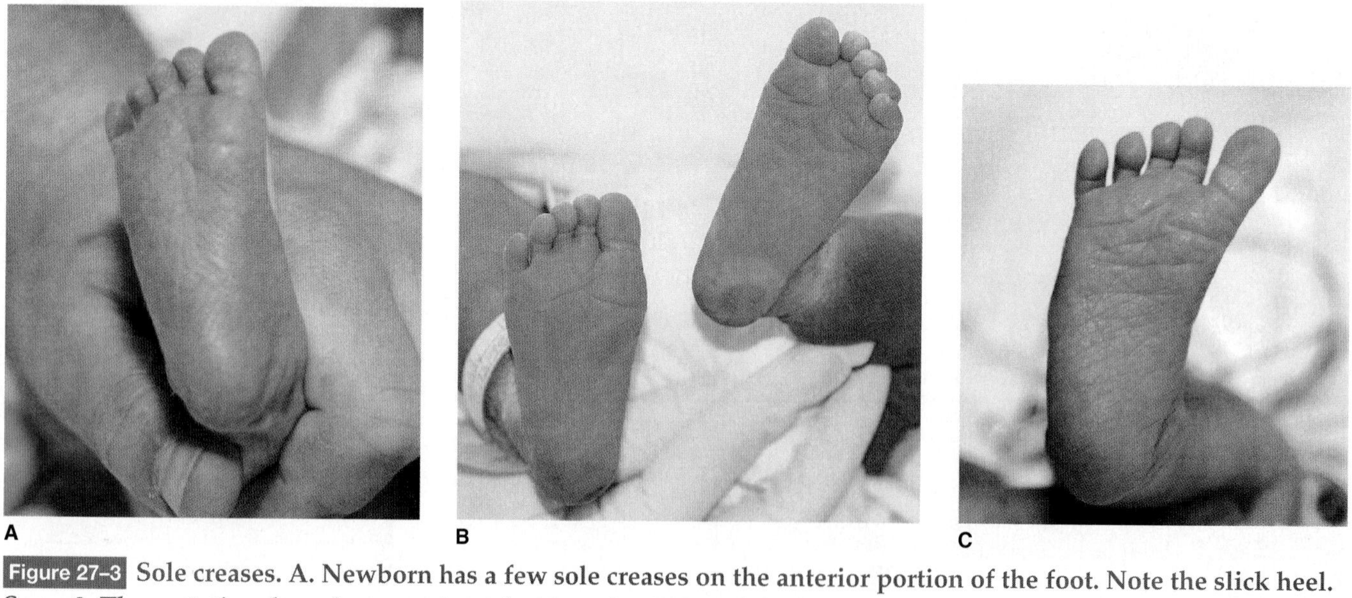

A B C

Figure 27–3 **Sole creases. A. Newborn has a few sole creases on the anterior portion of the foot. Note the slick heel. Score 2. The gestational age is approximately 35 weeks. B. Newborn has a deeper network of sole creases on the anterior two-thirds of the sole. Note the slick heel. Score 3. The gestational age is approximately 37 weeks. C. The full-term newborn has deep sole creases down to and including the heel as the skin loses fluid and dries after birth. Score 4. Sole (plantar) creases can be seen even in preterm newborns.**

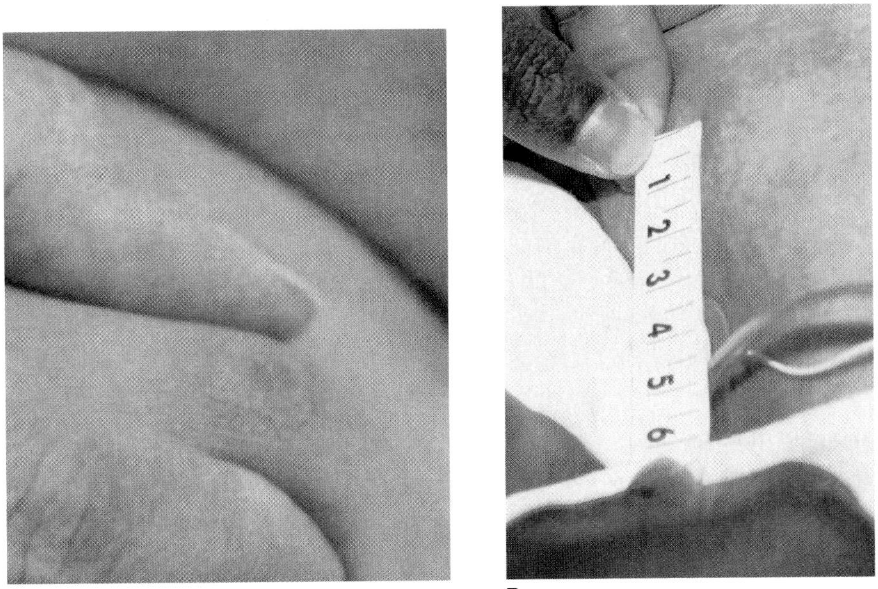

A B

Figure 27–4 Breast tissue. A. Newborn has a visible raised area greater than 0.75 cm diameter. Score 3. The gestational age is 38 weeks. B. Gently compress the tissue between the middle and index fingers, and measure the tissue in centimeters or millimeters. Absence of or decreased breast tissue often indicates premature or small-for-gestational-age newborn.

the head and releasing it, and then observing the response.) By term, the newborn's pinna is firm, stands away from the head, and springs back quickly from the folding.

7. *Male genitals* are evaluated for size of the scrotal sac, the presence of rugae (wrinkles and ridges in the scrotum), and descent of the testes (Figure 27–6). Before 36 weeks, the small scrotum has few rugae, and the testes are palpable in the inguinal canal. By 36 to 38 weeks, the testes are in the upper scrotum, and rugae have developed over the anterior portion of the scrotum. By term, the testes are generally in the lower scrotum, which is pendulous and covered with rugae.

8. The appearance of the *female genitals* depends in part on subcutaneous fat deposition and therefore relates to fetal nutritional status (Figure 27–7). The clitoris varies in size and occasionally is so large that it is difficult to identify the sex of the newborn. This swelling may be caused by adrenogenital syndrome, which causes the adrenals to secrete

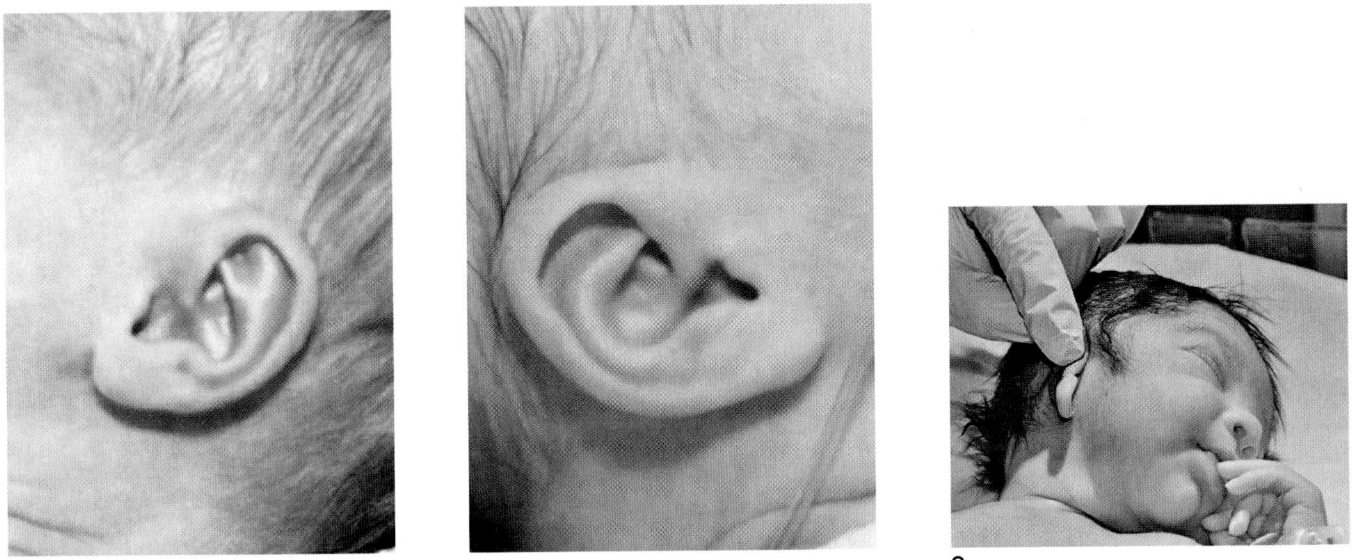

A B C

Figure 27–5 Ear form and cartilage. A. The ear of the newborn at approximately 36 weeks' gestation shows incurving of the upper two-thirds of the pinna. Score 2. B. Newborn at term shows well-defined incurving of the entire pinna. Score 3. C. The pinna is folded toward the face and released. If the auricle stays in the position in which it is pressed or returns slowly to its original position, it usually means that the gestational age is less than 38 weeks.

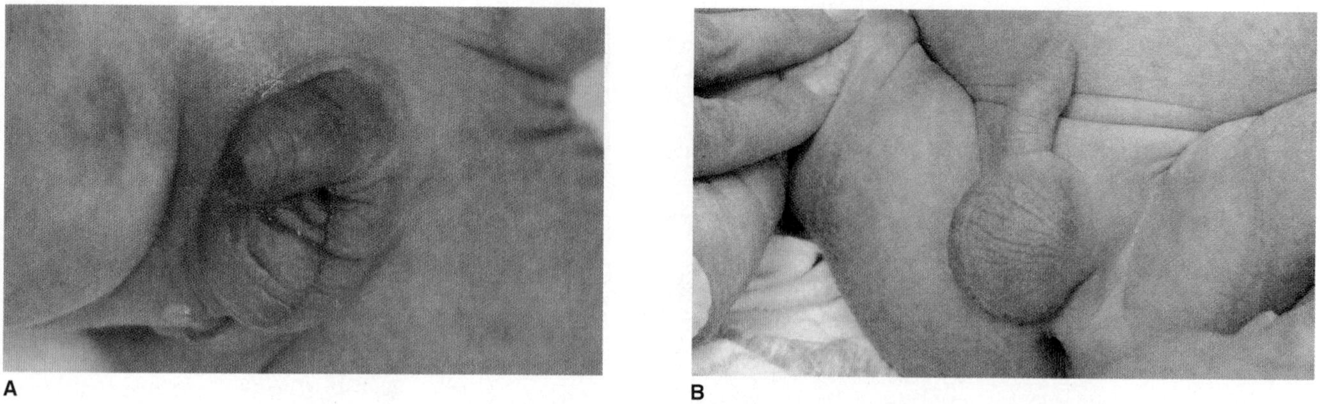

A B

Figure 27–6 Male genitals. A. Preterm newborn's testes are not within the scrotum. The scrotal surface has few rugae. Score 2. B. Term newborn's testes are generally fully descended. The entire surface of the scrotum is covered by rugae. Score 3.

excessive amounts of androgen and other hormones. At 30 to 32 weeks' gestation, the clitoris is prominent, and the labia majora are small and widely separated. As gestational age increases, the labia majora increase in size. At 36 to 40 weeks, they nearly cover the clitoris. At 40 weeks and beyond, the labia majora cover the labia minora and clitoris.

Other physical characteristics assessed by some gestational age scoring tools include:

1. *Vernix* covers the preterm newborn. The postterm newborn has no vernix. After noting vernix distribution, the birthing area nurse (wearing gloves) dries the newborn to prevent evaporative heat loss, thus disturbing the vernix and potentially altering this gestational age criterion. The birthing area nurse must communicate to the neonatal nurse the amount of vernix and the areas of vernix coverage.
2. *Hair* of the preterm newborn has the consistency of matted wool or fur and lies in bunches rather than in the silky, single strands of the term newborn's hair.
3. *Skull firmness* increases as the fetus matures. In a term newborn, the bones are hard, and the sutures are not easily displaced. The nurse should not attempt to displace the sutures forcibly.
4. *Nails* appear and cover the nail bed at about 20 weeks' gestation. Nails extending beyond the fingertips may indicate a postterm newborn.

Assessment of Neuromuscular Maturity Characteristics

The central nervous system of the human fetus matures at a fairly constant rate. Tests have been designed to evaluate neurologic status as manifested by development of neuromuscular tone. One significant neuromuscular change is that muscle tone

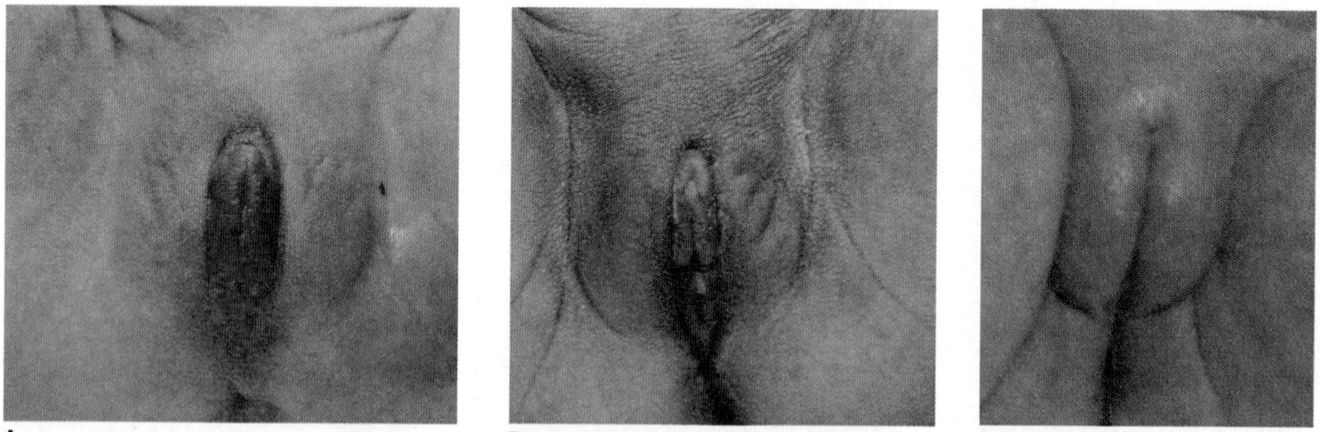

A B C

Figure 27–7 Female genitals. A. Newborn has a prominent clitoris. The labia majora are widely separated, and the labia minora, viewed laterally, would protrude beyond the labia majora. Score 1. The gestational age is 30 to 36 weeks. B. The clitoris is still visible. The labia minora are now covered by the larger labia majora. Score 2. The gestational age is 36 to 40 weeks. C. The term newborn has well-developed, large labia majora that cover both clitoris and labia minora. Score 3.

NOTE: The labia minora is often dark in some ethnic and racial groups of newborns.

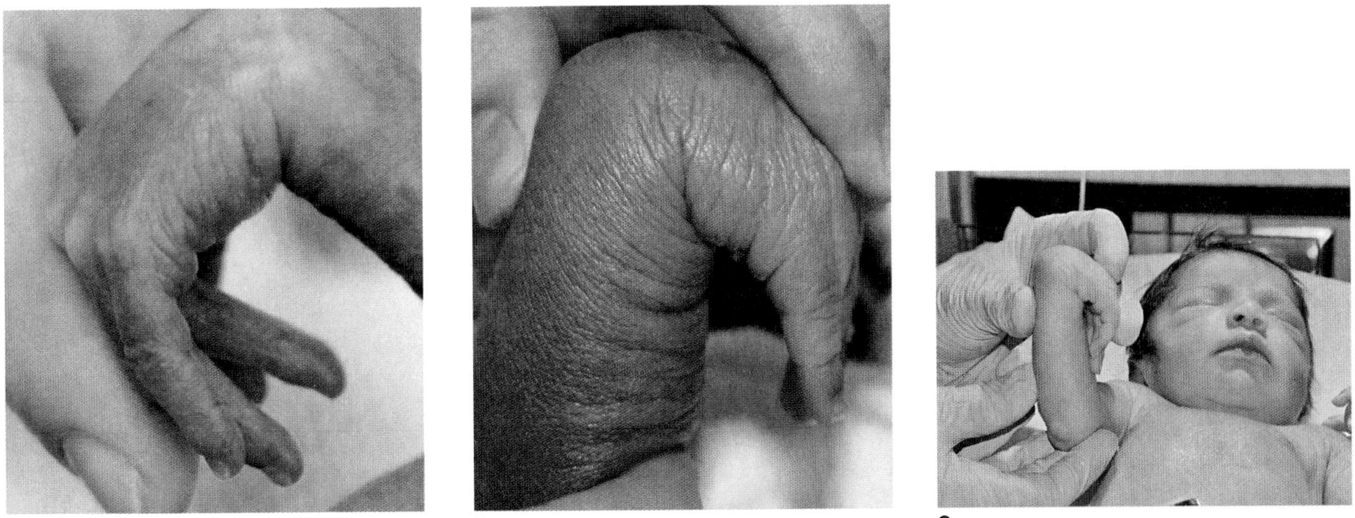

A B C

Figure 27–8 **Square window sign. A. This angle is 90 degrees and suggests an immature newborn of 28 to 32 weeks' gestation. Score 0. B. A 30- to 40-degree angle is commonly found in newborns from 38 to 40 weeks' gestation. Score 2–3. C. A 0- to 15-degree angle occurs in newborns from 40 to 42 weeks' gestation. Score 4.**

SOURCE: C. Vanessa Howell, RNC, MSN.

progresses from extensor tone to flexor tone and from lower to upper extremities as the neurologic system matures in a *caudocephalad* (tail-to-head) progression. The neuromuscular evaluation requires more manipulation and disturbances than the physical evaluation of the newborn. The neuromuscular evaluation is best performed when the baby has stabilized. The following characteristics are evaluated:

1. The *square window sign* is elicited by flexing the baby's hand toward the ventral forearm until resistance is felt. The angle formed at the wrist is measured (Figure 27–8).
2. *Recoil* is a test of flexion development. Because flexion first develops in the lower extremities, recoil is first tested in the legs. The nurse places the newborn on his or her back on a flat surface. With a hand on the newborn's knees and while manipulating the hip joint, the nurse places the baby's legs in flexion, and then extends them parallel to each other and flat on the surface. The response to this maneuver is recoil of the newborn's legs. According to gestational age, they may not move, or they may return slowly or quickly to the flexed position. Preterm newborns have less muscle tone than term newborns, so preterm babies have less recoil.

   Arm recoil is tested by flexion at the elbow and extension of the arms at the newborn's side. While the baby is in the supine position, the nurse completely flexes both elbows, holds them in this position for 5 seconds, extends the arms at the baby's side, and releases them. Upon release, the elbows of a full-term newborn form an angle of less than 90 degrees and rapidly recoil back to a flexed position (Figure 27–9). The elbows of preterm newborns have slower recoil time and form a greater than 90-degree angle. Arm recoil is also slower in healthy but fatigued newborns after birth; therefore, arm recoil is best elicited after the first hour of birth, when the baby has had time to recover from the stress of birth. The deep sleep state also decreases the arm recoil response. Assessment of arm recoil should be bilateral to rule out brachial palsy.
3. The *popliteal angle* (degree of knee flexion) is determined with the newborn flat on his or her back. The thigh is flexed on the abdomen and chest, and the nurse places the index finger of the other hand behind the newborn's ankle to extend the lower leg until resistance is met. The angle formed is then measured. Results vary from no resistance in the very immature newborn to an 80-degree angle in the term newborn.

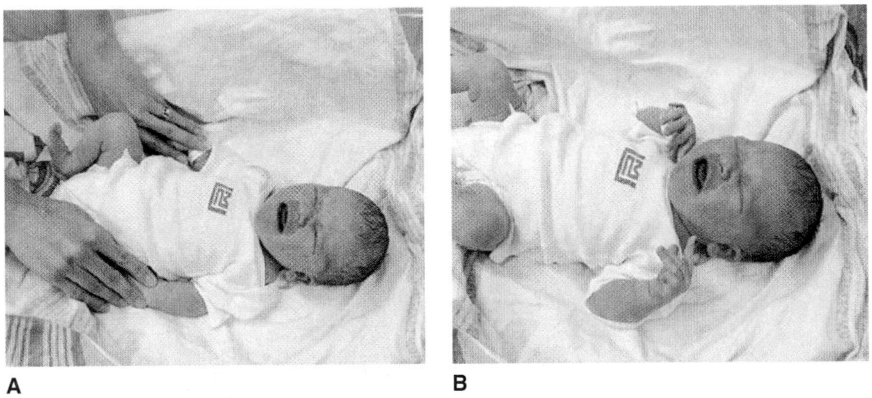

A B

Figure 27–9 **Arm recoil. A. Extend arms at elbows. B. Release arms to see recoil.**

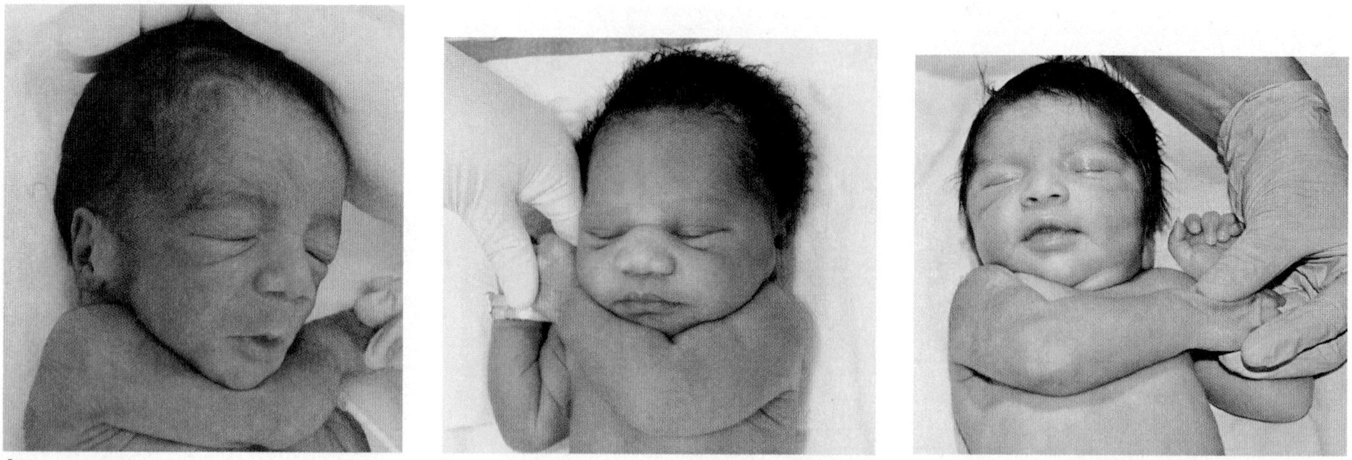

Figure 27–10 **Scarf sign. A. No resistance is noted until after 30 weeks' gestation. The elbow can be readily moved past the midline. Score 1. B. The elbow is at midline at 36 to 40 weeks' gestation. Score 2. C. Beyond 40 weeks' gestation, the elbow will not reach the midline. Score 4.**

SOURCE: C. Vanessa Howell, RN, MSN, NNP-BC.

4. The *scarf sign* is elicited by placing the newborn supine and drawing an arm across the chest toward the newborn's opposite shoulder until resistance is met. The location of the elbow is then noted in relation to the midline of the chest (Figure 27–10). A preterm newborn's elbow will cross the midline of the chest, whereas a full term newborn's elbow will not cross midline.
5. The *heel-to-ear extension* is performed by placing the newborn in a supine position and then gently drawing the foot toward the ear on the same side until resistance is felt (Figure 27–11). The nurse should allow the knee to bend during the test. It is important to hold the buttocks down to keep from rolling the baby. Both the proximity of foot to ear and degree of knee extension are assessed. The leg of a preterm, immature newborn remains straight and the foot goes to the ear or beyond. With advancing gestational age, the newborn demonstrates increasing resistance to this maneuver. Maneuvers involving the lower extremities of newborns who had frank breech presentation should be delayed to allow for resolution of leg positioning.
6. *Ankle dorsiflexion* is determined by flexing the ankle on the shin. The nurse uses a thumb to push on the sole of the newborn's foot while the fingers support the back of the leg. Then the angle formed by the foot and the interior leg is measured (Figure 27–12). This sign can be influenced by intrauterine position and congenital deformities.
7. *Head lag* (neck flexors) is measured by pulling the baby to a sitting position and noting the degree of head lag. Total lag is common in newborns up to 34 weeks' gestation, whereas the postmature newborn (42 or more weeks) will hold the head in front of the body line. Full-term newborns are able to support their heads momentarily.
8. *Ventral suspension* (horizontal position) is evaluated by holding the newborn prone on the examiner's hand. The position of head and back and degree of flexion in the arms and legs are then noted. Some flexion of arms and legs indicates 36 to 38 weeks' gestation; fully flexed extremities, with head and back even, are characteristic of a term newborn.

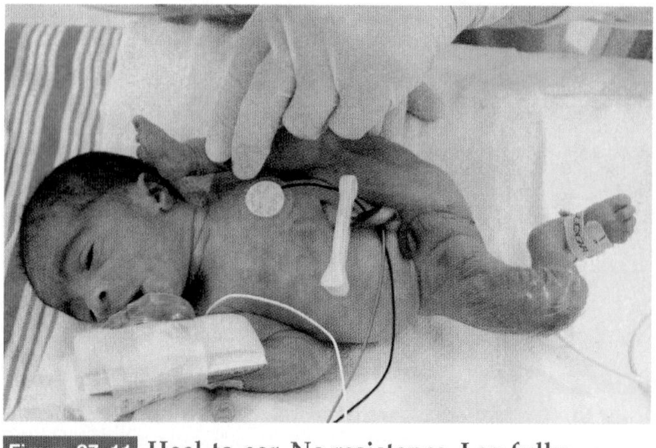

Figure 27–11 **Heel-to-ear. No resistance. Leg fully extended. Score 0.**

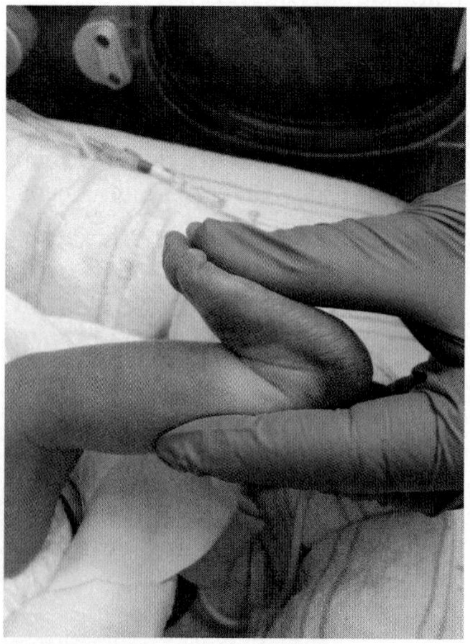

Figure 27–12 **Ankle dorsiflexion. A 45-degree angle indicates 32 to 36 weeks' gestation.**

SOURCE: Carol Harrigan, RNC, MSN, NNP-BC.

9. Major reflexes such as sucking, rooting, grasping, Moro, tonic neck, and others are also evaluated during the newborn exam. These reflexes are discussed later in the chapter and are shown in Table 27–1.

A supplementary method for estimating gestational age (done by the physician or nurse practitioner) is to view the vascular network of the cornea with an ophthalmoscope. The nurse should delay administration of prophylactic eye ointment until

TABLE 27–1 Common Newborn Reflexes

Tonic neck reflex (fencer position). Elicited when the newborn is supine and the head is turned to one side. In response, the extremities on the same side straighten, whereas on the opposite side they flex. This reflex may not be seen during the early newborn period, but once it appears it persists until about the third month.

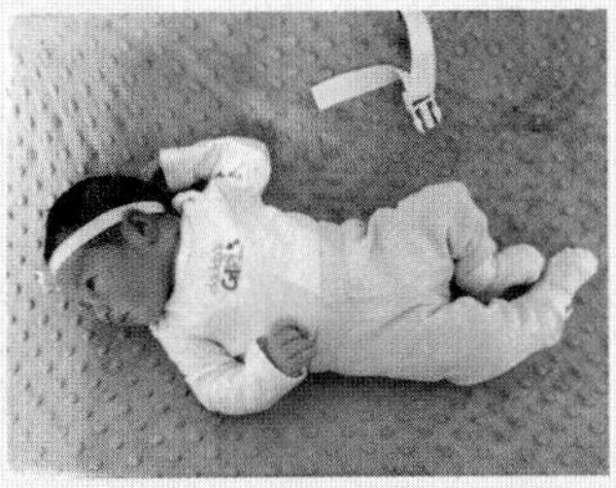

Tonic neck reflex.

SOURCE: Craig London.

Palmar grasping reflex. Elicited by stimulating the newborn's palm with a finger or object; the newborn grasps and holds the object or finger firmly enough to be lifted momentarily from the crib.

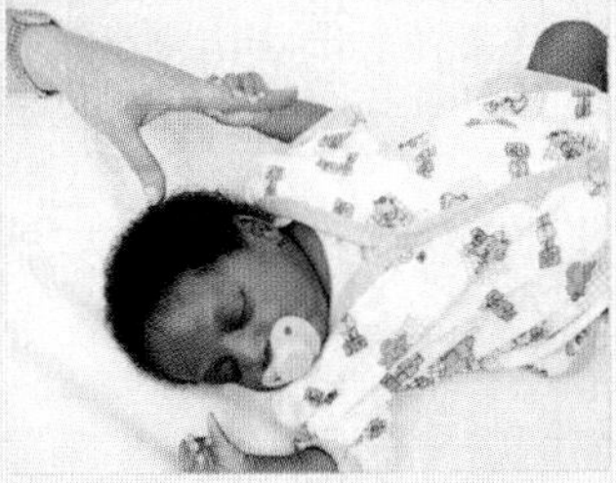

Palmar grasping reflex.

Moro reflex. Elicited when the newborn is startled by a loud noise or lifted slightly above the crib and then suddenly lowered. In response, the newborn straightens arms and hands outward while the knees flex. Slowly the arms return to the chest, as in an embrace. The fingers spread, forming a C, and the newborn may cry. This reflex may persist until about 6 months of age.

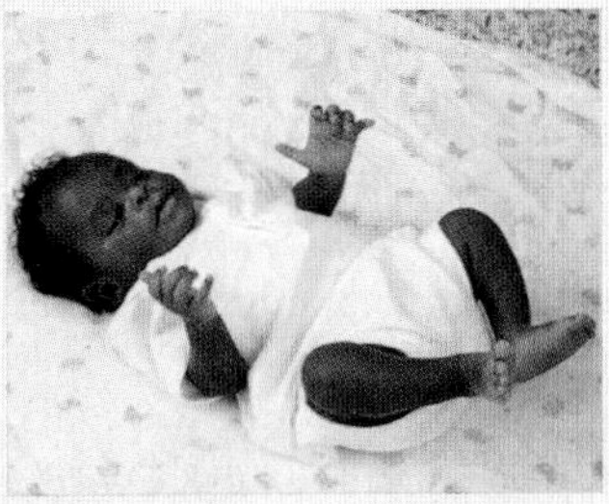

Moro reflex.

Rooting reflex. Elicited when the side of the newborn's mouth or cheek is touched. In response, the newborn turns toward that side and opens the lips to suck (if not fed recently).

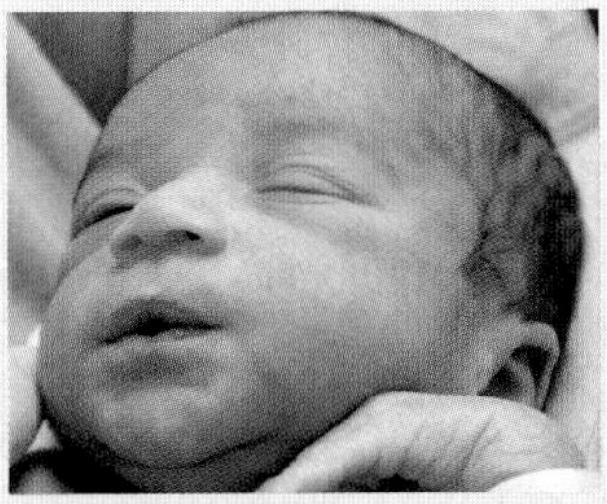

Rooting reflex.

Sucking reflex. Elicited when an object is placed in the newborn's mouth or anything touches the lips. Newborns suck even while sleeping; this is called *nonnutritive sucking*, and it can have a quieting effect on the baby. Disappears by 12 months.

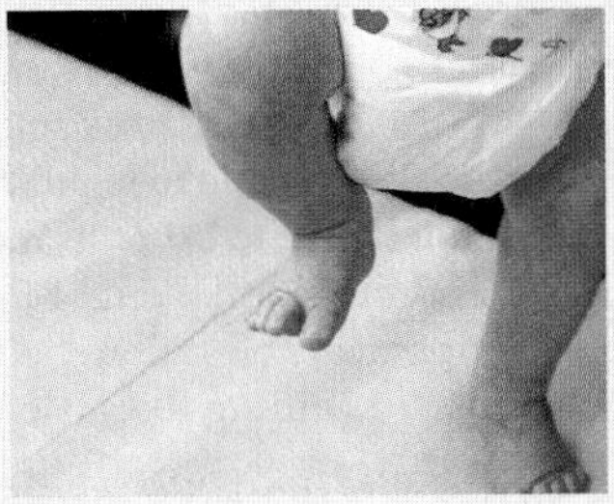

Sucking reflex.

SOURCE: Michele Davidson.

Stepping reflex. When held upright with one foot touching a flat surface, the newborn puts one foot in front of the other and "walks." This reflex is more pronounced at birth and is lost in 4 to 8 weeks.

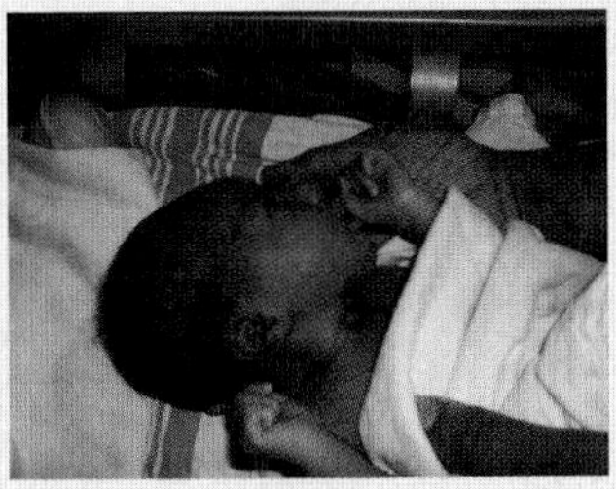

Stepping reflex.

SOURCE: Michele Davidson.

after the eye exam. The amount of vascularity present over the surface of the lens has excellent correlation with newborns of 27 through 34 weeks' gestational age. In babies less than 27 weeks' gestation, the cornea is cloudy, and the vascular network is not visible; after 34 weeks' gestation the vascular network has generally disappeared completely.

When the gestational age determination and birth weight are considered together, the newborn can be identified as one whose growth is:

- *Small for gestational age (SGA)* (below the 10th percentile)
- *Appropriate for gestational age (AGA)*
- *Large for gestational age (LGA)* (above the 90th percentile).

The nurse also plots the gestational age against the newborn's length, head circumference, and weight on the appropriate growth chart to determine if these measurements fall within the average range—the 10th to 90th percentile for the corresponding gestational age. These correlations further document the level of maturity and appropriate category for the newborn. (See Chapter 30 for further discussion of the various gestational age newborns.)

This determination (Figure 27–13) enables the nurse to anticipate possible physiologic problems. The growth information is used in conjunction with a complete physical examination to establish a plan of care appropriate for the individual newborn. For example, an SGA newborn often requires frequent glucose monitoring and early feedings. See Chapter 30 for a discussion of these categories and their potential problems.

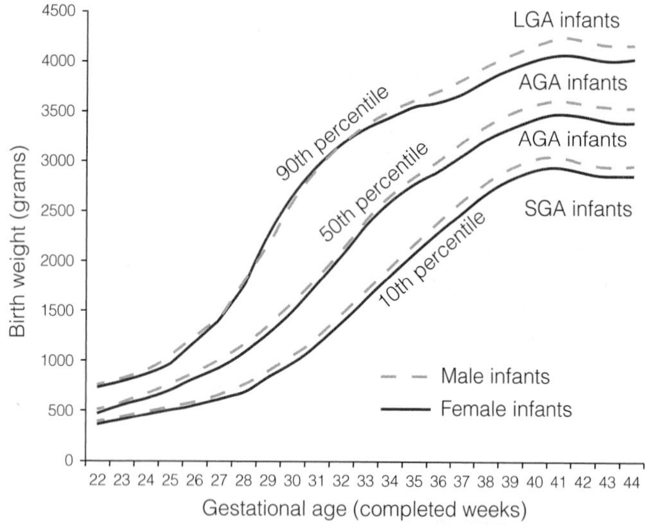

Figure 27–13 Select reference percentiles for birth weight at each gestational age from 22 to 44 completed weeks for male and female singleton newborns: 10th, 50th, and 90th percentiles. Data from 3,423,215 male and 3,267,502 female newborns in the 1999–2000 U.S. Natality datasets.

SOURCE: Oken, E., Kleinman, K. P., Rich-Edwards, J., & Gillman, M. W. (2003). A nearly continuous measure of birth weight for gestational age using a United States national reference. *BMC Pediatrics, 3,* 6. Retrieved from https://www.biomedcentral.com/1471-2431/3/6 © 2003 Oken et al.; licensee BioMed Central Ltd. This is an open access article: Verbatim copying and redistribution of this article are permitted in all media for any purpose, provided this notice is preserved along with the article's original URL.

Physical Assessment

After the initial determination of gestational age and related potential problems, the nurse carries out a more extensive physical assessment in a warm, well-lighted area that is free of drafts. Completing the physical assessment in the presence of the parents provides an opportunity to acquaint them with their newborn. The examination is performed in a systematic, head-to-toe manner, and all findings are recorded. When assessing the physical and neurologic status of the newborn, the nurse should first consider general appearance and then proceed to specific areas.

Assessment Guide: Newborn Physical Assessment, at the end of this chapter, outlines how to systematically assess the newborn. Normal findings, alterations, and related causes are presented and correlated with suggested nursing responses. The findings are typical for a full-term newborn.

General Appearance

The newborn's head is disproportionately large for the body. The neck looks short because the chin rests on the chest. Newborns have a prominent abdomen, sloping shoulders, narrow hips, and a rounded chest. The center of the baby's body is the umbilicus rather than the symphysis pubis, as in the adult. The body appears long and the extremities short.

Newborns tend to stay in a flexed position similar to the one maintained in utero and will offer resistance when the extremities are straightened. The flexed position that the newborn maintains contributes to the short appearance of the extremities. The hands are tightly clenched. After a breech birth, the feet are usually dorsiflexed, and it may take several weeks for the newborn to assume typical newborn posture.

Weight and Measurements

The normal full-term Caucasian newborn of European ancestry has an average birth weight of 3405 g (7 lb, 8 oz). Newborns of African, Asian, and Hispanic heritage are usually somewhat smaller at term. Other factors that influence weight are age and size of parents, health of mother (smoking and malnutrition decrease birth weight), and the interval between pregnancies (short intervals, such as every year, result in lower birth weight). After the first week and for the first 6 months, the newborn's weight will increase about 198 g (7 oz) weekly.

Approximately 70 to 75% of the newborn's body weight is water. During the initial newborn period (the first 3 or 4 days), term newborns have a physiologic weight loss of about 5 to 10% because of fluid shifts. This weight loss may reach 15% for preterm newborns. Large babies tend to lose more weight because of greater fluid loss in proportion to birth weight. If weight loss is greater than 10%, clinical reappraisal is necessary. Factors contributing to weight loss include small fluid intake resulting from delayed breastfeeding or a slow adjustment to formula, increased volume of meconium excreted, and urination. Weight loss may be marked in the presence of temperature elevation (because of associated dehydration) or consistent chilling (because of nonshivering thermogenesis).

The length of the normal newborn is difficult to measure because the legs are flexed and tensed. To measure length, the nurse should place newborns flat on their backs with legs extended as much as possible (Figure 27–14). The average length is 50 cm (20 in.), with the range being 46 to 56 cm (18 to 22 in.).

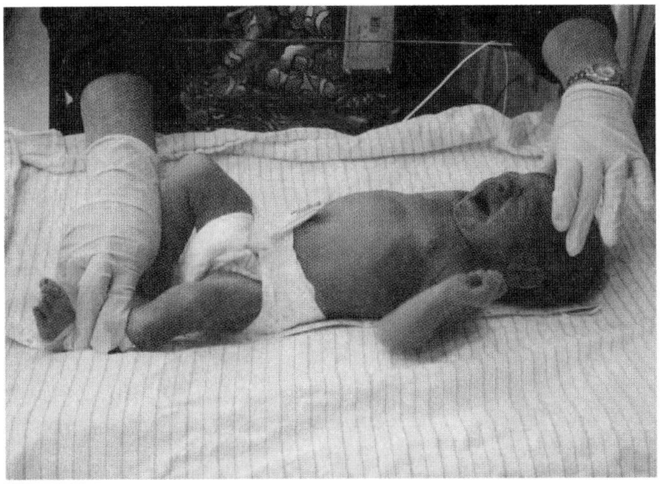

Figure 27–14 Measuring the length of the newborn.

The newborn will grow approximately 2.5 cm (1 in.) a month for the next 6 months. This is the period of most rapid growth.

At birth the newborn's head is one-fourth the size of an adult's head. The circumference of the newborn's head is 32 to 37 cm (12.6 to 14.6 in.). For accurate measurement, the nurse places the tape over the most prominent part of the occiput and brings it to just above the eyebrows (Figure 27–15A). The circumference of the newborn's head is approximately 2 cm (0.8 in.) greater than the circumference of the newborn's chest at birth and will remain in this proportion for the next few months. (Factors that alter this measurement are discussed under the *Head* section.) It is best to take another head circumference measurement on the second day if the newborn experienced significant head molding or caput from the birth process.

The average circumference of the chest at birth is 32 cm (12.6 in.) and ranges from 30 to 35 cm (11.8 to 13.4 in.). Chest measurements should be taken with the tape measure at the lower edge of the scapulas and brought around anteriorly directly over the nipple line (Figure 27–15B). The abdominal circumference or girth may also be measured at this time by placing the tape around the newborn's abdomen at the level of the umbilicus, with the bottom edge of the tape at the top edge of the umbilicus. Newborn measurements are summarized in *Key Facts to Remember: Newborn Measurements.*

Temperature

Initial assessment of the newborn's temperature is critical. In utero the temperature of the fetus is about the same as, or slightly higher than, the expectant mother's. When babies enter the outside world, their temperatures can suddenly drop as a result of exposure to cold drafts and the skin's heat-loss mechanisms.

If no heat conservation measures are initiated, the normal term newborn's core temperature falls 0.1°C (0.2°F) per minute; skin temperature decreases 0.3°C (0.5°F) per minute. Skin temperature markedly decreases within 10 minutes after exposure to room air. The temperature should stabilize within 8 to 12 hours. Temperature should be monitored when the newborn is admitted to the nursery and at least every 30 minutes until the newborn's status has remained stable for 2 hours (American Academy of Pediatrics [AAP] & American College of Obstetricians and Gynecologists [ACOG], 2017).

Thereafter the nurse should assess temperature at least once every 8 hours or according to institutional policy. In newborns who have been exposed to group B hemolytic streptococcus, more frequent temperature monitoring may be required. (See Chapter 26 for a discussion of the physiology of temperature regulation.)

Temperature can be assessed by the axillary skin method, by a continuous skin probe, or via the rectal route. Axillary temperature reflects body (core) temperature and the body's compensatory response to the thermal environment. Axillary temperatures are the preferred method and are considered to be a close estimation of the rectal temperature. In preterm and term newborns there is less than 0.1°C (0.2°F) difference between the two sites, and the axillary method is preferred. If the axillary method is used, the thermometer must remain in place at least 3 minutes, unless an electronic thermometer is used (Figure 27–16). Axillary temperature ranges from 36.5°C to 37.2°C (97.7°F to 99°F). Keep in mind that axillary temperatures can be misleading because the friction caused by apposition of the inner arm skin and upper chest wall and the nearness of brown fat to the probe may elevate the temperature.

Skin temperature is measured most accurately by continuous skin probe, especially for small newborns or newborns maintained in incubators or under radiant warmers. Normal skin temperature is 36°C to 36.5°C (96.8°F to 97.7°F). Assessing skin temperature allows time for interventions to be initiated before a more serious fall in core temperature occurs (Figure 27–17).

Rectal temperature is assumed to be the closest approximation to core temperature, but the accuracy of this method depends on the depth to which the thermometer is inserted. Normal rectal temperature is 36.6°C to 37.2°C (97.8°F to 99°F). The rectal route

Key Facts To Remember
Newborn Measurements

Weight	Length	Head Circumference	Chest Circumference
Average: 3405 g (7 lb, 8 oz)	Average: 50 cm (20 in.)	Average: 33–35 cm (13–14 in.)	Average: 32 cm (12.6 in.)
Range: 2500–4000 g (5 lb, 8 oz to 8 lb, 13 oz) Weight is influenced by a variety of factors and maternal age and size. Physiologic weight loss: 5–10% for term newborns, up to 15% for preterm newborns Growth: 198 g (7 oz) per week for first 6 months	Range: 46–56 cm (18–22 in.) Growth: 2.5 cm (1 in.) per month for first 6 months	Range: 32–37 cm (12.6–14.6 in.) Approximately 2 cm larger than chest circumference	Range: 30–35 cm (11.8–13.4 in.)

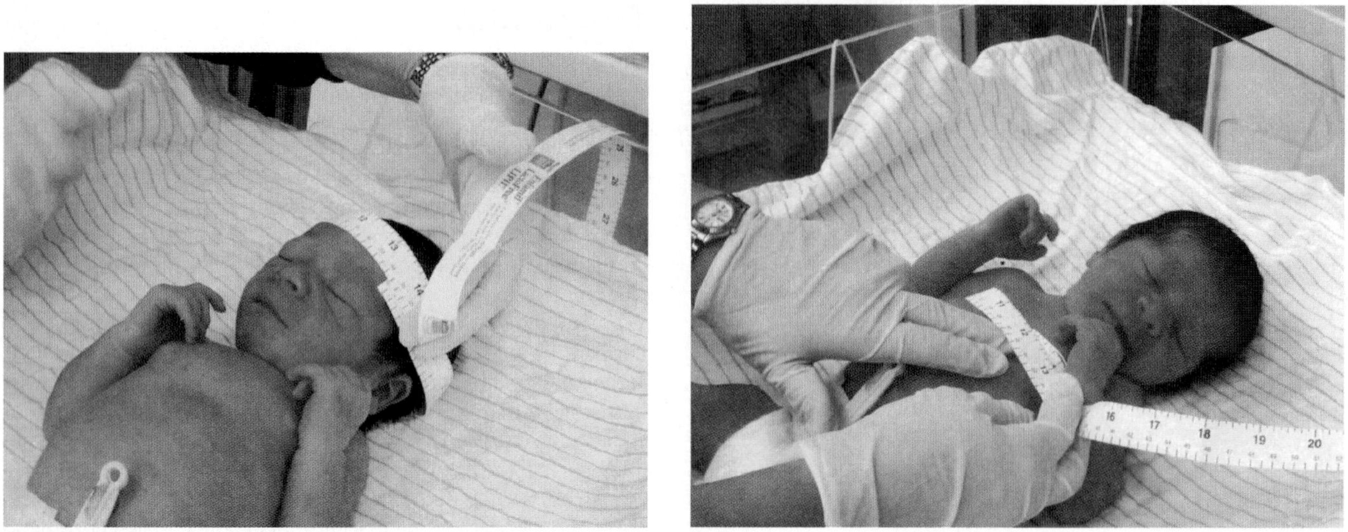

A B

Figure 27–15 A. Measuring the head circumference of the newborn. B. Measuring the chest circumference of the newborn.

is *not recommended* as a routine method unless done with a digital or electronic thermometer (AAP, 2015).

Temperature instability, a deviation of more than 1°C (2°F) from one reading to the next, or a subnormal temperature may indicate an infection. In contrast with an elevated temperature in older children, an increased temperature in a newborn may indicate a reaction to too many blankets, too hot a room, or dehydration. Dehydration, which tends to increase body temperature, occurs in newborns whose feedings have been delayed for any reason. Newborns respond to overheating (temperature greater than 37.5°C [99.5°F]) by increased restlessness and eventually by perspiration after 35 to 40 minutes of exposure. The perspiration is initially seen on the head and face, and then on the chest.

Many newborns initially cannot perspire, so they increase their respiratory and heart rates, which increases oxygen consumption. Whether the initial temperature is elevated or subnormal, the newborn must maintain a stable temperature per agency protocol before leaving the nursery. See *Developing Cultural Competence: Keeping Newborns Warm.*

Clinical Tip

Measuring weight and height often aggravates newborns and may alter their vital signs. For better accuracy, take the newborn's vital signs before weighing and measuring. In addition, assess the respiratory rate and heart rate before taking the temperature.

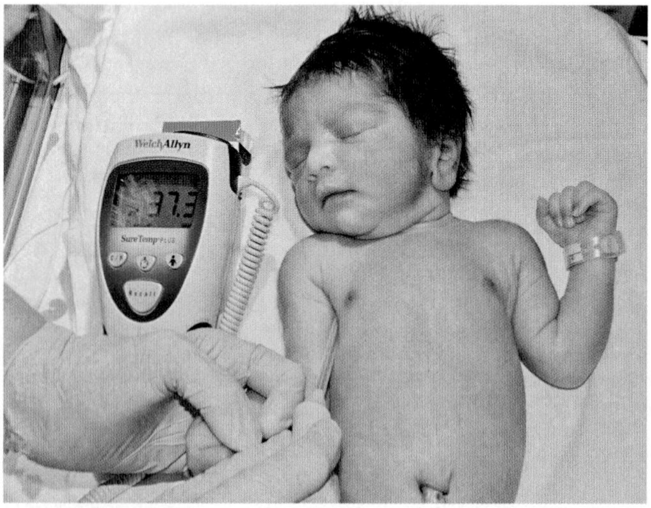

Figure 27–16 Axillary temperature measurement. The axillary temperature should be taken for 3 minutes. The newborn's arm should be tightly but gently pressed against the thermometer and the newborn's side, as illustrated.

SOURCE: Vanessa Howell, RN, MSN, NNP-BC.

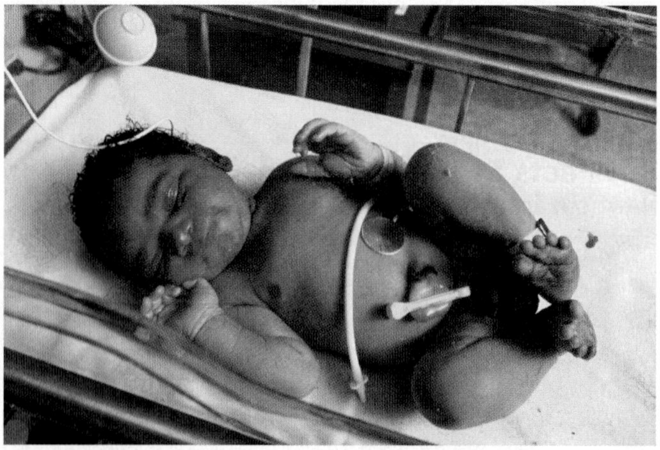

Figure 27–17 Temperature monitoring for the newborn. A skin thermal sensor is placed on the newborn's abdomen, upper thigh, or arm and secured with porous tape or a foil-covered foam pad.

SOURCE: Tom McCarthy/PhotoEdit.

Developing Cultural Competence Keeping Newborns Warm

In the Latino culture and others, parents may be overly concerned about keeping their newborn baby warm. Parents should be informed that overdressing babies while they are sleeping is related to a higher risk of sudden infant death syndrome and that bundling them excessively can be uncomfortable and lead to heat rash.

Note: It is unwise to attribute specific attitudes or beliefs to all members of a cultural group. The information in the Developing Cultural Competence boxes offers possible insights into caring for women from different cultural groups.

Skin Characteristics

Although the newborn's skin color varies with genetic background, all healthy newborns have a pink tinge to their skin. The ruddy hue results from increased red blood cell concentration in the blood vessels and from limited subcutaneous fat deposits.

Skin pigmentation is slight in the newborn period, so color changes may be seen even in darker-skinned babies. Caucasian American newborns have a pinkish-red skin tone a few hours after birth, and newborns of African descent have a skin color that is reddish-brown to pale pink, sometimes tinged with yellow. Newborns of Hispanic and Asian heritage can have a pink or rosy red to olive or yellow skin tone. Skin pigmentation deepens over time; therefore variations in skin color indicating illness are more difficult to evaluate in African American and Asian American newborns (Eichenwald et al., 2017).

A newborn who is cyanotic at rest and pink only when crying may have choanal atresia (congenital blockage of the passageway between the nose and pharynx). If crying increases the cyanosis, heart or lung problems should be suspected. Very pale newborns may be anemic or have *hypovolemia* (low blood volume and blood pressure [BP]) and should be evaluated for these problems.

Acrocyanosis (bluish discoloration of the hands and feet) may be present in the first 24 hours after birth (Figure 27–18). This condition is due to poor peripheral circulation, which results in vasomotor instability and capillary stasis, especially when the baby is exposed to cold. If the central circulation is adequate, the blood supply should return quickly (2 to 3 seconds) to the extremity after the skin is blanched with a finger. Blue hands and nails are a poor indicator of oxygenation in a newborn. The face and mucous membranes should be assessed for pinkness, reflecting adequate oxygenation.

Mottling (lacy pattern of dilated blood vessels under the skin) occurs as a result of general circulation fluctuations. It may last several hours to several weeks or may come and go periodically. Mottling may be related to chilling, prolonged apnea, sepsis, or hypothyroidism.

Harlequin sign (clown) color change is occasionally noted. A deep color develops over one side of the newborn's body while the other side remains pale, so that the skin resembles a clown's suit. This color change comes from the immaturity of the hypothalamic center and results in vasomotor disturbance in which blood vessels on one side dilate while the vessels on the other side constrict (Witt, 2019). It usually lasts from 1 to 30 minutes. Affected newborns may have single or multiple episodes, but they are transient and clinically insignificant. The nurse should document its occurrence (Figure 27–19).

Jaundice (yellowish discoloration of skin and mucous membranes) is first detectable on the face (where skin overlies cartilage) and the mucous membranes of the mouth (Eichenwald et al., 2017). Evaluation and determination of the cause of jaundice must be initiated immediately to prevent possibly serious sequelae. The jaundice may be related to immature liver function, hematomas, or poor feeding. It may also be caused by blood incompatibility, oxytocin (Pitocin) augmentation or induction, or a severe hemolysis process. Any jaundice noted before 24 hours of age should be reported to the healthcare provider. Breastfeeding is a possible cause of late-onset jaundice. See *Clinical Skill 27–1: Assessing Jaundice in the Newborn*. For a detailed discussion of the causes, assessment, and treatment of jaundice, see Chapter 31.

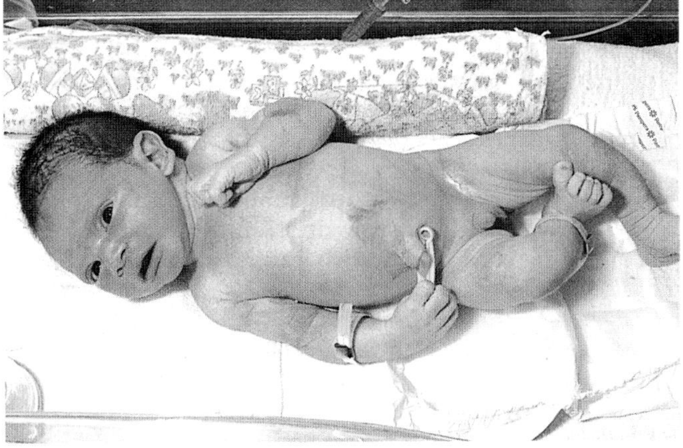

Figure 27–18 Acrocyanosis.

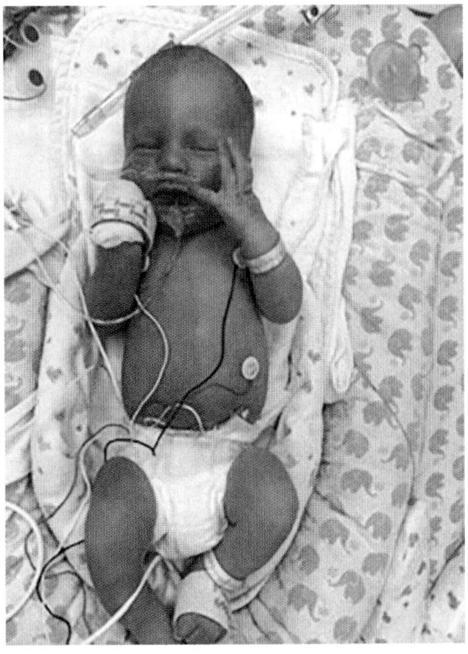

Figure 27–19 Harlequin sign.

SOURCE: Carol Harrigan, RNC, MSN, NNP-BC.

Clinical Skill 27–1

Assessing Jaundice in the Newborn

NURSING ACTION

Preparation

- Wash hands.
- Assemble equipment.

Equipment and Supplies

- Transcutaneous bilimeter

Procedure

1. Observe newborn in a well-lit room or near a window during daylight hours. Baby should be specifically checked for jaundice at least twice a shift or with every assessment.
2. Blanch skin on forehead, sternum, or gum line with digital pressure for 1 second and release. Observe for underlying yellow tinge to skin. If jaundice is observed on the sternum, also check palms and soles, and blanch skin below the knee. Another area to assess for jaundice is the sclera (whites of the eyes) or the inner aspect of the cheek in darker-skinned newborns.

   Rationale: *Progression of jaundice is head to toe (cephalocaudal progression). Jaundice is first seen in the face and neck when levels reach 4 to 8 mg/dL. Jaundice can be seen on palmar and plantar surfaces at levels greater than 15 mg/dL. Visual assessment is often an inaccurate predictor of bilirubin levels. Jaundice regresses in the opposite direction.*

3. If the newborn appears jaundiced, a total serum bilirubin or a transcutaneous bilirubin (TcB) level should be checked. TcB levels are monitored with a transcutaneous bilimeter. The device should be used according to manufacturer directions and calibrated as directed. The TcB measurement is obtained from the forehead or the sternum and plotted on a nomogram. A total serum bilirubin (TSB) level is still required when treatment with phototherapy or an exchange transfusion is being considered.

   Rationale: *A transcutaneous or total serum bilirubin level should be checked on all newborns who appear jaundiced in the first 24 hours of life. A TcB is as reliable as a TSB in most instances and is less invasive. The hour-specific nomogram recommended by the AAP provides guidelines for initiating phototherapy in hospitalized newborns of 35 weeks or greater gestational age. Full-term newborns receive phototherapy for bilirubin levels greater than 12 mg/dL. The recommended treatment levels for premature newborns are dependent on postnatal age, weight, and contributing factors.*

4. Assessment of jaundice risk requires gathering information about hydration status to include how the newborn is being fed, feeding tolerance, amount of urine and stool, and weight. Hemoglobin (Hgb) and hematocrit (Hct) levels are also helpful.

   Rationale: *Newborns who are not eating well are more prone to hyperbilirubinemia. Babies born at high altitude develop higher levels of bilirubin than babies born at sea level (related to elevated hematocrit and hypoxemia).*

5. The nurse assesses the newborn for early signs of bilirubin encephalopathy, which include poor feeding, hypotonia, and lethargy.
6. Document any physical findings and TcB levels, and report jaundice to the primary care practitioner.

Erythema toxicum is an eruption of lesions in the area surrounding a hair follicle that are firm, vary in size from 1 to 3 mm, and consist of a white or pale yellow papule or pustule with an erythematous base. It is often called *newborn rash* or *flea bite dermatitis*. The rash may appear suddenly, usually over the trunk and diaper area, and is frequently widespread (Figure 27–20). The lesions do not appear on the palms of the hands or the soles of the feet. The peak incidence is at 24 to 48 hours of life. The condition rarely presents at birth or after 5 days of life. The cause is unknown, and no treatment is necessary. Some clinicians feel it may be caused by irritation from clothing. The lesions disappear in a few hours or days. If a maculopapular rash (eruption consisting of both macules and papules) appears, a smear of the aspirated papule will show numerous eosinophils on staining; no bacteria will be cultured.

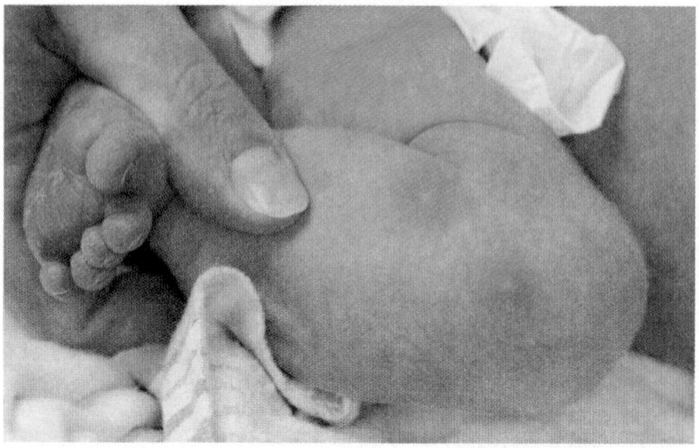

Figure 27–20 Erythema toxicum on leg.

Milia, which are exposed sebaceous glands, appear as raised white spots on the face, especially across the nose (Figure 27–21). No treatment is necessary because they will clear up spontaneously within the first month. Newborns of African heritage have a similar condition called *transient neonatal pustular melanosis*.

Skin turgor is assessed to determine hydration status, the need to initiate early feedings, and the presence of any infectious processes. The usual places to assess skin turgor are the abdomen, forearm, or thigh. Skin should be elastic and should return rapidly to its original shape.

Vernix caseosa, a whitish cheeselike substance, covers the fetus while in utero and lubricates the skin of the newborn. The skin of the term or postterm newborn has less vernix and is frequently dry; peeling is common, especially on the hands and feet.

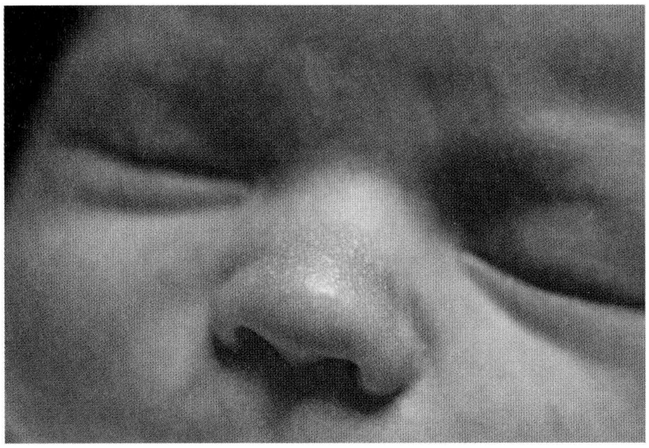

Figure 27–21 Facial milia over bridge of nose.

SOURCE: Jack Sullivan/Alamy Stock Photo.

Forceps marks may be present after a difficult forceps birth. The newborn may have reddened areas over the cheeks and jaws. It is important to reassure the parents that these will disappear, usually within 1 or 2 days. Transient facial paralysis resulting from the forceps pressure is a rare complication. Vacuum extractor suction marks on the vertex of the scalp are often seen when vacuum extractors are used to assist with the birth (Johnson, 2019). These are benign and do not indicate any underlying brain lesions.

Sucking blisters (vesicles or bullae) may appear on the lips, fingers, or hands of newborns as a result of vigorous sucking, either in utero or after birth. These sucking blisters (Figure 27–22) may be intact or ruptured and require no treatment.

Birthmarks

Telangiectatic nevi, sometimes called *stork bites*, appear as pale pink or red spots and are frequently found on the eyelids, nose, lower occipital bone, and nape of the neck (Figure 27–23). The lesions are common in light-complexioned newborns and are more noticeable during periods of crying. These areas have no clinical significance and usually fade by the second birthday.

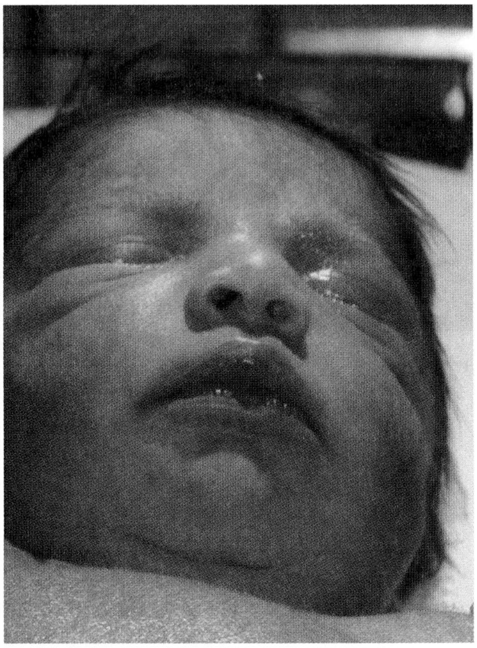

Figure 27–22 Sucking blister in middle of upper lip.

SOURCE: Vanessa Howell, RN, MSN, NNP-BC.

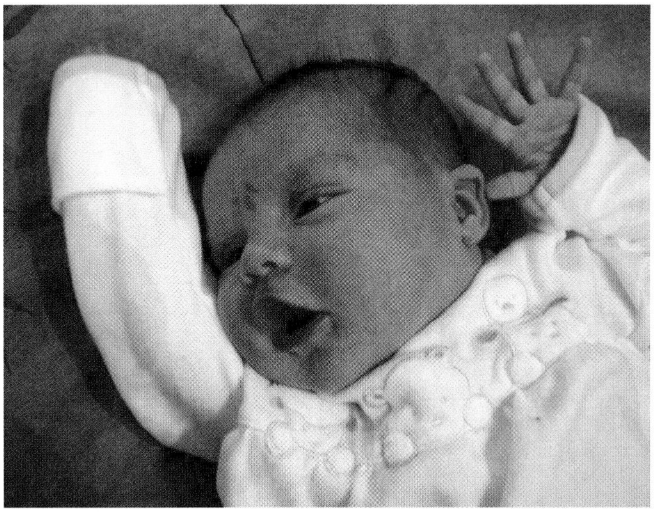

Figure 27–23 Stork bites over left eyelid and near right eyebrow.

SOURCE: Anne Garcia.

Congenital dermal melanocytosis, also called *Mongolian blue spots*, are macular areas of bluish-black or gray-blue pigmentation commonly found on the dorsal area and the buttocks but may be anywhere on the body (Figure 27–24). They are common in newborns of Asian, Hispanic, and African descent and can be seen in 1 to 9% of White newborns. They gradually fade during the first or second year of life. They may be mistaken for bruises and should be documented in the newborn's chart.

Nevus flammeus, also called *port wine stain*, is a capillary angioma directly below the epidermis. It is a nonelevated, sharply demarcated, red to purple area of dense capillaries (Figure 27–25). In newborns of African descent it may appear as a purple-black stain. The size and shape vary, but it commonly appears on the face. It does not grow in size, does not fade with time, and does not blanch as a rule. The birthmark may be concealed by using an opaque cosmetic cream. If convulsions and other neurologic problems accompany the nevus flammeus, the clinical picture is suggestive of *Sturge-Weber syndrome* with involvement of the fifth cranial nerve (the ophthalmic branch of the trigeminal nerve).

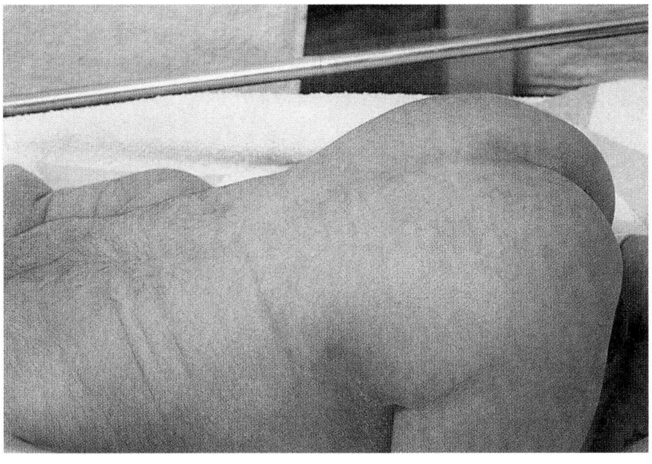

Figure 27–24 Mongolian spots.

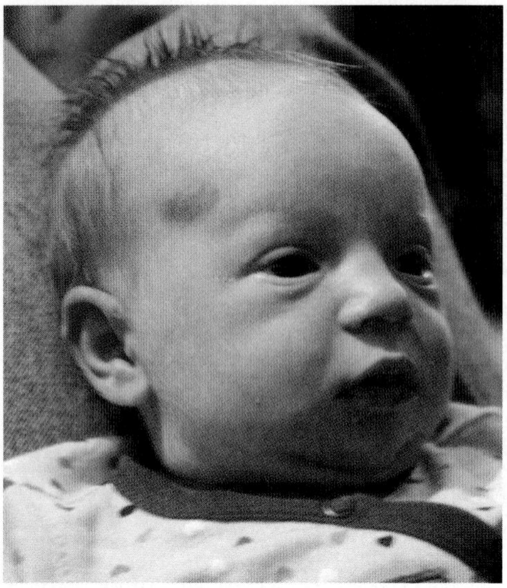

Figure 27-25 Port wine stain over temple area.

Nevus vasculosus, also called *strawberry mark,* is a capillary hemangioma. It consists of newly formed and enlarged capillaries in the dermal and subdermal layers. It is a raised, clearly delineated, dark red, rough-surfaced birthmark commonly found in the head region but can be anywhere on the body (Figure 27–26). Such marks usually begin to grow (often rapidly) during the second or third week of life and may not reach their full size until about 6 months of age (Witt, 2019). They begin to shrink and start to resolve spontaneously several weeks to months after they reach peak growth. A pale purple or gray spot on the surface of the hemangioma signals the start of resolution. The best cosmetic effect is achieved when the lesions are allowed to resolve spontaneously.

Clinical Tip

Birthmarks are frequently a cause of concern for parents. The mother may be especially anxious, fearing that she is to blame ("Is my baby marked because of something I did?"). Feelings of guilt are common in the presence of misconceptions about the cause. Birthmarks should be identified and explained to the parents. By providing appropriate information about the cause and course of birthmarks, the nurse frequently relieves the fears and anxieties of the family. The nurse should note any bruises, abrasions, or birthmarks seen on the newborn's admission to the nursery.

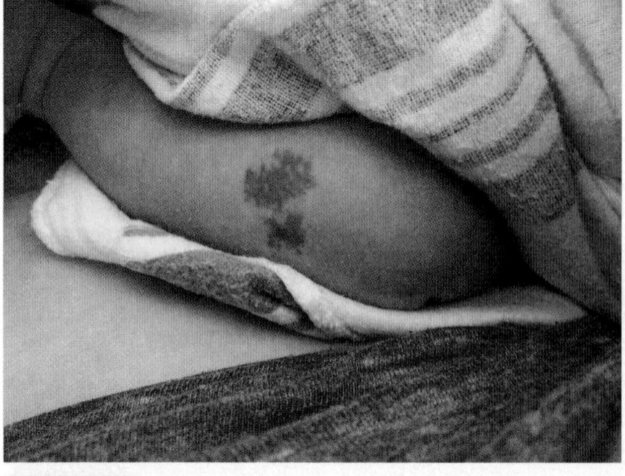

Figure 27-26 Nevus vasculosus, also called *strawberry mark,* on leg.

SOURCE: Craig London.

Head

GENERAL APPEARANCE

The newborn's head is large (approximately one-fourth of the body size), with soft, pliable skull bones. For most term newborns, the occipital-frontal circumference (OFC) is 32 to 37 cm (12.6 to 14.6 in.). The head may appear asymmetric in the newborn of a vertex presentation. This asymmetry, called **molding**, is caused by the overriding of the cranial bones during labor and birth (Figure 27–27). The degree of molding varies with the amount and length of pressure exerted on the head. Within a few days after birth, the overriding usually diminishes, and the suture lines become palpable. Because head measurements are affected by molding, a second measurement is indicated a few days after birth. The heads of breech-born newborns and those born by elective cesarean birth are characteristically round and well shaped because pressure was not exerted on them during birth. Any extreme differences in head size may indicate *microcephaly* (an abnormally small head) or *hydrocephalus* (an abnormal buildup of fluid in the brain). Variations in the shape, size, or appearance of the head may be due to *craniosynostosis* (premature closure of the cranial sutures), which needs to be corrected through surgery to allow brain growth, or *plagiocephaly* (asymmetry resulting in closure of sutures on one side caused by pressure on the fetal head during gestation) (Johnson, 2019).

Two *fontanelles* (also spelled *fontanels* and commonly called *soft spots*) may be palpated on the newborn's head. Fontanelles, which are openings at the juncture of the cranial bones, can be

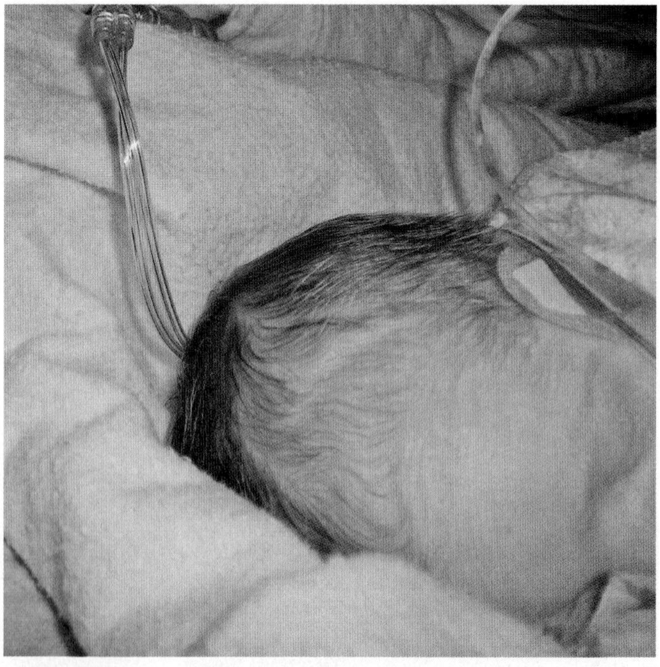

Figure 27-27 Overlapped cranial bones produce a visible ridge in a premature newborn. Easily visible overlapping does not occur often in term newborns.

SOURCE: Vanessa Howell, RN, MSN, NNP-BC.

measured with the fingers. Accurate measurement necessitates that the examiner's finger be measured in centimeters. The assessment should be carried out with the newborn in sitting position and not crying. The diamond-shaped *anterior fontanelle* is 3 to 4 cm (1.2 to 1.6 in.) long by 2 to 3 cm (0.8 to 1.2 in.) wide. It is located at the juncture of the frontal and parietal bones. The *posterior fontanelle,* smaller and triangular, is formed by the parietal bones and the occipital bone and is 0.5 cm by 1 cm. Because of molding, the fontanelles tend to be smaller immediately after birth than several days later. The anterior fontanelle closes within 18 months, whereas the posterior fontanelle closes within 2 to 3 months.

The fontanelles are a useful indicator of the newborn's condition. The anterior fontanelle may swell when the newborn cries or passes a stool or may pulsate with the heartbeat, which is normal. A bulging fontanelle usually signifies increased intracranial pressure, and a depressed fontanelle indicates dehydration. The sutures between the cranial bones should be palpated for amount of overlap. In newborns whose growth has been restricted, the sutures may be wider than normal, and the fontanelle may also be larger because of impaired fetal growth of the cranial bones. In addition to being inspected for degree of molding and size, the head should be evaluated for soft-tissue edema and bruising.

CEPHALOHEMATOMA

Cephalohematoma is a collection of blood resulting from ruptured blood vessels between the surface of a cranial bone (usually parietal) and the periosteal membrane (Figure 27–28). The scalp in these areas feels loose and slightly edematous. These areas emerge as defined hematomas between the first and second days. Although external pressure may cause the mass to fluctuate, it does not increase in size when the newborn cries. Cephalohematomas may be unilateral or bilateral and do not cross suture lines. They are relatively common in vertex births and disappear within 2 weeks to 3 months. They may be associated with physiologic jaundice because there are extra red blood cells being destroyed within the cephalohematoma. A large cephalohematoma can lead to anemia and hypotension.

CAPUT SUCCEDANEUM

Caput succedaneum is a localized, easily identifiable soft area of the scalp, generally resulting from a long and difficult labor or vacuum extraction (Figure 27–29). The sustained pressure of the presenting part against the cervix results in compression of local blood vessels, and venous return is slowed. Slowed venous return causes an increase in tissue fluids, an edematous swelling, and occasional bleeding under the periosteum. The caput may vary from a small area to a large area covering a severely elongated head. The fluid in the caput is reabsorbed within 12 hours to a few days after birth. Caputs resulting from vacuum extractors are sharply outlined, circular areas up to 2 cm (0.8 in.) thick. They disappear more slowly than naturally occurring edema. See *Key Facts to Remember: Comparison of Cephalohematoma and Caput Succedaneum*. See *Case Study: Angelina Newman*.

Hair

The term newborn's hair is smooth with texture variations depending on ethnic background. Scalp hair is usually high over the eyebrows. Assessment of the newborn's hair characteristics—such as color, quantity, hairlines, direction of growth, and hair whorls—can identify genetic, metabolic, and neurologic disorders (Johnson, 2019). For example, coarse, brittle, and dry hair may indicate hypothyroidism.

Face

The newborn's face is well designed to help the newborn suckle. Sucking (fat) pads are located in the cheeks and a labial tubercle (sucking callus) is frequently found in the center of the upper lip.

Key Facts To Remember
Comparison of Cephalohematoma and Caput Succedaneum

Cephalohematoma	Caput Succedaneum
Collection of blood between cranial (usually parietal) bone and periosteal membrane	Collection of fluid, edematous swelling of the scalp
Does not cross suture lines	Crosses suture lines
Appears between first and second day	Present at birth or shortly thereafter
Disappears after 2 to 3 weeks or may take months	Reabsorbed within 12 hours or a few days after birth

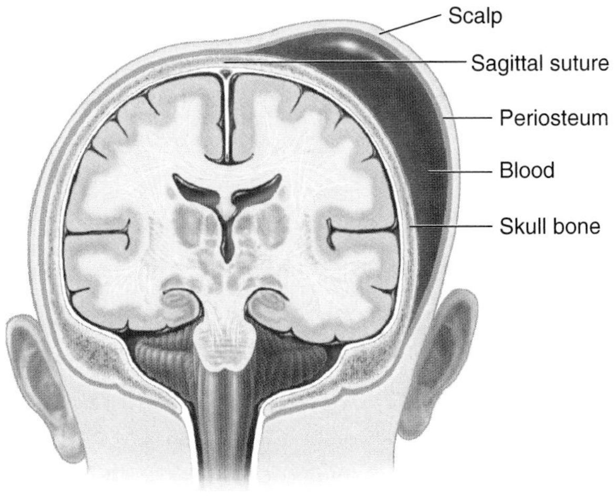

A

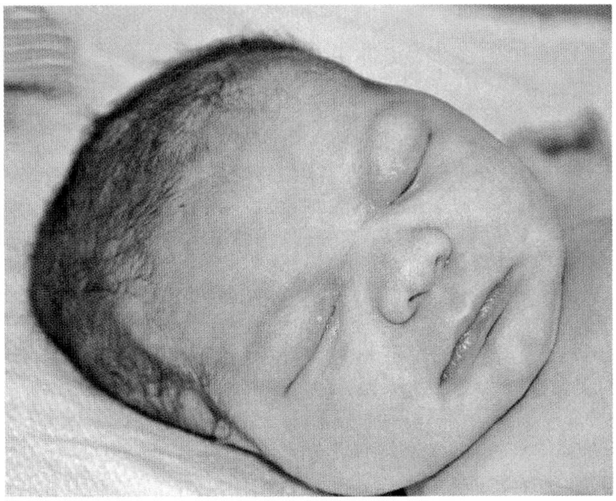

B

Figure 27–28 A. Cephalohematoma is a collection of blood between the surface of a cranial bone and the periosteal membrane. B. This is a cephalohematoma over the right parietal bone.

SOURCE: B. Vanessa Howell, RN, MSN, NNP-BC.

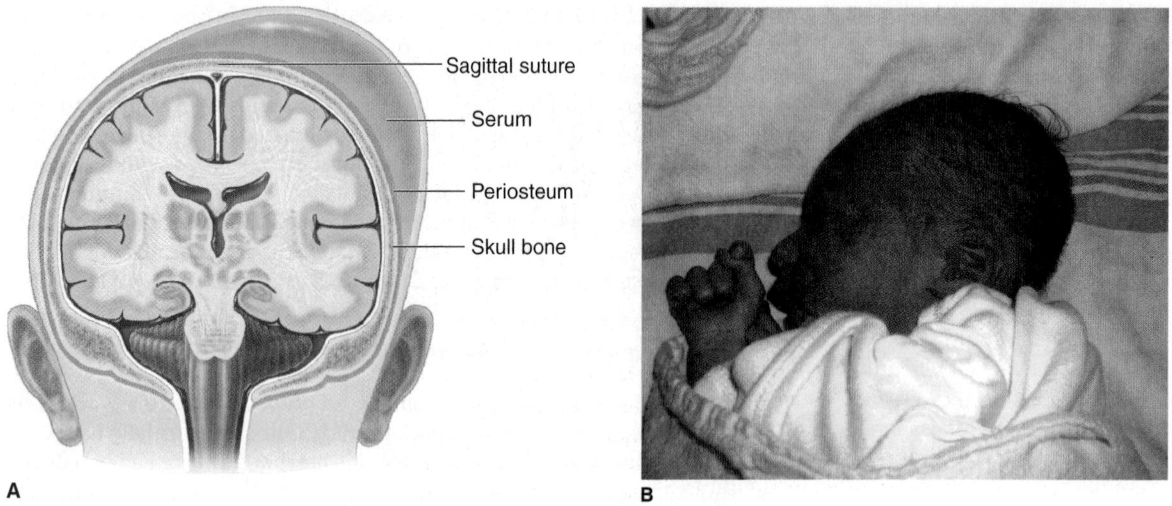

Figure 27–29 **A. Caput succedaneum is a collection of fluid (serum) under the scalp. B. Newborn with caput succedaneum.**

SOURCE: B. Michele Davidson.

The chin is recessed, and the nose is flattened. The lips are sensitive to touch, and the sucking reflex is easily initiated.

Symmetry of the eyes, nose, and ears is evaluated. See *Assessment Guide: Newborn Physical Assessment* at the end of this chapter for deviations in symmetry and variations in size, shape, and spacing of facial features. Facial movement symmetry should be assessed to determine the presence of facial palsy. Facial paralysis appears when the newborn cries; the affected side is immobile, and the palpebral (eyelid) fissure widens. Paralysis may result from forceps-assisted birth or pressure on the facial nerve from the maternal pelvis during birth. Facial paralysis usually disappears within a few days to 3 weeks, although in some cases it may be permanent.

Eyes

The eyes of newborns of northern European descent are a blue or slate blue-gray. Dark-skinned newborns tend to have dark eyes at birth. The scleral color tends to be white to bluish white because of the relative thinness of the sclera. A blue sclera is associated with osteogenesis imperfecta. The infant's eye color is usually established at approximately 3 months, but it may change any time up to 1 year.

The eyes should be checked for size, equality of pupil size, reaction of pupils to light, blink reflex to light, and edema and inflammation of the eyelids. The eyelids can be edematous during the first few days of life because of the pressure associated with birth.

Erythromycin and tetracycline (in some agencies) are used prophylactically and usually do not cause chemical irritation of the eye (see Chapter 28). The instillation of silver nitrate drops in the newborn's eyes may cause edema and **chemical conjunctivitis**, which may appear a few hours after instillation and disappear in 1 to 2 days (Eichenwald et al., 2017). If infectious conjunctivitis exists, the newborn has the same purulent (greenish-yellow) discharge as in chemical conjunctivitis, but it is caused by gonococcus, *Chlamydia*, staphylococci, or a variety of Gram-negative bacteria and requires treatment with ophthalmic antibiotics. Onset is usually after the second day. Edema of the orbits or eyelids may persist for several days until the newborn's kidneys can evacuate the fluid.

Small **subconjunctival hemorrhages** appear in about 10% of newborns and are commonly found on the sclera. These hemorrhages are caused by the changes in vascular tension or ocular pressure during birth. They will remain for a few weeks and are of no pathologic significance. Parents need reassurance that the baby is not bleeding from within the eye and that vision will not be impaired.

The newborn may demonstrate *transient strabismus (pseudostrabismus)* or squinting caused by neuromuscular control of eye muscles (Figure 27–30). It gradually regresses in 3 to 4 months. The "doll's-eye" phenomenon is also present for about

CASE STUDY: Angelina Newman

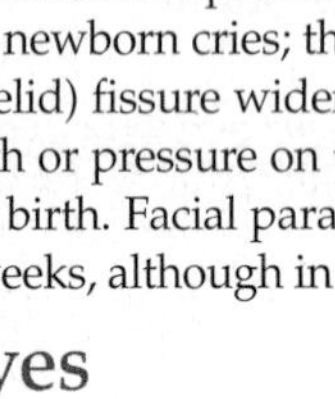

SOURCE: WAYHOME studio/Shutterstock.

Angelina and her boyfriend are watching the nurse perform a newborn assessment on their son. They observe that the nurse weighs the baby and takes measurements of the baby's length as well as the head and chest. During this assessment, they note the baby's head appears swollen and misshapen and worry the baby could have had some damage occur during the birth. The nurse explains that their baby has caput succedaneum, which commonly occurs as a result of a vaginal birth. As a nurse, it is important to differentiate between caput succedaneum and cephalhemotoma.

Questions to Ponder

How would you describe the difference between these two common head variations that are associated with vaginal birth? How can you reassure the parents that their baby will be fine?

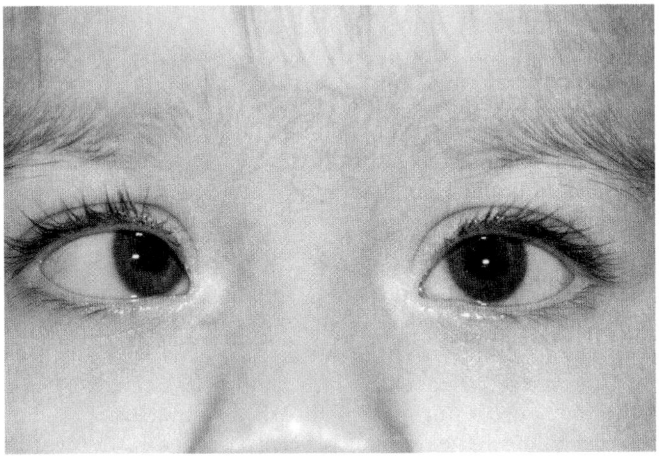

Figure 27–30 **Transient strabismus in the newborn may be due to poor neuromuscular control.**

SOURCE: Biophoto Associates/Science Source.

10 days after birth and results from underdeveloped integration of head–eye coordination. As the newborn's head position is changed to the left and then to the right, the eyes move to the opposite direction.

The nurse should observe the newborn's pupils for opacities or whiteness and for the absence of a normal red retinal reflex. Red retinal reflex is a red-orange flash of color observed when an ophthalmoscope light reflects off the retina. In a newborn with dark skin color, the retina may appear paler or more grayish. The color of the red reflex can also be abnormal with retinoblastoma. Absence of red reflex occurs with cataracts. Congenital cataracts should be suspected in newborns of mothers with a prenatal history of rubella, cytomegalic inclusion disease, or syphilis. Brushfield spots (black or white spots on the periphery of the iris) can be associated with trisomy 21 (Johnson, 2019).

The cry of the newborn is commonly tearless because the lacrimal structures are immature at birth and are not usually fully functional until the second month of life. However, some babies may produce tears during the newborn period.

Poor oculomotor coordination and absence of accommodation limit visual abilities, but newborns do have peripheral vision and can fixate on near objects (20.3 to 25.4 cm [8 to 10 in.]) in front of their faces for short periods, can accommodate to large objects (7.6 cm [3 in.] tall by 7.6 cm [3 in.] wide), and can seek out high-contrast geometric shapes. Newborns can perceive faces, shapes, and colors and begin to show visual preferences early. Newborns generally blink in response to bright lights, to a tap on the bridge of the nose (glabellar reflex), or to a light touch on the eyelids. Pupillary light reflex is also present. The eye is best examined by rocking the newborn from an upright position to the horizontal a few times or by other methods, such as diminishing overhead lights, which will elicit an opened-eye response.

Nose

The newborn's nose is small and narrow. Babies are characteristically nose breathers for the first few months of life. The newborn generally removes obstructions by sneezing. The nose is patent if the newborn breathes easily with the mouth closed. If respiratory difficulty occurs, the nurse checks for choanal atresia (congenital blockage of the passageway between the nose and pharynx). Historically, choanal atresia can be checked by attempting to gently pass a soft #5 French catheter into both nostrils. Because of possible trauma, alternately occlude each naris using gentle pressure (Caveliere & Sansoucie, 2014).

Newborns have the ability to smell after the nasal passages are cleared of amniotic fluid and mucus. They will turn their heads toward the milk source, whether bottle or breast. Newborns react to strong odors, such as alcohol, by turning their heads away or blinking.

Mouth

The lips of the newborn should be pink, and a touch on the lips should produce sucking motions. Saliva is normally scant. The taste buds are developed before birth, and the newborn can easily discriminate between sweet and bitter flavors.

The easiest way to examine the mouth completely is to stimulate babies to cry by gently depressing the tongue, thereby causing them to open the mouth fully. It is extremely important to observe the entire mouth to look for a cleft palate, which can be present even in the absence of a cleft lip. The examiner moves an unpowdered gloved index finger or pinky along the hard and soft palate to feel for any openings (Figure 27–31).

Occasionally, an examination of the gums will reveal *precocious teeth* over the area where the lower central incisor will erupt. If they appear loose, they should be removed to prevent aspiration. Gray-white lesions (inclusion cysts) on the gums may be confused with teeth. On the hard palate and gum margins, **Epstein pearls**, small glistening white specks (keratin-containing cysts) that feel hard to the touch, are often present. They usually disappear in a few weeks and are of no significance. **Thrush** may appear as white patches that look like milk curds adhering to the mucous membranes, and bleeding may occur when patches are removed. Thrush is caused by *Candida albicans*, often acquired from an infected vaginal tract during birth, antibiotic use, or poor handwashing when handling the newborn. Thrush is treated with nystatin (Mycostatin). The mother may also need to be treated at the same time.

A newborn who is tongue-tied has a ridge of frenulum tissue attached to the underside of the tongue at varying lengths from its base, causing a heart shape at the tip of the tongue. "Clipping

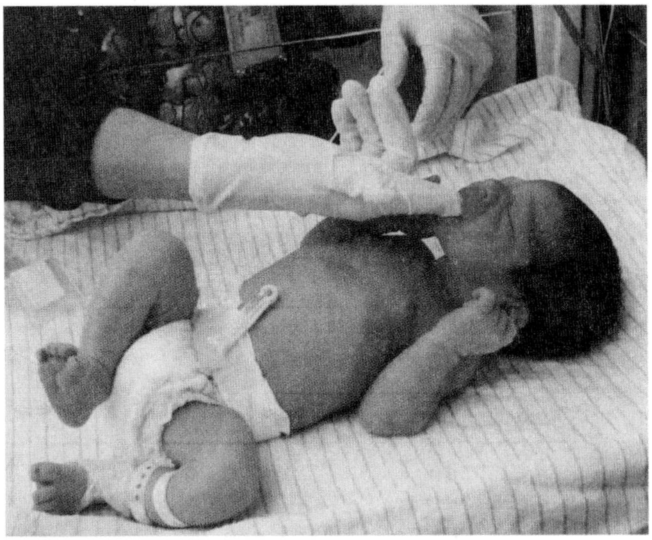

Figure 27–31 **The nurse inserts the index finger or pinky into the newborn's mouth and feels for any openings along the hard and soft palates.**

NOTE: Unpowdered gloves or a finger cot is always worn to examine the palate.

the tongue," or cutting the ridge of tissue, is not usually recommended unless the baby has trouble feeding. In this case the physician would perform a *frenotomy*. This ridge usually does not affect speech or eating, but cutting does create an entry for infection. Transient nerve paralysis resulting from birth trauma may be manifested by asymmetric mouth movements when the newborn cries or by difficulty with sucking and feeding.

Ears

The ears of the newborn are soft and pliable and should recoil readily when folded and released. In the normal newborn, the top of the ear (pinna) should be parallel to the outer and inner canthus of the eye. The ears should be inspected for shape, size, position, and firmness of ear cartilage. *Low-set ears* are characteristic of many syndromes and may indicate chromosomal abnormalities (especially trisomies 13 and 18), intellectual disability, or internal organ abnormalities such as bilateral renal agenesis as a result of embryologic developmental deviations (Figure 27–32). A *preauricular skin tag* may be present just in front of the ear. Visualization of the tympanic membranes is not usually done soon after birth because blood and vernix block the ear canal.

Following the first cry, the newborn's hearing becomes acute as mucus from the middle ear is absorbed, the eustachian tube is aerated, and the tympanic membrane becomes visible. The newborn's hearing can initially be evaluated by response to loud or moderately loud noises unaccompanied by vibrations; the sleeping newborn should stir or awaken in response. (This is not a very accurate test, but it may help to alert the examiner to possible problems.) The newborn can discriminate the individual characteristics of the human voice and is especially sensitive to sound levels within the normal conversation range. The newborn in a noisy nursery may be able to habituate to the sounds and not stir unless the sound is sudden or much louder than usual. AAP has endorsed universal newborn hearing screening (UNHS) in birthing units as the standard of care (AAP & ACOG, 2017; Johnson, 2019) (see Chapter 28 for further discussion).

Clinical Tip

Vital sign assessments are most accurate if the newborn is at rest, so measure pulse and respirations first if the baby is quiet. To soothe a crying baby, try placing your moistened, unpowdered, gloved finger in the baby's mouth, and then complete your assessment while the baby suckles.

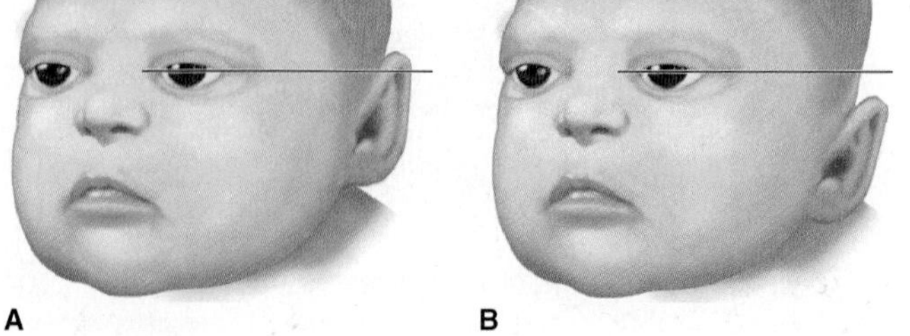

Figure 27–32 The position of the external ear may be assessed by drawing an imaginary line across the inner and outer canthus of the eye to the insertion of the ear. A. Normal position. B. True low-set position.

Neck

A short neck, creased with skin folds, is characteristic of the normal newborn. Because muscle tone is not well developed, the neck cannot support the full weight of the head, which rotates freely. The head lags considerably when the newborn is pulled up from a supine to a sitting position, but the prone newborn is able to raise the head slightly. The neck is palpated for masses and presence of lymph nodes and is inspected for webbing. Adequacy of range of motion and neck muscle function is determined by moving the head while supporting the newborn to prevent injury. Injury to the sternocleidomastoid muscle (congenital torticollis) must be considered in the presence of neck rigidity.

The clavicles are evaluated for evidence of fractures, which occasionally occur during difficult births or in newborns with broad shoulders. The normal clavicle is straight. If fractured, a lump and a grating sensation (crepitus) during movements may be palpated along the course of the side of the break. The Moro reflex (see Table 27–1 earlier in the chapter) is also elicited to evaluate bilateral equal movement of the arms. If the clavicle is fractured, this response will be demonstrated only on the unaffected side.

Chest

The thorax is cylindric and symmetric at birth, and the ribs are flexible. The general appearance of the chest should be assessed. A protrusion at the lower end of the sternum, called the *xiphoid cartilage*, is frequently seen. It is under the skin and will become less apparent after several weeks as the baby accumulates adipose tissue.

Engorged breasts occur frequently in both male and female newborns. This condition, which appears by the third day, is a result of maternal hormonal influences and may last up to 2 weeks (Figure 27–33). A whitish secretion from the nipples may also be noted. The baby's breast should not be massaged or squeezed because this practice may cause a breast abscess. Supernumerary nipples are occasionally noted below and medial to the true nipples. These harmless pink or brown spots vary in size and do not contain glandular tissue. Accessory nipples can be differentiated from a pigmented nevus (mole) by placing the fingertips alongside the accessory nipple and pulling the adjacent tissue laterally. The accessory nipple will appear dimpled.

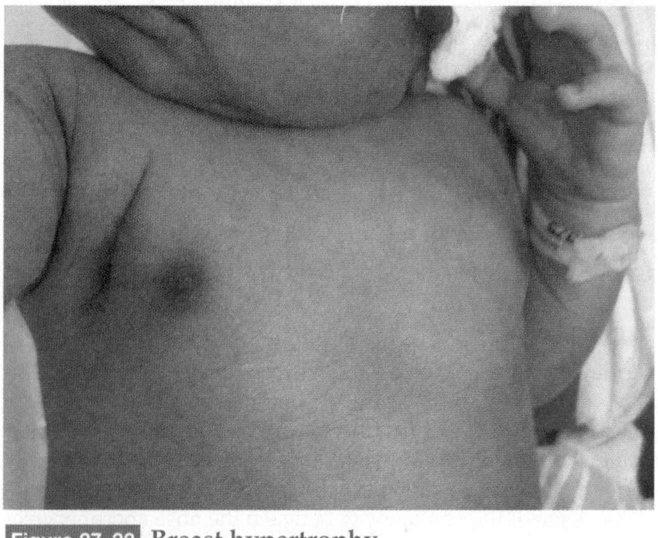

Figure 27–33 Breast hypertrophy.

SOURCE: Michele Davidson.

Cry

The newborn's cry should be strong, lusty, and of medium pitch. A high-pitched, shrill cry is abnormal and may indicate neurologic disorders or hypoglycemia. Periods of crying vary in length after consoling measures are used. A baby's cries are an important method of communication and alert caregivers to changes in the baby's condition and needs (see Chapter 26).

Respiration

Normal breathing for a term newborn is 30 to 60 respirations per minute and predominantly diaphragmatic, with associated rising and falling of the abdomen during inspiration and expiration. Any signs of respiratory distress, nasal flaring, intercostal or xiphoid retractions, expiratory grunting or sighing, seesaw respirations, or tachypnea (sustained or greater than 60 respirations per minute) should be noted. Hyperexpansion (chest appears high) or hypoexpansion (chest appears low) of the anteroposterior diameter of the chest should also be noted. Both the anterior and posterior chest are auscultated. Some breath sounds are heard best when the newborn is crying, but it is difficult to localize and identify breath sounds in the newborn. Upper airway noises and bowel sounds can be heard over the chest wall, making auscultation difficult. Because sounds may be transmitted from the unaffected lung to the affected lung, the absence of breath sounds may not be diagnosed. Air entry may be noisy in the first couple of hours until lung fluid resolves, especially in cesarean births. Brief periods of apnea (episodic breathing) may occur, but no color or heart rate changes occur in healthy, term newborns. Sepsis should be suspected in full-term newborns experiencing apneic episodes.

Clinical Tip

Always check breath sounds laterally under the arms because it may be easier to identify decreased breath sounds on one side, which can be indicative of a pneumothorax.

Heart

Heart rates can be as rapid as 180 beats per minute (beats/min) in newborns and fluctuate a great deal, especially if the baby moves or is startled. Normal range is 110 to 160 beats/min. Auscultation provides the nurse with valuable assessment data. The heart is examined for rate and rhythm, position of the apical impulse, and heart sound intensity. Dysrhythmias should be evaluated by the healthcare provider.

The pulse rate is variable and is influenced by physical activity, crying, state of wakefulness, and body temperature. Auscultation is performed over the entire heart region (precordium), below the left axilla, and below the scapula. Apical pulse rates are obtained by auscultation for a full minute, preferably when the newborn is asleep.

The placement of the heart in the chest should be determined when the newborn is in a quiet state. The heart is relatively large at birth and is located mid- to left chest and high in the chest, with its apex somewhere between the fourth and the fifth intercostal space.

A shift of heart tones in the mediastinal area to either side may indicate pneumothorax, dextrocardia (heart placement on the right side of the chest), or a diaphragmatic hernia. The experienced nurse can diagnose these and many other problems early with a stethoscope. Normally, the heartbeat has a "toc tic" sound. A slur or slushing sound (usually after the first sound) may indicate a murmur. Although 90% of all murmurs are transient and are considered normal, they should be monitored closely by a physician. Many murmurs are secondary to closing of patent ductus arteriosus or patent foramen ovale, which should close 1 to 2 days after birth. Occasionally, aortic or pulmonary stenosis or small ventricular septal defect murmurs are heard. See Chapter 30 for a discussion of congenital heart defects.

Peripheral pulses (brachial, femoral, pedal) are also evaluated to detect any lags or unusual characteristics. Brachial pulses are palpated bilaterally for equality and compared with the femoral pulses. Femoral pulses are palpated by applying gentle pressure with the middle finger over the femoral canal (Figure 27–34). Decreased or absent femoral pulses may indicate coarctation of the aorta or hypovolemia and require additional investigation. A wide difference in blood pressure between the upper and lower extremities also indicates coarctation of the aorta.

The measurement of BP is best accomplished by using a noninvasive blood pressure device (Figure 27–35). If a blood pressure cuff is used, the newborn's extremities must be immobilized during the assessment, and the cuff should cover two-thirds of the upper arm or upper leg. Movement, crying, and inappropriate cuff size can give inaccurate measurements of BP.

Blood pressure may not be measured routinely on healthy newborns but is an essential measurement in newborns who are having distress, are premature, or are suspected of having a cardiac anomaly, renal disease, or clinical signs of hypotension (Vargo, 2019). Newborns who have birth asphyxia and are on ventilators have significantly lower systolic and diastolic blood pressures than healthy newborns. If a cardiac anomaly is suspected, blood pressure is palpated in all four extremities. At birth, systolic values usually range from 70 to 50 mmHg and diastolic values from 45 to 30 mmHg. By the 10th day of life, blood pressure may rise to 90/50 mmHg. See *Key Facts to Remember: Newborn Vital Signs*.

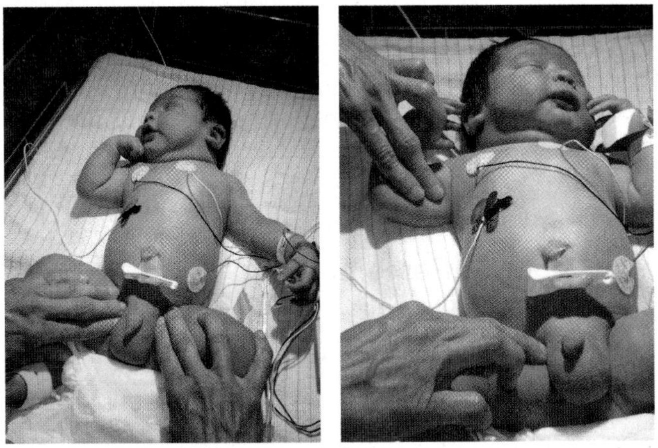

A B

Figure 27–34 A. Bilaterally palpate the femoral arteries for rate and intensity of the pulses. Press fingertip gently at the groin as shown. B. Compare the femoral pulses to the brachial pulses by palpating the pulses simultaneously for comparison of rate and intensity.

SOURCE: A.–B. Carol Harrigan, RNC, MSN, NNP-BC.

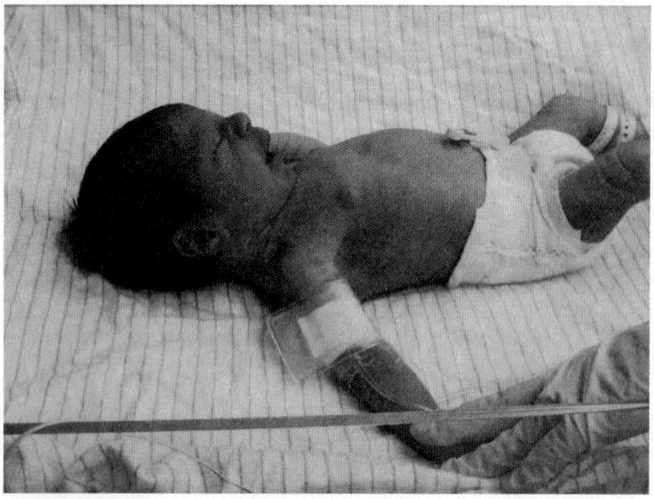

Figure 27-35 **Blood pressure measurement using the noninvasive Dinemapp and Doppler devices. The cuff can be applied to either the newborn's upper arm or the thigh.**

Clinical Tip

If possible, obtain BP measurement during quiet sleep or sleep state. Place cuff on arm or leg and give baby time to quiet. Obtain average of two to three measurements when making clinical decisions. Follow mean BP to monitor changes, as it is less likely to be erroneous. Noninvasive BP may overestimate BP in very low-birth-weight newborns.

Abdomen

The nurse can learn a great deal about the newborn's abdomen without disturbing the baby. The abdomen should be cylindrical, protrude slightly, and move with respiration. A certain amount of laxness of the abdominal muscles is normal. A scaphoid (hollow-shaped) appearance suggests the absence of abdominal contents, seen in diaphragmatic hernia. No cyanosis should be present, and few if any blood vessels should be apparent to the eye. There should be no gross distention or bulging. The more distended the abdomen, the tighter the skin becomes, and engorged vessels appear. Distention is the first sign of many of the gastrointestinal abnormalities.

Before palpation of the abdomen, the nurse should auscultate the presence or absence of bowel sounds in all four quadrants. Bowel sounds should be present by 1 hour after birth. Palpation can cause a transient decrease in bowel sound intensity.

Abdominal palpation should be carried out systematically. The nurse palpates each of the four abdominal quadrants, moving in a clockwise direction, checking for softness, tenderness, and the presence of masses. The nurse should place one hand under the back for support during palpation. When palpating the abdomen, the nurse may feel for the liver. The newborn's liver is large in proportion to the rest of the body and can usually be felt between 1 and 2 cm below the right costal margin (Cavaliere & Sansoucie, 2014).

Umbilical Cord

Initially, the umbilical cord is white and gelatinous in appearance, with the two umbilical arteries and one umbilical vein readily apparent. Because a single umbilical artery is frequently associated with congenital anomalies, the vessels should be counted as part of the newborn assessment. The cord begins drying within 1 or 2 hours after birth and is shriveled and blackened by the second or third day. (Care of the umbilical cord is discussed in Chapter 28.)

Developing Cultural Competence Native Americans and Umbilical Cord Care

In the Woodland Indian tribe, upon birth, the umbilical cord is tied and a small piece is saved. This section of the umbilical cord is sewn into a deerskin diamond-shaped pocket. The pocket is hung over the baby's crib to provide protection for the baby.

Cord bleeding is abnormal and may result from tension on the cord or clamp because the cord was inadvertently pulled or because the cord clamp was loosened. Foul-smelling drainage is also abnormal and is generally caused by infection, which requires immediate treatment to prevent septicemia. Serous or serosanguinous drainage that continues after the cord falls off

Key Facts To Remember
Newborn Vital Signs

Pulse	Respirations	Blood Pressure	Temperature
• 110–160 beats/min • During deep sleep, decrease to 70–90 beats/min; if crying, up to 180 beats/min (Vargo, 2019) • Apical pulse counted for 1 full minute	• 30–60 respirations/min • Predominantly diaphragmatic but synchronous with abdominal movements • Respirations are counted for 1 full minute	• 70–50/45–30 mmHg at birth • 90/50 mmHg at day 10	• Normal range: 36.5°C–37.5°C (97.7°F–99.4°F) • Axillary: 36.5°C–37.2°C (97.7°F–99°F) • Skin: 36°C–36.5°C (96.8°F–97.7°F) • Rectal: 36.6°C–37.2°C (97.8°F–99°F)

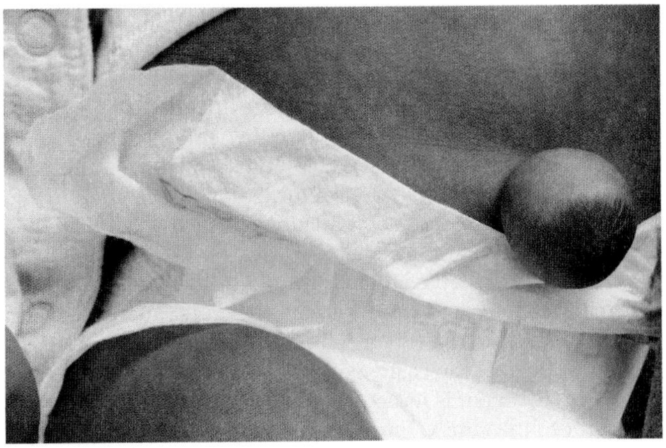

Figure 27–36 Umbilical hernia.

may indicate a granuloma. If the newborn has a patent urachus (abnormal connection between the umbilicus and bladder), moistness or draining urine may be apparent at the base of the cord. Another umbilical cord anomaly that can occur is umbilical cord hernia and associated patent omphalomesenteric duct (Figure 27–36). Umbilical hernias are more common in newborns of African descent than in newborns of European heritage (Goodwin, 2019). Umbilical hernias usually close spontaneously by 2 years of age.

Genitals

FEMALE NEWBORNS

The nurse examines the labia majora, labia minora, and clitoris, noting the size of each as appropriate for gestational age. A vaginal tag or hymenal tag is often evident and will usually disappear in a few weeks. During the first week of life, the female newborn may have a vaginal discharge composed of thick whitish mucus. This discharge, which can become tinged with blood, is referred to as **pseudomenstruation** and is caused by the withdrawal of maternal hormones. *Smegma*, a white cheeselike substance, is often present between the labia. Removing it may traumatize tender tissue.

MALE NEWBORNS

The penis is inspected to determine whether the urinary orifice is correctly positioned. *Hypospadias* occurs when the urinary meatus is located on the ventral surface of the penis; *epispadias* occurs when the meatus is located on the dorsal surface of the glans. Hypospadias occurs most commonly among people of Western European descent. *Phimosis* is a condition occurring in newborn males in which the opening of the foreskin (prepuce) is small and the foreskin cannot be pulled back over the glans at all. This condition may interfere with urination, so the adequacy of the urinary stream should be evaluated.

The scrotum is inspected for size and symmetry. Scrotal color variations are especially prominent in African American, Indian, and Hispanic newborns (Eichenwald et al., 2017). The scrotum should be palpated to verify the presence of both testes and to rule out *cryptorchidism* (failure of testes to descend). The testes are palpated separately between the thumb and forefinger, with the thumb and forefinger of the other hand placed together over the inguinal canal. Scrotal edema and discoloration are common in breech births. *Hydrocele* (a collection of fluid surrounding the testes in the scrotum) is common in newborns and should be identified. It usually resolves without intervention. The presence of a discolored or dusky scrotum and solid testis should raise the suspicion of testicular torsion, which is considered a surgical emergency and should be reported immediately.

Anus

The anal area is inspected to verify that it is patent and has no fissure. Imperforate anus and rectal atresia may be ruled out by observation. A digital examination, if necessary, is done by a physician or nurse practitioner. The passage of the first meconium stool is also noted. Atresia of the gastrointestinal tract or meconium ileus with resultant obstruction must be considered if the newborn does not pass meconium in the first 24 hours of life.

Extremities

Extremities are examined for gross deformities, extra digits or webbing, clubfoot, and range of motion. Normal newborn extremities appear short, are generally flexible, and move symmetrically.

ARMS AND HANDS

Nails extend beyond the fingertips in term newborns. Fingers and toes should be counted. *Polydactyly* is the presence of extra digits on either the hands or the feet. *Syndactyly* refers to fusion (webbing) of fingers or toes, which can be hereditary or associated with trisomy 21. Hands should be inspected for normal palmar creases. A single palmar crease is frequently present in children with trisomy 21.

Brachial palsy, a partial or complete paralysis of portions of the arm, results from trauma to the brachial plexus during a difficult birth. It occurs most commonly when strong traction is exerted on the head of the newborn in an attempt to deliver a shoulder lodged behind the symphysis pubis in the presence of shoulder dystocia. Brachial palsy may also occur during a breech birth if an arm becomes trapped over the head and traction is exerted.

The portion of the arm affected is determined by the nerves damaged. **Erb-Duchenne paralysis (Erb palsy)** involves damage to the upper arm (fifth and sixth cervical nerves) and is the most common type. Injury to the eighth cervical and first thoracic nerve roots and the lower portion of the plexus produces the relatively rare *lower arm injury*. The *whole arm type* results from damage to the entire plexus.

With Erb-Duchenne paralysis, the newborn's arm lies limply at the side. The elbow is held in extension, with the forearm pronated. The newborn is unable to elevate the arm, and therefore the Moro reflex cannot be elicited on the affected side. When a lower arm injury occurs, paralysis of the hand and wrist results; complete paralysis of the limb occurs with the whole arm type.

Prognosis is related to the degree of nerve damage resulting from trauma and hemorrhage within the nerve sheath. Complete recovery occurs within a few months with minimal trauma. Moderate trauma may result in some partial paralysis. Recovery is unlikely with severe trauma, and muscle wasting may develop.

Clinical Tip

Always examine more closely any newborn who is reluctant to move an extremity. Fractures are often asymptomatic in the newborn; paralytic injuries are characterized by immobility of an extremity. A fractured clavicle should be suspected when it is noted that the baby is moving only one arm.

LEGS AND FEET

The legs of the newborn should be of equal length, with symmetrical skinfolds. However, they may assume a fetal posture similar to the position in utero, and it may take several days for the legs and feet to relax into a normal position. The nurse should assess for asymmetry of inner thigh folds, limited hip abduction, and the *Allis sign* (an indication of fracture in the neck of the femur in which a finger easily sinks into the relaxed fascia between the great trochanter and the iliac crest) (Figure 27–37A).

To evaluate for hip dislocation or hip instability, the Barlow and Ortolani maneuvers are performed. The nurse (or, more commonly, the physician or nurse practitioner) examiner performs the **Barlow maneuver** (Figure 27–37B, C) to rule out the possibility of developmental dysplasic hip, also called *congenital hip dysplasia* (hip dislocatability). The examiner grasps and adducts the baby's thigh and applies gentle downward pressure. Dislocation is felt as the femoral head slips out of the acetabulum.

The **Ortolani maneuver** (Figure 27–37D) should be performed with the newborn relaxed and quiet on a firm surface. With the hips and knees flexed at a 90-degree angle, the examiner grasps the baby's thigh with the middle finger over the greater trochanter and lifts the thigh to bring the femoral head from its posterior position toward the acetabulum. With gentle abduction of the thigh, the femoral head is returned to the acetabulum and the examiner feels a sense of reduction or a "clunk." This reduction is palpable and may be heard.

The feet are then examined for evidence of a *talipes deformity* (clubfoot). Intrauterine position frequently causes the feet to appear to turn inward (Figure 27–38); this is termed a *positional clubfoot*. If the feet can easily be returned to midline by manipulation, no treatment is indicated. Range-of-motion exercises can be taught to the family. Further investigation is indicated when the foot will not turn to the midline position or align readily. This is considered the most severe type of *true clubfoot*, or talipes equinovarus.

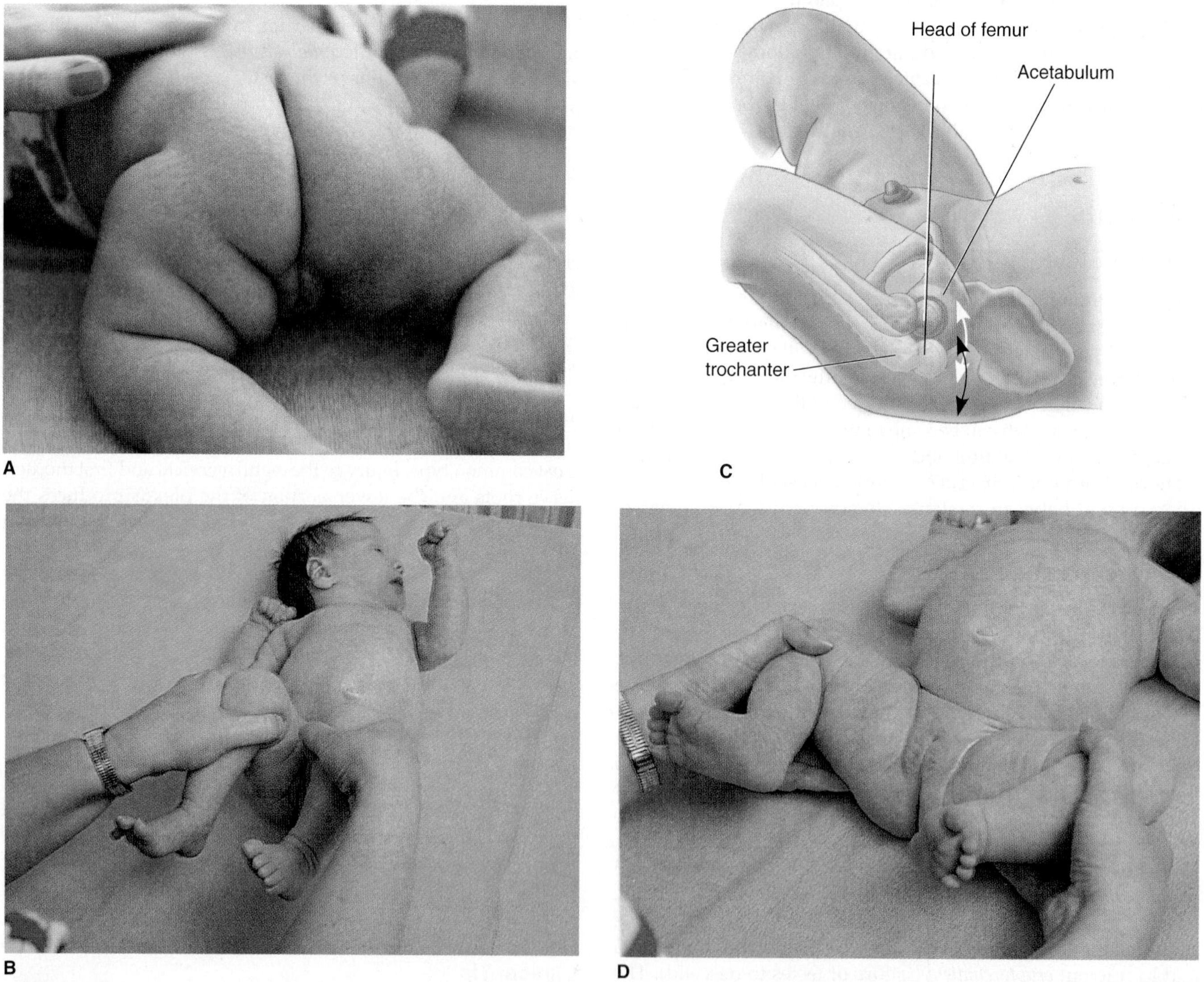

Figure 27–37 A. The asymmetry of gluteal and thigh fat folds seen in newborn with left developmental dysplasia of the hip. B. Barlow (dislocation) maneuver. Baby's thigh is grasped and adducted (placed together) with gentle downward pressure. C. Dislocation is palpable as femoral head slips out of acetabulum. D. Ortolani maneuver puts downward pressure on the hip and then inward rotation. If the hip is dislocated, this maneuver will force the femoral head back into the acetabular rim with a noticeable "clunk."

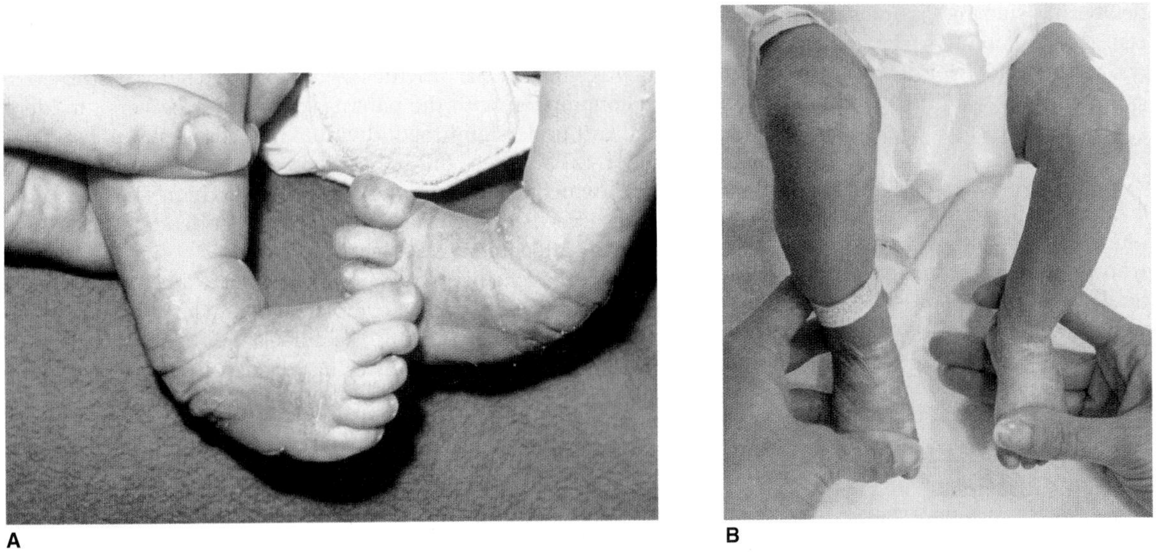

Figure 27–38 A. Bilateral talipes equinovarus (clubfoot). B. To determine the presence of clubfoot, the nurse moves the foot to the midline. Resistance indicates true clubfoot.

SOURCE: A. Jim Stevenson/Science Source.

Back

With the baby prone, the nurse examines the back. The spine should appear straight and flat because the lumbar and sacral curves do not develop until the infant begins to sit. The base of the spine is examined for a dermal sinus. A *nevus pilosus* ("hairy nevus") is occasionally found at the base of the spine in newborns. It is significant because it is frequently associated with spina bifida. A suspected pilonidal dimple should be reported to the healthcare provider to ascertain that there is no connection to the spinal canal.

Assessment of Neurologic Status

The nurse should begin the neurologic examination with a period of observation, noting the general physical characteristics and behavior of the newborn. Important behaviors to assess are:

- State of alertness
- Resting posture
- Cry
- Quality of muscle tone
- Motor activity.

The usual position of the newborn is partially flexed extremities with the legs abducted to the abdomen. When awake, the newborn may exhibit purposeless, uncoordinated bilateral movements of the extremities. If these movements are absent, minimal, or obviously asymmetric, neurologic dysfunction should be suspected. Eye movements are observable during the first few days of life. An alert newborn is able to fixate on faces and brightly colored objects. Shining a bright light in the newborn's eyes elicits the blinking response.

The nurse evaluates muscle tone by moving various parts of the newborn's body while the newborn's head remains in a neutral position. The newborn is somewhat *hypertonic*; that is, the newborn resists the examiner's attempts to extend the elbow and knee joints. Muscle tone should be symmetric. Diminished muscle tone and flaccidity require further evaluation.

Tremors or jitteriness (tremorlike movements) in the full-term newborn must be evaluated to differentiate the tremors from convulsions. Tremors may be related to hypoglycemia, hypocalcemia, or substance withdrawal. Environmental stimuli may initiate tremors. Jitteriness may be distinguished from tonic-clonic seizure activity because it can usually be stopped by the baby's sucking on the extremity or by the nurse holding or flexing the involved extremity. A fine jumping of the muscle is likely to be a central nervous system (CNS) disorder and requires further evaluation. Neonatal seizures may consist of no more than chewing or swallowing movements, deviations of the eyes, rigidity, or flaccidity because of CNS immaturity. In contrast to tremors, seizures are not usually initiated by stimuli and cannot be stopped by holding.

Specific deep tendon reflexes can be elicited in the newborn but have limited value unless they are obviously asymmetric. The knee jerk is brisk; a normal ankle clonus may involve three or four beats. Plantar flexion is present.

The immature CNS of the newborn is characterized by a variety of reflexes. Because the newborn's movements are uncoordinated, methods of communication are limited and control of body functions is restricted, so reflexes serve a variety of purposes. Some are protective (blink, gag, sneeze); some aid in feeding (rooting, sucking) and may not be very active if the baby has eaten recently; and some stimulate human interaction (grasping). In addition, newborns can *blink*, *gag*, *yawn*, *cough*, *sneeze*, and *draw back from pain* (protective reflexes). They can even move a little on their own. When placed on their stomachs, they push up and try to crawl (prone crawl). Absence or a variance in the response requires motor function evaluation by a specialist. Absence of the *plantar grasp* and *Galant (truncal) incurvation* reflexes require neurologic evaluation. The most common reflexes found in the normal newborn are shown in Table 27–1 earlier in the chapter.

The nurse uses the following steps to assess CNS integration:

1. Insert an unpowdered gloved finger into the newborn's mouth to elicit a sucking reflex.

2. As soon as the newborn is sucking vigorously, assess hearing and vision responses by noting sucking changes in the presence of a light, a rattle, and a voice.
3. The newborn should respond with a brief cessation of sucking followed by continuous sucking with repeated stimulation.

This examination demonstrates auditory and visual integrity as well as complex behavioral interactions. As healthcare providers carry out the newborn physical and neurologic assessment, they are always on the alert to recognize possible alterations and possible injuries related to the birth process that require further investigation and intervention. See Table 27–2 for potential birth injuries.

Newborn Behavioral Assessment

Two conflicting forces influence parents' perceptions of their newborn. One is the parents' preconceptions, based on hopes and fears, of what their newborn will be like. The other is their initial reaction to their baby's temperament, behaviors, and physical appearance. Nurses can assist parents in identifying their baby's specific behaviors.

“One of the newborn's first responses is to move into a quiet but alert state of consciousness. The baby is still; his body molds to yours; his hands touch your skin; his eyes open wide and are bright and shiny. He looks directly at you.

This special alert state, this innate ability to communicate, may be the initial preparation for becoming attached to other human beings. One feels awed by the intensity and appealing power of this little bud of humanity meeting the world for the first time.”

—Marshall H. Klaus & Phyllis H. Klaus, *The Amazing Newborn*

The Brazelton Neonatal Behavioral Assessment Scale

The **Brazelton Neonatal Behavioral Assessment Scale** is an assessment tool that identifies the newborn's repertoire of behavioral responses to the environment and also documents the newborn's neurologic adequacy and capabilities. (For a complete discussion of all test items and maneuvers, see Brazelton & Nugent, 2011.) It provides a way for the healthcare provider, in conjunction with the parents (primary caregivers), to identify and understand the individual newborn's states, temperament, capabilities, and individual behavior patterns. Families learn which responses, interventions, or activities best meet the special needs of their newborn, and this understanding fosters positive attachment experiences.

Because the first few days after birth are a period of behavioral disorganization, the complete assessment should be done on the third day after birth. The nurse should make every effort to elicit the best response. This may be accomplished by repeating tests at different times or by testing during situations that facilitate the best possible response, such as when parents are holding, cuddling, rocking, or singing to their baby.

The behavioral assessment of the newborn should be carried out initially in a quiet, dimly lighted room, if possible. The nurse should first determine the newborn's state of consciousness because scoring and introduction of the test items correlate with the sleep or awake state. The newborn's state depends on physiologic variables, such as the amount of time from the last feeding, positioning, environmental temperature, and health status; presence of such external stimuli as noises and bright lights; and the sleep–wake cycle of the baby. An important characteristic of the neonatal period is the pattern of states, as well as the transitions from one state to another. The pattern of states is a predictor of the newborn's receptivity and ability to respond to stimuli in a cognitive manner. Babies learn best in a quiet, alert state and in an environment that is supportive and protective and that provides appropriate stimuli.

The nurse should also observe the newborn's sleep–wake patterns (as discussed in Chapter 26) and the rapidity with which the newborn moves from one state to another, the newborn's ability to be consoled, and the newborn's ability to diminish the impact of disturbing stimuli. The following questions provide the nurse with a framework for assessment:

- Does the newborn's response style and ability to adapt to stimuli indicate a need for parental interventions that will alert the newborn to the environment so that the baby can grow socially and cognitively?
- Are parental interventions necessary to lessen the outside stimuli, as in the case of the baby who responds to sensory input with intensity?
- Can the baby control the amount of sensory input to be dealt with?

The behaviors and the sleep–wake states in which they are assessed are categorized as follows:

- ***Habituation.*** The newborn's ability to diminish or shut down innate responses to specific repeated stimuli, such as a rattle, bell, light, or pinprick to heel.
- ***Orientation to inanimate and animate visual and auditory assessment stimuli.*** How often and where the newborn attends to auditory and visual stimuli are observed. Orientation to the environment is determined by an ability to respond to cues given by others and by a natural ability to fix on and to follow a visual object horizontally and vertically. This capacity and parental appreciation of it are important for positive communication between baby and parents; the parents' visual (*en face*) and auditory (soft, continuous voice) presence stimulates their baby to orient to them. Inability or lack of response may indicate visual or

TABLE 27–2 Potential Birth Injuries

CLASSIFICATION	EXAMPLES*
Soft-tissue injuries	Lacerations, abrasions, bruising, fat necrosis
Skull injuries	Cephalohematoma, fractures*
Scalp laceration abscess	Fetal scalp electrode
Nasal injuries	Dislocation, fractures*
Intracranial hemorrhage	Subdural, subarachnoid
Eye injuries	Subconjunctival* and retinal hemorrhages
Bone fractures	Clavicle, facial bones*, humerus, femur
Dislocations	Hips
Cranial nerve injuries	Facial nerve, brachial plexus*, phrenic nerve*, recurrent laryngeal nerve (vocal cord paralysis), Horner syndrome

NOTE: *Most common birth injuries seen in newborns.

auditory problems. It is important for parents to know that their newborn can turn to voices soon after birth or by 3 days of age and can become alert at different times with a varying degree of intensity in response to sounds.

- *Motor activity.* Several components are evaluated. Motor tone of the newborn is assessed in the most characteristic state of responsiveness. This summary assessment includes overall use of tone as the newborn responds to being handled—whether during spontaneous activity, prone placement, or horizontal holding—and overall assessment of body tone as the newborn reacts to all stimuli.
- *Variations.* Frequency of alert states, state changes, color changes (throughout all states as examination progresses), activity, and peaks of excitement are assessed.
- *Self-quieting activity.* Assessment is based on how often, how quickly, and how effectively newborns can use their resources to quiet and console themselves when upset or distressed. Considered in this assessment are such self-consolatory activities as putting hand to mouth, sucking on a fist or the tongue, and attuning to an object or sound (Figure 27–39). The newborn's need for outside consolation must also be considered—for example, seeing a face; being rocked, held, or dressed; using a pacifier; and being swaddled.

  Neurologically impaired newborns are unable to use self-quieting activities and require more frequent comforting from caregivers when stimulated. For example, drug-positive newborns often exhibit abnormal sleep and feeding patterns and irritability. Swaddling newborns is a way to provide comfort and security. Swaddling also helps the newborn organize and control body movements and behaviors. Blanket swaddling should be loose and should allow the baby easy hand-to-mouth access to promote self-soothing abilities. Tight swaddling, "straitjacket" techniques with arms at sides, is not comforting and may further agitate the baby.
- *Cuddliness or social behaviors.* This area encompasses the newborn's need for and response to being held. Also considered is how often the newborn smiles. These behaviors influence the parents' self-esteem and feelings of acceptance or rejection. Cuddling also appears to be an indicator of personality. Cuddlers appear to enjoy, accept, and seek physical contact; are easier to placate; sleep more; and form earlier and more intense attachments. Noncuddlers are active and restless, have accelerated motor development, and are intolerant of physical restraint. Smiling, even as a grimace reflex, greatly influences parent–newborn feedback. Parents identify this response as positive.

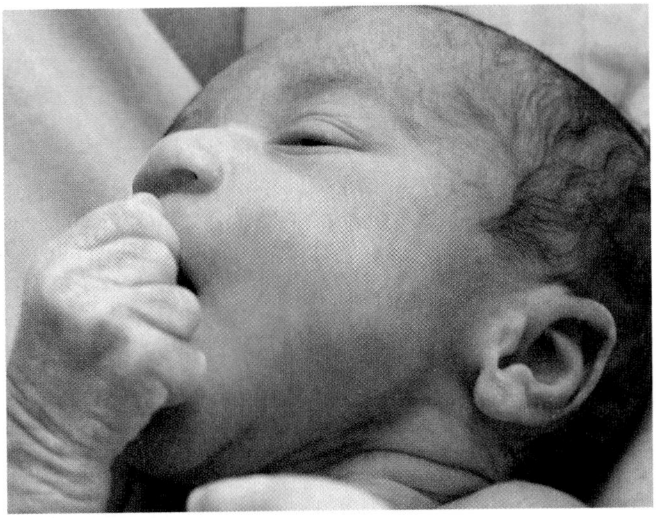

Figure 27–39 The newborn can bring hand to mouth as a self-soothing activity.

Newborn Physical Assessment Guide

Following is a guide for systematically assessing the newborn. Normal findings, alterations, and related causes are presented in correlation with suggested nursing responses. The findings are typical for a full-term newborn.

ASSESSMENT GUIDE | Newborn Physical Assessment

Physical Assessment/Normal Findings	Alterations and Possible Causes*	Nursing Responses to Data†
Vital Signs		
Blood pressure (BP): At birth: 70–50/45–30 mmHg	Low BP (hypovolemia, shock)	Monitor BP in all cases of distress, prematurity, or suspected anomaly.
Day 10: 90–60/50–40 mmHg (may be unable to measure diastolic pressure with standard sphygmomanometer)		Low BP: Refer to physician immediately so measures to improve circulation are begun.
Pulse: 110–160 beats/min (if in deep sleep, as low as 70 beats/min; if crying, up to 180 beats/min)	Weak pulse (decreased cardiac output) Bradycardia (severe asphyxia, arrhythmia) Tachycardia (over 160 beats/min at rest) (infection, central nervous system [CNS] problems, arrhythmia, stress, hypovolemia)	Assess skin perfusion by blanching (capillary refill test—normal: < 3 sec). Correlate finding with BP assessments; refer to physician. Carry out neurologic and thermoregulation assessments. Check blood pressure and hematocrit (Hct).

(continued)

ASSESSMENT GUIDE | Newborn Physical Assessment (*continued*)

Physical Assessment/Normal Findings	Alterations and Possible Causes*	Nursing Responses to Data†
Respirations: 30–60 breaths/min Synchronization of chest and abdominal movements Diaphragmatic and abdominal breathing	Tachypnea (pneumonia, respiratory distress syndrome [RDS]) Rapid, shallow breathing (hypermagnesemia due to large mg doses given to mothers with preeclampsia) Respirations below 30 breaths/min (maternal anesthesia or analgesia)	Identify sleep–wake state; correlate with respiratory pattern. Evaluate for all signs of respiratory distress; report findings to physician.
Transient tachypnea	Expiratory grunting; subcostal and substernal retractions; flaring of nares (respiratory distress); apnea (cold stress, respiratory disorder)	Evaluate for cold stress. Report findings to physician or neonatal nurse practitioner.
Crying: Strong and lusty Moderate tone and pitch	High pitched, shrill (neurologic disorder, hypoglycemia)	Discuss newborn's use of cry for communication. Assess and record abnormal cries.
Cries vary in length from 3 to 7 min after consoling measures are used	Weak or absent (CNS disorder, laryngeal problem)	Reduce environmental noises.
Temperature: Axilla 36.5°C–37.2°C (97.5°F –99°F)	Elevated temperature (room too warm, too much clothing or covers, dehydration, sepsis, brain damage)	Notify physician of elevation or drop in temperature.
	Subnormal temperature (brainstem involvement, cold, sepsis)	Counsel parents on possible causes of elevated or low temperatures, appropriate home care measures, when to call physician.
Heavier newborns tend to have higher body temperatures	Swings of more than 2°F from one reading to next or subnormal temperature (infection)	Teach parents how to take a rectal and/or axillary temperature; assess parents' knowledge regarding use of thermometer; provide teaching as needed.
Weight: 2500–4000 g (5 lb, 8 oz to 8 lb, 13 oz)	Less than 2748 g (less than 6 lb) = small for gestational age (SGA) or preterm Greater than 4050 g (greater than 9 lb) = large for gestational age (LGA) or newborns of mothers with diabetes	Plot weight and gestational age on growth chart to identify high-risk newborns. Ascertain body build of parents. Counsel parents regarding appropriate caloric intake.
Within first 3 to 4 days, normal weight loss of 5–10% Large babies tend to lose more due to greater fluid loss in proportion to birth weight except newborns of mothers with diabetes	Loss greater than 15% (low fluid intake, loss of meconium and urine, feeding difficulties, diabetes insipidus)	Notify physician of net losses or gains. Calculate fluid intake and losses from all sources (insensible water loss, radiant warmers, phototherapy lights). Daily weights and before discharge.
Length: 48–52 cm (18–22 in.)	Less than 45 cm (17.7 in.) (congenital dwarf)	Assess for other signs of dwarfism.
Grows 10 cm (3 in.) during first 3 months	Short/long bones proximally (achondroplasia) Short/long bones distally (Ellis-van Creveld syndrome)	Determine other signs of skeletal system adequacy. Plot progress at subsequent well-baby visits.
Posture		
Body usually flexed, hands may be tightly clenched, neck appears short because chin rests on chest	Only extension noted, inability to move from midline (trauma, hypoxia, immaturity)	Record spontaneity of motor activity and symmetry of movements.
In breech births, feet are usually dorsiflexed	Constant motion (maternal caffeine intake or drug withdrawal)	If parents express concern about newborn's movement patterns, reassure and further evaluate, if appropriate.

Physical Assessment/Normal Findings	Alterations and Possible Causes*	Nursing Responses to Data†
Skin		
Color: Color consistent with ethnic background	Pallor of face conjunctiva (anemia, hypothermia, anoxia)	Discuss with parents common skin color variations to allay fears. Skin color can vary widely in African American newborns.
Newborns of European descent: Pink-tinged or ruddy color over face, trunk, extremities Newborns of African or Native American descent: Pale pink with yellow or red tinge Newborns of Asian descent: Pink or rosy red to yellow tinge	Beefy red (hypoglycemia, immature vasomotor reflexes, polycythemia)	Document extent and time of occurrence of color change.
Common variations: Acrocyanosis, circumoral cyanosis, harlequin color change, or mongolian spots	Meconium staining (nonreassuring fetal status) Jaundice (hemolytic reaction from blood incompatibility within first 24 hours, sepsis)	Obtain Hgb and hematocrit values; obtain bilirubin levels. Assess for respiratory difficulty and temperature instability. Differentiate between physiologic and pathologic jaundice.
Mottled when undressed	Cyanosis (choanal atresia, CNS damage or trauma, respiratory or cardiac problem, cold stress)	Assess degree of (central or peripheral) cyanosis and possible causes; refer to physician.
Minor bruising over buttocks in breech presentation and over eyes and forehead in facial presentations		Discuss with parents cause and course of minor bruising related to labor and birth.
Texture: Smooth, soft, flexible; may have dry, peeling hands and feet	Generalized cracked or peeling skin (SGA or postterm; blood incompatibility; metabolic, kidney dysfunction)	Report to physician.
	Seborrheic-dermatitis (cradle cap) Absence of vernix (postmature) Yellow vernix (bilirubin staining)	Instruct parents to shampoo the scalp and anterior fontanelle areas daily with mild soap or baby shampoo; rinse well; avoid use of oil.
Turgor: Elastic, returns to normal shape after pinching	Maintains tent shape (dehydration)	Assess for other signs and symptoms of dehydration.
Pigmentation: Clear; milia across bridge of nose, forehead, or chin will disappear within a few weeks		Advise parents not to pinch or prick these pimple-like areas.
Café-au-lait spots (one or two)	Six or more spots (neurologic disorder such as von Recklinghausen disease, cutaneous neurofibromatosis)	If there are six or more café-au-lait spots, refer for genetic and neurologic consult.
Congenital dermal melanocytosis (Mongolian blue spots) common over dorsal area and buttocks in dark-skinned newborns		Assure parents of normality of this pigmentation; it will fade in first year or two.
Erythema toxicum	Impetigo (group A ß-hemolytic streptococcus or *Staphylococcus aureus* infection)	If impetigo occurs, instruct parents about handwashing and linen precautions during home care.
Telangiectatic nevi	Hemangiomas: Nevus flammeus (port-wine stain) Nevus vasculosus (strawberry hemangioma) Cavernous hemangiomas	Collaborate with physician. Counsel parents about birthmark's progression to allay misconceptions. Record size and shape of hemangiomas. Refer for follow-up at well-baby clinic.

(continued)

ASSESSMENT GUIDE | Newborn Physical Assessment (*continued*)

Physical Assessment/Normal Findings	Alterations and Possible Causes*	Nursing Responses to Data†
Rashes	Rashes (infection)	Assess location and type of rash (macular, papular, vesicular). Obtain history of onset, prenatal history, and related signs and symptoms.
Petechiae of head or neck (breech presentation, cord around neck)	Generalized petechiae (clotting abnormalities)	Determine cause; advise parents if further healthcare is needed.
Head		
General appearance, size, movement Round, symmetric, and moves easily from left to right and up and down; soft and pliable	Asymmetric, flattened occiput on either side of the head (plagiocephaly) Head held at angle (torticollis) Unable to move head side to side (neurologic trauma)	Instruct parents to change baby's positions frequently when awake. When awake, needs to spend "tummy time." Babies should be placed supine for sleep per "safe to sleep" guidelines (see Chapters 28 and 34). Determine adequacy of all neurologic signs.
Circumference: 32–37 cm (12.6–14.6 in.); 2 cm greater than chest circumference Head one-fourth of body size	Extreme differences in size may be due to microencephaly (Cornelia de Lange syndrome, cytomegalic inclusion disease [CID]), rubella, toxoplasmosis, chromosome abnormalities, hydrocephalus (meningomyelocele, achondroplasia), anencephaly (neural tube defect) Head is 3 cm (1.2 in.) or more larger than chest circumference (preterm, hydrocephalus)	Measure circumference from occiput to frontal area using metal or paper tape. Measure chest circumference using metal or paper tape and compare to head circumference. Record measurements on growth chart. Reevaluate at well-baby visits.
Common variations: Molding	Cephalohematoma (trauma during birth, may persist up to 3 months)	Evaluate neurologic response.
Breech and cesarean newborns' heads are round and well shaped	Caput succedaneum (long labor and birth; disappears in 1 week)	Observe for hyperbilirubinemia. Check Hct. Reassure parents regarding common manifestations due to birth process and when they should disappear.
Fontanelles: Palpation of juncture of cranial bones	Overlapping of anterior fontanelle (malnourished or preterm newborn)	Discuss normal closure times with parents and care of "soft spots" to allay misconceptions.
Anterior fontanelle; 3–4 cm (1.2–1.6 in.) long by 2–3 cm (0.8–1.2 in.) wide, diamond shaped	Premature closure of sutures (craniosynostosis)	Refer to physician. Assess fontanelles and sutures daily.
Posterior fontanelle: 1–2 cm (0.4–0.8 in.) at birth, triangle shaped	Late closure (hydrocephalus)	Observe for signs and symptoms of hydrocephalus.
Slight pulsation	Moderate to severe pulsation (vascular problems)	Refer to physician.
Moderate bulging noted with crying, stooling; pulsations with heartbeat	Bulging (increased intracranial pressure, meningitis) Sunken (dehydration)	Report to physician. Evaluate neurologic status. Evaluate hydration status.
HAIR		
Texture: Smooth with fine texture variations (*Note:* Variations depend on ethnic background.)	Coarse, brittle, dry hair (hypothyroidism) White forelock (Waardenburg syndrome)	Instruct parents regarding routine care of hair and scalp.

Physical Assessment/Normal Findings	Alterations and Possible Causes*	Nursing Responses to Data†
Distribution: Scalp hair high over eyebrows (Spanish, Mexican hairline begins midforehead and extends down back of neck)	Low forehead and posterior hairlines may indicate chromosomal disorders	Assess for other signs of chromosomal aberrations. Refer to physician.
FACE		
Symmetric movement of all facial features, normal hairline, eyebrows and eyelashes present		Assess and record symmetry of all parts, shape, regularity of features, sameness or differences in features.
Spacing of features: Eyes-ears at same level, nostrils equal size, cheeks full, and sucking pads present	Eyes wide apart—ocular hypertelorism (Apert syndrome, Cri-du-chat syndrome, Turner syndrome)	Observe for other signs and symptoms indicative of disease states or chromosomal aberrations.
Lips equal on both sides of midline	Abnormal face (trisomy 21 [Down syndrome], cretinism, gargoylism)	
Chin recedes when compared with other bones of face	Atypical small jaw—micrognathia (Pierre Robin syndrome, Treacher Collins syndrome)	Maintain airway; may do best in prone position. Initiate surgical consultation and referral.
Movement: Makes facial grimaces	Inability to suck, grimace, and close eyelids (cranial nerve injury)	Initiate neurologic assessment and consultation.
Symmetric when resting and crying	Asymmetry (paralysis of facial cranial nerve)	Assess and record symmetry of all parts, shape, regularity of features, and sameness or differences in features.
EYES		
General placement and appearance: Bright and clear; even placement; slight nystagmus (involuntary cyclic eye movements)	Gross nystagmus (damage to third, fourth, and sixth cranial nerves)	
Concomitant strabismus	Constant and fixed strabismus	Reassure parents that strabismus is considered normal up to 6 months.
Move in all directions	Lack of pigmentation (albinism)	Discuss with parents any necessary eye precautions.
Blue-gray or slate blue-gray	Brushfield spots may indicate trisomy 21 (a light or white speckling of the outer two-thirds of the iris)	Assess for other signs of trisomy 21.
Brown color at birth in dark-skinned newborns		Discuss with parents that permanent eye color is usually established by 3 months of age.
Eyelids: Position: above pupils but within iris, no drooping	Elevation or retraction of upper lid (hyperthyroidism). "Sunset sign" lid retraction and downward gaze (hydrocephalus), ptosis (congenital or paralysis of oculomotor muscle)	Assess for signs of hydrocephalus and hyperthyroidism. Evaluate interference with vision in subsequent well-baby visits.
Eyes on parallel plane	Upward slant in non-Asians (trisomy 21)	Assess for other signs of trisomy 21.
Epicanthal folds in Asian and 20% of newborns of northern European descent	Epicanthal folds (trisomy 21, Cri-du-chat syndrome)	
Movement: Blink reflex in response to light stimulus. Eyes open wide in dimly lighted room	Blink absent (CNS injury)	Evaluate neurologic status. Refer to physician.
Inspection: Edematous for first few days of life, resulting from birth; no lumps or redness	Purulent drainage (infection); infectious conjunctivitis (gonococcus, chlamydia, staphylococcus, or Gram-negative organisms) Marginal blepharitis (lid edges red, crusted, scaly)	Initiate good handwashing. Refer to physician. Evaluate newborn for seborrheic dermatitis; scales can be removed easily.

(continued)

ASSESSMENT GUIDE | Newborn Physical Assessment (*continued*)

Physical Assessment/Normal Findings	Alterations and Possible Causes*	Nursing Responses to Data†
Cornea: Clear	Ulceration (herpes infection); large cornea or corneas of unequal size (congenital glaucoma)	Refer to ophthalmologist.
Corneal reflex present	Clouding, opacity of lens (cataract)	Assess for other manifestations of congenital herpes; institute nursing care measures.
Sclera: May appear bluish in newborn, then white; slightly brownish color frequent in newborns of African descent	True blue sclera (osteogenesis imperfecta)	Refer to physician.
Pupils: Pupils equal in size, round, and react to light by accommodation	Anisocoria—unequal pupils (CNS damage) Dilation or constriction (intracranial damage, retinoblastoma, glaucoma) Pupils nonreactive to light or accommodation (brain injury)	Refer for neurologic examination.
Slight nystagmus in newborn who has not learned to focus	Nystagmus (labyrinthine disturbance, CNS disorder)	
Pupil light reflex demonstrated at birth or by 3 weeks of age		
Conjunctiva: Chemical conjunctivitis Subconjunctival hemorrhage	Pale color (anemia)	Obtain hematocrit and hemoglobin. Reassure parents that chemical conjunctivitis will subside in 1 to 2 days and subconjunctival hemorrhage disappears in a few weeks.
Palpebral conjunctival (red but not hyperemic)	Inflammation or edema (infection, blocked tear duct)	
Vision: 20/200 Tracks moving object to midline Fixed focus on objects at a distance of about 10–20 inches; may be difficult to evaluate in newborn Prefers faces, geometric designs, and black and white to colors	Cataracts (congenital infection)	Record any questions about visual acuity and initiate follow-up evaluation at first well-baby checkup. May suggest toys for parents to purchase.
Lashes and lacrimal glands: Presence of lashes (lashes may be absent in preterm newborns)	No lashes on inner two-thirds of lid (Treacher Collins syndrome), bushy lashes (Hurler syndrome), long lashes (Cornelia de Lange syndrome)	
Cry commonly tearless	Excessive tearing (plugged lacrimal duct, natal narcotic withdrawal), glaucoma	Demonstrate to parents how to milk blocked tear duct. Refer to ophthalmologist if tearing is excessive before third month of life.
NOSE		
Appearance of external nasal aspects: May appear flattened as a result of birth process	Continued flat or broad bridge of nose (trisomy 21)	Arrange consultation with specialist. May be normal racial variation—Asian or African ancestry.
Small and narrow in midline, even placement in relationship to eyes and mouth	Low bridge of nose, beaklike nose (Apert syndrome, Treacher Collins syndrome) Upturned (Cornelia de Lange syndrome)	Initiate evaluation of chromosomal abnormalities.
Patent nares bilaterally (nose breathers)	Blockage of nares (mucus or secretions), choanal atresia	Inspect for obstruction of nares.
Sneezing common to clear nasal passages	Flaring nares (respiratory distress)	Maintain oral airway until surgical correction is made.
Responds to odors, may smell breast milk	No response to stimulating odors	Inspect for obstruction of nares.

Physical Assessment/Normal Findings	Alterations and Possible Causes*	Nursing Responses to Data[†]
MOUTH		
Function of facial, hypoglossal, glossopharyngeal, and vagus nerves: Symmetry of movement and strength	Mouth draws to one side (transient seventh cranial nerve paralysis due to pressure in utero or trauma during birth, congenital paralysis)	Initiate neurologic consultation.
	Fishlike shape (Treacher Collins syndrome)	Administer artificial tears if eye on affected side of face is unable to close.
Presence of gag, swallowing, coordinated with sucking reflexes	Suppressed or absent reflexes	Evaluate other neurologic functions of these nerves.
Adequate salivation		
Palate (soft and hard): Hard palate dome shaped. Uvula midline with symmetric movement of soft palate	High-steepled palate (Treacher Collins syndrome), bifid uvula (congenital anomaly)	Assess for other congenital anomalies.
Palate intact, sucks well when stimulated	Clefts in either hard or soft palate (polygenic disorder)	Initiate a surgical consultation referral. Use special feeding devices.
Epithelial (Epstein) pearls appear on mucosa		Assure parents that these are normal and will disappear at 2 or 3 months of age.
Esophagus patent, some drooling common in newborn	Excessive drooling or bubbling (esophageal atresia)	Test for patency of esophagus.
Tongue: Free moving in all directions, midline	Lack of movement or asymmetric movement (neurologic damage)	Further assess neurologic functions.
	Tongue-tied Fasiculations (fine tremors) Spinal muscular atrophy	Test reflex elevation of tongue when depressed with tongue blade.
Pink color, smooth to rough texture, noncoated	Deviations from midline (cranial nerve damage)	Check for signs of weakness or deviation.
	White cheesy coating (thrush) Tongue has deep ridges	Differentiate between thrush and milk curds by wiping: If white patches don't come off easily, it is thrush.
		Reassure parents that tongue pattern may change from day to day.
Tongue proportional to mouth	Large tongue with short frenulum (cretinism, trisomy 21, other syndromes)	Evaluate in well-baby clinic to assess development delays. Initiate referrals.
Ears		
External ear: Without lesions, cysts, or nodules	Nodules, cysts, or sinus tracts in front of ear	Evaluate characteristics of lesions.
	Adherent earlobes	
	Low set (genetic abnormality or syndrome)	Counsel parents to clean external ear with washcloth only; discourage use of cotton-tipped applicators.
	Preauricular skin tags	Refer to physician for ligation.
Hearing: Eustachian tubes are cleared with first cry		
Absence of all risk factors	Presence of one or more risk factors	Assess history of risk factors for hearing loss.
Attends to sounds; sudden or loud noise elicits Moro reflex	No response to sound stimuli (deafness)	Test for Moro reflex.

(continued)

ASSESSMENT GUIDE | Newborn Physical Assessment (*continued*)

Physical Assessment/Normal Findings	Alterations and Possible Causes*	Nursing Responses to Data†
Neck		
Appearance: Short, straight, creased with skinfolds	Abnormally short neck (Turner syndrome)	Report findings to physician.
	Arching or inability to flex neck (meningitis, congenital anomaly)	
Posterior neck lacks loose extra folds of skin	Webbing of neck (Turner syndrome, trisomy 21, trisomy 18)	Assess for other signs of the syndromes.
Clavicles: Straight and intact	Knot or lump on clavicle (fracture during difficult birth)	Obtain detailed labor and birth history; apply figure-eight bandage. Consider oral analgesic.
Moro reflex elicitable	Unilateral Moro reflex response on unaffected side (fracture of clavicle, brachial palsy, Erb-Duchenne paralysis)	
Symmetric shoulders	Hypoplasia	
Chest		
Appearance and size: Circumference: 32.5 cm (12.8 in.), 1–2 cm (0.4–0.8 in.) less than head		Measure at level of nipples after exhalation.
Wider than it is long		
Normal shape without depressed or prominent sternum	Funnel chest (congenital or associated with Marfan syndrome)	Determine adequacy of other respiratory and circulatory signs.
Lower end of sternum (xiphoid cartilage) may be protruding; less apparent after several weeks	Continued protrusion of xiphoid cartilage (Marfan syndrome, "pigeon chest")	Assess for other signs and symptoms of various syndromes.
Sternum 8 cm (3.2 in.) long	Barrel chest	
Expansion and retraction: Bilateral expansion	Unequal chest expansion (pneumonia, pneumothorax, respiratory distress)	Assess respiratory effort regularity, flaring of nares, difficulty on both inspiration and expiration.
No intercostal, subcostal, or supraclavicular retractions	Retractions (respiratory distress)	
	Seesaw respirations (respiratory distress)	
Auscultation: Breath sounds are louder in newborns	Decreased breath sounds (decreased respiratory activity, atelectasis, pneumothorax)	Obtain transilluminator. Record findings and consult physician. Obtain a pulse oximetry reading.
Chest and axilla clear on crying	Increased breath sounds (resolving pneumonia or in cesarean births)	Perform assessment and report to physician any positive findings.
Bronchial breath sounds (heard where trachea and bronchi closest to chest wall, above sternum and between scapulae):		
Bronchial sounds bilaterally Air entry clear Rales may indicate normal newborn atelectasis Cough reflex absent at birth, appears in 2 or more days	Adventitious or abnormal sounds (respiratory disease or distress)	Evaluate color for pallor or cyanosis. Monitor every shift or more frequently. Report to physician.
Breasts: Flat with symmetric nipples	Lack of breast tissue (preterm or SGA)	
Breast tissue diameter 5 cm (2 in.) or more at term	Discharge	Evaluate for infection.
Average distance between nipples 8 cm (3.2 in.)	Breast abscesses	
Breast engorgement occurs on third day of life; liquid discharge may be expressed in term newborns	Enlargement	Reassure parents of normality of breast engorgement.
Nipples	Supernumerary nipples	No intervention is necessary.
	Dark-colored nipples	

Physical Assessment/Normal Findings	Alterations and Possible Causes*	Nursing Responses to Data†
Heart		
Auscultation: Location: lies horizontally, with left border extending to left of midclavicle		
Regular rhythm and rate	Arrhythmia (anoxia), tachycardia, bradycardia	Refer all arrhythmia and gallop rhythms. Initiate cardiac evaluation.
Determination of point of maximal impulse (PMI) Usually lateral to midclavicular line at third or fourth intercostal space	Malpositioning (enlargement, abnormal placement, pneumothorax, dextrocardia, diaphragmatic hernia)	
Functional murmurs No thrills	Location of murmurs (possible congenital cardiac anomaly)	Evaluate murmur: location, timing, and duration; observe for accompanying cardiac pathology symptoms; ascertain family history.
Horizontal groove at diaphragm shows flaring of rib cage to mild degree	Marked rib flaring (vitamin D deficiency) Inadequacy of respiratory movement	Initiate cardiopulmonary evaluation; assess pulses and blood pressures in all four extremities for equality and quality.
Abdomen		
Appearance: Cylindric, with some protrusion; appears large in relation to pelvis; some laxness of abdominal muscles	Distention, shiny abdomen with engorged vessels (gastrointestinal abnormalities, infection, congenital megacolon)	Examine abdomen thoroughly for mass or organomegaly. Measure abdominal girth.
No cyanosis, few vessels seen Diastasis recti—common in newborns of African heritage	Scaphoid abdominal appearance (diaphragmatic hernia)	Report deviations of abdominal size.
	Increased or decreased peristalsis (duodenal stenosis, small bowel obstruction)	Assess other signs and symptoms of obstruction.
	Localized flank bulging (enlarged kidneys, ascites, absent abdominal muscles)	Refer to physician.
Umbilicus: No protrusion of umbilicus (protrusion of umbilicus common in newborns of African heritage)	Umbilical hernia Patent urachus (congenital malformation)	Measure umbilical hernia by palpating the opening and record; it should close by 1 year of age; if not, refer to physician.
Bluish white color		Be aware of cultural practices. Taping or belly bands do not enhance closure.
	Omphalocele (covered defect) Gastroschisis (uncovered defect)	Cover omphalocele and gastroschisis with sterile, moist dressing or plastic sterile bag.
Cutis navel (umbilical cord projects), granulation tissue present in navel	Redness or exudate around cord (infection) Yellow discoloration (hemolytic disease, meconium staining)	Instruct parents on cord care and hygiene.
Two arteries and one vein apparent	Single umbilical artery (congenital anomalies)	Refer anomalies to physician.
Begins drying 1 to 2 hours after birth	Discharge or oozing of blood from the cord	
No bleeding		
Auscultation and percussion: Soft bowel sounds heard shortly after birth every 10–30 seconds	Bowel sounds in chest (diaphragmatic hernia) Absence of bowel sounds Hyperperistalsis (intestinal obstruction)	Collaborate with physician. Assess for other signs of dehydration or infection.

(continued)

ASSESSMENT GUIDE | Newborn Physical Assessment (*continued*)

Physical Assessment/Normal Findings	Alterations and Possible Causes*	Nursing Responses to Data†
Femoral pulses: Palpable, equal, bilateral	Absent or diminished femoral pulses (coarctation of aorta)	Monitor blood pressure in upper and lower extremities.
Inguinal area: No bulges along inguinal area	Inguinal hernia	Initiate referral.
No inguinal lymph nodes felt		Continue follow-up in well-baby clinic.
Bladder: Percusses 1–4 cm (0.4–1.6 in.) above symphysis	Failure to void within 24–48 hours after birth	Determine whether baby voided at birth.
Emptied about 3 hours after birth; if not, at time of birth	Exposure of bladder mucosa (exstrophy of bladder)	Consult with clinician. Cover exstrophy with sterile moist gauze.
Urine—inoffensive, mild odor	Foul odor (infection)	Obtain urine specimen if infection is suspected.
Genitals		
Gender clearly delineated	Ambiguous genitals	Refer for genetic consultation.
MALE		
Penis: Slender in appearance, about 2.5 cm (1 in.) long, 1 cm (0.4 in.) wide at birth	Micropenis (congenital anomaly) Meatal atresia	Observe and record first voiding.
Normal urinary orifice, urethral meatus at tip of penis	Hypospadias, epispadias	Collaborate with physician in presence of abnormality. Delay circumcision.
Noninflamed urethral opening	Urethritis (infection)	Palpate for enlarged inguinal lymph nodes and record painful urination.
Foreskin adheres to glans	Ulceration of meatal opening (infection, inflammation)	Evaluate whether ulcer is due to diaper rash; counsel regarding care.
Uncircumcised foreskin tight for 2 to 3 months	Phimosis—if still tight after 3 months	Instruct parents on how to care for uncircumcised penis.
Circumcised		Teach parents how to care for circumcision. Check for voiding after procedure and evaluate for excessive bleeding.
Erectile tissue present		
Scrotum: Skin loose and hanging or tight and small; extensive rugae and normal size	Large scrotum containing fluid (hydrocele) Red, shiny scrotal skin (orchitis)	Shine a light through scrotum (transilluminate) to verify diagnosis.
Normal skin color	Minimal rugae, small scrotum	Assess for prematurity.
Scrotal discoloration common in breech		
Testes: Descended by birth; not consistently found in scrotum	Undescended testes (cryptorchidism)	If testes cannot be felt in scrotum, gently palpate femoral, inguinal, perineal, and abdominal areas for presence.
Testes size 1.5–2 cm (0.6–0.8 in.) at birth	Enlarged testes (tumor) Small testes (Klinefelter syndrome or adrenal hyperplasia)	Refer to and collaborate with physician for further diagnostic studies.
FEMALE		
Mons: Normal skin color, area pigmented in dark-skinned newborns		

Physical Assessment/Normal Findings	Alterations and Possible Causes*	Nursing Responses to Data†
Labia majora cover labia minora in term and postterm newborns; symmetric size appropriate for gestational age	Hematoma, lesions (trauma) Labia minora prominent	Evaluate for recent trauma. Assess for prematurity.
Clitoris: Normally large in newborn Edema and bruising in breech birth	Hypertrophy (hermaphroditism)	Refer for genetic workup.
Vagina: Urinary meatus and vaginal orifice visible (0.5-cm (0.2 in.) circumference)	Inflammation; erythema and discharge (urethritis) Congenital absence of vagina	Collect urine specimen for laboratory examination. Refer to physician.
Discharge; smegma under labia	Foul-smelling discharge (infection)	Collect data and further evaluate reason for discharge.
Bloody or mucoid discharge (pseudomenstruation)	Excessive vaginal bleeding (blood coagulation defect)	
Buttocks and Anus		
Buttocks symmetric	Pilonidal dimple	Examine for possible sinus. Instruct parents about cleansing this area.
Anus patent and passage of meconium within 24–48 hours after birth	Imperforate anus, rectal atresia (congenital gastrointestinal defect)	Evaluate extent of problems. Initiate surgical consultation.
No fissures, tears, or skin tags	Fissures	Perform digital examination to ascertain patency if patency uncertain.
Extremities and Trunk		
Short and generally flexed; extremities move symmetrically through range of motion but lack full extension	Unilateral or absence of movement (spinal cord involvement) Fetal position continued or limp (anoxia, CNS problems, hypoglycemia)	Review birth record to assess possible cause.
All joints move spontaneously; good muscle tone, of flexor type, birth to 2 months	Spasticity when newborn begins using extensors (cerebral palsy, lack of muscle tone, "floppy baby" syndrome) Hypotonia (trisomy 21)	Collaborate with physician.
Arms: Equal in length Bilateral movement Flexed when quiet	Brachial palsy (difficult birth) Erb-Duchenne paralysis Muscle weakness, fractured clavicle Absence of limb or change of size (phocomelia, amelia)	Report to clinician.
Hands: Normal number of fingers	Polydactyly (Ellis-van Creveld syndrome) Syndactyly—one limb (developmental anomaly) Syndactyly—both limbs (genetic component)	Report to clinician.
Normal palmar crease	Single line on palm (trisomy 21)	Refer for genetic workup.
Normal-sized hands	Short fingers and broad hand (Hurler syndrome)	Evaluate for history of distress in utero.
Nails present and extend beyond fingertips in term newborn	Cyanosis and clubbing (cardiac anomalies) Nails long or yellow stained (postterm)	Carry out cardiac and respiratory assessments. Check pulse oximetry.
Spine: C-shaped spine	Spina bifida occulta (nevus pilosus)	Evaluate extent of neurologic damage; initiate care of spinal opening.
Flat and straight when prone	Dermal sinus	

(continued)

ASSESSMENT GUIDE | Newborn Physical Assessment (*continued*)

Physical Assessment/Normal Findings	Alterations and Possible Causes*	Nursing Responses to Data†
Slight lumbar lordosis	Myelomeningocele (incomplete closure of posterior spine)	
Easily flexed and intact when palpated	Head lag, limp, floppy trunk (neurologic problems)	
At least half of back devoid of lanugo		
Full-term newborn in ventral suspension should hold head at 45-degree angle, back straight		Elicit reflex to assess degree of involvement.
Hips: No sign of instability	Sensation of abnormal movement; jerk or snap of hip dislocation	Physician or nurse practitioner examines all newborns for dislocated hip prior to discharge from birthing center.
Hips abduct to more than 60 degrees		If this is suspected, refer to orthopedist for further evaluation. Reassess at well-baby visits.
Inguinal and buttock skin creases: Symmetric inguinal and buttock creases	Asymmetry (dislocated hips)	Refer to orthopedist for evaluation. Counsel parents regarding symptoms of concern and discuss therapy.
Legs: Legs equal in length	Shortened leg (dislocated hips)	Refer to orthopedist for evaluation.
Legs shorter than arms at birth	Lack of leg movement (fractures, spinal defects)	Counsel parents regarding symptoms of concern and discuss therapy.
Feet: Foot is in straight line	Talipes equinovarus (true clubfoot)	Discuss differences between positional and true clubfoot with parents.
Positional clubfoot—based on position in utero		Teach parents passive manipulation of foot. Refer to orthopedist if not corrected by 3 months of age.
Fat pads and creases on soles of feet	Incomplete sole creases in first 24 hours of life (premature)	
Talipes planus (flat feet) normal under 3 years of age		Reassure parents that flat feet are normal in newborns.
Neuromuscular		
Motor function: Symmetric movement and strength in all extremities	Limp, flaccid, or hypertonic (CNS disorders, infection, dehydration, fracture)	Appraise newborn's posture and motor functions by observing activities and motor characteristics.
May be jerky or have brief twitches	Tremors (hypoglycemia, hypocalcemia, infection, neurologic damage)	Evaluate for electrolyte imbalance, hypoglycemia, and neurologic functioning.
Head lag not over 45 degrees	Delayed or abnormal development (preterm, neurologic involvement)	
Neck control adequate to maintain head erect briefly	Asymmetry of tone or strength (neurologic damage)	Refer for genetic evaluation.

*Possible causes of alterations are placed in parentheses.

†This column provides guidelines for further assessment and initial nursing interventions.

Focus Your Study

- The three time frames for assessing newborns in the birth facility are (1) in the delivery room, (2) during the nursery admission examination, and (3) during the discharge examination.
- A perinatal history, determination of gestational age, physical examination, and behavioral assessment form the basis for complete newborn assessment.
- The common physical characteristics included in the gestational age assessment are skin, lanugo, sole (plantar) creases, breast tissue and size, ear form and cartilage, and genitals.
- The neuromuscular components of gestational age scoring tools are usually posture, square window sign, popliteal angle, arm recoil, heel-to-ear extension, and scarf sign.
- By assessing the physical and neuromuscular components specified in a gestational age tool, the nurse can determine the gestational age of the newborn.
- After determining the gestational age of the baby, the nurse can assess how the newborn will make the transition to extrauterine life and can anticipate potential physiologic problems.
- The nurse identifies the newborn as small for gestational age (SGA), appropriate for gestational age (AGA), or large for gestational age (LGA) and prioritizes individual needs.
- Normal ranges for vital signs assessed in newborns are heart rate of 110 to 160 beats per minute; respiratory rate of 30 to 60 respirations per minute; axillary temperature of 36.5°C to 37.2°C (97.7°F to 99°F); skin temperature of 36°C to 36.5°C (96.8°F to 97.7°F); rectal temperature of 36.6°C to 37.2°C (97.8°F to 99°F); and blood pressure of 70/45 to 50/30 mmHg (at birth).
- Normal newborn measurements include weight from 2500 to 4000 g (5 lb, 8 oz to 8 lb, 13 oz), with weight dependent on maternal size and age; length from 48 to 52 cm (18 to 22 in.); and head circumference from 32 to 37 cm (12.6 to 14.6 in.). Head circumference is approximately 2 cm (0.8 in.) larger than the chest circumference.
- Commonly elicited newborn reflexes are tonic neck, Moro, grasping, rooting, sucking, and blink.
- Newborn behavioral abilities include habituation, orientation to visual and auditory stimuli, motor activity, cuddliness, and self-quieting activity.
- An important role of the nurse during the physical and behavioral assessments of the newborn is to teach parents about their newborn and involve them in their baby's care. This facilitates the parents' identification of their newborn's uniqueness and allays their concerns.

References

American Academy of Pediatrics (AAP). (2015). *How to take a child's temperature.* Retrieved from https://www.healthychildren.org/English/health-issues/conditions/fever/Pages/How-to-Take-a-Childs-Temperature.aspx

American Academy of Pediatrics (AAP) Committee on Fetus and Newborn & American College of Obstetricians and Gynecologists (ACOG) Committee on Obstetrics. (2017). *Guidelines for perinatal care* (8th ed.). Evanston, IL: Author.

Ballard, J. L., Khoury, J. C., Wedig, K., Wang, L., Eilers-Walsman, B. L., & Lipp, R. (1991). New Ballard score, expanded to include extremely premature infants. *Journal of Pediatrics, 119*(3), 417–423.

Brazelton, T. B., & Nugent, J. K. (2011). *The Neonatal Behavioral Assessment Scale* (4th ed.). London, UK: MacKeith.

Cavaliere, T. A., & Sansoucie, D. A. (2014). Assessment of the newborn and infant. In C. Kenner & J. W. Lott (Eds.), *Comprehensive neonatal nursing care* (5th ed., pp. 71–112). New York, NY: Springer.

Eichenwald, E. C., Hansen, A. R., Martin, C. R., & Stark, A. R. (2017). *Cloherty and Stark's manual of neonatal care* (8th ed.). Philadelphia, PA: Lippincott Williams & Wilkins.

Garg, B., Sharma, D., & Farahbakhsh, N. (2018). Assessment of sickness severity of illness in neonates: Review of various neonatal illness scoring systems. *Journal of Maternal-Fetal & Neonatal Medicine, 31*(10), 1373–1380.

Goodwin, M. (2019). Abdominal assessment. In E. P. Tappero & M. E. Honeyfield (Eds.), *Physical assessment of the newborn* (6th ed., pp. 111–120). Petaluma, CA: NICU INK.

Johnson, D. (2019). Head, eyes, ears, mouth, and neck, assessment. In E. P. Tappero & M. E. Honeyfield (Eds.), *Physical assessment of the newborn* (6th ed., pp. 61–78). Petaluma, CA: NICU INK.

Vargo, L. (2019). Cardiovascular assessment. In E. P. Tappero & M. E. Honeyfield (Eds.), *Physical assessment of the newborn* (6th ed., pp. 93–110). Petaluma, CA: NICU INK.

Witt, C. (2019). Skin assessment. In E. P. Tappero & M. E. Honeyfield (Eds.), *Physical assessment of the newborn* (6th ed., pp. 45–60). Petaluma, CA: NICU INK.

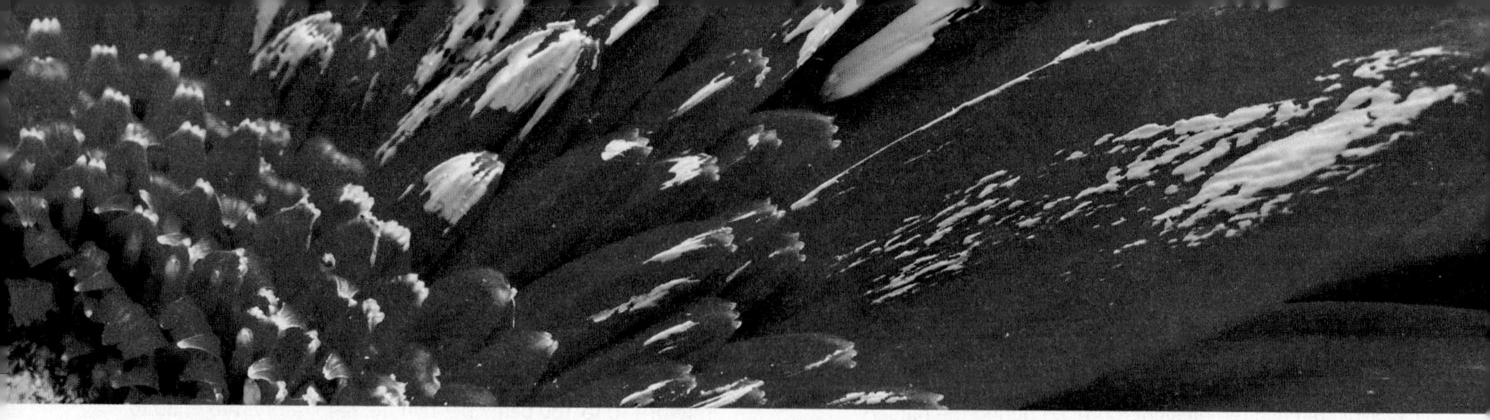

Chapter 28
The Normal Newborn: Needs and Care

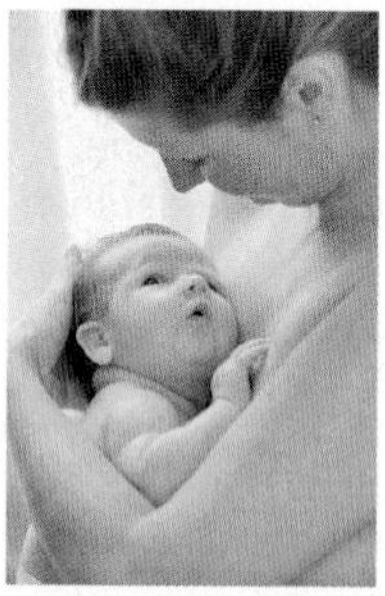

SOURCE: Blend Images/SuperStock.

"Now I believe in love at first sight!"
—A mother holding her newborn for the first time

Learning Outcomes

28.1 Summarize the essential areas of information to be obtained about a newborn's birth experience and immediate postnatal period.

28.2 Explain how the physiologic and behavioral responses of a newborn during the first 4 hours after birth (admission and transitional period) determine the newborn's nursing care.

28.3 Identify activities that should be included in a daily care plan for a normal newborn.

28.4 Discuss the common concerns of families regarding their newborns.

28.5 Describe the influence of cultural values on newborn care.

28.6 Identify opportunities to individualize parent teaching and enhance parents' abilities and confidence while providing newborn care in the birthing unit.

28.7 Discuss safety needs of the newborn that would ensure integration into the family unit.

Healthy People 2020

(MICH-20) Increase the proportion of infants who are put to sleep on their backs

(MICH-21.1) Increase the proportion of infants who are ever breastfed

At the moment of birth, numerous physiologic adaptations begin to take place in the newborn's body. Because of these dramatic changes, newborns require close observation to determine how smoothly they are making the transition to extrauterine life. Newborns also require special care that enhances their chances of making the transition successfully. The two broad goals of nursing care during this period are to:

1. Promote the physical well-being of the newborn by providing comprehensive care while in the mother–baby unit.
2. Support the establishment of a well-functioning family unit by teaching family members how to care for their new baby and by supporting their efforts so that they feel confident and competent.

The nurse must be knowledgeable about family adjustments that need to be made as well as the healthcare needs of the newborn. It is important that the family return home knowing that they have the support, information, and skills to care for their newborn. Equally important is the need for each member of the family to begin a unique relationship with the newborn. The cultural and social expectations of individual families and communities affect the way normal newborn care is carried out.

Chapters 26 and 27 present an informational database of the physiologic and behavioral changes occurring in the newborn and the pertinent nursing assessments that are needed. This chapter discusses nursing management while the newborn is in the birthing unit.

Admission and the First 4 Hours of Life

Immediately after birth, the baby is formally admitted to the healthcare facility.

●○● NURSING MANAGEMENT

For the Newborn During Admission and the First 4 Hours of Life

Nursing Assessment and Diagnosis

Before the birth of a baby, review the prenatal record of the mother for information concerning possible risk factors for the newborn. These include infectious disease screening results, drug or alcohol use by the mother, gestational diabetes, and any other data determined to be of use in anticipating the needs of the newborn. In addition, review the birth record for prolonged rupture of membranes, instrument or vacuum delivery, use of narcotic analgesia, presence of meconium, and any other data that may impact the newborn's ability to successfully transition to the extrauterine environment.

During the first hours after birth, carry out a preliminary physical examination, including an assessment of the newborn's physiologic adaptations. In many birthing units, the nurse performs and documents the initial head-to-toe physical assessment during the first hour of transition and is responsible for notifying the physician or nurse practitioner of any deviations from normal. A complete physical examination is also performed later by the physician or nurse practitioner, within the first 24 hours after birth and within 24 hours before discharge. This can be accomplished with one physical examination (American Academy of Pediatrics [AAP] & American College of Obstetricians and Gynecologists [ACOG], 2017). (See Chapter 27.)

Nursing diagnoses are based on an analysis of the assessment findings. Physiologic alterations of the newborn form the basis of many nursing diagnoses, as does the family's incorporation of them in caring for their new baby. Nursing diagnoses that may apply to newborns include:

- ***Airway Clearance, Ineffective,*** related to presence of mucus and retained lung fluid
- ***Body Temperature: Imbalanced, Risk for,*** related to evaporative, radiant, conductive, and convective heat losses
- ***Pain, Acute,*** related to heelsticks for glucose or hematocrit tests, vitamin K injection, or hepatitis B immunization

(NANDA-I © 2017)

As discussed in Chapter 26, the newborn's physiologic adaptation to extrauterine life occurs rapidly. All body systems are affected. Therefore, many of the nursing diagnoses and associated interventions must be identified and implemented in a very short period of time.

Planning and Implementation

Initiate newborn admission procedures and evaluate the newborn's need to remain under observation. This evaluation may take place in a special transition area or at the mother's bedside. It includes:

- Maternal and birth history
- Airway clearance
- Skin color
- Vital signs (body temperature, heart rate, respiratory rate)
- Measurements (head circumference, body length, body weight)
- Neurologic status (response to handling, muscle tone, level of consciousness, reflexes)
- Ability to feed
- Evidence of complications and/or illness
- Other evaluations as needed or directed by institution guidelines (blood pressure, oxygen saturation, capillary refill, oxygen requirement).

If the evaluation is normal, the baby is successfully making the transition to extrauterine life and may need less frequent observations. In some settings, this may also be a time for moving the mother and baby to another care unit.

Initiation of Admission Procedures

Admission procedures include a review of prenatal and birth information for possible risk factors, a gestational age assessment, and an assessment to ensure that the newborn's adaptation to extrauterine life is proceeding normally. This evaluation for risk factors and the status of the newborn must be done no later than 2 hours after birth (AAP & ACOG, 2017).

If the initial assessment indicates that the newborn is not at risk physiologically, you may perform many of the routine admission procedures in the presence of the parents and others in the birthing area. Some care measures indicated by the assessment findings may be performed by you or by family members under your guidance in an effort to educate and support the family. Other interventions might best be delayed if the newborn must be transferred to an observational nursery.

First check and confirm the newborn's identification with the mother's identification and then obtain and record all significant information. The essential data to be recorded as part of the newborn's chart includes:

1. ***Condition of the newborn.*** Pertinent information includes the newborn's Apgar scores at 1 and 5 minutes, resuscitative measures required in the birthing area, physical examination, vital signs, voidings, and passing of meconium. Complications to be noted include excessive mucus, delayed spontaneous respirations or responsiveness, abnormal number of cord vessels, abnormal vital signs, and obvious physical abnormalities.
2. ***Labor and birth record.*** A copy of the labor and birth record should be placed in the newborn's chart or be accessible on computer. The record contains all the significant data about the birth including duration, course, status of mother and fetus throughout labor and birth, and any analgesia or anesthesia administered to the mother. Particular care is taken to note any variation or difficulties such as prolonged rupture of membranes, abnormal fetal position, meconium-stained amniotic fluid, signs of nonreassuring fetal status during labor, nuchal cord (cord around the newborn's neck at birth),

precipitous birth, use of forceps or vacuum extraction-assisted device, maternal analgesia and anesthesia received within 1 hour of birth, and administration of antibiotics during labor.

3. ***Antepartum history***. Preexisting maternal conditions or any maternal problems that may have compromised the fetus in utero—such as preeclampsia, spotting, illness, recent infections, rubella status, serology results, hepatitis B screen results, colonization with group B streptococci, recent exposure to infectious disease, HIV status, or a history of maternal substance abuse—are of immediate concern in newborn assessment. The chart should also include information about maternal age, estimated date of birth (EDB), previous pregnancies, and presence of any congenital anomalies. An HIV test result, if obtained, is also relevant. State statutes vary as to who may have access to this information (AAP & ACOG, 2017).
4. ***Parent–newborn interaction information***. The nurse notes parents' interactions with their newborn and their desires regarding care, such as rooming-in, circumcision, and type of feeding. Information about other children in the home, available support systems, interactional patterns within each family unit, situations that compromise lactation (breast surgery, trauma, previous lactation failure), and any high-risk circumstances (adolescent mother, domestic violence, history of child abuse) help in providing comprehensive care (AAP & ACOG, 2017).

As part of the admission procedure, weigh the newborn in both grams and pounds (Figure 28–1). In the United States, most parents understand weights best when stated in pounds and ounces. Clean and cover the scale each time a newborn is weighed to prevent cross-infection and heat loss from conduction.

Measure the newborn, recording the measurements in both centimeters and inches. Three routine measurements are length, circumference of the head, and circumference of the chest. In some facilities, abdominal girth may also be measured (see *Key Facts to Remember: Newborn Measurements* in Chapter 27). Rapidly assess the baby's color, muscle tone, alertness, and general state. Remember that the first period of reactivity may have concluded, and the newborn may be in the sleep-inactive phase, which makes the baby hard to arouse. Perform basic assessments for estimating gestational age and complete the physical assessment. (For a detailed discussion of the process of newborn assessment, see Chapter 27.)

In addition to obtaining vital signs, perform hematocrit and blood glucose evaluations on at-risk newborns or as clinically indicated (such as for small-for-gestational-age [SGA] or large-for-gestational-age [LGA] newborns or if the newborn is jittery). These procedures may be done on admission or within the first 2 hours after birth (AAP & ACOG, 2017). (See *Clinical Skill 31–1: Performing a Heelstick on a Newborn* in Chapter 31.)

Maintenance of a Clear Airway and Stable Vital Signs

Free-flow oxygen should be readily available. Position the newborn on the back (or side, if the baby has copious secretions). If necessary, a bulb syringe or DeLee wall suction (see *Clinical Skill 21–1: Performing Nasal Pharyngeal Suctioning* in Chapter 21) can be used to remove mucus from the nasal passages and oral cavity. A DeLee catheter attached to suction may be used to remove mucus from the stomach to help prevent possible aspiration. When possible, this procedure should be delayed for 10 to 15 minutes after birth, reducing the potential for severe vasovagal reflex apnea.

In the absence of any newborn distress, continue with the admission by taking the newborn's vital signs. The initial temperature is taken by the axillary method (see Figure 27–16).

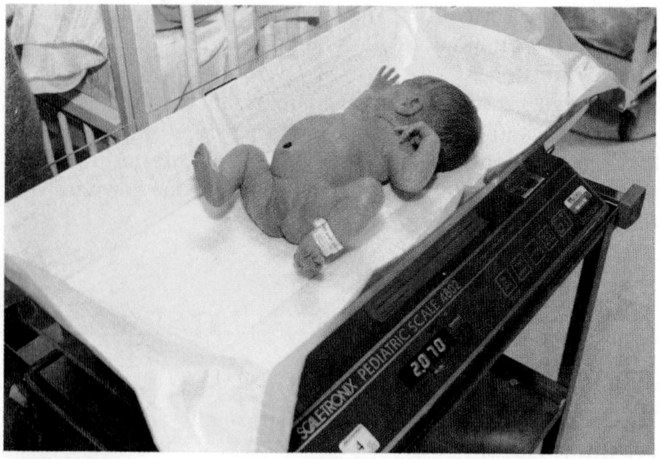

Figure 28–1 **Weighing a newborn. The scale is balanced before each weighing, with the protective pad in place.**

A wider range of normal exists for axillary temperature, specifically, 36.4°C to 37.2°C (97.5°F to 99°F).

Once the initial temperature is taken, monitor the core temperature either by obtaining axillary temperatures at intervals or by placing a skin sensor on the newborn for continuous reading. The vital signs for a healthy term newborn should be monitored at least every 30 minutes until the newborn's condition has remained stable for 2 hours (AAP & ACOG, 2017). The newborn's respirations may be irregular yet still be normal. Brief periods of apnea, lasting only 5 to 10 seconds with no color or heart rate changes, are considered normal. The normal pulse range is 110 to 160 beats per minute (beats/min), and the normal respiratory range is 30 to 60 respirations per minute.

Maintenance of a Neutral Thermal Environment

A neutral thermal environment is essential to minimize the newborn's need for increased oxygen consumption and use of calories to maintain body heat in the optimal range of 36.4°C to 37.2°C (97.5°F to 99°F). If the newborn becomes hypothermic, the body's response can lead to metabolic acidosis, hypoxia, and shock. See *Clinical Skill 28–1: Thermoregulation of the Newborn*.

A neutral thermal environment is best achieved by performing the assessment and interventions with a newborn unclothed and under a radiant warmer. The radiant warmer's thermostat is controlled by the thermal skin sensor taped to the newborn's abdomen, upper thigh, or arm (see Figure 27–17). The sensor indicates when the newborn's temperature exceeds or falls below the acceptable temperature range. Be aware that leaning over the newborn may block the radiant heat waves.

In light of early discharge practices (12 to 48 hours), healthy term newborns can be safely bathed immediately after the admission assessment is completed. It is recommended to wash off only the blood and fluid with the first bath and massage the vernix into the skin (AAP & ACOG, 2017). The baby is bathed while still under the radiant warmer; the bath should, when possible, take place in the parents' room or with parents present. Bathing the newborn offers an excellent opportunity for teaching and welcoming parent involvement in the care of their baby. If there is any doubt regarding the newborn's condition, the baby may be given a sponge bath when the newborn's temperature is normal and vital signs are stable (about 2 to 4 hours after birth), when the newborn's condition dictates, or when the parents wish to give the first bath.

Recheck the baby's temperature after the bath and, if it is stable, dress the newborn in a shirt, diaper, and cap; wrap

CLINICAL SKILL 28–1

Thermoregulation of the Newborn

NURSING ACTION

Preparation

- Prewarm the incubator or radiant warmer. Make sure warm towels and/or lightweight blankets are available.
- Maintain the temperature of the birthing room at 22°C (71°F), with a relative humidity of 60% to 65%.

Rationale: *The change from a warm, moist intrauterine environment to a cool, dry, drafty environment stresses the newborn's immature thermoregulation system.*

Equipment and Supplies

Prewarmed towels or blankets
Newborn stocking cap
Servocontrol probe
Newborn T-shirt and diaper
Open crib

Procedure: Clean Gloves

1. Don gloves.

   Rationale: *Gloves are worn whenever there is the possibility of contact with body fluids—in this case, a newborn wet with amniotic fluid, vernix, and maternal blood.*

2. Place the newborn under the radiant warmer. Wipe the newborn free of blood, fluid, and excess vernix, especially from the head, using prewarmed towels.

   Rationale: *The radiant warmer creates a heat-gaining environment. Drying is important to prevent the loss of body heat through evaporation.*

3. If the newborn is stable, wrap in a prewarmed blanket, apply a stocking cap, and carry the baby to the mother. The mother and her partner/support person can hold and enjoy the newborn together. Alternatively, carry the wrapped newborn to the mother, loosen the blanket, and place the baby skin to skin on the mother's chest under a warmed blanket.

   Rationale: *Use of a prewarmed blanket reduces convection heat loss and facilitates maternal–newborn contact without compromising the newborn's thermoregulation. Skin-to-skin contact with the mother or father/partner helps maintain the newborn's temperature.*

4. After the newborn has spent time with the parents, return the baby to the radiant warmer and apply a diaper. Leave the newborn uncovered (except for the cap and diaper) under the radiant warmer.

   Rationale: *Radiant heat warms the outer skin surface, so the skin needs to be exposed.*

5. Tape a servocontrol probe on the newborn's anterior abdominal wall, with the metal side next to the skin. Do not place it over the ribs. Secure the probe with porous tape or a foil-covered aluminum heat deflector patch. Figure 27–17 in Chapter 27 shows a newborn with a skin probe.

6. Turn the heater to servocontrol mode so that the abdominal skin temperature is maintained at 36.0°C to 36.5°C (96.8°F to 97.7°F).

7. Monitor the newborn's axillary and skin probe temperatures per agency protocol.

   Rationale: *The temperature indicator on the radiant warmer continually displays the newborn's probe temperature. The axillary temperature is checked to ensure that the machine is accurately recording the newborn's temperature.*

8. When the newborn's axillary temperature reaches 37°C (98.6°F), add a T-shirt, double-wrap the baby (two blankets), and place in an open crib.

9. Recheck the newborn's temperature in 1 hour and regularly thereafter according to agency policy.

   Rationale: *It is important to monitor the newborn's ability to maintain his or her own thermoregulation.*

10. If the newborn's temperature drops below 36.1°C (97°F), rewarm the baby gradually. Place the newborn (unclothed except for a diaper) under the radiant warmer with a servocontrol probe on the anterior abdominal wall.

    Rationale: *Rapid heating can lead to hyperthermia, which is associated with apnea, insensible water loss, and increased metabolic rate.*

11. Recheck the newborn's temperature in 30 minutes, and then hourly.

12. When the temperature reaches 37°C (98.6°F), dress the newborn, remove from the radiant warmer, double-wrap, and place in an open crib. Check the temperature hourly until stable, then regularly according to agency policy.

Note: A newborn who repeatedly requires rewarming should be observed for other signs and symptoms of illness and the healthcare provider notified because it may warrant screening for infection.

the baby; and place the baby in an open crib at room temperature. If the baby's axillary temperature is below 36.5°C (97.7°F), return the baby to the radiant warmer or place the newborn in skin-to-skin contact with the mother to rewarm and promote early bonding and breastfeeding. The rewarming process should be gradual to prevent the possibility of hyperthermia. (See Chapter 27 for information about temperature assessment and instability.) See *Key Facts to Remember: Maintaining a Stable Temperature in the Newborn* and *Case Study: Melissa Bond-James.*

CASE STUDY: Melissa Bond-James

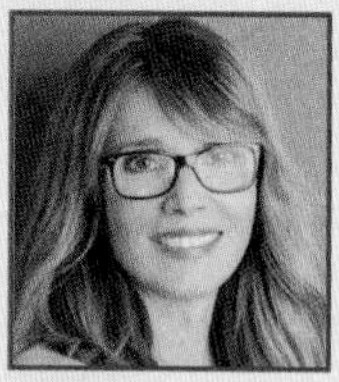
SOURCE: Kinga/ Shutterstock.

Melissa gives birth to a healthy baby girl with Apgar scores of 8 and 9. Within 15 minutes of giving birth, both sets of grandparents arrive to see the baby. Melissa is breastfeeding the baby and holding her skin-to-skin. Nancy's mother feels the newborn should be wrapped in blankets instead so she will not get a chill.

Question to Ponder

What education can you provide the family on heat loss while educating them on the benefits of skin-to-skin contact?

Key Facts To Remember
Maintaining a Stable Temperature in the Newborn

Take these actions to help the newborn maintain a stable temperature:

- Keep the newborn's clothing and bedding dry.
- Double-wrap and put a stocking cap on the newborn.
- Use the radiant warmer during procedures.
- Reduce the newborn's exposure to drafts.
- Warm objects that will be in contact with the newborn (e.g., stethoscopes, blankets).
- Encourage the mother to snuggle with the newborn under blankets or to breastfeed the newborn with stocking cap and light cover.

Prevention of Vitamin K Deficiency Bleeding

A prophylactic injection of vitamin K_1 (AquaMEPHYTON) is given to prevent hemorrhage, which can occur because of low prothrombin levels in the first few days of life (see *Drug Guide: Vitamin K_1 Phytonadione [AquaMEPHYTON]*). The potential for hemorrhage results from the absence of gut bacterial flora, which influences the production of vitamin K in the newborn (see Chapter 31 for further discussion). Current recommendations underscore the need for treatment in babies who are exclusively breastfed. Vitamin K injection can be delayed until first breastfeeding has occurred or up to 6 hours after birth (Wilson, Shannon, & Shields, 2018). It is often given in the labor and delivery unit before transfer to the newborn nursery.

Vitamin K injection is given intramuscularly in the vastus lateralis muscle that lies along the midanterior lateral aspect of the thigh (Figure 28–2). Before injecting, clean the newborn's skin site for the injection thoroughly with a small alcohol swab. Use a 25-gauge, 5/8-inch needle for the injection (Figure 28–3). An alternative site is the rectus femoris muscle in the anterior aspect of the thigh. However, this site is near the sciatic nerve and femoral artery and should be used with caution. If the mother received anticoagulants during pregnancy, an additional dose may be ordered by the healthcare provider and is given 6 to 8 hours after the first injection.

Prevention of Eye Infection

You are also responsible for giving the legally required prophylactic eye treatment for *Neisseria gonorrhoeae*, which may have infected the newborn of an infected mother during the birth

DRUG GUIDE

Vitamin K_1 Phytonadione (AquaMEPHYTON)

OVERVIEW OF NEONATAL ACTION

Phytonadione is used in prophylaxis and treatment of vitamin K deficiency bleeding (VKDB), formerly known as hemorrhagic disease of the newborn. It promotes liver formation of clotting factors II, VII, IX, and X. At birth, the newborn does not have the bacteria in the colon that are necessary for synthesizing fat-soluble vitamin K_1. Therefore, the newborn may have decreased levels of prothrombin during the first 5 to 8 days of life, reflected by a prolongation of prothrombin time.

ROUTE, DOSAGE, AND FREQUENCY

Intramuscular injection is given in the vastus lateralis thigh muscle. A one-time-only prophylactic dose of 0.5 to 1 mg is given intramuscularly in the birthing area or within 1 hour of birth or may be delayed until after first breastfeeding in the birthing area (Wilson et al., 2018).

If the mother received anticoagulants during pregnancy, an additional dose may be ordered by the physician and is given 6 to 8 hours after the first injection.

NEONATAL SIDE EFFECTS

Pain and edema may occur at the injection site. Allergic reactions, such as rash and urticaria, may also occur.

NURSING CONSIDERATIONS

- Protect the drug from light.
- Observe for signs of local inflammation.
- Observe for jaundice and kernicterus, especially in preterm newborns.
- Give vitamin K_1 before circumcision procedure.
- Observe for bleeding (usually occurs on second or third day). Bleeding may be seen as generalized ecchymoses or bleeding from the umbilical cord, circumcision site, nose, or gastrointestinal tract. Results of serial prothrombin time (PT) and international normalized ratio (INR) should be assessed.

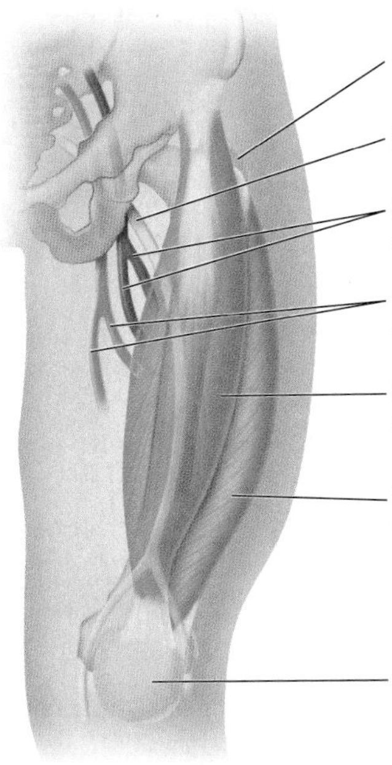

Figure 28–2 Injection sites. The middle third of the vastus lateralis muscle is the preferred site for intramuscular injection in the newborn. The middle third of the rectus femoris is an alternative site, but its proximity to major vessels and the sciatic nerve necessitates caution in using this site for injection.

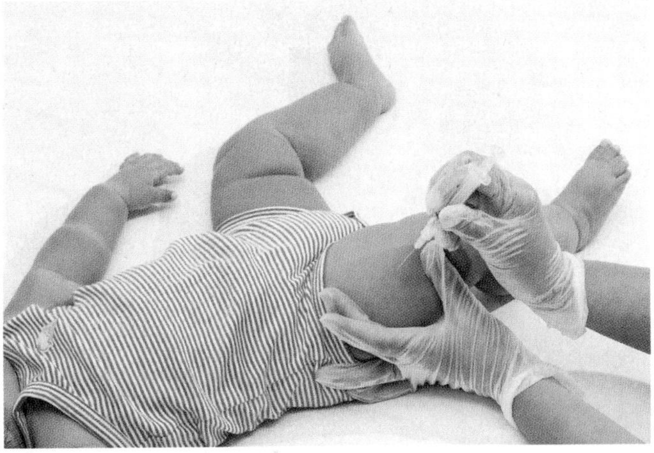

Figure 28–3 Procedure for vitamin K injection. Cleanse area thoroughly with alcohol swab and allow skin to dry. Bunch the tissue of the midanterior lateral aspect of the thigh (vastus lateralis muscle) and quickly insert a 25-gauge 5/8-inch needle at a 90-degree angle to the thigh. Aspirate, and then slowly inject the solution to distribute the medication evenly and minimize the baby's discomfort. Remove the needle and massage the site with an alcohol swab.

process. A variety of topical agents appear to be equally effective. Ophthalmic ointments that are used include 0.5% erythromycin (Ilotycin Ophthalmic) (see *Drug Guide: Erythromycin Ophthalmic Ointment [Ilotycin Ophthalmic]*), 1% tetracycline, or per agency protocol. All are also effective against chlamydia, which has a higher incidence rate than gonorrhea.

Successful eye prophylaxis requires that the medication be instilled into the lower conjunctival sac of each eye (Figure 28–4). Massage the eyelid gently to distribute the ointment. It is instilled only once in each eye (AAP & ACOG, 2017).

The resulting edema, inflammation, and discharge may cause concern if the parents have not been informed that the side effects will clear in 24 to 48 hours and that this prophylactic eye treatment is necessary for the newborn's well-being.

DRUG GUIDE

Erythromycin Ophthalmic Ointment (Ilotycin Ophthalmic)

OVERVIEW OF NEONATAL ACTION

Erythromycin (Ilotycin Ophthalmic) is used as prophylactic treatment of ophthalmia neonatorum, which is caused by the bacteria *Neisseria gonorrhoeae*. Preventive treatment of gonorrhea in the newborn is required by law. It is either bacteriostatic or bactericidal, depending on the organisms involved and the concentration of the drug.

ROUTE, DOSAGE, AND FREQUENCY

Ophthalmic ointment (0.5%) is instilled as a narrow ribbon or strand, 0.5 to 1 cm long, along the lower conjunctival surface of each eye, starting at the inner canthus. It is instilled only once in each eye. The ointment may be administered in the birthing area or, alternatively, later in the nursery so that eye contact between newborn and parent is facilitated and the bonding process immediately after birth is not interrupted. After administration, gently close the eye and manipulate to ensure spread of ointment (Wilson et al., 2018).

NEONATAL SIDE EFFECTS

Sensitivity reaction; may interfere with ability to focus and may cause edema and inflammation. Side effects usually disappear in 24 to 48 hours.

NURSING CONSIDERATIONS

- Use standard precautions before instillation to prevent introduction of bacteria if the baby has not been bathed yet.
- Do not irrigate the eyes after instillation. Use new tube or single-use container for ophthalmic ointment administration shortly after birth. May wipe away excess after 1 minute.
- Observe for hypersensitivity.
- Teach parents about need for eye prophylaxis. Educate them regarding side effects and signs that need to be reported to the healthcare provider.

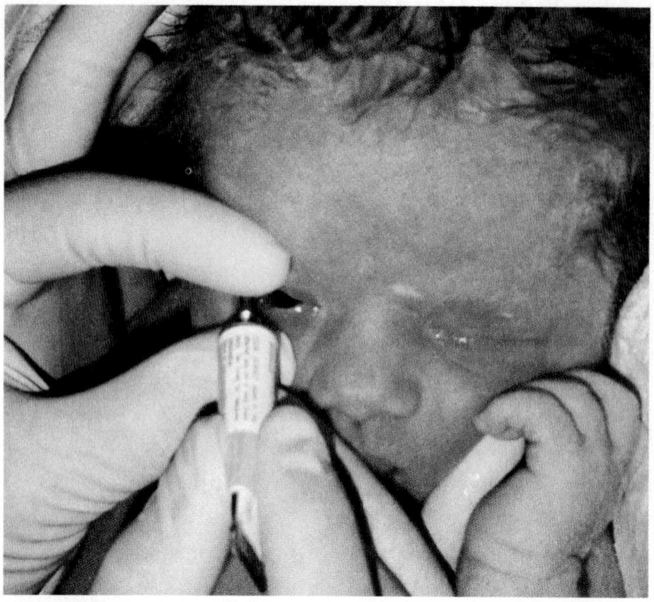

Figure 28–4 **Ophthalmic ointment. Retract lower eyelid outward to instill a 0.25-in. strand of ointment from a single-dose ampule along the lower conjunctival surface. Make sure that the tip of the tube does not touch the eye.**

Early Assessment of Neonatal Distress

During the first 24 hours of life, be constantly alert for signs of distress. If the newborn is with the parents during this period, take extra care to teach them how to maintain their newborn's temperature, recognize the hallmarks of newborn distress, and respond immediately to signs of respiratory problems. The parents should learn to observe the newborn for changes in skin color or activity, rapid breathing with chest retractions, nasal flaring, or facial grimacing. Their interventions should include nasal and oral suctioning with bulb syringe, positioning, and vigorous fingertip stroking of the newborn's spine to stimulate respiratory activity, if necessary. Be immediately available to provide appropriate interventions should the newborn develop distress (Table 28–1).

A common cause of neonatal distress is early-onset group B streptococcal (GBS) disease. Infected mothers transmit GBS infection to their babies during labor and birth; thus, it is recommended that at-risk mothers receive intrapartum antimicrobial prophylaxis (IAP) for GBS disease. All newborns of mothers identified as at risk should be assessed and observed for signs and symptoms of sepsis. (See Chapter 18 for discussion of maternal care and Chapter 31 for discussion of newborn care.) It is important to know the policy and procedures that your hospital follows for surveillance of at-risk newborns.

Initiation of First Feeding

The timing of the first feeding varies, depending on whether the newborn is to be breastfed or formula-fed and whether there were any complications during pregnancy or birth, such as maternal diabetes or intrauterine growth restriction (IUGR).

Mothers who choose to breastfeed their newborns should be encouraged to put their baby to breast during the first period of reactivity, while the baby is alert and responsive. (See Chapter 26 for further discussion of neonatal periods of reactivity.)

TABLE 28–1 Signs of Neonatal Distress

- Respiratory changes
  - Increased respiratory rate (more than 60/minute) or difficult respirations
  - Sternal, substernal, intercostal retractions
  - Nasal flaring
  - Excessive mucus
- Color change
  - Cyanosis (central: Skin, lips, tongue)
  - Pallor
  - Mottling
  - Plethora (ruddy skin)
  - Jaundice of the skin within 24 hours of birth or because of hemolytic process
- Abdominal distention or mass
- Vomiting of bile-stained material
- Absence of meconium elimination within 48 hours of birth
- Absence of urine elimination more than 24 hours after birth (AAP & ACOG, 2017)
- Temperature instability (hypothermia or hyperthermia)
- Jitteriness, irritability, or abnormal movements
- Difficult to waken, lethargy, or hypotonicity
- Weight change greater than 10% loss from birthweight

SOURCE: AAP & ACOG, 2017.

Placing the baby at mother's breast as soon as possible facilitates early latch and promotes successful breastfeeding. Breastfeeding should be initiated within the first hour of life unless medically contraindicated. Formula-fed newborns usually begin the first feeding by 5 hours of age, during the second period of reactivity, when they awaken and appear hungry.

Signs indicating newborn readiness for the first feeding are licking of the lips, placing a hand in or near the mouth, mouthing the blanket, active bowel sounds, absence of abdominal distention, and a lusty cry that quiets with rooting and sucking behaviors when a stimulus is placed near the lips. Observing the earlier, more subtle cues that baby is ready to nurse provides an opportunity to teach the parents to recognize these cues and respond before the baby is frustrated and crying.

Facilitation of Parent-Newborn Attachment

To facilitate **parent–newborn attachment**, eye-to-eye contact between parents and their newborn is extremely important during the early hours after birth, when the newborn is in the first period of reactivity. The newborn is alert during this time, the eyes are wide open, and direct eye contact is made with human faces within optimal range for visual acuity (7 to 8 inches) (see Figure 26–10 in Chapter 26). Eye contact is an important component of the emerging parent–baby bond (Klaus & Klaus, 1999). Consequently, the prophylactic eye medication is often delayed, but no more than 1 hour, to provide an opportunity for this period of eye contact between parents and their newborn, thus facilitating the attachment process (AAP & ACOG, 2017). Parents who cannot be with their newborns in this first period because of maternal or neonatal distress may need reassurance that the bonding process can proceed normally as soon as both mother and baby are stable.

PROFESSIONALISM IN PRACTICE Promoting Evidence-Based Clinical Practices

Many hospital units remove newborns from their mother following birth to allow convenient assessment and performance of procedures by hospital staff despite the preponderance of evidence that supports immediate skin-to-skin contact between mother (or father) and the newborn. Nurses are the professionals most often at the patient's bedside; they have the power and the obligation to serve as leaders and agents of change by promoting clinical practices that are supported by research evidence.

Another situation that can facilitate attachment is the interactive bath. While bathing their newborn for the first time, parents attend closely to their baby's behavior. Observe and point out behaviors, such as the baby attending to a parent's voice or making eye contact, and model appropriate responses. In this way, parents begin to learn the unique characteristics of their newborn.

Evaluation

When evaluating the nursing care provided during the period immediately after birth, the following outcomes may be anticipated:

- The newborn baby's adaptation to extrauterine life is supported and complete.
- The baby's physiologic and psychologic integrity is supported.
- Positive interactions between parent and newborn will be supported.

The Newborn Following Transition

Once healthy newborns have demonstrated successful adaptation to extrauterine life, they need appropriate observations for the first 6 to 12 hours after birth and the remainder of their stay in the birthing facility.

●○● NURSING MANAGEMENT

For the Newborn Following Transition

Nursing Assessment and Diagnosis

Examples of nursing diagnoses that may apply during daily care of the newborn include:

- *Breathing Pattern, Ineffective,* related to periodic breathing
- *Nutrition, Imbalanced: Less than Body Requirements,* related to limited nutritional and fluid intake and increased caloric expenditure
- *Urinary Elimination, Impaired,* related to meatal edema secondary to circumcision
- *Infection, Risk for,* related to umbilical cord healing, circumcision site, immature immune system, or potential birth trauma (forceps or vacuum extraction birth)
- *Knowledge, Readiness for Enhanced,* related to information about basic newborn care, male circumcision, and breastfeeding and/or formula-feeding
- *Family Processes, Readiness for Enhanced,* related to integration of newborn into family or demands of newborn care and feeding

(NANDA-I © 2017)

Planning and Implementation

Maintenance of Cardiopulmonary Function

Assess vital signs every 6 to 8 hours or more, depending on the newborn's status. The newborn should be placed on the back (supine) for sleeping. A bulb syringe is kept within easy reach should the baby need oral-nasal suctioning. If the newborn has respiratory difficulty, the airway is cleared. Vigorous fingertip stroking of the baby's spine will frequently stimulate respiratory activity. A cardiorespiratory monitor can be used on newborns who are not being observed at all times and are at risk for decreased respiratory or cardiac function. Indicators of risk are pallor, cyanosis, ruddy color, apnea, or other signs of instability. Changes in skin color may indicate the need for closer assessment of temperature, cardiopulmonary status, and hematocrit, glucose, and bilirubin levels.

Maintenance of a Neutral Thermal Environment

Make every effort to maintain the newborn's temperature within the normal range. Be certain the newborn is dried completely after the bath, dressed, and exposed to the air as little as possible. A head covering should be used initially and continued with the small newborn, who has less subcutaneous fat to act as insulation in maintaining body heat. Ambient temperature of the room where the newborn is kept should be monitored to prevent excessive cooling. Advise parents to dress the newborn in one more layer of clothing than is necessary for an adult to maintain thermal comfort. Layering of clothes allows for flexibility as the baby is moved from one area to another.

A newborn whose temperature falls below optimal levels will use calories to maintain body heat rather than for growth. Chilling also decreases the affinity of serum albumin for bilirubin, thereby increasing the likelihood of newborn jaundice. It also increases oxygen use and may cause respiratory distress. A newborn who is overheated will have increased respiratory and heart rates and may also become more active, burning up precious caloric reserves. The increase in respiratory rate also results in insensible fluid loss (Gardner & Hernandez, 2016).

Promotion of Adequate Hydration and Nutrition

Record the newborn's caloric and fluid intake and enhance adequate hydration by maintaining a neutral thermal environment and offering early and frequent feedings. Early feedings promote gastric emptying and increase peristalsis, thereby decreasing the degree of hyperbilirubinemia by limiting the amount of time fecal material is in contact with the enzyme β-glucuronidase in the small intestine. This enzyme acts to free the bilirubin from the stool, allowing bilirubin to be reabsorbed into the vascular system. (See Chapter 31 for a detailed discussion of hyperbilirubinemia.)

Record voiding and stooling patterns. The first voiding should occur within 24 hours and first passage of stool within 48 hours. When they do not occur, continue the normal observation routine while assessing for abdominal distention, bowel sounds, and hydration status.

The newborn should be weighed at the same time each day for accurate comparisons and must be kept warm during the weighing. A weight loss of up to 10% for term newborns is considered within normal limits during the first week of life (Eichenwald, Hansen, Martin, et al., 2017). This weight loss is the result of limited intake, loss of excess extracellular fluid, and passage of meconium. Parents should be told about the expected weight loss, the reason for it, and the expectations for regaining the birth weight. Birth weight should be regained by 2 weeks if feedings are adequate.

Excessive handling can cause an increase in the newborn's metabolic rate and calorie use and cause fatigue. Be alert to the baby's subtle cues of fatigue, including a decrease in muscle tension and activity in the extremities and neck, as well as loss of eye contact, which may be manifested by fluttering or closing the eyelids. Quickly cease stimulation when signs of fatigue appear and demonstrate to the parents the need to be aware of newborn cues of fatigue and to wait for periods of alertness for contact and stimulation. You are also responsible for assessing the woman's comfort and latching-on techniques, if breastfeeding, or bottle-feeding techniques. Newborn nutrition is addressed in depth in Chapter 29.

Promotion of Skin Integrity

Newborn skin care, including bathing, is important for the health and appearance of the individual newborn and for infection control within the nursery. Ongoing skin care involves cleansing the buttock and perianal areas with fresh water and cotton, or with mild soap and water, with diaper changes. If commercial baby wipes are used, those without alcohol should be selected. Wipes that are perfume- and latex-free are also available.

Assess the umbilical cord for signs of bleeding or infection. Removal of the cord clamp within 24 to 48 hours of birth reduces the chance of tension injury to the area. Keeping the umbilical stump clean and dry can reduce the chance for infection (AAP & ACOG, 2017) (Figure 28–5).

Many types of routine cord care are practiced, including the use of triple-dye or an antimicrobial agent such as bacitracin or application of 70% alcohol to the cord stump, but should not be encouraged. These practices are largely based on tradition rather than evidence-based findings. The skin absorption and toxicity of triple-dye agents in newborns have not been carefully studied. No single method of umbilical cord care has been proven to be superior in preventing colonization and infection (omphalitis) (AAP & ACOG, 2017). Folding the diaper down to prevent coverage of the cord stump can prevent contamination of the area and promote drying. You are responsible for cord care per agency policy. In developing countries, different standards of practice should be considered when standard hygiene practices are not being met (AAP & ACOG, 2017). The cord should look dark and dry up before falling off (Figure 28–6). It is also your responsibility to instruct parents in caring for the cord and observing for signs and symptoms of infection after discharge, such as foul smell, redness, greenish-yellow drainage, localized heat and tenderness, or bright red bleeding or if the area remains unhealed 2 to 3 days after the cord has sloughed off.

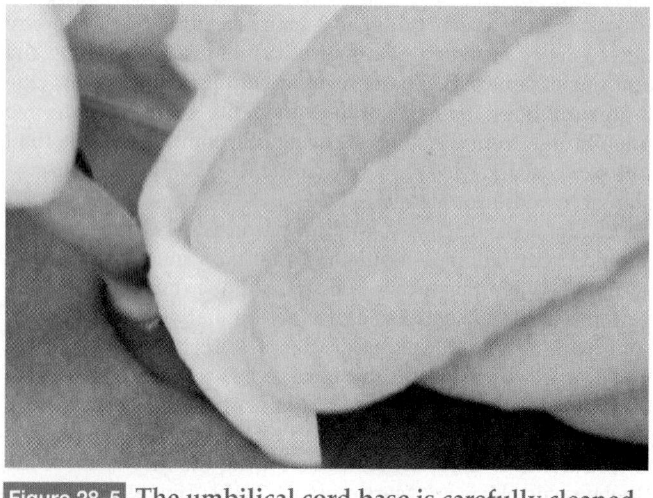

Figure 28–5 The umbilical cord base is carefully cleaned.

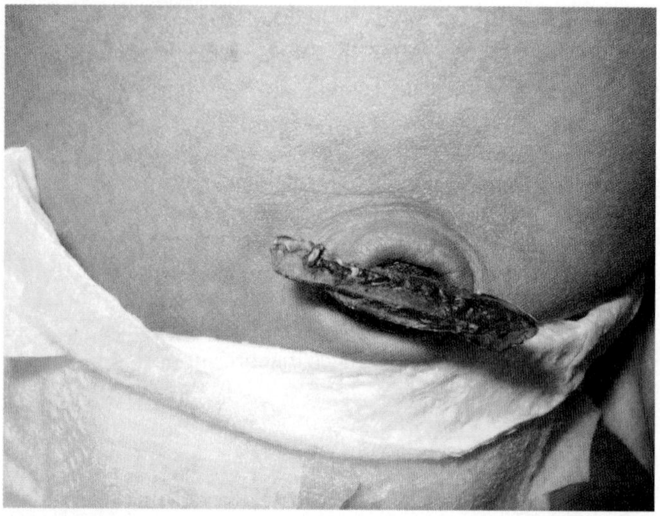

Figure 28–6 The umbilical cord looks dark and dries up prior to falling off.

SOURCE: Anna Garcia.

Promotion of Safety

The threat of abduction of the newborn requires that hospitals have active programs to prevent such an event (AAP & ACOG, 2017). Be aware of these policies and follow them rigorously. The Joint Commission (2018) mandated new newborn ID requirements for all JC-accredited hospitals and other facilities, which are effective as of January, 2019, and include:

- Use of the mother's first and last names and the newborn's gender (e.g., Brown, Ashley, girl)
- Use of standardized practices for identification banding (e.g., two body-site identification and bar coding)
- Establishment of identification-specific communication tools among staff.

Informing parents of their role in this process is part of a comprehensive safety plan. Parental measures to prevent abduction and promote newborn safety include:

Security

- Check that identification bands are in place as the parents care for their newborn and, if missing, ask that they be replaced immediately.
- If an electronically tagged band is used, keep the baby within the bounds of the system and notify the staff if the band becomes loose or comes off.
- Allow only people with proper birthing unit identification to remove the baby from the room. If parents do not know the staff person, they should call the nurse for assistance.
- Report the presence of any suspicious people on the birthing unit.

Safety

- Never leave the newborn alone in the room. If parents walk in the halls or take a shower, they should have a family member watch the newborn or they should return the newborn to the nursery.

- Never lift the newborn if feeling weak, faint, or unsteady on one's feet. Instead, the parent should call for assistance.
- Always keep an eye and hand on the newborn when he or she is out of the crib because babies can fall from beds and other surfaces if left alone.
- Protect from infection, even though newborns do possess some immunity. All caregivers should practice good hand hygiene before and after giving care. Parents should ask visitors to leave if they have a cold, diarrhea, discharge from sores, or a contagious disease.

Prevention of Complications

Newborns are at continued risk for the complications of hemorrhage, late-onset cardiac symptoms, jaundice, and infection. Pallor may be an early sign of hemorrhage and must be reported to the physician. The newborn is placed on a cardiorespiratory monitor to permit continuous assessment. Several newborn conditions or procedures such as circumcision put the newborn at risk for bleeding. Cyanosis that is not relieved by oxygen administration requires emergency intervention, may indicate a congenital cardiac condition or shock, and requires immediate and ongoing assessment.

Infection in the nursery is best prevented by requiring that all personnel having direct contact with newborns scrub for 2 to 3 minutes from fingertips to elbows at the beginning of each shift. The hands must be washed with soap and rubbed vigorously for 15 seconds, or a topical antimicrobial applied, before and after contact with every newborn or after touching any soiled surface, such as the floor or one's hair or face. Instruct parents to practice good handwashing and/or use an antiseptic hand cleaner before touching the baby. Also instruct them that anyone holding the baby should wash hands as well, even after the family returns home. In some clinical settings family members are requested to wear a gown (preferably disposable) over their street clothes during contact with newborns. These are good opportunities to reinforce the efficacy of good hand hygiene in preventing the spread of infection.

Jaundice occurs in most newborns. Generally jaundice is benign, but because of the potential toxicity of bilirubin, newborns must be monitored to identify those who might develop severe hyperbilirubinemia and, in rare cases, acute bilirubin encephalopathy or kernicterus (see Chapter 31 for a more detailed discussion) (AAP & ACOG, 2017). Current recommendations include obtaining a total serum bilirubin level in any newborn who is visibly jaundiced in the first 24 hours of life and obtaining either a serum or transcutaneous bilirubin level before discharge. Nomograms for evaluating risk factors based on bilirubin levels and age of baby are available (see Chapter 26 for discussion).

Circumcision

Circumcision is a surgical procedure in which the prepuce, an epithelial layer covering the tip of the penis, is separated from the glans penis and excised. This permits exposure of the glans for easier cleaning.

Scientific evidence demonstrates that the preventive health benefits of elective circumcision of newborn males outweigh the risks of this procedure (AAP & ACOG, 2017). Parents will need to weigh medical information in the context of their own religious, ethical, and cultural beliefs and practices, as it is the parents who must ultimately decide whether circumcision is in the best interest of their child (AAP & ACOG, 2017). To ensure informed consent, parents should be advised during the prenatal period about possible long-term medical effects of circumcision and noncircumcision.

Current Recommendations

AAP and ACOG (2017) do not recommend *routine* circumcision but acknowledge that medical indications for circumcision still exist. They recommend that analgesia (e.g., dorsal penile nerve block [DPNB], subcutaneous ring block, and eutectic mixture of local anesthetics [EMLA] cream) be used during circumcision to decrease procedural pain.

Circumcision *should not be performed* if the newborn is premature or compromised, has a known bleeding problem, or is born with a genitourinary defect, such as hypospadias or epispadias, which may necessitate the use of the foreskin in future surgical repairs.

CLINICAL TIP

A well-informed nurse can allay parents' anxiety by sharing information and allowing them to express their concerns. In order for parents to make a truly informed decision, they must be knowledgeable about the potential risks and outcomes of circumcision.

Care of the Uncircumcised Newborn

The parents of an uncircumcised male newborn require information about good hygiene practices. Tell them that the foreskin and glans are two similar layers of cells that separate from each other. The separation process begins prenatally and is normally completed at between 3 and 5 years of age. In the process of separation, sterile sloughed cells build up between the layers. This buildup looks similar to the smegma secreted after puberty, and it is harmless. Occasionally during the daily bath, the parents can gently test for retraction. If retraction has occurred, daily gentle washing of the glans with soap and water is sufficient to maintain adequate cleanliness. The parents should teach the child to incorporate this practice into his daily self-care activities. Most uncircumcised males have no difficulty doing so.

Care of the Circumcised Newborn

If circumcision is desired, the procedure should be performed after the newborn is well stabilized and has received his initial physical examination by a healthcare provider. Before a circumcision, ascertain that the physician has explained the procedure, determine whether the parents have any further questions about the procedure, and verify that the circumcision permit is signed. As with any surgical procedure, the identification band of the baby should be checked to verify his identity before the procedure begins. Gather the equipment and prepare the newborn by removing the diaper and placing him on a padded circumcision board or some other type of restraint, but restraining only the legs. These restraint measures along with the application of warm blankets to the upper body increase comfort during the procedure. In Jewish circumcision ceremonies, the baby is held by the father or grandfather and given wine before the procedure.

There are a variety of devices (Gomco clamp, Plastibell, Mogen clamp) used for circumcision (Figure 28–7 and Figure 28–8) and all produce minimal bleeding. Therefore, make special note of newborns with a family history of bleeding disorders or with mothers who took anticoagulants, including aspirin, prenatally. During the procedure, assess the newborn's response.

One important consideration is pain experienced by the newborn. The recommended acceptable methods of analgesia (DPNB, subcutaneous ring block, and EMLA cream) are to be

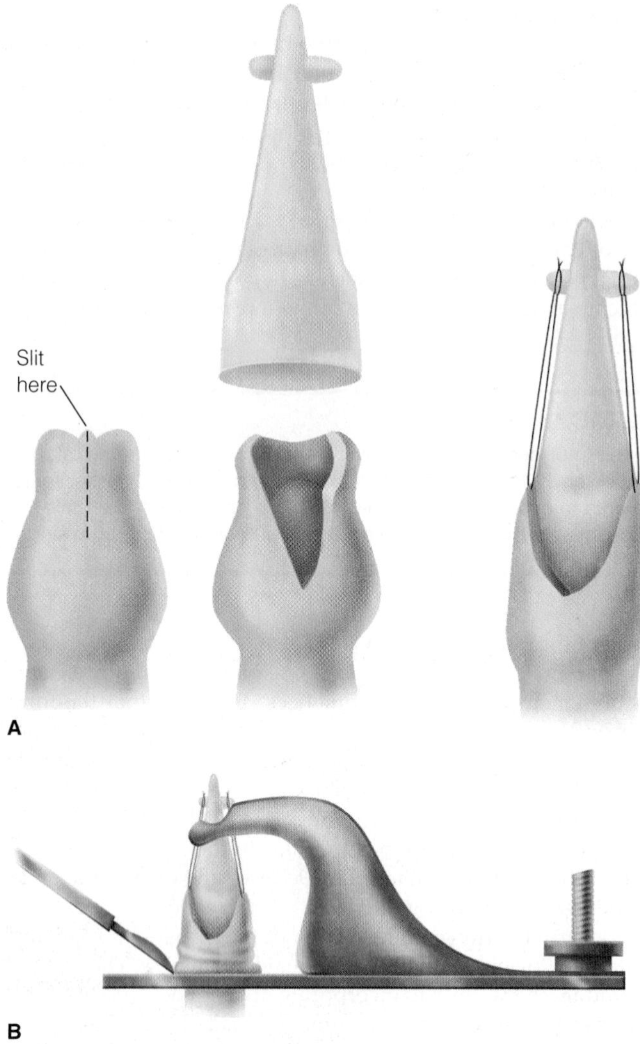

Figure 28-7 **Circumcision using the Yellen or Gomco clamp. A. The prepuce is drawn over the cone. B. The clamp is applied. Pressure is maintained for 3 to 4 minutes, and then excess prepuce is cut away.**

used during circumcision to decrease procedural pain (AAP & ACOG, 2017). The DPNB and subcutaneous ring block are the most effective options. The use of sucrose pacifiers has also been studied. Indications are that a combination of methods is most effective in reducing pain during circumcision (AAP & ACOG, 2017).

During the procedure, provide comfort measures such as lightly stroking the baby's head, providing a pacifier, and talking to him. Following the circumcision, the baby should be held and comforted by you or a family member. Be alert to any cues that these measures are overstimulating the newborn instead of comforting him. Such cues include turning away of the head, increased generalized body movement, skin color changes, hyperalertness, and hiccupping.

Ideally, the circumcision should be assessed for signs of hemorrhage and infection every 30 minutes for at least 2 hours following the procedure. It is important to observe for the first voiding after a circumcision to evaluate for urinary obstruction related to penile injury and/or edema. See *Health Promotion: Newborn Circumcision Care* and *Case Study: Angelina Newman.*

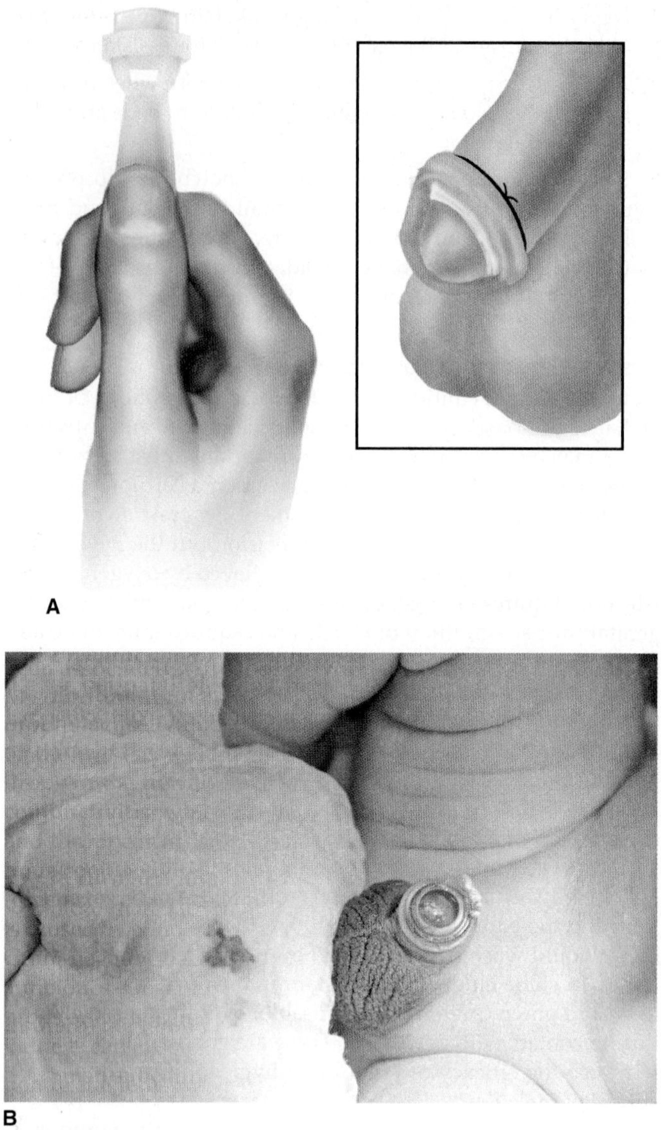

Figure 28-8 **Circumcision using the Plastibell. A. The bell is fitted over the glans. A suture is tied around the bell's rim, and the excess prepuce is cut away. The plastic rim remains in place for 3 to 4 days until healing occurs. The bell may be allowed to fall off; it is removed if still in place after 8 days. B. Plastibell.**

Health Promotion Newborn Circumcision Care

- Teach family members how to assess for unusual bleeding and how to respond if it is present.
- Stress to parents to report to the healthcare provider any signs or symptoms of infection, such as increasing swelling, pus drainage, and cessation of urination.
- Describe how to care for the newly circumcised penis.
- If the newborn's healthcare provider recommends oral analgesics, follow instructions for proper measuring and administration.
- Provide the following information to parents of newborns circumcised with a method other than Plastibell:

- Clean with warm water with each diaper change.
- Apply petroleum ointment for the next few diaper changes to help prevent further bleeding and to protect the healing tissue afterward (Figure 28–9).
- If bleeding does occur, apply light pressure with a sterile gauze pad to stop the bleeding within a short time. If this is not effective, contact the physician immediately or take the newborn to the healthcare provider.
- The glans normally has granulation tissue (a yellowish film) on it during healing. Continued application of a petroleum ointment (or ointment suggested by the healthcare provider) can help protect the granulation tissue that forms as the glans heals.
- When diapering, ensure that the diaper is neither too loose (causing rubbing with movement) nor too tight (causing pain).

- Provide the following information to parents of newborns circumcised using the Plastibell method:
  - The Plastibell should fall off within 8 days; if it remains on after 8 days, consult with the newborn's physician.
  - Though no ointments or creams should be used while the bell remains, application of petroleum ointment may protect the granulation tissue afterward (AAP & ACOG, 2017).

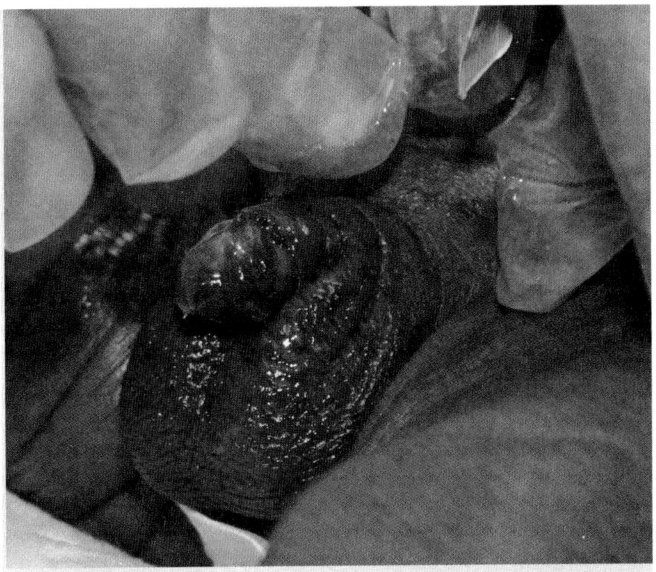

Figure 28–9 Following circumcision, petroleum ointment may be applied to the site for the next few diaper changes.

Enhancement of Parent–Newborn Attachment

Parent–newborn attachment is promoted by encouraging all family members to be involved with the new member of the family. Some specific interventions are examined in Chapters 21 and 33 and the accompanying *Teaching Highlights: What Parents Need to Know About Enhancing Attachment*.

Infant massage is a common childcare practice in many parts of the world, especially Africa and Asia, and has recently gained attention in the United States. Parents can be taught to use infant massage as a method to facilitate the bonding process and to reduce the stress and pain associated with teething, inoculations, constipation, and colic. Infant massage not only induces relaxation for the baby but also provides a calming and "feel-good" interaction for the parents, which fosters the development of warm, positive relationships. See *Developing Cultural Competence: Baby Naming in Africa*.

CASE STUDY: Angelina Newman

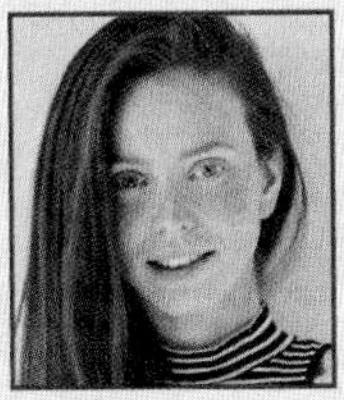

SOURCE: WAYHOME studio/Shutterstock.

Angelina decided to have her newborn son circumcised, and the nurse is now returning to her room with him after the procedure. He is a bit fussy, and Angelina wants to hold him to comfort him. She is concerned about changing his diaper since he now has a dressing over the circumcision site. After she feeds the baby, she calls the nurse and asks for assistance with changing him.

Questions to Ponder

How would you describe to Angelina the normal appearance of a circumcision? What care practices would you advise her to follow until the site appears to be healing?

TEACHING HIGHLIGHTS What Parents Need to Know About Enhancing Attachment

- Information on the periods of reactivity, expected newborn responses, and normal newborn physical characteristics.
- The gradual developmental nature of the bonding process and the reciprocal interactive nature of the process.
- The newborn's capabilities for interaction such as nonverbal communication abilities. Nonverbal communications include movement, gaze, touch, facial expressions, and vocalizations—including crying. Eye contact is considered one of the cardinal factors in developing newborn–parent attachment and will be integrated with touching and vocal behaviors.
- Touching, including stroking, patting, massaging, and kissing, will progress to interactive touch between parent and newborn; parents need to assimilate these and other comforting behaviors (talking, singing, swaddling, rocking) into daily routines with their baby.
- The newborn's behaviors will change as the baby matures, and it is important for parents to be consistent in response to their baby's cues and needs.
- Information about pamphlets, videos, and support groups in the community.

Developing Cultural Competence Baby Naming in Africa

In Africa, the naming of the child is an important event. Names are commonly selected to mirror important or current events. For example, a baby who is born while traveling may be given a name that means "wanderer" or "traveler." Other names may be chosen after a relative who is among the "living-dead" (deceased). It is believed that this results in a partial reincarnation of that relative, especially if the child has characteristics in common with that individual. It is also believed that there is a connection between newborns and the spirit world. In some parts of the country, the name is chosen when the child is crying. Different names of the living-dead are called, and if the child stops crying when a particular name is called, that becomes the child's given name. In some areas, the name is given on the third day and is marked by a celebration with feasting and rejoicing. On the fourth day, the father of the child commonly hangs an iron necklace on the child's neck. It is at this time that the baby is considered a full human being and the connection with the spirit world is lost (Arthur, 2016).

Note: It is unwise to attribute specific attitudes or beliefs to all members of a cultural group. The information in the Developing Cultural Competence boxes offers possible insights into caring for women from different cultural groups.

Discuss waking activities with the parents, such as talking with the baby while making eye contact, holding the baby in an upright position (sitting or standing), gently bending the baby back and forth while grasping under the knees and supporting the head and back with the other hand, and gently rubbing the baby's hands and feet. Quieting activities may include swaddling the baby to increase a sense of security; using slow, calming movements; and talking softly, singing, or humming to the baby.

Caring for newborns in the birthing setting means that you will have contact with patients from a wide variety of racial, religious, and cultural backgrounds. Though it may not be possible to be conversant with all cultures, you can demonstrate cultural competence with both colleagues and patients. Be sensitive to the cultural beliefs and values of the family and be aware of cultural variations in newborn care such as the timing of naming the newborn, giving compliments about the baby, and using good luck charms (see *Developing Cultural Competence: Examples of Cultural Beliefs and Practices Regarding Baby Care*).

Developing Cultural Competence Examples of Cultural Beliefs and Practices Regarding Baby Care

Umbilical Cord

- People of Latin American or Filipino cultural background may use an abdominal binder or bellyband to protect against dirt, injury, and umbilical hernia. They may also apply oils to the stump of the cord or tape metal to the umbilicus to ward off evil spirits (Purnell, 2013)
- People of northern European ancestry may expect a sterile cutting of the cord at birth. They may allow the stump to air-dry and discard the cord once it falls off.
- Women of India and Bangladesh may apply ashes, soot, powder, or dry cow dung on the umbilical cord (Coffey & Brown, 2017; Sujatha, 2014).
- In some cultures in India, Nepal, Bangladesh, and Tanzania some may cauterize the stump with a hot flame, hot coal, or the like (Coffey & Brown, 2017).
- In Zambia, Tanzania, Nepal, and Iran, women may express colostrum on the cord stump (Coffey & Brown, 2017; Sujatha, 2014).

Parent–Newborn Contact

- People of Asian ancestry may pick up the baby as soon as he or she cries, or they may carry the baby at all times.
- Some Native Americans, notably the Navajos, may use cradle boards so the baby can be with the family even during work (Andrews & Woodring, 2016).
- The Muslim father traditionally calls praise to Allah in the newborn's right ear and cleans the baby after birth (Purnell, 2013).

Circumcision

- People of Muslim and Jewish ancestry practice circumcision as a religious ritual (Morris, 2018; Purnell, 2013).
- The religions of Buddhism and Hinduism prohibit circumcision (Morris, 2018).
- Many native peoples of Africa and Australia practice circumcision as a puberty rite.
- Native Americans and people of Asian and South American cultures rarely perform circumcision (Morris, 2018).

Health and Illness

- Some people from Latin American cultural backgrounds may believe that touching the face or head of a baby when admiring it will ward off the "evil eye." They may also put off cutting the baby's nails to avoid nearsightedness and instead put mittens on the baby's hands to prevent scratching. They also may believe that fat babies are healthier (Andrews & Woodring, 2016).
- Some people of Asian heritage may not allow anyone to touch the baby's head without asking permission.
- Some Orthodox Jewish people believe that saying the baby's name before the formal naming ceremony will harm the baby.
- Some Asians and Haitians delay naming their babies (Purnell, 2013).
- Some people of Vietnamese ancestry believe that cutting a baby's hair or nails will cause illness.

Note: It is unwise to attribute specific attitudes or beliefs to all members of a cultural group. The information in the Developing Cultural Competence boxes offers possible insights into caring for women from different cultural groups.

Evaluation

When evaluating the nursing care provided during the newborn period, the following outcomes may be anticipated:

- The baby's physiologic and psychologic integrity is supported by maintaining stable vital signs and interactions based on normal newborn behaviors.
- The newborn feeding pattern will be satisfactorily established.
- The parents express understanding of the bonding process and display attachment behaviors.

Preparation for Discharge

Although the adjustment to parenting is a normal process, going home presents a critical transition for the family. The parents become the primary caregivers for the newborn and must provide a nurturing environment in which the emotional and physical needs of the newborn can be met. Nursing interventions focus on promoting health and preventing possible problems.

●○● NURSING MANAGEMENT

For the Newborn in Preparation for Discharge

Nursing Assessment and Diagnosis

When preparing for discharge, assess whether parents have realistic expectations of the newborn's behavior and the depth of their knowledge in caring for their newborn.

Nursing diagnoses that may apply to the newborn's family include:

- ***Parenting, Readiness for Enhanced,*** related to appropriate behavioral expectations for the newborn
- ***Family Processes, Readiness for Enhanced,*** related to integration of newborn into family unit or demands of newborn care and feeding

(NANDA-I © 2017)

Planning and Implementation

Parent Teaching

To meet parental needs for information, the nurse who is responsible for the daily care of the mother and newborn should assume the primary responsibility for parent education. Nearly every contact with the parents presents an opportunity for sharing information that can facilitate their sense of competence in newborn care. Recognize and respect the fact that there are many good ways to provide safe care. Unless their care methods are harmful to the newborn, the parents' methods of giving care should be reinforced rather than contradicted.

The information that follows is provided to increase your knowledge of newborn care and is used to meet parents' needs for information. Parents may be familiar with handling and caring for newborns or this may be their first time to interact with a newborn. If they are new parents, gently teach them by example and provide instructions geared to their needs and previous knowledge about the various aspects of newborn care.

Observe how parents interact with their baby during feeding and caregiving activities. Even during a short stay, there will be opportunities to provide information and evaluate whether the parents are comfortable with changing diapers and wrapping, handling, and feeding their newborn (Figure 28–10). Do both parents get involved in the baby's care? Is the mother depending on someone else to help her at home? Does the mother give excuses ("I am too tired," "My stitches hurt," or "I will learn later") for not wanting to be involved in her baby's care?

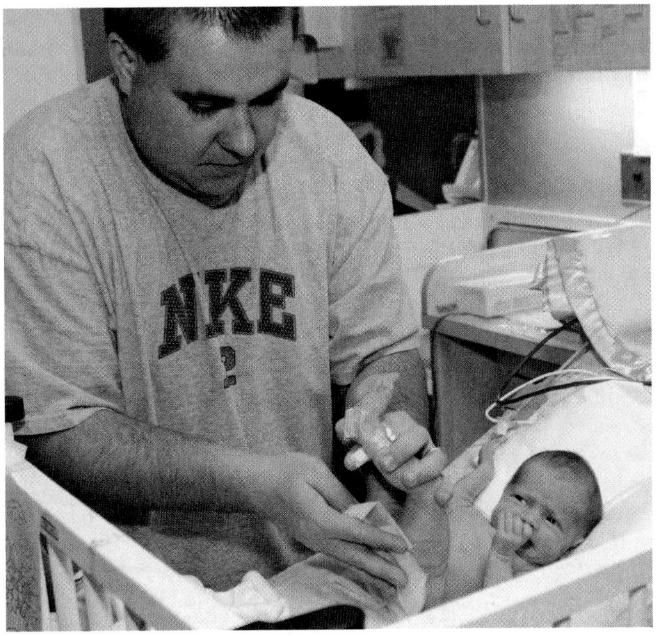

Figure 28–10 **A father demonstrates competence and confidence in diapering his newborn daughter.**

As the family provides care, enhance parental confidence by giving them positive feedback. If the family encounters problems, express confidence in the family's abilities to master the new skill or information, suggest alternatives, and serve as a role model. All these considerations need to be taken into account when evaluating the educational needs of the parents. Providing mother–baby care and home-care instruction on the night shift assists with education needs for early-discharge parents.

CLINICAL TIP

For patients who are hearing-impaired, videotapes with information in both spoken and signed formats are most helpful. Also, birthing centers should have handouts available for families who do not speak English, as well as either interpreters (not family members) or language interpreter phones.

One-on-one teaching while you are in the mother's room is shown to be the most effective educational model. Both first-time and experienced postpartum mothers rate individual teaching as the most effective method of instruction. Individual instruction is helpful both to answer specific questions and to clarify something that the parents may have found confusing in an educational video. With shorter stays, most teaching unfortunately tends to focus on newborn feeding and immediate physical needs of the mothers, with limited anticipatory guidance provided in other areas.

General Instructions for Newborn Care

One of the first concerns of anyone who has not had the experience of picking up a baby is how to do it correctly. The newborn is easily picked up by sliding one hand under the neck and shoulders and the other hand under the buttocks or between the legs, then gently lifting the newborn. This technique provides security and support for the head (which the baby is unable to consistently support until 3 or 4 months of age).

You can be an excellent role model for families in the area of safety. Safety topics include proper positioning of the newborn on the back to sleep and correct use of the bulb syringe. The baby should never be left alone anywhere but in the crib. Remind the mother that while she and the newborn are together in the birthing unit, she should never leave the baby alone for security reasons and because newborns spit up frequently the first day or two after birth. See previous discussion of safety. Other newborn safety measures are discussed in detail in Chapter 34.

Demonstrating a bath (see Chapter 34), cord care, and temperature assessment is the best way to provide information on these topics to parents.

Demonstrate and review the taking of an axillary or tympanic temperature with the family and discourage the use of mercury thermometers. It is important that families understand the differences and know how to select a thermometer. The newborn's temperature needs to be taken only when signs of illness are present. Advise parents to call their physician or pediatric nurse practitioner immediately if they observe any signs of illness. See *Women with Special Needs: Teaching Baby Care Practices*.

Women with Special Needs Teaching Baby Care Practices

The woman with a developmental disability may need to be shown how to carry out certain baby care practices and need repeated demonstrations and additional explanations. Teaching should be based on the woman's level of understanding with teaching methods customized for her individualized learning needs. Demonstration by the nurse with a return demonstration is an effective tool to ensure the skill is understood and done correctly.

Nasal and Oral Suctioning

Most newborns are obligatory nose breathers for the first months of life. They generally maintain air passage patency by coughing or sneezing. During the first few days of life, however, the newborn has increased mucus, and gentle suctioning with a bulb syringe may be indicated, but only in cases of obvious obstruction. The newborn's mouth should be suctioned first so that there is nothing to aspirate if the newborn gasps when the nose is suctioned (AAP & ACOG, 2017). Demonstrate the use of the bulb syringe in the mouth and nose and have the parents do a return demonstration. The parents should repeat this demonstration of suctioning and cleansing the bulb before discharge so they feel confident in performing the procedure. Care should be taken to apply only gentle suction to prevent nasal bleeding.

To suction the newborn, the bulb syringe is compressed and the tip is placed in the nostril. Take care not to occlude the passageway. The bulb is permitted to reexpand slowly by releasing the compression on the bulb (Figure 28–11). The bulb syringe is removed from the nostril, and drainage is then compressed out of the bulb onto a tissue. The bulb syringe may also be used in the mouth if the newborn is spitting up and unable to handle the excess secretions. The bulb is compressed, the tip of the bulb syringe is placed about 1 inch to one side of the newborn's mouth, and compression is released. This draws up the excess secretions. The procedure is repeated on the other side of the mouth. The roof of the mouth and back of the throat are avoided because suction in these areas might stimulate the gag reflex.

The bulb syringe should be washed in warm, soapy water and rinsed in warm water daily and as needed after use. Rinsing the inside with a half-strength white vinegar solution followed by clear water may help to extend the useful life of the bulb syringe by inhibiting bacterial growth. A bulb syringe should always be kept near the newborn. New parents and nurses who are inexperienced with babies may fear that the baby will choke and may be relieved if they know how to take action if such an event occurs. They should be advised to turn the newborn's head to the side or hold the newborn with the head down as soon as there is any indication of gagging or vomiting and to use the bulb syringe as needed.

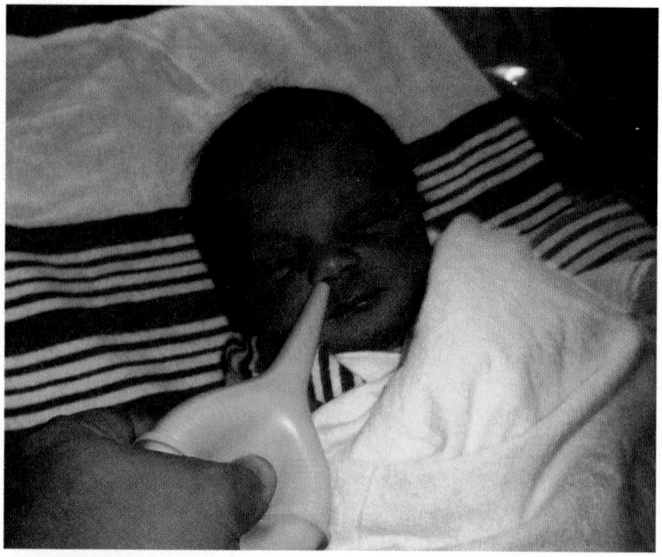

Figure 28–11 Nasal and oral suctioning. The bulb is compressed, the tip is placed in either the mouth or the nose, and the bulb is released.

SOURCE: Michele Davidson.

Some newborns may have transient edema of the nasal mucosa following suctioning of the airway after birth. Demonstrate the use of normal saline to loosen secretions and instruct parents in the gentle and moderate use of the bulb syringe to avoid further irritation of the mucous membranes. If parents will be using humidifiers at home, they should be instructed to follow the manufacturer's cleaning instructions carefully so that molds, spores, and bacteria from a dirty humidifier do not enter the baby's environment.

SAFETY ALERT!

You'll find that left-handed people tend to hold the baby over their right shoulder, and right-handed people do the opposite. This keeps the dominant hand free. However, most health personnel wear their name tags on the left side. To avoid scratching the baby's face, wear your name tag on the same side as your dominant hand.

Sleep and Activity

The National Institute of Child Health and Human Development and the American Academy of Pediatrics recommend that healthy term newborns be placed on their back to sleep. The crib or other sleeping space should be without pillow, toys, blankets, or other loose bedding. Parents are taught the importance of following "Safe to Sleep" guidelines to reduce the incidence of sudden infant death syndrome (SIDS) (AAP & ACOG, 2017). No evidence exists that newborns need to be placed on their sides initially because of secretions. Placing babies on their backs in the newborn period serves to educate parents regarding positioning of the baby. Studies indicate that parents position their babies in the same positions they observe in the hospital setting, so nurses must demonstrate this behavior to reduce the risk of SIDS. If exceptions are warranted, these should be explained to families so they do not misinterpret what they observe. The placement of babies in a prone position during wakeful play sessions ("tummy time") should be encouraged as well (AAP, 2017). Parents are also encouraged to hold their babies and not allow them to remain in infant carriers for prolonged periods of time. See *Genetic Facts: SIDS and the SCN_4A Gene.*

Genetic Facts SIDS and the SCN_4A Gene

Babies who die of SIDS may have a rare variant in their SCN_4A gene, which directly alters NaV1.4 function (control of skeletal muscle excitability). These variants contribute to skeletal muscle dysfunction and significantly alter muscle membrane excitability, thus compromising respiratory and laryngeal function (Männikkö et al., 2018).

Perhaps nothing is more individual to each baby than the sleep–activity cycle. It is important to recognize the individual variations of each newborn and to assist parents as they develop sensitivity to their baby's communication signals and rhythms of activity and sleep. See Chapter 27 for more detailed discussion of the sleep–activity cycle.

Car Safety Considerations

Half the children killed or injured in automobile accidents could have been protected by the use of a federally approved car seat. Newborns must go home from the birthing unit in a car seat adapted to fit newborns (Figure 28–12). Babies should never be in the front seat of a car equipped with a passenger-side air bag. The safest spot in any car is the middle of the back seat. The car seat should be positioned to face the rear of the car until the child reaches the highest weight or height allowed by the car seat's manufacturer (AAP, 2018).

Ensure that all parents are knowledgeable about the benefits of child safety seat use and proper installation. Encourage parents to have their infant safety seats checked by local groups trained specifically for that purpose. The Seat Check Initiative provides locations and information about child safety seats.

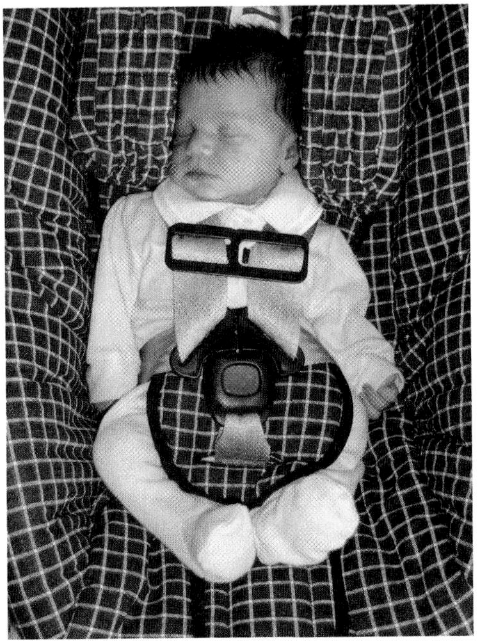

Figure 28–12 Infant car restraint for use from birth to about 12 months of age.

Newborn Screening and Immunization Program

Before the newborn and mother are discharged from the birthing unit, inform the parents about **newborn screening tests** and tell them when to return to the birthing center or clinic if further tests are needed. Newborn screening tests include:

- Blood spot screening, which allows for diagnosis of many disorders that might otherwise go unidentified and untreated in children (The number of disorders screened differs slightly from state to state.)
- Hearing screening
- Hyperbilirubinemia screening
- Critical congenital heart disease screening.

For information on the specific disorders tested for in your state, you can visit the newborn screening portal of the Centers for Disease Control (CDC, 2016). It is the responsibility of the nursing staff to see that these screening tests are completed by the time of discharge and that the parents understand the need for follow-up tests where indicated (Healthy Children, 2018).

Hearing loss is found in 1 to 3 per 1000 babies in the normal newborn population (Healthy Children, 2018). Hearing screenings before discharge are now conducted in all 50 states. The recommended initial newborn hearing screening should be accomplished before discharge from the birthing unit, with appropriate follow-up if the newborn fails to pass the initial screen in all hospitals providing obstetric services.

Sometimes newborns fail to pass these tests for reasons other than hearing loss. Amniotic fluid in the ear canals is a frequent cause of suboptimal test results. In these cases, babies are retested in a week or two. The current goal is to screen all babies by 1 month of age, confirm hearing loss with audiologic examination by 3 months of age, and treat with comprehensive early intervention services before 6 months of age (Healthy Children, 2018). Typically, screening programs use a two-stage screening approach (otoacoustic emissions [OAE] repeated twice, OAE followed by auditory brainstem response [ABR], or automated ABR repeated twice). Families need to be educated about appropriate interpretation of screening test results and appropriate steps for follow-up (Figure 28–13).

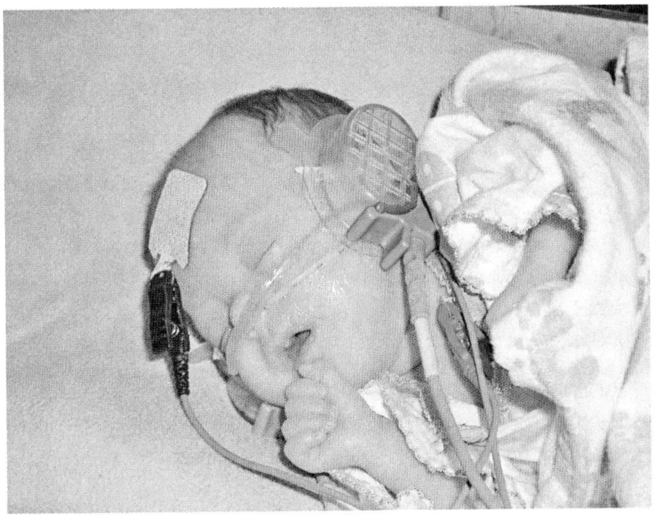

Figure 28–13 Newborn hearing screen.

SOURCE: Vanessa Howell, RN, MSN, NNP-BC.

Immunization programs against the hepatitis B virus during the newborn period and infancy are in place in many states, at least 20 countries, and high-incidence areas such as American Samoa. Universal vaccination of newborns and infants is recommended. See *Drug Guide: Hepatitis B Vaccine (Engerix-B, Recombivax HB)*. Advise parents as to whether their birthing center provides newborn hepatitis vaccination so that an adequate follow-up program can be set in motion (CDC, 2018).

Community-Based Nursing Care

Teach the family all necessary caregiving methods before discharge. A checklist may be helpful to determine whether the teaching has been completed and to verify the parents' knowledge on leaving the birthing unit (Figure 28–14). Review all areas for understanding or any outstanding questions with the mother and father, without rushing and taking time to answer all queries. Any concerns of the parents or nurse are noted.

Discuss with the parents ways to meet their newborn's needs, ensure safety, and appreciate the newborn's unique characteristics and behaviors. By assisting parents in establishing links with their community-based healthcare provider, you can get the new family off to a good start. Parents also need to know the signs of illness, how to reach the pediatrician or after-hours clinic, and the importance of follow-up after discharge. Parents should also check with their clinician for advice about over-the-counter medications to be kept in the medicine cabinet.

The family should have the care provider's phone number, address, and any specific instructions. Having the birthing unit or nursery phone number is also reassuring to a newborn's family. Encourage them to call with questions. Follow-up calls lend added support by providing another opportunity for parents to have their questions answered.

The follow-up newborn examination should occur within 48 hours of discharge. In some areas home visits are available to families in the period just following discharge. The home visit focuses on normal newborn care, assessment for hyperbilirubinemia (jaundice), extreme weight loss, feeding problems, and knowledge deficits related to newborn care and feeding within the family unit. (For detailed discussion of home care, see Chapter 34.)

Routine well-baby visits should be scheduled with the clinic, pediatric nurse practitioner, or physician. Regardless of the type of follow-up services available in the community, contribute to the newborn's health by stressing the importance of routine care and by helping families who have no follow-up plans to connect to local resources for care. See *Evidence-Based Practice: Improving Neonatal Outcomes*.

Evaluation

When evaluating the nursing care provided during the newborn period, the following outcomes may be anticipated:

- The parents demonstrate safe techniques for caring for their newborn.
- The parents verbalize developmentally appropriate behavioral expectations of their newborn and knowledge of community-based newborn follow-up care.

For a summary of neonatal care, see *Key Facts to Remember: What Parents Need to Know About Newborn Care*.**SOURCE:** WAYHOME studio/Shutterstock

DRUG GUIDE

Hepatitis B Vaccine (Engerix-B, Recombivax HB)

OVERVIEW OF NEONATAL ACTION

Recombinant hepatitis B vaccine is used as a prophylactic treatment against all subtypes of the hepatitis B virus. It provides passive immunization for newborns of HBsAg-negative and HBsAg-positive mothers. Hepatitis B can be transmitted across the placenta, but most newborns are infected during birth.

The vaccine is produced from baker's yeast and plasmid containing the HBsAg gene.

Hepatitis B (thimerosal-free) vaccine contains more than 95% HBsAg protein and is an inactivated (noninfective) product (AAP & ACOG, 2017). Universal immunization is recommended.

Newborns of HBsAg-positive mothers should concurrently receive 0.5 mL of hepatitis B immunoglobulin (HBIG) prophylaxis at separate injection sites (AAP & ACOG, 2017; CDC, 2018; Wilson et al., 2018).

ROUTE, DOSAGE, AND FREQUENCY

The first dose of 0.5 mL (10 mcg) is given intramuscularly into the anterolateral thigh within 24 hours of birth for babies born to HBsAg-positive mothers (AAP & ACOG, 2017). The second dose of vaccine is given at least 1 to 2 months after the first dose and is followed by a final dose at 6 months after the first dose (AAP & ACOG, 2017). Preterm babies based on weight have a different schedule.

Babies born to HBsAg-negative mothers receive their first dose of vaccine at birth, the second dose at 1 to 2 months, and the third dose at 6 to 18 months (CDC, 2018).

Newborns whose mother's HBsAg status is unknown should receive the same doses of vaccine as newborns born to HBsAg-positive mothers.

NEONATAL SIDE EFFECTS

The only common side effect is soreness at the injection site. Occasionally, there is erythema, swelling, warmth, and induration at the injection site; irritability; or a low-grade fever (37.7°C [99.8°F]).

NURSING CONSIDERATIONS

Delay administration during active infection; the vaccine will not prevent infection during its incubation period.

- The vaccine should be used as supplied. Do not dilute. Shake well.
- Do not inject intravenously or intradermally.
- Monitor for adverse reactions. Monitor temperature closely.
- Have epinephrine available to treat possible allergic reactions.
- Responsiveness to the vaccine is age dependent. Preterm newborns weighing less than 1000 g (2.2 lb.) have lower seroconversion rates. Consider delaying the first dose until the baby is term postconceptual age (PCA) or use a four-dose schedule.

NEWBORN CARE TEACHING CHECKLIST

Please read the *New Baby* booklet and view the film before completing this checklist. In the **Need Teaching** column, check off the areas in which you would like further instruction, advice, or demonstration.

	Need Teaching	Teaching Done	Nurse's Initials/Date
Breastfeeding			
Positioning			
Latching on			
Removing baby from nipple			
Let-down reflex			
Supply and demand concept			
How often and for how long			
Knowing if baby is getting enough			
Supplementing			
Expressing milk by hand			
Going back to work while breastfeeding			
Formula Feeding			
Feeding baby a bottle			
Cleaning bottles and nipples			
Choosing a formula			
Preparing formula			
Demand feeding			
Baby Care			
Positioning baby after feeding			
Burping			
Bathing			
Caring for circumcision/genital/umbilical area			
Taking baby's temperature—when to call the doctor			
Using a bulb syringe			
Elimination—what to expect			
Checking for signs of jaundice			
Caring for skin, rashes, milia			
Comforting crying baby			
Signs that baby is sick			
Positioning in crib (Safe to Sleep)			
Safety			
Baby is choking or gagging—what to do			
Shaken baby syndrome			
Newborn screening tests and immunizations			
Using infant car seat			

Other Concerns:	Language spoken by mother: ______
______	Was an interpreter used? ______
I understand the teaching instructions given on the specified topics and have no further questions.	Nurse's signature(s): ______ ______ ______
______ Mother's Signature	
Date:______	Date:______

Figure 28–14 A newborn teaching checklist is completed by the time of discharge.

SOURCE: Adapted from Presbyterian/St. Luke's Medical Center, Denver, CO.

EVIDENCE-BASED PRACTICE Improving Neonatal Outcomes

Clinical Question

Do community-based programs for new mothers improve neonatal outcomes?

The Evidence

While gains have been made, there are still an estimated 2.6 million neonatal deaths globally per year. Approaches based on community-building through empowerment and participation are attractive options for low- and middle-income mothers in emerging countries because of their low cost. Trials of these systems have focused on two approaches: Counseling via home visits and peer support groups. Hanson et al. (2018) undertook a study of the effectiveness of these two types of community-based approaches to improving neonatal survival. They used a meta-analysis, which is a statistically based analysis of the effect size of 17 aggregated studies. This type of systematic review is immune to most types of bias and is considered a gold standard as evidence for practice.

The greatest effect of community-based approaches seems to be among women with the fewest resources. These women experienced a 25% reduction in neonatal mortality in higher-risk settings. In lower-mortality settings, and in areas where a larger proportion of women deliver their babies in a facility, the community-based approaches had little effect (Hanson, Kujala, Waiswa, et al., 2018).

Best Practice

In settings with few resources and limited availability to healthcare practitioners and facilities, group interventions such as in-home counseling and peer support groups can reduce neonatal mortality. As mortality declines, though, the effect of these interventions becomes less significant (Hanson et al., 2018).

Clinical Reasoning

What are the characteristics of mothers in low-mortality settings that make them less likely to experience neonatal mortality? What roles can the nurse fill when providing community-based care in high-mortality settings?

Key Facts To Remember

What Parents Need to Know About Newborn Care

Immediate Safety Measures For The Newborn

- Watch for excessive mucus; use bulb syringe to remove mucus.
- Have baby sleep on his or her back in crib or in someone's arms.

VOIDING AND STOOL CHARACTERISTICS AND PATTERNS

- Urine is straw to amber color without foul smell. Small amounts of uric acid crystals are normal in the first days of life (may be mistaken by parents as blood in diaper because of reddish "brick dust" appearance).
- At least six to 10 wet diapers a day after the first few days of life.
- Normal progression of stool changes: (1) meconium (thick, tarry, dark green); (2) transitional stools (thin, brown to green); (3a) breastfed newborn: Yellow gold, soft or mushy stools; (3b) formula-fed newborn: Pale yellow, formed and pasty stools.
- Only one to two stools a day for formula-fed baby.
- Six to 10 small, loose yellow stools per day or only one stool every few days after breastfeeding is well established (after about 1 month).

CORD CARE

- Wash hands with clean water and soap before and after care. Keep the cord dry and exposed to air or loosely covered with clean clothes. (If cultural custom demands binding of the abdomen, a sanitary method such as the use of a clean piece of gauze can be recommended.)
- Clean cord and skin around base with a cotton swab or cotton ball. Clean two to three times a day or with each diaper change. Touching the cord, applying unclean substances to it, and applying bandages should be avoided. Do not give tub baths until cord falls off in 7 to 14 days.
- Fold diapers below umbilical cord to air-dry the cord (contact with wet or soiled diapers slows the drying process and increases the possibility of infection).
- Check cord each day for any odor, oozing of greenish-yellow material, or reddened areas around the cord. Expect tenderness around the cord and darkening and shriveling of cord. Report to healthcare provider any signs of infection.
- Normal changes in cord: Cord should look dark and dry up before falling off. A small drop of blood may be present when cord falls off.
- Never pull the cord or attempt to loosen it.

CARE REQUIRED FOR CIRCUMCISED AND UNCIRCUMCISED NEWBORNS

Circumcision Care

- Use a new, clean sponge or washcloth to squeeze warm water over circumcision site once a day.
- Rinse area off with warm water and pat dry.
- Apply small amount of petroleum jelly (unless a Plastibell is in place) with each diaper change.
- Fasten diaper over penis snugly enough so that it does not move and rub the tender glans.
- Because the glans is sensitive, avoid placing baby on his stomach for the first day after the procedure.
- Check for any foul-smelling drainage or bleeding at least once a day.
- Let Plastibell fall off by itself (about 8 days after circumcision).
- Plastibell should not be pulled off.
- Light, sticky, yellow drainage (part of healing process) may form over head of penis.

Uncircumcised Care

- Clean uncircumcised penis with warm water during diaper changes and with bath.
- Do not force foreskin back over the penis; foreskin will retract normally over time (may take 3 to 5 years).

TECHNIQUES FOR WAKING AND QUIETING NEWBORNS

Techniques for Waking Baby

- Loosen clothing, change diaper.
- Hand-express milk onto baby's lips.
- Talk with baby while making eye contact.
- Hold baby in upright position (sitting or standing).
- Have baby do sit-ups (gently and rhythmically bend baby back and forth while grasping the baby under his or her knees and supporting baby's head and back with your other hand).
- Play patty-cake with baby.
- Stimulate rooting reflex (brush one cheek with hand or nipple).
- Increase skin contact (gently rub hands and feet).

Techniques for Quieting Baby

- Check for soiled diaper.
- Swaddle or bundle baby (bring arms and legs into midline, which increases sense of security).
- Hold swaddled baby upright against midchest, supporting bottom and back of head. Baby can hear heartbeat, feel warmth, and hear your softly spoken words or calming sounds.
- Use slow, calming movements with baby.
- Softly talk, sing, or hum to baby.

WHEN PARENTS SHOULD CALL THEIR HEALTHCARE PROVIDER

- Temperature above 38°C (100.4°F) axillary or below 36.6°C (97.8°F) axillary
- Continual rise in temperature
- More than one episode of forceful vomiting or frequent vomiting over a 6-hour period
- Refusal of two feedings in a row
- Lethargy (listlessness), difficulty in awakening baby
- Cyanosis (bluish discoloration of skin) with or without a feeding
- Absence of breathing longer than 20 seconds
- Inconsolable baby (quieting techniques are not effective) or continuous high-pitched cry
- Discharge or bleeding from umbilical cord, circumcision, or any opening (except vaginal mucus or pseudomenstruation)
- Two consecutive green watery or black stools or increased frequency of stools
- No wet diapers for 18 to 24 hours or fewer than six to eight wet diapers per day after 4 days of age
- Development of eye drainage
- Yellowing of skin (jaundice)

Focus Your Study

- The overall goal of newborn nursing care is to provide comprehensive care while promoting the establishment of a well-functioning family unit.
- The period immediately following birth, during which adaptation to extrauterine life occurs, requires close monitoring to identify any deviations from normal.
- Nursing goals during the first hours after birth (admission and transitional period) are to maintain a clear airway, maintain a neutral thermal environment, prevent hemorrhage and infection, initiate oral feedings, and facilitate attachment.
- The newborn is routinely given prophylactic vitamin K to prevent possible hemorrhagic disease of the newborn.
- Prophylactic eye treatment for *Neisseria gonorrhoeae* is legally required on all newborns.
- Nursing goals in daily newborn care include maintaining cardiopulmonary function, maintaining a neutral thermal environment, promoting adequate hydration and nutrition, preventing complications, promoting safety, and enhancing attachment and family knowledge of child care.
- Essential daily care includes assessing vital signs, weight, overall color, intake and output, umbilical cord and circumcision, newborn nutrition, parent education, and attachment.
- Following a circumcision, the newborn must be observed closely for signs of bleeding, inability to void, and signs of infection.
- Signs of illness in newborns include temperature above 38°C (100.4°F) axillary or below 36.6°C (97.8°F) axillary, more than one episode of forceful vomiting, refusal of two feedings in a row, lethargy, cyanosis with or without a feeding, and absence of breathing for longer than 20 seconds.
- Newborn blood spot screening may be done on all newborns in the first 1 to 3 days. Hearing screening and critical congenital heart disease screening may be completed before discharge.

In order to make safe and effective judgments using NANDA-I © 2017 nursing diagnoses, it is essential that nurses refer to the definitions and defining characteristics of the diagnoses used in this text, which can be found in Appendix C.

References

American Academy of Pediatrics (AAP). (2017). *How to keep your sleeping baby safe: AAP policy explained.* Retrieved from https://www.healthychildren.org/English/ages-stages/baby/sleep/Pages/A-Parents-Guide-to-Safe-Sleep.aspx

American Academy of Pediatrics (AAP). (2018). *Car seats: Information for families.* Retrieved from https://www.healthychildren.org/English/safety-prevention/on-the-go/Pages/Car-Safety-Seats-Information-for-Families.aspx

American Academy of Pediatrics (AAP) Committee on Fetus and Newborn & American College of Obstetricians and Gynecologists (ACOG) Committee on Obstetrics. (2017). *Guidelines for perinatal care* (8th ed.). Evanston, IL: Author.

Andrews, M. M., & Woodring, B. C., (2016). Transcultural perspectives in the nursing care of children and adolescents. In M. M. Andrews & J. S. Boyle (Eds.), *Transcultural concepts in nursing care* (7th ed., pp. 153–185). Philadelphia, PA: Lippincott.

Arthur, A. (2016). *Africa's naming traditions: Nine ways to name your child.* Retrieved from https://www.bbc.com/news/world-africa-37912748

Centers for Disease Control and Prevention (CDC). (2016). *Newborn screening portal.* Retrieved from https://www.cdc.gov/newbornscreening

Centers for Disease Control and Prevention (CDC). (2018). *Recommended immunization schedule for children and adolescents aged 18 years or younger, UNITED STATES 2018.* Retrieved from https://www.cdc.gov/vaccines/schedules/hcp/child-adolescent.html

Coffey, P. S., & Brown, S. C. (2017). Umbilical cord-care practices in low- and middle-income countries: A systemic review. *BMC Pregnancy and Childbirth 17*(68). DOI: 10.1186/s12884-017-1250-7

Eichenwald, E. C., Hansen, A. R., Martin, C. R., & Stark, A. R. (2017). *Cloherty and Stark's manual of neonatal care* (8th ed.). Philadelphia, PA: Lippincott Williams & Wilkins.

Gardner, S. L., & Hernandez, J. A. (2016). Heat balance. In S. L. Gardner, B. S. Carter, M. Enzman Himes, & J. A. Hernandez (Eds), *Merenstein & Gardner's handbook of intensive care* (8th ed., pp. 105–125). St. Louis, MO: Elsevier.

Hanson, C., Kujala, S., Waiswa, P., Marchant, T., & Schellenberg, J. (2017) Community-based approaches for neonatal survival: Meta-analyses of randomized trial data. *Bulletin of the World Health Organization, 95*(6), 453–464C.

Healthy Children. (2018). *Purpose of newborn hearing screening.* Retrieved from https://www.healthychildren.org/English/ages-stages/baby/Pages/Newborn-Screening-Tests.aspx

Klaus, M., & Klaus, P. (1999). Your *amazing newborn.* Cambridge Park, MA: Pearson.

Männikkö, R., Wong, L., Tester, D. J., Thor, M. G., Sud, R., Kullmann, D. M., . . . Ackerman, M. J. (2018). Dysfunction of NaV1.4, a skeletal muscle voltage-gated sodium channel, in sudden infant death syndrome: A case-control study. *The Lancet. 391*(10129), 1483–1492.

Morris, B. J. (2018). *Circumcision—History and recent trends.* CircInfo.net. Retrieved from http://circinfo.net/history_and_recent_trends.html

Purnell, L. P. (2013). *Transcultural health care: A culturally competent approach* (4th ed.). Philadelphia, PA: F. A. Davis

Sujatha, R. (2014). Cultural practices and beliefs on newborn care among mothers in a selected hospital of Mangalore Taluk. *NUJHS 4*(2), 21–26.

The Joint Commission (2018). Distinct newborn identification requirements. *R3 report: Requirement, rationale, reference, 17*, 1–2.

Wilson, B. A., Shannon, M. T., & Shields, K. M. (2018). *Pearson nurse's drug guide 2019.* Hoboken, NJ: Pearson Education.

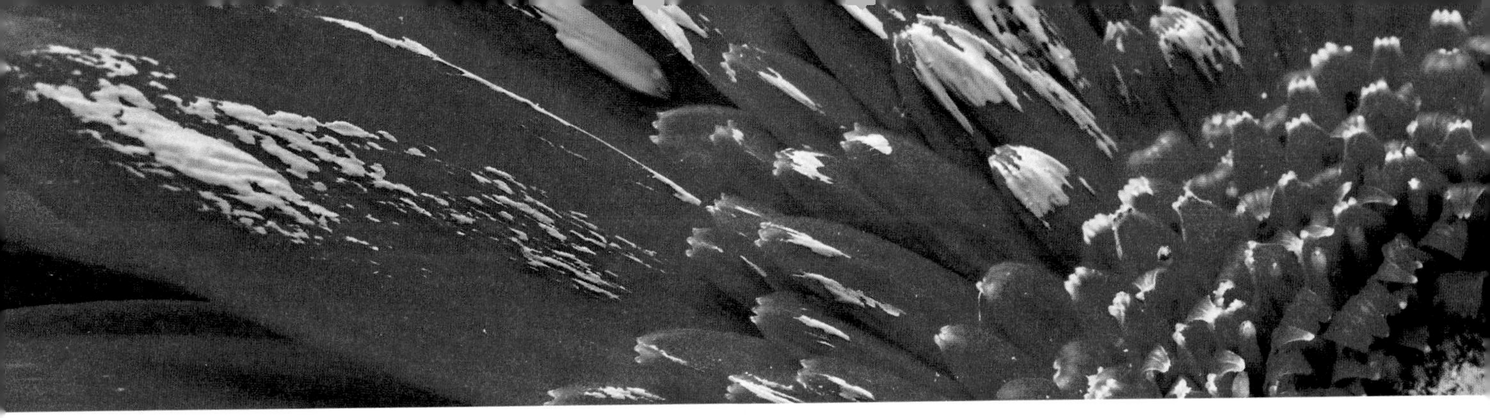

Chapter 29
Newborn Nutrition

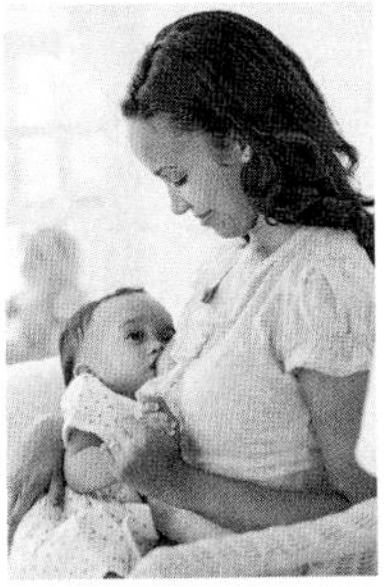

SOURCE: Blend Images /SuperStock.

I felt prepared for breastfeeding when my baby was born—I had taken a breastfeeding class and read several books. Breastfeeding started off well. I was a little surprised about the frequent feedings in the beginning, but we got through that just fine. The biggest surprise was that my baby developed allergy symptoms when she was 3 weeks old. It was determined that my daughter is allergic to cow's-milk protein. To continue feeding her just breast milk, I had to cut out milk and foods containing milk, which severely limited what I could eat. I did that because I was determined not to let anything stop me from nursing my child for my goal of at least the first year. Fortunately, the allergy is slowly going away as she grows older. At 9 months I can now have a little cheese in my diet again.

—Allyssa, age 25

Learning Outcomes

29.1 Compare the nutritional value and composition of human milk and formula preparations in relation to the nutritional needs of the newborn.

29.2 Explain the advantages and disadvantages of breastfeeding and formula-feeding in determining the nursing care of both mother/family and newborn.

29.3 Formulate guidelines for helping both breastfeeding and formula-feeding mothers to feed their newborns successfully in hospital and community-based settings.

29.4 Explain the influence of cultural values on newborn/infant feeding practices.

29.5 Explain the nutritional needs and normal growth patterns of newborns.

29.6 Describe ways to educate parents about their newborn's nutritional needs and normal growth patterns.

Healthy People 2020

(MICH-14) Increase the proportion of women of childbearing potential with intake of at least 400 μg of folic acid from fortified foods or dietary supplements

(MICH-21) Increase the proportion of infants who are breastfed

(MICH-21.1) Increase the proportion of infants who are ever breastfed (target 81.9%)

(MICH-21.2; 21.3) Increase the proportion of infants who are breastfed at 6 months (target 60.6%); at 1 year (target 34.1%)

(MICH-21.4; 21.5) Increase the proportion of infants who are breastfed exclusively through 3 months (target 46.2%); exclusively through 6 months (target 25.5%)

(MICH-22) Increase the proportion of employers that have worksite lactation support programs (target 38%)

(MICH-23) Reduce the proportion of breastfed newborns who receive formula supplementation within the first 2 days of life (target 14.2%)

(MICH-24) Increase the proportion of live births that occur in facilities that provide recommended care for lactating mothers and their babies (target 8.1%)

Newborn nutrition plays a vital part in the well-being of a baby. Adequate nutrition is essential for normal growth and development as well as brain development. In addition, newborn feeding itself is an important component of neonatal socialization that promotes cognitive and emotional development.

One of the first decisions parents will make is whether to breastfeed, formula-feed, or utilize a combination of both. It is important that the nurse is well informed about newborn/infant nutrition and feeding methods because the parents look to the nurse for this guidance. In this chapter we look at the nutritional needs of the full-term newborn of normal weight in the context of both breast milk and formula composition, discuss feeding methods, explore community-based nursing care, and look at a nutritional assessment of the newborn.

Nutritional Needs and Breast Milk/Formula Composition

The newborn's diet must supply all the nutrients required by the body to meet the rapid rate of physical and neurologic growth and development. A newborn's diet should provide adequate hydration and sufficient calories as well as protein, carbohydrates, fat, vitamins, and minerals. Exclusive breast milk is sufficient as the sole source of nutrition to meet the dietary needs of the newborn from birth up to 6 months of age. Thereafter, breastfeeding in combination with solid foods for the next 6 months is recommended. After the first year, breastfeeding may be continued for as long as mutually desired by mother and baby (Meek, 2017). Iron-fortified 20-calorie/ounce formula is also sufficient as the sole source of nutrition to meet the dietary needs of the newborn from birth up to 6 months of age. Solid foods are introduced in the next 6 months while the infant continues on formula until at least 12 months of age (Healthy Children, 2018). The following sections discuss the nutritional requirements of the newborn and evaluate human milk and standard cow's milk–based formula.

Dietary Reference Intakes

When discussing the nutritional needs of the newborn, the nurse should be familiar with the terms used. The term *dietary reference intake (DRI)* is an updated generic term that replaces the well-known nutritional reference term *recommended daily allowance (RDA)*. The dietary reference intake encompasses four aspects of nutrient-based reference values: (1) estimated average requirement (EAR), (2) recommended daily allowance (RDA), (3) adequate intake (AI), and (4) tolerable upper intake level (UL). The DRI represents a framework that links nutrition and health across the lifespan.

Growth

All newborns lose some percentage of their birth weight in the first few days after birth, which should cause no concern unless the loss approaches 7 to 10% of birth weight. Within 7 to 14 days newborns should regain their birth weight and consistently gain 35 grams (1.23 ounces) per day at 1 month if breastfed and 34.4 grams per day if formula-fed (Wambach & Riordan, 2016). The initial weight loss is attributed to a combination of the passage of meconium, loss of extracellular fluids, and low fluid intake, which is normal in the first few days while transitioning to feedings, especially among breastfed babies. This initial weight loss does not result in dehydration, as newborns draw on their extracellular water reserves.

As noted previously, breastfed and formula-fed babies have different growth rates. This is understandable because the compositions of human milk and formula are different. See Table 29–1 to compare the nutrients found in human milk and formula compositions. Based on the vast research evidence, breastfeeding is considered to be the "gold standard" for neonatal nutrition, and the outcomes associated with its use are the norm to which other forms of nutrition should be compared (Lawrence & Lawrence, 2016).

Formula-fed newborns tend to regain their birth weight earlier than breastfed newborns because of consistent fluid intake in the first few days of life, whereas the breastfed baby's fluid

TABLE 29–1 Comparison of Nutrients in Milk

NUTRIENT (PER 30 ML)	MATURE HUMAN MILK	SIMILAC PRO-ADVANCE 20	ENFAMIL PREMIUM NEWBORN	WHOLE MILK
Calories	20	20	20	19
Protein, grams	0.27	0.41	0.42	1.1
% of cal	6%	8%	8.5%	22%
Source	Human milk	Nonfat milk, whey protein	Nonfat milk, whey protein	Cow's milk
Whey: Casein	90:10 initially 50:50* late lactation	60:40	60:40	20:80
Fat, grams	1.2	1.1	1.1	1.1
% of cal	52%	49%	48%	49%
Source	Human milk (contains DHA, ARA**, etc.)	Safflower, soy, coconut DHA, ARA**	Palm, soy, coconut, sunflower, DHA, ARA**	Butterfat
Carbohydrate, grams	2.2	2.2	2.2	1.5
% of cal	42%	43%	43%	31%
Source	Lactose (human milk)	Lactose (nonfat milk)	Lactose (nonfat milk)	Lactose (whole milk)

TABLE 29–1 Comparison of Nutrients in Milk *(continued)*

NUTRIENT (PER 30 ML)	MATURE HUMAN MILK	SIMILAC PRO-ADVANCE 20	ENFAMIL PREMIUM NEWBORN	WHOLE MILK
Linoleic acid, mg	110.0	200.0	172.0	26.0
Calcium, mg	10.6	15.6	15.6	39.0
Phosphorus, mg	4.5	8.4	8.6	36.4
Iron, mcg	30.3	360.0	360.0	21.24
Copper, mcg	12.1	18.0	15.0	4.2
Selenium, mcg	0.4	0.4	0.6	0.0
Sodium, mg	4.6	4.8	5.4	17.8
Potassium, mg	17.2	21.0	21.6	43.9
Chloride, mg	12.1	13.0	12.6	32.7
Solute load, mOsm	2.9	3.7	3.8	10.0
Osmolality, mOsm/L	286	300	300	285
Vitamin A, international unit	84.8	60.0	60.0	54.5
Vitamin D, international unit	0.48	15.0	12.0	0.24
Vitamin E, mg	0.76	0.3	0.4	0.021
Vitamin K, mcg	0.45	1.6	1.6	1.8
Folate, mcg	0.04	3.0	3.2	0.039

* Whey: casein ratio in human milk changes after birth. In early lactation, the ratio is 90:10; later with mature milk, the ratio is 60:40; and in late lactation, the ratio is 50:50 (Lawrence & Lawrence, 2016).

Calculations of components converted from data reported per deciliter to 30 mL (1 ounce).

** Docosahexaenoic acid (DHA), arachidonic acid (ARA) additives derived from algae, mycotic sources.

SOURCES: Data from Abbott Nutrition, 2018; Lawrence & Lawrence, 2016; Mead-Johnson Nutritionals, 2018a.

intake depends on the mother's milk supply and breastfeeding efficiency. It is noteworthy that breastfed newborns born to multiparous mothers who have previously breastfed often do not lose as much weight as babies born to primiparous mothers because the multiparous mother's milk typically becomes more abundant sooner (Lawrence & Lawrence, 2016). If a newborn has a weight loss of 10% or greater, an evaluation, an intervention, and a follow-up weight check are indicated to assess for any breastfeeding problems or newborn-maternal risk factors contributing to inadequate milk production and/or milk transfer. Typically the weight loss in a breastfeeding newborn plateaus at 72 hours of age when milk production increases during the lactogenesis II phase, often termed the *milk coming in* (Lawrence & Lawrence, 2016).

Once feedings are established, growth rates for breastfed and formula-fed babies vary. Exclusively breastfed babies have the same or slightly higher weight gain than their formula-fed and combination-fed peers in the first 3 months. *Thereafter*, formula-fed and combination-fed infants have a greater weight gain pattern compared with breastfed infants. This characteristic weight gain pattern results in a leaner body build in the breastfed group by the latter half of the first year of life (Wambach & Riordan, 2016). Measurements of length and head circumference are similar in both groups. A baby typically grows 2.5 cm (1 inch) per month in the first 6 months, and then 1.3 cm (0.5 inch) for the next 6 months. Length has been shown to be a better indicator of growth than weight. Infants generally double their birth weight by 5 months, triple their birth weight by 1 year of age, and quadruple their birth weight by 2 years (Wambach & Riordan, 2016). The World Health Organization (WHO) growth charts are recommended by the Centers for Disease Control and Prevention (CDC) for monitoring growth for newborns, infants, and children from birth to 2 years of age (CDC, 2010). The CDC growth charts for tracking the weight, length, and head circumference of children 2 years of age and older can be downloaded from the CDC website. See *Key Facts to Remember: Newborn Caloric and Fluid Needs.*

Key Facts To Remember
Newborn Caloric and Fluid Needs

The following are newborn caloric and fluid needs:

- Caloric intake: 45.5 to 52.5 kcal/lb/day or 100 to 115 kcal/kg/day
- Fluid requirements: 64 to 73 mL/lb/day or 140 to 160 mL/kg/day
- Weight gain in the first few weeks: 1 oz/day (or about a half pound per week)

Fluid

Fluid requirements during the neonatal period are high (140 to 160 mL/kg/day). This is primarily due to the newborn's decreased ability to concentrate urine and increased overall metabolic rate. Although the newborn's total body water content is high (75 to 80%) compared with an adult's (60%), the newborn has an increased surface area-to-mass ratio and decreased renal absorptive capacity, which make the baby more susceptible to dehydration. Until the ability to retain body water through kidney function improves in the early months of life, the baby is at risk for dehydration. Dehydration may develop from insufficient fluid intake or increased fluid loss due to diarrhea, vomiting, or other source of fluid loss. Parents and caretakers should be aware of the signs of dehydration. See Box 29–1. In order to prevent dehydration, the newborn's fluid intake should be increased above the baseline fluid needs when the baby has a fever or is in a warm environment for an extended period of time. The increased fluid requirements should be met with additional breast milk or formula, rather than water, because the increased water can cause hyponatremia and may result in seizures if water consumption is excessive.

Box 29–1

Signs of Dehydration in the Newborn

- Depressed fontanelles
- Rapid, weak pulse
- Elevated low-grade temperature
- Dark, concentrated urine
- Dry, hard stools
- Dry skin with little turgor
- Elevated urine specific gravity (1.020)

SAFETY ALERT!

A newborn with a fever or with persistent diarrhea or vomiting should be evaluated by a healthcare provider in order to adequately diagnose and treat potential dehydration.

Energy

The *basal metabolic rate (BMR)* refers to the energy needed for thermoregulation, cardiorespiratory function, cellular activity, and growth. A baby requires 100 to 115 kcal/kg/day at 1 month and 85 to 95 kcal/kg/day from 6 to 12 months of age. When a newborn does not receive sufficient calories, the baby risks losing weight, may experience tissue breakdown, and is at risk for delayed growth and development (Wambach & Riordan, 2016).

Fats

Babies receive approximately 50% of their calories from fat. Fats help the body absorb the fat-soluble vitamins A, D, E, and K and are a precursor of prostaglandins and other hormones. Essential fatty acids and their derivatives, docosahexaenoic acid (DHA) and arachidonic acid (ARA), are major fatty acids found in the brain and retina. Both DHA and ARA are long-chain polyunsaturated fatty acids (LCPUFAs) derived from linoleic acid and α-linolenic acid. Along with oleic acid, these LCPUFAs are needed for myelination of the spinal cord and other nerves and play an important role in brain development. Research demonstrating better cognitive function in breastfed infants has led some to support the addition of ARA and DHA to infant formula because some studies have shown improved visual acuity and cognitive and behavioral functions in breastfed infants (Eichenwald, Hansen, Martin, et al., 2017).

Milk Composition. Approximately 98% of human milk fat is in the form of triglycerides, and a very small but clinically significant amount is from cholesterol. Cholesterol levels in breast milk may also stimulate the production of enzymes that lead to more efficient metabolism of cholesterol, thereby reducing its harmful long-term effects on the cardiovascular system.

Fat content is the most variable component in human milk, ranging from 12 grams/liter in colostrum and increasing to 30 to 50 grams/liter in mature milk. Fat content is influenced by maternal parity, duration of pregnancy, the stage of lactation, diurnal regulation, and changes in fat content even during a single feeding. Multiparous mothers produce milk with a lower content of fatty acids than primigravidas. The milk of a mother who delivers a preterm newborn has a higher percentage of fat and a greater concentration of DHA and ARA than does the milk of a mother who gives birth to a full-term baby. Preterm newborns receiving breast milk therefore receive the increased concentrations of DHA and ARA needed by the premature baby (Lawrence & Lawrence, 2016).

Phospholipids and cholesterol levels are higher in colostrum compared with mature milk, although overall fat content is higher in mature breast milk compared with colostrum. Fat content is generally higher in the evening and lower in the early morning. Within a single feeding session a baby initially receives the low-fat foremilk before receiving the higher-calorie, high-fat hindmilk, which has double the fat content (Wambach & Riordan, 2016). Finally, the fat content of breast milk is also affected by maternal diet and maternal fat stores. Mothers on low-fat diets have increased production of medium-chain fatty acids (C6–C10), and mothers with a higher weight gain in pregnancy produce breast milk with a higher fat content (Lawrence & Lawrence, 2016).

The fats in the milk-based formulas are modified to parallel the fat profile of human milk by removing the butterfat from cow's milk and adding vegetable oils. There are quite a few differences in the fat sources and amounts used among the major formula brands. Since 2002 infant formulas have been supplemented with DHA and ARA. However, breast milk also contains 167 other fatty acids of uncertain function, and these are absent from formula (Lawrence & Lawrence, 2016).

Carbohydrates

Carbohydrates (sugars) serve as the other main source of energy for the baby, providing about 40% of the calories in the baby's diet. By weight, both human milk and formula contain more carbohydrates than fat.

Milk Composition. The primary carbohydrate in breast milk is lactose. In addition to providing a cellular energy source especially for the brain in the form of glucose, lactose enhances the absorption of calcium and galactose facilitates the production of galactolipids, which are essential for central nervous system (CNS) development (Lawrence & Lawrence, 2016).

Human milk also contains trace amounts of other carbohydrates such as glucosamines and nitrogen-containing oligosaccharides. Glucosamines are one of the building blocks for connective tissues and help strengthen and hold together ligaments and tendons. Oligosaccharides promote the growth of *Lactobacillus bifidus*, which promotes an intestinal acidic environment creating a hostile environment for pathogens to thrive (Lawrence & Lawrence, 2016; Wambach & Riordan, 2016).

Proteins

Proteins are the building blocks for muscle and organ structure. They are key to almost every metabolic process in the body, including energy metabolism, cell-signaling, growth, and immune function.

Milk Composition. Milk proteins are often grouped into casein and whey proteins. Whey protein is the predominant dietary protein in human milk. During digestion this type of protein creates soft curds that are easily and quickly broken down. Because of this, breastfeeding babies digest their meals in 90 minutes and need to feed often, about 8 to 12 feedings per day. It is rare for exclusively breastfeeding babies to have constipation. Casein is the major phosphoprotein found in milk. Cow's milk contains a high amount of casein (a low ratio of whey to casein—approximately 20:80) compared with mature human milk (60:40). Because of its tendency to form curds, milk with high amounts of casein is less easily digested.

Cow's milk–based formulas are usually modified to get closer to the whey:casein ratio profile of mature human milk. It should also be noted that the whey and casein components in breast milk are not static and change over time to meet the needs of the growing infant. In early lactation, the whey:casein ratio is 90:10. As lactation progresses, the whey:casein ratio in mature breast milk is 60:40. Finally, during late lactation, the whey:casein ratio is 50:50 (Wambach & Riordan, 2016).

Whey protein in human milk is composed of five major components: (1) alpha-lactalbumin, (2) serum albumin, (3) lactoferrin, (4) immunoglobulins, and (5) lysozyme. The latter three components are believed to be nonnutritional proteins and serve immunologic functions in the body. Breast milk contains other nonnutritional proteins, such as other enzymes, growth modulators, and hormones (Wambach & Riordan, 2016).

Vitamins, Minerals, and Trace Elements

VITAMINS

The newborn's rapid growth makes the baby especially vulnerable to dietary inadequacies. Adequate vitamin intake is especially important to support normal growth and metabolism. When the mother is well nourished throughout her pregnancy, the full-term neonate can be expected to have adequate vitamin stores at birth.

Vitamins play an important role in the body's metabolic functions. The fat-soluble vitamins A, D, E, and K are absorbed in the presence of fat or bile and are stored in fat tissue and the liver for future use. Excessive intake of fat-soluble vitamins can result in toxicity; therefore, supplementation is not generally recommended, except in the case of vitamin D (see the following section for further discussion).

Milk Composition. Vitamins in human milk are influenced by the mother's vitamin intake, general nutritional status, and genetic differences and vary as lactation progresses. Many healthcare providers encourage new mothers to continue their prenatal vitamins after delivery and throughout the lactation period, unless the mother generally eats a well-balanced diet (Wambach & Riordan, 2016).

Human milk is naturally low in vitamin D (25 international units/L or less); therefore, breastfeeding newborns/infants who have limited sunlight exposure may be at risk for vitamin D deficiency. The American Academy of Pediatrics (2016c) recommends that all newborns/infants and children receive 400 international units of vitamin D daily, beginning within the first few days after birth, and that breastfed newborns/infants (including those receiving less than 32 ounces of vitamin D-fortified formula) should stay on vitamin D supplementation. Cow's milk-based formulas are currently supplemented with at least 400 international units of vitamin D per liter; the AAP recommends that formula-fed newborns/infants should receive additional supplementation until their intake reaches 1 liter (33.8 ounces) per day (generally about 3 months of age).

Vitamin K is present in human breast milk, but in small quantities. Vitamin K is also synthesized in the baby's intestinal tract by bacteria that are colonized there. Within a few days, newborns will generally have produced sufficient amounts of vitamin K to prevent excessive bleeding. To prevent vitamin K deficiency, it has been the standard of care to give vitamin K prophylaxis shortly after birth, but delayed until after the first breastfeeding in the delivery room and the baby becomes naturally vitamin K sufficient (American Academy of Pediatrics [AAP] & American College of Obstetricians and Gynecologists [ACOG], 2017).

The vitamin B complex and vitamin C (antioxidant) are water-soluble vitamins that pass readily from serum to breast milk. However, mothers who follow a strict vegetarian or macrobiotic diet may have insufficient vitamin B_{12} in their milk. In that case, the exclusively breastfed newborn/infant should receive vitamin B_{12} supplementation. Formula is fortified with adequate amounts of the water-soluble vitamins to meet the DRI. Unlike fat-soluble vitamins, any excess water-soluble vitamins ingested are simply excreted, so the threat of toxicity is low (Lawrence & Lawrence, 2016).

Vitamin A is needed for general maintenance of healthy skin, hair, nails, gums, glands, bones, and teeth. It also helps prevent infections. In developing countries where malnutrition is of great concern, human milk provides a vital source of vitamin A and helps prevent blindness (Lawrence & Lawrence, 2016).

Vitamin E (antioxidant and free radical scavenger) is naturally present in human milk, and mothers of preterm newborns produce a slightly higher level in their colostrum than mothers of term babies. This is particularly important to premature newborns in the neonatal intensive care unit (NICU), who may have damage to their lungs and retinas from oxygen toxicity.

MINERALS

Minerals have diverse regulatory functions throughout the body. For example, calcium is important in clotting mechanisms; phosphorus is a component in adenosine triphosphate (ATP), deoxyribonucleic acid (DNA), ribonucleic acid (RNA), and phospholipids; calcium and phosphorus are necessary for bone formation; sodium is involved in fluid balance; calcium, sodium, and potassium are needed for nerve and muscle function; chlorine is involved in acid–base balance; cobalt works with vitamin B_{12} to form blood cells; copper and iron aid in extracting energy from the citric acid cycle and are also involved in blood production; iodine is needed for thyroid hormone synthesis; and magnesium, manganese, and zinc are needed to help with many enzymatic processes. Calcium and iron are the two basic minerals that are of particular importance in maintaining adequate nutrition.

Milk Composition. Both human milk and infant formulas contain several major and trace minerals to satisfy the needs of the growing baby. The mineral content of human milk does not appear to be influenced by maternal diet. The vitamins and minerals among the formulas being compared are essentially the same, although all generally contain higher levels of minerals than human milk to compensate for their lower bioavailability.

The American Academy of Pediatrics (2016c) recommends against the use of low-iron-fortified formulas because of the increased risk for anemia associated with their use. Iron in human milk is much more completely absorbed—the baby receiving human milk absorbs 50 to 80% of the iron in human milk compared with less than 12% of the iron in formula. Healthy term babies with normal birth weights receiving breast milk or an iron-fortified infant formula during the first 5 to 6 months of life are unlikely to develop iron deficiency anemia because these infants have sufficient iron stores to sustain them until they start solid feedings in the second half of the first year of life (Wambach & Riordan, 2016). However, the late preterm newborn who is breastfeeding should receive routine iron supplementation (Academy of Breastfeeding Medicine [ABM], 2016). Preterm babies should receive 0.2 mg/kg/day of elemental iron upon discharge from the hospital (AAP & ACOG, 2017). Current recommendation for vitamin D for preterm babies is 400–1000 international units per kg per day (AAP & ACOG, 2017; Darmawikarta et al., 2016).

Nurses have a responsibility to educate parents and help them understand that the iron added to formula is in an ionic form and does not cause constipation. The casein in formula (which is different from the casein in human milk) creates firm, rubbery curds that are slow to metabolize and have been associated with constipation in formula-fed babies. In addition, palm olein oil is added to some formulas to provide palmitic acid in an attempt to match the natural palmitic acid profile in human milk. However, the chemical arrangements are different. Palmitic acid derived from olein oil is poorly absorbed. The unabsorbed palmitic acid in formula reacts with calcium to create insoluble soaps during digestion and contribute to constipation.

TRACE ELEMENTS

Other additives to formulas not yet mentioned include nucleotides (building blocks for DNA and RNA that appear to enhance the immune system, among other things), carnitine (functions include transport of fatty acids to the mitochondria for oxidation), and taurine (functions include contributing to growth and central nervous system and auditory function development). There are many other components in human milk not yet duplicated in formula, and not all components in breast milk have been identified. In general, though, formula companies strive to improve their products to develop the best "humanized" milk possible, and formulas available today are far superior to those of the past.

Feeding Intolerances

Often fussy breastfed or cow's milk-based formula-fed newborns are switched to a lactose-free formula because of concerns about lactose intolerance. It is important to distinguish true lactose intolerance from cow's-milk protein allergy or other source of feeding intolerance.

Many parents will assume that their baby has lactose intolerance because they or the child's older sibling has lactose intolerance. However, this is an age-related condition that develops after 2 to 5 years of age and is therefore not a condition affecting newborns.

Breastfeeding babies may not be allergic to the mother's milk but rather to the cow's-milk protein (an antigen) in the mother's milk. By eliminating the culprit (e.g., the bovine protein) from the mother's diet and therefore from the breast milk, the mother can continue to breastfeed, providing optimal nutrition and immune factors to her baby.

Specialty Formulas

AAP and ACOG (2017) recommend breastfeeding for all newborns/infants, with rare exceptions. When breastfeeding is not an option or is not chosen, then standard cow's milk-based formula is the first choice among the formulas. However, there are situations in which standard cow's milk-based formula is not tolerated, is contraindicated, or is not acceptable to the parents. Before switching to a specialty formula, the parents should first consult with their baby's healthcare provider (Abbott Nutrition, 2018).

MILK-BASED LACTOSE-FREE FORMULAS

Similac Sensitive is a milk-based formula containing milk protein isolate and is lactose-free. In place of lactose, the formula manufacturer substitutes a blend of corn syrup solids and sucrose. (Bear in mind that use of nonlactose products should be reserved for those rare newborns/infants with clinically proven lactose intolerance.)

SOY-BASED FORMULAS

Soy protein-based formula is not intended as a first-choice formula except for babies with primary lactase deficiency or galactosemia (which can be tested in newborn screens), for term babies of formula-feeding vegan parents (but breastfeeding is best), and for babies who develop secondary (transient) lactase deficiency following an acute bout with diarrhea (AAP, 2018a).

When a newborn is fussy and gassy, many parents mistakenly believe that their baby is "lactose intolerant" because an adult family member is lactose intolerant. Cow protein in standard cow's milk–based formula can cause colicky symptoms in sensitive babies. Switching to soy formula will not always solve the cause of the colic symptoms. The AAP recommends using hypoallergenic (hydrolyzed) formulas rather than soy formula for babies with documented cow's-milk allergy (AAP, 2018a).

HYDROLYZED (HYPOALLERGENIC) FORMULAS

For newborns who do not have cow's milk-based formula allergy but may have formula intolerance, the formula companies offer hydrolyzed or partially hydrolyzed formula. (*Note:* "Hydrolyzed" simply means the protein has been broken down into smaller components mimicking digestion.) Nestlé Good Start Gentle HMO provides 100% hydrolyzed whey protein (no casein protein) for easier digestion, and the carbohydrate requirement is met with a blend of lactose and corn maltodextrin. Fats come from a combination of vegetable oils (Nestlé Nutrition, 2016). Enfamil Neuro Pro Gentlease provides hydrolyzed whey and casein proteins with a profile similar to mature human milk, but the lactose amount is reduced to one-fifth the amount found in standard milk-based formula (Mead-Johnson Nutritionals, 2018a).

For newborns with documented cow's milk-based allergies or newborns with a metabolic disorder or malabsorption syndrome, the first-choice formula is a hypoallergenic formula such as Nutramigen or Alimenum. Both formulas use extensively hydrolyzed casein protein supplemented with a high percentage of free amino acids. Both are lactose-free and use a combination of vegetable fats to meet the fat requirement.

Choice of Feeding

Feeding their newborn is an exciting, satisfying, but often worrisome task for parents. Meeting this essential need of their new child helps parents strengthen their attachment to their child and fosters their self-images as nurturers and providers, yet carries great responsibility. Whether a woman chooses to breastfeed or formula-feed, she can be reassured that she can adequately meet her baby's needs. As questions about feeding arise, the nurse works with the woman to help her develop skill in her chosen method. In every interaction, it is the nurse's responsibility to support the parents and promote the family's sense of confidence.

The mother usually decides to breastfeed or formula-feed by the sixth month of pregnancy and often even before conception. However, she may not make her final decision until admission to the birth center. The decision is often influenced by relatives, especially the baby's father and the maternal grandmother (Meek, 2017), by friends, and by social customs rather than being based on knowledge about the nutritional and psychologic needs of the mother and her newborn.

Once the parents have made an informed choice of feeding method, the nurse's primary responsibilities are to support the family's decision and to help the family achieve a positive result. No woman should be made to feel either inadequate or superior because of her choice in feeding. There are advantages and disadvantages to breastfeeding and bottle-feeding, but positive bonds in parent–child relationships can be developed with either method.

Health Promotion *Healthy People 2020* Objectives for Exclusive Breastfeeding

The goals of the *Healthy People 2020* national health promotion and disease prevention program propose that at least 82% of all mothers will initiate breastfeeding (the current rate is 83.2); at least 61% will continue to breastfeed until their infants are 6 months old (the current rate is 57.6%); and at least 34% will continue to breastfeed until their infants are 12 months old (the current rate is 35.9%). The *Healthy People 2020* objective for exclusive breastfeeding at 3 months is 46% (the current rate is 46.9%); the objective at 6 months is 26% (the current rate is 24.9%) (CDC, 2018a).

There continue to be lower breastfeeding rates among racial and ethnic minority mothers in the United States. Lower breastfeeding rates are also associated with socioeconomic disparities, such as lower education level, poverty, young age, high body mass index, not abstaining from alcohol use, smoking within 6 weeks of delivery, and living in rural areas. It is the healthcare provider's responsibility to provide the parents with accurate information about the distinct advantages of breastfeeding to the mother and baby. Nurses and other healthcare professionals have a unique opportunity to promote and support breastfeeding, and their efforts can have a meaningful impact on the future health of the mother and child (Bunik, 2017; Jones, Power, Queenan, et al., 2015).

Breastfeeding

Breast Milk Production

The female breast is composed of glandular tissue containing lobules of alveolar clusters that contain the milk-secreting unit, the alveolus. The glandular tissue is embedded in fat tissue and is supported by connective tissue and ligaments. The majority of the glandular tissue is within 30 mm of the nipple. During lactation, milk is formed in the alveolus in these lobules and is transported through milk ducts that eventually branch closer to the nipple with a range of 4 to 18 milk ducts exiting the nipple. The alveolus is lined with epithelial cells surrounded by supportive connective tissue, blood vessels, and myoepithelial cells that contract in response to hormone stimulation to eject milk into the ducts. Oxytocin is the hormone that is responsible for stimulating these contractile cells, and this response is often termed the *milk ejection reflex* or *letdown*. The ductal system does not store milk; rather, it provides for the transport of milk from the units in the lobes (Blackburn, 2018). See Figure 29–1 to view the anatomy of the breast.

Physiologic and Endocrine Control of Lactogenesis

During pregnancy, increased levels of estrogen stimulate breast duct proliferation and development, and elevated progesterone levels promote the development of lobules and alveoli in preparation for lactation. Prolactin is responsible for the final preparation of the lobes and alveoli for milk production and the levels rise from approximately 10 ng/mL prepregnancy to 200 ng/mL at term. Even though these prolactin levels are elevated in pregnancy, lactation is suppressed by elevated progesterone levels secreted by the placenta. Once the placenta is expelled at birth, progesterone levels fall and the inhibition is removed, triggering milk production. **Lactogenesis II** is the period during which there is an increased volume of breast milk, called the *milk coming in*. This occurs whether the mother has breast stimulation or not. However, if by the third or fourth day breast emptying is not occurring, milk production will cease.

Initially, lactation is under endocrine control. The hormone **prolactin** is released from the anterior pituitary in response to breast stimulation from suckling or the use of a breast pump. Prolactin stimulates the milk-secreting cells in the alveoli to produce milk. Prolactin levels may range from 300 to 400 ng/mL in the first 10 days of lactation, then gradually decline to levels of 60 to 100 ng/mL by 3 months while still maintaining adequate milk supply. If more than approximately 3 hours occurs between breast stimulation, prolactin levels begin to drop below baseline. To reverse the overall decline in prolactin levels, the mother can be encouraged to breastfeed/pump more frequently (e.g., every 1.5 to 2 hours during day hours) for a few days to get baseline prolactin raised. This is especially important if the newborn is not an effective feeder or if the mother is separated from her newborn. Prolactin receptors are established during the first 2 weeks postpartum in response to frequency

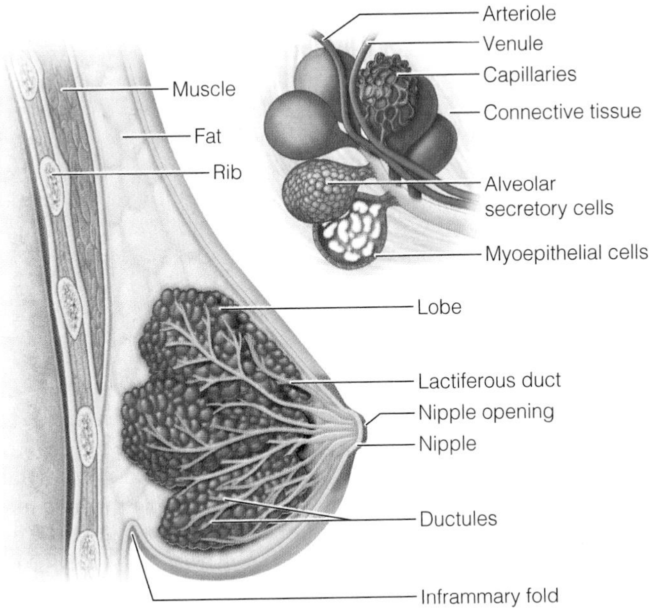

Figure 29–1 Anatomy of the breast.

of breast stimulation (Wambach & Riordan, 2016). Inadequate development of prolactin receptors during this time is likely to negatively impact the mother's long-term milk volume. By 2 weeks (14 days) postpartum, prolactin levels will be back to prepregnancy levels and milk production will cease if stimulation of the breasts by breastfeeding or pumping does not occur (Lawrence & Lawrence, 2016).

The milk that flows from the breast at the start of a feeding or pumping session is called **foremilk**. The foremilk is watery milk, high in lactose, high in protein, and low in fat (1 to 2%). This milk has trickled down from the alveoli between feedings to fill the lactiferous ducts. It is low-fat milk because the fat globules made in the alveoli stick to each other and to the walls of the alveoli and do not trickle down.

In addition to prolactin release, stretching of the nipple and compression of the areola signal the hypothalamus to trigger the posterior pituitary gland to release oxytocin. **Oxytocin** acts on the myoepithelial cells surrounding the alveoli in the breast tissue to contract, ejecting milk, including the fat globules present, into the ducts. This process is called the *milk-ejection reflex*, better known in lay terms as the **let-down reflex** response. The average initial let-down response occurs about 2 minutes after the newborn begins to suckle, and there will be several let-down responses during a feeding session. The milk that flows during let-down is called **hindmilk**. As noted, hindmilk is rich in fat (can exceed 10%) and therefore high in calories. In a sample of expressed human milk, the average total fat concentration is about 4% and the total caloric content is about 20 calories/ounce.

By 6 months of breastfeeding, prolactin levels are only 5 to 10 ng/mL, yet milk production continues. A whey protein called *feedback inhibitor of lactation (FIL)* has been identified as influencing milk production through a negative feedback loop. FIL is present in breast milk and functions to decrease milk production. The more milk that remains in the breast and the longer it remains, the more milk production is decreased. On the other hand, the more often the breasts are emptied, the lower the level of FIL and the faster milk is produced. This mechanism of regulating milk at the local level is called *autocrine control*. This process is key to understanding how a mother maintains or loses her milk supply (Lawrence & Lawrence, 2016).

There are a number of risk factors that can delay or impair lactogenesis. Maternal factors include cesarean birth, primiparity, long duration of the first or second stage of labor, postpartum hemorrhage, premature delivery, diabetes type 1, untreated hypothyroidism, obesity, polycystic ovary syndrome, vitamin B_6 deficiency, retained placenta fragments, history of previous breast surgery, insufficient glandular breast tissue, and significant stress (Wambach & Riordan, 2016). Other factors that can interfere with the breast milk supply include smoking and the use of alcohol and some prescription and over-the-counter medications (e.g., antihistamines, combined oral contraceptives [COCs]).

Stages of Human Milk

During the establishment of lactation there are three stages of human milk: Colostrum, transitional milk, and mature milk.

Colostrum is the initial milk that begins to be secreted during midpregnancy and is immediately available to the baby at delivery. The volume of colostrum is small, and this encourages the newborn to nurse frequently, helping to stimulate milk production. No supplementation with other fluids is necessary unless there is a medical indication. Colostrum is a thick, creamy, yellowish fluid with concentrated amounts of protein, fat-soluble vitamins, and minerals, and it has lower amounts of fat and lactose compared with mature milk. It also contains antioxidants and high levels of lactoferrin and secretory immunoglobulin A (IgA). It promotes the establishment of *Lactobacillus bifidus* flora in the digestive tract, which helps to protect the newborn from disease and illness. Colostrum also facilitates the passage of meconium stools, which in turn helps decrease hyperbilirubinemia. The volume of colostrum ranges from 7 to 20 mL per feeding in the first few days (Lawrence & Lawrence, 2016).

The onset of copious milk secretion begins between 48 and 96 hours postpartum. For most women this is observed on day 3. The milk produced during this period is called **transitional milk**. Transitional milk has qualities intermediate to colostrum and mature milk but may look indistinguishable from colostrum. It is still yellow in color like colostrum but is more copious and contains more fat, lactose, water-soluble vitamins, and calories (Figure 29–2). By day 5, most mothers are producing about 500 mL/day (Wambach & Riordan, 2016).

Mature milk is white or can be slightly blue-tinged in color. It is present by 2 weeks postpartum and continues thereafter until lactation ceases. Mature milk contains about 13% solids (carbohydrates, proteins, and fats) and 87% water. Although mature human milk appears similar in appearance to skim cow's milk and thus may cause mothers to question whether their milk is "rich enough," mothers should be reassured that this is the normal appearance of mature human milk and that it provides the newborn with all the necessary nutrients. Although gradual changes in composition do occur continuously over periods of weeks to accommodate the needs of the growing baby, in general the composition of mature milk is fairly consistent, with the exception of the fat content as noted previously. Milk production continues to increase slowly over the first month. By 6 months postpartum a mother produces about 800 mL/day (Wambach & Riordan, 2016).

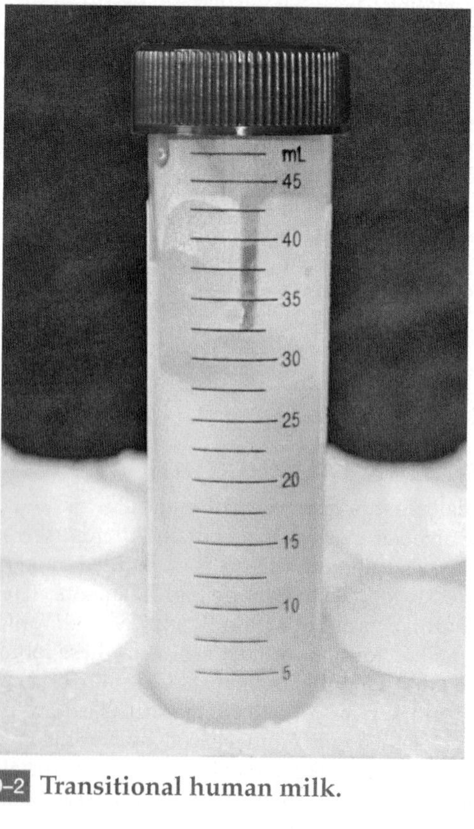

Figure 29–2 **Transitional human milk.**

Advantages of Human Milk

In its breastfeeding policy statement, the AAP recommends *exclusive* breastfeeding as the preferred feeding for all newborns/infants, with a few exceptions, for the first 6 months, with continuation of breastfeeding for 1 year or longer as mutually desired by mother and infant (AAP & ACOG, 2017). There is compelling scientific evidence that indicates that breastfeeding provides newborns/infants with specific nutritional, immunologic, and psychosocial advantages over formula feedings (AAP & ACOG, 2017).

NUTRITIONAL ADVANTAGES

Human milk provides optimum nutrition for the human baby because it is species specific. The macronutrients such as protein, fat, and carbohydrates (lactose) are synthesized by the mother in the alveoli of the breasts by specialized secretory cells. Micronutrient elements such as vitamins and minerals derive from the circulating maternal plasma. There are more than 200 distinct components in human milk, with more remaining to be identified (Lawrence & Lawrence, 2016).

Lactose is the primary carbohydrate in mammalian milk and plays a crucial role in the nourishment of our offspring. Human milk has a very high lactose content compared with the milk of other mammal species. After lactose is hydrolyzed into galactose and glucose, the galactose is used in the formation of cerebral galactolipids and contributes to brain and central nervous system (CNS) development. Glucose is used by many tissues, but especially by the brain, which consumes 20% of the body's energy requirements and derives this almost exclusively from glucose. In addition to providing a cellular energy source, lactose enhances the absorption of calcium, magnesium, and zinc (Lawrence & Lawrence, 2016).

The mineral content in human milk (colostrum) is a little higher for the first few days after birth, and then, after a slight decrease, the mineral content remains fairly constant thereafter. Maternal age, parity, and diet (even if the mother is receiving mineral supplement) has only a minimal influence on mineral content in breast milk. It is believed that the maternal body stores regulate the process. For example, if a mother's calcium intake in her diet is poor, the body will draw from its reserves (e.g., from bone) to provide a sufficient amount of calcium in her breast milk for her baby. Following weaning, through a feedback mechanism, transient bone loss normalizes.

The iron found in human milk, even though much lower in concentration than that of prepared formulas, is much more readily and fully absorbed and appears sufficient to meet the infant's iron needs for the first 6 months. Excess iron is not desirable because any extra iron that is not absorbed may promote the growth of pathogenic enteric bacteria as well as cause cellular oxidative injury. Lactoferrin, an iron-binding protein found only in breast milk, scavenges iron in the gut and enhances its absorption (Lawrence & Lawrence, 2016).

Health advantages for the breastfed baby include reduced risk of respiratory tract infections, otitis media, gastrointestinal infections, SIDS, type 1 or type 2 diabetes mellitus, lymphoma, childhood leukemia, Hodgkin disease, obesity, hypercholesterolemia, and allergic diseases such as asthma, food allergies, and dermatitis (Association of Women's Health, Obstetrics, and Neonatal Nurses [AWHONN], 2015). The reduced risk of gastrointestinal infections is related to receiving any human milk, whereas some of the advantages are dose related, indicating improved benefit with extended breastfeeding.

There are health benefits to the breastfeeding mother as well; when breastfeeding is initiated immediately after delivery, there is decreased risk for postpartum bleeding and more rapid uterine involution. Research has also shown that breastfeeding offers a protective function against premenopausal breast cancer and ovarian cancer and may be associated with a decrease in type 2 diabetes, rheumatoid arthritis, and cardiovascular disease (AAP, 2016a).

IMMUNOLOGIC ADVANTAGES

The immunologic advantages of human milk include varying degrees of protection from respiratory tract and gastrointestinal tract infections, urinary tract infections, otitis media, bacterial meningitis, bacteremia, and allergies (AAP, 2016b). The effects of transplacental passage of maternal immunoglobulin gradually diminishes over the first 6 months of life until the infant can begin to produce his or her own immunoglobulins. Human milk-derived immunologic protection helps supplement this protection.

Secretory IgA, an immunoglobulin present in colostrum and mature breast milk, has antiviral, antibacterial, and antigenic-inhibiting properties, specifically across mucosal surfaces such as the intestinal tract. Secretory IgA plays a role in decreasing the permeability of the small intestine to help prevent large protein molecules from triggering an allergic response. Other constituents of colostrum and mature breast milk that act to inhibit the growth of bacteria or viruses are *Lactobacillus bifidus,* lysozymes, lactoperoxidase, lactoferrin, transferrin, and various immunoglobulins.

All babies should receive vaccinations following a schedule as recommended by the CDC (2018a). Mothers may worry that their antibodies will inactivate the live poliovirus. But breastfeeding does not adversely affect immunization and is not a contraindication for any vaccine. Some mothers also wonder if it is safe for them to receive vaccinations while breastfeeding. Mothers should be reassured that most vaccines, with the exception of smallpox or yellow fever, can safely be taken during lactation (CDC, 2018b).

PSYCHOSOCIAL BENEFITS OF BREASTFEEDING

The psychosocial advantages of breastfeeding include increased self-esteem, enhanced bonding, and a decrease in stress for the mother and baby.

A mother's self-esteem is increased in knowing that she has provided the perfect food for her baby and provided protection with her antibodies. For many mothers breastfeeding takes effort, understanding, and an emotional commitment to endure the demands of this lifestyle choice. The mother's sense of accomplishment in being able to satisfy her baby's needs for nourishment and comfort can be a tremendous source of personal satisfaction. Women who breastfeed, by its nature, have close contact with their babies (Figure 29–3). Newborns are very responsive to touch, and touch is vital for the baby's emotional well-being. The tactile stimulation associated with breastfeeding can communicate warmth, closeness, and comfort and provide the opportunity for the mother and newborn to learn each other's behavioral cues and needs. From the release of prolactin and oxytocin while breastfeeding, mothers may feel more affectionate toward their newborns, have improved let-down response, and breastfeed more frequently and for longer periods of time (AAP, 2016a). Table 29–2 encompasses several factors for parents to consider when choosing between breastfeeding and formula-feeding.

Potential Challenges to Breastfeeding

Breastfeeding is a natural process but requires a certain knowledge base that once was passed along from generation to generation. With the decline in the extended family structure, this

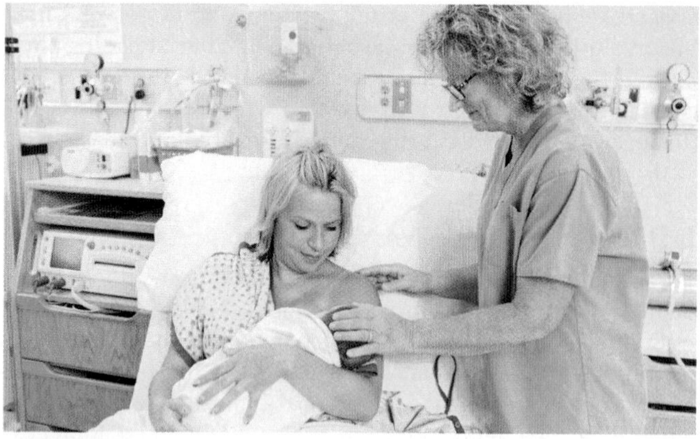

Figure 29–3 **Early breastfeeding assistance by the nurse helps to encourage close contact between mother and newborn.**

SOURCE: Tyler Olson/123RF.

source of knowledge and assistance is often missing for the new mother and can contribute to some of the following potential challenges to breastfeeding.

- ***Pain with breastfeeding.*** Nipple or breast pain can be one of the most common reasons for early weaning, therefore it needs to be addressed early in the plan of care. Nipple tenderness is a common source of discomfort and is usually related to improper positioning and/or not obtaining a deep areolar latch. Nipple pain can also result from mechanical trauma, infection, and anatomical variations in the baby's mouth. Common reasons for breast pain can be related to engorgement during lactogenesis II, plugged ducts, mastitis, or candidiasis. Breastfeeding should not be painful, therefore any reports of nipple or breast pain should include an assessment and referral to lactation support (Berens, Eglash, Malloy, et al., 2016).
- ***Concern over adequacy of milk volumes.*** Many mothers are concerned about the adequacy of their milk volumes, especially in the early days of breastfeeding when colostrum volumes are small, and they often ask, "Is my baby

TABLE 29–2 Comparison of Breastfeeding and Formula-Feeding

BREASTFEEDING	FORMULA-FEEDING (IRON ENRICHED)
Newborn/Infant Nutrition	
Species specific. An ideal balance of nutrients, efficiently absorbed. High bioavailability of iron leaves lower iron for bacterial growth, cell injury.	Derived from bovine milk and/or plant sources. Lower bioavailability of nutrients requires higher concentrations in milk. Additives may cause intolerance.
Higher levels of essential fatty acids, lactose, cystine, DHA, and cholesterol, necessary for brain and nerve growth.	Still missing numerous ingredients. Formulas do not contain cholesterol. Soy and hydrolysate formulas do not contain lactose. DHA and ARA now added.
Composition varies according to gestational age and stage of lactation, meeting changing nutritional needs.	Nutritional value not varied. Nutritional adequacy depends on proper preparation/dilution.
Long-term decreased incidence of diabetes, cancer, obesity, asthma.	
Contains unsaturated fats.	Contains saturated fats.
Babies determine the volume of milk consumed.	Parents or healthcare provider determine the volume consumed. Overfeeding may occur if caregiver is determined that baby empty bottle.
Frequency of feeding is determined by cues from the baby. May feed more frequently as milk digestion is faster.	Frequency of feeding is determined by cues from the baby. May feed less frequently as milk digestion is slower.
Immunologic Properties	
Contains immunoglobulins, enzymes, and leukocytes that protect against pathogens. Nutrients promote growth of *Lactobacillus*, protective bacteria. Lower rates of respiratory and gastrointestinal infections, otitis media, and other infectious diseases.	No anti-infective properties. Formula is linked to an increased incidence of gastrointestinal and respiratory tract infections.
Anti-infective properties present in the milk permit longer storage duration.	Potential for bacterial contamination exists during preparation and storage.
Breast milk is hypoallergenic, with minimal risk of protein allergy/intolerance.	Cow's-milk protein allergy relatively common.
Maternal Health	
Faster return to prepregnancy weight. Breastfeeding associated with lower risk of breast, type 2 diabetes, ovarian cancer.	Provides newborn/infant nutrition when breast milk not available because of maternal illness, medication/drug use, or lactation failure (breast surgery, endocrine disease).
Psychosocial Aspects	
Skin-to-skin contact enhances bonding.	Both parents can participate in positive parent–baby interaction during feeding.
Hormones of lactation promote maternal feelings and sense of well-being.	Father/partner can assume feeding responsibilities.

TABLE 29–2 Comparison of Breastfeeding and Formula-Feeding *(continued)*

BREASTFEEDING	FORMULA-FEEDING (IRON ENRICHED)
The value system of modern society can create barriers to successful breastfeeding.	
Some mothers may feel ashamed or embarrassed.	
Breastfeeding after returning to work may be difficult.	
Cost	
Healthy diet for mother; approximately $600 a year in additional nutritious food for mother.	Around $1,200 a year or more Up to $2,500 a year for hypoallergenic formulas Cost for bottles and other supplies
Savings for newborn/infant medical costs	Lost income when baby is ill (Ask Dr. Sears, 2018)
Cost of breast milk: $0.	
Ancillary costs: Nursing pads, nursing bras.	Ancillary costs: Bottles or bottle liners, nipples, cleaning costs.
A breast pump may be needed.	
Refrigeration is necessary for storing expressed milk.	Refrigeration is needed if preparing more than one bottle at a time.
Convenience	
Milk is always the perfect temperature. No preparation time is needed.	Formula must be purchased commercially. Preparation is time-consuming. Less convenient for traveling or for night feedings.
The mother must be available to feed or will need to provide expressed milk to be given in her absence.	Mother need not be present—anyone can feed the baby.
If she misses a feeding, the mother must express milk to maintain lactation.	
The mother may experience slight discomfort in the early days of lactation.	

getting enough to eat?" Early support by the nurse can assist in alleviating many of these concerns. The nurse can reinforce rooming-in, skin-to-skin contact, early feeding cues, and proper positioning and latch that will foster effective early feedings. The use of a feeding and elimination diary with daily goals can provide evidence that the newborn is meeting the necessary milestones, demonstrating effective feeding. The evidence is not clear on the percentage of mothers who truly have an insufficient milk supply, however, the number seems relatively small in practice. A thorough history of the mother and assessment of the mother–newborn dyad and effectiveness of the feeding should be done in newborns who are not meeting weight gain parameters. The key to initiating and maintaining milk supply in most cases is effective, regular breast emptying. The use of formula supplementation can contribute to a declining milk supply; therefore, formula supplementation in-hospital should not be used unless medically indicated (AAP & ACOG, 2017)

- ***Leaking milk.*** Some women will leak milk when their breasts are full and it is nearly time to breastfeed again or whenever they experience let-down, which can be triggered by hearing, seeing, or even thinking of their baby. If this causes concern to the mother, she can be instructed on how to apply gentle pressure directly over her nipple for a minute or so to stop the leaking momentarily. The mother can wear nursing pads inside her bra (with instructions to change wet pads frequently). Mothers should be given reassurance that this problem diminishes over time.
- ***Embarrassment.*** Breastfeeding in public is another frequently expressed concern that can create a barrier to achieving *Healthy People 2020* breastfeeding goals. Although people agree that breastfeeding is the most natural and healthy way to feed a baby, some mothers feel conflicted because in America breast exposure is often viewed in a sexual context and this may lead to disapproval of attempts to breastfeed in public. As national and state efforts are being made to promote breastfeeding duration to improve the health of mothers and babies, this barrier is slowly being broken down. This is not an easy issue to overcome. Public places are incorporating "mother rooms" to provide a comfortable, private area for the nursing mother. There is no state that prohibits breastfeeding in a public place, and currently all 50 states, the District of Columbia, and the Virgin Islands have created laws that specify that a woman is permitted to breastfeed in any location in which she is authorized to be (National Conference of State Legislatures, 2018). See *Professionalism in Practice: Breastfeeding Promotion Legislation—Breastfeeding in the Workplace*. Some mothers will feel more confident after learning how to breastfeed discreetly while in public. This is often taught at breastfeeding classes or mother-to-mother support groups. See Figure 29–4 to observe a mother discreetly breastfeeding. Some mothers may prefer a baby blanket or shawl to drape over their chests, which will provide more coverage. See *Case Study: Angelina Newman*. Finally, mothers who prefer not to breastfeed even discreetly in public can be encouraged to at least pump their breasts and feed the expressed milk in a bottle so they have the option of getting out of the house.
- ***Stress.*** Many mothers feel a lot of stress juggling work or school and the demands of home life. Some mothers cite this reason for wanting to wean. There are options to suggest for this concern. Mothers can learn about "double pumping" to save time. A double electric breast pump allows the mother to pump both breasts simultaneously, which cuts the pumping time in half. If a mother struggles to keep up her milk supply, she can try taking an herbal supplement to give her

Professionalism in Practice Breastfeeding Promotion Legislation—Breastfeeding in the Workplace

It is important to be a patient advocate and be involved in legislative initiatives on the national and local level. The Breastfeeding Promotion Act of 2009 was enacted into law on March 23, 2010, and acts to protect breastfeeding in the workplace by providing five provisions. These include:

- *Title I:* Amending the Civil Rights Act of 1964 to protect lactating women from being fired or discriminated against in the workplace.
- *Title II:* Giving tax incentives to businesses that establish a private space in the workplace for their employees to breastfeed or express their milk. Employers can also receive tax credits for supplying breastfeeding equipment and providing lactation consultation services for their employees.
- *Title III:* Establishing set standards for breast pumps to ensure that they are safe and effective.
- *Title IV:* Expanding the Internal Revenue Code definition of "medical care" to include breastfeeding equipment and lactation services as tax-deductible for families.
- *Title V:* Requiring employers with 50 or more employees to provide lactating employees break time and a private area to express their milk.

In addition, the U.S. Department of Labor (2011) enacted the Fair Labor Standards Act: Break Time for Nursing Mothers provision.

The Business Case for Breastfeeding program provides information for employers on the benefits (return on investment) of providing support to nursing mothers in the workplace. Under the Patient Protection and Affordable Care Act, most employers, with few exceptions, must offer a breastfeeding employee reasonable break times to pump for up to 1 year after her baby is born and a place other than a bathroom to comfortably, safely, and privately express breastmilk. Breastfeeding women also gain information about how to protect their right to breastfeed and how to create a lactation-friendly workplace as well as resources for support in the community (Office of Women's Health, 2017).

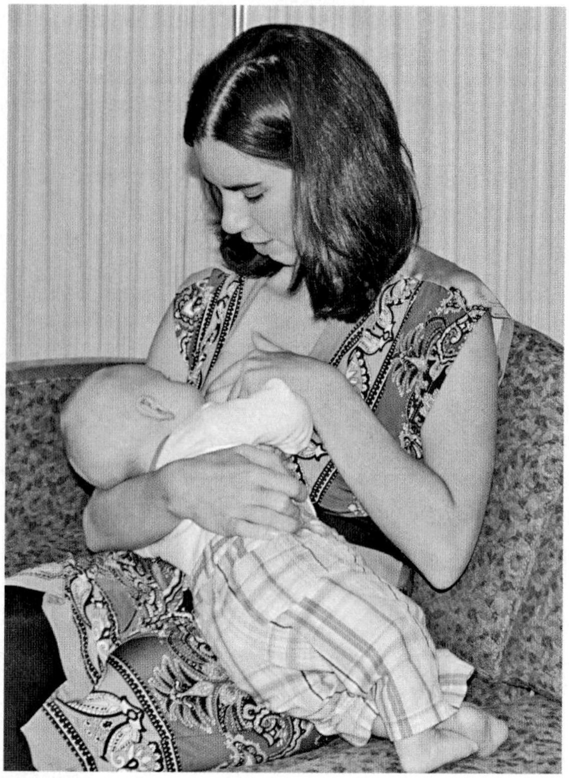

Figure 29–4 Breastfeeding discreetly.

milk supply a boost, unless contraindicated for her. Finally, it is still preferable to decrease the frequency of pumping rather than quitting altogether, if that makes things more manageable for the mother. Babies who get some breast milk are still receiving more of the benefits of breast milk than babies who do not receive any breast milk.

- ***Unequal feeding responsibilities.*** Some parents want feedings to be a shared responsibility. The parents should be informed that it is advisable for the father/partner to wait to bottle-feed the baby with expressed breast milk until after the milk supply and breastfeeding are established, generally when their baby is about 3 to 4 weeks old. In the meantime, encourage the father/partner to be supportive of the breastfeeding mother, to have a lot of skin-to-skin contact with the newborn, and to share the responsibilities of all other aspects of baby care (bathing, dressing, diapering, burping, rocking, etc.).
- ***Diet restriction.*** Some mothers think that they have to give up eating certain foods when they breastfeed. This is generally not true. Most mothers can still eat all the foods they are accustomed to eating. Mothers do need to restrict alcohol intake and keep caffeine to a minimum. In the uncommon case where a

CASE STUDY: Angelina Newman

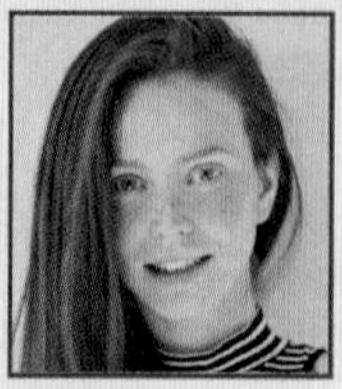

SOURCE: WAYHOME studio/Shutterstock.

Angelina says that she is interested in breastfeeding but feels uncomfortable breastfeeding in front of others. She is not sure learning to breastfeed will be worth the time because she will be returning to school in 8 weeks, at which time the baby will switch to formula. Angelina knows that breastfeeding offers the best nutrition for her new son, so she is conflicted and just not sure what the best option is for her and the baby.

Questions to Ponder

What education can you provide Angelina in how to breastfeed without embarrassment in different situations? Will breastfeeding for just 8 weeks be beneficial to the newborn?

baby has intolerance or allergy symptoms, the mother should consult with a lactation consultant or the baby's healthcare provider to help her work through this complication.

- ***Limited hormonal birth control options.*** Some mothers think that they cannot use a hormonal method of birth control while breastfeeding. Mothers should be informed that using birth control pills containing progesterone and estrogen can cause a decrease in milk volume and may affect the quality of breast milk. It is preferred that the mother who wants to use a hormonal birth control method consider using the progestin-only pill; receive Depo-Provera, a progestin-only injection administered every 90 days; or have a progestin-only implant. Although progestin-only hormonal birth control is compatible with lactation, it is recommended that the mother wait 6 weeks before taking the hormonal medication to ensure a good milk supply (ABM, 2015). Mothers can be reassured that barrier methods of birth control and natural family planning do not interfere with lactation at all and are good options to consider as well.
- ***Vaginal dryness associated with breastfeeding.*** Some mothers experience vaginal dryness related to a low level of estrogen while lactating. This is only a temporary side effect. A water-based lubricant such as K-Y Jelly or Astroglide can be used during intercourse until the woman weans the baby and estrogen levels increase again.

MEDICATIONS

Mothers can be reassured that most prescription and over-the-counter medications are safe for the breastfeeding baby. Medications taken by the breastfeeding mother may penetrate human milk to some degree. This is the primary reason that mothers cite for discontinuing breastfeeding. Having a basic understanding of the kinetics of drug entry into human milk, as well as factors influencing its availability to the baby (bioavailability), may help the nursing mother to continue safely breastfeeding her child.

It should be noted that (1) most drugs penetrate into human milk, (2) almost all medications appear in only small amounts in human milk (usually less than 1% of the maternal dosage), and (3) very few drugs are contraindicated for breastfeeding women (Briggs, Freeman, Towers, et al., 2017; Hale, 2019). See *Professionalism in Practice: FDA Clarification of Drug Risks for Pregnancy and Lactation.*

Professionalism in Practice FDA Clarification of Drug Risks for Pregnancy and Lactation

In 2015 the FDA made changes in the labeling of drugs that spell out the risks for pregnant and lactating women by including a risk summary, clinical considerations, and additional data on the drug, such as known and potential maternal or fetal adverse reactions and any dose adjustments that are needed during pregnancy and the postpartum period. This new labeling helps the healthcare provider make more informed evidence-based decisions (Pernia & DeMaagd, 2016).

SAFETY ALERT!

The mother should be advised to inform her healthcare provider and her baby's healthcare provider that she is breastfeeding when a drug is prescribed for her.

The healthcare provider should consider the following when prescribing a medication (Sachs & AAP Committee on Drugs, 2013):

- Mother's need for the medication
- Drug's potential effect on milk production
- Amount of drug excreted into the milk
- Extent of the baby's oral absorption of the drug
- Drug's potential adverse effects to the baby
- Baby's age and health.

The properties of a drug influence its passage into breast milk, as does the amount of the drug taken, the frequency and route of administration, and the timing of the dose in relationship to breastfeeding. The drug's effects are influenced by the baby's age, the feeding frequency, the volume of milk taken, and the degree of absorption through the gastrointestinal tract. LactMed is a database that has current data on individual medications.

Five adjustments should be made when administering drugs to a nursing mother to decrease the effects of the medication on the baby:

1. Avoid long-acting forms of drugs. The baby may have difficulty metabolizing and excreting them, and accumulation may be a problem.
2. Consider absorption rates and peak blood levels in scheduling the administration of the drugs. Less of the drug crosses into the milk if the baby is fed before the mother takes the oral medication.
3. Use preparations that can be given at longer intervals (once versus three to four times per day).
4. Select the drug that shows the least tendency to pass into breast milk when alternatives are available.
5. Use single-symptom drugs versus multi-symptom drugs (e.g., a decongestant for allergy rather than a multi-symptom drug, especially because liquid forms may contain alcohol).

Potential Contraindications to Breastfeeding

In some instances breastfeeding is or may be contraindicated:

- Mother is HIV positive or has AIDS and is counseled against breastfeeding, except in countries where the risk of neonatal death from diarrhea and other disease (excluding AIDS) is high (Wambach & Riordan, 2016).
- Mother has active, untreated tuberculosis, has varicella, is HTLV1-positive (human T-cell leukemia virus type 1), or has another illness, on a case-by-case basis.
- Mother has active herpes on her breast—the baby may still feed on the unaffected side until the lesion has healed.
- Mother uses illicit drugs (e.g., cocaine, heroin) or is an alcoholic.
- Mother smokes, posing health risks to herself and potential secondhand exposure risks to her baby. Research shows that smoking by breastfeeding mothers can significantly alter babies' sleep–wake cycles, causing them to sleep less; and smoking also affects milk flavor. Maternal smoking can result in breast milk concentrations of nicotine of 1.5 to 3 times the maternal plasma concentration. However, babies who receive breast milk from mothers who smoke are healthier than babies who receive formula and live in a household with smokers. Mothers who smoke cigarettes can breastfeed. To minimize effects on the baby, mothers should time their

smoking to immediately *after* breastfeeding and should not smoke in the same room as their baby (AAP & ACOG, 2017). Smoking has been associated with an increase in respiratory infections and allergies as well as being a considerable risk factor for low milk supply and poor weight gain in the baby (Wambach & Riordan, 2016).
- Mother takes specific medications (e.g., radioactive isotopes, antimetabolites, chemotherapy drugs). A mother with a diagnosis of breast cancer should not breastfeed so that she can begin treatment immediately (AAP & ACOG, 2017).
- Baby has galactosemia.

Clinical Tip

Because mothers are discharged from the birthing unit before breastfeeding is well established, they are frequently alone when they encounter challenges in the breastfeeding process. Many women stop nursing if the situations they encounter seem to pose problems. Nurses can offer anticipatory guidance regarding common breastfeeding phenomena and provide resources for the woman's use after discharge. (See Chapter 34 for a detailed discussion of self-care measures the nurse can suggest to a woman with a breastfeeding problem after discharge from the birthing unit.)

Cultural Considerations in Newborn/Infant Feeding

As healthcare professionals, we can learn about an individual patient's cultural background by engaging in discussions with the patient and asking questions in a sensitive and respectful way. This provides opportunity to validate healthy practices and to exert a positive influence on other matters (Callister, 2014). An occasion for this kind of dialogue might arise during interactions with a new mother who may have misconceptions about breastfeeding. For example, if a new mother says that she heard that getting upset or angry will spoil her milk, you can point out that this belief likely stems from the correct observation that the breastfeeding baby can sense maternal tension (which also may delay let-down) and may therefore act fussy as well, appearing to behave as if he or she were getting "spoiled milk." Then reassure the mother that there is no evidence that the milk composition itself is changed. This will allow you to focus on the real issues of bonding and relaxation technique. You may also note that simply understanding what is really going on may help the mother to be more relaxed.

Among some traditional cultures around the world, it is believed that colostrum is "unclean" or even harmful to a newborn. This belief is found among some groups of Asian, Hispanic, Native American, and Eastern European women (Wambach & Riordan, 2016).

Because of this ancient belief, some mothers even today discard their colostrum or wait 2 to 4 days to begin breastfeeding, when their "true milk" arrives. While waiting for their milk to come in, mothers feed their newborn a culturally specific colostrum substitute. These prelacteal feeds include cereal or gruel, animal milk, sugar water, and a variety of herbal teas (Tariku, Andargie, Wassie, et al., 2016). Not only are these newborns receiving an inferior quality food that is not appropriate for their development and possibly prepared with contaminated water, they are denied vital immunity-building substances; they also miss out on the laxative effect that colostrum provides to rid the body of bilirubin, which reduces the risk of jaundice. Nurses should be aware that some immigrant mothers may have this misconception about their colostrum. In a situation like this, in which a cultural custom is harmful or denies the newborn benefit, it is the nurse's responsibility to try to educate the family about the value of colostrum.

Whenever possible, it is best to have a female, non–family member translator present to interpret for a mother who does not speak English. For many Muslim women, it is culturally unacceptable for them to speak about intimate matters in front of their families. Therefore, it would be inappropriate to ask the new mother's husband or one of her children to be her interpreter. Even among those who speak English, language barriers and miscommunications still exist due in part to words having different meanings to people of different cultures. It is important to give enough explanation to ensure that the mother clearly understands the information provided. These are but a few of the numerous cultural influences related to feeding. (See *Developing Cultural Competence: Breastfeeding in Other Cultures*.) When nurses are faced with newborn/infant care practices different from the ones to which they are accustomed, they need to evaluate the effect of the practice. Different practices are not necessarily inferior. The nurse should intervene only if the practice is actually harmful to the mother or baby.

Developing Cultural Competence **Breastfeeding in Other Cultures**

Many Chinese women go through a 30-day period of home confinement ("doing the month" [zuo yue zi]) following delivery, during which they are not permitted to bathe or wash their hair (Callister, 2014). This is a centuries-old tradition to nurture the mother back to her prenatal state and to keep her body warm to ward off *fong* (flatulence) and other future health ailments. A *pui yuet* (companion) is hired to provide total care for the mother and newborn. The pui yuet will cook traditional confinement foods daily (provide "heating foods" and avoid "cooling foods"). Most foods must be cooked in sesame oil and old ginger. The mother drinks hot herbal tea with her meals and is not permitted to drink any water because it is thought to cause water retention (Callister, 2014).

Many Muslim women breastfeed until their children are 2 years of age. This is encouraged in the Koran. Although most Muslim women do not breastfeed in public, they will breastfeed in front of family members and relatives as long as the breast is not exposed (Yashmin, 2015).

Among traditional societies around the world, weaning from the breast occurs when a child is between 2 and 4 years of age. Some people of African ancestry may wean their babies after they begin to walk.

Some women of Asian heritage may breastfeed their babies for the first 1 to 2 years of life.

In sub-Indian cultures, some mothers may breastfeed female babies longer than male babies (Yashmin, 2015).

Haitian mothers may believe that "strong emotions" spoil breast milk, and that thick breast milk causes skin rashes and thin milk results in diarrhea (Callister, 2014).

To increase breast milk production, women from Ethiopia may have a special diet of milk and warm oat and honey gruel, women from the Middle East may eat lentil soup, and women from Korea may eat a special seaweed soup with beef broth (Callister, 2014).

Note: It is unwise to attribute specific attitudes or beliefs to all members of a cultural group. The information in the Developing Cultural Competence boxes offers possible insights into caring for women from different cultural groups.

Breastfeeding Technique

Breastfeeding is not instinctive, it is learned. It is a natural process, but it takes "know-how." Ideally, each breastfeeding mother should have a breastfeeding evaluation to determine any knowledge deficits, acknowledge any concerns, provide instructions, and assist with breastfeeding.

POSITIONING

There are multiple breastfeeding positions, but only the four classic breastfeeding positions are discussed in this text. In addition, there are minor variations of hand placement and body position even among the four classic positions. The four most widely used positions are the (1) cross-cradle position, (2) cradle position, (3) football (or clutch) hold position, and (4) side-lying position (Figures 29–5 through 29–8). After a mother has fed using one position, she can be encouraged to try a different position when she offers her second breast. Alternating positions facilitates drainage of the breasts and changes the pressure points on the breast. This will provide some relief to the mother with sore nipples. In addition to the classic position, "laid-back" breastfeeding is being advocated. This concept is based on biologic nursing (BN), a mother-centered approach, and purports that women can find the best position for themselves because breastfeeding initiation is intrinsic for both mother and baby (La Leche League International, 2018).

LATCHING ON

It is important to have the mother and baby positioned properly in order to achieve an optimal attachment. If, for example, the baby is lying flat on the back (supine position) to feed in the cross-cradle position, cradle position, or side-lying position, the baby can obtain only a shallow latch (not attached far back onto the areola). The baby's shoulder becomes an obstacle putting distance between the baby's mouth and the mother's breast.

Modified cradle position

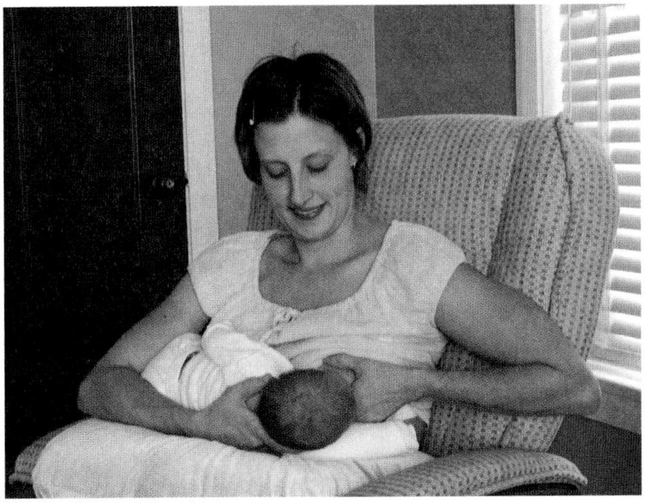

- Have mother sit comfortably in upright position using good body alignment. Use pillows for support (may use Boppy, body pillow, or standard bed pillows). Lap pillow should help bring baby up to breast level so mother does not lean over baby.
- Place baby on mother's lap and turn baby's entire body toward mother (baby is in side-lying position). Position baby's body so that the baby's nose lines up to the nipple. Maintain baby's body in a horizontal alignment.
- To feed at left breast, mother supports baby's head with her right hand at nape of baby's neck (allow head to slightly lag back), mother's right thumb by baby's left ear, and right forefinger near baby's right ear.
- With mother's free left hand, she can offer her left breast.

Figure 29–5 Cross-cradle position.

SOURCE: Brigitte Hall, RNC, MSN, IBCLC.

Cradle position

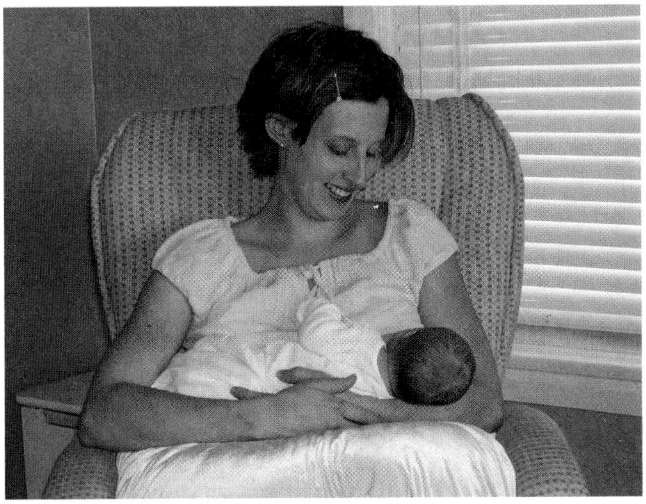

- Have mother sit comfortably in upright position using good body alignment. Use pillows for support (may use Boppy, body pillow, or standard bed pillows). Lap pillow should help bring baby up to breast level so mother does not lean over baby.
- Place baby on mother's lap and turn baby's entire body toward mother (baby is in side-lying position). Position baby's body so that the baby's nose lines up to the nipple. Maintain baby's body in a horizontal alignment.
- If feeding from the left breast, have mother cradle baby's head near the crook of her left arm while supporting her baby's body with her left forearm.
- With mother's free right hand, she can offer her left breast.

Figure 29–6 Cradle position.

SOURCE: Brigitte Hall, RNC, MSN, IBCLC.

Football hold position

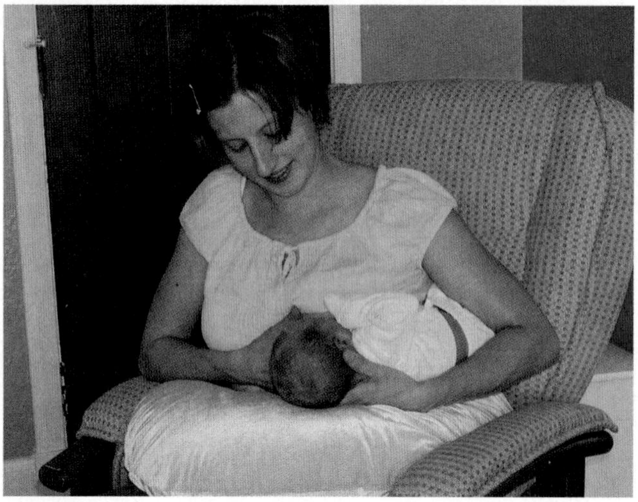

- Have mother sit comfortably and use pillows to raise baby's body to breast level. If using a Boppy and the Boppy is in "normal" position on mother's lap, turn it counterclockwise slightly (if feeding at left breast) to provide extended support for baby's body resting along mother's left side and near the back of mother's chair.
- If feeding at left breast, place baby on the left side of mother's body, heading baby into position feet first. Baby's bottom should rest on the pillow near mother's left elbow.
- Turn baby slightly on her side so that she faces the breast.
- Mother's left arm clutches baby's body close to mother's body. Baby's body should feel securely tucked in under mother's left arm.
- Have mother support baby's head with her left hand. With mother's free right hand, she can offer her breast. (Good position for mother with C-section).

Figure 29–7 **Football-hold position.**

SOURCE: Brigitte Hall, RNC, MSN, IBCLC.

Side-lying position

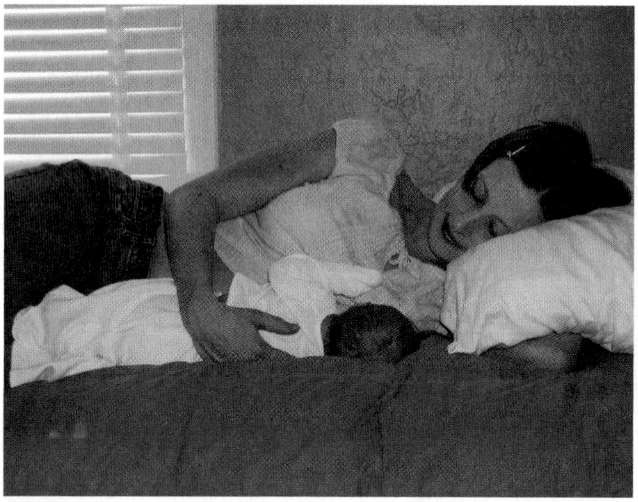

- Have mother rest comfortably lying on her side (left side for this demonstration). Use pillows to support mother's head and back, and provide support for mother's hips by placing a pillow between her bent knees.
- Place baby in side-lying position next to mother's body. Baby's body should face mother's body. Baby's nose should line up to mother's nipple. Place a roll behind baby's back, if desired.
- With mother's free right hand, she can offer her left breast. After baby is securely attached, mom can rest her right hand anywhere that is comfortable for her.

Figure 29–8 **Side-lying position.**

SOURCE: Brigitte Hall, RNC, MSN, IBCLC.

Anything that contributes to a shallow latch is going to cause sore nipples and other complications. Nipple trauma, although relatively common, is not normal. See Chapter 33 for a discussion of breastfeeding with inverted or flat nipples.

The baby needs to attach his or her lips onto the breast, far back onto the areola, not on the actual nipple. If the baby attaches just to the nipple, the mother will have sore nipples, and pain may inhibit the let-down reflex. To obtain a deep latch, the mother needs to be taught how to elicit the baby's rooting reflex, stimulating the baby to open the mouth as widely as possible (like a big yawn). Once the baby does this, the mother should quickly but gently draw her baby in toward her. During the first few days of life, the newborn typically only opens the mouth widely for a second or so, and then begins to close the mouth again. If the mother misses her chance to get her baby latched on, she simply needs to start over again.

Clinical Tip

As you assist new mothers with breastfeeding, it is important to create a relaxed environment and approach to breastfeeding. Encourage the mother to get into a comfortable position, well supported with pillows. Remind her to bring the baby to her breast rather than leaning forward to the baby.

Figures 29–9 through 29–14 demonstrate various positions and techniques used in latching on.

BREASTFEEDING ASSESSMENT

During the birthing unit stay, the nurse must carefully monitor the progress of the breastfeeding pair. A systematic assessment of several breastfeeding episodes provides the opportunity to teach the new mother about lactation and the breastfeeding process, provide anticipatory guidance, and evaluate the need for

C-hold hand position

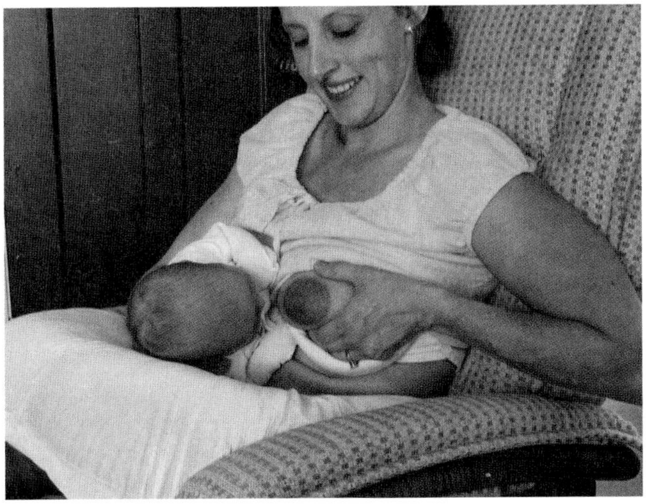

Figure 29–9 C-hold hand position.

SOURCE: Brigitte Hall, RNC, MSN, IBCLC.

To be ready to draw baby's mouth onto mother's breast, as soon as the baby opens her or his mouth widely enough, the mother needs to have her hand supporting her breast in ready position. She can use various hand holds, but she needs to keep her fingers well behind the areola. One such hand position is called the "C-hold." In this hold, the thumb is placed on top of the breast near 12 o'clock position and the other four fingers are placed on the underside of the breast near the 6 o'clock position (depends on mother's hand size and length of fingers). The key point is in keeping the fingers at least 1.5 inches back from the base of the nipple as the fingers support the breast. Mothers are not often aware of where they place their fingers, especially on the underside of the breast. If the fingers are too far forward (too close to the nipple), then the infant cannot grasp a large amount of areola in her or his mouth and this results in a "shallow" latch. A shallow latch is associated with nipple pain and ineffective drainage of the breast.

An alternate hand hold not shown is a "U-hold" hand position. The thumb and forefinger are near the 3 o'clock and 9 o'clock positions on the breast again with fingers at least 1.5 inches back from the base of the nipple; the body of the hand rests on the lower portion of the breast. Using this hand hold, the mother's arm position is down at her side rather than sticking outward as it is when supporting the breast using the C-hold position.

Scissor hold hand position

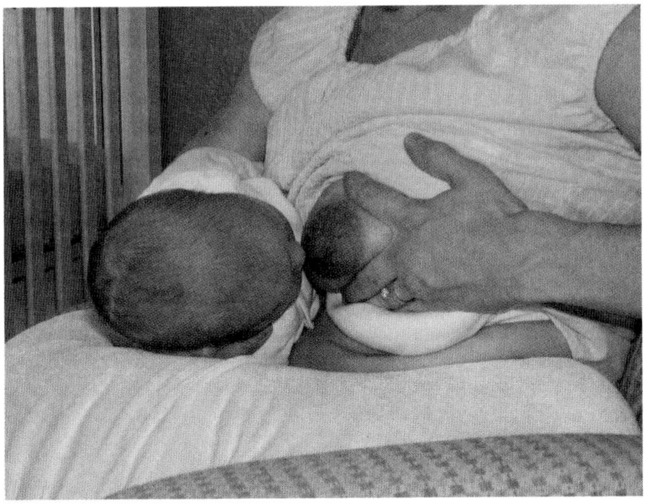

Figure 29–10 Scissor-hold hand position.

SOURCE: Brigitte Hall, RNC, MSN, IBCLC.

The scissor hold is often discouraged because mothers (especially mothers with small hands) have a difficult time keeping their fingers off the areola or at least 1.5 inches back from the base of the areola. Here, the mother is able to support her breast well without letting her fingers encroach onto the areola.

The mother should be instructed to gently support the breast and not press too deeply, which can obstruct the flow of milk through the ducts.

Nose to nipple

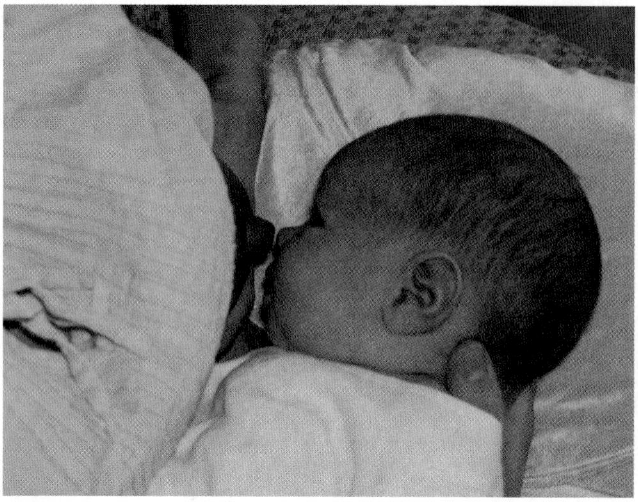

Before eliciting the rooting reflex, it is important to have the baby in good alignment. When the infant opens her or his mouth to latch on, the goal is to achieve a deep, asymmetric latch attachment. The goal is *not* to center the nipple in the baby's mouth. The rationale for this is to optimize oral-motor function. The jaw is a hinge joint. The upper jaw is immobile; the lower jaw compresses the breast. The breast is efficiently drained if more areola is drawn into the baby's mouth from the inferior aspect of the breast and a smaller amount drawn in from the superior aspect of the areola. Aligning the infant to the mother with baby's nose facing mother's nipple permits the jaw to be in a lower position. The next step is to let the infant drop his or her head back (head in "sniff position"), so that the infant leads into the breast with the chin.

Figure 29–11 Nose to nipple.

SOURCE: Brigitte Hall, RNC, MSN, IBCLC.

Initial attempt to elicit the rooting reflex

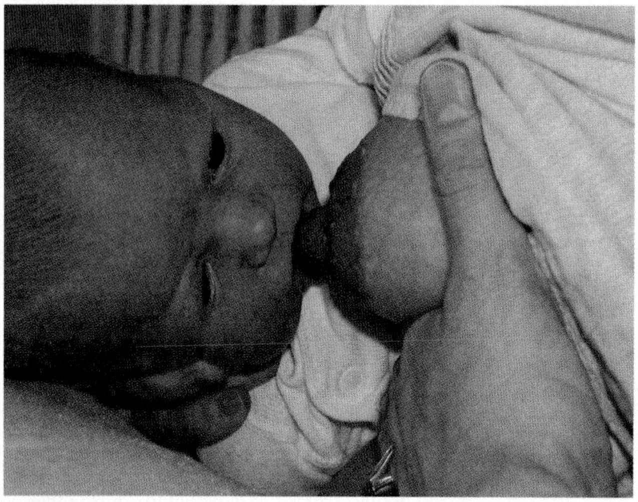

To trigger the rooting reflex, teach the mother to use her nipple to stroke downward in a vertical motion across the middle of baby's lower lip. Initially, the infant may respond by licking or smacking. This is a normal response to the stimulus. Encourage the mother to keep stimulating the infant's lower lip until the infant finally opens her or his mouth widely. If the infant is not responding at all, then the infant is probably too sleepy and may need help waking up. After trying wake up techniques, the infant may be ready to try breastfeeding again.

Figure 29–12 Initial attempt to elicit the rooting reflex.

SOURCE: Brigitte Hall, RNC, MSN, IBCLC.

Continued attempt to elicit rooting reflex

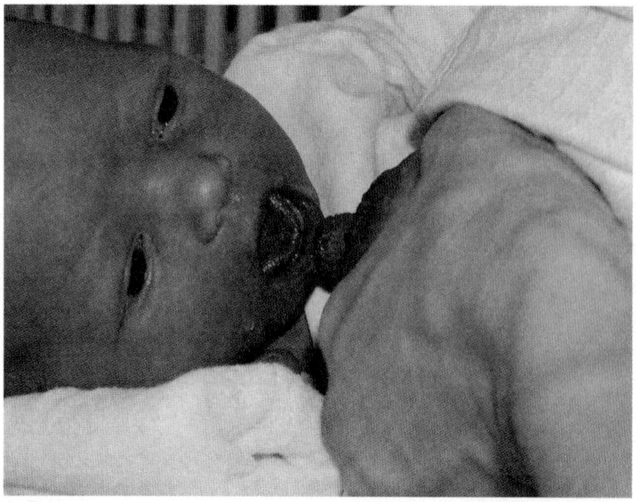

Teach the mother to be patient and wait for the infant's mouth to gape open as widely as possible. Here the infant needs to open the mouth even wider before the mother draws her baby toward the breast. The mother should be encouraged to continue stroking the infant's lip until the infant opens the mouth wider.

Figure 29–13 Continued attempt to elicit the rooting reflex.

SOURCE: Brigitte Hall, RNC, MSN, IBCLC.

Baby is latched-on

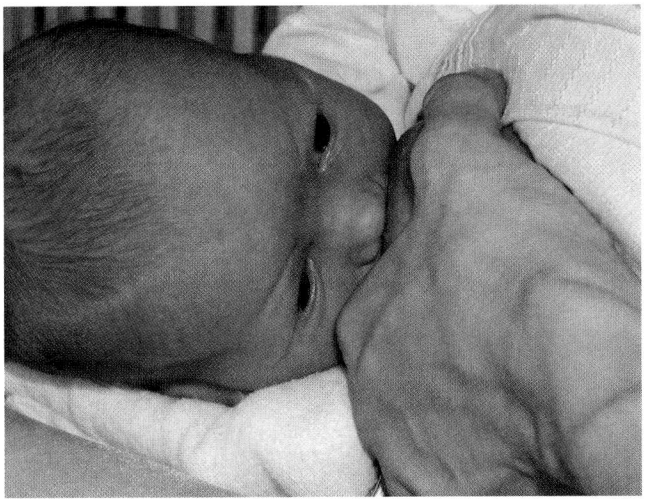

Once baby has latched onto the breast, the mother should check that baby is latched on properly. The infant's chin should be embedded into the mother's breast. The infant's nose should be very close but not actually touching the breast. The nose should be centered. If the mother feels a little pinch on her areola, she can slowly release the hand supporting her breast so she can have a free hand to attempt to move her baby's jaw gently downward. To do this maneuver, the mother needs to place her thumb or forefinger of her free hand (the hand that just released the breast) on baby's lower jaw (there is a horizontal groove to use as leverage—the groove on baby's chin is parallel with the baby's lips). With gentle downward pressure the mother should feel relief of any persistent tenderness. This procedure opens the jaw wider and it also helps to roll out the infant's lower lip that may have been inadvertently drawn into the baby's mouth. As the baby begins to suckle, there should be no dimpling of the infant's cheeks and no smacking or clicking noises.

Figure 29–14 Baby is latched on.

SOURCE: Brigitte Hall, RNC, MSN, IBCLC.

follow-up care after discharge. Criteria for evaluating a breastfeeding session include maternal response to newborn cues, latch-on technique, positioning, signs of active feeding, let-down response, nipple condition, maternal comfort during feeding, newborn's weight from previous measurement (usually from the night before), and report of newborn's intake and output. The literature provides various tools to guide the assessment and documentation of breastfeeding efforts, such as the LATCH Scoring Tool (Jensen, Wallace, & Kelsay, 1994). See *Women with Special Needs: Breastfeeding Assistance*.

Women with Special Needs Breastfeeding Assistance

For the woman with upper extremity impairment, breastfeeding may require assistance from a partner or care provider. Women with limited arm strength or manual dexterity may require wrist supports to maintain a proper latch-on. These women are also more prone to nipple soreness, cracking, and bleeding since when the baby slips off the nipple, it may be more difficult to reattach the baby properly. A lactation consultation should be performed on all women with upper extremity limitations.

BREASTFEEDING EFFICIENCY

Parents are often concerned because they have no visual assurance of the amount of breast milk consumed. The mother should be taught other signs of effective, active breastfeeding. The baby should have a rhythmic suckling pattern (the slight pause between jaw compressions on the breast permits the mouth to fill with milk before swallowing) with only brief pauses lasting seconds between spurts of active feeding. To assess if the jaw compressions are strong enough, the mother can observe or feel if there is movement at the temporomandibular joint located in front of the baby's ears.

The newborn should maintain a rhythmic feeding pattern with only brief pauses (lasting only seconds, not minutes) between spurts of active feeding, with the feeding session typically lasting for 10 to 20 minutes on the first breast. The baby may feed only a few minutes on the second breast or not at all, so the mother should alternate the first breast at the next feeding. The mother should visually observe for swallowing, and later, as her milk is abundant, she will hear the baby's swallows. Discourage the mother from watching the clock to determine when the baby needs to switch breast sides but rather encourage her to watch the newborn's feeding pattern to note when active feeding ceases. When satiated, the baby will either pull away from the breast or fall asleep. The baby will be extremely relaxed at the end of the feeding and will sleep until the next feeding is due (at least an hour). As the newborn matures, the feeding intervals will lengthen. Remind mothers to place their babies on their backs (supine) after feeding. See *Case Study: Angelina Newman*.

CASE STUDY: Angelina Newman

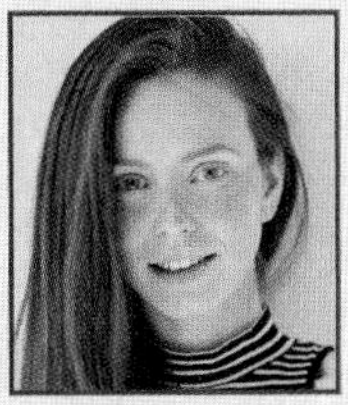

SOURCE: WAYHOME studio/Shutterstock.

Angelina gave birth yesterday and had difficulties breastfeeding her newborn overnight. This afternoon, her mother is visiting and attempting to help her breastfeed the baby when the nurse hears the women arguing and enters the room. Angela is irritated that her mother is telling her how to feed her own baby. She insists her mother is trying to take over and thinks her mother feels she can't do anything right. The mother confides that when she was pregnant with Angelina she never attended the childbirth education classes her parents paid for and she has no idea about breastfeeding.

Questions to Ponder

What steps can be taken to diffuse the situation? What education can you provide to help Angelina breastfeed successfully? What resources can be utilized to provide Angelina with the help she needs to successfully breastfeed her baby?

Clinical Tip

With a sleepy baby, unwrap the baby and place the baby skin-to-skin on the mother so the mother can recognize subtle early feeding cues. Encourage the mother to offer her breasts whenever she observes her baby's eyes fluttering under his or her eyelids, her baby beginning to stretch, lip smacking and rooting behavior, or hand-to-mouth activity.

Another indicator of breastfeeding efficiency is softening of the mother's breasts, although this is not a reliable indicator in the first few days postpartum while breast milk volume is low. Within a week, however, this is a good indicator of milk transfer.

The newborn who feeds well will have a characteristic output. Output is a reflection of intake. See Figure 29–15 for breastfeeding intake and output expectations.

In situations where there is a question regarding milk transfer effectiveness, it can be most reliably measured by obtaining pre- and postbreastfeeding weight checks using a baby scale that measures in grams. The difference between pre- and postfeed weights is the amount of milk (each gram increase reflects 1 mL) transferred to the newborn and may be useful with assessing breastfeeding efficiency and maternal milk volume. See *Key Facts to Remember: Successful Breastfeeding Evaluation*.

Key Facts To Remember
Successful Breastfeeding Evaluation

A newborn is probably getting enough milk if:

- The baby is nursing at least eight times in 24 hours.
- In a quiet room, the mother can hear her baby swallow while nursing, once her milk supply has become abundant.
- The mother's breasts appear to soften after breastfeeding once her milk has come in.
- The number of wet diapers increases daily by a minimum of one additional diaper until the fifth day after birth; after day 5, the newborn should have six to eight wet diapers daily.
- The newborn's stools are beginning to lighten in color by the third day after birth, or have changed to yellow no later than day 5.

  Note: Offering a supplemental bottle is not a reliable indicator because most newborns will take a few ounces even if they are getting enough breast milk.

Bottle-Feeding Expressed Breast Milk

There are a number of different reasons for bottle-feeding expressed breast milk. The nurse should evaluate the indications in order to recommend the best technique for the mother and her particular need.

HAND EXPRESSION

Hand expression should be taught to all breastfeeding mothers after delivery. By using hand expression, mothers can express drops of colostrum and apply to the nipple for skin care after each feeding (ABM, 2010). In addition, hand expression can be used prior to feeding to stimulate milk expression, can be used by the mother who is exclusively breast pumping to facilitate breast emptying after pumping, and can be used to relieve breast discomfort during engorgement. Some mothers prefer to hand-express their milk rather than use a breast pump, and many find that in the immediate postpartum period hand expression of milk may be a more effective method of removing drops of colostrum than using an electric breast pump. The mother should take care not to traumatize her breasts or nipples. Hand expression should not be painful. Most mothers will need assistance in learning this technique initially. Reassure the mother that it is a skill that is learned and that with practice, she can become an expert at hand expression (Figure 29–16). See Table 29–3 for pumping instructions and breast milk storage guidelines.

BREAST PUMPS

Although hand expression can be efficient, many mothers will choose to use a mechanical breast pump to express their milk. Not all breast pumps are of the same quality, even within the same category (see Table 29–4 and Figures 29–18 through 29–20). A desirable breast pump should be able to cycle from low to high suction at a frequency similar to that of a breastfeeding baby (about 45 to 60 cycles per minute). However, differences in the quality of the pump motor or the presence or absence of controls over suction pressure mean that some pumps will generate inadequate pressure or cycle too slowly to be effective, whereas others may exert too high a suction, which can cause injury. Breast flange fit and comfort are other variables to consider. Some good-quality pumps have multiple flange sizes available to accommodate the various nipple sizes of mothers. Excessive rubbing of the mother's nipple in the flange tunnel can cause discomfort and result in a decreased volume expressed. The nurse should refer the mother to a lactation consultant for help regarding the different breast pumps.

STORING BREAST MILK AND FORMULA

The guidelines for storage of expressed breast milk depends on whether the newborn is a healthy full-term baby or a newborn in the NICU. The guidelines in Table 29–5 are intended as a resource for the mother of a healthy, full-term newborn.

SUPPLEMENTARY FORMULA-FEEDING

Supplementary formula-feedings for the breastfeeding newborn after birth are not routinely recommended. Supplementation should be given only when medically indicated (AAP & ACOG, 2017). Routine supplements are not only unnecessary in the early days after birth, but bottle-feeding in itself may cause the newborn to develop an incorrect sucking pattern or may cause the baby to refuse the breast altogether (Wambach & Riordan, 2016). Early supplementation with formula may contribute to a delay in early maternal milk production, may result in maternal engorgement after the mother's milk production has increased, and may possibly sensitize an at-risk newborn for milk-protein allergy. These types of problems have been implicated in early breastfeeding terminations.

A newborn's refusal to breastfeed after receiving bottles in the early postdelivery period may be related to a phenomenon referred to as *nipple confusion* or, more accurately termed, *nipple preference*. This potential problem occurs because the techniques for breastfeeding and bottle-feeding are different. In breastfeeding, the baby has to open the mouth very wide in order to latch on to the breast. To transfer milk the baby has to extend the tongue forward, cupping the nipple and drawing the mother's nipple deep into the mouth until the teat reaches the "comfort zone" near the junction of the baby's hard and soft palate. After the baby creates suction from the tongue and cheeks and seals the latch with his or her lips, then the baby rhythmically compresses the breast with his or her jaw while the tongue moves in an undulating motion to move fluid toward the baby's pharynx before swallowing, in coordination with breathing. On average, it takes a couple of minutes before the breastfeeding mother's milk

- Infants should breastfeed 8 to 12 times per day and should appear relaxed after feeding.
- Colostrum is all that a newborn needs in the first few days of life in most cases.
- It is normal for an infant to lose up to 7% of birth weight in the first few days; however, up to 10% weight loss is tolerated if the mother's breasts are full, the infant is observed to breastfeed well, and the infant is not dehydrated.
- Infants should gain 10 grams/kg/day after the mother's milk supply is abundant (about day 4 of life).
- Infants should be back to their birth weight by 2 weeks of age.
- Infant's stool should change in color, consistency, and frequency during the first few days of life. The photo images noted below depict stool color progression. Some babies progress faster to yellow milk stools, as early as day 3.

Day 1

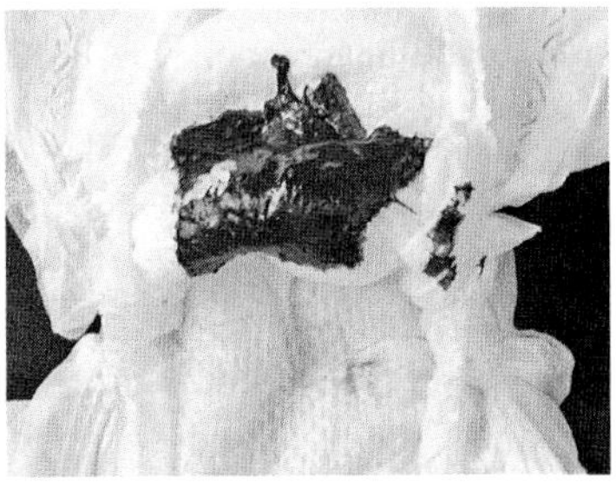

Minimum Output

On day 1, the infant should produce at least one wet diaper and one meconium stool by 24 hours of age.

Note the pinkish-red "brick dust" appearance on the diaper. The uric acid crystals produced by the kidneys is associated with concentrated urine. A red flag is raised if their presence is continued beyond day 2 or 3 of life.

Day 2

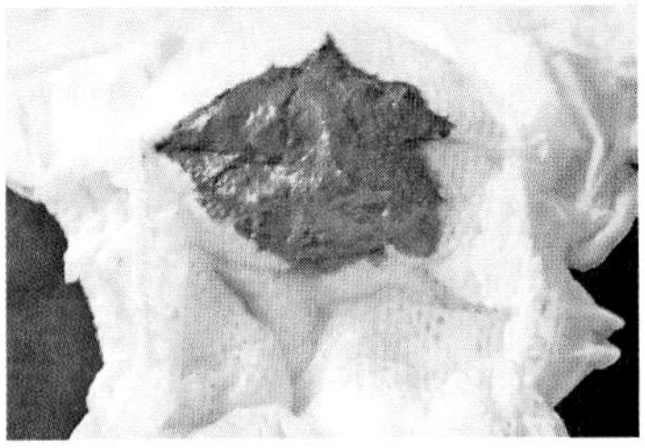

On day 2, the infant should produce at least two wet diapers and two early transitional stools in a 24-hour period by 48 hours of age.

Day 3

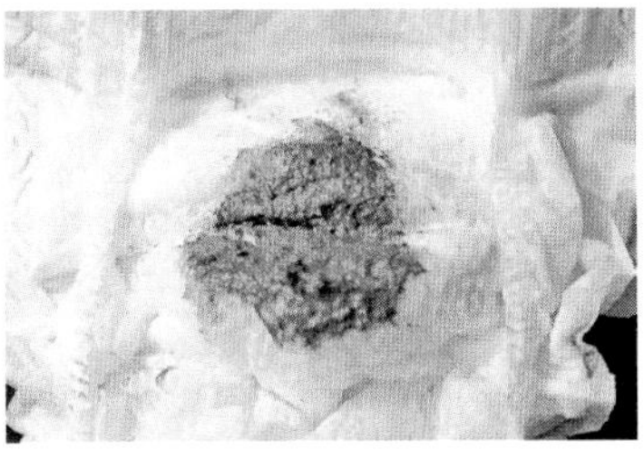

On day 3, the infant should produce at least three wet diapers and three transitional stools in a 24-hour period by 72 hours of age.

When a mother's milk supply is abundant on day 2, some babies will have transitioned to yellow milk stools as early as day 3.

Day 4

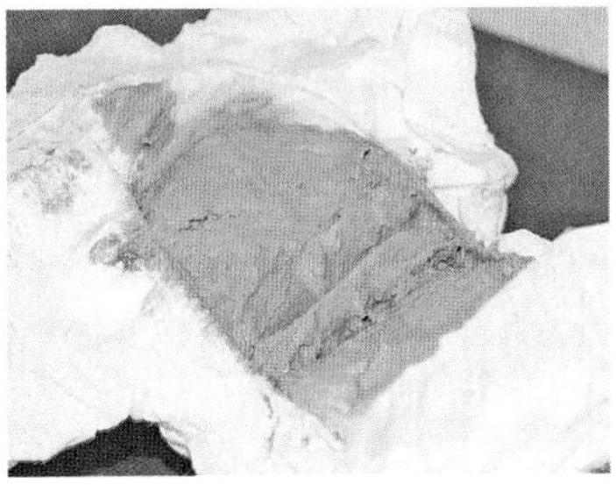

On day 4, the infant should produce at least four wet diapers and three to four yellow-green transitional stools or yellow milk stools in a 24-hour period by 96 hours of age.

Day 5

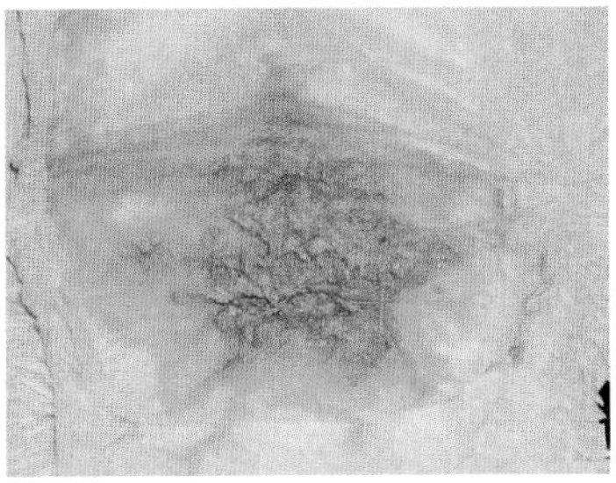

On day 5, the infant should produce at least five wet diapers and three to four yellow milk stools per day; the stools are typically explosive and have a curdy or seedy appearance.

Hereafter, breastfeeding infants will consistently produce at least six well-saturated wet diapers per day. These infants will typically continue to produce at least three to four yellow milk stools daily, but may have up to 10 stools per day until they are about a month old. Infants 4 weeks or older may suddenly decrease their stool frequency, even skipping days.

Figure 29–15 Breastfeeding intake and output expectations.

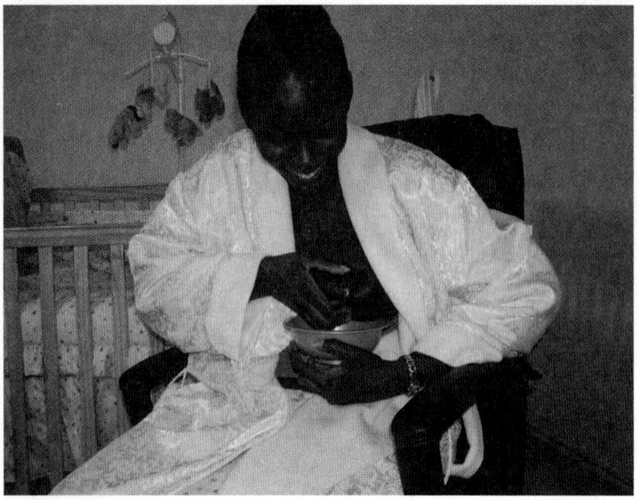

Figure 29–16 **Hand expression.**

SOURCE: Brigitte Hall, RNC, MSN, IBCLC.

flow increases during let-down. With bottle-feeding, the baby keeps the tongue retracted and uses the tip of the tongue to block the flow of milk, which otherwise drips continuously by gravity even when suction is not applied. The bottle-feeding baby merely needs to create suction with his or her mouth on the bottle nipple and the fluid flows easily.

When supplementation is indicated, the first choice is to use the mother's own milk (fresh, previously expressed, or frozen/thawed). If maternal milk is not available, pasteurized donor milk is the next choice, and then formula. Supplementation can be administered using various methods based on the particular situation, parental preference, and agency policy (ABM, 2017a). At times there are valid medical indications for supplementing a breastfeeding newborn in the early postpartum period. See Table 29–6 for a list of factors requiring consideration for supplementation.

TABLE 29–3 Pumping Instructions and Breast Milk Storage Guidelines

1.	Once a day rinse the breasts with water while bathing or showering. Avoid applying soap directly on the nipples.	**2.**	Wash hands well with soap and water before preparing to pump.
3.	Take a few minutes to massage the breasts and relax. Do some slow, deep breathing and think about or look at a picture of your baby. Being relaxed is very important for releasing milk from the breasts. (Stress can inhibit or delay let-down because stress hormones, such as cortisol and adrenalin, can block receptors for let-down.)	**4.**	Sit up straight or lean slightly forward. A pillow placed behind your back may facilitate the slightly tilted forward posture, as gravity aids in the flow of milk from the breasts.
For hand-expressing milk, use the Marmet technique, Steps 5–8			
5.	The mother will position her thumb at the 12 o'clock position on the top edge of the areola (about 1 to 1.5 inches back from the tip of her nipple) and her forefinger and middle finger pads at the 6 o'clock position on the bottom edge of the areola (about 1 to 1.5 inches from the tip of her nipple). If positioned correctly, an imaginary line between the thumb and fingers will cross through the nipple (refer to Figure 29–16).	**6.**	Next, the mother will stretch her areola back toward her chest wall without lifting her fingers off her breast.
7.	Now she should roll her thumb and fingers simultaneously forward. This action compresses the ducts beneath the areola and stimulates the breast to empty the breast both manually and by triggering the let-down reflex.	**8.**	The mother should repeat the sequence multiple times to completely drain her breasts. She should try to maintain a steady rhythm, cycling 45 to 60 times/minute. It is also more effective if the mother repositions her fingers to other positions on the same breast (3 and 9 o'clock, 1 and 7 o'clock, etc.) when the milk flow slows.
9.	For single-sided pumping, pump each breast for 10 to 20 minutes. Some mothers find that they empty their breasts more efficiently if they switch back and forth from one breast to the other as the milk flow diminishes, until they have stimulated each breast for 15 to 20 minutes. The entire pumping session will last 30 to 40 minutes.	**10.**	Pump the expressed milk preferably into glass or plastic bottles. Mothers of healthy babies may also use bottle bags or liners intended for human milk collection and storage; however, note that up to 60% of secretory IgA (SIgA) is lost when milk is stored in these kinds of containers for 48 hours because of the attraction of the antibodies to the polyethylene material used in making the bottle bags/liners (Lawrence & Lawrence, 2016). Because of the loss of antibodies that can occur with bottle bags or liners, mothers of preemies and fragile newborns should especially avoid using these kinds of storage containers. Do not fill milk storage containers more than three-quarters full, because milk expands during freezing.

TABLE 29–3 Pumping Instructions and Breast Milk Storage Guidelines *(continued)*

11.	Feed *freshly* expressed breast milk whenever there is a need to give a supplement, when possible. Reserve the stored milk for times when fresh milk is not available (e.g., when separated from baby). Fresh breast milk retains more nutrients than refrigerated or frozen milk, although these are still preferred over formula. Expressed human milk may be stored in the refrigerator for up to 8 days, but if intended to be frozen, this should be done within 48 hours of initial refrigeration. Avoid placing human milk in the freezer door or on the bottom of a self-defrosting freezer because the temperature fluctuates more in those areas.	**12.**	Store expressed human milk in volumes the baby is likely to consume at a single feeding or in a volume the baby will consume in a day.
13.	Human milk should never be thawed in a microwave oven or placed in a pan and warmed up on the stove. These methods may cause the milk to warm up too hot (and unevenly) and can burn a baby as well as cause heat-sensitive nutrients to be destroyed. Frozen milk can be thawed safely using one of two methods (13A & 13B).	**13.A**	For a quick thaw, remove the container of frozen milk from the freezer, place the container in a bowl in the sink, and run warm water over it for no longer than 15 minutes. Take care not to immerse the container in water because water may leach into the container of milk, possibly contaminating it and diluting it.
13.B	For a slow thaw overnight, take the frozen container of milk from the freezer the day before or several hours before it is needed and let it defrost in the refrigerator (not on the kitchen counter) over several hours. Breast milk that has been sitting for a while will normally separate (Figure 29–17). To remix, swirl the bottle (avoid vigorous shaking) until the milk is evenly mixed. Make certain that the fat that clings to the wall of the container has mixed into the milk. If the volume in the bottle is more than can be used in one feeding, pour only the amount needed into a clean bottle and put the rest of the milk immediately back in the refrigerator. Warm the bottle as described in 13.A.	**14.**	Check the temperature of the milk before feeding it. Babies will drink milk when the milk temperature is between room temperature and body temperature (roughly 65°F to 100°F).

SAFETY ALERT!

Any milk left over from a feeding should be discarded within an hour of starting the feeding. The reason for this is because saliva "back washes" into the bottle while nipple feeding, and the saliva contains bacteria that can multiply and potentially make a baby sick.

NOTE: Also see Table 29–5, Storage and Discard Guidelines for Breast Milk and Formula.

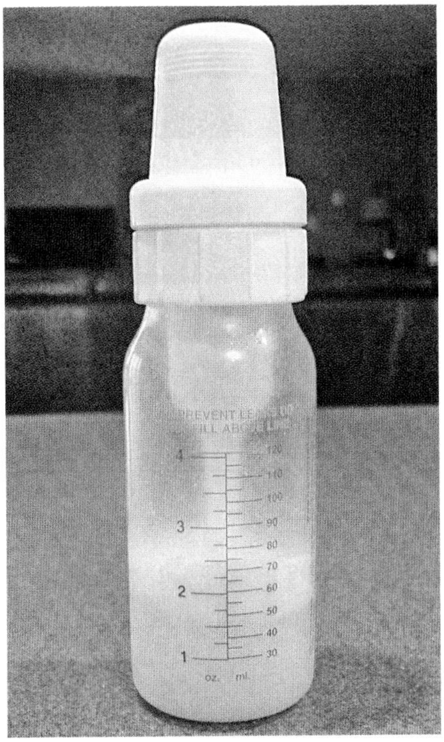

Figure 29–17 Expressed breast milk that has separated.

Timing of Newborn Feedings

The timing of newborn feedings, whether by breastfeeding or formula feeding, is ideally determined by physiologic and behavioral cues rather than a set schedule.

Initial Feeding

If there are no complications at the birth and the mother is receptive, the newborn should be placed on her chest (Figure 29–21). This skin-to-skin contact allows for breastfeeding immediately after birth, helps the baby maintain his or her body temperature, helps with self-regulation, increases maternal oxytocin levels, helps the mother to notice subtle feeding cues, and promotes bonding (AAP & ACOG, 2017).

Throughout the first 2 hours after birth, but especially during the first hour of life, most newborns are usually alert and ready to breastfeed. This first feeding should not be forced. Some babies are content just licking the nipple or nuzzling up against the breast initially. Early breastfeeding can enhance maternal–newborn bonding and facilitate release of oxytocin, which helps contract the uterus, expelling the placenta and decreasing the risk of postpartum hemorrhage.

Early breastfeeding benefits the newborn by preventing hypoglycemia, promoting the passage of meconium, providing immunologic protection from colostrum, and helping to stimulate further maternal milk production.

If the mother plans to formula-feed, she and her newborn can still enjoy and benefit from skin-to-skin contact initially after birth. Formula feedings are not typically initiated in the birthing room, but newborns are offered formula as soon as they show interest or feeding cues or per agency policy. For both breastfed and formula-fed newborns, early feeding stimulates peristalsis, which helps the newborn to eliminate the by-products of bilirubin conjugation that have been stored up in the bowel while in utero. Early passage of the meconium stool decreases the newborn's risk of jaundice.

TABLE 29–4 Types of Breast Pumps and Indications for Use

INDICATION	MANUAL BREAST PUMP (FIGURE 29–18)	SMALL BATTERY/ ELECTRIC BREAST PUMP	INDIVIDUAL DOUBLE ELECTRIC BREAST PUMP (FIGURE 29–19)	HOSPITAL-GRADE MULTI-USER DOUBLE ELECTRIC BREAST PUMP (FIGURE 29–20)
A missed feeding	■	■	■	
An evening out	■	■	■	
Working part time	■	■	■	
Convenience—occasional use	■	■	■	
Working full time			■	■
Premature/hospitalized newborn				■
Low milk supply				■
Sore nipples/engorgement		■	■	■
Latch-on problems/infection			■	■
Drawing out flattish nipples	■	■	■	■

Note: ■ Recommended

SOURCE: Data from Medela, 2016.

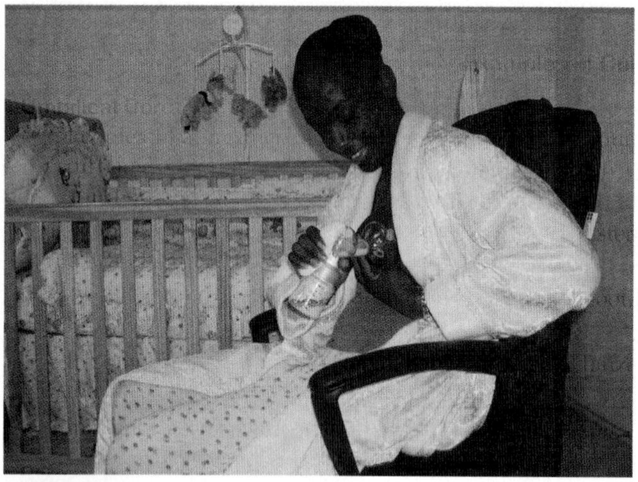

Figure 29–18 Manual breast pump.

SOURCE: Brigitte Hall, RNC, MSN, IBCLC.

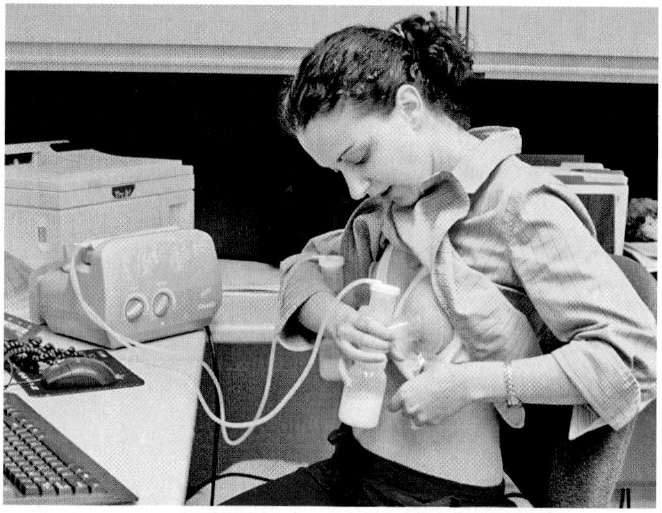

Figure 29–20 Hospital-grade multi-user breast pump.

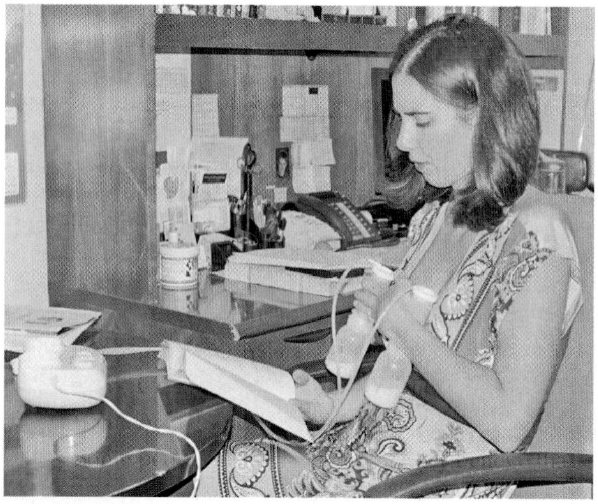

Figure 29–19 Individual double electric breast pump.

Assessment of the newborn's physiologic status is a primary and ongoing concern to the nurse throughout the first feeding. Newborns showing extreme fatigue coupled with tachypnea, who are dusky in color, and diaphoretic while feeding are most likely symptomatic for respiratory and/or cardiac problems or, rarely, esophageal anomalies (see Chapter 30). Findings associated with esophageal anomalies include maternal polyhydramnios and increased oral secretions in the newborn.

Although the nurse is always on the alert for any complications, keep in mind that it is not unusual for healthy newborns to regurgitate a small amount of mucus, fluid, or milk shortly after feeding or to develop hiccups. Most babies have "wet burps" at some point, and so virtually all have some degree of reflux. Holding the baby upright on the parent's chest for 15 to 20 minutes after a feeding and not placing the baby in a car seat or swing (which increases abdominal pressure) for that time can help decrease the incidence of reflux. Once the baby is tolerating feeding, the child's normal position after feeding is on his or her back.

TABLE 29–5 Storage and Discard Guidelines for Breast Milk and Formula

MILK	ENVIRONMENT	TIME UNTIL DISCARD	COMMENT
Breast milk **Formula (opened/reconstituted)**	Being fed	Finish feed within 1 hour	
Fresh breast milk	Room temperature 22.2°C (72°F) to 26.0°C (79°F)	4 hours	Containers should be covered with a cool towel as this may keep milk cooler for a longer period of time.
	Room temperature 18.1°C (66°F) to 22.2°C (72°F)	6–8 hours	
	Cooler w/ frozen ice packs 15°C (59°F)	24 hours	Keep ice packs in contact with milk containers at all times; limit opening cooler bag.
	Refrigerator	4–8 days	Store milk in the back of the main body of the refrigerator.
	Freezer	3–4 months	Store milk toward back of freezer, where temperature is most constant. Milk stored for longer time is safe, but some of the lipids in the milk undergo degradation, resulting in lower quality.
Thawed breast milk	Refrigerator	24 hours	
	Freezer less than −4°C (24.8°F)		Do not refreeze.
Formula, opened/reconstituted	Room temperature	2 hours	
	Refrigerator	24–48 hours (see label)	
Formula powder, opened can	Room temperature	1 month	
Formula/powder in sealed container	Avoid excessive heat	Printed expiration date	
Formula	Never freeze		

SOURCES: Data from ABM, 2017b; CDC, 2018d.

Establishing a Feeding Pattern

An "on-demand" feeding program facilitates each baby's own rhythm and helps a new mother establish lactation. Unrestricted feedings are best accomplished by hospitals that provide mother–baby rooming-in practices on a 24-hour basis. When the father/partner is able to room-in with the mother and new baby, it allows both parents to participate and learn how to care for their newborn; this has been shown to be important in the development of the family relationship. Having the father/partner room-in also allows the mother with a cesarean delivery to keep the baby in her room, thus allowing the parents to respond to their baby's needs more quickly than the nursery staff may be able to, resulting in less newborn crying, natural feeding intervals, and an adequate number of feedings in a 24-hour period.

Following the initial alert period (approximately the first 2 hours after birth), the newborn typically falls into a deep sleep for several hours. Mothers should be encouraged to rest during

TABLE 29–6 Factors Requiring Consideration of Supplementation

Risk Factors for Inadequate Intake

- Maternal/newborn separation
- Maternal barriers to breastfeeding (e.g., medications, fatigue, pain, cultural)
- Congenital malformation or illness interfering with ability to breastfeed
- Delayed lactogenesis after day 3 or 4
- Primary lactation failure (usually due to breast pathology or prior breast surgery)
- Low birth weight or newborn with illness/disorder requiring nutrient requirements that may exceed that available through breastfeeding

Signs of Potential Inadequate Intake

- Weight loss greater than 7% from birth weight
- Delayed bowel movements or continued meconium stools beyond day 2
- Hypoglycemia not responding to frequent breastfeeding attempts
- Hyperbilirubinemia due to breastfeeding jaundice

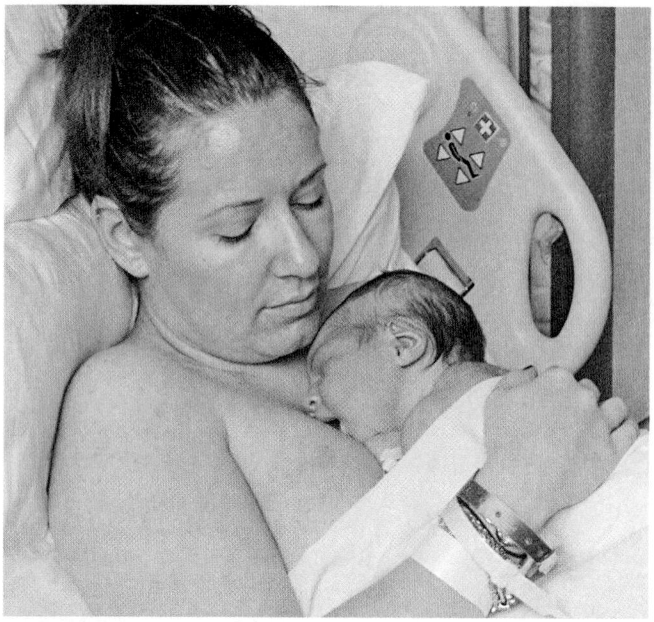

Figure 29–21 **Mother and newborn skin to skin.**

SOURCE: Brigitte Hall, RNC, MSN, IBCLC.

this time. When the newborn awakens, he or she will likely want to nurse frequently, alternating between relatively short periods of light sleep and quiet wakefulness. As wakefulness and interest in nursing increase, the baby will often cluster 5 to 10 feeding episodes over 2 to 3 hours (Wambach & Riordan, 2016). Mothers may misinterpret "cluster feedings" in the first few days of life to mean that her baby is not satisfied. The nurse should take this opportunity to reinforce the mother's perception that the newborn wants additional milk, but point out that cluster feeding is a normal and necessary pattern to stimulate mother's milk production. Formula supplementation is not indicated and will actually delay milk production.

Some healthy newborns are uninterested in nursing and just want to sleep for the first few days after birth. This pattern is noted in babies whose mothers have had a difficult labor, have had a prolonged pushing stage during delivery, or have had medication (especially multiple dosing) for labor pain or for a cesarean birth. In addition, male newborns who have undergone a circumcision procedure often become very sleepy after surgery.

Late-preterm newborns (born between 34 0/7 and 36 6/7 weeks' gestation) also tend to be very sleepy, have less stamina, have greater difficulty with latch, suck, and swallow for the first few days of life, and have more subtle feeding cues (ABM, 2016). These sleepy babies are at risk of losing an excessive amount of weight, becoming dehydrated, and developing exaggerated jaundice in just a few days after birth. In addition, mothers may develop pathologic engorgement if her baby does not wake up to breastfeed frequently and effectively during this time.

To avoid these complications, parents can be taught techniques to wake their sleepy baby whenever the newborn shows signs of being in the light state of sleep cycle. With a little help, this baby may be gently aroused to breastfeed. One method is to remove the baby's blanket and clothing so that the baby is wearing only a diaper and T-shirt. Babies feed better when they are not bundled, and they can achieve better attachment without the bulk of extra clothing and blankets. If the room is cool, have the mother apply a blanket over the top of her baby *after* the baby has attached to the breast. Another technique is to undo and check the baby's diaper. Sitting the baby in a burping position and gently "walking" fingers along the back will usually arouse the baby. Parents should also be encouraged to talk or sing to their baby while trying these techniques to further arouse their baby from sleep.

If the newborn falls asleep after the first few suckles, encourage the mother to use tactile stimulation while the newborn is still attached to the breast. The mother can also be encouraged to use breast compression or breast massage while the newborn is breastfeeding to keep milk trickling into the baby's mouth until the baby stimulates the mother to release her milk. If this is not sufficient to keep the baby actively feeding, suggest that the mother remove the baby from the breast momentarily and try to burp the newborn. The baby may not actually burp but the burping technique may help wake the baby.

A newborn's feeding pattern may change again when the mother's breasts become fuller. The breasts begin to look and feel noticeably heavier between the second and fourth day postpartum. When milk production has noticeably increased, the "cluster feeding" pattern ceases until the newborn has the first growth spurt at about 2 weeks of age. At this stage a baby generally feeds every 1.5 to 3 hours around the clock, or about 8 to 12 feedings per day. Feeding intervals are counted from the time of the start of one feeding to the start of the next feeding. During this engorgement phase of lactation some newborns may struggle initially with latch-on, especially if the mother allows greater than 3 hours to lapse between feedings. If the newborn is not breastfeeding often or effectively enough to soften the breasts, then the breasts may become quite firm and the mother's nipples may become less pliable; this can lead to a shallow latch attachment and sore nipples. If this occurs, the mother can try to express some milk to soften her areola before latching her newborn. When her baby breastfeeds on this fuller-than-usual breast, it is not uncommon for the baby to want to feed on just the one side. This feeding pattern usually does not last long, either. Within days the baby will be back to breastfeeding at both breasts.

Formula-fed newborns generally sleep longer at a stretch and awaken to feed every 3 to 4 hours, typically feeding only six to eight times per day. To compensate for sleeping longer between feedings, formula-fed newborns consume a larger volume at each feeding.

Regardless of whether a mother is breastfeeding or formula-feeding her newborn, many parents are distressed by their baby's erratic feeding pattern. Parents need to be informed about normal newborn/infant feeding and sleeping patterns and be aware that these patterns vary among babies and change over days, weeks, and months according to the baby's growth and development. In the beginning, the average newborn sleeps a total of 16 hours a day. Babies wake to feed and generally fall back to sleep within an hour. It will be awhile before the baby sleeps through the night.

Clinical Tip

Parents often ask "Does my breastfed baby need supplemental water in hot weather?" Exclusively breastfed babies do not require additional water when it is very hot outside, as long as the baby is allowed to nurse as needed. In hot weather a thirsty baby may want to breastfeed more often but for shorter periods.

Satiety behaviors are the same for formula-fed babies as for breastfed babies. These behaviors include longer pauses toward the end of the feeding, noticeable total body relaxation (the baby lies limp with hands down at his or her side and unclenched), the newborn may release his mother's nipple or the bottle nipple, and many fall asleep. If a baby is content following feedings, is meeting daily output expectations, and is gaining weight as

SAFETY ALERT!

Parents should be instructed never to put honey or corn syrup on their baby's pacifier to encourage the baby to accept it. Honey and possibly corn syrup may be contaminated with *Clostridium botulinum*, a bacterium that causes infantile botulism. Botulism is rare, but when it occurs it causes serious illness.

expected, then feedings are going well. On the other hand, if a breastfeeding baby awakens shortly after feeding and is exhibiting feeding cues, this baby should be offered the breast again regardless as to when he or she was last fed. The newborn may be cluster feeding or may not have fed efficiently at the previous feeding. Pacifier use in response to this early waking is not appropriate and needlessly postpones the feeding. The American Academy of Pediatrics recommends waiting to introduce a pacifier in the breastfeeding newborn until breastfeeding is well established, generally when the baby is 3 to 4 weeks old and only during naps or sleep time after breastfeeding. A formula-feeding newborn can be offered a pacifier any time after birth; it is thought to help reduce the risk for sudden infant death syndrome (AAP & ACOG, 2017).

Both breastfed and formula-fed newborns/infants experience growth spurts at certain times and require increased feeding volume. The breastfeeding mother may meet these increased demands by nursing more frequently to increase her milk supply. It takes up to 72 hours for the milk supply to increase adequately to meet the new demand. A slight increase in volume also meets the formula-fed baby's needs. Once the formula-feeding baby appears satiated, the baby should not be forced to continue to feed in order to finish the bottle.

Nourishing her newborn is a major concern of the new mother. Her feelings of success or failure may influence her self-concept as she assumes her maternal role. With proper instruction, support, and encouragement from professionals, feeding her baby becomes a source of pleasure and satisfaction to both the parents and baby.

Formula Feeding

With more attention placed on promoting and assisting breastfeeding mothers, the teaching needs of the mother who is formula feeding may inadvertently get overlooked. Nurses may assume that families can simply follow the formula preparation instructions on the side of the formula containers. Parents need to learn about the normal feeding pattern for a formula-feeding newborn and recognize symptoms of formula intolerance. They need to know intake and output expectations, the recommended type of formula for their baby, how to prepare and store formula, what equipment they will need, the feeding technique, and safety precautions.

Formula-Feeding Guidelines and Technique

Commercial formulas are available in three forms: Powder, concentrate, and ready-to-feed. There are situations in which one formula may be better to use than another, but, in general, convenience and cost usually influence the parents' decision.

- *Powdered formula* is the least expensive type of formula. This formula can be made up one bottle at a time, or multiple bottles can be prepared, but they must be used within 24 to 48 hours depending on the manufacturer's instructions. Standard powdered formula is made by adding one level *unpacked* scoop of powdered formula to 60 mL of water (the powder is added to the water). Powdered formulas are not sterile. Preparation of any newborn/infant formula, but especially powdered formulas, requires careful handling to avoid contamination with microorganisms, specifically *Cronobacter* (CDC, 2017). *Cronobacter* is a group of bacteria that can be found naturally in the environment and can live in dry foods, such as powdered baby formula and powdered milk. *Cronobacter* infections are rare, but they can be deadly in newborns.
- *Formula concentrate* is more expensive than powder but is not as expensive as ready-to-feed formula. Formula concentrate is commercially sterile. This formula requires being diluted with an equal part of water. By adding boiled water that has been cooled, sterility can be maintained.
- *Ready-to-feed formula* is the easiest to use because it does not require any mixing; however, this convenience comes at a cost—it is the most expensive formula. It is indicated for use when adequate water is not available, when the baby has a compromised immune system and requires commercially sterile (pasteurized) formula, when an inexperienced babysitter will be feeding the baby, and at other times simply for convenience.

Whichever type of formula they choose, parents will need to be briefed on safety precautions during formula preparation. A primary concern is proper mixing to reconstitute formula. Parents need clear instructions to avoid unintentional harm to their baby (Stockhausen, 2018). Parents should be instructed to follow the directions on the formula package label precisely as written. They should know that adding too much water during preparation (or supplementation with water) dilutes the nutrients and caloric density and may contribute to undernourishment, insufficient weight gain, and possibly water intoxication leading to hyponatremia and seizures (AAP, 2018b). Not adding enough water concentrates nutrients and calories and can damage a baby's immature kidneys and digestive system as well as cause dehydration.

Recommended sanitary precautions and additional safety precautions include:

- Check the expiration date on the formula container.
- Ensure good hand hygiene before preparing formula; never dip into the can without clean hands.
- Clean bottles, nipples, rings, disks, and bottle caps.
  - Wash in a dishwasher when available (small items and heat-sensitive items on top rack secured in a basket), or
  - Boil briefly (1 to 2 minutes) in a pot of water, or
  - Clean using a microwave sterilization kit, or
  - Clean using very warm soapy water and a nipple and bottle brush.
  - Inspect and replace bottle nipples as soon as they show wear—worn nipples can break apart and can become a choking hazard.
- Wash the top of the formula container before piercing the lid. Shake the liquid formulas well before pouring out desired amount.
- Shake prepared formula that has been sitting in the refrigerator before feeding.
- Use hot water (158°F [70°C] or higher) to make powdered formula.

- Use only the scoop supplied in the can of formula when formula preparation instructions call for a "scoop" of powdered formula. A scoop should not be "packed" and should be leveled off (e.g., with the back of a knife).
- Do not add anything else to the bottle, except under direction of baby's healthcare provider.
- Warm up formula in a bottle by placing the bottle in a bowl of warm tap water for no longer than 15 minutes. Do not fill the bowl with water higher than the rim of the bottle. (Infants can take cold formula, but most newborns will prefer it warm.)
- Allow freshly prepared (unused) formula to sit out at room temperature for no longer than 2 hours; use an insulated pack to transport formula. Milk left over in the bottle after a feeding should be discarded.
- In warm weather, transport reconstituted or formula concentrate from an open can in an insulated pack with frozen gel packs.
- Travel with water and formula separated—carry the premeasured water bottles and carry bottles with premeasured amounts of powdered formula, or carry premeasured commercially prepared formula packets, or have the can of formula available.
- Hold the baby during feedings (even later on when an older infant can hold the bottle for him- or herself) to promote bonding and prevent supine feedings.
- Do not allow the baby to bottle-feed in a supine position because this increases the risk of otitis media and dental caries in the older infant.
- Never prop a bottle—this is a choking hazard.
- Allow babies to take what they want *and* to stop when they want. Overfeeding can lead to obesity.

Parents need guidance about what kind of water to use to reconstitute formula (see Table 29–7 to review types of water sources) and should discuss with their baby's healthcare provider whether to boil the water before use. If boiled water is used, parents need to be instructed to heat the water until it reaches a rolling boil, continue to let the water boil for 1 to 2 minutes, and, most importantly, allow the water to cool before using it to reconstitute the formula. Parents should also be instructed not to let the water boil down to a low level in the pan because this can cause minerals in the water to become concentrated.

Use of distilled bottled water and filtered tap water raises concerns with regard to fluoride. The American Academy of Pediatrics recommends that no fluoride supplements be given to a baby before 6 months of age (AAP & ACOG, 2017). Parents should be encouraged to read the labels on bottled water to see if fluoride has been added and to determine if the water source is suitable for their baby depending on his or her age.

BOTTLES AND NIPPLES

Parents often have questions about the kind of bottles and nipples to purchase. Plastic, glass, or disposable bottle bags may all be used based on preference. Many newly designed bottles are marketed to lessen air intake while a baby feeds. There is not a particular bottle design that is best for all babies. A key point to emphasize to the families is feeding technique. Parents should try to avoid situations in which a baby is crying for a prolonged time. Crying results in increased ingestion of air even before the baby has started feeding. Babies who are very hungry also gulp more air. For these situations, instruct the parents to burp their baby frequently to prevent the baby from having a large emesis (Figure 29–22 and Figure 29–23). The parent may even want to attempt to pat the baby's back briefly before starting the feeding to calm a crying baby and possibly burp as well. Another tip to avoid excessive ingestion of air is to have the parent hold the baby cradled in his or her arms while bottle-feeding and tilting the bottle at a 45-degree angle in order for fluid to cover the nipple. This prevents the baby from sucking in air and swallowing it. The vented bottle design eliminates the negative effects of a vacuum and channels air through an internal vent system above the milk, avoiding air bubbles in the milk. See Figure 29–24 to view a baby bottle-feeding.

Parents will want to consider a slow-flow nipple for all newborns and for older breastfeeding babies learning to bottle-feed—over time the infant will graduate to medium-flow and high-flow nipples. Generally, nipple shape is of greater importance for breastfeeding babies receiving expressed breast milk or supplemental formula in a bottle. Breastfed babies transition best going from breast to bottle and back to breast again when using a bottle nipple that is not too firm, one that has a relatively wide base (to help maintain a wide-open latch), and one that has a medium nipple length. Nipples are generally made from either rubber or silicone. Families with a history of sensitivity to latex are advised to use the clear silicone nipples. Silicone nipples also have less of an odor, which may be an issue for some babies who are breastfed.

TABLE 29–7 Water Sources

TYPE	DESCRIPTION
Distilled water	Minerals and most other impurities have been removed. It will not contain any fluoride. An acceptable water source for reconstituting formula.
Filtered tap water	Some minerals and impurities removed during filtration, including fluoride. This is an acceptable water source for reconstituting formula.
Natural mineral water	Comes from protected groundwater and by law cannot be treated. Naturally contains high levels of minerals and sodium and so is not suitable for babies or for reconstituting formula.
Spring water	Comes from a single nonpolluted groundwater, but unlike natural mineral water, it can be further treated. Because there is no regulation requiring the mineral content to be printed on the bottle label, it is best to avoid this water source for reconstituting formula.
Tap water	Water from the municipal water supply and regulated by drinking water regulations. It is treated and considered safe for use in reconstituting formula.
Well water	Needs to be tested before use. Higher risk of nitrate poisoning. Untested water is not recommended for use in reconstituting formula.

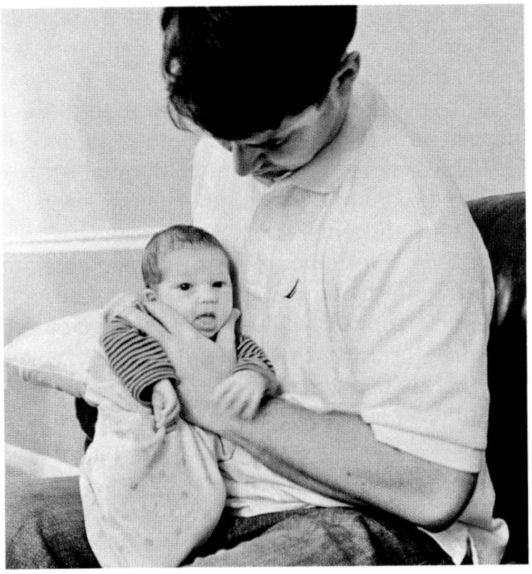

Figure 29–22 **Burping baby sitting up on lap.**

SOURCE: Brigitte Hall, RNC, MSN, IBCLC.

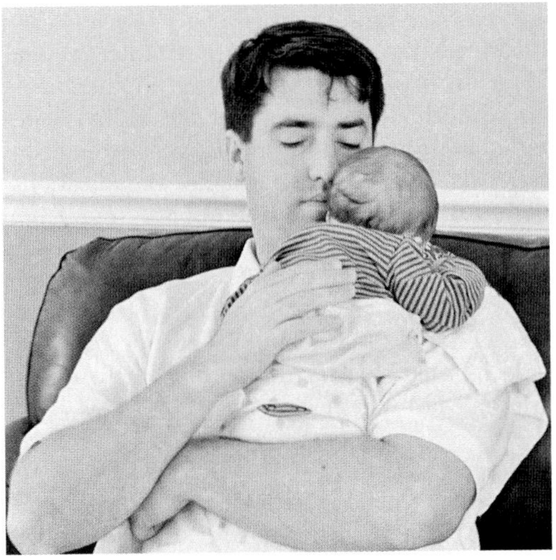

Figure 29–23 **Burping baby over the shoulder.**

SOURCE: Brigitte Hall, RNC, MSN, IBCLC.

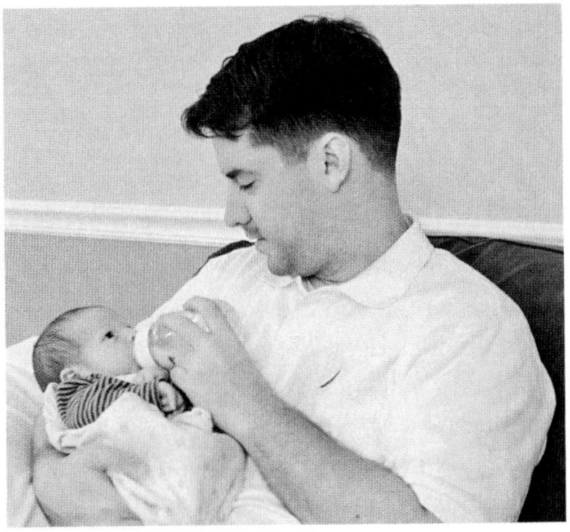

Figure 29–24 **Bottle-feeding.**

SOURCE: Brigitte Hall, RNC, MSN, IBCLC.

To know if a newborn is bottle-feeding well, the nurse needs to observe a bottle-feeding session. Parents should be informed that if the newborn is sucking effectively, they should observe bubbles rising in the fluid of standard bottles. (If a family is using vented bottles or bottles with liners that retract as fluid is removed, bubbles will not be detected.) No bubbles will be observed if the parent unintentionally places the bottle nipple under the baby's tongue, preventing the baby from sucking effectively. Some newborns, especially premature babies, raise their tongues to the roof of their mouths and so it is sometimes a challenge to place the nipple on top of the tongue. Newborns who persistently leak milk from the side of the mouth may be getting fluid too quickly. The nurse can suggest using a slower-flowing nipple. If symptoms persist, the newborn should have an oral evaluation. The baby could have a short lingual frenulum that is restricting tongue mobility (tongue-tied) and may not be able to properly cup the tongue under the nipple and channel fluid to the back of the throat, or the baby may have an oral-motor dysfunction and need speech therapy or occupational therapy evaluation.

There has been a growing concern regarding chemicals, specifically bisphenol-A (BPA), used in the manufacture of plastic baby bottles, the material used in lining formula cans, and soft plastics. Potential leaching from polycarbonate plastic used in the manufacturing of some baby bottles may transfer BPA into the baby's milk (National Institute of Environmental Health Sciences, 2017).

SAFETY ALERT!

Parents need to be instructed to read product labels to see if the merchandise they are purchasing is free of these potentially harmful chemicals. If product labels do not explicitly state that they are free of these chemicals, then it cannot be assumed that they are BPA-free, PVC-free, lead-free, and phthalates-free.

If parents cannot afford to purchase new BPA-free bottles, then encourage them to limit heating the bottles (avoid using the dishwasher and bottle warmers) and throw out old bottles with scratches. The harmful chemicals are leached most when the plastic is heated or damaged.

Involving Fathers and Partners

Our traditional view of the family following the birth of a child places most of the attention on the mother and newborn, oftentimes leaving the father or partner out. Nurses need to recognize this and make every effort to speak to both parents when entering the patient's room. Fathers/partners play a vital role in the family by providing support to the mother and care for their newborn. If a mother has chosen not to breastfeed, then the father/partner can be involved with bottle feedings from the start. However, if the mother is breastfeeding, it is important to ask the father/partner to wait to introduce a bottle until the mother's milk supply and breastfeeding are well established, generally by 3 to 4 weeks postdelivery. The father/partner can be encouraged to assist with breastfeeding in the meantime by helping the mother get in position and help tweak the baby's latch if the mother complains of any discomfort. The father/partner can also massage the mother's breasts during breastfeeding to help stimulate the sleepy baby to feed better and to relieve any engorgement.

The father/partner can help with other aspects, too, such as burping the baby, changing diapers, bathing, and comforting the baby. The father/partner can also provide skin-to-skin contact that enhances bonding, provides comfort to the newborn, and calms the baby down before offering the breast. One strategy is to hold the baby vertically on the father/partner's chest and let the baby suck on a clean finger for a minute or so (see Figure 29–25). These interactions promote family bonding and are important for paternal/maternal role development. See *Case Study: Melissa Bond-James*.

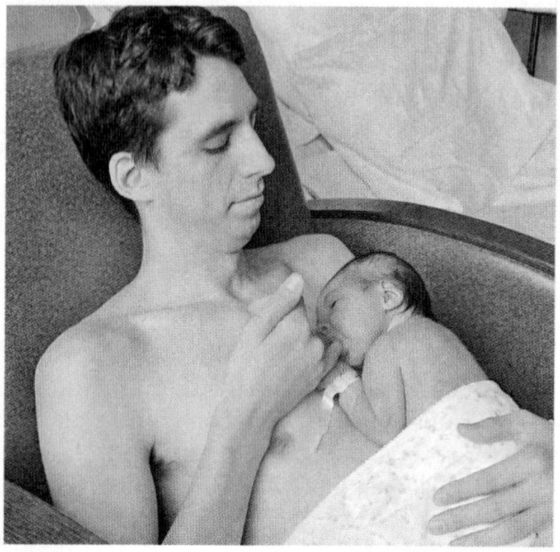

Figure 29–25 **Father and newborn skin to skin.**

SOURCE: Brigitte Hall, RNC, MSN, IBCLC.

Community-Based Nursing Care

Promotion of Successful Newborn/Infant Feeding

Childbirth and the beginning of motherhood are critical times in a woman's life, so physical, psychologic, and social supports are of paramount importance. The nurse needs to explore the family's social support base. The father or partner is the most important support person for her, although the baby can also provide some support in the form of positive feedback. Some families will have support from a large extended family group, friends, church, or other organization. However, that is not the case for everyone; as evidenced by the frequent discontinuing of breastfeeding in the early postpartum weeks, there is a need for assistance and follow-up in this area.

With the trend toward earlier discharge from the birthing center, there is limited time for inpatient education. Teaching moments, when they occur, may not be optimal because of the distraction of visitors and the mother being sleep-deprived, uncomfortable, or under the effects of an analgesic. It is important that parents receive verbal and written instructions and community resource information to which they can later refer.

To promote a supportive hospital environment for breastfeeding, the Baby-Friendly Hospital Initiative recognizes hospitals and birthing centers that offer optimal lactation services and comply with the 10 steps outlined in Box 29–2. Baby-Friendly designation is not easy to achieve. One obstacle to achieving Baby-Friendly status, among many, is having to agree not to accept free or low-cost formula. As of July 2018, there are approximately 529 hospitals in the United States with the Baby-Friendly designation, according to an update on the Baby-Friendly Hospital Initiative USA (2018) website.

COMMUNITY RESOURCES

Community-based support for breastfeeding mothers often focuses on breastfeeding support groups. **La Leche League International (LLLI)** is the first (not-for-profit international educational and service organization) mother-to-mother breastfeeding support group formally recognized in the United States. It also has expanded to provide educational breastfeeding conferences for professionals, and it is one of the few organizations to have a peer counselor breastfeeding training program, among other things. Encourage mothers to visit the International Lactation Consultant Association (ILCA) website to find lactation consultants in their geographic areas. Another professional organization, the Academy of Breastfeeding Medicine (ABM), provides many research-based breastfeeding protocols. To access the protocols, visit the ABM website.

WIC

The Supplemental Nutrition Program for Women, Infants, and Children (WIC) functions primarily to provide low-income women and children who are at risk for medical or nutritional problems with nutritious foods to supplement their diets, nutrition education and counseling, breastfeeding counseling, and screening and referrals to other health, welfare, and social programs. In a recent systematic review, the use of peer counselors was shown to have a positive impact on infant feeding behavior (U.S. Department of Agriculture, 2017). See Chapter 34 for further discussion of WIC services.

CASE STUDY: Melissa Bond-James

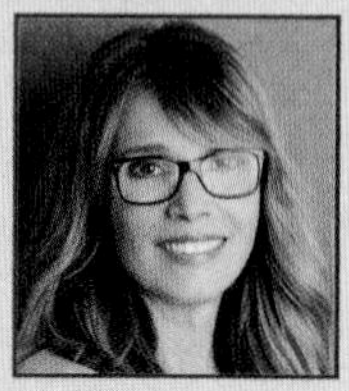

SOURCE: Kinga/Shutterstock.

Melissa is planning on breastfeeding and expressing milk via an electric breast pump so that Nancy can also participate in feeding their daughter. She asks if it is feasible to alternate nights when she pumps so she can sleep through every other night and not become sleep-deprived.

Questions to Ponder

What education would you provide to explain how milk production continues despite the baby being bottle-fed by someone else? Why is it important to ensure regular feedings or pumping on a routine basis? What other information is important to share with new mothers to ensure they maintain their milk supply when supplemental feedings are being given?

Box 29–2
Baby-Friendly Requirements

Ten Steps to Successful Breastfeeding (revised 2018)

Critical management procedures

1a. Comply fully with the *International Code of Marketing of Breast-milk Substitutes* and relevant World Health Assembly resolutions.
1b. Have a written infant feeding policy that is routinely communicated to staff and parents.
1c. Establish ongoing monitoring and data-management systems.
2. Ensure that staff has sufficient knowledge, competence, and skills to support breastfeeding.

Key clinical practices

3. Discuss the importance and management of breastfeeding with pregnant women and their families.
4. Facilitate immediate and uninterrupted skin-to-skin contact and support mothers to initiate breastfeeding as soon as possible after birth.
5. Support mothers to initiate and maintain breastfeeding and manage common difficulties.
6. Do not provide breastfed newborns any food or fluid other than breast milk, unless medically indicated.
7. Enable mothers and their infants to remain together and to practice rooming-in 24 hours a day.
8. Support mothers to recognize and respond to their infants' cues for feeding.
9. Counsel mothers on the use and risks of feeding bottles, teats, and pacifiers.
10. Coordinate discharge so that parents and their infants have timely access to ongoing support and care.

SOURCE: Reprinted from Implementation guidance: protecting, promoting and supporting breastfeeding in facilities providing maternity and newborn services – the revised Baby-friendly Hospital Initiative, Ten Steps to Successful Breastfeeding (revised 2018), Page No. 15, Geneva: World Health Organization; 2018.

Nutritional Assessment

A nutritional assessment is an integral part of a thorough health appraisal and is commonly performed by the newborn's primary care provider, a nurse, a lactation consultant, a registered dietitian, or a speech therapist. The nutritional assessment will include all or some of the following parameters to measure wellness and is an effective strategy for increasing breastfeeding rates.

Parents will be asked to present a feeding diary for the provider to review, or the parents will need to recall the newborn's feeding pattern over the last 24 to 48 hours. The parents will also be asked to describe the newborn's urine and stool output, including quantity and quality. The healthcare professional is interested in the baby's behavior pattern, especially during and immediately after feeding. If the newborn is not gaining sufficient weight, the baby's feeding history must be examined more closely. If the newborn is breastfeeding, a relevant maternal history is needed to determine if the mother is having breastfeeding difficulties and to help determine the root cause of the problem. If the newborn is formula-feeding, the healthcare professional will first want to investigate the family's formula-feeding practices (including formula preparation technique). While gathering these data, the healthcare professional should be sensitive to the family's cultural practices. However, if a cultural practice has harmful effects, then the provider needs to tactfully educate the family to that fact.

The provider should plot the newborn's measurements for length, head circumference, and weight on a growth chart, denoting the baby's individual percentile measurement compared with the general population. Because there are variations among newborns at the same age, it is important to monitor the baby's individual growth pattern over time. Ideally, the provider wants to see a newborn track along the same growth curve.

As the healthcare provider begins the newborn's physical exam, the provider first obtains a subjective impression of the baby's overall appearance. The provider performs a head-to-toe physical examination, carefully noting any deviations from normal. The physical exam helps identify any nutritional disorders. With all the data available, it is now possible to determine a newborn's nutritional status and potential risks. The following scenario and Nursing Management section show the effectiveness of these assessments and interventions.

> **Scenario:** Baby girl Smith was born at 37 weeks' gestation to an 18-year-old, G1P0 via cesarean section. The father of the baby was not present. Baby Smith is now 76 hours postpartum, and she and her mother are expected to go home today. While the nurse is weighing the newborn for a discharge weight, the mother mentions that she does not think her daughter is getting much breast milk when she feeds because her baby keeps falling asleep at the breast during the feeding. Baby Smith weighed 3542 grams at birth, and her present weight is 3173 grams. (The difference is 369 grams: $369/3542 = 0.104 \times 100 = 10.4\%$ weight loss.) An assessment of the mother's breasts reveals symmetric, soft breasts and normal-shaped nipples, with nipples intact. After contacting the newborn's healthcare provider to report the significant weight loss, the nurse is now ready to formulate a plan of care.

NURSING MANAGEMENT
For a Newborn with Significant Weight Loss

Nursing Assessment and Diagnosis

Nursing diagnoses that may apply include:

- ***Breastfeeding, Ineffective***, related to:
  - Mother's lack of knowledge about breastfeeding
  - Mother's not responding to newborn's feeding cues
  - Mother's inability to facilitate effective breastfeeding

As evidenced by a weight loss of 10.4% in baby.

- ***Breastfeeding, Ineffective***, related to:
  - Insufficient knowledge regarding newborn's reflexes and breastfeeding techniques
  - Lack of support by father of baby or other support persons
  - Lack of maternal self-confidence
  - Maternal fatigue
  - Possible maternal ambivalence
  - Poor newborn sucking reflex
  - Difficulty waking the sleepy baby

- *Nutrition, Imbalanced: Less Than Body Requirements,* related to:
  - Mother's increased caloric and nutrient needs status post-cesarean section
  - Newborn's inability to correctly latch on and transfer milk

(NANDA-I © 2017)

Nursing Plan and Implementation

1. Review the mother's history.
   - Maternal demographics—for example, mother's date of birth, parity, marital status, cultural feeding practices
   - Pregnancy history—for example, complications during pregnancy, gestation at delivery
   - Complications of delivery—for example, cesarean section, excessive blood loss
   - Current medical issues—for example, hypothyroidism? diabetes? polycystic ovary syndrome (PCOS)?
   - History of breast surgery or radiation—for example, breast reduction, breast augmentation, radiation to treat previous breast cancer
   - Use of prescribed or over-the-counter medications, herbs, alcohol, cigarettes
   - Psychosocial history—maternal support system, history of depression, and so on
   - History of previous breastfeeding experience
2. Maternal assessment
   - Assess the breasts and nipples.
   - Obtain a description of lochia drainage.
3. Newborn assessment
   - Obtain the newborn's weight and compare with previous weight measurements.
   - *Note:* If this were an older newborn, then it would be appropriate to obtain head circumference, length, and weight measurements and track the baby's trend on the growth chart; however, because this newborn is only 3 days old, daily tracking of the other growth parameters is not applicable for this situation.
   - Examine the newborn, with emphasis on oral anatomy and oral-motor function, reflexes, overall behavior, skin color (jaundice).
   - Assess the newborn for signs of dehydration.
4. Newborn feeding history
   - Diet
   - Feeding frequency and duration
   - History of supplementation
   - Review elimination pattern: Number of wet diapers, quality of urine, bowel movements, quality of stool.
5. Pre- and postbreastfeeding weight check
   - Calculate milk transfer during breastfeeding.

Note: Postfeed weight minus prefeed weight equals net breast milk transfer. You must use a digital electronic scale accurate within 2 grams. The baby does not have to be naked, but the clothing and diaper the baby is wearing cannot be changed during this next measurement.

6. Observation of breastfeeding technique
   - Positioning and latch-on technique, newborn responses, suckling pattern, satiated after feeding
7. Review feeding requirement/caloric requirement based on the newborn's birth weight (3542 g / 3.542 kg).
   - Fluid requirement: 140 to 160 mL/kg/day.
   - Should be up to full volume by day 6 or so; should then receive 496 to 567 mL/day. To convert milliliters to ounces: Take 496 mL/day, divide by 30 mL/oz; this equals 16.5 oz/day. For this scenario, the newborn should receive 16.5 to 18.9 oz/day.
   - The newborn should feed 8 to 12 times per day. If the newborn feeds 10 times per day, then the baby should receive 496/10 = 49.6 mL/feeding.
   - On day 3, the newborn will *not* be expected to feed approximately 50 mL/feeding (minimum *full* volume); based on physiologic stomach capacity, the baby may only feed about 30 mL/feeding on day 3 of life but will be increasing volume daily as tolerated until up to full volume in the next couple of days.
   - Caloric requirement 100 to 115 kcal/kg/day.
   - Should be up to full caloric requirement by about day 6; should receive 354 to 407 kcal/day. Human milk has 20 kcal/oz; standard formula has 20 kcal/oz. To determine how many ounces the newborn will require per day, take 354 kcal/day and divide by 20 kcal/oz, which equals 17.7 oz/day.

Note: The newborn should gradually be increasing her volume of milk each day and will soon be up to full volume.

8. Assess teaching needs and provide verbal and written instructions.
   - Review benefits of breastfeeding. Remind mother to provide frequent skin-to-skin contact.
   - Review breastfeeding technique (positioning and latch-on).
   - Watch the newborn for early feeding cues. If the baby is too sleepy to exhibit these feeding behaviors, then teach the mother to watch for signs that her baby is in a light state of sleep. When the newborn is in a light state of sleep, then the mother can try "wake-up techniques" to help her baby wake up at least every 3 hours to feed.
   - Provide breast pump instructions and review collection and storage.
   - May start pumping to increase breast stimulation. All expressed breast milk should be fed to the newborn. If the mother is not able to express enough milk, then the baby should be supplemented with formula.
   - Review the process of breastfeeding (principle of supply and demand) and practice proper breastfeeding technique. Encourage the mother to breastfeed as often as possible and observe for signs of effective breastfeeding.
   - Review newborn intake and output and weight gain expectations. Maintain a feeding diary to monitor the newborn's intake and output; call a lactation consultant or the baby's healthcare provider if the baby is not meeting expectations.
   - Provide information on maternal nutrition and fluid requirements. Encourage the mother to:
     - Rest as much as possible and be concerned only about self-care needs (i.e., prevention of engorgement, etc.) and caring for the newborn right now.
     - Eat healthy foods and drink plenty of fluids to quench thirst.
     - Plan for a follow-up weight check on newborn in 1 to 2 days to assess nutritional status.

Follow-up lactation consultation visit follows in 2 days to determine milk transfer efficiency and evaluate maternal milk production.

Evaluation

The expected outcomes of nursing care for the newborn include:

- Newborn will arouse to feed at least every 3 hours and will stay awake until the end of each feeding.
- The newborn will correctly latch on to the breasts and effectively breastfeed 8 to 12 times per day.
- The newborn will gain at least 10 g/kg/day and be back to birth weight no later than day 14 of life.
- The newborn will have four wet diapers, three to four bowel movements on day 4; five wet diapers, three to four bowel movements on day 5; and six to eight wet diapers, three to four bowel movements every day thereafter during the first month of life.
- Newborn's stools will transition from black to yellow by day 5 and will change in consistency from thick and sticky to loose and explosive with small curds or seedy appearance.
- Newborn will not have any uric-acid crystals in his or her diaper after day 3 or 4.
- Newborn will be satiated after feeding, as evidenced by relaxed muscle tone and sleepiness.

The expected outcomes of nursing care for the mother include:

- Mother will verbalize/demonstrate an understanding of breastfeeding technique, including positioning and latch-on, signs of adequate feeding, and self-care.
- Mother will breastfeed pain-free.
- Mother will express satisfaction with the breastfeeding experience.
- Mother will consume a nutritionally balanced diet with appropriate caloric and fluid intake to support breastfeeding.

Focus Your Study

- The dietary reference intake (DRI) for calories for the newborn is 100 to 115 kcal/kg/day and fluid intake is 140 to 160 mL/kg/day.
- A weight loss of more than 10% is excessive and requires an evaluation and follow-up. Newborns should be back to their birth weight by 10 to 14 days of age.
- The healthy full-term newborn gains approximately 10 g/kg/day for the first month of life. Exclusively breastfed newborns have the same or slightly greater weight gain in the first 3 to 4 months of life than mixed-fed and formula-fed newborns. Thereafter, formula-fed and mixed-fed newborns are heavier than breastfed newborns.
- Generally, newborns double their birth weight by 5 months, triple their birth weight by 1 year of age, and quadruple their birth weight by 2 years.
- Increases in body length and head circumference between breastfed and formula-fed newborns are the same. A baby gains 1 inch per month in the first 6 months, and then 0.5 inch per month for the following 6 months.
- The American Academy of Pediatrics (AAP) recommends exclusive breastfeeding for the first 6 months and continued breastfeeding until the infant is 1 year old or older.
- Human milk has immunologic and nutritional properties that make it the optimal food for the first year of life.
- The breastfed newborn's iron stores from in utero placental transfer is usually depleted by the time the infant is 6 months old. Breastfeeding infants over 6 months of age who are eating complementary foods rich in iron and infants consuming iron-enriched formula need no other vitamin or mineral supplements with the possible exception of vitamin D.
- Mature human milk and standard commercially prepared formulas provide 20 kcal/oz.
- There are five types of commercial infant formulas: (1) standard cow's milk-based formulas; (2) soy milk-based formulas; (3) partially hydrolyzed formulas; (4) extensively hydrolyzed hypoallergenic formulas; and (5) essentially nonallergenic amino acid–based formulas.
- Neither cow's milk nor soy milk should be given to infants before 1 year of age. The use of skim milk or low-fat cow's milk is not recommended for children under 2 years old.
- Most maternal medications are transmitted through human milk to some degree, but few are actually contraindicated. The bioavailability of transmitted drugs to the baby depends on a variety of factors, including route of administration, protein binding, degree of ionization, molecular weight, timing of the dose with respect to feeding time, and absorption across the baby's intestinal tract.
- Signs indicating a newborn's readiness to feed include hand-to-mouth movements, rooting, smacking, fussing, and crying (a late-feeding cue).
- Breastfeeding mothers should be taught to use proper positioning and latch-on technique. The mother should be advised to alternate feeding positions periodically to promote efficient drainage of all the ducts in the breast.
- During the first few days after birth, the minimum output expectations for an exclusively breastfeeding newborn are one wet/one stool on day 1; two wets/two stools on day 2; three wets/three to four stools on day 3; four wets/three to four stools on day 4; five wets/three to four stools on day 5. Thereafter, an exclusively breastfeeding newborn has a minimum of six to eight wet diapers and three to four yellow milk stools each day, generally during the first month of life.
- Newborns' stools start as black and sticky at birth and transition to yellow, curdy, or seedy by day 5, or sooner.

- The formula-feeding mother may need help learning about the types of formulas and how to prepare and store formula. Like the breastfeeding mother, she will benefit from understanding feeding cues and proper technique for feeding her newborn.
- Nutritional assessment of the newborn includes the baby's dietary history, anthropometric measurements, physical examination, and laboratory tests, if indicated.

In order to make safe and effective judgments using NANDA-I © 2017 nursing diagnoses, it is essential that nurses refer to the definitions and defining characteristics of the diagnoses used in this text, which can be found in Appendix C.

References

Abbott Nutrition. (2018). *Product information: Similac Pro-Advance™*. Columbus, OH: Abbott Laboratories. Retrieved from https://static.abbottnutrition.com/cms-prod/abbottnutrition-2016.com/img/Similac-Pro-Advance.pdf

Academy of Breastfeeding Medicine (ABM). (2010). Protocol #7: Model breastfeeding policy. *Breastfeeding Medicine, 5*(4), 173–178. DOI: 10.1089/bfm.2010.9986

Academy of Breastfeeding Medicine (ABM). (2015). Protocol #13: Contraception during breastfeeding. *Breastfeeding Medicine, 10*(1), 1–10. DOI: 10.1089/bfm.2015.9999

Academy of Breastfeeding Medicine (ABM). (2016). Protocol #10: Breastfeeding the late preterm (34–36 6/7 weeks of gestation) and early term infants (37–38 6/7 weeks of gestation), Second Revision 2016. *Breastfeeding Medicine, 11*(10), 1–10. DOI: 10.1089/bfm.2018.29031.egb

Academy of Breastfeeding Medicine (ABM). (2017a). Protocol #3: Supplementary feeding in the healthy term breastfed neonate, Revised 2017. *Breastfeeding Medicine, 12*(3), 1–10. DOI: 10.1089/bfm.2017.29038,ajk

Academy of Breastfeeding Medicine (ABM). (2017b). Protocol #8: Human milk storage information for home use for full-term infants, Revised 2017. *Breastfeeding Medicine, 12*(77), 1–10. DOI: 10.1089/bfm.2017.29047.aje

American Academy of Pediatrics (AAP). (2016a). *Benefits of breastfeeding for mom.* Retrieved from https://www.healthychildren.org/English/ages-stages/baby/breastfeeding/Pages/Benefits-of-Breastfeeding-for-Mom.aspx

American Academy of Pediatrics (AAP). (2016b). *Breastfeeding benefits your baby's immune system.* Retrieved from https://www.healthychildren.org/English/ages-stages/baby/breastfeeding/Pages/Breastfeeding-Benefits-Your-Baby%27s-Immune-System.aspx

American Academy of Pediatrics (AAP). (2016c). *Vitamin D & iron supplements for babies: AAP recommendations.* Retrieved from https://www.healthychildren.org/English/ages-stages/baby/feeding-nutrition/Pages/Vitamin-Iron-Supplements

American Academy of Pediatrics (AAP). (2018a). *Choosing a formula.* Retrieved from https://www.healthychildren.org/English/ages-stages/baby/feeding-nutrition/Pages/Choosing-a-Formula.aspx

American Academy of Pediatrics (AAP). (2018b). How to safely prepare formula with water. Retrieved from: https://www.healthychildren.org/English/ages-stages/baby/formula-feeding/Pages/How-to-Safely-Prepare-Formula-with-Water.aspx

American Academy of Pediatrics (AAP) Committee on Fetus and Newborn & American College of Obstetricians and Gynecologists (ACOG) Committee on Obstetrics. (2017). *Guidelines for perinatal care* (8th ed.). Evanston, IL: Author.

Ask Dr. Sears. (2018). *Comparison of human milk and formula.* Retrieved from https://www.askdrsears.com/topics/feeding-eating/bottle-feeding/comparision-formulas-and-breastmilk

Association of Women's Health, Obstetrics, and Neonatal Nurses (AWHONN). (2015). AWHONN position statement: Breastfeeding. *Journal of Obstetric, Gynecologic, & Neonatal Nursing, 44*(1), 145–150.

Baby-Friendly Hospital Initiative USA. (2016). *Implementing the UNICEF/WHO baby-friendly hospital initiative in the U.S.* Retrieved from https://www.babyfriendlyusa.org/get-started/the-guidelines-evaluation-criteria

Baby-Friendly Hospital Initiative USA. (2018). *Facilities in the U.S.* Retrieved from https://www.babyfriendlyusa.org/find-facilities

Berens, P., Eglash, A., Malloy, M., Steube, A., & Academy of Breastfeeding Medicine. (2016). ABM Protocol #26: Persistent pain with breastfeeding. *Breastfeeding Medicine, 11*(2). DOI: 10.1089/bfm.2016.29002.pjb

Backburn, S. T. (2018). *Maternal, fetal, neonatal physiology: A clinical perspective* (5th ed.). St. Louis, MO: Elsevier.

Briggs, G. G., Freeman, R. K., Towers, C. V., & Forinash, A. B. (2017). *Drugs in pregnancy and lactation: A reference guide to fetal and neonatal risk* (11th ed.). Philadelphia, PA: Wolters Kluwer Health.

Bunik, M. (2017). The pediatrician's role in encouraging exclusive breastfeeding. *Pediatrics in Review, 38*(8), 353–368.

Callister, L. C. (2014). Integrating cultural beliefs and practices when caring for childbearing women and families. In K. R. Simpson & P. A. Creehan (Eds.), *Perinatal nursing* (3rd ed., pp. 29–57). Philadelphia, PA: Lippincott Williams & Wilkins.

Centers for Disease Control and Prevention (CDC). (2010). *National Center for Health Statistics: WHO growth standards are recommended for use in the U.S. for infants and children 0 to 2 years of age.* Retrieved from http://www.cdc.gov/growthcharts/who_charts.htm

Centers for Disease Control and Prevention (CDC). (2017). *Learn about* Cronobacter *infection.* Retrieved from https://www.cdc.gov/features/cronobacter

Centers for Disease Control and Prevention (CDC). (2018a). *Breastfeeding report card progressing toward national breastfeeding goals 2018.* Retrieved from https://www.cdc.gov/breastfeeding/pdf/2018breastfeedingreportcard.pdf

Centers for Disease Control and Prevention (CDC). (2018b). *Breastfeeding: Vaccinations.* Retrieved from www.cdc.gov/breastfeeding/breastfeeding-special-circumstances/vaccinations-medications-drugs/vaccinations.html

Centers for Disease Control and Prevention (CDC). (2018c). *2018 recommended immunizations for children from birth through 6 years old.* Retrieved from https://www.cdc.gov/vaccines/parents/downloads/parent-ver-sch-0-6yrs.pdf

Centers for Disease Control and Prevention (CDC). (2018d). *Proper handling and storage of human milk.* Retrieved from https://www.cdc.gov/breastfeeding/recommendations/handling_breastmilk.htm

Darmawikarta, D., Chen, Y., Lebovic, G., Birken, C. S., Parkin, P. C., & Maguire, J. L. (2016). Total duration of breastfeeding, vitamin D supplementation, and serum levels of 25-hydroxyvitamin D. *American Journal of Public Health, 106*(4), 714–719. DOI: 10.2105/AJPH.2015.303021

Eichenwald, E. C., Hansen, A. R., Martin, C. R., & Stark, A. R. (2017). *Cloherty and Stark's manual of neonatal care* (8th ed.). Philadelphia, PA: Lippincott Williams & Wilkins.

Hale, T. W. (2019). *Medications and mothers' milk* (18th ed.). Amarillo, TX: Pharmasoft.

Healthy Children. (2018). Starting solid foods. Retrieved from https://www.healthychildren.org/English/ages-stages/baby/feeding-nutrition/Pages/Switching-To-Solid-Foods.aspx

Jensen, D., Wallace, S., & Kelsay, P. (1994). LATCH: A breastfeeding charting system and documentation tool. *Journal of Obstetric, Gynecologic, and Neonatal Nursing: JOGNN / NAACOG, 23*(1), 27–32.

Jones, K. M., Power, M. L., Queenan, J. T., & Schulkin, J. (2015). Racial and ethnic disparities in breastfeeding. *Breastfeeding Medicine 10*(4),186–196. DOI: 101089/bfm.2014.0152

La Leche League International. (2018). *Positioning.* Retrieved from https://www.llli.org/breastfeeding-info/positioning/

Lawrence, R. A., & Lawrence, R. M. (2016). *Breastfeeding: A guide for the medical profession* (8th ed.). Philadelphia, PA: Mosby.

Mead-Johnson Nutritionals. (2018a). Product Information: Enfamil NeuroPro Gentlease. Retrieved from https://www.meadjohnson.com/pediatrics/us-en/product-information/products/feeding-solution-formulas/enfamil-neuropro-gentlease#

Mead-Johnson Nutritionals (2018b). Product Information: Enfamil Premium Newborn. Retrieved from https://www.meadjohnson.com/pediatrics/us-en/

product-information/products/routine-infant-formulas/enfamil-premium-newborn#nutrients_facts

Meek, J. J. (2017). The American Academy of pediatrics new mother's guide to breastfeeding. (3rd ed.). New York, NY: Bantam Books.

Medela. (2016). *Breast pumps.*. Retrieved from https://www.medela.com.au/breastfeeding/products/breast-pumps

National Conference of State Legislatures. (2018). *Breastfeeding state laws.* Retrieved from https://www.ncsl.org/research/health/breastfeeding-state-laws.aspx

National Institute of Environmental Health Sciences (NIEHS). (2017). *Bisphenol A (BPA).* Retrieved from https://www.niehs.nih.gov/health/topics/agents/sya-bpa

Nestlé Nutrition. (2016). Gerber infant formulas & supplements. Retrieved from https://medical.gerber.com/products/formulas

Office of Women's Health. (2017). *Breastfeeding and going back to work.* Retrieved from https://www.womenshealth.gov/breastfeeding/breastfeeding-home-work-and-public/breastfeeding-and-going-back-work

Pernia, S., & DeMaagd, G. (2016). The new pregnancy and lactation labeling rule. *P.T.41*(11), 713–715.

Sachs, H. C., & American Academy of Pediatrics (AAP) Committee on Drugs. (2013). Transfer of drugs and therapeutics into human breast milk: An update on selected topics. *Pediatrics, 132*(3), e796–809.

Stockhausen, A. (2018). *How do I mix and serve infant formula for my baby?* Retrieved from https://www.healthychildren.org/English/tips-tools/ask-the-pediatrician/Pages/How-do-I-mix-and-serve-infant-formula-for-my-baby.aspx

Tariku, A., Andargie, G., Wassie, M. M., Gebeyehu, A., & Getie, A. A. (2016). Factors associated with prelacteal feeding in the rural population of northwest Ethiopia: A community cross-sectional study. *International Breastfeeding Journal, 11*(14). Retrieved from https://doi.org/10.1186/s13006-016-0074-9

U.S. Department of Agriculture, Food and Nutrition Service. (2017). *Women, infants, and children (WIC).* Retrieved from https://www.fns.usda.gov/wic/women-infants-and-children-wic

U.S. Department of Labor. (2011). *Section 7(r) of the Fair Labor Standards Act—Break time for nursing mothers provision.* Retrieved from https://www.dol.gov/whd/nursingmothers/Sec7rFLSA_btnm.htm

Wambach, K., & Riordan, J. (2016). *Breastfeeding and human lactation* (5th ed.). Burlington, MA: Jones & Bartlett.

Yashmin, S. (2015). *Islamic and cultural practices in breastfeeding.* Retrieved from https://www.llli.org/islamic-cultural-practices-breastfeeding-2/

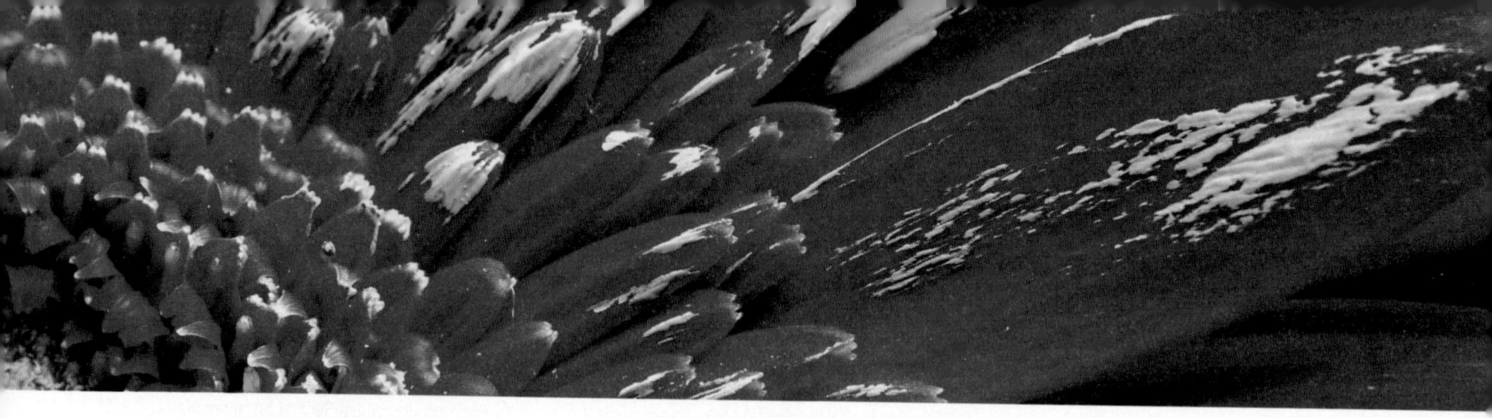

Chapter 30

The Newborn at Risk: Conditions Present at Birth

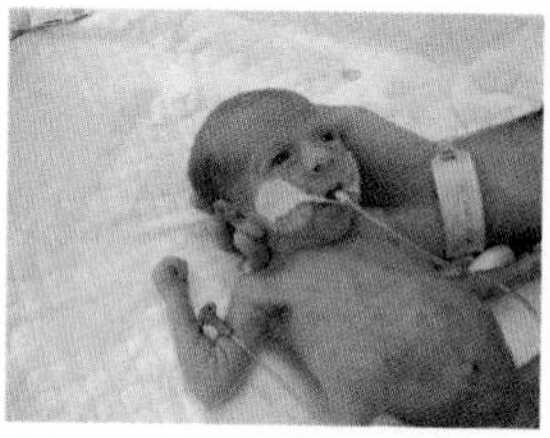

A baby fills a place in your heart that you never knew was there.
—Unknown

Learning Outcomes

30.1 Explain the factors present at birth that indicate an at-risk newborn.

30.2 Compare the underlying etiologies of the physiologic complications of small-for-gestational-age (SGA) newborns and preterm appropriate-for-gestational-age (Pr AGA) newborns and the nursing management for each.

30.3 Describe the potential complications for large-for-gestational-age (LGA) newborns.

30.4 Explain the impact of maternal diabetes mellitus on the newborn.

30.5 Compare the characteristics and potential complications that influence nursing management of the postterm newborn and the newborn with postmaturity syndrome.

30.6 Compare the physiologic and behavioral characteristics of the preterm newborn that predispose each body system to various complications and are used in the development of a plan of care that includes nutritional management.

30.7 Summarize the nursing assessments and initial interventions for a newborn born with selected congenital anomalies.

30.8 Identify physical examination findings during the early newborn period that would make the nurse suspect a congenital cardiac defect or congestive heart failure.

30.9 Explain the special care needed by an in utero alcohol- or drug-exposed newborn.

30.10 Relate the consequence of maternal HIV/AIDS to the management of and issues for caregivers of newborns at risk for HIV/AIDS in the neonatal period.

30.11 Explain the special care needed by a newborn with an inborn error of metabolism.

Healthy People 2020

(ENT-VSL-1.1) Increase the proportion of newborns who are screened for hearing loss no later than age 1 month

(MICU-20) Increase the proportion of infants who are put to sleep on their back

(MICH-1.7) Reduce the rate of infant deaths related to birth defects (congenital heart defects)

(MICH-11) Increase abstinence from alcohol, cigarettes, and illicit drugs among pregnant women

Many levels of neonatal care have evolved in response to increasing knowledge about at-risk newborns. Along with the newborn's parents, the nurse is an important caregiver in all these settings. As a member of the multidisciplinary healthcare team, the nurse is a technically competent professional who contributes the high-touch human care necessary in the high-tech perinatal environment. In addition to the availability of a high level of newborn care, various other factors influence the outcome of at-risk newborns, including:

- Birth weight
- Gestational age
- Type and length of newborn illness
- Environmental factors
- Maternal factors
- Maternal–newborn separation.

Identification of At-Risk Newborns

An at-risk newborn is one susceptible to illness (morbidity) or even death (mortality) because of dysmaturity, immaturity, physical disorders, or complications during or after birth. In most cases, the baby is the product of a pregnancy involving one or more predictable risk factors, including:

- Low socioeconomic level of the mother
- Limited access to health care or no prenatal care
- Exposure to environmental dangers, such as toxic chemicals and illicit drugs
- Preexisting maternal conditions such as heart disease, diabetes, hypertension, hyperthyroidism, and renal disease
- Maternal factors such as age and parity
- Medical conditions related to pregnancy and their associated complications
- Pregnancy complications such as abruptio placentae, placenta previa, oligohydramnios, preterm labor, premature rupture of membranes, preeclampsia, and uterine rupture.

Various prenatal risk factors and their specific effects on pregnancy outcomes are listed in Table 12–1. Because these factors and the perinatal risks associated with them are known, the birth of an at-risk newborn can often be anticipated. The pregnancy can be closely monitored, treatment can be started as necessary, and arrangements can be made for birth to occur at a facility with appropriate resources to care for both mother and baby.

Whether or not prenatal assessment indicates that the fetus is at risk, the course of labor and birth and the baby's ability to withstand the stress of labor cannot be predicted. Thus, the nurse's use of electronic fetal heart monitoring or fetal heart auscultation by Doppler plays a significant role in detecting stress or distress in the fetus. Immediately after birth the Apgar score (review Table 21–5) is a helpful tool for identifying the at-risk newborn, but it is not the only indicator of possible long-term outcomes.

The newborn classification and neonatal mortality risk chart is another useful tool for identifying newborns at risk. Before this classification tool was developed, a birth weight of less than 2500 g (5.5 lb) was the sole criterion for determining immaturity. Clinicians then recognized that a newborn could weigh more than 2500 g and still be immature. Conversely, a newborn weighing less than 2500 g might be functionally at term or beyond. Thus, birth weight and gestational age together are now the criteria used to assess neonatal maturity, morbidity, and mortality risk.

According to the newborn classification and neonatal mortality risk chart, gestation (postmenstrual age) is divided as follows (American College of Obstetricians and Gynecologists [ACOG] & Society for Maternal-Fetal Medicine [SMFM], 2015):

- Preterm: Less than or equal to 36 weeks, 6 days
- Late preterm: 34 to 36 weeks, 6 days
- Early term: 37 weeks, 0 days through 38 weeks, 6 days
- Full term: 39 weeks, 0 days through 40 weeks, 6 days
- Late term: 41 weeks, 0 through 6 days
- Postterm: 42 weeks, 0 days and beyond.

Late preterm is a new classification. These newborns have demonstrated increased incidences of morbidity and length of stay when compared to full-term newborns (Eichenwald, Hansen, Martin, et al., 2017). Morbidities associated with prematurity continue into early-term gestations and are compounded by socioeconomic status (Gill & Boyle, 2017).

Large-for-gestational-age (LGA) newborns are those who plot above the 90th percentile curve on intrauterine growth curves. *Appropriate-for-gestational-age (AGA)* newborns are those who plot between the 10th and the 90th percentile growth curves. **Small-for-gestational-age (SGA)** newborns are those who plot below the 10th percentile growth curve. A newborn is assigned to a category depending on birth weight, length, occipital–frontal head circumference, and gestational age. For example, a newborn classified as *Pr SGA* is preterm and small for gestational age. The full-term newborn whose weight is appropriate for gestational age is classified *F AGA*. It is important to note that intrauterine growth charts are influenced by altitude and the ethnicity of the newborn population used to create the chart. Also, the assigned newborn classification may vary according to the intrauterine growth curve chart used; therefore, the chart used should correlate with the characteristics of the patient population.

Neonatal mortality risk is the neonate's chance of death within the newborn period—that is, within the first 28 days of life. Seventy-five percent of all neonatal deaths occur within the first week, with the highest rates occurring during the first day of life. The neonatal mortality risk decreases as both gestational age and birth weight increase. Newborns who are Pr SGA have the highest neonatal mortality risk. The previously high mortality rates for LGA newborns have decreased at most perinatal centers because of improved management of diabetes in pregnancy and recognition of potential complications of LGA newborns.

Neonatal morbidity can be anticipated based on birth weight and gestational age. The neonatal morbidity by birth weight and gestational age tool assists in determining the needs of particular newborns for special observation and care. For example, a baby of 2000 g (4.4 lb) at 40 weeks' gestation should be carefully assessed for evidence of neonatal distress, hypoglycemia, congenital anomalies, congenital infection, and polycythemia.

Identifying the nursing care needs of the at-risk newborn depends on minute-to-minute observations of changes in the newborn's physiologic status. The organization of nursing care must be directed toward:

- Decreasing physiologically stressful situations
- Observing constantly for subtle signs of change in clinical condition

- Interpreting laboratory data and coordinating interventions
- Conserving the newborn's energy for healing and growth
- Providing for developmental stimulation and maintenance of sleep cycles
- Assisting the family in developing attachment behaviors
- Involving the family in planning and providing care.

Care of the Small-for-Gestational-Age/Intrauterine Growth Restriction Newborn

Currently newborns are considered SGA when they are less than the 10th percentile for birth weight; very small for gestational age is when they are two standard deviations below the population norm or less than the third percentile (Eichenwald et al., 2017) (Figure 30–1). When possible, the birth weight charts used to assign the SGA classification to a newborn should be based on the local population into which the newborn is born. An SGA newborn may be preterm, term, or postterm. An undergrown newborn may also be said to have **intrauterine growth restriction (IUGR)**, which describes pregnancy circumstances of advanced gestation and limited fetal growth. This classification of abnormal growth is also enhanced by looking at growth potential by adjusting birth weight reference limits for first-trimester maternal height, birth order, and newborn gender.

SGA newborns are commonly seen with mothers who smoke or have high blood pressure, causing these babies to have an increased incidence of perinatal asphyxia and perinatal mortality when compared with AGA newborns (ACOG, 2018). The incidence of polycythemia and hypoglycemia is also higher in this group.

Factors Contributing to IUGR

Intrauterine growth restriction may be caused by maternal, placental, or fetal factors and may not be apparent antenatally. Intrauterine growth is linear (follows expected growth line) in the normal pregnancy from approximately 28 to 38 weeks' gestation. After 38 weeks, growth is variable, depending on the growth potential of the fetus and placental function. The most common causes of growth restriction are:

- ***Maternal factors.*** Primiparity, grand multiparity, multiple-gestation pregnancy (twins and higher-order multiples), lack of prenatal care, age extremes (less than 16 years or more than 40 years), and low socioeconomic status (which can result in inadequate healthcare, education, and living conditions) affect IUGR (Eichenwald et al., 2017). Before the third trimester, the nutritional supply to the fetus far exceeds its needs. Only in the third trimester are maternal malnutrition and drug abuse limiting factors in fetal growth.
- ***Maternal disease.*** Maternal heart disease, substance abuse (drugs, tobacco, alcohol), sickle cell disease, phenylketonuria (PKU), lupus erythematosus, and asymptomatic pyelonephritis are associated with SGA. Complications associated with preeclampsia, chronic hypertensive vascular disease, and advanced diabetes mellitus can diminish blood flow to the uterus, thereby decreasing oxygen delivery to the fetus and minimizing organ growth.
- ***Environmental factors.*** High altitude, exposure to x-rays, excessive exercise, work-related exposure to toxins, hyperthermia, and maternal use of drugs that have teratogenic effects, such as nicotine, alcohol, antimetabolites, anticonvulsants, narcotics, and cocaine, affect fetal growth (Eichenwald et al., 2017).
- ***Placental factors.*** Placental conditions such as small placenta, infarcted areas, abnormal cord insertions, placenta previa, and thrombosis may affect circulation to the fetus, which becomes more deficient with increasing gestational age (Eichenwald et al., 2017).
- ***Fetal factors.*** Congenital infections such as TORCH infections (*t*oxoplasmosis, *o*ther, *r*ubella, *c*ytomegalovirus, *h*erpes simplex virus), syphilis, congenital malformations, discordant twins, gender of the fetus (females tend to be smaller), chromosomal syndromes (trisomies 13, 18, 21), two-vessel umbilical cord, and inborn errors of metabolism can predispose a fetus to fetal growth disturbances.

Identifying fetuses with IUGR is the first step in detecting common disorders associated with affected newborns. The perinatal history of maternal conditions, early dating of pregnancy by first-trimester ultrasound measurements, antepartum testing (nonstress test, contraction stress test, biophysical profile [see Chapter 16 for discussion of antepartum testing]), Doppler velocimetry of placenta, gestational age assessment, and the physical and neurologic assessment of the newborn are also important (Eichenwald et al., 2017).

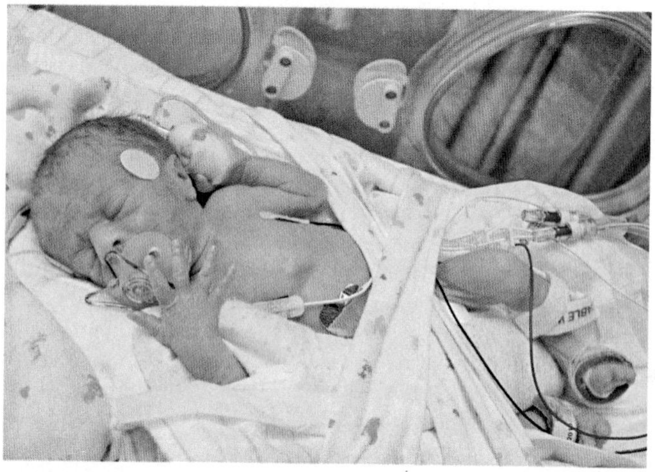

Figure 30–1 Thirty-one-week gestational age, SGA 2-day-old baby girl.

SOURCE: Carol Harrigan, RN, MSN, NNP-BC.

Clinical Tip

In assessing a growth-restricted newborn resulting from unexplained maternal etiology (e.g., hypertension, placental insufficiency), an in utero viral infection may be the answer.

Patterns of IUGR

Intrauterine growth occurs by an increase in both cell number and cell size. If insult occurs early during the critical period of organ development in the fetus, fewer new cells are formed, organs are small, and organ weight is subnormal. In contrast, growth failure that begins later in pregnancy does not affect the total number of cells, only their size. The organs are normal, but their size is diminished.

Symmetric (proportional) IUGR is caused by long-term maternal conditions (such as chronic hypertension, severe malnutrition, chronic intrauterine viral infection, substance abuse [drugs, alcohol, tobacco], anemia) or fetal genetic abnormalities (Hardy, D'Agata, & McGrath, 2016). *Asymmetric (disproportional) IUGR* is associated with an acute compromise of uteroplacental blood flow. Some associated causes are placental infarcts, preeclampsia, and poor weight gain in pregnancy.

Despite growth restriction, physiologic maturity develops according to gestational age. The SGA newborn's chances for survival are better than those of the preterm AGA newborn because of organ maturity, although this newborn still faces many potential difficulties.

Common Complications of the SGA or IUGR Newborn

The complications occurring most frequently in the SGA or IUGR newborn include:

- ***Fetal hypoxia.*** The SGA or IUGR newborn suffers from chronically lower-than-normal oxygen levels in utero, which leaves little reserve to withstand the demands of normal labor and birth. Thus, intrauterine asphyxia, and its potential systemic problems, can occur. Cesarean birth may be necessary because of worsening fetal compromise and intolerance to labor.
- ***Aspiration syndrome.*** In utero hypoxia can cause the fetus to gasp during birth, resulting in aspiration of amniotic fluid into the lower airways. It can also lead to relaxation of the anal sphincter and passage of meconium. This may result in aspiration of the meconium in utero or with the first breaths after birth.
- ***Hypothermia.*** Diminished subcutaneous fat (used for survival in utero), depletion of brown fat in utero, and a large surface area decrease the IUGR newborn's ability to conserve heat. The flexed position assumed by the term SGA newborn diminishes the effect of surface area.
- ***Hypoglycemia.*** An increase in metabolic rate in response to heat loss and poor hepatic glycogen stores causes hypoglycemia. In addition, the newborn is compromised by inadequate supplies of enzymes to activate gluconeogenesis (conversion of nonglucogen sources such as fatty acids and proteins to glucose).
- ***Polycythemia.*** The number of red blood cells is increased (central hematocrit greater than 65%) in the SGA newborn. This finding is considered a physiologic response to in utero chronic hypoxic stress. Polycythemia may contribute to hypoglycemia.

Newborns who have significant IUGR tend to have a poor prognosis, especially when born before 37 weeks' gestation. Factors contributing to poor outcome include:

- ***Congenital malformations.*** Congenital malformations occur in 5% of SGA newborns (Eichenwald et al., 2017). The more severe the IUGR, the greater the chance for malformation as a result of impaired mitotic activity and cellular hypoplasia.
- ***Intrauterine infections.*** When fetuses are exposed to intrauterine infections such as rubella and cytomegalovirus, they are profoundly affected by direct invasion of the brain and other vital organs by the offending virus.
- ***Continued growth difficulties.*** SGA newborns tend to be shorter than newborns of the same gestational age. Asymmetric IUGR newborns can be expected to catch up in weight and approach their inherited growth potential when given an optimal environment.
- ***Cognitive difficulties.*** Often SGA newborns can exhibit subsequent learning disabilities. The disabilities are characterized by hyperactivity, short attention span, and poor fine motor coordination (writing and drawing). Some hearing loss and speech defects also occur.

CLINICAL THERAPY

The goal of medical therapy for SGA/IUGR newborns is early recognition and implementation of the medical management of potential problems.

●○● NURSING MANAGEMENT

For the SGA/IUGR Newborn

Nursing Assessment and Diagnosis

You are responsible for assessing gestational age and identifying signs of potential complications associated with SGA newborns. All body parts of the symmetric IUGR newborn are in proportion (the head does not appear overly large or the length excessive in relation to the other body parts), but they are below normal size for the baby's gestational age. These newborns are generally vigorous.

The asymmetric IUGR newborn appears long, thin, and emaciated, with loss of subcutaneous fat tissue and muscle mass. The baby may have loose skin folds; dry, desquamating skin; and a thin and often meconium-stained cord. The head appears relatively large (although it approaches normal size) because the chest size and abdominal girth are decreased. The baby may have a vigorous cry and appear alert and wide eyed.

Nursing diagnoses that may apply to the SGA/IUGR newborn include those listed in the accompanying *Nursing Care Plan: For the Small-for-Gestational-Age Newborn* and include:

- ***Gas Exchange, Impaired,*** related to aspiration of amniotic fluid or meconium-stained fluid
- ***Injury, Risk for,*** related to decreased glycogen stores and impaired gluconeogenesis
- ***Tissue Perfusion: Peripheral, Ineffective,*** related to polycythemia and increased blood viscosity
- ***Parenting, Risk for Impaired,*** related to prolonged separation of newborn from parents secondary to illness

(NANDA-I © 2017)

Nursing Plan and Implementation

Hospital-Based Nursing Care

Hypoglycemia, the most common metabolic complication of SGA/IUGR, produces such sequelae as central nervous system (CNS) abnormalities and intellectual disability. Conditions such as asphyxia, hyperviscosity, and cold stress may also affect the baby's outcome. Meticulous attention to physiologic parameters is essential for immediate nursing management and reduction of long-term disorders.

Community-Based Nursing Care

The long-term needs of the SGA/IUGR newborn include careful follow-up evaluation of patterns of growth and possible disabilities that may later interfere with learning or motor functioning. Long-term follow-up care is essential for newborns with congenital malformations, congenital infections, and obvious sequelae from physiologic problems. Parents of the SGA/IUGR newborn need support because a positive atmosphere can enhance the baby's growth potential and the child's ultimate outcome.

Evaluation

Expected outcomes of nursing care include:

- The SGA/IUGR newborn is free from respiratory compromise.
- The SGA/IUGR newborn maintains a stable temperature.
- The SGA/IUGR newborn is free from hypoglycemic episodes and maintains glucose homeostasis.
- The SGA/IUGR newborn gains weight and takes breast or formula feedings without developing physiologic distress or fatigue.
- The parents verbalize their concerns about their baby's health problems and understand the rationale behind management of their newborn.

Nursing Care Plan: For The Small-For-Gestational-Age Newborn

1. Nursing Diagnosis: *Gas Exchange, Impaired*, related to amniotic fluid or meconium aspiration (NANDA-I © 2017)

Goal: The newborn's respiratory rate and effort will be within normal limits, with no periods of apnea or evidence of worsening distress.

INTERVENTION	RATIONALE
• Obtain maternal prenatal, labor, and delivery records.	• Provides information and clues of potential fetal stress that may have occurred during the antepartum and intrapartum period. In addition, the delivery record will provide information concerning the newborn's respiratory status at birth, such as the Apgar score.
• Maintain airway patency through judicious airway suctioning.	• Respiratory distress in SGA newborns is due to in utero hypoxia and aspiration of amniotic fluid or meconium-stained fluid.
• Observe for worsening signs of respiratory distress such as generalized cyanosis, increasing retractions, grunting, and nasal flaring (as evidenced by Silverman respiratory index), sustained tachypnea, apnea episodes, inequality of breath sounds, presence of rales and rhonchi.	
• Monitor and maintain adequate axillary body temperature (36.4°–37.2°C [97.5°–99.0°F]) to avoid increased oxygen consumption.	• Temperature elevation may cause metabolic rate and oxygen needs to increase when associated with meconium aspiration.
• Administer supplemental oxygen or other interventions (e.g., high-flow nasal cannula, nasal continuous positive airway pressure [CPAP], intubation with mechanical ventilation) per order for management of symptoms related to respiratory distress. (See Chapter 31 for nursing care and treatment of meconium aspiration and newborn resuscitation.)	• Provides healthcare personnel with information on cardiac and pulmonary status.
• Implement treatment plan for respiratory distress.	
• Monitor glucose levels.	• Respiratory distress increases consumption of glucose.
• **Collaborative:** Obtain blood gas (ABG or CBG) and pulse oximetry parameters, chest x-ray per healthcare provider orders.	
• Monitor newborn's cardiopulmonary status, pulse oximetry readings, and blood gas values.	• Oxygen demands increase with meconium aspiration. Obtaining serial blood gases and chest x-ray will provide medical personnel with baseline information of newborn's respiratory status and effective medical interventions can be initiated.

EXPECTED OUTCOMES: The newborn will maintain adequate respiratory gas exchange as evidenced by respirations of 30–60/min with pulse oximetry and blood gases within normal limits and will show no signs and symptoms of respiratory distress.

2. Nursing Diagnosis: *Thermoregulation, Ineffective*, secondary to decreased subcutaneous fat (NANDA-I © 2017)

Goal: The newborn's temperature will be stable and maintained within normal limits.

INTERVENTION	RATIONALE
• Provide neutral thermal environment (NTE) range for newborn based on postnatal weight.	• NTE charts used for preterm newborn are not reliable for weight of SGA newborn.

(continued)

Nursing Care Plan: For The Small-For-Gestational-Age Newborn *(continued)*

INTERVENTION	RATIONALE
• Place a skin probe to maintain newborn's temperature at 36.0°–36.5°C (96.8°–97.8°F).	• An NTE requires minimal oxygen consumption to maintain a normal core temperature.
• Obtain axillary temperatures and compare with registered skin probe temperature. If discrepancy exists, evaluate potential cause.	• Discrepancies between axillary and skin probe monitor temperatures may be due to mechanical causes or the burning of brown fat.
• Adjust and monitor incubator or radiant warmer to maintain set skin temperature, using the servocontrol mode.	
• Minimize heat losses and prevent cold stress by: 1. Warming and humidifying oxygen without blowing over face to avoid increasing oxygen consumption 2. Keeping skin dry, especially immediately following delivery 3. Keeping incubators, radiant warmers, and open cribs away from windows and cold external walls and out of drafts 4. Avoiding placing newborn on cold surrounding objects such as metal treatment tables, cold x-ray plates, and scales 5. Using radiant warmers during procedures 6. Wrapping the newborn in blankets and covering the head with a hat	• Physical principles of heat loss effects include: 1. Evaporation—loss of heat from newborn by water evaporation from the skin, especially seen immediately after birth 2. Convection—loss of heat from newborn to the surrounding air 3. Conduction—loss of heat from newborn to the surface with which the baby is in direct contact 4. Radiation—loss of heat from newborn to cooler, surrounding surfaces (not in direct contact)
• Observe for consequences of cold stress: Hypoglycemia, hypoxia, lethargy, pallor, metabolic acidosis (for further discussion, see Chapter 31).	• Hypothermia is a potential problem for an SGA newborn because: 1. SGA newborn has decreased brown fat stores available for thermogenesis because they have been used in utero for survival. 2. SGA newborn has poor insulation due to minimal subcutaneous tissues because they have been used in utero for survival.

EXPECTED OUTCOMES: The newborn will not exhibit consequences of hypothermia as evidenced by skin temperature maintenance of 36.0°–36.5°C (96.8°–97.8°F) and axillary temperature maintenance of 36.4°–37.2°C (97.5°–99.0°F).

3. Nursing Diagnosis: ***Injury, Risk for*, related to decreased glycogen stores and impaired gluconeogenesis (NANDA-I © 2017)**

Goal: Newborn will have a normal blood glucose level.

INTERVENTION	RATIONALE
• Monitor blood glucose levels per SGA protocol and report values less than 40 mg/dL. (The exact definition of hypoglycemia varies in the literature; it is best to follow your hospital's guidelines.)	• Combined with depletion of glycogen stores, impaired gluconeogenesis predisposes SGA newborns to profound hypoglycemia within first few hours of life.
• Observe, record, and report symptoms of hypoglycemia: Irritability, cyanosis, lethargy, hypotonia, poor feeding, temperature instability, tremors, jitteriness, seizure activity, and apnea.	• Target glucose screen greater than 40 mg/dL prior to routine feedings (Armentrout, 2015).
• Initiate feeding schedule for SGA newborns after screening for blood glucose level and symptoms of hypoglycemia per hospital protocol.	• Frequent monitoring of heelstick glucose assists in identifying decreased glucose levels.
• Provide glucose intake either through early enteral feeding (before 1 hr) and/or by intravenous (IV) per healthcare provider order.	• Provision of glucose through early feedings (begin within first hour of age) assists in maintaining glucose levels within the defined parameters. Always treat symptomatic hypoglycemia with IV glucose.

(See further discussion of hypoglycemia in Chapter 31.)

EXPECTED OUTCOME: The newborn will not exhibit signs and symptoms of hypoglycemia as evidenced by a euglycemic state and blood glucose greater than 45 mg/dL.

(continued)

Nursing Care Plan: For The Small-For-Gestational-Age Newborn *(continued)*

4. Nursing Diagnosis: *Nutrition, Imbalanced: Less than Body Requirements*, related to increased metabolic needs in the newborn (NANDA-I © 2017)

Goal: Newborn will show positive growth as evidenced by increased serial measurements of weight, length, and occipital–frontal circumference (OFC).

INTERVENTION	RATIONALE
• Assess suck, swallow, and breathe reflexes.	• Sterile water or breast milk may be used to test gag and swallow reflex because it causes fewer pulmonary complications in the presence of gastrointestinal tract abnormalities and/or aspiration of feeding.
• Assess for a nondistended, soft abdomen with active bowel sounds.	• Prevents feeding problems and assists in determining the best method of feeding for baby and feeding readiness.
• Initiate oral feeding per protocol at 1 hr of age; use expressed breast milk, if available, or commercially prepared formula based on hospital protocol.	• SGA newborns require more calories/kg for growth than AGA newborns because of increased metabolic activity and oxygen consumption secondary to increased percentage of body weight made up by visceral organs. • Human milk is preferred for feeding term, preterm, and sick babies.
• Supplement oral feedings with IV intake per orders. • Advance to concentrated formulas that supply more calories in less volume, such as 22 or 24 cal/oz.	• Small, frequent feedings of high-calorie formula are used because of limited gastric capacity and decreased gastric emptying.
• Promote growth by providing caloric intake of 110–140 cal/kg/day in small amounts.	• Growth is evaluated by increase in weight (about 15–30 g/day), length, and OFC.
• Observe, record, and report signs of feeding intolerance or fatigue occurring during breastfeeding or bottle-feedings.	• Decrease in exhaustion is an important consideration in feeding SGA newborn; gavage tube feeding may need to be initiated. • SGA newborns with in utero reversed or absent end-diastolic blood flow are at high risk for developing necrotizing enterocolitis. • Adequate nutritional intake promotes growth and prevents such complications as metabolic catabolism and hypoglycemia.
• Supplement gavage or nipple feedings with IV therapy per healthcare provider order until oral intake is sufficient to support growth.	• Gavage feedings require less energy expenditure on the part of the newborn.
• Establish a nipple-feeding program that is begun slowly and progresses slowly, such as this: Nipple-feed once per day, nipple-feed once per shift, progressing to nipple-feed every other feeding. • Initiate breastfeeding attempts when baby shows readiness.	• Cue-based feedings (based on engagement and hunger cues) allow the baby to become an active participant in the feeding process (Lubbe, 2017).
• Monitor daily weight with anticipation of small amount of weight loss when nipple feedings start.	• Nipple feeding, an active rather than passive intake of nutrition, requires energy expenditure and burning of calories by newborn.
• Weekly OFC and length measurements plotted on growth charts.	• Head circumference is an indicator for brain growth, at the rate of 0.5 cm/week.

EXPECTED OUTCOMES: The newborn will maintain consistent weight gain pattern as evidenced by less than 2%/day weight loss and tolerate enteral feedings.

Nursing Care Plan: For The Small-For-Gestational-Age Newborn *(continued)*

5. Nursing Diagnosis: ***Parenting, Impaired*****, related to lack of knowledge of newborn/infant care and prolonged separation of newborn and parents secondary to illness and prolonged hospitalization (NANDA-I © 2017)**

Goal: Parents will bond with their newborn and have realistic expectations about their baby. Parents are comfortable taking baby home. They are able to demonstrate normal newborn/infant care and assessments of possible complications and know when to return for follow-up.

INTERVENTION	RATIONALE
• Support emotionally the psychologic well-being of family, including positive parent–newborn attachment and sensory stimulation of baby.	• Parent–newborn attachment begins in first few hours or days following birth. SGA newborns may experience prolonged periods of separation from their parents, which necessitates intervention to ensure parent–newborn attachment.
• Include parents in determining newborn's plan of care and encourage their participation. Encourage parents to visit frequently. Provide opportunities for parents to touch, hold, talk to, and care for baby. Determine the type and amount of appropriate sensory stimulation and implement sensory stimulation program.	• Facilitating skin-to-skin care allows the newborn to be placed skin-to-skin with a parent, which contributes to the overall health and growth of the baby as well as providing crucial involvement by the parents (Charpak et al., 2016; Gardner, Voos, & Hills, 2016).
• Prepare for discharge by instructing parents in such areas as feeding techniques, formula preparation, and breastfeeding; bathing, diapering, and hygiene; temperature monitoring; administration of vitamins; care of complications and preventing exposure to infections; normal elimination patterns, normal reflexes and activity, and how to promote normal growth and development without being overprotective; returning for continued medical care; and availability of community resources, if indicated.	• Parents should receive the same postpartum teaching as any parent taking a newborn home. • Parents need to understand the changes to expect in color of the baby's stool and number of bowel movements plus odor from formula-feeding or breastfeeding to avoid unnecessary concern. SGA newborns usually do not require referral to community agencies such as visiting nurse associations unless there is a specific problem requiring assistance.

EXPECTED OUTCOMES: The parent will demonstrate ability to perform basic newborn/infant care tasks as evidenced by exhibiting appropriate attachment behaviors (e.g., talking to and holding baby), feeding and bathing baby.

Care of the Large-for-Gestational-Age Newborn

A newborn whose birth weight is at or above the 90th percentile on the intrauterine growth curve (at any week of gestation) is considered LGA. Some AGA newborns have been incorrectly categorized as LGA because of miscalculation of the date of conception caused by postconceptual bleeding. Careful gestational age assessment is essential to identify the potential needs and problems of these newborns.

The most well-known condition associated with excessive fetal growth is maternal diabetes; however, only a small fraction of large newborns are born to mothers who have diabetes. The cause of the majority of cases of LGA newborns is unclear, but certain factors or situations have been found to correlate with their birth (Eichenwald et al., 2017):

- Diabetes complications affect 3 to 10% of all pregnancies, it is estimated, with 60% of these women having gestational diabetes and 33% having insulin-dependent (type 1) diabetes.
- Macrosomia (increased size) affecting an LGA newborn of a mother with diabetes is directly proportional to high, unstable maternal glucose concentrations.
- Multiparous women have two to three times the number of LGA newborns as primigravidas.
- Male newborns are typically larger than female newborns.
- Babies with erythroblastosis fetalis, *Beckwith-Wiedemann syndrome* (a genetic condition associated with omphalocele, neonatal hypoglycemia, and hyperinsulinemia), or transposition of the great vessels are usually large.

The increase in the LGA newborn's body size is characteristically proportional, although head circumference and body length are in the upper limits of intrauterine growth. The exception to this rule is the baby of the mother with diabetes; such a newborn's body weight is higher, usually greater than 4 kg (8.8 lb), but the baby's length and head circumference may remain in the normal range. Macrosomic newborns have poor motor skills, feeding difficulties, and difficulty regulating behavioral states. LGA newborns tend to be more difficult to arouse to a quiet alert state.

Common Complications of the LGA Newborn

Complications of the LGA newborn can include:

- ***Birth trauma caused by cephalopelvic disproportion (CPD).*** Often LGA newborns have a biparietal diameter greater than 10 cm (4 in.) or are associated with a maternal fundal height measurement greater than 42 cm (16 in.) without the presence of polyhydramnios. Because of their excessive size, there are more breech presentations and shoulder dystocias. These complications may result in asphyxia, fractured clavicles, brachial palsy, facial paralysis, phrenic nerve palsy, depressed skull fractures, cephalohematoma, and intracranial hemorrhage caused by birth trauma.

- *Complications of hypoglycemia, polycythemia, and/or hyperviscosity.* These disorders are most often seen in newborns of mothers with diabetes and newborns with erythroblastosis fetalis or Beckwith-Wiedemann syndrome.

●○● NURSING MANAGEMENT

For the Large-for-Gestational-Age Newborn

The perinatal history, in conjunction with ultrasonic measurement of the fetal skull (biparietal diameter) and gestational age testing, is important in identifying an at-risk LGA newborn. Essential components of the nursing assessment are monitoring vital signs, screening for hypoglycemia and polycythemia, and observing for signs and symptoms related to birth trauma. Address parental concerns about the visual signs of birth trauma and the potential for continuation of the overweight pattern. Help parents learn to arouse and console their newborn and facilitate attachment behaviors. Mothers of LGA newborns with facial or head bruising may be reluctant to interact with their newborns because they fear hurting their babies. The nursing care involved in the complications associated with LGA newborns is similar to the care needed by the baby whose mother has diabetes and is discussed in the next section. See *Case Study: Angelina Newman.*

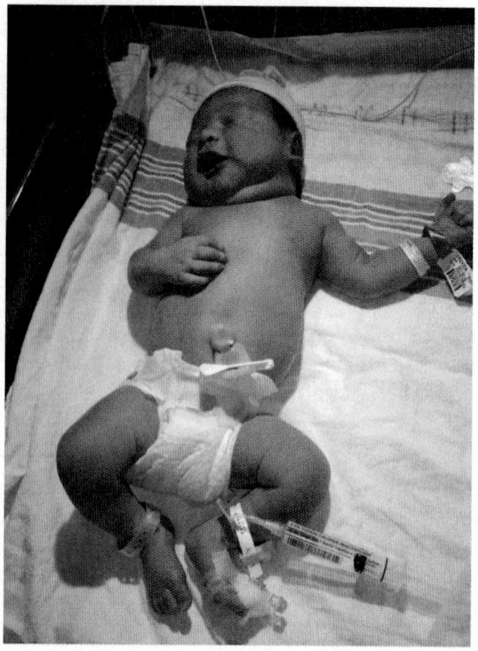

Figure 30–2 Macrosomic newborn of an undiagnosed gestational diabetic mother born at 35 weeks' gestation weighing 3775 g (8.3 lb). Note the peripheral IV in his foot placed to give a D10W bolus.

SOURCE: Carol Harrigan, RN, MSN, NNP-BC.

Care of the Newborn of a Mother with Diabetes

The newborn of a mother with diabetes, also called **infant of a diabetic mother (IDM)**, is considered at risk and requires close observation during the first few hours to the first few days of life. Mothers with severe diabetes or diabetes of long duration associated with vascular complications may give birth to SGA newborns. The typical IDM, when the diabetes is poorly controlled or is gestational, is LGA. The newborn is macrosomic, is ruddy in color, and has excessive adipose (fat) tissue (Figure 30–2). The umbilical cord is thick and the placenta is large. There is a higher incidence of macrosomic newborns born to certain ethnic groups in the United States, including Native Americans, Mexican Americans, African Americans, and Pacific Islanders.

Newborns of mothers with diabetes have decreased total body water, particularly in the extracellular spaces, and are therefore not edematous. Their excessive weight is a result of the increased weight of the visceral organs, cardiomegaly (hypertrophy), and increased body fat. The only organ not affected is the brain.

The excessive fetal growth of these babies is caused by exposure to high levels of maternal glucose, which readily crosses the placenta. The fetus responds to these high glucose levels with increased insulin production and hyperplasia of the pancreatic beta cells. The main action of the insulin is to facilitate the entry of glucose into muscle and fat cells. Once in the cells, glucose is converted to glycogen and stored. Insulin also inhibits the breakdown of fat to free fatty acids, thereby maintaining lipid synthesis; increases the uptake of amino acids; and promotes protein synthesis. Insulin is an important regulator of fetal metabolism and has a "growth hormone" effect that results in increased linear growth. IDMs may be obese as children (Eichenwald et al., 2017).

CASE STUDY: Angelina Newman

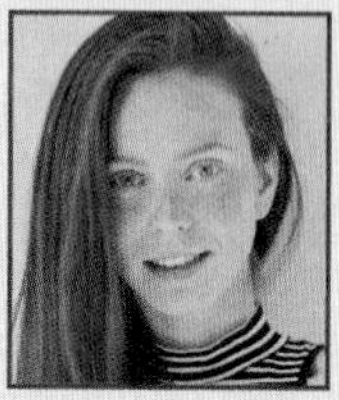

SOURCE: WAYHOME studio/Shutterstock.

Angelina gave birth after 32 hours of labor and felt proud that her baby boy weighed 9 lbs 3 oz. The nurse advises her that the baby needs to eat as soon as possible because his blood sugar is low. This is very surprising to the young couple because they assumed that with a large baby there would be fewer problems. They are very concerned that the baby has some facial bruising and are worried that there could be permanent damage due to birth trauma.

Questions to Ponder

What problems are common in newborns that are large for gestational age? What testing should be performed due to the LGA diagnosis?

Common Complications of the Infant of a Diabetic Mother

Although IDMs are usually large, they have immature physiologic functions and exhibit many of the problems of the preterm (premature) newborn. The complications most often seen in these newborns are:

- ***Hypoglycemia.*** Hypoglycemia is defined as a blood sugar less than 40 mg/dl. It occurs transiently in the immediate neonatal period for all newborns, but occurs sooner, with increased frequency, and to lower levels in IDMs (Eichenwald et al., 2017). Once the fetus is delivered and the maternal glucose supply is severed, the IDM continues to produce high levels of insulin, which deplete the newborn's blood glucose within hours after birth. IDMs also have less ability to release glucagon and catecholamines, which normally stimulate glucagon breakdown and glucose release. The incidence of hypoglycemia in IDMs varies according to the degree of success in controlling the maternal diabetes, the maternal blood sugar level at the time of birth, the length of labor, the class of maternal diabetes, and early versus late feedings of the newborn (Rozance, McGowan, Price-Douglas, et al., 2016). Signs and symptoms of hypoglycemia, which usually present within 1 to 2 hours following delivery, include tremors, cyanosis, apnea, temperature instability, poor feeding, and hypotonia. Seizures may occur in severe cases.
- ***Hypocalcemia.*** Tremors are the obvious clinical sign of hypocalcemia. They may be caused by the IDM's increased incidence of prematurity and by the stresses of difficult pregnancy, labor, and birth. Women with diabetes tend to have decreased serum magnesium levels at term secondary to increased urinary calcium excretion, which causes secondary hypoparathyroidism in their newborns. Other factors may include vitamin D antagonism, which results from elevated cortisol levels, hypophosphatemia from tissue catabolism, and decreased serum magnesium levels. Treatment is rarely necessary.
- ***Hyperbilirubinemia.*** This condition may be seen at 48 to 72 hours after birth. It may be caused by slightly decreased extracellular fluid volume, which increases the hematocrit level. This elevation facilitates an increase in red blood cell breakdown, thereby increasing bilirubin levels. The presence of hepatic immaturity may impair bilirubin conjugation. Enclosed hemorrhages resulting from complicated vaginal birth may also cause hyperbilirubinemia.
- ***Birth trauma.*** Because most newborns of mothers with diabetes are macrosomic, trauma may occur during labor and birth from shoulder dystocia.
- ***Polycythemia.*** Fetal hyperglycemia and hyperinsulinism result in increased oxygen consumption, which can lead to fetal hypoxia. Glycohemoglobin (HbA_{1c}) binds to oxygen, decreasing the oxygen available to the fetal tissues. This tissue hypoxia stimulates increased erythropoietin production, which increases both the hematocrit level and the potential for hyperbilirubinemia. See Chapter 17 for a discussion of HbA_{1c}.
- ***Respiratory distress syndrome (RDS).*** This complication occurs especially in newborns of mothers with diabetes whose diabetes is not well controlled (Eichenwald et al., 2017). Insulin antagonizes the cortisol-induced stimulation of lecithin synthesis that is necessary for lung maturation. Therefore, these newborns may have less mature lungs than expected for their gestational age. There is also a decrease in the phospholipid phosphatidylglycerol (PG), which stabilizes surfactant. The insufficiency of PG increases the incidence of RDS. Therefore, it is important to test for the presence of PG in the amniotic fluid before birth.

  RDS does not appear to be a problem for babies born of mothers with diabetes in White classifications D to F; instead, the stresses of poor uterine blood supply may lead to increased production of steroids, which accelerates lung maturation.
- ***Congenital birth defects.*** These may include congenital heart defects (transposition of the great vessels, ventricular septal defect, patent ductus arteriosus), small left colon syndrome, renal anomalies, neural tube defects, and sacral agenesis (caudal regression) (Eichenwald et al., 2017). Early close control of maternal glucose levels before and during pregnancy decreases the risk of birth defects. See Chapter 17 for more information on maternal diabetes.

CLINICAL THERAPY

Prenatal management is directed toward controlling maternal glucose levels, which minimizes the common complications of IDMs. Because the onset of hypoglycemia occurs between 1 and 3 hours after birth in these newborns (with a spontaneous rise to normal levels by 4 to 6 hours), blood glucose determinations should be done on cord blood or by heelstick hourly during the first 4 hours after birth and then at 4-hour intervals until the risk period (about 48 hours) has passed or per agency protocol (Figure 30–3).

Clinical Tip

When beginning fluids on a newborn of a mother with diabetes, it is sometimes best to start at a higher concentration of dextrose to avoid hypoglycemia episodes.

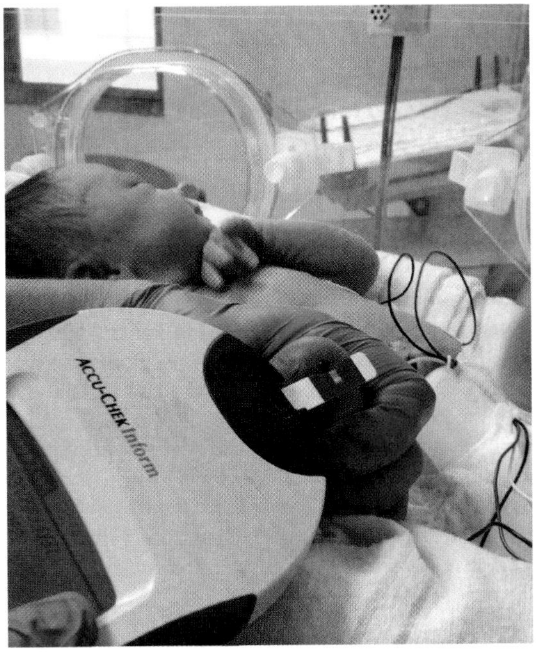

Figure 30–3 Nurse obtaining a bedside blood glucose.

SOURCE: Carol Harrigan, RN, MSN, NNP-BC.

IDMs whose serum glucose level falls below 40 mg/dL should have early feedings with formula or breast milk (colostrum). If normal glucose levels cannot be maintained with oral feedings, an IV infusion of glucose will be necessary. (See Chapter 31 for detailed discussion of hypoglycemia in the newborn.)

SAFETY ALERT!

When infusing either a $D_{10}W$ bolus or a constant infusion, be careful not to administer too much glucose too fast in order to prevent hyperglycemic-induced insulin secretion. When beginning IV fluids on a symptomatic IDM, it is best to start an IV glucose infusion at 4 to 6 mg/kg/min to avoid rebound hypoglycemia (Armentrout, 2015).

●○● NURSING MANAGEMENT

For the Infant of a Diabetic Mother

Nursing Assessment and Diagnosis

Do not be lulled into thinking that a big baby is a mature baby. In almost every case, because of the newborn's large size, the IDM will appear older than gestational age scoring indicates. Consider both the gestational age and whether the baby is AGA or LGA in planning and providing safe care. In caring for the IDM, assess for signs of respiratory distress, hyperbilirubinemia, hypocalcemia, birth trauma, and congenital anomalies.

Nursing diagnoses that may apply to IDMs include:

- *Nutrition, Imbalanced: Less than Body Requirements,* related to increased glucose metabolism secondary to hyperinsulinemia
- *Gas Exchange, Impaired,* related to respiratory distress secondary to impaired production of surfactant
- *Tissue Perfusion: Peripheral, Ineffective,* secondary to polycythemia related to increased synthesis of erythropoietin, chronic intrauterine hypoxia, and increased metabolic rate
- *Tissue Integrity, Impaired,* related to poor maternal metabolic control
- *Family Processes, Interrupted,* related to the illness of the baby

(NANDA-I © 2017)

Nursing Plan and Implementation

Nursing care of the IDM is directed toward early detection and ongoing monitoring of hypoglycemia (by performing glucose tests) and polycythemia (by obtaining central hematocrits), RDS, and hyperbilirubinemia. (These conditions are discussed in Chapter 31.) It is important to also assess for signs of birth trauma and congenital anomalies.

Parent teaching is directed toward preventing macrosomia and the resulting fetal/neonatal problems by instituting early and ongoing diabetic control. Advise parents that with early identification and care, most of these newborns' complications have no significant sequelae.

Evaluation

Expected outcomes of nursing care include:

- The newborn's respiratory distress and metabolic problems are minimized.
- The parents understand the effects of maternal diabetes on the baby's health and preventive steps they can initiate to decrease its impact on subsequent pregnancies.
- The parents verbalize their concerns about their baby's health problems and understand the rationale behind management of their newborn.

Care of the Postterm Newborn

The **postterm newborn** is any newborn born after 42 completed weeks of gestation. Postterm or prolonged pregnancy occurs in approximately 6% of all pregnancies (Eichenwald et al., 2017). The cause of postterm pregnancy is not completely understood, but several factors are known to be associated with it. (See Chapter 24 for a discussion of maternal factors.) Many pregnancies classified as prolonged are thought to be a result of inaccurate estimates of date of birth (EDB). Postterm pregnancy is more common in Australian, Greek, and Italian ethnic groups.

Most babies born as a result of prolonged pregnancy are of normal size and health; some continue growing and are over 4000 g (8.8 lb) at birth, which supports the contention that the postterm fetus can remain well nourished. Potential intrapartum problems for these healthy but large fetuses are CPD and shoulder dystocia (see Chapter 24 for discussion of the necessary assessments and interventions).

Common Complications of the Newborn with Postmaturity Syndrome

The term **postmaturity** applies only to the newborn that is born after 42 completed weeks of gestation and also demonstrates characteristics of *postmaturity syndrome.* Postterm newborns have begun to lose weight but usually have normal length and head circumference (ACOG, 2016; Eichenwald et al., 2017).

The characteristics of postmature newborns are primarily caused by a combination of advanced gestational age, placental aging and decreased placental function, and continued exposure to amniotic fluid. The truly postmature newborn is at high risk for morbidity and has a mortality rate two to three times greater than that of term newborns. Although today the percentages are extremely low, the majority of postmature fetal deaths occur during labor because the fetus uses up necessary body reserves.

The following are common disorders of the postmature newborn and characteristics of *postmaturity syndrome*:

- *Hypoglycemia,* from nutritional deprivation and depleted glycogen stores
- *Meconium aspiration* in response to in utero hypoxia as the stress of labor begins. The presence of oligohydramnios increases the danger of aspirating thick meconium. Severe meconium aspiration syndrome increases the baby's chance of developing persistent pulmonary hypertension, pneumothorax, and chemical pneumonitis.
- *Polycythemia* caused by increased production of red blood cells (RBCs) in response to hypoxia (impaired oxygenation)
- *Congenital anomalies* of unknown cause
- *Seizure* activity because of hypoxic insult
- *Cold stress* because of loss or poor development of subcutaneous fat.

CLINICAL THERAPY

The aim of antenatal management is to differentiate the fetus with postmaturity syndrome from the fetus who is large at birth, well nourished, alert, and tolerating the prolonged (postterm) pregnancy. Antenatal tests that are done to evaluate fetal status and determine obstetric management and their use in postterm pregnancy are discussed in more depth in Chapters 17 and 23. If the amniotic fluid is meconium stained, an amnioinfusion may be done during labor. This procedure dilutes the meconium by directly infusing either normal saline or Ringer lactate into the uterus, decreasing the risk of meconium aspiration syndrome. (For detailed discussion of clinical management and care of the newborn at risk for meconium aspiration, see Chapter 31.)

Hypoglycemia is monitored by serial glucose determinations per agency protocols. The baby may be placed on glucose infusions or given early feedings if respiratory distress is not present, but these measures must be instituted with caution because of the frequency of asphyxia in the first 24 hours. Postmature newborns are often voracious eaters.

For the SGA newborn who is postmature, peripheral and central hematocrits are tested to determine the presence of polycythemia. Fluid resuscitation can be initiated. In extreme cases a partial exchange transfusion may be necessary to prevent polycythemia and adverse sequelae such as hyperviscosity. Oxygen is provided for respiratory distress. In addition, temperature instability and excessive loss of heat can result from decreased liver glycogen stores. (See Chapter 31 for thermoregulation techniques.)

●○● NURSING MANAGEMENT

For the Newborn with Postmaturity Syndrome

Nursing Assessment and Diagnosis

The newborn with postmaturity syndrome appears alert. This wide-eyed, alert appearance is not necessarily a positive sign because it may indicate chronic intrauterine hypoxia. The newborn typically has dry, cracking, parchmentlike skin without vernix or lanugo (Figure 30–4). Fingernails are long, and scalp hair is profuse. The newborn's body appears long and thin. The wasting involves depletion of previously stored subcutaneous tissue, causing the skin to be loose. Fat layers are almost nonexistent.

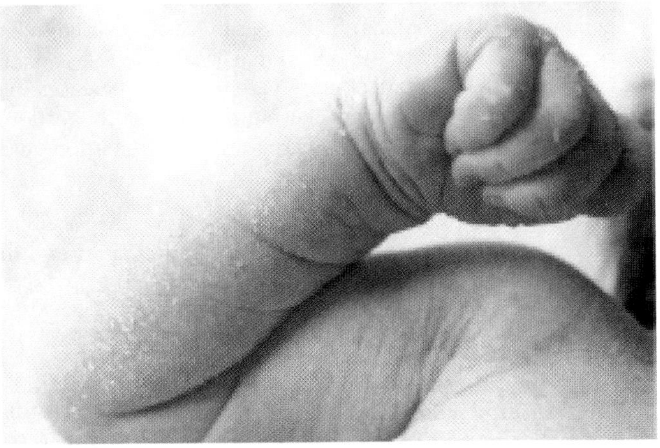

Figure 30–4 The skin of the postterm newborn exhibits deep cracking and peeling of skin.

SOURCE: Paolo Koch/Science Source.

Postmature newborns frequently have meconium staining, which colors the nails, skin, and umbilical cord. The varying shades (yellow to green) of meconium staining can give some clue as to whether the expulsion of meconium in utero was a recent or a chronic problem. Green coloring indicates a more recent event.

Nursing diagnoses that may apply to the postmature newborn include:

- ***Hypothermia*** related to decreased liver glycogen and brown fat stores
- ***Nutrition, Imbalanced: Less Than Body Requirements,*** related to increased use of glucose secondary to in utero stress and decreased placenta perfusion
- ***Gas Exchange, Impaired,*** related to airway obstruction from meconium aspiration
- ***Tissue Perfusion: Peripheral, Ineffective,*** related to increased blood viscosity caused by polycythemia

(NANDA-I © 2017)

Nursing Plan and Implementation

Nursing care of the postmature newborn is directed toward early detection and ongoing monitoring of hypothermia (by regulating thermoregulation), hypoglycemia (by performing glucose tests), polycythemia (by obtaining central hematocrits), and meconium aspiration and RDS (by monitoring cardiopulmonary status). (These conditions are discussed in Chapter 31.)

Encourage parents to express their feelings and fears about the newborn's condition and potential long-term problems. Give careful explanations of procedures, include the parents in the development of care plans for their baby, and encourage follow-up care as needed.

Evaluation

Expected outcomes of nursing care include:

- The postterm newborn establishes effective respiratory function.
- The postmature baby is free of metabolic alterations (hypoglycemia) and maintains a stable temperature.

Care of the Preterm (Premature) Newborn

A preterm newborn is any baby born too early, before 37 weeks of pregnancy have been completed (Figure 30–5). In 2016, preterm birth affected about 1 of every 10 neonates born in the United States. Preterm birth rates decreased overall from 2007 to 2014 (March of Dimes, 2016). Research shows that this decline is due, in part, to declines in the number of births to teens and young mothers (Centers for Disease Control and Prevention [CDC], 2017b). However, the preterm birth rate rose for the second straight year in 2016. Additionally, racial and ethnic differences in preterm birth rates remain. For example, in 2016, the rate of preterm birth among African American women was 14%; among Caucasian American women the rate was 9%. See *Professionalism in Practice: S.252 – PREEMIE Reauthorization Act (2013–2014).*

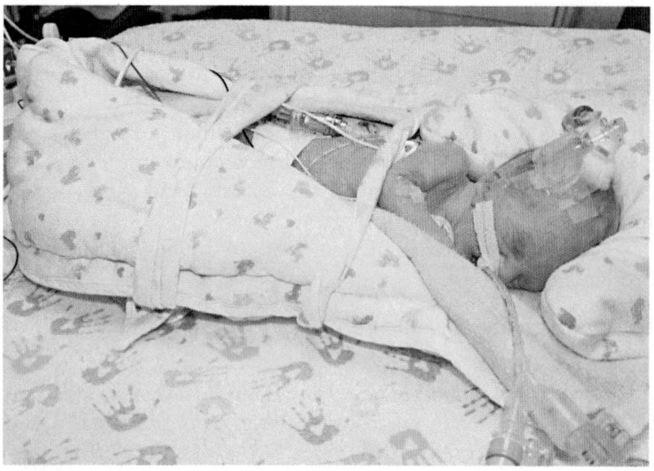

Figure 30-5 **A 6-day-old, 26-week gestational age, 960-g preterm newborn.**

SOURCE: Carol Harrigan, RN, MSN, NNP-BC.

The major problem of the preterm newborn is the variable immaturity of all systems. The degree of immaturity depends on the length of gestation. Because of immaturity, the premature newborn is ill equipped to smoothly traverse the same complex, interconnected pathways from intrauterine to extrauterine life. See *Genetic Facts: Gestational Duration and Preterm Birth.*

Genetic Facts Gestational Duration and Preterm Birth

Genes have been identified that are associated with preterm newborns. Three of the genes (EBF1, EEFSEC, AGTR2) are associated with gestational duration and spontaneous preterm birth and three of the genes (WNT4, ADCY5, RAP2C) are associated with gestational duration but not spontaneous preterm birth (Zang et al., 2017).

Professionalism in Practice S.252 – PREEMIE Reauthorization Act (2013–2014)

PREEMIE Act Reauthorization – Prematurity Research Expansion and Education for Mothers who Deliver Infants Early Reauthorization Act or the PREEMIE Reauthorization Act.

(Sec. 102). Amends the Prematurity Research Expansion and Education for Mothers who Deliver Infants Early Act to revise and reauthorize requirements for research on prematurity and preterm births.

(Sec. 103). Requires the Director of the Office for the Advancement of Telehealth to give preference in awarding grants to an eligible entity that proposes to use the grant funds to develop plans for, or to establish, telehealth networks that provide prenatal care for high-risk pregnancies.

Includes as activities under such projects programs to test and evaluate various strategies to provide information and education to health care providers and the public on: (1) the core risk factors for preterm labor and delivery, (2) medically indicated deliveries before full term, (3) the importance of preconception and prenatal care, (4) treatments and outcomes for premature infants, (5) meeting the informational needs of families during the stay of an infant in a neonatal intensive care unit, and (6) utilization of evidence-based strategies to prevent birth injuries.

Authorizes as additional activities under such projects the establishment of programs to increase the availability, awareness, and use of pregnancy and post-term information services that provide evidence-based, clinical information through counselors, community outreach efforts, electronic or telephonic communication, or other appropriate means regarding causes associated with prematurity, birth defects, or health risks to a post-term infant.

Source: S.252 – PREEMIE Reauthorization Act. (2013–2014). Retrieved from https://www.congress.gov/bill/113th-congress/senate-bill/252

Alteration in Respiratory and Cardiac Physiology

The preterm newborn is at risk for respiratory problems because of these critical factors in the development of respiratory distress:

1. The preterm newborn is unable to produce adequate amounts of surfactant. (See Chapter 26 for discussion of respiratory adaptation and development.) Inadequate surfactant lessens compliance (ability of the lung to fill with air easily), thereby increasing the inspiratory pressure needed to expand the lungs with air. This progressive atelectasis leads to an inability to develop a functional residual capacity (FRC), causing an ineffective exchange of oxygen and carbon dioxide. As a result, the baby becomes hypoxic, pulmonary blood flow is inefficient, and the preterm newborn's available energy is depleted.
2. The muscular coat of pulmonary blood vessels is incompletely developed. Consequently, the pulmonary arterioles do not constrict as well in response to decreased oxygen levels. This lowered pulmonary vascular resistance leads to left-to-right shunting of blood through the ductus arteriosus, which increases the blood flow back into the lungs.
3. Normally the ductus arteriosus responds to increasing oxygen levels and prostaglandin E levels by vasoconstriction; in the preterm newborn, who is more susceptible to hypoxia, the ductus may remain open. A patent ductus increases the blood volume to the lungs, causing pulmonary congestion, increased respiratory effort, carbon dioxide retention, and bounding femoral pulses.

The common complications of the cardiopulmonary system in preterm newborns are discussed later in this chapter and in Chapter 31.

Alteration in Thermoregulation

Heat loss is a major problem in preterm newborns. Two factors limiting heat production, however, are the decreased availability of glycogen in the liver and the limited amount of brown fat available for heat production, which appear in the third trimester. Because the muscle mass is small in preterm babies and muscular activity is diminished (they are unable to shiver), heat production is further limited.

Five physiologic and anatomic factors increase heat loss in the preterm newborn:

1. The preterm baby has a higher ratio of body surface to body weight. This means that the baby's ability to produce heat (based on body weight) is much less than the potential for losing heat (based on surface area). The loss of heat in a preterm newborn weighing 1500 g (3.3 lb) is five times greater per unit of body weight than in an adult.
2. The preterm baby has very little subcutaneous fat, which is the human body's insulation. Without adequate insulation, heat is easily conducted from the core of the body (warmer temperature) to the surface of the body (cooler temperature). Heat is lost from the body as the blood vessels, which lie close to the skin surface in the preterm newborn, transport blood from the body core to the subcutaneous tissues.
3. The preterm newborn has thinner, more permeable skin than the term baby. This increased permeability contributes to a greater insensible water loss as well as to heat loss.
4. Flexion of the extremities decreases the amount of surface area exposed to the environment. Extension increases the surface area exposed to the environment and thus increases heat loss. The gestational age of the newborn influences the amount of flexion, from completely hypotonic and extended at 28 weeks to strong flexion displayed by 36 weeks.
5. The preterm baby has a decreased ability to vasoconstrict superficial blood vessels and conserve heat in the body core.

In summary, gestational age is directly proportional to the ability to maintain thermoregulation; thus, the more preterm the newborn, the less able the baby is to maintain heat balance. Preventing heat loss by providing a neutral thermal environment using a servocontrol skin probe is one of the most important considerations in nursing management of the preterm baby. Other nursing interventions assisting in the thermoregulation of the preterm newborn include increasing the delivery room temperature, loosely covering the baby with polyethylene wrap, placing the baby in a plastic bag from feet to shoulders, and placing the baby on a chemical mattress. Cold stress, with its accompanying severe complications, can be prevented (see *Care of the Newborn with Cold Stress* in Chapter 31).

Alteration in Gastrointestinal Physiology

Maturation of the digestive and absorptive process is more variable, however, and occurs later in gestation. As a result of GI immaturity, the preterm newborn has the following ingestion, digestion, and absorption problems (Ditzenberger, 2015):

- A marked danger of aspiration and its associated complications because of the baby's poorly developed gag reflex, incompetent esophageal cardiac sphincter, and poor sucking and swallowing reflexes.
- Difficulty in meeting high caloric and fluid needs for growth because of small stomach capacity.
- Limited ability to convert certain essential amino acids to nonessential amino acids. Certain amino acids, such as histidine, taurine, and cysteine, are essential to the preterm newborn but not to the term newborn.
- Inability to handle the increased osmolarity of formula protein because of kidney immaturity. The preterm newborn requires a higher concentration of whey protein than of casein.
- Difficulty absorbing saturated fats because of decreased bile salts and pancreatic lipase. Severe illness of the newborn may also prevent intake of adequate nutrients.
- Difficulty with lactose digestion initially because processes may not be fully functional during the first few days of a preterm newborn's life. The preterm newborn can digest and absorb most simple sugars.
- Deficiency of calcium and phosphorus may exist because two-thirds of these minerals are deposited in the last trimester. Rickets and significant bone demineralization caused by deficiency of calcium and phosphorus, which are deposited primarily in the last trimester, are also problems.
- Increased basal metabolic rate and increased oxygen requirements caused by fatigue associated with sucking.
- Feeding intolerance and necrotizing enterocolitis (NEC) as a result of diminished blood flow and tissue perfusion to the intestinal tract because of a combination of contributing factors including prematurity, formula feeding, bacterial colonization, and hypoemia/ischemia events (Bradshaw, 2015).

Alteration in Hepatic and Hematologic Physiology

Immaturity of the preterm newborn's liver predisposes the baby to several problems:

- After birth, the glycogen stores in the liver are rapidly used for energy. Glycogen deposits are affected by asphyxia in utero and after birth by both asphyxia and cold stress. The baby born preterm has decreased glycogen stores at birth and frequently experiences stress, which rapidly uses up these limited stores. Therefore, the preterm newborn is at high risk for hypoglycemia and its complications.
- Iron is also stored in the liver, especially during the last trimester of pregnancy. Therefore, the preterm newborn is born with low iron stores. If subject to hemorrhage, rapid growth, and excessive blood sampling, the preterm baby is likely to become iron depleted more quickly than the term newborn. Many preterm babies require transfusions of packed cells to treat symptomatic anemia as a consequence of frequent blood sampling. An association between NEC and RBC transfusion has been a recent subject of major debate (Patel et al., 2016). As the premature baby grows and convalesces, oral iron supplementation may be started, as well as doses of erythropoietin, to enhance RBC production.
- Due to the relatively short half-life of the fetal hemoglobin molecule, bilirubin, the end-product of its breakdown, accumulates at a faster rate in the preterm newborn. It is within the liver that the bilirubin is bound to albumin and converted, or conjugated, to a more excretable form. However, conjugation of bilirubin in the liver is impaired in the preterm newborn. Thus, bilirubin levels increase more rapidly and to a higher level than in the full-term baby. Early clinical assessment of jaundice associated with indirect hyperbilirubinemia is more difficult in preterm newborns because they lack subcutaneous fat. All preterm newborns need to be monitored for development of jaundice. Clinical jaundice is evident usually in the face and progresses in a cephalocaudal manner. Preterm newborns with hyperbilirubinemia are often treated with phototherapy (Figure 30–6). (For a further discussion of the newborn with jaundice, see Chapter 31.)

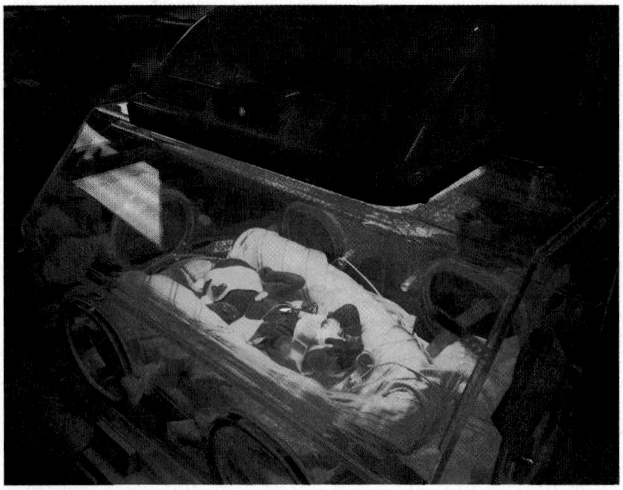

Figure 30–6 **A preterm, 4-day-old newborn, being treated with phototherapy for hyperbilirubinemia.**

SOURCE: Carol Harrigan, RN, MSN, NNP-BC.

- The normal cord hemoglobin in a newborn of 34 weeks' gestation is approximately 16.8 g/dL, and total blood volume ranges from 80 mL/kg to 100 mL/kg (Blackburn, 2018). Because of the small total blood volume, any blood loss is highly significant to the preterm newborn. Therefore, judicious blood draws and assessments of hemoglobin values are performed during the first several weeks of life.

Alteration in Renal Physiology

Specific characteristics of the preterm newborn that pose clinical problems in the management of fluid and electrolyte balance include:

- The glomerular filtration rate (GFR) is directly related to lower gestational age and increases steadily after 34 weeks postconceptual age (PCA). The GFR is also decreased in the presence of diseases or conditions that decrease the renal blood flow and perfusion, such as severe respiratory distress, hypotension, and asphyxia. Preterm newborns usually have some urine output during the first 24 hours of life. By day 3, urine output should be approximately 1 to 3 mL/kg/hr. A low systolic blood pressure can reflect any diseases that decrease cardiac output and affect renal blood flow. Systolic blood pressure (BP) varies with gestational age and PCA. See Table 30–1.

Clinical Tip

A gradual decline in urine may be associated with a drop in the newborn's blood pressure.

- The preterm newborn's kidneys are limited in their ability to concentrate urine or to excrete excess amounts of fluid because of a blunted response to antidiuretic hormone (ADH). This means that if excess fluid is administered, the baby is at risk for fluid retention and overhydration. If too little is administered, the baby will become dehydrated because of the inability to retain adequate fluid.
- The preterm newborn's kidneys begin excreting glucose (glycosuria) at a lower serum glucose level than that of the term newborn. Therefore, glycosuria with hyperglycemia can lead to osmotic diuresis and polyuria.
- The kidneys' buffering capacity is reduced, predisposing the newborn to metabolic acidosis. Bicarbonate is excreted at a lower serum level, and acid is excreted more slowly. Therefore, after periods of hypoxia or insult, the preterm baby's kidneys require a longer time to excrete the lactic acid that accumulates.
- The immaturity of the renal system affects the preterm newborn's ability to excrete drugs. Because excretion time is longer, many drugs are given over longer intervals (i.e., every 24 hours instead of every 12 hours). Urine output must be carefully monitored when the baby is receiving nephrotoxic drugs such as gentamicin and vancomycin. In the event that urine output is poor, drugs can become toxic in the baby much more quickly than in the adult.

TABLE 30–1 Systolic Blood Pressure Guidelines

	DAY OF LIFE #1		POSTCONCEPTUAL AGE		
GESTATIONAL AGE	RANGE SYSTOLIC BP	AVERAGE SYSTOLIC BP	WEEKS	RANGE SYSTOLIC BP	AVERAGE SYSTOLIC BP
23	23–55	39	24	35–67	48
24	26–58	42	26	38–70	52
26	29–61	45	28	41–73	56
28	32–65	48	30	45–77	60
30	35–68	51	32	49–81	64
32	38–71	54	34	52–84	68
34	41–75	57	36	56–88	72
36	44–78	60	38	60–91	76
38	47–81	63	40	63–94	80
40	51–85	67	42	66–97	83
42	54–88	71	44	70–100	87
			46	72–103	90

SOURCE: Data courtesy of NICU, Cardon Children's Hospital at Banner Desert Medical Center, Mesa, AZ, 2008.

Alteration in Immunologic Physiology

The preterm newborn has an increased susceptibility to infections acquired in utero that may have precipitated preterm labor and birth. However, all preterm newborns have immature specific and nonspecific immunity.

In utero the fetus receives passive immunity against a variety of infections from maternal IgG immunoglobulins, which cross the placenta. Most passive immunity is acquired in the last trimester of pregnancy; therefore, the preterm newborn has few antibodies at birth. The preterm newborn has less protection against infection and that protection becomes depleted earlier than in a full-term newborn. This may be a contributing factor in the higher incidence of recurrent bacterial infection during the first year of life as well as in the immediate neonatal period. (See *Care of the Newborn with Infection* in Chapter 31.)

The other immunoglobulin significant for the preterm newborn is secretory IgA, which does not cross the placenta but is found in breast milk. Breast milk's secretory IgA provides immunity to the mucosal surfaces of the GI tract, protecting the newborn from enteric infections such as those caused by *Escherichia coli* and *Shigella*.

In very small babies the skin is easily excoriated, and this factor, coupled with many invasive procedures, places the newborn at great risk for nosocomial infections. It is vital to use good hand hygiene techniques in the care of these babies to prevent unnecessary infection.

SAFETY ALERT!

The sudden onset of apnea and bradycardia, coupled with metabolic acidosis in an otherwise healthy, growing premature newborn, may be suggestive of bacterial sepsis, especially if there is a central line present.

Alteration in Neurologic Physiology

Because the period of most rapid brain growth and development occurs during the third trimester of pregnancy, the closer to term a baby is born, the better the neurologic prognosis. A common interruption of neurologic development in the preterm newborn is caused by intraventricular hemorrhage (IVH) and intracranial hemorrhage (ICH). Posthemorrhage hydrocephalus may develop as a consequence of an IVH caused by the obstruction at the cerebral aqueduct (Parsons, Seay, & Jacobson, 2016).

Alteration in Reactivity Periods and Behavioral States

The newborn's response to extrauterine life is characterized by two periods of reactivity (see Chapter 26). However, the preterm newborn's periods of reactivity are delayed. In the very ill newborn, these periods of reactivity may not be observed at all because the baby may be hypotonic and unreactive for several days after birth.

In general, stable preterm newborns do not demonstrate the same behavioral states as term newborns. Preterm babies tend to be more disorganized in their sleep–wake cycles and are unable to attend as well to the human face and objects in the environment. Neurologically, their responses (sucking, muscle tone, states of arousal) are weaker than full-term babies' responses.

Clinical Tip

After observing a newborn's pattern of behavior and responses, especially the sleep–wake states, use the time when the baby is alert and best able to attend to help parents learn about and provide newborn care and form a positive attachment with their child.

Management of Nutrition and Fluid Requirements

Early feedings are extremely valuable for the premature newborn in maintaining normal metabolism and lowering the possibility of such complications as hypoglycemia, hyperbilirubinemia, hyperkalemia, and osteopenia of prematurity and other digestive system problems.

NUTRITIONAL REQUIREMENTS

Oral (enteral) caloric intake necessary for growth in a healthy preterm newborn is 95 to 130 kcal/kg/day (Blackburn, 2018). Early feedings are associated with improved glucose homeostasis, immune functions, and weight gain patterns, ultimately resulting in early discharge home. Human milk is preferred for feeding the preterm newborn with significant benefits for the mother, baby, family, and society (American Academy of Pediatrics [AAP] & American College of Obstetricians and Gynecologists [ACOG], 2017).

Human donor milk from a milk bank is an available option for the high-risk newborn whose mother is unable to produce sufficient amounts of milk. Donor milk is provided by women who go through a screening process that includes blood tests for infections like hepatitis and HIV. All donated milk is then pasteurized, and banks routinely culture the pasteurized milk to look for bacterial contamination (Abrams, Landers, Noble, et al., 2017). The Human Milk Banking Association of North America (HMBANA) supervises many donor breast milk banks, which certify the quality of the milk (Zaichkin, Weiner, & Loren, 2017).

To meet the high caloric needs of the growing premature baby, breast milk may be fortified or special preterm formulas may be used. In addition to a higher calorie and protein formula, preterm newborns should receive supplemental multivitamins, including vitamins A, D, and E, iron, and trace minerals. However, the late preterm baby who is breastfeeding should also receive routine iron supplementation (Academy of Breastfeeding Medicine [ABM], 2016). Preterm newborns should receive 2 mg/kg/day of elemental iron upon discharge from the hospital (AAP & ACOG, 2017). The current recommendation for vitamin D for preterm babies is 400 to 1000 international units/kg/day (AAP & ACOG, 2017). A diet high in polyunsaturated fats (which preterm babies tolerate best) increases the requirement for vitamin E. Preterm newborns fed iron-fortified formulas have higher red cell hemolysis and lower vitamin E concentrations and thus require additional vitamin E. Preterm formulas also need to contain medium-chain triglycerides (MCTs) and additional amino acids such as cysteine, as well as calcium, phosphorus, and vitamin D supplements to increase mineralization of bones. Rickets and significant bone demineralization have been documented in very-low-birth-weight newborns and otherwise healthy preterm babies.

Whether breast milk or formula is used, feeding protocols are established based on the baby's weight and estimated stomach capacity. Nutritional intake is considered adequate when there is consistent weight gain of 20 to 30 g/day. Initially, no weight gain may be noted for several days, but total weight loss should not exceed 15% of the total birth weight or more than 1 to 2% per day. Some institutions add the criteria of head circumference growth and increase in body length of 1 cm (0.4 in.) per week, once the newborn is stable.

METHODS OF FEEDING

The preterm newborn is fed by various methods depending on the baby's gestational age, health and physical condition, and neurologic status. The three most common oral feeding methods are bottle, breast, and gavage.

Bottle-Feeding. Preterm newborns who have a coordinated as well as rhythmic suck–swallow–breathing pattern are usually between 35 and 36 weeks' postconception age and may be fed by bottle. Oral readiness to feed is best described by the following engagement and hunger cues (Lubbe, 2017):

- Bringing hands to the mouth
- Being alert
- Exhibiting fussiness
- Sucking on fingers or pacifier
- Exhibiting rooting behavior
- Showing relaxed facial expression and good tone.

To avoid excessive expenditure of energy, a soft, yellow, single-hole nipple is usually used (milk flow is less rapid). The baby is fed in a semisitting position and burped gently after each 0.5 to 1 oz. The feeding should take no longer than 15 to 20 minutes (nippling requires more energy than other methods). Premature newborns who are progressing from gavage feedings to bottle-feeding should be assessed for feeding readiness and started with one session of bottle-feeding a day. The number of times a day a bottle is offered should be increased slowly until the baby tolerates all feedings from a bottle (Figure 30–7).

Sucking may be affected by age, asphyxia, sepsis, intraventricular hemorrhage, or other neurologic insult. Before initiating nipple feeding, the nurse observes for signs of stress, such as tachypnea (more than 60 respirations per minute), respiratory distress, or hypothermia, which may increase the risk of aspiration. During the feeding the nurse observes the newborn for signs of feeding difficulty (tachypnea, decrease in oxygen saturation levels, bradycardia, lethargy, uncoordinated suck and swallow). Difficulty in bottle-feeding is often associated with a milk bolus that is too large for the baby's oral cavity, which can lead to aspiration. Demand feeding protocols, based on the baby's hunger cues, should be considered for a growing premature newborn only when there is sufficient caloric intake to promote consistent weight gain (Lubbe, 2017). See Table 30–2.

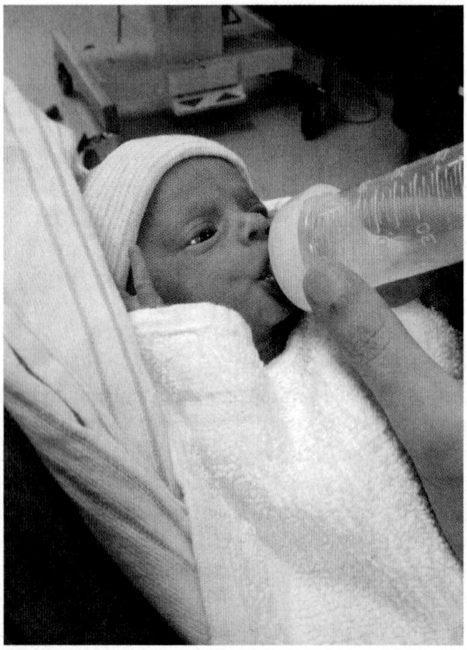

Figure 30–7 Mother bottle-feeding her premature newborn with expressed breast milk.

SOURCE: Carol Harrigan, RN, MSN, NNP-BC.

Clinical Tip

The more preterm the newborn is at birth, the longer it will take to reach the maturational state required to be successful at oral feedings.

Breastfeeding. Mothers who wish to breastfeed their preterm newborns are given the opportunity to put the baby to the breast as soon as the baby has demonstrated a coordinated suck and swallow reflex, is showing consistent weight gain, and can control body temperature outside of the incubator, regardless of weight. Preterm newborns tolerate breastfeeding with higher transcutaneous oxygen pressures and better maintenance of body temperature than during bottle-feeding. Besides breast milk's many benefits for the newborn, it allows the mother to contribute actively to the baby's well-being (Figure 30–8). The nurse should encourage mothers to breastfeed if they choose to do so. It is important for the nurse to be aware of the advantages of breastfeeding, as well as the possible disadvantages of breast milk as the sole source of food for the preterm newborn (see Chapter 29).

By initiating skin-to-skin holding of premature newborns in the early intensive care phase, mothers can significantly increase milk volume, thereby overcoming lactation problems. Many mothers of preterm newborns seem to find that the football hold (refer to Figure 29–7) is a convenient position for breastfeeding preterm babies. Feeding may take up to 45 minutes, and babies should be burped as they alternate breasts. Length of feeding time must be monitored so that the preterm newborn does not expend too many calories.

The nurse should coordinate a flexible feeding schedule so that babies can nurse during alert times and be allowed to set their own pace. Feedings should be on demand, but a maximum number of hours between feedings should be set. A similar regimen should be used for the baby who is progressing from gavage feeding to breastfeeding. The mother begins with one feeding at the breast and then gradually increases the number of times during the day that the baby breastfeeds. Even if the baby cannot be put to the breast, mothers can pump their breasts, and the breast milk can be given via gavage. A double-pumping system produces higher levels of prolactin than sequential pumping of the breasts. When breastfeeding is not possible because the baby is too small or too weak to suck at the breast, an option for the mother may be to express her breast milk into a cup. The milk touches the baby's lips and is lapped by the protruding motions of the tongue.

Gavage Feeding. The gavage feeding method is used with preterm newborns (less than 34 weeks' gestation) who lack or have a poorly coordinated suck and swallow reflex or are ill and ventilator dependent. Gavage feeding may be used as an adjunct to nipple feeding if the newborn tires easily or as an alternative if the baby is losing weight because of the energy expenditure required

TABLE 30–2 Cue-Based Feeding Readiness Scales

Feeding								
Readiness								
Quality								
Caregiver								
Time								
Quantity								
Nipple (circle breast or write nipple color)	Breast Nipple color	Breast Nipple color	Breast Nipple color	Breast Nipple color	Breast Nipple color	Breast Nipple color	Breast Nipple color	Breast Nipple color
Initial								

Readiness	
Breastfeed (Bottle)	
SCORE	DESCRIPTION
1	Drowsy, alert, or fussy prior to care. Rooting and/or hands to mouth/takes pacifier. Good tone.
2	Drowsy or alert once handled. Some rooting or takes pacifier. Adequate tone.
Breastfeed (No bottle)	
3	Briefly alert with care. No hunger behaviors. No change in tone.
4	Sleeping throughout care. No hunger cues. No change in tone.
Gavage only	
5	Needs increased O_2 with care. Apnea/bradycardia (A/B) with care. Tachypnea over baseline with care.
Caregiver Techniques	
SCORE	DESCRIPTION
A	Side-lying position
B	External pacing
C	Adding or increasing O_2 during feed
D	Imposed breaks
E	Stimulation for/recovery from A/B
F	Frequent burping
G	Nipple change
H	Other (specify)
Quality Breastfeeding	
SCORE	DESCRIPTION
1	Latched well with a strong coordinated suck for >15 min.
2	Latched well with a strong coordinated suck initially, but fatigues with progression. Active suck for 8–15 min.
3	Difficulty maintaining a strong, consistent latch. May be able to nurse intermittently but active for only <15 min.
4	Latch is weak/inconsistent, with a frequent need to relatch. Limited effort with inconsistent pattern. May be considered nonnutritional breastfeeding (NNBF).
5	Unable to latch to breast and achieve suck–swallow–breathe pattern. May have difficulty arousing to a state conducive to breastfeeding. Could result in frequent or significant A/Bs and/or tachypnea significantly above baseline with feeding.
Quality Bottle	
SCORE	DESCRIPTION
1	Nipples with a strong coordinated suck throughout feed.
2	Nipples with a strong coordinated suck initially, but fatigues with progression.
3	Nipples with consistent suck, but difficulty coordinating swallow; some loss of liquid or difficulty pacing. Benefits from external pacing.
4	Nipples with a weak/inconsistent suck. Little to no rhythm. May require some rest breaks.
5	Disorganized; unable to coordinate suck–swallow–breathe pattern. May result in frequent or significant A/Bs or large amounts of liquid loss and or tachypnea significantly above baseline with feeding.
6	Dysfunctional; abnormal or deviant oral motor patterns evidenced by inability to extract fluid from nipple.

SOURCES: Data from Baylor University Medical Center, Dallas, Texas; Lubbe, 2017; Ludwig & Weitzman, 2007.

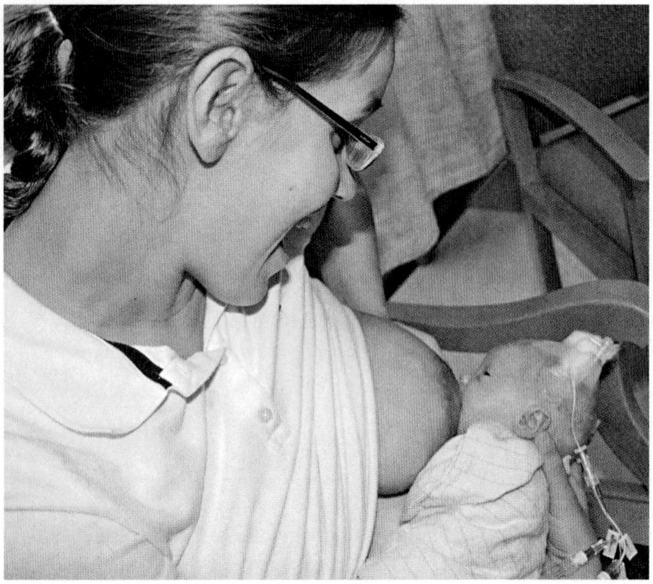

Figure 30–8 This mother is breastfeeding her premature newborn.

SOURCE: Carol Harrigan, RN, MSN, NNP-BC.

for nippling (see *Clinical Skill 30–1: Performing Gavage Feeding*). Gavage feedings are administered by the intermittent bolus or continuous drip method. In common practice, bolus gavage feedings are usually initiated, but if intolerance occurs, then the feedings are changed to infuse on a pump over a set amount of time (i.e., over an hour) or continuously. Gavage feeding is not without its consequences, including gastroesophageal reflux (GER), which can lead to significant emesis, food refusal, dysphagia, oral eversion, and aspiration (Eichenwald et al., 2017).

Early initiation of minimal enteral nutrition (MEN) via gavage is now advocated as a supplement to parenteral nutrition. MEN refers to small-volume feedings of formula or human milk (usually less than 24 mL/kg/day), which are designed to "prime" the intestinal tract, thereby stimulating many of its hormonal and enzymatic functions (Eichenwald et al., 2017). Benefits of early feeding (as early as 24 to 72 hours of life) include:

- No increase in the incidence of necrotizing enterocolitis
- Fewer days on total parenteral nutrition (TPN), thereby decreasing the incidence of cholestatic jaundice
- Increased weight gain
- Increased muscle maturation of the gut as well as muscle growth

Clinical Skill 30–1

Performing Gavage Feeding

NURSING ACTION

Preparation

- When choosing the catheter size, consider the size of the baby, the area of insertion (oral or nasal), and the desired rate of flow.

  Rationale: The size of the catheter will influence the rate of flow.
- Explain the procedure to the parents.
- Elevate the head of the bed and position the newborn on the back or side to allow easy passage of the tube.
- Measure the distance from the tip of the ear to the nose to the xiphoid process, and mark the point with a small piece of paper tape (Figure 30–9) to ensure enough tubing to enter the stomach.

Equipment and Supplies

- No. 5 or No. 8 Fr. feeding tube
- 3- to 5-mL syringe, for aspirating stomach contents
- 1/4-in. paper tape, to mark the tube for insertion depth and to secure the catheter during feeding
- Stethoscope, for auscultating the rush of air into the stomach when testing the tube placement
- Appropriate formula
- Small cup of sterile water to act as lubricant
- Clean gloves

Procedure: Clean Gloves

Inserting and Checking Placement of Tube

1. If inserting the tube nasally, lubricate the tip in a cup of sterile water. Use water instead of an oil-based lubricant,

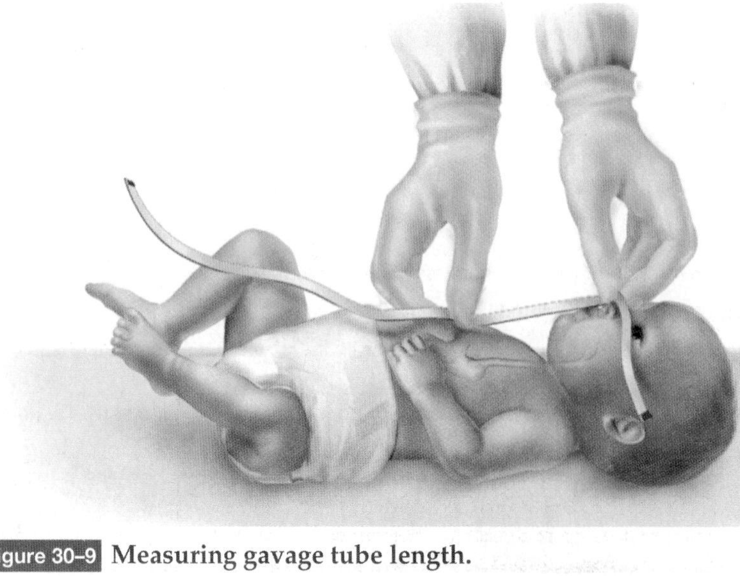

Figure 30–9 Measuring gavage tube length.

Clinical Skill 30–1 *(continued)*

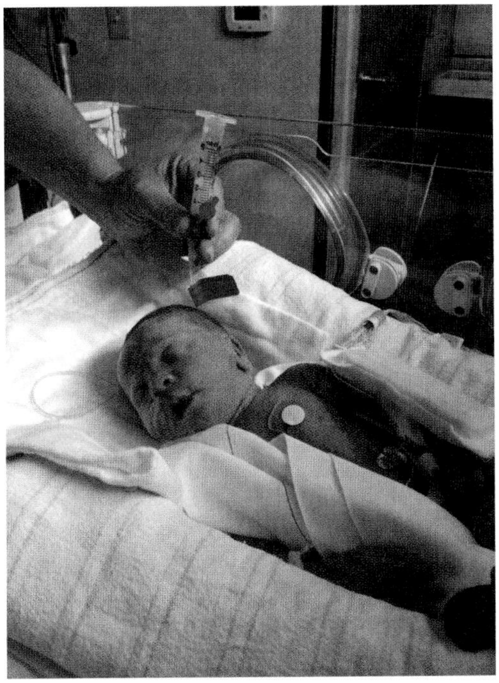

Figure 30–10 Gavage feeding a preterm newborn, flowing in by gravity.

SOURCE: Carol Harrigan, RN, MSN, NNP-BC.

in case the tube is inadvertently passed into a lung. Shake any excess drops to prevent aspiration.

2. If inserting the tube orally, the oral secretions are enough to lubricate the tube adequately.
3. Stabilize the baby's head with one hand and pass the tube via the mouth (or nose) into the stomach to the point previously marked. If the baby begins coughing or choking or becomes cyanotic or phonic, remove the tube immediately as the tube has probably entered the trachea.
4. If respiratory distress is not apparent, lightly tape the tube in position, draw up 0.5 to 1.0 mL of air in the syringe, and connect the syringe to the tubing. Place the stethoscope over the epigastrium and briskly inject the air (Figure 30–10). You will hear a sudden rush as the air enters the stomach.
5. Routine aspiration is now debated as an indication of food intolerance (Torrazza et al., 2015). Check agency protocol. If aspiration is ordered, aspirate the stomach contents with the syringe, and note the amount, color, and consistency. Return the residual to the stomach unless you are requested to discard it. It is usually not discarded because of the potential for electrolyte imbalance.

Administering the Feeding

1. Hold the baby for feeding or position the baby on the right or left side if regurgitation is present (Dutta et al., 2015).

   Rationale: This position decreases the risk of aspiration in case of emesis during feeding.

2. Separate the syringe from the tube, remove the plunger from the barrel, reconnect the barrel to the tube, and pour the formula into the syringe.
3. Elevate the syringe 6 to 8 inches over the baby's head, and allow the formula to flow by gravity at a slow, even rate. You may need to initiate the flow of formula by inserting the plunger of the syringe into the barrel just until you see formula enter the feeding tube. Do not use pressure.
4. Regulate the rate to prevent sudden stomach distention, leading to vomiting and aspiration. Continue adding formula to the syringe until the baby has absorbed the desired volume.

Clearing and Removing the Tube

1. Clear the tubing with 2 to 3 mL of air.

   Rationale: *This ensures that the baby has received all of the formula. If the tube is going to be left in place, clearing it will decrease the risk of occlusion and bacterial growth in the tube.*

2. To remove the tube, loosen the tape, fold the tube over on itself, and quickly withdraw the tube in one smooth motion to minimize the potential for fluid aspiration as the tube passes the epiglottis. If the tube is to be left in, position it so that the baby is unable to remove it. Replace the tube per hospital policy.

Maximize the Feeding Pleasure of the Baby

1. Whenever possible, hold the baby during gavage feeding. If it is too awkward to hold the baby during feeding, be sure to take time for holding after the feeding.

   Rationale: *Feeding time is important to the newborn's tactile sensory input.*

2. Offer a pacifier to the baby during the feeding.

   Rationale: *Sucking during feeding comforts and relaxes the newborn, making the formula flow more easily. Babies can lose their sucking reflexes when fed by gavage for long periods.*

3. Document procedure, including untoward complications, in the baby's medical record.

- Increased gut peristalsis and gut hormone levels, which can lead to improved feeding tolerance
- Shorter time required to reach full-volume enteral feedings
- Lower risk of osteopenia
- Possible decrease in the total number of hospital days in the neonatal intensive care unit (NICU).

SAFETY ALERT!

Orogastric gavage catheter placement is preferable to nasogastric because most newborns are obligatory nose breathers. If nasogastric is used, a #5 French catheter should be used to minimize airway obstruction.

Fluid Requirements. The calculation of fluid requirements must take into account the newborn's weight and postnatal age. Recommendations for fluid therapy in the preterm newborn weighing 1500 g (3.3 lb) are approximately 60 to 80 mL/kg/day for day 1; 80 to 120 mL/kg/day for day 2; and 120 to 160 mL/kg/day by day 3 of life. These amounts may be increased up to 190 mL/kg/day if the newborn is very small, receiving phototherapy, or under a radiant warmer because of the increased insensible water losses. Fluid losses can be minimized through the use of heat shields and added humidification in the incubator. Daily weights, and sometimes weights every 6 to 8 hours, are the best indicator of fluid status in the preterm newborn less than 1000 g (2.2 lb). The expected weight loss during the first 5 to 6 days of life in a preterm newborn is 15 to 20% of birth weight (Eichenwald et al., 2017). See *Case Study: Benita Cartier*.

Common Complications of Preterm Newborns and Their Clinical Management

The goals of medical and nursing care are to meet the preterm newborn's growth and development needs and to anticipate and manage the complications associated with prematurity. The most common complications associated with prematurity are:

- ***Apnea of prematurity.*** Apnea of prematurity refers to cessation of breathing for 20 seconds or longer or for less than 20 seconds when associated with cyanosis, pallor, and bradycardia. Apnea is a common problem in the preterm newborn less than 36 weeks, presenting between day 2 and day 7 of life. The etiology of apnea is multifactorial but is thought to be primarily a result of neuronal immaturity, a factor that contributes to the preterm newborn's irregular breathing patterns (central apnea). Obstructive apnea can occur when there is cessation of airflow associated with blockage of the upper airway (small airway diameter, increased pharyngeal secretions, altered body alignment and positioning). *Gastroesophageal reflux* is defined as a movement of gastric contents into the lower esophagus caused by poor esophageal sphincter tone, causing laryngospasm, which leads to bradycardia and apnea. Apnea of prematurity is then a diagnosis of exclusion.
- ***Patent ductus arteriosus (PDA).*** In the fetus, the ductus arteriosus shunts blood away from the fluid-filled lungs, which are nonfunctional during gestation, toward the placenta for gas exchange. The functional closure of the ductus arteriosus is related to birth weight; the incidence of a symptomatic PDA increases with a decrease in birth weight. For example, in newborns 30 weeks and less, functional closure may take several days to weeks to occur.

  Initially, as the pulmonary vascular resistance (PVR) falls and the systemic vascular resistance (SVR) rises, a left-to-right shunt via the PDA results. Blood flows from the aorta into the pulmonary artery, thereby increasing pulmonary blood flow. This leads to left-ventricular volume overload, pulmonary edema, and congestive failure. Oxygenation is compromised and ventilator requirements will increase, leading to the possible difficulty in weaning from the ventilator and long-term pulmonary sequelae. The ductus arteriosus fails to close because of decreased pulmonary arteriole musculature and hypoxemia.

  Clinical findings include a systolic murmur, tachypnea, hyperactive precordium, bounding peripheral pulses, hypotension, widened pulse pressure, tachycardia, and hepatomegaly. Symptomatic PDA is often seen around the time when premature newborns are recovering from RDS.

  Early identification and diagnosis of symptomatic newborns and prompt clinical intervention will minimize long-term complications. Initial medical management consists of providing adequate respiratory support, restricting fluids, and using diuretics (to decrease pulmonary edema) and perhaps digoxin (to treat congestive heart failure) while waiting for spontaneous closure of the ductus to occur. The administration of prostaglandin synthetase inhibitors, such as indomethacin (Indocin), impairs synthesis of the E series prostaglandins responsible for dilatation of the ductus and can cause ductal closure. Courses of indomethacin therapy vary; the standard, short course consists of three doses of indomethacin, 0.2 mg/kg IV every 12 hours. As an alternative, a long course of indomethacin may be chosen involving dosing over approximately 7 days. A decrease in renal side effects is thought to be the advantage of the longer dosing schedule. Indomethacin is effective, but it is not without side effects and must be used cautiously. Ibuprofen lysine (Neoprofen) is another pharmacologic agent used to close the ductus; the three-dose course consists of one dose of 10 mg/kg IV followed by two subsequent doses of 5 mg/kg IV at 24- and 48-hour intervals after the initial dose (Kenner, 2016). Adverse side effects of both medications include transient renal dysfunction, oliguria, platelet dysfunction, and GI bleeding.

Clinical Tip

For an otherwise healthy, growing premature newborn who is receiving total enteral intake and has started to experience apnea and bradycardia, one differential diagnosis to think about is reflux rather than sepsis, although sepsis may need to be ruled out.

CASE STUDY: BENITA CARTIER

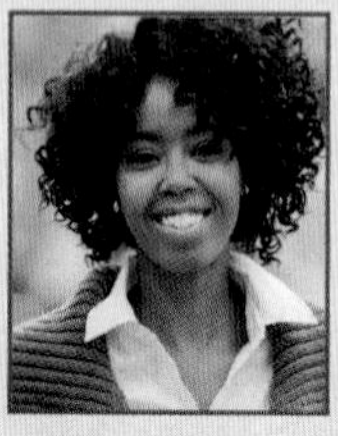

SOURCE: blvdone/Shutterstock.

Benita underwent an emergency cesarean birth for superimposed preeclampsia at 33 weeks' gestation. Her new daughter is currently admitted to the NICU with periods of apnea. She has been placed on an apnea monitor and is receiving oxygen therapy. Benita wants to breastfeed her baby, but at this time she is on a gavage feeding regimen. Benita's husband is distressed and asks for an explanation of why this is being done.

Questions to Ponder

How would you provide the rationale and explain the technique of gavage feeding to the parents? When Benita asks you why her newborn's appearance is different from a term baby's, how would you explain the characteristics associated with prematurity to her?

If medical and pharmacologic management is unsuccessful or contraindicated, then the ductus may need to be surgically ligated. PDA will often prolong the course of illness in a preterm newborn and may lead to chronic pulmonary dysfunction. However, the issues of whether to treat and when to treat are a continuing matter of controversy in the medical field.

Clinical Tip

A growing premature newborn showing clinical signs of worsening respiratory status (i.e., increased oxygen needs, increased ventilatory settings), acidosis, and hypotension may be exhibiting signs and symptoms of a PDA.

- *Respiratory distress syndrome (RDS).* Respiratory distress results from inadequate surfactant production (see Chapter 31).
- *Intraventricular hemorrhage.* Intraventricular hemorrhage is the most common type of intracranial hemorrhage in small preterm newborns, especially those weighing less than 1500 g (3.3 lb) or of less than 34 weeks' gestation. Up to 34 weeks' gestation, the preterm newborn's brain ventricles are lined by the germinal matrix, which is highly susceptible to hypoxic events such as respiratory distress, birth trauma, and birth asphyxia. The germinal matrix is highly vascular, and these blood vessels rupture in the presence of hypoxia.

SAFETY ALERT!

An extremely premature, low-birth-weight newborn who presents with a sudden drop in hemoglobin along with the onset of severe metabolic acidosis, a "waxy" color, and hypotension may have experienced an intracranial hemorrhage.

Other common problems of preterm newborns such as NEC are briefly discussed earlier in the physiologic sections. (For in-depth discussions of RDS, hyperbilirubinemia, hypoglycemia, anemia of prematurity, and sepsis, see Chapter 31.)

Long-Term Needs and Outcomes

The care of preterm newborns and their families does not stop on discharge from the nursery. Within the first year of life, low-birth-weight preterm babies face higher mortality rates than term babies. Causes of death include sudden infant death syndrome (SIDS)—which occurs about five times more frequently in the preterm baby—respiratory infections, and neurologic defects. Morbidity is also much higher among preterm babies, with those weighing less than 1500 g (3.3 lb) at highest risk for long-term complications. The most common long-term needs observed in preterm newborns include:

- *Retinopathy of prematurity (ROP).* Extremely premature newborns are particularly susceptible to injury of the delicate capillaries of the retina, causing characteristic retinal changes known as retinopathy of prematurity (ROP). It is this injury to the developing vascular system of the retina that leads to ischemia, resulting in hemorrhage, scarring, and, in extreme cases, retinal detachment, impaired vision, and eventual complete blindness. The disease is multifactorial in origin, with hyperoxemia (increased oxygen levels) as one factor. Other risk factors include in vitro fertilization (IVH), chronic lung disease (CLD), apnea, hypoxia, sepsis, acidosis, anemia, multiple gestation, exposure to bright lights, and blood transfusions. Increased survival of very-low-birth-weight newborns may be the most important factor in the increased incidence of ROP.

  Judicious use of supplemental oxygen therapy in the premature newborn has become the norm in NICUs across the country whereby oxygen saturations are maintained in set parameters in an attempt to reduce ROP (Table 30–3). Treatment of the acute stages of ROP with laser photocoagulation and cryotherapy is an option. Because most acute cases of ROP regress spontaneously with no long-term visual impairment, the possibility of regression must be weighed against the risk of an unfavorable outcome from treatment. For babies with bilateral traction and retinal detachment, surgical vitrectomy and scleral buckling are performed. A promising new medication yet to receive FDA approval for the NICU population, bevacizumab (Avastin), may offer an alternative or adjunct therapy for treatment of progressive ROP. The anti-VEGF (vascular endothelial growth factor) effects of Avastin suppress retinal neovascularization (an abnormal number and size of new vessels), which is responsible for ROP (Carter, Gratny, & Carter, 2016).

  Nursing care for the visually impaired newborn must concentrate on parental support and education. When the crisis of premature birth is quickly followed by the devastating news of suspected visual impairment (poor visual acuity, myopia, strabismus, amblyopia, and glaucoma) or blindness, the parents will need extensive support by all members of the interdisciplinary health team. The parents again experience overwhelming anxiety and uncertainty about their baby's future abilities. Premature babies with blindness due to ROP may be at increased risk of cognitive and emotional problems. The evidence suggests that this increased risk may be due to environmental factors rather than to inherent intellectual or neurologic factors.

SAFETY ALERT!

According to Carter et al. (2016), all newborns with a birth weight of less than or equal to 1500 g (3.3 lb) or gestational age of 30 weeks or less and selected newborns with a birth weight between 1500 and 2000 g (3.3 and 4.4 lb) or gestational age of more than 30 weeks with an unstable clinical course should have a retinal screening examination (see Figure 30–11).

- *Bronchopulmonary dysplasia (BPD).* Long-term lung disease is a result of damage to the alveolar epithelium secondary to positive pressure respiratory therapy and high oxygen concentration. These babies have long-term dependence on oxygen therapy and an increased incidence of respiratory infection during their first few years of life.
- *Speech defects.* The most frequently observed speech defects involve delayed development of receptive and expressive ability that may persist into the school-age years.

TABLE 30–3 Acceptable Oxygenation by Gestational Age

AGE	OXYGENATION
Less than 28 6/7 weeks' gestation	83–93%
29–33 6/7 weeks' gestation	85–95%
More than 34 weeks' gestation	90–98%

SOURCE: Data courtesy of the NICU, Banner Thunderbird Medical Center, Phoenix, AZ (2013).

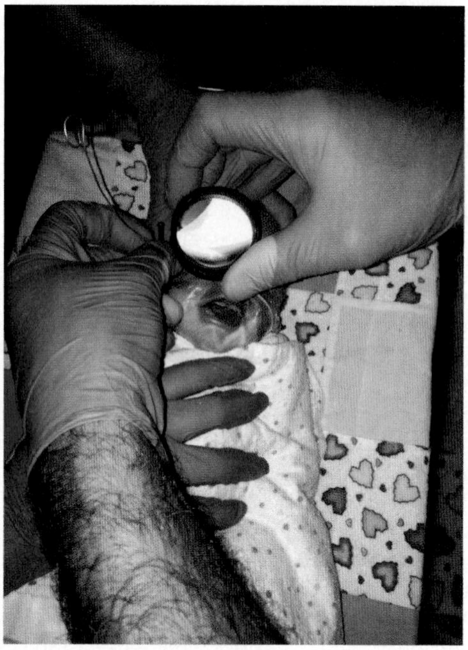

Figure 30–11 **A pediatric ophthalmologist performing an eye examination on a preterm newborn screening for ROP.**

SOURCE: Carol Harrigan, RN, MSN, NNP-BC.

- *Neurologic defects.* The most common neurologic defects include cerebral palsy, hydrocephalus, seizure disorders, lower IQ, and learning disabilities. However, the socioeconomic climate and family support systems are extremely important influences on the child's ultimate school performance in the absence of major neurologic defects. Families can be reminded that risk does not equal injury, injury does not equal damage, and description of damage does not allow a precise prediction about recovery or outcome.
- *Auditory defects.* Preterm newborns have a 1 to 4% incidence of moderate to profound hearing loss and should have a formal audiologic examination before discharge and at 3 to 6 months (corrected age). Tests currently used to measure hearing functions of the newborn are the evoked otoacoustic emissions (EOAE) or the automated auditory brain response (AABR) test (Figure 30–12). Any baby with repeated abnormal results should be referred to speech-language specialists.

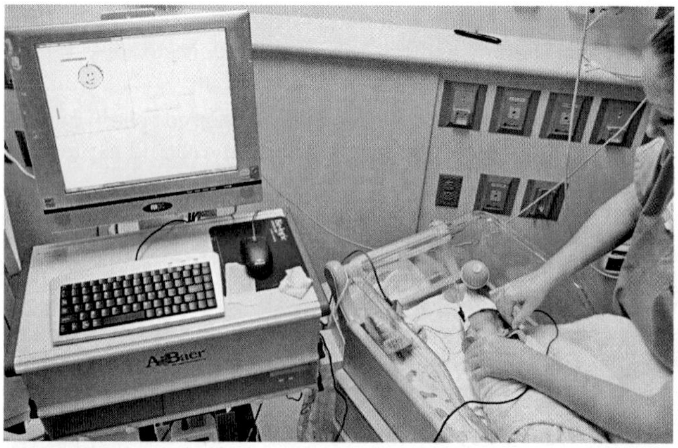

Figure 30–12 **Preterm newborns should have a formal hearing test prior to discharge.**

SOURCE: Carol Harrigan, RN, MSN, NNP-BC.

When evaluating the newborn's abilities and disabilities, parents must understand that developmental progress must be evaluated based on chronologic age from the expected date of birth, not from the actual date of birth (corrected age). In addition, the parents need the consistent support of healthcare professionals in the long-term management of their babies. Many new and ongoing concerns arise as the high-risk newborn grows and develops; the goal is to promote the highest quality of life possible.

●○● NURSING MANAGEMENT

For the Preterm Newborn

Nursing Assessment and Diagnosis

Assess the physical characteristics and gestational age of the preterm newborn accurately to anticipate the special needs and problems of the baby. Physical characteristics vary greatly depending on gestational age, but the following characteristics are frequently present:

- *Color.* Usually pink or ruddy but may be acrocyanotic (cyanosis, jaundice, and pallor are abnormal and should be noted)
- *Skin.* Reddened and translucent, blood vessels are readily apparent, lack of subcutaneous fat
- *Lanugo.* Plentiful and widely distributed
- *Head size.* Appears large in relation to the body
- *Skull.* Bones pliable, fontanelle smooth and flat, sutures approximated or overriding
- *Ears.* Minimal cartilage, pliable, folded over
- *Nails.* Soft, short
- *Genitals.* Male: Nonrugated, small scrotum; testes may or may not be descended or found in the inguinal canals. Female: Prominent clitoris and labia minora.
- *Posture.* Flaccid, froglike position
- *Cry.* Weak, feeble
- *Reflexes.* Poor suck, swallow, and gag; incomplete Moro
- *Activity.* Jerky, generalized movements (not seizure related), decreased tone

Determining gestational age in preterm newborns requires knowledge and experience in administering gestational assessment tools. The tool used should be specific, reliable, and valid. (For a discussion of gestational age assessment tools, see Chapter 27.)

Nursing diagnoses that may apply to the preterm newborn include:

- *Gas Exchange, Impaired,* related to immature pulmonary vasculature and inadequate surfactant production
- *Breathing Pattern, Ineffective,* related to immature central nervous system
- *Tissue Perfusion: Cardiac, Risk for Decreased,* related to hypotension due to decreased tissue perfusion secondary to PDA
- *Tissue Perfusion: Peripheral, Ineffective,* related to anemia of prematurity
- *Nutrition, Imbalanced: Less Than Body Requirements,* related to weak suck and swallow reflexes and decreased ability to absorb nutrients
- *Thermoregulation, Ineffective,* related to hypothermia secondary to decreased glycogen and brown fat stores

- ***Fluid Volume, Deficient,*** related to high insensible water losses and inability of kidneys to concentrate urine
- ***Family Processes, Dysfunctional,*** related to anger or guilt at having given birth to a premature baby

(NANDA-I © 2017)

Nursing Plan and Implementation

Maintenance of Respiratory Function

There is increased danger of respiratory obstruction in preterm newborns because their bronchi and trachea are so narrow that mucus can obstruct the airway. Maintain patency through judicious suctioning, but only on an as-needed basis.

Positioning can also affect respiratory function. If the baby is in the supine position, slightly elevate the baby's head to maintain the airway, being careful to avoid hyperextension of the neck because the trachea will collapse. Also, because the newborn has weak neck muscles and cannot control head movement, ensure that this head position is maintained by placing a small roll under the shoulders. Because the prone position splints the chest wall and decreases the amount of respiratory effort used to move the chest wall, it facilitates chest expansion and improves air entry and oxygenation. Weak or absent cough or gag reflexes increase the chance of aspiration in the premature newborn. Ensure that the newborn's position facilitates drainage of mucus or regurgitated formula.

Monitor heart and respiratory rates with cardiorespiratory monitors and observe the newborn to identify alterations in cardiopulmonary status. Signs of respiratory distress include:

- Cyanosis (serious sign when generalized)
- Tachypnea (sustained respiratory rate greater than 60/minute after first 4 hours of life)
- Retractions
- Expiratory grunting
- Nasal flaring
- Apneic episodes
- Presence of rales or rhonchi on auscultation
- Diminished air entry.

If respiratory distress occurs, administer oxygen per healthcare provider in order to relieve hypoxemia. If hypoxemia is not treated immediately, it may result in patent ductus arteriosus or metabolic acidosis. If oxygen is administered to the newborn, monitor the oxygen concentration with devices such as the transcutaneous oxygen monitor ($tcPO_2$) or the pulse oximeter. Periodic arterial blood gas sampling to monitor oxygen concentration in the baby's blood is essential because hyperoxemia may lead to ROP.

Consider respiratory function before initiation of feedings as well as during feeding to prevent aspiration as well as increased energy expenditure and oxygen consumption.

Maintenance of Neutral Thermal Environment

Providing a neutral thermal environment minimizes the oxygen consumption required to maintain a normal core temperature; it also prevents cold stress and facilitates growth by decreasing the calories needed to maintain body temperature. The preterm newborn's immature central nervous system, as well as small brown fat stores, provides poor temperature control. A small newborn (>1200 g [2.6 lb]) can lose 80 kcal/kg/day through radiation of body heat. Implement all the usual thermoregulation measures discussed in Chapter 28.

In addition, to minimize heat loss and temperature instability for preterm and low-birth-weight (LBW) newborns, do the following:

1. Allow **skin-to-skin contact (SSC)** (also called *kangaroo care*) between mother and newborn to maintain warmth and faster security.
2. Warm and humidify oxygen to minimize evaporative heat loss and decrease oxygen consumption.
3. Place the baby in a double-walled incubator or use a Plexiglas heat shield over small preterm babies in single-walled incubators to avoid radiative heat losses. Some institutions use radiant warmers and plastic wrap over the baby and pipe in humidity (swamping). Do not use Plexiglas shields on radiant warmer beds because they block the infrared heat.
4. Avoid placing the baby on cold surfaces such as metal treatment tables and cold x-ray plates (conductive heat loss). Pad cold surfaces with diapers and use radiant warmers during procedures, place the preterm newborn on prewarmed mattresses, and warm hands before handling the baby to prevent heat transfer via conduction.
5. Use warmed ambient humidity. Humidity can decrease insensible and transdermal water loss but the optimal level and duration is yet to be determined (Bagwell, Thomas, & Ryshen, 2016). Humidity, however, should be started only once the baby's temperature is within normal limits.
6. Keep the skin dry (evaporative heat loss) and place a cap on the baby's head. The head makes up 25% of the total body size.
7. Keep radiant warmers, incubators, and cribs away from windows and cold external walls (radiative heat loss) and out of drafts (conductive heat loss).
8. Open incubator portholes and doors only when necessary, and use plastic sleeves on portholes to decrease convective heat loss.
9. Use a skin probe to monitor the baby's skin temperature. Correlate ambient temperatures with the skin probe in the incubator using the servocontrol rather than the manual mode. The temperature should be 36° to 37°C (96.8° to 98.6°F). Temperature fluctuations indicate hypothermia or hyperthermia. Be careful not to place skin temperature probes over bony prominences, areas of brown fat, poorly vasoreactive areas such as extremities, or excoriated areas.
10. Warm formula or stored breast milk before feeding.
11. Use a reflector patch over the skin temperature probe when using a radiant warmer bed so that the probe does not sense the higher infrared temperature as the baby's skin temperature and therefore decrease the heater output.

Once preterm newborns are medically stable, they can be clothed with a double-thickness cap, cotton shirt, and diaper and, if possible, swaddled in a blanket. Be familiar with your individual institution's protocol for weaning a preterm newborn from an incubator to a crib. See *Concept Map: Hypothermia of Prematurity*.

Maintenance of Fluid and Electrolyte Status

Maintain hydration by providing adequate intake based on the newborn's weight, gestational age, chronologic age, and volume of sensible and insensible water losses. Adequate fluid intake should compensate for increased insensible losses and the amount needed for renal excretion of metabolic products. Insensible water losses can be minimized by providing high ambient humidity,

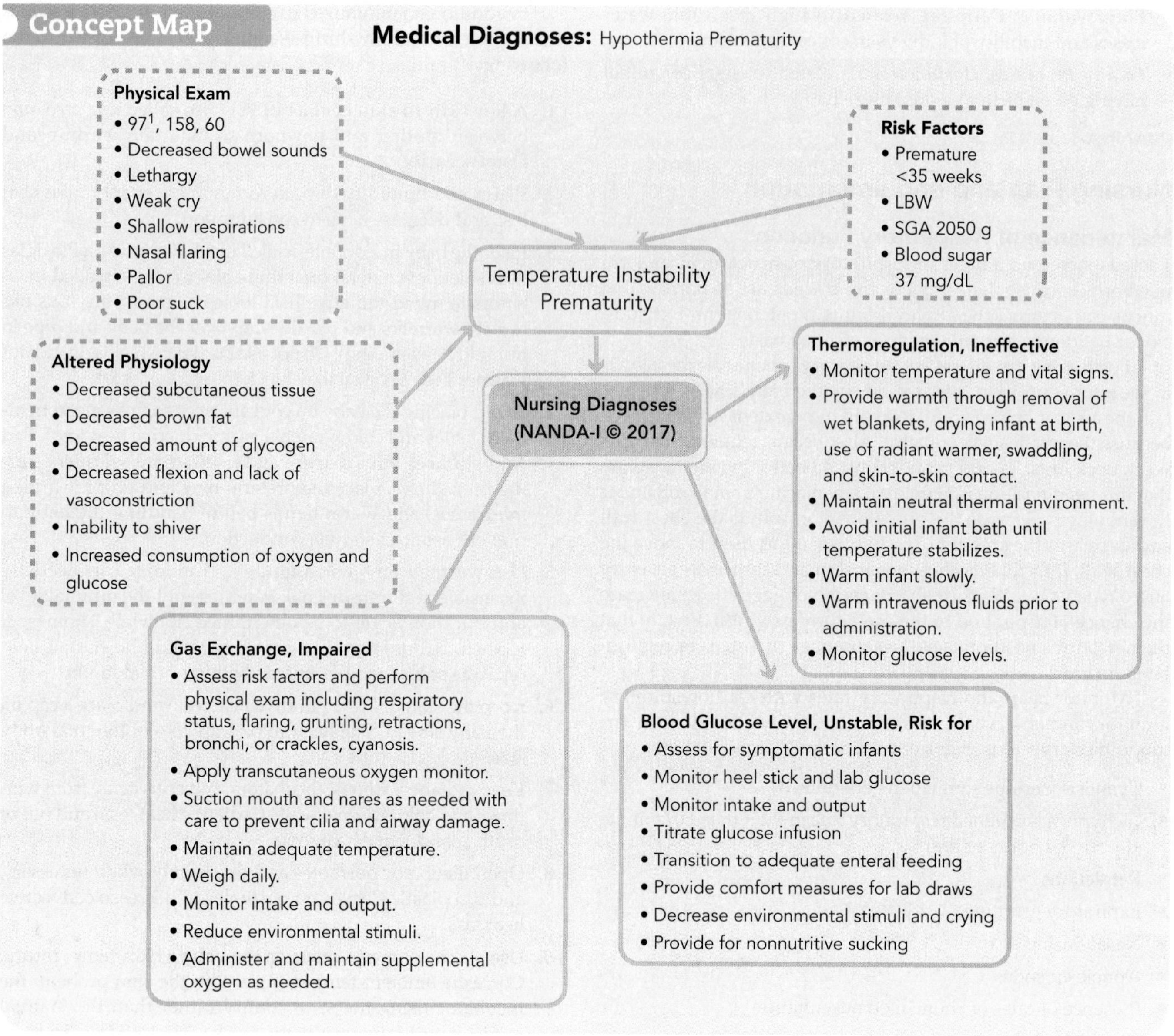

SOURCE: LADEWIG, PATRICIA W; LONDON, MARCIA L; DAVIDSON, MICHELE, CONTEMPORARY MATERNAL-NEWBORN NURSING, 9th Ed., ©2017. Reprinted and Electronically reproduced by permission of Pearson Education, Inc., New York, NY.

humidifying oxygen, using heat shields, covering the skin with plastic wrap, and placing the baby in a double-walled incubator.

Evaluate the hydration status of the baby by assessing and recording signs of dehydration. Be sure to identify signs of overhydration by observing the newborn for edema or excessive weight gain and by comparing urine output with fluid intake.

Weigh the preterm newborn at least once daily at the same time each day. Weight change is one of the most sensitive indicators of fluid balance. Weighing diapers is also important for accurate input and output measurement (1 mL = 1 g). A comparison of intake and output measurements over an 8- or 24-hour period provides important information about renal function and fluid balance. Assessment of patterns and whether they show a net gain or loss over several days is also essential to fluid management. In addition, monitor blood serum levels and pH to evaluate for electrolyte imbalances.

Accurate hourly intake calculations are needed when administering intravenous fluids. Because the preterm newborn is unable to excrete excess fluid, it is essential to maintain the correct amount of IV fluid to prevent overload. Accuracy can be ensured by using neonatal or pediatric infusion pumps. Periodically obtain urine-specific gravity and pH. Hydration is considered adequate when the urine output is 1 to 3 mL/kg/hr.

SAFETY ALERT!
To prevent electrolyte imbalance and dehydration, take care to give the correct IV solutions, as well as the correct volumes and concentrations of formulas.

Provision of Adequate Nutrition and Prevention of Fatigue During Feeding

The feeding method depends on the preterm newborn's feeding abilities and health status. Both nipple and gavage methods are initially supplemented with intravenous therapy until oral intake is sufficient to support growth. Early, small-volume enteral feedings called *minimal enteral nutrition via gavage* have proved to be of benefit to the VLBW newborn (see *Methods of Feeding* earlier in the chapter). Formula or breast milk (with or without fortifiers to increase caloric content) is incorporated into the feedings slowly. This is done to avoid overtaxing the digestive capacity of the preterm newborn.

Before each feeding, measure abdominal girth and auscultate the abdomen to determine the presence and quality of bowel sounds. Such assessments permit early detection of abdominal distention, visible bowel loops, and decreased peristaltic activity, which may indicate necrotizing enterocolitis (NEC) or paralytic ileus. Also check for residual formula in the stomach before feeding when the newborn is fed by gavage. The presence of increasing residual formula as an indication of intolerance to the type or amount of feeding or the increase in amount of feeding is debatable (Torrazza et al., 2015). Carefully watch for signs of feeding intolerance including guaiac-positive stools (occult blood in stools), lactose in stools (reducing substance in the stools), emesis, loose stools, and temperature instability.

Preterm newborns who are ill or who fatigue easily with nipple feedings are usually fed by gavage. The baby is essentially passive with these methods, thus conserving energy and calories. As the baby matures, gavage feedings are replaced with nipple (breast or formula) feedings to assist in strengthening the sucking reflex and in meeting oral and emotional needs. Signs that indicate readiness for oral feedings are a strong gag reflex, presence of nonnutritive sucking, and rooting behavior. Both low-birth-weight and preterm newborns nipple-feed more effectively in a quiet state. Establish a gradual nipple-feeding program, such as one nipple feeding per day, then one nipple feeding per shift, and then a nipple feeding every other feeding. Daily weights are monitored because often there is a small weight loss when nipple feedings are started. After feedings, place the baby on the right side (with support to maintain this position) or on the abdomen. These positions facilitate gastric emptying and decrease the chance of aspiration if regurgitation occurs. Gastroesophageal reflux is not uncommon in preterm newborns. Long-term gavage feeding may create nipple aversion that will require developmental occupational therapy interventions.

Involve the parents in feeding their preterm baby (Figure 30–13). This is essential to the development of attachment between parents and newborn. In addition, it increases parental knowledge about the care of their baby and helps them cope with the situation.

Prevention of Infection

You are responsible for minimizing the preterm newborn's exposure to pathogenic organisms. The preterm newborn is susceptible to infection because of an immature immune system and thin and permeable skin. Invasive procedures, techniques such as umbilical catheterization and mechanical ventilation, and prolonged hospitalization place the baby at greater risk for infection.

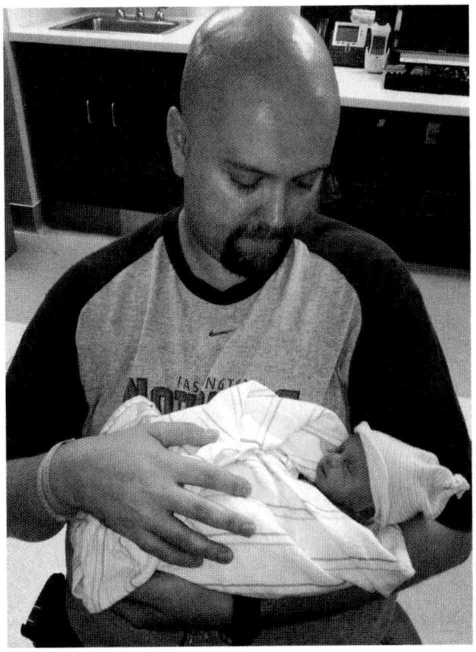

Figure 30–13 **Promotion of newborn attachment between father and his premature twin daughter.**

SOURCE: Carol Harrigan, RN, MSN, NNP-BC.

Strict hand hygiene and use of separate equipment for each baby help minimize the preterm newborn's exposure to infectious agents. Most nurseries have adopted the Centers for Disease Control and Prevention standard precautions of isolating every baby and The Joint Commission requirement that staff members have short-trimmed nails and no artificial nails. Staff members are required to complete a 2- to 3-minute scrub using iodine-containing antibacterial solutions, which inhibit growth of Gram-positive cocci and Gram-negative rod organisms. Other specific nursing interventions include limiting visitors, requiring visitors to wash their hands, maintaining strict aseptic practices when changing IV tubing and solutions (IV solutions and tubing should be changed every 24 hours or per agency protocols), administering parenteral fluids, and assisting with sterile procedures. Incubators and radiant warmers should be changed weekly. Prevent pressure-area breakdown by changing the baby's position regularly, doing range-of-motion exercises, and using water-bed pillows or an air mattress. To avoid skin tears, a protective transparent covering can be applied over vulnerable joints; however, this method is used sparingly (Blackburn, 2018). Chemical skin preps and tape may cause skin trauma and should be avoided as much as possible.

If infection (sepsis) occurs in the preterm newborn, you may be the first to identify its subtle clinical signs, such as lethargy and increased episodes of apnea and bradycardia. Inform the clinician of the findings immediately and implement the treatment plan per clinician orders in the presence of infection. (For specific nursing care required for the newborn with an infection, see Chapter 31.)

Clinical Tip

By 10 to 14 days of life, the skin integrity of the preterm newborn becomes mature and similar to that of a full-term baby.

Promotion of Parent–Newborn Attachment

Preterm newborns can be separated from their parents for prolonged periods after illness or complications that are detected in the first few hours or days following birth. The resultant interruption in parent–newborn bonding necessitates intervention to ensure successful attachment.

Measures need to be taken to promote positive parental feelings toward the preterm newborn. You can give photographs of the baby to parents to take home. These can also be given to the mother if she is in a different hospital or too ill to come to the nursery and visit. The newborn's first name is placed on the incubator as soon as it is known to help the parents feel that their baby is a unique and special person. Parents are given a weekly card with the baby's footprint, weight, and length, which helps to promote bonding. They are also given the telephone number of the nursery or intensive care unit and the names of staff members so that they have access to information about their baby at any time of the day or night. Encourage visits from siblings and grandparents to foster attachment.

Early involvement in the care of and decisions about their baby provides the parents with realistic expectations for their baby. The individual personality characteristics of the newborn and the parents influence bonding and contribute to the interactive process for the family. By observing a baby's patterns of behavior and responses, especially sleep–wake states, you can teach parents optimal times for interacting with their baby. Parents need education to develop caregiving skills and to understand the premature newborn's behavioral characteristics. Their daily participation (if possible) is encouraged, as are early and frequent visits.

Skin-to-skin care (also called *kangaroo care*) is defined as the practice of holding babies skin to skin next to a parent (Figure 30–14). The baby is usually naked, except for a diaper, and placed on the bare chest of the mother or father/partner. They are then both covered with a blanket. Benefits of skin-to-skin care as a developmental intervention include the following (Gardner, Voos, & Hills, 2016):

- Improved oxygenation as evidenced by an increase in transcutaneous oxygen levels
- Enhanced temperature regulation
- Decline in the episodes of apnea and bradycardia
- Increased periods of quiet sleep
- Stabilization of vital signs
- Positive interaction between parent and baby, which enhances attachment and bonding
- Increased growth parameters
- Early discharge.

Limitations to skin-to-skin care may be because of staff uneasiness and the lack of protocols or guidelines to safely maneuver, position, and hold the newborn.

You and the parents can plan nursing care around the times when the baby is alert and best able to attend. The more knowledge parents have about the meaning of their baby's responses, behaviors, and cues for interaction, the better prepared they will be to meet their newborn's needs and form a positive attachment with their child. Parental involvement in difficult care decisions is essential and is discussed in greater detail in Chapter 31.

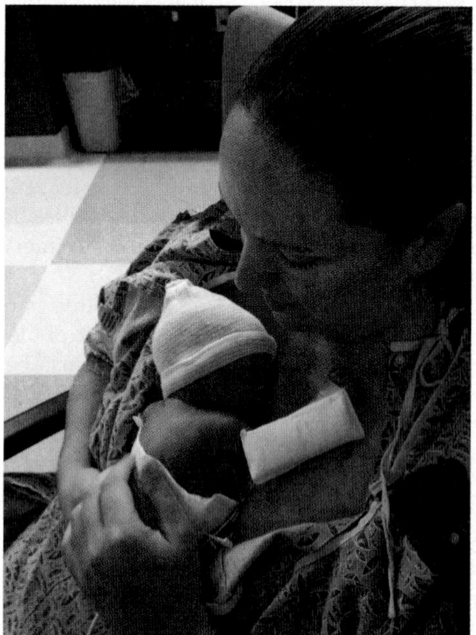

Figure 30–14 Kangaroo (skin-to-skin) care facilitates a closeness and attachment between mother and her premature newborn.

SOURCE: Carol Harrigan, RN, MSN, NNP-BC.

Some parents may progress easily to touching and cuddling their newborn; however, others will not. Parents need to know that their feelings are normal and that the progression of acquaintanceship is slow. Rooming-in can provide another opportunity for the stable preterm newborn and family to get acquainted; it offers both privacy and readily available help (Figure 30–15).

Promotion of Developmentally Supportive Care

Prolonged separation and the NICU environment necessitate individualized baby sensory stimulation programs. You can play a key role in determining the appropriate type and amount of visual, tactile, and auditory stimulation.

Some preterm newborns are not developmentally able to deal with more than one sensory input at a time. The Assessment of Preterm Infant Behavior (APIB) scale identifies individual preterm newborn behaviors according to five areas of development (Als, Butler, & Costa, 2005). The preterm baby's behavioral reactions to stimulation are observed, and developmental interventions are then based on reducing detrimental environmental stimuli to the lowest possible level and providing appropriate opportunities for development (Blackburn, 2018).

Providing developmentally supportive, as well as family-centered, care has been proven to improve the outcomes of the critically ill newborn. The NICU environment contains many detrimental stimuli that you can help reduce. Noise levels can be lowered by replacing alarms with lights. In addition, silencing alarms quickly and keeping conversations away from the baby's bedside can help. Dimmer switches should be used to shield the baby's eyes from bright lights, and blankets may be placed over the top portion of the incubator. Dimming the lights may encourage babies to open their eyes and be more responsive to their parents. Nursing care should be planned to decrease the number of times the baby is disturbed. Signs (e.g., "Quiet Please") can be placed near the bedside to allow the baby some periods of uninterrupted sleep (Blackburn, 2018). Some other developmentally supportive interventions include:

- Facilitate handling by using containment measures when turning or moving the newborn or doing procedures such as suctioning. Use your hands to hold the baby's arms and legs flexed close to the midline of the body. This helps stabilize the baby's motor and physiologic subsystems during stressful activities.

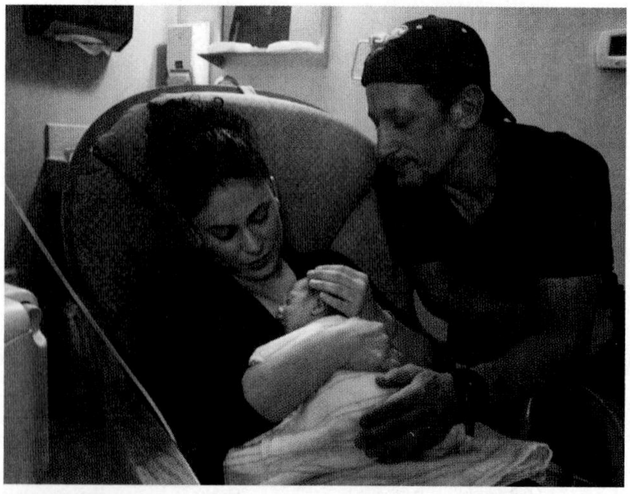

Figure 30–15 Family bonding occurs when parents have opportunities to spend time with their newborn.

SOURCE: Carol Harrigan, RN, MSN, NNP-BC.

- Touch the newborn gently and avoid sudden postural changes.
- Promote soothing activities, such as placing blanket rolls or approved manufactured devices next to the baby's sides and against the feet to provide "nesting." Swaddle the baby to maintain extremities in a flexed position while ensuring that the hands can reach the face. This permits the newborn to do hand-to-mouth activities. Also provide self-consoling objects for the baby to grasp (e.g., a piece of blanket, oxygen tubing, a finger) during caregiving (Figure 30–16).
- Simulate the kinesthetic advantages of the intrauterine environment by using sheepskin and approved water beds. Water bed and pillow use has been reported to improve sleep and decrease motor activity as well as lead to more mature motor behavior, fewer state changes, and a decreased heart rate.
- Provide opportunities for nonnutritive sucking with a pacifier. This improves transcutaneous oxygen saturation; decreases body movements; improves sleep, especially after feedings; and increases weight gain.

As NICUs become more and more developmentally supportive, complementary care has become an adjunct to that nurturing environment. This holistic approach in caring for the low-birth-weight/preterm newborn attempts not only to mimic the intrauterine environment, but also to foster parent–newborn bonding by simultaneously caring for the body, spirit, and mind. See *Complementary Health Approaches: Complementary Care in the NICU*.

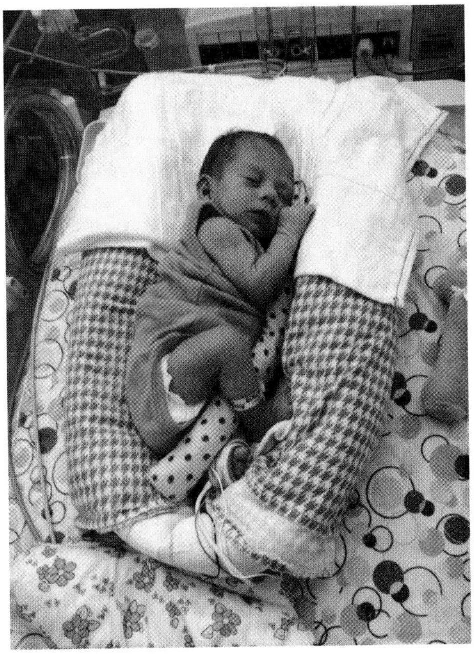

Figure 30–16 **A 3-week-old, 31 weeks' gestational age newborn is nested and developmentally positioned. Hand-to-mouth behavior facilitates self-consoling and soothing activities.**

SOURCE: Carol Harrigan, RN, MSN, NNP-BC.

Preparation for Home Care

Parents are often anxious when their premature newborn is transferred out of the NICU or is discharged home. Parents of preterm babies should receive the same postpartum teaching as any parent taking a newborn home. In preparing for discharge, encourage the parents to spend time caring directly for their baby. This familiarizes them with their baby's behavior patterns and helps them establish realistic expectations. Some hospitals have a special room near the nursery where parents can spend the night with their baby before discharge.

Discharge instruction includes breastfeeding and formula-feeding techniques, formula preparation, and vitamin administration. If the mother wishes to breastfeed, teach her to pump her

Complementary Health Approaches

Complementary Care in the NICU

- ***Aromatherapy*** is the use of scent to alter mood or behavior to produce a calming and sedating effect. There is an enhanced bonding process between mothers and newborns associated with the natural body odor emitted from the mother (Gardner, Goldson, & Hernandez, 2016). Aromatherapy is utilized in the NICU by placing an article of clothing belonging to the mother next to the newborn to produce a soothing and consoling effect on the baby in her absence. Researchers are also investigating other aromatherapies, including peppermint as a respiratory stimulant, chamomile as a method to regulate sleep–wake cycles, Brazilian guava for its analgesic effects, and lavender sitz baths for management of diaper rash.
- ***Music therapy*** as a noninvasive auditory stimulus has been shown to be advantageous in the premature newborn. The music used in NICUs includes primarily lullabies and soft acoustical pieces that are pleasant, soothing, and calming. Such music has been shown to affect newborn physiologic responses, such as improving oxygenation and increasing weight gain. It also has behavioral effects, leading to enhanced parental bonding and increased intervals of nonnutritive sucking periods. Language development is also enhanced if the music is live and sung by the mother or another female, which is preferential to the newborn. However, the overall noise level in the NICU needs to be considered before including any extra auditory stimulation, including music therapy (Gardner, Goldson, & Hernandez, 2016).
- ***Infant massage and gentle human touch (GHT)*** have been practiced for many centuries. The types of stimulation include massage with stroking, gentle touch without stroking, and therapeutic touch or "hands-on" containment. Practitioners report such physiologic benefits as stimulating blood and lymphatic flow, promoting weight gain in premature newborns, regulating sleep patterns, and many emotional and behavioral benefits. Massage demonstrates compassion while increasing parents' empathy and understanding of the baby. It helps parents learn to interpret their baby's behavioral cues such as facial expression, various crying patterns, and other body language. At the same time, it helps babies learn about their various body parts and boundaries and feel how they integrate into the whole. Therapeutic touch reduces motor activity and energy expenditure by the baby and also promotes comfort.

breasts to keep the milk flowing and provide milk even before discharge. Provide information on bathing, diapering, hygiene, and normal elimination patterns. Prepare the parents to expect changes in the color of the baby's stool, number of bowel movements, and timing of elimination when the baby is switched from formula-feeding to breastfeeding. This information can prevent unnecessary concern by the parents.

Discuss normal growth and development patterns, reflexes, and activities for preterm babies, especially signs and symptoms of overstimulation. In these discussions, emphasize ways to promote bonding behaviors and deal with newborn crying. Care of the preterm newborn with complications, preventing infections, recognizing signs of a sick baby, and the need for continued medical follow-up are other key issues. Family-care conferences with all the various disciplines involved in the care of the preterm newborn are often helpful just prior to discharge.

Families with preterm newborns usually do not need to be referred to community agencies, such as visiting nurse assistance. However, referral may be necessary if the baby has severe congenital abnormalities, feeding problems, or complications with infections or respiratory problems or if the parents seem unable to cope with an at-risk baby. In the weeks immediately following the birth of their babies, 40% of mothers and 36% of fathers experienced clinically significant symptoms of depression. This was compared to just 6% of mothers and 5% of fathers of healthy full-term babies (Pace, 2016). For many parents, the distress they feel after having a preterm baby does improve over the first few months. Parents of preterm newborns can benefit from meeting with others in a similar situation to share common experiences and concerns. Refer parents to support groups sponsored by the hospital or by others in the community and make connections for parents with early education intervention centers.

Preterm and LBW newborns are at greater risk of increased morbidity from vaccine-preventable diseases. Stable preterm newborns show consistently high rates of seroconversion following the first dose of hepatitis B vaccine even when the first dose is given as early as 1 month after birth (AAP & ACOG, 2017). The medically stable preterm newborn and the LBW newborn should receive full doses of diphtheria, tetanus, acellular pertussis, *Haemophilus influenzae* type b (Hib), hepatitis B, inactivated poliovirus, rotavirus, and pneumococcal conjugate vaccines (PCV) at a chronologic age consistent with the schedule recommended for full-term newborns. The influenza vaccine should be administered at 6 months of age before the beginning of and during the influenza season. The vaccine for immunoprophylaxis against respiratory syncytial virus (RSV) is given to those high-risk newborns prior to discharge from the NICU and monthly thereafter during local RSV season.

Evaluation

Expected outcomes of nursing care include:

- The preterm newborn is free of respiratory distress and establishes effective respiratory function.
- The preterm newborn gains weight and shows no signs of fatigue or aspiration during feedings.
- The preterm newborn demonstrates a serial head circumference growth rate of 1 cm (0.4 in.) per week.
- The parents are able to verbalize their anger and guilt feelings about the birth of a preterm baby and show attachment behavior such as frequent visits and growing confidence in their participatory care activities.

Care of the Newborn with Congenital Anomalies

The birth of a baby with a congenital defect places both newborn and family at risk. Many congenital anomalies can be life-threatening if not corrected within hours after birth; others are very visible and cause the families emotional distress. When one congenital anomaly is found, healthcare providers should look for others, particularly in body systems that develop at the same time during gestation. Table 30–4 identifies common anomalies and their early management and nursing care in the newborn period.

Care of the Newborn with Congenital Heart Defect

Congenital heart defect (CHD), the most common congenital defect, occurs in approximately 6 to 8 per 1000 live births (depending on severity of the structural defects). Only 25% of all cardiac lesions are identified on a prenatal ultrasound. Some newborns go home with their parents before their heart defect is detected. Of the babies with congenital heart defect, 3% have *critical congenital heart disease (CCHD)*, which results in death or requires cardiac surgery or cardiac catheterization in the first year of life (Diller, Kelleman, Kupke, et al., 2018). Of the cardiac lesions associated with death during the first 2 weeks of life, the most common are coarctation of the aorta, aortic valve stenosis, interrupted aortic arch, hypoplastic left heart syndrome, truncus arteriosus, and critical pulmonary stenosis.

These newborns can benefit from early treatment and can often be identified in their first days of life through pulse oximetry screening—a painless, readily available examination that is easy to incorporate into newborn assessments. This noninvasive test measures the percentage of hemoglobin in the blood that is saturated with oxygen and pulse rate. An oximetry probe placed on the foot (postductal) can transcutaneously measure the blood that is carrying oxygen. The oximetry probe includes a light source, detector, and microprocessor, which calculate the differences in the oxygen-rich versus oxygen-poor blood hemoglobin. Andrea (2015) proposes some activities to promote optimal accuracy of pulse oximetry readings that include:

- Placing the light probe emitter directly opposite the light emitter and wrapper provided by the manufacturer.
- Avoiding placing probes on an extremity with the automatic blood pressure cuff, which will impede blood flow and result in false readings. Blood flow is needed to get accurate readings and produce a waveform.
- Cleaning and drying skin prior to placement of the probe. Skin color and jaundice will not affect the reading, but dried blood under the probe will affect it.
- Covering the probe with an opaque covering in a bright environment. Bright lights such as bilirubin lights, surgical lights, and other infra lights can affect accuracy.

The addition of pulse oximetry to fetal ultrasound and physical examination as a screening tool can reduce the chance of overlooking CCHD in newborns (Andrea, 2015). CCHD screening with pulse oximetry should be done on babies over 35 weeks' gestation in the well-newborn nursery. The CCHD screening protocol is also applicable to newborns discharged from NICU.

TABLE 30–4 Congenital Anomalies: Identification and Care in the Newborn Period

CONGENITAL ANOMALY	NURSING ASSESSMENTS	NURSING GOALS AND INTERVENTIONS
Congenital Hydrocephalus (progressive ventricular enlargement due to a malformation and obstruction in the flow of the *cerebrospinal fluid [CSF]* pathways)	Enlarged or full fontanelles Split or widened sutures "Setting-sun" eyes Head circumference greater than 90% on growth chart Visibly distended scalp veins Behavioral state changes; may become increasingly irritable or lethargic	Assess presence of hydrocephalus: Measure and plot initial OFC measurement; then measure daily. Check fontanelle for bulging and sutures for widening. Obtain neurosurgery consult. Assist with imaging studies, to include cranial ultrasound, CT scan, and MRI. Maintain skin integrity: Change position frequently. Use gel pillow under head. Postoperatively, position head off operative site, watch for signs of infection.
Choanal Atresia (unilateral or bilateral bony occlusion of posterior nares)	Respiratory distress (cyanosis and retractions at rest) Noisy respirations Difficulty breathing during feeding (obligatory nose breathers) Obstruction by thick mucus	Assess patency of nares: Listen for breath sounds while holding baby's mouth closed and alternately compressing each nostril. Assist with passing a catheter through each naris to confirm diagnosis. Obtain ENT consult. Maintain respiratory function: Assist with taping airway in mouth to prevent respiratory distress. Position with head elevated to improve air exchange.
Cleft Lip (unilateral or bilateral visible defect) 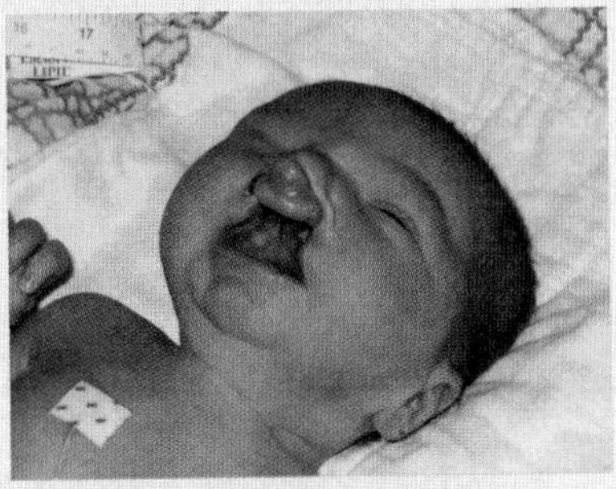 **Bilateral cleft lip with cleft abnormality involving both hard and soft palates.** **SOURCE:** Carol Harrigan, RN, MSN, NNP-BC.	May involve upper lip only or may involve external nares, nasal cartilage, nasal septum, and alveolar process Flattening or depression of midfacial contour	Provide nutrition: Feed with special nipple and bottle. Burp frequently (increased tendency to swallow air and reflex vomiting). Obtain craniofacial/ENT consult. Clean cleft with sterile water (to prevent crusting on cleft before repair). Support parental coping: Assist parents with grief over loss of idealized baby. Encourage verbalization of their feelings about visible defect.
Cleft Palate (fissure connecting oral and nasal cavity)	May involve uvula and soft palate May extend forward to nostril involving hard palate and maxillary alveolar ridge Difficulty in sucking Expulsion of formula through nose	Prevent aspiration/infection: Place in side-lying position to facilitate drainage. Obtain craniofacial/ENT consult. Feed in upright position (to prevent formula from flowing back into nasal passages, to aid swallowing and discourage aspiration). Provide nutrition: Feed with special nipple and bottle. Formula may escape through the nose, which is common (nasal regurgitation). Burp after each ounce (tendency to swallow large amounts of air). Plot weight gain patterns to assess adequacy of diet. Provide parental support: Refer parents to community agencies, support groups, and speech pathologists. Encourage verbalization of frustrations because feeding process is long and frustrating. Praise all parental efforts. Encourage parents to seek prompt treatment for upper respiratory infection (URI) and teach them ways to decrease URI.

(continued)

TABLE 30–4 Congenital Anomalies: Identification and Care in the Newborn Period *(continued)*

CONGENITAL ANOMALY	NURSING ASSESSMENTS	NURSING GOALS AND INTERVENTIONS
Tracheoesophageal Fistula (lower esophageal segment connects to the lower trachea with upper esophageal segment ending blindly [atresia]) 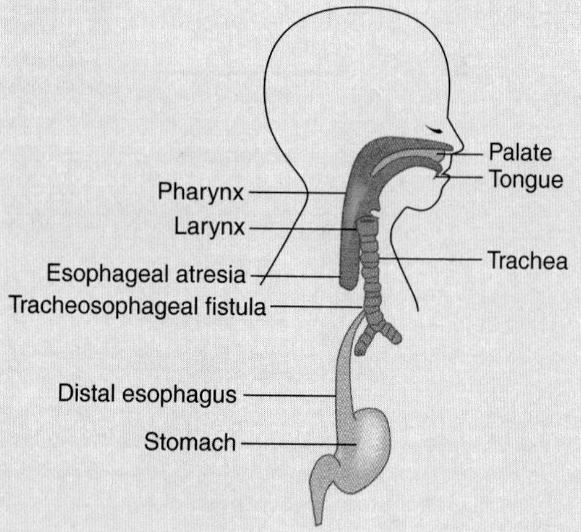 The most frequently seen type of congenital tracheoesophageal fistula with esophageal atresia. 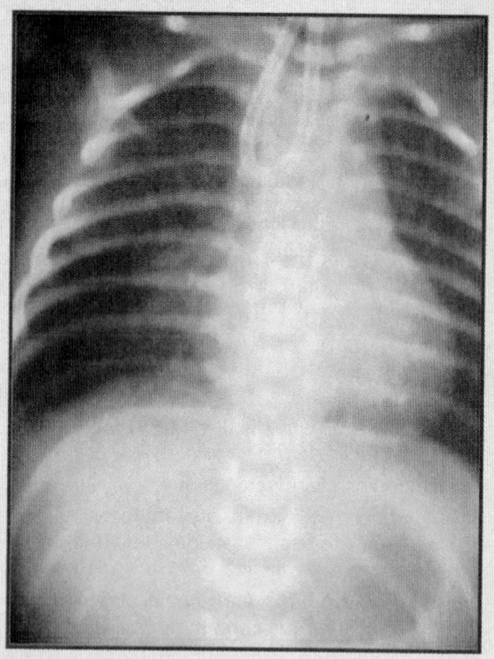 TEF with esophageal atresia. Note coiled NG tube and large stomach bubble. **SOURCE:** Carol Harrigan, RN, MSN, NNP-BC.	History of maternal polyhydramnios Excessive oral secretions Constant drooling Abdominal distention beginning soon after birth Periodic choking and cyanotic episodes Immediate regurgitation when feeding Aspiration of pharyngeal contents into trachea. Signs/symptoms: Tachypnea, retractions, rhonchi, decreased breath sounds, cyanotic spells Reflux of gastric contents into trachea leading to aspiration pneumonia Inability to pass nasogastric tube (will not pass beyond 10–15 cm from nares)	Maintain respiratory status and prevent aspiration. Withhold feeding until esophageal patency is determined by chest radiograph. Obtain a surgical consult. Place an indwelling Replogle tube attached to low intermittent suction to control saliva and mucus (to prevent aspiration pneumonia) in esophageal pouch. Elevate head of bed 20–40 degrees (to prevent reflux of gastric contents). Keep baby calm (crying causes air to pass through fistula and to distend intestines, causing compression of the diaphragm and respiratory embarrassment). Maintain fluid and electrolyte balance. Begin broad-spectrum antibiotics secondary to risk of aspiration pneumonia. Give fluids to replace esophageal drainage and maintain hydration. Provide parent education: Explain repair—primary or staged—provision of gastrostomy, ligation of fistula, repair of atresia. Keep parents informed; clarify and reinforce healthcare provider's explanations regarding malformation, surgical repair, preoperative and postoperative care, and prognosis.

TABLE 30–4 Congenital Anomalies: Identification and Care in the Newborn Period *(continued)*

CONGENITAL ANOMALY	NURSING ASSESSMENTS	NURSING GOALS AND INTERVENTIONS
Diaphragmatic Hernia (portion of intestines in the thoracic cavity through abnormal opening in diaphragm, occurring commonly on the left side) 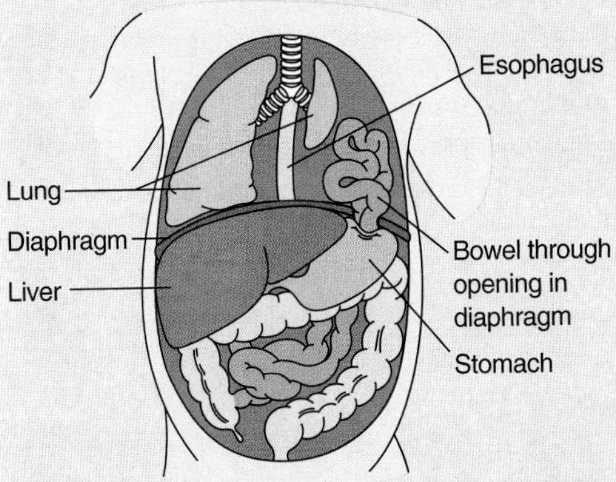 Diaphragmatic hernia. Note compression of the lung by the intestine on the affected side. **SOURCE:** Nancy Houck, RN, BSN, NNP-BC. 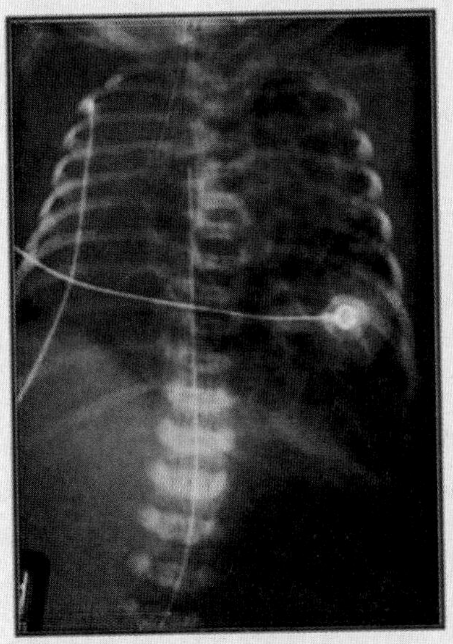 Diaphragmatic hernia. Note bowel gas pattern in the upper left chest with a shift in the mediastinum to the right. **SOURCE:** Carol Harrigan, RN, MSN, NNP-BC.	Difficulty initiating respirations secondary to hypoplastic lung on affected side, compression of lung on contralateral side Gasping respirations with nasal flaring and chest retractions Barrel chest and scaphoid abdomen Asymmetric chest expansion Breath sounds may be diminished or absent, usually on affected side Heart sounds displaced to contralateral side Bowel sounds may be heard in thoracic cavity	Nurse should never ventilate with bag and mask O_2 because the stomach and intestines will become air-filled and distended, further compressing the lungs. Obtain chest radiograph to confirm diagnosis. Obtain a surgical consult. Maintain respiratory status: Administer oxygen, prepare for intubation and ventilation (considered a respiratory emergency). Initiate gastric decompression by placing an indwelling Replogle tube attached to low intermittent suction. Place in high semi-Fowler position (to use gravity to keep abdominal organs' pressure off diaphragm). Turn onto affected side to allow unaffected lung expansion. Carry out interventions to alleviate respiratory and metabolic acidosis.

(continued)

TABLE 30–4 Congenital Anomalies: Identification and Care in the Newborn Period *(continued)*

CONGENITAL ANOMALY	NURSING ASSESSMENTS	NURSING GOALS AND INTERVENTIONS
Omphalocele (herniation of abdominal contents into base of umbilical cord) 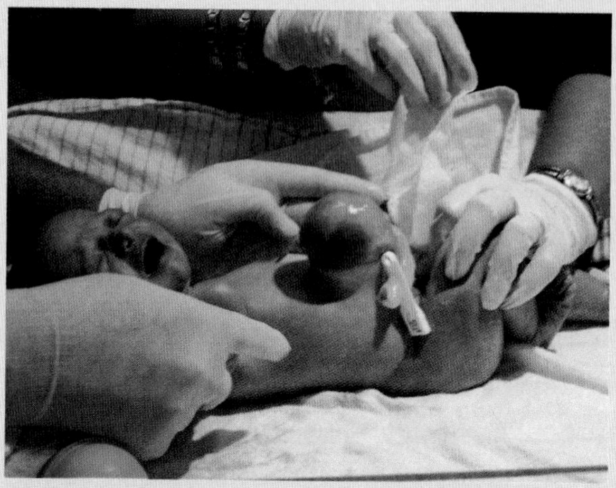 Newborn with omphalocele with ruptured umbilical cord. **SOURCE:** Carol Harrigan, RN, MSN, NNP-BC.	Abdominal contents may or may not remain encased in a protective, transparent membrane	Maintain hydration and temperature. Place baby in sterile bag up to and covering defect. Obtain surgical consult. Initiate gastric decompression by insertion of an indwelling Replogle tube attached to low suction (to prevent distention of lower bowel and impairment of blood flow). Position to prevent trauma to defect. Administer broad-spectrum antibiotics to prevent infection.
Gastroschisis (full-thickness defect in abdominal wall allowing viscera outside the body to the right of an intact umbilical cord) 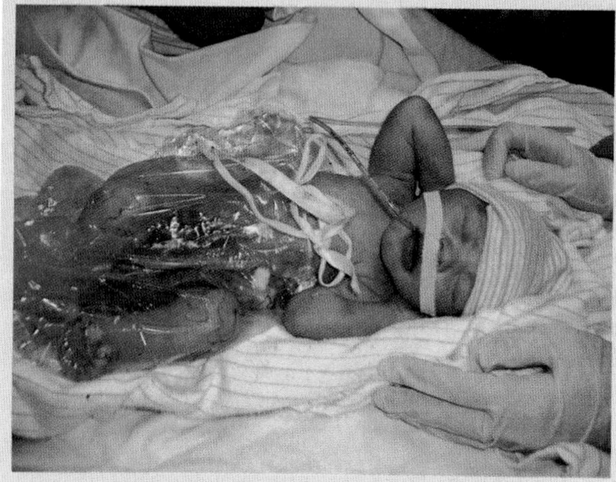 Term newborn with gastroschisis. Note the externalized loops of bowel visible through the bag. **SOURCE:** Carol Harrigan, RN, MSN, NNP-BC.	No protective covering Intestines exposed to the caustic amniotic fluid Associated with intestinal atresia, malrotation Large amount of evaporative fluid losses from exposed bowel	Maintain hydration and temperature. Provide normal saline for hypovolemia/fluid resuscitation. Place baby in sterile bag up to axilla in a side-lying position to prevent trauma of the bowel. *Do not cover defect with wet saline gauze.* Obtain surgical consult. Initiate gastric decompression by insertion of an indwelling Replogle tube attached to low suction; measure and replace gastric output. Administer broad-spectrum antibiotics to prevent infection of exposed bowel.

TABLE 30–4 Congenital Anomalies: Identification and Care in the Newborn Period *(continued)*

CONGENITAL ANOMALY	NURSING ASSESSMENTS	NURSING GOALS AND INTERVENTIONS
Prune Belly Syndrome (congenital absence of one or more layers of abdominal muscles) 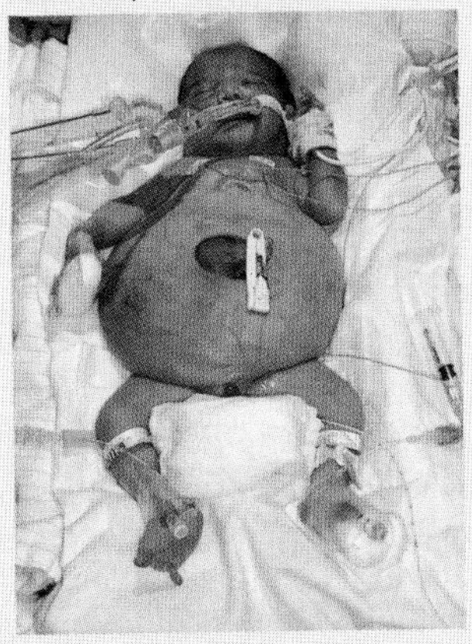 Prune belly syndrome. **SOURCE:** Carol Harrigan, RN, MSN, NNP-BC.	Oligohydramnios leading to pulmonary hypoplasia common Deficiency of the abdominal wall musculature causing the abdomen to be shapeless Skin hangs loosely and is wrinkled in appearance Associated with urinary abnormalities (urethral obstruction, renal dysplasia) In boys, cryptorchidism is common; rarely occurs in girls	Maintain respiratory status: May need to be immediately intubated and ventilated. Obtain surgical and urology consult. Prevent trauma and infection. Administer broad-spectrum antibiotics. Place a urinary catheter and monitor urinary output. Carry out interventions to alleviate respiratory and metabolic acidosis. Keep parents updated and informed about prognosis.
Myelomeningocele (saclike cyst containing meninges, spinal cord, and nerve roots in thoracic and/or lumbar area) 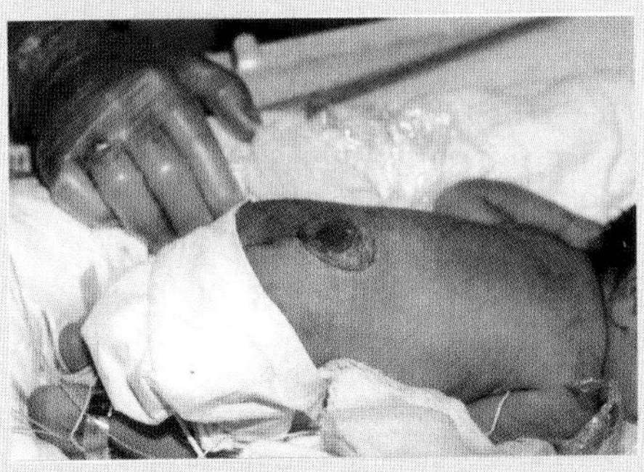 Newborn with lumbar myelomeningocele. **SOURCE:** Carol Harrigan, RN, MSN, NNP-BC.	Myelomeningocele directly connects to subarachnoid space so hydrocephalus often associated No response or varying response to sensation below level of defect May have constant dribbling of urine Incontinence or retention of stool Anal wink may or may not be present	Prevent trauma and infection. Position on abdomen or on side and restrain (to prevent pressure and trauma to sac). Obtain neurosurgery and urology consult. Meticulously clean buttocks and genitals after each void and stool (to prevent contamination and infection of sac). Cover with protective plastic wrap over sac (to prevent trauma, rupture, and drying). *Do not cover defect with wet saline gauze.* Administer broad-spectrum antibiotics to prevent infection. Observe sac for oozing of fluid. Credé bladder (apply downward pressure on bladder with thumbs, moving urine toward the urethra) as ordered to prevent urinary stasis. Assess amount of sensation and movement below defect. Obtain baseline OFC measurements; then measure head circumference daily (to detect hydrocephalus). Check fontanelle for fullness and bulging.
Imperforate Anus (absence of anal opening, may or may not have a fistula connection; boy: Fistula between rectum and urinary tract, scrotum, penis, perineum; girl: Fistula between rectum and vagina or perineum)	Inability to visualize rectal opening No meconium is passed Meconium passed through fistula or malpositioned anus Gradual abdominal distension if no fistula present	Inspect perineal area for presence of fistula. Initiate gastric decompression by insertion of an indwelling Replogle tube attached to low suction if no fistula present; measure and replace gastric output. Maintain fluid balance. Obtain surgical consult.
Congenital Dislocated Hip and Clubfoot	See discussion in Chapter 27	

Overview of Congenital Heart Defects

In the majority of cases of congenital heart malformations, the cause is multifactorial (a combination of multiple genes and the environment) with no specific trigger. Other factors that might influence development of congenital heart malformation can be classified as environmental or genetic. Infections of the pregnant woman, such as rubella, cytomegalovirus, coxsackie B, and influenza, have been implicated. Steroids, alcohol, lithium, and some anticonvulsants have been shown to cause malformations of the heart. Seasonal spraying of pesticides has also been linked to an increase in congenital heart defects. Clinicians are also beginning to see cardiac defects in babies of mothers with phenylketonuria (PKU) who do not follow their diets. Increased incidence and risk of recurrence of specific defects occur in families.

Genetic Facts Congenital Heart Disease

In the general population, about 1% of all children are born with congenital heart disease. There is an overall threefold increased risk for congenital heart disease when a first-degree relative has it (University of Rochester Medical Center, 2018). Congenital heart disease in the newborn increases the long-term risk of cardiovascular disease in the mother (Auger, Potter, Bilodeau-Bertrand, et al., 2018).

Babies with chromosomal abnormalities such as Down syndrome, Turner syndrome, Holt-Oram syndrome, trisomy 13, and trisomy 18 frequently have heart lesions or malformations. Chromosome analysis can be done from a small blood sample to look for a chromosome abnormality in a child with a congenital heart defect.

The most common cardiac defects seen in the first 6 days of life are left-ventricular outflow obstructions, such as mitral stenosis and aortic stenosis or atresia; hypoplastic left heart; coarctation of the aorta; PDA, which is the most common defect in premature newborns; transposition of the great vessels; tetralogy of Fallot; and large ventricular septal defect or atrial septal defects. Many cardiac defects may not manifest themselves until after discharge from the birthing unit.

Clinical Tip

When cyanosis occurs in an otherwise healthy 12- to-24-hour-old newborn displaying no respiratory symptoms other than a rapid respiratory rate without retractions or grunting and it is not resolved with oxygen, think about cardiac issues, especially a ductal-dependent lesion (termed *happy tachycardia*).

●○● NURSING MANAGEMENT

For the Newborn with a Cardiac Defect

The primary goals of the neonatal nurse are early identification of cardiac defects by a thorough physical examination and noninvasive tools to ensure quick intervention and referral to a cardiac specialist for a positive outcome. The physical assessment should include a visual inspection of the newborn's overall physical appearance; vital signs, including four-point blood pressures; and pre- and postductal oxygen saturations and pulse oximetry.

The three most common manifestations of a cardiac defect are central cyanosis, detectable heart murmur, and signs of congestive heart failure.

- *Central cyanosis* is defined as a visible, blue discoloration of the skin caused by decreased oxygen saturation levels.
- *Heart murmurs*, although not uncommon in the newborn period, are the result of turbulent blood flow within the heart and surrounding vessels and are described by their intensity or grading (Table 30–5) and timing. The timing of murmurs refers to whether the murmur is heard in systole (between first and second heart sound) or in diastole (during ventricular filling). Systolic murmurs are often innocent and are of no pathologic consequences. Diastolic murmurs, on the other hand, are often pathologic in nature and are often due to stenosis.
- *Congestive heart failure* (*CHF*) is the inability of the heart to pump adequate blood volumes needed by the body, typically caused by lesions with outflow obstructions (hypoplastic left heart syndrome) or volume overload of the left ventricle (PDA). Common symptoms seen with CHF include cardiomegaly, tachycardia, tachypnea, hepatomegaly, decreased peripheral pulses, peripheral edema, and low urinary output.

Table 30–6 presents the clinical manifestations and medical/surgical management of these cardiac defects.

Initial repair of heart defects in the newborn period is becoming more commonplace. The NICU staff is now more involved in both the preoperative and postoperative care of cardiac newborns. The benefits for the cardiac newborn of being cared for by NICU staff include the staff's knowledge of neonatal anatomy and physiology, experience in supporting the family, and an awareness of the developmental needs of the newborn

After the baby is stabilized, decisions are made about the special ongoing care needs. The parents need careful and complete explanations and the opportunity to take part in decision making. They also require ongoing emotional support. Families of all babies born with congenital abnormalities need genetic counseling regarding future conception. Parents need to verbalize their concern about their baby's health maintenance and to understand the rationale for follow-up care.

Ethics in Action!

With extensive counseling after the birth of a baby with hypoplastic left heart syndrome, the parents have decided to provide palliative care only for their newborn and not put her through numerous surgeries. What would you say to the parents regarding their decision?

TABLE 30–5 Grading of Heart Murmurs

Grade 1	Barely audible
Grade 2	Quiet
Grade 3	Moderately loud
Grade 4	Loud with palpable thrill
Grade 5	Very loud with palpable thrill; audible with stethoscope barely touching chest
Grade 6	Very loud with palpable thrill; audible without stethoscope touching chest

TABLE 30–6 Cardiac Defects of the Early Newborn Period

CONGENITAL HEART DEFECT	CLINICAL FINDINGS	MEDICAL/SURGICAL MANAGEMENT
INCREASED PULMONARY BLOOD FLOW		
Patent Ductus Arteriosus (PDA) ↑ in females, maternal rubella, RDS, less than 1500 g (3.3 lb) preterm newborns, high-altitude births	Harsh grade 2–3/6 machinery-type murmur heard at upper left sternal border (LSB) just beneath clavicle ↑ difference between systolic and diastolic pulse pressure Bounding peripheral pulses Hyperactive precordium Can lead to right-sided heart failure and pulmonary congestion ↑ left-atrial (LA) and left-ventricular (LV) enlargement, dilated ascending aorta ↑ pulmonary vascularity on x-ray Can be evident on day 2 or 3 of life	Indomethacin—0.2 mg/kg IV Q12 hr × 3 doses Neoprofen—10 mg/kg IV × 1 dose then 5 mg/kg IV at 24 and 48 hrs from first dose (both prostaglandin inhibitors) Surgical ligation, occlusion coil Use of O_2 therapy and blood transfusion to improve tissue oxygenation and perfusion Fluid restriction, digoxin, and diuretics to manage symptoms of CHF
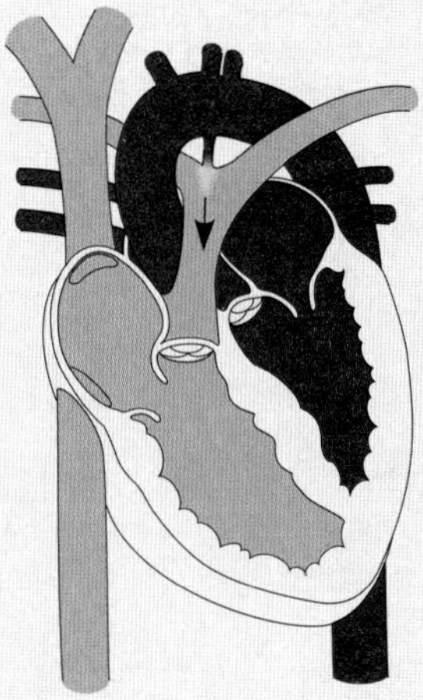	*The patent ductus arteriosus is a vascular connection that, during fetal life, bypasses the pulmonary vascular bed and directs blood from the pulmonary artery to the aorta. Postnatally, blood shunts through the ductus from the aorta to the pulmonary artery (left-to-right shunting).*	
Atrial Septal Defect (ASD) ↑ in females and Down syndrome	Initially frequently asymptomatic in the newborn period Systolic murmur grade 2–3/6 second heard at left sternal border left intercostal space (LICS) with splitting second heart sound (S2) With large ASD, diastolic rumbling murmur lower left sternal (LLS) border Failure to thrive, upper respiratory infection (URI), poor exercise tolerance	Surgical closure with patch or suture Umbrella occlude
Ventricular Septal Defect (VSD) ↑ in males Most common heart defect	Initially asymptomatic until end of first month or large enough to cause pulmonary edema Loud, blowing systolic murmur between the third and fourth intercostal space (ICS); pulmonary blood flow heard at lower left sternal border Right-ventricular hypertrophy Rapid respirations, growth failure, feeding difficulties Congestive right heart failure at 6 weeks–2 months of age Typically closes spontaneously during first 2 years of life	Follow medically—some spontaneously close Use of digoxin and diuretics to manage CHF Surgical closure with Dacron patch or umbrella occluder

(continued)

TABLE 30–6 Cardiac Defects of the Early Newborn Period *(continued)*

CONGENITAL HEART DEFECT	CLINICAL FINDINGS	MEDICAL/SURGICAL MANAGEMENT
OBSTRUCTION TO SYSTEMIC BLOOD FLOW		
Coarctation of Aorta Can be preductal or postductal 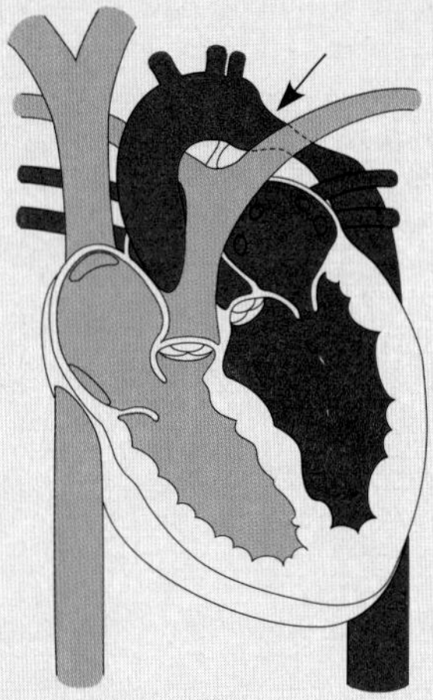	Blood pressure higher above the area of coarctation than below Absent or diminished femoral pulses Increased brachial pulses Late systolic ejection murmur Grade 1–2/6 heard at left intrascapular area, loudest in the back Systolic BP in lower extremities Enlarged left ventricle Can present in CHF at 7–21 days of life Progressive cyanosis as PDA closes *Coarctation of the aorta is characterized by a narrowed aortic lumen. The lesion produces an obstruction to the flow of blood through the aorta, causing an increased left-ventricular pressure and workload, minimizing systemic circulation of blood.*	Four-point blood pressure measurements Surgical resection of narrowed portion of aorta Prostaglandin E_1 (PGE_1) to maintain patency of PDA to ensure systemic blood flow No afterload reducer drugs
Hypoplastic Left Heart Syndrome	Normal at birth—cyanosis and shocklike congestive heart failure develop within a few hours to days Soft systolic murmur heard just left of the sternum Diminished pulses Aortic and/or mitral atresia Tiny, thick-walled left ventricle Large, dilated, hypertrophied right ventricle X-ray examination: Cardiac enlargement: Enlarged right atrium and ventricle and pulmonary venous congestion Hypoplastic left heart syndrome is the underdevelopment of the left side of the heart including aortic valve atresia, severe mitral valve stenosis, and small left ventricle	Prostaglandin E_1 (PGE_1) until treatment decision made Norwood procedure Fontan procedure Transplant Compassionate care
DECREASED PULMONARY BLOOD FLOW		
Tetralogy of Fallot (TOF) Pulmonary stenosis Ventricular septal defect (VSD) Overriding aorta Right-ventricular hypertrophy	May be cyanotic at birth or within first few months of life Harsh systolic murmur LSB Crying or feeding increases cyanosis and respiratory distress X-ray: "Boot-shaped" appearance secondary to small pulmonary artery Right-ventricular enlargement	Prevention of dehydration, intercurrent infections Alleviation of paroxysmal dyspneic attacks Palliative surgery to increase blood flow to the lungs Corrective surgery—resection of pulmonic stenosis, closure of VSD with Dacron patch

TABLE 30–6 Cardiac Defects of the Early Newborn Period *(continued)*

CONGENITAL HEART DEFECT	CLINICAL FINDINGS	MEDICAL/SURGICAL MANAGEMENT
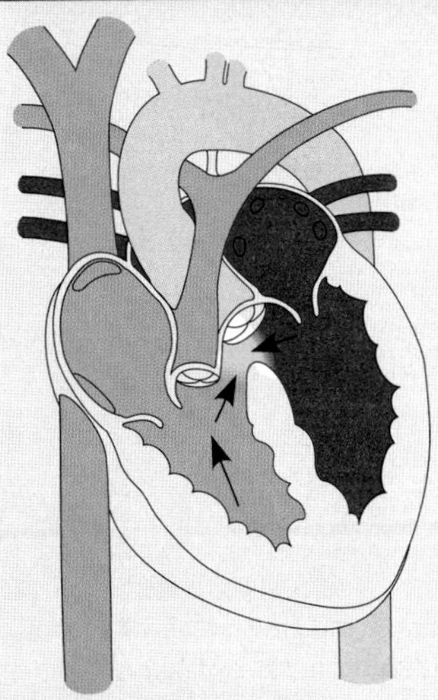	*In tetralogy of Fallot, the severity of symptoms depends on the degree of pulmonary stenosis, the size of the ventricular septal defect, and the degree to which the aorta overrides the septal defect.*	
MIXED DEFECTS*		
Transposition of Great Vessels (TGA) (Most common cyanotic heart defect) ↑ females, newborns of mothers with diabetes, LGAs	Significant cyanosis at birth or within 3 days as PDA closes Possible pulmonic stenosis murmur Right-ventricular hypertrophy Polycythemia X-ray: "Egg on its side" appearance	Prostaglandin E (PGE_1) to maintain patency of the PDA Initial surgery to create opening between right and left side of heart if none exists Total surgical repair—usually the arterial switch procedure—done within first few days of life
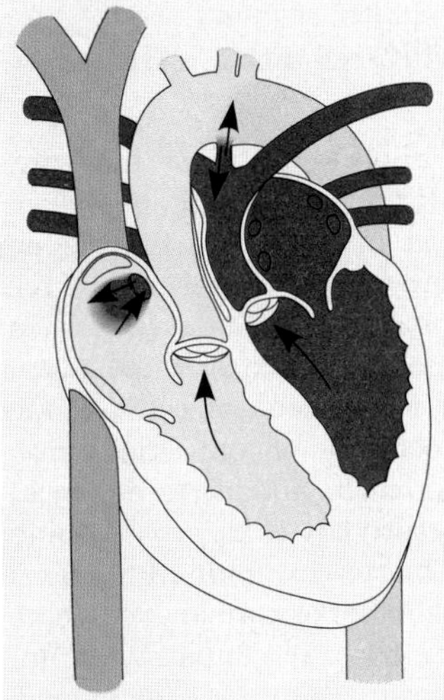	*Complete transposition of great vessels is an embryologic defect caused by a straight division of the bulbar trunk without normal spiraling. As a result, the aorta originates from the right ventricle and the pulmonary artery from the left ventricle, resulting in a parallel circulatory system. An abnormal communication between the two circulations must be present to sustain life.*	

*Mixed defects: Postnatal survival is dependent upon mixing of systemic and pulmonary blood flow.

SOURCE: LADEWIG, PATRICIA W; LONDON, MARCIA L; DAVIDSON, MICHELE, CONTEMPORARY MATERNAL-NEWBORN NURSING, 9th Ed., ©2017. Reprinted and Electronically reproduced by permission of Pearson Education, Inc., New York, NY.

Care of the Newborn of a Substance-Abusing Mother

Substance abuse during pregnancy is often undiagnosed and underestimated, putting the pregnant woman at high risk for maternal and fetal morbidity as well as significant neonatal withdrawal. Tetratogenicity, poor maternal nutrition, poor placental perfusion, and placental insufficiency leading to growth restriction in the fetus are common obstetric concerns for the substance-abusing mother. The drug or alcohol use of the substance-abusing mother may vary from infrequent, recreational use to daily use due to psychologic and physiologic addiction. An **infant of a substance-abusing mother (ISAM)** may be exposed to a number of licit and illicit drugs singularly or in combination (see Table 30–7). Identification of these intrauterine-drug-exposed newborns becomes essential not only to anticipate problems in the delivery room and in the nursery but also to recognize those babies at risk for long-term neurodevelopmental sequelae following discharge.

The Newborn with Fetal Alcohol Spectrum Disorders

Fetal alcohol syndrome (FAS), a leading cause of preventable, nongenetic intellectual disability, includes a group of physical, behavioral, and cognitive abnormalities frequently found in

TABLE 30–7 Common Drugs of Abuse

OPIOIDS/OPIATES	CNS STIMULANTS	CNS DEPRESSANTS/SEDATIVES	HALLUCINOGENS
Codeine	Amphetamines	Alcohol	Inhalants
Darvon	Cocaine	Barbiturates	LSD
Demerol	Methamphetamines	Benzodiazepines	Solvents and aerosols (glue, gasoline, paint, cleaning solutions)
Fentanyl	Nicotine	Chloral hydrate	
Heroin	Phencyclidines	Cannabinoids (marijuana)	
Hydrocodone (Lortab, Vicodin)	Ritalin		
Hydromorphone (Dilaudid)			
Methadone			
Morphine			
Oxycodone (Percocet, OxyContin)			

babies exposed to alcohol in utero. New guidelines for diagnosis and referral of newborns/infants and children with FAS have been developed. The term **fetal alcohol spectrum disorders (FASDs)** is now used to include all categories of prenatal alcohol exposure, including FAS. The diagnostic categories for FASDs take into consideration the various clinical manifestations of FAS, the social and family environment, and, if available, the maternal alcohol history. Current conservative estimates of FASD in U.S. populations ranges from 11.3 to 50% (May, Chambers, Kalberg, et al., 2018). Instances of FASD cross all races, ethnic groups, and socioeconomic levels.

Although it has been known that ethanol freely crosses the placenta to the fetus, it is now known that its by-products are equally responsible for the damage. There is also strong evidence that the amount of alcohol ingested is directly responsible for the neurodevelopmental outcomes of these babies; alcohol exposure includes at least six drinks during at least 2 weeks of pregnancy, or at least three drinks per occasion on two or more occasions while pregnant; or has documented alcohol-related social or legal problems during pregnancy (Hoyme et al., 2016). Often, the consumption of alcohol occurs during conception, when critical fetal organogenesis is most adversely affected. (Chapter 17 discusses alcohol abuse in pregnancy.) The effects of other substances often combined with alcohol—such as nicotine, diazepam (Valium), marijuana, and caffeine—as well as poor diet, enhance the likelihood of FAS. Newborns with FASDs show the following characteristics:

- *Abnormal structural development and CNS dysfunction.* These include irritability, hypotonia, microcephaly, and hyperactivity and cognitive disability in childhood.
- *Growth deficiencies.* The growth of babies with FAS is often restricted in regard to weight, length, and head circumference. These babies continue to show a persistent postnatal growth deficiency, with head circumference and linear growth most affected.
- *Distinctive facial abnormalities.* These include short palpebral fissures; epicanthal folds; broad nasal bridge; flattened midfaces; short, upturned, or beaklike nose; micrognathia (abnormally small lower jaw); hypoplastic maxilla; thin upper lip or vermilion border; and smooth philtrum (groove on upper lip) (Eichenwald et al., 2017).
- *Associated anomalies.* Abnormalities affecting the heart (primarily septal and valvular defects), eyes (optic nerve hypoplasia), ears (conductive and sensorineural hearing loss), kidneys, and skeletal system (especially involving joints, such as congenital dislocated hips) are often noted.

An alcohol-exposed newborn in the first week of life may show symptoms that include sleeplessness, excessive arousal states, inconsolable crying, abnormal reflexes, hyperactivity with little ability to maintain alertness and attentiveness to environment, jitteriness, abdominal distention, and exaggerated mouthing behaviors such as hyperactive rooting and increased nonnutritive sucking. Epilepsy may be common. These symptoms commonly persist throughout the first month of life but may continue longer (Hoyme et al., 2016). Alcohol dependence in the newborn is physiologic, not psychologic. Signs and symptoms of withdrawal often appear within 3 to 12 hours and can last up to 18 months (Eichenwald, 2017).

LONG-TERM COMPLICATIONS FOR THE NEWBORN WITH FASDS

Because of the failure-to-thrive appearance, many newborns with FASDs are often evaluated for deficiencies in organic and inorganic amino acids. These babies have a delay in oral feeding development but have a normal progression of oral–motor function. Many babies with FASDs nurse poorly and have persistent vomiting until 6 to 7 months of age. They have difficulty adjusting to solid foods and show little spontaneous interest in food.

CNS dysfunctions are the most common and serious problem associated with FASDs. Hypotonicity and increased placidity are seen in these babies. They also have a decreased ability to block out repetitive stimuli. Children exhibiting FASDs can have either severe intellectual disabilities or normal intelligence. These children show impulsivity, cognitive impairment, and speech and language abnormalities indicative of CNS involvement. As they progress through the adolescent years, they often change from very thin and underweight children to those who are overweight and even obese. Short stature and microcephaly (condition in which a baby's head is significantly smaller than expected, often due to abnormal brain development) persist.

●○● NURSING MANAGEMENT

For the Newborn with Fetal Alcohol Spectrum Disorders

Nursing care of the newborn with FASDs is aimed at avoiding heat loss, providing adequate nutrition, and reducing environmental stimuli. This baby is most comfortable in a quiet, dimly lit environment. Because of feeding problems, the newborn with FASDs requires extra time and patience during feedings. It is important to provide consistency in the staff working with the baby and the parents and to keep personnel and visitors to a minimum at any one time.

Inform the alcohol-dependent mother that breastfeeding is not contraindicated but that excessive alcohol consumption may intoxicate the newborn and inhibit the let-down reflex. Monitor the newborn's vital signs closely and observe for evidence of seizure activity and respiratory distress.

Babies affected by maternal alcohol abuse are also at risk psychologically. Restlessness, sleeplessness, agitation, resistance to cuddling or holding, and frequent crying can be frustrating to parents because their efforts to relieve the distress are unrewarded. Feeding difficulties can also result in frustrations for the caregiver and digestive upsets for the baby. Frustration may cause the parents to punish the baby or result in the unconscious desire to stay away from the baby. Either outcome may create an unstable family environment and result in failure to thrive.

Focus on providing support for the parents and reinforcing positive parenting activity. Before discharge, give parents opportunities to provide baby care so that they can feel confident in their interpretations of their baby's cues and ability to meet the baby's needs. Referring the family to social services and visiting nurse or public health nurse associations is essential for the well-being of the child. Follow-up care and teaching can strengthen the parents' skill and coping abilities and help them create a stable, healthy environment for their family. The baby with FASDs should be involved in intervention programs that monitor the child's developmental progress, health, and home environment. Having a medical home is recommended to ensure comprehensive and regular monitoring of health and developmental status.

Opiate Dependency

Patterns of abuse of opiates, including heroin, morphine, codeine, and prescription narcotics, in childbearing women have increased in the last several years (McQueen & Murphy-Oikonen, 2016). (See *Substances Commonly Abused During Pregnancy* in Chapter 17 for more discussion of maternal substance abuse.)

Almost all opioid drugs readily cross the placenta and enter the fetal circulation, resulting in problems in the fetus in utero or in the newborn following delivery. Because opioid receptors are primarily in the CNS and GI tract, the signs and symptoms reflect CNS irritability, autonomic irritability, and GI dysfunction. The effects of polydrug use on the newborn must always be taken into consideration. See Professionalism in Practice: HR 1462–Protecting Our Infants Act of 2015.

The greatest risks to the fetus of the drug-abusing mother include:

- ***Intrauterine asphyxia.*** Asphyxia is often a direct result of fetal withdrawal secondary to maternal withdrawal. Fetal withdrawal is accompanied by hyperactivity, with increased oxygen consumption. Insufficiency of oxygen can lead to fetal asphyxia. Moreover, women addicted to narcotics tend to have a higher incidence of preeclampsia, abruptio placentae, and placenta previa, resulting in placental insufficiency and fetal asphyxia.
- ***Intrauterine infection.*** Sexually transmitted infection, HIV infection, and hepatitis are often connected with the pregnant addict's lifestyle. In addition, intravenous drug abuse can predispose the mother to many infections including cellulitis, endocarditis, and chorioamnionitis (AAP & ACOG, 2017). Such infections can involve the fetus.
- ***Intrauterine growth restriction(IUGR).*** There is a high correlation between substance abuse and poor maternal nutrition. In addition, diminished placental function has been evident as an additional cause for compromised fetal growth including weight and OFC. This in turn contributes to the increased risk for stillbirths. Surveillance during the antenatal period, to include serial fetal ultrasounds, fundal height measurements, Doppler velometry readings, biophysical profiles, and nonstress tests (NSTs), will assist in diagnosing IUGR in the substance-abusing mother.
- ***Low Apgar scores.*** Low scores may be related to the intrauterine asphyxia or the medication the woman received during labor. The use of a narcotic antagonist (nalorphine or naloxone) to reverse respiratory depression is contraindicated because it may precipitate acute withdrawal in the newborn.

Professionalism in Practice HR 1462–Protecting Our Infants Act of 2015

(Sec. 3). This bill requires the Agency for Healthcare Research and Quality to report on prenatal opioid abuse and neonatal abstinence syndrome (symptoms of withdrawal in a newborn). The report must include:

- Assessment of existing research on neonatal abstinence syndrome
- Evaluation of the causes and barriers to treatment of opioid use disorders among women of reproductive age
- Evaluation of treatment for pregnant women with opioid use disorders and infants with neonatal abstinence syndrome
- Recommendations on preventing, identifying, and treating opioid dependency in women and neonatal abstinence syndrome.

(Sec. 4). The Department of Health and Human Services must review its activities related to prenatal opioid use and neonatal abstinence syndrome and develop a strategy to address gaps in research and programs.

(Sec. 5). The Centers for Disease Control and Prevention must provide technical assistance to states to improve neonatal abstinence syndrome surveillance and make surveillance data publicly available.

COMMON COMPLICATIONS OF THE DRUG-EXPOSED NEWBORN

The newborn of a woman who abused drugs during her pregnancy is predisposed to the following problems:

- ***Respiratory distress.*** The heroin-addicted newborn frequently suffers respiratory stress, mainly meconium-aspiration pneumonia and transient tachypnea. Meconium aspiration is usually secondary to increased oxygen consumption and activity experienced by the fetus during intrauterine withdrawal. Transient tachypnea may develop secondary to the inhibitory effects of narcotics on the reflex responsible for clearing the lungs. RDS, however, occurs less often in heroin-addicted newborns, even in those who are premature, because they have tissue-oxygen-unloading capabilities comparable to those of a 6-week-old term infant. In addition, heroin stimulates production of glucocorticoids via the anterior pituitary gland.
- ***Jaundice.*** Newborns of methadone-addicted women may develop jaundice because of prematurity. By contrast, babies of mothers addicted to heroin or cocaine have a lower incidence of hyperbilirubinemia because these substances contribute to early maturity of the liver.
- ***Congenital anomalies and growth restriction.*** Babies of cocaine-addicted mothers exhibit congenital malformations

involving bony skull defects, such as microcephaly, and symmetric IUGR, cardiac defects, and genitourinary defects. In addition, the incidence of SIDS is higher. Congenital anomalies, however, are rare. Newborns exposed to methamphetamines during gestation may show a higher incidence of cardiac anomalies, cleft lip and palate, microencephaly, and LBW (Blackburn, 2018). However, congenital anomalies are rare.

- ***Behavioral abnormalities.*** Babies exposed to cocaine have poor state organization. They exhibit decreased interactive behaviors when tested with the Brazelton Neonatal Behavioral Assessment Scale. These newborns also have difficulty moving through the various sleep–wake states and have problems attending to and actively engaging in auditory and visual stimuli.
- ***Withdrawal.*** The most significant postnatal problem of the drug-exposed newborn is opiate withdrawal (usually from heroin or methadone). The onset of withdrawal manifestations often begins within the first 24 to 48 hours of life; effects can be seen for as long as several days to a few weeks (ACOG, 2017). See Table 30–8 for the clinical manifestations of newborn withdrawal.

During the first 2 years of life, many cocaine-exposed infants demonstrate susceptibility to behavior lability and the inability to express strong feelings such as pleasure, anger, or distress, or even a strong reaction to being separated from their parents. As a result, these infants have poor social interaction skills; cannot habituate to external stimuli; and become easily overstimulated, having difficulty sleeping. Cocaine-exposed newborns are at higher risk for motor development problems, delays in expressive language skills, and feeding difficulties because of swallowing problems (Weiner & Finnegan, 2016). Behavioral state control is poorly developed in drug-exposed babies, who tend to rapidly progress from sleep to the awake state of crying without a smooth transition from one state to the next. Babies of drug-addicted mothers often demonstrate a higher incidence of gastrointestinal and respiratory illnesses related to the mother's lack of education regarding proper newborn/infant care, feeding, and hygiene. After birth the newborn born to a drug-dependent mother may also be subject to neglect or abuse, or both.

CLINICAL THERAPY

For optimal fetal and neonatal outcome, the heroin-addicted woman should receive complete prenatal care as early as possible to reduce maternal morbidity and mortality rates and to promote fetal stability and growth. Methadone maintenance programs have been the standard treatment for the heroin-addicted mother to combat the cravings and to prevent withdrawal, although evidence suggests that buprenorphine may be associated with less severe neonatal withdrawal than methadone (McQueen & Murphy-Oikonen, 2016). For those women dependent on narcotics, it is not recommended that they be withdrawn completely while pregnant because this induces fetal withdrawal with poor newborn outcomes.

Newborn treatment may include management of complications; serologic tests for syphilis, HIV, and hepatitis B; urine drug screen and meconium analysis; and social service referral. Screening of meconium provides a more comprehensive and accurate indication of exposure over a longer gestational period than does screening of neonatal urine and is comparable to umbilical cord tissue samples (Hamdan, 2017).

Pharmacologic management for opiate withdrawal may include oral morphine sulfate solution, paregoric, tincture of opium, oral methadone, phenobarbital (adjunct therapy) clonidine (adjunct therapy), and diazepam. In addition, the use of the mother's expressed breast milk or breastfeeding by women who are in methadone-assisted treatment programs has been beneficial for substance-exposed babies in decreasing the need for lengthy neonatal abstinence syndrome (NAS) treatment (ACOG, 2017). Nutritional support is important in light of the increase in energy expenditure that withdrawal may entail.

●○● NURSING MANAGEMENT

For the Substance-Exposed Newborn

Nursing Assessment and Diagnosis

Early identification of the newborn needing clinical or pharmacologic interventions decreases the incidence of neonatal mortality and morbidity. The identification of substance-exposed newborns is determined primarily by clinical indicators in the prenatal period including maternal presentation, history of substance use or abuse, medical history, or toxicology results. During the newborn period, nursing assessment focuses on:

- Discovering the mother's last drug intake and dosage level. Women may be reluctant to disclose this information; therefore, a nonjudgmental interview technique is essential (AAP & ACOG, 2017).

TABLE 30–8 Clinical Manifestations of Newborn Withdrawal

Central Nervous System Signs	Gastrointestinal Signs	AUTONOMIC SIGNS
• High-pitched cry • Hyperirritability, difficult to console, restlessness • Increased muscle tone • Exaggerated reflexes • Tremors, myoclonic jerks • Seizures • Sneezing, hiccups, yawning • Short, unquiet sleep **Cutaneous Signs** • Excoriated buttocks, knees, elbows • Facial scratches • Pressure-point abrasions	• Disorganized, vigorous suck • Excessive sucking • Vomiting • Poor weight gain • Sensitive gag reflex • Diarrhea • Poor feeding (less than 15 mL on first day of life; takes longer than 30 minutes per feeding)	• Stuffy nose, sneezing • Yawning • Mottled • Tachypnea (greater than 60 breaths/minute when quiet) • Sweating • Hyperthermia

- Assessing for congenital malformations and the complications related to intrauterine withdrawal such as SGA, asphyxia, meconium aspiration, and prematurity.
- Identifying the scoring system for signs and symptoms of newborn withdrawal or neonatal abstinence syndrome (see Table 30–9).

TABLE 30–9 Scoring of Neonatal Abstinence Syndrome Signs and Symptoms

Central Nervous System Disturbances	
Cry	• Continuous high-pitched cry
	• Excessive high-pitched cry
Sleep	• Sleeps less than 3 hours after feeding
	• Sleeps less than 2 hours after feeding
	• Sleeps less than 1 hour after feeding
Moro reflex	• Markedly hyperactive Moro reflex
	• Hyperactive Moro reflex
Tremors	• Moderate–severe tremors undisturbed
	• Mild tremors undisturbed
	• Moderate–severe tremors disturbed
	• Mild tremors disturbed
Convulsions	• Generalized convulsions
	• Myoclonic jerks
	• Increased muscle tone
	• Excoriation (specific area)
Metabolic Disturbances	
Thermo-regulation	• Sweating
	• Fever over 38.4°C (101°F)
	• Fever under 38.3°c (101°F) (37.2°–38.2°C [99°–100.8°F])
Vasomotor Disturbances	
	• Frequent yawning (more than 3–4 times/interval)
	• Mottling of the skin
	• Nasal stuffiness
	• Sneezing (more than 3–4 times/interval)
Respiratory Disturbances	
Respiration	• Nasal flaring
	• Respiratory rate more than 60 per minute with retractions
	• Respiratory rate more than 60 per minute
Gastrointestinal Disturbances	
Feeding	• Poor feeding
	• Excessive sucking
Vomiting	• Projectile vomiting
	• Regurgitation
Stooling	• Watery stools
	• Loose stools

NOTE:
- Signs and symptoms are listed in descending order of severity for each subgroup.
- Signs/symptoms are scored 1–5, with 5 being the most severe using a neonatal abstinence score sheet.
- The newborn should be evaluated every 4 hours and a daily weight noted.

SOURCES: Data from Finnegan, 1990; Zahorodny et al., 1998.

Although many of the signs and symptoms of drug withdrawal are similar to those seen with hypoglycemia and hypocalcemia, glucose and calcium values are reported to be within normal limits.

Neonatal abstinence syndrome includes both physiologic and behavioral responses. The severity of withdrawal can be assessed by a scoring system based on observations and measurement of the responses to neonatal abstinence such as the Finnegan scale. It evaluates the newborn every 4 hours on 31 potentially life-threatening signs, which are given a score from 1 to 5. A newer option, the Neonatal Withdrawal Inventory (NWI), is another tool that evaluates and scores seven prominent signs of withdrawal; each sign is given a predetermined weight of 1 to 4, with the highest total score of 19 (Hamdan, 2017; Zahorodny et al., 1998). Both NAS scoring tools help to guide the need for pharmacologic intervention; pharmacologic treatment is warranted for three consecutive Finnegan or NWI scores greater than 8. Many hospitals have modified existing scales and have created a scoring system of their own.

Nursing diagnoses that may apply to drug-dependent newborns include those below and in *Nursing Care Plan: For the Newborn of a Substance-Abusing Mother*.

- ***Infant Behavior: Disorganized,*** related to perinatal substance abuse
- ***Breathing Pattern, Ineffective,*** related to meconium aspiration syndrome due to fetal stress and hypoxia
- ***Skin Integrity, Impaired,*** related to constant activity, diarrhea
- ***Parenting, Impaired,*** related to hyperirritable behavior of the newborn and lack of knowledge of newborn/infant care

(NANDA-I © 2017)

Nursing Plan and Implementation

Hospital-Based Nursing Care

Care of the drug-dependent newborn is based on reducing withdrawal symptoms and promoting adequate respiration, temperature, and nutrition. See *Nursing Care Plan: For the Newborn of a Substance-Abusing Mother* for specific nursing measures. Some general nursery care measures include:

- Perform neonatal abstinence scoring per hospital protocol. (See *Professionalism in Practice: Newborns with Neonatal Abstinence Syndrome*.)
- Monitor temperature for hypothermia.
- Monitor pulse and respirations carefully every 15 minutes and pulse oximetry until stable.
- Provide small, frequent feedings, especially in the presence of vomiting, regurgitation, and diarrhea.
- Breastfeeding is recommended for women who are not using additional drugs or who are in methadone treatment programs (Reece-Stremtan, Marinelli, & Academy of Breastfeeding Medicine, 2015).
- Position on the right side-lying or semi-Fowler position to avoid possible aspiration of vomitus or secretions.
- Monitor weight-gain pattern daily to assess the need for increased calorie content of formula.
- Administer medications as ordered, such as oral morphine elixir, oral methadone, and sublingual buprenorphine (ACOG, 2017). Standardized administration protocols are instrumental in decreasing withdrawal time.
- Monitor frequency of diarrhea and vomiting and weigh newborn every 8 hours during withdrawal.

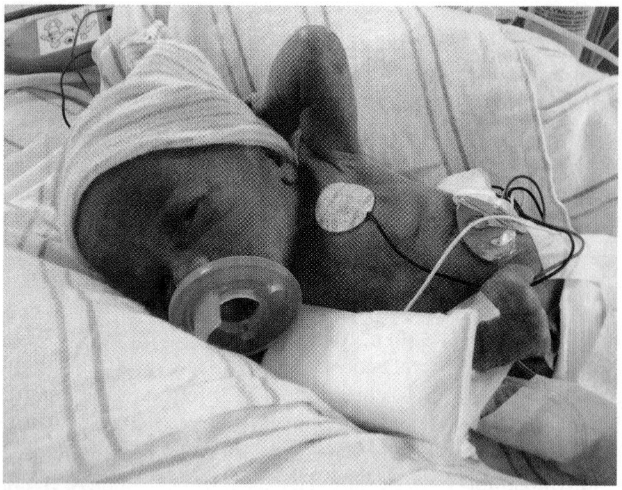

Figure 30–17 **Nonnutritive sucking on a pacifier has a calming effect on the preterm newborn and also facilitates readiness to bottle-feed.**

SOURCE: Carol Harrigan, RN, MSN, NNP-BC.

- Swaddle with hands near mouth to minimize injury and achieve more organized behavioral state. Offer breast or a pacifier for nonnutritive, excessive sucking (Figure 30–17). Gentle, vertical rocking can be successful in calming a baby who is out of control.
- Protect newborn's face and extremities from excoriation by using clothing with built-in mittens, as well as soft sheets or sheepskin. Apply protective skin emollient to the groin area with each diaper change. Breast milk lowers the pH of both the stool and urine, which could improve overall skin pH and assist in preventing diaper dermatitis (Bagwell et al., 2016).
- Place the newborn in a quiet, dimly lit area of the nursery. Research has shown that the more parental time spent at the baby's bedside decreases NAS severity (Howard, Schiff, Penwill, et al., 2017).

Professionalism In Practice Newborns with Neonatal Abstinence Syndrome

A multistate quality improvement collaborative focusing on newborns with NAS had increases in standardizing hospital patient care policies and decreases in healthcare utilization. There was a decrease in the proportion of newborns discharged on medication for NAS, and a standardized NAS scoring process was associated with a shorter length of stay (Patrick et al., 2016).

Community-Based Nursing Care

Parents need assistance to prepare for what they can expect for the first few months at home. At the time of discharge, the mother should be instructed to anticipate mild jitteriness and irritability in the newborn, which may persist from 6 days to 8 weeks, depending on the initial severity of the withdrawal (Blackburn, 2018). Babies with neonatal abstinence syndrome are at significantly higher risk for SIDS when the mother used heroin or cocaine. The baby should sleep supine and home apnea monitoring should be implemented. Help the mother learn feeding techniques, comforting measures, how to recognize newborn cues, and appropriate parenting responses. Counsel parents regarding available resources, such as support groups, as well as signs and symptoms that indicate the need for further care. Ongoing evaluation is necessary because of the potential for long-term problems. Follow-up on missed appointments can bring parents back into the healthcare system, thereby improving parent and baby outcomes and promoting a positive, interactive environment after birth (AAP & ACOG, 2017).

Evaluation

Expected outcomes of nursing care include:

- The newborn tolerates feedings, gains weight, and has a decreased incidence of diarrhea.
- The parents learn innovative ways to comfort their newborn.
- The parents are able to cope with their frustrations and begin to use outside resources as needed.

Newborns of Mothers Who Are Tobacco Dependent

Despite increased knowledge about the dangers to the fetus and newborn of smoking mothers, 1 in 10 women smokes in the 3 months before getting pregnant. The smoking rate overall during pregnancy was 8.4%, with 20.6% of women quitting by the third trimester (CDC, 2016). The common consequence of tobacco use is addiction to nicotine.

RISKS OF TOBACCO TO THE FETUS AND NEWBORN

Preconceptual cigarette smoking has been found to increase infertility. Fortunately, the reduction in fertility is reversible if the woman stops smoking. Smoking during pregnancy has been associated with spontaneous abortion, placenta previa, and abruptio placentae.

The most studied compound found in cigarette smoking that can adversely affect the intrauterine environment is carbon monoxide. Carbon monoxide binds hemoglobin to form carboxyhemoglobin, which reduces the oxygen-carrying capacity of the blood. It also increases the binding of hemoglobin to oxygen, which impairs the release of oxygen to the tissues. Therefore, the fetus can experience intrauterine hypoxia and ischemia. This chronic hypoxia causes the fetus to produce more red blood cells to increase available oxygen-carrying sites, resulting in polycythemia/hyperviscosity, which can further impair placental blood flow. Mothers who smoke during pregnancy are more likely to have IUGR and premature babies. These newborns typically weigh 150 to 250 g (0.3 to 0.5 lb) less than babies of nonsmokers (Eichenwald et al., 2017). The nicotine in cigarettes acts as a neuroteratogen that interferes with fetal development, specifically the developing nervous system. Additional risks to the fetus and newborn of the mother who smokes include (Pantoja & Enzman Hines, 2016):

- *Intrauterine distress* presenting as meconium staining and low Apgar scores
- *Neonatal neurobehavioral abnormalities* such as impaired habituation, orientation, consolability, orientation to sound
- *Hypertonia* or *hypotonia, increase in tremors, increased Moro reflex*
- *Signs of nicotine toxicity* (tachycardia, irritability, poor feeding)
- *Sudden infant death syndrome.*

Nursing Care Plan: For the Newborn of a Substance-Abusing Mother

1. Nursing Diagnosis: *Infant Behavior: Disorganized, Risk for*, related to perinatal substance abuse (NANDA-I © 2017)

GOAL: The newborn will be free of signs and symptoms of CNS effects from maternal substance abuse.

INTERVENTION	RATIONALE
• Obtain prenatal records and question the mother about history of drug use. Include type of drug or drugs used, duration, time and amount of last dose taken during pregnancy and during labor and delivery.	• Confirms what drugs, if any, were abused during pregnancy. If enrolled in a methadone-maintenance program, NAS withdrawal will be more significant and predictable. • Noting the mother's last drug ingestion will provide the medical staff with an approximate time frame to expect the newborn to exhibit withdrawal symptoms.
• Obtain meconium drug screen using newborn's first stool.	• Confirms what drugs, if any, were abused during pregnancy. Indications to test a newborn: History of drug abuse, no prenatal care, unexplained placental abruption, changes in behavioral state of newborn.
• Assess newborn for signs and symptoms of withdrawal (e.g., high-pitched shrill cry, sneezing, vomiting, diarrhea, hypertonicity, restlessness, and wakefulness) using neonatal abstinence scoring tool per hospital guidelines.	• The average symptoms of withdrawal occur 72 hr after birth; however, symptoms may appear as early as 6–24 hr after birth.
• Provide a quiet, calm, darkened environment. Swaddle baby tightly and place in a side-lying or prone position.	• Providing a quiet environment decreases stimuli, therefore reducing CNS symptoms.
• Carefully plan tests and/or treatments to avoid excessive stimuli.	• Planning care promotes rest and reduces external stimuli.
• Use soothing techniques such as rocking, cuddling, soft music, and soft tones when speaking.	• These activities promote comfort, security, and newborn bonding.
• Administer appropriate medications as ordered by healthcare provider. Monitor efficacy of these medications, as evidenced by a decrease in NAS scores.	• These medications aid the baby in minimizing symptoms related to withdrawal.

EXPECTED OUTCOME: Newborn will have no signs and symptoms of CNS effects of maternal substance abuse, as evidenced by reduced hyperactivity and irritability, normal sleep–wake pattern, no jitteriness, and no seizure activity.

2. Nursing Diagnosis: *Airway Clearance, Ineffective*, related to suppression of respiratory system (NANDA-I © 2017)

GOAL: Newborn will be free of signs and symptoms of respiratory distress after birth.

INTERVENTION	RATIONALE
• Obtain maternal prenatal, labor, and birth records.	• Provides information about fetal stress that may have occurred during the prenatal or intrapartum period. In addition, the birth record will provide information concerning the newborn's respiratory status at birth, for example, the Apgar score.
• Assess newborn's respiratory rate and effort, skin color, heart rate, presence or absence of cough reflex, and symptoms of respiratory distress.	• Maternal narcotic consumption may depress the cough reflex and respiratory center of the newborn after birth. Symptoms such as cyanosis, tachycardia, grunting, retractions, and nasal flaring may indicate hypoxia.
• Position baby in a side-lying or semi-Fowler position.	• Prevents aspiration.
• Monitor baby for temperature elevation.	• Temperature elevation may cause metabolic rate and oxygen needs to increase when associated with CNS stimulation.
• *Collaborative:* Obtain arterial blood gas (ABG) and chest radiograph as ordered by healthcare provider.	• Oxygen demands increase with drug withdrawal. Obtaining an ABG and chest radiograph will provide healthcare personnel baseline information on newborn's respiratory status, and effective medical interventions can be initiated.
• Monitor newborn's cardiac status and pulmonary status using electrocardiogram (ECG) and pulse oximetry.	• Provides healthcare personnel with cardiac and pulmonary status.

(continued)

Nursing Care Plan: For the Newborn of a Substance-Abusing Mother *(continued)*

EXPECTED OUTCOME: The newborn will maintain adequate respiratory effort as evidenced by respirations of 30–60/min; no signs of retractions, grunting, or cyanosis; arterial blood gas values within normal range; and normal pulse oximetry saturations for gestational age.

3. Nursing Diagnosis: ***Nutrition, Imbalanced: Less than Body Requirements*, related to vomiting and diarrhea, uncoordinated suck and swallow reflex, and hypertonia secondary to withdrawal (NANDA-I © 2017)**

GOAL: The newborn will maintain a consistent weight gain pattern.

INTERVENTION	RATIONALE
• Review gestational age assessment.	
• Assess newborn's sucking and swallowing reflexes.	
• Monitor regurgitation, vomiting, diarrhea.	• Gastrointestinal (GI) hypermobility, irritation, and CNS stimulation can increase nutritional needs.
• Use bulb syringe judiciously before feedings if newborn is having problems with nasal stuffiness and congestion.	• Allows newborn to breathe easier by ridding the nasal passages of excessive mucus.
• Initiate appropriate feedings per healthcare provider orders (e.g., nipple and/or gavage); may need supplemental IV fluids.	• Oral feeding may be difficult because of CNS hyperactivity and GI hypermobility.
• Provide small, frequent feedings of a high-calorie formula.	• Facilitates nutritional intake because SGA newborns require 110–140 kcal/kg/day for adequate nutrition.
• Position baby on right side after feedings.	• Prevents regurgitation and promotes gastric emptying.
• Monitor newborn's weight and document on graph.	• Identifies abnormalities in weight gain/loss and allows for early intervention when necessary.
• Offer pacifier between feedings for nonnutritive sucking.	• Nonnutritive sucking allows for sucking practice, management of pain, and self-consoling behaviors.

EXPECTED OUTCOMES: The newborn will tolerate feedings and maintain consistent weight gain pattern evidenced by no regurgitation or aspiration of feedings and adequate weight gain according to weight graph.

4. Nursing Diagnosis: ***Parenting, Risk for Impaired*, related to lack of knowledge of newborn/infant care (NANDA-I © 2017)**

GOAL: The parent will demonstrate ability to independently provide newborn/infant care.

INTERVENTION	RATIONALE
• Assess mother's desire to learn newborn/infant care tasks as well as evaluate her present physical and emotional stability.	• Provides knowledge of mother's ability to care for newborn.
• Instruct mother on coping strategies (e.g., exercise, listening to music, and discussing concerns openly) to manage stressful situations.	• Gives mother the tools to handle stress, thereby decreasing the chances of exhibiting abusive behavior.
• Assess mother's insight into her own chemical dependency.	• Assistance in enrollment into a chemical dependency program may be necessary before mother can independently care for baby.
• Instruct mother on signs and symptoms of withdrawal and treatment interventions.	• Assists the mother in understanding newborn's behaviors and gives her the tools to intervene without feeling anxious.
• Offer a night of "nesting in" with baby before discharge.	• Assists parents to care for baby by themselves, but with nursing support nearby.
• Encourage mother and family members to perform basic newborn/infant care tasks.	• Facilitates attachment and increases parenting competence.
• Initiate social service consult.	

EXPECTED OUTCOME: The parent will demonstrate the ability to perform basic newborn/infant care tasks, as evidenced by exhibiting appropriate attachment behaviors (e.g., talking to and holding baby), and feeding and bathing baby.

CLINICAL THERAPY

Inquiry into tobacco and smoke exposure should be a routine part of the prenatal history. Preconception and prenatal counseling about the effects of cigarette smoking on pregnancy and the fetus should occur. An estimated 5% reduction in perinatal mortality would occur if smoking during pregnancy were eliminated (AAP & ACOG, 2017). Mothers should be counseled that eliminating or reducing smoking even late in pregnancy can improve fetal growth. The use of nicotine patches (instead of smoking) reduces the absorption of nicotine and thereby may increase the birth weight of the fetus. See Tobacco in Chapter 13 for further discussion of prenatal smoking cessation and other intervention programs.

Cotinine, a metabolite of nicotine, has been found in fetal body fluids. There is also a positive correlation between the number of cigarettes smoked per day and the concentration of cotinine in maternal urine. Other factors that influence fetal and maternal serum cotinine concentrations are nicotine content of the cigarette and the time elapsed between the last cigarette smoked and the sampling. These findings indicate that cotinine may be used as a marker of maternal–fetal tobacco exposure during pregnancy (Fischer et al., 2017).

Newborns of mothers who are tobacco dependent may be screened with the NICU Network Neurobehavioral Scale (NNNS) to assess their neurologic, behavioral, and stress/abstinence neurobehavioral function.

The potential for long-term respiratory problems such as asthma, as well as cognitive and receptive language delays that may persist into school age, should be evaluated. Hearing impairment in the newborn is associated with prenatal and postnatal smoking (Wilunda,Yoshida, Tanaka, et al., 2018).

Care of the Newborn Exposed to HIV/AIDS

Approximately 36.9 million people around the world live with HIV (Eichenwald et al., 2017). In the United States, the CDC estimates that each year 100 to 200 babies with HIV infections are born (Eichenwald et al., 2017). Preventive strategies, including prenatal testing, antiretroviral therapy, viral load measurements, and scheduled cesarean sections, have reduced the risk of maternal–child transmission of HIV to approximately 1% or less (CDC, 2017a). Most HIV transmissions during the perinatal and newborn periods occur across the placenta, across the amniotic membranes, or through breast milk or contaminated blood (Eichenwald et al., 2017). The risk of vertical transmission in mothers not receiving an antiretroviral (ARV) drug regimen such as oral zidovudine (ZDV) (also known as azidothymidine [AZT]) during gestation is 25 to 40% in the United States (Rivera, 2017). Pregnant women should be universally tested (with patient notification) for HIV infection as part of the routine battery of prenatal blood tests unless they decline the test (i.e., opt-out approach) as permitted by local and state regulations. Refusal of testing should be documented. (For discussion of maternal and fetal HIV/AIDS, see Chapter 17.) Some babies infected by maternal–fetal transmission suffer from severe immunodeficiency, with HIV disease progressing more rapidly during the first year of life.

Early identification of babies with or at risk for HIV/AIDS is essential during the newborn period in addition to a consultation with a pediatric HIV specialist. Currently available HIV serologic tests (enzyme-linked immunosorbent assay [ELISA] and Western blot test) cannot distinguish between maternal and infant antibodies; therefore, they are inappropriate for babies less than 15 months of age. It may take up to 15 months for infected infants to form their own antibodies to HIV (Eichenwald et al., 2017). The preferred test for diagnosis of HIV infection in newborns is the bDNA polymerase chain reaction (PCR) assay and HIV RNA assays (Eichenwald et al., 2017). A positive result by 3 days of age suggests in utero transmission, thus allowing early identification and treatment. If testing is performed at birth, umbilical cord blood should not be used as it may be contaminated with maternal blood, leading to a false-positive result. A repeat, confirmatory HIV DNA PCR is done at 14 to 21 days, 1 to 2 months, and 4 to 6 months postnatally (National Institutes of Health [NIH], 2017).

For full-term newborns, a 4-week ZDV/AZT prophylactic regimen should begin as soon after birth as possible and continue for 6 weeks. If the HIV DNA PCR is positive, the National Institutes of Health (2017) recommends changing to combination antiretroviral therapy; this has been shown to decrease the rate of servoconversion of babies born to mothers infected with HIV. Breastfeeding in developed countries, where there are accessible alternative feeding methods, should be avoided with an HIV-positive mother, as transmission of the HIV virus to the newborn in breast milk is well documented (NIH, 2017). A baseline complete blood count (CBC) with differential and platelets is obtained because anemia is one of the side effects of ZDV/AZT therapy (NIH, 2017).

●○● NURSING MANAGEMENT

For the Newborn Exposed to HIV/AIDS

Nursing Assessment and Diagnosis

Many newborns exposed to HIV/AIDS are premature or SGA, or both, and show evidence of failure to thrive during neonatal and infant periods. They can show signs and symptoms of disease within days of birth. Signs that may be seen in the neonatal and early infancy periods include enlarged spleen and liver, swollen glands, recurrent respiratory infections, rhinorrhea, interstitial pneumonia (rarely seen in adults), recurrent GI (diarrhea and weight loss) and urinary system infections, persistent or recurrent oral candidiasis infections, and loss of achieved developmental milestones. There is also a high risk of acquiring *Pneumocystis jirovecii* pneumonia. Opportunistic diseases such as Gram-negative sepsis and problems associated with prematurity are the primary causes of mortality in babies with HIV infection (NIH, 2017).

Nursing diagnoses that may apply to a newborn exposed to HIV/AIDS include:

- ***Nutrition, Imbalanced: Less than Body Requirements,*** related to formula intolerance and inadequate intake
- ***Skin Integrity, Impaired,*** related to chronic diarrhea
- ***Infection, Risk for,*** related to perinatal exposure and immunoregulation suppression secondary to HIV/AIDS
- ***Mobility: Physical, Impaired,*** related to decreased neuromuscular development
- ***Development: Delayed, Risk for,*** related to lack of attachment and stimulation
- ***Parenting, Impaired,*** related to diagnosis of HIV/AIDS and fear of future outcome

(NANDA-I © 2017)

Nursing Plan and Implementation

Hospital-Based Nursing Care

Nursing care of the newborn exposed to HIV/AIDS includes all the care normally given to any newborn in a nursery. In addition, you must include care for a newborn suspected of having a bloodborne infection, as with hepatitis B. See *Health Promotion: Preventing Infection*. See Table 30–10 for some general issues for all nurses and healthcare providers of the newborn at risk for HIV/AIDS.

SAFETY ALERT!

Standard precautions should be used when caring for the newborn immediately after birth and when obtaining blood samples via vein puncture or heelstick. The blood of all newborns must be considered potentially infectious because the status of the baby's blood is often not known until after the baby is discharged.

Health Promotion Preventing Infection

Most institutions recommend that their healthcare provider wear gloves during all diaper changes, especially in the presence of diarrhea because blood may be in the stool, and during examination of the newborn. There is a window of time before seroconversion occurs when the baby is still considered infectious. Provide for comfort; keep the newborn properly nourished and protected from opportunistic infections; provide good skin care to prevent skin rashes; and facilitate growth, development, and attachment.

Community-Based Nursing Care

Hand hygiene is crucial when caring for newborns at risk for AIDS. Parents should be taught proper handwashing technique. Nutrition is essential because failure to thrive and weight loss are common. Small, frequent feedings and food supplementation are helpful. Discuss with parents sanitary techniques for preparing formula. Inform the parents that the baby should not be put to bed with juice or formula because of potential bacterial growth. Parents need to be alert to the signs of feeding intolerance, such as increasing regurgitation, abdominal distention, and loose stools. The newborn should be weighed three times a week.

The baby should have his or her own skin care items, towels, and washcloths. Most clothing and linens can be washed with other household laundry. Linens that are visibly soiled with blood or body fluids should be washed separately in hot, sudsy water with household bleach. Prompt diaper changing and perineal care can prevent or minimize diaper rash and promote comfort.

The diaper-changing area in the home should be separate from the food preparation and serving areas. Soiled diapers should be placed in plastic bags, sealed, and disposed of daily. Diaper-changing areas should be cleaned with a 1:10 dilution of household bleach after each diaper change. Toys should be kept as clean as possible, not shared with other children, and checked for sharp edges to prevent scratches.

Instruct the parents about signs of infection to be alert to and when to call their healthcare provider. The inability to feed without pain may indicate esophageal yeast infection and may require administration of nystatin (Mycostatin) for oral thrush. Topical Mycostatin or Desitin ointment is used for diaper rashes. If diarrhea occurs, the baby needs frequent perineal care as well

TABLE 30–10 Issues for Caregivers of Newborns at Risk for HIV/AIDS

Resuscitation	For suctioning use a bulb syringe, mucus extractor, or meconium aspirator with wall suction on low setting. Use masks, goggles, and gloves.
Admission care	To remove blood from baby's skin, give warm water/mild soap bath using gloves as soon as possible after admission.
Hand hygiene	Thorough handwashing is indicated before and after caring for baby. Hands must be washed immediately if contaminated with blood or body fluids. Wash hands after removal of gloves.
Gloves	Gloves are indicated with touching blood or other high-risk fluids. Gloves should also be worn when handling newborns before and during their initial baths, cord care, eye prophylactics, and vitamin K administration.
Mask, goggle, and gown	Not routinely needed unless coming in contact with placenta or the blood and amniotic fluid on the skin of the newborn.
Needles and syringes	Used needles should not be recapped or bent; they should be disposed of in a puncture-resistant plastic container belonging specifically to that baby. After the newborn is discharged, the container is discarded.
Specimens	Blood and other specimens should be double-bagged and/or sealed in an impervious container and labeled according to agency protocol.
Equipment and linens	Articles contaminated with blood or body fluids should be discarded or bagged according to isolation or institution protocol.
Body fluid spills	Blood and body fluids should be cleaned promptly with a solution of 5.25% sodium hypochlorite (household bleach) diluted 1:10 with water. Apply for at least 30 seconds then wipe after the minimum contact time.
Education and support	Provide education and psychologic support for family and staff. Nurses and healthcare providers who avoid contact with a baby at risk or who overdress in unnecessary isolation garb subtly exacerbate an already difficult family situation. Information resources include the National AIDS Hotline (1-800-232-4636) and the AIDS Clinical Trials Information Service (1-800-TRIALS-A).
Exempted personnel	Immunologically compromised staff (pregnant women may be included in this group) and possibly infectious staff members should not care for these newborns.

SOURCES: Data from CDC, 2017a; Smith & Carley, 2014.

as fluid replacement. Antidiarrheal medications are often ineffective. Irritability may be the first sign of fever. Fluids, antipyretics, and sponging with tepid water are of use in managing fever. Preventive care for exposed newborns includes routine immunizations, except the combined measles–mumps–rubella–varicella (MMRV) vaccine. HIV-1 exposed and infected infants should receive the rotavirus vaccine at 2, 4, and 6 months of age.

Parents and family members need to be reassured that there are no documented cases of people contracting HIV/AIDS from routine care of infected babies. Emotional support for family members is essential because of the stress and social isolation they may face. Because of these stresses, parents may not bond with the baby or they may fail to provide the baby with enough sensory and tactile stimulation. Encourage the parents to hold the baby during feedings because the baby benefits from frequent, gentle touch. Auditory stimulation may also be provided by using music or tapes of parents' voices. Offer families information about support groups, available counseling, and information resources.

All newborns born to HIV-positive mothers require regular clinical, immunologic, and virologic monitoring. At 1 month of age the baby's physical examination should include a developmental assessment and complete blood count, including differential blood count, CD4+ count, and platelet count. Prophylaxis for *Pneumocystis jirovecii* pneumonia for all babies born to women who are HIV infected should be initiated following completion of the ZDV/AZT prophylaxis regimen (NIH, 2017). Pediatric HIV disease raises many healthcare issues for the family. The parents, depending on their health status, may or may not be able to care for their baby, and they must deal with many psychosocial and economic issues.

Evaluation

Expected outcomes of nursing care include:

- Parents are able to bond with their newborn and have realistic expectations about the baby.
- Potential opportunistic infections are identified early and treated promptly.
- Parents verbalize their concerns about their baby's existing and potential health problems and long-term care needs and accept outside assistance as needed.

Care of the Newborn with an Inborn Error of Metabolism

Inborn errors of metabolism (IEM) are a group of hereditary disorders transmitted by mutant genes. Each causes an enzyme defect that blocks a metabolic pathway and leads to an accumulation of toxic metabolites. Some of the inborn errors of metabolism (especially those associated with intellectual disability) are now detected neonatally through newborn screening programs. All states require screening of newborns for phenylketonuria, congenital hypothyroidism, sickle cell disease, congenital adrenal hypoplasia, s-beta thalassemia, and galactosemia (Matthews & Robin, 2016). Mandatory newborn screening for other inborn errors of metabolism varies among states and often includes maple syrup urine disease (MSUD), homocystinuria, and cystic fibrosis (CF). With new laboratory technology and the introduction of tandem mass spectrometry (MS/MS), a spot of blood from a newborn can be used to detect more than 50 inborn errors of metabolism (Matthews & Robin, 2016).

Genetic Facts Inborn Errors of Metabolism

Most inborn error of metabolism disorders are transmitted by an autosomal recessive gene, requiring two heterozygous parents to produce a homozygous child with the disorder. Possible clues to inborn errors can include newborn presenting with hypoglycemia and ketouria, acidosis with recurrent vomiting and hyperammonemia, and acidosis that is difficult to correct and is out of proportion to the clinical state (Matthews & Robin, 2016). Heterozygous parents carrying some inborn errors of metabolism disorders can be identified by special tests, and some inborn errors of metabolism can be detected and treated in utero.

Selected Inborn Errors of Metabolism

Phenylketonuria (PKU) is the most common of the amino acid disorders. Newborn screenings show its incidence at about 1 in 10,000 to 15,000 live births in the United States; however, the incidence varies considerably among ethnic groups (Sampson, Groshong, & Wall, 2016). The highest incidence is noted in Caucasian populations from northern Europe and the United States. It is rarely observed in people of African, Hispanic, Chinese, or Japanese descent (Sampson et al., 2016).

Phenylalanine is an essential amino acid (found in dietary protein) used by the body for growth. In the normal individual any excess is converted to tyrosine. The newborn with PKU lacks this converting ability, which results in an accumulation of phenylalanine in the blood. Phenylalanine produces two abnormal metabolites, phenylpyruvic acid and phenylacetic acid. These are eliminated in the urine, producing a musty odor. Excessive accumulation of phenylalanine and its abnormal metabolites in the brain tissue leads to progressive intellectual disability.

The Guthrie blood test for PKU, required for all newborns before discharge, uses a drop of blood collected from a heelstick and placed on filter paper (Figure 30–18). Because phenylalanine metabolites begin to build up in the PKU baby once milk feedings have begun, the test is done at least 24 hours after the initiation of feedings containing the usual amounts of breast milk or formula. At-risk newborns should receive a 60% milk intake, with no more than 40% of their total intake from nonprotein intravenous fluids. The PKU testing of at-risk newborns should be deferred for at least 48 hours after hyperalimentation is initiated. It is vital that the parents understand the need for the screening procedure; a follow-up check is necessary to confirm that the test was done.

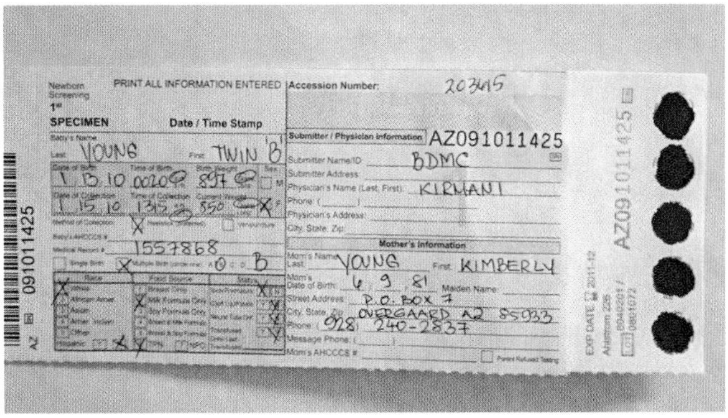

Figure 30–18 Guthrie card for newborn testing.

SOURCE: Carol Harrigan, RN, MSN, NNP-BC.

Another disorder frequently included in mandatory newborn screening blood tests is *congenital hypothyroidism (CH)*. An inborn enzymatic defect, lack of maternal dietary iodine, or maternal ingestion of drugs that depress or destroy thyroid tissue can cause CH. An elevated thyroid-stimulating hormone (TSH) and low T_4 level are commonly seen in the premature newborn following birth; it may be necessary to repeat levels at 2 to 6 weeks of age. Congenital hypothyroidism occurs more often in Hispanic and Native American/Alaska Native people. Babies with Down syndrome are also at increased risk of having CH (Eichenwald et al., 2017).

The incidence of metabolic errors is relatively low, but for affected newborns and their families these disorders pose a threat to the baby's survival. If they survive, these children frequently require lifelong treatment.

CLINICAL THERAPY

Identification via newborn screening and early clinical intervention for some inborn errors of metabolism has become more difficult with the advent of early discharge of newborns. If the initial specimen is obtained before the newborn is 24 hours of age, then a second specimen should be obtained between 48 and 72 hours of age (Eichenwald et al., 2017). Early collection of specimens may yield false-positive results for certain metabolic disorders. Conversely, other metabolic disorders may go undetected. Newborns in the NICU who require interhospital transfers and early-discharge healthy newborns are at risk for nonscreening. Newborn screen specimens are always collected before a blood transfusion.

●○● NURSING MANAGEMENT

For the Newborn with an Inborn Error of Metabolism

Assess the newborn for signs of inborn errors of metabolism and carry out state-mandated newborn screening tests. Refer parents of affected newborns to support groups. Ensure that parents are informed about centers that can provide information about biochemical genetics and dietary management.

Nursing Plan and Implementation

Newborn with Phenylketonuria

Typically, a baby with PKU is a normal-appearing newborn, most often with blond hair, blue eyes, and fair complexion. Decreased pigmentation may be related to the competition between phenylalanine and tyrosine for the available enzyme tyrosinase. Tyrosine is needed for the formation of melanin pigment and the hormones epinephrine and thyroxine. Without treatment, the baby fails to thrive and develops vomiting and eczematous rashes. By about 6 months of age, the infant exhibits behaviors indicative of intellectual disability and other CNS involvement, including seizures and abnormal electroencephalogram (EEG) patterns.

Advise parents that once identified, a baby with PKU can be treated with a special diet that limits ingestion of phenylalanine. A combination of breast milk and low phenylalanine formula can give the newborn the benefits of breast milk (Sampson et al., 2016). Special formulas low in phenylalanine, such as Phenyl-Free 1 and Phenex-1, are available. Special food lists are helpful for parents of a child with PKU. If treatment is begun before 1 month of age, CNS damage can be minimized. There is an increased risk of producing a child with intellectual disability if the mother with PKU is not on a low-phenylalanine diet during pregnancy. It is recommended that the woman reinstate her low-phenylalanine diet before becoming pregnant again (AAP & ACOG, 2017).

Newborn with Congenital Hypothyroidism

Approximately 5% of newborns with CH, generally those who are more severely affected, have recognizable features at birth, including a large tongue, umbilical hernia, cool and mottled skin, low hairline, hypotonia, and large fontanelles (especially the posterior fontanelle in term newborns) (Eichenwald et al., 2017). Early symptoms include prolonged neonatal jaundice, poor feeding, constipation, low-pitched cry, poor weight gain, inactivity, early sleeping through the night, and delayed motor development. In addition, premature newborns of less than 30 weeks' gestation frequently have lower T_4 and TSH values than those of term babies. This difference may reflect the premature newborn's inability to bind thyroid and a risk for hypothyroidism.

Babies with CH need frequent follow-up laboratory monitoring and adjustment of thyroid medication to accommodate the child's growth and development. With adequate treatment, children remain free of symptoms, but if the condition is left untreated, stunted growth (slowed linear growth) and intellectual disability occur.

Evaluation

Expected outcomes of nursing care include:

- Newborns at risk for inborn errors of metabolism are promptly identified and receive early intervention.
- Parents verbalize their concerns about their baby's nutritional status, health problems, long-term care needs, and potential outcomes.
- Parents are aware of available community health resources and use them as indicated.

Focus Your Study

- Early identification of potential high-risk fetuses through assessment of preconception, prenatal, and intrapartum factors facilitates strategically timed nursing observations and interventions.
- High-risk newborns—whether they are premature, small for gestational age (SGA), large for gestational age (LGA), postterm, infant of a diabetic mother (IDM), or infant of a substance-abusing mother (ISAM)—have many similar problems, although their problems are based on different physiologic processes.
- SGA newborns are at risk for perinatal asphyxia and resulting aspiration syndrome, hypothermia, hypoglycemia,

hypocalcemia, polycythemia, congenital anomalies, and intrauterine infections. Long-term problems include continued growth and learning difficulties.

- LGA newborns are at risk for birth trauma as a result of cephalopelvic disproportion, hypoglycemia, polycythemia, and hyperviscosity.
- IDMs are at risk for hypoglycemia, hypocalcemia, hyperbilirubinemia, polycythemia, and respiratory distress caused by delayed maturation of their lungs.
- Postterm newborns often encounter intrapartum problems such as cephalopelvic disproportion (CPD) (shoulder dystocia) and birth traumas, hypoglycemia, polycythemia, meconium aspiration, cold stress, and possible seizure activity. Long-term complications may involve poor weight gain and low IQ scores.
- The common problems of the preterm newborn are a result of the baby's immature body systems. Potential problems include respiratory distress syndrome (RDS), patent ductus arteriosus (PDA), hypothermia and cold stress, feeding difficulties and necrotizing enterocolitis (NEC), marked insensible water loss and loss of buffering agents through the kidneys, infection, anemia of prematurity, apnea, intraventricular hemorrhage, retinopathy of prematurity, and behavioral state disorganization. Long-term needs and problems include bronchopulmonary dysplasia, speech defects, sensorineural hearing loss, and neurologic sequelae.
- Cardiac defects are a significant cause of morbidity and mortality in the newborn period. Early identification and nursing and medical care of newborns with cardiac defects are essential to improve the outcomes for these babies. Care is directed toward lessening the workload of the heart and decreasing oxygen and energy consumption.
- Newborns of alcohol-dependent mothers are at risk for physical characteristic alterations and the long-term complications of feeding problems; CNS dysfunction, including low IQ, hyperactivity, and language abnormalities; and congenital anomalies.
- Newborns of drug-dependent mothers experience drug withdrawal as well as respiratory distress, jaundice, congenital anomalies, and behavioral abnormalities. With early recognition and intervention, the potential long-term physiologic and emotional consequences of these difficulties can be avoided or at least lessened in severity.
- Newborns of mothers with HIV/AIDS require early recognition and treatment so that the physiologic and emotional consequences may be lessened in severity and CDC guidelines implemented.
- Inborn errors of metabolism such as phenylketonuria (PKU) and congenital hypothyroidism (CH) are usually included in a newborn screening program designed to prevent intellectual disability through dietary management and medication.
- The nursing care of the newborn with special problems involves the understanding of normal physiology, the pathophysiology of the disease process, clinical manifestations, and supportive or corrective therapies. Only with this theoretical background can the nurse make appropriate observations about responses to therapy and development of complications.
- The nurse facilitates interprofessional communication with the parents. Parents of at-risk newborns need support from nurses and healthcare providers to understand the special needs of their babies and feel confident in their ability to care for them at home.

In order to make safe and effective judgments using NANDA-I © 2017 nursing diagnoses, it is essential that nurses refer to the definitions and defining characteristics of the diagnoses used in this text, which can be found in Appendix C.

References

Abrams, S. A., Landers, S., Noble, L. M., & Pointexter, B. B. (2017). Donor human milk for the high-risk infant: Preparation, safety, and usage options in the United States. *Pediatrics, 139*(1), e20163440. DOI: 10.1542/peds.2016-3440

Academy of Breastfeeding Medicine (ABM). (2016). Protocol #10: Breastfeeding the late preterm (34–36 6/7 weeks of gestation) and early term infants (37–38 6/7 weeks of gestation), Second Revision 2016. *Breastfeeding Medicine, 11*(10), 1–10. DOI: 10.1089/bfm.2018.29031.egb

Als, H., Butler, S., & Kosta, S. (2005). The assessment of preterm infant's behavior (APIB): Furthering the understanding and measurement of neurodevelopmental competence in preterm and full-term infants. *Mental Retardation and Developmental Disabilities Research Reviews, 11*(1), 94–102. DOI: 10.1002/mrdd.20053

American Academy of Pediatrics (AAP) & American College of Obstetricians and Gynecologists (ACOG). (2017). *Guidelines for perinatal care* (8th ed.). Elk Grove Village, IL: Author.

American College of Obstetricians and Gynecologists (ACOG). (2000, reaffirmed 2018). Fetal growth restriction (ACOG Practice Bulletin No.134). *Obstetrics & Gynecology, 121,* 1122–1133.

American College of Obstetricians and Gynecologists (ACOG). (2017). Statement on opioid use during pregnancy (ACOG Committee Opinion No. 711). *Obstetrics & Gynecology, 130,* 281–94.

American College of Obstetricians and Gynecologists (ACOG). (2014, reaffirmed 2016). Management of late-term and postterm pregnancies (ACOG Practice Bulletin No.146). *Obstetrics & Gynecology, 124,* 390–396.

American College of Obstetricians and Gynecologists (ACOG) & Society for Maternal-Fetal Medicine. (2013, reaffirmed 2015). Definition of term pregnancy (Committee Opinion No. 579). *Obstetrics & Gynecology, 122,* 1139–1140.

Andrea, J. (2015). Implications of using pulse oximetry to screen for critical congenital heart disease in newborns. *Nursing for Women's Health 19*(4), 314–323. DOI: 10.1111/1751-486X.12217

Armentrout, D. (2015). Glucose management. In M. T. Verklan & M. Walden (Eds.), *Core curriculum for neonatal intensive care nursing* (5th ed., pp. 162–171). St. Louis, MO: Saunders.

Auger, N., Potter, B. J., Bilodeau-Bertrand, M., & Paradis, G. (2018). Long-term risk of cardiovascular disease in women who have had infants with heart defects. *Circulation, 137*(22), 2321–2331. DOI: 10.1161/CIRCULATIONAHA.117.030277

Bagwell, G. A., Thomas, A., & Ryshen, G. (2016). Improving skin integrity in babies diagnosed with neonatal abstinence syndrome. *Neonatal Network 35*(5), 1–7. DOI: 10.1891/0730-0832.35.S1.1

Blackburn, S. (2018). *Maternal, fetal, neonatal physiology: A clinical perspective* (5th ed.). Philadelphia, PA: Saunders

Bradshaw, W. T. (2015). Gastrointestinal disorders. In M. T. Verklan & M. Walden (Eds.), *Core curriculum for neonatal intensive care nursing* (5th ed., pp. 583–631). St. Louis, MO: Saunders.

Carter, A., Gratny, L., & Carter, B. S. (2016). Discharge planning and follow-up of the neonatal intensive care unit infant. In S. L. Gardner, B. S. Carter, M. Enzman Hines, & J. A. Hernandez (Eds.), *Merenstein & Gardner's handbook of neonatal intensive care* (8th ed., pp. 903–923). St. Louis, MO: Mosby

Centers for Disease Control and Prevention (CDC). (2016). Smoking prevalence and cessation before and during pregnancy: Data from the birth certificate, 2014. *National Vial Statistics Reports, 85*(1), 1–13.

Centers for Disease Control and Prevention (CDC). (2017a). *HIV among pregnant women, infants, and children.* Retrieved from https://www.cdc.gov/hiv/risk/gender/pregnantwomen/facts

Centers for Disease Control and Prevention (CDC). (2017b). *Preterm.* Retrieved from https://www.cdc.gov/reproductivehealth/maternalinfanthealth/pretermbirth.htm

Charpak, N., Tessier, R., Ruiz, J. G., Hernandez, J. T., Uriza, F., Villegas, J., . . . Maldonado, D. (2016). Twenty-year follow-up of kangaroo mother care versus traditional care. *Pediatrics, 139*(1). Retrieved from https://www.ncbi.nlm.nih.gov/pubmed/27965377

Ditzenberger, G. R. (2015). Nutritional management. In M. T. Verklan & M. Walden (Eds.), *Core curriculum for neonatal intensive care nursing* (5th ed., pp. 172–196). St. Louis, MO: Saunders.

Diller, C. L., Kelleman, M. S., Kupke, K. G., Quary, S. C., Kochilas, L. K., Oster, M. E. (2018). A modified algorithm for critical congenital heart disease screening using pulse oximetry. *Pediatrics, 141*(5). Retrieved from http://pediatrics.aappublications.org/content/141/5/e20174065

Dutta, S., Singh, B., Chessell, L., Wilson, J., James, M., Kimberly, M., . . . Fusch, C. (2015). Guidelines for feeding low birth weight infants. *Nutrients, 7*(1), 423–442. DOI: 10.3390/nu7010432

Eichenwald, E. C., Hansen, A. R., Martin, C. R., & Stark, A. R. (2017). *Cloherty and Stark's manual of neonatal care* (8th ed.). Philadelphia, PA: Lippincott Williams & Wilkins.

Finnegan, L. P. (1990). Neonatal abstinence syndrome. In N. Nelson (Ed.), *Current therapy in neonatal-perinatal medicine* (2nd ed., pp. 314–340). Philadelphia, PA: B. C. Decker.

Fischer, S. T., Loukia, N. L., Li, S., Tran, V. T., Stewart, K. B., Schwartz, C. E., . . . Fridovich-Keil, J. L. (2017). Low-level maternal exposure to nicotine associates with significant metabolic perturbations in second-trimester amniotic fluid. *Environment International, 107*, 227–234. DOI: 10.1016/j.envint.2017.07.019

Gardner, S. L., Goldson, E., & Henandez, J.A. (2016). The neonate and the environment: Impact on development. In S. L. Gardner, B. S. Carter, M. Enzman Hines, & J. A. Hernandez, (Eds.), *Merenstein & Gardner's handbook of neonatal intensive care* (8th ed., pp. 262–314). St. Louis, MO: Mosby.

Gardner, S. L., Voos, K., & Hills, P. (2016). Families in crisis: Theoretic and practical considerations. In S. L. Gardner, B. S. Carter, M. Enzman Himes, & J. A. Hernandez (Eds.), *Merenstein & Gardner's handbook of neonatal intensive care* (8th ed., pp. 821–864). St. Louis, MO: Mosby.

Gill, J. V., & Boyle, E. M. (2017). Outcomes of infants born near term. *Archives of Disease in Children, 102,* 194–198.

Hamdan, A. H. (2017). *Neonatal abstinence syndrome.* Retrieved from https://emedicine.medscape.com/article/978763-overview

Hardy, W., D'Agata, A., & McGrath, J. M. (2016). The infant at risk. In S. Mattson & J. E. Smith (Eds.), *AWHONN core curriculum for maternal-newborn nursing* (5th ed., pp. 363–416). St. Louis, MO: Mosby Elsevier.

Howard, M. B., Schiff, D. M., Penwill, N., Si, W., Rai, A., Wolfgang, T., Moses, J. M., Wachman, E. M. (2017). Impact of parental presence at infants' bedside on neonatal abstinence syndrome. *Hospital Pediatrics, 7*(2), 63–69. DOI: 10.1542/hpeds.2016-0147

Hoyme, H. E., Kalberg, W. O., Ellicott, A. J., Blankenship, J., Buckley, D., Marais, A-S., . . . May, P. A. (2016). Updated clinical guidelines for diagnosing fetal alcohol spectrum disorders. *Pediatrics 138*(2), e20154256. Retrieved from http://pediatrics.aappublications.org/content/138/2/e20154256

Kenner, C. (2016). Hematologic and immune system. In C. Kenner & J. W. Lott (Eds.), *Neonatal nursing care handbook: An evidence-based approach to conclusions and procedures* (2nd ed., pp. 236–243). New York, NY: Springer.

Lubbe, W. (2017). Clinicians guide for cue-based transition to oral feeding in preterm infants: An easy-to-use clinical guide. *Journal of Evaluation in Clinical Practice 23*(5), 903–1131. DOI: 10.1111/jep.12721

Ludwig, S. M., & Weitzman, K. A. (2007). Changing feeding documentation to reflect infant-driven feeding practice. *Newborn and Infant Nursing Reviews, 7,* 155–160.

March of Dimes. (2016). *2016 Premature birth report card.* Retrieved from https://www.marchofdimes.org/materials/premature-birth-report-card-united-states.pdf

Matthews, A., & Robin, N. H. (2016). Genetic disorders, malformation, and inborn errors of metabolism. In S. L. Gardner, B. S. Carter, M. Enzman Hines, & J. A. Hernandez (Eds.), *Merenstein & Gardner's handbook of neonatal intensive care* (8th ed., pp. 763–786). St. Louis, MO: Mosby.

May, P. A., Chambers, C. D., Walberg, W. O., Zellner, J., Haruna Feldman, H., Buckley, D., . . . Hoyme, H. E. (2018). Prevalence of fetal alcohol spectrum disorders in 4 US communities. *JAMA, 319*(5), 474–482. DOI:10.1001/jama.2017.21896

McQueen, K., & Murphy-Oikonen, J. (2016). Neonatal abstinence syndrome. *New England Journal of Medicine, 375*(24), 68–79. DOI: 10.1056/NEJMra1600879

National Institutes of Health (NIH). (2017). *Recommendations for use of antiretroviral drugs in pregnant HIV-1-infected women for maternal health and interventions to reduce perinatal HIV transmission in the United States.* Retrieved from https://aidsinfo.nih.gov/guidelines/brief-html/3/perinatal/0

Pace, C. (2016). *Mums and dads of very preterm babies more likely to be depressed.* The Conversation. Retrieved from https://theconversation.com/mums-and-dads-of-very-preterm-babies-more-likely-to-be-depressed-62545

Pantoja, A. F., & Enzman Hines, M. (2016). Evidence-based clinical practice. In S. L. Gardner, B. S. Carter, M. Enzman Hines, & J. A. Hernandez (Eds.), *Merenstein & Gardner's handbook of neonatal intensive care* (8th ed., pp. 1–10). St. Louis, MO: Mosby.

Parsons, J. A., Seay, A. R., & Jacobson, M. (2016). Neurologic disorders. In S. L. Gardner, B. S. Carter, M. Enzman Hines, & J. A. Hernandez (Eds.), *Merenstein & Gardner's handbook of neonatal intensive care* (8th ed., pp.727–762). St. Louis, MO: Mosby.

Patel, R. M., Knezevic, A., Shenvi, N., Hinkes, M., Keene, S., Roback, J. D., . . . Josephson, C. D. (2016). Association of red blood cell transfusion, anemia, and necrotizing enterocolitis in very low-birth-weight infants. *Journal of the American Medical Association, 315*(9), 889–897. DOI: 10.1001/jama.2016.1204

Patrick, S. W., Schumacher, R. E., Horbar, J. D., Buus-Frank, M. E., Edwards, E. M., Morrow, K. A., . . . Soll, R. F. (2016). Improving care for neonatal abstinence syndrome. *Pediatrics 137*(5), 1–5. DOI: 10.1542/peds.2015-3835

PREEMIE Reauthorization Act (S.252). (2013–2014). Retrieved from https://www.congress.gov/bill/113th-congress/senate-bill/252

Protecting Our Infants Act of 2015 (S. 799/H.R. 1462). (2015). Retrieved from https://www.congress.gov/bill/114th-congress/house-bill/1462

Reece-Stremtan, S., Marinelli, K. A., & Academy of Breastfeeding Medicine (ABM). (2015). ABM Clinical Protocol #21: Guidelines for breastfeeding and substance use or substance use disorder, revised 2015. *Breastfeeding Medicine 10*(3), 135–141. DOI: 10.1089/bfm.2015.9992.

Rivera, D. M. (2017). *Pediatric HIV infection.* Retrieved from: https://emedicine.medscape.com/article/965086-overview2

Rozance, P. J., McGowan, J. E., Price-Douglas, W., & Hay, W. W. (2016). Glucose homeostasis. In S. L. Gardner, B. S. Carter, M. Enzman Hines, & J. A. Hernandez (Eds.), *Merenstein & Gardner's handbook of neonatal intensive care* (8th ed., pp. 337–359). St. Louis, MO: Mosby.

Sampson, J., Groshong, M., & Wall, D. M. (2016). What nurses need to know about PKU. *Nursing, 46*(8), 66–67.

Smith, J. R., & Carley, A. (2014). Common neonatal complications. In K. R. Simpson & P. A. Creehan (Eds.), *AWHONN's perinatal nursing* (4th ed., pp. 662–698). Philadelphia, PA: Lippincott Williams & Wilkins.

Torrazza, R. M., Parker, L. A., Li, Y., Talaga, E., Schuster, J., & Neu, J. (2015). The value of routine evaluation of gastric residuals in very low birth weight infants. *Journal of Perinatology, 35*(1), 57–60.

University of Rochester Medical Center. (2018). *Health encyclopedia: Factors contributing to congenital heart disease.* Retrieved from https://www.urmc.rochester.edu/encyclopedia/content.aspx?contenttypeid=90&contentid=p01788

Weiner, S. M., & Finnegan, L. P. (2016). Drug withdrawal in the neonate. In S. L. Gardner, B. S. Carter, M. Enzman Hines, & J. A. Hernandez (Eds.), *Merenstein & Gardner's handbook of neonatal intensive care* (8th ed., pp. 199–217). St. Louis, MO: Mosby.

Wilunda, C., Yoshida, S., Tanaka, S., Kanazawa, Y., Kimura, T., & Kawakami, K. (2018). Exposure to tobacco smoke prenatally and during infancy and risk of hearing impairment among children in Japan: A retrospective cohort study. *Paediatric and Perinatal Epidemiology.* Retrieved from https://doi.org/10.1111/ppe.12477

Zahorodny, W., Rom, C., Whitney, W., Giddens, S., Samuel, M., Maichuk, G., & Marshall, R. (1998). The neonatal withdrawal inventory: A simplified score of newborn withdrawal. *Developmental and Behavioral Pediatrics, 19*(2), 89–93. DOI: 10.1097/00004703-199804000-00004

Zaichkin, J., Weiner, G., & Loren, D. (2017). *Understanding the NICU: What parents of preemies and other hospitalized newborns need to know.* Elk Grove Village, IL: American Academy of Pediatrics.

Zang, G., Feenstra, B., Bacelis, J., Liu, X., Muglia, L. M., Juodakis, J., Miller, D. E., ... Muglia, L. J. (2017). Genetic associations with gestational duration and spontaneous preterm birth. *New England Journal of Medicine, 377*, 1156–1167. DOI: 10.1056/NEJMoa1612665

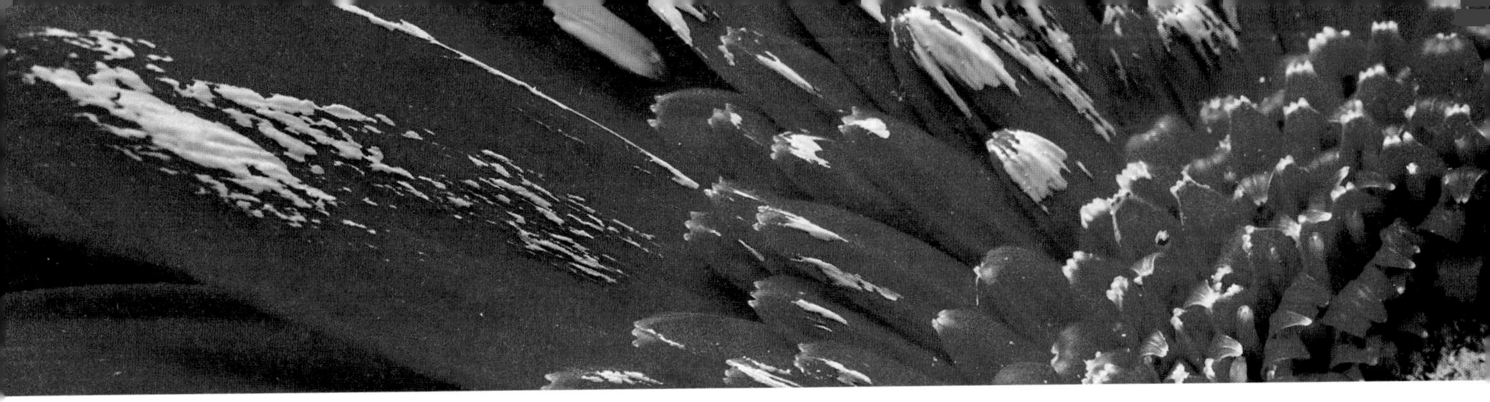

Chapter 31

The Newborn at Risk: Birth-Related Stressors

I watched her breathe every precious breath on the respirator. I saw her covered with wires and tubes. I kept watch. She was special to me and I would tell her over and over, "Daddy is here. Daddy loves you." The three days she lived were hell—not knowing if she would make it, uncertain about what plans we should make. Somehow, I thought she would live; I was hopeful. When she died, at least I was there with her. The grief was unbearable. But there was also a sense of relief. The uncertainty, the waiting, were finally over.

—**Susan Borg,** *When Pregnancy Fails*

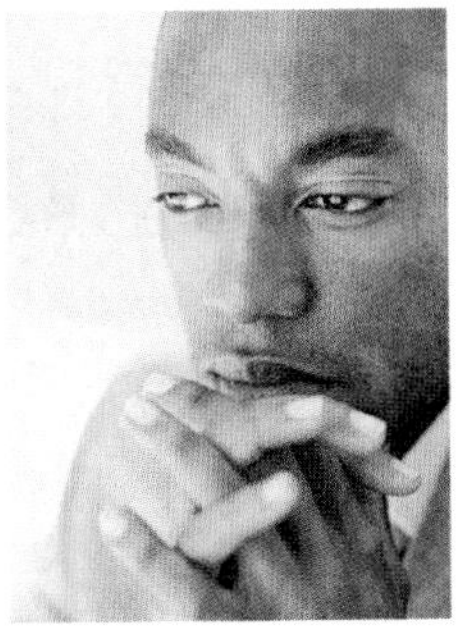

SOURCE: Exactostock/SuperStock.

Learning Outcomes

31.1 Describe how to identify newborns in need of resuscitation and the appropriate method of resuscitation based on the prenatal/labor record and observable physiologic indicators.

31.2 Differentiate, based on clinical manifestations, among the various types of respiratory distress (respiratory distress syndrome, transient tachypnea of the newborn, meconium aspiration syndrome, and persistent pulmonary hypertension) in the newborn and the nursing care required.

31.3 Discuss the types of metabolic abnormalities (cold stress, asphyxia, and hypoglycemia), the effects on the newborn, and the nursing implications.

31.4 Differentiate between physiologic and pathologic jaundice according to timing of onset (age in hours), etiology, possible sequelae, and specific management.

31.5 Explain how Rh incompatibility or ABO incompatibility can lead to the development of hyperbilirubinemia.

31.6 Identify the nursing responsibilities in caring for the newborn receiving phototherapy.

31.7 Explain the etiology and the nursing care of newborns with anemia.

31.8 Describe the clinical manifestations that would lead the nurse to suspect newborn sepsis.

31.9 Delineate the nursing care of the newborn with an infection.

31.10 Relate the consequences of maternally transmitted infections, such as maternal syphilis, gonorrhea, herpesviridae family (HSV or CMV), and chlamydia, to the management of the newborn in the neonatal period.

31.11 Describe interventions to facilitate parental attachment and meet the special initial and long-term needs of parents of at-risk newborns.

Healthy People 2020

(MICH-1.2) Decrease fetal and infant deaths during perinatal period (28 weeks of gestation to 7 days after birth)

(MICH-1.4) Decrease neonatal deaths (within the first 28 days of life)

(MICH-33) Increase the proportion of very-low-birth-weight (VLBW) infants born at Level III hospitals or subspecialty perinatal centers

(HAI-1) Reduce central line–associated bloodstream infections (CLABSI)

(HAI-2) Reduce invasive healthcare-associated methicillin-resistant *Staphylococcus aureus* (MRSA) infections

Marked homeostatic changes occur during the transition from fetal to newborn life. The most rapid anatomic and physiologic changes of this period occur in the cardiopulmonary system. Major problems in transition of the newborn are usually related to this system. These problems include asphyxia, respiratory distress caused by a number of different physiologic problems, and cardiac defects that interrupt blood flow. Cold stress, jaundice, hemolytic disease, anemia, and infection can also cause alterations in adaptation for the neonate. Ideally, problems are anticipated and identified prenatally, some treatment may be initiated in the prenatal/intrapartum period, and appropriate intervention measures are begun prior to, at, or immediately after birth. Mothers carrying fetuses with known cardiac or genetic diagnoses should be referred for delivery at a facility capable of offering surgical management and cardiac intensive neonatal care.

Care of the Newborn at Risk Due to Asphyxia

Neonatal asphyxia, which is the deprivation of oxygen to the baby's brain and organs during the birth process, can cause long-term disabilities and developmental delays in the child. Also called *perinatal asphyxia* or *birth asphyxia*, neonatal asphyxia results from circulatory, respiratory, and biochemical factors and occurs in approximately 1 to 3 per 1000 live term births in developed countries. It can lead to hypoxic-ischemic encephalopathy (HIE), a brain injury caused by oxygen deprivation (Shea & Palanisamy, 2015).

Circulatory patterns that accompany asphyxia indicate an inability to make the transition to extrauterine circulation—in effect, a return to fetal circulatory patterns, with the majority of the blood bypassing the lungs, thus failing to become oxygenated. Failure of lung expansion and establishment of respiration rapidly produce serious biochemical changes, including hypoxemia (decreased oxygen in blood), metabolic acidosis (increased acidity of blood reflected by low pH), and hypercapnia (excess levels of carbon dioxide in the blood). The incidence of acidosis increases with the decrease in gestational age. In the United States, newborns with respiratory failure requiring intubation and mechanical ventilation (MV) comprise approximately 18 in 1000 live births (Lakshminrusimha & Saugstad, 2016).

The failure of normal neonatal transition following clamping of the umbilical cord leads to subsequent biochemical changes that can produce these results:

- Pulmonary vasoconstriction and high pulmonary vascular resistance in relation to lower systemic vascular resistance (following birth the pulmonary vascular resistance should be markedly lower than the systemic vascular resistance)
- Hypoperfusion of the lungs, leading to failure to achieve functional residual capacity (FRC), which is the air remaining in the lungs at the end of a breath
- A large right-to-left shunt (from the right side of the heart to the left side of the heart) through the ductus arteriosus, bypassing the lungs and impeding oxygenation of the blood.

As right-atrial pressure exceeds left-atrial pressure, the foramen ovale reopens, and blood flows from right to left. See Chapter 26 for a review of normal newborn cardiopulmonary adaptation.

However, the most serious biochemical abnormality caused by hypoxia (oxygen starvation at the tissue level) is a change from aerobic to anaerobic metabolism. This change results in the buildup of lactate, combining with hydrogen to form lactic acid, and subsequently developing metabolic acidosis. Lactic acidosis can develop after prolonged tissue hypoxia as active cells rely on anaerobic metabolism.

Simultaneously, respiratory acidosis may also occur in response to a rapid increase in carbon dioxide (PCO_2) during asphyxia. In response to hypoxia and anaerobic metabolism, the amounts of free fatty acids (FFA) and glycerol in the blood increase. Glycogen stores are mobilized to provide a continuous glucose source for the brain. Hepatic and cardiac stores of glycogen may be used up rapidly during an asphyxial incident. Monitoring and treatment of hypoglycemia is also critical in the asphyxiated newborn, as this affects the neonatal brain.

The newborn has several protective mechanisms against hypoxic insults:

- Relatively immature brain
- Resting metabolic rate lower than that observed in the adult
- Ability to mobilize substances within the body for anaerobic metabolism and to use the energy more efficiently
- Intact circulatory system able to redistribute lactate and hydrogen ions in tissues still being perfused.

Severe prolonged hypoxia will overcome these protective mechanisms, resulting in the buildup of lactate and eventual brain damage from the initial insult of acidosis or from the reperfusion injury that can occur following the resuscitative efforts of the newborn. The asphyxia or reperfusion injury can ultimately lead to HIE, which is one of the leading causes of death or disability in the neonatal population worldwide and can lead to a lifelong burden on the healthcare system as well as the family (Shea & Palanisamy, 2015).

The newborn suffering apnea or ineffective ventilation requires immediate resuscitative efforts. The need for resuscitation can be anticipated if specific risk factors are present during the pregnancy or labor and birth period.

Risk Factors Predisposing to Asphyxia

Identification of the newborn in need of resuscitation may be anticipated and acted upon if the mother demonstrates the antepartum and intrapartum risk factors described in Table 12–1 in Chapter 12 and Table 20–1 in Chapter 20. Fetal/neonatal risk factors are (American Academy of Pediatrics [AAP] & American Heart Association [AHA], 2016; Ariff, Lee, Lawn, et al., 2016):

- Nonreassuring fetal heart rate (FHR) pattern/sustained bradycardia
- Impairment of maternal oxygenation (maternal asthma/cardiac disease)
- Alteration of blood flow through the placenta or cord
- Significant intrapartum bleeding
- Pregnancy-induced hypertension or preeclampsia
- Difficult birth, prolonged labor, malposition, prolonged rupture of membranes
- Narcotic use in labor, illicit drug use in pregnancy
- History of meconium or blood in amniotic fluid
- Prematurity
- Male newborn
- Intrauterine growth restriction (IUGR)

- Small for gestational age (SGA)
- Newborn of a mother with diabetes
- Large for gestational age (LGA) or macrosomia
- Multiples
- Structural lung abnormality/oligohydramnios (congenital diaphragmatic hernia, lung hypoplasia)
- Congenital heart disease
- Maternal fever
- Anemia: Isoimmunization, intrapartum hemorrhage, maternal viral illness.

Risk factors are not always apparent prenatally. Particular attention must be paid to all at-risk pregnancies during the intrapartum period. Certain aspects of labor and birth challenge the oxygen supply to the fetus, and often the at-risk fetus has less tolerance to the stress of labor (indicated by decelerations, a fixed baseline heart rate, or lack of variability of the FHR) and the birth presentation (AAP & AHA, 2016). Antenatal neuroprotection is being studied and magnesium sulfate administration is thought to have a significant benefit (Shea & Palanisamy, 2015).

CLINICAL THERAPY

The primary goal is to identify the fetus at risk for asphyxia so that resuscitative efforts can begin at birth.

Fetal biophysical assessment (see Chapter 16) combined with FHRs and fetal oximetry, if available, during the intrapartum period may help identify the presence of nonreassuring fetal status. If nonreassuring fetal status is present, appropriate measures can be taken to deliver the fetus immediately, before acidosis occurs, and to treat the asphyxiated newborn. The stress of labor causes an intermittent decrease in exchange of gases in the placental intervillous space, which causes the fall in pH and fetal acidosis. The fetal acidosis is primarily metabolic via three factors: (1) excess CO_2, which converts to carbonic acid; (2) lactic, uric, or keto acids; or (3) both carbonic and noncarbonic acids. CO_2 quickly transfers across the placenta and maternal kidneys, if they are healthy. Noncarbonic acids are slower to diffuse across the placenta and continue in fetal circulation (Rainaldi & Perlman, 2016). However, low fetal pH without associated hypoxia can be caused by maternal acidosis secondary to prolonged labor, dehydration, maternal lactate production, and infection.

Assessment of the newborn's need for resuscitation begins at the time of birth by assessing color, heart rate, and respirations/respiratory effort of the newborn. The nurse should note the time of the first gasp, first cry, and onset of sustained respirations in order of occurrence. The Apgar score (see Chapter 21) may be helpful in describing the status of the newborn at birth and the baby's subsequent adaptation to the extrauterine environment, but *should not be used* to determine whether certain steps need to be taken during resuscitation. The Apgar can serve as a measure of the neonate's response to effective resuscitation and clinical status. If indicated, resuscitation should be started before the 1-minute Apgar score is calculated. An assisted Apgar scoring system is recommended by the AAP Committee on the Fetus and Newborn (COFN), which documents the assistance the newborn is receiving at the time the Apgar score is assigned (American Academy of Pediatrics [AAP] & American College of Obstetricians and Gynecologists [ACOG], 2017). The Apgar score at 1 minute tends to relate to intrapartum depression, an ischemic or hypoxic event in utero, and umbilical cord blood pH, and subsequent scores relate to the response of the newborn to the resuscitative efforts. Retrospective Apgar scores are likely to be assigned when stabilizing critically ill newborns. A score of less than 7 at 5 minutes following birth requires that additional scores be assigned every 5 minutes up to 20 minutes (AAP & AHA, 2016). A score of less than 5 at 5 minutes indicates that a newborn should be evaluated for some form of resuscitation. The expanded Apgar form provides space for recording Apgar scores and resuscitation efforts at 1, 5, 10, 15, and 20 minutes and a space for additional information such as cord clamping (AAP & ACOG, 2017).

Resuscitative efforts are required by 10% of all newborns to initiate breathing and assist with circulation. Fewer than 1% of all newborns require more extensive resuscitative efforts, such as chest compressions, intubation, medications, or therapeutic cooling (AAP & AHA, 2016; Ariff et al., 2016). Immediate care of every high-risk newborn should be given by at least one healthcare provider with the skills and knowledge provided by the Neonatal Resuscitation Program (AAP & AHA, 2016). Identification of newborns that may require resuscitation is accomplished by carrying out a rapid assessment of four characteristics by asking these questions:

1. What is the gestational age?
2. Is the amniotic fluid clear of meconium and evidence of infection?
3. How many babies are expected?
4. Are there any other risk factors?

Following birth, these three questions need to be posed:

1. Is the baby term?
2. Is the baby breathing and crying?
3. Does the baby have good muscle tone?

If the answers to these questions are "yes," then the baby does not need resuscitation and should not be separated from the mother. If the answer to *any* of the previous questions is "no," then the newborn should receive resuscitative evaluation for assistance (AAP & AHA, 2016). The newborn should receive one or more of these categories of action:

- Initial steps in stabilization (warming, positioning, clearing the airway as necessary, drying, stimulating, and repositioning)
- Oxygen administration with continuous monitoring of the pulse oximeter, preferably on the right hand or wrist because it will be measuring the amount of oxygen available to the brain (AAP & AHA, 2016)
- Positive pressure ventilation/intubation
- Chest compressions, with simultaneous cardio/respiratory (CR) monitor to ensure appropriate assessment of heart rate (HR) (AAP & AHA, 2016)
- Administration of epinephrine, volume expansion, or both as needed (AAP & AHA, 2016)
- Neonatal therapeutic hypothermia (therapeutic cooling [TC]): A relatively new treatment option in which a newborn's body temperature is reduced shortly after birth in order to lessen the chances of severe brain damage and disability in late premature and term babies (AAP & AHA, 2016).
- Newborn blood gas to follow up cord gas values and response to resuscitation efforts.

SAFETY ALERT!

In the birthing room, exposure to blood or other body fluids is inevitable. Standard precautions must be practiced by wearing caps, goggles or glasses, gloves, and impervious gowns until the cord is cut and the newborn is dried and wrapped.

Resuscitation Management

Suctioning (clearing the airway mouth first, then nose) should be considered if the newborn is still struggling with secretions after adequately clearing the mouth and nose with a bulb syringe. Clearing the nasal and oral passages of obstructive fluids establishes a patent airway. Vigorous suctioning of the posterior pharynx should be avoided because it can produce significant reflex bradycardia and damage the oral mucosa (AAP & AHA, 2016). When a suction catheter is utilized it should be connected to low continuous suction.

The stable newborn may be placed on the mother's chest or abdomen skin-to-skin as another heat source. When further resuscitative efforts are warranted, the nurse places the newborn in a level position under a preheated radiant heat source and dries the baby quickly with warm blankets to maintain abdominal skin temperature at about 36.5°C (97.7°F). If a premature newborn is expected, it is recommended that the temperature of the delivery room be raised to 23° to 25°C (74° to 77°F) (AAP & AHA, 2016). The extremely preterm newborn (less than 28 weeks estimated gestational age [EGA] or less than 1000 grams [2.2 lb]) may be covered with a plastic wrap or placed in a plastic bag up to the neck to attempt to prevent evaporative heat loss under the radiant warmer (AAP & AHA, 2016). Warming pads that are chemically activated may be used under extremely premature newborns (AAP & AHA, 2016). Drying is also a good stimulus for breathing. Heat loss through evaporation, convection, and conduction is tremendous during the first few minutes of life. The use of a polyethylene lined or woolen hat, not cotton, placed over the scalp of an extremely-low-birth-weight (ELBW) newborn may help reduce the amount of heat lost through the head. Newborns' temperatures may decrease quickly during the first 10 to 20 minutes following birth if they are not thermally protected (Vali, Mathew, & Lakshminrusimha, 2015). Hypothermia increases oxygen consumption and vasoconstriction, leading to decreased oxygen to the tissues, increased glucose utilization, and ultimately decreased glycogen stores. Additionally, hypothermia can result in worsening respiratory distress, leading to pulmonary vasoconstriction because the pulmonary bed is reactive to oxygen levels in the body.

Ventilation is established by employing the simplest form of resuscitative measures initially, with progression to more complicated methods, as required. For example:

1. Position and clear airway as necessary. Simple stimulation is provided by tapping the soles of the feet, gently rubbing the back with a blanket or towel, while simultaneously drying the newborn.
2. If respirations have not been initiated or are inadequate (gasping or occasional respirations), the lungs must be inflated with positive pressure via bag mask ventilation (BMV) or continuous positive airway pressure (CPAP) (Niermeyer, Clark, & Hernandez, 2016). The proper-sized mask is positioned securely on the face (over the nose and mouth, avoiding the eyes) with the newborn's head in a *sniffing* or neutral position (Figure 31–1). Hyperextension of the newborn's neck will obstruct the trachea and must be avoided.

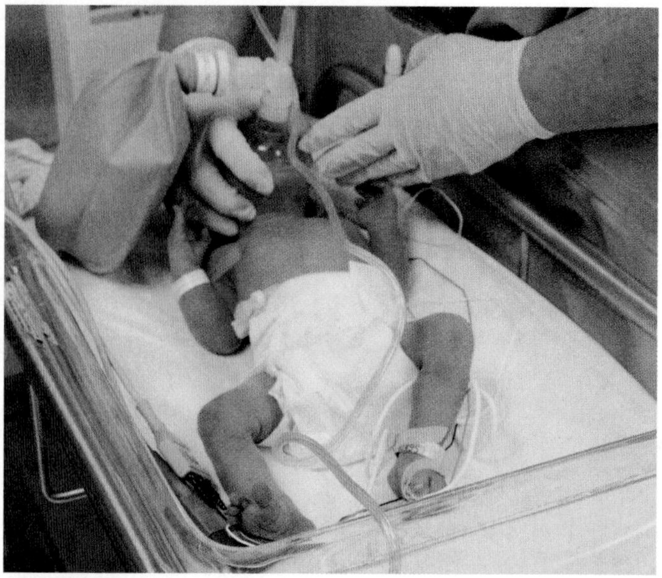

Figure 31–1 **Demonstration of resuscitation of a newborn with flow inflating/anesthesia bag and mask. Note that the mask covers the nose and mouth and that the head is in a neutral position. The resuscitation bag is placed to the side of the baby so that chest movement can be seen.**

An airtight connection is made between the baby's face and the mask (thus allowing the flow inflating bag to inflate). The lungs are inflated rhythmically by squeezing the bag.

All devices utilized for ventilation of newborns during resuscitation should have a pressure gauge/manometer in place. These devices include:

- Self-inflating bag
- Flow inflating/anesthesia bag
- T-Piece resuscitator (AAP & AHA, 2016; Vali et al., 2015).

Supplemental oxygen is not utilized when initiating resuscitation on a term newborn. The amount of oxygen administered is titrated from 21 (room air) to 100% based on clinical assessment and pulse oximeter measurement of the newborn (AAP & AHA, 2016). Oxygen is a medication, and it is only administered in the presence of central cyanosis or when the pulse oximeter readings are less than expected for the age of the newborn. Too much oxygen can actually cause long-term detrimental outcomes. Oxygen saturation of the neonate in utero is approximately 60%, and it typically increases to greater than 90% during the first 10 minutes following birth. An anesthesia bag with an attached manometer or modified self-inflating bag and adequate liter flow of 8–10 L/min is utilized for neonatal resuscitation (AAP & AHA, 2016).

3. Chest movement is observed for proper ventilation. Bilateral equal air entry and the presence of breath sounds in the lung bases are important to assess for air leak and function of lungs in the preterm newborn. HR may be quickly checked by auscultation or by palpating the base of the umbilical cord stump and counting the pulsations for 6 seconds and then multiplying by 10. Cardiopulmonary monitoring is recommended for all births at gestational ages less than 32 weeks as well as high-risk births (AAP & AHA, 2016). Manual resuscitation is coordinated with any voluntary efforts. During positive pressure ventilation, the resuscitation bag is squeezed just enough to see visible chest rise, improved HR, color, and muscle tone,

at a rate of 40 to 60 breaths per minute. The pressure gauge (manometer) must be in place to avoid overdistention of the newborn's lungs and other problems such as pneumothorax or abdominal distention. An inspiratory pressure of approximately 20 to 25 cm H_2O should be adequate to start. Increasing the pressure by 5 to 10 cm H_2O increments is occasionally necessary if there is no improvement in heart rate, color, and muscle tone; however, the amount of pressure should never exceed 40 cm H_2O (AAP & AHA, 2016). If ventilation is adequate, the chest moves symmetrically with each inspiration, bilateral breath sounds are audible, and the lips and mucous membranes become pink. Distention of the stomach is controlled by inserting a nasogastric tube for decompression.

4. Endotracheal intubation (Figure 31–2) may be needed. However, most newborns, except for very-low-birth-weight (VLBW) (less than 1500 g) newborns, can be effectively resuscitated by bag-and-mask ventilation. An increasing HR and CO_2 detection are the primary methods for confirming endotracheal tube placement. This positioning will be later confirmed by chest x-ray.

Once breathing has been established, the HR should increase to over 100 beats/min. If the HR is absent or the HR remains less than 60 beats/min after 30 seconds of effective positive pressure with oxygen concentration of 100%, external cardiac massage (chest compression) is begun (AAP & AHA, 2016). See Table 31–1.

SAFETY ALERT!

Establishing effective ventilation is the highest priority in neonatal resuscitation. Do not start chest compressions without first establishing effective ventilation, as evidenced by audible bilateral breath sounds and chest movement. Although resuscitation is started at 21%, it is recommended to increase oxygen concentration to 100% if chest compressions are initiated (AAP & AHA, 2016).

Chest compressions are started immediately after 30 seconds of adequate ventilation if there is no detectable heartbeat or a heart rate less than 60 beats/min. The procedure for performing chest compression is as follows:

1. The newborn is positioned properly on a firm surface.
2. The resuscitator stands at the foot or head of the newborn and places both thumbs over the lower third of the sternum (just below an imaginary line drawn between the nipples) with

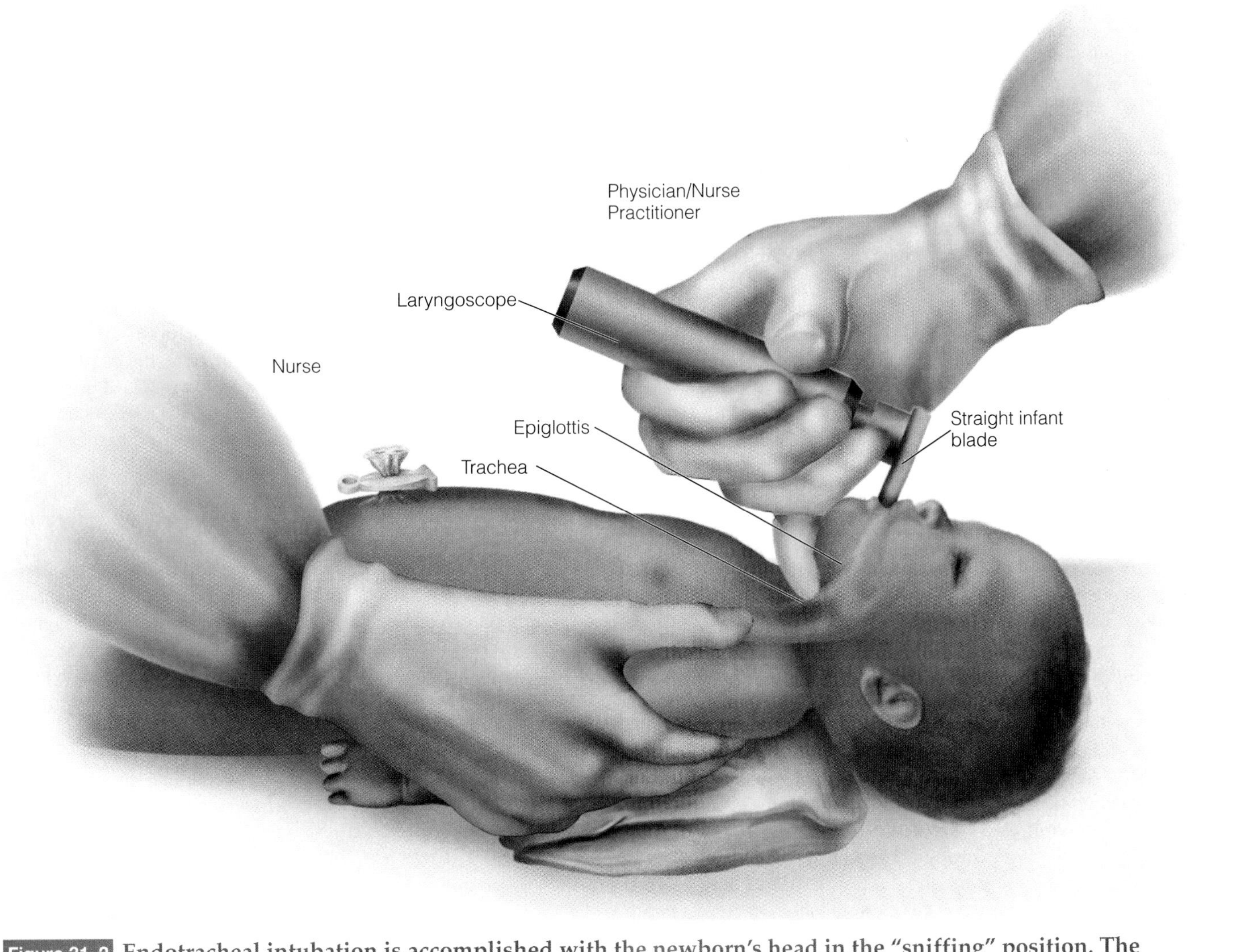

Figure 31–2 Endotracheal intubation is accomplished with the newborn's head in the "sniffing" position. The clinician places the fifth finger under the chin to hold the tongue forward and inserts the laryngoscope blade. Once the blade is in position as shown, an endotracheal tube is inserted through the groove in the laryngoscope blade. The endotracheal tube is not seen in this illustration.

TABLE 31–1 Oxygen Saturation Target Range

TIME	S_pO^2
1 min	60–65%
2 min	65–70%
3 min	70–75%
4 min	75–80%
5 min	80–85%
10 min	85–95%

SOURCE: Data from AAP & AHA, 2016.

the fingers wrapped around and supporting the back (Figure 31–3). The two-thumb method is preferred because it may provide better coronary perfusion pressure and a more consistent and controlled depth of compression. Thumbs should remain in contact with the chest at all times, and compressions must be done from head of bed during access to the umbilical cord for medication administration (AAP & AHA, 2016). Alternatively, the examiner can use two fingers instead of the thumbs, but this method is no longer recommended.

3. The sternum is depressed to sufficient depth to generate a palpable pulse or approximately one-third of the anterior–posterior depth of the chest, with effective release of pressure for refill of the heart at a rate of 90 beats/min (AAP & AHA, 2016). Use a 3:1 ratio of heartbeat to assisted ventilation, 90 chest compressions:30 breaths/min (AAP & AHA, 2016).

SAFETY ALERT!

Remember to say, "One and two and three and breathe, and one and two and three and breathe" out loud so all members of the resuscitation team are aware of where they are in the cycle. There are five cycles in 10 seconds. Getting the speed and rhythm right takes practice, good teamwork, and communication.

Drugs that should be available in the birthing area include those needed in the treatment of shock and cardiac failure. Oxygen is the drug used most often because of its effectiveness in ventilation. After 30 seconds of ventilation and coordinated cardiac compression on 100% oxygen, the newborn's cardiopulmonary status is reassessed by palpating the umbilical cord for a pulse, auscultation of HR, and presence of HR on a cardiorespiratory (CR) monitor. If the newborn has not responded with spontaneous respirations and an HR above 60 beats/min, resuscitative medications are necessary (AAP & AHA, 2016).

The most accessible route for administering medications is the umbilical vein (intravenous [IV]), although intraosseous (IO) insertion (injecting into the marrow of a bone) is recommended when necessary. When the HR remains below 60 beats/min, despite 30 seconds of assisted ventilation followed by another 30 seconds of coordinated chest compression, epinephrine, a cardiac stimulant, is indicated. If persistent bradycardia is present, epinephrine (0.1 to 0.3 mL/kg of a 1:10,000 solution [0.1 mg/mL]) is given through the umbilical vein catheter as rapidly as possible. Endotracheal administration may be considered while IV/IO access is being established. When epinephrine is administered by endotracheal tube, consider a higher dose (0.5–1 mL/kg or 0.05–0.1 mg/kg) (AAP & AHA, 2016). See *Drug Guide: Epinephrine Hydrochloride (Adrenaline Chloride)*.

If shock is suspected due to hypovolemia (e.g., low BP, pallor, poor peripheral perfusion, known cord compression, or

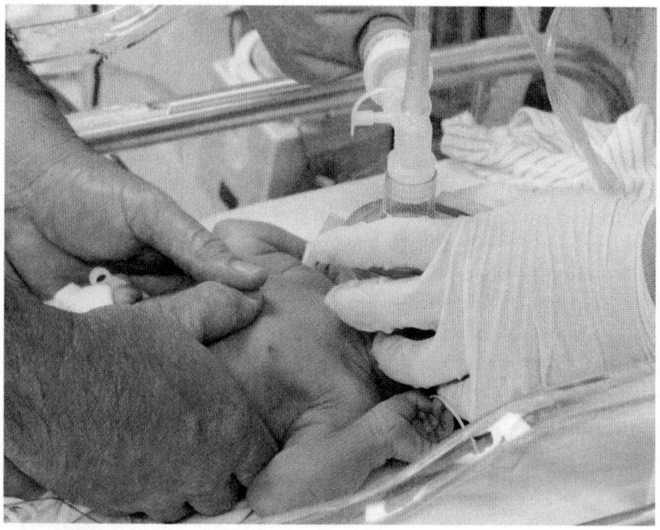

Figure 31–3 External cardiac massage. The lower third of the sternum is compressed with two thumbs at a rate of 90 beats per minute. The fingers support the newborn's back and both thumbs compress the sternum.

loss of blood in birth process), the baby may be given a volume expander such as normal saline (0.9 nacl solution) in a dose of 10 ml/kg via umbilical vein route. If there is a known fetal hemorrhage or fetal anemia, whole blood or packed red blood cells (PRBCS) 10 to 15 ml/kg (O Rh-negative emergency, non-cross-matched against the mother's blood) given over a 5- to 10-minute period can be used for volume expansion and treatment of hypovolemic shock. see *Case Study: Melissa Bond-James*.

Neonatal therapeutic hypothermia, also called *therapeutic cooling (TC)*, is a therapy embraced by the International Liaison Committee on Resuscitation (ILCOR) as a standard of care in the newborn with asphyxia to decrease injury to the brain during reperfusion, preventing cell death (or apoptosis) and improving long-term neurodevelopmental outcomes. This therapy has been shown to improve long-term outcomes in the mild to moderately asphyxiated newborn.

The newborn is placed on a cooling blanket filled with continuously circulating cold water. This is called *whole body cooling (WBC)*. The newborn is monitored over several days while the baby's metabolic processes slow down. Alternatively, *head cooling (HC)* may be utilized, in which a head cooling cap is placed on the newborn's head. Some believe that head cooling is more effective than full-body cooling, and that it reduces negative side effects associated with whole body cooling. Currently, however, both practices are utilized as there is no direct evidence supporting one as a significant benefit over the other (Chiang, Jong, & Lin, 2017). Often, the newborn must be transported to a tertiary care center for WBC or HC. During transport, *passive cooling*, which is simply turning off all external heat sources to the baby's isolette, is frequently used.

Minimal criteria for consideration for passive cooling and further assessment at a center that provides therapeutic cooling by WBC or HC are:

- 5-minute Apgar of 5 or less
- Cord pH or newborn pH of less than 7.0 or base deficit of −15 or greater
- Abnormal neurologic exam.

Drug Guide

Epinephrine Hydrochloride (Adrenaline Chloride)

OVERVIEW OF NEONATAL ACTION

Epinephrine (adrenaline) is used during resuscitation and with severe bradycardia, systemic hypotension, and cardiovascular collapse. It is the primary hormone secreted by the adrenal medulla. Epinephrine increases the strength and rate of cardiac contractions and causes peripheral vasoconstriction, thus improving oxygen delivery to the brain and heart (Vali et al., 2015).

ROUTE, DOSAGE, AND FREQUENCY

The dose is 0.1 to 0.3 mL/kg of 1:10,000 concentration (0.01–0.03 mg/kg). The drug is usually given through the umbilical vein or intraosseous route. If IV/IO access is not immediately available it can be given via the endotracheal tube (ET); the dose is 0.5 to 1 mL/kg when given via this route (AAP & AHA, 2016).

NEONATAL SIDE EFFECTS

Tachycardia may occur as well as premature ventricular contractions (PVCs); bolus doses may be associated with renal vascular ischemia, hypertension, and intracranial hemorrhage. If it infiltrates in a peripheral vein it can cause tissue necrosis and ischemia. Low dosages are associated with pulmonary and systemic vasodilation, and higher doses have a direct stimulating effect on the heart, causing an increase in blood pressure.

NURSING CONSIDERATIONS

- Always use the correct concentration 1:10,000 (0.1 mg/mL).
- Protect from light.
- Epinephrine should be given rapidly.
- When given via the IV/IO route, follow the drug dose with 0.5–1 mL of normal saline flush.
- When given via the ET route, several positive pressure breaths should be given to ensure even distribution throughout the lungs.
- Monitor heart rate and blood pressure continually with a CR monitor.
- Chest compressions must continue with administration for effective utilization and circulation within the body.

TC should be initiated within 6 hours of delivery, which typically includes transport time to a tertiary center, if necessary. The newborn is cooled to a core temperature of 33.5°C (92.3°F) for 72 hours and then slow warming over 4 hours is allowed to occur. Newborns have magnetic resonance imaging and an electrocardiogram following the warming period to assist the team in giving predictive outcome data to parents (Thoresen, 2015). Particular care should be utilized to avoid hyperthermia as this can be detrimental to neurons in the brain, causing premature cellular death.

●○● NURSING MANAGEMENT

For the Newborn Needing Resuscitation

Nursing Assessment and Diagnosis

Communication between the obstetric office or clinic and the birthing area nurse helps in the identification of newborns who may need resuscitation. When the woman arrives in the birthing area, assess the prenatal/antepartum record, any contributory prenatal history factors, and present fetal status. As labor progresses, nursing assessments include ongoing monitoring of fetal heartbeat and its response to contractions and observing for the presence of meconium in the amniotic fluid, when ruptured, to help identify possible fetal asphyxia. In addition, alert the interdisciplinary resuscitation team and the practitioner responsible for the care of the newborn of any potential high-risk laboring women.

Nursing diagnoses that may apply to the newborn with asphyxia and the newborn's parents include:

- ***Breathing Pattern, Ineffective,*** related to lack of spontaneous respirations at birth secondary to in utero asphyxia
- ***Cardiac Output, Decreased,*** related to impaired oxygenation
- ***Coping: Family, Compromised,*** related to baby's lack of spontaneous respirations at birth, continued care needed in NICU, possible transfer to tertiary care center, and parents' fear of losing their newborn

(NANDA-I © 2017)

Nursing Plan and Implementation

Hospital-Based Nursing Care

Following identification of possible high-risk situations, the next step in effective resuscitation is assembling the necessary equipment and ensuring proper functioning.

Check and maintain equipment to ensure its reliability before an emergency arises. The equipment must be cleaned or replaced and restocked immediately after each use and rechecked before every birth. Inspect all equipment—bag and mask, pressure

CASE STUDY: Melissa Bond-James

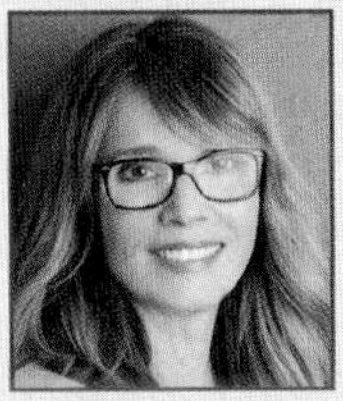

SOURCE: Kinga/Shutterstock.

Melissa has given birth to a 7 pound, 5 ounce baby girl after a prolonged second stage. Upon birth, the newborn has a heart rate of 90, is blue in color, and her respirations are limited. She exhibits nasal flaring, poor muscle tone, and is gasping. The midwife clamps and cuts the cord and hands the baby to the nurse for evaluation and possible resuscitation.

Questions to Ponder

What are the next steps in evaluation of this newborn? If resuscitation measures are needed, what would be the steps in starting those efforts?

manometer, oxygen and flow meter, pulse oximeter, laryngoscope bulb/battery, and suction machine—for damaged or nonfunctioning parts before a birth or when setting up an admission bed. A systematic check of the emergency cart and equipment is a routine responsibility of each shift. Gather equipment for pH and blood gas determination as well.

During resuscitation, it is essential that the newborn is kept warm unless the healthcare provider determines that the baby may benefit from passive cooling or other form of cooling therapy. Dry the newborn quickly with prewarmed towels or blankets and put a hat on the baby to prevent evaporative heat loss. Place the newborn under a prewarmed radiant warmer with servocontrol set at 36.5°C (97.7°F). The radiant warmer provides an overhead radiant heat source (a thermostatic mechanism that is secured to the newborn's abdomen, over a solid organ like the liver, triggers the radiant warmer to turn on or off to maintain a constant temperature). An open bed is necessary for easy access to the newborn.

Training and knowledge about resuscitation are vital to personnel in the birth setting for both normal and high-risk births. Neonatal Resuscitation Program (NRP) certification is renewed every 2 years for personnel working with newborns. Resuscitation is at least a two-person effort, and additional support should be called for as needed. One member of the collaborative care team must have the skill to perform airway management, line placement, and ventilation (AAP & AHA, 2016). The resuscitative efforts are recorded on the newborn's chart so that all members of the interprofessional healthcare team will have access to this information.

Supporting Parents

Family members may be present during resuscitation in the birthing room or in the neonatal intensive care unit (NICU), and the procedure is distressing for the parents. When resuscitation is anticipated, assure the parents that a collaborative care team will be present at the birth specifically for their newborn. A support person such as a chaplain or a social worker can be made available for the parents. As soon as the newborn's condition has been stabilized, a member of the collaborative care team will discuss the baby's condition with the parents. The parents often have many fears about the reasons for resuscitation and the short-term and long-term condition of their baby following the resuscitation. The individual leading the resuscitation team is often a good person to help with this discussion.

Ethics in Action!

When a newborn is expected who is on the cusp of the medical definition of viability or who is found to have a potentially lethal condition, who should make the decisions about resuscitation? Should it be the parents? Should it be the medical team?

Evaluation

Expected outcomes of nursing care include:

- The newborn requiring resuscitation is promptly identified, and intervention is started early.
- The newborn's metabolic and physiologic processes are stabilized, and recovery proceeds without complications.
- The parents can verbalize the reason for resuscitation and what was done to resuscitate their newborn.
- The parents can verbalize their fears about the resuscitation process and potential implications for their baby's future.

Care of the Newborn with Respiratory Distress

One of the most severe conditions a newborn can experience is respiratory distress or respiratory failure—an inappropriate respiratory adaptation to extrauterine life. Respiratory distress occurs in 5% of near-term newborns, 30% of newborns less than 30 weeks' gestation, and 60% of premature newborns of gestational age less than 28 weeks (Pramanik, Rangaswamy, & Gates, 2015). The nurse caring for a baby with respiratory distress needs to understand the normal pulmonary and circulatory physiology (see Chapter 26), the pathophysiology of the disease process, clinical manifestations, and supportive and corrective therapies. Only with this knowledge can the nurse make appropriate observations concerning responses to therapy and anticipate development of complications. Unlike the verbalizing adult patient, the newborn communicates needs only by exhibiting behaviors or physiologic parameters that must be interpreted by the NICU nurse. The neonatal nurse interprets this behavior as clues about the individual newborn's condition. In this section, respiratory distress syndrome, transient tachypnea of the newborn, meconium aspiration syndrome, and persistent pulmonary hypertension are discussed. While the pathophysiology differs, the nursing care of these conditions are similar and detailed in Table 31–3 later in this section.

Respiratory Distress Syndrome

Respiratory distress syndrome (RDS), formerly called *hyaline membrane disease (HMD)*, is the result of a primary absence, deficiency, or alteration in the production of pulmonary surfactant, a substance produced in the lungs that keeps alveoli from collapsing on expiration. The first hour of a premature newborn's life, which is sometimes called the "golden hour," is when the baby needs to achieve a successful transition to birth with inflation of the lungs and clearing of fluid and retention of FRC without hypoxia or hyperoxia or drastic changes in cerebral blood flow that can cause neurologic damage. RDS is generally higher in newborns who are exposed to infection in utero and those born without the benefit of antenatal steroids.

All the factors precipitating the pathologic changes of RDS have not been determined, but the main factors associated with its development are:

1. ***Prematurity.*** All preterm newborns—no matter their size—and especially newborns of mothers with diabetes are at risk for RDS. The incidence of RDS increases with the degree of prematurity, with most deaths occurring in newborns weighing less than 1500 g (3.3 lb). The maternal and fetal factors resulting in preterm labor and birth, complications of pregnancy, indications for cesarean birth, and familial tendency are all associated with RDS.
2. ***Surfactant deficiency disease.*** Normal pulmonary adaptation requires adequate surfactant, a lipoprotein that coats the inner surface of the alveoli. Surfactant provides alveolar stability by decreasing the alveoli's surface tension and tendency for collapse. Surfactant is produced by type II alveolar cells starting at about 24 weeks' gestation. In the normal or mature newborn lung, it is continuously synthesized, oxidized during breathing, and replenished. Adequate surfactant levels lead to better lung compliance and permit breathing with less work. The degree of development of RDS in a newborn is due to alterations in surfactant quantity, composition, function, or production. The production and

adequacy of surfactant can be altered in conditions such as aspiration (of blood or meconium), infection, and prematurity (Adamkin, 2017).

Clinical Tip

You can help parents understand their baby's respiratory distress by having them think of the alveolus as a small balloon filled with water and no air. When the balloon is emptied, the water droplets that remain inside the balloon increase the surface tension. As a result, the sides of the balloon stick together. The increased surface tension makes reinflation very difficult and requires an increased amount of energy. If there is no air left in the alveolus at the end of expiration, this is a failure to achieve functional residual capacity.

Development of RDS indicates a failure to synthesize adequate surfactant, which is required to maintain alveolar stability (see discussion in Chapter 25). Upon expiration, the instability increases *atelectasis* (collapse of part or all of a lung), which decreases diffusion of CO_2 across the blood vessels in the lungs, thereby causing hypoxia and acidosis. These conditions further inhibit surfactant production and cause pulmonary vasoconstriction. The resulting lung instability causes the biochemical problems of hypoxemia (decreased PO_2), hypercarbia (increased PCO_2), and acidemia (decreased pH), which further increases pulmonary vasoconstriction and hypoperfusion; alveolar endothelial and epithelial damage; and subsequent protein-rich interstitial and alveolar edema. The cycle of events of RDS leading to eventual respiratory failure is diagrammed in Figure 31–4.

Because of these pathophysiologic conditions, the newborn must expend increasing amounts of energy to reopen the collapsed alveoli with every breath, so that each breath becomes more difficult than the last. The progressive expiratory atelectasis upsets the physiologic homeostasis of the pulmonary and cardiovascular systems and prevents adequate gas exchange. Breathing becomes progressively harder as lung compliance decreases, which makes it more difficult for the newborn to inflate the lungs and breathe. The physiologic alterations of RDS produce these complications:

1. ***Hypoxia.*** As a result of hypoxia, the pulmonary vasculature constricts, pulmonary vascular resistance increases, and pulmonary blood flow is reduced. Increased pulmonary vascular resistance may precipitate a return to fetal circulation as the ductus arteriosus is typically still open and blood flow is shunted at times toward the lungs and at times away from the lungs, depending on the pulmonary pressures and pressures in the body (systemic pressures). This shunting increases the hypoxia and further decreases pulmonary perfusion. Hypoxia also causes impairment or absence of metabolic response to cold; reversion to anaerobic metabolism, resulting in lactate accumulation (acidosis); and impaired cardiac output, which decreases perfusion to vital organs.
2. ***Respiratory acidosis.*** Increased PCO_2 and decreased pH are results of alveolar hypoventilation. A persistent rise in PCO_2 is a poor prognostic sign of pulmonary function and adequacy because increased PCO_2 and decreased pH are results of alveolar hypoventilation.
3. ***Metabolic acidosis.*** Because cells lack oxygen, the newborn begins an anaerobic pathway of metabolism, with an increase in lactate levels and a resulting base deficit (loss of bicarbonate). As the lactate levels increase, the pH decreases in an attempt to maintain acid–base homeostasis.

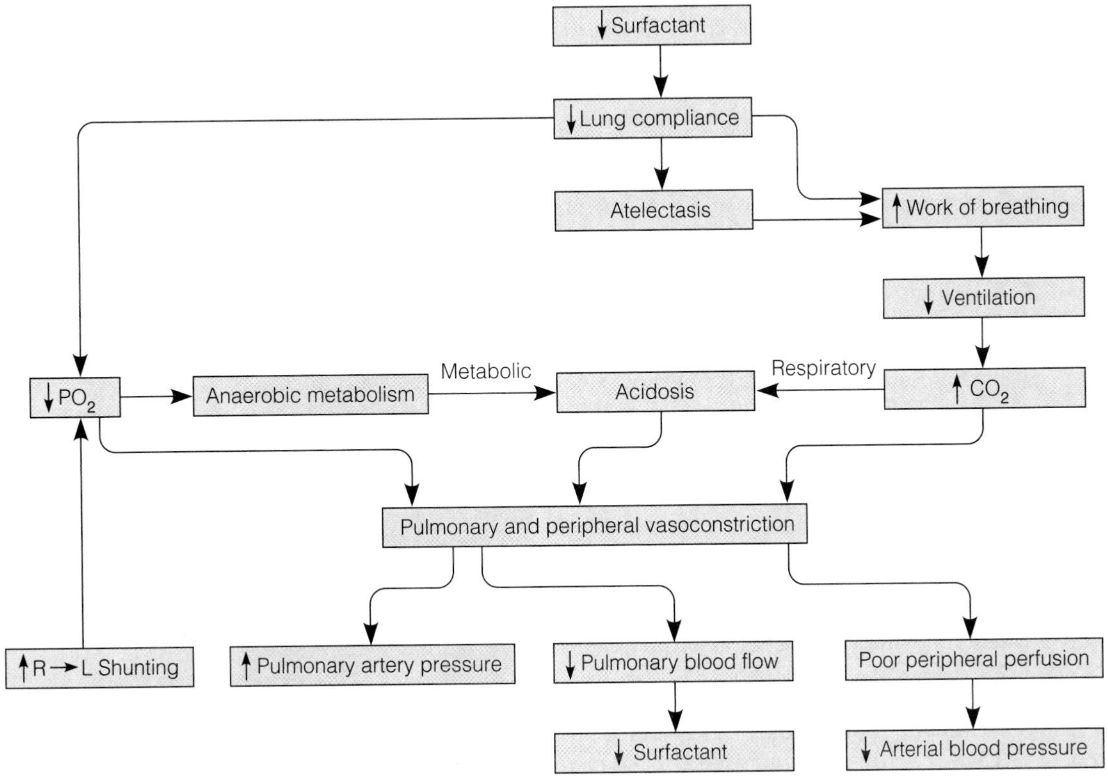

Figure 31–4 **Cycle of events of RDS leading to eventual respiratory failure.**

SOURCE: Modified from Gluck & Kulovich, 1973.

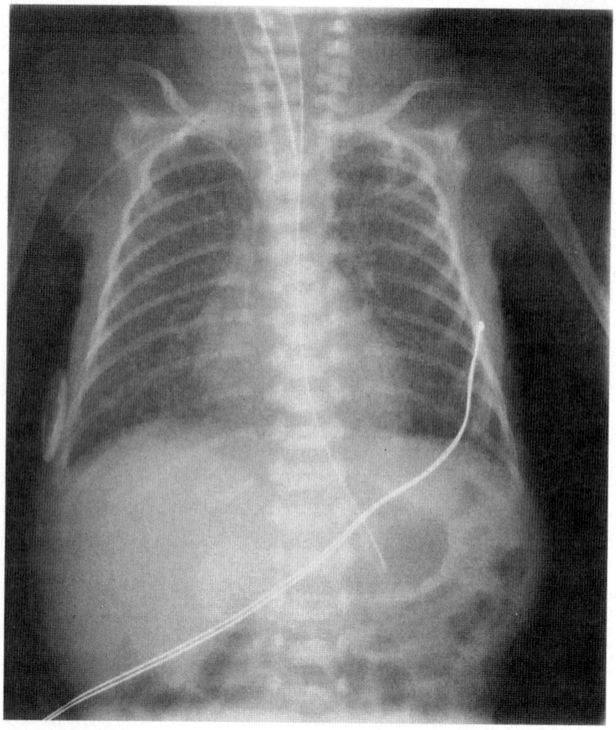

Figure 31–5 RDS chest X-ray. Chest radiograph of respiratory distress syndrome characterized by a reticulogranular pattern with areas of microatelectasis of uniform opacity and air bronchograms.

SOURCE: Carol Harrigan, RN, MSN, NNP-BC.

The classic radiologic picture of RDS is diffuse bilateral reticulogranular (ground glass appearance) density, with portions of the air-filled tracheobronchial tree (air bronchogram) outlined by the opaque ("white-out") lungs with widespread atelectasis, potentially obliterating the heart borders (Gallacher, Hart, & Kotcha, 2016; Pramanik et al., 2015) (Figure 31–5). Opacification of the lungs on x-ray image may be due to massive atelectasis, diffuse alveolar infiltrate, or pulmonary edema. The progression of x-ray findings parallels the pattern of resolution, which usually occurs in 4 to 10 days, and the time of surfactant reappearance, unless surfactant replacement therapy has been used. Echocardiography is a valuable tool in diagnosing vascular shunts that shunt blood either away from, right to left reverting to a fetal pattern, or toward the lungs. If a neonate doesn't improve with surfactant treatment and mechanical ventilation (MV), a patent ductus arteriosus (PDA) should be evaluated (Pramanik et al., 2015).

CLINICAL THERAPY

The primary goal of prenatal management is to prevent preterm birth through aggressive antenatal treatment of preterm labor and administration of steroids to enhance fetal lung development if birth is imminent (see Chapter 18). Antenatal steroids reduce the incidence and severity of RDS and improve survivability of the 24 to 34 weeks' gestation and extremely low-birth-weight newborn (less than 1250 g [2.8 lb]).

Postnatal surfactant replacement therapy, given as prophylaxis or rescue treatment, is available for newborns to decrease the severity of RDS in low-birth-weight babies. Unfortunately, babies born at less than 30 weeks' gestation who receive prophylactic surfactant show no decrease in chronic lung disease (AAP & ACOG, 2017). Surfactant replacement therapy is delivered when necessary through an endotracheal tube and may be given either in the birthing room or in the nursery, as indicated by the severity of respiratory failure. Repeat doses are often required. The most frequently reported response to treatment is rapidly improved oxygenation and decreased need for ventilatory support, sometimes occurring quite quickly after the dose is administered. Newborns with RDS vary greatly in their presentation and degree of respiratory failure and need to be managed according to their individual needs (Hardy, D'Agata, & McGrath, 2016).

Supportive medical management consists of establishing positive end expiratory pressure (PEEP) when assisting a newborn who is starting the transition to developing FRC (the air left in the alveoli after an exhaled breath). Ventilatory therapy, blood gas monitoring, pulse oximetry monitoring, correction of acid–base imbalance, environmental temperature regulation, adequate nutrition, and protection from infection are additional therapies needed. Ventilatory therapy is directed toward preventing hypoventilation and hypoxia.

Mild cases of RDS may require only increased humidified oxygen concentrations. Use of CPAP from birth may be the best therapy in newborns born early; up to 50% required no further intervention. Heated high-flow nasal cannula at 2 liters with blended oxygen has also shown to be effective at distending airway pressure in the preterm newborn (Jeon, 2016). Newborns with severe cases of RDS require mechanical ventilatory assistance from a respirator (Figure 31–6). The pressure-controlled volume ventilation setting on the respirator is the most ideal because it automatically adapts to the baby's lungs as they become more compliant, thereby reducing ventilator-associated lung injury (VALI) (Keszler & Sant'Anna, 2015). This also allows for the ventilator to adapt pressures to the baby when lung compliance improves following the administration of surfactant.

High-frequency ventilation (HFV) can be tried when conventional ventilator therapy is not successful, and it sometimes can be the primary mode of ventilation to minimize lung injury in very small and/or sick newborns (Keszler & Sant'Anna, 2015). In some institutions, morphine or fentanyl is used for its analgesic and sedative effects while using this respiratory modality.

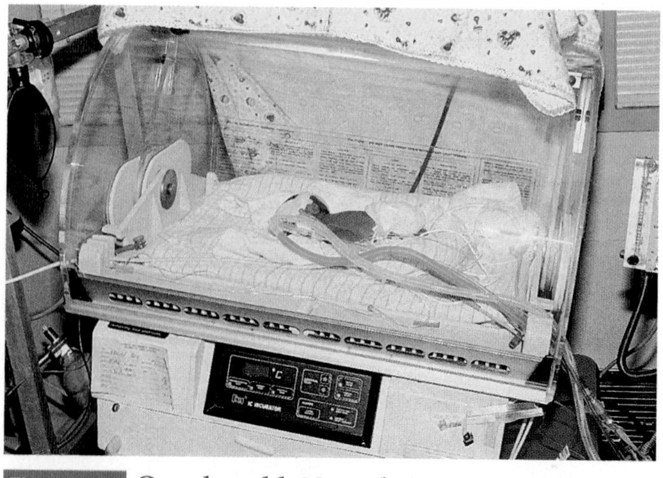

Figure 31–6 One-day-old, 29 weeks' gestational age, 1450 g (3.2 lb) baby on respirator and in isolette.

SOURCE: Carol Harrigan, RN, MSN, NNP-BC.

Clinical Tip

In babies with RDS who are on ventilators, increased urination/diuresis (determined by weighing diapers) may be an early clue that the baby's condition is improving (usually in the second to fourth day). As fluid moves out of the lungs into the bloodstream, alveoli open and kidney perfusion increases; this results in increased voiding. At this point, the nurse must monitor chest expansion closely. If chest expansion is increasing, pulmonary compliance is improving and ventilator settings may have to be decreased, sometimes quite soon after surfactant dosing. Too high a ventilator setting may overinflate the lung, only to have it collapse and then burst, resulting in pneumothorax.

●○● NURSING MANAGEMENT

For the Newborn with Respiratory Distress Syndrome

Nursing Assessment and Diagnosis

Characteristics of RDS that should be looked for are known prematurity, increasing cyanosis, tachypnea (greater than 60 respirations per minute), grunting respirations, nasal flaring, significant retractions, and apnea. Table 31–2 reviews clinical findings associated with respiratory distress in general. These clinical findings may lead a healthcare provider to evaluate a chest x-ray and a blood gas on the newborn. Many of the subtle findings on chest x-ray will lead to a more definitive diagnosis of the neonate with respiratory distress.

Based on clinical parameters, the neonatal nurse implements therapeutic approaches to provide the newborn with respiratory distress with a very supportive environment (Figure 31–7) that includes maintaining thermoregulation to decrease respiratory effort and decrease infection secondary to invasive procedures and using standard precautions. (See *Nursing Care Plan: The Newborn with Respiratory Distress Syndrome.*) Newborns with severe respiratory distress are cared for in NICUs where they can be continuously observed on a CR monitor by nurses with advanced knowledge and training.

Nursing interventions and criteria for instituting mechanical ventilatory assistance are done per institutional protocol. Noninvasive oxygen monitoring, as well as CO_2 monitors, provide real-time information that is particularly useful in newborns showing frequent changes in PaO_2 and oxygen saturation. These methods (pulse oximetry, transcutaneous oxygen, and CO_2 monitor) can also reduce the frequency of blood gas sampling. Methods of noninvasive oxygen monitoring and nursing interventions are

TABLE 31–2 Clinical Assessments Associated with Respiratory Distress

CLINICAL PICTURE	SIGNIFICANCE
Skin Color	
Pallor or mottling	These represent poor peripheral circulation caused by systemic hypotension and vasoconstriction and pooling of independent areas (usually in conjunction with severe hypoxia).
Cyanosis (bluish tint)	Depending on hemoglobin concentration, peripheral circulation, intensity and quality of viewing light, and acuity of observer's color vision, this is frankly visible in advanced hypoxia. Central cyanosis is most easily detected by examination of mucous membranes and tongue.
Jaundice (yellow discoloration of skin and mucous membranes caused by presence of unconjugated [indirect] bilirubin)	Metabolic alterations (acidosis, hypercarbia, asphyxia, sepsis) of respiratory distress predispose a newborn to dissociation of bilirubin from albumin-binding sites and deposition in the skin and central nervous system.
Edema (presents as slick, shiny, taut skin)	This is characteristic of preterm newborns because their total protein concentration is low, with a decrease in colloidal osmotic pressure and transudation of fluid. Edema of hands and feet is frequently seen within first 24 hours and resolved by fifth day in newborns with severe RDS.
Respiratory System	
Tachypnea (normal respiratory rate 30 to 60/minute, sustained, elevated respiratory rate 60+/minute)	Increased respiratory rate is the easiest detectable sign of respiratory distress after birth. Because of the premature newborn's very compliant chest wall, it is more energy efficient to increase the respiratory rate than the depth of respirations. This compensatory mechanism attempts to increase respiratory dead space to maintain alveolar ventilation and gas exchange in the face of an increase in mechanical resistance. As a decompensatory mechanism it increases workload and energy output by increasing respiratory rate, which causes increased metabolic demand for oxygen and thus increases alveolar ventilation on an already overstressed system. During shallow, rapid respirations, there is an increase in dead space ventilation, thus decreasing alveolar ventilation.
Apnea (episode of nonbreathing for more than 20 seconds; periodic breathing, a common "normal" occurrence in preterm newborns, is defined as apnea of 5 to 10 seconds alternating with 10 to 15 seconds of ventilation) that is sometimes quite rapid	This poor prognostic sign indicates cardiorespiratory disease, CNS disease, metabolic alterations, intracranial hemorrhage, sepsis, or immaturity. Physiologic alterations include decreased oxygen saturation, respiratory acidosis, and bradycardia.

(continued)

TABLE 31–2 Clinical Assessments Associated with Respiratory Distress *(continued)*

CLINICAL PICTURE	SIGNIFICANCE
Chest	
Chest movement	Inspection of the thoracic cage includes shape, size, and symmetry of movement. Respiratory movements should be symmetrical and diaphragmatic; asymmetry such as seesaw-like movements reflects pathology (pneumothorax, diaphragmatic hernia). Increased anteroposterior diameter indicates air trapping (meconium aspiration syndrome).
Labored respirations indicate severity of retractions (see below), grunting, and nasal flaring, which are signs of labored respirations	Indicates marked increase in the work of breathing.
Retractions (inward pulling of soft parts of the chest cage—suprasternal [above the sternum], substernal, intercostals [between the ribs]—at inspiration)	These reflect the significant increase in negative intrathoracic pressure necessary to inflate stiff, noncompliant lungs. Newborns attempt to increase lung compliance by using accessory muscles. Lung expansion markedly decreases. Seesaw respirations are seen when the chest flattens with inspiration and the abdomen bulges. Retractions increase the work of breathing and O_2 need. As a result, assisted ventilation may be necessary because of exhaustion.
Nasal flaring (inspiratory dilation of nostrils)	This compensatory mechanism attempts to lessen the resistance of the narrow nasal passage.
Expiratory grunt (Valsalva maneuver in which the newborn exhales against a partially closed glottis, thus producing an audible moan)	This increases intrapulmonary pressure, which decreases or prevents atelectasis, thus improving oxygenation and alveolar ventilation and allowing more time for the passage of oxygen into the circulatory system. Intubation should only be attempted if the newborn's condition is rapidly deteriorating because it may cause the alveoli to collapse.
Rhythmic body movement with labored respirations (chin tug, head bobbing, retractions of anal area)	This is a result of using abdominal and other respiratory accessory muscles during prolonged forced respirations.
Auscultation of chest reveals decreased air exchange, with harsh breath sounds or fine inspiratory rales; rhonchi may be present	Decrease in breath sounds and distant quality may indicate interstitial or intrapleural air or fluid.
Cardiovascular System	
Continuous systolic murmur may be audible	Patent ductus arteriosus is a common occurrence with hypoxia, pulmonary vasoconstriction, right-to-left shunting, and congestive heart failure.
Heart rate usually within normal limits (fixed heart rate may occur with a rate of 110 to 120 beats/min)	A fixed heart rate indicates a decrease in vagal control.
Point of maximal impulse usually located at fourth to fifth intercostal space, left sternal border	Displacement may reflect dextrocardia, pneumothorax, or diaphragmatic hernia.
Hypothermia	This is inadequate functioning of metabolic processes that require oxygen to produce necessary body heat.
Muscle Tone	
Flaccid, hypotonic, unresponsive to stimuli Hypertonia and/or seizure activity	These may indicate deterioration in the newborn's condition and possible CNS damage caused by hypoxia, acidemia, or hemorrhage.

described in Table 31–3. (The nursing care of newborns on ventilators or with umbilical vein and artery catheters is not discussed here. These babies have severe respiratory distress and are cared for in NICUs by nurses with advanced knowledge and training.) Ventilatory assistance with high-frequency ventilators has shown positive results. The parents of a baby born having respiratory distress will need a very supportive environment and team of professionals.

Transient Tachypnea of the Newborn

Some newborns, primarily large-for-gestational-age (LGA), term, and late preterm newborns, may develop progressive respiratory distress that can resemble classic RDS; this is called *transient tachypnea of the newborn (TTN)*. Risk factors for TTN include maternal diabetes and asthma, male sex of the fetus, macrosomia (possibly related to maternal diabetes), and cesarean section delivery, especially elective cesarean sections without spontaneous labor. Some of these babies with progressively worsening respiratory distress may benefit from exogenous surfactant (Gardner, Enzman-Hines, & Nyp, 2016).

Typically, supplemental oxygen of less than 40% will alleviate the hypoxia (Eichenwald, Hansen, Martin, et al., 2017). The fetus may have had intrauterine or intrapartum asphyxia due to maternal oversedation or poor uterine perfusion, maternal bleeding, prolapsed cord, or breech presentation. The newborn then

TABLE 31–3 Ventilation Monitors Utilized in the Newborn

TYPE	FUNCTION AND RATIONALE	NURSING INTERVENTIONS
Pulse Oximetry—SpO_pO_2		
Estimates beat-to-beat arterial oxygen saturation.	Calibration is automatic.	Understand and use oxyhemoglobin dissociation curve.
Microprocessor measures saturation by the absorption of red and infrared light as it passes through tissue.	Less dependent on perfusion than $TcPO_2$ and $TcPCO_2$; however, functions poorly if peripheral perfusion is decreased because of low cardiac output.	Monitor trends over time and correlate with arterial blood gases. Check disposable sensor at least every 8 hr.
Changes in absorption related to blood pulsation through vessel determine saturation and pulse rate.	Much more rapid response time than $TcPO_2$—offers real-time readings. Can be located on extremity, digit, or palm of hand, leaving chest free; not affected by skin characteristics. Requires understanding of oxyhemoglobin dissociation curve. Pulse oximeter reading of 88 to 93% reflects a PaO_2 of 50–80 mm Hg Extreme sensitivity to movement; decreases if average of 7th or 14th beat is selected rather than beat to beat. Poor correlation with extreme hyperoxia.	Use disposable cuffs (reusable cuffs allow too much ambient light to enter, and readings may be inaccurate).
Transcutaneous Oxygen Monitor—$TcPO_2$		
Measures oxygen diffusion across the skin. Clark electrode is heated to 43°C [109.4°F] (preterm) or 44°C [111.2°F] (term) to warm the skin beneath the electrode and promote diffusion of oxygen across the skin surface. Po_2 is measured when oxygen diffuses across the capillary membrane, skin, and electrode membrane.	When transcutaneous monitors are properly calibrated and electrodes are appropriately positioned, they will provide reliable, continuous, noninvasive measurements of PO_2, PCO_2, and oxygen saturation. Readings vary when skin perfusion is decreased. Reliable as trend monitor. Frequent calibration necessary to overcome mechanical drift. Following membrane change, machine must "warm up" 1 hour prior to initial calibration; otherwise, after turning it on, it must equilibrate for 30 minutes prior to calibration. When placed on newborn, values will be low until skin is heated; approximately 15 minutes required to stabilize. Second-degree burns are rare but can occur if electrodes remain in place too long. Decreased correlations noted with older babies (related to skin thickness), with babies with low cardiac output (decreased skin perfusion), and with hyperoxic babies. The adhesive that attaches the electrode may abrade the fragile skin of the preterm newborn. May be used for both preductal and postductal monitoring of oxygenation for observations of shunting.	Measures oxygen diffusion across the skin. Clark electrode is heated to 43°C [109.4°F] (preterm) or 44°C [111.2°F] (term) to warm the skin beneath the electrode and promote diffusion of oxygen across the skin surface. Po_2 is measured when oxygen diffuses across the capillary membrane, skin, and electrode membrane.

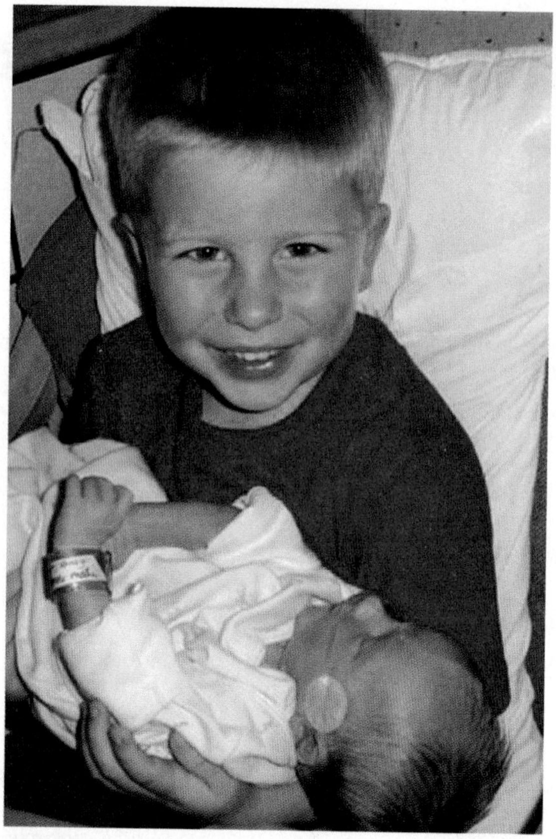

Figure 31–7 This baby born at 36 weeks' gestational age had severe RDS. He has ongoing oxygen needs provided by a nasal cannula but still can be held by his proud big brother.

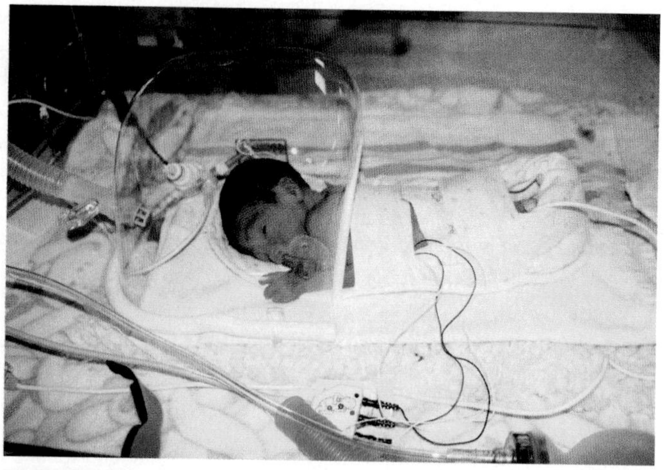

Figure 31–8 Premature newborn under oxygen hood. Baby is nested and has a nonnutritive sucking pacifier.

fails to clear the airway of lung fluid, mucus, and other debris or an excess of fluid in the lungs due to aspiration of amniotic or tracheal fluid. TTN is also more prevalent in cesarean birth newborns who have not had the *thoracic squeeze* that occurs during vaginal birth and removes some of the lung fluid.

Usually the newborn experiences little or no difficulty at the onset of breathing. However, shortly after birth, expiratory grunting, flaring of the nares, subcostal retractions, desaturation, and mild cyanosis may be noted in the newborn that is breathing room air (Gardner et al., 2016). Air will become trapped and an increase in the anterior–posterior diameter of the chest may be observed. Tachypnea is usually present by 6 hours of age, with respiratory rates consistently greater than 60 breaths/min, and possibly reaching 80–100 breaths/min and higher, with a requirement of oxygen. Mild respiratory and metabolic acidosis may be present within the first 6 hours. These clinical signs usually improve within 12 to 24 hours. In mild TTN, the signs can improve within 24 hours but may continue for 48 to 72 hours when more severe and possibly last up to 1 week (Eichenwald et al., 2017).

CLINICAL THERAPY

Initial x-ray findings may be identical to those showing RDS within the first 3 hours. However, radiographs of newborns with transient tachypnea usually reveal a generalized overexpansion of the lungs (hyperaeration of alveoli), which is identifiable principally by flattened contours of the diaphragm. Dense streaks (increased vascularity) radiate from the hilar region and represent engorgement of the lymphatic vessels, which clear alveolar fluid on initiation of air breathing. Within 48 hours the chest x-ray examination is generally normal, with the exception of perihilar markings, which may remain visible for 3 to 7 days due to remaining fluid in the periarterial tissue.

Ambient oxygen concentrations of 30 to 50%, usually under an oxyhood, may be required to correct the hypoxemia (Figure 31–8).

When hypoxemia is severe and tachypnea continues, persistent pulmonary hypertension of the newborn (PPHN) must be considered and treatment measures initiated. Newborns with TTN are often suspected initially of pneumonia, and antibiotics are generally administered prophylactically while a blood culture and placental culture is evaluated. For nursing actions, see *Nursing Care Plan: For the Newborn with Respiratory Distress Related to RDS and TTN.*

Persistent Pulmonary Hypertension of the Newborn

Persistent pulmonary hypertension of the newborn (PPHN) is a serious disorder that primarily affects on average 1 to 2 of 1000 liveborn newborns annually, and the mortality rate is between 4 and 33% (Lakshminrusimha & Saugstad, 2016). The fetus late in gestation needs to increase the pulmonary expression of nitric oxide (NO) synthases and soluble guanylate cyclase, so that normal pulmonary vasodilation occurs. The newborn has exposure to oxygen, which stimulates the pulmonary bed, and the cascade effect causes the pulmonary endothelium to release these mediators, such as prostacyclin and inhaled nitric oxide (iNO). These mediators cause the cardiopulmonary transition to be successful in the newborn. If there is an alteration in the development of these mediators or the release of them, the transition is blunted and the cycle of pulmonary constriction starts. This leads to right-to-left (R-L) shunting of blood away from the lungs and through the fetal ductus arteriosus and patent foramen ovale, consequently bypassing the lungs and the ability to be oxygenated, causing worsening hypoxemia and acidosis (Lakshminrusimha & Saugstad, 2016). The hypoxemia and acidosis are the most potent stimulants of pulmonary vasoconstriction and increased PVR. Once this process has begun, it is self-perpetuating and difficult to interrupt. Clinical deterioration is rapid and difficult to reverse. In the presence of continued pulmonary vasoconstriction, vascular changes can occur and lead to remodeling of the vascular bed within the lungs, leading to the continued cycle of hypoxia and acidosis.

Nursing Care Plan: For the Newborn with Respiratory Distress Related to RDS and TTN

1. Nursing Diagnosis: *Breathing Pattern, Ineffective*, related to immature lung development or inadequate lung surfactant (NANDA-I © 2017)

Goal: The newborn will maintain an effective breathing pattern.

INTERVENTION	RATIONALE
• Review maternal birth records, noting medications given to mother before birth and the newborn's condition at birth such as Apgar scores and resuscitative measures.	• Several drugs suppress respiratory function in the newborn.
• Administer surfactant replacement therapy as ordered.	
• Surfactant replacement therapy may be administered via endotracheal tube either in the birthing room or in the nursery.	• Surfactant improves lung compliance; therefore, the need for ventilatory support may be decreased. Surfactant provides alveolar stability by decreasing the alveoli's surface tension and tendency to collapse. Alterations in surfactant quantity, composition, function, or production result in respiratory distress syndrome.
• Initiate cardiac and respiratory monitoring and calibrate these monitors every 8 hours or per protocol	• Close monitoring detects periodic apneic spells and allows for medical intervention, if necessary.
• Monitor newborn's respiratory rate and rhythm, pulse, blood pressure, chest movement, and activity.	• Increases in respiratory rate and pulse and alteration in rhythm and blood pressure may indicate respiratory distress.
• Assess skin color; note signs of cyanosis, duskiness, and pallor.	• Any changes in the normal skin color may indicate a physiologic change occurring.
• Clear newborn's airway by suctioning PRN with bulb syringe.	• Opens airway by clearing mucus and allows maximum respiratory effort.
• Administer warmed, humidified oxygen by oxygen hood and monitor the oxygen concentrations every 30 minutes.	• Prevents mucosal dryness and insensible water loss in the preterm newborn and maintains an even level of oxygen administration.
• Oxygen may be administered to the newborn experiencing mild respiratory distress via nasal cannula or oxygen hood. With severe respiratory distress, mechanical ventilatory assistance from a respirator may be necessary.	• Oxygenation and ventilatory therapy may prevent hypoventilation and hypoxia. Mild cases of respiratory distress may require only increased humidified oxygen concentrations, whereas more severe cases may require CPAP.
	• Allowing oxyhood to touch newborn's face may cause apnea by stimulating the facial nerve.
• **Collaborative:** Obtain arterial blood gases (ABGs) per healthcare provider orders.	• Obtaining ABGs is essential in managing a newborn receiving oxygen.
• Maintain constant O_2 concentration for 15–30 minutes before sample is obtained. • Avoid stimulating newborn for 15 minutes before obtaining sample.	• Failure to synthesize surfactant increases atelectasis, which causes hypoxia and acidosis caused by lack of gas exchange. Lung compliance will deteriorate and result in difficulty of inflation, labored respirations, and increased work of breathing. Progressive hypoxia may be seen when ABG levels are compared and evaluated.
• Avoid suctioning newborn before obtaining sample.	• Suctioning may cause a discrepancy in ABG readings and should be avoided within 30 minutes of sample.
• Obtain sample in heparinized tuberculin syringe and maintain the temperature of the sample. • Assess the patency of the arterial line to prevent clot formation, and then replace blood used to clear line. • Flush line with 2 mL heparinized solution before restarting flow of IV fluids.	
• Attach pulse oximeter to newborn's extremity to measure tissue oxygenation	• Oxygen saturation should be kept at approximately 88 to 92% (Eichenwald et al., 2017). Avoid excessive oxygenation, which can increase the risk of developing chronic lung disease and retinopathy of prematurity.

(continued)

Nursing Care Plan: For the Newborn with Respiratory Distress Related to RDS and TTN (*continued*)

INTERVENTION	RATIONALE
• Monitor transcutaneous pulse oximeter and transcutaneous CO_2 monitor as utilized, continuously or hourly, and record. Rotate sensor site every 3–4 hours.	
• Assess newborn's need for mechanical ventilation: Apnea present, hypoxia (PaO_2 less than 50 mmHg), hypercapnia ($PaCO_2$ greater than 60 mmHg), respiratory acidosis (pH less than 7.2).	• Mechanical ventilation improves oxygenation and ventilation, resulting in rise in PaO_2 and decrease in $PaCO_2$.
• Administer mechanical ventilation per hospital protocol.	• CPAP or PEEP can be administered by nasal prongs, nasopharyngeal or oral intubation.

EXPECTED OUTCOMES: The newborn will maintain an effective breathing pattern as evidenced by respirations of 30–60 breaths/min, arterial blood gases are within normal range, newborn is free of signs of retractions or nasal flaring, and blood pH is 7.35–7.45.

2. Nursing Diagnosis: ***Thermoregulation, Ineffective*, related to increased respiratory effort (NANDA-I © 2017)**

Goal: **The newborn will exhibit no signs of hypothermia.**

INTERVENTION	RATIONALE
• Review maternal prenatal and intrapartum records. Note any medications mother received during these times.	• Medications such as Demerol and magnesium sulfate used by the mother during the prenatal or intrapartum periods significantly interfere with the newborn's ability to retain heat.
• Assess newborn's temperature frequently. Place servo probe on newborn's skin over a solid organ.	• Hypothermia leads to pulmonary vasoconstriction because of the increase in oxygen consumption. Cold stress leads to increased oxygen needs; consequently, brown fat is used to maintain body temperature.
• Observe for signs of increased oxygen consumption and metabolic acidosis.	• Hypoxia and acidosis further depress surfactant production.
• Warm and humidify all inspired gases and record temperature of delivered gases.	• Cold air/oxygen blown in face of newborn is stimulus for consumption of oxygen and glucose and increased metabolic rate.
• Use radiant warmers or incubators with servo controls and open cribs with appropriate clothing.	• Maintains neutral thermal environment.
• Note signs and symptoms of respiratory distress, including tachypnea, apnea, cyanosis, acrocyanosis, bradycardia, lethargy, weak cry, and hypotonia.	• These signs can predispose the newborn to metabolic acidosis.

EXPECTED OUTCOMES: The newborn will not exhibit signs and symptoms of hypothermia as evidenced by temperature maintenance of 97.7°F–99.1°F and no signs and symptoms of respiratory distress.

3. Nursing Diagnosis: ***Nutrition, Imbalanced: Less Than Body Requirements*, related to increased metabolic needs in the newborn (NANDA-I © 2017)**

Goal: **The newborn will maintain normal electrolytes and establish appropriate weight gain.**

INTERVENTION	RATIONALE
• Assess suck, swallow, gag, and cough reflexes.	• Prevents feeding problems and assists in determining the best individualized method of feeding for newborn.
• Assess respiratory status of newborn. If any problems are noted, notify physician/neonatal nurse practitioner (NNP).	• In the presence of respiratory distress, avoid oral fluids and initiate oral gastric (OG) feedings or parenteral nutrition by IV route, per physician's orders.
• Monitor IV rates per infusion pump (starting at 80 mL/kg/day) as ordered by physician.	• Allows for close monitoring of fluid intake, as well as frequent checks of fragile veins.
• Record hourly intake and output (I&O) and daily weights.	• IV fluids are administered to replace sensible and insensible water loss, as well as evaporative water loss secondary to respiratory distress. Monitoring I&O will prevent circulatory system overload that can lead to pulmonary edema and cardiac problems.
• Provide total parenteral nutrition (TPN) when indicated.	• TPN is used as nutritional alternative if bowel sounds are not present and/or newborn remains in acute distress.

Nursing Care Plan: For the Newborn with Respiratory Distress Related to RDS and TTN (*continued*)

Intervention	Rationale
• Advance, based on tolerance, from IV to gastrointestinal (GI) feedings. Gavage or nipple feedings are used, and IV is used as supplement (discontinued when enteral intake is sufficient).	• If IV is discontinued before enteral intake is established, baby will not receive adequate calories. • Formula or breast milk stimulates GI hormones necessary for a functional absorptive GI tract.
• Provide adequate caloric intake: Consider amount of intake, type of formula, route of administration, and need for supplementation of intake by other routes.	• Calories are essential to prevent catabolism of body proteins and metabolic acidosis due to starvation or inadequate caloric intake. This can be achieved with nasogastric (NG) or OG feedings or with TPN.
• Assess infusion site for signs and symptoms of infection, including erythema, edema, and drainage with a foul odor.	• Appropriate intervention can be initiated when signs and symptoms of infection are detected early. Treatment may avoid infection and sepsis in the newborn.

EXPECTED OUTCOMES: The newborn will maintain normal electrolytes and establish steady weight gain as evidenced by no more than 2%/day weight loss, tolerate oral feedings, and urine output of 1–3 mL/kg/hour.

4. Nursing Diagnosis: *Fluid Volume: Risk for Imbalanced,* related to increased insensible water losses (NANDA-I © 2017)

Goal: The newborn will not exhibit signs of dehydration and will display appropriate weight gain.

INTERVENTION	RATIONALE
• Observe for weight fluctuations by obtaining daily or twice-daily weights.	• Fluctuations in weight may indicate water imbalance or inadequate caloric intake.
• Consider humidity therapy in isolette for newborns less than 28 weeks' gestation.	• Prevention of fluid loss through permeable skin of the preterm neonate.
• Document cumulative balances of intake (IV fluid administration and feedings) and output (urine collection bags, weighing or counting diapers) hourly.	• Balanced fluid intake and output suggest homeostasis.
• Follow urine output in weight-based measures (ml/kg/hour).	• Electrolytes and urinary output (UOP) (minimum of 1 ml/kg/hr) are specific indicators of fluid balance in the preterm or ill neonate with respiratory distress.
• Monitor vital signs including blood pressure, pulse, temperature, and mean arterial pressure (MAP).	• MAP of less than gestational age may indicate hypotension.
• Assess patient for signs of dehydration (i.e., poor skin turgor, pale mucous membranes, and sunken anterior fontanelle).	• Detecting signs and symptoms of dehydration early in the newborn is important because early interventions are vital to prevent further damage.
• Assess IV site for signs of infection (erythema and edema) and infiltration.	• If signs and symptoms of infection are noted, intervention is necessary and IV site should be changed.
• **Collaborative:** Obtain labs for hematocrit (Hct), serum calcium, serum magnesium, serum potassium, blood urea nitrogen (BUN), creatinine, and uric acid levels.	• Determines necessity for supportive care with TPN administration.
• Administer fluids, blood products, and electrolytes as ordered by physician/NNP.	• Replaces low nutrient stores and treats anemia, if present.

EXPECTED OUTCOMES: The newborn will be free of signs and symptoms of dehydration as evidenced by intake equaling output and a weight gain after the first week of life of at least 20–30 grams/day.

CLINICAL THERAPY

Diagnosis of PPHN in the cyanotic term or postterm newborn includes clinical assessment, and definitive diagnosis, if available, occurs with the use of an echocardiogram (ECG). ECG will exclude structural anomalies and will exhibit the diagnostic hemodynamic shunting of unoxygenated blood passing from the right to the left side of the heart, through the fetal ducts (foramen ovale and ductus arteriosus) (Gallacher et al., 2016; Lakshminrusimha & Saugstad, 2016).

Perinatal asphyxia, as discussed previously, is a known predisposing factor to PPHN and utilizing appropriate resuscitation techniques is essential. Oxygen is a potent pulmonary vasodilator and the recommendation for pulse oximeter use in the delivery room will help the nurse to respond to individual needs for each newborn. Excessive oxygen has a role in exacerbation of PPHN and possibly of HIE (Lakshminrusimha & Saugstad, 2016). ECG with Doppler flow can show a prolonged ratio of right-ventricular ejection period, with right-to-left shunting sending deoxygenated blood to the body in newborns with PPHN. The goal of therapeutic intervention is to lower the pulmonary vascular resistance and reverse the process of shunting. This can be accomplished with excellent ventilation (the management of acidosis), elevated oxygenation (as evidenced by goal PaO_2), and, when diagnosed on ECG, with a right-to-left shunt, a dose of

20 ppm of iNO. Volume expanders and drug therapy—such as analgesics or sedatives, vasopressors (dopamine, epinephrine, dobutamine, milrinone), hydrocortisone, and afterload reducers—may be used adjunctively until the PaO_2 can be consistently maintained. There are some newborns who do not respond to iNO, but these babies do respond at times to inhaled or systemic vasodilators such as prostaglandins and milrinone. When failure occurs with these therapies, *extracorporal membrane oxygenation (ECMO)*, a procedure in which the blood is removed, oxygenated externally, and then replaced, is life-saving in babies with PPHN (Lakshminrusimha & Saugstad, 2016).

●○● NURSING MANAGEMENT

For the Newborn with Persistent Pulmonary Hypertension

Assess for the onset of symptoms, which usually occur in the first few hours of life. Affected newborns exhibit signs of respiratory distress (grunting, nasal flaring, tachypnea), with increased anteroposterior diameter and cyanosis. They typically fail to respond to conventional methods of oxygenation and ventilation. Significant unexplained hypoxemia exists in the absence of congenital heart disease. The chest radiograph might show little or no evidence of pulmonary parenchymal disease (depending on the underlying disease). The hypoxemia and cyanosis associated with PPHN are characteristic of extreme reactivity. Marked, rapid changes in PaO_2 and color are seen with agitation, stimulation, therapeutic intervention (suctioning), or rapid changes in ambient oxygen. There is typically a gradient or a difference of 10 to 15 points when measuring pre- and postductal saturations.

Newborns with PPHN are critically ill and require experienced, highly skilled nurses to provide optimal care with minimal manipulation/stimulation. Any disturbance may cause agitation, which leads to hypoxemia. If a paralyzing agent is used, nursing care includes monitoring the newborn's response to artificial oxygenation and mechanical ventilation. Ensure that the oxygen is delivered in correct amounts and route and record the percentage of oxygen flow. The ventilator settings should be checked frequently and recorded per unit policy. Carefully suction the endotracheal tube only as necessary while assessing the effect of the procedure on the baby's oxygenation and perfusion. The amount and type of secretions should be noted. Carefully assess arterial blood gases and notify the clinician if the results are out of the acceptable range. Oxygen monitoring is essential for identifying activities that may compromise the newborn's status. (Nursing interventions required for noninvasive oxygen monitoring are discussed in Table 31–3.) Continuous monitoring of vital signs, blood pressure, and perfusion is required, and careful inspection of the skin during positioning is necessary to avoid pressure necrosis. Aggressive ventilation poses a potential risk for pneumothorax. Many of these babies need to be transferred to a NICU familiar with this disease process and with access to services such as surgery and ECMO care.

Many newborns suffering PPHN are born at or near term at a time when parents least expect problems—especially life-threatening problems—to occur. The magnitude of the baby's illness and the rapid deterioration may be overwhelming to parents. Attachment becomes difficult when the newborn responds poorly to stimulation such as physical touch (as seen by decreased SaO_2 or PaO_2). Encourage parents to talk very softly to their baby because this will usually not compromise the baby's condition. Assess the parents' level of understanding and assist them by providing information about their newborn's condition and therapies in easily understandable terms. Continuity of nursing care is helpful because of the trust relationship that occurs with a smaller group of nurses.

Care of the Newborn with Meconium Aspiration Syndrome

Because the body's physiologic response to asphyxia/hypoxia is increased intestinal peristalsis and relaxation of the anal sphincter, the presence of meconium in the amniotic fluid indicates that the fetus may be suffering from asphyxia, either in the immediate period during labor or perhaps some time in the recent past (Pramanik et al., 2015). However, if the fetus is in a breech position, the presence of meconium in the amniotic fluid does not necessarily indicate asphyxia.

In approximately 10 to 15% of all live births, the babies are born through meconium-stained amniotic fluid (MSAF) and 4 to 5% of those neonates will develop **meconium aspiration syndrome (MAS)** (Pramanik et al., 2015).This fluid may be aspirated into the tracheobronchial tree by the fetus in utero or during the breaths taken by the newborn. Meconium in the lungs can lead to the mechanical obstruction of airways by ball-valve action (air is allowed in but not exhaled), so that alveoli overdistend, with oxygen and carbon dioxide trapping and hyperinflation; chemical pneumonitis; and inactivation of natural surfactant.

Clinical Manifestations of MAS

Clinical manifestations of MAS include (1) fetal hypoxia in utero a few days or a few minutes before birth, indicated by a sudden increase in fetal activity followed by diminished activity, slowing of fetal heart rate (FHR) or weak and irregular heartbeat, loss of beat-to-beat variability, and meconium staining of amniotic fluid or particulate meconium; and (2) presence of signs of distress at birth, such as pallor, cyanosis, apnea, slow heartbeat, and occasionally low Apgar scores. Newborns with intrauterine asphyxia, meconium-stained newborns, or newborns who have aspirated particulate meconium often have respiratory depression at birth and require resuscitation to establish adequate respiratory effort. Some, however, have a slower decline, requiring only a small amount of oxygen in a hood at first, then progressing to respiratory distress and then respiratory failure over the first few hours of life.

After the initial resuscitation, the severity of clinical symptoms correlates with the extent of aspiration. Many newborns require mechanical ventilation at birth because of immediate signs of distress (generalized cyanosis, tachypnea, and severe retractions). An overdistended, barrel-shaped chest with increased anteroposterior diameter is common. Auscultation reveals diminished air movement with prominent rales and rhonchi. Abdominal palpation may reveal a displaced liver caused by diaphragmatic depression resulting from the overexpansion of the lungs. Yellowish/pale green staining of the skin, nails, and umbilical cord is usually present, especially if the incident occurred sometime before birth.

The MAS chest x-ray film reveals asymmetric, coarse, patchy densities/infiltrates, with possible hyperinflation (9- to 11-rib expansion) and atelectasis, which may predispose the newborn to air leak syndromes such as pneumothorax or pneumomediastinum (Pramanik et al., 2015). These newborns have serious biochemical alterations, which include:

- Metabolic acidosis resulting from the cardiopulmonary shunting (bypassing the lungs) and hypoperfusion
- Respiratory acidosis due to shunting and alveolar hypoventilation
- Hypoxia, even in 100% O_2 concentrations and with ventilatory assistance

- Meconium with pH of 7.0–7.2; the inhalation of it causes chemical pneumonitis and leads to an inflammatory process within the lungs
- Meconium is full of bile acids and these inactivate the natural surfactant in the newborn
- Hypoxia continues the cardiopulmonary shunting and can lead to PPHN.

CLINICAL THERAPY

The combined efforts of the maternity and pediatric team are needed to prevent MAS. Previously, the most effective form of preventive management was intrapartum and postpartum suctioning after the head of the newborn was delivered but the shoulders and chest were still in the birth canal. Current evidence does not support this practice, as routine intrapartum oropharyngeal and nasopharyngeal suctioning does not prevent or alter the course of MAS (AAP & ACOG, 2017).

If the newborn is vigorous, even if there is meconium-stained amniotic fluid, no subsequent special resuscitation is indicated, and the newborn can often stay with the mother and do skin-to-skin time. If it is necessary, the steps of resuscitation will be the same as those previously discussed with the newborn who is asphyxiated. If the baby requires intubation and the airway has secretions visible, the healthcare provider may determine suctioning is warranted. A meconium aspirator should always be available for these newborns. A low-pressure wall suction device not to exceed 100 mmHg must also be ready. Literature has reinforced that the majority of newborns affected by MAS have aspirated in utero prior to delivery; the delay in electively intubating for suctioning can delay resuscitation as well as cause vagal response (AAP & AHA, 2016). Resuscitated newborns should be immediately transferred to the nursery for closer observation. The baby should be maintained in a neutral thermal environment, unless it is determined that the baby would benefit from cooling therapy, and tactile stimulation should be minimized. An umbilical arterial line may be used for direct monitoring of arterial blood pressures and blood sampling for pH and blood gases. An umbilical venous catheter may be placed for infusion of IV fluids, blood, or medications.

Treatment usually involves delivery of high oxygen concentrations and high-pressure ventilation. Low PEEPs (4–7 cm H_2O) are preferred to avoid air leaks such as pneumothorax. Unfortunately, high pressures may be needed to cause sufficient expiratory expansion of the obstructed terminal airways or to stabilize airways that are weakened by inflammation so that the most distal atelectatic (collapsed) alveoli are ventilated. Naturally occurring surfactant may be inactivated by the presence of meconium and the subsequent inflammatory response that occurs. Surfactant replacement therapy is most effective when given as a prophylactic measure. Providing exogenous surfactant possibly decreases the need for heart–lung bypass or extracorporeal membrane oxygenation (ECMO) and may prevent worsening respiratory distress (Eichenwald et al., 2017).

Systemic blood pressure and pulmonary blood flow must be maintained for both circulatory benefits and the balance of pulmonary pressures. Dopamine or dobutamine (volume expanders), or both, may be used to maintain systemic blood pressure.

Newborns with respiratory failure who are not responding to conventional ventilator therapy may require treatment with high-frequency ventilation and/or nitric oxide therapy if they are found to have PPHN. Inhaled nitric oxide has proven successful for newborns with meconium aspiration, pneumonia, and PPHN who are not responding to traditional treatment methods. These therapies should be utilized only if a center capable of providing ECMO is readily available. ECMO may be utilized in newborns greater than 1.8 kg (4.0 lb) and 34 weeks EGA if adequate ventilation and iNO fails (Lakshminrusimha, Mathew, & Leach, 2016).

Treatment includes minimized handling of the neonate in combination with sedation, prophylactic antibiotics, and metabolic acidosis correction, as well as expert ventilation management. Serial ABGs, chest x-rays, and transcutaneous monitoring is helpful in the management of the critically ill newborn. Mortality in term and postterm newborns with MAS is very high because the cycle of hypoxemia and acidemia is difficult to break.

●○● NURSING MANAGEMENT

For the Newborn with Meconium Aspiration Syndrome

Nursing Assessment and Diagnosis

During the intrapartum period, observe for signs of fetal hypoxia and meconium staining of amniotic fluid. At birth, assess the newborn for signs of distress. During the ongoing assessment of the newborn, carefully observe for complications such as pulmonary air leaks; anoxic cerebral injury manifested by seizures/convulsions; myocardial injury evidenced by congestive heart failure or cardiomegaly; disseminated intravascular coagulation (DIC) resulting from hypoxic hepatic damage with depression of liver-dependent clotting factors; anoxic renal damage demonstrated by hematuria, oliguria, or anuria; fluid overload; sepsis secondary to bacterial pneumonia; and any signs of intestinal necrosis from ischemia, including GI obstruction or hemorrhage.

Nursing diagnoses that may apply to the newborn with MAS and the family include:

- ***Gas Exchange, Impaired***, related to aspiration of meconium and amniotic fluid
- ***Nutrition, Imbalanced: Less Than Body Requirements***, related to respiratory distress and increased energy requirements
- ***Coping: Family, Compromised***, related to life-threatening illness in a term newborn

(NANDA-I © 2017)

Nursing Plan and Implementation

Hospital-Based Nursing Care

Initial interventions are aimed at early identification of meconium aspiration. When significant aspiration occurs, therapy is supportive with the primary goals of maintaining appropriate gas exchange and minimizing complications. Nursing interventions after resuscitation should include maintaining adequate oxygenation and ventilation, regulating temperature, performing glucose testing by glucometer to check for hypoglycemia, observing IV fluids, calculating necessary fluids (which may be restricted in the first 48 to 72 hours because of cerebral edema), providing caloric requirements possibly with TPN, keeping the environment quiet and decreasing interventions as much as possible, and monitoring IV antibiotic therapy.

Evaluation

Expected outcomes of nursing care include:

- The newborn at risk of MAS is promptly identified and early intervention is initiated.
- The newborn is free of respiratory distress and metabolic alterations.
- The parents verbalize their concerns about their baby's health problem and survival and understand the rationale behind management of their newborn.

Care of the Newborn with Complications Due to Respiratory Therapy

Oxygen and mechanical ventilation (MV), although required as therapeutic interventions to reduce hypoxia, hypercarbia, ischemia, and infarction to vital organs, may also have harmful effects. The concentrations of ambient oxygen administered to the newborn must be titrated according to oxygen tension within arterial blood to avoid development of retinopathy of prematurity or bronchopulmonary dysplasia/chronic lung disease. Because lungs develop in five stages and this development continues until the age of 8 years, damage to the lungs can occur because of arrested or modified development. Ventilator-associated lung injury (VALI) is damage to the lungs as a result of *barotrauma* (pressure-related damage), *volutrauma* (caused by overdistention), or *atelectrauma* (damage from under inflation or atelectasis) from MV (Keszler & Sant'Anna, 2015). Some of the complications of MV are discussed below.

Pulmonary Interstitial Emphysema

Pulmonary interstitial emphysema (PIE) is the accumulation of air in lung tissues occurring predominantly in VLBW neonates who are on mechanical ventilators for pulmonary disorders for an extended period of time. Overdistention of alveoli may cause blebs to form and can progress to PIE when rupture occurs and air escapes and becomes trapped in the interstitial spaces. Air moves along perivascular spaces, but not into the pleural space or mediastinum. As the air collections increase, blood vessels are constricted, and blood oxygenation and ventilation are impaired; thus, hypoxia and hypercarbia may develop. The air does not decrease on expiration. This condition is highly associated with subsequent bronchopulmonary dysplasia (BPD) and should be considered in newborns with recurrent air leaks. Incidence of PIE has decreased with the use of surfactant and improved ventilation strategies in the preterm or VLBW newborn. Treatment involves positioning, if it is unilateral, with the affected side down; intubation of only one lung; or, rarely, surgical resection.

Pneumothorax

Pneumothorax, a common complication of respiratory therapy, is an accumulation of air in the thoracic cavity between the parietal and visceral pleura, typically caused by overexpansion and rupture of the alveolar wall with air subsequently leaking from the intra-alveolar space to outside locations. Spontaneous pneumothorax occurs in up to 1% of term newborns, with the incidence increasing to 3 to 9% of VLBW newborns (Bruschettini et al., 2016). In addition, pulmonary air leaks occur in significant numbers of mechanically ventilated newborns. The cause is postulated to be due to use of tidal volumes and peak inspiratory pressures greater than required by the neonate, pulmonary hypoplasia, and/or surfactant deficiency or inactivation. Vigilant continual assessment by the healthcare team is needed to prevent the overventilation or expansion.

Pneumothorax in the newborn causes several physiologic changes: Collapse of the lung, compression of the heart and lungs, compromise of venous return to the right heart with mediastinal air, and development of tension in the pleural space. Symptoms of pneumothorax include:

- Sudden, unexplained deterioration in the newborn's condition
- Decreased breath sounds
- Apnea
- Bradycardia
- Tachypnea
- Nasal flaring
- Grunting
- Palpable liver or spleen
- Cyanosis
- Increased oxygen requirements
- Higher PCO_2
- Decrease in pH
- Mottled, asymmetric chest expansion
- Decreased arterial blood pressure
- Shocklike appearance
- Shift of the apical cardiac impulses to the side opposite the pneumothorax, often with muffled heart sounds.

Transillumination of the chest is used for rapid evaluation of pneumothorax. However, x-ray examination is the main method of diagnosing this complication (Figure 31–9). Pneumothorax is a potentially life-threatening situation for the newborn who is hemodynamically unstable and may demand immediate removal

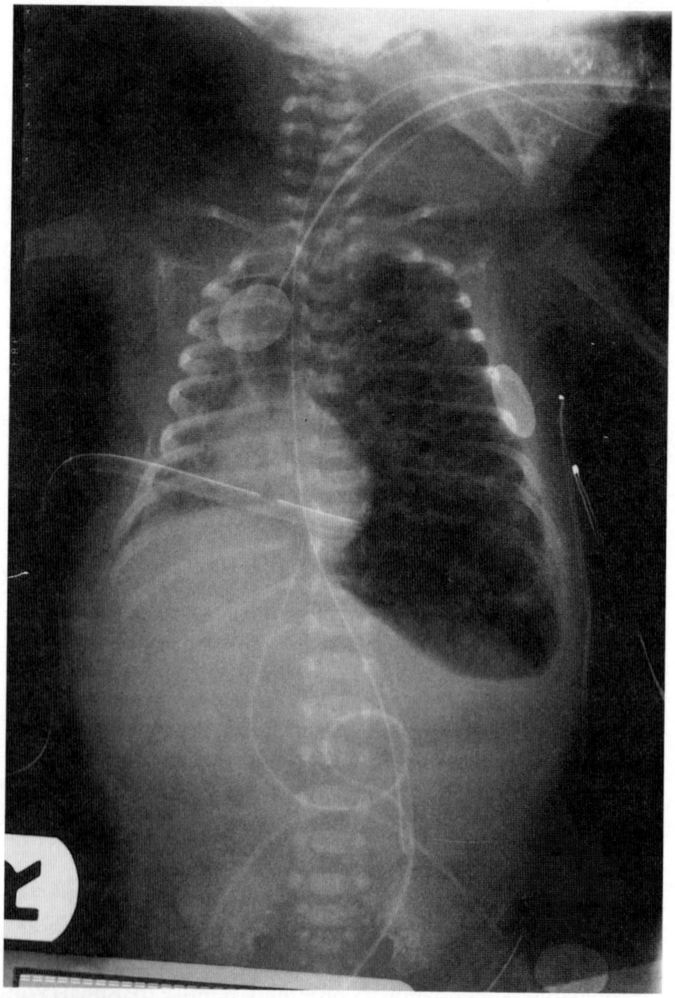

Figure 31–9 Chest X-ray of a left-sided pneumothorax. A rupture of the alveoli sacs allows air to leak through the pleura, forming collections of air outside the lung (air shows on X-ray as dark area over lung).

SOURCE: Carol Harrigan, RN, MSN, NNP-BC.

of the accumulated air with needle aspiration or possible placement of a chest tube. Only skilled and specifically trained personnel should perform a thoracentesis (pleural tap), which is usually done with a needle and syringe. A thoracostomy, or placement of a chest tube, may be necessary for continued air accumulation. For some pneumothorax that is not hemodynamically significant, time and close observation may be all that is warranted.

Bronchopulmonary Dysplasia/ Chronic Lung Disease

Bronchopulmonary dysplasia (BPD), also known as *chronic lung disease (CLD) of prematurity*, most commonly occurs in 23% of VLBW and 40% of ELBW newborns (Eichenwald et al., 2017). The majority of ELBW newborns and newborns with primary respiratory disease—such as neonatal pneumonia, meconium aspiration syndrome (MAS), persistent pulmonary hypertension (PPHN), or congenital heart disease (patent ductus arteriosus [PDA]) and other congenital anomalies—may require oxygen therapy with MV, which can cause a variety of injuries to the lung (Keszler & Sant'Anna, 2015).

BPD is now thought to occur from an inflammatory response to premature delivery before complete development of the fetal pulmonary architecture and tends to be worse in newborns not treated with antenatal steroids. Low-grade or asymptomatic pulmonary infection with *Ureaplasma urealyticum*, the microorganism frequently located in the amniotic fluid and pulmonary secretions after birth in the preterm newborn, are implicated in the development of BPD. A history of maternal chorioamnionitis or other infectious process is seen in many newborns who develop BPD (Keszler & Sant'Anna, 2015). In addition, literature documents the presence of inflammatory markers in the newborn who develops BPD, as evidenced by CRP elevation and inflammatory mediators in tracheal aspirates (Hascoët et al., 2016)

The definition of BPD is dependence on oxygen at or longer than 28 days of age following mechanical ventilation with subsequent x-ray changes and dependence on supplemental oxygen longer than 36 weeks corrected gestational age (Hascoët et al., 2016). The process of BPD is one of continuous lung tissue injury and repair, delaying both lung maturation and body growth. The continuum of degree of illness varies greatly with regard to mild to severe BPD. BPD or CLD is an important factor to consider as the baby grows, as this can set the child up for long-term pathology in the lungs even into adulthood (Balany & Bhandari, 2015).

CLINICAL THERAPY

The goals of therapeutic intervention for the newborn with BPD are to provide adequate oxygenation and ventilation, prevent further lung damage, promote optimal nutrition, and give supportive care to ensure adequate rates of growth and development. Because of the chronic nature of BPD, therapeutic intervention must be individualized to meet the specific needs of the newborn. Supplemental oxygen levels are adjusted to consistently keep O_2 saturations at a percentage between the low- and mid-90s, depending on associated clinical problems such as poor growth, recurrent bradycardia, and pulmonary hypertension. Diuretics and fluid restriction are frequently used to control pulmonary fluid retention and to improve lung function; electrolyte supplements are necessary to offset the results of chronic diuretics. In addition, bronchodilators are indicated to decrease airway resistance and to control bronchospasm. The baby with chronic lung disease is often on long-term steroids, sometimes even through childhood. Serial echocardiography is used to monitor cardiac response to the chronic pulmonary disease.

●○● NURSING MANAGEMENT

For the Newborn with Complications Due to Respiratory Therapy

Hospital-Based Nursing Care

Carefully observe for any changes in the newborn's oxygenation, giving special attention to maintaining the prescribed oxygen concentration, based on clinical assessments and pulse oximetry parameters, during all activities, especially during periods of stress such as when the baby is crying, care times, when blood is drawn, while starting an IV infusion, suctioning, chest physiotherapy (CPT), and even feeding.

Obtain blood gases based on the institution's chronic blood gas protocol—for example, every 3 days, 20 minutes after a permanent change in ambient oxygen concentration (FiO_2), or more frequently if the newborn experiences increasing respiratory distress or increasing lethargy. Maintain the baby's body temperature because hypothermia or hyperthermia will increase oxygen consumption and may increase oxygen requirements. Bronchodilators such as albuterol, diuretics, steroids, and electrolyte supplements may be used in the clinical management of the BPD newborn. Many of the side effects of these drugs, such as hypokalemia and mineral losses (fractures), can be avoided by giving the diuretics every other day.

Providing for adequate nutrition enhances growth and formation of new alveoli and enlargement of the airway diameter. The more severely ill the newborn is, the more difficulty the baby will have with feedings, and therefore a higher caloric need will exist to meet the greater expenditure of energy for survival and healing. As soon as tolerated, a 24 kcal/oz formula or fortified breast milk for preterm newborns is started, especially if the baby is on fluid restriction. More oxygen may be required during feeding, and the least energy-consuming feeding method should be used (Figure 31–10). If the feeding schedule is too stressful, smaller, more frequent feedings may be initiated.

A newborn with BPD is very susceptible to infection, especially if on long-term steroids; therefore, it is important to discourage anyone with early signs of infectious disease from having contact with the neonate. Monitor the baby's behavior and vital signs for changes that might indicate early-developing

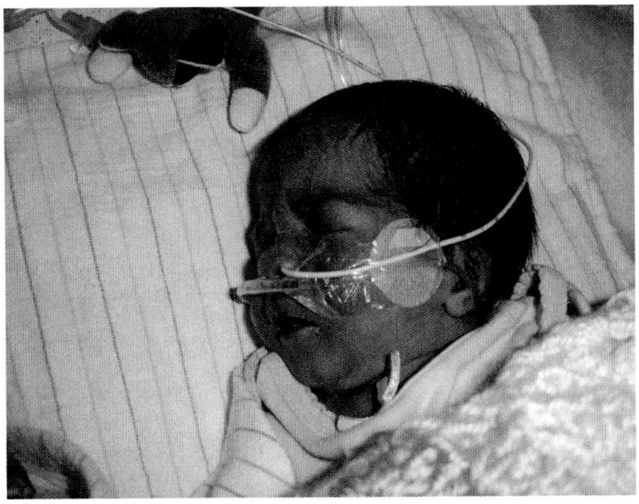

Figure 31–10 **A baby with BPD requires oxygen at greater than 36 weeks' gestational age. She still needs to be fed through a nasogastric tube because she tires with nipple feeds.**

infection. Note and report any changes in color, quantity, or quality of pulmonary secretions. The frequency of CPT and suctioning may need to be increased.

When the newborn develops BPD and the family members become aware of the implications of chronic illness and prolonged hospitalization, they may experience despair and find it difficult to cope with this added burden. Help family members cope by involving them in the plan of care and encouraging them to take an active role in their baby's daily activities. Their involvement will help dispel feelings of inadequacy and prepare them to perform the unique tasks necessary to meet their baby's needs. Continued use of a collaborative healthcare team—usually including counseling, occupational and physical therapies, a home health nurse, a respiratory caregiver, as well as the primary care provider—can aid in optimizing outcomes for the newborn and the family.

Parents need to demonstrate their ability to provide all the care their child will require at home before leaving the hospital. This may include feeding, adjusting O_2 support, O_2 saturation monitoring, suctioning and airway management, CPT, bathing, and giving medications. They also need to know when to call the home health nurse who is providing care. Teach parents how to assess the newborn's respiratory condition and understand the BPD baseline respiratory pattern (frequency of respiration, rhythm, degree of retractions, and color of skin and mucous membranes). Illness limits the tolerance level for activity, and parents must be taught to evaluate their newborn's tolerance of activities and to recognize signs of distress due to poor oxygenation, inadequate ventilation, infection, fluid retention, and bronchospasm. Give special attention to formulating a program of early stimulation activities because psychomotor delays are frequently seen.

Care of the Newborn with Cold Stress

Cold stress occurs when newborns lose more heat than their bodies can produce. Excessive heat loss in newborns causes them to utilize stores of energy to compensate and attempt to maintain core temperatures in the normal range. Newborns utilize nonshivering thermogenesis (NST) and brown fat to compensate for hypothermia. Heat loss that results in cold stress occurs in the newborn through the mechanisms of evaporation, convection, conduction, and radiation. (See Chapter 26 for a detailed discussion of thermoregulation.) Heat loss at birth that leads to cold stress can play a significant role in the severity of RDS and the ultimate outcome for the newborn. Moderate hypothermia, 32° to 35.9°C (89.6° to 96.6°F), is also implicated in intraventricular hemorrhage and higher mortality (Lyu et al., 2015). Preterm and growth-restricted newborns are at increased risk for cold stress because they have decreased adipose tissue, brown fat stores, and glycogen available for metabolism.

As discussed in Chapter 26, the newborn's major source of heat production in NST is brown fat metabolism. The ability of a newborn to respond to cold stress by NST is impaired in the presence of several conditions:

- Hypoxemia (PO_2 less than 50 torr)
- Intracranial hemorrhage or any CNS abnormality
- Hypoglycemia (blood glucose less than 45 mg/dL) (AAP & ACOG, 2017).

When these conditions occur, the newborn's temperature should be monitored more closely and the neutral thermal environment conscientiously maintained with ambient feedback tools such as an isolette or radiant warmer. The nurse must recognize these conditions and treat them as soon as possible. The metabolic consequences of cold stress, caused by activation of the sympathetic nervous system, can be devastating and potentially fatal to a newborn. Oxygen requirements increase; even before noting a change in body temperature, glucose use increases; acids are released into the bloodstream; cardiac output is decreased, which can have an effect on pulmonary blood flow and therefore PPHN; and surfactant production decreases. The effects are graphically depicted in Figure 31–11.

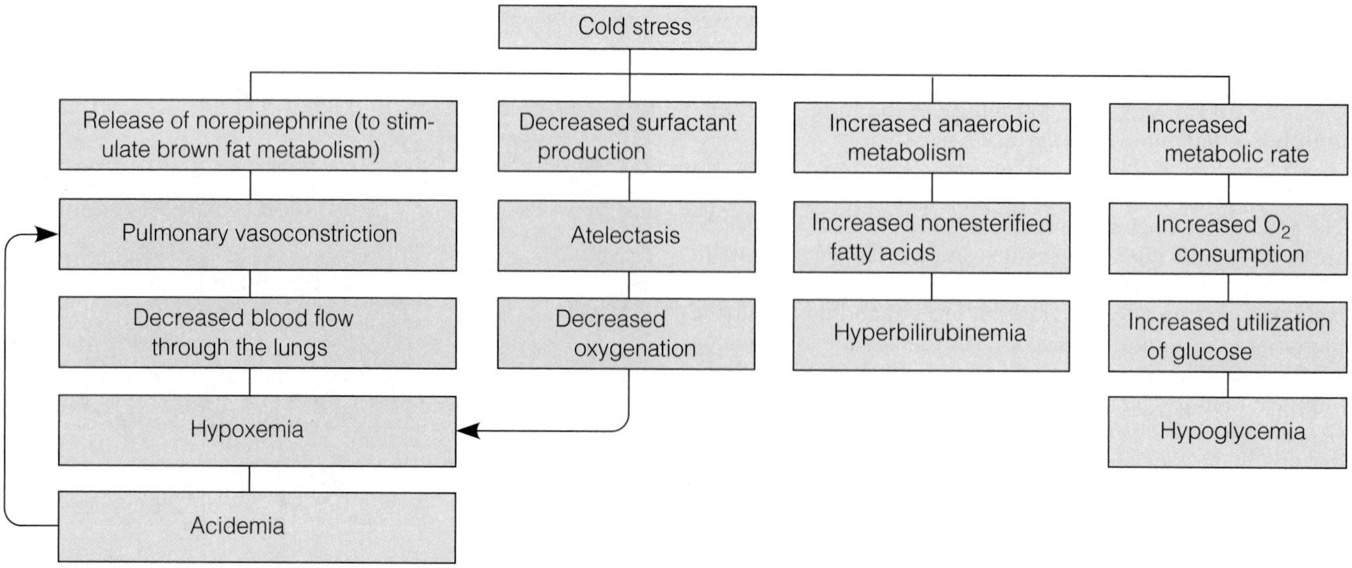

Figure 31–11 Cold stress chain of events. The hypothermic, or cold-stressed, newborn attempts to compensate by conserving heat and increasing heat production. These physiologic compensatory mechanisms initiate a series of metabolic events that result in hypoxemia and altered surfactant production, metabolic acidosis, hypoglycemia, and hyperbilirubinemia.

●○● NURSING MANAGEMENT

For the Newborn with Cold Stress

The amount of heat lost by a newborn depends to a large extent on the actions of the nurse or caregiver. Prevention of hypothermia is especially critical in the VLBW or ELBW newborn. Placing the VLBW or ELBW newborn in a polyethylene wrapping or the use of a chemically activated warming mattress immediately following birth can decrease the postnatal fall in temperature that normally occurs (AAP & ACOG, 2017). Convective, radiant, and evaporative heat loss can all be reduced by utilizing skin-to-skin care when able, polyethylene wraps and/or swaddling, non-cotton-lined hats, and warming the delivery room to the recommended 23° to 25°C (74° to 77°F) (AAP & ACOG, 2017; Vali et al., 2015). Swaddling and nesting maintain flexion, which reduces exposed surface area and thus convective and radiant losses.

Observe the newborn for signs of cold stress. These include increased movements and respirations, decreased skin temperature and peripheral perfusion, development of hypoglycemia, and, possibly, development of metabolic acidosis. Vasoconstriction is the initial response to cold stress; because it initially decreases skin temperature, monitor and assess skin temperature instead of rectal temperature. By monitoring skin temperature, a possible decrease in temperature will become apparent before the newborn's core temperature is affected.

When a decrease in skin temperature is noted, determine whether hypoglycemia is present. Hypoglycemia is a result of the metabolic effects of cold stress and is suggested by glucometer values below 40–50 mg/dL, tremors, irritability or lethargy, apnea, or seizure activity. (Treatment of hypoglycemia is discussed in the next section.)

Many interventions are done to prevent a newborn from experiencing hypothermia, but if it occurs, these nursing interventions should be initiated:

- Warm the newborn slowly because rapid temperature elevation may cause hypotension, cerebral hemorrhage, seizures, and apnea. Goal for rewarming is to increase the baby's temperature by 0.5°C (0.9°F) per hour.
- Increase the air temperature in hourly increments of 0.5°C (0.9°F) if on a radiant warmer or in an isolette until the newborn's temperature is normal.
- Monitor temperature every 15 to 30 minutes to determine whether the newborn's temperature is increasing, assessing the temperature with the use of a skin probe attached to the baby and axillary measurement (most commonly utilized method). Continue to follow the baby's temperature until it is stable for 1 hour.
- Remove plastic wrap, caps, and heat shields while rewarming the newborn so that cool air as well as warm air is not trapped.
- Warm IV fluids before infusion and warm oxygen sources to which the newborn is connected.
- Once the newborn is rewarmed, continue efforts to block heat loss by evaporation, radiation, convection, and conduction. Maintain the newborn in a neutral thermal environment (NTE), which is the temperature range at which heat production is at the minimum needed to maintain normal body temperature.

Attempts to burn brown fat increase oxygen consumption, lactic acid levels, and metabolic acidosis. Assess and treat any metabolic acidosis.

Care of the Newborn with Hypoglycemia

Hypoglycemia, or low blood sugar, in the neonate may cause long-term poor developmental outcomes ranging from learning disabilities to cerebral palsy, recurrent seizure disorders, and intellectual disability. The incidence is dependent on the pathophysiology of cause. A threshold for intervention in newborn hypoglycemia is a plasma glucose concentration of less than 45 to 47 mg/dL at any time in any newborn (Adamkin, 2017). Within the first hours to days of life, normal asymptomatic newborns may have a transient glucose level that will increase either spontaneously with gluconeogenesis, glycogenolysis, ketogenesis, or external support with feedings or IV fluids (Stanley et al., 2015). Plasma glucose values less than 20 to 25 mg/dL should be treated with parenteral glucose $D_{10}W$, regardless of the age or gestation, to raise plasma glucose to greater than 45 mg/dL. There is no absolute threshold that can be applied to all babies; a level of 45 mg/dL may be normal for one newborn and another may show symptoms of hypoglycemia at that level. Glucose concentrations must be looked at in conjunction with risk assessment and clinical manifestations. Newborns who show symptoms at any level should have intervention. Obtaining follow-up glucose measurement to document normal values after intervention is imperative (AAP & ACOG, 2017).

Hypoglycemia screening should occur in the following populations at most risk (Adamkin, 2017):

- Symptomatic newborn
- Newborns of mothers with diabetes
- LGA newborn
- SGA or IUGR newborns
- Neonates born with perinatal stress (e.g., MAS, polycythemia, hypothermia, birth asphyxia, cesarean birth for fetal distress, preterm, postmature, or born to mothers with preeclampsia or hypertension).

The pathophysiology of hypoglycemia differs for each underlying etiology. Preterm newborns have not been in utero a sufficient time to store glycogen and fat. As a result, they have a decreased ability to carry out gluconeogenesis. This situation is further aggravated by increased use of glucose by the tissues (especially the brain and heart) during stress and illness (hypothermia, asphyxia, sepsis, and RDS). See *Genetic Facts: Genetic Involvement in Hypoglycemia*.

Genetic Facts Genetic Involvement in Hypoglycemia

Babies who have hypoglycemia due to hyperinsulinemia (often newborns of mothers with diabetes) may have mutations of the pancreatic beta-cells in the ATP-sensitive potassium channel genes. In addition, an increase in insulin can be seen with loss of function of the *HNF4A* gene (Eichenwald et al., 2017).

Newborns of White's classifications A through C or type 1 diabetic mothers (women with diagnosed or gestational diabetes) have increased stores of glycogen and fat (see Chapters 17 and 30 for more information on mothers with diabetes and their newborns). Circulating insulin and insulin responsiveness are also higher when compared with other newborns. Because the high glucose loads present in utero stop at birth, and the newborn continues to produce high levels of insulin from its pancreatic beta cells, the newborn experiences rapid and profound hypoglycemia that can last for several days to a week (Adamkin, 2017).

The SGA newborn has used up glycogen and fat stores because of intrauterine malnutrition and has a blunted hepatic enzymatic response with which to produce and use glucose. Any newborn stressed at birth from asphyxia or cold also quickly uses up available glucose stores and becomes hypoglycemic.

CLINICAL THERAPY

The goal of medical management includes early identification of hypoglycemia through observation and screening of newborns at risk (Adamkin, 2017). The baby may be asymptomatic, or any of these symptoms of hypoglycemia may occur:

- Lethargy, sleepiness, and limpness
- Poor feeding, poor/inadequate sucking reflex, vomiting
- Hypothermia or temperature instability
- Pallor, cyanosis
- Apnea, irregular respirations, respiratory distress, cyanosis, tachypnea
- Hypotonia, possible loss of swallowing reflex
- Tremors, jerkiness, jitteriness, seizure activity, irritability, eye rolling
- High-pitched cry (Eichenwald et al., 2017)
- Exaggerated Moro reflex
- Temperature instability.

Universal blood glucose screening before clinical signs develop is not recommended by the AAP (Adamkin, 2017). Aggressive treatment is recommended after a single low blood glucose value if the newborn shows any of the symptoms of hypoglycemia. At-risk newborns should be fed by 1 hour of age and screened 30 minutes after feeding. In at-risk newborns, routine screening should be done frequently during the first hours of life and then whenever any of the noted clinical manifestations appears or at 1- to 4-hour intervals until the risk period has passed. Screening criteria will vary depending on at-risk category; the nurse should check agency protocol. Several blood glucose results should be obtained before or after feedings and during fasting (Adamkin, 2017).

Symptomatic newborns with recurrent episodes of hypoglycemia may have long-term neurologic deficits on the continuum from learning disabilities to recurrent seizure disorders to intellectual disability (AAP & ACOG, 2017).

Blood glucose sampling techniques can significantly affect the accuracy of the blood glucose value. Point of care (POC) glucose testing meters were developed for the adult population and correlate nicely when the newborn is normoglycemic or at a level greater than 70. A newborn is considered by most to be hypoglycemic at 47 or less. At these levels, POC devices provide estimates at best and typically vary by 10 to 15 mL/dL from serum samples run in the laboratory (Eichenwald et al., 2017). Often the population at risk is polycythemic, and elevated hematocrit (HCT) can interfere with accuracy as well. Treatment of the newborn in response to the low glucose reading from the POC device should not be delayed while waiting for the serum lab sample value (AAP & ACOG, 2017). See *Clinical Skill 31–1: Performing a Heelstick on a Newborn.*

Clinical Tip

Venous blood samples for the laboratory should be placed on ice and analyzed within 30 minutes of drawing to prevent the red blood cells (RBCs) from continuing to metabolize glucose and giving a falsely low reading. Avoid transporting the blood in tubes containing a glycolytic inhibitor such as fluoride. Transport blood samples on ice and analyze quickly (Eichenwald et al., 2017).

Adequate caloric intake is important. Early breastfeeding or formula-feeding is one of the major preventive approaches. If early feeding or IV glucose is started to meet the recommended fluid and caloric needs, the blood glucose is likely to remain above the hypoglycemic level. During the first hours after birth, asymptomatic newborns may be given oral glucose contained in formula or breast milk (glucose water should not be used because it causes a rapid increase in glucose followed by an abrupt decrease), and then another plasma glucose measurement is obtained within 30 to 60 minutes after feeding.

IV infusions of a dextrose solution D_5W to $D_{10}W$ (5 to 10%) begun immediately after birth in the at-risk newborn should prevent hypoglycemia. Plasma glucose levels are obtained when the parenteral infusion is started. However, in the SGA or VLBW newborn, infusions of 10% dextrose solution may cause hyperglycemia to develop, requiring an alteration in the glucose concentration. Any IV glucose solution, as with other medications in the neonate, should be calculated based on body weight of the baby in mg/kg/min and fluid requirements in ml/kg/day and correlated with blood glucose tests to determine adequacy of the infusion treatment (AAP & ACOG, 2017)

In more severe cases of hypoglycemia, glucagon (rarely used), drugs (such as diazoxide or octeotide), or corticosteroids may be administered (Eichenwald et al., 2017). Insulin and cortisol levels in addition to a few other hormone levels, such as beta hydroxybuterate and growth hormone, can be drawn with serum glucose levels to assist in the proper etiology of the hypoglycemia. This is usually done if hypoglycemia persists past the 24- to 48-hour mark or if the glucose demands appear out of proportion to presumed etiology. Some institutions may use steroids, which seem to enhance gluconeogenesis from noncarbohydrate protein sources and can be helpful if cortisol levels are low (Eichenwald et al., 2017). Additionally, promising research is emerging on glucose gels in the assistance of treating hypoglycemia in the neonate (Makker et al., 2018).

●○● NURSING MANAGEMENT

For the Newborn with Hypoglycemia

Nursing Assessment and Diagnosis

The objective of nursing assessment is to identify newborns at risk and to screen symptomatic newborns. For newborns diagnosed with hypoglycemia, assessment is ongoing with careful monitoring of glucose values. Glucose strips, urine electrolytes, and urine volume (monitor only if above 1 to 3 mL/kg/hr) are evaluated frequently for osmotic diuresis and glycosuria.

Nursing diagnoses that may apply to the newborn with hypoglycemia include:

- ***Nutrition, Imbalanced: Less Than Body Requirements***, related to increased glucose use secondary to physiologic stress
- ***Breathing Pattern, Ineffective***, related to tachypnea and apnea
- ***Pain, Acute***, related to frequent heelsticks for glucose monitoring

Clinical Skill 31–1

Performing a Heelstick on a Newborn

NURSING ACTION

Preparation

- Explain to parents what will be done.
- Select a clear, previously unpunctured site.

  Rationale: *The selection of a previously unpunctured site minimizes the risk of infection and excessive scar formation.*
- The newborn's lateral heel is the site of choice because it precludes damaging the posterior tibial nerve and artery, the plantar artery, and the important longitudinally oriented fat pad of the heel, which in later years could impede walking (Figure 31–12). This is especially important for babies undergoing multiple heelstick procedures.

Equipment and Supplies

- Microlancet (do not use a needle)
- Alcohol swabs or other skin prep per agency protocol
- 2 × 2 sterile gauze squares
- Small bandage (may not use on premature newborn with extremely sensitive skin; instead, hold pressure until bleeding ceases)
- Glucose reagent strips or reflectance meters
- Gloves

Procedure: Clean Gloves

1. Apply gloves.

   Rationale: *A needle may nick the periosteum. Gloves are used to implement standard precautions and prevent nosocomial infections.*
2. Warming the baby's heel is typically performed by commercially available chemical warmer for controlled warming. Check agency policy.

Performing the Heelstick

1. Grasp the newborn's foot in your nondominant hand so as to impede venous return slightly. Support the dorsum of the foot with your thumb and the ankle with your other fingers. This will facilitate extraction of the blood sample (Figure 31–13).
2. Clean the site by rubbing vigorously with 70% isopropyl alcohol swab or skin prep per agency.

   Rationale: *Friction produces local heat, which aids vasodilation.*
3. Blot the site dry completely with a dry sterile gauze square before lancing.

   Rationale: *Alcohol is irritating to injured tissue and it may also produce hemolysis, as well as cause a false low reading.*
4. With a quick, piercing motion, puncture the lateral heel with a microlancet. Be careful not to puncture too deeply. Optimal penetration is 4 mm.
5. Wipe the first drop of blood away with the gauze.

   Rationale: *The first drop may be contaminated by skin contact and the blood cells may have been traumatized during the stick. Blood glucose may be lowered by residual alcohol.*

Collecting the Blood Sample

1. Place a drop of blood on glucose reflectance meter or directly onto the Glucometer test strip.

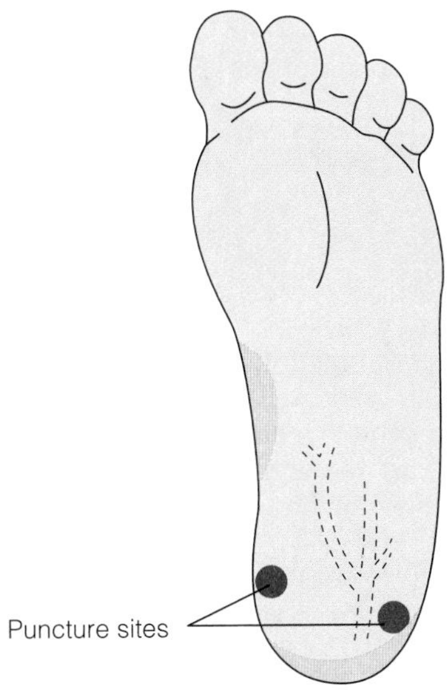

Figure 31–12 Potential sites for heelsticks. Avoid shaded areas to prevent injury to arteries and nerves in the foot and the important longitudinally oriented fat pad of the heel, which in later years could impede walking.

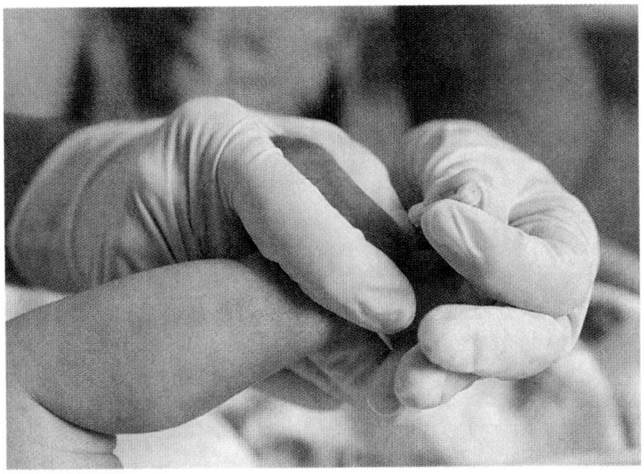

Figure 31–13 Heelstick. With a quick, piercing motion, puncture the lateral heel with a microlancet. Be careful not to puncture too deeply.

(continued)

Clinical Skill 31–1 *(continued)*

2. Use appropriate capillary tubes for hematocrit alternative testing, if ordered.

Preventing Excessive Bleeding

1. Apply a folded gauze square to the puncture site and secure it firmly with a bandage, or hold pressure until bleeding stops.
2. Check the puncture site frequently for the first hour after sampling.

Documentation: Record the lab values and the intervention in the newborn's electronic health record.

- *Coping: Family, Compromised,* related to need for nursery admission secondary to hypoglycemia
- *Parenting, Risk for Impaired,* related to deficient knowledge of newborn care and prolonged separation of baby and parents secondary to illness

(NANDA-I © 2017)

Nursing Plan and Implementation

Monitor all at-risk groups within 30 to 60 minutes after birth and before feedings or whenever there are abnormal signs. Once an at-risk newborn's blood sugar level is stable, glucose testing every 2 to 4 hours (or per agency protocol), or before feedings, adequately monitors glucose levels. Refer to *Clinical Skill 31–1: Performing a Heelstick on a Newborn*. See *Complementary Health Approaches: Pain Relief in the NICU.*

The method of feeding greatly influences glucose and energy requirements; thus, carefully calculating glucose requirements and attention to glucose monitoring is required during the transition from IV to oral feedings. Titration of IV glucose may be required until the newborn is able to take adequate amounts of formula or breast milk to maintain a normal blood sugar level. Titrate by decreasing the concentration of parenteral glucose gradually to 10% ($D_{10}W$), and then reducing the rate of infusion (mg/kg/min), and slowly discontinuing it as preprandial glucoses are sampled. At-risk asymptomatic newborns should be fed every 2 to 3 hours and screened before feeding. Target goal is plasma glucose greater than or equal to 45 mg per dL before feeding (AAP & ACOG, 2017). Enteral feeds are increased to maintain an adequate glucose and caloric intake and maintain normal blood glucose levels. Titration of breastfeeding versus bottle-feeding may need to occur as well, as measured amounts are not available.

Care of the Newborn with Jaundice

The most common abnormal physical finding in newborns is jaundice (*icterus neonatorum*). Some degree of newborn jaundice, resulting from elevated unconjugated bilirubinemia, with total serum bilirubin levels greater than 6 to 9 mg/dL, occurs in up to 80% of healthy newborns in the first 7 days following birth (Flaherman, Maisels, & Academy of Breastfeeding Medicine, 2017). **Jaundice** is a yellowish coloration of the skin and sclera of the eyes that develops from the deposit of yellow pigment bilirubin in lipid/fat-containing tissues, as described in Chapter 26. Fetal unconjugated bilirubin is normally cleared by the placenta in utero, so total bilirubin at birth is usually less than 3 mg/L unless an abnormal hemolytic process has been present. Postnatally, the

Complementary Health Approaches

Pain Relief in the NICU

The newborn relies on the nurse's observational, assessment, and interventional skills for prompt, safe, and effective pain relief. It is vital that the nurse assist newborns to cope with and recover from necessary painful clinical procedures. A variety of nonpharmacologic pain prevention and relief techniques have been shown to be effective in reducing pain from minor procedures in newborns.

Any unnecessary stimuli (i.e., noise, visual, tactile, and vestibular) of the newborn should be avoided, if possible. Developmental care—which includes limiting environmental stimuli, developmental appropriate positioning, skin-to-skin care, the use of supportive bedding, swaddling, nonnutritive sucking (NNS), and attention to behavioral cues—assists the newborn to cope with painful procedures (AAP & ACOG, 2017; Marko & Dickerson, 2017).

Containment with swaddling or facilitated tucking (holding the arms and legs in a flexed position) is effective in reducing excessive immature motor responses. Swaddling also may provide comfort through other senses, such as thermal, tactile, and proprioceptive senses. Breastfeeding and skin-to-skin contact/kangaroo care with the mother during the painful procedure may help to relieve pain (Marko & Dickerson, 2017).

NNS refers to the provision of a pacifier into the newborn's mouth to promote sucking without the provision of breast milk or formula for nutrition. NNS is thought to produce analgesia through stimulation of orotactile and mechanoreceptors when the pacifier is placed into the baby's mouth. Allowing NNS with a pacifier aids in the reduction of procedural pain and stress (Marko & Dickerson, 2017).

A wide range of oral sucrose doses has been used for procedural pain relief (heelsticks, venipuncture, IM injections), and while no optimal dose has been established, a solution of 24% sucrose solution is agreed upon (AAP, 2016). The sweetness of the sucrose, a disaccharide, elevates the pain threshold through endogenous opioid release in the CNS and produces a calming effect (AAP, 2016).

newborn must conjugate bilirubin (convert a lipid-soluble pigment into a water-soluble pigment that can be excreted) in the liver.

The rate and amount of conjugation of bilirubin depend on the rate of hemolysis, the bilirubin load, the maturity of the liver, and the presence of albumin-binding sites. See Chapter 26 for discussion of conjugation of bilirubin. A normal, healthy, full-term newborn's liver is usually mature enough and produces enough glucuronyl transferase that the total serum bilirubin concentration does not reach a pathologic level. The diagnosis of *pathologic jaundice* is given to newborns who exhibit jaundice within the first 24 hours of life, have a total serum bilirubin concentration increase of greater than 0.2 mg/dL/hour, surpass the 95th percentile on the nomogram of bilirubin risk for age in hours, or have persistent visible jaundice after 2 weeks of age in term newborns (Eichenwald et al., 2017).

Physiologic Jaundice

Physiologic or *neonatal jaundice* is a normal process that occurs during transition from intrauterine to extrauterine life and appears after 24 hours of life. This form of jaundice is typically due to the newborn's increased red cell mass, shorter red cell lifespan (90 days as compared with 120 days in the adult), slower uptake of bilirubin by the liver, lack of intestinal bacteria, and/or poorly established hydration from initial breastfeeding, coupled with decreased stooling. Total bilirubin levels peak in a full-term newborn around 3 to 5 days after birth, usually after discharge from the hospital (Eichenwald et al., 2017).

The pattern of physiologic jaundice differs between breastfed and formula-fed newborns. (For further discussion of physiologic jaundice, see Chapter 26.) Physiologic jaundice remains a common problem for the term newborn and may require treatment with phototherapy.

Pathophysiology of Hyperbilirubinemia

Hyperbilirubinemia is a condition in which the total serum bilirubin level in the blood is increased. Serum albumin-binding sites are usually able to conjugate enough bilirubin to meet the demands of the normal newborn. However, certain conditions tend to decrease the number or quality of available binding sites. Fetal or neonatal asphyxia and neonatal drugs such as indomethacin decrease the binding affinity of bilirubin to albumin because acidosis impairs the capacity of albumin to hold bilirubin. Hypothermia and hypoglycemia release free fatty acids (FFAs) that dislocate bilirubin from albumin. Maternal use of sulfa drugs and salicylates interferes with conjugation or with serum albumin-binding sites by competing with bilirubin for these sites. Finally, premature newborns have less albumin available for binding with bilirubin. Neurotoxicity is possible because unconjugated bilirubin has a high affinity for extravascular tissue, such as fatty tissue (subcutaneous tissue) and cerebral tissue.

Bilirubin not bound to albumin, unconjugated, is free to cross the blood–brain barrier, damaging cells of the CNS. Toxicity involves deposition of unconjugated bilirubin in the cells of the brainstem and basal ganglia (i.e., bilirubin-induced neurologic damage [BIND]). BIND is called *kernicterus* when seen at autopsy (AAP & ACOG, 2017; Eichenwald et al., 2017). The main host protection against BIND is extracellular albumin.

The classic bilirubin encephalopathy most commonly found with Rh and ABO blood group incompatibility is less common today because of aggressive treatment with phototherapy and exchange transfusions (described later in this section). With the early discharge of newborns, there is an increased concern for developing bilirubin encephalopathy due to dehydration (a result of discharge before mother's milk is established when breastfeeding). Unfortunately, current therapy cannot distinguish all newborns who are at risk. It is recommended that *all* newborns be screened for bilirubin level prior to leaving the hospital using either total serum bilirubin (TSB) or transcutaneous bilirubin (TcB) (Eichenwald et al., 2017). See *Genetic Facts: Genetic Variations and Jaundice.*

Genetic Facts Genetic Variations and Jaundice

Newborns of East Asian descent (Japanese, Chinese, and Filipino ethnic groups) have a higher occurrence of hyperbilirubinemia than Caucasian newborns. Other ethnic groups at risk for increased neonatal bilirubinemia are Navajo, Eskimo, and Sioux Native American; Greek; Sephardic-Jewish; and some Hispanic groups. The incidence is lower in African Americans (Gomella, 2013).

Causes of Hyperbilirubinemia

A primary cause of pathologic hyperbilirubinemia is **hemolytic disease of the newborn**. All pregnant women who are Rh negative or who have blood type O (possible ABO incompatibility) should be asked about outcomes of any previous pregnancies, including abortions, and history of blood transfusion. Prenatal amniocentesis with spectrophotographic examination may be indicated in some cases. Cord blood from newborns is evaluated for bilirubin level, which normally does not exceed 5 mg/dL. Newborns of Rh-negative and O blood type mothers are carefully assessed for blood type status, appearance of jaundice, and levels of serum bilirubin.

Erythroblastosis fetalis, also known as *alloimmune hemolytic disease*, occurs when an Rh-negative mother is pregnant with an Rh-positive fetus and maternal antibodies cross the placenta. Maternal antibodies enter the fetal circulation, then attach to and destroy the fetal RBCs. The fetal system responds by increasing RBC production. Jaundice, anemia, and compensatory erythropoiesis result. A marked increase in immature RBCs (erythroblasts) also occurs, hence the designation erythroblastosis fetalis. Because of the widespread use of Rh immune globulin (RhoGAM), also called *anti-D*, the incidence of erythroblastosis fetalis has dropped dramatically.

Hydrops fetalis, the most severe form of erythroblastosis fetalis, occurs when maternal antibodies attach to the Rh site on the fetal RBCs, making them susceptible to destruction; severe anemia and multiple organ system failure result. Cardiomegaly with severe cardiac decompensation (heart failure) and *hepatosplenomegaly* (simultaneous enlargement of both the liver and the spleen) occur. Severe generalized massive edema (anasarca) and generalized fluid effusion into the pleural cavity (hydrothorax), pericardial sac, and peritoneal cavity (ascites) develop. Jaundice is not present until the newborn period because the bilirubin pigments for the fetus are being excreted through the placenta into the maternal circulation. The hydropic hemolytic disease process is also characterized by hyperplasia of the adrenal cortex and pancreatic islets, which predisposes the newborn to neonatal hypoglycemia similar to that of babies of mothers with diabetes. These newborns also have increased bleeding tendencies due to associated thrombocytopenia and hypoxic damage to the capillaries. Hydrops is a frequent cause of intrauterine death among fetuses with Rh disease.

ABO incompatibility (the mother is blood type O and the baby is blood type A or B) may result in jaundice, although it rarely results in hemolytic disease severe enough to be clinically diagnosed and treated. Hepatosplenomegaly may be found occasionally in newborns with ABO incompatibility, but hydrops fetalis and stillbirth are rare.

During pregnancy, predisposing maternal conditions include hereditary spherocytosis, diabetes, intrauterine infections, Gram-negative bacilli infections that stimulate production of maternal alloimmune antibodies, drug ingestion (such as sulfas, salicylates, novobiocin, and diazepam), and oxytocin administration. Early prenatal identification of the fetus at risk for Rh or ABO incompatibility allows prompt treatment. (See Chapter 18 for discussion of in utero management of this condition.) Table 31–4 presents risk factors for development of severe hyperbilirubinemia.

The prognosis for a newborn with hyperbilirubinemia depends on the extent of the hemolytic process and the underlying cause. Severe hemolytic disease may result in fetal or early neonatal death from the effects of anemia—cardiac decompensation, edema, ascites, and hydrothorax. Hyperbilirubinemia may lead to kernicterus if not aggressively treated. Continuing worsening progression includes neurologic damage, which may cause death, cerebral palsy, cognitive impairment, or hearing loss/nerve deafness, or, to a lesser degree, perceptual impairment, delayed speech development, hyperactivity, muscle incoordination, or learning difficulties (Kamath-Rayne, Thio, Deacon, et al., 2016).

LABORATORY AND DIAGNOSTIC ASSESSMENTS

When one or more of the predisposing factors or the appearance of early jaundice is present, the maternal and neonatal blood should be tested in the laboratory for blood type and antibodies, and a direct antiglobulin test (DAT) performed. Other necessary laboratory evaluations include Coombs test, serum bilirubin levels (direct and total), hemoglobin, reticulocyte percentage, white blood cell count, and positive smear for cellular morphology.

Neonatal hyperbilirubinemia must be considered pathologic if any of these criteria are met:

- Clinically evident jaundice appearing before 24 hours of life or if jaundice seems excessive for the newborn's age in hours
- TSB concentration or TcB rising by more than 0.2 mg/dL per hour
- Symptoms of primary illness
- Elevation of TB that requires phototherapy based on management algorithm

TABLE 31–4 Risk Factors for Development of Severe Hyperbilirubinemia in Newborns of 35 or More Weeks' Gestation*

Major Risk Factors

- Predischarge TSB or TcB level in the high-risk or high intermediate zone
- Jaundice observed in the first 24 hours after birth
- Blood group incompatibility with positive direct antiglobulin test, other known hemolytic disease (e.g., glucose-6-phosphate dehydrogenase [G6PD] deficiency), elevated $ETCO_2$ (end-tidal carbon dioxide level)
- Gestational age 35–36 weeks (late preterm gestational age)
- Previous sibling received phototherapy
- Cephalohematoma/significant bruising
- Unrecognized hemolysis such as ABO blood type incompatibility or Rh incompatibility
- Infection
- Exclusive breastfeeding, particularly if nursing is not going well and excessive weight loss is experienced
- East Asian or Mediterranean heritage**

Minor Risk Factors

- Predischarge TSB or TcB level in the high intermediate risk zone
- Gestational age 37–38 weeks
- Jaundice observed before discharge
- Previous sibling with jaundice
- Macrosomic baby of a mother with diabetes
- Maternal age equal to or greater than 25 years
- Male gender

Decreased Risk

(These factors are associated with decreased risk of significant jaundice, listed in order of decreasing importance.)

- TSB or TcB level in the low-risk zone
- Gestational age greater than or equal to 41 weeks
- Exclusive bottle-feeding
- African heritage**
- Discharge from hospital after 72 hours

* In approximate order of importance.

** Heritage as defined by mother's description.

SOURCES: Data from American Academy of Pediatrics, Subcommittee on Hyperbilirubinemia, 2004, Table 2, p. 301; Bhutani & Committee on the Fetus and Newborn, 2011.

- Clinical jaundice persisting for more than 14 days in a term newborn (Eichenwald et al., 2017).

Initial diagnostic procedures are aimed at differentiating jaundice resulting from increased bilirubin production, impaired conjugation or excretion, increased intestinal reabsorption, or a combination of these factors.

TcB measurements are a noninvasive method of assessing bilirubin levels and may be used for risk assessment (Figure 31–14). A TcB can be performed quickly and painlessly, and repeated measures are easily obtained. TcB can quantify the amount of bilirubin pigment in the newborn's skin. Nurses need to measure bilirubin levels to confirm the presence, absence, or suspicion of jaundice. However, it is important to remember that total serum bilirubin levels remain the standard of care for confirmation or diagnosis of hyperbilirubinemia (AAP & ACOG, 2017).

Because of the shorter lifespan of red blood cells in the newborn, a significant bilirubin load is produced. When bilirubin breaks down, carbon monoxide (CO) is released. This production of carbon monoxide is being investigated as a marker in the study of bilirubin production.

Clinical Tip

Risk zone and phototherapy nomograms are available from the AAP, and the bedside RN has the ability to calculate the number of hours of age of the newborn and plot on these nomograms. The time to the next sample needed is a part of this AAP statement as well. Risk factors as previously described should be considered when evaluating a newborn's level on the nomogram (AAP & ACOG, 2017; Bhutani & Committee on the Fetus and Newborn, 2011).

Essential laboratory evaluations are Coombs test, serum bilirubin levels (direct and total), hemoglobin, reticulocyte percentage, white cell count, and positive smear for cellular morphology.

The Coombs test (DAT-direct antiglobin) helps to determine whether jaundice is due to Rh, ABO, or other antibody incompatibility. The indirect Coombs test measures the amount of Rh-positive antibodies in the mother's blood. Rh-positive RBCs are added to the maternal blood sample. If the mother's serum contains antibodies, the Rh-positive RBCs will agglutinate (clump) when rabbit immune antiglobulin is added, which is a positive test result. The direct Coombs test reveals the presence of antibody-coated (sensitized) Rh-positive RBCs in the newborn. Rabbit immune antiglobulin is added to the specimen of neonatal blood cells. If the neonatal RBCs agglutinate, they have been coated with maternal antibodies, a positive result.

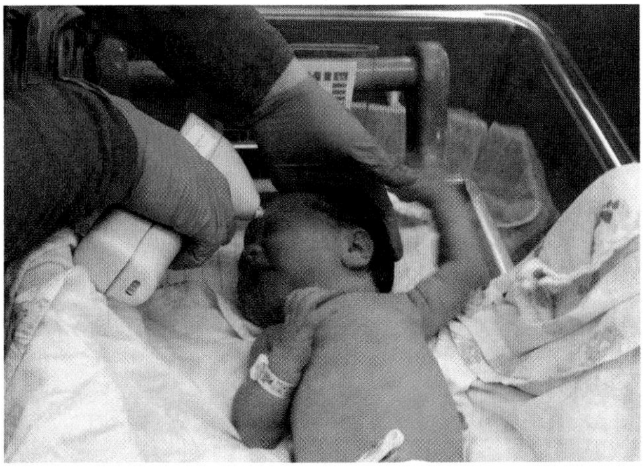

Figure 31–14 **A newborn being screened with a transcutaneous bilirubinometer.**

If the hemolytic process is due to Rh sensitization, laboratory findings reveal (1) an Rh-positive newborn with a positive Coombs test; (2) increased erythropoiesis with many immature circulating RBCs (nucleated blastocysts); (3) anemia, in most cases; (4) elevated levels (5 mg/dL or more) of bilirubin in cord blood; and (5) a reduction in albumin binding capacity. Maternal data may include an elevated anti-Rh titer and spectrophotometric evidence of fetal hemolytic process.

If the hemolytic process is due to ABO incompatibility, laboratory findings reveal an increase in reticulocytes. The resulting anemia is usually not significant during the newborn period and is rare later on. The direct Coombs test may be negative or mildly positive, whereas the indirect Coombs test may be strongly positive. Newborns with a positive direct Coombs test have increased incidence of jaundice with bilirubin levels in excess of 10 mg/dL. Increased numbers of spherocytes (spherical, plump, mature erythrocytes) are seen on a peripheral blood smear. Increased numbers of spherocytes are not seen on blood smears from Rh disease newborns.

CLINICAL THERAPY

The best treatment for hemolytic disease is prevention. Prenatal identification of the fetus at risk for Rh or ABO incompatibility, along with other, lesser-known antibodies like anti-Kell and anti-C, will allow prompt treatment. See Chapter 18 for discussion of in utero management of this condition.

Whatever the cause of hyperbilirubinemia, management of these newborns is directed toward alleviating anemia, removing maternal antibodies and sensitized erythrocytes, reducing serum bilirubin levels, and minimizing the consequences of hyperbilirubinemia. Early discharge of newborns from birthing centers has significantly influenced the diagnosis and management of neonatal jaundice, increasing the emphasis on outpatient and home care management.

Hemolytic disease may be treated with phototherapy, exchange transfusion, and drug therapy. When determining the appropriate management of hyperbilirubinemia due to hemolytic disease, the three variables that must be taken into account are the newborn's (1) gestational age at birth, (2) serum bilirubin level, and (3) age in hours. If a newborn is 35 weeks' gestational age, has hemolysis with an unconjugated bilirubin level of 14 mg/dL, weighs less than 2500 g (5.5 lb) (birth weight), and is 24 hours old or less, a dose of intravenous immunoglobulin (IVIG) or ultimately an exchange transfusion may be the best management. However, if that same newborn is over 24 hours old, which is past the time where an increase in bilirubin would result from pathologic causes, phototherapy may be the treatment of choice to prevent the possible complications of kernicterus.

PHOTOTHERAPY

Phototherapy is the exposure of the newborn to high-intensity light to reduce serum bilirubin levels. It may be used alone or in conjunction with exchange transfusion. Exposure of the newborn to high-intensity light (a bank of fluorescent light bulbs, LEDs, or bulbs in the blue-light spectrum) decreases serum bilirubin levels in the skin by facilitating biliary excretion of unconjugated bilirubin. Phototherapy decreases serum bilirubin levels by changing bilirubin from the non-water-soluble (lipophilic) form to water-soluble by-products that can then be excreted via urine and bile.

Photoisomerization occurs when the natural form of bilirubin is exposed to light at a certain wavelength and the bilirubin is converted to a less toxic form. The new isomer, photobilirubin, is created rapidly but is quite unstable. The photobilirubin is bound to albumin, transported to the liver, and incorporated into bile. If it is not quickly eliminated from the bowel, it can convert back to its original form and return to the bloodstream. In addition, the photodegradation products formed when light oxidizes bilirubin can be excreted in the urine.

Phototherapy is a primary intervention that is used more for the prevention of hyperbilirubinemia, that is, to halt bilirubin levels from climbing dangerously high. The decision to start phototherapy is based on three factors: Gestational age, age in hours, and level of total bilirubin or unconjugated bilirubin. Phototherapy is most effective with measured flux of light intensity above 8 to 10 for standard phototherapy and above 35 for high-intensity phototherapy. Phototherapy does not alter the underlying cause of jaundice, and hemolysis may continue to produce anemia. See *Case Study: Benita Cartier*.

Clinical Tip

When excreted, the newborn's urine will be much darker in color/appearance due to the excreted higher-conjugated bilirubin content. Newborns also excrete bilirubin in their stools, so it is important that the stooling pattern be established; babies may need glycerin suppositories in some instances to avoid constipation.

Phototherapy can be provided by conventional banks of phototherapy lights, a fiberoptic blanket attached to a halogen light source around the trunk of the newborn, LEDs (light-emitting diodes), or a combination of these delivery methods. Conventional banks of phototherapy lights are the most effective source available but can mask cyanosis and cause dizziness and nausea in the parents and staff. Bilirubin levels should continue to decline when phototherapy covers a wider surface area. If a drop in levels is not reached, then an exchange transfusion should be considered. Disadvantages of lights are that they create a difficult work environment and can distort a baby's color. See *Clinical Skill 31–2: Newborn Receiving Phototherapy*.

CASE STUDY: Benita Cartier

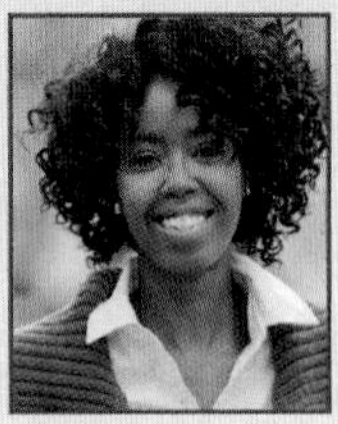

SOURCE: blvdone/ Shutterstock.

The neonatologist informs Benita and her husband that their newborn needs phototherapy for jaundice. The Coombs test is positive and their baby's bilirubin level is 16 mg/dL. The doctor recommends phototherapy in the NICU. Benita and her husband are upset and anxiously question the nurse about this therapy after the doctor leaves the room.

Questions to Ponder

How would you explain to the couple how phototherapy will reduce the bilirubin levels in their baby? What interventions are needed for newborns receiving phototherapy?

Clinical Skill 31–2

Newborn Receiving Phototherapy

NURSING ACTION

Preparation

- Explain the purpose of phototherapy, the procedure itself (including the need to use eye patches and keep groin covered), and possible side effects such as dehydration and skin breakdown from more frequent stooling.
- Note evidence of jaundice in the skin, sclera, and mucous membranes (in newborns with darkly pigmented skin). Be sure that recent serum bilirubin levels are available.

Rationale: *The decision to use phototherapy is based on a careful assessment of the newborn's condition over a period of time. The most recent results before starting therapy serve as a baseline to evaluate the effectiveness of therapy.*

Equipment and Supplies

- Bank of phototherapy lights or Bili Bed or Blanket as ordered
- Eye patches
- Small scale to weigh diapers
- White sheet or foil to line bed if high intensity is ordered
- Bili meter to measure irradiance

Procedure

1. Obtain vital signs including axillary temperature.

Rationale: *Provides baseline data.*

2. Remove all of the baby's clothing except the diaper (keep genitals covered).

Rationale: *Exposure of the newborn to high-intensity light (a bank of fluorescent light bulbs or bulbs in the blue-white spectrum) decreases serum bilirubin levels in the skin by aiding biliary excretion of unconjugated bilirubin. Because the tissue absorbs the light, best results are obtained when there is maximum skin surface exposure.*

3. Apply eye coverings (eye patches or a Bili Mask) to the baby according to agency policy (Figure 31–15).

Rationale: *Eye coverings are used because it is not known if phototherapy injures delicate eye structures, particularly the retina.*

Clinical Skill 31–2 *(continued)*

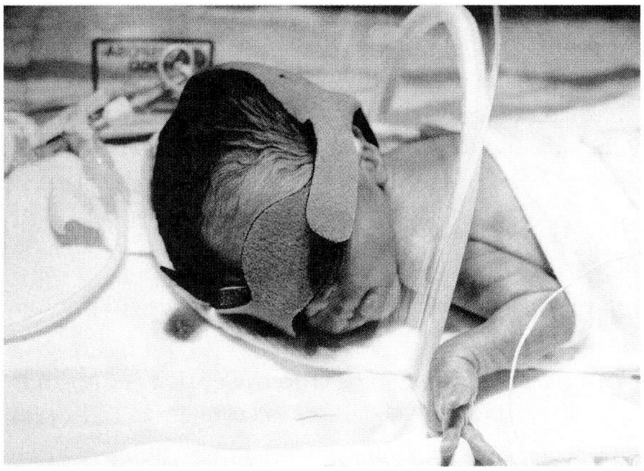

Figure 31–15 **Newborn receiving phototherapy. The phototherapy light is positioned over the incubator. Bilateral eye patches are always used during photo light therapy to protect the baby's eyes.**

4. Place the newborn in an open crib or isolette (more commonly used in preterm babies and babies who are sicker) about 45 to 50 cm below the bank of phototherapy lights. Reposition if high intensity is ordered (Bhutani et al., 2013).

Rationale: *The isolette helps the newborn maintain body temperature while undressed. Repositioning exposes different areas of skin to the lights, prevents the development of pressure areas on the skin, and varies the stimulation the baby receives.*

5. Monitor vital signs every 4 hours with axillary temperatures.

Rationale: *Temperature assessment is indicated to detect hypothermia or hyperthermia. Deviation in pulse and respirations may indicate developing complications.*

6. Check the lights using a bilimeter to ensure safe, effective treatment.
7. Cluster care activities.
8. Discontinue phototherapy and remove eye patches at least every 2 to 3 hours when feeding the baby and when the parents visit.

Rationale: *Care activities are clustered to help ensure that the newborn has maximum time under the lights. Eye patches are removed to assess for signs of complications such as excessive pressure, discharge, or conjunctivitis. Patches are also removed to provide some social stimulation and to promote parental attachment.*

9. Maintain adequate fluid intake. Evaluate need for IV fluids.
10. Monitor I&O carefully. Weigh diapers before discarding. Record quantity and characteristics of each stool.

Rationale: *Newborns undergoing phototherapy treatment have increased water loss and loose stools as a result of bilirubin excretion. This increases their risk of dehydration.*

11. Weigh newborn daily.

Rationale: *Weight loss is also a sign of fluid balance and an indicator of developing dehydration in the newborn.*

12. Observe the baby for signs of perianal excoriation and institute therapy if it develops.

Rationale: *Perianal excoriation may develop because of the irritating effect of diarrhea stools.*

13. Ensure that serum bilirubin levels are drawn regularly according to orders or agency policy. Turn the phototherapy lights off while the blood is drawn.

Rationale: *Serum bilirubin levels provide the most accurate indication of the effectiveness of phototherapy. They are generally drawn every 12 hours but at least once daily. The phototherapy lights are turned off to ensure accurate serum bilirubin levels.*

14. Examine the newborn's skin regularly for signs of developing pressure areas, bronzing, maculopapular rash, and changes in degree of jaundice.

Rationale: *Pressure areas may develop if the baby lies in one position for an extended period. A benign, transient bronze discoloration of the skin may occur with phototherapy when the newborn has elevated direct serum bilirubin levels or liver disease. A maculopapular rash is another transient side effect of phototherapy that develops occasionally.*

15. Avoid using lotion or ointment on the exposed skin.

Rationale: *Lotions and ointments on a newborn receiving phototherapy may cause skin burns.*

16. Provide parents with opportunities to hold the newborn and assist in the baby's care. Answer their questions accurately and keep them informed of developments or changes.

Rationale: *A sick newborn is a source of great anxiety for parents. Information helps them deal with their anxiety. Moreover, they have a right to be kept well informed of their baby's status so that they are able to make informed decisions as needed.*

17. May also provide phototherapy using lightweight, fiberoptic blankets (Bili Blankets). The baby is wrapped in the blanket, which is plugged into an outlet (Figure 31–16).

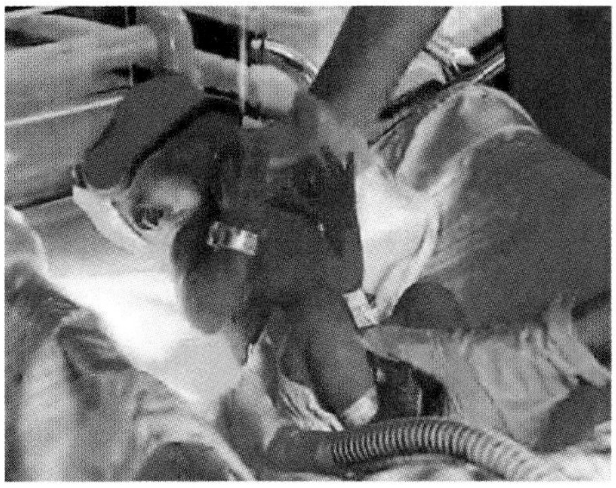

Figure 31–16 **Newborn on fiberoptic Bili Bed and under phototherapy lights.**

NOTE: The color is distorted because of the reflection of the Bili Bed.

Rationale: *With fiberoptic beds and blankets the newborn is readily accessible for care, feedings, and diaper changes. The baby does not get overheated, and fluid and weight loss are not complications of this system. The baby is accessible to the parents and the procedure seems less alarming to parents than standard phototherapy.*

EXCHANGE TRANSFUSION

Exchange transfusion is the withdrawal and replacement of the newborn's blood containing high levels of bilirubin with donor blood containing much lower levels. It is used to treat anemia with RBCs that are not susceptible to maternal antibodies, remove sensitized RBCs that would be lysed soon, remove serum bilirubin, and provide bilirubin-free albumin and increase the binding sites for bilirubin. Concerns over doing an exchange transfusion are related to the use of blood products and associated potential for HIV infection and hepatitis. Additionally, electrolyte imbalances can be fatal with exchange transfusions and should be monitored closely. If the TSB is at or approaching the exchange level, the nurse should send blood for immediate type, cross-match, and electrolyte testing. Blood for exchange transfusion is modified whole blood (red cells and plasma) cross-matched against the mother and compatible with the newborn. A blood warmer is often utilized to maintain thermoregulation.

Many exchange transfusions have been avoided with the use of intravenous immunoglobulin (IVIG), which binds to the antibody sites on the red cell and causes a decrease in the hemolysis that the newborn is experiencing. The dose for IVIG is 1 gram per kg over 4 hours and repeat in 12 hours if required. If after having tried IVIG the newborn has symptoms of abnormal neurologic exam (poor feeding, shrill cry, posturing) and a serum bilirubin level above line on the nomogram for exchange level, an acute intervention of an exchange transfusion should be performed.

●○● NURSING MANAGEMENT

For the Newborn with Jaundice

Nursing Assessment and Diagnosis

Assessment is aimed at identifying prenatal and perinatal factors that predispose to development of jaundice and identifying jaundice as soon as it is apparent. Significant hyperbilirubinemia in the neonatal population is often due to a multitude of causes including gestational age, blood type, and a genetic basis. Clinically, ABO incompatibility presents as jaundice and occasionally as hepatosplenomegaly. Fetal hydrops or erythroblastosis fetalis is rare (see Chapter 18). Hemolytic disease of the newborn is suspected if one or more of the following are evident:

- The placenta is enlarged.
- The newborn is edematous, with pleural and pericardial effusion plus ascites.
- Pallor or jaundice is noted during the first 24 to 36 hours.
- Hemolytic anemia is diagnosed.
- The spleen and liver are enlarged.

Changes in behavior should be carefully noted; observe for evidence of bleeding. If laboratory tests indicate elevated bilirubin levels, check the newborn for jaundice about every 2 hours and record observations.

To check for jaundice in lighter-skinned babies, blanch the skin over a bony prominence (forehead, nose, or sternum) by pressing firmly with the thumb. After pressure is released, if jaundice is present, the area appears yellow before normal color returns. Check oral mucosa and the posterior portion of the hard palate and conjunctival sacs for yellow pigmentation in darker-skinned babies. Jaundice progresses in a cephalocaudal direction from the head to the trunk and then to the lower extremities. The overall progression of jaundice should be noted. Assessment in daylight or bright fluorescent light gives the best results because pink walls and surroundings may mask yellowish tints, and yellow light makes differentiation of jaundice difficult. The time at onset of jaundice is recorded and reported. If jaundice appears, careful observation of the increase in depth of color and of the newborn's behavior is mandatory. Advocating for a serum level assessment is warranted anytime jaundice appears before 24 hours of life or when jaundice appears to be worsening rapidly.

Nursing diagnoses that may apply to a newborn with jaundice include the diagnoses in the nursing care plan and these diagnoses:

- ***Fluid Volume: Risk for Deficient***, related to increased insensible water loss and frequent loose stools
- ***Injury, Risk for***, related to jaundice and use of phototherapy and eye mask
- ***Neurovascular Dysfunction: Peripheral, Risk for***, related to neurologic damage secondary to kernicterus
- ***Parenting, Risk for Impaired***, related to deficient knowledge of newborn care and prolonged separation of newborn and parents secondary to illness

(NANDA-I © 2017)

Nursing Plan and Implementation

Hospital-Based Nursing Care

Hospital-based care is described in *Nursing Care Plan: For the Newborn with Hyperbilirubinemia*. Phototherapy success is measured every 12 hours or daily by serum bilirubin levels (more frequently if there is hemolysis or a higher level before initiation of phototherapy). The phototherapy lights must be turned off while drawing blood for serum bilirubin levels. Because it is not known whether phototherapy injures the delicate eye structures, particularly the retina, apply eye patches over the newborn's closed eyes during exposure to banks of phototherapy lights (refer to Figure 31–15 in *Clinical Skill 31–2: Newborn Receiving Phototherapy*). Discontinue conventional phototherapy and remove the eye patches at least once per shift to assess the eyes and promote eye contact during feeding times. This social stimulation is important for both newborn and parent bonding.

Most phototherapy units will provide the following levels of irradiance: 8 to 10 | mu | W/cm^2/nm below the lamps for conventional phototherapy and greater than 30 | mu | W/cm^2/nm in the 430–490 nm band for intensive phototherapy (Sawyer, 2015). A photometer can be used to measure and maintain desired irradiance levels. Lotions and ointments should be avoided under bilirubin lights because they may cause burns.

Some parents may feel guilty about their baby's condition and think they have caused the problem. Under stress, parents may not be able to understand the healthcare provider's first explanations. Expect the parents to need explanations repeated and clarified. Coach parents when they visit the baby and encourage eye and tactile contact with the newborn. After the mother's discharge, keep parents informed of their baby's condition and encourage them to return to the hospital or to telephone at any time so that they can be fully involved in the care of their newborn. Tell parents that they can expect a rebound after discontinuation of phototherapy and that a follow-up bilirubin test is typically done prior to discharge and an outpatient test may also be done (Eichenwald et al., 2017).

While the mother is still hospitalized, phototherapy can also be carried out in the parents' room if the only problem is physiologic hyperbilirubinemia and the parents agree to these actions:

- Keep the baby in the room for 24 hours a day.
- Take emergency action (e.g., for choking) if necessary.
- Complete instruction checklists.
- Sign a consent form per agency protocol.

Nursing Care Plan: For the Newborn with Hyperbilirubinemia

1. Nursing Diagnosis: *Tissue Integrity, Impaired*, related to predisposing factors associated with hyperbilirubinemia (NANDA-I © 2017)

Goal: Babies at risk for jaundice and early signs of jaundice will be identified.

INTERVENTION	RATIONALE
• Evaluate baby's history for predisposing factors for hyperbilirubinemia.	• Early identification of risk factors enables the nurse to monitor babies for early signs of hyperbilirubinemia. Acidosis, hypoxia, and hypothermia increase the risk of hyperbilirubinemia at lower bilirubin levels.
• Observe color of amniotic fluid at time of rupture of membranes.	• Amber-colored amniotic fluid indicates hyperbilirubinemia.
• Assess baby for developing jaundice in daylight, if possible.	• Early detection is affected by nursery environment. Artificial lights (with pink tint) may mask beginning of jaundice.
1. Observe sclera.	1. Most visible sign of hyperbilirubinemia is jaundice noted in skin, sclera, or oral mucosa. Onset is first seen on face and then progresses down the trunk.
2. Observe skin color and assess by blanching.	2. Blanching leaves a yellow color to the skin immediately after pressure is released.
3. Check oral mucosa, posterior portion of hard palate, and conjunctival sacs for yellow pigmentation in dark-skinned newborns.	3. Underlying pigment of dark-skinned newborns may normally appear yellow.
• Report jaundice occurring within 24 hours of birth.	

EXPECTED OUTCOMES: Baby's jaundice is identified early.

2. Nursing Diagnosis: *Fluid Volume: Imbalanced, Risk for*, related to phototherapy (NANDA-I © 2017)

Goal: The newborn will not exhibit signs of dehydration and will display appropriate weight gain.

INTERVENTION	RATIONALE
• Offer feedings every 2 to 3 hours.	• Adequate hydration increases peristalsis and excretion of bilirubin.
• Breastfeed on demand with no supplementation unless excessive weight loss or increasing TSB with adequate feeding.	
• Provide 25% extra fluid intake.	• Replace fluid losses due to watery stools, if under phototherapy.
• Assess for dehydration: 1. Poor skin turgor 2. Depressed fontanelles 3. Sunken eyes 4. Decreased urine output 5. Weight loss 6. Changes in electrolytes	• Phototherapy treatment may cause liquid stools and increased insensible water loss, which increases risk of dehydration.
• Monitor I&O.	
• Weigh daily.	
• Report signs of dehydration.	
• Administer IV fluids:	• Prevents fluid overload.
1. Monitor flow rates. 2. Assess insertion sites for signs of infection.	• IV fluids may be used if baby is dehydrated or in presence of other complications. IV may be started if exchange transfusion is to be done.

EXPECTED OUTCOMES: Baby will have good skin turgor, clear amber urine output of 1–3 mL/kg/hr, six to eight wet diapers/day, and maintain weight.

3. Nursing Diagnosis: *Injury, Risk for*, related to hyperbilirubinemia and use of phototherapy (NANDA-I © 2017)

Goal: Baby will not have any corneal irritation/drainage, skin breakdown, or major fluctuations in temperature.

(continued)

Nursing Care Plan: For the Newborn with Hyperbilirubinemia (*continued*)

INTERVENTION	RATIONALE
• Cover baby's eyes with eye patches while under phototherapy lights. Cover testes/penis in male newborns.	• Protects retina from damage due to high-intensity light and testes from damage due to heat.
• Make certain that eyelids are closed before applying eye patches.	• Prevents corneal abrasions.
• Remove baby from under phototherapy and remove eye patches during feedings.	• Provides visual stimulation and facilitates attachment behaviors.
• Inspect eyes each shift for conjunctivitis, drainage, and corneal abrasions due to irritation from eye patches.	• Prevents or facilitates prompt treatment of purulent conjunctivitis.
• Administer thorough perianal cleansing with each stool or change of perianal protective covering.	• Frequent stooling increases risk of skin breakdown. Prevents infection.
• Provide minimal coverage—only of diaper area.	• Provides maximal exposure. Shielded areas become more jaundiced, so maximum exposure is essential.
• Avoid the use of oily applications on the skin.	• Prevents superficial burns to skin.
• Reposition baby every 2 hours.	• Provides equal exposure of all skin areas and prevents pressure areas.
• Observe for bronzing of skin.	• Bronzing is related to use of phototherapy with increased direct bilirubin levels or liver damage; may last for 2 to 4 months.
• Place Plexiglas shield between baby and light.	• Hypothermia and hyperthermia are common complications of phototherapy.
• Monitor baby's skin and core temperature frequently until temperature is stable.	• Hypothermia results from exposure to lights, subsequent radiation, and convection losses.
• Check axillary temperature with readings on servo-controlled unit on incubator.	• Hyperthermia may result from the increased environmental heat.
• Regulate incubator temperature as needed.	• Additional heat from phototherapy lights frequently causes a rise in the baby's and incubator's temperatures.
	• Fluctuations in temperature may occur in response to radiation and convection.

EXPECTED OUTCOMES: Baby's eyes are protected, skin is intact, and baby maintains a stable temperature.

4. Nursing Diagnosis: ***Parenting, Risk for Impaired*, related to deficient knowledge of newborn care and prolonged separation of newborn and parents secondary to illness (NANDA-I © 2017)**

Goals: Parents will bond with newborn and have realistic expectations about their newborn. Parents are comfortable taking their newborn home. They are able to demonstrate normal newborn care and assessments of possible complications, and they know when to return for follow-up.

INTERVENTION	RATIONALE
• Encourage parents to provide tactile stimulation during feeding and diaper changes.	• Newborn has normal needs for tactile stimulation. • Presence of equipment may discourage parents from interacting with newborn.
• Encourage cuddling and eye contact during feedings.	• Provides opportunity for parents to bond with their newborn.

• Offer suggestions to comfort restless newborn:
  • Nesting when beneath bili lights
  • Talking softly and singing quietly to baby
  • Taped music or tape recording of evening activities from home
  • Rhythmic patting of buttocks
  • Firm, nonstroking touch, assisting with control of extremities
  • Pacifier for nonnutritive sucking
	• Provides comfort and decreases sensory deprivation.

• Encourage family/friend support of mother/parents (i.e., meals, rest, child care for siblings, allow expressions of concerns/feelings).	• Decreases strain on mother/parents by assisting with other responsibilities and allows for additional time with newborn for bonding, care, etc.
• Evaluate additional psychosocial needs.	• Parents may not understand what is happening or why.

Nursing Care Plan: For the Newborn with Hyperbilirubinemia (*continued*)

• Discuss rationale for treatment and possible side effects of phototherapy with family (stool changes, increased fluid loss, possible temp instability, slight lethargy, rash, altered sleep–wake patterns).
• Instruct family on newborn's care while undergoing phototherapy:
  • Safety precautions—Bili Mask (to protect eyes), incubator door closed and latched, covering genitalia per policy.
  • Skin care, cord care, circumcision care as appropriate.
  • Lab draws, rationale I&O.
• Encourage parent/partner/sibling involvement in newborn care as possible.
• Give explanation of equipment being used and changes in bilirubin levels. Allow parents an opportunity to ask questions; reinforce or clarify information as needed.
• Evaluate family's understanding of information.
	• Physician preference of treatment modalities may vary. Parents may not understand why their newborn is not receiving a treatment that another with the same condition is receiving.

• As necessary, review role of pumping breasts and offering formula for limited time.	• The etiology of breast milk jaundice remains uncertain. The serum bilirubin levels begin to fall within 48 hours after discontinuation of breastfeeding. Opinion of physicians varies regarding the need for discontinuing breastfeeding.
• Assist mother to pump her breasts to maintain milk supply.	• If breastfeeding is temporarily discontinued, assess mother's knowledge of pumping her breasts in regular increments (q 2–3 hours), and provide information and support as needed.

EXPECTED OUTCOMES: The parent will demonstrate ability to perform basic newborn care tasks as evidenced by exhibiting appropriate attachment behaviors (i.e., talking and holding baby, feeding baby, and caring for baby under home bili therapy).

Parents verbalize understanding of rationale and possible side effects from phototherapy; parents/family demonstrate safety precautions when caring for newborn; parents get meals and rest and verbalize support given.

Give the instructions to the parents but also continue to monitor the newborn's temperature, activity, I&O, and positioning of eye patches (if conventional light banks are used) at regular intervals.

Community-Based Nursing Care

Some studies have shown that with early discharge of newborns and their mothers comes an increase in hospital readmission and elevated risk of pathologic hyperbilirubinemia. Home phototherapy use is recommended only if the newborn is having physiologic hyperbilirubinemia. Home phototherapy is not recommended by the AAP for hemolytic hyperbilirubinemia (Bhutani & Committee on the Fetus and Newborn, 2011). Any newborn with a level in the higher range should be hospitalized for continual phototherapy and have serum bilirubin levels closely monitored on a regular schedule.

Jaundice and its phototherapy treatment can be very disturbing to parents and may generate feelings of guilt and fear. The parents' perception of and/or misconceptions about jaundice can affect parent–newborn interactions. Explain the causes of jaundice and emphasize that it is usually a transient problem and one to which all newborns must adapt after birth. Reassurance and support are vital, especially for the breastfeeding mother, who may question her ability to adequately nourish her newborn.

It is essential that the impact of cultural beliefs be considered. Some Latina women believe that showing strong maternal emotions during pregnancy and breastfeeding can be detrimental. *Bilis* associated with anger may be blamed by some Latina women for jaundice. Cultural beliefs lead mothers to interpret illness within their cultural framework, especially when left without clear and understood explanations. Maternal reactions can be lessened by offering careful explanations to the mothers about the diagnosis, prognosis, duration, and management options for jaundice and about the possibility of its recurrence.

If the baby is to receive phototherapy at home, teach the parents to record the newborn's temperature, weight, fluid I&O, stools, and feedings and to use the phototherapy equipment. In addition, if phototherapy lights are being used, parents must agree that the baby will be exposed to the lights for long periods of time; that they will hold the baby for only short periods for feedings, comforting, and cleansing of the perineal area; and that the room temperature will be regulated to minimize heat loss. Fiberoptic phototherapy blankets eliminate the need for eye patches, decrease heat loss because the baby is clothed, and provide more opportunities for interaction between the baby and parents. Ongoing monitoring of bilirubin levels is essential with home phototherapy and can be measured as an outpatient in the follow-up lab or in the clinician's office.

Evaluation

Expected outcomes of nursing care include:

- The newborn at risk for development of hyperbilirubinemia is identified, and action is taken to minimize the potential impact of hyperbilirubinemia.

- The newborn will not have any corneal irritation or drainage, skin breakdown, or major fluctuations in temperature.
- The newborn will not experience further dehydration.
- Parents understand the rationale for, goal of, and expected outcome of therapy.
- Parents verbalize their concerns about their baby's condition and identify how they can facilitate their baby's improvement.

Care of the Newborn with Anemia

Neonatal anemia is often difficult to recognize by clinical evaluation alone. Babies are born with hemoglobin that is generous and then falls over time, unless there is a peripartum reason for anemia.

A condition known as **physiologic anemia of infancy** exists as a result of the normal gradual drop in hemoglobin; theoretically, the bone marrow stops production of RBCs in response to higher oxygen levels resulting from initiation of breathing, reaching the lowest point, or nadir, of less than 11 mg/dL of hemoglobin by 8 to 12 weeks of age for term-born and 8 to 11 g/dL by 4 to 8 weeks for preterm-born babies depending on weight. At that point the bone marrow begins production of RBCs again, and the anemia disappears (Colombatti, Sainati, & Trevisanuto, 2016). The normal hemoglobin concentration in newborns weighing less than 2000 grams (4.4 lb) is 12 to 19 g/dL, and in full-term newborns it is 13 to 16 g/dL (Colombatti et al., 2016).

The preterm baby's hemoglobin reaches a nadir sooner than does a term newborn's because a preterm newborn's RBC survival time is shorter than that of a term newborn. This difference is a result of several factors: The preterm newborn's rapid growth rate, decreased iron stores, and an inadequate production of erythropoietin. Iatrogenic causes occur more in preterm newborns or newborns that are critically ill, as their conditions require more laboratory assessments and therefore more blood draws.

Some peripartum examples of blood loss (hypovolemia) occur in utero from placental bleeding (placenta previa or abruptio placentae); during the intrapartum period blood loss may be fetomaternal, fetofetal, or the result of umbilical cord bleeding; following delivery it may be caused by birth trauma to abdominal organs (adrenal hemorrhage) or the cranium (subgaleal bleed). Cerebral bleeding, especially in preterm newborns, may occur because of hypoxia, hypercapnia, fluctuations of blood pressure, and reperfusion injury.

Anemia can also be a result of hemolysis (the breakdown of RBCs) or the underproduction of RBCs. Maternal viral illness, such as parvovirus, Epstein-Barr, and cytomegalovirus, can cause anemia in the newborn. Thalassemias and spherocytosis (genetic inherited blood abnormalities) cause anemia as well because the cell life is shorter in duration due to the fragility of the cells. Excessive hemolysis of red cells is usually a result of blood group incompatibilities (most often ABO), the treatment of Rh disease with Rho(D), and can also be due to antibodies Kell, FyJk, C, and E, as well as infection (Colombatti et al., 2016; Noronha, 2016). The most common cause of impaired red cell production is a genetically transmitted deficiency in glucose-6-phosphate dehydrogenase (G6PD). Anemia and jaundice are typically the presenting signs in about 33% of neonatal jaundice cases but typically present later in the child with elevated unconjugated bilirubin problems (Noronha, 2016).

CLINICAL THERAPY

Clinical management depends on the severity of the anemia, whether blood loss is acute or chronic, clinical manifestations, and whether it was anticipated based on the pregnancy history. The age at which anemia is first noted is also of diagnostic value. Clinically, light-skinned anemic newborns are very pale when they do not have other symptoms of shock and usually have abnormally low RBC counts. In acute blood loss, symptoms of shock may be present, such as pallor, low arterial blood pressure, and a decreasing hematocrit value.

The initial laboratory workup should include determination of:

- Hemoglobin and hematocrit measurements
- Reticulocyte count
- Examination of maternal blood smear for fetal erythrocytes (Kleihauer-Betke test) (if maternal/fetal hemorrhage suspected)
- Bilirubin levels (in hemolytic disease).

Mild or chronic anemia in a newborn may be treated adequately with iron supplements alone or with iron-fortified formulas. Folate and vitamin E may have to be supplemented depending on the type of formula ingested.

In severe cases of anemia, transfusions with O-negative or typed and cross-matched packed red cells are the preferred method of treatment. Guidelines describe characteristics to consider to avoid undue exposure to blood products; they also provide clear indications when a newborn might need a life-saving transfusion, such as anemia in the first 24 hours, acute blood loss and shock, cardiac defects with anemia, and for newborns requiring oxygen (Colombatti et al., 2016).

Management of anemia of prematurity includes treating the causative factor (e.g., antibiotics or antivirals used for infection, steroid therapy for disorders of erythrocyte production) and supplemental iron. Iron is essential in the formation of RBCs. In the preterm newborn, third-trimester transplacental infusion of iron stores is interrupted, thus stores in general are low (Kling & Coe, 2016). Blood transfusions, in spite of dedicated units for newborns, should be avoided if possible.

Use of recombinant human erythropoietin (rEPO) in preterm neonates can be beneficial in decreasing blood transfusions by stimulating the baby's own RBC production (Ohls et al., 2016). There is data to support giving darbepoetin alfa as needed in the newborn population as well; the benefit is once-weekly dosing. Both erythropoietin- and darbepoetin alfa–treated preterm newborns had better mental and developmental outcomes at evaluations at 3 to 4 years of age than those treated with placebo (Ohls et al., 2016)

NURSING MANAGEMENT

For the Newborn with Anemia

Assess the newborn for symptoms of anemia. If the blood loss is acute, the baby may exhibit these signs of shock:

- Capillary filling time greater than 3 seconds
- Decreased pulses
- Tachycardia
- Low blood pressure.

Signs of longer-term compromise include:

- Poor weight gain
- Pallor
- New onset of jaundice or recurrent jaundice
- Tachycardia
- Tachypnea
- Apneic episodes.

The newborn should be placed on continuous cardiac and respiratory monitoring. Any symptoms indicating anemia or shock should be promptly reported to the healthcare provider. Continued observations will be necessary to identify physiologic anemia as the preterm newborn grows. Babies who receive transfusions often have elevated ferritin levels and do not need supplemental iron. Babies who receive erythropoietin or darbepoetin alfa need additional iron. Administration of iron and multivitamins to support the newborn's ability to produce RBCs is important. Teaching the parents why it is needed helps with compliance and continued supplementation after discharge.

Care of the Newborn with Infection

Newborns up to 1 month of age are particularly susceptible to infection, referred to as **sepsis neonatorum**, caused by organisms that do not typically cause significant disease in older children. Once any infection occurs in the newborn, it can spread rapidly through the bloodstream, regardless of its primary site. Despite the great advances in neonatal medicine and intrapartum management, sepsis remains the leading cause of morbidity and mortality in the newborn. Overall incidence of sepsis is 1 to 5 per 1000, and the mortality rate of those newborns is 5 to 10% (Deleon, Shattuck, & Jain, 2015). The incidence of *early-onset neonatal sepsis (EONS)* is 0.98 per 1000 live births, but among VLBW newborns it is 10.96 per 1000 (Deleon et al., 2015). EONS, seen in the first 7 days of life but present at birth, is caused primarily by vertical transmission of maternal organisms. *E. coli* and group B streptococcus (GBS) remain the most common causative organisms. With the utilization of the Centers of Disease Control and Prevention recommendations, GBS sepsis has declined, but at the cost of significant use of antibiotics, which in this time of focus on antibiotic stewardship is not without risk.

Neonatal *late-onset sepsis (LOS)* occurs in a baby older than 72 hours and is typically caused by a host of other organisms. Nosocomial infections are infections acquired while a baby is in the NICU and are usually caused by organisms introduced during procedures or on equipment such as ventilators or central lines required to care for the neonate. The general debilitation and underlying illness often associated with prematurity and respiratory distress necessitate invasive procedures such as umbilical catheterization, intubation, resuscitation, ventilatory support, monitoring, parenteral alimentation, and broad-spectrum antibiotic therapy. Methicillin-resistant *Staphylococcus aureus* (MRSA), pseudomonas, and *Candida*, which cause late-onset sepsis, are some of the most common pathogens causing hospital-acquired infections in the NICU population. Hospitals that admit from referral hospitals swab for MRSA on admission and maintain strict isolation until the results of the swab are known.

Full-term newborns are also susceptible to infection because their immunologic systems are immature (Figure 31–17). They lack the complex factors involved in effective phagocytosis and the ability to localize infection or to respond with a well-defined recognizable inflammatory response. In addition, newborns lack IgM immunoglobulin, which is necessary to protect against bacteria, because it does not cross the placenta (refer to Chapter 26 for immunologic adaptations in the newborn period).

Most nosocomial infections in the NICU present as bacteremia/sepsis, urinary tract infections, meningitis, or pneumonia. Maternal antepartum infections such as rubella,

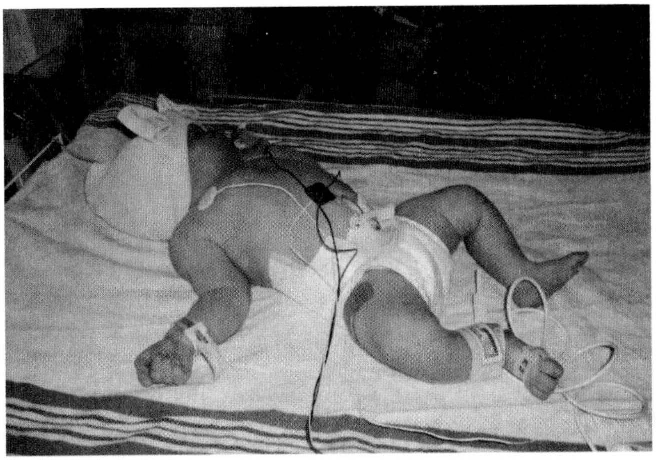

Figure 31–17 Term newborn with suspected sepsis.

SOURCE: © by Valentina Mescolotto. Used by permission of Valentina Mescolotto.

toxoplasmosis, cytomegalic inclusion disease, and herpes may cause congenital infections and resulting disorders in the newborn. Intrapartum maternal infections, such as amnionitis and those resulting from premature rupture of membranes (PROM) and precipitous birth, are sources of neonatal infection. (See Chapter 18 for more detailed information.) Passage through the birth canal and contact with microorganisms in the vaginal flora (β-hemolytic streptococci, herpes, *Listeria*, and gonococci) expose the neonate to infection (Table 31–5). With infection anywhere in the fetus or newborn, the adjacent tissues or organs are very easily penetrated, and the blood–brain barrier is ineffective in protecting from infection. Rates of infection are more common in preterm newborns, especially those who are VLBW, and in newborns of African heritage (Stoll, 2016).

Gram-positive organisms account for 70% of neonatal sepsis; Gram-negative organisms cause 15 to 20%; and the remaining 10% result from fungus (Fraser, 2016). *Staphylococcus aureus* and *Staphylococcus epidermidis* are responsible for the majority of late-onset infections in many neonatal units. Other commonly isolated organisms are coagulase negative staphylococci, E coli, group B streptococcus, Klebsiella, enterococcus, and pseudomonas. There is no good consensus on what antibiotics are recommended in LOS, but broad-spectrum antibiotics are generally used (Fraser, 2016).

Protection of the newborn from infections starts prenatally and continues throughout pregnancy and birth. Prenatal prevention should include maternal screening for sexually transmitted infections and monitoring of rubella titers in women who test negative. Sterile technique during intrapartum care is essential. Viral cultures are definitive tests but take time to get results. Visual exam of the lesions is often reported on the labor and birth record to identify a patient with herpes. Placental and amniotic fluid cultures and pathology on the placenta are obtained if amnionitis is suspected. Local eye treatment with an antibiotic ophthalmic ointment is given to all newborns to prevent damage from gonococcal (occurring 3 days following birth) and possibly chlamydial (occurring 7 to 10 days after birth) infections. Prophylactic antibiotic therapy for asymptomatic women who test positive for GBS during the intrapartum period helps prevent EONS. There has been a decrease in clinical neonatal sepsis rates due to the use of prenatal prophylactic antibiotic therapy recommended by the CDC (Stoll, 2016). See *Health Promotion: Preventing Newborn Infections*.

TABLE 31–5 Maternally Transmitted Newborn Infections

INFECTION	NURSING ASSESSMENT OF THE NEWBORN	NURSING PLAN AND IMPLEMENTATION
Group B Streptococcus		
1–2% colonized, with 1 in 10 developing disease Early onset—usually within hours of birth to 48 hours of life Late onset—72 hours to 3 months (Deleon et al., 2015; Eichenwald et al., 2017)	Severe respiratory distress (grunting and cyanosis) May become apneic or demonstrate symptoms of shock Meconium-stained amniotic fluid seen at birth	Early assessment of clinical signs necessary. Assist with x-ray examination—shows aspiration pneumonia or respiratory distress syndrome. Immediately obtain blood, gastric aspirate, external ear canal, and nasopharynx cultures. Administer antibiotics, usually aqueous penicillin or ampicillin combined with gentamicin, as soon as cultures are obtained. Early assessment and intervention are essential to survival.
Congenital Syphilis		
Spirochetes cross placenta after 16th–18th week of gestation The more recent the maternal infection, the higher the likelihood of transmission; titers should be monitored in pregnancy Most are asymptomatic at birth but develop symptoms within first 3 months of life	Assess newborn for: Elevated cord serum IgM and FTA-ABS (fluorescent treponemal antibody absorbed) IgM Rhinitis (snuffles) Fissures on mouth corners and excoriated upper lip Red rash around mouth and anus Copper-colored rash over face, palms, and soles Irritability, generalized edema, particularly over joints; bone lesions; painful extremities, hepatosplenomegaly, jaundice, congenital cataracts, SGA, and failure to thrive	Refer to evaluate for blindness, deafness, learning or behavioral problems. Initiate standard and contact precautions. Administer penicillin for 10 days. Provide emotional support for parents because of their feelings about mode of transmission and potential long-term sequelae.
Gonorrhea		
Approximately 30–35% of newborns born vaginally to infected mothers acquire the infection	Assess for: Ophthalmia neonatorum (conjunctivitis) Purulent discharge and corneal ulcerations Neonatal sepsis with temperature instability, poor feeding response, and/or hypotonia, jaundice	Administer ophthalmic antibiotic ointment or penicillin. If positive maternal test, initiate single-dose systemic antibiotic therapy. Make a follow-up referral to evaluate any loss of vision.
Herpes Type 2		
Usually transmitted during vaginal birth; a few cases of in utero transmission have been reported.	Check perinatal history for active herpes genital lesions. Small-cluster vesicular skin lesions over whole body about 6 to 9 days of life Disseminated form—DIC, pneumonia, hepatitis with jaundice, hepatosplenomegaly, and neurologic abnormalities Without skin lesions, assess for fever or subnormal temperature, respiratory congestion, tachypnea, and tachycardia.	Carry out careful handwashing and contact precautions (gown and glove isolation with linen precautions). Obtain skin, eye, and mucocutaneous membrane lesion and cerebrospinal fluid (CSF) cultures to identify herpes virus type 2 antigen-specific antibodies in serum. Cultures positive in 24–48 hours. Administer intravenous acyclovir from initiation of workup. Make a follow-up referral to evaluate potential sequelae of microcephaly, spasticity, seizures, deafness, or blindness. Encourage parental rooming-in and touching of their newborn. Show parents appropriate hand-washing procedures and precautions to be used at home if mother's lesions are active.

TABLE 31–5 Maternally Transmitted Newborn Infections *(continued)*

INFECTION	NURSING ASSESSMENT OF THE NEWBORN	NURSING PLAN AND IMPLEMENTATION
Cytomegalovirus (Cmv)		
Most common cause of congenital infection in the United States—approximately 1% of all newborns (Eichenwald et al., 2017) Transmission occurs in utero or during labor, or may happen postnatally through breast milk	Congenital CMV disease, including intrauterine growth retardation, jaundice, hepatosplenomegaly, petechiae or purpura (blueberry muffin spots), thrombocytopenia, and pneumonia CNS manifestations are very common and include lethargy and poor feeding, hypertonia or hypotonia, microcephaly, intracranial calcifications, chorioretinitis, and sensorineural deafness.	Diagnosis of congenital CMV infection is established by isolating virus from urine, saliva, or tissue obtained during the first 3 weeks of life. All newborns in whom the diagnosis is suspected should have a viral culture performed; a CT scan of the brain is particularly important to document the extent of CNS involvement; perform eye examination and hearing test; close long-term follow-up evaluation is needed for developmental effects. Gancyclovir is also utilized in this population for the goal of preservation of hearing.
Oral Candidal Infection (Thrush)		
Acquired during passage through birth canal	Assess newborn's buccal mucosa, tongue, gums, and inside the cheeks for white plaques (seen 5–7 days of age). Check diaper area for bright-red, well-demarcated eruptions. Assess for thrush periodically when newborn is on long-term antibiotic therapy.	Differentiate white plaque areas from milk curds by using cotton-tipped applicator (if it is thrush, removal is quite difficult and may cause rawness and bleeding in some areas, whereas milk curds wipe off easily). Maintain cleanliness of hands, linens, clothing, diapers, and feeding apparatus. Instruct breastfeeding mothers on treating their nipples with nystatin. Administer nystatin swabbed on oral lesions 1 hour after feeding or nystatin instilled in baby's oral cavity and on mucosa. Swab skin lesions with topical nystatin.
Congenital Zika Syndrome		
Caused by flavivirus (single-stranded RNA virus) via mosquito Perinatal transplacental/or placental inflammation; some peripartum transmission	Assess newborn for: Severe microcephaly (smaller-than-normal head (>3 SD below mean) Brain internal structural abnormalities Ocular (macular scarring, focal pigmentary retinal mottling, optic nerve atrophy/hypoplasia) Congenital contractures Neurological impairments: Early hyperactivity/spasticity, motor and cognitive disabilities, swallowing dysfunction, vision and hearing impairment, excessive crying, epilepsy No hepatomegaly, rash, and hematologic, renal, or hepatic abnormalities	Vision screening including ABR test. Monitor growth parameters and physical and intellectual development. Monitor for difficulty breathing and swallowing. Monitor for hydrocephaly. Keep updated via the CDC website. Referral for multidisciplinary care in medical home environment.
Chlamydia Trachomatis		
Acquired during passage through birth canal.	Assess for perinatal history of preterm birth. Symptomatic newborns present with pneumonia; chlamydial conjunctivitis presents with inflammation, yellow discharge, and eyelid swelling 5 to 14 days after birth Assess for chronic follicular conjunctivitis (corneal neovascularization and conjunctival scarring).	Treat chlamydial conjunctivitis or pneumonia with oral erythromycin for 14 days (Eichenwald et al., 2017). Monitor for hypertrophic pyloric stenosis. Initiate follow-up referral for eye complications and late development of pneumonia at 4–11 weeks postnatally.

Health Promotion Preventing Newborn Infections

The following measures will help to prevent newborn infections.

During the prenatal period:

- Group B strep swab between 35 and 37 weeks' gestation.
- Conduct maternal screening and treatment for sexually transmitted infections (STIs).
- Monitor rubella titers in women who test negative.

During the intrapartum period:

- Sterile technique is essential.
- Visual exam of any lesions should be reported on the labor and birth record to identify a patient with herpes; a cesarean section is the recommended birth process if any active lesions are identified.
- Placental and amniotic fluid cultures are obtained if maternal infection is suspected.
- Prenatal prophylactic antibiotic therapy for asymptomatic women who test positive for GBS helps prevent early-onset sepsis and has shown a decrease in clinical neonatal sepsis rates (Stoll, 2016).

During the postpartum period:

- Local eye treatment with an antibiotic ophthalmic ointment is given to all newborns to prevent damage from gonococcal infections (occurring 3 days following birth) and the possibility of chlamydial infection (occurring 7 to 10 days after birth).
- Sterile technique at all times with central lines, including when changing fluids.
- Education of parents and visitors on adequate hand hygiene.

CLINICAL THERAPY

Newborns with a history of possible exposure to infection in utero (e.g., PROM more than 24 hours before birth or questionable maternal history of infection, maternal fever, chorioamnionitis, or high-risk behavior [such as multiple sexual partners or illicit drug use]) should have cultures taken as soon as possible once concern for infection presents. Cultures are obtained before antibiotic therapy is begun (Bennett, 2017; Polin & Committee on the Fetus and Newborn, 2012):

1. Anaerobic and aerobic blood culture is taken from a peripheral site or umbilical vessel. The skin or the hub of the catheter is prepared by cleaning with a unit-specified antiseptic solution and allowed to dry; the specimen is obtained with a sterile needle/syringe. Correct sterile technique will lessen the likelihood of contamination.
2. Spinal fluid culture is done following a spinal tap/lumbar puncture if there are concerns about CNS symptoms/pathology. The fluid can be analyzed for cell count, cell smear, culture and Gram stain, as well as for viral presence.
3. The specimen for urine culture is best obtained by a suprapubic bladder aspiration or sterile catheterization.
4. Skin or mucus membrane cultures are taken of any lesions or drainage from lesions or reddened areas.
5. Tracheal aspirate cultures, if intubated, may be obtained.
6. Placental cultures and pathology may be helpful.

Other laboratory investigations include a complete blood count (CBC), C-reactive protein (CRP), procalcitonin (PCT), chest X-ray examination, serology, and Gram stains of cerebrospinal fluid, urine, skin exudate, and umbilicus. White blood cell (WBC) count with differential may indicate the presence or absence of sepsis. A level of 30,000 to 40,000 mm^3 WBC may be normal in the first 24 hours of life, whereas low WBC (less than 5000 to 7500/mm^3) may be indicative of sepsis. A low neutrophil count and high band (immature white cell) count can indicate that an infection is present. CRP, an acute-phase reactant protein synthesized in response to inflammation, is generally reflective of maternal inflammatory response until 12 to 24 hours after delivery. Other inflammatory responses may cause an elevation in the CRP, so it should not be used as the only indicator of infection. A CRP in combination with a CBC may be helpful in watching for improvement once antibiotic therapy is initiated or for determining length of therapy (Beltempo, Veil-Theriault, Thibeault, et al., 2018). PCT is used as a biomarker for the diagnosis of sepsis. It is most diagnostic in newborns, with high specificity and sensitivity for septicemia, as it rises in the first 48 hours, but it is not always readily available in laboratories (Hasan, Khan, Maharoof, et al., 2017).

Serum IgM levels are elevated (normal level less than 20 mg/dL) in response to transplacental infections. If available, counterimmunoelectrophoresis tests for specific bacterial antigens are performed. Repetitive sequence-based polymerase chain reactions (rep-PCR) can be used to identify specific infectious organisms within hours instead of days. Evidence of congenital infections may be seen on skull x-rays, ultrasound, or CT scans for cerebral calcifications (cytomegalovirus or toxoplasmosis), on bone x-rays (syphilis or cytomegalovirus), and in serum-specific IgM levels (rubella). Cytomegalovirus infection is best diagnosed by buccal swab or urine protein:creatinine ratio (PCR), and should be checked if a hearing screen has failed on a growth-restricted newborn or in the presence of low platelet count. A newborn exposed to maternal viral illness can have significant lifelong difficulties and may receive special services in many states if documented.

Neonatal infection often correlates with high mortality, therefore therapy is instituted while the sepsis workup is ongoing. A combination of two broad-spectrum antibiotics, such as ampicillin and gentamicin, is given in large doses until a culture with sensitivities results is obtained.

After the pathogen and its sensitivities are determined, appropriate specific antibiotic therapy is begun. Rotating aminoglycosides has been suggested to prevent development of resistance. Use of cephalosporins and, in particular, cefotaxime has emerged as an alternative to aminoglycoside therapy in the treatment of neonatal infections for infants 1 to 3 months of age. For newborns, third-generation cephalosporins are not currently recommended as single-agent therapy (Schrag et al., 2016). Duration of therapy varies from 7 to 14 days unless meningitis is suspected and then a longer course of therapy will be necessary (Table 31–6). However, if cultures are negative and symptoms subside, antibiotics may be discontinued after 2 days/48 hours of negative blood cultures. A normal CRP at 24 to 48 hours also supports discontinuing antibiotics if clinical presentation improves and blood cultures are negative. Supportive physiologic care may be required to maintain respiratory, hemodynamic, nutritional, and metabolic homeostasis.

TABLE 31–6 Neonatal Sepsis Antibiotic/Antiviral Therapy

DRUG	DOSE (MG/KG) TOTAL DAILY DOSE	SCHEDULE FOR DIVIDED DOSES	ROUTE	COMMENTS
Acyclovir (Zovirax)	20 mg/kg	q 8 hr	IV	Length of treatment is 14 days for skin/eye/mouth (SEM) or 21 days for CNS and disseminated disease, *herpes simplex virus*
Ampicillin	25–50 mg/kg/dose (100 mg/kg/dose if treating meningitis and severe group B streptococcal sepsis)	q 12 hr* q 8 hr† q 6 hr**	IM or IV	Effective against Gram-positive microorganisms, *Listeria*, and most *Escherichia coli* strains; higher doses indicated for meningitis; used with aminoglycoside for synergy
Cefotaxime	50 mg/kg/dose (25 mg/kg/dose gonococcal infection)	q 12 hr* q 8 hr q 6 hr**	IM or IV	Active against most major pathogens in babies; effective against aminoglycoside-resistant organisms; achieves CSF bactericidal activity; lack of ototoxicity and nephrotoxicity; wide therapeutic index (levels not required); resistant organisms can develop rapidly if used extensively; ineffective against *Pseudomonas*, *Listeria*
Gentamicin	4–5 mg/kg/dose 4–5 mg/kg/dose (first week of life)	q 24–48 hr‡*** q 24–48 hr	IM or IV	Effective against Gram-negative rods and staphylococci; may be used instead of kanamycin against penicillin-resistant staphylococci and *E. coli* strains and *Pseudomonas aeruginosa*. May cause neurotoxicity, ototoxicity, and nephrotoxicity. Need to follow serum levels. Must never be given as IV push. Must be given over at least 30–60 minutes. In presence of oliguria or anuria, dose must be decreased or discontinued. In newborns less than 1000 g (2.2 lb) or 29 weeks, lower dosage to 2.5–3 mg/kg/day. Monitor serum levels before administration of second dose. Peak: 5–10 mcg/mL Trough: 1–2 mcg/mL
Vancomycin	10–20 mg/kg 30 mg/kg/day	q 12–24 hr*‡ q 8 hr†	IV	Effective for methicillin-resistant strains (*Staphylococcus epidermidis*); must be administered by slow IV infusion to avoid prolonged cutaneous eruption. For smaller newborns (less than 1200 g [2.7 lb], less than 29 weeks), smaller dosages and longer intervals between doses. Nephrotoxic, especially in combination with aminoglycosides. Slow IV infusion over at least 60 minutes. Peak: 25–40 mcg/mL Trough: 5–10 mcg/Ml

* Up to 7 days of age.

** Greater than 45 weeks postmenstrual age.

† Greater than 7 days of age.

‡ Dependent on gestational age.

*** Dependent on postnatal age.

●○● NURSING MANAGEMENT

For the Newborn with Infection

Nursing Assessment and Diagnosis

Symptoms of infection are most often noticed by the nurse during daily care of the newborn. The newborn may deteriorate rapidly in the first 4 to 6 hours after birth if β-hemolytic streptococcal infection is present, with signs and symptoms mimicking RDS. In other cases, the onset of sepsis may be gradual, with more subtle signs and symptoms. The most common symptoms include:

- Subtle behavioral changes—the baby "isn't doing well," the mother states. "Something isn't right with my baby." The newborn is often lethargic or irritable (especially after the first 24 hours), hypotonic, and hypotensive. Color changes may include pallor, duskiness, cyanosis, or a "shocky" appearance. The skin may be cool, mottled, and clammy.
- Temperature instability, manifested most commonly by hypothermia (recognized by a decrease in skin temperature) or, rarely in newborns, hyperthermia (elevation of skin temperature), necessitates a corresponding increase or decrease in incubator temperature to maintain a neutral thermal environment.
- Feeding intolerance is evidenced by a decrease in total intake, an increase in residuals if NG tube feeding is used, abdominal distention, vomiting, poor sucking, lack of interest in feeding, and diarrhea.

- Hyperbilirubinemia, petechial hemorrhages, hepatosplenomegaly.
- Tachycardia initially, followed by spells of apnea/bradycardia.

Signs and symptoms may suggest CNS disease (jitteriness, tremors, seizure activity). A differential diagnosis is necessary because of the similarity of symptoms to other, more specific conditions.

Nursing diagnoses that may apply to the newborn with suspected sepsis neonatorum and the family include:

- ***Infection, Risk for***, related to newborn's immature immunologic system
- ***Fluid Volume: Deficient***, related to feeding intolerance
- ***Coping: Family, Compromised***, related to present illness resulting in prolonged hospital stay for the newborn

(NANDA-I © 2017)

Nursing Plan and Implementation

In the nursery, controlling the environment and preventing acquired infection are the responsibilities of the neonatal nurse. An infected newborn can be isolated effectively in an isolette and receive close observation. Promote strict handwashing technique for all who enter the nursery, including nursing colleagues; physicians; laboratory, x-ray, and respiratory therapists; and parents. Visits to the nursery area by unnecessary personnel should be discouraged. Assist in the aseptic collection of specimens for laboratory tests. Scrupulous care of equipment—changing and cleaning incubators at least every 3 to 7 days, removing and sterilizing wet equipment every 24 hours, preventing cross-use of linens and other equipment, cleaning sink-side equipment such as soap containers periodically, and taking special care with open radiant warmers (access without prior handwashing is much more likely to occur than with the closed incubator)—will prevent contamination.

Administration of Antibiotic Therapy

Administer antibiotics as ordered by the healthcare provider. Knowledge of the following is critical:

- The proper dose to be administered, based on the weight of the newborn and desired peak and trough levels
- The appropriate route, method, and timing of administration
- Admixture incompatibilities; some antibiotics precipitate in IV solutions when mixed with other antibiotics
- Side effects and signs of toxicity.

Provision of Supportive Care

In addition to antibiotic therapy, physiologic supportive care is essential in caring for a septic newborn. These actions should be carried out:

- Observe for resolution of symptoms or development of other symptoms of sepsis.
- Maintain a neutral thermal environment with accurate regulation of humidity and oxygen administration.
- Provide respiratory support: Administer oxygen and observe and monitor respiratory effort.
- Provide cardiovascular support: Observe and monitor pulse and blood pressure; observe for hyperbilirubinemia, anemia, and hemorrhagic symptoms.
- Provide adequate calories by IV or OG, if needed, because oral feedings may be discontinued due to increased mucus, abdominal distention, vomiting, or aspiration.
- Provide fluids and electrolytes to maintain homeostasis. Monitor weight changes, urine output, and urine specific gravity.
- Observe for the development of hypoglycemia, hyperglycemia, acidosis, hyponatremia, and hypocalcemia.

Restricting parental visits has not been shown to have any effect on the rate of infection and may be harmful to the newborn's psychologic development. With instruction and guidance from the nursing staff, both parents should be allowed to handle the baby and participate in daily care. Support of the parents is crucial. They need to be informed of the newborn's prognosis as treatment continues and to be involved in care as much as possible. They also need to understand how infection is transmitted.

Evaluation

Expected outcomes of nursing care include:

- The risks for development of sepsis are identified early, and immediate action is taken to minimize the development of the illness.
- Appropriate use of aseptic technique protects the newborn from further exposure to illness.
- The baby's symptoms are relieved, and the infection is treated.
- The parents verbalize their concerns about their newborn's illness and understand the rationale behind the management of their baby.

Care of the Family with Birth of an At-Risk Newborn

The birth of a newborn who is preterm or ill or has a congenital anomaly is an unanticipated event that can quickly launch a family into an altered state of function. Throughout the pregnancy, both parents, together and separately, have felt excitement, experienced thoughts of acceptance, and pictured how their baby would look and act. Both parents have wished for a perfect baby and may or may not have imagined a damaged, unhealthy one. Janvier et al. (2016) was written by a group of healthcare professionals that works daily in the NICU, and each contributor also had the experience of having a loved one in the NICU. They put words to this stressful experience in a firsthand way that also balances their knowledge as healthcare providers. They describe the event as being psychologically traumatic and anxiety provoking, and they report experiencing insomnia and feelings of being out of control (Janvier et al., 2016)

Parental Responses

Family members have acute grief reactions to the loss of the idealized baby they have envisioned. In a preterm birth, the mother is denied the last few weeks of pregnancy that seem to prepare her psychologically for the stress of birth and the attachment process. Attachment at this time is fragile, and interruption of the process by separation can affect the future mother–child relationship. Parents express grief as shock and disbelief, denial of reality, anger toward self and others, guilt, blame, and concern for the future. Self-esteem and feelings of self-worth are jeopardized (Janvier et al., 2016).

Feelings of guilt and failure often plague mothers of preterm newborns. They may ask themselves, "Why did labor start? What did I do (or not do)?" A woman may have guilt fantasies and wonder what she may have done to cause the early labor: "Was it because I had sex with my husband [a week, 3 days, a day] ago?" "Was it because I carried three loads of laundry up from the basement?" "Am I being punished for something I did in the past—even in childhood?"

The period of waiting between suspicion and confirmation of abnormality or dysfunction is a very anxious one for parents because it is difficult, if not impossible, to begin attachment to the baby if the newborn's future is questionable. During the waiting period, parents need support and acknowledgment that this is an anxious time. When results become available, the best approach is to tell both parents about the diagnosis at the same time and with the baby present. By first pointing out the positives, a caregiver shows acceptance of the baby as a person and a loved one of the family. An honest discussion of the diagnosis and anticipatory management at the earliest possible time by healthcare professionals can help the parents (1) initiate bonding with the newborn as the primary caregivers and decision makers, (2) maintain trust in the physician and nurse, (3) appreciate the reality of the situation by dispelling fantasy and misconception, (4) begin the grieving and eventual acceptance process, and (5) mobilize internal and external support.

Nurses need to be aware that anger can be, as one of the stages of grief, a normal response and that it is best directed outward. Anger, aggression, hostility, and irritability may be exhibited and directed unjustifiably at the physician and/or nurse, at the food, at nursing care, or at hospital regulations and routines (Janvier et al., 2016). Parents rarely show anger with the baby, and such responses can precipitate guilt feelings. Perceived maternal stress may be lessened if information is provided regarding preterm behavioral cues. This empowers the mother and allows her to better care for her child. Mothers of preterm newborns who have to spend time in the NICU suffer from psychologic distress similar to posttraumatic stress disorder (PTSD) (Janvier et al., 2016). Nurses working with mothers in the NICU setting have the opportunity to encourage maternal competence and confidence, both during and after hospitalization, by teaching interpretation of their child's behavioral cues, prompting maternal care of the baby while in the NICU, and facilitating expression of their feeling (for more detailed discussion of PTSD, see Chapter 35).

Solnit and Stark (1961) postulated that grief and mourning of the loss of the loved object—the idealized child—mark parental reactions to a newborn with abnormalities. *Grief work*, the emotional reaction to significant loss, must occur before adequate attachment to the actual baby is possible. Parental detachment precedes parental attachment. The parents must first grieve the loss of the wished-for perfect child, if they haven't already after learning the prenatal diagnosis, and then adopt the imperfect child as the new love object.

Some degree of postpartum depression occurs in new mothers up to 15% of the time, and rates can be as high as 32 to 63% in mothers with babies in the NICU. Depression in mothers and family members can have a negative impact on their ability to bond with the baby as well as on family dynamics. Although reactions and steps of attachment are altered by the birth of these newborns, a healthy parent–child relationship can occur. Other relationships may suffer, however, if the challenges are not approached as a family (Janvier et al., 2016).

Developmental Consequences

The baby born prematurely or with illness, malformation, or disorder is at risk for emotional, intellectual, and cognitive development delays. The risk is directly proportional to the seriousness of the problem and the length of treatment. The necessary physical separation of family and newborn and the tremendous emotional and financial burdens adversely affect the parent–child relationship. The recent trend to involve the parents with the newborn early, repeatedly, and over protracted periods of time through family-centered care has done much to facilitate positive parent–child relationships, as well as positive relationships with the caregivers (Janvier et al., 2016).

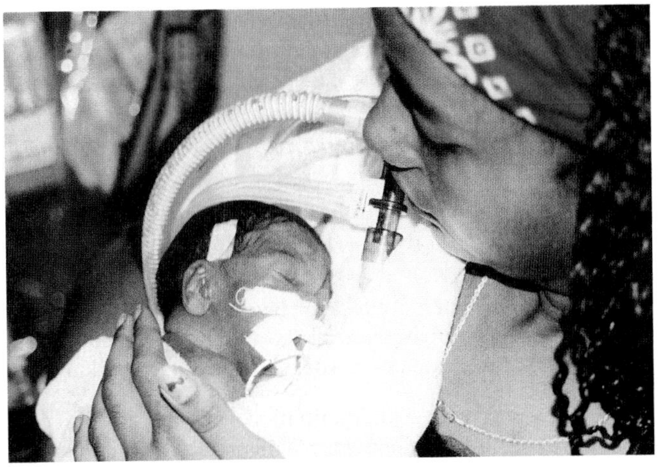

Figure 31–18 Mother of a 26-week gestational age newborn with respiratory distress syndrome on a ventilator is getting acquainted with her baby. Physical contact is vital to the bonding process and should be encouraged whenever possible.

The parents must have a clear picture of the reality of the disability and the types of developmental hurdles ahead. Unexpected behaviors and responses from the newborn because of the problem or disorder can be upsetting and frightening. The demands of care for the child and disputes regarding management or behavior stress family relationships. The entire interprofessional care team may need to pool their resources and expertise to help parents of children born with problems or disorders so that both parents and children can thrive. Daily involvement of the parents in rounds can be a valuable tool to enhance their feelings of inclusion in the care and decision-making process of their newborn in the NICU.

Early and continued involvement may only mean opportunities to look at or touch the newborn (Figure 31–18). Later, when the mother's and newborn's conditions warrant it, the parents should participate in the baby's care (to the extent they are willing) and in planning for the future. This type of involvement facilitates early bonding, attachment, and emotional investment (O'Brien et al., 2015; Zaichkin, Weiner, & Loren, 2017). The parents need a sense of personal success, self-worth, self-esteem, and confidence from the knowledge that they can cope with the situation.

●○● NURSING MANAGEMENT

For the Family of an At-Risk Newborn

Nursing Assessment and Diagnosis

A concurrent illness of the mother or other family members or other concurrent stress (lack of health insurance, loss of job, age of parents) may change the family response to the newborn. Feelings of apprehension, guilt, failure, and grief that are verbally or nonverbally expressed are important aspects of the nursing history. These observations enable all professionals to be aware of the parental state, coping behaviors, and readiness for attachment, bonding, and caretaking. Appropriate nursing assessments during interviewing and relating to the family include:

1. **Level of understanding.** Observations concerning the family's ability to assimilate information given and to ask appropriate questions; the need for constant repetition of information.
2. **Behavioral responses.** Appropriateness of behavior in relation to information given; lack of response; flat affect.
3. **Difficulties with communication.** Deafness (reads lips only); blindness; dysphasia; understanding only a non-English language.
4. **Paternal and maternal education level.** Parents who are unable to read or write; parents with eighth-grade-level education; parents with a graduate-level degree or healthcare background.

Documentation of such information, gathered through continuing contact and development of a therapeutic family relationship, allows all professionals to understand and use the nursing history to provide continuous individualized care.

A record of visits, caretaking procedures, affect (in relating to the newborn), and telephone calls indicate the level or lack of parental attachment. Serial observations, rather than just isolated observations that cause concern, must be obtained. Grant (1978) developed a conceptual framework depicting adaptive and maladaptive responses to parenting of a preterm or less-than-perfect baby (Table 31–7).

If a pattern of distancing behaviors evolves, institute appropriate interventions such as social work assistance, counseling, or even child protective services (CPS) involvement if there are significant concerns for safety. Follow-up studies have found that a statistically significant number of preterm, sick, and congenitally defective newborns suffer from failure to thrive, battering, or other disorders of parenting. Early detection and intervention may prevent these aberrations in parenting behaviors from leading to irreparable damage or death.

Nursing diagnoses that may apply to the family of a newborn at risk include:

- *Grieving, Complicated*, related to loss of idealized newborn
- *Fear* related to emotional involvement with an at-risk newborn
- *Parenting, Impaired*, related to impaired bonding secondary to feelings of inadequacy about caretaking activities

(NANDA-I © 2017)

Nursing Plan and Implementation

Hospital-Based Nursing Care

In their sensitive and vulnerable state, parents are acutely perceptive about others' responses and reactions (particularly nonverbal) to the child. Parents can be expected to identify with the responses of others. Therefore, it is imperative that medical and nursing staff be fully aware of the parents' feelings and come to terms with their own feelings so that they are comfortable and at ease with the newborn and the grieving family.

Nurses may feel uncomfortable, not know what to say to parents, or may fear confronting their own feelings as well as those of the parents. Each nurse must work out personal reactions with instructors, peers, clergy, parents, or significant others.

TABLE 31–7 Adaptive and Nonadaptive Parental Responses to a Newborn's Health Crisis

Parental tasks at this time include:

- Understanding the newborn's medical condition and needs
- Adapting to the NICU environment
- Assuming the main caretaking role
- Taking responsibility for the baby after discharge
- Coping with the death of the baby

Adaptive Responses	Nonadaptive Responses
• Frequent visits to baby and calls to the unit	• Failure to visit baby or communicate with unit
• Emotional involvement with baby	• Emotional withdrawal from baby
• Positive interaction with baby during hospitalization	• Lack of interaction with baby during hospitalization
• Eagerness to assume caretaking during baby's hospitalization	• Resistance to providing care of the baby during hospitalization
• Increasing sense of parental competence	• Lack of a sense of parental competence
• Growing attachment to baby	• Failure to achieve attachment to baby
• Realistic interpretation of medical information	• Inability to understand or accept medical information
• Acceptance of baby's condition	• Unhealthy preoccupation with baby's condition
• Understanding of the causes of baby's condition	• Blaming others for baby's condition
• Eagerness to assume total responsibility for baby	• Fear of going home with baby
• Realistic understanding of baby's needs at discharge	• Negative view of baby and his or her needs at discharge
• Open discussion of concerns and needs to staff and family	• Inability to discuss needs and concerns with staff and family
• Fair and realistic expectations of staff	• Distrustful and hostile attitude toward staff
Positive Outcome	**Negative Outcome**
• Healthy parent–child relationship	• Poor parent–child relationship
• Marital and family equilibrium is maintained	• Failure to thrive
	• Vulnerable child syndrome
	• Marital and family equilibrium is compromised

Source: Data from Grant, 1978.

It is helpful to have a stockpile of therapeutic questions and statements to initiate meaningful dialog with parents. Opening statements can be as follows:

"You must be wondering what could have caused this."

"This environment feels really overwhelming to many parents. Is there anything that you have questions about?"

"How can I help?"

"What tools do you and your family have to help you manage?"

Avoid statements such as:

"It could have been worse."

"It's God's will."

"You have other children."

"You are still young and can have more."

"I understand how you feel."

Always remember that grief is individual and this child and this situation are important now.

Support of Parents in Initial Viewing of the Newborn

In preparation for the first visit to the NICU, present the parents with a positive, realistic attitude regarding the newborn. An overly negative, fatalistic attitude further alienates the parents from their baby and represses attachment behaviors. Instead of beginning to bond with their child, the parents will anticipate their loss and the process of grieving. Once started, this process is very difficult to reverse.

Before preparing parents for the first view of their newborn, observe the baby. All babies exhibit strengths as well as deficiencies; prepare the parents to see both the deviations and the normal aspects of their baby. You might say something like this: *"Your baby is small, about the length of my two hands. She weighs 2 lb 3 oz but is very active and cries when we disturb her. She is having some difficulty breathing but is breathing without assistance and in only 35% oxygen and room air is 21%."*

Many NICUs have booklets for parents to read before entering the unit. Through explanations and pictures, the parents can be better prepared to deal with the feelings they may experience when they see their baby for the first time (Figure 31–19). Describe the equipment being used for the at-risk newborn and its purpose before entering the unit.

Upon entering the unit, parents may be overwhelmed by the sounds of monitors, alarms, and respirators, as well as by the unfamiliar language and "foreign" atmosphere. Preparing the parents by having the same healthcare professional(s) accompany them to the unit can be reassuring. The primary nurse and physician caring for the newborn should be with the parents when they first visit the baby. Parental reactions vary, but there is usually an element of initial shock. Providing them with chairs and time to regain composure will assist the parents. Slow, complete, and simple explanations—first about the baby and then about the equipment—allay fear and anxiety.

Concern about the baby's physical appearance is common, yet may remain unvoiced. Parents may express such concerns as, *"He looks so small and red—like a drowned rat." "Why do her genitals look so abnormal?" "Will that awful-looking mouth* [cleft lip and palate] *ever be normal?"* Such questions need to be anticipated and addressed. Use of pictures, such as a photo of a baby after cleft lip repair, may be reassuring to doubting parents. Knowledge of the development of a "normal" preterm baby will allow you to make reassuring statements such as, *"The baby's skin may look very red and transparent with lots of visible veins, but it is normal for her maturity. As she grows, subcutaneous fat will be laid down, and these superficial veins will begin to disappear."*

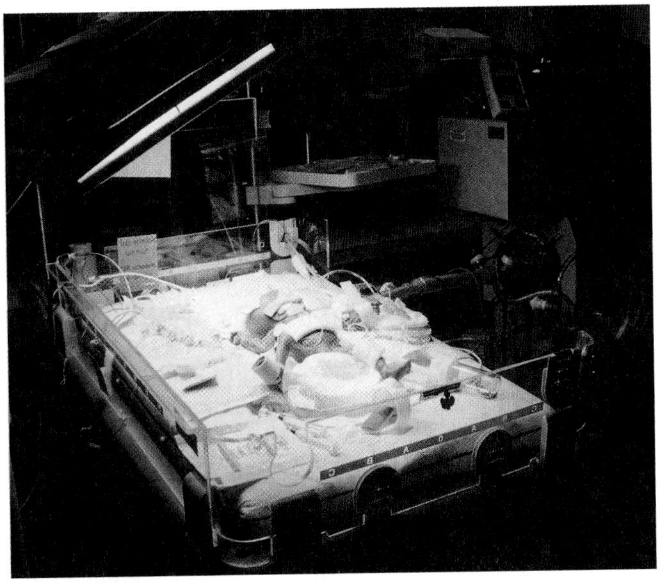

Figure 31–19 **This 25-week gestational age newborn with respiratory distress syndrome may be frightening for her parents to see for the first time because of the technology that is attached to her.**

The nursing staff sets the tone of the NICU. Nurses foster the development of a safe, trusting environment by viewing the parents as essential caregivers, not as visitors or nuisances in the unit. It is important to provide parents privacy when needed and easy access to staff and facilities. An uncrowded and welcoming atmosphere lets parents know, "You are welcome here." However, even in crowded physical surroundings, it is possible to convey an attitude of openness and trust.

A trusting relationship is essential for collaborative efforts in caring for the newborn. Use your responses therapeutically to relate to the parents on a one-to-one basis. Each individual has different needs, different ways of adapting to crises, and different means of support. Professionals must use techniques that are real and spontaneous to them and avoid adopting words or actions that are foreign to them. Gauge your interventions to match the parents' pace and needs.

Implementation of family-centered care—a collaborative care team approach with healthcare professionals and the family, in which the mother, father or partner, and other family members are vital elements of the team—is important to bonding and development of the family (Stevens, Munson, & Khan, 2016). It is important to show concern and support by planning time to spend with the parents, by being psychologically as well as physically present, by encouraging open discussion and grieving, by repetitious explanations (as necessary), by providing privacy as needed, and by encouraging contact with the newborn. Identifying and clarifying feelings and fears decrease distortions in perception, thinking, and feeling. The NICU nurse is in an important position to assess the mother for perinatal depression and recommend the introduction of services or interventions. When you provide meticulous care to the newborn, talk and coo (especially in the face-to-face position) while holding or providing care to the newborn, and relate the newborn's activities (*"He took a whole ounce of formula"* or *"She took hold of the blanket and just wouldn't let go"*), you invest the baby with value in the eyes of the parents. Note the "normal" characteristics and capabilities of each newborn as well as the newborn's needs. Learn the baby's name and refer to him or her by name. When the newborn is physiologically stable and of an appropriate weight, allowing the baby to be dressed in clothes has been determined to aid the mother's perception of the baby as a "person" or "actual baby."

Facilitation of Attachment if Neonatal Transport Occurs

Transport to a regional referral center some distance from the parents' community may be necessary. It is essential that the mother see and touch her newborn before the baby is transported. Bringing the mother to the nursery or taking the baby in a warmed transport incubator to the mother's bedside will allow her to see the baby before transportation to the center. When the newborn reaches the referral center, a staff member should call the parents with information about the baby's condition during transport, safe arrival at the center, and present condition.

Support of parents, with explanations from the professional staff, is crucial. Occasionally, the mother may be unable to see the baby before transport, for example, if she is still under general anesthesia or experiencing postpartum complications such as shock, hemorrhage, or seizures. In these cases, photographs of the baby can be provided to give the mother a visual explanation of the baby's condition and problems and a detailed image of the baby's characteristics to facilitate the attachment process until the mother can visit. An additional photograph is also helpful for the father/partner to share with siblings or extended family. If the mother is hospitalized apart from the newborn, the first person to visit the baby should relay information regarding the baby's care and condition to the mother and family. Because the mother has had minimal contact, if any, with her baby she may mistrust all those who provide information (the father/partner, nurse, physician, or extended family) until she sees the baby for herself. This can put tremendous stress on the relationship between spouses and family members.

With the increased attention to improved fetal outcome, prenatal maternal transports, rather than neonatal transports, are occurring more frequently. This practice gives the mother of an at-risk newborn the opportunity to visit and care for her baby in the same facility during the early postpartum period.

Promotion of Touching and Parental Caretaking

Parents visiting a small or sick newborn may need several visits to become comfortable and confident in their abilities to touch the baby without causing injury. Barriers such as incubators, incisions, monitor electrodes, and tubes may delay the mother's development of comfort in touching the newborn.

The premature baby's brain response to gentle touch is different from full-term newborns and can affect how the brain will continue to develop (Maitre et al., 2017). Neurodevelopment relies on gentle touch, which is the cornerstone of interpersonal interactions and sensory-cognitive development. Klaus and Kennell (1982) found a significant difference in the amount of eye contact and touching behaviors of mothers of normal newborns and mothers of preterm newborns. Whereas mothers of normal newborns progress within minutes to palm contact of the baby's trunk, the mother of a preterm newborn is slower to progress from fingertip to palm contact and from the extremities to the trunk. The progression to palm contact with the baby's trunk may take several visits to the nursery.

Through use of support, reassurance, and encouragement, you can facilitate the mother's positive feelings about her ability and her importance to her newborn. Touching facilitates "getting to know" the baby and thus establishes a bond with the baby. Touching as well as seeing the newborn helps the mother to realize the "normals" and potentials of her baby (Figure 31–20).

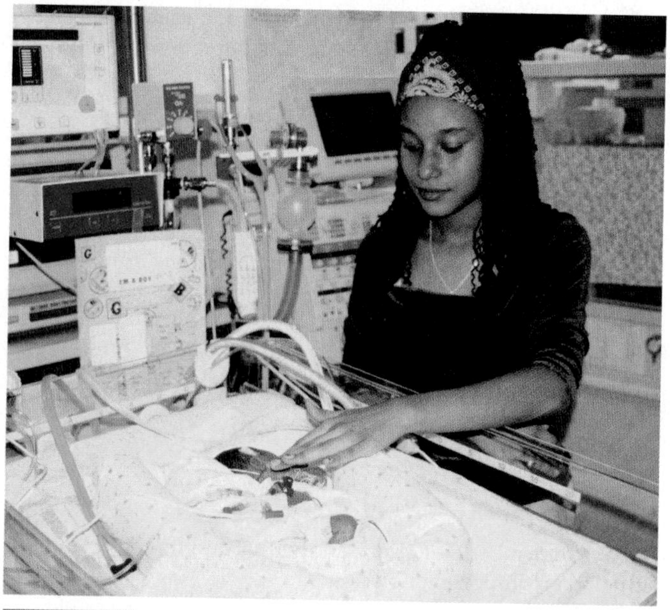

Figure 31–20 Mother of this 26-week gestational age 600 g (1.3 lb) baby begins attachment through fingertip touch.

Encourage parents to meet their newborn's need for stimulation. Touching, rocking, cuddling, singing, and talking should be an integral part of the parents' caretaking responsibilities when tolerated by their newborn. Bonding can be facilitated by encouraging parents to visit and become involved in their baby's care (Figure 31–21). Skin-to-skin contact (kangaroo care), usually between the mother, father/partner, or surrogate (another person instead of the parents) and the neonate, was first introduced over 40 years ago. Kangaroo care is now utilized to enhance bonding and impacts positively in both the behavior and physiology of the newborn (AAP & ACOG, 2017). Something as simple as softly reading a book, singing a song, or using hands for gentle containment for the baby can help during this time. When visiting is impossible, the parents should feel free to phone whenever they wish to receive an update on their newborn. Showing a warm, receptive attitude provides support. Facilitate parenting by personalizing a baby to the parents, by referring to the baby by name, or by relating personal behavioral characteristics.

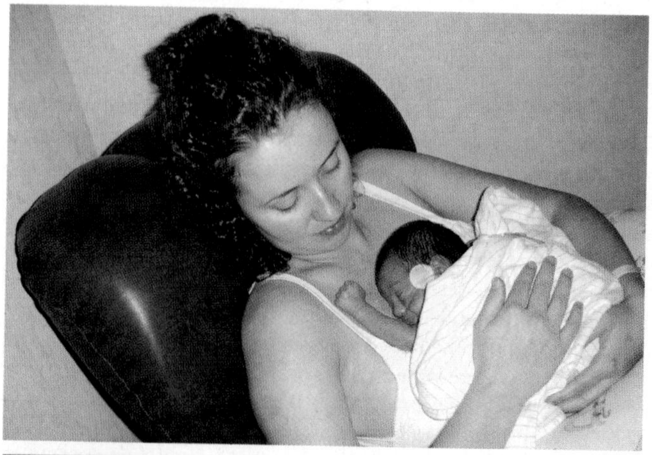

Figure 31–21 This mother of a 31-week gestational age newborn with respiratory distress syndrome is spending time with her newborn and meeting the baby's need for cuddling. This is an example of kangaroo care.

Statements such as, *"Jenny loves her pacifier,"* help make the baby seem individual and unique.

The variety of equipment needed for life support is hardly conducive to anxiety-free caretaking by the parents. However, even the sickest newborn may be cared for, if only in a small way, by the parents. Incorporating the family into the plan of care is beneficial and should promote the parents' success (AAP & ACOG, 2017). Demonstration and explanation, followed by support of the parents in initial caretaking behaviors, positively reinforce this behavior. Changing the baby's diaper, taking a temperature, giving their baby skin care or oral care, or helping to turn the baby may at first be anxiety provoking for the parents, but confidence in caretaking and bonding between parents and newborn is enhanced (Janvier et al., 2016). Cues that the parents are ready to become involved with the child's care include their reference to the baby by name and their questioning as to amount of feeding taken, sleeping patterns, appearance today, and the like. Simple inclusion of the parents in providing comfort care for their baby is an early step in transferring care from the medical staff to the parents (Feeley, Genest, Niela-Vilén, et al., 2016; Janvier et al., 2016). Another way of inclusion is to request input on critical care decision making by "providing options" rather than "making recommendations" (Shaw, Stokoe, Gallagher, et al., 2016).

> "Being the parent of a NICU patient is overwhelming. I found what helped me remember and comprehend things was to keep a paper and pen close to me. I wrote everything down. I was stressed and hormonal and couldn't remember everything I was told or even understand some of the words used. I would take notes and then ask questions. If someone doesn't explain well enough to you, or you still don't understand, ask someone else again. The NICU world was all new to me and everyone was so patient to explain things to me."
>
> —Nicole Peterson, mother of 28-week newborn

Sometimes parents of high-risk newborns have ambivalent feelings toward the healthcare team. These feelings may take the form of criticism of the care of the baby, manipulation of staff, or personal guilt. Accept this behavior but continue to remind the parents that it is okay and natural to feel disappointment, a sense of failure, helplessness, or anger about the birth. Overprotectiveness and overoptimism are defense mechanisms. To deny the negative feelings only entrenches them further, delays their resolution, and delays realistic planning. Recognize and accept such feelings by the parents and intervene appropriately to enhance mother–newborn attachment. Encourage the family to look for areas where they are developing strength and resilience together (Janvier et al., 2016). Verbalizations that improve parental self-esteem are essential and easily shared. Point out that, in addition to physiologic use, breast milk is important because of the emotional investment of the mother. Pumping, storing, labeling, and delivering quantities of breast milk is time-consuming and a "labor of love" for mothers. Positive remarks regarding breast milk reinforce the maternal behavior of caretaking and providing for her baby: *"Breast milk is something that only you can give your baby"* or *"You really have brought a lot of milk today"* or *"Every drop of milk is important, and look how rich it is."*

If the newborn begins to gain weight while being fed breast milk, it is important to point this correlation out to the mother. Parents should also be advised that initial weight loss with beginning nipple feedings is common because of the increased energy expended when the baby begins active rather than passive nutritional intake.

During quiet time it may help to encourage the parents to talk about their hopes and fears and to facilitate their involvement in parent groups. Encourage parents to provide care for their newborn even if the baby is very sick and likely to die. Detachment is easier after attachment because the parents are comforted by the knowledge that they did all they could for their child while he or she was alive.

Facilitation of Family Adjustment

During crisis, maintaining close interpersonal relationships is difficult. Yet in a newborn intensive care area, the parents are expected to relate to many different care providers. It is important that parents have as few professionals as possible relaying information to them. A primary nurse should coordinate and provide continuity for parents. Care providers are individuals and thus will use different terms, inflections, and attitudes. These subtle differences are monumental to parents and only confuse, confound, and produce anxiety. The transfer of the baby from the NICU to a step-down unit or a "regular nursery" or transport back to the home hospital is very anxiety producing for the parents because they must now deal with new healthcare professionals. They may feel that their newborn is not being cared for as proficiently because the nurses are not at the bedside as often as they were in the NICU. The nurse functions as a fulcrum of sorts by supporting the parents, advocating for the newborn and the parents, and coordinating between many different disciplines in the medical field.

Encourage the parents to deal with the crisis with help from their support system. The support system attempts to meet the emotional needs and provide support for the family members in crisis and stress situations. Biologic kinship is not the only valid criterion for a support system; an emotional kinship is the most important factor. In our mobile society of isolated nuclear families, the support system may be a next-door neighbor, a best friend, or perhaps a schoolmate. You may have to search out the significant people in the lives of the parents and help them understand the problems so that they can support the parents.

The impact of the crisis on the family is individual and varied. You can obtain information about the couple's ability to adapt to the situation through the relationship with the family. To institute appropriate interventions, try to view the birth of the newborn (normal newborn, preterm newborn, or newborn with illness or congenital anomaly) as defined by the family. Because the family is a unit composed of individuals who must deal with the situation, it is important to encourage open, intrafamily communication. Discourage the family from keeping secrets from one another, especially between spouses, because secrets undermine the trust of their relationship. Well-meaning rationales such as, "I want to protect her" and "I don't want him to worry about it" can be destructive to open communication and to the basic element of a relationship—trust.

The needs of siblings should not be overlooked. Siblings have been looking forward to the new baby, and they too suffer a degree of loss. Young children may react with hostility and older ones with shame at the birth of a baby with an anomaly. Both reactions make them feel guilty. Parents, preoccupied with working through their own feelings, often cannot give the other children the attention and support they need. Sometimes another child becomes the focus of family tension. Anxiety thus directed can take the form of finding fault or of overconcern. This is a form of denial; the parents cannot face the real worry—the newborn at risk. After observing and assessing the situation, you might try to see to it that another family member or friend steps in and gives the needed support to the siblings of the affected newborn. Counseling support is also valuable in this situation.

Always respect and facilitate the desires and needs of the individuals involved; differences are tolerable and should be able to exist side by side. You can easily elicit the parents' feelings and the meaning of this experience to them by asking, *"How are **you** doing?"* The emphasis is on "you," and the interest must be sincere. Taking the time to sit in their presence additionally shows an effort to take the time to listen and be empathic.

Parents from foreign cultures must deal with language barriers and cultural differences that can make feelings of isolation and uncertainty more acute. Healthcare providers have the professional responsibility to be aware of cultural needs of all patients and to ensure that their needs are met. Feelings of isolation and uncertainty influence not only the parents' emotional responses to the ill newborn, but also their use of services and their interaction with health professionals. Hospital cultural interpreter programs can assist families in interactions with staff and provide translation during family meetings, multidisciplinary family conferences, and parent support groups.

Families with children in the NICU often become friends and support one another. To encourage the development of these friendships and to provide support, many units have established parent support groups. The core of the groups consists of parents who previously have had newborns in the intensive care unit. Most groups will make contact with a new NICU family within a day or two of a baby's admission to the unit through either phone calls or visits to the hospital. Early one-on-one parent contacts are more effective than discussion groups in helping parents work through their feelings. This personalized method gives the grieving parents an opportunity to share personal feelings about the pregnancy, labor, and birth and their "different from expected" baby with others who have experienced the same feelings and with whom they can identify.

Community-Based Nursing Care

Predischarge planning begins once the newborn's condition becomes stable and it seems likely the newborn will survive. The medically fragile baby may remain vulnerable for several years (Balany & Bhandari, 2015). Discharge preparation and care conferences should involve a collaborative care team approach. NICU nursing staff plays an essential role in the transitioning of the high-risk newborn from the intensive care unit to the home. Effective open communication with the parents during the entire discharge planning phase of care empowers them to assume the role of primary caregivers for the child. Adequate predischarge teaching helps parents transform any feelings of inadequacy they may have into feelings of self-assurance and attachment.

SAFETY ALERT!

The high incidence of prematurity and low birth weight in multiple-birth babies and the corresponding risks for sudden infant death syndrome (SIDS) should be considered. As with all families at discharge, parents of multiples should be taught SIDS risk-reduction practices, which includes flat supine positioning, babies sleeping in parents' room but not co-sleeping with parents or siblings, firm bedding surface, and no loose coverings or stuffed items in the crib or bassinet.

Provide home care instructions in an optimal environment for parental learning. Learning should take place over time, to avoid the necessity of bombarding the parents with instructions in the day or hour before discharge. Teaching that occurs on the day of discharge by the NICU staff is not always perceived by the family as adequate, and the stress levels of the family while in the NICU can be a barrier to a learning environment. The involvement of the parents in daily care-giving activities and preparation for discharge starting at admission with teaching and return demonstrations help parents to learn over a period of time. Multiple return demonstrations by both parents are helpful (AAP & ACOG, 2017; Janvier et al., 2016).

Parents often enjoy doing minimal caretaking tasks with gradual expansion of their role. Many NICUs provide facilities for parents to room-in with their newborn for a few days before discharge. This allows parents a degree of independence in the care of their baby with the security of nursing help nearby. This practice is particularly helpful for anxious parents, parents who have not had the opportunity to spend extended time with their baby, or parents who will be giving complex physical care at home, such as gastrostomy feeding and care. In this way, the parents are able to interact with the staff while gradually transitioning to sole caretakers of their medically complex, high-risk newborn.

The basic elements of discharge and home care instruction include:

1. Teach parents routine well-baby care, such as bathing, taking a temperature, preparing formula, and/or breastfeeding.
2. Help parents learn to do special procedures as needed by the newborn, such as gavage or gastrostomy feedings, tracheostomy or enterostomy care, medication administration, cardiopulmonary resuscitation (CPR), and operation of an apnea monitor or any required medical equipment. Before discharge, the parents should be as comfortable as possible with these tasks and should demonstrate independence. Written tools and instructions are useful for parents to refer to once they are home with the newborn, but they should not replace actual predischarge participation in the baby's care.
3. Make sure that all applicable screening (metabolic, vision, hearing) tests, immunizations, and respiratory syncytial virus (RSV) prophylaxis are done before discharge and that all records are given to the primary care provider and parents.
4. Refer parents to community health and support organizations. The Visiting Nurses Association, public health nurses, or social services can assist the parents in the stressful transition from hospital to home by providing predischarge home visits and then the necessary home teaching and support. Some NICUs have their own parent support groups to help bridge the gap between hospital and home care. Parents can also find support from a variety of community support organizations, such as mothers of twins groups, March of Dimes Birth Defects Foundation, handicapped children services, and teen mother and child programs. Each community has numerous agencies capable of assisting the family in adapting emotionally, physically, and financially to the chronically ill newborn. The nurse should be familiar with community resources and help the parents identify which agencies may benefit them.
5. Help parents recognize the growth and development needs of their newborn. A developmental care program begun in the hospital can be continued at home, or parents may be referred to a developmental program in the community. Earliest interventions are the most successful for the baby as well as the family.

6. Arrange medical follow-up care before discharge. The newborn will need to be followed up by a family pediatrician, a well-baby clinic, or a specialty clinic. The first appointment should be made before the baby is discharged from the hospital.
7. Evaluate the need for durable medical equipment for newborn care (such as a respirator, oxygen, apnea monitor, feeding pump) in the home. Any extra equipment or supplies should be placed in the home before the baby's discharge.
8. Arrange for neonatal hospice for parents of the medically fragile baby, as needed.

When preparing to discharge a medically fragile newborn to home, schedule a predischarge home visit by a public health nurse or home health agency. This predischarge visit evaluates the home for any possible issues that may complicate the parents' ability to care for their at-risk newborn, especially if there are multiple monitoring equipment needs. Another supportive measure is to establish when the follow-up physician will be seeing the baby and make a phone call to the physician as a follow-up to the discharge summary. The parents will experience a nicer transition if they know the NICU team and the healthcare provider have been in communication. Furthermore, they will not feel responsible for fully "briefing" the healthcare provider on their recently discharged baby.

Further evaluation after the newborn has gone home is useful in determining whether the crisis has been resolved satisfactorily. The parents are usually given the intensive care nursery's telephone number to call for support and advice. The staff can follow up each family with visits or telephone calls at intervals for several weeks to assess and evaluate the baby's (and parents') progress. Akbarian, Dashti, and Baraz (2017) found that doing telephone consultations was an affordable way to engage and support mothers of premature babies. Such consultations also decreased readmission rates because they improved the mothers' understanding of follow-up care after discharge. (Figure 31–22).

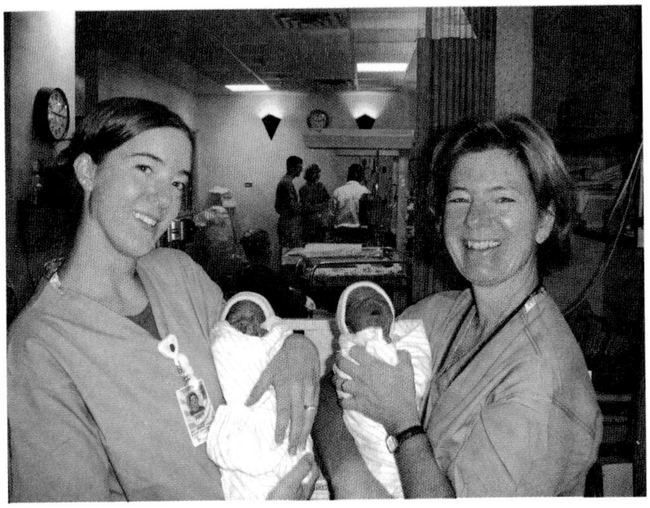

Figure 31–22 Twins on the happy day of discharge, being held by staff in the NICU. This is what is so rewarding about working in the NICU: Healthy babies going home to their families.

Evaluation

Expected outcomes of nursing care include:

- The parents are able to verbalize their feelings of grief and loss.
- The parents verbalize their concerns about their newborn's health problems, care needs, and potential outcome.
- The parents are able to participate in their newborn's care and show attachment behaviors.

Considerations for the Nurse Who Works with At-Risk Newborns

The birth of a baby with an alteration in transition or a deformity is a traumatic event with the potential for either disruption or growth of the involved family. The NICU staff nurses may never see the long-term results of the specialized, sensitive care they give to parents and their newborns. Their only immediate evidence of effective care may be the beginning of resolution of parental grief, with plans for continued care and counseling, or the discharge of a recovered, thriving baby to the care of parents who can adequately bond and care for their child, and the beginning of reintegration of family life.

Nurses cannot provide support unless they themselves are supported. Working in an emotional environment of "lots of living and lots of dying" takes its toll on staff. NICUs are among the most stressful areas in healthcare for patients, families, and nurses. Nurses bear most of the stress and largely determine the atmosphere of the NICU. The nurse's ability to cope with stress is the key to creating an emotionally healthy environment and a positive working atmosphere. The emotional needs and feelings of the staff must be recognized and dealt with to enable them to support the parents. An environment of openness to feelings and support in dealing with their own human needs and emotions is essential for the staff.

As caregivers, nurses may be unaware of their need to grieve for their own losses in the NICU. Working with babies and their families for hours, days, weeks, and sometimes months can foster intimate attachments to them by the nurses. Nurses must be comfortable with the process of grief and be comfortable with their own feelings about death to effectively assist parents with this process. Techniques such as group meetings, individual support, and doing primary care nursing may assist in maintaining staff mental health. Hospital-supported reunions and memorials in some nurseries are beneficial for the families and nurses so they are able to see the children and/or families after discharge.

Focus Your Study

- The sick newborn—whether preterm, term, or postterm—must be managed within narrow physiologic parameters.
- These parameters (respiratory, cardiovascular, and thermal regulation) will maintain physiologic homeostasis and prevent introduction of iatrogenic stress to the already stressed newborn.
- The nursing care of the newborn with special problems involves understanding normal physiology, the pathophysiology of the disease process, clinical manifestations, and supportive or corrective therapies. Only with this theoretic background can the nurse make appropriate observations concerning responses to therapy and development of complications.
- Asphyxia results in significant circulatory, respiratory, and biochemical changes in the newborn that make the successful transition to extrauterine life difficult. Asphyxia requires early identification and resuscitative management.
- Newborn conditions that commonly present with respiratory distress and require oxygen and ventilatory assistance are respiratory distress syndrome (RDS), transient tachypnea of the newborn, meconium aspiration syndrome (MAS), and persistent pulmonary hypertension of the newborn (PPHN).
- Management of respiratory problems can result in further respiratory compromising conditions such as pulmonary interstitial emphysema, pneumothorax, and bronchopulmonary dysplasia (BPD) / chronic lung disease (CLD).
- Cold stress sets up the chain of physiologic events of hypoglycemia, pulmonary vasoconstriction, hyperbilirubinemia, respiratory distress, and metabolic acidosis.
- Nurses are responsible for early assessment and detection and initiation of treatment for hypoglycemia.
- Differentiation between pathologic and physiologic jaundice is key to early and successful intervention.
- Anemia (decreased amount of red blood cell volume) places the newborn at risk for alterations in blood flow and the oxygen-carrying capacity of the blood.
- Nursing assessment of the septic newborn involves identifying very subtle clinical signs that are also seen in other clinical disease states.
- The nurse is the facilitator for interdisciplinary communication with the parents, identifying their understanding of their baby's care and their needs for emotional support.
- Parents of at-risk newborns need support from nurses and healthcare providers to understand and meet the special needs of their babies and to feel comfortable in overwhelming and often unfamiliar environments.

In order to make safe and effective judgments using NANDA-I © 2017 nursing diagnoses, it is essential that nurses refer to the definitions and defining characteristics of the diagnoses used in this text, which can be found in Appendix C.

References

Akbarian, M., Dashti, F., & Baraz, S. (2017). The effect of phone counseling for mothers of premature infants discharged from the hospital on infant's readmission. *International Journal of Pediatrics, 5*(8), 5441–5450. DOI: https://doi.org/10.22038/ijp.2017.24329.2054

Adamkin, D. H. (2017). Neonatal hypoglycemia. *Seminars in Fetal & Neonatal Medicine, 22*(1), 36–41. Retrieved from http://dx.doi.org/10.1016/j.siny.2016.08.007

American Academy of Pediatrics (AAP) & American Heart Association (AHA). (2016). *Textbook of neonatal resuscitation* (7th ed.). Elk Grove Village, IL: Author.

American Academy of Pediatrics (AAP), Committee on the Fetus and Newborn, & American College of Obstetricians and Gynecologists (ACOG), Committee on Obstetric Practice. (2017). *Guidelines for perinatal care* (8th ed.). Elk Grove Village, IL: Author.

American Academy of Pediatrics (AAP), Committee on Fetus and Newborn and Section on Anesthesiology and Pain Medicine. (2016). Prevention and management of procedural pain in the neonate: An update. *Pediatrics 137*(2). Retrieved from http://pediatrics.aappublications.org/content/pediatrics/137/2/e20154271.full.pdf

American Academy of Pediatrics, Subcommittee on Hyperbilirubinemia. (2004). Management of hyperbilirubinemia in the newborn 35 or more weeks of gestation. *Pediatrics, 114*(1), 297–316.

Ariff, S., Lee, A., Lawn, J., & Bhutta, Z. A. (2016). Global burden, epidemiologic trends, and prevention of intrapartum-related deaths in low resource settings. *Clinics in Perinatology, 43*(3), 593–608.

Balany, J., & Bhandari, V. (2015). Understanding the impact of infection, inflammation, and their persistence in the pathogenesis of bronchopulmonary dysplasia. *Frontiers in Medicine, 2*(90), 1–10. DOI: 10.3389/fmed.2015.00090

Beltempo, M., Viel-Thériault, I., Thibeault, R., Julien, A. S., & Piedboeuf, B. (2018). C-reactive protein for late-onset sepsis diagnosis in very low birth weight infants. *BMC Pediatrics 18*(16). DOI: 10.1186/s12887-018-1002-5

Bennett, N. J. (2017). Bacteremia. In *Medscape reference: Drugs, diseases and procedures.* Retrieved from https://emedicine.medscape.com/article/961169-overview

Bhutani, V. K., & Committee on the Fetus and Newborn. (2011). Phototherapy to prevent severe neonatal hyperbilirubinemia in the newborn infant 35 or more weeks of gestation. *Pediatrics 128*, e1046–1052. DOI: 10.1542/peds.2011-1494

Bhutani, V. K., Stark, A. R., Lazzeroni, L. C., Poland, R., Gourley, G. R., Kazmierczak, S., . . . & Initial Clinical Testing Evaluation and Risk Assessment for Universal Screening for Hyperbilirubinemia Study Group. (2013). Predischarge screening for severe neonatal hyperbilirubinemia identifies infants who need phototherapy. *The Journal of Pediatrics, 162*(3), 477–482.

Bruschettini, M., Romantsik, O., Ramenghi, L. A., Zappettini, S., O'Donnell, C. P. F., & Calevo, M. G. (2016). Needle aspiration versus intercostal tube drainage for pneumothorax in the newborn. *Cochrane Database of Systematic Reviews, 1*, 1–6. DOI: 10.1002/14651858.CD011724.pub2

Chiang, M-C., Jong, Y-J., & Lin, C-H. (2017). Therapeutic hypothermia for neonates with hypoxic ischemic encephalopathy. *Pediatrics and Neonatology, 58*(6), 475–483. Retrieved from https://www.pediatr-neonatol.com/article/S1875-9572(17)30175-4/fulltext

Colombatti, R, Sainati, L., Trevisanuto, D. (2016). Anemia and transfusion in the neonate. *Seminars in Fetal & Neonatal Medicine, 21*, 2–9.

Deleon, C., Shattuck, K., & Jain, S. (2015). Biomarkers of neonatal sepsis. *NeoReviews, 16*(5), e297–e308.

Eichenwald, E. C., Hansen, A. R., Martin, C. R., & Stark, A. R. (2017). *Manual of neonatal care* (8th ed.). Philadelphia, PA: Lippincott Williams & Wilkins.

Feeley, N., Genest, C., Niela-Vilén, H., Charbonneau, L., & Axelin, A. (2016). Parents and nurses balancing parent-infant closeness and separation: A qualitative study of NICU nurses perceptions. *BMC Pediatrics 16*(134). Retrieved from https://www.ncbi.nlm.nih.gov/pubmed/27543122

Flaherman, V. J., Maisels, M. J., & Academy of Breastfeeding Medicine. (2017). ABM Clinical Protocol #22: Guidelines for management of jaundice in the breastfeeding infant 35 weeks or more of gestation–Revised 2017. *Breastfeeding Medicine 12*(5), 250–257.

Fraser, D. (2016). *Infection in the neonate: A comprehensive guide to assessment, management, and nursing care* (2nd ed.). Petaluma, CA: NICU INK.

Gallacher, D. J., Hart, K., & Kotecha, S. (2016). Common respiratory conditions of the newborn. *Breathe 12*(1), 30–42. DOI: 10.1183/2d0734735.000716

Gardner, S. L., Enzman-Hines, M., & Nyp, M. (2016). Respiratory diseases. In S. L. Gardner, B. S. Carter, M. Enzman-Hines, & J. A. Hernandez (Eds.), *Merenstein & Gardner's handbook of neonatal intensive care* (8th ed., pp. 565–648). St. Louis. MO: Mosby Elsevier.

Gluck, L., & Kulovich, M. V. (1973). Fetal lung development. *Pediatric Clinics of North America, 20*, 375.

Gomella, T. L. (2013). *Neonatology: Management, procedures, on-call problems, diseases, and drugs* (7th ed.). New York, NY: Lange Medical Books/McGraw-Hill.

Grant, P. (1978). Psychological needs of families of high risk infants. *Family and Community Health, 1*(3), 91–102.

Hardy, W., D'Agata, A., & McGrath, J. M. (2016). The infant at risk. In S. Mattson & J. E. Smith (Eds), *AWHONN core curriculum for maternal-newborn nursing* (5th ed., pp. 363–416). St. Louis, MO: Mosby Elsevier.

Hasan, F., Khan, S. A., Maharoof, M. K., & Muhammed, N. (2018). Role of procalcitonin in early diagnosis of neonatal sepsis. *International Journal of Contemporary Pediatrics, 4*(2), 383–389. DOI: http://dx.doi.org/10.18203/2349-3291.ijcp20170477

Hascoët, J. M., Piccaud, J. C., Ligi, I., Blanc, T., Moreau, F., Pinturier, M. F., . . . Vieux, R. (2016). Late surfactant administration in very preterm neonates with prolonged respiratory distress and pulmonary outcome at 1 year of age: A randomized clinical trial. *Journal of the American Medical Association Pediatrics, 170*(4), 365–372.

Janvier, A., Lantos, J., Aschner, J., Barrington, K., Batton, B., Batton, D., . . . Spitzer, A. R. (2016). Stronger and more vulnerable: A balanced view of the impacts of the NICU experience on parents. *Pediatrics, 138*(3), e20160655. DOI: 10.1542/peds.2016-0655

Jeon, G. (2016). Respiratory support with heated humidified high flow nasal cannula in preterm infants. *Korean Journal of Pediatrics, 59*(10), 389–394.

Kamath-Rayne, B. D., Thio, E. H., Deacon, J., & Hernandez J. J. (2016). Neonatal hyperbilirubinemia. In S. L. Gardner, B. S. Carter, M. Enzman-Hines, & J. A. Hernandez (Eds.), *Merenstein & Gardner's handbook of neonatal intensive care* (8th ed., pp. 511–536). St. Louis, MO: Mosby Elsevier.

Keszler, M., & Sant'Anna, G. (2015). Mechanical ventilation and bronchopulmonary dysplasia. *Clinics in Perinatology, 42*(4), 781–796. Retrieved from https://doi.org/10.1016/j.clp.2015.08.006

Klaus, M. H., & Kennell, J. H. (1982). *Maternal-infant bonding* (2nd ed.). St. Louis, MO: Mosby.

Kling, P. J., & Coe, C. L. (2016). Iron homeostasis in pregnancy, the fetus, and the neonate. *NeoReviews, 17*(11), e657–e664. DOI: 10.1542/neo.17-11-e657

Lakshminrusimha, S., Mathew, B., & Leach, C. L. (2016). Pharmacological strategies in neonatal pulmonary hypertension other than nitric oxide. *Seminars in Perinatology, 40*(3), 160–173.

Lakshminrusimha, S., & Saugstad, O. D. (2016). The fetal circulation, pathophysiology of hypoxic respiratory failure and pulmonary hypertension in neonates, and the role of oxygen therapy. *Journal of Perinatology, 36*, S3–S11.

Lyu, Y., Shah, P., Ye, X. Y., Warre, R., Deshpandey, A., & Canadian Neonatal Network. (2015). Association between admission temperature and mortality and major morbidity in preterm infants born at fewer than 33 weeks' gestation. *Journal of the American Medical Association Pediatrics, 169*(4). DOI: 10.1001/jamapediatrics.2015.0277

Maitre, N. L., Key, A. P., Choma, C. D., Slaughter, J. C., Matusz, P. J., Wallace, M. T., & Murrary, M. M. (2017). The dual nature of early life experience on somatosensory processing in the human infant brain. *Current Biology, 27*(7), 1048–1054. DOI: http://dx.doi.org/1016/j.pub.201702.038

Makker, K., Alissa, R., Dudek, C., Travers L., Smotherman, C., & Hudak, M. L. (2018). Glucose gel in infants at risk for transitional neonatal hypoglycemia. *American Journal of Perinatology*. DOI: 10.1055/s-0038-1639338. [Epub ahead of print]. Retrieved from https://www.ncbi.nlm.nih.gov/pubmed/29579758

Marko, T., & Dickerson, M. L. (2017). *Clinical handbook of neonatal pain management for nurses*. New York, NY: Springer.

Niermeyer, S., Clarke, S. B., & Hernandez J. J. (2016). Delivery room care. In S. L. Gardner, B. S. Carter, M. Enzman-Hines, & J. A. Hernandez (Eds.), *Merenstein & Gardner's handbook of neonatal intensive care* (8th ed., pp. 47–70). St. Louis, MO: Mosby Elsevier.

Noronha, S. (2016). Acquired and congenital hemolytic anemia. *Pediatrics in Review, 37*(6), 235–246. DOI: 10.1542/pir.2015-005

O'Brien, K. O., Bracht, M., Robson, K., Ye, X. Y., Mirea, L., Cruz, L., . . . Lee, S. K. (2016). Evaluation of the family integrated care model of neonatal intensive care: A cluster randomized controlled trial in Canada and Australia. *BioMed Central Pediatrics, 15*, 210. DOI: 10.1186/s12887-015-0527-0

Ohls, R. K., Cannon, D. C., Phillips, J., Caprihan, A., Patel, S., Winter, S., . . . & Lowe, J. (2016). Preschool assessment of preterm infants treated with darbepoetin and erythropoietin. *Pediatrics, 137*(3), 1–9. Retrieved from http://pediatrics.aappublications.org/content/pediatrics/137/3/e20153859.full.pdf

Polin, R. A., & Committee on the Fetus and Newborn. (2012). Management of neonates with suspected or proven early-onset bacterial sepsis. *Pediatrics, 129*, 1006–1015.

Pramanik, A. K., Rangaswamy, N., & Gates, T. (2015). Neonatal respiratory distress: A practical approach to its diagnosis and management. *Pediatric Clinics of North America, 62*(2), 453–469. DOI: 10.1016/j.pcl.2014.11.008

Rainaldi, M. A., & Perlman, J. M. (2016). Pathophysiology of birth asphyxia. *Clinics in Perinatology, 43*(3), 409–422.

Sawyer, T. L. (2015). *Jaundice.* Medscape Reference. Retrieved from http://emedicine.medscape.com/article/189477-overview.#2

Schrag, S. J., Farley, M. M., Petit, S., Reinold, A., Weston, E. J., Pondo,T., . . . Lynfield, R. (2016). Epidemiology of invasive early-onset neonatal sepsis, 2005 to 2014. *Pediatrics, 138*(6), e2016–3038. DOI: 10:1542/pds.2016-3038

Shaw, C., Stokoe, E., Gallagher, K., Aladangady, N., & Marlow, N. (2016). Parental involvement in neonatal critical care decision-making. *Sociology of Health & Illness, 38*(8), 1217–1242. DOI: 10.1111/1467-9566.12455

Shea, K., & Palanisamy, A. (2015). What can you do to protect the newborn brain? *Obstetric and Gynecological Anesthesia, 28*(3), 261–266.

Solnit, A., & Stark, M. (1961). Mourning and the birth of a defective child. *Psychoanalytic Study of the Child, 16*, 505.

Stanley, C., Rozance, P., Thornton, P. S., De Leon, D. D., Harris, D., Haymond, M. W., . . . Wolfsdorf, J. I. (2015). Re-evaluating "transitional neonatal hypoglycemia": Mechanism and implications for management. *Journal of Pediatrics, 166*(6), 1520–1525.

Stevens, D. C., Munson, D. P., & Khan, M. A. (2016). The single-family room neonatal intensive care environment. *NeoReviews, 17*(12), e687–697. DOI: 10.1542/neo.17-12e687

Stoll, B. J. (2016). Early-onset neonatal sepsis: A continuing problem in need of novel prevention strategies. *Pediatrics, 138*(6), e2016–3038. DOI: 10:1542/pds.2016-3038

Thoresen, M. (2015). Who should we cool after perinatal asphyxia? *Seminars in Fetal & Neonatal Medicine, 20*(2), 66–71.

Vali, P., Mathew, B., & Lakshminrusimha, S. (2015). Neonatal resuscitation: Evolving strategies. *Maternal Health, Neonatology, and Perinatology, 1*(4). DOI: 10.1186/s40748-014-0003-0

Zaichkin, J., Weiner, G., & Loren, D. (2017). *Understanding the NICU: What parents of preemies and other hospitalized newborns need to know.* Elk Grove Village, IL: American Academy of Pediatrics.

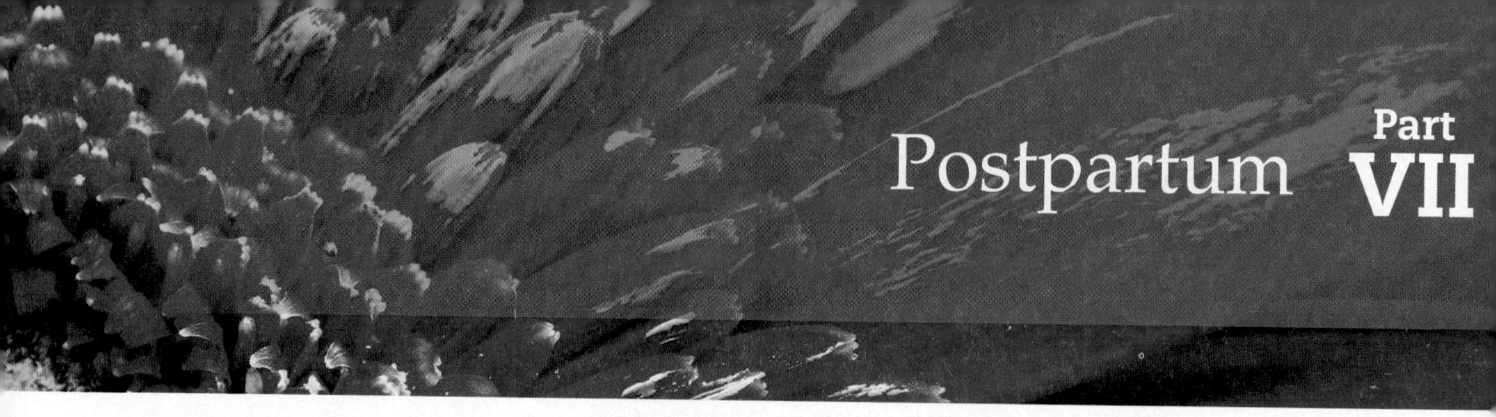

Part VII Postpartum

Chapter 32

Postpartum Adaptation and Nursing Assessment

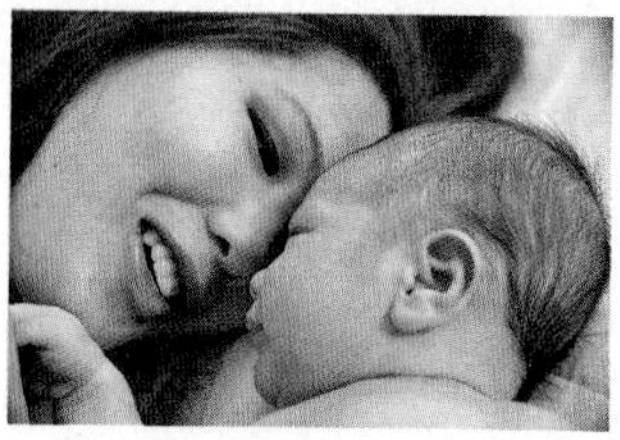

SOURCE: Diane Macdonald/ Exactostock/SuperStock.

I had heard about the negatives—the fatigue, the loneliness, loss of self. But nobody told me about the wonderful parts: Holding my baby close to me, seeing her first smile, watching her grow and become more responsive day by day. How can I describe the way I felt when she stroked my breast while nursing, or looked into my eyes or arched her eyebrows like an opera singer? This was the deepest connection I'd felt to anybody. Sometimes the intensity almost frightened me. For the first time I cared about somebody else more than myself, and I would do anything to nurture and protect her.

—**The Boston Women's Health Collective,** *The New Our Bodies, Ourselves*

Learning Outcomes

32.1 Delineate the basic physiologic changes that occur in the postpartum period as a woman's body returns to its prepregnant state.

32.2 Describe the psychologic adjustments that normally occur during the postpartum period.

32.3 Differentiate the physiologic and psychosocial components of a postpartum assessment.

32.4 Describe the common concerns of the mother that are considered in a postpartum assessment.

32.5 Examine the physical and developmental tasks that the mother must accomplish during the postpartum period.

32.6 Explain the impact of cultural influence upon the postpartum period.

32.7 Identify the factors that influence the development of parent–newborn attachment in the nursing assessment of early attachment.

The **puerperium**, or postpartum period, is the period during which the woman readjusts, physically and psychologically, from pregnancy and birth. It begins immediately after birth and continues for approximately 6 weeks or until the body has returned to a near nonpregnant state.

This chapter describes the physiologic and psychologic changes and adaptations that occur postpartum and the basic aspects of a thorough postpartum assessment.

Postpartum Physical Adaptations

Comprehensive nursing assessment is based on a sound understanding of the normal anatomic and physiologic processes of the puerperium. These processes involve the reproductive organs and other major body systems.

Reproductive System

INVOLUTION OF THE UTERUS

The term **involution** is used to describe the rapid reduction in size of the uterus and its return to a condition similar to its nonpregnant state, although it remains slightly larger than it was before the first pregnancy. Following separation of the placenta, the decidua of the uterus is irregular, jagged, and varied in thickness. The spongy layer of the decidua is cast off as lochia, and the basal layer of the decidua remains in the uterus to become differentiated into two layers within the first 48 to 72 hours after birth. The outermost layer becomes necrotic and is sloughed off in the lochia. The layer closest to the myometrium contains the fundi of the uterine endometrial glands, and these glands lay the foundation for the new endometrium. Except at the placental site, this process is completed in approximately 3 weeks. The placental site can take up to 6 weeks to completely heal (King, 2019). Bleeding from the larger uterine vessels of the placental site is controlled by compression of the retracted uterine muscle fibers. The clotted blood is gradually absorbed by the body. Some of these vessels are eventually obliterated and replaced by new vessels with smaller lumens.

The placental site heals by a process of exfoliation and growth of endometrial tissue. The placental site is undermined by the growth of the endometrial tissue, both from the margins of the site and from the fundi of the endometrial glands left in the basal layer of the site. The infarcted superficial tissue then becomes necrotic and is sloughed off (Blackburn, 2018). *Exfoliation* is one of the most important aspects of involution. If the healing of the placental site left a fibrous scar, the area available for further implantation would be limited, as would the number of possible pregnancies.

Factors that enhance involution include an uncomplicated labor and birth, complete expulsion of the amniotic membranes and the placenta, manual removal of the placenta during a cesarean birth, breastfeeding, and early ambulation. Factors that slow uterine involution and the rationale for each factor are listed in Table 32–1.

CHANGES IN FUNDAL POSITION

The **fundus** (top portion of the uterus) is situated in the midline of the abdomen, midway between the symphysis pubis and the umbilicus (Figure 32–1). Immediately following the expulsion of the placenta, the uterus contracts firmly to the size of a large grapefruit. The walls of the contracted uterus are in close proximity, and the uterine blood vessels are firmly compressed by the myometrium. Within 6 to 12 hours after birth, the fundus of the uterus rises to the level of the umbilicus because of blood and clots that remain within the uterus and changes in support of the uterus by the ligaments. A fundus that is above the umbilicus and boggy (feels soft and spongy rather than firm and well contracted) is associated with excessive uterine bleeding. As blood collects and forms clots within the uterus, the fundus rises; firm contractions of the uterine muscle are interrupted, causing a **boggy uterus (uterine atony)**.

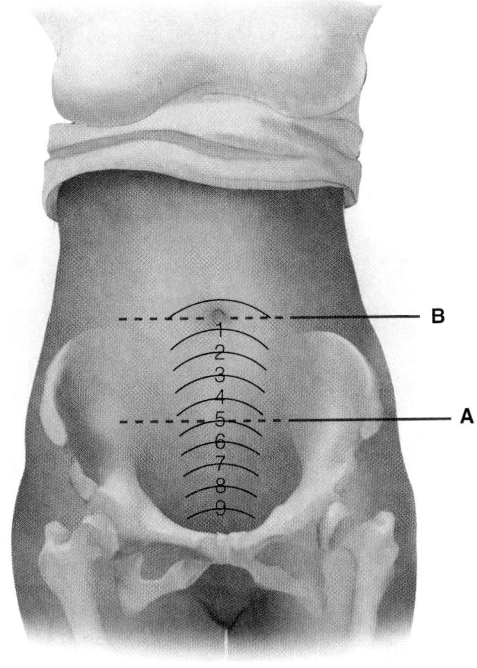

Figure 32–1 Involution of the uterus. A. Immediately after delivery of the placenta, the top of the fundus is in the midline and approximately two-thirds to three-fourths of the way between the symphysis pubis and the umbilicus B. About 6 to 12 hours after birth, the fundus is at the level of (or one fingerbreadth below) the umbilicus. The height of the fundus then decreases about one fingerbreadth (approximately 1 cm) each day.

When the fundus is higher than expected and is not in midline (usually deviated to the right), distention of the bladder should be

TABLE 32–1 Factors That Slow Uterine Involution

FACTOR	RATIONALE
Prolonged labor	Muscles relax because of prolonged time of contraction during labor.
Anesthesia	Muscle relaxation results in a boggy uterus.
Difficult birth	The uterus is manipulated excessively, causing fatigue.
Grandmultiparity	Repeated distention of uterus during pregnancy and labor leads to muscle stretching, diminished tone, and muscle relaxation.
Full bladder	As the uterus is pushed up and usually to the right, pressure on it interferes with effective uterine contraction.
Incomplete expulsion of placenta or membranes	The presence of even small amounts of tissue interferes with ability of uterus to remain firmly contracted.
Infection	Inflammation interferes with uterine muscle's ability to contract effectively.
Overdistention of uterus	Overstretching of uterine muscles with conditions such as multiple gestation, polyhydramnios, or a very large baby may set the stage for slower uterine involution.

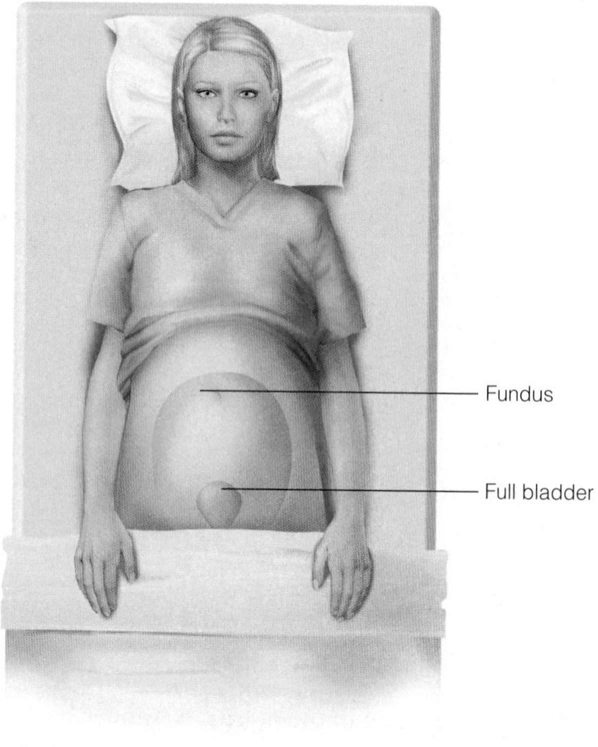

Figure 32–2 **The uterus becomes displaced and deviated to the right when the bladder is full.**

suspected and the bladder should be emptied immediately and the uterus remeasured (Figure 32–2). If the woman is unable to void, in-and-out catheterization of the bladder may be required. In the immediate postpartum period many women may not be aware of a full bladder. Because the uterine ligaments are still stretched, a full bladder can move the uterus. By the end of the puerperium these ligaments have regained their nonpregnant length and tension.

After birth the top of the fundus remains at the level of the umbilicus for about half a day. On the first postpartum day, the top of the fundus is located about 1 cm (0.4 in.) below the umbilicus. On day 3 after delivery, the fundus is 3 cm (1.18 in.) below the umbilicus (Blackburn, 2018). The top of the fundus descends approximately one fingerbreadth (width of index, second, or third finger), or 1 cm, per day until it descends into the pelvis on about day 10. By 6 to 8 weeks, the uterus weighs 60 grams (2 oz) (Whitmer, 2016).

If the mother is breastfeeding, the release of endogenous oxytocin from the posterior pituitary in response to suckling may hasten this process. Barring complications, such as infection or retained placental fragments, the uterus approaches its prepregnant size and location by 5 to 6 weeks. In women who had an oversized uterus during the pregnancy (hydramnios, birth of a large-for-gestational-age [LGA] newborn, or multiple gestation), the time frame for immediate uterine involution process is lengthened. If intrauterine infection is present, in addition to the presence of foul-smelling lochia or vaginal discharge, the uterine fundus descends much more slowly. When infection is suspected, other clinical signs such as fever and tachycardia in addition to delay in involution must be assessed. Any slowing of fundal descent is called **subinvolution** (for further discussion of subinvolution, see Chapter 35).

LOCHIA

The uterus rids itself of the debris remaining after birth through a discharge called **lochia**, which is classified according to its appearance and contents.

- **Lochia rubra**, named for the Latin word for *red*, is dark red in color. It is present for the first 2 to 3 days postpartum and contains epithelial cells, erythrocytes, leukocytes, bacteria, shreds of the decidua, and, occasionally, fetal meconium, lanugo, and vernix caseosa. Clotting is often the result of pooling of blood in the upper portion of the vagina. A few small clots (no larger than a nickel) are common, particularly in the first few days after birth. However, lochia should not contain large (plum-sized) clots; if it does, the cause should be investigated without delay.
- **Lochia serosa** is a pinkish color. It follows from about the third to the tenth day. Lochia serosa is composed of serous exudate (hence, the name), shreds of degenerating decidua, erythrocytes, leukocytes, cervical mucus, and numerous microorganisms (Blackburn, 2018). The red blood cell (RBC) component decreases gradually, and a creamy or yellowish discharge persists for an additional week or two.
- **Lochia alba**, from the Latin word for *white*, is the final discharge and is composed primarily of leukocytes, decidual cells, epithelial cells, fat, cervical mucus, cholesterol crystals, and bacteria.

Recent studies examining lochia patterns have found that the lochia rubra phase lasts longer than generally assumed and that it varies according to breastfeeding practice and parity (Cunningham et al., 2018). Variation in the duration of lochia discharge is not uncommon; however, the trend should be toward a lighter amount of flow and a lighter color of discharge (Blackburn, 2018). When the lochia stops, the cervix is considered closed, and chances of infection ascending from the vagina to the uterus decrease.

Like menstrual discharge, lochia has a musty, stale odor that is not offensive. Microorganisms are always present in the vaginal lochia, and by the second day following birth the uterus is contaminated with the vaginal bacteria. It is thought that infection does not develop because the organisms involved are relatively nonvirulent. In addition, by the time the bacteria reach the raw, exposed surface of the uterus, the process of granulation has begun, forming a protective barrier. Any foul smell to the lochia or used perineal pads suggests infection and the need for prompt additional assessment, such as white blood cell (WBC) count and differential and assessment for uterine tenderness and fever.

The total volume of lochia is approximately 225 mL, and the daily volume decreases gradually. Discharge is greater in the morning because of pooling in the vagina and uterus while the mother lies sleeping. The amount of lochia may also be increased by exertion or breastfeeding. Multiparous women usually have more lochia than first-time mothers. Women who undergo a cesarean birth typically have less lochia than women who give birth vaginally (King, 2019).

Evaluation of lochia is necessary not only to determine the presence of hemorrhage but also to assess uterine involution. The type, amount, and consistency of lochia determine the state of healing of the placental site, and a progressive color change from bright red at birth to dark red to pink to white or clear should be observed. Persistent discharge of lochia rubra or a return to lochia rubra indicates subinvolution or late postpartum hemorrhage (see Chapter 35).

The nurse should exercise caution in evaluating bleeding immediately after birth. The continuous seepage of blood is more consistent with cervical or vaginal lacerations and may be effectively diagnosed when the bleeding is evaluated in conjunction with the consistency of the uterus. Lacerations should be suspected if the uterus is firm and of expected size and if no clots can be expressed.

CERVICAL CHANGES

Following birth, the cervix is spongy, flabby, and formless and may appear bruised. The lateral aspects of the external os are frequently lacerated during the birth process (Cunningham et al., 2018). The external os is markedly irregular and closes slowly. It admits two fingers for a few days following birth, but by the end of the first week it will admit only a fingertip.

The shape of the external os is permanently changed by the first childbearing. The characteristic dimple-like os of the nullipara changes to the lateral slit os of the multipara. After significant cervical laceration or several lacerations, the cervix may appear lopsided. Because of the slight change in the size of the cervix, a diaphragm or cervical cap will need to be refitted if the woman is using one of these methods of contraception.

VAGINAL CHANGES

Following birth, the vagina appears edematous and gaping and may be bruised. Small superficial lacerations may be evident, and the rugae have been obliterated. The apparent bruising of the vagina is due to pelvic congestion and trauma and will quickly disappear. The hymen, torn and jagged, heals irregularly, leaving small tags called the *carunculae myrtiformes*.

The size of the vagina decreases, and rugae begin to return within 3 to 4 weeks (Blackburn, 2018). This facilitates the gradual return to smaller, although not to nulliparous, dimensions. By 6 weeks, the nonlactating woman's vagina usually appears normal. The lactating woman is in a hypoestrogenic state because of ovarian suppression, and her vaginal mucosa may be pale and without rugae. This may lead to dyspareunia (painful intercourse), which may be reduced by the addition of a water-soluble personal lubricant. Tone and contractibility of the vaginal opening may be improved by perineal tightening exercises such as Kegel exercises (see Chapter 13), which may begin soon after birth. The labia majora and labia minora are looser in the woman who has borne a child than in the nullipara woman.

PERINEAL CHANGES

During the early postpartum period, the soft tissue in and around the perineum may appear edematous with some bruising. If an episiotomy or laceration is present, the edges should be approximated. Occasionally, ecchymosis occurs, and this may delay healing. Initial healing of the episiotomy or laceration occurs in 2 to 3 weeks after the birth, although complete healing may take up to 4 to 6 months. Perineal discomfort may be present during this time.

RECURRENCE OF OVULATION AND MENSTRUATION

The return of menstruation and ovulation varies for each postpartum woman. Menstruation generally returns as soon as 7 weeks in 70% and by 12 weeks in all nonlactating mothers or as late as 3 years in 70% of breastfeeding mothers. The return of ovulation is directly associated with a rise in the serum progesterone level. In nonlactating women the average time to first ovulation can occur within 70 to 75 days, with a mean time of 6 months (Isley & Katz, 2017).

The return of menstruation and ovulation in breastfeeding mothers is usually prolonged and is associated with the length of time the woman breastfeeds and whether formula supplements are used. If a mother breastfeeds for less than 1 month, the return of menstruation and ovulation is similar to the nonbreastfeeding mother. In women who exclusively breastfeed, menstruation is usually delayed for at least 3 months. Sucking by the baby typically results in alterations in the gonadotropin-releasing hormone (GnRH) production, which is thought to be the cause of amenorrhea (Blackburn, 2018). Although exclusive breastfeeding helps to reduce the risk of pregnancy for the first 6 months after delivery, it should be relied upon only temporarily and if it meets the observed criteria for lactational amenorrhea method (LAM). Furthermore, because ovulation precedes menstruation and women often supplement breastfeeding with bottles and pacifiers, breastfeeding is not considered a reliable means of contraception.

Abdomen

The uterine ligaments (notably the round and broad ligaments) are stretched and require the length of the puerperium to recover. The stretched abdominal wall appears loose and flabby, but it will respond to exercise within 2 to 3 months. **Diastasis recti abdominis**, a separation of the rectus abdominis muscles, may occur with pregnancy, especially in women with poor abdominal muscle tone (Figure 32–3). If diastasis occurs, part of the abdominal wall has no muscular support but is formed only by skin, subcutaneous fat, fascia, and peritoneum. This may be especially pronounced in women who have undergone a cesarean section, as the rectus abdominis muscles are manually separated to access the uterine muscle. Improvement depends on the physical condition of the mother, the total number of pregnancies, pregnancy spacing, and the type and amount of physical exercise. This may result in a pendulous abdomen and increased maternal backache. Fortunately, diastasis usually responds well to exercise, and abdominal muscle tone can improve significantly.

The striae (stretch marks), which occurred as a result of stretching and rupture of the elastic fibers of the skin, take on different colors based on the mother's skin color. The striae of mothers with white skin are red to purple at the time of birth and gradually fade to silver or white. The striae of mothers with darker skin are darker than the surrounding skin and remain darker. These marks gradually fade after a time but remain visible.

Lactation

During pregnancy, the breasts develop in preparation for lactation as a result of the influence of both estrogen and progesterone. After birth, the interplay of maternal hormones leads to the establishment of milk production (see Chapter 29).

Gastrointestinal System

Hunger following birth is common, and the mother may enjoy a light meal. Frequently, she is thirsty and will drink large amounts of fluids. Drinking fluids helps replace fluid lost during labor, in the urine, and through perspiration.

The bowels tend to be sluggish after birth because of the lingering effects of progesterone, decreased abdominal muscle tone, and bowel evacuation associated with the labor and birth process (Whitmer, 2016). Women who have had an episiotomy, lacerations, or hemorrhoids may tend to delay elimination for fear of increasing their pain or in the belief that their stitches will be torn if they bear down. In resisting or delaying the bowel movement, the woman may cause increased constipation and more pain when elimination finally occurs.

The woman with a cesarean birth may receive clear liquids shortly after surgery. Once bowel sounds are present, the diet is quickly advanced to solid food. In addition, the woman may experience some initial discomfort from flatulence, which is relieved by early ambulation and use of antiflatulent medications. Chamomile tea and peppermint tea may also be helpful in reducing discomfort from flatulence. It may take a few days for the bowel to regain its tone. The woman who has had a cesarean or a difficult birth may benefit from stool softeners.

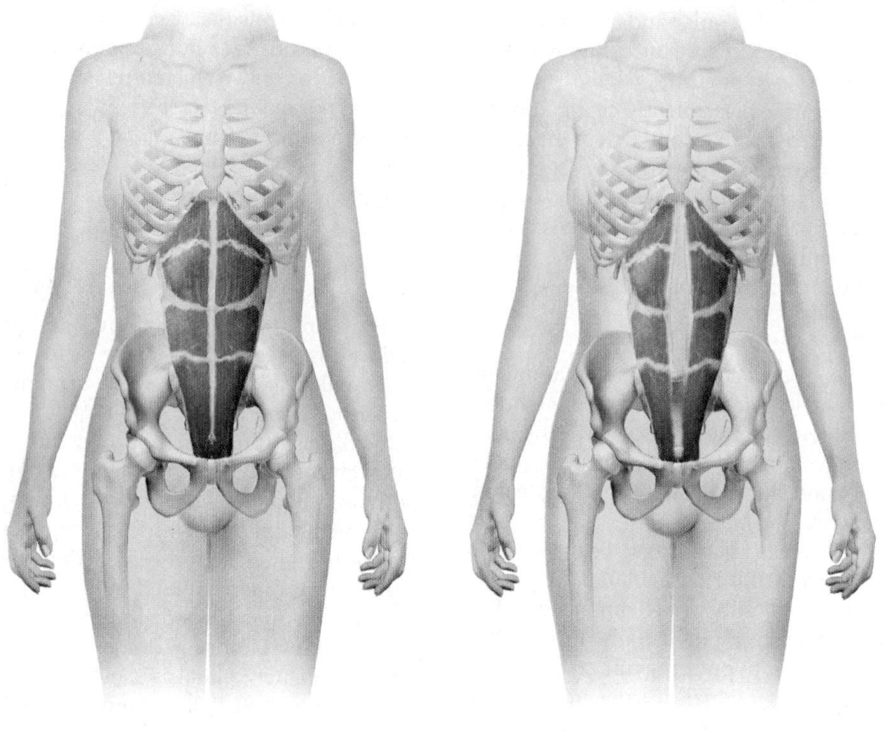

Figure 32–3 **Diastasis recti abdominis, a separation of the musculature, commonly occurs after pregnancy.**

Urinary Tract

The postpartum woman has an increased bladder capacity, swelling and bruising of the tissues around the urethra, decreased sensitivity to fluid pressure, and decreased sensation of bladder filling. Consequently, she is at risk for overdistention, incomplete emptying, and buildup of residual urine. Women who have had an anesthetic block have inhibited neural functioning of the bladder and are more susceptible to bladder distention, difficulty voiding, and bladder infections. In addition, immediate postpartum use of oxytocin to facilitate uterine contractions following expulsion of the placenta has an antidiuretic effect. Following cessation of the oxytocin the woman will experience rapid bladder filling.

Urinary output increases during the early postpartum period (first 12 to 24 hours) because of *puerperal diuresis*. The kidneys must eliminate an estimated 2000 to 3000 mL of extracellular fluid with a normal pregnancy, which causes rapid filling of the bladder. Thus, adequate bladder elimination is an immediate concern. Women with preeclampsia, chronic hypertension, and diabetes experience even greater fluid retention, and postpartum diuresis is increased accordingly.

If urine stasis exists, chances increase for urinary tract infection because of bacteriuria and the presence of dilated ureters and renal pelves, which persist for about 6 weeks after birth. A full bladder may also increase the tendency of the uterus to relax by displacing the uterus and interfering with its contractility, leading to hemorrhage. In the absence of infection, the dilated ureters and renal pelves return to prepregnant size by the end of the sixth week.

Hematuria, resulting from bladder or urethral trauma, may occasionally occur after birth, but the presence of lochia may mask this sign. If hematuria occurs in the second or third postpartum week, there may be a bladder infection. Acetone may be present in the urine of women with diabetes or of women with prolonged labor and dehydration. Slight (1+) proteinuria may occur during the first week following birth. However, proteinuria may be associated with an infectious process (cystitis, pyelitis), so it should be evaluated further. A urine specimen contaminated with lochia may falsely indicate proteinuria, so any specimen should be obtained as a midstream or a catheterized specimen.

Vital Signs

During the postpartum period, with the exception of the first 24 hours, the woman should be afebrile. A maternal temperature of up to 38°C (100.4°F) may occur up to 24 hours after birth as a result of the exertion and dehydration of labor. An increase in temperature to between 37.8° and 39°C (100° and 100.2°F) may also occur during the first 24 hours after the mother's milk comes in (Cunningham et al., 2018). However, in women not meeting these criteria, infection must be considered in the presence of an increased temperature (see Chapter 35).

Immediately following delivery, many women experience a transient rise in both systolic and diastolic blood pressure, which spontaneously returns to the prepregnancy baseline over the next few days (American Academy of Pediatrics (AAP) & American College of Obstetricians and Gynecologists (ACOG), 2017). A decrease may indicate physiologic readjustment to decreased intrapelvic pressure or it may be related to uterine hemorrhage. Orthostatic hypotension, as indicated by feelings of faintness or dizziness immediately after standing up, can develop in the first 48 hours as a result of abdominal engorgement that may occur after birth. A low or decreasing blood pressure may reflect hypovolemia secondary to hemorrhage, but it is a late sign. Blood pressure elevations may result from excessive use of oxytocin or vasopressor medications. Because preeclampsia can persist into or occur first in the postpartum period, routine evaluation of blood pressure is needed. If a woman complains of headache, hypertension must be ruled out before analgesics are administered.

Puerperal bradycardia with rates of 50 to 70 beats per minute (beats/min) commonly occurs during the first 6 to 10 days of the postpartum period. It may be related to decreased cardiac strain, the decreased blood volume following placental separation, contraction of the uterus, and increased stroke volume. A pulse rate greater than 100 beats/min may be indicative of hypovolemia, infection, fear, or pain and requires further assessment (Whitmer, 2016).

Blood Values

Blood values should return to the prepregnant state by the end of the postpartum period. Pregnancy-associated activation of coagulation factors may continue for variable amounts of time after birth. This condition, in conjunction with trauma, immobility, or sepsis, predisposes the woman to development of thromboembolism. The incidence of thromboembolism is reduced by early mobilization.

Nonpathologic leukocytosis often occurs during labor and in the immediate postpartum period, with WBC counts up to 20,000 to 25,000/mm^3. WBC values typically return to normal levels by the end of the first postpartum week (Blackburn, 2018). Leukocytosis combined with the normal increase in erythrocyte sedimentation rate may obscure the diagnosis of acute infection at this time (Whitmer, 2016).

Hemoglobin and hematocrit levels may be difficult to interpret in the first 2 days after birth because of the changing blood volume. This loss in blood in the first 24 hours accounts for half of the RBC volume gained during the course of the pregnancy. Blood loss averages 200 to 500 mL with a vaginal birth and 1000 mL or more with a cesarean birth (King, 2019). Lochia constitutes less than 25% of this blood loss. As extracellular fluid is excreted, hemoconcentration occurs, with a concomitant rise in hematocrit. A drop in values indicates an abnormal blood loss. The following is a convenient rule to remember: A 2 to 3 percentage point drop in hematocrit equals a blood loss of 500 mL (Whitmer, 2016). After 3 to 4 days, mobilization of interstitial fluid leads to a slight increase in plasma volume (Blackburn, 2018). This hemodilution leads to a decrease in hemoglobin, hematocrit, and plasma protein by the end of the first postpartum week.

Platelet levels typically fall as a result of placental separation. They then begin to increase by the third to fourth postpartum day, gradually returning to normal by the sixth postpartum week. Fibrinolytic activity typically returns to normal during the hours following the birth. The hemostatic system as a whole reaches its normal pregnant status by 3 to 4 weeks postpartum; however, the diameter of deep veins can take up to 6 weeks to return to prepregnant levels (King, 2019). This is why there is a prolonged risk of thromboembolism in the first 6 weeks following birth.

Cardiovascular Changes

The cardiovascular system undergoes dramatic changes during birth that can result in cardiovascular instability due to an increase in cardiac output. The cardiac output typically stabilizes and returns to prepregnancy levels within an hour following birth (Blackburn, 2018). Maternal hypervolemia typically occurs immediately following birth because the maternal circulation has an increase in blood volume that no longer travels through the placenta. Maternal hypervolemia acts to protect the mother from excessive blood loss. Cardiac output declines by 30% in the first 2 weeks and reaches normal levels by 6 to 12 weeks (Blackburn, 2018). Diuresis in the first week after birth helps to decrease the extracellular fluid and results in a weight loss of 3 kg (6.6 lb) (Blackburn, 2018). Failure to diurese in the immediate postpartum period can lead to pulmonary edema and subsequent cardiac problems. This is seen more commonly in women with a history of preeclampsia or preexisting cardiac problems.

Neurologic Changes and Conditions

Neurologic problems and disorders can predispose women to higher rates of morbidity and mortality during pregnancy and in the postpartum period. Headaches are the most common neurologic symptoms encountered by postpartum women. Headaches can result from fluid shifts in the first week after birth, leakage of cerebrospinal fluid into the extradural space during spinal anesthesia, pregnancy-induced hypertension, fluid and electrolyte imbalance, or stress (Blackburn, 2018). It is estimated that up to 40% of postpartum women develop headaches within the first week following birth when estrogen drops precipitously. There may be an increased incidence in headache if the woman had spinal or epidural anesthesia. Migraine headaches, although less frequent during pregnancy, tend to resume in the postpartum period (Isley & Katz, 2017). Women with epilepsy are nine times more likely to have a seizure during labor or in the first 24 hours after birth than during pregnancy (Gerard & Samuels, 2017). The postpartum epileptic woman is more likely to be diagnosed with depression and referral to a therapist or support group should be made. The physiologic changes of pregnancy that may have required increasing antiepileptic drug (AED) dosage are now removed, and retitration of the AEDs is required to prevent toxicity. Women with multiple sclerosis (MS) and Guillain-Barré syndrome are more likely to have symptoms in the postpartum period than during pregnancy (Gerard & Samuels, 2017).

Weight Loss

An initial weight loss of 10 to 12 lb occurs as a result of the birth of the baby and placenta and release of amniotic fluid. Puerperal diuresis accounts for the loss of an additional 5 lb during the early puerperium. By the sixth to eighth week after birth, many women have returned to approximately prepregnant weight if they gained the average 25 to 30 lb. Women often express concern about the slow pace of their postpartum weight loss. Multiparas tend to have a more positive outlook than primiparas, probably because the multipara's previous experience has prepared her for the fact that the body does not immediately return to a prepregnant state.

Postpartum Chill

Frequently the mother experiences intense tremors that resemble shivering from a chill immediately after birth. Several theories have been offered to explain this shivering: The result of sudden release of pressure on the pelvic nerves after birth, a response to a fetus-to-mother transfusion that occurred during placental separation, a reaction to maternal adrenaline production during labor and birth, or a reaction to epidural anesthesia. If not followed by fever, this chill is of no clinical concern, but it is uncomfortable for the woman. The nurse can increase the woman's comfort by covering her with a warmed blanket and reassuring her that the shivering is a common, self-limiting situation. The nurse may also hold the woman's hand and place her other hand on the woman's shoulder and, speaking softly, urge the woman to breathe slowly while relaxing her shoulders. This will quickly decrease the shaking if not completely eliminate it. As the woman begins to shake again, she can gently be reminded to relax her shoulders.

Postpartum Diaphoresis

The elimination of excess fluid and waste products via the skin during the puerperium greatly increases perspiration. Diaphoretic (sweating) episodes frequently occur at night, and the woman may awaken drenched with perspiration. This perspiration is not significant clinically, but the mother should be protected from chilling.

Afterpains

Afterpains occur more commonly in multiparas than in primiparas and are caused by intermittent uterine contractions. Although the uterus of the primipara usually remains consistently contracted, the lost tone of the uterus of the multipara results in alternate contraction and relaxation. This phenomenon also occurs if the uterus has been markedly distended, as with multiple-gestation pregnancies or polyhydramnios, or if clots or placental fragments were retained. These afterpains may cause the mother severe discomfort for 2 to 3 days following birth. The administration of oxytocic agents (intravenous infusion with Pitocin or oral administration of Methergine) stimulates uterine contraction and increases the discomfort of the afterpains. Because endogenous oxytocin is released when the baby suckles, breastfeeding also increases the severity of the afterpains. A warm water bottle placed against the low abdomen may reduce the discomfort of afterpains. In addition, the breastfeeding mother may find it helpful to take a mild analgesic agent approximately 1 hour before feeding her baby. The nurse can assure the mother that the prescribed analgesic agents are not harmful to the newborn and help improve the quality of the breastfeeding experience. An analgesic agent such as ibuprofen is also helpful at bedtime if the afterpains interfere with the mother's rest. See Chapter 33 for a further discussion of afterpains.

Postpartum Psychologic Adaptations

The postpartum period is a time of readjustment and adaptation for the entire childbearing family but especially for the mother. The woman experiences a variety of responses as she adjusts to a new family member, postpartum discomforts, changes in her body image, and the reality that she is no longer pregnant. One young mother described her responses well:

> "I feel like it's the day after Christmas. I'm relieved that everything went well and I have a fine baby, but I feel so let down. I had an image of what childbirth would be like, but everything was a little different. I figured that as soon as I gave birth, I would feel fine. Why didn't someone tell me I would still be sore? The pain didn't magically disappear! When I was pregnant, everyone treated me as though I was a little fragile. Now when people call or visit, all they talk about is the baby. I don't think I'm really jealous, but I do miss the attention. During this past day I've started to realize that my life will never, ever be the same again. I've always wanted to be a mother, but I'm not really sure how to do it. Isn't that strange?"

Taking-In and Taking-Hold Periods

Soon after birth during the *taking-in* period, the woman tends to be passive and somewhat dependent. She follows suggestions, hesitates about making decisions, and is still rather preoccupied with her needs (Rubin, 1984). She may have a great need to talk about her perceptions of her labor and birth. This helps her work through the process, sort out the reality from her fantasized experience, and clarify anything that she did not understand. Food and sleep are major needs.

By the second or third day after birth, the new mother may be observed to be ready to resume control of her body, her mothering, and her life in general. Rubin (1984) labeled this phase as *taking hold*. If she is breastfeeding, the mother may worry about her technique or the quality of her milk. If her baby spits up following feeding, she may view it as a personal failure. She may also feel demoralized by the fact that the nurse or an older family member handles her baby proficiently while she feels unsure and tentative. She requires assurance that she is doing well as a mother. Today's mothers seem to be more independent and adjust more rapidly, exhibiting behaviors of "taking in" and "taking hold" in shorter time periods than those previously identified.

BECOMING A MOTHER

Maternal role attainment (MRA) is the process by which a woman learns mothering behaviors and becomes comfortable with her identity as a mother. As the mother grows to know this child and forms a relationship with her or him, the mother's maternal identity gradually and systematically evolves, and she "binds in" to the infant (Rubin, 1984). In most cases, maternal role attainment occurs within 3 to 10 months following birth.

Mercer proposed replacing the term *maternal role attainment* with the term **becoming a mother (BAM)**. She stated that BAM "more accurately encompasses the dynamic transformation and evolution of a woman's persona than does MRA, and the term MRA should be discontinued" (2004, p. 226). BAM more accurately reflects the transition process of becoming a mother that changes throughout the maternal–child relationship.

Postpartum nurses need to be aware of the long-term adjustments and stresses that the mother faces as she adjusts to new and different roles. Nursing interventions that foster the process of becoming a mother include:

- Instructing about newborn/infant caregiving
- Building awareness of and responsiveness to newborn/infant interactive capabilities
- Promoting maternal–newborn attachment
- Preparing the woman for the maternal social role
- Encouraging interactive therapeutic nurse–patient relationships.

Maternal/social role preparation and interactive therapeutic nurse–patient relationships have a greater impact on the progress of becoming a mother than formal teaching (see Chapter 33 for further discussion).

Professionalism in Practice Enhancing Patient-Centered Care

Mercer (2006) emphasized the importance of individualized dialogue between the mother and the nurse, which involves "a mutual identification by the mother and the nurse of the mother's needs and the available resources among the mother's family and friends, her community, and the larger society. With the mother's input about her preferences for available assistance . . . . Appropriate referrals may be made" (p. 650). Professional nurses who follow Mercer's recommendations enhance the process of a mother and engage in patient-centered care.

Postpartum Blues

The **postpartum blues** consist of a transient period of depression that occurs during the first few days of the puerperium. Symptoms may include mood swings, anger, weepiness, anorexia, difficulty sleeping, and a feeling of letdown. This mood change frequently occurs while the woman is still hospitalized, but it may occur at home as well. Changing hormone levels are certainly a factor; an unsupportive environment and insecurity also have been identified as potential causes. In addition, fatigue, discomfort, and overstimulation may play a part. Postpartum pain can be a result of both vaginal and cesarean births and has been shown to be associated with postpartum depression (ACOG, 2018). Managing acute postpartum pain supports the new mother's ability to emotionally attach and care for her baby. See *Developing Cultural Competence: Postpartum Depression.*

Postpartum blues usually resolve naturally within 10 to 14 days, but if they persist or if symptoms worsen, the woman may need evaluation for postpartum depression. Ideally a depression assessment should be completed each trimester to update a pregnant woman's risk status (Hart & Flynn, 2016). If not done previously, the nurse assesses the woman for predisposing factors during labor and the postpartum stay. Several depression scales are available for assessing postpartum depression (see Chapter 35 for further discussion).

Importance of Social Support

After the birth of a baby, a woman and her partner may find that family relationships become increasingly important. The attention that their baby receives from family members is a source of satisfaction to the new parents. In many cases, the ties to the woman's family become especially good. Fathers may report that their relationships with their in-laws become far more positive and supportive. However, the increased family interaction can be a source of stress, especially for the new mother, who often tends to have more contact with both families.

The new parents may also have increasing contact with other parents of small children, although contact with other friends and coworkers may decline. Of great concern are women and their partners, or single mothers, who have no family or friends with whom to form a social network. Isolation at a time when the woman feels an increased need for support can result in tremendous stress and is often a contributing factor in situations of postpartum depression, child neglect, or abuse. New mother support groups are helpful for women who lack a social support system.

Postpartum doulas are professionals trained to help the new mother after the birth of the baby. As a "mother's helper," postpartum doula services are tailored to help the new mother feel as rested and well nourished as possible and to keep her household in good order so that she can focus her energy on her new baby. See *Developing Cultural Competence: Initial Postpartum Experience within the Muslim Family.*

Development of Family Attachment

Some parents may lack any experience with babies and may feel overwhelmed by the newborn. Bonding is a series of steps in which the mother, father, and baby develop relationships.

Developing Cultural Competence Postpartum Depression

Nurses should take cultural and ethnic influences into account when assessing for the signs of postpartum depression (PPD). In a Pregnancy Risk Assessment Monitoring System (PRAMS) survey, socioeconomic variables (SES) accounted for increased rates of depressed mood and anhedonia (a psychological condition characterized by the inability to experience pleasure in normally pleasurable acts) among African American and Hispanic women compared with Caucasian White women. Women of Asian/Pacific Islander descent had more than 2.1 times the rate of anhedonia after controlling for SES and were more likely to be diagnosed with PPD after the birth of a female baby (Liu & Tronick, 2014). Some characteristics, such as the baby's gender, are not commonly thought of as predictors for depression, but are predictive in specific ethnic groups. Middle Eastern culture has a combination of symptoms that mimic PPD called *Jinn*; the postpartum care includes support through the family and community but no medications (Lauderdale, 2016). Across all the ethnic and racial groups, prenatal depression is a strong predictor of PPD and assessment for signs of depression both before and after the birth is best practice.

Note: It is unwise to attribute specific attitudes or beliefs to all members of a cultural group. The information in the Developing Cultural Competence boxes offers possible insights into caring for women from different cultural groups.

Developing Cultural Competence Initial Postpartum Experience within the Muslim Family

Traditionally in the Muslim community, labor and delivery is the business of women with *dayahs* (midwives). Therefore, all-female attendants are preferred at the birth, whether they be doctors, nurses, midwives, doulas, or female relatives (Lauderdale, 2016). However, it is permissible in Islam for male doctors to attend to a pregnant woman. There is no Islamic teaching that prohibits fathers from attending the birth of their child; this is left up to personal choice.

The Call to Prayer (*Adhan*) are the beautiful words that call the Muslim community to prayer five times a day and are also the first words the Muslim baby will hear. The father or a family elder will whisper these words in the baby's ear shortly after its birth.

One of the very first duties that parents have toward a new child, besides physical care and love, is to give the child a meaningful Islamic name. The children are usually named within 7 days of their birth. The new mother is in convalescence for a period of 40 days, during which friends and relatives will often provide the family with meals. It is common for close family members to visit right away and for other visitors to wait until a week or more after birth in order to protect the child from exposure to illnesses. Among Muslims, visiting and assisting the indisposed is a basic form of worship to bring one closer to God (Huda, 2017).

Note: It is unwise to attribute specific attitudes or beliefs to all members of a cultural group. The information in the Developing Cultural Competence boxes offers possible insights into caring for women from different cultural groups.

Maternal–Newborn Attachment Behavior

A mother's first interaction with her newborn is influenced by many factors, including her family of origin, her relationships, the stability of her home environment, the communication patterns she has developed, and the degree of nurturing she received as a child. These factors have shaped the person she has become. The following personal characteristics are also important:

- ***Level of trust.*** What level of trust has this mother developed in response to her life experiences? What is her philosophy of childrearing? Will she be able to treat her baby as a unique individual with changing needs that should be met as much as possible?
- ***Level of self-esteem.*** How much does she value herself as a woman and as a mother? Does she feel generally able to cope with the adjustments of life?
- ***Capacity for enjoying herself.*** Is the mother able to find pleasure in everyday activities and human relationships?
- ***Adequacy of knowledge about childbearing and childrearing.*** What beliefs about the course of pregnancy, the capacities of newborns, previous experiences with infants or children, and the nature of her emotions may influence her behavior at first contact with her newborn and later?
- ***Prevailing mood or usual feeling tone.*** Is the woman predominantly content, angry, depressed, or anxious? Is she sensitive to her own feelings and those of others? Will she be able to accept her own needs and to obtain support in meeting them?
- ***Reactions to the present pregnancy.*** Was the pregnancy planned? Did it go smoothly? Were there ongoing life events that enhanced her pregnancy or depleted her reserves of energy? How were other life roles changed because of her pregnancy and motherhood?

By the time of birth, each mother has developed an emotional orientation of some kind to the baby based on these factors.

Initial Attachment Behavior

After labor and birth, a new mother demonstrates a fairly regular pattern of maternal behaviors as she continues to familiarize herself with her newborn. In a progression of touching activities, the mother proceeds from fingertip exploration of the newborn's extremities toward palmar contact with larger body areas and finally to enfolding the baby with the whole hand and arms. The time taken to accomplish these steps varies from minutes to days. The mother also increases the proportion of time spent in the *en face* position (Figure 32–4), in which she arranges herself and the newborn so that they have direct face-to-face and eye-to-eye contact. There is an intense interest in having the baby's eyes open. When the eyes are open, the mother characteristically greets the newborn and talks in high-pitched tones to the baby.

In most instances the mother relies heavily on her senses of sight, touch, and hearing in getting to know what her baby is really like. She also tends to respond verbally to any sounds emitted by the newborn, such as cries, coughs, sneezes, and grunts. The sense of smell may be involved as well.

While interacting with her newborn, the mother may be experiencing shock, disbelief, and denial. She may state, "I can't believe she's finally here" or "I felt he was a stranger." However, the mother may express feelings of connectedness between the newborn and the rest of the family, either in positive or in negative terms: "She's got your cute nose, Daddy" or "Oh, no! He looks just like my first one, and he was an impossible baby." A mother's facial expression or the frequency and content of her questions may demonstrate concerns about the newborn's general condition or normality, especially if her pregnancy was complicated or if a previously born baby was not healthy.

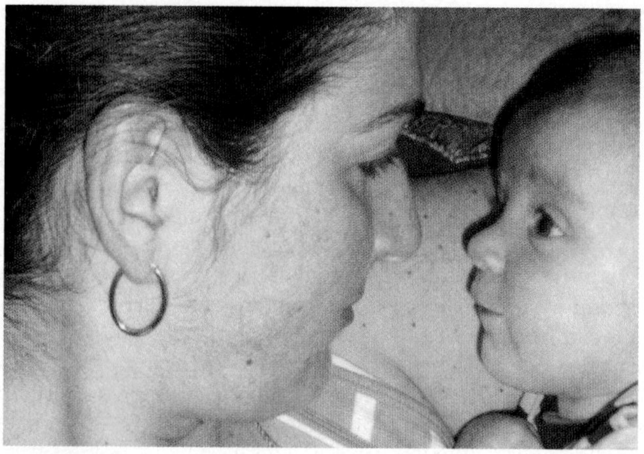

Figure 32–4 The mother has direct face-to-face and eye-to-eye contact in the *en face* position.

SOURCE: Joanna Allen.

During the first few days after her child's birth, the new mother applies herself to the task of getting to know her baby. This is termed the *acquaintance phase*. If the newborn gives clear behavioral cues about needs, the baby's responses to mothering will be predictable, which will make the mother feel effective and competent. Other behaviors that make a baby more attractive to caretakers are smiling, grasping a finger, breastfeeding eagerly, cuddling, and being easy to console.

During this time the newborn is also becoming acquainted. Within a few days after birth, babies show signs of recognizing recurrent situations and responding to changes in routine. To the extent that their mother is their world, they are actively acquainting themselves with her.

During the *mutual regulation phase*, mother and newborn seek to deal with the degree of control to be exerted by each in their relationship. In this phase of adjustment, a balance is sought between the needs of the mother and the needs of the baby. The most important consideration is that each should obtain a good measure of enjoyment from the interaction. During the mutual adjustment phase, negative maternal feelings are likely to surface or intensify. Because "everyone knows that mothers love their babies," these negative feelings often go unexpressed and are allowed to build up. If they are expressed, the response of friends, relatives, or healthcare personnel is often to deny the feelings to the mother: "You don't mean that." Some negative feelings are normal in the first few days after birth, and the nurse should be supportive when the mother vocalizes these feelings.

When mutual regulation arrives at the point where both mother and baby primarily enjoy each other's company, reciprocity has been achieved. **Reciprocity** is an interactional cycle that occurs simultaneously between mother and baby. It involves mutual cuing behaviors, expectancy, rhythmicity, and synchrony. The mother develops a new relationship with an individual who has a unique character and evokes a response entirely different from the fantasy response of pregnancy. When reciprocity is synchronous, the interaction between mother and baby is mutually gratifying and is sought and initiated by both partners (Feldman, 2017; Kim, Chow, Bray, et al., 2017).

Clinical Tip

Newborns are sometimes taken from their parents immediately after birth and placed in a special care or intensive care nursery. This separation can interfere with the normal attachment process. If this occurs, parents should be brought to the nursery as soon as possible to interact with their newborns and should be allowed to hold and care for their babies as much as possible. If a newborn is in an incubator and cannot be held, encourage the parents to stroke the baby's hand, foot, or cheek. Provide reassurance that this will not hurt the baby and is in fact beneficial.

FATHER–NEWBORN INTERACTIONS

In Western cultures, commitment to family-centered maternity care has fostered interest in understanding the feelings and experiences of the new father. Evidence suggests that the father has a strong attraction to his newborn and that the feelings he experiences are similar to the mother's feelings of attachment (Figure 32–5). The characteristic sense of absorption, preoccupation, and interest in the baby demonstrated by fathers during early contact has been termed **engrossment**. Differences in involvement still exist among fathers in Western culture and may be influenced by factors other than culture (e.g., previous experience with paternal role or exposure to male/father role models). See *Professionalism in Practice: Promoting Skin-to-Skin Contact*.

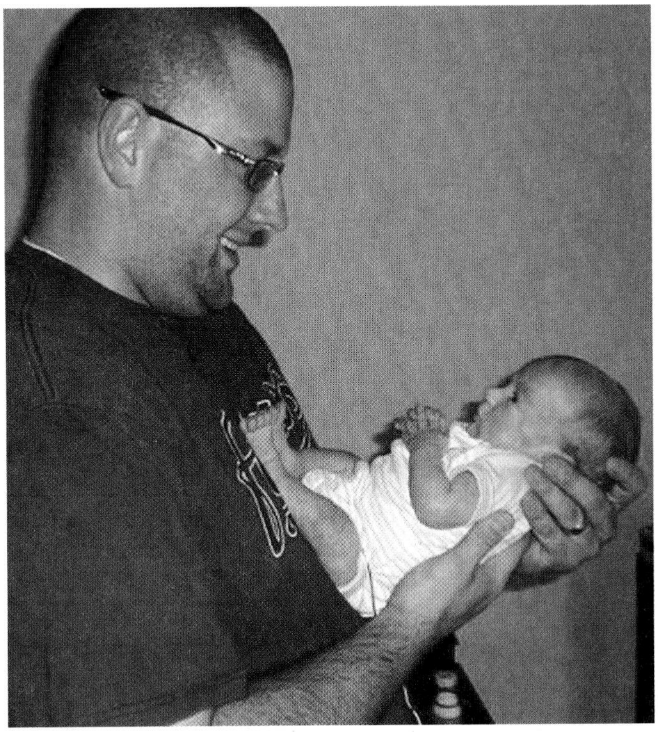

Figure 32–5 The father experiences strong feelings of attraction during engrossment.

SOURCE: Joanna and Christopher Allen.

SIBLINGS AND OTHERS

Babies are capable of maintaining a number of strong attachments without loss of quality. These attachments may include siblings, grandparents, aunts, and uncles. The social setting and personality of the individual seem to be significant factors in the development of multiple attachments. Birth centers are especially geared toward the inclusion of the family in the birth process. In the hospital setting, the advent of open visiting hours and rooming-in permits siblings and grandparents to participate in the attachment process.

Cultural Influences in the Postpartum Period

Whereas Western culture places primary emphasis on the events of birth, many other cultures place greater emphasis on the postpartum period. For women not of the dominant American culture, the new mother's primary culture, personal values, and level of acculturation can influence her beliefs about her postpartum care. Her expectations regarding food, fluids, rest, hygiene, medications, relief measures, support, and counsel—as well as other aspects of her life—will be influenced by the beliefs and values of her family and cultural group. Sometimes a new mother's wishes will differ from the expectations of the healthcare provider or nurse. (See Chapter 2 for an in-depth discussion of family and culture.)

All nurses belong to their particular ethnoculture and also share in the culture of healthcare. As a part of the healthcare cultural group, nurses implement practices that support their general beliefs, such as offering food in the recovery period following birth, providing iced fluids, expecting the woman to ambulate as soon as possible, and assuming the woman will want to shower and perhaps wash her hair soon after birth. It is important for nurses to recognize that they are approaching their patient's care from their own perspective and that, to individualize care for each mother, they need to assess the woman's preferences, her level of acculturation and assimilation to Western culture, her linguistic abilities, and her educational level (Lauderdale, 2016; Spector, 2017). In addition, the nurse should have the mother exercise her choices when possible and support those choices, with the help of cultural awareness and a sound knowledge base.

The woman of European heritage may expect to eat a full meal and have a large amount of iced fluids following the birth, in the belief that the food restores energy and the fluids help replace fluid lost during labor. She may want to ambulate shortly after the birth, shower, wash her hair, and put on a fresh gown. She may expect a relatively short stay in the hospital and may or may not be interested in educational classes. A woman of the Islamic faith may have specific modesty requirements; she must be completely covered, with only her feet and hands exposed, and no man, other than her husband or a family member, may be alone with her (Lauderdale, 2016).

Professionalism in Practice Promoting Skin-to-Skin Contact

Many hospital units remove newborns from their mothers following birth to allow convenient assessment and performance of procedures by hospital staff despite a preponderance of evidence that supports immediate skin-to-skin contact (SSC) between mother (or father) and the newborn. Nurses are the professionals most often at the patient's bedside; they have the power and an obligation to serve as leaders and change agents by promoting clinical practices that are supported by research evidence. After both vaginal and cesarean births, SSC should be continued throughout the postpartum period as needed, including during procedures that are painful for the newborn such as injections or heelsticks.

Some cultures emphasize certain postpartum routines or rituals for mother and baby that are designed to restore the hot–cold balance of the body. Some women of Hispanic, African, and Asian cultures may avoid cold after birth. This prohibition includes cold air, wind, and all water (even if heated). On the other hand, some traditional Mexican women may avoid eating "hot" foods, such as pork, just after the birth of a baby (considered a "hot" experience). It is important to note that each individual or cultural group may define hot and cold conditions as well as hot and cold foods differently. The nurse should ask each woman what she can eat and what foods she thinks would be helpful for healing. The nurse may encourage family members to bring preferred food and drink for the mother. See *Developing Cultural Competence: Caring for the Orthodox Jewish Couple.*

In many cultures, the extended family plays an essential role during the puerperium. The grandmother is often the primary helper to the mother and newborn. She brings wisdom and experience, allowing the new mother time to rest as well as giving her ready access to someone who can help with problems and concerns as they arise. African American mothers may model their mothering skills after their older female relatives. In addition, these same older female relatives often provide child care as needed (Spector, 2017).

It is important to ensure access of all family members during the postpartum period. Visiting rules may be waived to allow family members or authority figures access to the mother and newborn. These practices show respect and foster a blending of old and new behaviors to meet the goals of all concerned (Giger, 2017; Lauderdale, 2016; Spector, 2017).

Developing Cultural Competence **Caring for the Orthodox Jewish Couple**

The orthodox Jewish couple's beliefs and practices are strictly adhered to in their dress, communication, dietary practices, and activities of daily living in the postpartum time. Jewish patients may request a kosher diet. The nurse should assist the woman in maintaining her modesty in her dress and keeping her hair covered at all times. For the first 7 days after delivery the woman will be given special treatment and will be cared for by family members (Lauderdale, 2016).

Some traditional Jewish couples avoid physical contact while the woman is experiencing any vaginal discharge; as a result, unfortunately, the man may be viewed as unsupportive by the staff during the postpartum period (Lauderdale, 2016).

Resting after childbirth is considered crucial for the first 6 weeks. The woman will breastfeed her newborn. The baby will not be named and the newborn male will not be circumcised until a later date after discharge from the hospital. The Sabbath is sacred and begins at sundown on Friday evening and ends after dark on Saturday. During this time neither the man nor the woman will use electricity, travel, or write. They will not tear or cut anything. So if the woman is in the hospital during the Sabbath, the nurse should be sensitive to the fact that any forms that may need to be signed will have to be signed before or after the Sabbath. The woman will need the nurse to adjust an electric bed, turn off/on lights, and tear pieces of toilet paper for her to use. The woman will not leave the hospital and travel home until after the Sabbath (Lauderdale, 2016).

Note: It is unwise to attribute specific attitudes or beliefs to all members of a cultural group. The information in the Developing Cultural Competence boxes offers possible insights into caring for women from different cultural groups.

Postpartum Nursing Assessment

Comprehensive care is based on a thorough assessment, with identification of individual needs or potential problems.

Risk Factors

Ongoing assessment and patient education during the puerperium are designed to meet the needs of the childbearing family and to detect and treat possible complications. Table 32–2 identifies factors that may place the new mother at risk during the postpartum period. The nurse uses this knowledge during the assessment and is particularly alert for possible complications that may occur in an individual because of identified risk factors.

Physical Assessment

There are several principles to remember in preparing for and completing an assessment of the postpartum woman:

- Select the time that will provide the most accurate data. Palpating the fundus when the woman has a full bladder, for example, may give false information about the progress of involution. Ask the woman to void before assessment.
- Consider the patient's need for possible premedication before any painful assessments such as fundal massage.
- Provide an explanation of the purposes of regular assessment to the woman.
- Ensure that the woman is relaxed before starting; perform the procedures as gently as possible to avoid unnecessary discomfort.
- Document and report the results according to hospital/unit policy.
- Take appropriate precautions to prevent exposure to body fluids.

The physical assessment is an excellent opportunity for patient teaching. For example, when assessing the breasts of a lactating woman, the nurse can discuss breast care, breast milk production, the let-down reflex, and breast self-examination. A new mother may be very receptive to instruction on postpartum abdominal tightening exercises when the nurse assesses the woman's fundal height and diastasis. The assessment also provides an excellent time to provide information about the body's postpartum physical and anatomic changes as well as danger signs to report. See *Key Facts to Remember: Common Postpartum Concerns*.

Because the time the woman spends in the postpartum unit is limited, nurses should use every available opportunity for patient teaching regarding self-care. To assist nurses in recognizing these opportunities, examples of patient teaching during the assessment have been provided throughout the following discussion.

VITAL SIGNS

The nurse may organize the physical assessment in a variety of ways. Many nurses choose to begin by assessing vital signs because the findings are more accurate when they are obtained with the woman at rest. In addition, establishing whether the vital

TABLE 32–2 Postpartum High-Risk Factors

FACTOR	MATERNAL IMPLICATION
Preeclampsia	Blood pressure ↑ CNS irritability → ↑ risk for seizure ↑ Need for bedrest → ↑ Risk of thrombophlebitis
Diabetes	Need for insulin regulation Episodes of hypoglycemia or hyperglycemia ↓ Healing
Cardiac disease	↑ Maternal exhaustion
Cesarean birth	↑ Healing needs ↑ Pain from incision ↑ Risk of infection ↑ Length of hospitalization Exacerbation of carpal tunnel syndrome
Overdistention of uterus (multiple gestation, polyhydramnios)	↑ Risk of thrombophlebitis (cesarean section [C/S] risk) ↑ Risk of problems breastfeeding (C/S risk) ↑ Risk of hemorrhage ↑ Risk of anemia ↑ Stretching of abdominal muscles ↑ Incidence and severity of afterpains
Abruptio placentae, placenta previa	Hemorrhage → anemia ↓ Uterine contractility after birth→ ↑ Infection risk
Precipitous labor (less than 3 hours)	↑ Risk of lacerations to birth canal → hemorrhage
Prolonged labor (greater than 24 hours)	Exhaustion ↑ Risk of hemorrhage Nutritional and fluid depletion ↑ Bladder atony and/or trauma ↑ Pain and bruising from prolonged time in stirrups
Difficult birth	Exhaustion ↑ Risk of perineal lacerations ↑ Risk of hematomas ↑ Risk of hemorrhage → anemia
Extended period of time in stirrups at birth	↑ Risk of thrombophlebitis
Retained placenta	↑ Risk of hemorrhage ↑ Risk of infection

signs are within the expected normal range will assist the nurse in determining other assessments that might be needed. For instance, if the temperature is elevated, the nurse considers the time since birth and begins to gather information to determine whether the woman is dehydrated or whether an infection is developing.

Temperature elevations (less than 38°C [100.4°F]) due to normal processes should last for only 24 hours. The nurse should evaluate any temperature elevation in light of other signs and symptoms and should carefully review the woman's history to identify other factors, such as premature rupture of membranes (PROM) or prolonged labor, that might increase the incidence of infection in the genital tract.

Alterations in vital signs may indicate complications, so they are assessed at regular intervals. After an immediate, transient rise after birth, the blood pressure should remain stable. The pulse often shows a characteristic slowness that is no cause for alarm. Pulse rates return to prepregnant norms very quickly unless complications arise.

SAFETY ALERT!

During the first few hours after birth, the woman may have some orthostatic hypotension. This will cause her to have a lower blood pressure reading in a sitting position. For the most accurate reading, measure her blood pressure with the woman in the same position each time, preferably lying on her back with her arm at her side. Because of the propensity for hypotension, the nurse should assist the mother the first few times she attempts to ambulate after childbirth.

The nurse informs the woman of the results of the vital signs assessment, providing information regarding the normal changes in blood pressure and pulse. This may also be an opportunity to assess whether the mother knows how to take her own and her baby's temperatures, how to read a thermometer, and how to select a thermometer from the wide variety now available (see discussion in Chapter 34).

Key Facts To Remember

Common Postpartum Concerns

Several postpartum occurrences cause special concern for mothers. The nurse will frequently be asked about the following events.

Source of Concern	Explanation
Gush of blood that sometimes occurs when she first arises	There is a normal pooling of blood in the vagina when the woman lies down to rest or sleep. Gravity causes blood to flow out when she stands.
Passing clots	Blood pools at the top of the vagina and forms clots that are passed upon rising or sitting on the toilet.
Night sweats	Normal physiologic occurrence that results as body attempts to eliminate excess fluids that were present during pregnancy. May be aggravated by plastic mattress pad.
Afterpains	More common in multiparas. Caused by contraction and relaxation of uterus. Increased by oxytocin, breastfeeding. Relieved with mild analgesics and time.
"Large stomach" after birth and failure to lose all weight gained during pregnancy	The baby, amniotic fluid, and placenta account for only a portion of the weight gained during pregnancy. The remainder takes approximately 6 weeks to lose. Abdomen also appears large because of decreased muscle tone. Postpartum exercises will help.

AUSCULTATION OF LUNGS

The breath sounds should be clear. Women who have been treated for preterm labor or preeclampsia are especially at risk for pulmonary edema (see discussion in Chapter 18).

BREASTS

Before examining the breasts, the nurse dons gloves and then assesses the fit and support of the woman's bra. The nurse provides information about how to select a bra. A properly fitting bra provides support to the breasts and helps maintain breast shape by limiting stretching of supporting ligaments and connective tissue. If the mother is breastfeeding, the straps of the bra should be cloth, not elastic (because cloth has less stretch and provides more support) and easily adjustable. The back should be wide and have at least three rows of hooks to adjust for fit. Traditional nursing bras have a fixed inner cup and a separate half-cup that can be unhooked for breastfeeding while continuing to support the breast. Purchasing a nursing bra one size too large during pregnancy will usually result in a good fit because the breasts increase in size with milk production.

The nurse asks the woman to remove her bra so the breasts can be examined. It is important to note the size and shape of the breasts and any abnormalities, reddened areas, or engorgement. The nurse also palpates the breasts lightly for softness, slight firmness associated with filling, or firmness associated with engorgement, warmth, or tenderness. The nipples are assessed for fissures, cracks, soreness, or inversion. The nurse teaches the woman the characteristics of the breast and explains how to recognize problems such as fissures or cracks in the nipples.

The nurse assesses the nonbreastfeeding mother for evidence of breast discomfort and provides relief measures, if necessary. (See discussion of lactation suppression in the nonbreastfeeding mother in Chapter 33.) Breast assessment findings for a nonbreastfeeding woman may be recorded as follows: "Breasts soft, filling, no evidence of nipple tenderness or cracking, nipples everted."

Clinical Tip

An easy way to remember the components specific to the postpartum examination is to remember the term *BUBBLEHE*: B: breast, U: uterus, B: bladder, B: bowel, L: lochia, E: episiotomy/laceration, H: Homans/hemorrhoids, and E: emotional.

ABDOMEN AND FUNDUS

The woman should void before her abdomen is examined. This practice ensures that a full bladder is not causing displacement of the uterus or any uterine atony; if atony is present, other causes (such as uterine relaxation associated with a regional block, overstretched uterus, or distended bladder) must be investigated.

The nurse determines the relationship of the fundus to the umbilicus and also assesses the firmness of the fundus. The top of the fundus is measured in centimeters (cm) above, below, or at the umbilicus. The nurse notes whether the fundus is in the midline or displaced to either side of the abdomen. If not midline, the uterus position should be located. The most common cause of displacement is a full bladder; thus, this finding requires further assessment. If the fundus is in the midline but higher than expected, it is usually associated with clots within the uterus. The results of the assessment should then be recorded. (See *Clinical Skill 32–1: Assessing the Status of the Uterine Fundus After Vaginal or Cesarean Birth.*)

While completing the assessment, the nurse teaches the woman about fundal position and how to determine firmness. The mother can be taught to massage her fundus gently if it is not firm.

In the woman who has had a cesarean birth, the abdominal incision is extremely tender. The nurse should palpate the fundus with extreme care and inspect the abdominal incision for signs of healing, such as approximation (edges of incision appear "glued" together), bleeding, and any signs of infection, including drainage, foul odor, or redness. The nurse should document whether internal sutures, Steri-Strips, or staples are intact. The nurse can also review characteristics of normal healing and incision care and discuss signs of infection.

Clinical Tip

Assessing the status of the uterine fundus may be uncomfortable. In addition to explaining the importance of the assessment to the mother, you can show her how to perform frequent light massage of the fundus herself to promote uterine involution. She may be delighted to be able to feel the difference between where the fundus is now and where the top of the uterus was just prior to delivery. Involving her in her own care encourages her participation. In addition, having her massage her own uterus may lessen bleeding and reduce the need for more thorough massage.

Clinical Skill 32–1

Assessing the Status of the Uterine Fundus After Vaginal or Cesarean Birth

NURSING ACTION

Preparation

- Consider offering to premedicate 30 to 45 minutes before assessing the fundus, especially if the woman has had a cesarean section.

  Rationale: *The postoperative area will be very tender, and she may be very fearful of the potential pain.*
- Explain the procedure, the information it provides, and what it might feel like.
- Ask the woman to void.

  Rationale: *A full bladder can cause uterine atony.*
- Have the woman lie flat in bed with her head on a pillow. If the procedure is uncomfortable, she may find that it helps to flex her legs. Flexing the legs and providing support under them with folded pillows is especially helpful with women who have had a cesarean.

  Rationale: *The supine position prevents a falsely high assessment of fundal height. Flexing the legs relaxes the abdominal muscles.*

Equipment and Supplies

- Clean perineal pad
- Clean gloves

CLINICAL TIP

Gloves may be put on before assessing the abdomen and fundus and must be worn when you are ready to assess the perineum and lochia.

Procedure

1. Gently place one hand on the lower segment of the uterus. Using the side of the other hand, palpate the abdomen until you locate the top of the fundus.

   Rationale: *One hand stabilizes the uterus while the other hand locates the top of the fundus. (Support of the uterus prevents stretching of the ligaments that support the uterus.)*
2. Determine whether the fundus is firm. If it is, it will feel like a hard round object (similar to a grapefruit) in the abdomen. If it is not firm, massage the abdomen lightly until the fundus is firm, then check for bleeding.

   Rationale: *A firm fundus indicates that the uterine muscles are contracted and bleeding will not occur.*
3. Measure the top of the fundus in fingerbreadths above, below, or at the fundus (Figure 32–6).

   Rationale: *Fundal height gives information about the progress of involution.*
4. Determine the position of the fundus in relation to the midline of the body. If it is not in the midline, locate it and then evaluate the bladder for distention.

   Rationale: *The fundus may deviate from the midline when the bladder is full because the enlarged bladder pushes the uterus aside.*
5. If the bladder is distended, use nursing measures to help the woman void. If she is not able to void after a specified period of time, catheterization may be necessary.
6. Measure urine output for the next few hours until normal elimination is established.

   Rationale: *During the postpartum period as diuresis occurs, the bladder may fill far more rapidly than normal, putting the woman at risk for uterine atony and hemorrhage. (Diminished tone of the uterus may cause loss of the urge to void.)*
7. Assess the lochia (see *Clinical Skill 32–2: Evaluating Lochia*).
8. During the first few hours postpartum, if the fundus becomes boggy frequently or is located high above the umbilicus and the woman's bladder is empty, the uterine cavity may be filled with clots of blood. In this case, do the following:
   - Release the front of the perineal pad and lay it back so that you can see the perineum and the pad lying between the woman's legs.
   - Massage the uterine fundus until it is firm.
   - Keep one hand in position, stabilizing the lower portion of the uterus. With the hand you used to massage the fundus, put steady pressure on the top of the now-firm fundus and see if you are able to express any clots. (Watch the pad between her legs for clots to pass from the vagina.)

   Rationale: *If the woman's uterus is filled with blood, it acts as an irritant and the uterus will not remain contracted. When the muscle fibers relax, bleeding results, further aggravating the problem. Pushing on a uterus that is not firm is dangerous because it is possible to cause the uterus to invert, a true emergency.*
9. If measurement of the blood loss is needed, the perineal pads and absorbent pad can be weighed.
10. Provide the woman with a clean perineal pad.

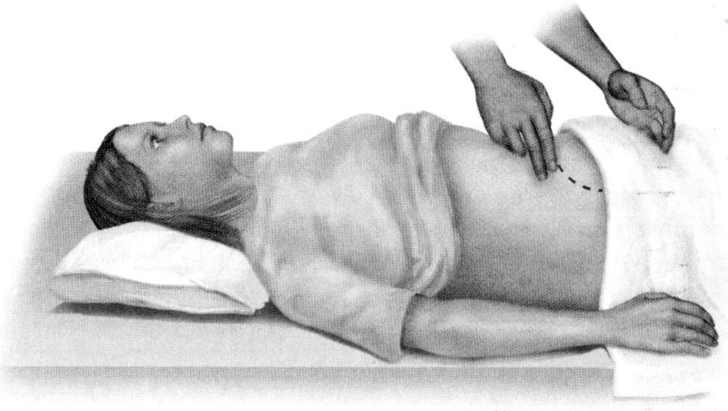

Figure 32–6 **Determining the position of the fundus for the woman with a vaginal birth. The fundus is located 2 cm (two fingerbreadths) below the umbilicus. Always support the bottom of the uterus during any assessment of the fundus.**

(continued)

Clinical Skill 32–1 *(continued)*

11. Record findings. Fundal height is recorded in fingerbreadths (e.g., "2 FB ↑ U" or "1 FB ↑ U"). If fundal massage was necessary, note that fact: "Uterus boggy → firm with light massage."
12. Communicate bogginess or heavy flow to primary provider.
13. If the woman is post–cesarean section, inspect the abdominal incision for signs of healing, such as approximation or bleeding, and for any signs of infection, including drainage, edema, foul odor, or redness. Observe whether internal sutures, Steri-Strips, or staples are intact. If dressing is in place over the incision, observe for the dressing to be clean, dry, and intact.

    Rationale: *If drainage is present on the dressing, mark the outline of the drainage and reevaluate 30 minutes later for further bleeding or drainage.*
14. Document findings according to hospital or unit policy.
15. Communicate active bleeding, increasing drainage, redness, foul odor, or incision edges not approximated to primary care provider.

A well-contracted uterus feels as firm as the uterus does during a strong labor contraction. If handled gently, the uterus should not be overly tender. Excessive pain in the uterus during postpartum examination should alert the nurse to possible uterine infection. If the uterus is not firm, the nurse should gently massage the fundus with the fingertips of the examining hand, and then assess the results. If the uterus becomes firm, the chart should read: "Uterus: boggy → firm with light massage." A good habit for the nurse to develop during the postpartum examination is to have the woman lie flat on her back with her head on a pillow and legs flexed. Then the nurse can release the perineal pad to observe the results of uterine massage based on the amount of expelled blood. Occasionally, oxytocic agents, such as an intravenous Pitocin infusion or methylergonovine maleate (Methergine), need to be administered postpartum to maintain uterine contraction and prevent or treat hemorrhage (see *Drug Guide: Methylergonovine Maleate [Methergine]* in Chapter 33).

Clinical Tip

During postpartum assessment, a firm uterus typically feels like a grapefruit because the muscles are well contracted. If the uterus loses its ability to contract and begins to relax, it is called *boggy*. A boggy uterus feels softer, like a sponge, or may become so relaxed that you cannot feel it at all. If the uterus is boggy but you can still feel it, massage it until it becomes firm. If you cannot feel it at all, place the side of one hand just above the woman's symphysis pubis to provide stability. Then place the other hand at the level of the umbilicus. (The fundus may have risen to this level because it is relaxed and filling with blood.) Press deeply into the abdomen and massage in a circular motion. You will usually feel the uterus begin to firm up under your hand. If you do not, move your hand slightly lower on the abdomen, and repeat the process.

A boggy uterus that does not contract with light, gentle massage may need more vigorous massage. The nurse assesses the amount and character of any expelled blood obtained while massaging the fundus. When a woman has postpartum uterine atony (the uterus does not remain firm), the nurse should:

1. Reevaluate for full bladder; if the bladder is full, have the woman void.
2. Question the woman on her bleeding history since the birth or last examination. How heavy does her flow seem? Has she passed any clots? How frequently has she changed pads? Were the pads saturated? Look at the discarded pads.
3. For the breastfeeding mother, put the newborn to the mother's breast for feeding to stimulate oxytocin production.
4. Assess maternal blood pressure and pulse to identify hypotension.
5. Reassess the fundus; if the fundus is still boggy, alert the physician/CNM immediately because further interventions, such as intravenous fluids and an oxytocic medication, are needed.

LOCHIA

Lochia is assessed for character, amount, odor, and the presence of clots. The nurse must wear disposable gloves when assessing the perineum and lochia. Nurses may put on the gloves before beginning the assessment, just before assessing the abdomen and fundus, or when they are ready to assess the perineum and lochia. During the first 1 to 3 days, the lochia should be rubra. A few small clots are normal and occur as a result of blood pooling in the vagina. However, the passage of numerous or large clots is abnormal, and the cause should be investigated immediately. After 2 to 3 days, the lochia becomes serosa.

Lochia should never exceed a moderate amount, such as that needed to partially saturate four to eight peripads daily, with an average of six. However, because this number is influenced by an individual woman's pad-changing practices, as well as the absorbency of the pad, the nurse must consider the length of time the current pad has been in use, the parity, and the size of the baby and ask whether the amount is normal compared with her typical menstrual period and whether any clots were passed before the examination, such as during voiding. If heavy bleeding is reported but not seen, the nurse asks the woman to put on a clean perineal pad and reassesses the discharge in 1 hour (see *Clinical Skill 32–2: Evaluating Lochia* and Figure 32–7).

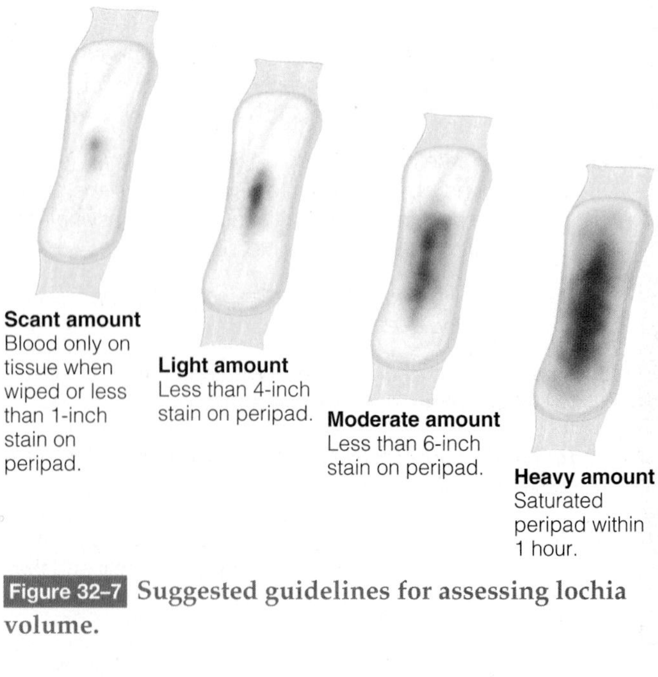

Figure 32–7 Suggested guidelines for assessing lochia volume.

Clinical Skill 32–2

Evaluating Lochia

NURSING ACTION

Preparation

- Explain why lochia occurs, why it is assessed, how it is assessed, and how it changes during the postpartum period.
- Ask the woman to void.

  Rationale: *A full bladder can cause uterine atony and increase the amount of lochia.*
- Complete the assessment of uterine fundal height and firmness.

  Rationale: *In almost all cases, fundal height and firmness are evaluated with an assessment of lochia. This practice provides a more thorough assessment.*
- If she has not already done so for the fundal assessment, ask the woman to flex her legs. Then ask her to spread her legs apart. Use the bed sheet as a drape to preserve her modesty.

  Rationale: *This position allows you to see the perineum and the perineal pad more effectively.*

Equipment and Supplies

- Clean gloves
- Clean perineal pad

Procedure

1. Don gloves before assessing the perineum and lochia.
2. Lower the perineal pad and observe the amount of lochia on the pad. Because women's pad-changing practices vary, ask her about the length of time the current pad has been in use, whether the amount is normal, and whether any clots were passed before this examination, such as during voiding.

   Rationale: *During the first 1 to 3 days, the woman's lochia should be rubra, which is dark red in color. A few small clots are normal and occur as a result of pooling of blood in the vagina when the woman is lying down. The passage of large clots is abnormal and the cause should be investigated immediately.*
3. If the woman reports heavy bleeding or clots, ask her to put on a clean perineal pad and then reassess the pad in 1 hour. Also ask her to call you before flushing any clots she passes into the toilet during voiding.
4. When the uterine fundus is firm and stabilized with the nondominant hand, press down on it with the dominant hand while watching to see if any clots are expelled (see *Clinical Skill 32–1: Assessing the Status of the Uterine Fundus After Vaginal or Cesarean Birth*, Step 8).
5. Determine the amount of lochia, using the following guide (refer to Figure 32–7):
   - Heavy amount—Perineal pad has a stain larger than 6 inches in length within 1 hour; 30 to 80 mL lochia.
   - Moderate amount—Perineal pad has a stain less than 6 inches in length within 1 hour; 25 to 50 mL lochia.
   - Small (light) amount—Perineal pad has a stain less than 4 inches in length after 1 hour; 10 to 25 mL lochia.
   - Scant amount—Perineal pad has a stain less than 1 inch in length after 1 hour or lochia is only on tissue when the woman wipes.

   Rationale: *Lochia should never exceed a moderate amount such as four to eight partially saturated perineal pads daily. Using a consistent standard for measuring lochia improves the accuracy of the information charted and conveyed to others.*
6. In most cases, a woman is discharged while her lochia is still rubra. Provide her with information about lochia serosa and lochia alba.

   Rationale: *Accurate discharge information enables the woman to assess herself more accurately and enables her to judge better when to contact her caregiver.*
7. Document the findings according to hospital/unit policy. For example, "Uterus firm, 1 FB ↓ U. Lochia: Moderate rubra, no clots passed."

SAFETY ALERT!

If blood loss exceeds the guidelines given in this chapter, weigh the perineal pads and the absorbent pads to estimate the blood loss more accurately. Typically, 1 g = 1 mL blood. Because blood can pool below the woman on the absorbent pad, make sure you elevate the buttocks as part of your assessment.

Clots and heavy bleeding may be caused by uterine relaxation (atony), retained placental fragments, or, rarely, an unknown cervical laceration (seen as heavy bleeding but with firm fundus) that may require further assessment (see *Key Facts to Remember: Changes in Lochia That Cause Concern*). Because of the evacuation of the uterine cavity during cesarean birth, women with such surgery usually have less lochia after the first 24 hours than mothers who give birth vaginally. If the woman is at increased risk for bleeding or is actually experiencing heavy flow of lochia rubra, her blood pressure, pulse, and uterus need to be assessed frequently, and the physician may prescribe oxytocin (Pitocin), methylergonovine maleate (Methergine), or misoprostol (Cytotec).

Key Facts To Remember

Changes in Lochia That Cause Concern

Change	Possible Problem	Nursing Action
Presence of clots	Inadequate uterine contractions that allow bleeding from vessels at the placental site.	Assess location and firmness of fundus. Assess voiding pattern. Record and report findings.
Persistent lochia rubra	Inadequate uterine contractions; retained placental fragments; infection; undetected cervical laceration.	Assess location and firmness of fundus. Assess activity pattern. Assess for signs of infection. Record and report findings.

Clinical Tip

The parity, length of time since delivery, method of delivery, size of baby/gestation (and other factors that could cause hyperextension of the uterus such as multiple gestation, polyhydramnios, large for gestational age, etc.) *must* be considered when deciding whether the amount and color of the lochia is appropriate.

The odor of the lochia is nonoffensive and never foul. If foul odor is present, so is an infection. When using narrative nursing notes, document the amount of lochia first, followed by character. For example:

- Lochia: Moderate rubra
- Lochia: Small rubra/serosa.

Health Promotion Teaching Hygienic Practices

Teaching during assessment of the lochia may center on normal changes, the effect of position changes, or what can be expected in the amount and color of the flow. Hygienic measures, such as wiping the perineum from front to back and washing hands after toileting and changing pads, may be reviewed, if appropriate. The nurse should approach the timing of teaching hygienic practices delicately, along with the content to be included. By establishing positive goals for the teaching—promoting comfort, enhancing tissue healing, and preventing infection—the nurse can avoid value-laden statements regarding personal beliefs about the need for cleanliness or control of body odor. The nurse should review with the mother the need to notify a healthcare professional if there is regression in the lochia flow pattern (i.e., color or amount).

PERINEUM

The perineum is inspected with the woman lying in Sims position. The buttock is lifted to expose the perineum and anus.

If an episiotomy was performed or a laceration required suturing, the nurse assesses the wound. To evaluate the state of healing, the nurse inspects the wound using the REEDA scale: *R*edness, *e*dema, *e*cchymosis, *d*ischarge, and *a*pproximation. After 24 hours, some edema may still be present, but the skin edges should be approximated ("glued" together) so that gentle pressure does not separate them. Gentle palpation should elicit minimal tenderness, and there should be no hardened areas suggesting infection. Ecchymosis interferes with normal healing, as does infection. Foul odors associated with drainage indicate infection. Hematomas sometimes occur, although these are considered abnormal.

The nurse next assesses whether hemorrhoids are present around the anus. If present, they are assessed for size, number, and pain or tenderness (see *Clinical Skill 32–3: Postpartum Perineal Assessment* and Figure 32–8).

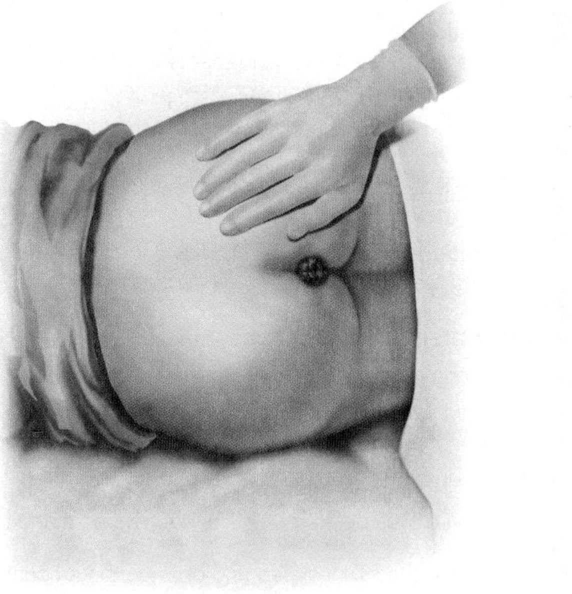

Figure 32–8 Intact perineum with hemorrhoids.

Clinical Skill 32–3

Postpartum Perineal Assessment

NURSING ACTION

Preparation

- Explain the purpose of and the procedure for assessing the perineum during the postpartum period.
- Complete the assessment of fundal height and lochia as described in *Clinical Skill 32–1: Assessing the Status of the Uterine Fundus After Vaginal or Cesarean Birth* and *Clinical Skill 32–2: Evaluating Lochia*.

  Rationale: *Typically, perineal assessment follows the fundal and lochial assessments.*
- At this point in a postpartum assessment, the woman is lying on her back with her knees flexed. Her perineal pad has already been lifted away from her perineum to permit inspection of the lochia. If an episiotomy was performed or if the birth was difficult, the woman may be using an ice pack on her perineum to reduce swelling. The ice pack should also be removed for inspection of the lochia.
- Ask her to turn onto her side with her upper knee drawn forward and resting on the bed (Sims position).

  Rationale: *When the woman is supine, even with her knees flexed, it is very difficult to expose the posterior portion of the perineum. Thus, Sims position makes it easiest to inspect the perineum and anal area.*

Equipment and Supplies

- Clean perineal pad; clean ice pack, if desired or needed
- Small light source such as a penlight may be necessary

Procedure: Clean Gloves

1. Use a systematic approach to assessment.

   Rationale: *A systematic approach helps ensure that you do not overlook a significant finding.*

Clinical Skill 32–3 *(continued)*

2. In evaluating the perineum, begin by asking about the woman's perceptions. How does she describe her discomfort? Does it seem excessive to her? Has it become worse since the birth? Does it seem more severe than you would expect?

   Rationale: *Information from the woman herself often helps identify developing problems.*

Note: Pain that seems disproportionately severe may indicate that the woman is developing a vulvar hematoma.

3. After talking with the woman, assess the condition of the tissue. To allow for full visualization, it may be helpful to ask the woman to lift the knee of her upper leg to expose her perineum more fully. In some cases it may help to use the nondominant gloved hand to lift the buttocks and tissue. Note any swelling (edema) and bruising (ecchymosis). (Use the REEDA scale to recall what to assess.)

   Rationale: *The tissue is often traumatized by the birth and mild bruising is not unusual. However, excessive bruising may indicate that a hematoma is developing.*

CLINICAL TIP

In evaluating the perineum, use the REEDA scale as a quick reminder of what to assess.

Specifically:

R = redness
E = edema or swelling
E = ecchymosis or bruising
D = drainage
A = approximation (how well the edges of an incision—the episiotomy—or a repaired laceration seem to be holding together) Be prepared to respond appropriately to findings.

4. Evaluate the episiotomy, if there is one, or any repaired laceration for its state of healing. Is it reddened? Note the edges of the incision. Are they well approximated? Tell the woman that you are going to palpate the incision gently, then do so. Note any areas of hardness. Note whether the incision is warmer to the touch than the surrounding tissue.

   Rationale: *Gentle palpation should elicit minimal tenderness and there should be no redness, warmth, or areas of hardness, which suggest infection. Both bruising and infection interfere with normal healing. Typically, within 24 hours the edges of the incision should be "glued" together (well approximated).*

5. During the assessment be alert for odors. Typically the lochia has an earthy, but not unpleasant, smell that is easily identifiable.

   Rationale: *A foul odor associated with drainage often indicates infection.*

6. Finally, assess for hemorrhoids. To visualize the anal area, lift the upper buttocks to fully expose the anal area (refer to Figure 32–8). If hemorrhoids are present, note the size, number, and pain or tenderness.

   Rationale: *Hemorrhoids often develop during pregnancy or labor and can cause considerable discomfort. If hemorrhoids are present, the woman may benefit from available comfort measures.*

7. During the assessment, talk to the woman about the effectiveness of comfort measures being used. Provide teaching about care of the episiotomy, hemorrhoids, and the like.

   Rationale: *Health teaching is an important part of nursing care. Many women have concerns about the episiotomy and may not know, for example, that the suture used is dissolvable. This is an excellent time to provide information about good healthcare practices in both the short and the long term.*

8. Provide the woman with a clean perineal pad. Replenish the ice pack if necessary.

9. Document findings according to hospital or unit policy. For example: "Midline episiotomy; no edema, ecchymosis, or tenderness. Skin edges well approximated. Woman reports pain relief measures are controlling discomfort" or "Perineal repair is approximated, minimal edema, no ecchymosis or tenderness; ice pack to perineum relieves pain."

During the assessment, the nurse talks with the woman to determine the effectiveness of comfort measures that have been used. The nurse provides teaching about the episiotomy or perineal laceration. Some women do not thoroughly understand what an episiotomy is and where it is and may believe that the stitches must be removed, as with other types of surgery. Frequently, when women fear that the stitches must be removed manually, they are afraid to ask about them. While explaining the findings of the assessment, the nurse can provide information about the episiotomy, its location, and signs that are being assessed. In addition, the nurse can casually add that the sutures are special and will dissolve slowly over the next few weeks as the tissues heal. By the time the sutures are dissolved, the tissues are strong, and the incision edges will not separate. This is also an opportunity to teach comfort measures that may be used and reinforce the need to consult with the healthcare provider before

Complementary Health Approaches

Lysine Following Episiotomy

Lysine, an essential amino acid, has been identified as a supplement that decreases the incidence of pain following an episiotomy. Lysine is available as a supplement. The recommended adult dosage is 12 mg/kg of body weight per day. It is present in dietary sources, including meat, cheese, fish, eggs, soybeans, and nuts.

using over-the-counter (OTC) medications or supplements if breastfeeding (see discussion in Chapter 33).

An example of documentation of a perineal assessment might read "Midline episiotomy; no edema, tenderness, or ecchymosis present. Skin edges are approximated" or, if a perineal laceration repair, "Skin edges intact, no edema, tenderness, or ecchymosis, pain meds helpful. Woman reports sitz bath and astringent wipes or pain relief measures are controlling discomfort."

LOWER EXTREMITIES

Postpartum women are at increased risk for thrombophlebitis, thrombus formation, and inflammation involving a vein (see discussion in Chapter 35). If thrombophlebitis occurs, the most likely site will be the woman's legs. Conditions that predispose a patient for thrombophlebitis are hypercoagulability, severe anemia, obesity, and traumatic delivery. To assess for thrombophlebitis, the nurse should have the woman stretch her legs out, with the knees slightly flexed and the legs relaxed. The nurse then grasps the foot and dorsiflexes it sharply (Figure 32–9). The second leg is assessed in the same way. No discomfort or pain should be present. If pain is elicited, the nurse notifies the healthcare provider that the woman has a positive Homans sign. The pain is caused by inflammation of a vessel. The nurse also evaluates the legs for edema by comparing both legs because usually only one leg is involved. Any areas of redness, tenderness, and increased skin temperature are also noted.

Some facilities have discontinued performing a Homans sign in the nursing assessment, stating that it is not diagnostic and could lead to an embolus if the clot is dislodged during assessment. Supporters advocate its use as a screening tool, and there are no published reports of an embolus occurring as a result of performing a Homans sign. In the event of a positive Homans sign, diagnosis is made by compression or duplex ultrasonography. Low-dose heparin therapy is used in postpartum women who develop a deep vein thrombosis (Ambesh, Obiagwu, & Shetty, 2017; Cunningham et al., 2018).

Early ambulation is an important aspect of preventing thrombophlebitis. Most women are able to get up shortly after birth or once they have fully recovered from the effects of the regional anesthetic agent, if one has been used. The mother's legs should be assessed for return of sensation following regional anesthesia. The cesarean birth patient requires passive range-of-motion exercises until she is ambulating more freely. If the mother is unable to get up soon after delivery, sequential compression devices may be used.

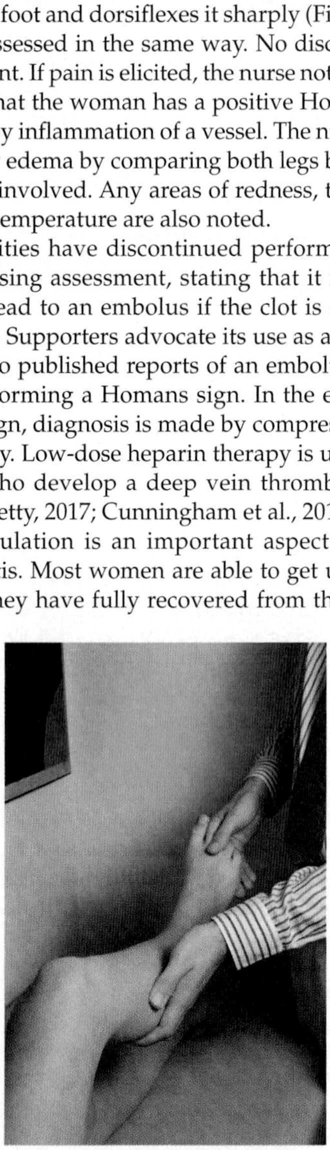

Figure 32–9 Homans sign. With the woman's knees flexed, the nurse dorsiflexes the foot. Pain in the foot or leg is a positive Homans sign.

SOURCE: Image Source/Getty Images.

Patient teaching associated with assessment of the lower extremities focuses on the signs and symptoms of thrombophlebitis. In addition, the nurse may review self-care measures to promote circulation and prevent thrombophlebitis, such as leg exercises that may be performed in bed, dorsiflexion on an hourly basis while on bedrest, ambulation, avoiding pressure behind the knees, and avoiding crossing the legs.

Usually, the nurse records the results of the assessment on a flowsheet or a summary nursing note. If tenderness and warmth have been noted, they might be recorded as: "Tenderness, warmth, slight edema, and slight redness noted on posterior aspect of left calf—positive Homans. Woman advised to avoid pressure to this area; lower leg elevated and moist heat applied per agency protocol. Call placed to Dr. Garcia to report findings."

ELIMINATION

During the hours after birth, the nurse carefully monitors a new mother's bladder status. A boggy uterus, displaced uterus, or palpable bladder is a sign of bladder distention and requires nursing intervention.

The postpartum woman can quickly show signs of bladder distention, possibly as soon as 1 to 2 hours after childbirth. This distention results because of normal postpartum diuresis. The nurse should assess the bladder for distention frequently until the woman is able to completely empty her bladder with each voiding. The nurse may employ techniques to facilitate voiding, such as helping the woman out of bed to void, pouring warm water on the vulva, running water in the sink, and encouraging the woman to relax and take deep breaths. The healthcare provider will order catheterization when the bladder is distended and the woman cannot void, when she is voiding small amounts (less than 100 mL) frequently, or when no voiding has occurred in 8 hours. Although many healthcare providers write orders stating that the woman can be catheterized in 8 hours if she has not voided, the nurse needs to assess the bladder and any voiding pattern frequently before the end of the 8-hour period. Some women may require catheterization sooner. The cesarean birth mother may have an indwelling catheter inserted prophylactically. The nurse should perform the same assessments in evaluating bladder emptying once the catheter is removed.

The nurse elicits information from the woman regarding the adequacy of her fluid intake, whether she feels she is emptying her bladder completely when she voids, and any signs of urinary tract infection (UTI) she may be experiencing.

In the same way, the nurse obtains information about the new mother's intestinal elimination and any concerns she may have about it. Many mothers fear that the first bowel movement will be painful and possibly even damaging if an episiotomy has been performed. Often, women defecate during labor or childbirth; therefore, bowel movements normally return within 2 to 3 days after a vaginal childbirth. Stool softeners may be ordered to increase bulk and moisture in the fecal material and to allow more comfortable and complete evacuation. Constipation may cause pressure on sutures and increase discomfort. Encouraging ambulation, forcing fluids (up to 2000 mL/day or more), and providing fresh fruits and roughage in the diet enhance bowel elimination and help the woman reestablish her normal bowel pattern.

During the assessment, the nurse may provide information regarding postpartum diuresis, explaining why the woman may be emptying her bladder so frequently. Information about the need for additional fluid intake, with suggestions of specific amounts, may be helpful. The woman should drink at least eight 8-oz glasses of water or juice in addition to other fluids. Breastfeeding mothers will have a higher requirement. The nurse discusses signs of retention and overflow voiding and reviews symptoms of UTI with the mother at this time if it seems an appropriate moment for teaching. The nurse can also review methods of assisting bowel elimination and provide opportunities for the woman to ask questions.

REST AND SLEEP STATUS

Physical fatigue often affects other adjustments and functions of the new mother. The mother requires energy to make the psychologic adjustments to a new baby and to assume new roles. Fatigue is often a highly significant factor in a new mother's apparent disinterest in her newborn. Frequently the woman is so tired from a long labor and birth that everything seems to be an effort.

To avoid inadvertently classifying a very tired mother as one with a potential attachment problem, the nurse should do a psychologic assessment on more than one occasion. After a nap the new mother is often far more receptive to her baby and her surroundings. As part of the postpartum assessment, the nurse evaluates the amount of rest the new mother is getting. If the woman reports difficulty sleeping at night, the nurse should try to determine the cause. If it is simply the strange environment, a warm drink, backrub, or mild sedative may prove helpful. Appropriate nursing measures are indicated if the woman is bothered by normal postpartum discomforts such as afterpains, diaphoresis, or episiotomy or hemorrhoidal pain. The impact of rooming-in on the mother's ability to rest should be assessed. See Chapter 33 for more detailed discussion of comfort and pain relief measures.

A daily rest period should be encouraged, and hospital activities should be scheduled to allow time for napping. The nurse can also provide information about the fatigue a new mother experiences, strategies to promote rest and sleep at home, and the impact fatigue can have on a woman's emotions and sense of control. See *Developing Cultural Competence: Rest, Seclusion, and Dietary Restraint in Non-Western Cultures.*

Developing Cultural Competence Rest, Seclusion, and Dietary Restraint in Non-Western Cultures

Rest, seclusion, and dietary restraint practices in many non-Western traditional cultures (African, traditional Mexican, Chinese, Japanese, South Asian groups) are designed to assist the woman and her baby during postpartum vulnerable periods. The period of postpartum vulnerability and seclusion varies between 7 and 40 days. In Ghana, for instance, new mothers are relieved from all chores, told to abstain from sex, and not allowed to leave the home (Holtz & Grisdale, 2017; Lauderdale, 2016). Decreased activity and seclusion practices are designed to lessen the influence of spirits or of spreading evil and misfortune. The time of seclusion coincides with the period of lochial flow or postpartum bleeding.

NUTRITION

During pregnancy the daily recommended dietary allowances call for increases in calories, proteins, and most vitamins and minerals. After birth the nonbreastfeeding mother's dietary requirements return to prepregnancy levels, whereas the lactating mother's requirements increase. The nonbreastfeeding mother should be advised about the need to reduce her caloric intake by about 300 kcal and to return to prepregnancy levels for other nutrients. The breastfeeding mother should increase her caloric intake by about 200 kcal over pregnancy requirements, or a total of 500 kcal over the nonpregnant requirement. Iron supplements may be prescribed after birth. The hemoglobin and hematocrit values are then checked at the postpartum visit to detect any anemia.

Basic discussion will usually prove helpful, followed by referral as needed. In all cases, the nurse should provide literature on nutrition so that the woman will have a source of information following discharge. The nurse should inform the dietitian of any mother who is a vegetarian, who has food allergies or lactose intolerance, or whose cultural or religious beliefs require specific foods. Appropriate meals can then be prepared for her. Many women, especially those who gained more than the recommended number of pounds, are interested in losing weight after birth. The dietitian can design weight-reduction diets to meet nutritional needs and food preferences. The nurse may also refer women with unusual eating habits or numerous questions about good nutrition to the dietitian. See the discussion of postpartum nutrition in Chapter 14.

Psychologic Assessment

During the first several postpartum weeks, the new mother must accomplish certain physical and developmental tasks, including:

- Restore physical condition
- Develop competence in caring for and meeting the needs of her baby
- Establish a relationship with her new child
- Adapt to altered lifestyles and family structure resulting from the addition of a new member.

Adequate assessment of the mother's psychologic adjustment is an integral part of postpartum evaluation. Some new mothers have little or no experience with newborns and may feel totally overwhelmed. They may show these feelings by asking questions and reading all available material or by becoming passive and quiet because they simply cannot deal with their feelings of inadequacy. Unless a nurse questions the woman about her plans and previous experience in a supportive, nonjudgmental way, the nurse might conclude that the woman is uninterested, withdrawn, or depressed. Clues that may indicate a problem include excessive, continued fatigue; marked depression; excessive preoccupation with physical status or discomfort; evidence of low self-esteem; lack of support systems; marital or relationship problems; inability to care for or nurture the newborn; and current family crises (such as illness or unemployment). These characteristics frequently indicate a potential for maladaptive parenting, which may lead to child abuse or neglect (physical, emotional, intellectual), and cannot be ignored. Referrals to public health nurses or other available community resources may provide greatly needed assistance and alleviate potentially dangerous situations.

Assessment of Early Attachment

The nurse in any of the various postpartum settings should periodically observe and note the mother's progress toward attachment. The assessment should include both parents when possible; however, in this section, the behaviors focus primarily on the mother's attachment process. As discussed previously, research shows that fathers experience attachment feelings similar to those experienced by mothers. These questions can be addressed in the course of nurse–patient interaction:

- Is the mother attracted to her newborn? To what extent does she seek face-to-face contact and eye contact? Has she progressed from fingertip touch to palmar contact to enfolding the baby close to her own body? Is attraction increasing or decreasing? If the mother does not exhibit increasing attraction, why not? Do the reasons lie primarily within her, in the baby, or in the environment?
- Is the mother inclined to nurture her newborn? Is she progressing in her interactions with her baby?
- Does the mother act consistently? If not, is the source of unpredictability within her or her newborn?
- Is her mothering consistently carried out? Does she seek information and evaluate it objectively? Does she develop solutions based on adequate knowledge of valid data? Does she evaluate the effectiveness of her maternal care and make appropriate adjustments?
- Is she sensitive to the newborn's needs as they arise? How quickly does she interpret her baby's behavior and react to cues? Does she seem happy and satisfied with the baby's responses to her efforts? Is she pleased with feeding behaviors? How much of this ability and willingness to respond is related to the baby's nature, and how much to her own?
- Does she seem pleased with her baby's appearance and sex? Is she experiencing pleasure in interaction with her newborn? What interferes with the enjoyment? Does she speak to the baby frequently and affectionately? Does she call him or her by name? Does she point out family traits or characteristics she sees in the newborn?
- Are there any cultural factors that might modify the mother's response? For instance, is it customary for the grandmother to assume most of the childcare responsibilities while the mother recovers from childbirth?

Once these questions are addressed and the facts are assembled, the nurse can combine the information with personal intuition and knowledge to answer three more unspoken questions: Is there a problem in attachment? What is the problem? What is its source? The nurse can then devise a creative approach to the problem as it presents itself in the context of a unique, developing mother–newborn relationship. See *Assessment Guide: Postpartum—First 24 Hours After Birth.*

ASSESSMENT GUIDE | Postpartum—First 24 Hours After Birth

Physical Assessment/Normal Findings	Alterations and Possible Causes*	Nursing Responses to Data[†]
Vital Signs		
Blood Pressure (BP): Should remain consistent with baseline BP during pregnancy	High BP (preeclampsia, essential hypertension, renal disease, anxiety)	Evaluate history of preexisting disorders and check for other signs of preeclampsia (edema, proteinuria).
	Drop in BP (may be normal; uterine hemorrhage)	Assess for other signs of hemorrhage.
Pulse: 50–90 beats/min; may be bradycardia if 50–70 beats/min	Tachycardia (difficult labor and birth, hemorrhage)	(↑ pulse, cool clammy skin) Evaluate for other signs of hemorrhage.
	Marked tachypnea (respiratory disease)	(↓ BP, cool clammy skin)
Respirations: 16–24/min	Diminished respirations (long-acting epidural narcotics)	Assess for other signs of respiratory disease.
Temperature: 36.2°C to 38°C (97.1°F to 100.4°F)	After first 24 hours, temperature of 38°C (100.4°F) or above suggests infection	Assess for other signs of infection; notify healthcare provider.
Breasts		
General appearance: Smooth, even pigmentation, changes of pregnancy still apparent: One may appear larger	Reddened area (mastitis)	Assess further for signs of infection.
Palpation: Depending on postpartum day, may be soft, filling, full, or engorged	Palpable mass (caked breast, mastitis)	Assess for other signs of infection; if blocked duct, consider heat, massage, position change for breastfeeding.
	Engorgement (venous stasis)	Assess for further signs.
	Tenderness, heat, edema (engorgement, caked breast, mastitis)	Report mastitis to physician or CNM.
Nipples: Supple, pigmented, intact; become erect when stimulated	Fissures, cracks, soreness (problems with breastfeeding), not erectile with stimulation (inverted nipples)	Reassess technique: Recommend appropriate interventions.

ASSESSMENT GUIDE Postpartum—First 24 Hours After Birth (*continued*)

Physical Assessment/Normal Findings	Alterations and Possible Causes*	Nursing Responses to Data†
Lungs		
Sounds: Clear to bases bilaterally	Diminished (fluid overload, asthma, pulmonary embolus, pulmonary edema)	Assess for other signs of respiratory distress.
Abdomen		
Musculature: Abdomen may be soft, have a "doughy" texture; rectus muscle intact	Separation in musculature (diastasis recti abdominis)	Evaluate size of diastasis: Teach appropriate exercises for decreasing the separation.
Fundus: Firm, midline; following expected process of involution	Boggy (full bladder, uterine bleeding, deviation from midline)	Massage until firm; assess bladder and have woman void, if needed; attempt to express clots when firm. If bogginess remains or recurs, report to healthcare provider.
May be tender when palpated	Constant tenderness (infection)	Assess for evidence of endometritis.
Cesarean section incision dressing; dry and intact	Moderate to large amount of blood or serosanguineous drainage on dressing	Assess for hemorrhage; reinforce dressing and notify healthcare provider.
Lochia		
Scant to moderate amount, earthy odor; no clots	Large amount, clots (hemorrhage)	Assess for firmness, express additional clots; begin peripad count.
	Foul-smelling lochia (infection)	Assess for other signs of infection; report to healthcare provider.
Normal progression: First 1–3 days: Rubra **Following rubra:** Days 3–10: Serosa (alba seldom seen in hospital)	Failure to progress normally or return to rubra from serosa (subinvolution)	Report to healthcare provider.
Perineum		
Slight edema and bruising in intact perineum	Marked fullness, bruising, pain (vulvar hematoma)	Assess size; apply ice glove or ice pack, analgesic and anesthetic sprays; report to healthcare provider.
Episiotomy: No redness, edema, ecchymosis, or discharge, edges well approximated	Redness, edema, ecchymosis, discharge, or gaping stitches (infection)	Encourage sitz baths; review perineal care, appropriate wiping techniques.
Hemorrhoids: None present; if present, should be small and nontender	Full, tender, inflamed hemorrhoids	Encourage sitz baths, side-lying position; astringent wipes, anesthetic ointments, manual replacement of hemorrhoids, stool softeners, increased fluid intake.
Costovertebral Angle (CVA) Tenderness		
None	Present (kidney infection)	Assess for other symptoms of UTI; obtain clean-catch urine sample; report to healthcare provider.
Lower Extremities		
No pain with palpation; negative Homans sign	Positive findings (thrombophlebitis)	Report to healthcare provider.
Elimination		
Urinary output: Voiding in sufficient quantities at least every 4–6 hours; bladder not palpable	Inability to void (urinary retention); urgency, frequency, dysuria (UTI)	Employ nursing interventions to promote voiding; if not successful, obtain order for catheterization. Report symptoms of UTI to healthcare provider.

(*continued*)

ASSESSMENT GUIDE | Postpartum—First 24 Hours After Birth (*continued*)

Physical Assessment/Normal Findings	Alterations and Possible Causes*	Nursing Responses to Data†
Bowel elimination: Should have normal bowel movement by second or third day after birth	Inability to pass feces or hard, small amount of stool (constipation due to fear of pain from episiotomy, hemorrhoids, perineal trauma)	Encourage fluids, ambulation, roughage in diet; sitz baths to promote healing of perineum; obtain order for stool softener.
Cultural Assessment‡	**Variations to Consider***	**Nursing Responses to Data†**
Determine customs and practices regarding postpartum care.	Individual preference may include:	Provide for specific request, if possible.
Ask the mother whether she would like fluids and ask what temperature she prefers.	• Room-temperature or warmed fluids rather than iced drinks.	If woman is unable to provide specific information, the nurse may draw from general information regarding cultural variation.
Ask the mother what foods or fluids she would like.	• Special foods or fluids to hasten healing after childbirth.	Mexican women may want food and fluids that restore hot–cold balance to the body. Women of European background may ask for iced fluids.
Ask the mother whether she would prefer to be alone during breastfeeding.	• Some women may be hesitant to have someone with them when their breast is exposed.	Provide privacy as desired by mother.
Psychologic Adaptation		
During first 24 hours: Passive; preoccupied with own needs; may talk about her labor and birth experience; may be talkative, elated, or very quiet	Very quiet and passive; sleeps frequently (fatigue from long labor; feelings of disappointment about some aspect of the experience; may be following cultural expectation)	Provide opportunities for adequate rest; provide physical comfort measures; provide nutritious meals and snacks that are consistent with what the woman desires to eat and drink; provide opportunities to discuss birth experience in nonjudgmental atmosphere if the woman desires to do so.
Usually by 12 hours; beginning to assume responsibility; some women eager to learn; others easily feel overwhelmed	Excessive weepiness, mood swings, pronounced irritability (postpartum blues; feelings of inadequacy); culturally prescribed behavior	Explain postpartum blues; provide supportive atmosphere; determine support available for mother; consider referral for evidence of profound depression.
Attachment		
En face position; holds baby close; cuddles and soothes; calls by name; identifies characteristics of family members in baby; may be awkward in providing care	Continued expressions of disappointment in sex, appearance of baby; refusal to care for baby; derogatory comments; lack of bonding behaviors (difficulty in attachment, following expectations of cultural/ethnic group)	Provide reinforcement and support for newborn/infant caretaking behaviors; maintain nonjudgmental approach and gather more information if caretaking behaviors are not evident.
Initially may express disappointment over sex or appearance of baby but within 1–2 days demonstrates attachment behaviors		
Patient Education		
Demonstrates basic understanding of self-care activities and newborn/infant care needs; can identify signs of complications that should be reported	Unable to demonstrate basic self-care and newborn/infant care activities (knowledge deficit; postpartum blues; following prescribed cultural behavior and will be cared for by grandmother or other family member)	Identify predominant learning style. Determine whether woman understands English and provide interpreter, if needed; provide reinforcement of information through conversation and through written material (remember that some women and their families may not be able to understand written materials because of language difficulties or inability to read); provide information regarding newborn/infant care skills that are culturally consistent; give woman opportunity to express her feelings and demonstrate skills taught; consider social service home referral for women who have no family or other support, are unable to take in information about self-care and newborn/infant care, and demonstrate no caretaking activities.

‡ These are only a few suggestions. It is not our intent to imply this is a comprehensive cultural assessment.

* Possible causes of alterations are identified in parentheses.

† This column provides guidelines for further assessment and initial nursing action.

Discharge Assessment and Follow-Up

The final discharge assessment should include a physical examination and appropriate discharge teaching that includes both maternal and newborn care guidelines. The optimal time for a home visit or follow-up phone call is 3 to 4 days after birth; this provides opportunities for further assessment of mothers and their newborns and teaching. See *Assessment Guide: Postpartum—First Home Visit and Anticipated Progress at Six Weeks* in Chapter 34.

During this time period, infections, hypertensive issues, substance abuse, depression, poor newborn feeding, excessive weight loss, jaundice, and other problems become apparent (AAP & ACOG, 2017). The follow-up phone call is often initiated by a nurse from the postpartum unit of the agency where the mother gave birth. It is made soon after discharge and is designed to provide assessment and, if necessary, care; to reinforce knowledge and provide additional teaching; and to make referrals, if indicated. Alternatively, a follow-up phone call from a nurse from the healthcare provider's office can provide new mothers with a source of support and an opportunity to ask questions. Women who appear to be having adjustment problems should be scheduled for an appointment for further evaluation. See *Women with Special Needs: Specialized Equipment*.

Women with Special Needs Specialized Equipment

For the woman with a mobility disorder, specialized equipment will be needed in order for her to care for the baby. Modifications should include a lower crib and changing table height, arrangement of care supplies in an area she can adequately reach, and space in the nursery or designated sleep location of the baby for a wheelchair or walker to move easily, if used.

In ideal situations, a family approach involving the father/partner, newborn, and other siblings permits a total evaluation and provides an opportunity for all family members to ask questions and express concerns. In addition, a family approach can sometimes enable the nurse to identify disturbed family patterns more readily and suggest, or even institute, therapeutic measures to prevent future problems of neglect or abuse.

Focus Your Study

- The uterus involutes rapidly, primarily through a reduction in cell size.
- Involution is assessed by measuring fundal height. The fundus is at the level of the umbilicus within a few hours after birth and should decrease by approximately one fingerbreadth per day.
- The placental site heals by a process of exfoliation, so no scar formation occurs.
- Lochia progresses from rubra to serosa to alba and is assessed in terms of type, quantity, and characteristics.
- The abdomen may have decreased muscle tone (flabby consistency) initially. The nurse should assess for diastasis recti abdominis, separation of the rectus abdominis muscles.
- Constipation may develop postpartum because of decreased tone in the abdominal muscles, limited diet, and denial of the urge to defecate because of fear of pain.
- Decreased bladder sensitivity, increased capacity, and postpartum diuresis may lead to problems with bladder elimination. Frequent assessment and prompt intervention are indicated. A fundus that is boggy but does not respond to massage, is higher than expected, or deviates to the side usually indicates a full bladder.
- Postpartum, a healthy woman should be normotensive and afebrile.
- The white blood cell (WBC) count is often elevated postpartum. Activation of clotting factors predisposes the woman to thrombus formation.
- Psychologic adaptations of the postpartum woman are traditionally described as "taking in" and "taking hold."
- Postpartum "blues" is a common occurrence, and ways to prevent and cope with it should be discussed not only with the mother but also with her significant other(s). Signs of postpartum depression should be discussed as well.
- In consideration of the patient's background, the nurse should recognize and respect cultural variations and individual preferences.
- Postpartum assessment should be completed in a systematic way, usually head to toe, and should include assessment of rest and sleep, nutrition, and attachment. The assessment provides opportunities for informal patient teaching.
- In the weeks following birth, the woman's physical condition returns to a nonpregnant state, and she gains competence in caregiving and confidence in herself as a parent.

References

Ambesh, P., Obiagwu, C., & Shetty, V. (2017). Homan's sign for deep vein thrombosis: A grain of salt? *Indian Heart Journal, 69*(3), 418–419.

American Academy of Pediatrics (AAP), Committee on the Fetus and Newborn, & American College of Obstetricians and Gynecologists (ACOG), Committee on Obstetric Practice. (2017). *Guidelines for perinatal care* (8th ed.). Elk Grove Village, IL: Author.

American College of Obstetricians and Gynecologists (ACOG). (2018). *Postpartum pain* (ACOG Committee Opinion No. 742). *Obstetrics & Gynecology 132*(1), e1–e9.

Blackburn, S. T. (2018). *Maternal, fetal, and neonatal physiology: A clinical perspective* (5th ed.). St. Louis, MO: Saunders.

Cunningham, F. G., Leveno, K. J., Bloom, S. L., Dashe, J. S., Hoffman, B. L., . . . Spong, C. Y (2018). *Williams obstetrics* (25th ed.). New York, NY: McGraw-Hill.

Ding, T., Wang, D., Qu, Y., Chen, Q., & Zhu, S. (2014). Epidural labor analgesia is associated with a decreased risk of postpartum depression: A prospective cohort study. *Anesthesia and Analgesia, 119*(2), 383–392.

Dodge, H. (2017, September 2). *Common practices of Islamic birth rites*. Retrieved from https://www.thoughtco.com/islamic-birth-rites-2004500

Feldman, R. (2017). The neurobiology of human attachments. *Trends in Cognitive Sciences, 21*(2), 80–99.

Gerard, E. E., & Samuels, P. (2017). Neurologic disorders. In S. G. Gabbe, J. R. Niebyl, & J. L. Simpson (Eds.), *Obstetrics: Normal and problem pregnancies* (7th ed., pp. 1030–1056). Philadelphia, PA: Churchill Livingstone/Elsevier.

Giger, J. N. (2017). *Transcultural nursing: Assessment and intervention* (7th ed.). St. Louis, MO: Elsevier.

Hart, K. J., & Flynn, H. A. (2016). Screening, assessment and diagnosis of mood and anxiety disorders during pregnancy and the postpartum period. In A. Wenzel (Ed.), *The Oxford handbook of perinatal psychology* (pp. 319–340). Oxford, UK: Oxford University Press.

Holtz, C., & Grisdale, S. (2017). Global health in reproduction and infants. In C. Holtz (Ed.), *Global health care: Issues and policies* (3rd ed., pp. 453–461). Boston, MA: Jones & Bartlett.

Isley, M. M., & Katz, V. L. (2017). Postpartum care and long-term health considerations. In S. G. Gabbe, J. R. Niebyl, & J. L. Simpson (Eds.), *Obstetrics: Normal and problem pregnancies* (7th ed., pp. 499–516). Philadelphia, PA: Churchill Livingston/Elsevier.

Kim, B. R., Chow, S. M., Bray, B., & Teti, D. M. (2017). Trajectories of mothers' emotional availability: Relations with infant temperament in predicting attachment security. *Journal of Attachment and Human Development, 19*(1), 38–57.

King, T. L. (2019). Anatomy and physiology of postpartum. In T. L. King, M. C. Brucker, K. Osborne, & C. M. Jevitt (Eds.), *Varney's midwifery* (6th ed., pp. 1169–1182), Burlington, MA: Jones & Bartlett Learning.

Lauderdale, J. (2016). Transcultural perspectives in childbearing. In M. M. Andrews & J. S. Boyle (Eds.), *Transcultural concepts in nursing care* (7th ed., pp. 120–152). Philadelphia, PA: Lippincott Williams & Wilkins.

Lui, C. H., & Tronick, E. (2014). Prevalence and predictors of maternal postpartum depressed mood and anhedonia by race and ethnicity. *Epidemiology and Psychiatric Sciences, 23*(2), 201–209.

Mercer, R. T. (2004). Becoming a mother versus maternal role attainment. *Journal of Nursing Scholarship, 36*(3), 226–232.

Mercer, R. T. (2006). Nursing support of the process of becoming a mother. *JOGNN: Journal of Obstetric, Gynecologic, & Neonatal Nursing, 35*(5), 649–651. DOI: 10.1111/J.1552-6909.2006.00086.x

Rubin, R. (1984). *Maternal identity and the maternal experience.* New York, NY: Springer.

Spector, R. E. (2017). *Cultural diversity in health and illness* (9th ed.). Hoboken, NJ: Pearson.

Whitmer, T. (2016). Physical and psychologic changes after childbirth. In AWOHNN, S. Mattson, & J. E. Smith (Eds.), *Core curriculum for maternal-newborn nursing* (6th ed., pp. 297–313). Philadelphia, PA: Mosby.

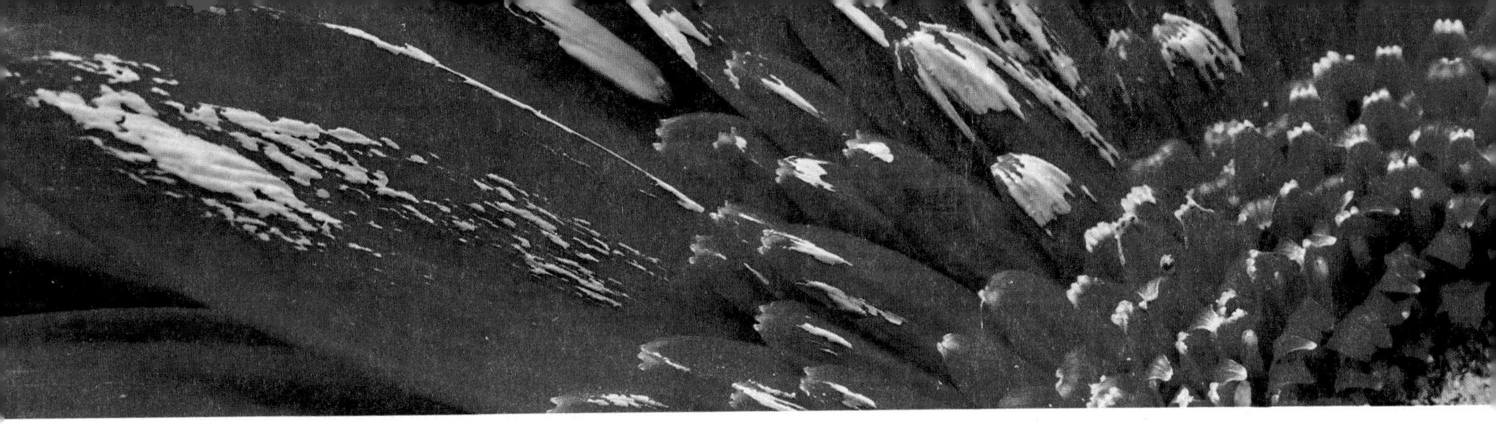

Chapter 33

The Postpartum Family: Needs and Care

Providing family-centered postpartum care is a challenge that requires creativity, patience, and a sincere desire to help families grow and thrive. Individual families come to the unit with a unique set of values, beliefs, life experiences, challenges, gifts, and expectations. The nurse needs to personalize care to meet their special needs in a manner that helps them to nurture one another and their newborn within the context of their family, their community, and the world. It has been helpful to remember that while it is simply another day of work for me, it is probably one of the most important days in the lives of my patients and their families. The care that I provide shapes their memories of this special time and may affect their health and family processes for many years to come.

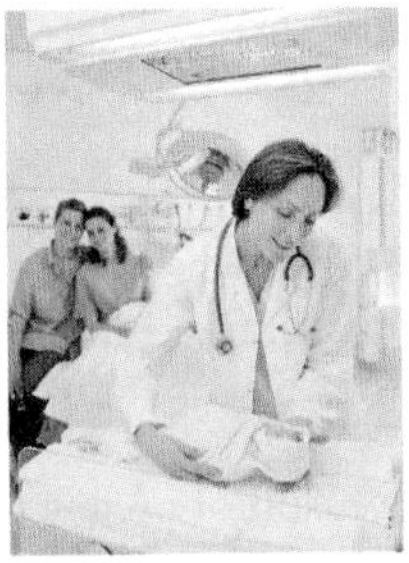

SOURCE: OJO Images/Exactostock/SuperStock

Learning Outcomes

33.1 Delineate nursing responsibilities for patient teaching during the early postpartum period.

33.2 Discuss appropriate nursing interventions to promote maternal comfort and well-being.

33.3 Describe the nurse's role in promoting maternal rest and helping the mother to gradually resume an appropriate level of activity.

33.4 Identify patient teaching topics for promoting postpartum family wellness.

33.5 Compare the nursing needs of a woman who experienced a cesarean birth with the needs of a woman who gave birth vaginally.

33.6 Identify critical physiologic, psychosocial, and safety needs related to the care of obese and morbidly obese postpartum women.

33.7 Summarize the nursing needs of the childbearing adolescent during the postpartum period.

33.8 Describe possible approaches to sensitive, holistic nursing care for targeted populations of childbearing patients: Lesbian birth mothers and co-mothers, women with special needs, women who have experienced abuse, and women relinquishing their newborns.

33.9 Delineate the nurse's responsibilities related to early postpartum discharge.

33.10 Describe the nurse's role related to promoting safety for the postpartum patient and family.

Healthy People 2020

(FP-5) Reduce the proportion of pregnancies conceived within 18 months of a prior birth

(MICH 7-2) Reduce cesarean births among low-risk women giving birth with a prior cesarean birth

(MICH-19) Increase the proportion of women giving birth who attend a postpartum care visit with a health worker

The following premises form the basis of effective nursing care during the postpartum period.

- The best postpartum care is family centered and disrupts the family unit as little as possible. This approach uses the family's resources to support adjustment to the newborn by all family members.
- Knowledge of the range of normal physiologic and psychologic adaptations occurring during the postpartum period allows the nurse to recognize alterations and initiate interventions. Communicating information about postpartum adaptations to the family facilitates their adjustment.

- Nursing care is aimed at accomplishing specific goals that ultimately meet individual needs. These goals are formulated after assessment and consideration of factors that could influence the outcome of care.
- Nursing care must include patient education that prepares the woman and her family to recognize signs of life-threatening postpartum or newborn complications and to seek care accordingly.

Chapter 32 provides a thorough discussion of postpartum assessment. This chapter describes nursing care during the immediate postpartum period, focusing on specific nursing responses to the mother's physical needs and the family's psychosociocultural needs.

Nursing Care During the Early Postpartum Period

For most postpartum women, physical recovery proceeds smoothly and is considered a healthy process. Some women, however, experience life-threatening complications and even death after childbirth. Although the global *maternal mortality ratios (MMRs)* (maternal deaths per 100,000 live births) have declined in recent decades, hundreds of thousands of women still die as a result of pregnancy and childbearing complications each year (World Health Organization [WHO], 2015). There has been an increase in **late maternal mortality**, or "maternal deaths that occur more than 42 days but less than one year after termination of pregnancy" (WHO, 2015, p. 26) in a number of countries. Although it decreased globally, the MMR in the United States rose between 1990 and 2015 (WHO, 2015). Therefore, postpartum nursing care should focus on health promotion as well as the prevention, recognition, and timely intervention for complications such as hemorrhage, infection, thrombosis, mental health disorders, and hypertensive disorders. Postpartum women and their families must be educated about recognition and follow-up of complications that may occur during the 12 months after childbirth.

Nursing Diagnoses

The postpartum family's needs, which should be identified during assessment, are the basis for developing nursing diagnoses. Once a nursing diagnosis is made and recorded, systematic action, as delineated in a nursing care plan, can be used to meet the identified need.

Nursing schools and agencies frequently use NANDA International–approved diagnoses. Examples of diagnoses with defining characteristics and related factors commonly found in postpartum patients include:

- ***Urinary Elimination, Impaired.*** Defining characteristics may include dysuria, hesitancy, frequency, retention, urgency, incontinence, or nocturia. Related factors may include anatomic obstruction (urethral swelling), sensory motor impairment (spinal or epidural anesthesia), multiple causality, or urinary tract infection.
- ***Skin Integrity, Impaired.*** Defining characteristics may include alteration in skin integrity and foreign matter piercing skin. Related factors may include mechanical factors (tearing/shearing forces during delivery).
- ***Pain, Acute.*** Defining characteristics may include guarding behavior, change in physiological parameter, expressive behavior, positioning to avoid pain, protective behavior, or self-report of pain. Related factors may include physical injury agent (trauma during labor and birth) or biological injury agent (infection, ischemia).
- ***Infection, Risk for.*** Risk factors may include inadequate primary defenses (alterations in integrity such as surgical incision, lacerations, or abrasions; open cervix; premature or prolonged rupture of amniotic membranes; and others), inadequate secondary defenses (decreased hemoglobin), and invasive procedures (history of cervical exams or instrumentation during labor and delivery).
- ***Constipation, Risk for.*** Risk factors may include physiologic (decreased motility of gastrointestinal tract), pharmacologic (opiates), or mechanical (hemorrhoids).

(NANDA-I © 2017)

Wellness diagnoses related to family coping, instructional needs, and newborn/infant nutrition are also used frequently. Examples of these diagnoses and defining characteristics commonly found in postpartum patients include:

- ***Knowledge, Readiness for Enhanced.*** Defining characteristic is expressed desire to enhance learning.
- ***Coping: Readiness for Enhanced.*** Defining characteristics may include desire to enhance knowledge of stress management strategies, to enhance social support, and to enhance use of spiritual resources.
- ***Breastfeeding, Readiness for Enhanced.*** Defining characteristics include the mother expressing the desire to enhance her ability to provide breast milk for the child's nutritional needs and to enhance her ability to exclusively breastfeed.

(NANDA-I © 2017)

After completing the assessment and diagnosis steps of the nursing process, the nurse identifies desired outcomes and selects nursing interventions that will promote these outcomes.

Nursing Plan and Implementation

Nursing management is individualized to meet the needs of each postpartum woman, her newborn, and her family. The plan of care needs to consider the newborn's schedule of activities during the day, such as feeding times, because they frequently determine the mother's schedule. Flexibility is crucial because most breastfeeding babies feed on demand at frequent intervals.

An important component of nursing care is patient teaching, which is designed to help the woman and her family learn how to perform self-care and provide effective newborn care. Detailed forms and technological resources are often available to assist in health teaching. Such tools are useful but cannot take the place of the nurse's patient-centered plan. As part of patient teaching, the nurse should discuss cultural beliefs, desired outcomes, and goals with the mother as soon as possible after her arrival in the postpartum unit. Examples of these desired patient outcomes include:

- Mother and baby remain healthy, safe, and free of injury or complications.
- Mother verbalizes comfort.
- Mother tells birth story and verbalizes feelings and concerns regarding the event.
- Mother reviews educational resources for self- and newborn/infant care.
- Mother performs appropriate self- and newborn/infant care.
- Parent(s) and newborn demonstrate positive bonding behaviors.
- Parents practice principles of newborn/infant safety.
- Mother verbalizes understanding of and demonstrates successful breastfeeding and breast care or mother describes

accurate preparation of formula, demonstrates safe bottle-feeding techniques, and verbalizes understanding of lactation suppression care.

- Mother verbalizes sources of support to assist in newborn care and family responsibilities.
- Mother states plan for follow-up healthcare for self and newborn.
- Mother identifies signs and symptoms of maternal or newborn complications and reasons to seek care before routine follow-up visits.

Additional outcomes for the cesarean birth mother include:

- Mother expresses understanding of the reason for the cesarean birth and verbalizes feelings related to the event.
- Mother maintains desired comfort level (pain level less than 4 on 1 to 10 scale).
- Mother maintains mobility (up in chair within 12 hours; ambulates within 24).

In summary, all components of nursing care management are designed to achieve the desired outcomes identified for the woman and her family. If the mother is unable to meet all of the educational outcomes prior to discharge, the father, partner, or a family caregiver should verbalize and/or demonstrate understanding of outcomes related to maternal and newborn/infant health and safety.

For a brief summary of postpartum assessment, see *Key Facts to Remember: Postpartum Assessment*.

Key Facts To Remember
Postpartum Assessment

- BP and HR q 15 minutes × 8, then q 4 hours
- Temperature q 4 hours × 2, then q 8 hours
- Fundus, lochia, bladder, and perineum q 15 minutes × 4, then every 30 minutes × 2, then q 4 hours

Community-Based Nursing Care

Various services are available to meet the needs of the childbearing family during the immediate postpartum period and beyond. Educational opportunities include:

- Nutrition counseling
- Breastfeeding assistance
- Maternal exercise
- Newborn/infant care
- Newborn/infant development
- Parenting courses.

Other healthcare program opportunities should be discussed with the family, including:

- Well-baby clinics
- Immunization clinics
- Lactation centers
- Family planning agencies
- New mother support groups.

Services may be offered by the birthing unit, private caregivers, volunteer and charitable organizations, or publicly funded agencies. In all cases, the goal is consistent: To meet the health, safety, and psychosocial needs of the mother, the newborn, and the family.

Home healthcare is one of the most important forms of community-based nursing care offered to postpartum families. Home care visits and phone contacts (telephone follow-up) help ensure that families have the necessary skills and resources to care for a baby and to meet their own health needs. Because of its importance today in caring for childbearing families, home care is discussed in depth in Chapter 34. See *Evidence-Based Practice: Postnatal Support from the Midwife*.

EVIDENCE-BASED PRACTICE | Postnatal Support from the Midwife

Clinical Question

What kind of postnatal support can be provided by a midwife that will ensure healthy outcomes for mother and baby?

The Evidence

The postnatal period is one of change and recovery for the new mother and baby. The mother is also learning how to carry out her new role for the care and nurturing of a baby. Early discharge from the hospital is common, limiting the time that healthcare professionals have contact with new mothers. This postnatal period is often not given as much attention as the prenatal period, and yet it is a critical time for the mother's and baby's health and growth. A systematic review by Panagopoulou, Hancock, and Tziaferi (2017) investigated what types of postnatal support provided by midwives were effective in helping the mother adapt to motherhood in a way that was healthy for both mother and baby. Many articles (355) were included in this review, representing the strongest level of evidence for practice.

The research evidence is consistent that early discharge can be cost-effective when coupled with early prenatal intervention by a midwife. In some cases, satisfaction, health, and wellness of both mother and baby were better than that of mothers who stayed longer in the hospital. The optimal practices included weekly visits by a midwife for the first 5 weeks. Also deemed effective was the use of technology including text messages, emails, telephone calls, and social networks. The services provided included guidance regarding newborn care and parenting, reducing the mother's isolation, and promoting exclusive breastfeeding. Although technology facilitated communication between the mother and midwife, personal contact was determined to be the most effective and was associated with the best health outcomes (Panagopoulou et al., 2017).

Best Practice

In mothers with early discharge after birth, a midwife can provide valuable support in adapting to motherhood and caring for the baby. Midwives can be cost-effective providers of maternal support. Personal attention and weekly visits for at least 5 weeks provides optimal benefit.

Clinical Reasoning

What might be a teaching plan for each of the 5 weeks of a midwife visit? In what other ways might the midwife be helpful in the immediate postpartum visits?

Health Promotion Education

Meeting the educational needs of the new mother and her family is one of the primary responsibilities of the postpartum nurse. Each woman's educational needs vary according to age, background, culture, experience, and expectations. The mother spends only a brief period of time in the postpartum area, so identifying and addressing individual instructional needs can be difficult. Effective education provides the childbearing family members with sufficient knowledge to meet many of their own health needs and to seek assistance, if necessary.

The nurse assesses the learning needs of the new mother through observation, sensitivity to nonverbal clues, and tactfully phrased questions. For example, "What plans have you made for handling things when you get home?" will elicit a more detailed response than, "Will someone be available to help you at home?" To assess learning needs, some agencies provide a patient handout listing frequently identified areas of concern for new mothers. The mother checks those that apply to her or writes in concerns not included. The nurse should plan and implement learning experiences in a logical, nonthreatening way based on knowledge of and respect for the family's cultural values and beliefs.

Timing and Methods of Teaching

Childbearing nursing units must provide education efficiently and effectively in today's healthcare environment, which is characterized by shortened postpartum stays. Assessment of learning needs and patient education should begin when the woman first accesses the healthcare system and should continue throughout the postpartum period.

Nursing units should offer a variety of educational options including the following:

- Structured group classes
- Individualized instruction
- Printed materials
- Online materials
- Educational television channels
- Approved streaming videos produced by professional organizations.

The use of standardized, comprehensive postpartum educational materials that can be streamlined to meet the specific needs of individual patients fosters consistency of teaching and efficiently meets the needs of diverse patients, many of whom may have limited *health literacy*. "Health literacy is the degree to which individuals have the capacity to obtain, process, and understand basic health information and services needed to make appropriate health decisions" (National Institutes of Health, 2016, para. 12).

Educational materials should be written at a level that is easily understood and should be clear and simple. Pictures, diagrams, wide margins, conversational language, large font, and headings increase understandability. The Agency for Healthcare Research and Quality (AHRQ) offers professional resources to assist with the development of patient education materials, such as the *Patient Education Materials Assessment Tool (PEMAT) and User's Guide* (AHRQ, 2016) and the *AHRQ Health Literacy Universal Precautions Toolkit* (Brega et al., 2015).

Most learners absorb more information when printed materials are accompanied by verbal explanations. Observation followed by hands-on practice increases learning and promotes patient confidence when performing self- and newborn care. Opportunities for continued learning include the following methods:

- Home visits
- Telephone advice lines
- Postpartum education and support groups
- Outpatient nurse consultation, especially for those who are discharged within 24 to 48 hours following delivery
- Online professional patient-oriented websites
- Professionally moderated social media sites.

Clinical Tip

Discuss online and social media sources as a source of patient education. Ensure women understand how to determine if a website or social media site is from a reliable source. Websites from government offices, such as the Centers for Disease Control and Prevention and the National Institutes of Health, or from professional nursing or medical organizations are recommended. Some social media sites are moderated or monitored by professionals, which increase their accuracy.

Nurses should determine whether the patient has access to and uses the technology required for ongoing communication and education after discharge in order to plan delivery of the material by the most appropriate method.

Content of Teaching

Postpartum patients should receive information about the following health promotion issues (American Academy of Pediatrics [AAP], Committee on the Fetus and Newborn, & American College of Obstetricians and Gynecologists [ACOG], Committee on Obstetric Practice, 2017; Association of Women's Health, Obstetric, & Neonatal Nurses [AWHONN], 2016; James, 2013):

- Expected physiologic changes
- Activity level
- Self-care
- Maternal nutrition
- Exercise
- Sexuality and contraception
- Emotional responses to childbearing
- Newborn care
- Newborn safety
- Newborn immunizations
- Signs of maternal and newborn complications
- Emergency contact information
- Psychosocial support
- Specific follow-up for high-risk patients (gestational diabetes mellitus, etc.)
- Healthcare team roles and recommended follow-up appointments.

The nurse should tailor education after conducting a needs assessment of the patient and family, which will vary depending on the mother's age and whether she is a primipara or multipara.

Teaching should not be limited to "how-to" activities. Anticipatory guidance is essential in assisting the family to cope with role changes, the realities of a new baby, and potential complications such as a baby with colic or postpartum health issues. Small-group discussions provide a chance for the new parents to talk about fears and expectations. Questions may arise about sexuality, contraception, childcare, and even the grief associated with giving up the fantasized baby in order to accept the actual one.

Although childbearing is generally considered a natural and healthy experience, the incidence of complications and discomforts in the first year postpartum is common. Women may experience pain, fatigue, urinary incontinence, sleep deprivation, and changes in mental health status. Complications during hospitalization and the first postpartum year are responsible for the rising MMR in the United States. Effective patient education is essential in the prevention of maternal deaths. AWHONN and the National Partnership for Maternal Safety are determining best practices related to provision of education that prepares patients and families to recognize and seek care for signs and symptoms of life-threatening postpartum complications such as hemorrhage, thromboembolism, hypertension, infection, and depression. Nurses should educate every postpartum woman about the following critical concepts prior to discharge, and the father, partner, or a family member should be present during the teaching:

- Headache
- Leg pain
- Abnormal vaginal bleeding
- Swelling of face or extremities
- Chest pain or shortness of breath
- Thoughts of harming self or baby
- Oral temperature of 100.4°F or higher
- Excessive incisional pain or discharge.

Additionally, all postpartum women should be informed that every time they seek healthcare for any reason during the 12 months after giving birth, they need to inform the provider that they have recently been pregnant (D'Oria, Myers, & Logsdon, 2016).

Adolescent mothers, patients with cesarean delivery, and parents of newborns with congenital anomalies or adverse clinical courses will have special concerns, as will patients with special needs related to their own physical, mental, or emotional health and abilities. Postpartum nurses should ensure that special needs families have additional support in place from home care nurses, social workers, chaplains, and other professionals before discharge.

Table 33–1 presents a form that identifies important topic areas to be included in postpartum patient teaching. Methods and validation can be checked off as they occur.

TABLE 33–1 Areas to Include in Postpartum Teaching

	TEACHING METHOD			PATIENT VALIDATION	
KNOWLEDGE AND SKILLS TO BE TAUGHT	PRINTED MATERIALS	INDICATE VIDEO, ONLINE, OR DEMO	VERBAL INSTRUCTION	VERBALIZES UNDERSTANDING	RETURN DEMONSTRATION
Care Of The Mother					
Signs of complications and when to seek immediate care					
Breast care					
Breastfeeding or lactation suppression					
Possible problems and care					
Involutional changes					
Position of fundus					
Afterpains					
Changes in lochia					
Signs of possible problems					
Bladder function					
Fluid needs					
Signs of possible problems					
Bowel function					
Normal patterns					
Dietary assistance					
Perineal care					
Expected healing changes in episiotomy/laceration					
Comfort measures (rinsing with warm water, use of cooling packs, use of analgesic/anesthetic spray, sitz bath, tucks), home care					
Signs of possible problems					
Rest and activity					
Scheduling rest periods, postpartum fatigue					

(continued)

TABLE 33–1 Areas to Include in Postpartum Teaching *(continued)*

KNOWLEDGE AND SKILLS TO BE TAUGHT	TEACHING METHOD: PRINTED MATERIALS	TEACHING METHOD: INDICATE VIDEO, ONLINE, OR DEMO	TEACHING METHOD: VERBAL INSTRUCTION	PATIENT VALIDATION: VERBALIZES UNDERSTANDING	PATIENT VALIDATION: RETURN DEMONSTRATION
Ambulation					
Watching for circulatory problems in legs					
Emotional changes					
Changes in mood, crying, anxiety, "baby blues," postpartum depression, psychosis					
Care of the Father/Partner					
Emotional changes					
Emotional changes and challenges that may occur					
Encouragement to seek support as needed					
Physiologic and psychologic changes that may occur in the mother and newborn					
Newborn care concerns					
Possible supportive measures for the new family					
Care of the Baby					
Newborn safety and security measures					
Observing the baby					
General appearance					
Newborn vision					
Newborn hearing					
Vital signs					
Normal parameters					
How to take a temperature					
Skin					
Coloring					
Normal rashes					
Diaper care					
Elimination cycles of stool/urine					
Normal characteristics					
Signs of diarrhea and treatment					
Signs of constipation and treatment					
Emotional and comforting needs					
Protective reflexes					
Blinking					
Sneezing					
Swallowing					
Normal reflexes					

TABLE 33–1 Areas to Include in Postpartum Teaching *(continued)*

	TEACHING METHOD			PATIENT VALIDATION	
KNOWLEDGE AND SKILLS TO BE TAUGHT	PRINTED MATERIALS	INDICATE VIDEO, ONLINE, OR DEMO	VERBAL INSTRUCTION	VERBALIZES UNDERSTANDING	RETURN DEMONSTRATION
Feeding the baby					
Schedule					
Breastfeeding					
Positioning, latch, initiating and ending feeding					
Newborn cues for feeding					
Identifying problem areas and possible solutions					
Signs of dehydration					
Signs of adequate breastfeeding (output, satiation, weight)					
Formula-feeding					
Positioning					
Preparation of bottles and formula					
Burping or bubbling the baby					
Holding, wrapping, and diapering the baby					
Various holds (cradle, football)					
Securing baby in blanket to provide warmth					
Diapering					
Perineal skin care					
Circumcision care					
"Safe to sleep!"					
Bathing the baby					
Supplies					
Method					
Safety					
Use of bulb syringe and care if choking					
Sudden infant death syndrome (SIDS) prevention (home *and* child care)					
Prevention of abusive head trauma (battering/shaken baby injuries)					
Prevention of falls					
Childproofing the home					
Positioning					
Car seat/vehicle safety					
Health promotion					
When to call healthcare provider					
Temperature					
Diarrhea					

(continued)

TABLE 33–1 Areas to Include in Postpartum Teaching *(continued)*

	TEACHING METHOD			PATIENT VALIDATION	
KNOWLEDGE AND SKILLS TO BE TAUGHT	PRINTED MATERIALS	INDICATE VIDEO, ONLINE, OR DEMO	VERBAL INSTRUCTION	VERBALIZES UNDERSTANDING	RETURN DEMONSTRATION
Poor feeding/feeding intolerance					
Malaise/lethargy/"not acting right"					
Protecting baby from infections					
Immunization schedule					
Hearing and metabolic screening					
Aspects of Parenting					
Adjustment to motherhood					
Stressors related to motherhood					
Interaction with newborn					
Newborn behavioral states					
Newborn cues and capacity for interaction					
Baby with colic					
Acquaintance with individual characteristics of their newborn and possible techniques to use					
Resources available					

Evaluating Learning

Methods for evaluating learning vary according to the objectives and teaching methods. The nurse should validate the knowledge of self- and newborn care through patient discussion and return demonstration. Follow-up is indicated if learning needs related to maternal and newborn care and safety are not validated as met prior to discharge.

Evaluation of attitudinal or less concrete learning is more difficult. For example, a mother's ability to express her frustrations over an unanticipated cesarean birth or difficulties with breastfeeding as opposed to her desired and expected experience may be the nurse's only clues that learning has occurred. Follow-up phone calls and home visits after discharge may provide additional evaluative information and continue the helping process as the nurse assesses the family's current educational needs and begins planning accordingly.

Promotion of Maternal Comfort and Well-Being

The nurse promotes and restores maternal physical well-being by assessing the patient on a regular basis and providing essential care. Maternal blood pressure and pulse should be monitored every 15 minutes for the first 2 hours and then every 4 hours; maternal temperature should be monitored every 4 hours for the first 8 hours and then every 8 hours (Gabbe et al., 2017).

Although there is a lack of definitive research data indicating how often maternal status should be assessed, most institutions have assessment protocols for the focused postpartum assessment. At a minimum, the uterine fundus, the perineum, lochia, and urinary output or need to void are assessed at least every 15 minutes for the first hour following delivery of the placenta, every 30 minutes for the second hour, and then every 4 hours for 24 hours (Gabbe et al., 2017).

The nurse performs nursing activities aimed at relieving specific discomforts, such as an edematous perineum or a distended bladder. In addition, medications may be needed to promote comfort, treat anemia, enhance immunity to infectious diseases, and prevent development of antibodies in the nonsensitized Rh-negative woman. Finally, the woman may require care for alterations in her emotional well-being.

Monitoring Uterine Status

The nurse completes an assessment of the uterus as discussed in Chapter 32 and described in detail in *Clinical Skill 32–1*. The nurse should follow institutional protocol regarding frequency of assessments and use professional judgment to decide when maternal status requires more frequent checks or additional assessments to determine:

- Presence of **bogginess** (softening of the uterus due to inadequate contraction of the muscle tissue)
- Positioning out of midline
- Heavy lochial flow
- Presence of clots
- Formation of a hematoma.

The amount, consistency, color, and odor of the lochia are monitored on an ongoing basis. Increased bleeding is most often related to uterine atony and responds to fundal massage, expression of any clots, and emptying the bladder. Nipple stimulation can also be utilized to promote contraction of the uterus. Breastfeeding is an ideal and natural way to stimulate oxytocin release and contract a boggy uterus. Bleeding that does not respond readily requires additional evaluation to rule out complications such as retained placenta, lacerations, coagulation defects, or uterine inversion. Changes in lochia that need to be assessed further, documented, and reported to the physician/CNM are discussed in Chapter 32 and presented in detail in *Clinical Skill 32–2: Evaluating Lochia*. See *Professionalism in Practice: Using Critical Thinking to Anticipate Postpartum Hemorrhage*.

Professionalism in Practice Using Critical Thinking to Anticipate Postpartum Hemorrhage

The nurse uses critical thinking skills to anticipate a postpartum hemorrhage and remains sensitive to a uterus that becomes boggy or to increases in lochial flow. The astute nurse will also be aware of risk factors, such as prolonged second stage, macrosomia, manual removal of the placenta, use of magnesium sulfate, cesarean during second stage, chorioamnionitis, or multiparity. The nurse will monitor closely, maintain intravenous access, know recent vital signs, and make certain that oxytocic drugs are readily available when caring for patients at increased risk for postpartum hemorrhage. Accurate visual estimation should be accompanied by weighing pads in the patient with heavy lochia and in patients at high risk. The nurse should be aware that vaginal bleeding in the presence of a firm fundus may be related to internal lacerations requiring repair. Optimal communication between the nurse and other members of the healthcare team is essential to the prevention and treatment of this potentially life-threatening complication.

Resources:

- The AWHONN Postpartum Hemorrhage Project (AWHONN, 2014) developed guidance to assist nurses in the prevention, recognition, and timely treatment of postpartum hemorrhage. Bedside nurse leaders should advocate for the display of resources such as the Postpartum Hemorrhage Project—Recognition, Readiness & Response poster on nursing units.
- See Behling and Renaud (2015) for description of an obstetric vital sign alert initiative to improve quality and safety for postpartum patients.

Intravenous oxytocin (Pitocin) remains the first-line drug for prevention and treatment of excessive bleeding related to postpartum uterine atony. Methylergonovine maleate (Methergine) may also be prescribed to promote uterine contractions in the presence of atony, but a Cochrane Review did not find evidence to support its prophylactic use (Gabbe et al., 2017; Yaju, Kataoka, Eto, et al., 2013). See *Drug Guide: Methylergonovine Maleate (Methergine)* in this chapter and *Drug Guide: Oxytocin (Pitocin)* in Chapter 25. Carboprost (Hemabate) may be used for uterine atony resistant to Pitocin and Methergine. See Table 35–1 regarding the use of uterine stimulants. Misoprostol is not supported as a first-line drug for postpartum hemorrhage (Gabbe et al, 2017; Mousa, Blum, Abou El Senoun, et al., 2014).

Teaching for Self-Care. Teach the woman to assess her fundus for firmness and position and to massage the fundus gently to promote uterine contraction. In addition, instruct her to monitor the amount and color of the lochia. Being aware of normal involutional changes will help the woman identify problems. Discharge instructions should specify that the woman call her healthcare provider if her bleeding is saturating more than one standard-sized sanitary pad per hour.

Relief of Perineal Discomfort

Many nursing interventions are available for relieving perineal discomfort. Before selecting a method, the nurse needs to assess the perineum to determine the degree of edema and other problems. It is also important to ask the woman whether there are special measures that she feels will be particularly effective and to offer her choices when possible. For instance, some cultures believe that the use of "cold" versus "hot" may alter the recovery or spirit of the new mother (see Chapter 32). These beliefs will affect the choices made by the new mother. The nurse uses disposable gloves while applying all relief measures and washes hands before and after using the gloves. The nurse should be aware that severe perineal discomfort that does not respond to comfort measures may be indicative of a complication such as hematoma and warrants further investigation.

It is important to use good hygienic practices, such as moving from the front (area of the symphysis pubis) to the back (area around the anus) of the perineum. The nurse should follow this principle when placing cooling packs and perineal pads and applying topical anesthetic agents or pain relief products. Avoiding contamination between the anal area and the urethral-vaginal area minimizes the risk of infection.

Clinical Tip

You may be surprised by how quickly the postpartum woman shows signs of bladder distention, possibly as soon as 1 to 2 hours after childbirth. This is because of normal postpartum diuresis. You can help prevent distention by palpating the woman's bladder frequently and encouraging her to void. Some women, particularly those who had epidural anesthesia, may not feel an urge to void when the bladder is full. Others may feel the urge to urinate but be unable to begin the flow of urine. Possible interventions include turning on a faucet to produce the sound of running water, having the patient place a hand or foot in a basin of warm water, squirting warm water over her perineum using a peri bottle, and placing a few drops of peppermint oil in the urine collection device ("hat"). The first few voids should be measured and documented according to agency policy. The amount should be at least 150 to 200 mL. If the woman is still unable to void and catheterization becomes necessary, be prepared for difficulty in visualizing the urethra because of localized swelling and discomfort. If a patient requires more than one straight catheterization during the postpartum period, the provider may order an indwelling catheter for at least 8 to 12 hours to allow the swelling to subside.

PERINEAL CARE

Perineal care after each elimination (urination or defecation) cleanses the perineum and helps to promote comfort. Many agencies provide "peri bottles" that the woman can use to squirt warm tap water over her perineum following elimination. To cleanse her perineum, the woman may also use a handheld shower head, moist antiseptic towelettes, or toilet paper in a blotting (patting) motion. She should be taught to start at the front (area just under the symphysis pubis) and proceed toward the back (area around

Drug Guide

Methylergonovine Maleate (Methergine)

OVERVIEW OF ACTION

Methylergonovine maleate (Methergine) is an oxytocic ergot alkaloid that stimulates uterine and vascular smooth muscle. It is used postpartum to stimulate the uterus to contract. Sustained contraction clamps off uterine blood vessels, decreases blood loss, and promotes involution. The drug has a vasoconstrictive effect on all blood vessels, especially the larger arteries. This may result in hypertension, particularly in a woman whose blood pressure is already elevated.

ROUTE, DOSAGE, AND FREQUENCY

Methergine has a rapid onset of action and may be given orally or intramuscularly.

Usual IM dose: 200 mcg (0.2 mg) following expulsion of the placenta. It may be administered after delivery of the anterior shoulder, but only under direct supervision of the obstetric provider. The dose may be repeated every 2–4 hours if necessary. Usual onset is 2–5 minutes.

Usual oral dose: 200 mcg (0.2 mg) three or four times a day for up to 7 days. Usual onset is 5–10 minutes.

Not for IV use except in life-threatening emergency—severe hypertension and vasoconstriction may result. Give no more than 0.2 mg/min IV. Do not mix with other drugs in syringe or IV line.

MATERNAL CONTRAINDICATIONS

Pregnancy, hypersensitivity, preeclampsia, hypertension, lactation. Use caution in hepatic or renal disease, cardiac disease, and sepsis. Administration during the third stage of labor should occur only under direct supervision of the obstetric provider. Women should not breastfeed during Methergine treatment and should wait 12 hours after treatment is discontinued to breastfeed. Discard any milk pumped during this time period.

MATERNAL SIDE EFFECTS

Hypertension is the most common adverse reaction. Some patients experience nausea and vomiting, headaches, and severe uterine cramping. Dizziness, tinnitus, palpitations, arrhythmias, diaphoresis, dyspnea, chest pain, and allergic reactions may occur.

Rare and severe reactions include hypertension with seizures, encephalopathy, water intoxication, stroke, myocardial infarction, and pulmonary edema. Hypotension may occur in some women.

EFFECTS ON FETUS OR NEWBORN

Because Methergine has a long duration of action and can thus produce tetanic contractions, it *should never be used during pregnancy or before delivery of the fetus*, when a sustained uterine contraction could cause injury or death to the mother and/or fetus.

SAFETY ALERT!

Methergine should never be administered to a newborn as it can cause life-threatening complications; store in a separate location from newborn medications to avoid accidental administration (Corbett, O'Connell, Boutin, et al., 2016).

NURSING CONSIDERATIONS

- Monitor fundal height location and consistency and the amount and character of the lochia.
- Notify provider if uterus remains boggy despite Methergine administration.
- Assess the blood pressure before and routinely throughout drug administration.
- Inform patient that Methergine may cause severe menstrual-like cramps.
- Observe for adverse effects or symptoms of ergot toxicity (ergotism) such as nausea and vomiting, headache, muscle pain, tingling of extremities, cold or numb fingers and toes, chest pain, and general weakness.
- Provide patient and family teaching regarding importance of not smoking during Methergine administration (nicotine from cigarettes constricts vessels and may lead to hypertension), signs of toxicity.

Sources: Akorn, Inc., 2015; Vallerand, Sanoski, & Deglin, 2017.

the anus) to prevent contamination from the anal area. In addition, to prevent contamination, the perineal pad should be applied from front to back, placing the front portion against the perineum first. Perineal pads should be changed regularly to prevent infection.

Women with Special Needs Perineal Hygiene

The woman who is visually impaired may need assistance with perineal hygiene initially since she is unable to visualize her pad. The nurse can suggest a regular schedule to ensure proper hygiene is performed to reduce the risk of infection.

Teaching for Self-Care. The nurse demonstrates how to cleanse the perineum and assists the woman as necessary, for example, by offering additional information regarding the use of perineal pads. Some women may need instruction on the proper use of perineal pads during the postpartum period. (See *Teaching Highlights: Episiotomy Care*.) Some women may prefer to use pads designed for urinary incontinence. The pads are also highly absorbent and are usually self-adherent.

LOCAL PERINEAL COOLING

If an episiotomy is performed at the time of birth or if a laceration occurs, local cooling is generally applied to reduce edema and numb the tissues, which promotes comfort. Many agencies offer commercial cooling packs or cold gel pads, which should be used according to the manufacturer's instructions. The nurse should ask the woman for permission before using perineal cooling and should consider cultural norms. Use of perineal cooling measures may be continued for as long as necessary. Cooling is most often used during the first 24 hours postpartum.

A Cochrane Review (East, Begg, Henshall, et al., 2012) found that local perineal cooling had no effect on healing and found limited evidence for the use of local cooling for perineal pain. Cooling packs are commonly applied for 10 to 20 minutes with no adverse effects, and women in some studies experienced increased comfort (Lu, Su, Gau, et al., 2015). Paiva and

TEACHING HIGHLIGHTS | Episiotomy Care

- Describe the process of wound healing.
- Discuss the risks of contamination of the episiotomy by bacteria from the anal area.
- Describe techniques that are used to keep the episiotomy clean and promote healing and comfort:
  - Sitz bath
  - Use of peri-bottle following each voiding or defecation
  - Use of premoistened antiseptic wipes
  - Pad change following each elimination and at regular intervals
  - Ice pack or ice-filled glove to perineum immediately following childbirth
  - Judicious use of analgesics or topical anesthetics
  - Tightening buttocks before sitting.
- Identify signs of episiotomy infection (redness, edema, drainage, incomplete approximation of the edges).
- Advise the woman to contact her healthcare provider if signs of infection develop.

colleagues (2016) evaluated 50 Brazilian women who applied ice packs for 20-minute intervals and found that women noted pain relief for up to 2 hours after they were removed. In the Cochrane Review, optimal times and length of application have not been established, and women under the effects of epidural anesthesia may be at risk for localized trauma from too much cooling. The authors noted that analgesics, topical anesthetics, witch hazel application, and pulsed electromagnetic energy may also be effective alone or in combination with perineal cooling, and more research is needed (East et al., 2012).

Teaching for Self-Care. The nurse provides information about the purpose of perineal cooling, anticipated effects, benefits, and possible problems.

SITZ BATH

The warmth of the water in the sitz bath provides comfort, decreases pain, and increases circulation to the tissues, which promotes healing and reduces the incidence of infection (Figure 33–1). Sitz baths may be used PRN. The nurse teaches the mother to fill the disposable sitz bath with water at a temperature (warm or cool) that is comfortable for her. The nurse instructs the woman to remain in the sitz bath for 20 minutes. It is important for the woman to have a clean towel to pat dry her perineum after the sitz bath and to have a clean perineal pad ready to apply. The woman should rinse the sitz bath with clean warm water after each use. See *Clinical Skill 33–1: Use of Perineal Hygiene, Perineal Cooling, and Sitz Baths.*

Teaching for Self-Care. The nurse provides information about the purpose and use of the sitz bath, anticipated effects, benefits, possible problems, and safety measures to prevent injury from possible slipping or extreme water temperature. Home use of sitz baths may be recommended for the woman with an extensive episiotomy or laceration; the woman may use either the disposable sitz bath from the birthing unit or a clean bathtub. When using a bathtub, the woman should draw 4 to 6 inches of water, assess the temperature of the water, and soak in the water for 15 to 20 minutes. If other family members use the bathtub, it should be cleaned prior to her use. The use of a handheld showerhead to irrigate the perineum is another way to cleanse and soothe the traumatized tissue. See *Complementary Health Approaches: Promotion of Perineal Comfort*.

TOPICAL AGENTS AND ORAL ANALGESICS

Topical anesthetic agents may be used to relieve perineal discomfort. The woman is advised to apply the anesthetic agent after a sitz bath or perineal care. Anesthetic sprays, foams, ointments, or

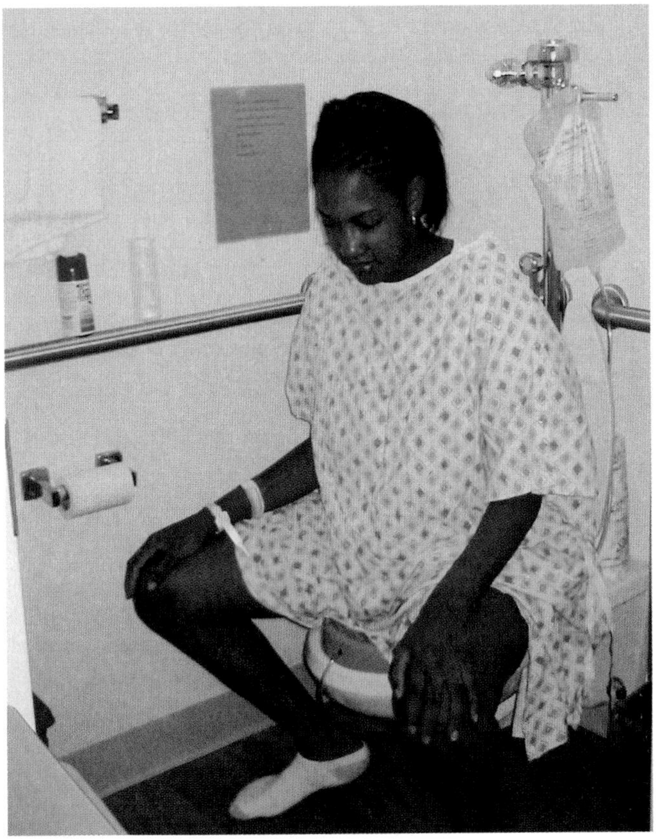

Figure 33–1 **A sitz bath promotes healing and provides relief from perineal discomfort during the initial weeks following birth.**

SOURCE: Michele Davidson.

Complementary Health Approaches

Promotion of Perineal Comfort

Transcutaneous electrical nerve stimulation (TENS), dry cupping, and ear acupressure are complementary and alternative therapies that have been used to promote perineal comfort (Akbarzade et al., 2016; Kwan & Li, 2014; Pitangui, Araújo, Bezerra, et al., 2014). There is a need for ongoing research about complementary and alternative treatments for postpartum perineal pain.

Clinical Skill 33-1

Use of Perineal Hygiene, Perineal Cooling, and Sitz Baths

NURSING ACTION

Preparation

- Explain the importance and benefits of perineal care. These methods can be used for the woman who has had any type of perineal trauma such as an episiotomy, laceration, extension of the episiotomy, or edema from an extended period of pushing.

Rationale: *Perineal care promotes healing, prevents infection, and relieves discomfort in the perineal area following a vaginal birth. It may be needed after a cesarean birth if the woman had perineal trauma before having to advance to a cesarean delivery.*

Equipment and Supplies

- Peri bottle or squirt bottle
- Commercial cooling packs *or* latex-free exam glove filled with ice chips, tied at top, powder rinsed off and covered with clean cloth
- Sitz bath as provided by the facility
- Clean towel for drying perineum and one placed on floor around toilet to prevent slipping on wet floor

Rationale: *The woman may need only one of these procedures or she may need to use a combination of two or three. At the very least, the use of peri bottles should be encouraged after each urination or defecation.*

Procedure

Peri Bottle

1. Explain the purpose and use of the peri bottle as well as the benefits. Its use can enhance cleanliness, provide comfort, prevent infection, and promote healing.
2. Demonstrate and assist the patient as needed to fill a small plastic peri bottle with warm water and reapply the cap. Have patient feel water to assure it is at a comfortably warm temperature. Open the top of the cap and gently squirt the warm water on the entire perineal, urethral, and anal area.

Rationale: *The warm water increases blood flow, which promotes healing, and will loosen dried blood that may be present, which aids in cleansing.*

3. Have the woman dry the perineal area with a clean towel, patting dry, beginning at the front (urethral area) and ending at the back (anal area). Apply new peri-pad, cooling pack (if using), and underwear.

Rationale: *Instruct the woman to perform this procedure and apply a new peri-pad after each urination and defecation.*

Perineal Cooling Measures

1. Explain the purpose and use of the perineal cooling and expected results, as well as benefits and possible problems.

Rationale: *Cool packs or cooling gel pads are used to reduce edema due to perineal trauma. Many women find that localized perineal cooling relieves the discomfort by temporarily numbing the area. For edema, the cooling packs will usually be used for 12–24 hours or until the mother no longer feels a need for it.*

2. If commercial cooling packs are used, activate the pack according to the manufacturer's instructions.
3. If commercial cooling packs are not available, nurses at some facilities use a latex-free exam glove filled with ice chips and tied off the top of the glove like a balloon. Rinse any powder off the glove and wrap with a clean cloth. Do not apply the glove directly to the skin, as it may cause irritation or burns from the extreme cold.
4. The cooling pack should be placed directly on the perineum; larger, more absorbent peri-pads can be placed between the cooling pack and the patient's underwear.
5. The cooling pack can remain in place for up to 20 minutes at a time.

Rationale: *Document use of perineal cooling measures per agency guidelines. Report and document any adverse event related to the use of perineal cooling measures.*

Sitz Baths

1. Explain the purpose and use of the sitz bath, anticipated effects, benefits, possible problems, and safety measures to prevent slipping or an injury from hot water. The sitz bath will last approximately 20 minutes.

Rationale: *The nurse may compare the sitz bath to "sitting in a gentle whirlpool for 20 minutes."*

2. Raise the toilet seat on the toilet.
3. Insert large infusion bag or tube into the back of the sitz bath basin, anchoring it to the bottom of the basin with the small opening at the end of the tubing facing upward, toward the ceiling. Follow manufacturer's instructions on the package.
4. Close the clamp on the tubing.
5. Fill the drainage bag with warm or cool water up to the top line as indicated on the bag (have bag as full as possible without spilling when carried from the top).

Rationale: *Warm water (102°F to 105°F or to touch) provides comfort and cleansing and increases circulation, which promotes healing and the prevention of infection. Cool water is effective in reducing edema and decreases pain when used in the first 24 to 48 hours. Offer both choices and allow the woman to choose which temperature she wants.*

6. Place the basin in the toilet with the side marked "front" facing the front of the toilet.
7. Secure the drainage bag from handle or hook above the toilet.
8. After placing towels on the floor around the toilet, assist the woman to sit directly on the basin edges as if it were the toilet seat.

Rationale: *When the woman sits on the basin, excess water may overflow onto the floor around the toilet, thus the need for towels on the floor.*

9. Open the clamp on the tubing. The water will drain from the bag into the basin, which already has water in it, thus producing a gentle swirling movement of the water in the basin and on the perineal area. Water from the basin or bag will flow into the toilet through holes in the sides of the basin.

Clinical Skill 33-1 *(continued)*

10. Once the sitz bath is complete, instruct the woman to close the clamp on the tubing, dry the perineum with a clean towel, and apply a new peri-pad.

11. Rinse the basin and place the tubing and bag inside and set it aside for the next use.

12. Take care to wipe up any spilled water from the floor to avoid slippage and injury.

13. Document the use of the sitz bath as per agency documentation guidelines. Document and report any adverse events related to the use of the sitz bath.

Tucks pads may be ordered for relief of both perineal and hemorrhoidal pain. It is important for the nurse to emphasize that the woman should wash her hands before and after using the topical treatments. A Cochrane Review found that administering an oral nonsteroidal anti-inflammatory drug (NSAID) decreased perineal pain within the first 6 hours after delivery (Wuytack, Smith, & Cleary, 2016). The nurse should offer an analgesic as ordered and should instruct the woman to request additional doses as needed. See *Professionalism in Practice: Managing Postpartum Perineal Trauma.*

Professionalism in Practice Managing Postpartum Perineal Trauma

The nurse should be aware that approaches to management of postpartum perineal trauma vary between facilities and regions of the country. It is important for baccalaureate-prepared nurses to be familiar with online databases such as the Cochrane Library, to periodically review current literature, and to participate in the development of agency policies and procedures that promote the use of interventions substantiated by research. Nurses who do this are engaged in the Quality and Safety Education in Nursing (QSEN) competency of evidence-based practice.

Teaching for Self-Care. The nurse provides information about the prescribed analgesic, anesthetic spray, or topical agent. The woman needs to understand the purpose, use, anticipated effects, benefits, and possible problems associated with the product. The nurse can combine an explanation with a demonstration of correct application of sprays or topical agents. A return demonstration is a useful method of evaluating the woman's understanding. Directions for self-application should be provided in the woman's primary language and should include instructions to keep the products away from children. Some facilities post instructions with text and photos in postpartum patient restrooms.

Relief of Hemorrhoidal Discomfort

Some mothers experience hemorrhoidal pain after giving birth. Relief measures include the use of sitz baths, topical anesthetics, cool packs, or witch hazel pads (Tucks) applied directly to the anal area. Short-term use of topical creams or rectal suppositories containing hydrocortisone is often helpful. Increasing fiber and fluids in the diet, exercising moderately, and using stool softeners as needed prevents straining (Lamb & Sanders, 2015). Women who have had a fourth-degree laceration during birth should not use rectal suppositories.

Teaching for Self-Care. The woman should know that she may find it helpful to maintain a side-lying position when possible or to tighten her buttocks when sitting down to reduce contact of the perineum with the seat and to avoid prolonged sitting. The mother is encouraged to continue a high-fiber diet, maintain adequate fluid intake, and begin moderate exercise such as walking. The nurse can reassure her that hemorrhoids usually disappear a few weeks after birth if the woman did not have them before her pregnancy. See *Case Study: Azia Askari.*

Relief of Afterpains

Afterpains are the pain associated with intermittent uterine contractions that occur when the uterus contracts as it returns to its prepregnant state (see Chapter 32). A primipara may not notice afterpains because her uterus is able to maintain a contracted state. Multiparous women and those who have had an overdistended uterus (due to multiple gestation or hydramnios) frequently experience discomfort from afterpains as the uterus intermittently contracts more vigorously. Breastfeeding women are also more likely to experience afterpains than formula-feeding

CASE STUDY: Azia Askari

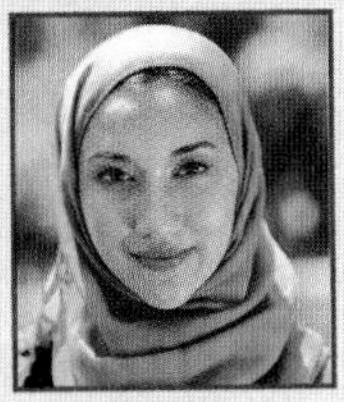

SOURCE: HONGQI ZHANG/123RF

Azia has given birth to a boy, to the delight of her husband and extended family. After a prolonged labor and difficult birth, Azia appears uncomfortable and is grimacing when you begin to examine her. As you are about to begin, you ask her family to leave the room. Azia's exam reveals soft breasts with colostrum present, a firm fundus 2 centimeters below the umbilicus, swelling of the perineal area and labia, slight bruising on the right labia, and a laceration that is well approximated. A 2 cm hemorrhoid is also present and her bleeding is moderately heavy rubra without clots.

Questions to Ponder

What comfort measures can you provide to help with her perineal discomfort? What cultural factors would you consider when providing comfort measures throughout the shift?

women because of the release of oxytocin when the baby suckles. The nurse can suggest the woman lie prone with a small pillow under the lower abdomen, explaining that the discomfort may be intensified for about 5 minutes but then will diminish greatly. The prone position applies pressure to the uterus and therefore stimulates contractions. When the uterus maintains a constant contraction, the afterpains cease. Additional nursing interventions include positioning, ambulation, or administration of an analgesic agent.

The mother's description of the type and severity of her pain is usually the most reliable method of determining which analgesic agent will best promote the comfort she desires. Many women who are breastfeeding have concerns about the effects of medications on the baby. It is helpful to point out to concerned mothers that mild analgesics such as acetaminophen and ibuprofen pose little risk to their newborns when used judiciously in the short term to allow them the ability to bond and breastfeed in comfort. Short-term use of prescription narcotic agents may be necessary for pain that does not respond to ibuprofen or acetaminophen. Nurses can use references such as the Drugs and Lactation Database (LactMed) when advising breastfeeding mothers about use of analgesics.

Teaching for Self-Care. The nurse provides information about the cause of afterpains and methods to decrease discomfort. The nurse also explains any medications that are ordered, expected effect, benefits, possible side effects, and any special considerations such as the possibility of dizziness or sleepiness with particular medications. The nurse must inform patients who take acetaminophen about the risks of accidental overdose. Patients should be instructed to carefully read the labels of any drugs they take concurrently for the presence of acetaminophen.

Relief of Discomfort from Immobility and Muscle Strain

Discomfort may also be caused by immobility and muscle strain. The woman who pushed for a long time during labor may experience muscular aches. It is not unusual for women to experience joint pain and discomfort in both arms and legs, depending on the effort they exerted during the second stage of labor. Early ambulation is encouraged to help reduce the incidence of complications such as constipation and thrombophlebitis. It also helps promote a general feeling of well-being.

The nurse assists the woman the first few times she gets up during the postpartum period. Fatigue, effects of medications, loss of blood, and possibly even lack of food may cause feelings of dizziness when the woman stands up. The nurse ensures that the new mother feels steady and is able to stand without assistance before the initial shower. The nurse should provide a chair if a built-in shower seat is not present, in case the woman feels dizzy. The nurse instructs the woman in the use of the emergency call button in the bathroom prior to the first shower, so the new mother can call for assistance, if needed. Dizziness may be aggravated by standing still and by the warmth of the water, so it is best to wait until the woman has eaten and has shown stability when ambulating. The first shower should be brief. Some women may prefer for a family member to be present. On many postpartum units, ammonia inhalants (referred to as "smelling salts") are available for use in case of fainting.

Teaching for Self-Care. The nurse provides information about ambulation and the importance of monitoring any signs of dizziness or weakness. If she becomes dizzy, the woman should sit down and call for assistance.

Postpartum Diaphoresis

Postpartum diaphoresis (excessive perspiration) may cause discomfort for new mothers. The nurse can offer a fresh dry gown and bed linens to enhance comfort.

Some women may feel refreshed by a shower. It is important to consider cultural practices and realize that some women may prefer not to shower in the first few days following birth. For example, some Hispanic and Asian women prefer to delay showering. Nurses can offer these women a wet washcloth to increase maternal comfort. Because diaphoresis may also lead to increased thirst, the nurse can offer fluids as the woman desires. Again, cultural practices are important to consider. Women of Western European background may prefer ice water; women of Asian background may prefer hot water or water at room temperature. The nurse should ascertain the woman's wishes rather than operate solely from the nurse's own values or cultural belief system.

Teaching for Self-Care. The nurse provides information about the normal physiologic changes that cause diaphoresis and methods to increase comfort.

Suppression of Lactation in the Nonbreastfeeding Mother

Many women who do not breastfeed experience some degree of engorgement, accompanied by milk leakage and discomfort. Some women report relief from nonpharmacologic means of suppression such as wearing a support bra continuously for the first week except when showering, avoiding breast stimulation, applying cold packs, or applying cabbage leaves. Although binding the breasts was used in the past, it is no longer recommended. Signs of engorgement usually peak by day 4 and spontaneously resolve by the 10th day postpartum, regardless of treatment. Analgesics such as acetaminophen and ibuprofen can be used until the discomfort subsides (Gagandeep, Sagar, Mamta, et al., 2013; Smith, 2016). Drugs such as Bromocriptine are no longer used in the United States for lactation suppression due to concerns related to the rare possibility of adverse cardiovascular events. Acupuncture, acupressure, ultrasound, and Gua Sha scraping therapy are used in some settings (Mangesi & Zakarija-Grkovic, 2016). According to recent Cochrane Reviews, there is a lack of adequate research regarding side effects of pharmacologic suppression and the efficacy of nonpharmacologic approaches. Further research is needed to build an evidence base (Mangesi & Zakarija-Grkovic, 2016). Breastfeeding difficulties, postpartum breast care, and breast problems, such as engorgement and plugged ducts, after discharge are discussed in detail in Chapter 34; mastitis is discussed in Chapter 35.

Teaching for Self-Care. Nurses should advise the nonbreastfeeding mother to avoid any stimulation of her breasts and nipples by her baby, herself, breast pumps, or her sexual partner until the sensation of fullness has passed (usually in 7 to 10 days). Such stimulation will increase milk production and delay the suppression process. Heat is avoided for the same reason, and the mother is encouraged to let shower water flow over her back rather than her breasts. The wearing of a 24-hour support bra, the use of analgesics as prescribed, and the use of cabbage leaves and/or cold compresses should be helpful during this period of time (AAP & ACOG, 2017). Suppression takes only a few days in most cases.

Ethics in Action!

How do you respond to the postpartum woman who tells you she doesn't have time to breastfeed because of her busy work and social schedule?

Pharmacologic Interventions

Pharmacologic preparations, including immunizations, Rh immune globulin, and pain medications, are frequently administered in the postpartum period.

IMMUNIZATIONS

Optimal timing for the tetanus toxoid, reduced diphtheria toxoid, and acellular pertussis (Tdap) administration is between 27 and 36 weeks' gestation of each pregnancy, as that maximizes maternal and child protection. However, postpartum women who have never received Tdap should receive it during the immediate postpartum period (Centers for Disease Control and Prevention [CDC], 2015). While optimal timing for the influenza immunization is during pregnancy, women not currently immunized for influenza who deliver during influenza season should be offered the vaccine prior to discharge (AAP & ACOG, 2017; CDC, 2016).

RUBELLA VIRUS VACCINE

Women who are not rubella immune as determined by lab studies should receive the rubella vaccine early in the postpartum period, preferably prior to discharge. The AAP and ACOG also recommend varicella immunization for susceptible women in the postpartum period.

Administering live virus vaccines shortly after childbirth is advantageous because the woman is definitely not pregnant and typically does not want another pregnancy in the near future. Although the CDC and AAP and ACOG recommend immunization for measles, mumps, and rubella and for varicella even if breastfeeding, the manufacturers note that caution should be exercised when administering these drugs to nursing mothers (Merck Sharpe & Dohme Corp., 2015).

Teaching for Self-Care. The nurse needs to ensure that the woman understands the purpose of the vaccine(s) and that the manufacturer recommends avoiding pregnancy for 3 months (the CDC recommends 1 month) after receiving live virus vaccines such as those for varicella and rubella. The nurse should provide the patient with the vaccine information statement and answer any questions before the patient signs the informed consent for administration. Because avoiding pregnancy is so important after live virus vaccines, counseling regarding contraception is necessary. The nurse should emphasize the need for all family members to have current immunizations and should refer them to local agencies or programs as available. See *Case Study: Benita Cartier*.

Rh_O(D) IMMUNE GLOBULIN

All Rh_o(D)-negative women with Rh_o(D)-positive babies should receive Rh_o(D) immune globulin (RhoGAM or a similar formulation) within 72 hours after childbirth to prevent sensitization from a fetomaternal transfusion of Rh-positive fetal red blood cells (Moise, 2018). See discussion of criteria in *Clinical Skill 18–2: Intramuscular Administration of Rh Immune Globulin (RhoGAM, WinRho-SDF)* in Chapter 18. The Rh-negative woman needs to understand the implications of her Rh-negative status in future pregnancies. (See Chapter 18 for a detailed discussion.) The nurse provides opportunities for questions during teaching. (See Table 33–2 for further information about postpartum immunizations.) See *Professionalism in Practice: How to Address Differing Drug Recommendations*.

Professionalism in Practice How to Address Differing Drug Recommendations

The nurse will find that sources sometimes vary regarding recommendations for certain drugs. For example, some sources recommend delaying pregnancy for a minimum of 1 month following rubella immunization (CDC, 2016), but the manufacturer recommends delaying pregnancy for 3 months (Merck Sharp & Dohme Corp., 2015). Both the AAP and ACOG and the manufacturer noted that the risk of congenital rubella syndrome from the vaccine is theoretical and emphasized that cases have not occurred despite accidental administration during pregnancy. The professional nurse should discuss issues such as these with providers, be aware of professional organization recommendations, and read current literature in order to give accurate advice to patients.

CASE STUDY: Benita Cartier

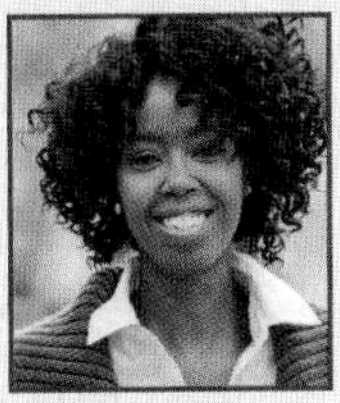

SOURCE: blvdone/Shutterstock

Benita has been visiting her newborn daily in the NICU after her emergency cesarean. She becomes upset when the nurse informs her that she will need a rubella vaccination prior to discharge. Benita is concerned about getting a live vaccine because she is pumping and feeding her milk to the baby. She also feels her baby could be at risk to get rubella because the baby is preterm.

Questions to Ponder

What information would you provide to Benita to ease her concerns about receiving a vaccine so soon after giving birth? Why is the immediate postpartum period an ideal time to vaccinate non-immune women?

TABLE 33–2 Essential Information for Postpartum Immunizations

RUBELLA VIRUS VACCINE, LIVE MMR II (MEASLES, MUMPS, AND RUBELLA VIRUS VACCINE LIVE)

Dose/Route: Single-dose vial of 0.5 mL; inject subcutaneously in outer aspect of the upper arm.

Primary Indication: Stimulate active immunity against rubella virus in the postpartum woman who is susceptible to rubella in order to protect future pregnancies.

Adverse Effects: Burning, pain, or stinging at the injection site; fever; rash; arthritis/arthralgia; encephalitis; allergic reactions

Nursing Implications: The nurse should not administer the immunization and should notify the healthcare provider if the woman has any of the following.

- History of anaphylactic hypersensitivity to neomycin, eggs, or gelatin
- Febrile illness
- Blood dyscrasia
- Neoplasm of the bone marrow or lymphatic system
- Thrombocytopenia
- History of convulsions or cerebral injury
- Immunosuppression.

It is possible that blood transfusions or administration of $Rh_o(D)$ immune globulin in the postpartum period may interfere with the desired immune response. The immunization is contraindicated during pregnancy, and the manufacturer recommends that patients not become pregnant for 3 months after receiving the vaccine. The nurse needs to provide the patient with the MMR Vaccine Information Statement (CDC, 2012), obtain the patient's informed consent prior to administration, and document the vaccine as required by the healthcare facility. As with any immunization, epinephrine should be available in case of anaphylactic reaction.

Patient Teaching: Name of drug, expected effect, possible adverse effects, comfort measures to use if adverse effects occur; instruct the woman to *avoid pregnancy for 3 months* following immunization. (*Note:* CDC recommends 1 month.) Provide information regarding contraceptives and their use.

Nursing Diagnoses Related to Drug Therapy:

- ***Pain, Acute.*** Defining characteristics may include guarding behavior, positioning to ease pain, or self-report of pain during or following subcutaneous administration of immunization.
- ***Health Management, Readiness for Enhanced.*** Defining characteristics may include expressed desire to enhance immunization/ vaccination status.

(NANDA-I © 2017)

$RH_o(D)$ IMMUNE GLOBULIN (RH IMMUNE GLOBULIN SPECIFIC FOR D ANTIGEN)

Standard intramuscular (IM) formulations include **RhoGAM** or **HyperRHO S/D Full Dose**

Microdose IM formulations include **HyperRHO S/D Mini-Dose**, **MICRhoGAM**. (IM formulations are not intended for IV administration.)

Dose/Route:

Postpartum administration: One vial (300 mcg) IM (deltoid) within 72 hours of birth to the $Rh_o(D)$-negative woman who has delivered an $Rh_o(D)$-positive baby. Additional vials may be necessary after significant (more than 15 mL) fetal-maternal hemorrhage as indicated by lab results (Kleihauer-Betke test). A 300-mcg dose is also administered to the $Rh_o(D)$-negative woman following the early termination of pregnancy at 13 weeks or beyond. A 50-mcg minidose is administered to the $Rh_o(D)$-negative woman following the termination of pregnancy prior to 13 weeks (includes spontaneous or elective abortion, ectopic, etc.). (Antepartum administration is discussed in Chapter 18.)

Additional formulations are available. *WinRho® SDF* and *Rhophylac®* are IV formulations, and the dose for WinRho may differ from the information above. Rhophylac may only be given IV, and WinRho may be given IV or IM. As always, refer to manufacturer's current recommendations for safe administration.

Indication: Prevention of sensitization in $Rh_o(D)$-negative women by preventing production of anti-$Rh_o(D)$ antibodies following exposure to $Rh_o(D)$-positive blood. Mother must be Rh-negative, not previously sensitized to Rh factor. Newborn must be Rh-positive, direct antiglobulin negative. Given during pregnancy to prevent erythroblastosis fetalis if fetus is $Rh_o(D)$-positive in current and/or future pregnancies. Given postpartum to protect future pregnancies.

Adverse Effects: Pain at injection site, anemia, fever. May decrease response to live virus vaccines such as rubella or varicella. Severe systemic reactions such as intravascular hemolysis (IVH) are rare in $Rh_o(D)$-negative patients treated for prevention of isoimmunization, but the patient should be observed during and for 20 minutes following administration. There is a risk of infectious agent transmission, as the formulations are made from human plasma.

Nursing Implications: Contraindicated in patients with documented hypersensitivity to human immune globulins, IgA-deficient patients, and those with history of sensitivity to the $Rh_o(D)$ formulation. Confirm criteria for administration are present. Review type and cross-match of mother's and newborn's blood and any other labs, as dosage and administration depend on results. Do not confuse IM and IV formulations. If using a prefilled syringe, allow it to come to room temperature before IM administration. If the mother is $Rh_o(D)$-negative, and there is a delay in determining the newborn's blood type, RhoGAM should be administered to the mother within 72 hours of giving birth. *Do not administer to newborn.* Review manufacturer's current recommendations prior to administration.

Patient Teaching: Name of drug, expected action, possible side effects; report soreness at injection site to nurse; woman should carry information regarding Rh status and dates of $Rh_o(D)$ immune globulin injections with her at all times; explain relevance to subsequent pregnancies.

Nursing Diagnoses Related to Drug Therapy:

- ***Pain, Acute.*** Defining characteristics may include guarding behavior, positioning to ease pain, or self-report of pain during or following intramuscular administration of immunization.
- ***Health Management, Readiness for Enhanced.*** Defining characteristics may include expressed desire to enhance immunization/ vaccination status.

(NANDA-I © 2017)

SOURCES: AAP & ACOG, 2017; Aptevo BioTherapeutics, 2016; CDC, 2012, 2016; CSL Behring AG, 2016; Kedrion Melville, Inc., 2014; Merck Sharpe & Dohme Corp., 2015; Vallerand et al., 2017.
Note: See detailed manufacturers' guidelines prior to administration, and review CDC (2016) guidelines for questions about any other immunizations for pregnant and lactating women.

ANALGESICS

A variety of drugs are used alone or in combination to provide relief of postpartum pain. Options include acetaminophen, nonsteroidal anti-inflammatory agents such as ibuprofen and ketorolac, and narcotic analgesics such as tramadol and hydrocodone. The nurse should assess pain before and 1 hour after administration and should assess level of consciousness, blood pressure, pulse, and respirations before and periodically during treatment. As always, the nurse should clarify allergies prior to administration, inform patients of possible side effects, and monitor for side effects throughout treatment. Detailed information and instructions from manufacturers and the FDA are found on package inserts, in resources accessed through agency electronic health record systems, and at Daily Med, a publication of the National Library of Medicine.

Clinical Tip

Use of narcotic analgesics may cause respiratory depression, sedation, gastrointestinal upset, constipation, and urinary retention. The nurse should do the following:

- Inform the postpartum patient of the risks and assess for respiratory depression, particularly if narcotic analgesics are given with barbiturates, with sedative/hypnotics, or after epidural morphine.
- Monitor bowel sounds and urine output.
- Instruct patient to take narcotic analgesics with food, increase fluids and fiber, and use a stool softener.
- Warn patients that narcotic analgesics may cause sedation; assistance with newborn care and ambulation may be necessary.
- Offer NSAIDS as ordered and encourage use of nonpharmacologic pain control. Managing pain with other methods may decrease the need for narcotics.

SAFETY ALERT!

Prescription combination drugs such as Lortab or Vicodin (hydrocodone and acetaminophen) and Percocet (oxycodone and acetaminophen) are commonly used for postpartum discomfort. In 2011 the Food and Drug Administration (FDA, 2011, 2017) asked manufacturers of combination drugs to limit the dose of acetaminophen in each tablet or capsule to 325 mg or less to decrease the risk of fatal liver damage from the drug. Manufacturers are also required to warn consumers of the risk of severe liver damage. In 2015, the FDA released information from two studies indicating that Tylenol use in pregnancy could be associated with increased risk of attention-deficit/hyperactivity disorder (ADHD) and hyperkinetic disorder (HKD). The FDA estimates that 60 to 70% of women have taken Tylenol during pregnancy and adverse outcomes were associated with women who took the medication throughout pregnancy on a regular basis (FDA, 2017). Nurses should inform postpartum patients of the risks of using prescription and/or over-the-counter drugs including acetaminophen, encourage them to read labels carefully to ensure that they don't consume more than 4 grams of acetaminophen in any 24-hour period, and highlight risks related to using over-the-counter and prescription analgesics containing acetaminophen at the same time.

Support of Maternal Psychosocial Well-Being

The birth of a child, with the role changes and increased responsibilities it produces, is a time of emotional stress for the new mother. This stress is increased by the tremendous physiologic changes that occur as her body adjusts to a nonpregnant state. Nurses working in maternal-child care should read the works of Rubin (1984) and Mercer (1986, 2004, 2006), two key theorists who have researched and written about the process of developing a maternal identity. Mercer recommended changing the previous terminology, *maternal role attainment (MRA)*, to *becoming a mother (BAM)* in 2004. Their work is also discussed in Chapter 32.

Mercer (2004) described BAM as a life-transforming process through which mothers establish maternal identity, including:

- Commitment, attachment, and preparation (pregnancy)
- Acquaintance, learning, and physical restoration (first 2 to 6 weeks following birth)
- Moving toward a new normal (2 weeks to 4 months)
- Achievement of the maternal identity (around 4 months).

Interactive nurse–patient relationships are necessary to support this transition. Reisz, Jacobvitz, and George (2015) discovered a relationship between maternal perception of a positive birth experience and maternal self-esteem. Nurses can influence the patient's subjective experience by validating the mother's perceptions and offering supportive care.

Although agencies may use technological approaches to patient education, a portion of patient education and support needs to be offered through individualized patient–nurse interaction.

Immediately following the birth (*taking-in period*), the mother may be dependent and inwardly focused on bodily concerns. Although the mother will benefit from rest at some point early in the postpartum period, there is a preponderance of evidence that immediate **skin-to-skin contact (SSC)** between mother and newborn has many positive effects for both (Klaus, 2009; Moore, Anderson, Bergman, et al., 2012). Nurses should encourage SSC for all couplets, including those who experienced cesarean births (Moran-Peters, Zauderer, Goldman, et al., 2014; Stone, Prater, & Spencer, 2015), unless complications prevent it. Many women are focused on their own needs during the immediate postpartum period. Once the woman's self-care needs have been met, her focus will shift to the care of her newborn and her ability as a parent (*taking-hold period*). During this time the mother is usually receptive to teaching, and tactful instructions and demonstrations assist her in developing mothering skills. By functioning as an adviser and allowing the mother to perform the actual care, the nurse demonstrates confidence in the mother's skill and ability, which in turn increases the mother's self-confidence about her effectiveness as a parent. See *Developing Cultural Competence: Becoming a Mother*.

The mother may benefit from the opportunity to tell her birth story during the hours and days following birth. During the postpartum period, the mother must adjust to the loss of her fantasized child and accept the child she has borne. This may be more difficult if the child is not of the desired sex or has birth defects. Parents of newborns requiring special care due to congenital anomalies or prematurity will require extra attention and opportunities to share their concerns, fears, and disappointment.

Mood disturbances, including depression, are problematic for many postpartum women. Significantly, new mothers are often discharged before the onset of mental health disorders associated with the postpartum period. Many women experience some mild depressive symptoms, referred to as *postpartum baby blues*, for up to 2 weeks following delivery, but maternal

Developing Cultural Competence Becoming a Mother

The process of becoming a mother is influenced by many variables, including culture, religion, and societal norms. Afiyanti and Solberg (2015) researched the transition to motherhood among 13 rural Indonesian women and two main themes emerged: (1) "trying to be a good mother" and (2) "confirming my destiny as a woman" (p. 494). The theme of *confirming my destiny as a woman* included reframing losses as well as adhering to traditional postpartum prohibitions and practices, even if the woman perceived them as restrictive or uncomfortable. According to the participants, motherhood conferred a positive identity within the village that aligned with local gender expectations. The challenge of *trying to be a good mother* has been reported in Western cultures, and for the Indonesian women in this study, it encompassed caring for the entire family in addition to mothering the newborn. As in studies of women in Western cultures, the new Indonesian mothers felt unprepared to optimally fulfill the maternal role, and they verbalized needs for assistance and support.

The nurse should listen to each patient and not assume that the experience will be the same from woman to woman, even for new mothers within the same cultural group. Nurses can begin by asking, "What should I know about you and your family in order to provide the best nursing care possible for you and your baby?"

Note: *It is unwise to attribute specific attitudes or beliefs to all members of a cultural group. The information in the Developing Cultural Competence boxes offers possible insights into caring for women from different cultural groups.*

mood during the hospital stay is often predictive of postpartum depression (AAP & ACOG, 2017; Kansky, 2016). Therefore, the nurse needs to individually assess all postpartum patients for mood disorders and coordinate follow-up care for women who exhibit postpartum baby blues prior to discharge. Women who experience depressive symptoms during their hospital stays should be reevaluated at 2 weeks postpartum using a two-phase screening approach (Kansky, 2016). Postpartum baby blues, postpartum depression, and postpartum psychosis are discussed in detail, as are assessment and screening tools, in Chapter 35.

Teaching for Self-Care. The nurse should advise the mother that physical, psychologic, and hormonal factors all influence an individual's response to childbirth. It is often helpful to discuss normal adaptations in the postpartum period with both the mother and her partner or another family member. This ensures that someone close to her will be aware of the normal patterns of psychologic responses in the early postpartum period. Normal responses include a brief period of irritability, mood swings, crying spells, and other mood-related symptoms associated with postpartum baby blues. Symptoms are relatively mild and self-limiting, usually resolving within 10 days. Women who experience severe symptoms or symptoms that extend beyond the second postpartum week should be advised to contact their physician/CNM. The nurse should advise families about symptoms of postpartum depression and emphasize the importance of seeking help should they occur (Liu & Tronick, 2013). See *Case Study: Benita Cartier.*

Promotion of Maternal Nutrition, Rest, and Activity

Promotion of Nutrition

The mother may be hungry and thirsty immediately following delivery, particularly if she had limited oral intake during a prolonged labor. She should be allowed to eat and drink as desired, unless complications prevent it. All postpartum women should be encouraged to eat a healthy, well-balanced diet. A breastfeeding mother will require 500 kcal/day above what is ordinarily recommended for a woman of her age. Nonbreastfeeding women may return to normal caloric requirements for their age. Many women continue prenatal vitamin and iron supplementation until the postpartum checkup, and breastfeeding mothers may continue supplementation throughout lactation. See Chapter 14 for more information about postpartum maternal nutrition.

Relief of Fatigue

Following birth, some women feel exhausted and want to rest. Other women are euphoric and full of energy, ready to retell their experience of birth repeatedly. The nurse evaluates individual needs, always with the goal of providing opportunities for rest (see Chapter 32 for information on assessing rest and sleep status). This may include limiting visitors and providing a comfortable place for the woman's husband or partner to sleep.

Fatigue is a common occurrence, which should be expected to resolve over the first few postpartum weeks. Women who experience long labors, complicated deliveries, or cesarean births are at high risk for postpartum fatigue, which can affect the ability to develop attachment and to care for the baby in the

CASE STUDY: Benita Cartier

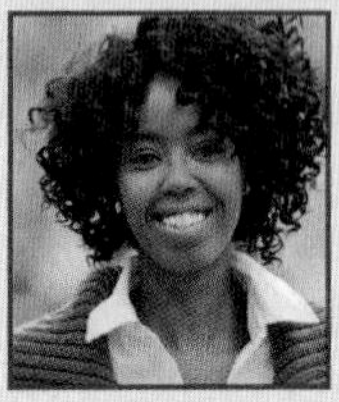

SOURCE: blvdone/Shutterstock.

Benita is preparing for discharge and is tearful because her daughter has to remain a few more days in the NICU. She tells the nurse she feels very guilty that the baby won't be going home with her and can't stop crying. She asks the nurse if she thinks she has postpartum depression because she feels sad and anxious about leaving the baby behind.

Question to Ponder

Do Benita's symptoms seem consistent with postpartum depression or do you feel it is a normal grief response related to having to leave her baby in the NICU?

immediate postpartum period (Lai, Hung, Stocker, et al., 2015). Additive sleep deprivation related to pregnancy discomforts, labor and delivery, and caring for a newborn, especially if there are other young children in the home, contributes to the problem. Adequate rest is essential to a smooth postpartum transition. The nurse can encourage rest by organizing activities to avoid frequent interruptions for the woman. Ideally, one person close to the mother will be in the room to watch the newborn when the mother sleeps. If this is not possible, the newborn may return to the nursery for a period of time to ensure that the baby remains safe while the mother is sleeping soundly.

Postpartum fatigue can be severe and extended in some women, complicating the recovery process. Fatigue is a health problem frequently reported by parents of young children. Parental fatigue can have a negative impact on parental self-efficacy and parenting behaviors. The Wide Awake Parenting (WAP) psychoeducational intervention increases maternal prioritization of self-care to manage fatigue and promote mental health by using professionally led telephone support for postpartum mothers (Giallo, Cooklin, Dunning, et al., 2014).

Teaching for Self-Care. Nearly all new mothers experience some degree of fatigue or sleep deprivation during the postpartum period. Women who have had a cesarean birth are coping with both the constant demands of the baby and their own recovery needs. Some women feel self-induced pressure to take care of household chores while the baby is napping. Fatigue and worry about unaccomplished tasks can become continuous and cyclical. Mothers should be counseled to sleep when the baby sleeps, to utilize family and friends for support, and to delegate or postpone unnecessary chores and activities. Additionally, they should be advised to contact their healthcare provider if they experience signs of infection, anemia, thyroid dysfunction, or unrelenting postpartum fatigue that persists beyond the initial postpartum period. See *Developing Cultural Competence: Rest and Activity in the Postpartum Period.*

Developing Cultural Competence Rest and Activity in the Postpartum Period

Some cultures have distinct customs regarding rest and activity in the postpartum period. For example, Chinese women may follow a traditional recuperation strategy of *doing-the-month (zuo yue zi)*, which requires rest, seclusion, and protective rituals such as not washing their hair for the first month postpartum. Holroyd, Lopez, and Chan (2011) discovered that although the current generation of Chinese mothers modified the restrictions more than their mothers did, the practices promoted recuperation and encouraged help from other female relatives for both generations of new mothers. Liu, Maloni, and Petrini (2014), however, discovered that the traditional practice correlated negatively with aerobic endurance and correlated positively with depression at 6 weeks postpartum. Most cultural customs can be accommodated if they are not harmful, and nurses should support women's beliefs about postpartum self-protection. The nurse should inform the mother of the health benefits of early postpartum ambulation and resumption of physical activity. Ongoing research into traditional cultural practices within the context of current scientific evidence is needed.

Note: *It is unwise to attribute specific attitudes or beliefs to all members of a cultural group. The information in the Developing Cultural Competence boxes offers possible insights into caring for women from different cultural groups.*

Resumption of Activity

Ambulation and activity may gradually increase after discharge. The new mother should avoid heavy lifting, excessive stair climbing, and strenuous activity. One or two daily naps are essential and are most easily achieved if the mother sleeps when her baby does.

By the second week at home, the new mother may begin some light housekeeping activities. Although it is customary to delay the return to work outside the home for 6 weeks, most women are physically able to resume nearly all activities in 4 to 5 weeks when the lochial flow has stopped. Delaying the return to work until after the final postpartum examination will minimize the possibility of problems.

Teaching for Self-Care. The nurse can provide the new mother with suggestions for resuming her normal level of activity. Women should be encouraged to limit the number of activities to prevent excessive fatigue, increase in lochia, and negative psychologic reactions, such as feeling overwhelmed. If excessive fatigue or an increase in lochia occurs, the woman should increase rest periods and decrease extra activities.

SAFETY ALERT!

Postpartum women are at high risk for falls, especially during their first attempts at ambulation following delivery. Pain medications, significant blood loss, epidural anesthesia, and cesarean delivery intensify the risk. Educating patients and family members, providing verbal and visual reminders of the risk, and answering call bells rapidly can decrease falls. See Lockwood and Anderson (2013) and Ainsworth, Summerlin-Long, and Mog (2016) for initiatives designed to prevent maternal and newborn falls.

Postpartum Exercise

The nurse should encourage the woman to begin simple exercises while in the birthing unit and continue them at home, advising her that increased lochia or pain means she should reevaluate her activity and make necessary reductions. Most agencies provide a booklet describing suggested postpartum activities. (Exercise routines vary for women undergoing tubal ligation following birth and for cesarean birth patients.) The postpartum woman is more likely to have positive views of her own well-being and less fatigue if she continues to do stretching and/or her own programmed pattern of exercise.

Teaching for Self-Care. The nurse should advise the woman to begin Kegel exercises immediately after birth (see Chapter 13 and Figure 13–15). The nurse can explain that these exercises will assist in returning vaginal tone and preventing urinary leakage. If no complications exist, normal exercise can be initiated at 2 weeks after birth. Women should be advised to take short walks outside if the weather is appropriate. Abdominal exercises can be suggested to retone the abdominal muscles. A regular exercise program including vigorous activities such as running, weightlifting, or competitive sports can usually be initiated after her 6-week postpartum examination or when approved by her physician/CNM.

Promotion of Family Wellness and Shared Parenting

A satisfactory maternity experience may have a positive impact on the entire family. The new or expanding family that receives appropriate information and has adequate time to interact with its newest member in a supportive environment will feel more comfortable and secure at home.

In the past, newborns were typically separated from their parents immediately after birth. Today most facilities support **family-centered care**, which is focused on keeping the mother and baby together as much as the mother desires. **Mother-baby care**, or **couplet care** (care of both the mother and her baby), is an important part of the family-centered care approach, in which the baby remains at the mother's bedside and both are cared for by the same nurse. Couplet care allows the nurse to teach and role-model and to integrate the entire family into the care of the woman and her newborn. It also enables the mother to have time to bond with her baby and learn to care for him or her in a supportive environment.

The nurse should encourage immediate SSC following delivery of healthy term and late preterm newborns if stable. When initiating SSC, the nurse should place the unclothed newborn directly on the mother's bare chest and place a hat on the newborn's head and a warm blanket over his or her back. Mother and newborn can rest comfortably together under close nursing supervision; immediate newborn care such as Apgar scoring and assessment of vital signs can be performed in this position. Weighing, measuring, and administering eye prophylaxis and vitamin K can be completed after breastfeeding has occurred, within 1 to 2 hours of birth (Phillips, 2013). The father/partner can participate in SSC if the couple prefers or if the mother is unable to begin SSC immediately following birth. See *Professionalism in Practice: Family-Centered Care During the Immediate Postpartum Period*.

In a mother-baby unit, the newborn's crib is placed near the mother's bed, where she can see her baby easily (Figure 33–2). The crib should be a self-contained unit stocked with items the parents might require in providing care. A bulb syringe for suctioning the mouth or nares should always be accessible, and the mother and father/partner should be familiar with its use. The mother-baby unit is conducive to an on-demand feeding schedule for both breastfeeding and formula-feeding newborns.

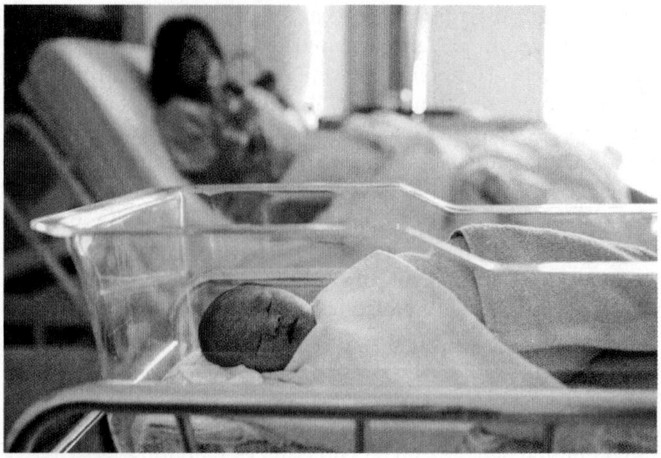

Figure 33–2 **The mother and her newborn room together in a mother-baby unit.**

SOURCE: Phattana Stock/Shutterstock.

Mothers are frequently very tired after birth, so the responsibility for providing total newborn care could be overwhelming. The mother-baby policy must be flexible enough to permit the mother to return the baby to the nursery if she finds it necessary because of fatigue or physical discomfort. Many agencies have unlimited visiting hours for the father/partner. These opportunities to hold and care for the child promote parental self-confidence and foster parental attachment. Encouraging fathers/partners to spend the night allows parents to share initial newborn care responsibilities while they still have the support of nursing staff if questions arise.

Although our culture idealistically and theoretically supports involved fathers/partners, they often lack role models, support, and resources. It is imperative that all teaching in the family-centered care unit be directed to both parents at times that are convenient for both and that fathers/partners be encouraged to share their feelings and be actively involved in the childbearing experience. It is also helpful to provide anticipatory guidance for fathers/partners regarding the feelings and situations they may experience, particularly if their baby is breastfed. Encouraging fathers/partners to be involved in bathing the baby, the bedtime routine, holding, cuddling, and playing will allow them to develop a relationship and reap the rewards they desire.

Professionalism in Practice **Family-Centered Care During the Immediate Postpartum Period**

Nurses who initiate SSC are engaging in the Quality and Safety Education in Nursing (QSEN) competencies of patient-centered care and evidence-based practice. However, it is important to recognize that some newborn care practices are mandated by state law. For example, some states require administration of eye prophylaxis within 1 to 2 hours of birth. Other states, such as New York in 2014, amended the law to require administration within 6 hours of birth—aligning the law with current scientific evidence and recommendations of the American Academy of Pediatrics. As bedside leaders, baccalaureate-prepared nurses need to be aware of state laws, clinical facility protocols, current scientific evidence, and recommendations of professional organizations. Nurses who collaborate with other healthcare providers, facility administrators, and legislators to promote alignment between scientific evidence, local protocols, and state laws are fulfilling the role of the nurse as a member of the profession.

Reactions of Siblings

Sibling visitation helps meet the needs of both the siblings and their mother. A visit to the hospital reassures children that their mother is well and still loves them. The mother has the opportunity to introduce her older children to the newest family member. It also provides an opportunity for the children to become familiar with the new baby.

Most agencies now recognize the importance of providing siblings with opportunities to see their mother and meet the baby during the early postpartum period (Figure 33–3). Approaches to this issue vary from specified visiting hours for siblings to unlimited visiting privileges.

Although the parents have prepared the child(ren) for the presence of a new brother or sister, the actual arrival of the baby requires some adjustments. Some children may be present for the

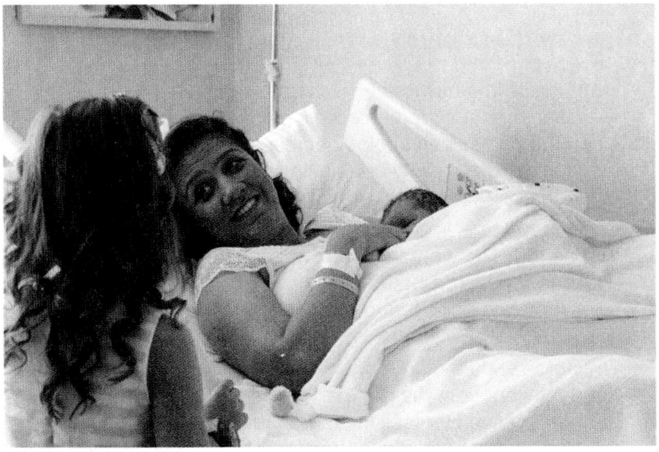

Figure 33–3 This young girl visits her mother in the hospital and becomes acquainted with her new sibling.

SOURCE: martin81/Shutterstock.

birth and have an opportunity to spend time with their new sibling and their parents immediately following the birth. They may even remain throughout the woman's hospitalization, especially if it is brief, and all go home as a family.

For the mother who is returning home to small children, it is often helpful to have the father/partner carry the new baby inside (Figure 33–4). This practice keeps the mother's arms free to immediately hug and hold her older children, reaffirming her love for them. Many mothers have found that bringing a doll home with them for an older child is helpful. The child cares for the doll alongside his or her parents, thereby identifying with the parent. This identification helps decrease anger and the need to regress to get attention.

Older children often enjoy working with the parents to care for the newborn. Involvement in care helps the older child develop a sense of closeness to the baby. It also helps the child learn acceptable behavior toward the newborn, feel a sense of accomplishment, and develop tenderness and caring. With constant supervision and assistance as necessary, even very young children can hold the baby or a bottle during feeding.

Regression is a common occurrence even when siblings have been well prepared. The nurse can provide anticipatory guidance so that parents are not surprised or upset if their previously

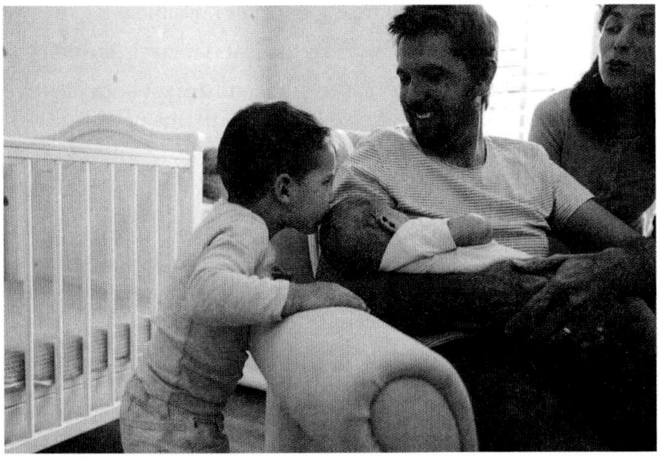

Figure 33–4 Father takes the lead in introducing big brother to his new sister.

SOURCE: Cathy Yeulet/123RF.

toilet-trained child begins to have accidents or if an older sibling requests a bottle or the breast.

Regardless of age, an older sibling needs reassurance that he or she is still special to the parents, a truly loved and valued family member. Words of love and praise coupled with hugs and kisses are very important. So, too, is special parent–child time. Both parents should spend quality one-on-one time with each of their older children. This may require some careful planning, but its worth cannot be overestimated. It confirms the parents' love for the child and often helps the child accept the new baby.

The child, especially one of the opposite gender from the newborn, may raise queries about the appearance of the genitals as compared to his or her own. A simple explanation, such as, "That's what little girls (boys) look like," is often sufficient.

Resumption of Sexual Activity

Nursing interventions in the postpartum period acknowledge that each parent is also a sexual being. It is not uncommon for couples to delay resumption of sexual activity due to a variety of factors including cesarean birth, operative vaginal delivery, episiotomy, lacerations, fatigue, breastfeeding, lack of desire on the part of one or both partners, fear of discomfort or pain, or presence of the newborn in the parents' bedroom.

A study of 188 postpartum women documented a wide range of variation in the time that elapsed before participants resumed various penetrative, nonpenetrative, solitary, and dyadic sexual practices after childbirth. Women's relationship satisfaction and their perceptions of partner desire were associated with the return to sexual activity (Cappell, MacDonald, & Pukall, 2016).

Couples were formerly discouraged from engaging in sexual intercourse until 6 weeks postpartum. Although the earliest time at which the couple can safely resume intercourse has not been demonstrated by research, the risks of hemorrhage and infection are minimal after 2 weeks postpartum (AAP & ACOG, 2017). Currently, couples are advised to abstain from intercourse until the perineum is healed and the lochial flow has stopped (usually by the third to sixth week postpartum). During this period, couples can be encouraged to express their sexuality through nonpenetrative activities. Since postpartum women often experience vaginal dryness due to hormonal changes, the use of a water-based lubricant, such as K-Y Jelly or Astroglide, may initially be necessary during intercourse. Vaginal dryness may continue throughout the period of lactation in breastfeeding mothers because of lower estrogen levels. The female-superior or side-by-side positions for coitus may be preferable because they enable the woman to control the depth of penile penetration.

Breastfeeding women should be forewarned that during orgasm, milk may spurt from the nipples because of the release of oxytocin. Some couples find this pleasurable or amusing; other couples choose to have the woman wear a bra during sexual activity. Breastfeeding the baby before lovemaking may reduce the chance of milk release.

Other factors may inhibit satisfactory sexual experience. The baby's crying may "spoil the mood," the woman's changed body may be unattractive to her or to her partner, and maternal sleep deprivation may interfere with a mutually satisfying experience. The woman may experience decreased libido or changes in her physiologic response to sexual stimulation, which may persist for several months due to hormonal alterations. Maternal fatigue is often a significant factor limiting the resumption of sexual intercourse. Consequently, couples should be encouraged to find a time for lovemaking when both are interested and

TEACHING HIGHLIGHTS | Resuming Sexual Activity After Childbirth

- Delay intercourse until no lochia is present because lochia indicates that healing is not yet complete.
- Tenderness of the vagina and perineum may cause discomfort. The partner may test the woman's level of comfort by slipping a lubricated finger inside her vagina. The female-superior and side-lying positions may be preferable because they let the woman control the depth of penetration of the penis.
- Vaginal dryness may occur because the vagina is "hormone poor." Discomfort as a result of dryness can be avoided by using a water-soluble lubricant.
- Based on the amount of breast engorgement and tenderness present, the partner may need to avoid breast stimulation during foreplay or use a very gentle approach.
- Escape of milk during sexual activity can be minimized by breastfeeding immediately beforehand.
- Fatigue and the new baby's schedule may have a negative impact on the woman's feelings of desire. Napping when the baby sleeps helps decrease fatigue. However, fatigue may be a reality couples need to accept during the early postpartum months.
- Contraception is important even during the early postpartum period. The woman's body needs adequate time to heal and recover from the stress of pregnancy and childbirth. Couples opposed to contraception may choose abstinence at this time.
- The nurse should discuss normal sexual changes that frequently occur in the postpartum period with both partners, which can facilitate an open dialogue between them and can provide an opportunity for questions and answers.

awake. Although interest and desire vary, most couples resume sexual activity within 3 months.

Anticipatory guidance during the prenatal and postnatal periods can alert couples to the temporary changes in sexuality that are experienced by many new parents. See *Teaching Highlights: Resuming Sexual Activity After Childbirth.*

Contraception

Because some couples resume sexual activity before the postpartum examination, family-planning information should be made available before discharge. In choosing a specific method, consistency of use outweighs the absolute reliability of a given method. The nurse must identify risk factors and contraindications of the various methods to help the couple select a contraceptive method that has practical application and is compatible with the couple's health and physical needs. The currently available contraceptive methods are discussed in detail in Chapter 4.

The nurse should discuss available contraceptive methods with both partners before discharge. Written information should also be provided for the couple to refer to at a later time. The nurse should stress the fact that pregnancy can occur before the first menstrual period returns and that contraception before that time is necessary to avoid pregnancy. According to the National Survey of Family Growth, 33.1% of pregnancies occurred within 18 months postpartum between 2006 and 2010. The target goal of *Healthy People 2020* is a 10% decrease to 29.8% by 2020 (U.S. Department of Health and Human Services [HHS], 2013).

Parent–Newborn Attachment

Nursing interventions to enhance the quality of parent–newborn attachment should be designed to promote feelings of well-being, comfort, and satisfaction. Table 33–3 describes parental attachment behaviors and those that require further assessment (see Chapter 32 for ways to assess maternal–newborn attachment). Following are some suggestions for ways of achieving parent–newborn attachment.

- Determine the childbearing and childrearing goals of the newborn's mother and father/partner and incorporate them when planning nursing care for the family, including cultural preferences for their initial interactions with the baby.
- Postpone eye prophylaxis for 1 hour (or as allowed by state law) after birth to facilitate eye contact between parents and their newborn (eye ointment further clouds the newborn's vision and makes eye contact difficult for the baby).
- Provide private time in the first hour after birth for the new family to become acquainted. Encourage skin-to-skin contact between mother (or father/partner) and baby to promote breastfeeding and bonding.
- Arrange the healthcare setting so that the individual nurse–patient relationship can be developed and maintained. A primary nurse can develop rapport and assess the mother's strengths and needs.
- Encourage the mother to tell her birth story. Clarify information for the mother as necessary.
- Encourage the parents to involve the siblings in integrating the baby into the family by bringing them to the birthing center for sibling visits.
- Use anticipatory guidance from conception through the postpartum period to prepare the parents for expected problems of adjustment.
- Include parents in any nursing intervention, planning, and/or evaluation. Give choices whenever possible.
- Initiate and support measures to alleviate fatigue in the parents.
- Help parents identify, understand, and accept both positive and negative feelings related to the birth, the newborn, and the overall parenting experience.
- Support and assist parents in determining the personality and unique needs of their newborn.

Whenever possible and culturally acceptable, the mother and father/partner should be allowed to care for their baby. This practice gives them a chance to learn their newborn's normal patterns and develop confidence in caring for him or her. It also allows them to spend more uninterrupted time with their baby in the first days of life. Early discharge may be advantageous if mother and baby are doing well, help is available for the mother at home, and the family and healthcare provider agree that both patients are healthy and ready for discharge.

The nurse may observe beginnings of parent–newborn attachment in the first few hours after birth and when continuing

TABLE 33–3 Parental Attachment Behaviors

ASSESSMENT AREA	ATTACHMENT	BEHAVIOR REQUIRING ASSESSMENT AND INFORMATION
Caretaking	Talks with baby. Demonstrates and seeks eye-to-eye contact. Touches and holds baby *en face*. Changes diapers when needed. Baby is clean. Clothing is appropriate for room temperature. Feeds baby as needed, and baby is gaining weight by the end of the first week of life. Positions baby comfortably and checks on baby.	Does not refer or speak to baby. Completes activities without addressing the baby or looking at the baby. Lack of interaction. Does not recognize need for or demonstrate concern for baby's comfort or needs. Feeding occurs intermittently. Baby does not gain weight. Waits for baby to cry and then hesitates to respond.
Perception of the baby	Has knowledge of expected child development. Understands that the baby is dependent and cannot meet parent's needs. Accepts gender of child and characteristics.	Has unrealistic expectations of the baby's abilities and behaviors. Expects love and interaction from the baby. Believes that the baby will fulfill parent's needs. Is distressed about gender of baby or feels that some aspect of the baby is unacceptable.
Support	Has friends who are available for support. Seems to be comfortable with being a parent. Has a realistic belief of parenting role.	Is alone or isolated. Is on edge, tense, anxious, and hesitant with the baby. Demonstrates difficulty incorporating parenting with own wants and needs.

Note: These are a few of the behaviors that may be associated with attachment. It is vitally important for the nurse to observe the parents on more than one occasion and to take into consideration individual characteristics, values, beliefs, and customs.

assessments during home visits after discharge. As the nurse assesses attachment, it is important to remember that cultural values, beliefs, and practices will direct child-care activities and self-care practices. For example, preparing for the baby prior to delivery is viewed as a sign of acceptance and attachment in many cultures. Nurses should respect cultural norms and incorporate them into the care of the newborn whenever possible. Chapter 32 discusses this and other cultural practices in the postpartum period.

Some parents, especially first-time parents, may feel awkward in their new role. It is helpful for the nurse to advise parents that they may experience feelings of uncertainty as they grow into the parental role and alter their family processes to accommodate the new family member. The nurse should also provide reassurance and advise new parents of normal newborn behavior and activity. The nurse assesses attachment before discharge. If the nurse identifies a possible alteration in attachment, the parents can be referred to a new parent support group, parenting classes, or counseling to assist them with their transition into their new roles. The nurse can explain that new attachments are being formed and, like all new relationships, both the baby and the parents are discovering each other. The nurse should inform families to seek help if the new mother experiences an inability or a lack of desire to care for the baby.

Nursing Care Following Cesarean Birth

Approximately 32% of women delivered their newborns by cesarean section in the United States in 2014 (Hamilton, Martin, Osterman, et al., 2015). Nurses need to be adept at addressing the special needs of this population of patients. After a cesarean birth, the new mother has postpartum needs similar to those of women who gave birth vaginally. Because she has undergone major abdominal surgery, however, the woman also has nursing care needs similar to those of other surgical patients.

Promotion of Maternal Physical Well-Being After Cesarean Birth

Care of the patient following cesarean delivery is similar to the care of patients who deliver vaginally, but also includes consideration of the postoperative condition. Nursing interventions will focus on promotion of maternal comfort, promotion of maternal and newborn safety, and prevention of postoperative complications. The nurse will monitor neurologic and neuromuscular status closely until effects of anesthesia have worn off. Routine postpartum assessments will include inspection of the dressing or incision for intactness and signs of complications or infection, as well as increased attention to lung sounds, gastrointestinal status, and genitourinary status.

Immobility after the use of narcotic and sedative agents and alterations in the immune response of postoperative patients increase the chances of pulmonary infection. For this reason, the woman is encouraged to cough and breathe deeply and to use incentive spirometry every 2 to 4 hours while awake for the first few days following cesarean birth.

Immobility increases the risk of abdominal distention and discomfort, deep vein thrombosis, and pulmonary embolism. The patient may wear sequential compression devices (SCDs) until she is ambulating. Within the first 12 hours postoperatively, unless medically contraindicated, the woman should be assisted to dangle her legs on the side of the bed. Once she is awake, alert, and has complete sensation and strength in her lower extremities, the woman should be assisted out of bed. Ambulation should begin no later than 24 hours postoperatively and should be encouraged at least 2 to 3 times a day.

The nurse continues to assess the woman's pain level and provide relief measures as needed. Sources of pain include incisional pain, gas pain, referred shoulder pain, periodic uterine contractions (afterpains), and pain associated with voiding, defecation, or constipation.

Nursing interventions are oriented toward preventing or alleviating pain or helping the woman cope with pain. The nurse should undertake the following measures:

- Administer analgesic medications as needed and ordered, especially during the first 24 to 72 hours. Their use will relieve the woman's pain and enable her to be more mobile and active.
- Promote comfort through proper positioning, backrubs, oral care, and the reduction of noxious stimuli, such as noise and unpleasant odors.
- Encourage the presence of the father/partner and the newborn. This may provide distraction from the painful sensations and help reduce the woman's fear and anxiety. A loved one can provide a watchful presence over the newborn, allowing the baby to stay in the room with the mother while she may not be alert or comfortable enough to be responsible for the newborn if left alone.
- Encourage the use of breathing, relaxation, and distraction techniques (for example, stimulation of cutaneous tissue) taught in childbirth preparation class.
- Instruct the woman to splint her incision with a pillow when changing positions, coughing, deep-breathing, or sneezing.
- Encourage adequate rest periods. This may include limiting excessive visitors and phone calls.
- Encourage early ambulation to prevent abdominal distention that can occur with excess accumulation of gas in the intestines.
- Allow the woman to begin judiciously consuming food and fluids as desired when awake and alert. Although some institutions still withhold oral intake until bowel sounds return, there is no research evidence to support this practice.

Neuraxial analgesia administered just after the cesarean birth is an effective method of pain relief for most women in the first 24 hours following birth (see *Drug Guide: Postpartum Neuraxial Morphine*).

The physician may prescribe **patient-controlled analgesia (PCA)**. With this approach, the woman is given a bolus of analgesia, often morphine, at the beginning of therapy. Using a special intravenous (IV) pump system, the woman presses a button to self-administer small doses of the medication as needed. For safety, the pump is preset with a time lockout so that the pump cannot deliver another dose until a specified time has elapsed. Women using PCA feel less anxious and have a greater sense of control with less dependence on the nursing staff. The frequent, smaller doses help the woman experience rapid pain relief without grogginess and also eliminate the discomfort of injections. As with any drug therapy, the nurse should monitor the patient for side effects and intervene as necessary.

Oral analgesics are often used to manage postoperative pain related to cesarean section as well. Some women tolerate oral pain relievers, while others experience nausea and vomiting and drowsiness. More research is needed to determine the safest and most effective oral pain management regimens (Mkontwana & Novikova, 2015)

If general anesthesia was used, abdominal distention from the accumulation of gas in the intestines may produce discomfort for the woman during the first postpartum days. Additional measures to prevent or minimize gas pains include leg exercises, abdominal tightening, avoiding carbonated or very hot or cold beverages, and avoiding the use of straws. The woman may find it helpful to lie prone or on her left side. Lying on the left side allows gas to rise from the descending colon to the sigmoid colon so that it can be expelled more readily. Other women report that a rocking chair helps them obtain relief. Medical interventions for gas pain include the use of antiflatulents (such as Mylicon), suppositories, and enemas. A number of studies found that chewing gum may promote the return of normal bowel function in patients after cesarean section (Pereira Gomes Morais et al., 2016).

The nurse can minimize discomfort and promote satisfaction as the mother assumes the activities of her new role. Instruction and assistance in assuming comfortable positions when holding or breastfeeding the baby will do much to increase the mother's sense of competence and comfort. Sitting in a chair or sitting with legs bent and crossed in bed, leaning slightly forward with the baby propped on a pillow in her lap, will prevent irritation to the incision. Use of the football hold and side-lying positions may be most comfortable for breastfeeding during the initial postoperative course. See Chapter 29 for breastfeeding positions.

By the first or second day after the cesarean birth, the mother is usually receptive to learning how to care for herself and her newborn. Demonstration of proper body mechanics in getting out of bed without the use of a side rail and ways of caring for the baby that prevent strain and torsion on the incision are also indicated. The nurse needs to place special emphasis on home management, encouraging the woman to let others assume responsibility for housekeeping and cooking. Fatigue not only prolongs recovery but also interferes with breastfeeding and mother–baby interaction.

SAFETY ALERT!

Mothers who have experienced cesareans, particularly unanticipated ones that follow lengthy labors, may be fatigued, sleep deprived, and under the influence of medications that alter their level of consciousness. Nurses should monitor the mother's level of consciousness and ability to stay awake when holding her baby, providing care, and breastfeeding. Some mothers will require constant support and observation to complete these activities safely. Nursing units should have risk management guidelines in place to assist nurses in their assessment and support of these vulnerable patients.

The woman usually does extremely well postoperatively. If neuraxial anesthesia was used, the side effects of general anesthesia are absent. Even after general anesthesia, however, most women are ambulating by the day after the surgery. Usually the woman can shower by the first or second postpartum day, which seems to provide a mental as well as physical lift. The incision can be covered with plastic if the dressing is still in place. If staples have been used, the incision is sometimes left open to the air, and showering is permitted without covering it. Most women are discharged on the second or third postoperative day.

Teaching for Self-Care. The nurse can assist the woman in identifying interventions to relieve discomfort or pain. The woman should be encouraged to take pain medication regularly, engage in frequent rest periods, avoid prolonged activity, and observe for signs of "overdoing it" (such as discomfort and fatigue). The nurse should advise the woman that recovery after a surgical procedure involves healing time and that fatigue and soreness are common symptoms of too much activity too quickly. The nurse can assist the family in identifying resources for assisting the new mother at home, such as assistance from friends and family, cleaning services, or food delivery services.

Drug Guide

Postpartum Neuraxial Morphine

OVERVIEW OF OBSTETRIC ACTION

Neuraxial administration (epidural or intrathecal) of morphine is used to provide relief of pain associated with cesarean births, extensive episiotomies, or third- and fourth-degree lacerations. Neuraxial administration is associated with better pain control, earlier ambulation, and earlier bowel function in postoperative cesarean patients when compared to intravenous administration (Gabbe et al., 2017). There is minimal motor, sensory, or sympathetic blockade. Morphine binds to opiate receptors in the central nervous system, thereby altering both the perception of and emotional response to pain. Women experience little or no discomfort or pain during recovery and for up to 24 hours following epidural or intrathecal administration of morphine. This may be extended to 48 hours with the use of extended-release epidural morphine (EREM), such as Depodur.

ROUTE, DOSAGE, AND FREQUENCY

Morphine (preservative-free formulation) is administered intrathecally or epidurally by the anesthesia provider. If a subsequent postoperative dose is required, the anesthesia provider, not the nurse, administers it. Patient-controlled epidural administration (PCEA) may be used as well.

MATERNAL CONTRAINDICATIONS

Allergy/hypersensitivity to morphine.

MATERNAL SIDE EFFECTS

Most common: Confusion, sedation, constipation, hypotension, pruritus, urinary retention, and nausea and vomiting.

Early-onset respiratory depression (< 2 hours after administration) and late-onset respiratory depression (> 2 hours after administration) are rare in young, healthy obstetric patients but can result in irreversible neurologic injury or death. Women who are morbidly obese, who are concurrently receiving magnesium sulfate, or who have obstructive sleep apnea or coexisting disease such as diabetes, are at increased risk for respiratory depression. Respiratory depression is managed by administration of naloxone (Narcan), mask ventilation, and endotracheal intubation with mechanical ventilation, if necessary.

NURSING CONSIDERATIONS

- Obtain history: Sensitivity (allergy) to morphine.
- Assess vital signs, orientation, level of consciousness, motor function, sensation, reflexes, skin color, breath sounds, depth and rate of respirations, epidural catheter insertion site, and ability to void (unless indwelling urinary catheter in place). Notify anesthesia provider of abnormal assessments or complications.
- Monitor and evaluate analgesic effect. Ask patient about comfort level and notify anesthesia provider of inadequate pain relief.
- Check epidural catheter (if still present) to ensure it is intact and not leaking.
- Assess for pruritus (scratching and rubbing, especially around face and neck).
- Administer comfort measures for narcotic-induced pruritus, such as lotion, backrubs, cool or warm packs, or diversional activities. Administer prescribed medications PRN.
- If adverse reaction (urticaria, edema, or respiratory difficulties) occurs, administer PRN medications per provider standing order. Have drugs immediately available.
- Provide comfort measures for nausea or vomiting, such as frequent oral hygiene or gradual increase of activity; administer prescribed PRN medications as needed.
- Assess level of consciousness, lower extremity sensation and strength, postural blood pressure, and heart rate before ambulation.
- Assist patient with her first ambulation and then PRN.
- Provide assistance and supervision with newborn care.
- According to guidelines approved by the American Society of Anesthesiologists Task Force and the American Society of Regional Anesthesia and Pain Medicine in 2016, respiratory status should be assessed at least hourly for the first 12 hours and at least every other hour for the second 12 hours (12 to 24 hours) following a single administration of neuraxial morphine. Respiratory status should continue to be assessed every 4 hours for the next 24 hours—until 48 hours following administration of EREM. Patients receiving continuous morphine or PCEA should be assessed throughout the duration of administration. Monitoring after discontinuation of PCEA should be continued as appropriate, depending on the patient's condition and any concurrent medications. Supplemental oxygen, reversal agents such as naloxone, and equipment needed to provide noninvasive positive pressure ventilation should be readily available. Intravenous access should be maintained throughout the monitoring periods described above.

SAFETY ALERT!

Nursing care must include assessment of oxygenation (pulse oximetry), ventilation (rate and depth of respirations), and level of consciousness. Pulse oximetry and apnea monitors are sometimes employed as adjuncts, but they cannot take the place of a thorough nursing assessment. Pulse oximetry is not sensitive to hypercarbia, and neither tool is sensitive to hypoventilation. Naloxone and supplemental oxygen should be readily available. Use of naloxone for reversal of respiratory depression may negate the analgesic effects of morphine. Rebound respiratory depression may occur after naloxone.

- Assess bladder for distention if unable to void. Assist patient to void. Catheterization may be necessary if unresolved.
- Inform patient that headaches related to epidurals are uncommon but occasionally occur 2 to 5 days after administration. Bedrest in a quiet dark room, caffeine, and hydration may help. Call anesthesia provider as needed. Blood patch can be administered by anesthesia if unresolved.

Sources: American Society of Anesthesiologists Task Force and the American Society of Regional Anesthesia and Pain Medicine, 2016; Tawfic & Faris, 2015; Vallerand et al., 2017.

Promotion of Parent–Newborn Interaction After Cesarean Birth

Many factors associated with cesarean birth may hinder successful and frequent maternal–newborn interaction. These include the physical condition of the mother and newborn and maternal reactions to stress, anesthesia, and medications. The mother and her baby may be separated after birth because of hospital routines, prematurity, or neonatal complications. A healthy baby born by an uncomplicated cesarean birth is no more fragile than a baby born vaginally. Many agencies are beginning to provide time for the family together in the operating room if the mother's and baby's conditions permit. As noted earlier in the chapter, if skin-to-skin contact (SSC) with the mother is not possible immediately following cesarean delivery of a healthy newborn, the nurses should offer SSC with the father/partner.

Signs of depression, anger, or withdrawal in the mother following cesarean birth may indicate a grief response to the loss of the fantasized vaginal birth experience. Fathers/partners as well as mothers may experience feelings of "missing out," or guilt that the surgery was the result of something they did "wrong." The couple may also feel guilty that they are considering their personal needs and not simply the welfare of the baby.

The nurse can support the parents in a variety of ways. Initially, nurses must work through their own feelings about cesarean birth. The nurse who considers a vaginal birth "normal" and refers to it as such implies that a cesarean birth is "abnormal," rather than simply an alternative method. Thus, language and terminology can convey significant messages to the couple about their cesarean birth experience.

The nurse should offer positive support to the couple. They may need the opportunity to tell their story repeatedly to work through their feelings. The nurse can provide factual information about their situation and support the couple's effective coping behaviors. The nurse should provide the parents with choices by allowing them to participate in decision making about the options available to them.

The presence of the father/partner during the birth process may positively influence the woman's perception of the birth event. He or she can take pictures, hold the baby, and foster the discovery process by directing the mother's attention to details about her newborn. The father/partner can help the mother to relive the experience and fill in any gaps or missing pieces later. This is especially valuable if the mother has had general anesthesia.

The perception of and reactions to a cesarean birth experience depend on how the woman defines that experience. If the woman's attitude is more positive than negative, successful resolution of subsequent stressful events is more likely. Often the mothering role is perceived as an extension of the childbearing role, and inability to fulfill expected childbearing behavior (vaginal birth) might lead to parental feelings of failure and frustration. The nurse can help families alter their negative definitions of cesarean birth and encourage positive perceptions.

According to the National Vital Statistics System, 90.8% of low-risk women with a prior cesarean delivered by cesarean again. The target goal of *Healthy People 2020* is a 10% reduction to 81.7% by 2020 (HHS, 2013). Nurses can encourage patients to discuss the possibility of a vaginal birth after cesarean (VBAC) (see Chapter 25) with their providers if they become pregnant again.

Teaching for Self-Care. The nurse should advise the mother that she is able to hold, cuddle, lift, and feed her baby despite her surgical incision. The nurse can assist the woman in finding positions that are comfortable for holding and feeding the baby

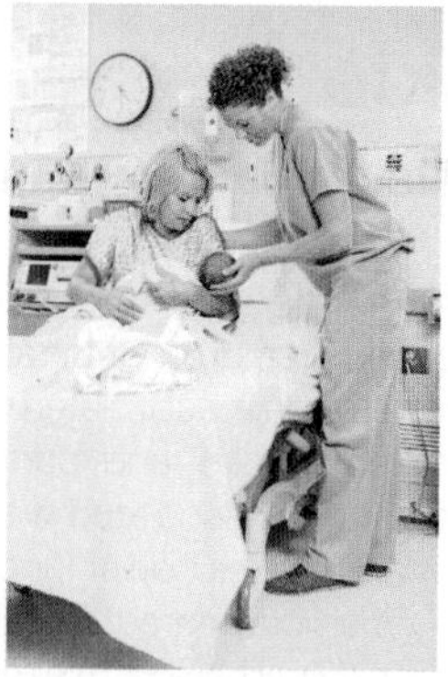

Figure 33–5 The nurse assists the postcesarean mother find comfortable ways to hold and care for her newborn.

SOURCE: Tyler Olson/123RF.

(Figure 33–5). Upon discharge, the woman should be encouraged to care for the baby and to allow family members or friends to assist with other household duties.

Nursing Care of the Obese Postpartum Mother

Obesity is increasing in the United States, and the postpartum nurse will care for a growing number of obese and morbidly obese patients. The obese mother has needs similar to all postpartum patients, but she needs special attention to prevent injury, respiratory complications, thromboembolic disease, and infection, for which she is at high risk.

Obesity may double the woman's risk for postpartum hemorrhage, regardless of the method of delivery, and it increases the risk of postpartum mortality (Creanga et al., 2015). Therefore, the obese patient requires vigilant assessment of her fundus and lochia. The nurse should also carefully assess the woman for airway obstruction and hypoxia, particularly if she received opioids. Ambulation should be encouraged as soon as possible to prevent pneumonia. The use of sequential compression devices (SCDs) and early ambulation are essential to the prevention of deep vein thrombosis, especially if the patient had a cesarean birth. If mechanical vacuum devices are used to facilitate drainage from her incision following a cesarean birth, the patient should be educated about them. The mother should demonstrate how to see, clean, and completely dry her incision prior to discharge. The use of a mirror may be helpful. She needs to recognize and report signs of infection or dehiscence of her surgical incision or episiotomy repair promptly.

SAFETY ALERT!

The obese patient has special safety concerns. The nurse needs to utilize adequate personnel and appropriate assistive devices to maintain safety for both the patient and staff members during position changes, transport, and ambulation. Additionally, the new mother may need extra supervision and assistance when breastfeeding her baby to ensure newborn safety.

In addition to the health and safety risks, obese women sometimes experience prejudice, psychologic distress, and humiliation when in the healthcare setting (Heslehurst et al., 2015; Wahedi, 2016). The nurse needs to be sensitive to special needs in order to promote the woman's dignity. Advance communication and coordination that ensures the woman will have the correct-sized bed, blood pressure cuff, transport equipment, gown, and assistive equipment for ambulation is essential to efficient, compassionate, and respectful patient-centered nursing care.

Teaching for Self- and Family-Care. The nurse should advise the mother to ambulate as early as possible to avoid medical complications. The mother is taught symptoms of infection and should report these symptoms immediately to her healthcare provider.

Children of obese mothers are at risk for obesity, impaired glucose tolerance, and cardiometabolic complications. Nurses should educate the obese mother on the importance of breastfeeding, as it decreases the child's risk of obesity. The patient should receive information about healthy food choices for families and/or a referral to a professional or an agency that promotes healthy nutrition for families prior to discharge (Purnell & MacKenzie, 2016).

Nursing Care of the Adolescent Postpartum Mother

The postpartum nurse will provide care for adolescent mothers, some of whom are very young. Chapter 15 discusses adolescent pregnancy in depth. The transition to motherhood can be stressful for adult women. Teen mothers have fewer life experiences and fewer social, educational, and financial resources to help with the transition than do older mothers. They experience higher rates of postpartum depression accompanied by inadequate evaluation and treatment (Logsdon et al., 2015). Their newborns are also more likely to suffer from low birth weight, preterm birth, and death in infancy than those born to adult women (Jeha, Usta, Ghulmiyyah, et al., 2015). Additional teaching, support, referrals, and follow-up may be required, particularly if the young woman has delivered a baby with special concerns due to prematurity, low birth weight, or other complications.

Adolescent mothers have the same basic physical care needs as older mothers. They usually recover without difficulty, as they are young and generally healthy. Some adolescents, however, may not have a working knowledge of their own anatomy and physiology or the related terminology, and they may require special assistance with postpartum hygiene and care. Some may never have had a gynecologic exam prior to pregnancy, and they may feel embarrassed or intimidated by the experience of being examined by a variety of healthcare professionals. The nurse should be sensitive to the patient's needs and ensure that she understands the reason for assessments, demonstrates appropriate self- and newborn care, and feels comfortable to ask questions. The nurse should offer detailed teaching on contraception, as the young woman may have no prior experience with it and may not feel comfortable requesting this information.

The nurse has many opportunities for teaching adolescent parents about their newborn in the postpartum unit and serves as a role model for new parents when responding to and caring for the newborn. The father, if he is involved, should be included as much as possible. Although the grandmother or another family member may plan to assist with or provide much of the newborn care in some cases, the nurse should always ensure that the adolescent mother has the knowledge and demonstrates the skills to provide care for her newborn before discharge. The young mother will usually appreciate positive feedback about her newborn and her developing maternal responses. This praise and encouragement will increase her confidence and self-esteem.

A newborn physical examination performed at the bedside gives the parent(s) immediate feedback about the newborn's health and demonstrates methods of handling a baby. The nurse can teach as the examination progresses, giving the new mother information about the fontanelles, cradle cap, shampooing the newborn's hair, and so on. The nurse might also use this time to teach the young parent(s) about providing auditory and visual stimulation for their newborn. Performing an examination at the bedside gives the adolescent permission to explore her baby, which she may have been hesitant to do. A Brazelton neonatal assessment (see Chapter 27) will help the mother understand the newborn's response to stimuli, a key factor in the adolescent's response to the individuality of her newborn once she goes home. Parents who have some idea of what to expect from their newborn will be less frustrated with the baby's behavior. See *Professionalism in Practice: Pregnancy in Adolescents of Diverse Sexual Orientations*.

Group classes for adolescent mothers should include newborn/infant care skills and information about growth and development, newborn/infant feeding, well-baby care, and danger signals in the ill baby. If classes are offered in the hospital during the postpartum stay, the adolescent mother and father should be strongly encouraged to attend and participate. The nurse can correct misconceptions and unrealistic expectations about growth and development.

During the postpartum period, adolescents may have special needs, depending on their level of maturity, support systems, and cultural backgrounds. Nurses should be aware of local programs offered through schools and healthcare organizations and assist teen parents to access these services prior to discharge whenever possible. Adolescent parenting clinics, school-based programs, support groups, case management services, and home visit programs are options for the teen parent. There is a need for ongoing evaluation of programs and strategies to develop an evidence base that optimizes care for this population. See *Case Study: Angelina Newman*.

Professionalism in Practice Pregnancy in Adolescents of Diverse Sexual Orientations

Recent research shows that adolescents who identify as lesbian or bisexual are at an increased risk for teen pregnancy. These adolescents are more likely to initiate sexual activity at a younger age and because of their identification as lesbian or bisexual, are more unlikely to use contraception (Lindley & Walsemann, 2015). It is important for nurses not to assume an adolescent mother's sexual orientation. The nurse can ask the young mother if there will be another parent involved. Avoiding terminology like *boyfriend* or *father of the baby* conveys openness to young mothers who may be reluctant to disclose their sexual orientation. Maternal child nurses should maintain a respectful, nonjudgmental attitude and listen to the young woman to learn of her individual needs. Nurse leaders can coordinate educational programs and opportunities for staff members to engage with community experts, develop protocols for the care of adolescent mothers, and communicate an expectation of high-quality care in order to optimize outcomes for teen mothers and their newborns (Charlton et al., 2016).

Nursing Care of LGBTQ Postpartum Mothers

The body of literature regarding the nursing care of lesbian, gay, bisexual, transgender, and queer (LGBTQ) individuals and families is growing. In one study, lesbian mothers described encountering healthcare professionals who made heterosexual assumptions about childbearing, asked inappropriate questions, and excluded the nonbirth mother (Hayman, Wilkes, Halcomb, et al., 2013). Nonbiological lesbian co-mothers reported feeling different and described a sense of isolation and being left out in healthcare settings designed to include fathers (Hayman et al., 2013; Wojnar & Katzenmeyer, 2014). In one study, midwives expressed a desire to fully engage in caring relationships with the women, yet they expressed ambivalence about the best way to achieve this. Most took cues from the couple and followed their professional instincts when developing a relationship with the couple. The midwives highlighted respectful acknowledgment and culturally sensitive communication as priorities for care (Goldburg, 2017). The researchers noted that additional studies are needed, particularly on the role and needs of co-mothers, to guide nurses who care for lesbian childbearing couples.

The nurse should maintain an attitude that is respectful, caring, and open to sexual diversity when working with all patients. Providing quality patient-centered care for any postpartum woman involves acknowledging, welcoming, and involving her intimate partner in care and decision making. The nurse should ask the patient for guidance regarding any special needs or requests that she or her partner may have. At the unit and facility level, policies and forms should be designed to facilitate inclusive care (Hayman et al., 2013; Pharris, Bucchio, Dotson, et al., 2016; Wojnar & Katzenmeyer, 2014). Standardized postpartum instructions, particularly those related to intercourse and contraception, need to be individualized and amended.

Nursing Care of the Postpartum Mother with Special Needs

The postpartum time period is one of great growth in the maternal mothering role. New mothers are faced with various challenges and different learning opportunities. Women with physical, developmental, or intellectual disabilities, as well as those suffering from chronic health conditions, are at particular risk during this time period. A needs assessment should be performed to determine the special needs of the mother and family, and care should be coordinated accordingly. Community and private resources should be available to make the transition to the postpartum period as flawless as possible.

Nursing Care of the Postpartum Mother with a History of Sexual Abuse

Women who have been previously sexually abused may experience more anxiety and stress related to hospital procedures, interactions with unfamiliar staff, and being touched. The postpartum woman who has a history of sexual abuse may have difficulty establishing trust and may feel uncomfortable when asked to share private information or when subjected to physical examinations. The nurse should ensure privacy and safety and work to build trust with the patient.

Twelve percent of women in a study of more than 1000 postpartum women reported a history of physical or sexual abuse before becoming pregnant; 17% of participants screened positive for postpartum depression (PPD). A number of recent studies have found an association between prior abuse, posttraumatic stress disorder (PTSD), and PPD, and more research is needed (LaCoursiere, Hirst, & Barrett-Connor, 2012; Seng et al., 2013; Wosu, Gelaye, & Williams, 2015).

Postpartum patients with a history of abuse should be thoroughly screened for PPD prior to discharge and at follow-up visits. Support groups may offer the mother with a history of sexual abuse a safe haven in which to share her experiences and to consider the impact of the abuse on her mothering. Nurses should privately question all postpartum patients as to whether they feel safe returning to their home environment prior to discharge.

Nursing Care of the Woman Who Relinquishes her Newborn

A **relinquishing mother** is one who chooses to place her newborn for adoption or one who has conceived via traditional or gestational means and is acting as a surrogate mother with the intention of placement of the newborn with another family. Traditional surrogacy typically uses the biological mother's egg and sperm donation, often from the intended adoptive father or sometimes from a sperm donor. In LGBTQ families, the sperm donor may be someone who is known or an anonymous donor

CASE STUDY: Angelina Newman

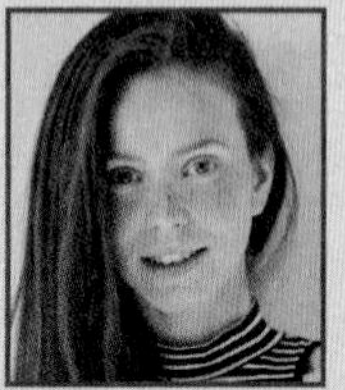

SOURCE: WAYHOME studio/Shutterstock.

Angelina expresses feeling overwhelmed with caring for the baby, her lack of sleep, and her inexperience with babies. The nurse refers her for a social work consult due to her young age. Angelina reveals that her parents are supportive and hopes her boyfriend will be involved after she returns home. Angelina tells you that none of her friends have experience with babies and that they seem to be more distant the last few months. Her best friend complains that all she ever talks about is the baby. Her boyfriend seems indifferent to her and the baby. She feels they are drifting apart.

Questions to Ponder

What referral sources are appropriate to help Angelina build social support networks? What social service referrals are appropriate for this young mother?

via a sperm bank. In gestational surrogacy, the egg comes from the intended mother and in vitro fertilization (IVF) is performed to achieve pregnancy; the woman carrying the pregnancy is not related biologically to the child she is carrying.

Traditional adoption, in which the birth mother terminates her parental rights and gives consent for another person or persons to adopt her child, is becoming increasingly rare in modern society. The adoption rate in the United States decreased 24% from 2001 to 2012, according to available statistics (Child Welfare Information Gateway, 2016). It is difficult, however, to determine how many mothers actually pursue this option each year, as information regarding the characteristics of children adopted independently or through private agencies is not always readily available, and there is no single tracking agency or source for this data.

In 2014, 40.2% of births were to unmarried women (Hamilton et al., 2015). Historically, adoption was the only option for young, unmarried women with an unplanned pregnancy; however, single parenthood is no longer as stigmatized as it once was. There are still a small number of mothers who pursue adoption for a variety of reasons, including an inability to care for the child financially, multiple children in the family already, or life circumstances; and there are women who simply do not wish to be mothers. Complex psychosocial issues such as rape, incest, conception outside the woman's current intimate relationship, intimate partner violence, cultural norms, family disapproval, or threat of abandonment by her intimate partner or family if the mother keeps the child are sometimes factors. Some women may not want to share this personal information, while others may view the nurse as the only safe person she can talk with about her feelings and decision. The nurse can support the mother by encouraging her to share her feelings, by listening actively, and by being present for her.

Adoption may be facilitated by private independent agreements, private agencies, and public agencies. Adoptions may be termed open, semi-open, or closed, according to the information shared between parties and future contact desired. In some cases, the birth parents select the adoptive parents. If the adoptive parents are involved during the postpartum period, it is important to remember that the birth mother is the legal guardian and her preferences should be supported until paperwork is completed and she is discharged home.

Adoptive parents may be openly involved in the labor and birth process, whereas others may be present but not reveal the relationship between the birth mother and themselves. Surrogacy laws differ from state to state within the United States. Some states prohibit surrogacy under any conditions, while others prohibit the exchange of money to surrogate mothers. Many states do not have specific laws to address surrogacy, some states have regulations, and others have specific laws related to surrogacy.

Clinical Tip

It is important to know the state laws governing surrogacy in the state in which you work to ensure that all actions are in adherence with HIPAA and that discharge of the newborn is in compliance with state statues.

For a woman relinquishing her baby, both sets of parents may be present for the delivery and throughout the immediate postpartum period. The nurse may work with all members of the group, including the birth parents, the adoptive parents, surrogate parents, and the newborn. Nursing interventions may include psychosocial support, therapeutic communication, advocacy, patient education, coordinating referrals, and physical care. Psychosocial support may facilitate grieving on the part of a birth mother.

Critical thinking and flexibility are required in order to respond to the complex needs of all parents involved. The nurse may collaborate with social workers, adoption agency personnel, surrogacy agencies, or attorneys. Providing care may be stressful for the nurse if controversies occur between the parties or if unfamiliar situations arise.

Many states have laws in place to guide the process of surrogacy and voluntary relinquishment and to promote informed decision making by birth mothers. Laws vary and some states may have specific requirements for counseling, waiting periods, chain of custody, or revocation of the decision to relinquish. Birthing units should have policies and resources available to guide the care of relinquishing mothers according to state laws, and nurses should consult with facility resource experts if they are uncertain how to proceed in a given situation.

The postpartum nurse's primary responsibility is to provide compassionate patient-centered care that supports the birth mother's relinquishment plan and promotes a positive experience for her. The nurse should make certain that the plan is clear and communicated to other staff members. If no support person is present, the nurse acts as the primary support person. Following birth, the amount of contact the birth mother chooses to have with her newborn should be respected. When the birth father and/or prospective or intended adoptive parents are present, the nurse should take cues from the birth mother as to how to best provide support for all. Nurses should have a familiarity with the rights of birth fathers within their state and provide support to the father whenever possible as well (Karst & Lindsey, 2012; Shaw, 2016).

Respectful communication that involves choosing words thoughtfully and accurately is important when caring for women who are relinquishing their newborns. Professional organizations recommend use of the phrases "choosing an adoption plan" or "finding a family to parent your child" rather than terms such as "giving away," "giving up your child," or "putting your child up for adoption."

Finally, the nurse needs to acknowledge the significance of the birth mother's experience. Birth mothers and fathers may experience complex and conflicted emotions—including grief, loss, and guilt—despite believing that they made the right decision (Child Welfare Information Gateway, 2013; Clutter, 2014). Surrogate mothers who become pregnant knowing they will be giving up the child at birth may also have mixed emotions and experience a sense of ambivalence or loss. The nurse can support the relinquishing mother by acknowledging her relationship with the newborn, validating her loss, supporting her decision, offering her the opportunity to spend time with the baby to create memories, and giving her time to say goodbye. Nurses should inform relinquishing mothers of resources prior to discharge. The Child Welfare Information Gateway and the National Council for Adoption offer resources for birth parents, adoptive families, and adopted children. Many surrogacy agencies offer ongoing support and counseling for surrogate mothers. The mother may benefit from a referral to an organization, a support group, a therapist who specializes in the care of relinquishing mothers, or a clergy member (Child Welfare Information Gateway, 2013). For additional information regarding nursing care of parents experiencing grief and loss, see Chapter 36.

Discharge Information

Healthy postpartum women and newborns are frequently discharged within 24 to 48 hours of delivery, before many of their important healthcare and educational needs have been addressed. These include establishing breastfeeding, ruling out infections, supporting newborn–family bonding, and patient teaching. Home health services are increasingly being recognized as a cost-effective means of meeting the postbirth needs of mothers and newborns. Home care of the postpartum family is the subject of Chapter 34.

Ideally, preparation for discharge begins the moment a woman initially enters the healthcare system for prenatal care. Nursing efforts should be directed toward assessing the couple's knowledge, expectations, and beliefs and then providing anticipatory guidance and teaching accordingly (refer to Table 33–1). Because teaching is one of the primary responsibilities of the postpartum nurse, many agencies have elaborate teaching programs and classes. Before the actual discharge, however, the nurse should spend private time with the woman (or couple) to determine whether they have any last-minute questions (Figure 33–6). See *Key Facts to Remember: Discharge Teaching*.

The nurse can reassure the couple of their ability to be successful parents, stressing the baby's need to feel loved and secure. The nurse can also urge parents to talk to each other and work together to solve any problems that may arise.

Postpartum nurses should ensure that the patient has access to follow-up care, coordinate the postpartum appointment when possible, and inform the patient and her family of the importance

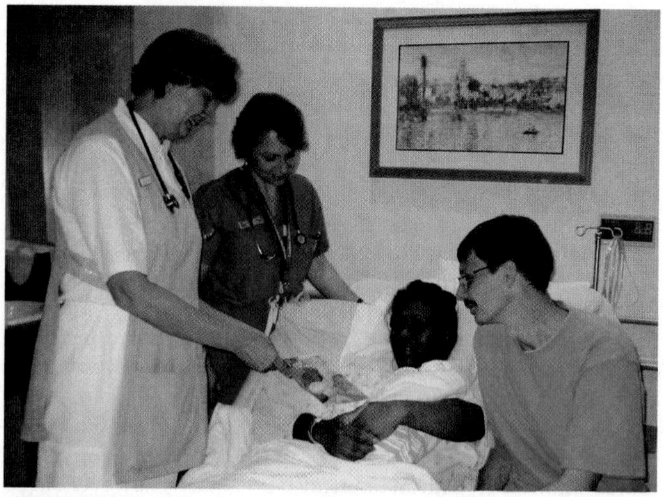

Figure 33–6 **The nurse provides discharge instructions to the mother and father before discharge.**

SOURCE: Michele Davidson.

Key Facts To Remember
Discharge Teaching

1. The woman should contact her caregiver if she develops any of the signs of possible complications:
   - Sudden, persistent, or spiking fever (greater than 100.4°F) or chills
   - Change in the character of the lochia—foul smell, return to bright red bleeding, excessive amount (more than one pad per hour after 24 hours)
   - Evidence of mastitis, such as breast tenderness, reddened areas, malaise, fever, chills
   - Evidence of thrombophlebitis, such as calf pain, tenderness, redness, or pain with walking
   - Evidence of urinary tract infection, such as urgency, frequency, burning on urination
   - Evidence of infection in an incision (either episiotomy or cesarean), such as redness, edema, pain or discomfort, discharge, or lack of approximation
   - Continued mood changes or signs of postpartum depression, inability to care for self or baby, feelings of self-harm, thoughts of harming the newborn, or anxiety
   - Severe pelvic pain or abdominal tenderness
   - Chest pain or shortness of breath
   - Signs of preeclampsia such as headache or swelling of the face or extremities.
2. The woman should review the literature she has received that explains recommended postpartum exercises, the need for adequate rest, the need to avoid overexertion, and the recommendation to abstain from sexual intercourse until lochia has ceased. The woman may take a shower and may continue sitz baths at home if she desires.
3. The woman should be given the phone numbers of the postpartum unit, lactation consultant, and nursery and should be encouraged to call if she has any questions.
4. The woman should receive information on local agencies or support groups that might be of particular assistance to her.
5. Both breastfeeding and formula-feeding mothers should receive information geared to their specific nutritional needs. They should also be told to continue their vitamin and iron supplements until their postpartum examination.
6. The woman should have a scheduled appointment for her postpartum examination and for her baby's first well-baby examination before they are discharged.
7. The mother should clearly understand the correct procedure for obtaining copies of her baby's birth certificate.
8. The new parents should be able to provide home care for their baby and should know when to anticipate that the cord will fall off, when the baby will need his or her immunizations, and so on. They should also be comfortable feeding and handling the baby and should be aware of basic safety considerations, including the need to use a car seat whenever the baby is in a car, SIDS prevention, and prevention of shaken-baby injuries.
9. The parents should be aware of signs and symptoms in the baby that indicate possible problems and who to contact if problems occur.
10. The parents should be given information about postpartum mood and anxiety disorders, how to monitor for them, who to call, and how to receive medical services should they occur.

of returning for the follow-up visit. If not already discussed, teaching about family planning is appropriate at this time, and the nurse can provide information regarding contraception.

In ideal situations, a family approach involving the father/partner, newborn, and possibly other siblings would permit a total evaluation and provide an opportunity for all family members to ask questions and express concerns. In addition, a family approach can enable the nurse to identify disturbed family patterns more readily and initiate interventions to prevent future problems of neglect or abuse. See *Professionalism in Practice: Caring for a Complex Patient Population*.

Professionalism in Practice Caring for a Complex Patient Population

Nursing students will work with a variety of patients in the postpartum setting, including women at the far ends of the childbearing age spectrum; women across the socioeconomic spectrum; women who abuse substances; women who have experienced a variety of assistive reproductive techniques; women who will return to prison after childbirth; women with a history of trauma, intimate partner violence, or abuse; and women who are homeless or otherwise disenfranchised. This responsibility may initially be overwhelming to students, particularly as they worry about the future of the woman and/or her newborn. It may also be difficult for students to imagine a professional lifetime of caring for such a complex patient population. Postconference conversations with faculty members, peers, and staff nurses, if possible, are the appropriate time to discuss such concerns. There are no easy answers, but it is helpful to view problematic issues within the context of guiding principles such as the American Nurses Association (ANA, 2015) Code of Ethics for Nurses, the Association of Women's Health, Obstetric, and Neonatal Nurses (AWHONN, 2009) Standards for Professional Nursing Practice in the Care of Women and Newborns, and the mission of the university, hospital, or nursing school.

Evaluation of the Postpartum Family

Anticipated outcomes of comprehensive nursing care of the postpartum family include:

- The mother and newborn remain healthy, safe, and free of injury or complications.
- The mother verbalizes comfort and uses self-comfort measures as appropriate.
- The mother verbalizes feelings and concerns related to the birth event and her newborn.
- The mother performs appropriate self-care measures.
- The new parents demonstrate safe and effective care of their baby.
- The parents and newborn display positive bonding behaviors.
- The mother–newborn dyad demonstrates successful breastfeeding (or parents describe safe formula preparation and demonstrate safe bottle-feeding). Mothers describe breast care as appropriate.
- The mother is rested and verbalizes understanding of the importance of gradual return to activities.
- The mother identifies sources of support to assist with newborn care and family responsibilities.
- The mother states plan for follow-up healthcare for herself and her newborn.
- The mother identifies signs and symptoms of maternal–newborn complications and reasons to seek care before routine follow-up visits.
- The cesarean birth mother states in her own words the reason for the cesarean birth and verbalizes feelings.
- The cesarean birth mother verbalizes comfort and maintains mobility.
- The obese patient remains free of injury or complications.
- The adolescent mother expresses her feelings about the childbearing experience and verbalizes knowledge of resources for continued support.
- The woman relinquishing her newborn expresses her feelings, verbalizes knowledge of resources for continued support, and demonstrates acceptance of her decision.
- All mothers and fathers/partners report that they have been supported regarding their cultures (may include special considerations related to age, sexual preference, religion, ethnic background), their abilities, and their histories.
- The mother and father/partner are aware of symptoms of postpartum mood and anxiety disorders.

In summary, all components of nursing care are designed to achieve the desired outcomes identified for the woman and her family.

Focus Your Study

- Effective parent learning requires precise timing of teaching, as well as choice of a teaching method that is effective for the family, such as written material, DVDs, online streaming videos, and return demonstration. Content on self-care, newborn/infant care, and anticipatory guidance is important.
- Postpartum discomfort may be due to a variety of factors, including an edematous perineum, an episiotomy or extension, engorged hemorrhoids, hematoma formation, afterpains, immobility, diaphoresis, sore nipples, or engorged breasts. Various self-care approaches are helpful to promote comfort. Cultural values are incorporated in providing care to the new family.

- Lactation occurs in response to breast stimulation. Nursing support is essential for effective breastfeeding.
- A variety of techniques may be helpful to relieve discomfort during suppression of lactation if breastfeeding is not planned.
- The first day or two following birth are marked by maternal behaviors that are more dependent and oriented to the woman's comfort. Thereafter the woman becomes more independent and ready to assume responsibility.
- The new mother requires opportunities to discuss her childbirth experience with an empathetic listener.
- Initiation of skin-to-skin contact (SSC) immediately after birth benefits mom and newborn.
- Maternal rest is promoted by advising the woman to take frequent rest periods, nap when the baby is napping, avoid unnecessary activities, and use her social support system. Ambulation and activity should be resumed gradually.
- Rooming-in provides the childbearing family with opportunities to interact with their newborn during the first hours and days of life. This enables the family to develop some confidence and skill in a "safe" environment.
- Sexual intercourse may resume once the episiotomy has healed and lochia has stopped. Couples should be forewarned of possible changes; for example, the vagina may be "dry," fatigue may inhibit the level of desire, or the woman's breasts may leak milk during orgasm.
- Following cesarean birth, a woman has the nursing care needs of a surgical patient in addition to her needs as a postpartum patient. She may also require assistance in working through her feelings if the cesarean birth was unexpected.
- Following vaginal or cesarean birth, obese and morbidly obese women are at high risk for injury and complications. These new mothers have special physiologic, safety, and psychosocial needs.
- Postpartum, the nurse evaluates the adolescent mother in terms of her level of maturity, available support systems, cultural background, and existing knowledge, and then plans care accordingly.
- The lesbian mother and her wife/partner value the same treatment as other couples. Nurses should acknowledge, accept, and involve the wife/partner in care and decision making.
- Mothers with special needs will require additional support and access to external resources.
- Women who have a history of sexual abuse often have difficulty with physical examinations and are at risk for PTSD and PPD.
- The mother who decides to relinquish her baby needs emotional support and validation of her loss. She should decide whether to see and hold her baby and should have any special requests regarding the birth honored.
- Before discharge, the nurse should give the patient and her primary support person all information necessary for the woman to provide appropriate self-care. They should demonstrate beginning skill in caring for the newborn and should be able to verbalize warning signs of possible complications for mother or baby. Printed information is valuable for reference, as couples will have questions after discharge.
- The woman should receive education regarding symptoms of life-threatening postpartum complications for which she needs to seek immediate care. The nurse should educate her to inform providers that she has recently given birth during all healthcare encounters for 1 year.
- Because of the trend toward early discharge, follow-up care is more important than ever. Many approaches are used, especially home visits and telephone contact.

In order to make safe and effective judgments using NANDA-I © 2017 nursing diagnoses, it is essential that nurses refer to the definitions and defining characteristics of the diagnoses used in this text, which can be found in Appendix C.

References

Afiyanti, Y., & Solberg, S. M. (2015). "It is my destiny as a woman": On becoming a new mother in Indonesia. *Journal of Transcultural Nursing, 26*(5), 491–498. DOI: 10.1177/1043659614526243

Agency for Healthcare Research and Quality (AHRQ). (2016). *The patient education materials assessment tool (PEMAT) and user's guide: An instrument to assess the understandability and actionability of print and audiovisual patient education materials.* Retrieved from https://www.ahrq.gov/professionals/prevention-chronic-care/improve/self-mgmt/pemat/index.html

Ainsworth, R. M., Summerlin-Long, S., & Mog, C. (2016). A comprehensive initiative to prevent falls among newborns. *Nursing for Women's Health, 20*(3), 247–257. DOI: 10.1016/j.nwh.2016.04.025

Akbarzade, M., Ghaemmaghami, M., Yazdanpanahi, Z., Zare, N., Mohagheghzadeh, A., & Azizi, A. (2016). Comparison of the effect of dry cupping therapy and acupressure at BL23 point on intensity of postpartum perineal pain based on the short form of McGill Pain Questionnaire. *Journal of Reproduction & Infertility, 17*(1), 39–46.

Akorn, Inc. (2015). Methylergonovine Maleate. National Library of Medicine *Daily Med.* Retrieved from https://dailymed.nlm.nih.gov/dailymed/drugInfo.cfm?setid=b4c5f70e-da62-4d1d-a3e0-6fe5e-45bb65b

American Academy of Pediatrics (AAP), Committee on the Fetus and Newborn, & American College of Obstetricians and Gynecologists (ACOG), Committee on Obstetric Practice. (2017). *Guidelines for perinatal care* (8th ed.). Elk Grove Village, IL: Author.

American Nurses Association (ANA). (2015). *Code of ethics for nurses with interpretive statements.* Silver Spring, MD: Author.

American Society of Anesthesiologists Task Force and the American Society of Regional Anesthesia and Pain Medicine. (2016). Practice guidelines for the prevention, detection, and management of respiratory depression associated with neuraxial opioid administration: An updated report by the American Society of Anesthesiologists Task Force on Neuraxial Opioids and the American Society of Regional Anesthesia and Pain Medicine. *Anesthesiology, 124*(3), 535–552. DOI: 10.1097/ALN.0000000000000975

Aptevo BioTherapeutics. (2016). WinRho® SDF [Rh_0(D) Immune Globulin Intravenous (Human)]. *Solution for intravenous or intramuscular injection.* Retrieved from http://www.winrho.com/pdfs/WinRho_SDF_PI_Aptevo.pdf

Association of Women's Health, Obstetric, and Neonatal Nurses (AWHONN). (2009). *Standards for professional nursing practice in the care of women and newborns* (7th ed.). Washington, DC: Author.

Association of Women's Health, Obstetric, and Neonatal Nurses (AWHONN). (2014). *AWHONN postpartum hemorrhage (PPH) project.* Retrieved from https://www.awhonn.org/?page=PPH

Association of Women's Health, Obstetric, and Neonatal Nurses (AWHONN). (2016). *AWHONN's save your life: Post-birth warning signs.* Retrieved from https://cdn.ymaws.com/www.awhonn.org/resource/resmgr/files/Post-Birth_Warning_signs_160.pdf

Behling, D. J., & Renaud, M. (2015). Development of an obstetric vital sign alert to improve outcomes in acute care obstetrics. *Nursing for Women's Health, 19*(2), 128–141. DOI: 10.1111/1751-486X.12185

Brega, A. G., Barnard, J., Mabachi, N. M., Weiss, B. D., DeWalt, D. A., Brach, C., . . . West, D. R. (2015). *AHRQ health literacy universal precautions toolkit* (2nd ed.). Rockville, MD: Agency for Healthcare Research and Quality. Retrieved from https://www.ahrq.gov/sites/default/files/publications/files/healthlittoolkit2_4.pdf

Cappell, J., MacDonald, T. K., & Pukall, C. F. (2016). For new mothers, the relationship matters: Relationship characteristics and postpartum sexuality. *Canadian Journal of Human Sexuality, 25*(2), 126–137. DOI: 10.3138/cjhs.252-A5

Centers for Disease Control and Prevention (CDC). (2012). *MMR vaccine: What you need to know.* Retrieved from https://www.immunize.org/vis/mmr.pdf

Centers for Disease Control and Prevention (CDC). (2015). *Pregnancy and whooping cough.* Retrieved from https://www.cdc.gov/pertussis/pregnant/hcp/pregnant-patients.html

Centers for Disease Control and Prevention (CDC). (2016). *Guidelines for vaccinating pregnant women.* Retrieved from https://www.cdc.gov/vaccines/pregnancy/hcp/guidelines.html

Charlton, B. M., Rosario, M., Roberts, A. L., Katz-Wise, S., Spiegelman, D., & Autin, S. B. (2016). Teen pregnancy risk factors among female adolescents of diverse sexual orientations. *Journal of Pediatric and Adolescent Gynecology, 29*(2), 195–196. DOI: http://dx.doi.org/10.1016/j.jpag.2016.01.088

Child Welfare Information Gateway. (2013). *Impact of adoption on birth parents.* Washington, DC: U.S. Department of Health and Human Services. Retrieved from https://www.childwelfare.gov/pubpdfs/f_impact.pdf

Child Welfare Information Gateway. (2016). *Trends in U.S. adoptions: 2008–2012.* Washington, DC: U.S. Department of Health and Human Services. Retrieved from https://www.childwelfare.gov/pubPDFs/adopted0812.pdf

Clutter, L. B. (2014). Adult birth mothers who made open infant adoption placements after adolescent unplanned pregnancy. *JOGNN: Journal of Obstetric, Gynecologic & Neonatal Nursing, 43*(2), 190–199. DOI: 10.1111/1552-6909.12280

Corbett, B. M., O'Connell, C., Boutin, M. A., Fatayerji, N. I., & Sauer, C. W. (2016). Inadvertent methylergonovine administration to a neonate. *American Journal of Case Reports, 17*, 770–773. DOI: 10.12659/AJCR.900263

Creanga, A. A., Berg, C. J., Syverson, C., Seed, K., Bruce, C., & Callaghan, W. M. (2015). Pregnancy-related mortality in the United States, 2006–2010. *Obstetrics & Gynecology, 125*(1), 5–12. DOI: 10.1097/AOG.0000000000000564

CSL Behring AG. (2016). RHOPHYLAC- human rho(d) immune globulin solution. In National Library of Medicine *Daily Med.* Retrieved from https://dailymed.nlm.nih.gov/dailymed/drugInfo.cfm?setid=c1b5d801-336f-4541-a7d9-a8d4a110a4cc&audience=consumer

D'Oria, R. Myers, J., & Logsdon, M. D. (2016). Strategies to reduce maternal mortality during the first year after birth. *Journal of Obstetric, Gynecologic, and Neonatal Nursing, 45*(6), 885–893. DOI: 10.1016/j.jogn.2016.04.013

East, C. E., Begg, L., Henshall, N. E., Marchant P. R., & Wallace, K. (2012). Local cooling for relieving pain from perineal trauma sustained during childbirth. *Cochrane Database of Systematic Reviews*, Issue 5, Article No. CD006304. DOI: 10.1002/14651858.CD006304.pub3

Food and Drug Administration (FDA). (2011). *FDA limits acetaminophen in prescription combination products; requires liver toxicity warnings.* Retrieved from https://www.fda.gov/Drugs/DrugSafety/ucm239821.htm

Food and Drug Administration (FDA). (2017). *Acetaminophen: Avoiding liver damage.* Retrieved from https://www.fda.gov/ForConsumers/ConsumerUpdates/ucm168830.htm

Gabbe, S. G., Niebyl, J. R., Simpson, J. L., & Landon, M. B., Galan, H. L., Jauniaux, E. R. M., . . . Grobman, W. A. (2017). *Obstetrics: Normal and problem pregnancies* (7th ed.). Philadelphia, PA: Saunders.

Gagandeep, Sagar, N., Mamta, & Kaur, J. (2013). Efficacy of cabbage leaves in relief of breast engorgement among postnatal mothers. *International Journal of Nursing Education, 5*(2), 76–79. DOI: 10.5958/j.0974-9357.5.2.068

Giallo, R., Cooklin, A., Dunning, M., & Seymour, M. (2014). The efficacy of an intervention for the management of postpartum fatigue. *JOGNN: Journal of Obstetric, Gynecologic, and Neonatal Nursing, 43*(5), 598–613. DOI: 10.1111/1552-6909.12489

Goldburg, A. E. (2017). *The Sage encyclopedia of LGBTQ studies.* Oxford, UK: Sage.

Hamilton, B. E., Martin, J. A., Osterman, M. J. K., Curtin, S. C., & Mathews, T. J. (2015). Births: Final data for 2014. *National Vital Statistics Reports, 64*(12), 1–64. Retrieved from https://www.cdc.gov/nchs/data/nvsr/nvsr64/nvsr64_12.pdf

Hayman, B., Wilkes, L., Halcomb, E. J., & Jackson, D. (2013). Marginalised mothers: Lesbian women negotiating heteronormative healthcare services. *Contemporary Nurse: A Journal for the Australian Nursing Profession, 44*(1), 120–127. DOI: 10.5172/conu.2013.44.1.120

Heslehurst, N., Russell, S., Brandon, H., Johnston, C., Summerbell, C., & Rankin, J. (2015). Women's perspectives are required to inform the development of maternal obesity services: A qualitative study of obese pregnant women's experiences. *Health Expectations, 18*(5), 969–981. DOI: 10.1111/hex.12070

Holroyd, E., Lopez, V., & Chan, S. W. (2011). Negotiating "doing the month": An ethnographic study examining the postnatal practices of two generations of Chinese women. *Nursing and Health Sciences, 13*(1), 47–52. DOI: 10.1111/j.1442-2018.2011.00575.x

James, D. C. (2013). Postpartum care. In K. R. Simpson & P. A. Creehan (Eds.), *AWHONN's perinatal nursing* (4th ed., pp. 530–580). Philadelphia, PA: AWHONN.

Jeha, D., Usta, I., Ghulmiyyah, L., & Nassar, A. (2015). A review of the risks and consequences of adolescent pregnancy. *Journal of Neonatal–Perinatal Medicine, 8*(1), 1–8. DOI: 10.3233/NPM-15814038

Kansky, C. (2016*). Normal and abnormal puerperium.* Medscape. Retrieved from https://emedicine.medscape.com/article/260187-overview#a7

Karst, D., & Lindsey, M. (2012). Educating hospitals about adoption: How hospital staff can support parents considering an adoption plan. *Adoption Advocate, No. 52.* Retrieved from https://www.adoptioncouncil.org/images/stories/documents/NCFA_ADOPTION_ADVOCATE_NO52.pdf

Kedrion Melville, Inc. (2014). RhoGAM Ultra-Filtered Plus. MICRhoGAM Ultra-Filtered Plus. In National Library of Medicine *Daily Med.* Retrieved from https://dailymed.nlm.nih.gov/dailymed/lookup.cfm?setid=d87e4d0b-2442-4135-b3f9-5c4f74845b87

Klaus, M. (2009). Commentary: An early, short, and useful sensitive period in the human infant. *Birth, 36*(2), 110–112. DOI: 10.1111/j.1523-536X.2009.00315.x

Kwan, W. S. C., & Li, W. W. H. (2014). Effect of ear acupressure on acute postpartum perineal pain: A randomized controlled study, *Journal of Clinical Nursing, 23*(7–8), 1153–1164. DOI: 10.1111/jocn.12281

LaCoursiere, D. Y., Hirst, K. P., & Barrett-Connor, E. (2012). Depression and pregnancy stressors affect the association between abuse and postpartum depression. *Maternal Child Health Journal, 16*(4), 929–935. DOI: 10.1007/s10995-011-0816-7

Lai, Y. L., Hung, C. H., Stocker, J., Chan, T. F., & Liu, Y. (2015). Postpartum fatigue, baby-care activities, and maternal-infant attachment of vaginal and cesarean births following rooming-in. *Applied Nursing Research, 28*(2), 116–120. DOI: 10.1016/j.apnr.2014.08.002

Lamb, K., & Sanders, R. (2015). Constipation and haemorrhoids: A midwifery perspective for the childbearing continuum. *British Journal of Midwifery, 23*,(3), 171–177. DOI: 10.12968/bjom.2015.23.3.171

Lindley, L. L., & Walsemann, K. M. (2015). Sexual orientation and risk of pregnancy among New York City high-school students. *American Journal of Public Health, 105*(7), 1379–1386. DOI: 10.2105/AJ PH.2015.302553

Liu, C. H., & Tronick, E. (2013). Rates and predictors of postpartum depression by race and ethnicity: Results from the 2004 to 2007 New York City PRAMS survey (Pregnancy Risk Assessment Monitoring System). *Maternal and Child Health Journal, 17*(9), 1599–1610. DOI: 10.1007/s10995-012-1171-z

Liu, Y. Q., Maloni, J. A., & Petrini, M. A. (2014). Effect of postpartum practices of doing the month on Chinese women's physical and psychological health. *Biological Research for Nursing, 16*(1), 55–63. DOI: 10.1177/1099800412465107

Lockwood, S., & Anderson, K. (2013). Postpartum safety: A patient-centered approach to fall prevention. *MCN: American Journal of Maternal/Child Nursing, 38*(1), 15–18. DOI: 10.1097/NMC.0b013e31826bae4b

Logsdon, M. C., Martin, V. H., Stikes, R., Davis, D., Ryan, L., Yang, I., & . . . Rushton, J. (2015). Lessons learned from adolescent mothers: Advice on recruitment. *Journal of Nursing Scholarship, 47*(4), 294–299. DOI: 10.1111/jnu.12142

Lu, Y. Y., Su, M. L., Gau, M. L., Lin, K. C., & Au, H. K. (2015). The efficacy of cold-gel packing for relieving episiotomy pain—A quasi-randomised control trial. *Contemporary Nurse: A Journal for the Australian Nursing Profession, 50*(1), 26–35. DOI: 10.1080/10376178.2015.1010257

Mangesi, L., & Zakarija-Grkovic, I. (2016). Treatments for breast engorgement during lactation. *Cochrane Database of Systematic Reviews*, Issue 6, Article No. CD006946. DOI: 10.1002/14651858.CD006946.pub3

Mercer, R. T. (1986). *First-time motherhood: Experiences from teens to forties.* New York, NY: Springer.

Mercer, R. T. (2004). Becoming a mother versus maternal role attainment. *Journal of Nursing Scholarship, 36*(3), 226–232. DOI: 10.1111/j.1547-5069.2004.04042.x

Mercer, R. T. (2006). Nursing support of the process of becoming a mother. *JOGNN: Journal of Obstetric, Gynecologic, & Neonatal Nursing, 35*(5), 649–651. DOI: 10.1111/J.1552-6909.2006.00086.x

Merck Sharp & Dohme Corp. (2015). M-M-R® II (Measles, Mumps, and Rubella Virus Vaccine Live). Retrieved from https://www.merck.com/product/usa/pi_circulars/m/mmr_ii/mmr_ii_pi.pdf

Mkontwana, N., & Novikova, N. (2015). Oral analgesia for relieving post-caesarean pain. *Cochrane Database of Systematic Reviews*, Issue 3, Article No. CD010450. DOI: 10.1002/14651858.CD010450.pub2

Moise, K. J. (2018). *Prevention of Rhesus (D) alloimmunization in pregnancy.* Retrieved from https://www.uptodate.com/contents/prevention-of-rhesus-d-alloimmunization-in-pregnancy?search=prevention-of-rhesus-dalloimmunization-in-pregnancy&source=search_result&selectedTitle=2~150&usage_type=default&display_rank=2

Moore, E. R., Anderson, G. C., Bergman, N., & Dowswell, T. (2012). Early skin-to-skin contact for mothers and their healthy newborn infants. *Cochrane Database of Systematic Reviews*, Issue 5, Article No. CD003519. DOI: 10.1002/14651858.CD003519.pub3

Moran-Peters, J. A., Zauderer, C. R., Goldman, S., Baierlein, J., & Smith, A. E. (2014). A quality improvement project focused on women's perceptions of skin-to-skin contact after cesarean birth. *Nursing for Women's Health, 18*(4), 294–303. DOI: 10.1111/1751-486X.12135

Mousa, H. A., Blum, J., Abou El Senoun, G., Shakur, H., & Alfirevic, Z. (2014). Treatment for primary postpartum haemorrhage. *Cochrane Database of Systematic Reviews*, Issue 2, Article No. CD003249. DOI: 10.1002/14651858.CD003249.pub3

National Institutes of Health (NIH). (2016). *Clear communication.* Retrieved from https://www.nih.gov/institutes-nih/nih-office-director/office-communications-public-liaison/clear-communication

Paiva, C. D. S. B., de Oliveira, S. M. J. V., Francisco, A. A., da Silva, R. L., Mendes, E. D. P. B., & Steen, M. (2016). Length of perineal pain relief after ice pack application: A quasi-experimental study. *Women and Birth, 29*(2), 117–122. DOI: http://dx.doi.org/10.1016/j.wombi.2015.09.002

Panagopoulou, V., Hancock, J., & Tziaferi, S. (2017). Midwifery in the postnatal period: A systematic review of the literature. *Hellenic Journal of Nursing, 56*(2), 125–137.

Pereira Gomes Morais, E., Riera, R., Porfírio, G. J. M., Macedo, C. R., Sarmento Vasconcelos, V., de Souza Pedrosa, A., & Torloni, M. R. (2016). Chewing gum for enhancing early recovery of bowel function after caesarean section. *Cochrane Database of Systematic Reviews*, Issue 10, Article No. CD011562. DOI: 10.1002/14651858.CD011562.pub2

Pharris, A., Bucchio, J., Dotson, C., & Davidson, W. (2016). Supporting lesbian couples during pregnancy. *International Journal of Childbirth Education, 31*(3), 23–24.

Phillips, R. (2013). The sacred hour: Uninterrupted skin-to-skin contact immediately after birth. *Newborn & Infant Nursing Reviews, 13*(2), 67–72. DOI: 10.1053/j.nainr.2013.04.001

Pitangui, A. C. R., Araújo, R. C., Bezerra, M. J. S., Ribeiro, C. O., & Nakano, A. M. S. (2014). Low and high-frequency TENS in post-episiotomy pain relief: A randomized, double-blind clinical trial. *Brazilian Journal of Physical Therapy, 18*(1), 72–78. DOI: 10.1590/S1413-35552012005000143

Purnell, M. C., & MacKenzie, M. A. (2016). The intergenerational cycle of obesity and its implications for nursing care of childbearing women. *Nursing for Women's Health, 20*(3), 289–297. DOI: 10.1016/j.nwh.2016.03.003

Reisz, S., Jacobvitz, D., & George, C. (2015). Birth and motherhood: Childbirth experience and mothers' perceptions of themselves and their babies. *Infant Mental Health Journal, 36*(2), 167–178. DOI:10.1002/imhj.21500

Rubin, R. (1984). *Maternal identity and the maternal experience.* New York, NY: Springer.

Seng, J. S., Sperlich, M., Low, L. K., Ronis, D. L., Muzik, M., & Liberzon, I. (2013). Childhood abuse history, posttraumatic stress disorder, postpartum mental health, and bonding: A prospective cohort study. *Journal of Midwifery & Women's Health, 58*(1), 57–68. DOI: 10.1111/j.1542-2011.2012.00237.x

Shaw, R. (2016). Considering birth fathers: Ensuring right and inclusion for fathers before adoption placement. *Adoption Advocate No. 96.* Retrieved from https://www.adoptioncouncil.org/files/large/bed26063416cc19

Smith, E. (2016). If it's natural, why does it hurt?: Examining the reasons mom may feel pain with breastfeeding. *International Journal of Childbirth Education, 31*(4), 40–43.

Stone, S., Prater, L., & Spencer, R. (2015). Facilitating skin-to-skin contact in the operating room after cesarean birth. *Nursing For Women's Health, 18*(6), 486–499. DOI: 10.1111/1751-486X.12161

Tawfic, Q. A., & Faris, A. S. (2015). Acute pain service: Past, present and future. *Pain Management, 5*(1), 47–58. DOI: 10.2217/pmt.14.48

U. S. Department of Health and Human Services (HHS). (2013). *Healthy People 2020.* Retrieved from https://www.healthypeople.gov/2020/

Vallerand, A. H., Sanoski, C. A., & Deglin, J. H. (2017). *Davis's drug guide for nurses* (15th ed.). Philadelphia, PA: F. A. Davis.

Wahedi, M. (2016). Should midwives consider associated psychological factors when caring for women who are obese? *British Journal of Midwifery, 24*(10), 724–735. DOI: 10.12968/bjom.2016.24.10.724

Wojnar, D. M., & Katzenmeyer, A. (2014). Experiences of preconception, pregnancy, and new motherhood for lesbian nonbiological mothers. *JOGNN: Journal of Obstetric, Gynecologic & Neonatal Nursing, 43*(1), 50–60. DOI: 10.1111/1552-6909.12270

World Health Organization (WHO). (2015). *Trends in maternal mortality: 1990 to 2015.* Geneva, Switzerland: Author.

Wosu, A., Gelaye, B., & Williams, M. (2015). History of childhood sexual abuse and risk of prenatal and postpartum depression or depressive symptoms: An epidemiologic review. *Archives of Women's Mental Health, 18*(5), 659–671. DOI: 10.1007/s00737-015-0533-0

Wuytack, F., Smith V., & Cleary B. J. (2016). Oral non-steroidal anti-inflammatory drugs (single dose) for perineal pain in the early postpartum period. *Cochrane Database of Systematic Reviews*, Issue 7, Article No. CD011352. DOI: 10.1002/14651858.CD011352.pub2

Yaju, Y., Kataoka, Y., Eto, H., Horiuchi, S., & Mori, R. (2013). Prophylactic interventions after delivery of placenta for reducing bleeding during the postnatal period. *Cochrane Database of Systematic Reviews*, Issue 11, Article No. CD009328. DOI: 10.1002/14651858.CD009328.pub2

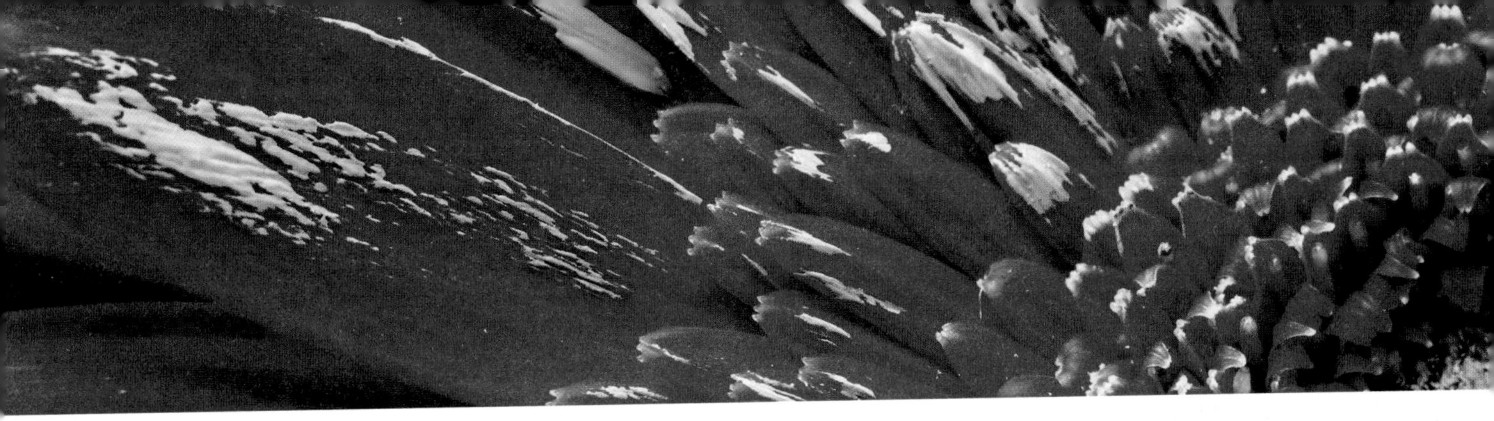

Chapter 34

Home Care of the Postpartum Family

Working as a home care nurse with an early discharge program is the most fulfilling job I have ever had. It is an honor and a privilege to be allowed into the home to share this special time with childbearing families. When I offer breastfeeding support, help new parents to access the resources they need, or recognize a problem and ensure timely follow-up, I know that I am making a difference in their lives. The appreciation expressed by the families and the healthcare providers with whom I work is a gift that I receive.

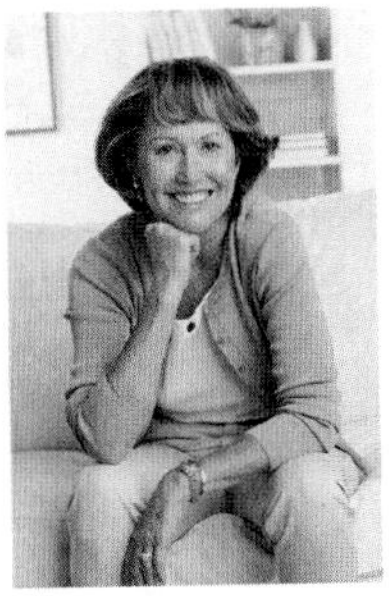

SOURCE: Corbis/SuperStock.

Learning Outcomes

34.1 Discuss the components of postpartum home care.

34.2 Identify the main purposes of home visits during the postpartum period.

34.3 Summarize actions the nurse should take to ensure personal safety during a home visit.

34.4 Delineate aspects of fostering a caring relationship in the home.

34.5 Describe assessment, care of the newborn, and reinforcement of parent teaching in the home.

34.6 Discuss maternal and family assessment and anticipated progress after birth.

34.7 Describe appropriate nursing interventions for women who are experiencing breastfeeding difficulties.

34.8 Identify postpartum resources that are available to new families.

Healthy People 2020

(MICH-20) Increase the proportion of infants who are put to sleep on their backs

(MICH-21) Increase the proportion of infants who are breastfed

(MICH-22) Increase the proportion of employers that have worksite lactation support programs

Role of Length of Stay and Professional Guidelines for Discharge

The Newborns' and Mothers' Health Protection Act (NMHPA) was signed into law in 1997 and took effect in January 1998. Although the bill does not prohibit earlier discharge, it provides for a guaranteed minimum length of stay (LOS) of up to 48 hours following an uncomplicated vaginal birth and 96 hours following an uncomplicated cesarean birth at the discretion of the new mother and her healthcare provider (American Academy of Pediatrics [AAP], Committee on Fetus and Newborn, 2010; U.S. Department of Labor, Employee Benefits Security Administration, 2008). The health of the mother and baby, the mother's ability and confidence regarding self- and newborn care, support systems available, and access to follow-up care should form the basis of the discharge decision. Whenever possible, the mother and baby should be discharged at the same time to support breastfeeding (Benitz, 2015).

As the member of the interprofessional healthcare team who likely spends the most time with the family, the professional nurse can contribute valuable input to inform the decision, advocating on the patient's behalf as appropriate.

Recommended discharge criteria for healthy term newborns and recommendations for follow-up after early discharge are found in Table 34–1.

Newborns discharged prior to 48 hours of age should be examined by a healthcare professional "competent in newborn assessment" (AAP & ACOG, 2017) within 48 hours of discharge. A qualified nurse can accomplish the visit in a clinical setting or in the home, provided that the results are reported to the newborn's healthcare provider that day.

Considerations for the Home Visit

In the United States, less than 60% of women attend a postpartum visit between 4 and 6 weeks after giving birth (ACOG, 2018). The frequency of home health visits is even rarer, but there is no data on the subject. In planning a home visit, the nurse should

TABLE 34–1 Minimal Criteria for Discharge of Healthy Term Newborns

1. Newborn's vital signs are normal and stable for 12 hours before discharge
   - Respiratory rate less than 60/min; absence of respiratory distress
   - Heart rate 100–190/min when awake
   - Axillary temperature of 36.5°C to 37.4°C (97.7°F to 99.3°F) in an open crib with appropriate clothing
2. Newborn has urinated and passed at least one spontaneous stool
3. Newborn has completed at least two successful feedings
   - Documented effective breastfeeding to include latch, swallowing, and newborn satiety by a caregiver qualified to assess
   - Documented ability of the bottle-feeding newborn to coordinate sucking, swallowing, and breathing while feeding
4. Physical exam reveals no abnormalities requiring a longer hospital stay
5. No evidence of excessive bleeding from the circumcision site for the previous 2 hours
6. Clinical significance of any jaundice has been determined, and appropriate management and follow-up are in place
7. Mother's knowledge, ability, and confidence to care for the newborn are documented to include teaching of the following:
   - Condition of the newborn
   - Benefits of breastfeeding
   - Appropriate newborn output (urine and stools)
   - Care of the cord, skin, and genitals as well as temperature assessment and measurement
   - Maternal knowledge of signs of illness and common problems, including jaundice
   - Instruction in newborn safety to include car seat use, positioning for sleep, smoke-free environment, and sleeping nearby without bed sharing
   - Handwashing hygiene
8. Appropriate car seat that meets Federal Motor Vehicle Safety Standard 213 is available
9. Support persons and healthcare providers are available during the first few days following discharge; providers must be knowledgeable about lactation and able to detect jaundice and dehydration
10. Instructions given to follow in the event of a complication or emergency
11. Lab data have been reviewed to include maternal syphilis, hepatitis B virus surface antigen, and HIV; umbilical cord or newborn blood type and direct Coombs, if indicated
12. Required metabolic, hearing, and pulse oximetry screening tests have been accomplished; if a metabolic test was performed before 24 hours of milk feeding, a plan for repeat must be in place in accordance with local or state policy
13. Initial hepatitis B vaccine has been administered
14. Sepsis evaluation accomplished
15. A physician-directed source of continuing medical care for both mother and baby has been identified and mother can access it; appropriate follow-up within 48 hours by a person qualified to assess the newborn is scheduled
16. Family, environmental, and social risk factors have been assessed. If present, the discharge should be delayed until resolved or a plan is in place to keep the baby safe. Factors may include but not be limited to untreated parental substance use, positive maternal or newborn toxicology results, history of child abuse or neglect, mental illness in a parent or other individual who is in the home, lack of social support, no fixed home, history of domestic violence, adolescent mother—especially with other risk factors and barriers to follow-up (lack of access to telephone, transportation issues, non-English-speaking parents).
17. Mother received tetanus toxoid, reduced diphtheria toxoid, and acellular pertussis (Tdap) and/or influenza vaccine if not currently immunized; family and close contacts educated to get Tdap as well

Recommended follow-up for newborns includes the following (needs to occur within 48 hours of discharge if the baby is discharged prior to 48 hours of age):

- Weigh the baby
- Assess the newborn's general health, hydration, and degree of jaundice; identify any new problems
- Review feeding pattern and technique; encourage and observe breastfeeding for adequate position, latch-on, and swallowing; refer for lactation support as appropriate
- Assess historical evidence of stool and urine patterns for adequacy
- Assess quality of mother–newborn interaction and details of newborn behavior
- Reinforce maternal or family education in neonatal care, to include feeding, sleep position, no bed-sharing, and car seat safety
- Review results of laboratory tests performed at discharge
- Perform screening tests as required by the state and others as clinically indicated (bilirubin level for jaundice)
- Identify a plan for healthcare maintenance, including a method for obtaining emergency services, preventive care and immunizations, periodic evaluations and physical examinations, and screenings
- Assess parental well-being (postpartum depression screening)

Note: Criteria apply to a healthy term (37 0/7 weeks to 41 6/7 weeks of gestation) newborn whose mother experienced an uncomplicated pregnancy, labor, and delivery. Late preterm (34 0/7 to 36 6/7 weeks) newborns should meet additional criteria prior to discharge, such as maintaining 93% or more of birth weight, passing the car seat safety test, and 24 hours of documented successful feedings (American Academy of Pediatrics [AAP] & the American College of Obstetricians and Gynecologists [ACOG], 2017).

SOURCES: Data from AAP & ACOG, 2017; Benitz, 2015.

clearly understand the purpose of the visit and the amount of content to be covered. Other considerations include ways of creating and fostering relationships with families, preplanning and executing the visit, maintaining safety, documenting the visit, and ensuring follow-up and referrals as appropriate.

The postpartum home visit differs from community health visits in that only one or two visits are typically planned, and long-term follow-up in the home is not anticipated. The aim of the visit is the postpartum family's needs and care. Family well-being should be determined through a comprehensive assessment that includes physical, emotional, and social functioning.

Because of the established guidelines for discharge of the mother and baby (see Table 34–1), the nurse can expect to find certain levels of health and wellness and should assess for deviations from the norm.

Purpose and Timing of the Home Visit

The postpartum home visit focuses on family assessment, teaching, and counseling and often occurs on the third to sixth day postpartum, depending on the timing of discharge. This time frame encompasses the potential peak times for newborn jaundice, weight loss, dehydration, and gastrointestinal obstruction or cardiac lesions that often occur after the first 2 days of life (Kliegman, Stanton, Geme, et al., 2015). This coincides with the mother's milk coming in so that a breastfeeding assessment can be performed. In addition, parents have now provided care on their own and often have questions at this stage.

Postpartum home care provides opportunities for expanding information and reinforcing self- and newborn care techniques in a more relaxed environment, where the family has control of the setting. A safety assessment of the home environment can be performed in a setting where the nurse can help the family identify unique needs and develop creative options.

Fostering a Caring Relationship with the Family

The most essential component of the home care visit is to develop a trusting relationship with the family that shows respect, to communicate a willingness to listen, and to help the family identify knowledge gaps. It is important to establish regard for patients, genuineness, empathy, and establishment of trust and rapport (Table 34–2).

Planning the Home Visit

Prior to the visit, it is important to identify the purpose of the visit and gather anticipated materials and equipment. The nurse should obtain a copy of inpatient records and any prenatal history that would warrant follow-up care in the postpartum period. The nurse schedules the visit via phone, informing the family of the purpose, goals, and approximate length of the visit.

Maintaining Safety

Nurses may be exposed to safety hazards traveling to and during home visits. Risks related to bloodborne pathogens, ergonomics, latex, and patient lifting are present across multiple healthcare settings. Additional risks may include isolated locations, illegal drugs, threatening animals, gangs, vandalism, inadequate lighting, guns, verbal abuse, robberies, inappropriate sexual comments, patients with unpredictable behavior due to mental illness or cognitive impairments, adverse weather and road conditions, dilapidated or pest-infested buildings, unsanitary conditions, and violent lifestyles (Yonemoto, Dowswell, Nagai, et al., 2017). It is important to follow some basic safety rules, including:

- Confirm the address.
- Outline the route via a GPS device, if available.
- Provide a schedule of visits with patient addresses and phone numbers to supervisors.
- Notify a supervisor when leaving for a visit and check in once completed.
- Carry a charged cell phone.
- Carry a hard copy of agency phone numbers that are also programmed into the cell phone, in case of emergency (ICE).
- Ensure that the vehicle used for visits is well maintained and has sufficient fuel.
- Wear a name tag and carry identification.

TABLE 34–2 Fostering a Caring Relationship

DEMONSTRATED GOAL	APPROACHES TO ACHIEVE GOAL
Regard	• Introduce yourself to the family. Call the family members by their surnames until you have been invited to use the given or a less formal name. • Ask to be introduced to other members of the family who are present. Allow the mother or spokesperson to assume this role. Remember, in some cultures, it may be a male figure or a mother figure who assumes the primary role. Use active listening. Maintain objectiveness. • Ask permission before sitting.
Genuineness	• Mean what you say. Make sure that your verbal and nonverbal messages are congruent. • Be nonjudgmental. Do not make assumptions about individuals or settings. • Always strive to demonstrate caring behaviors. • Be prepared for the visit, honestly answer questions and provide information, and be truthful. If you do not know the answer to a question, tell the patient you will find the information and report back.
Empathy	• Listen to the mother and family "where they are" without judgment. Be attentive to what the birthing experience is for them so that you will understand from their perspective. • Remember that empathy denotes understanding, not sympathy.
Trust and rapport	• Do what you say you will do. • Be prepared for the visit and be on time. • Follow-up on any areas that are needed.

- Carry a flashlight or use smartphone flashlight, particularly for night visits.
- Avoid wearing any jewelry.
- Lock personal belongings in the trunk of the car, out of sight, before starting out (or before arriving at the home).
- Call patient to confirm appointment prior to leaving for visit.
- Identify all individuals present in the home at the start of the visit.
- Pay attention to the body language throughout the visit.
- If any threatening, sexually inappropriate behavior, presence of weapons, threatening pets, illegal substance use, or issues that make the nurse feel unsafe occur, terminate visit.
- Be aware of personal body language and how it might be interpreted (e.g., avoid crossing arms or shoving hands in pockets; remain calm and convey a sense of respect at all times).
- Have car keys in hand before returning to the vehicle.
- Lock the doors and drive away upon return to the vehicle at the completion of visits.
- Inform the supervisor immediately of any threatening situation, assault, or injury.
- Notify authorities if a crime has been committed.

It may be helpful to drive around neighborhoods known to be unsafe before making an initial visit to identify potential cues to violence and to determine whether extra security is necessary. If the visit is in an area that seems very unsafe, it may be wise for the nurse to be accompanied by a security officer. Nurses should avoid entering areas where violence is in progress. In such cases, they should return to the car and contact the appropriate authorities by calling 911. If violence erupts while in the home and the nurse is unable to safely exit, the nurse should stay in a secure room with the door locked, if possible, and call 911.

The Occupational Safety and Health Administration (OSHA, 2015) and the National Institute for Occupational Safety and Health (NIOSH, 2010, 2012, 2014) offer guidance about the hazards of home care, rights of employees, and responsibilities of employers in the home care environment. Employers must have policies in place and must provide safety education for workers. Nurses should ask about and review the violence protection plan of a home care agency to ensure that their safety will be protected to the extent possible before accepting employment. Nurses may also wish to enroll in further personal safety training independently. Because postpartum home care frequently involves only one visit, it may be helpful to discuss safety expectations during the previsit telephone contact. Home care nurses should be familiar with their agency policies and notify supervisors if safety issues requiring agency support are present.

Most people are more comfortable in familiar settings and have some hesitation when entering other residential areas. It is important for nurses to be aware of their surroundings and the people who are nearby. First home visits may feel uncomfortable because they are unfamiliar, but comfort increases with experience (Figure 34–1).

Ethics in Action!

Concerned that the baby of a single, adolescent mother is dehydrated, you enter the home and see that the baby is visibly jaundiced. Immediately, the patient's brother and his friends begin making sexually threatening comments to you. Do you attend to the sick newborn despite the risk, or do you protect yourself by immediately leaving the home?

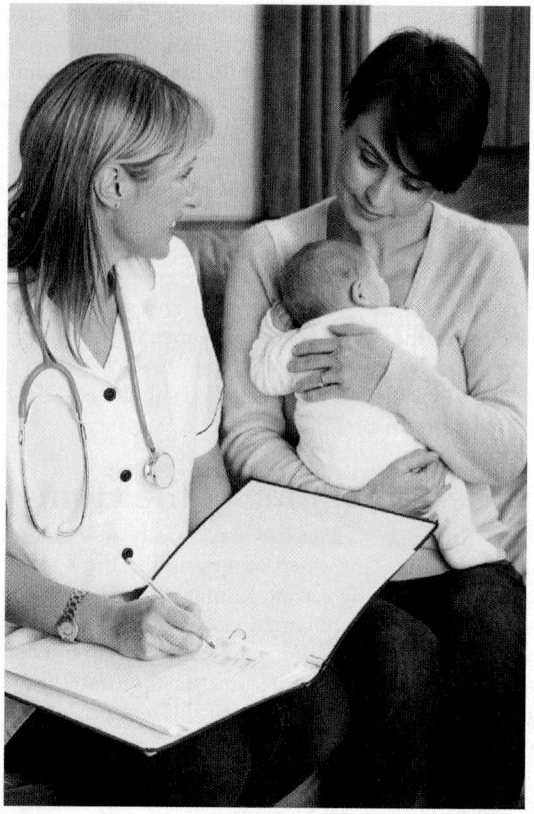

Figure 34–1 Nurse providing care and teaching to a new mother and baby at the home visit.

SOURCE: Monkey Business Images/Shutterstock.

Carrying Out the Home Visit

The nurse should introduce herself or himself to all persons present and confirm that the location is correct upon arrival. If a place to sit is not indicated, the nurse may inquire, "Where is the best place to sit so that we can talk for a while?" The nurse should follow cues from the patient regarding family and cultural norms. For example, many Asian families do not wear shoes in their homes. The nurse may want to carry indoor slippers for this situation.

Many agencies have developed a uniform assessment tool to be used during postpartum home visits that includes a physical assessment of the mother and newborn; assesses feeding; obtains maternal and newborn weight; evaluates maternal psychosocial adjustment, parental bonding, parenting behaviors, family adaptation, and coping skills; and determines environmental strengths and risk factors. A postpartum depression screening tool, such as the Edinburgh Postpartum Depression Inventory, should be performed to assess for postpartum mood and anxiety disorders. Based on these assessments the nurse may do any of the following:

- Provide direct physical care.
- Conduct patient and family teaching.
- Consult with the physician, midwife, or a specialist, such as a lactation consultant. *Note:* The term *lactation consultant* in this chapter refers to an international board-certified lactation consultant (IBCLC).
- Refer the woman or family to appropriate community agencies.
- Schedule additional home visits or telephone follow-up.

Because the home may be geographically isolated, the nurse needs to have excellent assessment skills, identify signs that indicate variations from the norm, and utilize critical thinking and problem-solving skills. See *Professionalism in Practice: Reporting Unsanitary Conditions in the Home*. Effective communication with the families and healthcare providers is essential to coordinate care and appropriate follow-up. The remainder of the chapter focuses on specific aspects of newborn and maternal care that are assessed, addressed, and evaluated during the home visit.

Professionalism in Practice Reporting Unsanitary Conditions in the Home

As healthcare professionals, nurses are required to report neglect or abuse of a child. When practicing in private homes, the nurse will be exposed to a wide range of home management practices with regard to aesthetics and sanitation. For example, the nurse will need to distinguish a home that is simply messy from a home that is unsanitary. It is important to develop rapport with the parents and to provide education as needed when sanitation issues are present. In certain cases, a follow-up visit is warranted. In cases of extreme filth or severe pest infestations, the nurse will need to use critical thinking skills to determine whether the most vulnerable patient—the baby—is at risk for injury. If that is the case, the nurse should notify the appropriate authorities and follow the home care agency plan for such contingencies. If in doubt, the nurse should call upon resource persons and supervisors for assistance.

Home Care: The Newborn

The nurse provides positive feedback to the family members as they provide care for the newborn. The nurse offers guidance, suggests alternatives, provides feedback, and serves as a role model. Each newborn has variations in normal physiologic responses and in growth and development patterns. Parents need to learn to interpret these changes in their child. A home visit and 24-hour telephone access to the birthing unit nursing staff are invaluable resources, providing additional support and consultation during the first few days at home.

The family should have been taught all necessary caregiving methods before discharge. Many nurses utilize a checklist to ensure the content is understood and determine if additional demonstration is needed. Parents are frequently overwhelmed, sensory overloaded, and exhausted during their short hospital stay and will require a review of initial teaching.

Parents often have questions regarding newborn/infant care, feeding, and signs of illness, which can be reviewed at the visit along with specific instructions and contact information for their healthcare providers. The family should be encouraged to call with any questions.

Home visits are associated with a reduction in adverse undetected health issues and cost savings. Increasingly, modern technology has been utilized to provide interventions to improve continuity of care, reduce adverse health outcomes, and decrease healthcare costs. Telemedicine has been shown to be an effective tool for providing home visits. In one study, nurse practitioners utilized cell phone technology to text and call new mothers during the first 6 months postpartum. This intervention was associated with greater perceived social support, earlier newborn follow-up, higher immunization rates at the appropriate time intervals, and lower infant morbidity rates compared to a control group (Hannan, Brooton, Page, et al., 2016). This study is promising in that it shows the use of technology can be successfully utilized to provide high-tech care, resulting in positive health outcomes at a cost savings, especially when families are reluctant or fail to schedule home visits.

This chapter identifies a number of printed and online resources for nurses and families. The nurse must assess each family's education level, primary language, literacy level, financial resources, and access to technology when determining the teaching needs and plan. Educational resources should be provided in ways that are understandable and accessible for the family.

Physical Assessment of the Newborn at Home

In the home, a newborn physical exam is performed to assess general appearance and vital signs and assess the skin, respiratory, cardiovascular, gastrointestinal, genitourinary, musculoskeletal, and neurologic body systems. The baby's behavioral state and parent–newborn interaction should also be assessed. An exam of the baby's fontanelles, eyes, ears, mouth, nose, neck, color, evidence of jaundice, umbilical cord, circumcision if done, reflexes, hydration, nutritional status and feeding history, elimination of urine and stool, activity, sleep–wake cycles, weight, and percentage of change from birth weight should be documented. See Chapter 27 for a complete, step-by-step newborn assessment.

The nurse should ensure that appropriate screening exams as required by the state have been accomplished and to obtain the blood for screening, if still needed. If the newborn did not pass a universal hearing screen before discharge, the nurse should ensure that the parents have a plan to accomplish the required screening or audiology follow-up. The nurse will also assess and reinforce parental knowledge related to newborn/infant care as detailed in the following sections.

ASSESSMENT OF LATE PRETERM NEWBORNS

Late preterm newborns, born between 34 0/7 and 36 6/7 gestational weeks, accounted for 6.87% of total births in the United States in 2015, according to preliminary data (Centers for Disease Control and Prevention [CDC], 2016a). Late preterm newborns have higher morbidity and mortality rates than term babies, as they experience more respiratory complications, apnea, sepsis, jaundice, hypoglycemia, temperature instability, and feeding difficulties (Aly, Hoffman, El-Dib, et al., 2015; Bulut, Gürsoy, & Ovali, 2016). Because of a greater risk for complications, these newborns should be evaluated within 24 to 48 hours of discharge and receive additional follow-up as needed to monitor feeding and weight gain (AAP & ACOG, 2017). A home health nurse visit is an optimal way to meet this need.

A large population-based study discovered that mothers of late preterm newborns were more likely to smoke, less likely to place the newborn on the back to sleep, and less likely to initiate and continue breastfeeding. Despite the AAP recommendations for a follow-up visit 24 to 48 hours after discharge, 11% of late preterm newborns were not seen in the first week after discharge (Hwang et al., 2015). The home health nurse can conduct the recommended visit, report findings to the provider, and reinforce the importance of a smoke-free environment and supine sleep, while also providing breastfeeding support.

Late preterm newborns who are breastfed are more likely to be readmitted to the hospital for jaundice, weight loss, and dehydration than those that are bottle-fed. Although breastfeeding is extremely beneficial for this population, many late preterm newborns are sleepier and lack the developmental maturity to breastfeed efficiently and effectively. They may tire easily, have a weak suck, and have trouble coordinating sucking, swallowing, and breathing. Therefore, they need frequent monitoring, and their mothers require additional assistance to breastfeed effectively and build up their milk supply (Goyal, Attanasio, & Kozhimannil, 2014).

A home health nurse with expertise in breastfeeding support can provide the assistance needed for newborn hydration, growth, and safety. The nurse should talk with the mother about her desires related to feeding. If the newborn is formula-fed, the nurse should observe the mother complete a feeding and note the newborn's behavior during the feeding. Similarly, the breastfeeding couplet should be assessed throughout a feeding for effectiveness and efficiency. See Chapter 29 for details regarding assessment of breastfeeding.

Assessment of intake, output, weight, and hydration status is imperative. Parent education should include the signs of dehydration, adequate feeding parameters, expected urinary/stool output, and the symptoms of jaundice. Parents should be instructed to awaken the late preterm newborn every 2 to 3 hours for breastfeeding and every 3 to 4 hours if formula-feeding. They should keep a record of feedings, voids, and stools. Follow-up visits are indicated to assess ongoing weight gain patterns at least weekly until the newborn is 40 weeks postconception or is thriving (gaining 20 to 30 g/day).

Clinical Tip

If the newborn has lost between 7 and 10% of birth weight at the time of the visit (often on day 3 or 4), assess further by observing and evaluating a breastfeeding. If the mother's milk has come in, the newborn is latching and nursing well, and you hear swallowing, increasing breastfeeding frequency may be all that is needed. Ideally, weigh the breastfeeding newborn before and after the feeding, with the newborn wearing the same diaper (and no other clothing), using a scale that is accurate to within 5 g. This will indicate the approximate amount of breast milk ingested. A weight gain of 30 g (1 ounce) or more following the feeding is reassuring. If the mother's milk has not come in or if the newborn is unable to transfer milk effectively, notify the healthcare provider, as it is likely that temporary supplementation after each breastfeeding will be required to avoid dehydration. Instruct the mother to pump in order to build up her milk supply, and the pumped milk is the first choice for supplementation. If her milk has not come in, supplemental formula may be needed following each breastfeeding in the interim.

If you do not have a highly accurate scale or do not have the expertise to effectively assess breastfeeding, the newborn should be seen by the healthcare provider or by a lactation consultant the same day. Newborns who have lost 10% or more of birth weight need supplementation and should be seen by the healthcare provider.

Late preterm newborns are more likely to develop hyperbilirubinemia (see Chapter 31). If the newborn appears jaundiced, the nurse should assess using a transcutaneous bilirubin screening device (see Figure 31–14) or collect a blood sample for serum bilirubin, if ordered (Lain, Roberts, Bowen, et al., 2015). The Bilitool™ (Bilitool, Inc., 2004–2016) is a reputable online resource that the healthcare team can use to assess risk related to newborn bilirubin levels. Some babies may be undergoing home phototherapy. In these cases, the nurse assesses the baby's color; collects a blood sample, if indicated; and ensures that phototherapy equipment is being used properly.

Late preterm babies are also more likely to acquire infections (see Chapter 31); thus, the nurse should instruct the family members to use good hand hygiene techniques, avoid exposure to individuals with infections or illnesses, and avoid taking the baby out in public. Although later preterm newborns may be similar in size and appearance to term newborns, they require ongoing assessment and care from the family and the healthcare team. Close observation and intervention can help prevent readmission to the hospital and long-term complications.

Positioning and Handling of the Newborn

The nurse demonstrates methods of positioning and handling the newborn as needed. When the newborn is out of the crib, one of the following holds can be used (Figure 34–2). The *cradle hold* is frequently used during feeding. It provides a sense of warmth and closeness, permits eye contact, frees one of the adult's hands, and provides security because the cradling protects the newborn's body. Extra security is provided by gripping the thigh with the hand while the arm supports the newborn's body. The *upright position* provides security and a sense of closeness and is ideal for burping. One hand should support the neck and shoulders while the other hand holds the buttocks or is placed between the newborn's legs. The newborn may also be held upright in a cloth sling carrier that gently holds the baby against the mother's or father's chest and frees the hands for other tasks. The *football hold* frees one of the caregiver's hands and permits eye contact. This hold is ideal for shampooing, carrying, or breastfeeding.

Skin Care and Bathing

The skin maintains temperature and serves as a barrier between the newborn and the environment, but is also a potential portal of entry for environmental toxins and infectious agents. Keeping the skin healthy and intact can be ensured by ongoing frequent assessment, effective cleansing, effective moisturizing, and maintenance of an effective barrier against external irritants.

An actual bath demonstration is the best way for the nurse to provide information to parents. Immersion bathing, in which the newborn is placed in a small tub with the caregiver keeping the head and neck above water, results in less heat loss than sponge bathing, and it is safe prior to cord separation provided the cord is dried at the end of the bath. Water temperature should be 38° to 40°C (100.4° to 104°F) (Ball & Bindler, 2016). The room should be warm and free of drafts to maintain the newborn's temperature during the bath.

Excess bathing and use of soap removes natural skin oils and dries out the newborn's sensitive skin; therefore, bathing should be limited to every other day and to 10 minutes in length. Mild liquid cleansing agents with a neutral to mildly acidic pH (5.5 to 7.0) that are fragrance- and preservative-free are recommended if soap is used. Because cleansers can be drying to the skin, they should be used sparingly and thoroughly removed by rinsing. Antimicrobial soaps should be avoided, as they may disturb the baby's normal skin colonization. Products containing chlorhexidine and alcohol should be avoided as well (Association of Women's Health, Obstetric, and Neonatal Nursing [AWHONN], 2013; Ness et al., 2013; Visscher, Adam, & Brink, 2015).

Many birthing units and agencies provide specialty television channels for parents to watch before bathing their baby for the first time, as a home visit does not usually allow time for a nurse demonstration and a parent return demonstration of a bath. See *Women with Special Needs: Newborn Care* and *Teaching Highlights: Newborn Bathing*.

Supplies can be kept in a plastic bag or container for convenience (Box 34–1). At home, the family may want to use a small plastic dishpan, a clean kitchen or bathroom sink, or a large bowl

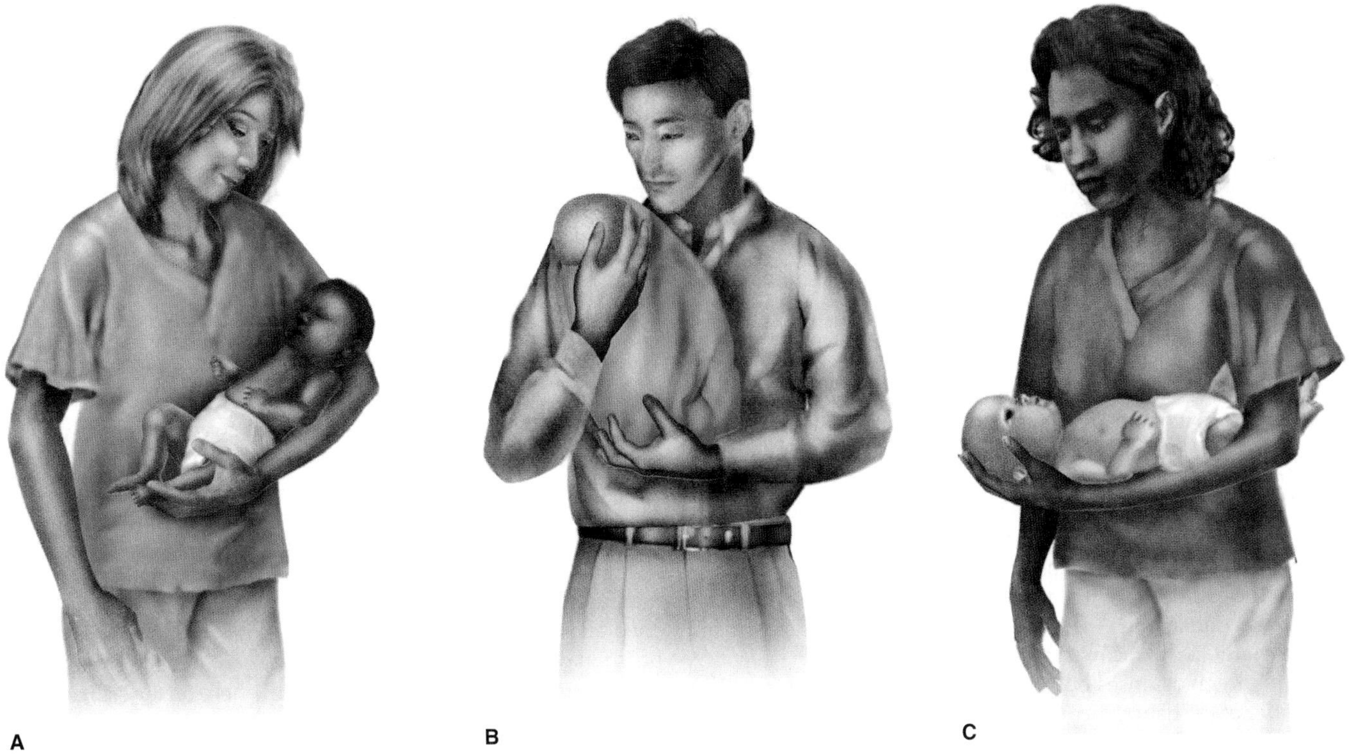

Figure 34–2 Various positions for holding a newborn. A. Cradle hold. B. Upright position. C. Football hold.

Women with Special Needs Newborn Care

Women with multiple sclerosis (MS) are typically asymptomatic during pregnancy but may develop worsening MS symptoms after birth. The nurses should evaluate the woman's level of functioning. Some modifications or assistance with newborn care such as bathing may be needed for these women.

Box 34-1
Bath Supplies

- Washcloths (2)
- Towels (2)
- Blankets (2)
- Unperfumed mild skin cleanser
- Shampoo
- Petrolatum product or diaper ointment, if indicated
- Diapers
- Clean clothes

as the baby's tub. Commercial plastic baby tubs are not necessary, but some parents prefer to purchase them.

SPONGE BATH

After the supplies are gathered, the tub (or any of the containers mentioned) is filled with approximately 5 inches of water that is warm to the touch. Parents can test the water temperature against their forearm or use a thermometer to help them determine when the bath water is comfortable and safe to use (38° to 40°C [100.4° to 104°F]).

Clinical Tip

Remind parents to never leave a baby unattended to answer the phone or door. Initial bathing can be performed when another adult is available to retrieve forgotten items, attend to interruptions, and provide support. Advise the parents to gather supplies before beginning. Advise parents to maintain at least one hand on the baby at all times.

TEACHING HIGHLIGHTS | Newborn Bathing

- Describe the proper environment (including safety factors) for sponge and tub bathing for newborns.
- Identify proper bathing supplies that are needed for both sponge and tub baths and encourage the mother to assemble supplies before beginning the newborn bath to avoid cold exposure and ensure that proper supplies are being used.
- Explain the need for neutral-pH, fragrance-free, and dye-free cleansing products for newborn use.
- Demonstrate sponge bathing.
- Discuss and demonstrate tub bathing using a newborn model.
- Encourage the family to ask questions as they arise. Help instill confidence in new parents.

The newborn is placed on a flat protected surface, such as a counter covered in towels or in a bassinet adjacent to the container of water for a sponge bath. The newborn should be wrapped in a blanket, with a T-shirt and diaper on, to provide warmth and security. Parents should be reminded never to leave a baby unattended on an elevated surface or near any amount of water. Parents should be encouraged to keep one hand on their baby at all times and to keep their eyes on their baby at all times while positioned for a bath.

To start the sponge bath, the adult wraps the dampened washcloth around the index finger once. Each eye is gently wiped from inner to outer canthus. This direction prevents the potential for clogging the tear duct at the inner canthus, where the eye naturally drains. A different portion of the washcloth is used for each eye to prevent cross-contamination. Some eye swelling and drainage may be present the first few days after birth as a result of the eye prophylaxis.

The bath giver washes the ears next by wrapping the washcloth once around an index finger and gently cleaning the external ear and behind the ear. Cotton swabs (Q-tips) are never used in the ear canal because it is possible to put a swab too far into the ear and damage the eardrum. In addition, a swab may push any discharge farther down into the ear canal.

The caregiver rinses out the washcloth and then wipes the remainder of the baby's face with the warm, dampened soap-free washcloth. The face should be washed every day, and the mouth and chin should be wiped off after each feeding.

The neck is washed carefully but thoroughly with the washcloth. A mild soap may now be used if skin is visibly soiled. Formula or breast milk and lint collect in the skin folds of the neck, so it may be helpful to sit the newborn up, supporting the neck and shoulders with one hand while washing the neck with the other hand.

When sponge-bathing, the bath giver will want to bathe the upper and lower body separately to minimize heat loss. Once the face and neck are clean and dry, the bath giver unwraps the blanket, removes the T-shirt, and wets the chest, back, and arms with the washcloth. The bath giver may then lather his or her hands with a mild infant skin cleanser and wash the baby's chest, back, and arms. Soap is rinsed off with the wet washcloth, and the upper part of the body is dried with a towel or blanket. The newborn's upper body is then wrapped with a clean, dry blanket to prevent heat loss.

Next, the bath giver unwraps the newborn's legs, wets them with the washcloth, and lathers, rinses, and dries them well. If the newborn has dry skin, a small amount of an emollient such as petrolatum may be used. Baby oil is not recommended because it clogs skin pores. Families need to be aware that baby powder should be avoided, as it can cause serious respiratory problems if the baby inhales it. The genital area is cleansed after each wet or dirty diaper. Females are washed from the front of the genital area toward the rectum to avoid fecal contamination of the urethra and the bladder. Newborn females often have a thick, white mucous discharge or a slight bloody discharge from the vaginal area. This discharge is normal for the first 1 to 2 weeks after birth. The mucus may come off if wiped gently after diaper changes but should not be intentionally scrubbed off.

Parents of uncircumcised males should cleanse the penis daily. Retraction of the foreskin is not advised (see in-depth discussion of care of uncircumcised and circumcised male babies in Chapter 28). Males who have been circumcised also need their penises cleansed daily. A very wet washcloth is squeezed above the baby's penis, allowing clear water to run over the circumcision site. The area is gently patted or fanned dry. Soap is not used around the penis for the first 3 to 4 days following circumcision, as it can be irritating to the tissues. A small amount of an emollient such as petrolatum or petrolatum-impregnated gauze strips may be applied during each diaper change for the first 24 to 48 hours. Emollients promote comfort and healing and prevent adherence of the diaper to the site. It is important to avoid using ointments if a Plastibell is in place because ointments may cause the Plastibell ring to slip off the penis too early. The Plastibell usually falls off within 5 to 8 days. If it does not, the family needs to call the healthcare provider (AAP & ACOG, 2017). For more information, see *Health Promotion: Newborn Circumcision Care* in Chapter 28.

The newborn should be wrapped in a terry cloth bath towel or bath blanket and gently patted dry at the end of the bath to promote skin integrity and prevent heat loss. It is particularly important that the cord be thoroughly dried if it has become wet during the bath.

The last step in bathing is washing the hair (although some prefer to do this step first). The newborn is swaddled in a dry blanket, leaving only the head exposed, and held in the football hold with the head tilted slightly downward. A cup or cupped hand may be used to pour warm water over the newborn's head, taking care to avoid the eyes and ear canals. Parents should avoid placing the baby's head directly under running water, as changes in water temperature could cause burns or discomfort. The hair is moistened and lathered with a small amount of shampoo. A very soft brush may be used to massage the shampoo over the entire head, including the fontanelles, which families often call the "soft spots." The hair is then rinsed and toweled dry. Oils or lotions are not used on the newborn's head unless prescribed by a healthcare provider.

TUB BATHS

When tub-bathing, the bath can be completed efficiently with the newborn's trunk and lower extremities underwater. The newborn's face, eyes, ears, and neck can be washed and dried as described before undressing him or her for the tub bath. A large, clean kitchen or bathroom sink, plastic container, or commercial tub that allows the baby to be immersed to the neck may be used as the bathing tub. A washcloth can be placed in the bottom of the bathing tub to prevent slippage. The baby should be held securely at all times (Figure 34–3). Commercial tubs often

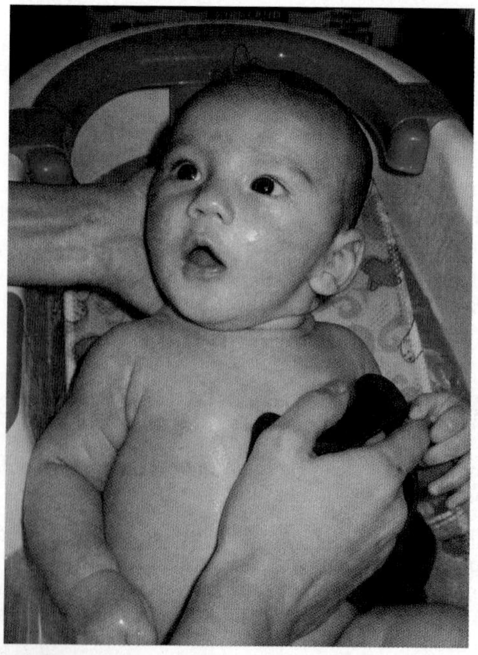

Figure 34–3 **When bathing the newborn, the caregiver must support the head. Wet babies are very slippery.**

SOURCE: Michele Davidson.

support the baby's head and neck. If desired by the parents and if time allows, the nurse can demonstrate how to securely support the baby while giving an immersion bath.

Because wet newborns are slippery, some parents pull a cotton sock (with holes cut out for the fingers) over the supporting arm to provide a "nonskid" surface. The newborn's body is washed with a soapy washcloth or hand. To wash the back, the bath giver places the noncradling hand on the newborn's chest with the thumb under the newborn's arm closest to the adult. Gently tipping the newborn forward onto the supporting hand frees the cradling arm to wash the back. After the bath, the newborn is lifted out of the tub in the cradle position, dried well, and wrapped in a dry blanket. If the cord has not fallen off, it should be thoroughly dried before re-covering with clothing. The hair is then washed in the same way as for a sponge bath.

Once the bath is complete, the parents can double-blanket the newborn in clean dry blankets and a hat for approximately 10 minutes. Once the baby is totally dry, they may dress the baby and apply a clean, dry hat and blanket. The nurse must educate parents that babies and young children can drown even in small amounts of water. It is paramount that adults not allow the baby to be immersed above the neck and that they keep the baby safe by maintaining hand, arm, and eye contact with the baby at all times during the tub bath.

Cord Care

The parents should be instructed to allow the cord to dry naturally. They should be taught to:

- Wash their hands before and after handling the cord.
- Keep the cord clean and dry.
- Keep the cord exposed to air or covered only loosely by clean clothes.
- Keep the diaper folded below the cord to prevent contamination.
- Clean the cord if it becomes soiled with urine or stool.
- Dry the cord thoroughly after each cleansing.

There is no evidence to support the routine application of topical agents such as alcohol or triple dye to the cord in developed countries (AAP & ACOG, 2017). Application of antiseptics delayed the time to cord separation when compared with dry cord care in a number of studies (AAP & ACOG, 2017). Although a 2015 Cochrane Review found that application of chlorhexidine to neonatal skin and to the umbilical cord decreased life-threatening infections in some countries, ongoing research is needed related to the absorption and safety of chlorhexidine in newborns (Sinha, Sazawal, Pradhan, et al., 2015).

The nurse should teach the parents to inspect the cord during each diaper change and bath. Parents can be reassured that the stump may smell earthy as it necroses. Although a small amount of mucous may be present, the parents should consult their healthcare provider immediately if they notice drainage from the stump or at the point of attachment, if the cord or drainage smells foul, or if they notice redness, swelling, or other discoloration of the surrounding skin. This could indicate *omphalitis* (infection of the umbilical cord stump) or *necrotizing fasciitis* (soft tissue infection), potentially fatal complications (AAP & ACOG, 2017). Signs of systemic infection such as fever, inability to maintain temperature, poor feeding, or lethargy should always be reported. Parents should also notify the provider if the cord doesn't fall off within 15 days or if the area fails to heal within 2 or 3 days of separation.

Nail Care

During the first days of life, the nails may adhere to the skin of the fingers, and cutting is contraindicated. Within a week the nails separate from the skin and frequently break off. If the nails are long or if the newborn is scratching his or her face, the nails may be gently filed using a newborn file. This is most easily done while the baby is asleep. Newborn socks or mittens may be used to cover the newborn's hands and prevent facial scratching.

Dressing the Newborn

Newborns need to wear a T-shirt, diaper (diaper cover if using cloth diapers), and a sleeper. At home, the temperature determines the amount of clothing the newborn wears. Families who maintain their home at 60° to 69°F should dress the baby more warmly than those who maintain a temperature of 70°F or higher.

Clinical Tip

Dressing a newborn with a T-shirt can be quite a challenge. First, pull the T-shirt over the baby's head. The next challenge is getting the arms in the sleeves because the newborn grasps at the fabric of the T-shirt as you try to pull it over the hands and arms. It helps to put your hand through the right sleeve of the T-shirt and hold the baby's right hand. Then pull the sleeve over your hand. Repeat the same movements for the left sleeve.

Newborns should wear a head covering outdoors to protect their sensitive ears from drafts and to prevent heat loss. Parents can wrap a blanket around the baby, leaving one corner free to place over the head for added protection while outdoors or in crowds. The nurse must advise families about the ease with which a newborn's skin can burn when exposed to the sun. To prevent sunburn, the newborn should remain shaded, wear a light layer of clothing, or be protected with sunscreen specifically formulated for babies. Many healthcare professionals, however, recommend avoiding sunscreen until the infant is at least 6 months old.

Diaper shapes vary and are subject to personal preference. Prefolded and disposable diapers are usually rectangular. Cloth diapers may also be triangular or kite-folded. Extra material is placed in front for males and toward the back for females to increase absorbency. See Figure 34–4. Although some parents prefer to use traditional cloth diapers, the use of super-absorbent disposable diapers decreases the incidence of diaper dermatitis (Harfmann, Chen, & Whitman, 2017).

Baby clothing should be laundered separately with a mild soap or detergent. Diapers are generally presoaked before washing. All clothing should be rinsed twice to remove soap and residue and to decrease the possibility of rash. Some newborns may not tolerate clothing treated with fabric softeners added to the washer or dryer.

SWADDLING THE NEWBORN

Swaddling (wrapping) helps the newborn maintain body temperature, provides a feeling of closeness and security, and may be effective in quieting a crying baby by having the newborn's hands near the mouth to allow for sucking (Davidson, 2014). If the baby is not resting, placing its hands at its sides then swaddling reduces the amount of stimulation of hand-to-mouth movement and may allow the child to rest. When wrapping the baby, a blanket is placed on the crib (or secure surface) in the shape of a diamond. The top corner of the blanket is folded down slightly,

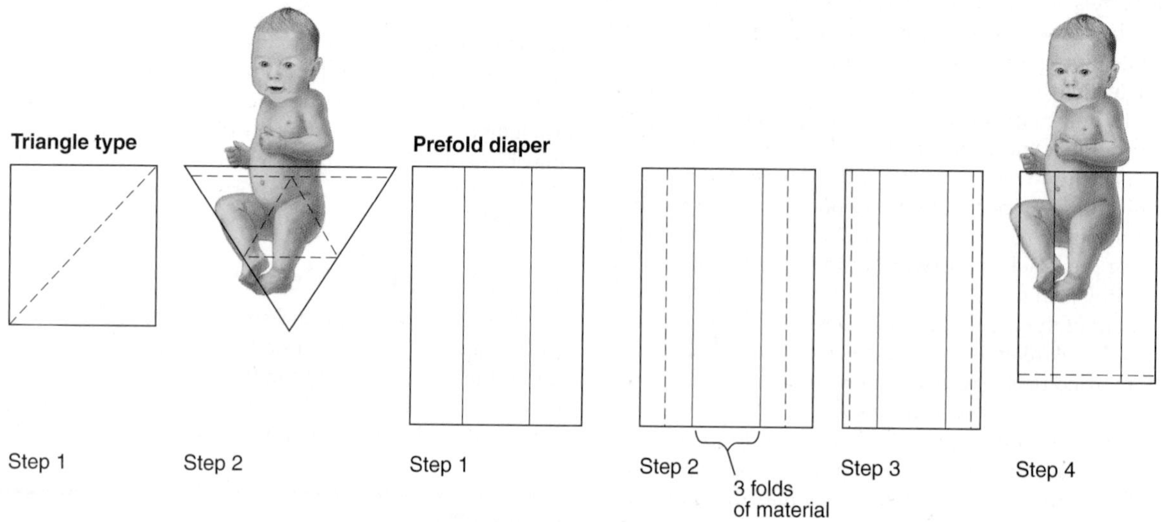

Figure 34–4 **Two basic cloth diaper shapes. Dotted lines indicate folds.**

and the newborn's body is placed with the head at the upper edge of the blanket. The right corner of the blanket is wrapped around the baby and tucked under the left side (not too tightly—newborns need a little room to move and to allow for hands to get to the mouth). The bottom corner is then pulled up to the chest, and the left corner is wrapped around the baby's right side (Figure 34–5). The nurse can show this wrapping technique to a new mother so she will feel more skilled in handling her baby.

Temperature Assessment, Fever, and Illness

As the nurse prepares to teach parents about taking their baby's temperature, it is important to provide opportunities for discussion and demonstration. Families often need a review of how to take their baby's temperature and when to call their primary healthcare provider.

Parents need to take the newborn's temperature only when signs of illness are present. Axillary temperatures are used to determine temperature stability and readiness for discharge in healthy newborns, and a newborn axillary temperature of 36.5° to 37.4°C (97.7° to 99.3°F) is considered normal (AAP & ACOG, 2017). Although the axillary temperature doesn't correlate closely with the rectal temperature, this method is convenient, easy for parents to employ, and poses low risk to the newborn. See Figure 27–16.

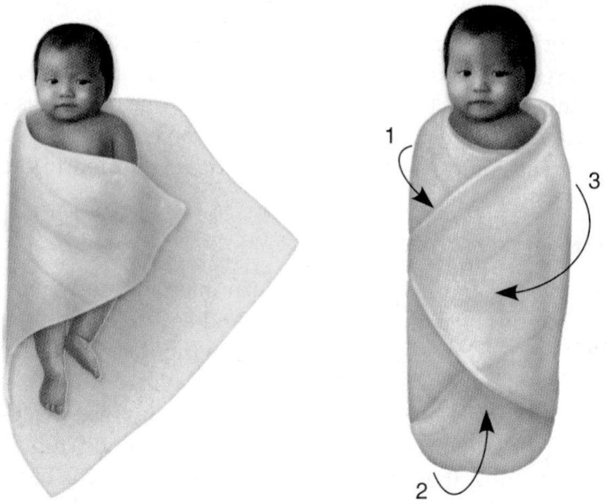

Figure 34–5 **Steps in wrapping a baby.**

The rectal method was once considered the gold standard for measuring temperatures of febrile babies, as rectal temperature is closer to the true core temperature found in the pulmonary artery, but it carries the risk of rectal trauma, which can result in rare but life-threatening complications (Syrkin-Nikolau, Johnson, Colaizy, et al., 2017). Recent research has shown that temporal artery thermometers are accurate when used in an open crib to obtain newborn temperature. It should be noted that some studies have found that when readings are obtained from newborns in an isolette, these readings may become less accurate due to the controlled internal temperature in closed environments (Syrkin-Nikolau et al., 2017). Thermometers that use infrared scanning to measure temporal artery temperature are commercially available and have become more common in both healthcare settings and in the home environment. These devices are placed on the newborn's forehead and a reading is displayed within a few seconds (Syrkin-Nikolau et al., 2017).

Measuring the axillary temperature with an electronic thermometer is a safe screening method for a baby less than 4 weeks of age. Because an absolute fixed conversion isn't possible, the approximate rectal temperature can be determined by adding 0.4°C to the axillary temperature of a term newborn (Lantz & Ottosson, 2015). Tympanic thermometer measurements are not recommended, as they have not been found to be accurate in young babies.

Some parents use skin palpation to determine temperature. This is not a reliable way to measure fevers in young babies, yet parents are often able to detect the presence or absence of a fever with palpation. In the absence of one best answer, the nurse can recommend that parents purchase a new thermometer that is designed to measure temperature in babies. It is helpful for nurses to periodically check thermometer availability at local and online retailers and to review current academic and manufacturers' literature. The parents may also want to discuss their choice of temperature measurement location and type of thermometer with their primary healthcare provider.

The nurse should ensure that parents do not plan to use a mercury thermometer. Breakage of mercury thermometers has caused symptomatic mercury poisoning in children and adults, and improper disposal contributes to environmental contamination. Mercury thermometers should not be used or kept in homes and should be disposed of at a hazardous waste collection site (U.S. Environmental Protection Agency [EPA], 2016). Parents can contact their local health department or review websites for the EPA or CDC if they need additional information.

Parents should use the same thermometer and measurement site during the course of one illness in order to more accurately monitor trends in the baby's temperature. The parents should inform the pediatric healthcare provider of the temperature, the site, and the type of thermometer used. Most healthcare providers will verify temperature with a rectal measurement when evaluating a baby for fever.

Traditionally, a rectal temperature of 38°C (100.4°F) has been considered a fever. Because babies under 90 days of age, and particularly those under 30 days of age, are at high risk for serious bacterial infections, the nurse should tell parents to see their healthcare provider if their newborn has an axillary temperature of 37.4°C (99.4°F) or greater. It will be important for the parents to document the measured temperature, time of measurement, and the method used. Parents can expect that their baby will be admitted and receive a febrile workup, including blood and urine cultures, urinalysis, complete blood count, chest x-ray, and lumbar puncture if he or she has a fever before 1 month of age. Infants between 1 and 3 months of age will receive the febrile evaluation and may or may not be admitted, depending on symptoms (DePorre, Aronson, & McCulloh, 2017). Parents need to be informed that newborns with systemic infection may not be febrile but may exhibit more subtle manifestations such as temperature instability, poor feeding, abdominal distention, inability to tolerate feedings, apnea, or alterations in behavior such as irritability or lethargy. A baby who is feeding poorly or just not acting right, even in the absence of a fever, may be exhibiting signs of potentially serious infection. Therefore, parents of young babies should call their primary care provider immediately for any signs of illness and/or fever, rather than treating the baby at home. Although acetaminophen and ibuprofen are not contraindicated in babies, a baby who experiences symptoms requiring these medications needs to be evaluated by a healthcare provider.

SAFETY ALERT!

Parents should not administer any over-the-counter (OTC) cough or cold medications to their baby. OTC antihistamine and decongestant preparations have not been demonstrated to be helpful in young children and are potentially harmful to them. The AAP (2003) and the Food and Drug Administration (FDA, 2016) have issued warnings against their use in children under the age of 2 years. Additionally, parents should never give young children any medication designed for adult use, and parents should not give more than one medication concurrently to their child unless prescribed by their provider.

Stools and Urine

The appearance and frequency of a newborn's stools can cause concern for parents. The nurse prepares them by discussing and showing pictures of meconium stools and transitional stools and by describing the difference between breast milk and formula stools. Although each baby develops his or her own stooling patterns, parents can get an idea of what to expect (see Figure 29–15).

- Babies can be expected to have at least one meconium stool on the first day of life and at least one or two during the second 24 hours. For breastfed babies, one to four stools can be expected each day by 3 to 4 days of age, and three to five per day by 1 week of age. Stools progress from meconium on the first 2 days to transitional (greenish-brown) stools to mushy yellow and seedy by day 4. Once breastfeeding is well established, usually by 1 month of age, individual babies vary in their stooling patterns. Constipation is unlikely to occur in newborns receiving only breast milk. Infrequent stooling in the first few weeks may indicate inadequate milk intake (Koehn & Dowling, 2016; Smith, 2016).
- Formula-fed babies may have only one or two stools a day; their stools are more formed and may be darker yellow or brown in color.

The nurse can show parents pictures of a constipated stool (small, pellet-like) and diarrhea (watery, loose, green). Families should understand that a green color is common in transitional stools so that they do not mistake transitional stools for diarrhea during the first week of a newborn's life.

Babies normally void (urinate) at least once in the first 24 hours and at least twice in the second 24 hours. At least three to five daily voids can be expected on days 3 through 5. By the fifth day of life and thereafter, the newborn can be expected to have five or more wet diapers per day. A breastfeeding newborn who has six or more urine-soaked diapers and five or more yellow stools per day by 1 week of age is likely well hydrated and getting enough milk (Smith, 2016). Fewer may indicate that the newborn needs more fluids. Parents who use super-absorbent single-use disposable diapers may have difficulty determining voiding patterns because the surface of the diaper feels dry. The liquid pools inside the filling of the diaper. Parents can pull the top layer off to check whether the filling is saturated. Although pink or orange uric acid crystals may be found in the diaper during the first few days of life, the presence of crystals beyond the third or fourth day may indicate inadequate hydration.

DIAPER AREA CARE

The diaper area should be cleansed and well dried with each diaper change. Frequent diaper changes minimize contact between the skin and urine or stool and decrease the risk of *diaper dermatitis (DD)*—often referred to by parents as diaper rash. It is also helpful to allow the baby to spend short periods of time air-drying with the diaper off in order to prevent maceration and irritation. Minimal soap is required when cleaning the diaper area, and scrubbing should be avoided. If the parents use commercial diaper wipes, they should be alcohol-free. If an emollient with petrolatum is routinely used as a barrier to protect the skin in the diaper area, the parents do not need to scrub all of it off with each diaper change (Reich, Psomadakis, & Buka, 2017).

Even with proper care, many babies experience some type of diaper rash. This can take the form of a contact dermatitis, otherwise known as *irritant diaper dermatitis (IDD)*, a localized, nonimmunologic reaction to the friction, occlusion, moisture, urine, feces, and chemicals in the diaper environment. Moisturizers such as petrolatum provide protection from wetness and promote healing of mildly irritated skin. If diaper rash occurs, parents should also apply a protective skin barrier containing zinc oxide to prevent further injury. A thin layer of petrolatum can be placed on top of the zinc oxide layer to prevent the diaper from sticking. Fecal material and urine should be removed with each diaper change, but the skin barrier should be maintained if possible and reapplied as necessary.

A variety of commercial newborn care barrier products are available, which contain either petrolatum or zinc oxide. Some products also contain lanolin, which protects the skin but may be allergenic to some babies. The nurse can recommend a commercial product or tell the parents to choose one with petrolatum and another with zinc oxide. Baby powder and cornstarch should not be used as they are considered an inhalation risk.

When the rash is severe or persists beyond 2 to 3 days despite the treatment above, the parents should contact their healthcare provider. DD is frequently complicated by *Candida albicans*. If this is the case, the provider can prescribe a topical agent containing an antifungal such as miconazole, zinc oxide, and petrolatum (Reich et al., 2017).

Sleeping

When, where, and for how long their baby sleeps are common concerns of parents. The following sections address prevention of sudden infant death syndrome and sudden unexpected infant death, crib safety, and the proper positioning of a baby for sleep. The newborn's sleep–wake states are then described.

SIDS AND SUID PREVENTION

Sudden infant death syndrome (SIDS) is defined as a sudden death in a child less than 12 months of age that is not explained by autopsy, site investigation, and clinical history. **Sudden unexpected infant death (SUID)** includes SIDS as well as deaths that are explained by a thorough investigation. The incidence of SIDS decreased dramatically as a result of the AAP's 1992 "Back to Sleep" campaign, but the number of SUIDs that occurred during sleep increased in recent years. The AAP expanded the "Back to Sleep" guidelines in 2011 and again in 2016 (now called "Safe to Sleep") to decrease the risk of SUID related to asphyxiation, suffocation, and/or entrapment during sleep.

Nurses should educate parents about the following AAP (2016) recommendations to promote a safe sleep environment and decrease the risk of SIDS and SUID in infants less than 12 months of age:

- Babies should sleep on their backs every time they are put down for sleep (Figure 34–6); all caregivers should be informed that side positioning is unsafe.

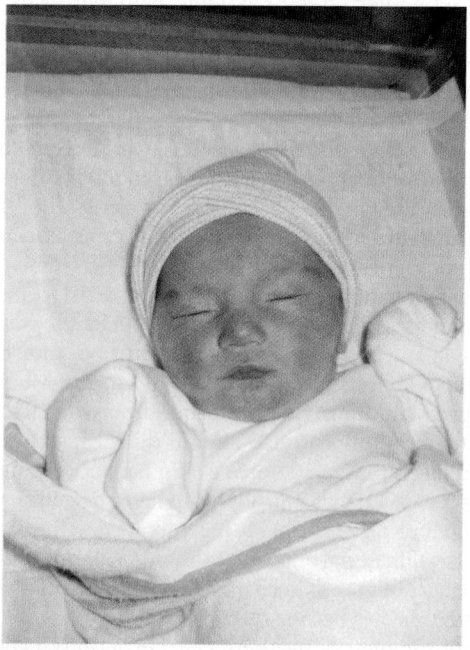

Figure 34–6 Babies should be placed on their backs when sleeping.

SOURCE: Michele Davidson.

- Babies should sleep on a firm surface, preferably in a crib or bassinet that meets Consumer Product Safety Commission requirements.
- Babies should sleep in the same room as their parent(s) or an adult care provider, but they should *not* share the bed with anyone. Bed-sharing before 4 months of months of age—with individuals who smoke, with individuals other than parents, with individuals who use sedating substances, on soft surfaces, or with soft pillows—is particularly dangerous.
- Babies' cribs should have no loose bedding (blankets, quilts, pillows, etc.) or soft objects (toys, crib bumpers, etc.) during sleep time.
- Babies should not be exposed to smoking before or after birth.
- Babies should not be exposed to alcohol or illicit drugs during pregnancy or through breastfeeding.
- Babies should be breastfed unless contraindicated. Exclusive breastfeeding for at least 6 months is ideal, but any amount is better than none.
- Babies should be offered a pacifier while falling asleep.
- Babies should not be overheated by the use of too many covers during sleep.
- Babies should receive their immunizations on time as recommended by the CDC. Immunizations do not cause SIDS, and they may protect against it.
- Babies should not sleep with commercial devices marketed to maintain position. Safety has not been established.
- Babies should not sleep attached to cardiorespiratory monitors unless prescribed by their healthcare provider for a specific health condition. Monitors have not been demonstrated to reduce the risk of SUID.
- Babies should have "tummy time" when they are awake and observed by an adult to prevent positional plagiocephaly and to promote motor development.
- Pregnant women should follow the recommended schedule for prenatal care, as regular prenatal care reduces the risk of SIDS.

Clinical Tip

Explain and expand on the AAP (2016) safe sleep environment guidelines to make them understandable for families and caregivers. For example, describe plagiocephaly as a flattened area on the head and recommend that parents alternate their baby's head position between the right and the left side when placing the baby supine for sleep. Placing the baby's head at alternate ends of the crib every few days is helpful as well. The baby commonly turns the head toward the activity in the room. Alternating the orientation of the baby in the crib to the location of usual activity in the room will limit the time spent in a given resting position and will decrease the risk of positional plagiocephaly. Demonstrate these positions for the parents, reinforce the importance of supine sleep in relation to SIDS and SUID prevention, and give parents other ideas for carrying and positioning, such as the safe use of front packs, backpacks, and slings.

The AAP guidelines are for healthy babies, and parents should follow them unless otherwise directed by their healthcare provider in response to a particular medical condition. Nurses have the opportunity to assess for risk factors in the home environment and to educate families, particularly patients in groups

EVIDENCE-BASED PRACTICE | Bed-Sharing and the Risk of Sudden Infant Death Syndrome

Clinical Question

Why do mothers continue the practice of bed-sharing in the face of evidence that it is associated with a higher risk of SIDS?

The Evidence

Multiple studies have demonstrated the association between bed-sharing with a neonate and the incidence of SIDS. These risks are the greatest for the neonate who is not yet 4 months old (AAP, 2016). Yet women continue to bed-share with their newborns/infants even when informed that the practice is risky. Nurse researchers conducted a study to determine the reasons why mothers continue the practice. They interviewed 56 mothers about their plans and actual practices related to newborn sleep locations. Approximately 11% of participants originally planned to sleep with their newborns because of convenience in provision of newborn care, personal preference, or lack of a bassinet. However, nearly 48% reported bed-sharing during the first month of the newborn's life. The most common reason cited for bed-sharing was the baby's fussiness. Other reasons included maternal preference for closeness to the baby, desire to monitor newborn well-being, and feeding convenience (Tully, Holditch-Davis, & Brandon, 2015).

Best Practice

Parents and caregivers should be cautioned not to share a bed, sofa, chair, or any other surface with a baby for sleep. Sharing a sleep surface with a baby after consuming drugs or alcohol is particularly hazardous. Nurses should inform new parents that the risk of SIDS decreases by up to 50% in babies who sleep on a surface designed for newborns/infants that is separate from, yet close to, the parents' bed (Moon & AAP Task Force, 2016). Anticipatory discussions about the importance of room-sharing without bed-sharing and plans for responding to fussy infants and frequent feedings may assist new parents to consider safety and nighttime responses in advance.

Clinical Reasoning

What alternatives can be taught to the mother to get the baby to sleep other than bed sharing? How can the mother protect the baby if she does bring the baby to her bed?

at high risk for SIDS and SUID. Parents can be encouraged to attend infant cardiopulmonary resuscitation (CPR) classes, especially if there is a family history of SIDS, SUID, prematurity, or another health problem. See *Evidence-Based Practice: Bed-Sharing and the Risk of Sudden Infant Death Syndrome.*

Nurses and parents can find additional free information about the Safe to Sleep Campaign in English and Spanish at the National Institute of Child Health and Human Development (NICHD) website. See *Case Study: Azia Askari.*

CRIB SAFETY

During the home visit, the nurse discusses with the family their newborn's sleeping arrangements and observes the crib, bassinet, cradle, mat, or other devices. The crib should be a recent model with a mattress that fits snugly and is designed to prevent entrapment and suffocation. If possible, the nurse should observe the baby while sleeping to ensure all safety precautions are being followed. The Consumer Product Safety Commission (CPSC) updated its requirements for crib safety in 2011. Although a full discussion of the requirements is beyond the scope of this chapter, nurses and families can access additional information about safety related to cribs and other infant products at the CPSC website. Some new parents find helpful information regarding infant product safety through consumer or parenting magazines, online websites, and apps. The nurse can assist parents to determine the credibility of specific resources.

The newborn/infant should always be placed on the back from the time of birth. Some nurses may turn a blind eye to safety risks such as bed-sharing or the placement of stuffed animals and fluffy blankets in newborn bassinets and cribs. Nurses should begin modeling safe practice for parents on the newborn's first day of life by placing the newborn directly on the back whenever skin-to-skin care (SSC) isn't in progress. Full endorsement by nurses of evidence-based, safe-to-sleep practices for babies is essential to prevent parental confusion and to promote safety for the baby. See *Professionalism in Practice: Professional Nurse Endorsement of Safe to Sleep Guidelines.*

Proper Positioning

Some parents may resist supine positioning due to fears about aspiration. The nurse can encourage parents to hold their babies upright for 10 to 15 minutes following feedings. Additionally, nurses can reassure parents that the newborn gag reflex is

CASE STUDY: Azia Askari

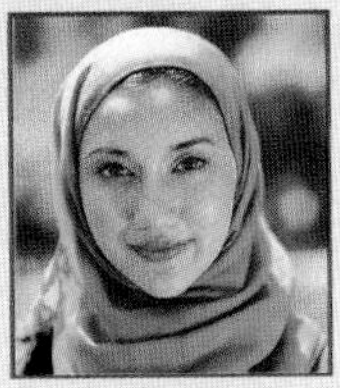

SOURCE: HONGQI ZHANG/123RF.

Azia is scheduled for a home visit from a local postpartum nursing agency. She is breastfeeding her newborn and states the family is adjusting well. Her other children are adjusting well to their new brother. Azia tells you she often plays games with her older children while the baby naps to ensure they feel they are getting enough attention. During naps, she places the baby on his back in the crib. She says that at night the baby sleeps with her and her husband so she can avoid having to get up throughout the night.

Questions to Ponder

How would you educate this couple on proper sleeping conditions for babies? What is the preferred position and sleep location for babies?

Professionalism in Practice **Professional Nurse Endorsement of Safe to Sleep Guidelines**

In addition to the recommendations for the home sleep environment, the AAP (2016) included guidelines that apply to healthcare providers and other professionals.

- Healthcare professionals should endorse and model the guidelines designed to prevent SUID and SIDS beginning at birth.
- Manufacturers should follow the guidelines in all marketing and advertising.
- The campaign should expand beyond SIDS reduction to the promotion of an overall safe sleep environment.

Abney-Roberts (2015) described enhanced modeling of newborn/infant safe sleep practices on a nursing unit as a result of staff education and introduction of Safe to Sleep protocols. Professional nurses should initiate quality improvement related to clinical practice and parental education in healthcare settings.

protective and that choking and aspiration are less likely to occur in the supine position. Many mothers return to the workforce during the first year of their newborn's life, so the nurse should remind parents to educate family members and others who will care for the newborn in their absence about the importance of supine sleep positioning and insist that it is practiced with their child. See *Case Study: Melissa Bond-James.*

Sleep–Wake States

The newborn demonstrates several different sleep–wake states after the initial periods of reactivity. It is not uncommon for a newborn to sleep almost continuously for the first 2 to 3 days following birth, awakening only for feedings every 3 to 4 hours. Some newborns bypass this stage of deep sleep and require only 12 to 16 hours of sleep, but most require at least 16 to 18 hours of sleep each day. The parents need to know that this is normal.

Sleep states include deep sleep and light sleep. During **deep sleep** (also referred to as *quiet sleep*) the baby will be nearly still except for occasional startles. It is characterized by slow and regular heart rate and regular respirations. Eyes are closed and eye movement is absent. The newborn will arouse to intense stimuli, but care and feeding at this time will be frustrating. **Light sleep** (also referred to as *active sleep*) makes up the highest proportion of newborn sleep and usually precedes awakening. It is characterized by some body movements, rapid eye movements (REM), more variation in heart and respiratory rates, and brief fussing or crying (Brazelton & Nugent, 2011). The baby may rouse, remain in light sleep, or return to deep sleep in response to stimuli. Babies are not usually ready to feed in this state.

Awake states include drowsy, quiet alert, active alert, and crying states. During the **drowsy state**, newborns open and close their eyes, but the eyes appear dull and the face is often still. They may return to sleep or awaken further in response to stimuli. The **quiet alert state** (also called *wide awake state*) is characterized by a brightening of the eyes and face. Newborns are most attentive to their environment in this state and provide positive feedback to caregivers (Brazelton & Nugent, 2011; McGrath & Vittner, 2015). Quiet alert is an optimal state during which to initiate breastfeedings (Koehn & Dowling, 2016). The **active alert state** (also called *active awake state*) brings about an increase in facial and body movement, with periods of fussiness occurring. The newborn in this state has increased sensitivity to disturbing stimuli, and intervention to console the baby at this point is beneficial. The **crying state** is evidenced by increased motor activity, grimaces, eyes tightly closed or open, and extreme responsiveness to stimuli (Brazelton & Nugent, 2011; McGrath & Vittner, 2015). Babies may be able to console themselves, or they may require consoling from a caregiver.

For newborns, crying is a spontaneous response to unpleasant stimuli and their only means of expressing their needs vocally. After 2 or 3 days, newborns settle into individual patterns and families learn to distinguish different tones and qualities of their newborn's cry. The amount of crying is also highly individual. Some newborns cry as little as 15 to 30 minutes in 24 hours, others as long as 2 or more hours. When crying continues after causes such as discomfort and hunger are eliminated, the newborn may be comforted by swaddling, rocking, or other reassuring activities. There is some indication that newborns who are held more tend to be calmer and cry less when not being held. Some parents may be afraid that holding will "spoil" the newborn and need reassurance that this is not the case. On the contrary, picking babies up when they cry teaches them that adults

> "It was so exciting to go home with our new baby. That first day went quite well, and Joe and I felt that we were on our way as new parents. Our son had been fed and diapered a number of times, and it was now time for bed. When we snuggled him in his bassinet, he lay quietly and didn't cry. Then we looked at each other and at the same time said, "What if we don't hear him in the middle of the night?" We went on to bed but with much trepidation. Our baby's first cry in the night woke us immediately. We both sat up and simultaneously said, "There he is!"
>
> After a few weeks, we could laugh at the anxiety we had during those first few days. I'm sure all new parents must have had similar experiences."

CASE STUDY: Melissa Bond-James

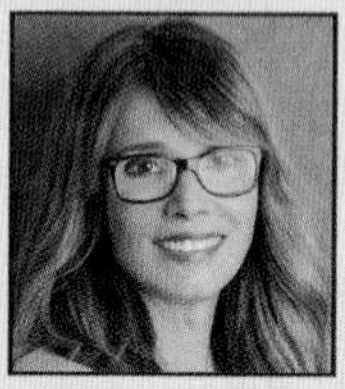

SOURCE: Kinga/Shutterstock.

Melissa and Nancy are concerned about placing their newborn on her back and prefer to put the baby to sleep on the stomach. They feel that if the baby spits up, she will be less likely to aspirate her secretions.

Question to Ponder

What educational materials and key points should the nurse review with the couple to ensure that the baby is placed in a proper sleeping position to reduce the risk of SIDS?

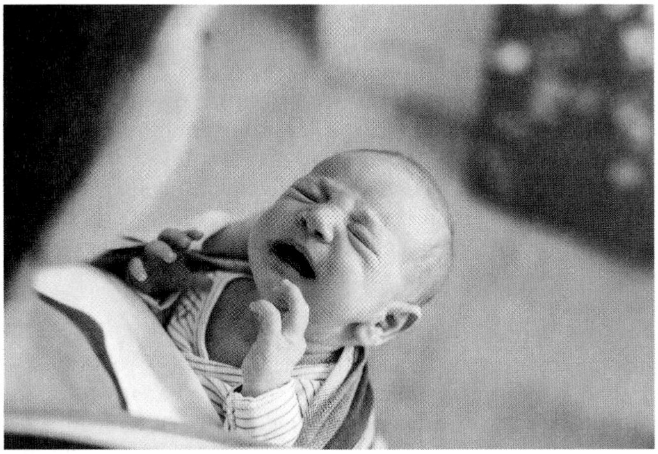

Figure 34–7 **Picking up babies and consoling them when they cry teaches them that adults are responsive to them.**

SOURCE: Halfpoint/Shutterstock.

are responsive to them (Figure 34–7). This helps build a sense of trust. The nurse documents and assesses any crying and provides teaching and referrals as necessary.

Injury Prevention

Accidental injuries were the fifth leading cause of death in infants under 1 year of age in the United States in 2013 and 2014 (Kochanek, Murphy, Xu, et al., 2016; Mathews, MacDorman, & Thoma, 2015). The most common fatal injuries in infants under 1 year of age in 2014 included suffocation, homicide, motor vehicle accidents, drowning, fire/burns, and natural/environmental (National Center for Injury Prevention and Control, CDC, 2016a). The most common nonfatal accidental injuries in infants under 1 year of age in 2014 were falls, strikes, bites or stings, foreign bodies, inhalation/suffocation, other, and fires/burns (National Center for Injury Prevention and Control, CDC, 2016b). It is helpful to keep these causes of injury in mind when counseling new parents regarding safety in the home.

During the home visit, the nurse can share information regarding common injuries and accidents that happen to babies as well as how to prevent them. The parents should have been instructed on car seat safety before leaving the birthing unit, and the nurse can confirm this (see Figure 28–12). It is essential that the parents understand never to leave a baby unattended on any elevated surface, near water, or near pets or other children who may unintentionally harm them.

If time allows, the nurse observes the environment and identifies future changes that need to be made to childproof the home. Safety related to electrical outlets, appliances, and sources of danger in kitchens and bathrooms will need to be addressed as the infant becomes mobile. Poisonous substances and medications should be secured. It is important for nurses to be aware of the impact they can have on the safety of families through home visits.

ABUSIVE HEAD TRAUMA

Abusive head trauma (AHT), previously called *shaken baby syndrome (SBS)*, is a non-accidental traumatic brain injury that results from violent shaking, with or without contact between the baby's head and an exterior surface. Swelling, increased intracranial pressure, and bleeding (subdural hematomas and retinal hemorrhages) result, and the baby may sustain permanent neurologic damage. AHT is the most common cause of injury and death related to child abuse; it results in death in approximately 25% of cases, and survivors usually have permanent neurologic injuries requiring some level of lifelong care. The most common trigger for AHT is crying by the baby. Parental risk factors include male caregiver; less educated, young, substance-abusing, poorly supported, or single parent; history of poor impulse control; history of prior military service; history of abuse as a child; and living in poverty (Barr, 2014; Mian, Shah, Dalpiaz, et al., 2015; Stadtlander, 2016; Thomas, 2016). The Shaken Baby Syndrome Prevention Act of 2010 was introduced in the United States' 111th Congress, but it was not enacted. However, a number of states have passed legislative preventive programs (Govtrack, 2010; National Conference of State Legislatures, 2015).

An educational program devised by the National Center on Shaken Baby Syndrome (NCSBS, 2017) called "The Period of PURPLE Crying," is designed to prevent AHT. The program addresses the modifiable risk factor, which is the caregiver's response to crying by the baby. Using a three-pronged approach that aims to educate adults on the normality of crying for many babies during the first few months of life, the program includes (1) parental education prior to discharge home about newborn/infant crying patterns, coping strategies, and the hazards of shaking; (2) family support and education during home visits by nurses and in the clinic with providers; and (3) a public media campaign designed to alter the culture of adult response to a well but crying baby (Barr, 2014). The acronym PURPLE derives from the character of the crying that some healthy infants experience between 2 and 4 months of age (Reese, Heiden, Kim, et al., 2014, p. 753) (Figure 34–8):

- **P:** Peak of crying
- **U:** Unexpected/unexplained
- **R:** Resists soothing
- **P:** Pain-like face
- **L:** Long lasting
- **E:** Evening and late afternoon

Reese et al. (2014) evaluated a PURPLE Crying intervention that was led by nurses in five birthing centers. NCSBS provides evidence-based resources for healthcare professionals and for families in multiple languages and formats.

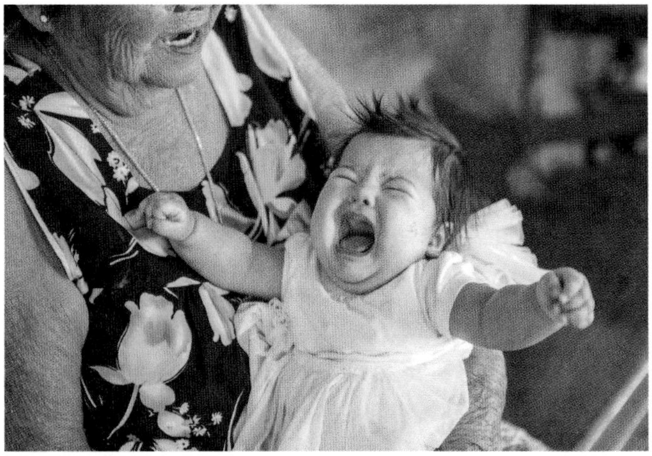

Figure 34–8 **Some healthy babies experience unexplained and long-lasting periods of intense crying.**

SOURCE: Witthaya Phonsawat/123RF.

Home visits provide an excellent opportunity to educate parents regarding safety and injury prevention, shaken baby injuries, and the hazards of abuse and neglect. Nurses need to directly inform parents to never shake a baby. Nurses can educate parents to implement techniques such as singing, swaddling, gentle rhythmic movements, white noise, and offering a pacifier before the baby is crying vigorously (Stadtlander, 2016; Thomas, 2016). Home visits are also the ideal time to provide appropriate resources and referrals to local preventive educational and support programs. See *Professionalism in Practice: Reporting Cases of AHT*.

Professionalism in Practice Reporting Cases of AHT

Suspected cases of AHT should be reported to Child Protective Services (within the county) or law enforcement for an immediate evaluation, ongoing follow-up, home visits, and possible legal intervention. Nurses are mandatory reporters and are required to report suspected child abuse or neglect.

COLIC AS A PARENTAL STRESSOR

Newborn/infant colic is manifested by persistent, unexplained, inconsolable crying that can continue for several hours each day, often occurring in the evening. The baby may have flatulence, arch the back, or draw up the knees. It is a source of great distress and anxiety to new parents, as the colicky baby does not respond to usual methods of soothing. Wessel et al. (1954) cited diagnostic criteria for colic that included 3 or more hours of crying per day that occurred on 3 or more days per week and lasted for 3 weeks or longer. More than 6 decades later, the diagnosis and management of colic in babies remain elusive. There is still no gold standard for diagnosis, and further research is needed to build an evidence base regarding optimal management.

Colic can emerge by 2 to 3 weeks of age, often peaks at 6 to 8 weeks, and can continue until the infant is 4 to 6 months of age. The etiology is unknown, but is believed by many to be gastrointestinal in nature. Colic leads to parental exhaustion and has been associated with postpartum depression, early cessation of breastfeeding, and decreased maternal interaction with the baby. It carries a risk for child abuse, particularly AHT (Yangyang et al., 2018). A variety of treatments have been tried and researched. A maternal hypoallergenic diet may be helpful for breastfed babies, and switching from cow's-milk formula to a soy or hydrolyzed formula may be helpful for those who are formula-fed. However, more research is needed regarding specific dietary approaches (Iacovou et al, 2017).

Recent Cochrane Reviews found inadequate evidence to recommend infant massage (Bennett, Underdown, & Barlow, 2013), manipulative techniques (Dobson et al., 2012), or pain relievers such as simethicone, herbal agents, sugar dicyclomine, or cimetropium bromide (Biagioli, Tarasco, Lingua, et al., 2016) in the treatment of colic. Ongoing research includes studies about gastrointestinal microbes, allergens, connections between colic and childhood migraines, maternal acupuncture, use of probiotics, and a variety of other etiologies and treatments for newborn colic. Nurses should periodically review the literature for new information.

It is important for nurses to provide new parents with anticipatory guidance regarding the symptoms of colic and the strain that it can cause in family relationships. Parents will want to see their baby's healthcare provider to rule out other causes for prolonged crying. If no physiologic etiology is found, the parents should be supported and educated regarding the risks of child abuse. Nurses should remind parents to simply lay the baby down safely in the crib and take a break if they become frustrated with the crying. Parents should be encouraged to ask family and friends for help. It is important to reassure parents that the condition does resolve in time and that newborns go on to develop normally. Home care nurses can share information about local and online resources for colic with all new parents. See *Case Study: Benita Cartier*.

Newborn Screening and Immunization Program

Newborn screening tests use a few drops of the newborn's blood to detect disorders that are often asymptomatic at birth but cause irreversible harm if not detected early. Profound physical, intellectual, and developmental complications and even death can result from many of the conditions for which newborns are screened prior to discharge. The home care nurse answers parents' questions about screening, ensures that the blood specimens have been obtained, and may obtain a specimen as necessary. Parents should be instructed that a second blood specimen will often be required from the newborn after 7 to 14 days. Nurses should clarify that an abnormal test result is not diagnostic and additional definitive tests are required to verify the results. It is important to follow protocols that incorporate state laws about newborn testing, as the required screening and protocols vary between states. The CDC website offers information that nurses can use to supplement the information the parents received from the birthing unit or their healthcare provider. See Chapter 28 for more information regarding newborn screening.

CASE STUDY: Benita Cartier

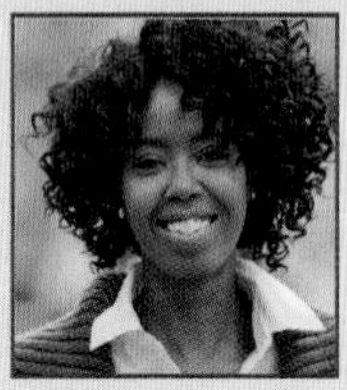

SOURCE: blvdone/Shutterstock.

Benita and her husband, Gerald, advise the nurse at the home visit that they recently brought their newborn home from the NICU and that the baby frequently cries and pulls her legs up while screaming. They note their first child was a good sleeper and wonder if the baby may have colic.

Questions to Ponder

What recommendations can the nurse provide to decrease parental anxiety related to colic? How would you address the parents' questions regarding specific interventions to treat colic?

The newborn hearing screening is usually administered prior to discharge as well. The nurse should verify that it was accomplished and should arrange for the screening if it was not. Parents may have questions, particularly if their baby had an abnormal result.

The nurse should ensure that the family has information regarding the current childhood immunization schedule and has plans to begin or continue immunizations. If the newborn did not receive the initial hepatitis B vaccine prior to discharge, the nurse should ensure that it is planned for the first well-baby visit with the provider.

The nurse should verify that the mother received the tetanus toxoid, reduced diphtheria toxoid, and acellular pertussis vaccine (Tdap) during pregnancy or the immediate postpartum period. The nurse can emphasize the need for other family members and caregivers to have current pertussis protection to protect the newborn against whooping cough.

Home Care: The Mother and Family

Home care of the mother and family involves performing an assessment of the mother and family as well as discussing breastfeeding concerns.

Assessment of the Mother and Family at Home

During the home visit, the nurse will continue the ongoing postpartum assessment that started prior to discharge. The initial goal is to assess the woman's perceptions of her current circumstances, her recovery from childbirth, her adjustment and that of her partner to parenthood, the newborn's condition, family–newborn bonding, and any problems or concerns the woman may have. The nurse asks specifically about the following areas:

- Progression of lochia (color, amount of flow, presence of foul odor or clots)
- Fever or malaise
- Dysuria or difficulty voiding
- Pain in the pelvis or perineum
- Painful, reddened hot spots or shooting pains in the breasts during or between feedings
- Areas of redness, edema, tenderness, or warmth in the legs.

The nurse also talks with the mother about her diet, fatigue level, ability to rest and sleep, pain management, signs of postpartum complications, activity level, sexuality issues, self-care ability, social support system, and any pertinent cultural or religious practices related to postpartum or newborn care. Before performing the physical assessment, the nurse ensures privacy. The physical assessment focuses on maternal physical adaptation, which is assessed by evaluating vital signs, heart and lungs, breasts, abdominal musculature, bowel and bladder elimination patterns, fundal height and location, the perineum, lochia, edema, extremities, and laboratory values.

The psychologic assessment focuses on attachment, adjustment to the parental role, maternal emotions, sibling adjustment, and educational needs. When appropriate, the nurse mentions available community resources, including the public health department, which can be used for follow-up visits. A family approach involving the presence of the spouse/partner and any siblings provides an opportunity to observe family interactions and opportunities for all family members to ask questions and express concerns. In multigenerational households, inclusion of grandparents is important because they may play a key role in childrearing and care of the newborn. In addition, this approach may bring to the surface any questionable family interaction pattern, such as one suggestive of abuse or neglect; the nurse can consider further referral, if needed. See *Assessment Guide: Postpartum—First Home Visit and Anticipated Progress at Six Weeks*.

During the home visit, the nurse continues to provide teaching to the mother and her family and describes self-care measures as needed. The nurse also reviews the signs of developing illness. If signs of potential complications are present, the nurse completes a more in-depth evaluation and determines whether it is necessary for the woman to see her primary care provider. If information about family-planning options has not been given previously, the nurse provides it at this time and answers any questions the woman or her spouse/partner may have about methods of birth control and their sexual relationship. See *Professionalism in Practice: Privacy During Postpartum Home Care Visit*.

Professionalism in Practice Privacy During Postpartum Home Care Visit

Childbearing women should be asked and informed about postpartum depression at every healthcare encounter, and the home visit is no exception. It is helpful for the nurse to include other family members in this discussion, so everyone is aware of the symptoms. However, the patient may share things with the nurse in private that she would not share in front of others, so it is important that the nurse request at least a few minutes alone with her. Asking others to leave briefly during the perineal exam is one option for the nurse. The private interaction also allows the nurse to screen the patient for intimate partner violence, which often escalates during the childbearing period.

Postpartum Fatigue

Postpartum fatigue is a major concern that may trouble new mothers for as long as 19 months postpartum. It is characterized by feelings of exhaustion and decreased capacity for physical and mental work. Chapter 33 includes a discussion on postpartum fatigue, including complications and management.

The home care nurse should inform mothers that fatigue may be a significant problem, which can increase the risk of postpartum depression. The nurse can emphasize the benefits of good nutrition and periods of uninterrupted sleep. The mother should be encouraged to ask family and friends for assistance with responsibilities, limit visitors, and use an answering machine or voicemail to allow for more rest. The nurse can also reinforce the need for continued use of prescribed prenatal vitamins and iron, particularly if the patient is breastfeeding.

Breastfeeding Concerns Following Discharge

Healthy People 2020 aims to increase the proportion of newborns/infants ever breastfed from 74 to 89.1%. Specific goals include increasing the proportion of babies breastfed exclusively until

ASSESSMENT GUIDE | Postpartum—First Home Visit and Anticipated Progress at Six Weeks

Physical Assessment/Normal Findings	Alterations and Possible Causes*	Nursing Responses to Data†
Vital Signs		
Blood Pressure: Return to normal prepregnant level	Elevated blood pressure (anxiety, essential hypertension, renal disease), preeclampsia (can occur postpartum)	Review history, evaluate normal baseline; refer to physician/certified nurse midwife (CNM), if necessary.
Pulse: 60–90 beats/min (or prepregnant normal rate)	Increased pulse rate, tachycardia, chest pain (excitement, anxiety, blood loss, cardiac disorders)	Count pulse for full minute, note irregularities; marked tachycardia or beat irregularities require additional assessment and possible physician/CNM referral.
Respirations: 12–24/min	Marked tachypnea or abnormal patterns (respiratory or cardiac disorders)	Evaluate for respiratory disease or cardiac complications; refer to physician/CNM, if necessary.
Temperature: 36.6°C–37.6°C (98°F–99.6°F)	Increased temperature (infection or engorgement)	Assess for signs and symptoms of infection or disease state.
Weight		
2 days: Possible weight loss of 12–20+ lb	Minimal weight loss (fluid retention, preeclampsia)	Evaluate for fluid retention, edema, deep tendon reflexes, and blood pressure elevation.
6 weeks: Returning to normal prepregnant weight	Retained weight (excessive caloric intake)	Determine amount of daily exercise. Provide dietary teaching. Refer to dietitian, if necessary, for additional dietary counseling.
	Extreme weight loss (excessive dieting, inadequate caloric intake)	Discuss appropriate diets, refer to dietitian for additional counseling, if necessary; reinforce need for up to 500 additional kcal/day when breastfeeding.
Breasts		
Nonbreastfeeding: 2 days: May have mild discomfort; small amount of milk may be expressed	Some engorgement (incomplete suppression of lactation)	Engorgement may be seen in nonbreastfeeding mothers. Advise patient to wear a supportive, well-fitting bra, avoid very warm showers, avoid pumping or any stimulation of breasts, use cooling packs for comfort; evaluate for signs and symptoms of mastitis.
6 weeks: Soft, with no tenderness; return to prepregnant size	Redness; hardened area, marked tenderness (mastitis)	Counsel about nipple care. Observe newborn feeding.
	Palpable mass (tumor)	Evaluate patient condition, evidence of fever; refer to physician/CNM, if indicated. A breastfeeding mother should examine her breasts monthly, after feeding, when breasts are empty; if palpable mass is felt, refer to physician for further evaluation.
Breastfeeding: Full, with prominent nipples; lactation established	Cracked, fissured nipples (improper latch); redness, marked tenderness, hardened area (mastitis or abscess); palpable mass (plugged milk duct, tumor)	For breast engorgement accompanied by erythema, instruct the mother to: **1.** Keep breast empty by frequent feeding. **2.** Rest when possible with breasts elevated. **3.** Take prescribed pain relief medication(s). **4.** Drink adequate fluids. If symptoms persist for more than 24 hours, or if accompanied by fever greater than 100.4°F, flulike symptoms, or redness, instruct her to call her physician/CNM.

ASSESSMENT GUIDE | Postpartum—First Home Visit and Anticipated Progress at Six Weeks (*continued*)

Physical Assessment/Normal Findings	Alterations and Possible Causes*	Nursing Responses to Data†
Abdominal Musculature		
2 days: Improved firmness, although "bread dough" consistency is not unusual, especially in multipara Striae pink and obvious	Marked relaxation of muscles	Evaluate exercise level; provide information on appropriate exercise program.
Cesarean incision healing	Drainage, redness, tenderness, pain, edema (infection)	Evaluate for infection; refer to physician/CNM, if necessary.
6 weeks: Muscle tone continues to improve; striae may be beginning to fade; linea nigra fading		
Elimination Pattern		
Urinary tract: Return to prepregnant urinary elimination routine	Urinary incontinence, especially when lifting, coughing, laughing, and so on (urethral/perineal trauma, hormonal influences, cystocele)	Assess for cystocele; instruct in appropriate muscle tightening exercises; refer to physician/CNM.
	Pain or burning when voiding, urgency and/or frequency, pus or white blood cells (WBCs) in urine, pathogenic organisms in culture (stinging may be due to lacerations or episiotomy; urinary tract infection [UTI])	Evaluate for urinary tract infection; obtain clean-catch urine; refer to physician/CNM for treatment, if indicated.
Routine urinalysis within normal limits (proteinuria disappeared)	Sugar or ketone in urine—may be some lactose present in urine of breastfeeding mothers (diabetes)	Evaluate diet; assess for signs and symptoms of diabetes; refer to physician/CNM.
Bowel habits: 2 days: May have some discomfort with defecation, especially if patient had severe hemorrhoids or third- or fourth-degree tear	Severe constipation or pain when defecating (trauma or hemorrhoids)	Discuss dietary patterns; encourage fluid, adequate roughage. Continue use of stool softener if necessary to prevent pain associated with straining; continue sitz baths, periods of rest for severe hemorrhoids; assess healing of episiotomy and/or lacerations; severe constipation may require administration of laxatives, stool softeners, and an enema if not contraindicated (check with physician/CNM).
6 weeks: Return to normal prepregnancy bowel elimination	Marked constipation (inadequate fluid and/or fiber intake)	See previously discussed interventions.
	Fecal incontinence or constipation (rectocele)	Assess for evidence of rectocele; instruct in muscle-tightening exercises; refer to physician/CNM.
Reproductive Tract		
Lochia: 2 days: Lochia rubra or lochia serosa, scant amounts, fleshy odor	Excessive amounts and/or large clots (nonfirm uterus), foul odor (infection), passing tissue (retained placenta)	Assess for evidence of infection and/or failure of the uterus to descend and decrease in size; refer to physician/CNM.
6 weeks: No lochia or return to normal menstruation pattern	See above.	See above.
Fundus and perineum: 2 days: Fundus is at least two fingerbreadths below the umbilicus; uterine muscles still somewhat lax; introitus of vagina lacks tone—gapes when intra-abdominal pressure is increased by coughing or straining	Uterus not decreasing in size appropriately or extremely tender (infection)	Assess fundus for firmness and/or signs of infection; refer to physician/CNM, if indicated.
Episiotomy and/or lacerations healing; no signs of infection; may have some bruising and tenderness	Evidence of redness, severe pain, poor tissue approximation in episiotomy and/or laceration (wound infection)	Continue perineal hygiene care; refer to physician or CNM, if necessary.

(continued)

ASSESSMENT GUIDE | Postpartum—First Home Visit and Anticipated Progress at Six Weeks (*continued*)

Physical Assessment/Normal Findings	Alterations and Possible Causes*	Nursing Responses to Data†
6 weeks: Uterus almost returned to prepregnant size with almost completely restored muscle tone	Continued flow of lochia, failure to decrease appropriately in size (subinvolution)	Assess for evidence of subinvolution and/or infection; refer to physician or CNM for further evaluation and treatment, if necessary.
Hemoglobin and Hematocrit Levels		
6 weeks: Hemoglobin (Hb) 12 g/dL; Hematocrit (Hct) 37% ± 5%	Hb less than 12 g/dL; Hct less than 32% (anemia)	Assess nutritional status, assess for signs or symptoms of anemia, instruct on high-iron foods and supplemental iron; for marked anemia (Hb less than or equal to 9 g/dL), additional assessment and/or physician/CNM referral may be necessary.
Attachment		
Bonding process demonstrated by soothing, cuddling, and talking to baby; appropriate feeding techniques; eye-to-eye contact; touching; calling baby by name	Absence of behaviors associated with bonding process; calling baby by nickname that promotes ridicule; inadequate weight gain; baby is dirty; hygienic measures are not maintained; severe diaper rash; failure to obtain adequate supplies for baby	Provide counseling; talk with the woman about her feelings regarding the baby; provide support for the caretaking activities that are being performed; refer to public health nurse or social worker for continued home visits; refer to Child Protective Services if abuse or neglect is suspected.
Parent interacts with baby and provides soothing, caretaking activities	Parent is unable to respond to baby's needs (inability to recognize needs, inadequate education and support, substance abuse, fear, family stress)	Provide support for caretaking activities observed; provide information regarding caretaking activities, such as responding to baby's cry; methods of wrapping baby; methods of soothing the baby such as swaddling, rocking, increasing stimuli by singing to the baby or decreasing stimuli by putting baby to rest in quiet room; methods of holding the baby; differences in the cry. Identify support system; provide information regarding community resources and support groups; reinforce "Never shake a baby."
Parents express feelings of comfort and success with the parent role	Evidence of stress and anxiety (difficulty moving into or dealing with the parent role)	Provide support and encouragement; provide information regarding progression into parent role and assist parents in talking through their feelings; refer to community resources and support groups.
Woman is in the informal or personal stage of maternal role attainment	Woman is still greatly influenced by others, has not developed an image or style of her own (woman remains in the anticipatory stage)	Provide role-modeling for the woman in working through problem solving with the baby; provide encouragement as she thinks through decisions and develops her sense of problem solving; encourage her to make decisions regarding baby care; provide positive reinforcement.
Adjustment to Parental Role		
Parents are coping with new roles in terms of division of labor, financial status, communication, readjustment of sexual relations, and adjusting to new daily tasks	Inability to adjust to new roles (immaturity, extremes of maternal age, inadequate education and preparation, ineffective communication patterns, inadequate support, current family crisis)	Provide counseling and anticipatory guidance; refer to parent groups.

ASSESSMENT GUIDE Postpartum—First Home Visit and Anticipated Progress at Six Weeks (*continued*)

Physical Assessment/Normal Findings	Alterations and Possible Causes*	Nursing Responses to Data†
Emotional/ Psychologic		
Mother screens negative for postpartum depression or postpartum mood and anxiety disorders	Severe depression, unable to care for self and/or baby, significant anxiety, postpartum trauma or evidence of post-traumatic stress disorder, paranoia, inability to sleep, delusions, or hallucinations	All mothers should be screened for postpartum mood and anxiety disorder. Provide postpartum depression screening administration to all women. Refer to mental health practitioner, screen for postpartum depression, mood, and anxiety disorders, pharmacologic intervention as needed. Screen for suicidal thoughts and ideations. Postpartum psychosis warrants immediate psychiatric hospitalization.
Education		
Mother understands self-care measures	Inadequate knowledge of self-care (inadequate education)	Provide education and counseling.
Parents are knowledgeable regarding baby care	Inadequate knowledge of baby care (inadequate education)	
Siblings are adjusting to new baby	Excessive sibling rivalry	
Parents have a method of contraception	Birth control method not chosen	

*Possible causes of alterations are placed in parentheses.

†This column provides guidelines for further assessment and initial nursing intervention.

3 and 6 months, as well as the proportion of infants who are still breastfed at 6 and 12 months of age (U.S. Department of Health and Human Services [HHS], 2013). Most mothers are discharged before breastfeeding is well established, however, and many require anticipatory guidance and support in order to continue once they go home. The home visit is the ideal time to promote continuation of breastfeeding. The home care nurse has the opportunity to reinforce initial breastfeeding teaching, answer questions, and observe an episode of breastfeeding in the home environment. Guidance and support can be individualized according to the mother's specific needs and living situation.

AAP and ACOG (2017) recommend that all breastfeeding newborns be seen by a pediatrician or other knowledgeable healthcare professional at 3 to 5 days of age to assess weight and to have a physical exam to include assessment of jaundice and hydration, maternal breastfeeding status, newborn elimination, and formal observation of a breastfeeding session. A home nurse visit meets these requirements and can identify at-risk newborns at a time when intervention can correct most breastfeeding problems before they become complicated by insufficient milk. The home health nurse can assess the baby and the breastfeeding process, provide appropriate education to promote breastfeeding, and initiate referrals to a lactation consultant or primary healthcare provider as needed. Additionally, the nurse can provide individualized support and encouragement as desired by the patient.

BREASTFEEDING ASSESSMENT

The nurse should observe a feeding episode, if possible, to assess for correct position, latch-on, let-down, sucking pattern, nipple condition, and the response of baby and mother. The nurse can assess the parents' ability to identify feeding cues such as rooting, hand-to-mouth movements, sucking, opening of mouth in response to stimulation, and transition of the baby from sleep to drowsy awake to quiet alert states. Various tools are available to assess the breastfeeding session, including the LATCH Scoring Tool (Jensen, Wallace, & Kelsay, 1994).

CONCERNS RELATED TO THE BREASTFEEDING BABY

According to AAP criteria, the newborn's weight should remain within 10% of the birth weight, and the baby should be evaluated for breastfeeding problems if weight loss exceeds 7%. A study of more than 100,000 racially diverse and exclusively breastfed newborns in California determined that babies born by cesarean section experienced more weight loss than those born by vaginal delivery. Median loss at 72 hours was 6.4% for those born vaginally and 8.6% for those born by cesarean. Although the newborns typically began gaining weight back by 48 to 72 hours of age, those with higher weight loss began regaining later than those with lower weight loss. The researchers developed expected weight loss nomograms based on the findings, as well as a weight loss tool (Newborn Weight Tool [NEWT]), which can be found online (Flaherman et al., 2015; Penn State Hershey Medical Center, 2017).

The nurse can assist the couplet experiencing a 7 to 9% newborn weight loss with techniques to increase milk production and promote better milk transfer. The nurse will provide assistance with breastfeeding techniques as needed, encourage breastfeeding every 2 hours for the next 24 hours, and recheck the newborn's weight the next day. If breastfeeding technique is correct and the milk is just starting to come in, the newborn generally begins gaining weight back within hours. Lactation problems beyond the expertise of the nurse require a lactation consultant and/or provider referral.

The nurse should discuss the clinical picture of the newborn experiencing more than 7% weight loss with the healthcare provider. Babies experiencing breastfeeding difficulties whose weight loss is greater than 7% may need supplementation. A newborn with a weight loss of 10% or more will almost always need supplementation. Because it is important to begin rehydrating the newborn as soon as possible, the home care nurse may need to help a patient who has planned only to feed from the breast to formulate an interim contingency plan. The nurse can assist her with pumping or hand-expressing.

Expressed breast milk is the ideal intervention. However, if the mother does not have enough breast milk, the nurse may need to assist the mother with preparation of formula until her supply is adequate and the baby is rehydrated. The use of infant formula is discussed later in this chapter and in greater detail in Chapter 29. The mother may need to begin pumping to increase her milk supply as well. Walker (2016) offered guidance regarding pumping and the use of feeding tube devices that support breastfeeding in the event that supplementation is required.

Newborns frequently require assistance in awakening to feed at least eight times a day during the first week of life. The quiet alert state is ideal for latch-on, and parents should be taught to recognize this state as well as the presence of early feeding cues. The quiet alert baby has bright eyes and is responsive to stimuli. Early feeding cues include sucking motions, bringing the hands to the mouth, rooting, extending the tongue, turning the head to the side, and whimpering (Koehn & Dowling, 2016). Techniques that are helpful in arousing a sleepy baby to the quiet alert state include undressing the baby, changing the diaper, lightly touching, speaking, turning on lights, placing the baby skin-to-skin on the mother's chest, and gently rocking the baby. Newborns who are crying or who exhibit behaviors such as tightly closed eyes and uncoordinated movements of extremities require calming techniques to bring them to a quiet alert state. Changing the diaper, comforting, holding, swaddling, gently rocking, and talking softly will assist the newborn to return to the quiet alert state so the breast can be offered (Hoover, 2016; Koehn & Dowling, 2016).

Many mothers have concerns related to their breast milk supply. The nurse can educate and reassure the mother regarding the signs of adequate transfer during the first week of life:

- Baby swallows audibly during feedings.
- Mother's nipple is moist after feedings.
- Baby has moist mucous membranes and skin is elastic.
- Mother and baby both appear satisfied and comfortable after feedings.
- Baby passes three to five loose yellow stools per day by day 4 or 5.
- Six or more diapers are saturated with clear urine each day by the end of the first week.
- Baby actively suckles eight or more times in 24 hours for a total of 140 minutes or more.

Additionally, the baby should return to birth weight by the 2-week well-baby visit. The satiated baby will be content at the end of feedings with arms extended and relaxed. A small amount of milk may be visible at the side of the mouth. If all of the previous criteria are met, the nurse can feel confident in telling the mother that the baby is "getting enough" and reminding her that exclusive breastfeeding is the ideal diet for the baby until 6 months of age (Powers, 2016; Smith, 2016).

Recommendations at this point would be to continue nursing on demand, at least every 3 hours, and to expect the baby to demand more frequent feedings during growth spurts. The mother can allow the baby who is actively sucking and swallowing to nurse for as long as desired on the first side and then for as long as the baby desires on the second side to encourage consumption of the high-fat hind milk. See *Case Study: Angelina Newman*.

CONCERNS RELATED TO MATERNAL BREASTFEEDING DIFFICULTIES

In addition to problems with milk transfer and concerns about milk supply, many new mothers have breastfeeding difficulties, including discomfort, cracked nipples, breast engorgement, and plugged ducts. The nurse can assess for these complications at the home visit and provide interventions to decrease maternal discomfort.

Nipple Soreness. Mothers should be counseled to expect sensations of massaging and stretching as the baby elongates the nipple during nursing. This may be uncomfortable when the

CASE STUDY: Angelina Newman

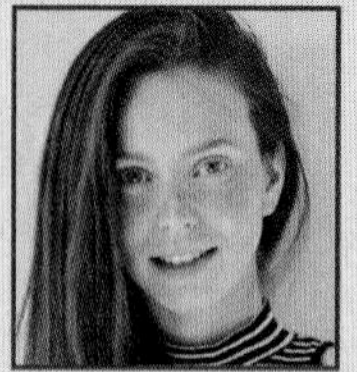

SOURCE: WAYHOME studio/Shutterstock.

Angelina gave birth to a healthy son 3 days ago and was discharged home yesterday. She had decided to breastfeed early in the pregnancy with her aunt's encouragement. Her aunt is a newborn nursery nurse and stressed the health benefits to the baby and Angelina's likelihood to lose weight more quickly. Angelina had initial difficulties but with the help of the nursery nurse and the lactation consultant was able to latch the baby on and feed fairly well in the hospital. You are conducting a home health visit when Angelina opens the door tearful and says, "It's not working now, it's not going to work." You calm her down and she states that now that the milk is coming in, she can't get the baby to latch on anymore.

Questions to Ponder

What initial steps do you perform in assessing the mother and baby? What instructional steps can you provide to demonstrate proper latch-on and ensure the baby is getting enough to eat?

baby initially latches for feedings, but the discomfort should decrease after the first few seconds of nursing. Nipple soreness is a common complaint and frequent reason for early discontinuation of breastfeeding. The nipples may exhibit erythema, edema, abrasions, fissures, cracks, bruises, blisters, and bleeding. This early transient discomfort is usually due to mechanical trauma; it is often apparent by day 3 and resolves by day 6. Poor latch and/or suck are the primary causes of mechanical trauma. Therefore, observation of feeding and assistance with proper positioning and latching technique are essential to the prevention and treatment of soreness (Bainbridge, 2015; da Silva Santos et al., 2016).

The baby's position at the breast is a critical factor in nipple soreness. (See Figures 29–5 through 29–14 for correct positioning.) Encouraging the mother to rotate positions when feeding the baby may decrease nipple soreness. Changing positions alters the focus of greatest stress and promotes more complete breast emptying. Although some mothers are initially hesitant to try the side-lying position, this is frequently a helpful position to use when difficulty in latching is encountered. An observation of the feeding should assess the baby's oral cavity for anatomic concerns as well as the ability to open the mouth wide enough to attain a deep latch. When latched, the lips should be flanged out, and the newborn should cover as much of the areola as possible. Turning the lips under can cause pain and inadequate transfer of milk. The mother can be taught to observe this and to apply gentle upward pressure on the newborn's upper lip and gentle downward pressure on the baby's chin to correct the position as needed. To prevent trauma, the mother should also be taught to gently insert her finger between the baby's gums to break the latch before removing the baby from the breast.

While nursing, the baby can be expected to suck rapidly at the beginning and more slowly toward the end of a feeding. Sucking should be quiet, with swallowing heard every two to three sucks. The baby's cheeks should be full and rounded. Movement should be seen at the jawline. Dimpling at the cheek may be indicative of a poor or shallow latch or an unusual movement of the tongue. Finally, the mother's nipple will be elongated at the end of a feeding, but it should be the same shape as at the beginning. Abnormal sounds, distorted nipple appearance after feedings, or nipple pain that persists after correcting the latch requires additional evaluation (Smith, 2016).

The nurse can instruct the mother in a number of measures to promote comfort and healing and to prevent skin breakdown. Washing the breasts with warm water and avoiding drying soaps are recommended. Simply keeping the nipples clean and dry is adequate for many mothers. Alternatively, warm water compresses can be applied followed by air-drying (Figure 34–9). Gently massaging or manually expressing some milk before feedings stimulates let-down and may be helpful in decreasing initial latch-on pain related to vigorous nursing (Smith, 2016).

The application of highly purified anhydrous (HPA) lanolin and/or breast milk accompanied by air-drying at the end of feedings has been shown to be safe for treating nipple pain. Neither needs to be washed off prior to the next feeding. A Cochrane Review did not find evidence to support the use of any specific products and determined that application of breast milk or nothing may be as effective as lanolin (Dennis, Jackson, & Watson, 2014). It is essential that the nurse read the product literature and current research on products recommended by the providers and lactation consultants in the local area.

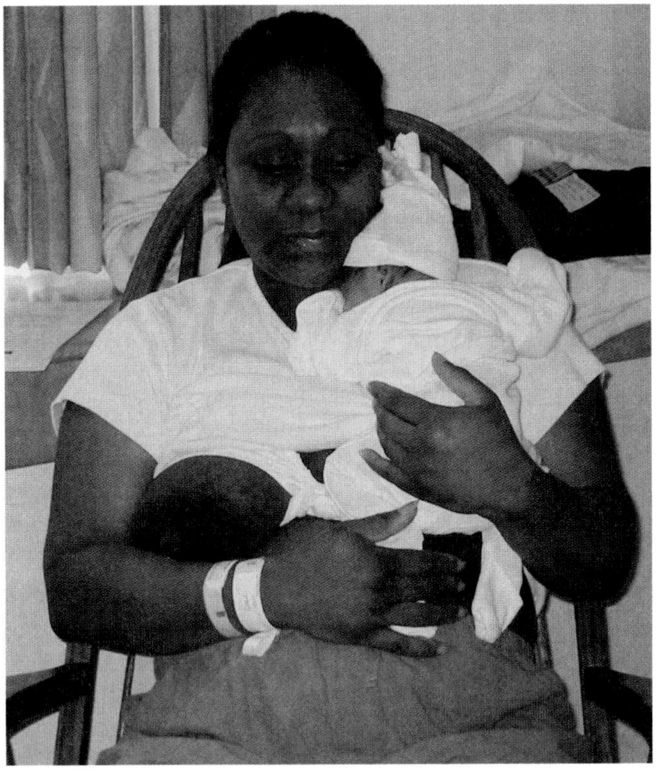

Figure 34–9 **Air-drying the nipples can help prevent cracking and fissures.**

SOURCE: Michele Davidson.

Additionally, the nurse should remind the mother that small amounts of any product applied to her nipples will be ingested by her newborn. Therefore, she will want to consult her healthcare provider or a lactation consultant before applying commercial products. Nipple pain that does not resolve after a few days may indicate infection or other problems and should be referred to a healthcare provider so the appropriate therapy can be prescribed. An antifungal agent may be needed for nipple pain related to candidiasis (Wambach, 2016). Fortunately, nipple pain diminishes significantly for most women by 10 days postpartum (Dennis et al., 2014).

Flat or Inverted Nipples. Many women with flat or inverted nipples have the fear that they will be unable to breastfeed. This is not usually the case. Pregnancy and previous breastfeeding often lessen the inversion to the point that it is not an issue with subsequent babies. Breastfeeding mothers with flat or inverted nipples may experience difficulties after discharge if breastfeeding was not successfully established before leaving the hospital. Frequently, positioning the baby well back on the areola will be enough to promote the suckling that stretches and elongates the nipple during feedings. The nurse can teach the mother to stimulate and shape the nipple just before feeding. A cold pack will evert a flat nipple. Inverted nipples that can be everted can be shaped by the mother by placing her thumb 1½ to 2 inches behind the nipple and pulling back into her chest. Use of the side-lying position is helpful as well (Walker, 2016).

The nurse can also recommend use of a pump to evert the nipple just before latch-on. Experienced nurses may feel comfortable assisting mothers to use a thin silicone nipple shield during the initial latch. The shield can be removed once the baby has suckled enough to elongate the nipple. Inverted nipples that are not easily everted by the measures above should be referred to a lactation consultant. The nurse should talk with a lactation consultant or provider if the patient requires temporary use of a thin silicone nipple shield and/or pumping rather than nursing. Nipple shields should be used only under close monitoring, as they can potentially affect milk transfer. They should not substitute for nursing assessment and interventions related to the underlying issue (Walker, 2016).

Breast Engorgement. A distinction exists between breast fullness and engorgement. All lactating women experience a transitional fullness at first, initially because of venous congestion and later because of accumulating milk. However, this fullness generally lasts only 24 hours, the breasts remain soft enough for the newborn to suckle, and there is no pain. Severely engorged breasts are hard, painful, and warm, and may appear taut and shiny. Engorgement can be accompanied by a fever up to 101°F (38.6°C). Engorgement may occur as a result of infrequent feedings, delayed initiation of feedings, improper latch, use of supplements, time-limited feedings, and too quickly removing the baby from the first side to ensure feeding from both breasts at each feeding (Hoover, 2016; Mangesi & Zakarija-Grkovic, 2016).

Treatments employed for engorgement may include warm compresses or showers for a short time just before nursing, cold compresses applied to breasts after feedings, cabbage compresses, breast massage and milk expression, ultrasound, anti-inflammatory medications, oxytocin spray, acupuncture, acupressure, Gua-Sha therapy (alternative therapy that involves scraping your skin with a massage tool to improve your circulation), and pumping. Although women have reported symptomatic relief from a number of these interventions, a Cochrane Review concluded that there is not enough evidence to recommend one treatment over the others (Mangesi & Zakarija-Grkovic, 2016). Unrelieved engorgement and stasis are not necessarily associated with mastitis, but they do lead to involution and decreased milk synthesis. Frequent feedings for a minimum of approximately 160 minutes of nursing every 24 hours are essential to the treatment of engorgement. Although pumping is sometimes discouraged in this situation for fear that it will increase milk production, it is necessary to manually express or pump if the baby is unable to nurse to empty the breasts (Berens, Brodribb, & Academy of Breastfeeding Medicine, 2016; Hoover, 2016; Smith, 2016). See *Nursing Care Plan: For the Woman with Engorgement*.

Plugged Ducts. Some mothers experience plugging of one or more ducts. Manifested as an area of tenderness, redness, and heat or a palpable lump in an otherwise well woman, plugging may be relieved by the use of massage and frequent feedings. The nurse can encourage the mother to massage her breasts from her chest wall forward to the nipple while standing in a warm shower or following the application of moist heat to the breast. The mother should then breastfeed her baby, starting on the affected breast to promote drainage. Frequent breastfeeding and the use of a variety of positions to ensure complete emptying help to prevent and to resolve the problem. The nurse should also encourage the patient to wear a comfortable bra and loose, nonrestrictive clothing (Wambach, 2016).

Mastitis. Plugged ducts and milk stasis increase the risk for *mastitis*, an inflammatory condition of the breast. Stress and fatigue, cracked nipples, and an abundant milk supply are associated with mastitis as well. Symptoms of mastitis include fever (greater than 100.4°F [38°C]); a hot, red, tender area on the breast; and flulike symptoms. Treatment of mastitis includes continued breastfeeding, application of moist heat, increased fluids, rest, analgesics, and antibiotics as prescribed if necessary (Wambach, 2016). For more information about mastitis, see Chapter 35 and Figure 35–2.

Effect of Medications and Alcohol. Analgesics are appropriate as directed by a primary healthcare provider. Avoidance of breastfeeding while the drug levels are peaking in maternal plasma minimizes the amount received by the baby. The peak concentration varies from drug to drug, and it may be difficult to time this during the first week of breastfeeding. Nursing ideally occurs frequently, and the mother may require analgesics to nurse comfortably, particularly if she experiences afterpains (see Chapter 33) during breastfeeding.

Acetaminophen and nonsteroidal anti-inflammatory drugs (NSAIDs) are generally safe for use during breastfeeding. Short-term use of opioids for pain unrelieved by NSAIDs or acetaminophen is safe according to some experts, but newborn adverse reactions following maternal opioid use have been reported, and babies less than 2 months of age seem to be at highest risk for complications (Anderson, Manoguerra, & Valdés, 2016; Carroll, 2015; Dalal, 2015; Darnall & Schatman, 2015a, 2015b). Because most drugs do pass into the breast milk, the mother should check with her provider before taking medications. The nurse can use the references listed in Table 34–3 to check recommendations regarding use of specific drugs during lactation.

Alcohol passes into the breast milk, and the concentration in the breast milk parallels that in the maternal blood. Although a review of the literature found that babies are exposed to minute amounts of alcohol from social drinking (Haastrup, Pottegård, & Damkier, 2014), a recent study discovered significant deficits in physical and neurological development among 6- to 8-year-olds whose mothers consumed alcohol during the breastfeeding period (May et al., 2016). Alcohol intake can also have a negative impact on milk production, ejection, and intake. Therefore, it is not recommended for breastfeeding women. Mothers who do occasionally drink while lactating should be advised to consume the alcohol after a breastfeeding episode in order to minimize the amount the baby receives (Hale & Rowe, 2017; Powers, 2016; Reece-Stremtan, Marinelli, & Academy of Breastfeeding Medicine, 2015).

Breastfeeding and the Working Mother. Many mothers return to work while still breastfeeding. The home care nurse can help the woman to explore options and solve problems related to breastfeeding in the workplace to promote continuation. The earlier the breastfeeding mother returns to work, the more often she will need to pump her breasts to express the breast milk (see Chapter 29 for more information). Recommendations for mothers who are using a breast pump can be found in Table 29–4. Because milk production follows the principle of supply and demand, if breasts are not pumped, the milk supply will decrease. The nurse can review pumping and storage of breast milk with the mother, as the mother will want to begin pumping at least a week or two before returning to work. The mother will also want to introduce her baby to expressed milk from a bottle or cup prior to her return. An electric pump and double collection system is optimal for the working mother (see Figures 29–18 through 29–20 in Chapter 29). Breastfeeding mothers can obtain printed

Nursing Care Plan: For the Woman with Engorgement

Nursing Diagnosis: *Pain, Acute*, related to increased breast fullness secondary to increased blood supply to breast tissue causing swelling of tissue around milk ducts (NANDA-I © 2017)

Goal: Patient will remain free of breast fullness and pain.

INTERVENTION	RATIONALE
• Instruct patient to nurse frequently.	• Engorgement may be a result of infrequent or missed feedings. Frequent feedings will prevent the breast from becoming increasingly full, which in turn decreases pain caused by engorgement. The newborn should be offered the breast at least 8 to 10 times in a 24-hour period.
• Instruct patient to nurse at least 10 to 15 minutes on each breast per feeding.	• Hind milk may be brought forward when the newborn is able to suckle for 10 to 15 minutes per breast. This will allow the breast ducts to empty with each feeding.
• Assist patient to pre-express milk onto nipple or baby's lips.	• Engorgement may be the result of newborns who are too sleepy to suck at each feeding or not eager to nurse vigorously. Expressing some milk onto the nipple may entice the newborn to nurse more aggressively.
• Initiate pumping or manually express milk at the beginning of the feeding.	• Engorgement may be the result of the breast not emptying at each feeding. Pumping or manually expressing the breast will allow the breast to empty. Pumping or hand-expressing the milk at the beginning of each feeding will help soften the breast so the newborn can latch on to the nipple and facilitate letdown.
• Instruct patient to pump, hand-express, or massage to empty breast when feedings are missed.	• If patient develops a feeling of fullness in the breast, or the newborn has missed a feeding, then pumping or hand-expressing the milk will help keep the milk ducts empty. When the milk ducts become backed up, milk production can be inhibited, eventually decreasing the milk supply. Pumping during engorgement should not affect the milk supply.
• Administer analgesics before nursing.	• Acetaminophen and ibuprofen alone or in combination with codeine may be administered just before nursing to relieve pain and discomfort. The medication will reach the milk within 30 minutes.
• Apply warm and/or cold compresses before nursing.	• Warm compresses may be applied before nursing to stimulate let-down or soften the breast. This will allow the newborn to grasp the areola. A proper latch-on will help prevent plugged ducts and assist in emptying the breast to reduce breast fullness and pain associated with engorgement. Relaxing in the shower with warm water running over the breast may have the same effect. Cold compresses may also be used to help reduce pain.
• Apply fresh cabbage leaves to the breast between feedings.	• Placing fresh cabbage leaves inside the bra is a home remedy that may relieve edema associated with engorgement, thereby reducing pain. Relief may be experienced within 30 minutes. Prolonged application of cabbage leaves may reduce the milk supply.

EXPECTED OUTCOMES: There will be no evidence of swelling found in breast tissue. The woman's pain will have decreased, and her breast tissue will be soft and without tenderness.

materials on pumping, storage, working while breastfeeding, breastfeeding legislation, and related issues from lactation consultants, breastfeeding support groups, La Leche League, and the Special Supplemental Nutrition Program for Women, Infants, and Children (WIC) (Rojjanasrirat & Wambach, 2016). The CDC (2016b) offers free online resources as well.

The nurse can suggest methods of maintaining breast milk supply such as relaxation, stress reduction, proper nutrition, adequate fluid intake, and frequent nursing during the evenings, in the mornings, and on days off. The nurse and patient can explore options such as pumping at work, visiting the baby or having the baby brought to work during the mother's lunch, and having the childcare provider give expressed breast milk or formula (Rojjanasrirat & Wambach, 2016).

Use of the side-lying position is less fatiguing and may allow the mother to relax when she does have the opportunity to breastfeed her baby before and after work. Night breastfeeding may help a working mother maintain her milk supply, but it may also contribute to fatigue. Depending on the rigidity and demands of the mother's work schedule, the nurse can explore options with the mother to promote the continuation of breastfeeding as much as possible during the first year of life.

Many women experience anxiety, guilt, or doubt about returning to work. Women should be reassured that these feelings are normal and that the mothering role will continue to evolve and grow even when separation occurs. The home health nurse provides a resource for the working mother and can deliver ongoing support. See *Professionalism in Practice: Workplace Issues Related to Breastfeeding*.

Weaning. Weaning is a process that begins with the introduction of sources of nutrition other than breast milk and ends when the child no longer breastfeeds and receives all nutrition from other sources. The decision to wean the baby from the breast may be

Professionalism in Practice Workplace Issues Related to Breastfeeding

Nurses can engage in public education campaigns related to the benefits of breastfeeding in the workplace, such as less absenteeism related to illness in the baby. *The Surgeon General's Call to Action to Support Breastfeeding* (U.S. Department of Health and Human Services, 2011) recommends implementation strategies to educate employers about breastfeeding and to help them establish high-quality lactation programs. Nurses need to conduct research that investigates the effects of corporate lactation support programs and work cultures that are supportive of breastfeeding.

Many working mothers may not be aware of their right to continue breastfeeding after they return to work. The professional nurse can advocate for patients by informing and encouraging them to discuss breastfeeding and the law with their employers. Nurses need to be familiar with current breastfeeding legislation. Comprehensive information about U.S. and global laws related to breastfeeding is available through La Leche League International (2018).

made for a variety of reasons, including family or cultural pressures, changes in the home situation, work schedules, pressure from the woman's partner, or a personal opinion about when weaning should occur.

The home care nurse will likely visit the mother early in the postpartum period, and it is important to provide anticipatory guidance and support to the mother in order to extend breastfeeding for as long as possible to benefit mother and baby. Education about how to establish and maintain sufficient milk supply and how to respond to infant growth spurts is essential. The woman should also receive contact information for support groups and lactation consultants in her local area.

Although some women need to wean abruptly due to medical or logistical reasons, a gradual approach is physically and emotionally comfortable for many mothers and their babies. The mother may wish to start by substituting one or two breastfeedings with other sources of nutrition and cup feedings each day. Eventually, the mother may want to breastfeed only once or twice a day prior to stopping entirely.

Nurses should inform mothers that lactation consultants will help them with weaning issues in addition to providing support for establishing and continuing lactation. The nurse can also share resources with breastfeeding mothers (see Table 34–3). See *Developing Cultural Competence: Breastfeeding Initiation Rates.*

Clinical Tip

Many women have strong feelings regarding weaning, especially women who will likely not have more children. The mother must adjust to this developmental milestone and may experience some regret and sadness during this time. Reassuring women that this is normal enables them to express their emotions in a safe environment.

Developing Cultural Competence Breastfeeding Initiation Rates

According to the CDC (2016c), approximate breastfeeding rates* among babies at 6 months in the United States during 2013 were:

- Non-Hispanic Asians – 64.4%
- Non-Hispanic Whites – 57.9%
- Two or more races – 51%
- Non-Hispanic Hawaiian/Pacific Islander – 50.2%
- Hispanics – 45.6%
- Non-Hispanic Native American/Alaska Native – 41.3%
- Non-Hispanic Blacks – 39.1%

Cultures vary in their initiation of breastfeeding, support persons important to the continuation of breastfeeding, and weaning practices. It is important for the home care nurse to individualize care for all women by incorporating their cultural beliefs and practices related to breastfeeding. Peer, spouse/partner, and family support is important to all breastfeeding women, and support is essential to increasing the rates of breastfeeding in women of African heritage, which still fall behind those of other demographic groups (Currie, 2013; Eastin & Sharma, 2015). The home care nurse should ensure that the woman is connected to a source of support. Reaching Our Sisters Everywhere (ROSE) is a nonprofit breastfeeding support organization directed toward African American women.

*Percentages reflect any amount of continued breastfeeding.

Note: *It is unwise to attribute specific attitudes or beliefs to all members of a cultural group. The information in the Developing Cultural Competence boxes offers possible insights into caring for women from different cultural groups.*

Breastfeeding Referrals and Social Support. Support from the woman's family and social contacts is very important with regard to the initiation and continuation of breastfeeding, as is support from healthcare professionals. Providers of care need to be

TABLE 34–3 References for Nurses Who Work with Breastfeeding Patients

- Academy of Breastfeeding Medicine (ABM).
- Association of Women's Health, Obstetric, and Neonatal Nursing (AWHONN). (2015). *AWHONN position statement: Breastfeeding.*
- BiliTool, Inc. (2004–2016). *BiliTool*™.
- Drugs and Lactation Database (LactMed).
- Goldbas, A. (2015). Breastfeeding: What's law got to do with it? *International Journal of Childbirth Education, 30*(4), 21–24.
- Hale, T. D., & Rowe, H. E. (2017). *Medications and mothers' milk* (17th ed.). New York, NY: Springer.
- La Leche League International (LLLI) (2018).
- Wambach, K., & Riordan, J. (2016). *Breastfeeding and human lactation* (5th ed.). Burlington, MA: Jones & Bartlett.
- U.S. Department of Health and Human Services. (2011). *The Surgeon General's call to action to support breastfeeding.* Washington, DC: U.S. Department of Health and Human Services, Office of the Surgeon General.

educated about breastfeeding physiology and resources in order to educate and support patients. Family members require information and education from professionals in order to support breastfeeding women as well. The home care nurse should be familiar with local lay support groups and arrange for the initial contact.

Formula Feeding

The AAP recommends that parents use a commercially prepared, iron-fortified infant formula until 1 year of age if the baby is not breastfed (AAP & ACOG, 2017). Some mothers need or choose to feed their babies formula because of their own health status or personal preference. If the mother does not have a health history that precludes her from breastfeeding, it may be helpful to explore the reasons for her decision. Some mothers choose formula because of lack of education about the benefits of breastfeeding, misconceptions about breastfeeding, or lack of support. If that is the case and the mother desires help with breastfeeding, lactation can still be established at this time with proper support. If the mother needs or chooses to use formula, it is important for the nurse to respect her choice and provide information related to safe formula-feeding.

Most human milk substitutes in this country are available in ready-to-feed, liquid concentrate, and powder forms. Many parents reconstitute the powder, as it is the most economical formulation. Chronic overconcentration can result in hypernatremic dehydration, whereas underconcentration can result in water intoxication and undernourishment. Therefore, it is important to emphasize the importance of mixing the formula exactly as the package directs.

The World Health Organization (WHO) published guidelines for the preparation of powdered formula in 2007, due to concerns regarding *Enterobacter sakazakii* and *Salmonella enterica*. The FDA and CDC published additional guidance after a number of U.S. babies developed *Cronobacter* infection in 2011 (FDA, 2018). Home care nurses should be aware that there are significant education gaps regarding the safe preparation and storage of infant formula. The home visit is an excellent time to assess the parents' understanding and to inspect the area where the formula will be prepared and stored. The WHO (2007) developed pamphlets describing safe formula preparation, which offer explicit instructions in multiple languages. Pamphlets can be downloaded from the WHO website. See Chapter 29 for a detailed discussion of the safe preparation of formula and formula-feeding.

Other Types of Follow-Up Care

Other types of follow-up care may include return home visits, telephone follow-up, and postpartum classes or support groups.

Return Visits

If the mother and family and physician/CNM have chosen discharge earlier than 48 hours after vaginal birth, the mother may, in some states, request a total of three visits. In such cases, the nurse would schedule the first visit about 24 hours after discharge and then space out the other two visits over the next week. In other instances, the nurse may schedule additional home visits based on the findings of the first home visit and the follow-up phone call.

Telephone Follow-Up

The postpartum home care nurse usually makes a follow-up phone call a few days after the home visit. During the call, the nurse may provide additional information, address questions or areas of confusion, and make referrals.

Some families may be offered or may request a telephone follow-up at the time of discharge. A mutually agreeable time is set for the call, typically within 3 days of discharge, or earlier if desired. Calls typically last about 10 to 20 minutes and are preplanned and goal directed.

To perform an effective telephone assessment, the nurse must be able to project a caring attitude, listen skillfully, use open-ended questions, and wait for answers. When assessment reveals signs of an initial or recurring postpartum complication, the nurse refers the woman to her primary care provider for further evaluation.

The plan of care developed and implemented during a telephone conversation is limited to supportive counseling, teaching, and referral. The new mother may have many questions, especially about newborn care, and is generally at a high level of learning readiness. The nurse can answer the woman's questions and use the questions as a stepping-stone for further teaching. Many communities have established 24-hour advice lines for new parents to call when they have questions or need support. In areas where helplines are not available, parents may be directed to call the birthing center. If birthing center nurses field parent phone calls, they should follow established protocols regarding the advice to be given and the documentation required. In either case, the home care nurse provides the number so that it is readily accessible for the family.

Postpartum Classes and Support Groups

Postpartum classes are becoming more common as caregivers recognize the continuing needs of the childbearing family. In many instances, classes are prepared to meet the specific needs of a variety of families so that, for example, single mothers and adolescent mothers can attend class with peers. A series of structured classes may focus on topics such as parenting, postpartum exercise, or nutrition, or there may be loosely structured group sessions that address mothers' concerns as they arise. Such classes offer chances for the new mother to socialize, share her concerns, and receive encouragement.

Some cities offer breastfeeding or new-parent support groups through birthing centers or hospitals or as a community effort, providing an opportunity for parents to interact with one another and to share information and experiences. New-mother support groups can provide a peer group for mothers as they evolve in the parenting role. Women in peer support groups have the opportunity to discuss physical, emotional, and social changes that occur for the childbearing family. Postpartum depression groups can be a tremendous support for women suffering from postpartum mood and anxiety disorders, providing an opportunity to share their experiences and have a supportive environment to discuss their feelings and symptoms.

Support Programs Utilizing Technology

Technology plays a central role in communication today, and the use of phone apps, online support groups, internet discussion boards, social media, and peer-support online technologies will continue to provide information and support for new mothers and their families. The nurse should encourage mothers to evaluate the online information source to ensure the content is up-to-date and research-based and to confirm the expertise of the author. It is important to remind new mothers that peer-support groups, discussion boards, and other internet sites often represent opinions and individual experiences and are not a replacement for professional medical advice. New mothers should be encouraged to view websites affiliated with government organizations, universities, or healthcare organizations because such sites are usually credible.

Focus Your Study

- The Newborns' and Mothers' Health Protection Act took effect in January 1998 and provides for a guaranteed minimum stay of up to 48 hours following an uncomplicated vaginal birth and up to 96 hours following an uncomplicated cesarean birth. The AAP recommends that all newborns discharged before 48 hours be examined within 48 hours after discharge, and, ideally, that all newborns be seen at the 3- to 5-day point for weight, hydration, intake and output, and jaundice screening. Home care nursing meets this requirement.
- The overall goal of postpartum home visits is to enhance opportunities for smooth transition of the new family. The home visit provides opportunities for assessment, teaching, breastfeeding support, and fostering a caring relationship with new families.
- In planning the home visit, the nurse needs to take precautions to maintain safety, such as carrying a cell phone, notifying supervisors of the location of the visit, keeping personal belongings out of sight, assessing the neighborhood and home for signs of danger, and, if danger is present, terminating the visit.
- Physical assessment of the newborn during a home visit includes assessments of vital signs, weight, overall color including jaundice, body systems, intake/output, hydration, umbilical cord and circumcision, newborn nutrition, newborn safety, parent education, and attachment.
- Teaching goals during home visits include reinforcing daily newborn care, including demonstrations of positioning and handling, sponge and tub bathing, nail care, and dressing; discussing temperature assessment and signs of illness; assisting with newborn feeding; discussing expected newborn output; discussing newborn behavioral states; promoting a safe sleep environment for the newborn, including SIDS and SUID prevention; promoting crib safety; encouraging childproofing of the home environment; discussing prevention of unintentional injuries and abuse; and facilitating newborn screening and immunization.
- The physician or pediatric nurse practitioner should be notified if there is evidence of redness around the newborn's umbilicus, if there is bright red bleeding or puslike drainage near the cord stump, or if the umbilical site remains unhealed.
- A primary risk factor for sudden infant death syndrome (SIDS) is sleeping in the prone position. Babies should sleep on their backs in a crib that is near the parents' bed. Babies should not be exposed to secondhand smoke and should not sleep in a bed with anyone. Use of a pacifier as the baby is falling asleep may help to prevent SIDS.
- State-mandated screening is performed on all newborns in the first 1 to 3 days. States vary regarding the conditions for which they screen.
- Universal hearing screening is performed on all newborns. Newborns who do not pass the screening should receive diagnostic testing by age 3 months and interventions by age 6 months as necessary.
- Signs of illness in mothers include pain or burning with urination, passage of clots or placental tissue, excessive pelvic or perineal pain, chest pain, difficulty breathing, excessive or foul-smelling lochia, failure of fundus to descend at the anticipated rate, temperature of 100.4°F (38°C) or higher, elevation of blood pressure, tenderness, redness, or pain in the legs or breasts, and feelings consistent with postpartum depression.
- Difficulties with breastfeeding include sore, cracked, flat, or inverted nipples; breast engorgement; plugged ducts; and mastitis.
- Breastfeeding mothers require information on effects of alcohol and various medications on breast milk, pumping, weaning, and breastfeeding referrals and social support.
- Parents who feed their newborn with a human milk substitute need information about safe preparation, storage, handling, and feeding of infant formula.
- Return visits, telephone follow-up, classes, support groups, and online resources can provide valuable information and support to new mothers and their families.

In order to make safe and effective judgments using NANDA-I © 2017 nursing diagnoses, it is essential that nurses refer to the definitions and defining characteristics of the diagnoses used in this text, which can be found in Appendix C.

References

Abney-Roberts, S. E. (2015). A successful quality improvement project to improve infant safe sleep practice. *JOGNN: Journal of Obstetric, Gynecologic & Neonatal Nursing, 44*(s1), S43. DOI: 10.1111/1552-6909.12599

Aly, H., Hoffman, H., El-Dib, M., Said, L., & Mohamed, M. (2015). Factor affecting length of stay in late preterm infants: An US national database study. *Journal of Maternal-Fetal & Neonatal Medicine 28*(5), 598–604. DOI: 10.3109/14767058.2014.927428

American Academy of Pediatrics (AAP). (2013). *Five things physicians and patients should question.* Retrieved from http://www.choosingwisely.org/wp-content/uploads/2015/02/AAP-Choosing-Wisely-List.pdf

American Academy of Pediatrics (AAP). (2016). Taskforce on SIDS and other sleep-related infant deaths: Updated 2016 recommendations for a safe infant sleeping environment. *Pediatrics, 138*(5). DOI: 10.1542/peds.2016-2938

American Academy of Pediatrics (AAP), Committee on Fetus and Newborn. (2010). Hospital stay for healthy term newborns. *Pediatrics, 125(2),* 405–409. DOI: 10.1542/peds.2009-3119

American Academy of Pediatrics (AAP) & American College of Obstetricians and Gynecologists (ACOG). (2017). *Guidelines for perinatal care* (8th ed.). Elk Grove Village, IL: Author.

American College of Obstetricians and Gynecologists (ACOG). (2018). *Optimizing postpartum care* (ACOG Committee Opinion No. 736). Washington, DC: Author.

Anderson, P. O., Manoguerra, A. S., & Valdés, V. (2016). A review of adverse reactions in infants from medications in breastmilk. *Clinical Pediatrics, 55*(3), 236–244. DOI: 10.1177/0009922815594586

Association of Women's Health, Obstetric, and Neonatal Nurses (AWHONN). (2013). *Neonatal skin care evidence-based clinical practice guideline* (3rd ed.). Washington, DC: Author.

Bainbridge, J. (2015). Dealing with breast and nipple soreness when breastfeeding. *British Journal of Midwifery, 13*(9), 552–556

Ball, J., Bindler, R., Cowen, K., & Shaw, M. (2016). *Principles of pediatric nursing* (6th ed., pp. 154–165). Hoboken, NJ: Pearson.

Barr, R. (2014). Crying as a trigger for abusive head trauma: A key to prevention. *Pediatric Radiology, 44*(4), S559–564. DOI: 10.1007/s00247-014-3100-3

Benitz, W. E. (2015). Hospital stay for healthy term newborn infants. *Pediatrics, 135*(5), 948–953. DOI: 10.1542/peds.2015-0699

Bennett C., Underdown A., & Barlow J. (2013). Massage for promoting mental and physical health in typically developing infants under the age of six months. *Cochrane Database of Systematic Reviews,* (Issue 4), Article No. CD005038. DOI: 10.1002/14651858.CD005038.pub3

Berens, P., Brodribb, W., & Academy of Breastfeeding Medicine. (2016). ABM clinical protocol #20: Engorgement, revised 2016. *Breastfeeding Medicine, 11,* 159–163. DOI: 10.1089/bfm.2016.29008.pjb

Biagioli, E., Tarasco, V., Lingua, C., Moja, L., & Savino, F. (2016) Pain-relieving agents for infantile colic. *Cochrane Database of Systematic Reviews,* Issue 9, Article No. CD009999. DOI: 10.1002/14651858.CD009999.pub2

BiliTool, Inc. (2004–2016). *BiliTool™.* Retrieved from http://bilitool.info

Brazelton, T. B., & Nugent, J. K. (2011). *Neonatal Behavioral Assessment Scale* (4th ed.). London, UK: Mac Keith Press.

Bulut, C., Gürsoy, T., & Ovali, F. (2016). Short-term outcomes and mortality of late preterm infants. *Balkan Medical Journal, 33*(2), 198–203. DOI: 10.5152/balkanmedj.2016.16721

Carroll, I. R. (2015). Opioids and lactation: Insufficient evidence of safety. *Pain Medicine, 16*(4), 628–630. DOI: 10.1111/pme.12718_2

Centers for Disease Control and Prevention (CDC). (2016a). Births: Preliminary data for 2015. *National Vital Statistics Reports, 65*(3). Retrieved from https://www.cdc.gov/nchs/data/nvsr/nvsr65/nvsr65_03_tables.pdf

Centers for Disease Control and Prevention (CDC). (2016b). *Breastfeeding: Proper handling and storage of human milk.* Retrieved from https://www.cdc.gov/breastfeeding/recommendations/handling_breastmilk.htm

Centers for Disease Control and Prevention (CDC). (2016c). *Rates of any and exclusive breastfeeding by socio-demographics among children born in 2013.* Retrieved from https://www.cdc.gov/breastfeeding/data/nis_data/rates-any-exclusive-bf-socio-dem-2013.htm

Currie, D. (2013). Breastfeeding rates for black US women increase but lag overall. *The Nation's Health, 43*(3), 1–20.

da Silva Santos, K. J., Silva Santana, G., de Oliveira Vieira, T., de Souza Teles Santos, C. A., Justo Giugliani, E. R., & Vieira, G. O. (2016). Prevalence and factors associated with cracked nipples in the first month postpartum. *BMC Pregnancy & Childbirth, 16,* 1–8. DOI: 10.1186/s12884-016-0999-4

Dalal, P. G. (2015). The need to treat maternal pain in the breastfeeding mother: Are opioids safe? *Pain Medicine, 16*(4), 630–631. DOI: 10.1111/pme.12718_3

Darnall, B. D., & Schatman, M. E. (2015a). Opioid use and lactation: Protecting the child in the context of maternal pain care. *Pain Medicine, 16*(4), 628. DOI: 10.1111/pme.12718

Darnall, B. D., & Schatman, M. E. (2015b). Protecting the infant from unknown risks. *Pain Medicine, 16*(4), 631–632. DOI: 10.1111/pme.12718_4

Davidson, M. R. (2014). *Fast facts for the neonatal nurse: An orientation for neonatal and high-neonatal nurses.* New York, NY: Springer.

Dennis, C. L., Jackson, K., & Watson, J. (2014). Interventions for treating painful nipples among breastfeeding women. *Cochrane Database of Systematic Reviews,* Issue 12, Article No. CD007366. DOI: 10.1002/14651858.CD007366.pub2

DePorre, A. G., Aronson, P. L., & McCulloh, R. J. (2017). Facing the ongoing challenge of the febrile young infant. *Critical Care, 21*(1), 68. DOI: 10.1186/s13054-017-1646-9

Dobson, D., Lucassen, P. L. B. J., Miller, J. J., Vlieger, A. M., Prescott, P., & Lewith, G. (2012). Manipulative therapies for infant colic. *Cochrane Database of Systematic Reviews,* Issue 12, Article No. CD004796. DOI: 10.1002/14651858.CD004796.pub2

Eastin, A., & Sharma, M. (2015). Using social cognitive theory to predict breastfeeding in African-American women. *American Journal of Health Studies, 30*(4), 196–202.

Flaherman, V. J., Schaefer, E. W., Kuzniewicz, M. W., Li, S. X., Walsh, E. M., & Paul, I. M. (2015). Early weight loss nomograms for exclusively breastfed newborns. *Pediatrics, 135*(1), e16–e23. DOI: 10.1542/peds.2014-1532

Food and Drug Administration (FDA). (2016). *Use caution when giving cough and cold products to kids.* Retrieved from http://www.fda.gov/Drugs/ResourcesForYou/SpecialFeatures/ucm263948.htm

Food and Drug Administration (FDA). (2018). *FDA takes final step on infant formula protections.* Retrieved from https://www.fda.gov/ForConsumers/ConsumerUpdates/ucm048694.htm

Govtrack. (2010). *H. R. 4642: Shaken Baby Syndrome Prevention Act of 2010.* Retrieved from https://www.govtrack.us/congress/bills/111/hr4642

Goyal, N. K., Attanasio, L. B., & Kozhimannil, K. B. (2014). Hospital care and early breastfeeding outcomes among late preterm, early-term, and term infants. *Birth: Issues in Perinatal Care, 41*(4), 330–338. DOI: 10.1111/birt.12135

Haastrup, M. B., Pottegård, A., & Damkier, P. (2014). Alcohol and breastfeeding. *Basic & Clinical Pharmacology & Toxicology, 114*(2), 168–173. DOI: 10.1111/bcpt.12149

Hale, T. D., & Rowe, H. E. (2017). *Medications and mothers' milk* (17th ed.). New York, NY: Springer.

Hannan, J., Brooten, D., Page, T., Galindo, A., & Torres, M. (2016). Low-income first-time mothers: Effects of APN follow-up using mobile technology on maternal and infant outcomes. *Global Pediatric Health, 3,* 2333794X16660234. DOI: 10.1177/2333794X16660234

Harfmann, K., Chen, A. Y., & Witman, P. (2017). Bullous diaper dermatitis with cloth diaper use. *Pediatric Dermatology, 34*(6), e309–e312. DOI: 10.1111/pde.13263

Hoover, K. (2016). Perinatal and intrapartum care. In K. Wambach & J. Riordan (Eds.), *Breastfeeding and human lactation* (5th ed., pp. 227–271). Burlington, MA: Jones & Bartlett.

Hwang, S. S., Lu, E., Cui, X., Diop, H., Barfield, W. D., & Manning, S. E. (2015). Home care practices for preterm and term infants after hospital discharge in Massachusetts, 2007 to 2010. *Journal of Perinatology, 35,* 880–884. DOI: 10.1038/jp.2015.90

Iacovou, M., Mulcahy, E. C., Truby, H., Barrett, J. S., Gibson, P. R., & Muir, J. G. (2017). Reducing the maternal dietary intake of indigestible and slowly absorbed short-chain carbohydrates is associated with improved infantile colic: A proof-of-concept study. *Journal of Human Nutrition and Dietetics, 31*(2), 149–285. DOI: 10.1111/jhn.12488

Jensen, D., Wallace, S., & Kelsay, P. (1994). LATCH: A breastfeeding charting system and documentation tool. *Journal of Obstetric, Gynecologic, and Neonatal Nursing: JOGNN / NAACOG, 23*(1), 27–32.

Kliegman, R. M., Stanton, B., Geme, J., & Schor, N. F. (2015). *Nelson textbook of pediatrics* (20th ed.). Philadelphia, PA: Elsevier.

Kochanek, K. D., Murphy, S. L., Xu, J., & Tejada-Vera, B. (2016). Deaths: Final data for 2014. *National Vital Statistics Reports, 65*(4). Retrieved from https://www.cdc.gov/nchs/data/nvsr/nvsr65/nvsr65_04.pdf

Koehn, M., & Dowling, J. (2016). Infant assessment. In K. Wambach & J. Riordan (Eds.), *Breastfeeding and human lactation* (5th ed., pp. 775–812). Burlington, MA: Jones & Bartlett.

La Leche League International (2018). *Breastfeeding and the law.* Retrieved from https://www.llli.org/resources/

Lain, S. J., Roberts, C. L., Bowen, J. R., & Nassar, N. (2015). Early discharge of infants and risk of readmission for jaundice. *Pediatrics, 135*(2), 314–321. DOI: 10.1542/peds.2014-2388

Lantz, B., & Ottosson, C. (2015). Using axillary temperature to approximate rectal temperature in newborns. *Acta Paediatrica, 104*(8), 766–770. DOI: 10.1111/apa.13009

Mangesi, L., & Zakarija-Grkovic I. (2016). Treatments for breast engorgement during lactation. *Cochrane Database of Systematic Reviews*, Issue 6, Article No. CD006946. DOI: 10.1002/14651858.CD006946.pub3

Mathews, T. J., MacDorman, M. F., & Thoma, M. E. (2015). Infant mortality statistics from the 2013 period linked birth/infant death data set. *National Vital Statistics Reports, 64*(9). Retrieved from https://www.cdc.gov/nchs/data/nvsr/nvsr64/nvsr64_09.pdf

May, P. A., Hasken, J. M., Blankenship, J., Marais, A., Joubert, B., Cloete, M., & . . . Seedat, S. (2016). Breastfeeding and maternal alcohol use: Prevalence and effects on child outcomes and fetal alcohol spectrum disorders. *Reproductive Toxicology, 63,* 13–21. DOI: 10.1016/j.reprotox.2016.05.002

McGrath, J. M., & Vittner, D. (2015). Behavioral assessment. In E. P. Tappero & M. E. Honeyfield (Eds.), *Physical assessment of the newborn* (5th ed., pp. 193–219). Petaluma, CA: NICU INK.

Mian, M., Shah, J., Dalpiaz, A., Schwamb, R., Miao, Y., Warren, K., & Khan, S. (2015). Shaken baby syndrome: A review. *Fetal & Pediatric Pathology, 34*(3), 169–175. DOI: 10.3109/15513815.2014.999394

Moon, R. Y., & American Academy of Pediatrics (AAP) Task Force on Sudden Infant Death Syndrome. (2016). SIDS and other sleep-related infant deaths: Updated 2016 recommendations for a safe infant sleeping environment. *Pediatrics, 138*(5), 1–12. DOI: 10.1542/peds.2016-2938

National Center for Injury Prevention and Control, Centers for Disease Control and Prevention. (2016a). *10 leading causes of injury deaths by age group highlighting unintentional injury deaths, United States—2014.* Retrieved from https://www.cdc.gov/injury/wisqars/pdf/leading_causes_of_injury_deaths_highlighting_unintentional_injury_2014-a.pdf

National Center for Injury Prevention and Control, Centers for Disease Control and Prevention. (2016b). *10 leading causes of nonfatal injury, United States—2014.* Retrieved from https://webapp.cdc.gov/cgi-bin/broker.exe?_PROGRAM=wisqnf.nfilead.sas&_SERVICE=v8prod&log=0&rept=nfil&year1=2014&year2=2014&Racethn=0&Sex=0&disp=0&ranking=10&PRTFMT=FRIENDLY&lcnifmt=lcd1age&intent=0&c_age1=0&c_age2=0&_debug=0

National Center on Shaken Baby Syndrome. (2017). *The period of purple crying.* Retrieved from https://www.dontshake.org/purple-crying

National Conference of State Legislatures. (2015). *Shaken baby syndrome prevention legislation.* Retrieved from http://www.ncsl.org/research/health/injury-and-violence-prevention-resources.aspx

National Institute for Occupational Safety and Health (NIOSH). (2010). *NIOSH hazard review: Occupational hazards in home healthcare.* Retrieved from https://www.cdc.gov/niosh/docs/2010-125/pdfs/2010-125.pdf

National Institute for Occupational Safety and Health (NIOSH). (2012). *Home healthcare workers: How to prevent violence on the job.* Retrieved from https://www.cdc.gov/niosh/docs/2012-118/pdfs/2012-118.pdf

National Institute for Occupational Safety and Health (NIOSH). (2014). *Caring for yourself while caring for others.* Retrieved from https://www.cdc.gov/niosh/docs/2015-103/pdf/2015-103.pdf

Ness, M. J., Davis, D. M. R., & Carey, W. A. (2013). Neonatal skin care: A concise review. *International Journal of Dermatology, 52*(1), 14–22. DOI:10.1111/j.1365-4632.2012.05687.x

Occupational Safety and Health Administration (OSHA). (2015). *Guidelines for preventing workplace violence for healthcare and social service workers.* Retrieved from https://www.osha.gov/Publications/osha3148.pdf

Penn State Hershey Medical Center. (2017). *NEWT: Newborn weight tool.* Retrieved from https://www.newbornweight.org

Powers, N. G. (2016). Low intake in the breastfed infant: Maternal and infant considerations. In K. Wambach & J. Riordan (Eds.), *Breastfeeding and human lactation* (5th ed., pp. 359–404). Burlington, MA: Jones & Bartlett.

Reece-Stremtan, S., Marinelli, K. A., & Academy of Breastfeeding Medicine (ABM). (2015). ABM clinical protocol #21: Guidelines for breastfeeding and substance use or substance use disorder, revised 2015. *Breastfeeding Medicine, 10*(3), 135–141. DOI: 10.1089/bfm.2015.9992

Reese, L. S., Heiden, E. O., Kim, K. Q., & Yang, J. (2014). Evaluation of period of PURPLE crying, an abusive head trauma prevention program. *Journal of Obstetric, Gynecologic, and Neonatal Nursing, 43*(6), 752–761. DOI: 10.1111/1552-6909.12495

Reich, D., Psomadakis, C. E., & Buka, B. (2017). Diaper dermatitis. In *Top 50 dermatology case studies for primary care* (pp. 191–198). Cham, Switzerland: Springer. DOI: https://doi.org/10.1007/978-3-319-18627-6_31

Rojjanasrirat, W., & Wambach, K. (2016). Maternal employment and breastfeeding. In K. Wambach & J. Riordan (Eds.), *Breastfeeding and human lactation* (5th ed., pp. 635–666). Burlington, MA: Jones & Bartlett.

Sinha, A., Sazawal, S., Pradhan, A., Ramji, S., & Opiyo, N. (2015). Chlorhexidine skin or cord care for prevention of mortality and infections in neonates. *Cochrane Database of Systematic Reviews,* Issue 3, Article No. CD007835. DOI: 10.1002/14651858.CD007835.pub2

Smith, L. J. (2016). Postpartum care. In K. Wambach & J. Riordan (Eds.), *Breastfeeding and human lactation* (5th ed., pp. 273–318). Burlington, MA: Jones & Bartlett.

Stadtlander, L. (2016). Sensory-based calming strategies for infants. *International Journal of Childbirth Education, 31*(4), 18–20.

Syrkin-Nikolau, M. E., Johnson, K. J., Colaizy, T. T., Schrock, R., & Bell, E. F. (2017). Temporal artery temperature measurement in the neonate. *American Journal of Perinatology, 34*(10), 1026–1031. DOI: 10.1055/s-0037-1601440

Thomas, S. (2016). Soothing crying babies and preventing shaken baby syndrome. *International Journal of Nursing Education, 8*(2), 34–38. DOI: 10.5958/0974-9357.2016.00043.X

Tully, K. P., Holditch-Davis, D., & Brandon, D. (2015). The relationship between planned and reported home infant sleep locations among mothers of late preterm and term infants. *Maternal Child Health Journal, 19*(7), 1616–1623. DOI: 10.1007/s10995-015-1672-7

U.S. Department of Health and Human Services (HHS). (2011). *The Surgeon General's call to action to support breastfeeding.* Washington, DC: U.S. Department of Health and Human Services, Office of the Surgeon General. Retrieved from https://www.surgeongeneral.gov/library/calls/breastfeeding/calltoactiontosupportbreastfeeding.pdf

U.S. Department of Health and Human Services (HHS). (2013). *Healthy People 2020.* Retrieved from https://www.healthypeople.gov/2020

U.S. Department of Labor, Employee Benefits Security Administration. (2008). *Protections for newborns, adopted children, and new parents: The newborns' and mothers' health protection act of 1996.* Retrieved from https://www.dol.gov/agencies/ebsa/about-ebsa/our-activities/resource-center/faqs/nmhpa

U.S. Environmental Protection Agency (EPA). (2016). *Mercury thermometers.* Retrieved from https://www.epa.gov/mercury/mercury-thermometers

Visscher, M. O., Adam, R., Brink, S., & Odio, M. (2015). Newborn infant skin: Physiology, development, and care. *Clinics in Dermatology, 33*(3), 271–280. DOI: 10.1016/j.clindermatol.2014.12.003

Walker, M. (2016). Breast pumps and other technologies. In K. Wambach & J. Riordan (Eds.), *Breastfeeding and human lactation* (5th ed., pp. 419–468). Burlington, MA: Jones & Bartlett.

Wambach, K. (2016). Breast-related problems. In K. Wambach & J. Riordan (Eds.), *Breastfeeding and human lactation* (5th ed., pp. 319–356). Burlington, MA: Jones & Bartlett.

Wessel, M. A., Cobb, J. C., Jackson E. B., Harris, G. S., & Detwiller, A.C. (1954). Paroxysmal fussing in infancy: Sometimes called colic. *Pediatrics, 14*(5), 421–435.

World Health Organization (WHO). (2007). *Safe preparation, storage, and handling of powdered infant formula guidelines.* Retrieved from https://www.who.int/foodsafety/publications/micro/pif_guidelines.pdf

Yangyang, R. Y., DeMello, A. S., Greeley, C. S., Cox, C. S., Naik-Mathuria, B. J., & Wesson, D. E. (2018). Injury patterns of child abuse: Experience of two level 1 pediatric trauma centers. *Journal of Pediatric Surgery, 53*(5), 1028–1032. DOI: 10.1016/j.jpedsurg.2018.02.043

Yonemoto, N., Dowswell, T., Nagai, S., & Mori, R. (2017). Schedules for home visits in the early postpartum period. *Cochrane Database of Systematic Reviews,* Issue 8, Article No. CD009326. DOI: 10.1002/14651858.CD009326.pub3

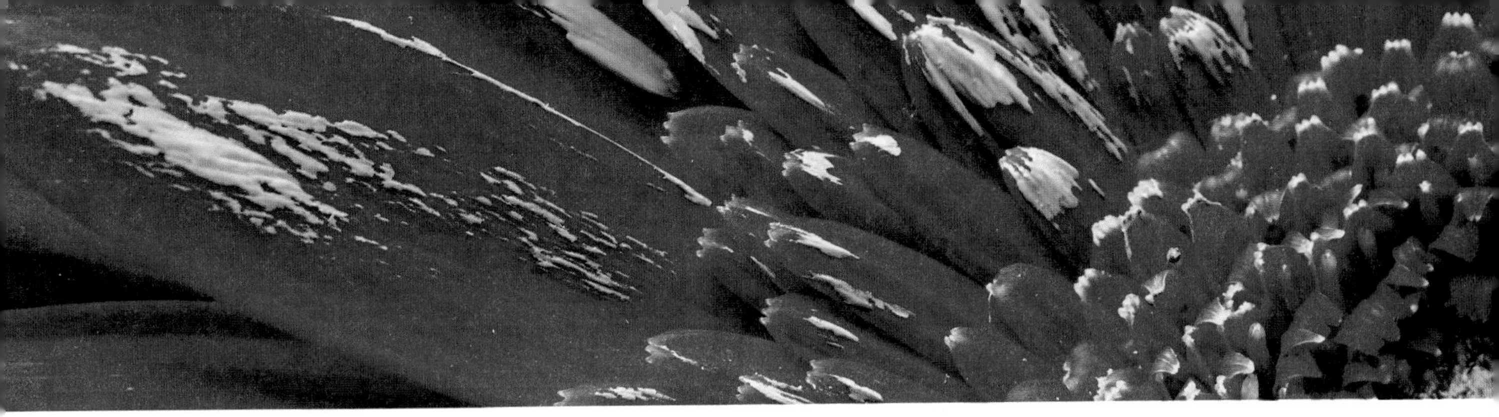

Chapter 35

The Postpartum Family at Risk

We are surviving. Just. Why don't they give the Croix de Guerre to people who can go without more than 2 hours total daily sleep for 5 weeks? I thought babies ate at 6–10–2–6–10–2—mine does. He also eats at 5–7–9–11 and 4–8–12. I am getting rather used to going around with my breasts hanging out. They are either drying from the last feed or getting ready for the next one. But the love—I never knew, never imagined that I would love him like this. This incredible feeling of boundless, endless love—a wish to protect his innocence from ever being hurt or wounded or scratched. And that awful, horrible, mad feeling in the first week that you'll never be able to keep anything so precious and so vulnerable alive.

—The Boston Women's Health Collective, *The New Our Bodies, Ourselves*

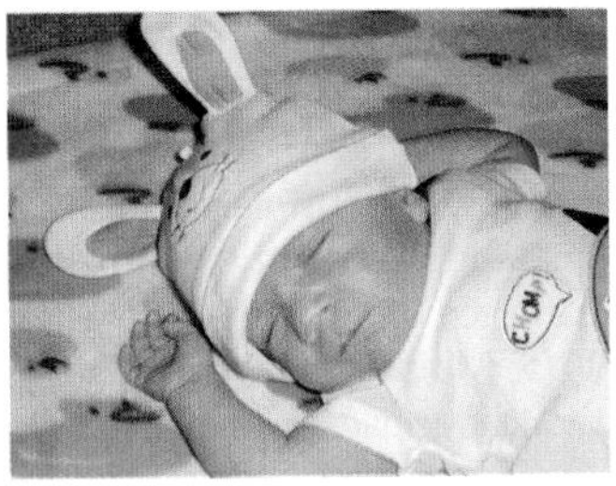

Learning Outcomes

35.1 Identify the causes, contributing factors, signs and symptoms, clinical therapy, and nursing interventions for early and late hemorrhage during the postpartum period.

35.2 Identify the causes, contributing factors, signs and symptoms, clinical therapy, and nursing interventions for reproductive tract infection.

35.3 Develop a nursing care plan that reflects knowledge of etiology, pathophysiology, current clinical therapy, and nursing and preventive management for the woman experiencing:

- Urinary tract infection
- Lactation mastitis
- Thromboembolic disease
- Postpartum psychiatric disorder.

35.4 Identify the woman's knowledge of self-care measures, signs of complications to be reported to the primary care provider, and measures that can be taken to prevent recurrence of complications.

Healthy People 2020

(MICH-5) Reduce the rate of maternal mortality to 11.4 maternal deaths per 100,000 live births

(MICH-6) Reduce maternal illness and complications due to pregnancy (complications during hospitalized labor and delivery) to 28.0%

The postpartum period is typically viewed as a smooth, uneventful transition time—and often it is, even with the challenges of new parenthood and the integration of a new person into the family. However, it is important for the nurse to be aware of physical or emotional complications that may develop postpartum. The nurse should teach the family the signs of postpartum complications, findings to report to the physician/certified nurse midwife (CNM), and preventive measures, if available.

Early postpartum discharge challenges the nurse to impart anticipatory information about normal postpartum recovery and self-care for the mother and her newborn, as well as be vigilant about recognizing when things go wrong. Postpartum complications can be life-threatening to the mother and require immediate collaborative management. These complications sometimes necessitate readmission of the woman to the hospital, thereby disrupting the family and adding concerns not only about her health but also about the way in which care of the newborn will be managed. The most common complications of the postpartum period are hemorrhage, infection, thromboembolic disease, and postpartum psychiatric disorders. These complications are the major focus of this chapter.

Care of the Woman with Postpartum Hemorrhage

The American College of Obstetricians and Gyncologists' reVITALize program's definition of **postpartum hemorrhage (PPH)** is a "cumulative blood loss greater than or equal to 1,000 mL or blood loss accompanied by signs or symptoms of hypovolemia within 24 hours after the birth process (includes intrapartum blood loss) regardless of route of delivery" (ACOG, 2017a, p. e168). The traditional definition of postpartum hemorrhage is a blood loss greater than 500 mL following a vaginal delivery and 1000 mL following a cesarean delivery. This definition is being questioned because quantification studies indicate that these numbers are close to the average blood loss during vaginal and cesarean births; however, these numbers are still abnormal and require careful monitoring (ACOG, 2017a; American Academy of Pediatrics [AAP] & ACOG, 2017; Dildy, 2018; Main et al., 2015). Therefore, practitioners use the definitive diagnoses of a drop in maternal hematocrit levels of 10% or more from predelivery baseline or excessive bleeding that causes hemodynamic instability or the need for a blood transfusion (ACOG, 2017a).

PPH is described as either early (immediate or primary) or late (delayed or secondary) postpartum hemorrhage. *Early (primary) postpartum hemorrhage* occurs in the first 24 hours after childbirth and is the more common of the two. *Late (secondary) postpartum hemorrhage* occurs from 24 hours after delivery to 12 weeks after birth (ACOG, 2017a). Postpartum hemorrhage accounts for more than 10% of the significant maternal mortality and morbidity in the United States. The decrease in mortality and morbidity has been attributed to better management of uterine atony, the primary cause of PPH. Worldwide, PPH is the leading cause of pregnancy-related deaths (Dildy, 2018).

Estimation of blood loss at childbirth may be difficult because blood mixes with amniotic fluid and is obscured as it oozes onto drapes or is sponged away and thus is often underestimated by as much as 50% (Cunningham et al., 2018). As the amount of blood loss increases, as in the case of hemorrhage, estimates are likely to be even less accurate than those associated with normal childbirth. Given the increased blood volume of pregnancy, the clinical signs of hemorrhage—such as decreased blood pressure (BP), increasing pulse, widening pulse pressure, thirst, restlessness, and decreasing urinary output—may not appear until significant blood loss (approximately 1,500 mL or more, or 25% of blood volume) has occurred (ACOG, 2017a). Visual estimation of blood loss (with education) has been shown to improve in accuracy (ACOG, 2017a).

SAFETY ALERT!

To meet the standard of care in cases of postpartum hemorrhage, *rapid response systems* are needed in every obstetric setting that will enable nurses to respond quickly to independently implement certain actions based on evidence-based protocols, similar to a call for coding someone experiencing a cardiac arrest. This multidisciplinary team approach helps to organize roles and prioritize care to stabilize the patient in a timely manner, thus averting massive hemorrhage.

Early (Primary) Postpartum Hemorrhage

When the placenta separates from the uterine wall, the many uterine vessels that have carried blood to and from the placenta are severed abruptly. The normal mechanism for hemostasis after expulsion of the placenta is contraction of the interlacing uterine muscles to occlude the open sinuses that previously brought blood into the placenta. Absence of prompt and sustained uterine contraction (uterine atony) can cause significant blood loss. Other causes of hemorrhage include laceration of the genital tract; episiotomy; retained placental fragments; vulvar, vaginal, or subperitoneal hematomas; uterine inversion; uterine rupture; problems of placental implantation; and coagulation disorders.

UTERINE ATONY

Uterine atony (relaxation of the uterus) is the leading cause of early postpartum hemorrhage, accounting for over 80% of PPH cases (ACOG, 2017a). Although uterine atony can occur after any childbirth, its contributing factors include (Cunningham et al., 2018):

- Overdistention of the uterus due to multiple gestation, hydramnios, or a large baby (macrosomia)
- Prolonged or precipitous labor
- Oxytocin augmentation or induction of labor
- Grandmultiparity because stretched uterine musculature contracts less vigorously
- Use of anesthesia (especially halothane) or other drugs such as magnesium sulfate, calcium channel blockers such as nifedipine, or tocolytics like terbutaline (Brethine), any of which cause the uterus to relax
- Prolonged third stage of labor—more than 30 minutes
- Preeclampsia
- Asian or Hispanic heritage
- Operative birth (includes vacuum extraction or forceps-assisted births)
- Retained placental fragments
- Placenta previa or accreta; placental abruption
- Obesity.

When evaluating a patient who is bleeding, it may be helpful to consider the "**4 Ts**" mnemonic device: *Tone, trauma, tissue,* and *thrombin* (ACOG, 2017a). Hemorrhage from uterine atony may be slow and steady or sudden and massive. The blood may escape vaginally or collect in the uterus, evident as large clots. The uterine cavity may distend with up to 1000 mL or more of blood, while the perineal pad and linen protectors remain suspiciously dry. A treacherous feature of postpartum hemorrhage is that maternal vital signs may not change until significant blood loss has occurred because of the increased blood volume associated with pregnancy.

SAFETY ALERT!

It is critical to remember that a woman with no identifiable risk factors may hemorrhage after childbirth.

Ideally, PPH is prevented, beginning with adequate prenatal care, good nutrition, avoidance of traumatic procedures, risk assessment, early recognition, and management of complications as they arise. Review of maternal records for risk factors will help nurses to plan assessment timelines to maximize early identification and management of excessive bleeding. There are many risk assessments available and they are able to identify 60 to 85% of patients who will experience significant hemorrhaging (ACOG, 2017a).

There is evidence that active management of the third stage of labor through administration of an oxytocic drug after delivery, controlled traction on the umbilical cord, and uterine massage after birth could prevent many cases of postpartum hemorrhage (ACOG, 2017a). Any woman at risk should be typed and cross-matched for blood transfusion. Postpartum women must be assessed at frequent intervals, especially in the initial hours after delivery of the placenta, when most deaths from hemorrhage occur.

CLINICAL THERAPY

The goals of medical management of PPH are to stop the hemorrhage, correct hypovolemia, and treat the underlying cause. After expulsion of the placenta, the fundus is palpated to ensure that it is firmly contracted. If it is not firm, gentle fundal massage is performed until the uterus contracts. Fundal massage is uncomfortable for the woman who has not received regional anesthesia; she will need an explanation for why this procedure is necessary and support as massage is initiated. When excessive bleeding continues despite external uterine massage, the physician may elect to do a bimanual massage (Figure 35–1A). Bimanual massage compresses the body of the uterus from below while the abdominal hand massages the fundus from above.

If uterine massage is not effective, uterine stimulants (uterotonic agents) will be administered to contract the atonic musculature. Oxytocin, ergotamine, prostaglandin analog, and misoprostol are most often used. Prophylactic oxytocin, by dilute intravenous infusion (bolus dose of 10 units) or intramuscular injection (10 units) by itself, is the most effective medication (ACOG, 2017a). Oxytocin can be administered after delayed cord clamping, with delivery anterior shoulder or with placental delivery. Table 35–1 summarizes critical nursing information about the use of uterine stimulants to control bleeding. The need for IV fluid replacement and blood transfusion is determined on the basis of hemoglobin and hematocrit results as well as coagulation studies.

Management By Uterine Tamponade. If uterotonic agents are unsuccessful at correcting uterine atony, the physician may use uterine tamponade as a temporizing measure, buying time for fluid and blood replacement. One technique of uterine tamponade is the use of the Bakri balloon, which is inserted into the uterine cavity and inflated with 300–500 mL of isotonic saline to provide pressure against the uterine walls. The tube has an open tip, which permits any continuous bleeding from the uterus to be visualized. If bleeding is controlled, the tamponade is removed after 24 hours (Cunningham et al., 2018). Alternatively, the uterine cavity may be packed tightly with 4-inch-wide sterile gauze (ACOG, 2017a).

Management By Uterine Artery Embolization. If uterotonic agents or tamponade efforts are unsuccessful, uterine artery embolization (UAE) may be considered using a percutaneous catheter to embolize bleeding vessels. The woman must be hemodynamically stable as the procedure itself takes approximately 30 minutes. UAE is performed by an interventional radiologist in a facility with this capability, thus it may not be available in rural settings or small community hospitals. However, this procedure has been successful as a method of controlling PPH when traditional therapies fail and is an alternative to hysterectomy in preserving future fertility (Francois & Foley, 2017).

Surgical Management Of Postpartum Hemorrhage. An exploratory laparotomy may be performed, with a variety of uterine compression techniques attempted.

One technique of uterine compression sutures is the B-Lynch compression (brace suture) procedure, which is used as a secondary treatment (ACOG, 2017a). When tied, the suture creates "suspenders" to compress the uterus (Francois & Foley, 2017). For non-life-threatening levels of hemorrhage, the uterine artery may be surgically ligated to diminish uterine perfusion and control bleeding, especially when excessive bleeding occurs during cesarean childbirth. There are a variety of techniques.

When all conservative efforts to control hemorrhage fail, a hysterectomy provides definitive surgical treatment of uterine bleeding; however, it also carries serious surgical complications (e.g., bladder and ureteral injuries). Because it ends childbearing for the woman, it is often considered a procedure of last resort (ACOG, 2017a). The new mother may experience emotional distress related to loss of fertility and need opportunities to discuss those feelings candidly with a caring professional.

LACERATIONS OF THE GENITAL TRACT

Early postpartum hemorrhage may also be associated with lacerations of the perineum, vagina, or cervix. Several factors predispose women to higher risk of reproductive tract lacerations:

- Nulliparity
- Epidural anesthesia
- Precipitous childbirth (less than 3 hours)
- Macrosomia
- Forceps- or vacuum-assisted birth
- Use of oxytocin.

Genital tract lacerations should be suspected when bright red vaginal bleeding persists in the presence of a firmly contracted uterus. The nurse who suspects a laceration should notify the clinician so that the laceration can be immediately sutured to control hemorrhage and repair the integrity of the reproductive tract (Francois & Foley, 2017). The woman may be moved to a delivery or surgical area for access to special lighting to facilitate treatment.

Episiotomies can be an underappreciated source of postpartum blood loss because of slow, steady bleeding, especially if it was done early in the birth process. To fully assess the episiotomy site, the nurse must position the woman on her side. See discussion of episiotomy in Chapter 25.

RETAINED PLACENTAL FRAGMENTS

Retained placental fragments can be a cause of early postpartum hemorrhage; however, they are generally the most common cause of late hemorrhage. Retention of fragments is usually attributable to partial separation of the placenta during massage of the fundus before spontaneous placental separation, so this practice should be avoided.

Following birth, the placenta should always be inspected for intactness and evidence of missing fragments or cotyledons on the maternal side and for vessels that traverse to the edge of the placenta outward along the membranes of the fetal side. The latter finding may indicate succenturiate placenta and a retained lobe. Uterine exploration by the physician may be required at that time to remove missing fragments (see Figure 35–1B). This cause should be immediately suspected if bleeding persists and no lacerations are noted. Sonography may be used to diagnose retained placental fragments (ACOG, 2017a). Treatment options for retained placenta include uterotonic agents or curettage (Francois & Foley, 2017).

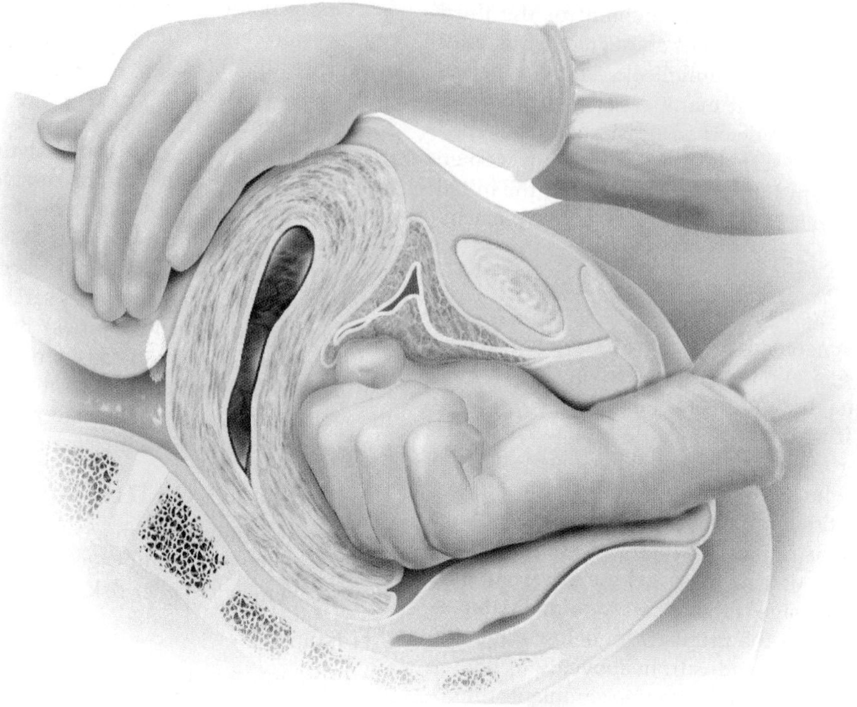

A

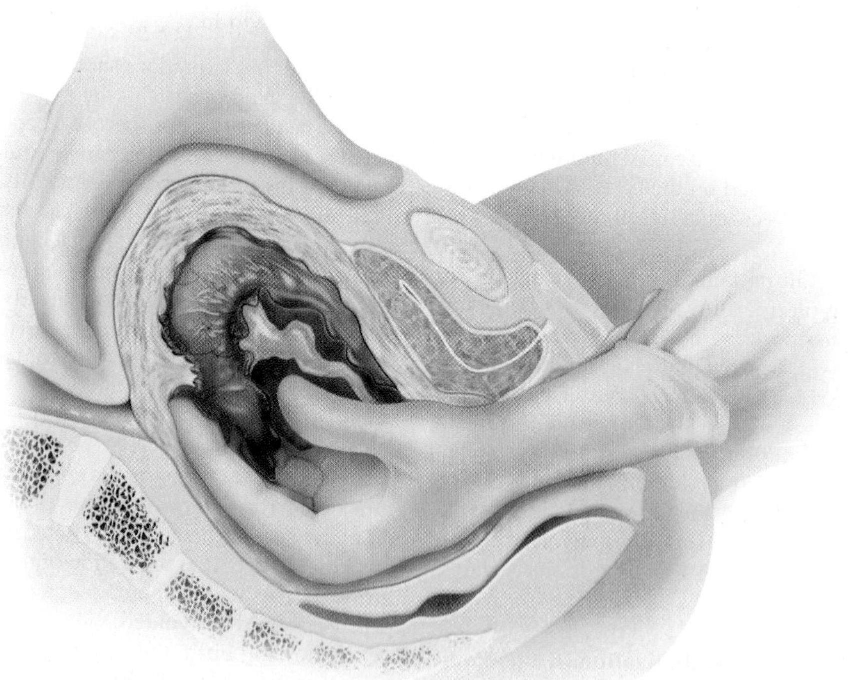

B

Figure 35–1 A. Manual compression of the uterus and massage with the abdominal hand will usually effectively control hemorrhage from uterine atony. B. Manual removal of placenta. The fingers are alternately abducted, adducted, and advanced until the placenta is completely detached. Both procedures are performed only by the medical clinician.

TABLE 35–1 Uterine Stimulants Used to Prevent and Manage Uterine Atony

DRUG	DOSING INFORMATION	CONTRAINDICATIONS	EXPECTED EFFECTS	SIDE EFFECTS
Oxytocin (Pitocin, Syntocinon)	IV use: 10–40 units in 500–1000 mL crystalloid fluid at 50 milliunits/min continuous administration rate. Onset: Immediate. Duration: 1 hr. **IV bolus administration not recommended.** IM use: 10 units. Onset: 3–5 min. Duration: 2–3 hr.	Rare hypersensitivity to medication.	Rhythmic uterine contractions that help to prevent or reverse postpartum hemorrhage caused by uterine atony.	Usually none. Uterine hyperstimulation, nausea and vomiting, mild transient hypertension, hyponatremia with prolonged dosing. Avoid undiluted rapid IV infusion, which causes hypotension.
Misoprostol (Cytotec)	800–1000 mcg Rectally, orally, or sublingually. One dose only. Rapid effects, contractions within minutes.	Rare. History of allergies to prostaglandins.	Used to prevent and treat uterine atony after failed attempts to control bleeding with oxytocics.	Nausea and vomiting, diarrhea, shivering, abdominal pain, headache.
Methylergonovine maleate (Methergine)	IM use: 0.2 mg every 2–4 hr. Onset: 2–5 min. Duration: 3 hr (for five-dose maximum). PO use: 0.2 mg every 4 hr (for six doses). Onset: 7–15 min. Duration: 3 hr (for 1 week). **IV administration not recommended—can cause dangerous hypertension and stroke.**	Hypertension. Preeclampsia. Women with known sensitivity to drug, cardiac disease, scleroderma, and Raynaud disease. Use with caution during lactation.	Sustained uterine contractions that help to prevent or reverse postpartum hemorrhage caused by uterine atony. Management of postpartum subinvolution.	Severe hypertension, particularly when given IV. Nausea and vomiting, headache (migraine), hypotension.
Prostaglandin (15-methyl PGF_{2a}, Prostin/15M)	IM use: 0.25 mg repeated every 15–90 min, up to eight doses max. Physician may elect to administer by direct intramyometrial injection.	Women with active cardiovascular, renal, liver disease, or asthma, or with known hypersensitivity to drug.	Control of refractory cases of postpartum hemorrhage caused by uterine atony. Generally used after failed attempts at control of hemorrhage with oxytocic agents.	Nausea and vomiting, diarrhea, headache, flushing, bronchospasm, wheezing, cough, chills, transient fever.
Dinoprostone (Prostin E_2)	Vaginal or rectal suppository 20 mg every 2 hr. Stored in frozen form—must be thawed to room temperature.	Avoid if woman is hypotensive or has asthma or acute inflammatory disease. Hypotension.	Stimulate uterine contractions.	Fever is common and occurs within 15 to 45 min of insertion. Headache, chills diarrhea, nausea and vomiting.

Nursing Implications with Uterine Stimulants

- Note expected duration of action of drug being administered and take care to recheck fundus at that time for adequate tone.
- When the drug is ineffective and the fundus remains atonic (boggy or uncontracted) and bleeding continues, massage the fundus. If massage fails to cause sustained contraction, consider the status of the urinary bladder. If uterine tone is not restored after the bladder is empty and fundal massage has been performed, notify the physician/CNM immediately.
- Monitor woman for signs of known side effects of the drug; report to healthcare provider if side effects occur.
- Remind the woman and her support person that uterine cramping is an expected result of these drugs and that medication is available for discomfort. Administer analgesic medications as needed for pain relief. Provide nonpharmacologic comfort measures. If analgesic medication ordered is insufficient for pain relief, notify the healthcare provider.
- Provide information to the woman and her family regarding the importance of not smoking during Methergine administration (nicotine from cigarettes leads to constricted vessels and may lead to hypertension) and signs of toxicity.

When Prostaglandin Is Used

- Check temperature every 1–2 hours. Administer antipyretic medication as ordered for prostaglandin-induced fever.
- Auscultate breath sounds frequently for signs of adverse respiratory effects.
- Assess for nausea and vomiting and diarrhea. Administer antiemetic and antidiarrheal medications as ordered. (In some settings, women are premedicated with these drugs.)

SOURCES: Data from ACOG, 2017a; Francois & Foley, 2017; Rhode, 2016.

SAFETY ALERT!

Postpartum nurses need to bear in mind that most deaths from postpartum hemorrhage are not caused by catastrophic bleeding episodes but by ineffective management of slow, steady blood loss.

VULVAR, VAGINAL, AND PELVIC HEMATOMAS

Hematomas occur as a result of injury to a blood vessel from birth trauma, often without noticeable trauma to the superficial tissue, or from inadequate hemostasis at the site of repair of an incision or laceration. The soft tissue in the area offers little resistance, and hematomas containing 250 to 500 mL of blood may develop rapidly. Hematomas may be vulvar, vaginal, vulvovaginal, or subperitoneal. The latter are rare but most dangerous because of the large amount of blood loss that can occur without clinical symptoms until the woman becomes hemodynamically unstable. Subperitoneal hematomas involve the uterine artery branches or vessels in the broad ligaments and require laparotomy for surgical correction.

Risk factors for hematomas include episiotomy, forceps- or vacuum-assisted birth, and genital tract laceration. Other associated risk factors are primiparity, macrosomia, prolonged second stage, preeclampsia, clotting disorder, and history of vulvar varicosities. Hematomas less than 3 cm in size and nonexpanding are managed expectantly with ice packs and analgesia. Heat may be used after 24 hours to facilitate absorption of the blood within the hematoma. Small hematomas usually resolve over several days. For larger hematomas and those that expand, surgical management is usually required: The hematoma is evacuated using incision and drainage. The bleeding vessel is ligated and the wound closed, with or without vaginal packing.

The hematoma site is an ideal medium for the growth of flora normally present in the genital tract. Consequently, broad-spectrum antibiotics are usually ordered to prevent infection or abscess.

UTERINE INVERSION

Uterine inversion, a prolapse of the uterine fundus to or through the cervix so that the uterus is, in effect, turned inside out after birth, is a rare but life-threatening cause of associated postpartum hemorrhage. Although not always preventable, uterine inversion is often associated with abnormal adherence of the placenta, weakness of the uterine musculature or other uterine abnormalities, rapid labor, uterine relaxation secondary to anesthesia or drugs such as magnesium sulfate, and excess traction on the umbilical cord or vigorous manual removal of the placenta. Most cases of uterine inversion are managed by immediate repositioning of the uterus within the pelvis by the physician under intravenous tocolysis or general anesthesia (ACOG, 2017a).

COAGULATION DISORDERS

Coagulation disorders, such as von Willebrand disease or thrombocytopenia, are associated with PPH and should be suspected when postpartum bleeding persists with no identifiable cause. A consumptive coagulopathy, such as disseminated intravascular coagulation (DIC), can lead to PPH. DIC may occur during pregnancy or postpartum as a result of preeclampsia, amniotic fluid embolism, sepsis, abruptio placentae, or prolonged intrauterine fetal demise syndrome (Francois & Foley, 2017).

Late Postpartum Hemorrhage

Although early postpartum hemorrhage most often occurs within hours of birth, delayed hemorrhage occurs more than 24 hours to 12 weeks after childbirth, most frequently as a result of **subinvolution** (failure to return to normal size) of the placental site or retention of placental tissue. Blood loss at this time may be excessive but rarely poses the same risk as that from immediate postpartum hemorrhage. Late postpartum hemorrhage occurs in 1% of pregnancies and can be extremely stressful for the woman and her family who are at home by this time (ACOG, 2017a).

With subinvolution, the postpartum fundal height is greater than expected, often discovered 4 to 6 weeks after birth. In addition, lochia often fails to progress normally from rubra to serosa to alba. Some women report scant brown lochia or irregular heavy bleeding. Leukorrhea, backache, and foul-smelling lochia may occur if infection is a cause. There may be a history of heavy early postpartum bleeding or difficulty in expulsion of the placenta during the third stage of labor. When portions of the placenta have been retained in the uterus, bleeding continues because normal uterine contraction that constricts the bleeding site is prohibited. Presence of placental tissue within the uterus can be confirmed by pelvic ultrasonography.

Treatment includes oral administration of methylergonovine maleate (Methergine) 0.2 mg every 3 to 4 hours for 24 to 48 hours (see Table 35–1). When uterine infection is present, antibiotics are also administered. If retained placenta is suspected or other treatment is ineffective, curettage may be indicated (ACOG, 2017a).

●○● NURSING MANAGEMENT

For the Woman with Postpartum Hemorrhage

Nursing Assessment and Diagnosis

Careful and ongoing assessment of the woman during labor and birth and evaluation of her prenatal history will help identify factors that put her at risk for PPH. However, it is critical to remember that PPH may occur without any risk factors, so all women must be monitored. Regular and frequent assessment of fundal position and tone or contractility will alert you to the possible development of hemorrhage.

Monitoring the bladder for increasing distention, with immediate intervention, can prevent excessive bleeding that occurs when a full bladder displaces the uterus and interferes with contractility. Assessment for bleeding can be done visually, by pad counts, or by weighing the perineal pads or other items that have absorbed blood. In cases of excessive bleeding, be alert for signs of impending hypovolemic shock and the development of coagulation problems, such as disseminated intravascular coagulation (DIC) (see Chapter 24 for a discussion of DIC).

For all complaints of perineal pain, examine the perineal area for signs of hematomas: Ecchymosis, edema, tenseness of tissue overlying the hematoma, a fluctuant mass bulging at the introitus, and extreme tenderness to palpation. Estimating the size on first assessment of the perineum enables you to better identify increases in size and the potential blood loss. Notify the physician/CNM if a hematoma is suspected. The risk of vulvar or vaginal hematoma can be decreased by applying an ice pack to the woman's perineum during the first hour after birth and intermittently thereafter for the next 8 to 12 hours. If a small hematoma develops despite preventive measures, a sitz bath after the first 12 hours will aid fluid absorption once bleeding has stopped and will promote comfort, as will the judicious use of analgesic agents (see Chapter 33).

In cases of excess bleeding, be alert for signs of impending hypovolemic shock. Frequent noninvasive monitoring should continue: Heart rate, blood pressure, auscultation of heart sounds and breath sounds, oxygen saturation, skin turgor, color, temperature, color and moisture of mucous membranes, capillary refill, level of consciousness, and urinary output, possibly with Foley catheter/urometer, and electrocardiogram (ECG) readings. With severe hemorrhage, anticipate the addition of invasive monitoring for a more objective evaluation of status: Central venous pressure (CVP) monitoring via a peripheral line and/or Swan-Ganz central line insertion for pulmonary artery wedge pressure monitoring and arterial blood gases to ascertain acidosis and hypoxia. In some settings, the woman needing invasive hemodynamic monitoring may be transported to an intensive care unit.

Development of a rapid response team is a patient safety initiative. When obstetric postpartum hemorrhage occurs, the interprofessional perinatal rapid response team needs to work collaboratively to treat the underlying cause, manage the blood loss, and lessen the risk to the mother (ACOG, 2017a).

Nursing diagnoses that may apply when a woman experiences postpartum hemorrhage include:

- *Fluid Volume: Deficient*, related to blood loss secondary to uterine atony, lacerations, hematomas, or retained placental fragments
- *Tissue Perfusion: Peripheral, Risk for Ineffective*, related to hypovolemia
- *Bleeding, Risk for*, related to lack of information about signs of delayed postpartum hemorrhage

(NANDA-I © 2017)

Nursing Plan and Implementation

Hospital-Based Nursing Care

If a soft, boggy uterus is detected, massage it until firm. If the uterus is not contracting well and appears larger than anticipated, clots may be expressed during fundal massage. Once clots are removed, the uterus tends to contract more effectively. Overly aggressive massage should be avoided so as not to injure the vessels in the broad ligaments or cause reactive relaxation of the musculature.

If the woman seems to have a slow, steady, free flow of blood, begin weighing the perineal pads (1 mL = 1 g) (Rhode, 2016). Monitor the woman's vital signs at least every 15 minutes, more frequently if indicated. If the fundus is displaced upward or to one side because of a full bladder, encourage the woman to empty her bladder—or catheterize her if she is unable to void—to allow for efficient uterine contractions. Excessive bleeding or uterine atony despite fundal massage necessitates prompt notification to the healthcare provider.

Clinical Tip

A boggy uterus indicates that the uterus is not well contracted. This results in increased uterine bleeding, which may remain in the uterus and form clots or may result in increased flow. To assess the amount of blood loss, you must first massage the uterus until it is firm and then express clots. Even though the woman may have a firm uterus, significant bleeding can occur from causes other than uterine atony. To accurately determine the amount of blood loss, it is not sufficient to assess only the peri-pad. You should also ask the woman to turn on her side so you can assess underneath her for pooling of blood. Be sure to have a good light source.

When there are risk factors for postpartum hemorrhage or frequent fundal massage has been necessary to sustain uterine contractions, maintain the vascular access (the IV line) initiated during labor in case additional fluid or blood becomes necessary. If blood has been cross-matched earlier, check that blood is available in the blood bank.

As the woman's blood volume becomes depleted, positioning her with her legs elevated to 30 degrees facilitates venous return and promotes oxygenation. Unlike the Trendelenberg position used in the past for shock, this position does not impede breathing or cardiac function and promotes cerebral circulation. Supplemental oxygen may be necessary to keep peripheral tissues oxygenated when blood is shunted to protect vital organs like the brain and kidneys. See *Key Facts to Remember: Nursing Actions During Postpartum Hemorrhage*.

Key Facts To Remember
Nursing Actions During Postpartum Hemorrhage

- Call for help. Initiate response team as per hospital protocol.
- Massage uterus until firm.
- Administer prescribed medications.
- Ensure large-bore (14-, 16-, or 18-gauge) needle IV access (consider starting a second line).
- Replace volume with normal saline or lactated Ringer solution.
- Apply pulse oximeter and administer oxygen according to agency protocol.
- Insert a Foley catheter to empty the bladder and accurately measure output.
- Maintain accurate intake and output measurements.
- Assess blood loss; weigh peri-pads or Chux dressing for objective estimate of blood loss.
- Monitor pulse and blood pressure every 15 minutes or more often as indicated.
- Assess for shock.
- Elevate the legs to a 20- to 30-degree angle to increase venous return.
- Draw blood for complete blood count (CBC), type and cross-match, coagulation studies (PT, PTT, fibrinogen), and blood chemistry.
- Notify blood bank that transfusion may be necessary; administer blood products as ordered.
- Continuous electrocardiogram (ECG) monitoring may be indicated for hypotension, continuous bleeding, tachycardia, or shock.
- Prepare for additional interventions such as uterine tamponade, exploratory laparotomy, or uterine artery embolization.
- Anticipate pain management needs for fundal massage and uterotonic medications.
- Provide emotional support for the woman and her family.

Sources: Data from Francois & Foley, 2017; Rhode, 2016.

Fluid Replacement and Transfusion

Rapid administration of crystalloid fluids (normal saline and lactated Ringer solution) is necessary with excessive blood loss. Intravascular volume is replaced initially with rapid administration of warmed crystalloid solutions, in a 3 mL solution per 1 mL of estimated blood lost ratio. With rapid attempts to replace depleted blood volume, you must carefully monitor the woman for evidence of fluid overload. When blood loss is significant and vital signs become unstable, crystalloid fluid replacement can no longer compensate for the loss, and transfusion of blood products becomes necessary. When blood products are transfused, watch for transfusion reactions and respond promptly according to hospital procedures. Normal saline must be hung prior to administration of blood since dextrose causes hemolysis and lactated Ringer solution causes agglutination of cells. Blood products such as red blood cells (RBCs) are often transfused to replace depleted oxygen-carrying red cells. If platelets decrease significantly, fresh frozen plasma may be added. Evidence is emerging that the use of recombinant activated factor VIIa is an effective adjunctive measure for massive hemorrhage and coagulopathy. Factor VIIa is a precursor for the extrinsic clotting cascade and becomes depleted with massive hemorrhage (ACOG, 2017a). Frequent laboratory testing of hemoglobin, hematocrit, platelets, and a coagulation panel should be monitored. During bleeding episodes, it is important to appreciate that hemoglobin and hematocrit levels will not reflect the volume lost until after plasma volume equilibrates. Table 35–2 provides basic information about blood products used with women experiencing PPH.

Women who require blood products may be concerned about the associated risks. Provide assurance that follow-up care will monitor for untoward consequences of blood replacement. Adherence to strict clinical protocols while accessing blood products from the lab and administering blood products is imperative to maximize patient safety. More immediately evident transfusion reactions range from a nonhemolytic and self-limited febrile response to life-threatening hemolytic reactions with blood group incompatibility, often because of error. Assess for any type of transfusion reaction and notify the physician immediately. In the case of the hemolytic reaction, the uninfused blood is returned to the lab for evaluation.

Ethics in Action!

How does the nurse respond when a patient's religious beliefs do not allow her to receive blood products? When is the ideal time to discuss this with the patient and family?

Keeping the woman as comfortable as possible with perineal care and frequent changes of disposable pads is important, but her position cannot be allowed to compromise venous return or oxygenation. She will be kept NPO in case surgery is needed, so oral care is important for comfort. There are many interruptions when the patient is experiencing a complication, so you will need to seek opportunities to promote rest whenever possible. Any intervention to help with maternal–newborn bonding in the interval of separation is of great value to the woman. These include providing photographs or videotapes of the newborn, direct reports from the nursery staff, and brief visits to the room if her condition allows. Encourage the father/partner to visit the newborn and bring information to the mother.

If assessment reveals that the woman's condition is deteriorating, anticipate that more intensive monitoring will be necessary in an intensive care setting. If the woman will remain on the obstetrical unit, anticipate and request necessary resources and personnel to ensure the patient's safety and well-being. In urgent situations, such as escalating postpartum bleeding, it is easy for the woman and her family to feel as if they are the center of attention but not to understand what is happening—only that something is going "badly wrong." The need to provide them with ongoing information about her status and each procedure and its rationale in understandable terms is a critical dimension of quality nursing care. A calm, competent approach goes a long way toward calming the woman and her family, as does offering them opportunities to verbalize their feelings and ask questions or seek clarification.

Clearly, the care of the woman experiencing postpartum hemorrhage depends on good nursing assessment and prompt reporting of nonreassuring findings to the physician. Direct treatment methods, however, require the collaboration of a physician and, in some cases, radiography or surgical staff. You will become an important liaison between these departments, keeping the necessary individuals apprised of the woman's status. For example, if additional transfusions of whole blood or blood products are anticipated, you will need to keep the hospital laboratory informed to facilitate timely response. Care may well include the preprocedural preparation of the woman for surgery or for procedures such as arterial embolization performed by a radiologist.

TABLE 35–2 Blood Products for Managing Postpartum Hemorrhage

BLOOD PRODUCT	USE IN PPH	VOLUME/UNIT	INFUSION INFORMATION
Cryoprecipitate	Corrects deficiencies of factor VIII, XIII, von Willebrand factor + fibrinogen.	10–15 mL	Increases fibrinogen levels 5–10 mg/dL per unit transfused.
Fresh frozen plasma	Contains all clotting factors.	250 ML	Thawed for use. Must use within 24 hours of thaw. Infuse with blood filter or component filter. May give at 200 mL/hour unless fluid overload.
Packed red blood cells	Contain RBCs and plasma. Increase oxygen-carrying capacity of blood without adding volume—used for acute blood loss.	300 ML	Filter required for administration. Infusion rate +/– 4 hours/unit within 1 hour (ACOG, 2017a). Expected to increase hemoglobin by 1 g/dL and hematocrit by 3% per unit transfused.
Platelets (single donor pooled)	Control or prevent blood loss associated with deficiency in platelets and for prophylactic use for those with platelet counts <10,000.	300 mL (6U)	Give within 4 hours of preparation. Use component filter for administration. Increases platelets by 30,000–60,000^3 per unit transfused.

SOURCES: Data from ACOG, 2017a; Francois & Foley, 2017.

After a postpartum hemorrhage, evaluate the woman for signs of anemia, such as fatigue, pallor, headache, thirst, and orthostatic changes in pulse or BP, and review the results of all hematocrit determinations. All medical interventions, IV infusions, blood transfusions, oxygen therapy, and medications such as uterine stimulants are monitored as necessary and evaluated for effectiveness. Urinary output should be monitored to determine adequacy of fluid replacement and renal perfusion, with amounts less than 30 mL/hr reported to the physician (Rhode, 2016).

Help the woman plan activities so that adequate rest is possible. The woman who is experiencing anemia and fatigue may need assistance with self-care and progressive ambulation for several days. When she is able to be out of bed to shower, use of a shower chair permits independence while providing a measure of safety should the woman experience weakness or dizziness.

SAFETY ALERT!
The emergency call light should be easily accessible to the patient whenever nurses have left the bedside, even temporarily.

Once her condition has stabilized somewhat, the mother may find it difficult to care for her newborn because of the fatigue associated with blood loss and may require additional assistance in caring for her baby. If she has IV lines in place, even carrying the newborn may be awkward.

If the father/partner is involved in the birth experience, including that person in the plan of care is a productive strategy. This person can support the mother's recovery by helping to meet her physical needs while encouraging her to rest. The mother is likely to feel less concern over her limited opportunities for the newborn's care if she can witness the father/partner interacting with and caring for the newborn. Hospitals providing family-centered care will accommodate the father, partner, or other family member to stay in the hospital room so that rooming-in with the newborn is still an option. See *Health Promotion: Preventing Postpartum Bleeding*.

Health Promotion Preventing Postpartum Bleeding

The woman and her family or other support persons should receive clear, preferably written, explanations of the normal postpartum course, including changes in the lochia and fundus and signs of abnormal bleeding. Instructions for the prevention of bleeding should include fundal massage, ways to assess the fundal height and consistency, and inspection of any episiotomy and lacerations, if present. The woman should receive instruction in perineal care (see discussion on perineal care in Chapter 33). The mother and her family are advised to contact her healthcare provider if any of the signs of postpartum hemorrhage occur (see *Key Facts to Remember: Signs of Postpartum Hemorrhage*). If iron supplementation is ordered, instructions for proper dosage should be provided along with client teaching to enhance absorption and avoid constipation and nausea.

SAFETY ALERT!
Good hand hygiene using standard precautions throughout the hospitalization and emphasizing to the patient proper handwashing for home care is important to minimize risk of postpartum infection.

Key Facts To Remember
Signs of Postpartum Hemorrhage

- Excessive or bright red bleeding (saturation of more than one pad per hour)
- A boggy fundus that does not respond to massage
- Abnormal clots
- High temperature
- Any unusual pelvic discomfort or backache
- Persistent bleeding in the presence of a firmly contracted uterus
- Rise in the level of the fundus of the uterus
- Increased pulse or decreased BP
- Hematoma formation or bulging/shiny skin in the perineal area
- Decreased level of consciousness.

Community-Based Nursing Care

When a telephone follow-up or an examination at the home visit provides evidence of a developing complication, share these findings or impressions with the woman and mutually plan an appropriate next step. In the case of telephone follow-up, counsel the woman to notify her healthcare provider and be prepared to schedule an appointment immediately if risk assessment indicates. If a complication is identified at the home visit, you will need to communicate the clinical findings to the healthcare provider and document them and any interventions for the permanent record. See Chapter 34 for a more detailed discussion of home care for the postpartum family.

For most postpartum women, routine discharge instructions include advice such as "You take care of the baby, and let someone else care for you, the family, and the household." Because of her fatigue and weakened condition, the woman who experienced postpartum hemorrhage may be unable even to care for her newborn without assistance. The caregivers at home need clear, concise explanations of her condition and needs for recovery. For example, all should understand the woman's need to rest and to be given extra time to rest after any necessary activity. See *Complementary Health Approaches: Adjunct Therapy for Controlling Postpartum Bleeding*.

To ensure her safety, advise the woman to rise slowly to minimize the likelihood of orthostatic hypotension. Until she regains strength, the mother should be seated when holding the newborn.

The person who assumes responsibility for grocery shopping and meal preparation will need advice about the importance of including foods high in iron in the daily menus. Explain the rationale for continuing medications containing iron and remind the woman that vitamin C–containing fluids maximize absorption of iron, and tea or milk products prevent absorption.

The woman should continue to count perineal pads for several days so she can recognize any recurring problem with excessive blood loss (hypovolemia). Invasive procedures, her debilitated condition, and anemia associated with hemorrhage increase the woman's risk of puerperal infection. She and her caregivers should use good handwashing technique and minimize exposure to infection in the home. They should be given a list of signs of infection and should understand the importance of alerting her healthcare provider immediately should signs occur.

In addition to meeting the woman's physical needs, assess the couple's coping strategies and resources for dealing with unanticipated complications. Providing realistic information and exploring effective coping strategies can be of immeasurable value as they try to maintain a sense of balance in this difficult situation. A sense of emergency often exists in the event of late postpartum

Complementary Health Approaches

Adjunct Therapy for Controlling Postpartum Bleeding

The herb shepherd's purse can be used in tea or tincture form to help control postpartum bleeding. Yarrow is often used with shepherd's purse as a homeostatic agent. Cinnamon and cayenne have also been used. Always report bleeding to a healthcare provider.

hemorrhage. Because it commonly occurs 1 to 2 weeks after birth, the couple is generally at home, involved in the day-to-day activities demanded by their new roles, when the unexpected, excessive bleeding begins. Quick decisions about child care arrangements must often be made so that the mother can return to the hospital. Both mother and father/partner are likely to be alarmed by the excessive bleeding and concerned about her prognosis. There will be additional worries about separation from the newborn, especially when the mother is breastfeeding. The father/partner may find himself torn between the needs of the mother and those of the newborn and any other children. Ideally, arrangements can be made to minimize separation of the family members.

Evaluation

Expected outcomes of nursing care include:

- Signs of postpartum hemorrhage are detected quickly and managed effectively.
- Maternal–newborn attachment is maintained successfully.
- The woman is able to identify abnormal changes that might occur following discharge and understands the importance of notifying her healthcare provider if they develop.

Care of the Woman with a Reproductive Tract Infection or Wound Infection

Puerperal infection is an infection of the reproductive tract associated with childbirth that occurs at any time up to 6 weeks postpartum. The most common postpartum infection is endometritis (metritis), which is infection limited to the uterine lining. However, infection can spread by way of the lymphatic and circulatory systems to become a progressive disease resulting in parametrial cellulitis and **peritonitis** (infection involving the peritoneal cavity). The cause of postpartum fever is presumed to be endometritis until proven otherwise. Other causes of postpartum fever should be considered: Respiratory complications such as atelectasis or pneumonia, acute pyelonephritis, thrombophlebitis, or breast engorgement, which rarely lasts more than 24 hours (Duff & Birsner, 2017).

Although the death rate from postpartum infection is low in the United States, infection accounts for 11% of pregnancy-related deaths. Uterine infections are relatively uncommon following uncomplicated vaginal births, but they continue to be a major source of morbidity for women who give birth by cesarean section. Routine antibiotic prophylaxis for cesarean childbirth in conjunction with aseptic technique, fewer traumatic operative births, a better understanding of labor dystocia, improved surgical intervention, and a population that is generally at less risk from malnutrition and chronic debilitative disease have contributed to a reduction in overall postpartum morbidity and mortality.

The standard definition of **puerperal morbidity** established by The Joint Committee on Maternal Welfare is a temperature of 38°C (100.4°F) or higher (taken by mouth four times a day) on any 2 of the first 10 days after birth, not including the first 24 hours. During today's short obstetric hospital stays, the temperature is often measured every 6 hours, consistent with the definition for puerperal morbidity. However, serious infections can occur in the first 24 hours or may cause only persistent low-grade temperatures. Therefore, careful assessment of all postpartum women with elevated temperatures is essential.

The normal vaginal flora of a healthy pregnant woman contains microorganisms that can be the source of infection to the upper genital tract and peritoneal cavity. Although the uterus is considered a sterile cavity before rupture of the fetal membranes, bacterial contamination of amniotic fluid with the membranes still intact at term is more common than previously believed and may contribute to premature labor. Following rupture of the membranes and during labor, contamination of the uterine cavity by vaginal or cervical bacteria can easily occur. Other factors must also be present for infection to occur, such as the change to an alkaline pH postpartum that favors growth of aerobes.

Because shortened inpatient stays are the norm in maternity care, women will likely be discharged following childbirth before clinical signs of puerperal infection are evident. Consequently, perinatal nurses are challenged to analyze the woman's history and clinical course for risk assessment and to recognize the early subtle signs of infection so that discharge may be delayed as needed. Before discharge, the nurse advises the woman about preventive measures, including scrupulous handwashing, and signs of infection. Nurses should educate the patient and her family about the risk of infection and how to recognize and respond appropriately, should it occur.

Postpartum Endometritis

Postpartum endometritis (metritis), an inflammation of the endometrium portion of the uterine lining, may occur postpartum in 1 to 3% of women who give birth vaginally and in 30 to 35% of those who give birth by cesarean after an extended period of labor and ruptured membranes (Duff & Birsner, 2017; Rhode, 2016).

Postpartum infection from vaginal delivery primarily affects the placental implantation site, the decidua, and adjacent myometrium. Bacteria that colonize the cervix and vagina gain access to the amniotic fluid during labor and postpartum and begin to invade devitalized tissue (the lower uterine segment, lacerations, and incisions). The same pathogenesis, polymicrobial proliferation and tissue invasion, is associated with cesarean delivery, but surgical trauma, additional devitalization of tissue, blood and serum accumulation, and foreign bodies (sutures, staples) provide additional favorable anaerobic bacterial conditions.

Clinical findings of metritis in the initial 24 to 36 hours postpartum tend to be related to group B streptococcus (GBS). Late-onset postpartum endometritis/metritis is most commonly associated with genital mycoplasmas and *Chlamydia trachomatis* (Duff & Birsner, 2017).

Risk factors for postpartum uterine infection include:

- Cesarean birth is the single most significant risk, especially when it occurs after an extended labor with ruptured membranes; the incidence of infection can be as high as 35% without antibiotic prophylaxis and 20% or less with prophylactic coverage (Duff & Birsner, 2017; Rhode, 2016).
- Premature rupture of the amniotic membranes (PROM)
- Prolonged labor preceding cesarean birth
- Multiple vaginal examinations during labor
- Compromised health status (low socioeconomic status, anemia, obesity, smoking, use of illicit drugs or alcohol, poor nutritional state)
- Use of fetal scalp electrode or intrauterine pressure catheter for internal monitoring during labor
- Obstetric trauma—episiotomy; laceration of perineum, vagina, or cervix
- Chorioamnionitis—infection of placenta, chorion, and amnion
- Preexisting bacterial vaginosis or *Chlamydia trachomatis* infection
- Instrument-assisted childbirth—vacuum or forceps
- Manual removal of the placenta or uterine exploration after delivery
- Retained placental fragments
- Lapses in aseptic technique by surgical staff
- Diabetes mellitus
- Immunocompromised status.

Assessment findings consistent with endometritis are foul-smelling lochia, fever (usually between 38.3° and 40°C [101° and 104°F]), uterine tenderness on palpation, lower abdominal pain, tachycardia, and chills (Duff & Birsner, 2017).

Prophylactic antibiotics during cesarean section decreases the incidence of endometritis by as much as 60%, particularly after prolonged labor or ruptured membranes. Traditionally, antibiotics are given to the mother during surgery after the umbilical cord is cut, thus avoiding difficulties in evaluating the baby for sepsis should the baby develop symptoms of infection (Duff & Birsner, 2017; Rhode, 2016).

Postpartum Wound Infections

Infections can occur at the episiotomy or repaired laceration site or at the site of a cesarean incision. Perineal wound infections are more likely to occur following a vaginal birth with a third- or fourth-degree laceration of the episiotomy due to bacterial contamination from the rectum (Duff & Birsner, 2017). It is recognized by the classic signs of redness, warmth, edema, purulent drainage, and, later, gaping of the previously approximated wound. Local pain may be severe.

After cesarean delivery, wound infection is most often associated with concurrent endometritis. The wound is typically red, indurated, tender at the margins, and draining purulent exudate. Some women have cellulitis without actual purulent drainage. Clinical exam is usually sufficient for diagnosis, but culture of the exudate should be routinely done when community-acquired methicillin-resistant *Staphylococcus aureus* (CA-MRSA) infections are possible (Cunningham et al., 2018).

CLINICAL THERAPY

The infection site and causative organism(s) are diagnosed by careful history, complete physical examination, and blood tests; aerobic and anaerobic endometrial cultures are no longer routinely performed because multiple organisms are usually present (Duff & Birsner, 2017; Rhode, 2016).

Localized wound infection is treated with broad-spectrum antibiotics, sitz baths, and analgesics as necessary for pain relief (see Chapter 33). Wounds with evidence of pus or serosanguineous effusion or an infected stitch site are opened and drained completely. Once the incision and drainage (I&D) of the wound is complete, it should be irrigated with warm saline two to three times daily and a clean dressing should be applied. It is then allowed to heal by secondary intention (Duff & Birsner, 2017). Alternatively, it may be packed with saline-dampened gauze, repacked two to three times daily, and covered with clean gauze using aseptic technique. This allows removal of necrotic debris when packing is removed. Antibiotics with coverage against *Staphylococcus aureus* should be given. Antibiotics are typically continued until the wound base is clean and any signs of cellulitis have resolved.

Endometritis is treated with intravenous antibiotics, such as cephalosporins and penicillins or carbapenem antibiotics. Women generally improve within 2 days of initiating antibiotics, which are continued until the patient has been afebrile and asymptomatic for 24 hours. If fever continues at 48 hours after antibiotic therapy, an additional workup is necessary to check for refractory pelvic infection. Approximately 90 to 95% of women with postpartum infection respond quickly to antibiotic therapy or drainage of abscesses and have a complete recovery and no long-term sequelae (Duff & Birsner, 2017).

●○● NURSING MANAGEMENT

For the Postpartum Woman with Puerperal Infection

Nursing Assessment and Diagnosis

After the initial postpartum inspections, inspect the woman's perineum or abdominal wound site every 8 to 12 hours for signs of early infection. The REEDA scale helps you remember to consider *r*edness, *e*dema, *e*cchymosis, *d*ischarge, and *a*pproximation of either the perineal or surgical wound. Any degree of induration (hardening) should be immediately reported to the clinician.

Fever, malaise, abdominal pain, foul-smelling lochia, larger-than-expected uterus, tachycardia, and other signs of infection should be noted and reported immediately so that treatment can begin. The white blood cell (WBC) count, a usual objective measure of infection, cannot be used reliably because of the normal increase in WBCs during the postpartum period; a postpartum WBC count of 14,000 to 16,000/mm^3 is not an unusual finding. An increase in WBC level of more than 30% in a 6-hour period, however, is indicative of infection.

Nursing diagnoses that may apply to the woman with a puerperal infection include:

- ***Injury, Risk for,*** related to the spread of infection
- ***Pain, Acute,*** related to the presence of infection
- ***Parenting, Risk for Impaired,*** related to delayed parent–newborn attachment secondary to woman's pain and other symptoms of infection as well as possible separation of the newborn from the mother

(NANDA-I © 2017)

Nursing Plan and Implementation

Hospital-Based Nursing Care

Careful attention to standard precautions and aseptic techniques during labor, birth, and postpartum is essential. In caring for a woman during the postpartum period, you are responsible for teaching her self-care measures that are helpful in preventing infection. If the woman has a draining wound or purulent lochia, it is especially important that those in contact with soiled items and linens practice good handwashing hygiene. Provide clear, concise instructions about wound care and how to discard soiled dressings appropriately to safeguard the woman and her caregivers.

If the woman is seriously ill, ongoing assessment of urine specific gravity and intake and output is necessary. Carefully administer antibiotics as ordered and regulate the IV fluids rate. Ongoing assessment of the woman's condition is vital to detect subtle changes in her health status. Be sure to recognize the woman's comfort needs related to hygiene, positioning, oral care, and pain relief. See *Nursing Care Plan: For the Woman with a Puerperal Infection* for specific nursing care measures.

Nursing Care Plan: For the Woman with a Puerperal Infection

1. Nursing Diagnosis: *Infection, Risk for*, related to traumatized tissues (NANDA-I © 2017)

Goal: The woman will be free of complications associated with infection.

INTERVENTION	RATIONALE
• Encourage the woman, staff, and family members to adhere to a strict hand-hygiene policy.	• Handwashing kills bacteria and prevents cross-contamination.
• Review the woman's prenatal, intrapartum, and postpartum records for underlying problems that could contribute to poor wound healing or increased risk for spread of infection.	• Identifying underlying problems gives the caregiver an opportunity to initiate preventive measures that will promote healthy wound healing and stop the spread of infection.
• Monitor blood pressure, pulse, respiration, and temperature.	• Obtain baseline data; signs and symptoms of septic shock produce a decrease in blood pressure and an increase in respirations. Temperature increase of 38°C/100.4°F or greater on any 2 days after the first 24 hours indicates infection.
• Instruct the woman on proper perineal care including wiping perineum from front to back after voiding, washing the perineum after voiding and defecating, and changing peri-pads frequently.	• Proper perineal care techniques enhance good hygiene and assist in removing urine and fecal contaminants from perineum. Changing peri-pads frequently decreases skin contact with a moist medium that favors bacteria growth.
• Encourage a well-balanced diet with adequate protein, calories, and vitamin C.	• Protein and vitamin C are essential nutrients for tissue healing and repair.
• Continue prenatal vitamins and iron as ordered	
• Encourage the woman to consume 2000 mL of fluid a day.	• Maintains hydration and increases circulating volume. Dilutes organisms that are eliminated with voiding.
• Encourage use of the sitz bath, Surgigator, or the perineal light two to four times a day for at least 10–15 minutes.	• Moist or dry heat to the perineum increases localized blood flow, promotes healing, and provides comfort.
• Encourage early ambulation.	• Enhances circulation and drainage of lochia.
• Assess and report signs and symptoms of infection in perineum including redness, erythema, edema, discharge, approximation of wound edges (REEDA), and pain.	• Identifying signs and symptoms of infection early allows for prompt treatment and healing.
• **Collaborative:** Obtain labwork as ordered by the physician including culture and sensitivity, CBC with differential, and WBC count.	• Identifies abnormal lab values for early intervention. In addition, identifies infection and its causative organism for appropriate antibiotic treatment.
• Administer antibiotic therapy as ordered by the physician.	• Fights infection and helps prevent ascension of organisms into further tissue.
• Promote wound drainage by assisting physician in opening the wound, if necessary. Also, if the wound is greater than 2–3 cm, pack with iodoform gauze.	• Iodoform gauze is used to maintain patency of wound opening. This promotes drainage and prevents abscesses from developing.
• Report signs and symptoms of severe infections: Foul-smelling lochia, uterine subinvolution, uterine tenderness, severe lower abdominal pain, elevated temperature, elevated WBC count, general malaise, chills, lethargy, tachycardia, nausea and vomiting, and abdominal rigidity.	• Reporting signs and symptoms of severe infections early allows for initiation of appropriate therapy by the physician and prevents further spread of the invading pathogen.

EXPECTED OUTCOME: The woman will be free of complications associated with infection as evidenced by practicing behaviors that prevent the spread of infection and promote timely wound healing.

Nursing Care Plan: For the Woman with a Puerperal Infection *(continued)*

2. Nursing Diagnosis: *Pain, Acute*, related to the infection process (NANDA-I © 2017)

Goal: The woman will be free of pain or have a level of relief that is acceptable.

INTERVENTION	RATIONALE
• Assess pain location and intensity; have the woman describe on a scale from 1 (mild) to 10 (severe). Assess nonverbal signs of pain, including facial grimacing and agitation.	• Assesses the need for pain management and evaluates interventions already implemented.
• Encourage the woman to discuss anxiety and fears.	• Reduces anxiety/fear and may decrease the woman's perception of pain.
• Encourage frequent rest periods and decrease disturbing environmental stimuli.	• Frequent rest periods will conserve woman's energy. Excessive environmental stimuli may increase woman's pain perception.
• Promote relaxation by encouraging diversionary activities and the use of exercises including radio/television, reading, guided imagery, deep-breathing techniques, massage, visualization, and meditation.	• Promotes relaxation and refocuses woman's attention away from the intensity of pain.
• **Collaborative:** Administer analgesics as ordered by the physician, evaluating the response to the analgesic and any adverse effects in a timely manner.	• Relieves pain and interrupts the pain–fear–tension cycle to facilitate relaxation.

EXPECTED OUTCOME: Woman is free of pain or has an acceptable level of pain as evidenced by verbalization of pain relief and the exhibition of a relaxed demeanor.

3. Nursing Diagnosis: *Parenting, Risk for Impaired*, related to pain secondary to maternal infection and/or separation from newborn to minimize exposure (NANDA-I © 2017)

Goal: Mother will have no problems bonding with newborn and assuming responsibility for the care of the baby with assistance and later independently.

INTERVENTION	RATIONALE
• Provide quality time for mother and newborn contact.	• Aids in the bonding process.
• Encourage the partner or family members to give the woman videos and pictures of the baby if the mother's condition requires separation from the baby.	• Promotes bonding and gives the mother reassurance that the baby is being cared for.
• Encourage the partner and family members to become involved with the care of the baby and verbalize interaction to the mother.	• Allows the mother to feel as though she is involved in the care of the baby.
• Encourage the mother to feed (breast or bottle) baby if her condition is stable. If the mother is unable to breastfeed, encourage and assist her in pumping her breasts to maintain milk production.	• Hands-on participation in the baby's care gives mother a positive outlook.
• Assess maternal support systems.	• As the mother is recovering, she will need assistance in household organization and personal care.
• **Collaborative:** Offer referrals to home health services, doula services, lactation services, and/or support groups.	• Ensures the woman's well-being and identifies problems that may require intervention.

EXPECTED OUTCOME: Mother will bond with the newborn as evidenced by exhibiting appropriate attachment behaviors when interacting with baby, providing care to self and baby, and verbalization of understanding of the parenting role.

Generally, breastfeeding is not contraindicated with postpartum infections. However, if the mother is seriously ill and is unable to nurse the baby, lactation should be supported with frequent pumping as tolerated. The partner of a seriously ill woman will be concerned about her condition and torn about spending time with her or with their newborn. Because maternal–newborn bonding may be compromised, father/partner–newborn bonding can be especially important. Allow the mother time to discuss her feelings and concerns (Rhode, 2016).

Community-Based Nursing Care

The woman with a puerperal infection needs assistance when she is discharged from the hospital. If the family cannot provide this home assistance, a referral to home care services is needed. Home care services should be contacted as soon as puerperal infection is diagnosed so that a nurse can meet with the woman for a family and home assessment and development of a home care plan.

The family needs instruction in the care of a newborn, including feeding, bathing, cord care, immunizations, and significant observations that should be reported. Breastfeeding mothers receiving antibiotics should be instructed to inspect the baby's mouth for signs of thrush and to report the finding to their physician.

The mother should be instructed regarding activity, rest, medications, fluids, diet, and signs and symptoms of recurrent infection and complications, and she should be scheduled for a return medical visit. Breastfeeding mothers need to know the importance of taking the entire course of prescribed antibiotics even though they may begin to feel better before the bottle is empty. She also needs to be informed about the importance of pelvic rest; that is, she should not use tampons or douches or have intercourse until she has been examined by the physician and told it is safe to resume those activities. See *Case Study: Benita Cartier*.

Evaluation

Expected outcomes of nursing care include:

- The infection is quickly assessed, and treatment is instituted successfully without further complications.
- The woman understands the nature of the infection and the purpose of therapy; she carries out any ongoing antibiotic therapy necessary after discharge.
- Maternal–newborn attachment is maintained.

Care of the Woman with a Urinary Tract Infection

The postpartum woman is at increased risk of developing urinary tract problems because of the normal postpartum diuresis, increased bladder capacity, decreased bladder sensitivity from stretching or trauma, bacterial shedding with urinary stasis, and possible inhibited neural control of the bladder following the use of general or regional anesthesia and contamination from catheterization. It is important that the mother empty her bladder completely with each voiding.

Overdistention of the Bladder

Overdistention occurs postpartum when the woman is unable to empty her bladder, usually because of trauma or the effects of anesthesia. Women who have not sufficiently recovered from the effects of anesthesia cannot void spontaneously, and catheterization is necessary. Other risk factors for urinary retention after childbirth include nulliparity, instrumental childbirth, and prolonged labor. Delay in recognizing and managing urinary retention increases the woman's risk of developing a urinary tract infection (UTI) (Stanley & Conner, 2015).

Clinical Tip

Postpartum urinary retention is often defined as "the absence of spontaneous urination within 6 hours of a vaginal delivery or within 6 hours after removal of an indwelling catheter post-cesarean delivery." The astute nurse will watch the woman's bladder for signs of retention—not the clock! As urinary retention promotes uterine atony and a subsequent increase in bleeding and also contributes to the possibility of UTI, timely intervention is crucial.

CLINICAL THERAPY

Overdistention in the early postpartum period is often managed by draining the bladder with a straight catheter as a one-time measure. If the overdistention recurs or is diagnosed later in the postpartum period, an indwelling catheter may be ordered for 24 hours. An alternate urinary retention protocol involves bladder ultrasound scans with intervention based on the amount of urine volume.

NURSING MANAGEMENT

For the Postpartum Woman with a Urinary Tract Infection

Nursing Assessment and Diagnosis

The overdistended bladder appears as a large mass, reaching sometimes to the umbilicus and displacing the uterine fundus upward and to one side. There is increased vaginal bleeding, the fundus is boggy, and the woman may complain of cramping as the uterus attempts to contract. Some women also experience backache and restlessness.

Nursing diagnoses that may apply when a woman has difficulties due to overdistention include:

- ***Infection, Risk for***, related to urinary stasis secondary to overdistention of the bladder
- ***Urinary Retention***, related to decreased bladder sensitivity and normal postpartum diuresis

(NANDA-I © 2017)

CASE STUDY: Benita Cartier

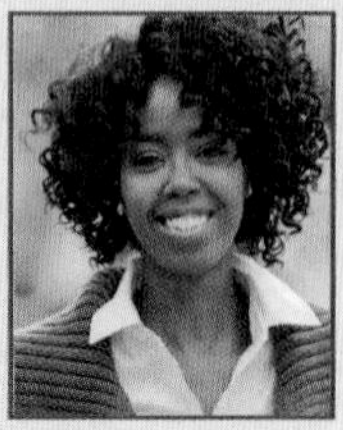

SOURCE: blvdone/Shutterstock.

Benita is still recovering after her emergency cesarean birth. This afternoon she notes she feels feverish and her incision is really uncomfortable, more so than yesterday. She is advised to come in to see the doctor. Her physical exam reveals that her incision appears red, tender with palpation, and is draining purulent drainage. There is a centimeter area adjacent to the left edge that appears to be opened and actively draining, no bright red is noted. Upon uterine palpation, she screams out in pain. The uterus appears to be firm, but it is hard to do any additional uterine assessment. Her vitals are T 101.3°F, HR 92, P 22, and BP 132/82.

Questions to Ponder

What would be your next step if you were caring for Benita? What labs would the healthcare provider be likely to order?

Nursing Plan and Implementation

Diligent monitoring of the bladder during the recovery period and preventive health measures greatly reduce the chance for overdistention of the bladder. Encouraging the mother to void spontaneously and helping her use the toilet, if possible, or the bedpan if she has received conductive anesthesia, prevents overdistention in most cases. Assist the woman to a normal position for voiding (i.e., sitting with the legs and feet lower than the trunk) and provide privacy to encourage voiding. The woman should be medicated for whatever pain she may be having before attempting to void because pain may cause a reflex spasm of the urethra. Perineal ice packs applied after birth will minimize any edema, which may interfere with voiding. Pouring warm water over the perineum or having the woman void in a sitz bath may also be effective. Some women note that hearing running water nearby, blowing bubbles through a straw into a glass of water, or voiding onto a bedpan into which a few drops of tincture of peppermint have been added helps stimulate voiding.

If catheterization becomes necessary, a careful, meticulous, aseptic technique should be employed during catheter insertion. The vagina and vulva are traumatized to some degree by vaginal birth, and edema is common. This edema may obscure the urinary meatus; therefore, be extremely careful in cleansing the vulva and inserting the catheter. It is imperative to discard a catheter that has inadvertently been introduced into the vagina and thus contaminated. Because catheterization is an uncomfortable procedure as a result of the postpartum trauma and edema of the tissue, be careful and gentle not only in inserting the catheter but also in handling and cleaning the perineal area.

If the amount of urine drained from the bladder reaches 800 mL, the catheter should be clamped and taped firmly to the woman's leg. Carefully document the procedure, including taking the woman's vital signs before and after the procedure and noting her responses. After an hour, the catheter may be unclamped and placed on gravity drainage. This technique protects the bladder and avoids rapid intra-abdominal decompression. When the indwelling catheter is removed, a urine specimen is often sent to the laboratory. The tip of the catheter is also removed and may be sent for culture.

Evaluation

Expected outcomes of nursing care include:

- The woman voids adequately to meet the demands of the increased fluid shifts during the postpartum period.
- The woman does not develop infection due to stasis of urine.
- The woman actively incorporates self-care measures to decrease bladder overdistention.

Cystitis (Lower Urinary Tract Infection)

Retention of residual urine, bacteria introduced at the time of catheterization, and a bladder traumatized by childbirth combine to provide an excellent environment for the development of cystitis (lower urinary tract infection). *Escherichia coli* has been demonstrated to be the causative agent in most cases of postpartum cystitis and pyelonephritis (upper urinary tract infection). In most cases, the infection ascends the urinary tract from the urethra to the bladder. If cystitis is not treated, the infection can spread to the kidneys (pyelonephritis) because vesicoureteral reflux (backward flow of urine) forces contaminated urine into the renal pelvis.

CLINICAL THERAPY

When cystitis is suspected, a clean-catch, midstream urine sample is obtained for microscopic examination, culture, and sensitivity tests. The specimen may require collection by the nurse with the woman on a bedpan because few postpartum women can collect a true midstream, clean-catch specimen without contaminating the specimen with lochia. A catheterized specimen is avoided when possible because of the increased risk of infection. When the bacterial concentration is greater than 100,000 colonies of the same organism per milliliter of fresh urine, infection is generally present (Duff & Birsner, 2017). Counts between 10,000 and 100,000 may also suggest infection, particularly if clinical symptoms are noted.

In the clinical setting, antibiotic therapy is often begun before culture and sensitivity reports are available. Frequently used antibiotics include a preparation of trimethoprim-sulfamethoxazole–double strength (Bactrim DS, Septra DS), one of the short-acting sulfonamides, nitrofurantoin (Macrodantin), or, in the case of sulfa allergy, ampicillin or amoxicillin-clavulanic acid. The antibiotic is changed later, if indicated by the results of the sensitivity report. Antispasmodic or urinary analgesic agents, such as phenazopyridine hydrochloride (Pyridium), may be given to relieve discomfort.

NURSING MANAGEMENT

For the Postpartum Woman with Cystitis

Nursing Assessment and Diagnosis

Women should be encouraged to void every 2 to 4 hours to prevent urinary stasis and to report any sensations of incomplete emptying of the bladder or dysuria. Symptoms of cystitis often appear 2 to 3 days after childbirth and may include frequency, dysuria, urgency, hesitancy and dribbling, nocturia, and suprapubic pain. Gross hematuria may be noted, but high fever and systemic symptoms are not expected.

When a UTI progresses to pyelonephritis, systemic symptoms usually occur and the woman becomes acutely ill. Symptoms include high fever, chills, flank pain (unilateral or bilateral), and nausea and vomiting, in addition to the signs of lower UTI. Costovertebral angle (CVA) tenderness may be noted on exam but is not required for diagnosis. Clean-catch urine specimens show large numbers of WBCs and are positive for infection (bacterial growth more than 100,000 colonies/mL) (Duff & Birsner, 2017).

Nursing diagnoses that may apply if a woman develops a UTI postpartum include:

- ***Pain, Acute,*** with voiding related to dysuria secondary to infection
- ***Health Management, Ineffective,*** related to need for information about self-care measures to prevent UTI

(NANDA-I © 2017)

Nursing Plan and Implementation

Encourage frequent emptying of the bladder during labor and postpartum to prevent overdistention and trauma to the bladder. Catheterization technique and nursing actions to prevent overdistention (previously discussed) also apply. The woman with pyelonephritis must understand the importance of follow-up care after discharge to prevent recurrence or further complications. See *Health Promotion: Avoiding Postpartum UTIs.*

Health Promotion Avoiding Postpartum UTIs

Advise the postpartum woman to continue good perineal hygiene after discharge. Also advise the woman to maintain a good fluid intake (at least eight to ten 8-oz glasses daily), especially of water, and to empty her bladder whenever she feels the urge to void, but at least every 2 to 4 hours while awake. Once sexual intercourse is resumed, the new mother should void before (to prevent bladder trauma) and following intercourse (to wash contaminants from the vicinity of the urinary meatus). Wearing underwear with a cotton crotch to facilitate air circulation also reduces the risk of UTI. Acidification of the urine is thought to aid in preventing and managing UTI but it is controversial. Therefore, advise the woman to avoid carbonated beverages, coffee, citrus fruits, tomatoes, and chocolate, which increase the alkalinity of urine, and to drink low-sugar juices such as cranberry, plum, apricot, and prune and take vitamin C, which increase the acidity of urine.

Evaluation

Expected outcomes of nursing care include:

- The woman identifies the signs of UTI, and her condition is treated successfully.
- The woman uses self-care measures to prevent the recurrence of UTI as part of her personal hygiene routine.
- The woman continues with any long-term therapy or follow-up as appropriate for the diagnosis.
- Maternal–newborn attachment is maintained; the woman is able to care for her newborn effectively.

Care of the Woman with Postpartum Mastitis

Mastitis is an inflammation of the breast, with or without bacterial infection, that occurs primarily in lactating women. Onset is usually between the third and fourth week postpartum or any other time that nursing frequency decreases (Cunningham et al., 2018). It ranges in severity from local inflammation to abscess and septicemia. The incidence of mastitis is estimated to be as high as 20% in breastfeeding mothers (Newton, 2017).

With infective mastitis, the usual causative organism is *Staphylococcus aureus*, especially methicillin-resistant *Staphylococcus aureus* (MRSA) (Cunningham e al., 2018). Infective mastitis is a serious infection, with fever, chills, headache, flulike muscle aches and malaise because of myalgia, and a warm, reddened, painful area of the breast, often wedge-shaped because of connective tissue septal distribution of the breast (Newton, 2017) (Figure 35–2).

The infection usually begins when bacteria invade the breast tissue after it has been traumatized in some way (see the factors commonly associated with mastitis Table 35–3). Milk serves as a favorable medium for the invasive bacteria to multiply; thus, milk stasis is another risk factor. (See *Concept Map: Milk Stasis.*) The most common source of the causative organism is the baby's nose and throat, although other sources include the hands of the mother or hospital staff and the woman's circulating blood.

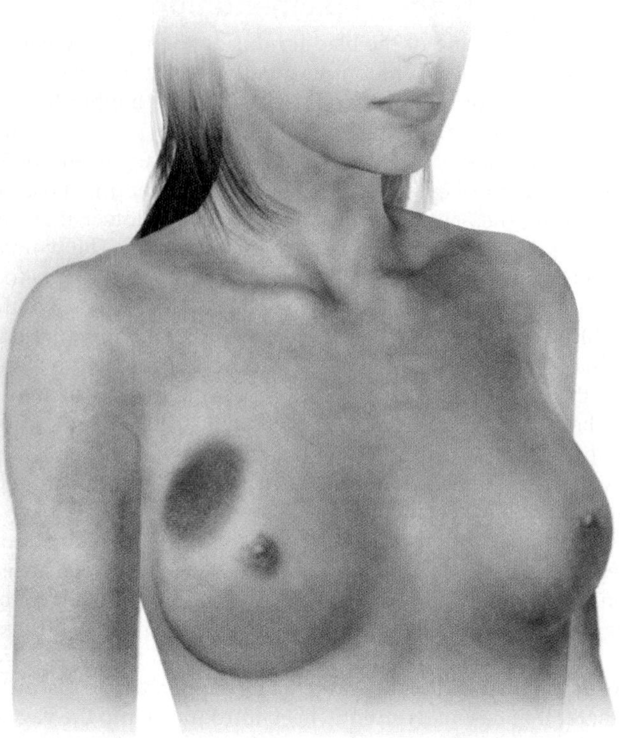

Figure 35–2 Mastitis. Erythema and swelling are present in the upper outer quadrant of the breast. Axillary lymph nodes are often enlarged and tender. The segmental anatomy of the breast accounts for the demarcated, often V-shaped wedge of inflammation.

Babies of women with mastitis generally remain well unless the causative organism is *Candida albicans*.

When *Candida albicans* is the causative organism of mastitis, entering the breast through a small fissure or abrasion on the nipple, the baby will often have thrush, a candidal infection of the mouth. There may be a history of a recent course of antibiotics in the woman. Signs include late-onset nipple pain, followed by shooting pain between feedings, often radiating to the chest wall (Newton, 2017). Eventually, the skin of the affected breast may become pink, flaking, and pruritic. Women may notice a yeasty odor to their milk. Unless the mother and her newborn are treated for *Candida*, recolonization will occur when breastfeeding is resumed.

CLINICAL THERAPY

The diagnosis of mastitis is usually made based on clinical signs and symptoms. Culture and sensitivity of the breast milk may be done in cases where the patient does not respond to antibiotics or has a severe, unusual, or recurring case of mastitis. If a culture of the breast milk is ordered, it is collected with a midstream-type process. The nipple is washed first; then the first 3 mL of breast milk are manually expressed and discarded, after which the actual specimen is collected (Newton, 2017). If the culture shows greater than 100,000 leukocytes/mL and greater than 1,000 bacteria/mL, it is considered to be mastitis (Newton, 2017).

Treatment of mastitis primarily includes frequent and complete emptying of the breasts, as well as antibiotic coverage. Supportive measures such as rest, increased fluid intake (at least 2 to 2.5 L/day), a supportive bra, local application of warm, moist

TABLE 35–3 Factors Affecting Development of Postpartum Mastitis

Milk Stasis
• Failure to change position of baby to allow emptying of all lobes
• Failure to alternate breasts at feedings
• Poor suck
• Poor let-down
Actions that Promote Access/Multiplication of Bacteria
• Poor hand hygiene technique
• Improper breast hygiene
• Failure to air-dry breasts after breastfeeding
• Use of plastic-lined breast pads that trap moisture against nipple
Breast/Nipple Trauma
• Incorrect positioning for breastfeeding
• Poor latch-on
• Failure to rotate position on nipple
• Incorrect or aggressive pumping technique
• Cracked nipples
Obstruction of Ducts
• Restrictive clothing
• Constricting bra
• Underwire bra
Change in Number of Feedings/Failure to Empty Breasts
• Attempted weaning
• Missed feeding
• Prolonged sleeping of baby, including sleeping through the night
• Favoring side of nipple soreness
Lowered Maternal Defenses
• Fatigue
• Stress
• Poor diet

heat prior to feeding and ice packs after, and analgesics should also be implemented. Nonsteroidal anti-inflammatory agents are recommended to treat both fever and inflammation. The preferred antibiotics are usually penicillinase-resistant penicillins, such as dicloxacillin 500 mg every 6 hours orally for 14 days (Cunningham et al., 2018; Newton, 2017). The woman should continue to breastfeed; in fact, regular drainage of both breasts actually helps by preventing milk stasis and abscess formation, and there is virtually no risk to the newborn. If there has been no change in symptomatology in 48 hours, modification of the antibiotic therapy will be considered. There have been increasing cases of MRSA mastitis. When a woman does not respond to first-line antibiotics, MRSA should be considered and a breast milk culture and antibiotic sensitivity should be ordered (Newton, 2017).

Candidal infections should be suspected with complaints of burning nipple pain or radiating breast pain and can be especially stubborn. Antifungal medications are used for treatment of candida (Newton, 2017).

Abscess formation is a complication of mastitis, resulting from delayed treatment, treatment failure, or abrupt weaning of the baby. Abscesses are usually in the upper outer quadrants of the breast and will show a localized area of erythema, exquisite tenderness, and induration. Breast abscess may require incision and drainage. Breastfeeding can usually continue on the affected breast, as long as the incision is well away from the areola and the cellulitis resolves about 4 to 7 days into treatment. The baby can continue to nurse on the unaffected breast (Newton, 2017).

The breasts should continue to be emptied by either breastfeeding or pumping in order to decrease duration of symptoms and to reduce the chance of a breast abscess. Thus, continued breastfeeding is recommended in the process of mastitis. The plan of care should include contacting the woman within 24 hours of initiation of treatment to ensure that symptoms are subsiding.

●○● NURSING MANAGEMENT

For the Postpartum Woman with Mastitis

Nursing Assessment and Diagnosis

Daily assessment of breast consistency, skin color, surface temperature, nipple condition, and presence of pain is essential to detect early signs of problems that may predispose to mastitis. Observe the mother breastfeeding her baby to ensure use of proper technique for positioning, latch-on, and disengagement of the baby from the nipple (see Chapter 29). Consultation with a lactation specialist can be of great value, especially for first-time mothers.

If an infection has developed, assess for contributing factors such as cracked nipples, poor hygiene, engorgement, supplemental feedings, change in routine or feeding pattern, abrupt weaning, or lack of proper breast support so that these factors may be corrected as part of the treatment plan.

Nursing diagnoses that may apply to the woman with mastitis include:

- ***Trauma, Risk for,*** related to lack of information about appropriate breastfeeding practices
- ***Breastfeeding, Ineffective,*** related to pain secondary to development of mastitis

(NANDA-I © 2017)

Nursing Plan and Implementation

Preventing mastitis is far simpler than treating it. Ideally, mothers should be instructed in proper breastfeeding technique prenatally. Help the mother breastfeed soon after birth and review correct technique. Referral to a lactation specialist is necessary with continued latch problems. All women, even those not breastfeeding, are encouraged to wear a good supportive bra at all times to avoid milk stasis, especially in the lower lobes, and are advised to change breast pads frequently. (Chapter 34 discusses the breastfeeding difficulties of the woman with mastitis.)

Meticulous handwashing by the breastfeeding mother and all personnel is the primary measure for preventing epidemic nursery infections and subsequent maternal mastitis. Prompt attention to mothers who have blocked milk ducts eliminates stagnant milk as a growth medium for bacteria or the development of cracks and fissures, a common portal for bacterial entry. If the mother finds that one area of her breast feels distended or lumpy, she can rotate the position of her baby for breastfeeding, manually express milk remaining in the breast after feeding (usually only necessary if the baby is not sucking well), or massage the lumpy area toward the nipple as the baby nurses. Mothers who have developed mastitis can apply warm, moist compresses to the affected area before breastfeeding. Encourage the mother to breastfeed frequently, starting with the unaffected breast until

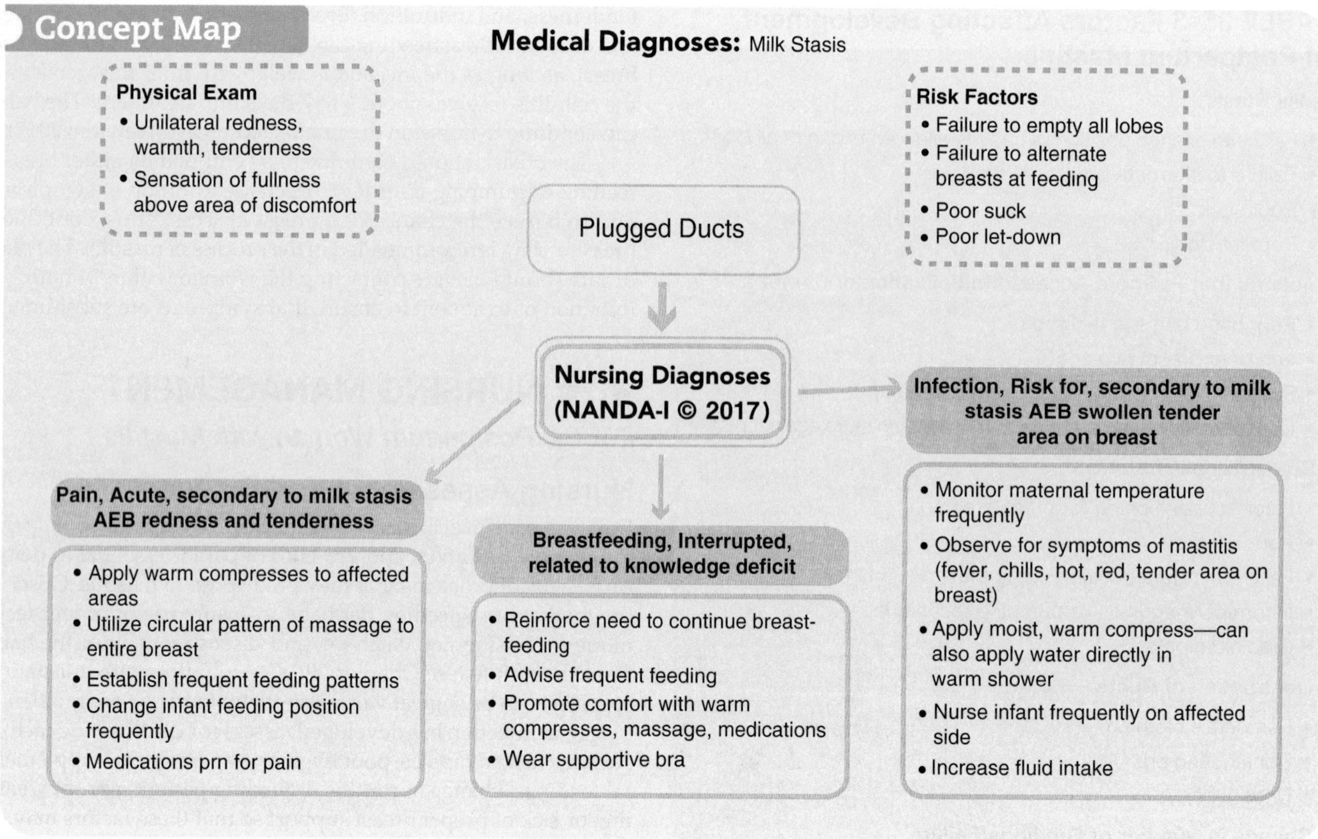

let-down occurs in the affected breast, and then encourage feeding from the affected breast until it is emptied completely. After nursing, the mother can leave a small amount of milk on each nipple to prevent cracking and allow nipples to air-dry and apply cold packs to reduce pain and edema. Early identification of and intervention for sore nipples are also essential, as is prompt assessment of the breastfeeding mother's breasts when thrush is discovered in her newborn's mouth. For a detailed discussion of breastfeeding issues, see *Breastfeeding Concerns Following Discharge* in Chapter 34.

Discharge Planning and Home Care Teaching

The woman should be aware of the importance of regular, complete emptying of the breasts to prevent engorgement and stasis. She should also understand the role of letdown in successful breastfeeding, correct positioning of the baby on the nipple, proper latch-on, and the principles of supply and demand. If the mother is taking antibiotics, she needs to understand the importance of completing the full course of antibiotics, even if the infection seems to clear quickly. Postpartum women need to be advised that mastitis may recur. Breastfeeding mothers who will be returning to work outside the home need information on how to do so successfully. Because mastitis tends to develop following discharge, it is important to include information about signs and symptoms in the discharge teaching and printed materials (Table 35–4). All flulike symptoms should be considered a sign of mastitis until proven otherwise. If symptoms develop, the woman should contact her healthcare provider immediately because prompt treatment helps to avoid abscess formation. See *Complementary Health Approaches: Probiotics*.

TABLE 35–4 Symptoms of Engorgement, Plugged Duct, and Mastitis

ONSET	LOCATION	HEAT/SWELLING	TEMPERATURE	PAIN	GENERAL SYMPTOMS
Engorgement					
Gradual; postpartum	Entire breast	Breast is hot and swollen	Less than 38.4°C (101.1°F)	Entire breast	None
Plugged Duct					
Gradual; after feedings	One side of breast	Little or no heat; there may be swelling	Less than 38.4°C (101.1°F)	Mild pain on affected side	None
Mastitis					
Sudden; usually after about 10 days	Generally one side of breast	Swelling on affected side; skin is red and hot	Greater than 38.4°C (101.1°F)	Intense pain on affected side	Similar to flu

SOURCE: Data from Lawrence & Lawrence, 2016.

Complementary Health Approaches

Probiotics

Probiotics are a category of dietary supplements consisting of beneficial microorganisms (*pro* means "for" and *biotic* means "life"; compare to *antibiotic*, which literally means "against life"). Probiotics compete with disease-causing microorganisms in the gastrointestinal tract. When antibiotics are taken, they kill many of the beneficial bacteria that exist naturally in the digestive tract. Supplementing with probiotics after a course of antibiotics is frequently prescribed by nutritionists and complementary practitioners. Commonly used probiotics include *Lactobacillus acidophilus* and *Bifidobacterium bifidum*; there are other species of *Lactobacillus* and *Bifidobacterium* that have been shown to be effective in such conditions as diarrhea and vaginal infections. *Bifidobacterium* also competes against *Candida albicans*. Probiotics can be taken in the form of powders, capsules, and suppositories or in fermented milk products such as yogurt or *kefir*.

Other complementary therapies used for mastitis include belladonna, acupuncture, oxytocin nasal spray to improve milk ejection, a traditional Chinese herb known as extracts of *Fructus gleditsiae*, and application of cabbage leaves over the affected area to relieve engorgement.

Community-Based Nursing Care

Because symptoms seldom occur before the second to fourth week postpartum, perinatal nurses are often not fully aware of how uncomfortable and acutely ill the woman can be. If you suspect mastitis on the basis of assessment findings, refer the woman to her healthcare provider.

If the mother feels too ill to breastfeed or develops an abscess that prevents breastfeeding, help the mother obtain an appropriate breast pump to help her maintain lactation. Provide opportunities for demonstration and return demonstration of pumping. Assist the mother to deal with her feelings about temporarily being unable to breastfeed. Referral to a lactation consultant or to La Leche League can be invaluable to the woman's physical and emotional adjustment to mastitis. See *Case Study: Azia Askari*.

Evaluation

Expected outcomes of nursing care include:

- The woman is aware of the signs and symptoms of mastitis.
- The woman reports her signs and symptoms of mastitis early, and it is treated successfully.
- The woman can continue breastfeeding if she chooses.
- The woman understands self-care measures she can use to prevent recurrence of mastitis.

Care of the Woman with Postpartum Thromboembolic Disease

Thromboembolic disease may occur during pregnancy and postpartum. **Venous thromboembolism (VTE)** is a term that includes *deep vein thrombosis (DVT)* and *pulmonary embolism (PE)*. *Venous thrombosis* refers to formation of a blood clot (thrombus formation) at an area of impeded blood flow in a superficial or deep vein. When the thrombus is formed in response to inflammation in the vein wall, it is termed **thrombophlebitis**. Pulmonary embolism, a rare but life-threatening condition, occurs when thrombi formed in the deep leg veins are carried to the pulmonary artery, obstructing pulmonary blood flow to one or both lungs. Pulmonary embolism is rare, but accounts for 9% of maternal mortality in the United States (AAP & ACOG, 2017).

Three major causes of thromboembolic disease, often referred to as *Virchow's Triad*, are hypercoagulability of blood, venous stasis, and injury to the epithelium of the blood vessel. Changes in the woman's coagulation system in pregnancy contribute to hypercoagulability, and compression of the common iliac vein by the gravid uterus leads to venous stasis. These factors increase the risk of thromboembolic disease by fourfold to fivefold when compared to non-pregnant women (AAP & ACOG, 2017).

Risk factors associated with increased risk of thromboembolic disease include:

- Cesarean birth
- Immobility (prolonged)
- Obesity
- Cigarette smoking
- Previous thromboembolic disease or strong family history
- Trauma to extremity (can include injury from incorrect positioning or prolonged interval in stirrups during labor)
- Varicose veins
- Diabetes mellitus
- Advanced maternal age
- Multiparity

CASE STUDY: Azia Askari

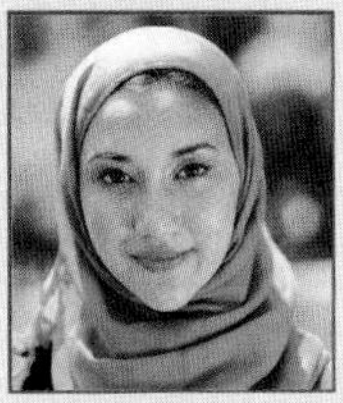
SOURCE: HONGQI ZHANG/123RF

Azia awakes with flulike symptoms and a temperature of 102.5°F. She calls the nurse at her healthcare provider's office and says that her left breast is red, swollen, and warm to the touch. She is concerned she has mastitis and asks if she should refrain from feeding the baby.

Questions to Ponder

What treatment would be warranted for Azia? What information would you give her regarding feeding her baby while being treated for mastitis? What education would you provide to prevent mastitis in the future?

- Anemia
- Malignancy
- Inherited coagulation pathway deficiency
- Proteins C and S deficiency.

Factors contributing directly to the development of postpartum thromboembolic disease include (1) increased amounts of certain blood clotting factors; (2) postpartum thrombocytosis (increased quantity of circulating platelets and their increased adhesiveness); (3) release of thromboplastin substances from the tissue of the decidua, placenta, and fetal membranes; and (4) increased amounts of fibrinolysis inhibitors. These same factors protect childbearing women from exsanguinating from blood loss at delivery. Because all women are at risk for thromboembolic disease during the childbearing period, attention should be given to measures that decrease risk of thromboembolic disease (Table 35–5).

Superficial Vein Disease

Superficial thrombophlebitis is far more common in postpartum women than in pregnant women. Often the clot involves the saphenous veins. This disorder is more common in women with pre-existing varices (enlarged veins), although it is not limited to that group. Superficial vein disease (SVD) may also occur as a sequelae to IV catheterization. Symptoms—tenderness in a portion of the vein, local heat and redness, normal temperature or low-grade fever, and, occasionally, slight elevation of the pulse—usually become apparent about the third or fourth postpartum day. A tender palpable cord may be noted along a portion of the vein. Treatment involves application of local heat, elevation of the affected limb, and analgesic agents. Anticoagulants are usually not necessary unless complications develop. Pulmonary embolism is extremely rare.

Deep Vein Thrombosis

Deep vein thrombosis (DVT) or thrombophlebitis is more frequently seen in women with a history of thrombosis. Obstetric complications such as polyhydramnios, preeclampsia, and operative birth are associated with an increased incidence. After a clinical diagnosis of DVT, a woman's risk in a subsequent pregnancy increases. See *Women with Special Needs: Lupus and Thromboembolic Disease.*

Women with Special Needs **Lupus and Thromboembolic Disease**

Women with lupus have a higher incidence of thromboembolic disease and need close observation for the development of DVT and PE. Early ambulation and frequent leg exercises should be encouraged. Symptoms of thromboembolic disease should be reviewed. Hormonal contraceptives that contain estrogen are contraindicated in these women.

Clinical manifestations may include edema of the ankle and leg and an initial low-grade fever often followed by high temperature and chills. Other findings include tenderness or pain, a palpable cord, changes in limb color, and difference in limb circumference of more than 2 cm (0.8 in.). Depending on the vein involved, the woman may complain of pain in the popliteal and lateral tibial areas (popliteal vein), entire lower leg and foot (anterior and posterior tibial veins), inguinal tenderness (femoral vein), or the lower abdomen (iliofemoral vein). Homans sign (refer to Chapter 32 and Figure 32–9) may or may not be positive. Most DVTs occur in the left leg. Because of reflex arterial spasm, sometimes the limb is pale and cool to the touch, and the dorsalis pedis pulse may be diminished or difficult to palpate. These signs and symptoms have less than 50% specificity, however, and diagnosis of DVT is usually confirmed by objective testing (venous ultrasound and D-dimer assays) (Pettker & Lockwood, 2017).

Pulmonary Embolism

Pulmonary embolism (PE) occurs when a thrombus from a lower extremity or the pelvis lodges in the pulmonary vascular bed and restricts circulation to the corresponding area of the lung vasculature. The size of the clot may be microscopic or large enough to occlude the branches of the pulmonary artery, affect

TABLE 35–5 Measures to Decrease Risk of Thromboembolic Disease in Childbearing Women

ANTEPARTUM MEASURES	INTRAPARTUM MEASURES	POSTPARTUM MEASURES
• Advise woman to avoid sedentary lifestyle and to exercise as much as possible (walking is ideal). • Recommend plenty of fluids to avoid dehydration. • Advise to quit smoking. • Teach to avoid prolonged standing or sitting in one position or sitting with legs crossed. • Encourage elevation of legs when sitting. • Teach to avoid tight knee-high hose or other constrictive garments. • Encourage frequent breaks during long car trips to walk around, thereby preventing prolonged venous stasis.	• Encourage ambulation unless contraindicated in early labor. • Later, encourage leg exercises. • Do not gatch bed or use pillows under knees. • Pad stirrups. • Ensure correct positioning in stirrups that minimizes pressure on the popliteal area. • Limit time in stirrups as much as possible. • After cesarean birth, initiate leg and foot exercises as soon as possible (in recovery). • Use antiembolism stockings for women at risk of DVT.	• Encourage early ambulation. • For women on bedrest, advise or assist with turning and leg exercises every 2 hours (woman may be encouraged to rotate ankles and to "write baby's name in air with toes"). • Encourage fluids to avoid dehydration. • Advise no smoking. • Use antiembolism stockings with those at risk. Pneumatic compression stockings may be ordered after cesarean birth until ambulation occurs. • Advise against prolonged sitting and crossing legs. • Avoid knee gatch in hospital bed. • Encourage elevation of legs while sitting.

the hemodynamic response, and possibly result in cardiovascular collapse (Rhode, 2016). Pulmonary embolism is a particularly catastrophic event with a high mortality rate; most fatalities occur within 30 to 60 minutes. However, early recognition and prompt action can decrease the mortality rate significantly, and treatment of DVT can often prevent this complication. Although the incidence of DVT in pregnancy is now believed to be almost comparable with that of postpartum DVT, PE develops most commonly in postpartum women. The most common risk factors are proximal DVT and recurrent thromboembolic disease. Diagnosis may be difficult because the most common clinical findings include nonspecific signs and symptoms such as dyspnea, pleuritic chest pain, cough with or without hemoptysis, cyanosis, tachypnea and tachycardia, panic, syncope, or sudden hypotension. Physical assessment may also reveal diaphoresis, friction rub, and wheezing or rales. A compression venous ultrasonography (VUS) with or without contrast color Doppler is used when a DVT is suspected (Pettker & Lockwood, 2017). An MRI can also be used, especially if a centralized (pelvic, iliac, or femoral) DVT is suspected. Abnormal findings on an ECG may also be present (Pettker & Lockwood, 2017). The nurse who recognizes the clinical findings of this emergency, especially in a woman at risk, should alert the woman's healthcare provider and rapid response team immediately, as time can be critical. Elevating the head of the woman's bed may facilitate ease of breathing; oxygen by facemask at 8 to 10 L per minute is initiated. Narcotics may be ordered for pain and to decrease anxiety, thereby decreasing the respiratory effort. Several imaging tests are available to assist in diagnosing pulmonary embolism; the choices depend on availability, the woman's condition, and the element of time. The woman with pulmonary embolism will be transferred to an intensive care setting where cardiovascular and respiratory status can be monitored closely.

CLINICAL THERAPY

Treatment of acute DVT or pulmonary embolus involves the immediate administration of anticoagulants. Unfractionated heparin (UFH) or low-molecular-weight heparin (LMWH) are the drugs of choice. Heparin therapy is continued until the international normalized ratio (INR) with oral warfarin is achieved at 2.0–3.0 for 2 successive days (Pettker & Lockwood, 2017). An advantage of LMWH is a safe profile and dosing not reliant on monitoring the activated partial thromboplastin time (aPTT) at a laboratory (Pettker & Lockwood, 2017). Postpartum women who require more than 6 weeks of anticoagulation therapy may be bridged to warfarin sodium (Coumadin) or a direct oral anticoagulant if not breastfeeding. Warfarin can be started concurrently with heparin compounds during the postpartum period. Maintenance with warfarin sodium (Coumadin) is started at 1 to 5 days for these women. The woman with a mechanical heart valve will restart warfarin 24 hours after delivery (ACOG, 2018). In some cases, thrombolytics (streptokinase or urokinase) or an embolectomy may be used.

Strict bedrest and elevation of the affected leg are required, and analgesics are given as necessary to relieve discomfort. Graduated compression stockings and a pneumatic compression device should be left on until symptoms subside (usually in several days), patient is walking with elastic support stockings, and anticoagulation therapy is restarted (AAP & ACOG, 2017). While taking warfarin sodium, prothrombin times and INR are assessed periodically to maintain correct dosage levels. Periodic assessment for signs of bleeding is essential, including those for hematuria and fecal occult blood.

●○● NURSING MANAGEMENT

For the Postpartum Woman with Thromboembolic Disease

Nursing Assessment and Diagnosis

Carefully assess the woman's history for factors predisposing to development of thrombosis or thrombophlebitis. In addition, as part of regular postpartum assessment, be alert to any patient complaints of pain in the leg, inguinal area, or lower abdomen because such pain may indicate DVT. Assess the woman's legs for evidence of edema, temperature change, or pain with palpation.

Nursing diagnoses that may apply to a postpartum woman with thromboembolic disease include:

- ***Tissue Perfusion: Peripheral, Ineffective,*** related to obstructed venous return
- ***Pain, Acute,*** related to tissue hypoxia and edema secondary to vascular obstruction
- ***Parenting, Risk for Impaired,*** related to decreased maternal–newborn interaction secondary to bedrest and intravenous lines
- ***Family Processes, Interrupted,*** related to illness of family member
- ***Knowledge, Deficient,*** related to self-care after discharge on anticoagulant therapy

(NANDA-I © 2017)

Nursing Plan and Implementation

Hospital-Based Nursing Care

Women with varicosities should be evaluated for the need for support hose during labor and postpartum.

Once the diagnosis of DVT is made, maintain the heparin therapy, provide for appropriate comfort measures, and monitor the woman closely for signs of PE. Assess for evidence of bleeding related to heparin and keep the antagonist for heparin, protamine sulfate, readily available.

Instruct the woman to avoid prolonged standing or sitting because these positions contribute to venous stasis. Also instruct her to avoid crossing her legs because of the pressure it causes. Advise her to take frequent breaks, such as when taking car trips and while working if she sits most of the day. Walking is acceptable because it promotes venous return. Remind the woman to identify her history of thrombosis or thrombophlebitis to her physician during subsequent pregnancies so that preventive measures may be instituted early because she is at increased risk for recurrence (Pettker & Lockwood, 2017).

Women discharged on warfarin sodium (Coumadin) should be taught about the drug and the safety factors associated with its use. *See Teaching Highlights: What the Postpartum Woman Taking Warfarin Needs to Know.*

See *Nursing Care Plan: The Woman with Thromboembolic Disease* for specific nursing care measures.

Community-Based Nursing Care

Because the mother with postpartum thromboembolic disease will depend on others for much of her initial home care, it is helpful for the father/partner to be involved in preparations for discharge. Provide ample opportunities to answer questions and clarify instructions, verbally and in writing. Evaluate the extent to which both mother and father/partner have understood instructions regarding the plan of care. It is especially important before discharge

TEACHING HIGHLIGHTS | What the Postpartum Woman Taking Warfarin Needs to Know

- Warfarin is compatible with breastfeeding (Pettker & Lockwood, 2017).
- Foods high in vitamin K lessen warfarin's effectiveness, thus you will need to strive for consistent daily intake so that accurate dosage of the drug can be achieved. If intake of vitamin K decreases significantly, there is a risk of bleeding.
- Foods high in vitamin K include cauliflower, soybean and canola oil, mayonnaise, broccoli, green and black tea, peppers, and spinach, collard, and other leafy greens. Many multivitamins contain vitamin K; you may take them but should do so consistently.
- Cranberry juice increases the effects of warfarin and, if desired, should be consumed in moderation and with consistency.
- Binge alcohol use inhibits warfarin metabolism; an occasional alcoholic beverage does not affect coagulation adversely.
- Several herbals affect the efficacy of warfarin sodium; for example, garlic, ginger, and ginkgo prolong prothrombin time (PT) and should be avoided.
- Vitamin C doses up to 500 mg per day and vitamin E doses up to 400 international units per day are considered safe; higher doses can affect coagulation.
- Certain medications such as aspirin and other nonsteroidal anti-inflammatory drugs increase anticoagulant activity and should be avoided.
- Be alert for signs of bleeding, such as bleeding gums, epistaxis, petechiae or ecchymosis, and evidence of blood in the urine or stool.
- Check for possible medication interaction with warfarin before taking any other medication.
- Be cautious about using sharp objects such as knives or razor blades to avoid injury.
- Avoid risky behaviors that could contribute to falls.
- Wear protective gloves during gardening or heavy housework, and always wear shoes, to keep hands and feet safe from injury.
- Carry a MedicAlert card or wear a bracelet stating that you are taking warfarin in case of emergency.
- Inform all healthcare providers (including dentists) that you are taking anticoagulants and to have vitamin K available in case of bleeding.
- Bleeding should be reported if it fails to stop within 10 minutes.
- Keep scheduled appointments for PT assessment to guide dosing.
- Consider utilizing point-of-care testing, which decreases the inconvenience of going to the laboratory. Home self-testing involves a single capillary fingerstick (CoaguChek, ProTime, Avocet) to test thromboplastin-mediated clotting expressed as PT or INR. The therapeutic range of INR is 2–3, and the risk of bleeding increases significantly when the INR is 3 or greater (Pettker & Lockwood, 2017). Bleeding should be reported if it fails to stop within 10 minutes.

Nursing Care Plan: The Woman with Thromboembolic Disease

1. Nursing Diagnosis: *Tissue Perfusion: Peripheral, Ineffective*, related to interruption of venous blood flow secondary to complications of labor and birth (NANDA-I © 2017)

Goal: The woman's presenting signs and symptoms are relieved.

INTERVENTION	RATIONALE
• Assess, record, and report signs of thrombophlebitis.	• Early detection of developing thrombophlebitis permits prompt treatment. As the thrombus increases in size, signs of obstruction also increase.
• Assess leg for edema, peripheral pulse, temperature, color, and tenderness every 8 hours. Initially note presence of palpable cord. Homans sign may be assessed, but is only positive in less than 50% of patients with DVT (Pettker & Lockwood, 2017).	• Edema/swelling, diminished or absent peripheral pulse, pallor, cool skin temperature, and tenderness are symptoms of DVT and indicate dysfunction of peripheral circulation in the lower extremities. Measure circumference of lower leg to monitor for swelling. Peripheral pulses in both legs should be palpated for pulse rate and pulse strength to allow for comparison. A lower extremity cool to the touch may be due to reflex arterial spasm.
• Maintain bedrest during the acute phase.	• Bedrest is ordered to decrease the possibility that a portion of the clot will dislodge and result in pulmonary embolism.
• Provide warm, moist soaks as ordered.	• Warmth promotes blood flow to affected area.

Nursing Care Plan: The Woman with Thromboembolic Disease *(continued)*

Intervention	Rationale
• Maintain limb in elevated position.	• Elevation of affected limb promotes venous return and helps decrease edema.
• Initiate progressive ambulation following the acute phase and provide properly fitting compression stockings before ambulation. These should be properly measured.	• Elastic compression stockings or "TEDs" help prevent pooling of venous blood in lower extremities. Stockings should be carefully measured according to guidelines to ensure proper pressure gradient and avoid "garter-like" roll at top. • Woman may begin to ambulate within a few days when symptoms subside.
• **Collaborative:** Administer unfractionated heparin as ordered, by continuous IV drip, heparin lock, or subcutaneously, or administer LMWH subcutaneously as ordered, including: 1. Monitor IV or heparin lock site (if in use) for patency, signs of infiltration, or signs of infection. 2. Obtain INR and partial thromboplastin time PTT per physician order and review before administering heparin. 3. Observe for signs of anticoagulant overdose with resultant bleeding, including: a. Hematuria b. Epistaxis c. Ecchymosis or petechiae d. Bleeding gums	• Heparin does not dissolve the blood clot but is administered to prevent further clotting and improve tissue perfusion. It is safe for breastfeeding mothers because heparin is not excreted in breast milk.
4. Provide protamine sulfate, per physician order, to combat bleeding problems related to heparin overdose.	• Protamine sulfate is a heparin antagonist, given intravenously, which is almost immediately effective in counteracting bleeding complications caused by heparin overdose.
5. Monitor and report any signs of PE.	• PE is a major complication of DVT/thrombophlebitis.
6. Initiate or support any emergency treatment.	• Signs and symptoms may occur suddenly and require immediate emergency treatment; prognosis is related to size and location of embolism.
7. PT/INR and review before beginning warfarin. Repeat periodically per physician order.	• The INR is the universal monitoring index based on PT.

EXPECTED OUTCOME: Woman will have increased venous return from lower leg as evidenced by decreased edema, negative Homans sign, and no pain or tenderness in lower leg.

2. Nursing Diagnosis: *Pain, Acute*, related to tissue hypoxia and edema secondary to vascular obstruction (NANDA-I © 2017)

Goal: Woman will obtain relief of pain or experience level of pain that is acceptable.

INTERVENTION	RATIONALE
• Administer analgesics per physician order. Notify physician if pain is not relieved.	• Analgesics act to relieve pain and enable the woman to rest. Aspirin or ibuprofen products are contraindicated because they inhibit platelet adhesiveness. Acetaminophen may be ordered by the physician.
• Observe or report disruptive effects of pain on emotions and behavior. • Provide supportive nursing comfort measures such as backrubs, provision of quiet time for sleep, diversional activities, or imagery.	• Once pain decreases, woman is more likely to ambulate, which will help increase venous return and decrease edema.

EXPECTED OUTCOME: Woman will have reduction in pain as evidenced by a pain level less than 5 at all times.

(continued)

Nursing Care Plan: The Woman with Thromboembolic Disease *(continued)*

3. Nursing Diagnosis: *Parenting, Risk for Impaired*, related to decreased maternal–newborn interaction secondary to bedrest and IVS (NANDA-I © 2017)

Goal: Woman will demonstrate evidence of positive physical and social interaction with newborn.

INTERVENTION	RATIONALE
• Maintain mother–newborn attachment when mother is on bedrest: 1. Provide frequent contacts for mother and baby; provide modified rooming-in, if possible, by having the crib placed close to the mother's bed; conduct nurse checks often to help mother lift or move baby. 2. Encourage mother to continue feeding baby.	• Mother–newborn attachment is enhanced by frequent contact and opportunities to interact.

EXPECTED OUTCOME: Woman will develop attachment bonds as evidenced by physical interactions: Good eye contact, touching the baby, holding baby close, attempting to comfort baby, and kissing baby, and social interactions: Calling baby by name, making positive comments about baby, asking questions about baby, asking questions about baby care, and talking to baby.

4. Nursing Diagnosis: *Family Processes, Interrupted*, related to illness of family member (NANDA-I © 2017)

Goal: Woman and her family will cope effectively with her illness.

INTERVENTION	RATIONALE
• Encourage woman to express her concerns to her partner. Assist couple in planning ways to manage while woman is hospitalized and after her discharge. • Encourage partner or support person to bring other children to the hospital to visit mother and meet new sibling. • Encourage partner or support person to bring in family pictures and notes from other children. Encourage phone calls. • Contact social services, if indicated, to obtain additional assistance for family, if needed.	• Illness of any family member impacts the entire family. This is especially true when the family situation is such that the mother is the primary nurturer and she is absent. Family members attempt to continue their own roles while also assuming the tasks of the missing mother. This can result in crisis.

EXPECTED OUTCOMES: Woman expresses assurance that her family misses her but is coping effectively as evidenced by:

- Family visits woman frequently.
- Woman and family verbalize plan for division of family tasks while the woman is hospitalized and exhibit understanding of potential needs of woman once released from hospital.

5. Nursing Diagnosis: *Bleeding, Risk for*, related to lack of information about DVT/thrombophlebitis, its treatment, preventive measures, and the medication warfarin sodium (Coumadin) (NANDA-I © 2017).

Goal: Woman will understand her condition, its treatment, safety during treatment, and long-term implications.

INTERVENTION	RATIONALE
• Provide information (both verbal and written supplements) about the woman's condition, its treatment regimen, the importance of compliance, and safety factors. Provide contact information that the woman can access 24/7.	• Such discussion is essential to help the woman understand the condition, her medication, and its implications. She must have a clear understanding to be able to provide effective self-care.
• Discuss ways of avoiding circulatory stasis such as avoiding prolonged standing, sitting, crossing legs, and wearing restrictive clothing.	• Prolonged sitting, standing, and crossing legs should be avoided, as these activities decrease venous return.

Nursing Care Plan: The Woman with Thromboembolic Disease *(continued)*

• Review need to wear support stockings and to plan for rest periods with legs elevated.	
• In the presence of DVT, discuss:	
1. The use of warfarin, its side effects, possible interactions with other medications, and the need to have dosage assessed through periodic checks of the prothrombin time.	• Patient placed on warfarin (Coumadin) therapy for 2–6 months at home.
2. Signs of bleeding, which may be associated with warfarin sodium, need to be reported immediately. Signs include: Hematuria, epistaxis, ecchymosis, bleeding gums, and rectal bleeding.	
3. Monitor menstrual flow: Bleeding may be heavier.	
4. Review need for woman to eat a consistent amount of leafy green vegetables (lettuce, cabbage, brussels sprouts, broccoli) every day.	• These foods are high in vitamin K and will affect balance between dose of warfarin and prothrombin.
5. Instruct the woman to report any bleeding that continues more than 10 minutes.	
6. Instruct the woman to: • Routinely inspect the body for bruising. • Carry medical alert card indicating she is on anticoagulant therapy. • Use electric razor to avoid scratching skin. • Use soft-bristled toothbrush. • Avoid binge alcohol intake or keep at minimum. • Avoid taking certain herbs such as ginger, garlic, and ginkgo, and any other drugs that can prolong PT without checking with the physician. • Note that stools may change color to pink, red, or black as a result of anticoagulant use. • Advise all health providers, including dentists, that she is taking anticoagulants.	

EXPECTED OUTCOMES: Woman has health promotion knowledge as evidenced by:

- Woman verbalizes understanding of ways to avoid circulatory stasis, need to wear supportive stockings, medication dosage and side effects, and the importance of a balanced diet.
- Woman verbalizes understanding of signs and symptoms of bleeding that need to be reported to healthcare provider.

to assess the couple's plans to ensure bedrest for the mother, if ordered. They might explore ways for her to maintain bedrest and still spend quality time with her newborn and any other children. For example, young children can sit on the bed for storytelling or play quiet games, and the newborn's crib can be placed adjacent to the mother's bed. The father/partner may be assuming multiple roles during this time—household manager, parent, worker, and caregiver. There may be financial concerns as a result of prolonged health care or extended time away from work to care for the family. It is valuable to provide the family with an accessible resource and to plan telephone or home visit follow-up care. Signs of postpartum thrombophlebitis may not occur until after discharge from the birthing unit. Consequently, all couples must be taught about the signs and symptoms and to appreciate the importance of reporting them immediately and of not massaging the affected leg. If signs and symptoms occur after discharge, a short readmission might be required. Every effort is made in that case to allow mother, father/partner, and newborn to remain together.

After DVT, some women continue to have leg pain, edema, and dermatitis of the affected extremity for prolonged periods caused by a residual venous abnormality that can significantly affect one's quality of life. Continuing use of compression stockings can help prevent thrombus formation.

Evaluation

Expected outcomes of nursing care include:

- The woman seeks treatment for her thrombophlebitis early and is managed successfully without further complications.
- At discharge, the woman is able to explain the purpose, dosage regimen, and necessary precautions associated with any prescribed medications, such as anticoagulants.
- The woman can discuss self-care measures and ongoing therapies (such as the use of compression stockings) that are indicated.
- The woman has bonded successfully with her newborn and is able to care for the baby effectively.

Care of the Woman with a Postpartum Psychiatric Disorder

The postpartum period can be a time of increased emotional lability for women. Some women will develop postpartum psychiatric disorders, which can have serious and long-lasting negative consequences for the woman, child, and family. Postpartum depression can impair maternal–newborn/infant bonding and can cause developmental and cognitive delays in the child (Rhode, 2016).

Types of Postpartum Psychiatric Disorders

Many types of psychiatric problems may occur postpartum. The classification of postpartum psychiatric disorders is a subject of some controversy. The fifth edition of the *Diagnostic and Statistical Manual of Mental Disorders* (*DSM-5*) American Psychiatric Association [APA], 2013) has added a peripartum-onset specifier to the mood disorder diagnostic category of psychiatric disorders. It is proposed that postpartum psychiatric disorders be considered one diagnosable syndrome with three subclasses: (1) adjustment reaction with depressed mood, (2) postpartum mood episodes with psychotic features, and (3) peripartum major mood episodes (also known as postpartum depression). The incidence, etiology, symptoms, treatment, and prognosis vary with each subclass.

ADJUSTMENT REACTION WITH DEPRESSED MOOD

Adjustment reaction with depressed mood is the mildest condition of disrupted mood and is commonly known as **postpartum blues**, or as *maternal* or *baby blues*. It occurs in as many as 85% of mothers and is characterized by mood lability and emotional hypersensitivity, but does not consistently affect the woman's ability to function. Postpartum blues typically begins within 2 to 4 days after the baby's birth and is self-limiting, lasting from a few hours to 1 to 14 days. The condition is more severe in primiparas than in multiparas and seems related to the rapid alteration of estrogen, progesterone, and prolactin levels after birth, challenges of new motherhood, fatigue, and lifestyle adjustments. New mothers experiencing postpartum blues commonly report feeling overwhelmed, unable to cope, fatigued, anxious, irritable, and oversensitive. A key feature is episodic tearfulness and rapid mood shifts, often without an identifiable reason. Not uncommonly, when asked why she is crying, this woman responds that she does not know. Cunningham et al. (2018) identifies several factors that contribute to the "blues":

- Emotional letdown that follows labor and childbirth
- Physical discomfort typical in early postpartum
- Fatigue
- Anxiety about caring for the newborn after discharge
- Depression during pregnancy or previous depression unrelated to pregnancy
- Severe PMS (premenstrual syndrome).

Validating the existence of this phenomenon, labeling it as a real but normal adjustment reaction, and providing reassurance can offer a measure of relief. Assistance with self- and baby care, rest, good nutrition, information, and family support aids recovery. Helping the new mother anticipate a transient emotional letdown after discharge is important guidance from the nurse, as is talking with her about her view of the "perfect mother." Trying to achieve that image can contribute to fatigue and exacerbate the letdown feeling. The partner should be encouraged to watch for and report signs that the new mother is not returning to a more normal mood but is instead slipping into a deeper depression or that happier times are no longer interspersed with the blues.

PERIPARTUM MAJOR MOOD EPISODES

Peripartum major mood episodes, also known as **postpartum depression (PPD)**, is clinical depression, categorized by DSM-5 as Major Depressive Disorder with Peripartum Onset (APA, 2013). Research shows that nationally about 1 in 9 women experience symptoms of postpartum depression and approximately 4% of fathers experience depression in the first year after their child's birth (Centers for Disease Control and Prevention [CDC], 2018).

Risk factors for postpartum depression include:

- History of major depression
- Depression during pregnancy
- History of postpartum depression or bipolar illness (recurrence rates are ≥ 20%)
- Stressful life events
- Primiparity
- Ambivalence about maintaining the pregnancy
- Occurrence of postpartum blues
- Lack of social support
- Lack of a stable and supportive relationship with parents (especially her father, as a child) or partner
- The woman's dissatisfaction with herself, including body image problems and eating disorders
- Complications of delivery
- Loss of newborn
- Age (adolescence increases risk).

Although it may occur at any time during the first postpartum year, the periods of greatest risk occur around the fourth week, just before the initiation of menses, and upon weaning (Figure 35–3). It is not always associated with depression during pregnancy, although gestational depression is a strong predictor of PPD. Women with postpartum depression are at risk for suicide, most prominently as they enter or exit the deeply depressed state. In a deep depression, the woman is unlikely to be able to plan and carry out suicide. For that reason, signs of improvement in depression should be celebrated with some caution. Whereas the woman with postpartum psychosis may attempt suicide because of illogical thought processes, the woman with major depression attempts suicide because her suffering is so great that dying seems a more favorable option than continuing to live in such pain. She may also attempt suicide to save her newborn from some perceived or real threat—including the possibility that she

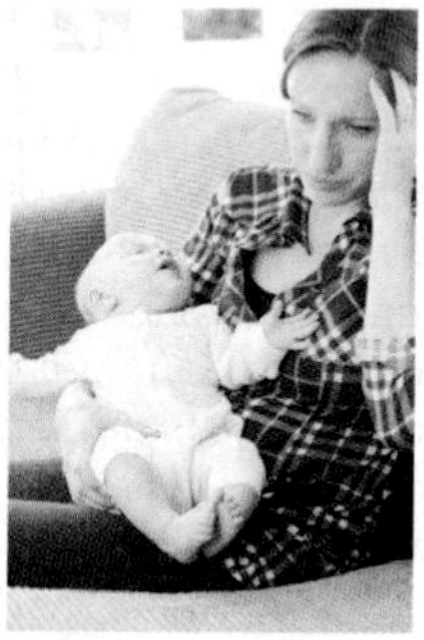

Figure 35–3 **Postpartum depression occurs in 10 to 20% of all postpartum women.**

SOURCE: SpeedKingz/Shutterstock.

herself might harm the baby. The risk of suicide is greater in those who have attempted suicide previously, have a specific plan, and can access the means or weapon identified within the plan. The more specific the plan, the greater the probability of an attempt.

For women considered to be at high risk, telephone follow-up after delivery or a clinic appointment earlier than 6 weeks may be helpful. Community health nurses who are seeing other members of the family or parish nurses who know new mothers in their congregation can observe for evidence of depression. The Postpartum Depression Screening Scale (PDSS) and the Edinburgh Postnatal Depression Scale (EPDS) are useful and validated for screening for postpartum depression.

The woman's safety, and that of her child(ren), is a priority. Inquiring about suicidal ideas and assessment for thoughts and feelings toward the baby, hallucinations and delusions, and impulsiveness that might put the baby and siblings at risk are critical. The woman and her family need information about the illness and its expected course, including the risk of recurrence, as well as comprehensive information about the treatment plan. They need opportunities to clarify misconceptions about mental illness and to have their questions answered. Referral to local or online support groups may be helpful.

Treatment options for PPD include individual or group psychotherapy, antidepressants, or a combination of both (ACOG, 2017b; AAP & ACOG, 2017). The expected outcomes for mild to moderate depression treated with antidepressants and psychotherapy are good; recurrence rates are increased after each episode of depression. Serotonin reuptake inhibitors (SSRIs) are used most often, as well as tricyclic antidepressants. Monoamine oxidase inhibitors (MAOIs) are rarely used in the treatment of PPD because these drugs have a high profile of interacting with other medications. Women typically continue antidepressants for 1 year after symptoms abate. Reoccurrence rates for women with PPD who had only the usual hospital visit after their first birth had a 46 times higher reoccurrence rate of PPD following a second birth, whereas women using antidepressants had a 27 times higher reoccurrence rate of PPD following a second birth (Rasmussen, Strøm, Wohlfahrt, et al., 2017).

All current antidepressant agents are excreted into breast milk. However, most SSRIs and tricyclic antidepressants are considered safe with breastfeeding. Because of its prolonged half-life, fluoxetine (Prozac) is usually not recommended for nursing mothers as a first choice (Lawrence & Lawrence, 2016). Physicians need to educate their breastfeeding postpartum patients who need antidepressants about the different alternatives and help them to balance the risks and benefits with the safety profiles. The final decision about continuing to breastfeed and to take antidepressants is the informed woman's. To help in making the decision, she and her husband or partner need to be helped to consider how she will respond without pharmacologic therapy and how unmedicated depression will affect the maternal–newborn/infant relationship and the baby's well-being and development. An invaluable online resource for prescribers with current information on drug safety and toxic effects during pregnancy and lactation is the LactMed Database. See *Evidence-Based Practice: Psychosocial and Psychologic Interventions for Preventing Postpartum Depression*.

POSTPARTUM MOOD EPISODES WITH PSYCHOTIC FEATURES

The most serious of postpartum psychiatric disorders is **postpartum mood episodes with psychotic features**, also called **postpartum psychosis**. Although relatively rare (1–2/1000), this disorder gains considerable national attention in the media and is considered an emergency, given the risk of infanticide or suicide. Symptoms usually become evident within the first few days after birth. Clinical features progress rapidly and include:

- Sleep disturbances—the woman is unable to sleep, even when her baby is sleeping

EVIDENCE-BASED PRACTICE | Psychosocial and Psychologic Interventions for Preventing Postpartum Depression

Clinical Question

What kinds of psychosocial and psychologic interventions may be helpful in the prevention of postpartum depression?

The Evidence

There is substantial evidence identifying the risk factors for the development of postpartum depression. It has been theorized that these risk factors could serve as the basis for designing psychosocial and psychologic interventions that could be offered during pregnancy and the immediate postpartum period to prevent the occurrence of this serious condition. Two researchers conducted a systematic review to first discover if these types of interventions are effective preventive measures. A secondary goal of the review was to determine the specific aspects of these interventions that were effective, such as professional versus lay-based interventions; individual versus group-based interventions; effects of interventions on onset and duration of depression; and relationship of treatment and specific risk factors. This review was structured and peer reviewed and published in the rigorous *Cochrane Database of Systematic Reviews*, which forms the strongest level of evidence. Twenty-eight studies with samples totaling almost 17,000 women were represented in this review.

Women who received psychosocial and/or psychologic interventions were considerably less likely to experience postpartum depression (Dennis & Dowswell, 2014). The most promising interventions were the provision of intensive, individualized postpartum home visits provided by nurses or nurse-midwives. These women had nearly half the rate of postpartum depression as women without this support. Peer-provided telephone support by lay women was also successful, as was interpersonal psychotherapy provided by professional counselors. Using risk factors to identify mothers who were most likely to develop postpartum depression aided in its prevention.

Best Practice

Psychosocial and psychologic interventions are clearly effective in preventing postpartum depression. Mothers should be assessed for risk factors and interventions should be applied accordingly. These interventions can be provided through professionally based home visits or psychotherapy or by lay peers via telephone consultation.

Clinical Reasoning

What are some of the prenatal risk factors that might help identify women who should receive interventions for prevention of postpartum depression? What might be the major components of a psychosocial or psychologic intervention?

- Depersonalization—seemingly unaware of or distant from the immediate environment and individuals within it
- Confusion; irrational or disorganized thinking; bizarre behaviors
- Hallucinations; delusions
- Psychomotor disturbances—stupor or agitated state sometimes accompanied by rapid and incoherent speech.

Significant risk factors include previous postpartum psychosis and/or a history of bipolar disorder. Family history of postpartum psychosis and bipolar disorder have also been found to increase the risk (Wesseloo et al., 2016).

The psychotic woman experiences delusions and/or visual, auditory, or tactile hallucinations. In some women, these symptoms support her perceptions that the baby should not be allowed to live or that she should commit suicide. For example, she may believe that her newborn is evil, is some form of "changeling," and will harm her or others, or she may believe that her newborn would be "better off dead" than living in such an evil world. She may contemplate suicide because she believes that her child would be better off without a mother than with her as such a "terrible, crazy mother." Illogical thinking or evidence of bonding difficulties may serve as cues to infanticide and suicide risk; however, this assessment is often challenging because of periods of lucidity seen in some psychotic women. Nurses in various clinical settings who come in contact with this woman may note that the child has been neglected or that the woman is practicing unsafe behaviors because of her cognitive impairment. For example, a pediatric nurse noticed that one mother placed her newborn across the room at the edge of the narrow exam table while she paced back and forth across the room, muttering to herself, appearing not to notice the baby. This same woman came to her appointment during heavy snow with both her baby and herself underdressed for warmth. See *Women with Special Needs: Bipolar Disorder*.

Women with Special Needs Bipolar Disorder

Women with a history of bipolar disorder have a 100 times higher risk of developing postpartum psychosis. A complete assessment should include administering the PPD and assessing the woman for symptoms that would be considered atypical and may be an indicator of psychosis. The woman and her support persons should be educated about symptoms that warrant immediate medical intervention.

An assessment for a family history of psychiatric disorders, especially bipolar disorder, should be done. This assessment can identify an important risk factor for postpartum psychiatric disorders. Questions related to female and male first-degree relatives with bipolar disorder are of the highest importance and should be added to routine clinical screening guidelines to improve prediction of risk (Bauer et al., 2018).

Provisions for safety of the woman and baby are paramount. This woman needs immediate referral to psychiatric care, usually requiring admission to an inpatient psychiatric hospital. Continued assessment of her symptomatology, safety, and functional capacity is a major nursing role in the setting. An initial history, physical examination, and labwork will help to rule out an organic cause of acute psychosis.

A dilemma exists for breastfeeding women for whom lithium or psychotropic medication is being considered. Because babies have immature hepatic and renal systems and a more permeable blood–brain barrier, they may be vulnerable to side effects, especially when younger than 2 months of age, premature, or exposed to these medications in utero. With the exception of lithium (which is rated a category 5 [use with caution] by the American Academy of Pediatrics), the amount of psychotropic drugs excreted into breast milk appears to be modest and not to compromise growth and development (Lawrence & Lawrence, 2016). Parents of a baby need to be educated to consider these factors in making a decision about the use of psychotropic medications: (1) severity of symptoms and their effect on the baby if medications are not used; (2) benefits of breastfeeding to the baby; (3) potential risks to the baby if psychotropics are used; and (4) preferences of the woman. If psychotropics are prescribed, the lowest dose possible of monotherapy should be used, and the baby should be monitored carefully by a pediatrician for difficulty being aroused from sleep, rigidity, tremors, irritability, poor hydration, and poor feeding with failure to gain weight (Lawrence & Lawrence, 2016).

POSTTRAUMATIC STRESS DISORDER

Many women envision their own labor and delivery unfolding in a particular way and may experience angst if their labor reality fails to match their expectations. Labor and birth that go awry, including those associated with complications, may cause **posttraumatic stress disorder (PTSD)**, which DSM-5 (APA, 2013) describes as "the development of characteristic symptoms following exposure to one or more traumatic events." Traumatic events during childbirth may include emergency cesarean sections, surgery or medical interventions without adequate anesthesia, or the loss of a baby. The prevalence of full-blown postpartum PTSD is 4 to 6% (Yildiz, Ayers, & Phillips, 2017). At particular risk for PTSD are women who have histories of prior trauma and/or prior psychiatric histories and women who undergo emergency cesarean sections.

Clinical features of PTSD include feeling numb, seeming dazed and unaware of her environment, intrusive thoughts and flashbacks to the threatening event, difficulty thinking, difficulty sleeping, irritability, and avoidance of others and reminders of the traumatic event. These signs and symptoms may not be evident until after the woman has left the birth setting. Distress associated with the original traumatic event can recur at anniversaries, and some women are hesitant to consider future pregnancies because of this birth trauma (Yildiz et al., 2017).

CLINICAL THERAPY

Women with a history of postpartum psychosis or depression or other risk factors may benefit from a referral to a mental health professional for counseling during pregnancy or postpartum. Medication, individual or group psychotherapy, and practical assistance with child care and other demands of daily life are common treatment measures for both disorders; however, the specific therapies used may vary. It is important for the nurse to realize that many of the drugs used in treating postpartum psychiatric conditions are contraindicated in breastfeeding women.

Treatment of postpartum psychosis is directed at the specific type of psychotic symptoms displayed and may include lithium, antipsychotics, or electroconvulsive therapy in combination with psychotherapy, removal of the baby, and social support.

Support groups are successful adjuncts to the previously discussed treatments. Within a support group of postpartum women and their partners, a couple may feel consolation that they are not alone in their experience. Moreover, the group provides a forum for exchanging information about postpartum depression, learning stress-reduction measures, and experiencing renewed self-esteem and support.

●○● NURSING MANAGEMENT

For the Postpartum Woman with a Psychiatric Disorder

Nursing Assessment and Diagnosis

Assessment for factors predisposing a woman to postpartum depression or psychosis should begin prenatally. Questions designed to detect problems can be included as part of the routine prenatal history interview or questionnaire. Women with a personal or family history of psychiatric disease, particularly postpartum depression or psychosis, need prenatal instructions on the signs and symptoms of depression and may need additional emotional support. Assess the woman for predisposing factors during her labor and postpartum stay.

New mothers and their families expect a challenging adjustment period after bringing home a new baby; they may not realize that their experiences are outside the norm. There is general anticipation that motherhood will be a happy occasion; a woman may not be able to admit her unhappiness out of shame or embarrassment that she is somehow different as a mother. The woman might be concerned that telling someone, even a professional, about her symptoms makes her sound "crazy" and that her baby might be taken away.

Several screening tools are available for assessing postpartum depression. The routine use of a screening tool in a matter-of-fact approach significantly increases the diagnosis because the woman does not feel singled out. The Edinburgh Postnatal Depression Scale is likely the most widely used screening tool for postpartum depression in large populations of women. The tool has been validated, computerized, and used in telephone screening. Mothers who score above 12 on the EPDS are likely to be suffering from postpartum depression. The Postpartum Depression Screening Scale is another widely used and validated tool and has the highest sensitivity. No matter what approach used to assess for postpartum depression, enabling the woman's voice to be heard about her feelings of maternal role transition and how she is adjusting in this vulnerable time is of great value. Listening to her story provides a critical emic (insider's) view of her circumstances as opposed to an etic (outsider's) view.

In providing daily care, observe the woman for objective signs of depression—anxiety, irritability, poor concentration, forgetfulness, sleeping difficulties, appetite change, fatigue, and tearfulness—and listen for statements indicating feelings of failure and self-accusation. Severity and duration of symptoms should be noted. Behavior and verbalization that are bizarre or seem to indicate a potential for violence against herself or others, including the baby, need to be reported as soon as possible for further evaluation. Be aware that many normal physiologic changes of the puerperium are similar to symptoms of depression (lack of interest in sex, indecisiveness, appetite change, sleep disturbance, and fatigue). It is essential that observations be as specific and as objective as possible, as well as carefully documented.

A central challenge for nursing is identifying women at risk of suicide. Family members of the depressed woman should also be alert to signals that she may be intent on self-harm; advise them that threats should always be taken seriously. Tell family members to be especially vigilant for suicide when the woman seems to be feeling better.

If a woman admits that she has thought of hurting herself, assessment of the risk that she will follow through is imperative. The mnemonic *SAL* is useful for risk assessment:

- Is there a *S*pecific plan with a designated time?
- Is there an *A*ccessible weapon or other means?
- How *L*ethal is the method identified in the plan?

A specific plan that identifies a highly lethal method that is immediately accessible is evidence of very high risk of suicide. Immediate intervention is critical; emergency psychiatric hospitalization is likely necessary. Those considered a threat to themselves or others may be admitted to involuntary hospitalization for a minimum of 48 hours until further evaluation is complete.

Family members of the depressed woman should also be alert to signals that she may be intent on self-harm; they must be advised that threats should always be taken seriously. Clues to suicide that might be noted by family are comments such as "I don't deserve to live," "Life is no longer worth living," or "You won't have to worry about me for long." Someone who is considering suicide may also telephone or write family or friends to say good-bye or give away prized possessions. Family members should be told to be especially vigilant for suicide when the woman seems to be feeling better.

Possible nursing diagnoses that may apply to a woman with a postpartum psychiatric disorder include:

- ***Coping, Ineffective***, related to postpartum depression
- ***Parenting, Risk for Impaired***, related to postpartum mental illness
- ***Violence: Self-Directed, Risk for***, against self (suicide), newborn, and other children related to depression

(NANDA-I © 2017)

Nursing Plan and Implementation

Nurses working in antepartum settings or teaching childbirth classes play indispensable roles in helping prospective parents appreciate the lifestyle changes and role demands associated with parenthood. Offering realistic information and anticipatory guidance and debunking myths about the perfect mother or perfect newborn may help prevent postpartum depression. Social support teaching guides are available to assist you in helping postpartum women explore their needs for postpartum support.

Alert the mother, partner, and other family members to the possibility of postpartum blues in the early days after birth and reassure them of the short-term nature of the condition. Symptoms of postpartum depression should be described and the mother encouraged to call her healthcare provider if symptoms become severe, if they fail to subside quickly, or if at any time she feels she is unable to function. Encouraging the mother to plan how she will manage at home and providing concrete suggestions on how to cope will aid in her adjustment to motherhood. *Teaching Highlights: Primary Prevention Strategies for Postpartum Depression* provides suggestions for the mother that serve as primary prevention for postpartum depression.

Information, emotional support, and assistance in providing or obtaining care for the baby may be needed. Assist family members by identifying community resources and making referrals to public health nursing services and social services. Postpartum follow-up is especially important, as well as visits from a psychiatric home-health nurse.

Community-Based Nursing Care

Home visits, especially for early-discharge families, are invaluable in fostering positive adjustments for the new family. Telephone follow-up at 2 to 3 weeks postpartum to ask whether the mother is experiencing difficulties is also helpful. Monitoring for signs of depression or performing brief screening at well-child follow-ups also can be valuable for early identification and timely intervention (van der Zee-van den Berg, Boere-Boonekamp, Ijzerman, et al., 2017).

Depression does appear to interfere with optimal mothering; there is less interaction between mother and child, lower rates

TEACHING HIGHLIGHTS | Primary Prevention Strategies for Postpartum Depression

1. Celebrate childbirth but appreciate that it is a life-changing transition that can be stressful—at times it can seem overwhelming. Share your feelings with each other and/or others.
2. Consider keeping a journal where you write down feelings. Not only is it emotionally cathartic, it provides a great memory book.
3. Appreciate that you do not have to know everything to be a good parent—it is okay to seek advice during this transition.
4. Connect to others who are parents—use them as a support and information network.
5. Set a daily schedule and follow it even if you do not feel like it. Structuring activity helps counteract inertia that comes with feeling sad or unsettled.
6. Prioritize daily tasks. Decide what must be done and what can wait. Try to get one major thing done every day. Remember that you do not always have to look like a magazine fashion model.
7. Remember that you do not have to entertain or care for everyone who drops by. Doing something for someone else, however, often tends to make you feel better.
8. If someone volunteers to help you with tasks or baby care, take them up on it. While your volunteer is in action, do something pleasurable or get some rest.
9. Maintain outside interests. Plan some time every day—even if it's just 15 minutes—to do something exclusively for "you" that is pleasurable.
10. Eat a healthful diet. Limit alcohol. Quit smoking. Get some exercise. (All of these can positively affect the immune system.)
11. Get as much sleep as possible. Rest whenever you can, such as when the baby is napping. If you have other young children, bring them onto your bed to read or play quietly while you lie down.
12. Limit major changes (moves, job changes, etc.) the first year insofar as possible.
13. Spend time with others.
14. If things get overwhelming, and you feel yourself slipping into depression, reach out to someone for help.
15. Attend a postpartum support group if one is available. Consider also an international program.

Source: Data from Postpartum Support International (PSI).

of initiation and shorter duration of breastfeeding, more mood and cognitive development problems, and more visits to the doctor in these children. A diagnosis of postpartum depression or other psychiatric disorder may pose problems for the family, especially the father/partner. The symptoms of these disorders are difficult to witness and may be harder to understand than physical problems such as hemorrhage or infection. The father/partner may feel hurt by the mother's hostility and may worry that she is becoming insane or be baffled by her mood swings and lack of concern about herself, the newborn, or household responsibilities. The couple's lack of intimacy or deteriorating communication may be troubling. Certainly, there is cause for concern about how the newborn and any other children are being affected. There may be very real practical matters to handle—running the household; managing the children, including the totally dependent newborn; and caring for the mother—added to the usual routines and work responsibilities of the father/partner. It is not surprising that even in the most supportive families, relationships may suffer in response to these circumstances. It is often a family member who in desperation makes contact with the healthcare agency. This is especially difficult when the mother is reluctant to admit she is suffering emotional difficulty or is too ill to recognize her own needs.

Netsi, Pearson, and Murray (2018), in an observational study in the United Kingdom, found that children of women with persistent and severe depression are at increased risk for behavioral problems by age 3.5 years, as well as lower mathematics grades and depression during adolescence. The integration of the newborn into the family and care of the newborn and other children can be further compromised by concurrent postpartum depression in fathers/partners. With both parents having depressive symptomatology, the baby and other children are further at risk.

Evaluation

Expected outcomes of nursing care include:

- The woman's signs of depression are identified and she receives therapy quickly.
- The newborn is cared for effectively by the father/partner or another support person until the mother is able to provide care.
- The mother and newborn will remain safe.
- The newborn is integrated into the family.

Focus Your Study

- Nursing assessment and intervention play a large role in preventing postpartum complications.
- The main causes of early postpartum hemorrhage are uterine atony, lacerations of the vagina and cervix, and retained placental fragments. Late postpartum hemorrhage most often originates from retained placental fragments and, though not usually as catastrophic as early hemorrhage, may require readmission.
- The most common postpartum infection is metritis, which is limited to the uterine cavity.

- A postpartum woman is at increased risk for developing urinary tract problems because of normal postpartum diuresis, increased bladder capacity, decreased bladder sensitivity from stretching or trauma, and possibly inhibited neural control of the bladder following the use of anesthetic agents.
- Mastitis is an inflammation of the breast primarily seen in breastfeeding women. Symptoms seldom occur before the second to fourth postpartum week. Continuation of breastfeeding is recommended as part of the treatment plan.
- Thromboembolic disease originating in the veins of the leg, thigh, or pelvis may occur antepartum or postpartum and carries with it the potential for creating a life-threatening pulmonary embolus.
- Although many different types of psychiatric problems may be encountered in the postpartum period, postpartum blues is the most common. Postpartum blues episodes occur frequently in the week after birth, are associated with hormonal fluctuations, and are typically transient.
- Risk factors for postpartum depression should be screened for routinely during pregnancy and the postpartum period. Nurses should be alert to the risk of suicide and infanticide in cases of severe postpartum depression or psychosis.
- Telephone calls and home visits are effective measures for extending comprehensive care into the home setting of the postpartum family at risk. Support groups in which child care is available also can be an invaluable community service by professional nurses.

In order to make safe and effective judgments using NANDA-I © 2017 nursing diagnoses, it is essential that nurses refer to the definitions and defining characteristics of the diagnoses used in this text, which can be found in Appendix C.

References

American Academy of Pediatrics (AAP), Committee on the Fetus and Newborn, & American College of Obstetricians and Gynecologists (ACOG), Committee on Obstetric Practice. (2017). *Guidelines for perinatal care* (8th ed.). Elk Grove Village, IL: Author

American College of Obstetrics & Gynecology (ACOG). (2017a). Postpartum hemorrhage (ACOG Practice Bulletin No. 183). *Obstetrics & Gynecology, 130*(4), e168–e186.

American College of Obstetrics & Gynecology (ACOG). (reaffirmed 2017b). Use of psychiatric medications during pregnancy and lactation (ACOG Practice Bulletin No. 87). *Obstetrics & Gynecology, 111*(4), 1001–1020.

American College of Obstetrics & Gynecology (ACOG). (2018). Thromboembolism in pregnancy (ACOG Practice Bulletin No. 196). *Obstetrics & Gynecology, 132*(1), e1–e16.

American Psychiatric Association (APA). (2013). *Diagnostic and statistical manual of mental disorders* (5th ed.). Arlington, VA: American Psychiatric Association.

Bauer, A. E., Maegbaek, M. L., Liu, X., Wray, N. R., Sullivan, P. F., Miller, W. C., ... Munk-Olsen, T. (2018). Familiality of psychiatric disorders and risk of postpartum psychiatric episodes: A population-based cohort study. *American Journal of Psychiatry, 175*(8), 701–783.

Centers for Disease Control and Prevention (CDC). (2018). *Depression among women.* Retrieved from https://www.cdc.gov/reproductivehealth/depression/index.htm

Cunningham, F. G., Leveno, K. J., Bloom, S. L., Dashe, J. S., Hoffman, B. L., Casey, B. M., & Spong, C. Y. (2018). *Williams obstetrics* (25th ed.). New York, NY: McGraw-Hill.

Dennis, C., & Dowswell, T. (2014). Psychosocial and psychological interventions for preventing postpartum depression. *Cochrane Database of Systematic Reviews*, Issue 2, Article No. CD001134.

Dildy, G. A. (2018). How to prepare for postpartum hemorrhage: Lapses in safety culture play a significant role in maternal mortality. *Contemporary OB/GYN.* Retrieved from http://www.contemporaryobgyn.net/modern-medicine-feature-articles/how-prepare-postpartum-hemorrhage

Duff, P., & Birsner, M. (2017). Maternal and fetal infectious disorders. In S. G. Gabbe, J. R. Niebyl, & J. L. Simpson (Eds.), *Obstetrics: Normal and problem pregnancies* (7th ed. pp. 1130–1146). Philadelphia, PA: Churchill Livingston/Elsevier.

Francois, K. E., & Foley, M. R. (2017). Antepartum and postpartum hemorrhage. In S. G. Gabbe, J. R. Niebyl, & J. L. Simpson (Eds.), *Obstetrics: Normal and problem pregnancies* (7th ed. pp. 395–424). Philadelphia, PA: Churchill Livingston/Elsevier.

Lawrence, R. M., & Lawrence, R. A. (2016). *Breastfeeding: A guide for the medical profession.* (8th ed). Maryland Heights, MO: Mosby.

Main, E. K., Goffman, D., Scavone, B. M., Low, L. K., Bingham, D., Fontaine, P. L., & . . . Levy, B. S. (2015). National partnership for maternal safety consensus bundle on obstetric hemorrhage. *Journal of Midwifery & Women's Health, 60*(4), 458–464. DOI: 10.1111/jmwh.12345

Netsi, E., Pearson, R. M., & Murray, L. (2018). Association of persistent and severe postnatal depression with child outcomes. *JAMA Psychiatry, 75*(3), 247–253. DOI:10.1001/jamapsychiatry.2017.4363

Newton, E. R. (2017). Lactation and breastfeeding. In S. G. Gabbe, J. R. Niebyl, & J. L. Simpson (Eds.), *Obstetrics: Normal and problem pregnancies* (7th ed. pp. 517–548). Philadelphia, PA: Churchill Livingston/Elsevier.

Pettker, C. M., & Lockwood, C. J. (2017). Thromboembolic disorders in pregnancy. In S. G. Gabbe, J. R. Niebyl, & J. L. Simpson (Eds.), *Obstetrics: Normal and problem pregnancies* (7th ed. pp. 965–980). Philadelphia, PA: Churchill Livingston/Elsevier.

Rasmussen, M. H., Strøm, M., Wohlfahrt, J., Videbech, P., & Melbye, M. (2017). Risk, treatment duration, and reoccurrence risk of postpartum affective disorder in women with no prior psychiatric history: A population-based cohort study. *PLOS.* Retrieved from https://journals.plos.org/plosmedicine/article?id=10.1371/journal.pmed.1002392

Rhode, M. A. (2016). Postpartum complications. In S. Mattson & J. E. Smith (Eds.), *AWHONN core curriculum for maternal-newborn nursing* (5th ed., pp. 645–661). St. Louis, MO: Elsevier.

Stanley, A. Y., & Conner, B. T. (2015). Implementing a clinical practice guideline to manage postpartum urinary retention. *Journal of Nursing Care Quality, 30*(2), 175–180. DOI: 10.1097/NCQ.0000000000000087

van der Zee-van den Berg, A. I.. Boere-Boonekamp, M. M., Ijzerman, M. J., Haasnoot-Smallegange, R. M. E., & Reijneveld, S. A. (2017). Screening for postpartum depression in well-baby care settings: A systematic review. *Maternal and Child Health Journal, 21*(1), 9–21. DOI: 10.1007/s10995-016-2088-8

Wesseloo, R., Kamperman, A. M., Munk-Olsen, T., Pop, V. J., Kushner, S. A., & Bergink, V. (2016). Risk of postpartum relapse in bipolar disorder and postpartum psychosis: A systematic review and meta-analysis. *American Journal of Psychiatry, 173*(2), 117–127. DOI: 10.1176/appi.ajp.2015.15010124

Whitner, T. (2016). Physical and psychologic changes after childbirth. In S. Mattson & J. E. Smith (Eds.), *AWHONN core curriculum for maternal-newborn nursing* (5th ed. pp. 297–313). St. Louis, MO: Elsevier.

Yildiz, P. D., Ayers, S., & Phillips, L. (2017). The prevalence of posttraumatic stress disorder in pregnancy and after birth: A systematic review and meta-analysis. *Journal of Affective Disorders 208,* 634–645. DOI: 10.1016/j.jad.2016.10.009

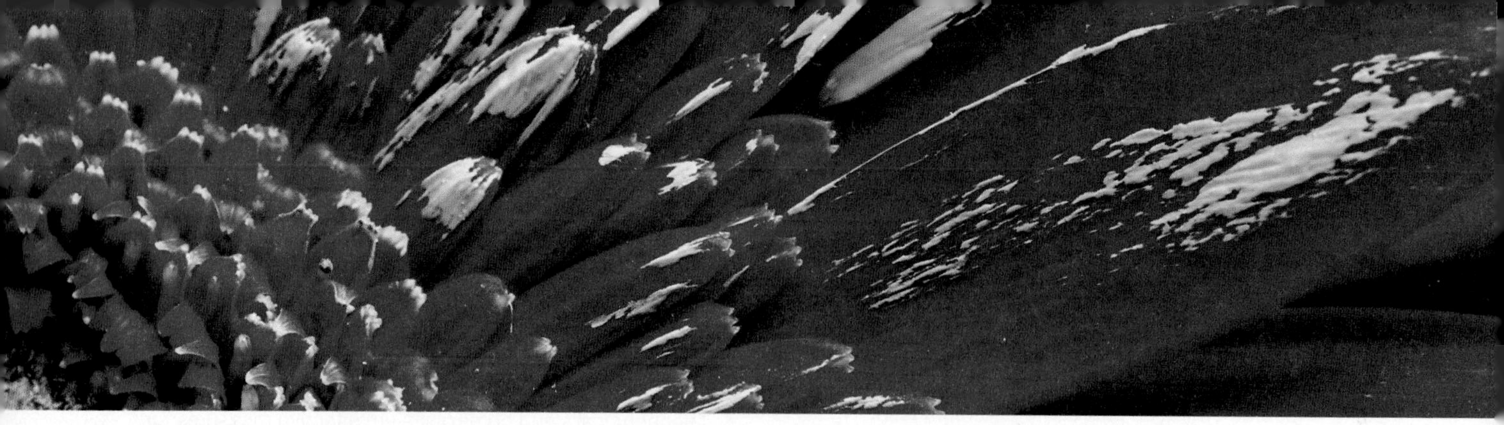

Chapter 36
Grief and Loss in the Childbearing Family

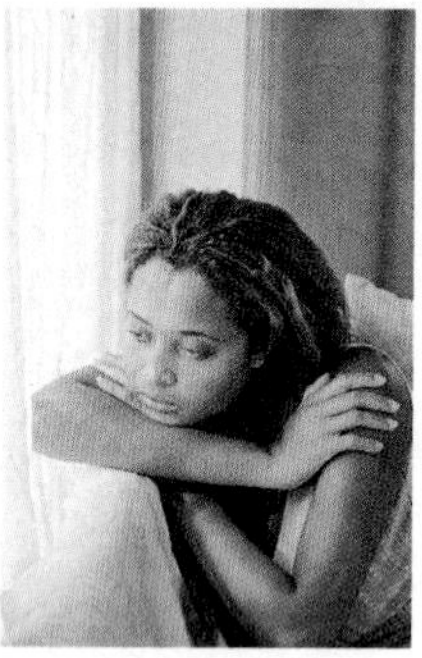

SOURCE: Stockbyte/Getty Images.

"You have a beautiful baby," the ultrasound technician said quietly. She was studying the flickering images on her screen, staring intently at the shadows of the tiny heart. I think she had already seen that our baby was going to die.
—Amy Kuebelbeck*

Learning Outcomes

36.1 Discuss perinatal loss including etiology, diagnosis, and the nurse's role in facilitating the family's mourning process.

36.2 Describe the physical, cognitive, emotional, behavioral, and spiritual responses experienced by parents during grieving associated with perinatal loss.

36.3 Delineate the personal, societal, and cultural issues that may complicate responses to perinatal loss.

36.4 Identify nursing diagnoses and interventions to meet the special needs of parents and their families related to perinatal loss and grief.

36.5 Differentiate between helpful and nonhelpful responses in caring for families experiencing perinatal loss.

Healthy People 2020

(MICH-1.1) Reduce the rate of fetal deaths at 20 or more weeks of gestation to 5.6 per 1000 live births from baseline of 6.2 fetal deaths

(MICH-1.2) Reduce the rate of fetal and infant deaths during perinatal period (28 weeks of gestation to less than 7 days after birth)

(MICH-5) Reduce the rate of maternal mortality to 11.4 maternal deaths per 100,000 live births

Perinatal loss is the death of a fetus or newborn from the time of conception through the end of the neonatal period 28 days after birth. This chapter discusses grief and loss in the childbearing family and the nurse's role in facilitating the family's mourning process. Although the primary focus is stillbirth, care of the family experiencing the death of a baby in the newborn period is inclusive. Causes and clinical aspects of spontaneous abortion (miscarriage) in the antepartum period are discussed in Chapter 18, and Chapter 24 discusses labor-related complications that can lead to

*Excerpt from *Waiting with Gabriel: A Story of Cherishing a Baby's Brief Life* by Amy Kuebelbeck (Loyola Press, 2003). Reprinted with permission of Loyola Press. To order copies call 1-800-621-1008 or go to https://www.loyolapress.com.

fetal demise; this chapter discusses causes and clinical aspects of *intrauterine fetal death (IUFD)* after 20 weeks' gestation, often referred to as *stillbirth* or *fetal demise*. Maternal death is any death that occurs during pregnancy or within 42 days of the termination of a pregnancy.

Perinatal loss is a tragic event for the couple experiencing it and the family members who love them. Compounding the tragedy are many misconceptions surrounding perinatal loss, a lack of grief education afforded healthcare personnel, and clinical interventions that are out of step with current research. One of the biggest misconceptions about perinatal loss is that it is not as relevant as other losses because of the lack of interaction with the baby. In reality, this could not be further from the truth. Additionally, the grief for parents is lifelong and nonlinear, often described as the grief that never goes away.

Studies assessing the comfort level of nurses assisting families experiencing perinatal loss clearly demonstrate that many nurses are uncomfortable with death and dying and that more education is needed and, indeed, greatly desired (Steen, 2015). The level of comfort, or lack thereof, observed in the study was mostly dependent upon the nature of thinking on a more hopeful level, length of experience in nursing, and palliative care education, with palliative care education making the most significant difference (Kingdon, O'Donnell, Givens, et al., 2015).

Lastly, concerning research and practice, in recent years there has been a paradigm shift in the field of grief and bereavement regarding the components of a "normal" mourning process as well as when, where, and how much intervention is warranted. Much of what has become the traditional standard of care for bereaved individuals has come into question as new research sheds light on the inefficacy of predetermined early and intense intervention. This chapter focuses on providing frameworks for understanding grief and loss, guidelines for effectively responding to a grieving family, and specific nursing interventions for the family experiencing perinatal loss in the clinical setting.

Common Causes of Perinatal Loss

The *National Vital Statistics Reports*' most recent compilation of fetal mortality statistics occurred in 2013, and for the first time in decades there was a slight reversal to the trend of declining fetal mortality rates from 2011 to 2013. In the United States, the incidence of fetal death after 20 weeks' gestation decreased to 5.96 per 1000 total births (MacDorman & Gregory, 2015).

The *perinatal mortality rate (PMR)* is defined by the National Center for Health Statistics as late fetal deaths (over 28 gestational weeks) and neonatal deaths that occur up to 7 days after birth (MacDorman & Gregory, 2015). Perinatal deaths may be related to fetal, maternal, or placental factors or may have no apparent cause (MacDorman & Gregory, 2015).

The cause of fetal death may be unknown, or it may result from any of a number of physiologic maladaptations including asphyxia; congenital malformations; and superimposed pregnancy complications including preeclampsia or eclampsia, diabetes, systemic lupus erythematosus, renal disease, thyroid disorders, cholestasis of pregnancy, abruptio placentae, placenta previa, diabetes, renal disease, cord accidents, fetal growth restriction, and alloimmunization (MacDorman & Gregory, 2015).

Perinatal losses have occurred because of inaccurate gestational age designation which resulted in inappropriate interventions. A decline in the neonatal mortality rate can largely be attributed to changes in the gestational age distribution rather than to gestational age–specific mortality. This finding may be due to pregnancies delivered at 39 to 40 weeks that previously would have been unnecessarily delivered earlier, leaving fetuses at higher risk for mortality at other gestational ages (Ananth, Goldenberg, Friedman, et al., 2018). Perinatal loss can also occur due to infections. Perinatal loss is increased in women with multiple gestations and among women who smoke, have lower education attainment levels, are advanced maternal age, and are obese. Women who have had other pregnancies affected by stillbirth or growth restriction are at greater risk for having a stillborn baby (Romero & Lockwood, 2016). Perinatal loss associated with birth defects can occur as a result of congenital anomalies or may occur if the fetus is exposed to teratogens late in the pregnancy.

Although the cause is often unknown, several risk factors elevate the chances of stillbirth, including maternal race or ethnicity, age, multiple gestation, and number of previous pregnancies (with nulliparas at highest risk). Most disturbing is the continuing disparity in race and ethnicity.

Per 1000 births, African American women have fetal mortality rates of 10.53%, Native Americans 6.22%, Hispanic Americans 5.22%, Caucasian Americans 4.88%, and Asian/Pacific Islanders 4.68% (MacDorman & Gregory, 2015). African American women have higher rates of stillbirth (due to prematurity [20 to 27 weeks' gestation]) (MacDorman & Gregory, 2015).

Fetal mortality rates were higher than average for teenagers, unmarried women, women ages 45 and over, and women with multiple pregnancies. Twin pregnancies demonstrated a mortality rate 2.5 times higher than singleton pregnancies, and triplets or higher multiples were at five times the singleton rate. Pregnancies conceived by in vitro fertilization have higher rates of pregnancy complications and loss; multiple gestations related to infertility treatments have a lower rate of loss because these procedures commonly result in dichorionic twins. Monochorionic twins, which are most often conceived naturally, have a higher incidence of loss (Richards, Graham, Embleton, et al., 2015). Advanced maternal age appeared to be an independent risk factor even when concurrent medical conditions were factored out (MacDorman & Gregory, 2015).

Perinatal loss has declined as a result of early diagnosis of congenital anomalies and advances in genetic testing techniques. Although the incidence is extremely low, certain diagnostic testing options can contribute to fetal deaths, including amniocentesis and chorionic villus sampling (CVS).

In developing countries, infection plays a significant role in fetal mortality. These may include:

- *Escherichia coli*
- Group B streptococci
- *Ureaplasma urealyticum*
- Parvovirus
- Coxsackievirus
- *Toxoplasma gondii*
- *Listeria monocytogenes*
- Leptospirosis
- Q fever
- Lyme disease.

Certain maternal conditions can also be associated with higher rates of fetal death. Past maternal exposure to some bacterial and viral antigens can produce an autoimmune response that can result in fetal death. Women with acquired and immune thrombophilia have higher rates of miscarriage and fetal demise than those without hematologic alterations (Romero & Lockwood, 2016).

Maternal medical conditions contributing to the incidence of stillbirth include (Mattingly, 2016):

- Hypertensive disorders
- Diabetes mellitus
- Thyroid, renal, or liver disease
- Connective tissue disease (such as systemic lupus erythematosus [SLE])
- Cholestasis.

Other maladaptations that can cause stillbirth are:

- Antiphospholipid syndrome
- Heritable thrombophilias
- Red cell and/or platelet alloimmunization
- Congenital anomaly and malformations
- Chromosomal abnormalities including confined placental mosaicism
- Fetomaternal hemorrhage
- Fetal growth restriction
- Placental abnormalities including vasa previa and placental abruption
- Umbilical cord pathology including velamentous insertion, prolapse, occlusion, and entanglement
- Multifetal gestation including twin–twin transfusion syndrome/twin reverses arterial perfusion
- Amniotic band sequence
- Central nervous system lesions.

Maternal Physiologic Implications

The greatest maternal risk occurs when there is prolonged retention of the deceased fetus. These risks may include (Gold, Mozurkewich, Puder, et al., 2016):

- Disseminated intravascular coagulation (DIC)
- Infection
- Endometritis
- Sepsis
- Acute renal failure
- Shock or hypotension
- Maternal death.

Induction is commonly scheduled immediately upon diagnosis but may be delayed if the mother refuses or if it is a multiple gestation. When delays occur, fibrinogen levels are monitored weekly or biweekly to identify progressive coagulopathy. In cases of fetal death in the presence of a multiple gestation, coagulation labs may be obtained. DIC rarely occurs in cases of multiple gestations where the remaining fetus(es) are allowed to grow and mature (Mattingly, 2016).

Clinical Therapy

Many women first report an absence of fetal activity, although some women may fail to recognize this change. Diagnosis of IUFD is confirmed by visualization of the fetal heart with absence of heart action on ultrasound (American College of Obstetricians & Gynecologists [ACOG], 2017). Some practitioners routinely have a second ultrasound performed or have a second practitioner verify the absence of cardiac activity before making the diagnosis. When a fetal demise occurs, maternal estriol levels fall. In most cases, spontaneous labor begins within 2 weeks of fetal death without medical intervention. Because complications increase with delayed birth and identification of the cause of death becomes more difficult the longer pregnancy continues, labor is typically induced as soon as possible.

In modern practice, women with a diagnosed fetal demise are given the option of waiting a few days or weeks until emotionally prepared or scheduling an induction procedure immediately. The majority of women with a fetal demise will select a time to schedule an induction and most will elect for an induction immediately, although some women may wish to arrange for family members or other support persons to be present, which may necessitate a brief waiting period. The mode of induction is dependent on the gestational age, cervical readiness, and the type of incision if a cesarean was previously performed (ACOG, 2016). In women who have had previous cesarean births, a trial of labor is favored unless unusual circumstances exist (ACOG, 2016).

Women with an unfavorable cervix may be given vaginal prostaglandin agents, misoprostol, or laminaria tents. Women whose gestations are less than 16 gestational weeks may have a laminaria tent inserted into the cervix before a dilatation and extraction procedure. *Laminaria tents* are made from the stems of brown seaweed, which are cut, shaped, dried, sterilized, and packaged in specific sizes. Laminaria tents work by drawing water out of the cervical tissue, allowing the cervix to soften and dilate, and are most often used in preterm gestation. Sagiv and colleagues (2015) compared the efficiency of misoprostol and laminaria tents and found both were equally effective. Laminaria tents were associated with more pain and discomfort at the time of placement while misoprostol was associated with more side effects (Sagiv et al., 2015). Both may be placed before surgical procedures or inductions of labor. Transcervical Foley catheter placement or oxytocin (Pitocin) induction can also be used in women with an unfavorable cervix.

Women less than 28 weeks' gestation are typically given prostaglandin E2 vaginal suppositories (10–20 mg q 4–6 h), misoprostol 800 mcg vaginally (repeated for second dose no earlier than 3 hours and typically within 7 days if no response to first dose), and/or oxytocin (preferred in women with prior uterine surgery) until spontaneous labor occurs (ACOG, 2017; Mattingly, 2016). Women who are term and have not had a previous cesarean birth or other uterine scar may undergo an induction of labor. Women with an unfavorable cervix may be given cervical ripening agents, such as vaginal prostaglandin agents or misoprostol.

In women who have had a previous low transverse incision cesarean birth over 28 gestational weeks, cervical ripening and transcervical Foley catheter are recommended. Misoprostol 400 mcg every 6 hours has been given to women between 24 and 28 weeks with a previous uterine incision (Mattingly, 2016). Management of women with a previous classical incision or uterine surgery is limited and the method of birth should be individualized.

Postbirth Evaluation

Identifying the causative factor of fetal loss assists many families in progressing through the grieving process. Postmortem examination or studies can provide information related to the cause of the fetal death and risk of reoccurrence, and assist with future preconception counseling, prenatal screening procedures, and pregnancy management, as well as provide closure for the

TABLE 36–1 Tests to Determine Cause of Fetal Loss

FETAL TESTING	MATERNAL TESTING	PLACENTAL TESTING
• Blood tests and x-rays • Ultrasound • Autopsy or MRI • Cultures (IgG and IgM if specific infections suspected) • Chromosomal studies (if indicated)	• Fasting postpartum glucose level and hemoglobin A1C • CBC with platelet count • Rh testing • Kleihauer-Betke test • Abnormal antibody testing (lupus anticoagulant, anticardiolipin antibodies) • TSH levels • Infectious disease testing (rubella, syphilis, malaria, toxoplasmosis, cytomegalovirus, human parvovirus 19) • Hereditary thrombophilia testing • Toxicology testing • Protein S and C activity	• Placental studies (IgG and IgM if specific infections suspected) • Pathology

couple (ACOG, 2016). The types of studies and tests performed depend on the parents' past history, medical history, pregnancy course, appearance of the fetus, and the couple's preferences for the testing. Fetal, maternal, and placental testing are performed (Table 36–1).

A visual inspection of the baby determines obvious defects or abnormalities. The placenta and membranes are inspected. The umbilical cord should be inspected for true knots, a velamentous insertion, lack of Wharton jelly, or a short cord to determine if a cord accident was the cause. An autopsy is the best mechanism to determine the cause of death; however, in the event that the parents decline an autopsy, magnetic resonance imaging (MRI) can also provide detailed information (ACOG, 2016).

The Experience of Loss

The term **bereavement** comes from a root term meaning to be "deprived of something" or to be left "desolate or alone." To be bereaved simply means to have suffered the *event of loss*. **Grief** is an individual's *reaction to the loss*, including physical symptoms, thoughts, feelings, functional limitations, and spiritual responses. Grief reactions may be immediate or delayed, heightened or stunted, and highly variable. Though often used interchangeably, **mourning** is the *process* by which individuals incorporate the experience into their lives. Mourning is influenced by many factors, including personality, gender, family dynamics, and social, religious, and cultural norms. Mourning may be manifested by certain behaviors and rituals, such as weeping or visiting a gravesite, which help the person experience, accept, and adjust to the loss. The unanticipated loss of an expected child can be devastating and traumatic for parents. Though most people eventually regain a sense of purpose and adjust well, some suffer long-lasting and destructive consequences. Allahdadian and Iraipour (2015) suggest that there is nothing in a person's background to prepare him or her for the abrupt transition from a joyous event to the sorrow of perinatal loss. Perinatal loss is also unique in that the parents have not had experiences with the child that was to be, and attachment is based mostly on hopes and dreams for the future relationship.

Society typically does not offer the kind of support for perinatal loss that is offered for other, more recognized losses. This places perinatal loss in the category of disenfranchised grief. **Disenfranchised grief**, as defined by Kenneth Doka (2016), is grief that is not supported by the usual societal customs. Perinatal loss is sometimes referred to as a "silent loss" because of this phenomenon of disenfranchising grief (Bhat & Byatt, 2016). People are uncomfortable discussing the loss with the parents and often pull away when their support is most needed. "The loss of a child and all the child has to offer, compounded with the societal attitude discounting the loss and the potential withdrawal of social support, may leave the bereaved parents feeling distraught and alone at a time that was supposed to be full of happiness" (Bennett, Litz, Lee, et al., 2005, p. 181). Parents struggle to come to terms with the devastation of the loss and are often confused and bewildered as to how to make that happen. The nurse caring for a family experiencing perinatal loss can take positive steps to help facilitate the family's mourning process and help them begin their journey to recovery.

Frameworks for Understanding Perinatal Loss

There have been a plethora of models and theories postulated over the years attempting to explain patterns of grief and loss, and there is no consensus for which models should serve as the cornerstones of theory and teaching. There has been some very enlightening research in the last decade, however, that is presenting a vastly different perspective of bereavement than previously offered. For instance, in natural deaths, whether expected or unexpected, acceptance and sense making were the predominant emotions throughout the first 24 months, rather than the previous stage model where the acceptance stage followed the depression stage close to the end of the first year (Neimeyer, 2016). Current evidence-based research supports the belief that the grieving process is entirely variable and dependent upon many factors, such as the type of death, age of the deceased, and age of the griever. It is nonlinear and more easily understood when simply thought of as a process that encompasses the need of the griever to remain connected to the deceased, while simultaneously finding a way to exist in a changed world without the deceased (Neimeyer, 2016). For a mother who loses a baby, this might be phrased as "Am I still a mother? Who am I now?" The *intensity* to which the grief will be experienced is best understood from the aspect of the level of attachment the grieving person had to the deceased and usually entails finding personal meaning in the loss for successful integration into the grieving person's life. Several models explain these concepts.

Worth noting is the **dual process model**, a view of grief encompassing two competing spheres: Loss and restoration. The loss orientation is concerned with the individual's need to confront the reality of the loss, and the restoration orientation seeks to regain balance and temper the pain of grief. Both spheres of orientation are important; some people may gravitate more toward the loss side and some more toward the restoration side. The dual process model can be helpful as the griever comes to understand that he or she has the choice to consciously shift between spheres, allowing grief in the safer moments while recognizing the necessity of change (Neimeyer, 2016).

With respect to perinatal loss specifically, there are two theories that may provide the best framework for the nurse seeking to understand and assess the grieving family in his or her care. **Attachment theory**, first developed by Bowlby (1969) and revisited by Brier (2009), begins with the basic premise that human beings are biologically predisposed to bond with emotionally significant persons in their lives. The grief response as seen through the lens of attachment theory is a state of separation anxiety brought on by the disruption in the attachment bond. The intensity of the grief response displayed by parents experiencing perinatal loss can be assessed to some extent by determining the level of attachment to the anticipated baby. For mothers, nine events are important to the formation of attachment to her baby (Bennett et al., 2005; Klaus & Kennell, 1976):

1. Planning the pregnancy
2. Confirming the pregnancy
3. Accepting the pregnancy
4. Feeling fetal movement
5. Accepting the fetus as an individual
6. Giving birth
7. Seeing the baby
8. Touching the baby
9. Giving care to the baby.

Helpful questions to assess the first five levels of attachment could include topics such as naming of the baby, future plans, nursery preparations, and personal stories of the pregnancy. Additionally, there are psychologic processes related to becoming a parent that can help to identify those parents who have a strong level of attachment. These are noted in Table 36–2.

TABLE 36–2 Psychologic Process of Becoming a Parent

- Feelings of procreativity or generativity
- A sense of continuity through the generations
- Responses to quickening and bodily changes
- Fears and expectations about the coming baby
- The impact of this exciting process on expectant parents' relationship at home
- Changes that the baby will bring to their careers and to their lives in general
- Attachment to real and idealized aspects of the baby
- Self-esteem building

SOURCE: Reprinted from *Loss during pregnancy or in the newborn period: Principles of care with clinical cases and analyses*, 1997, p. 7. Reprinted with permission of the publisher, Jannetti Publications, Inc., East Holly Avenue, Box 56, Pitman, NJ 08071-0056. Phone (856) 256-2300; Fax (856) 589-7463.

Several researchers and theorists have demonstrated the need for continuing bonds as a means to remain connected to the deceased baby (Gold, Leon, Boggs, et al., 2016). Therefore, the goal of recovery, as related to attachment theory, is for the grieving parent to find a way to maintain the bond with the deceased baby while at the same time acknowledging that the baby is not physically present for future interactions.

The second theory centers on a search for meaning and is probably the most prevalent theme for bereaved parents. Robert Neimeyer (2016) proposes that meaning reconstruction is one of the most important aspects of the grieving process for bereaved individuals. Simply put, **meaning reconstruction** focuses on redefining ourselves and our interactions with the world after a significant loss. There is no question that the unexpected loss of a baby can precipitate a crisis of meaning for the parents. Are they still parents? How do they readapt to the world without their child in it? (Neimeyer, 2016). A large percentage of parents (61%) are troubled by the question "Why me?" and 70 to 85% find themselves searching for meaning early in the loss. Evidence supporting the conceptualization of parental bereavement as a crisis of meaning is plentiful (Neimeyer, 2016). However, it has also been suggested that some individuals do not seek meaning; that of those who do, less than half are able to find it; and that even when they do, the tendency is to continue searching (Neimeyer, 2016). Other studies showed that a significant factor of influence is the particular meaning construct the person places on the loss. People who tend to find positive constructs within the loss fare better than those who tend toward negative constructs. Neimeyer concluded, partly in response to the Davis study, that when parents are struggling with making meaning of their loss, it is important to facilitate the process; but if they are not, the caregiver should not initiate the process. The goal of recovery, as related to meaning reconstruction, is a positive change in self-identity by assigning the loss a meaning, thereby allowing the individual to assimilate the loss into her or his world.

Once there is an understanding of the frameworks for the mourning process, or the rationale behind the grief, common manifestations of grief can be explored. It is important to note that for purposes of this discussion, only the possible early responses are identified, as these are the ones the nurse is most likely to encounter in the clinical care setting. Initial grief reactions can include shock, numbness, denial, protest, disorientation, guilt, and confusion. In the initial grief reaction, there is a protective brain mechanism at work that activates to prevent us from taking in too much damaging information at one time and going into "meltdown." For a couple experiencing perinatal loss, this might manifest itself in *denial* of the impending or actual death of the fetus or baby. Even when the initial healthcare provider suspects fetal demise, the couple is hoping that a second opinion may be different. Some couples may not be convinced of the death until they see and hold the dead baby after birth. The couple may move rapidly from shock, confusion, and denial into very intense emotions. Anger—resulting from feelings of loss, loneliness, and, perhaps, guilt—is a common reaction, as is despair and an intense longing for the event not to have occurred. Anger may be projected at significant others and/or healthcare team members. The mother may attempt to identify a specific event that caused the death and may blame herself for the death. As the couple and their families begin to confront the pain of their loss, many normal manifestations of grief may be present. The nurse should be familiar with these normal reactions, so that abnormal or complicated reactions can be identified when present. See Table 36–3. See *Evidence-Based Practice: Perinatal Grief Intensity Scale.*

EVIDENCE-BASED PRACTICE | Perinatal Grief Intensity Scale

Clinical Question

Can the Perinatal Grief Intensity Scale (PGIS) accurately identify and predict intense grief and the need for follow-up after perinatal loss?

The Evidence

Perinatal loss occurs in 25% of all pregnancies. This includes miscarriages, stillbirths, and neonatal deaths. Families experience a wide range of responses to the grief of perinatal loss. Mothers may experience normal grief reactions, but about a fourth of women will have significant, prolonged, highly intense, and complicated grief that negatively affects their quality of life. These high-intensity grief reactions may be associated with other serious mental illnesses in the perinatal period, such as depression and posttraumatic stress disorder. There may also be detrimental effects on the relationship between mother and father, with a divorce rate four times higher among these families (Hutti et al., 2017). There is a need to identify those mothers who will encounter such an intense grief response so that supportive and timely help can be offered. These authors tested an instrument, the Perinatal Grief Intensity Scale, to determine if it is a reliable, valid predictor of intense grief response. The sample size for this instrumentation study was adequate, and its statistical results were acceptable. This type of study, while not an experiment, can produce moderately strong evidence for nursing practice in determining which instruments can be used for appropriate assessment.

The PGIS was found to be reliable and valid. It was assessed as a low-response burden and could provide the nurse with good predictive information about a mother's risk of serious, intense grief from perinatal loss (Hutti et al., 2017).

Best Practice

The PGIS can be used by the nurse to predict which mothers are more likely to experience life-altering intense grief. This should be administered to mothers who experience perinatal grief to identify those who could benefit from types of added support. These supports may prevent escalation of the grief into mental illness and interference with the mother's relationships.

Clinical Reasoning

When would be the optimal time to administer the PGIS? How could this instrument be incorporated into the nursing assessment of a family with perinatal loss?

TABLE 36–3 Normal Physical, Cognitive, Emotional, Behavioral, and Spiritual Early Responses to Loss

PHYSICAL	COGNITIVE	EMOTIONAL	BEHAVIORAL	SPIRITUAL
Physical signs and symptoms of shock	Denial, disbelief	Sadness	Withdrawal	Blaming God
Palpitations	Confusion	Anger/rage	Dependence	Hostility toward God
Shortness of breath	Sense of unreality	Guilt/self-reproach	Fear of being alone	Lack of meaning or direction
Difficulty sleeping	Disorientation	Anxiety	Memorializing the loss	Wishing to join the deceased
Nausea/vomiting	Time confusion	Numbness	Disorientation	Isolation
Loss of appetite	Vigilance or obliviousness	Flat affect	Sleep and appetite disturbances	Feelings of betrayal
Dry mouth	Focused or detached	Indifference	Absent-minded behavior	Hopelessness
Feeling of emptiness in the pit of the stomach	Poor concentration	Withdrawn or explosive	Dreams of the deceased	Destruction or strengthening of beliefs
Weakness/lethargy	Preoccupation	Repetitive storytelling	Crying/sighing	Feelings of being punished
Tightness in throat	Sense of presence	Loneliness	Restlessness	Acceptance as "divine will"
Sighing	Hallucinations of the deceased baby	Yearning/nostalgia	Avoidant behaviors	Assigning of deceased baby as "angel" in heaven
Fatigue			Treasuring of mementos	
Oversensitivity to light and sound				
"Aching" arms				

SOURCES: Data from DeSpelder & Strickland, 2005; Eutsey & Di Lima, 2001; Schneider, 1994; Worden & Winokuer, 2011.

Special Issues for Consideration

Many factors will influence a couple's response to perinatal loss, including individual factors such as age, gender, and personality type. A teenage couple is going to react very differently than a couple in their 30s, men and women tend to respond differently, and emotional personalities will display differently than stoic personalities. Family dynamics will greatly factor into the grief response. Is the family chaotic in nature? Is there a family leader? Do they have open communication or closed and guarded interactions? Do they deny the reality of the event and pretend it isn't happening? Answers to these questions can greatly assist the nurse who is caring for the family. Cultural and religious beliefs also influence the couple's reaction in a negative or positive manner. Socioeconomic status will play a role, in that for some people, grief is a luxury. If the grieving parent(s) are more concerned with children at home or putting food on the table, their grief will most likely be delayed to a time when they have the resources to deal with it. Finally, there are special circumstances that will influence the grief response. Early pregnancy loss has a special form of grief attached, fetal reduction and multifetal pregnancy loss entail separate and distinct issues, and grief from infertility is a largely ignored segment of the grieving population. Each of these components bears further discussion.

Individual and Family Issues

AGE

Age plays a major role in grief reactions. Couples in their 30s may feel that they are running out of time for childbearing; however, they are most likely to have living children at the time of the loss, which may eventually soften the blow somewhat. Couples in their 20s may be experiencing their first significant death, yet often have the sense that they still have time to have another child. With regard to age, however, adolescent parents probably pose the greatest challenge to nursing interventions.

The birth rates for females ages 15 to 19 was 24.2% higher than for women ages 30 to 34 (lowest risk group) (MacDorman & Gregory, 2015). The adolescent who attaches meaning to her pregnancy has the highest rate of grief reaction and life impact. Wheeler's (1997) landmark study showed that grief responses of adolescents were also affected by age of the adolescent, the gestational age at the time of the loss, and the length of time since the loss. The younger the adolescent, the more physical and emotional responses to the loss were experienced as compared to older adolescents (Wheeler & Sefton, 2016). Though adolescents have a mature concept of death, it is often clouded by their sense of invulnerability, an "It can't happen to me" mentality. Adolescents rely heavily on peer support and have a natural mistrust of authority figures, which can make assisting them more difficult. It is important to remember that adolescents are already experiencing major life changes, and the death of a baby can have a profound impact on their development. For many adolescents, a pregnancy loss may be the first time they are experiencing the psychologic impact of grief, and normal adolescent growth and development must be taken into consideration when assessing the impact of grief responses (Wheeler & Sefton, 2016). Nursing care of the adolescent parent experiencing perinatal loss requires patience and understanding on the part of the nurse. Adolescent parents should be treated with respect and offered the same consideration as adult grievers. They should not be forced into any particular mode of response but allowed to dictate their own needs within the experience. Gentle and honest guidance are often all that are needed to ensure a healthy nurse–patient interaction.

FAMILY DYNAMIC

Family dynamics and the presence or lack of cohesion will greatly factor into a couple's grief response. Families who are chaotic and have poor interfamily communication skills are often fractured and of little support to the couple experiencing the loss. Families who demonstrate strong familial ties and open group interaction tend to fare better in the long run. The most difficult family dynamic to assess and assist is the "lie and deny" family. This family deals with bad news and loss events as though they have not occurred. If they do not talk about it, it did not happen. Because a necessary component for the beginning of a healthy mourning process is to accept the reality of the death, the nurse is placed in the tenuous position of mediator between medical personnel and the family members, who do not want to hear anything negative. It is important to discern the possible causes for denial before proceeding. Denial is a normal and necessary process in the beginning of the mourning process, and the family may just need more time to assimilate the difficult information. Persistent denial, however, can be addressed by a gentle review of the facts of the situation with an emphasis on past-tense verbiage when discussing the baby.

GENDER ISSUES

Historically, most of the research regarding grief and bereavement has been done on women. As a result, many stereotypes developed regarding how men and women cope with loss. Hallmark research by Doka and Martin (2010) identified a new model for the two major coping styles and reveals a more effective means of supporting the griever. The model identified the two dominant styles of coping as "intuitive" and "instrumental." People with **intuitive styles of coping** generally feel their way through loss and prefer care with an emphasis on emotional and psychosocial support. People with **instrumental styles of coping** generally use more cognitive skills to navigate loss and value care that includes an emphasis on problem solving (Martin & Doka, 2011). It is important for the nurse to be aware that although gender *influences* mourning, it does not *determine* the experience for the bereaved.

For intuitive grievers, the nurse may initiate discussion of thoughts and feelings concerning the loss. Mobilization of support from nonjudgmental family and friends is generally appreciated, and providing resource materials that include support groups and the opportunity for networking is usually welcome. The nurse should share with the intuitive griever that enlisting the support of others with whom he or she can talk rather than relying solely on the spouse is favorable for both partners. The nurse should also share that spouses are commonly unable to be emotionally available to each other following loss. The nurse should normalize the lack of emotional accessibility and provide reassurance that the relationship is not doomed to fail because of the death of the baby.

For the instrumental griever, the nurse should specifically address the fact that a parent who seems detached and unaffected by the loss is not uncaring. It is more common for men to fall into this category, as they frequently experience pregnancy through the woman and, when traditionally raised, believe they are not supposed to be emotional but be strong for their partner (Beckett & Dykeman, 2015). The parent who is an instrumental griever may not mention the baby, talk about the loss, or view pictures. The instrumental griever may resist when the partner shows emotion or attempts to engage in conversation regarding the loss. Instrumental grievers tend to be more active as well as more vocal in assigning blame and commonly use explosive emotion to obtain desired results. Contrary to traditional thought, instrumental grievers' responses to loss are not unhealthy, yet they are often criticized for their behaviors. Because of their perceived strength, they rarely receive validation and support from others. In supporting instrumental grievers, the nurse should keep in mind that they value acceptance, acknowledgment of their pain, information regarding the loss, what to expect in the aftermath, and tasks that are connected to the loss.

The nurse should inform bereaved couples that both styles of grieving are acceptable and should be honored. Intuitive grievers (most often women) should understand that instrumental grievers may not show emotion or wish to talk about the loss, but are mourning in their own way. Instrumental grievers (most often men) should understand that intuitive grievers will need to talk about the event and help to provide avenues for that outlet. The nurse can instill a measure of hope by reassuring parents that although they may feel as if they cannot bear the pain of the loss, it will not always remain so intense. Parents who experience the stillbirth together often feel that their relationship has been strengthened by grieving together (Alghamdi & Jarrett, 2016).

OTHER FEATURES OF BEREAVED INDIVIDUALS

In addition to age, family traits, and gender issues, Parkes and Weiss (1983) identified overall features of bereaved individuals that place them at increased risk for pathologic or complicated grief reactions. These features include insecurity, anxiety, or low self-esteem; previous psychiatric history; excessive anger and guilt; a physical disability or illness; previous unresolved losses; inability to express emotion; and concurrent problems of living. Parkes and Weiss also identified features of bereaved individuals' circumstances that will put them at risk; these include an unsupportive or unavailable family, lack of social/religious or other supports, and low socioeconomic status.

Societal Issues

SPIRITUALITY

In times of crisis, spirituality brings comfort and strength to some people, and for some it is the single most important factor in quality of life. For others, a life crisis may precipitate a spiritual crisis and catalyze a complete redefining of the belief system, though the new belief system is often stronger than the one previously ascribed to (Neimeyer, 2016).

Religion and spirituality are not one and the same. **Spirituality** is defined as the human search for meaning and connectedness to life, others, God, the universe, and transcendence. **Religion** is defined as structured efforts conducted in a systematic approach to attain holiness. Religious practices are based on the level of a person's assimilation into the particular religion and are too varied and numerous to define for standards of care. With regard to specific religious practices, it is prudent for the nurse simply to ask the family how they can best be assisted in meeting their religious needs.

One study identified six themes affecting the spiritual needs of bereaved parents: Honest exchange of information, empathy and presence, continuing bonds, spiritual rites, attachment with others, and grief support (Adzich et al., 2016). The nurse can facilitate the spiritual needs of the couple by providing an atmosphere of acceptance regarding spiritual rites and encouraging the couple's use of spiritual writings, prayers, and observances. Questions that solicit the spiritual viewpoint of the couple regarding the loss can allow release of parental distress concerning spiritual matters. It is important for the nurse not to answer rhetorical questions, but allow the parents to process their own thoughts and feelings concerning meaning, purpose, and significance of the life and death of their baby. It is also important for the nurse to distinguish between his or her own personal beliefs and those of the parents. Some healthcare professionals get defensive and critical when the spiritual needs of the parents conflict with their own spiritual viewpoint. Recognition of personal limitations is healthy, and providing care is not exclusive to direct delivery. The nurse acts as a family advocate by offering to contact the couple's clergyperson, spiritual advisor, or the hospital chaplain. Research confirms that providing effective spiritual care to a parent during loss and bereavement is valuable in facilitating healthy parental mourning (Adzich et al., 2016).

Clinical Tip

It is vitally important to respect the family's religious beliefs and not interject your own preferences into the situation. Baptizing a baby whose parents have not requested such is a violation of their rights and disrespecting of their wishes. Allow the parents to dictate all spiritual aspects of their baby's care.

CULTURE

Keeping in mind that while the family is the most reliable source of information about its own beliefs and how to best assist it, there *are* some commonalities within culture groups that the nurse should be aware of in anticipation of meeting the parents' and family's needs (Table 36–4). The way many cultures experience grieving and death rituals is often heavily influenced by their religious beliefs and therefore addressed in the table as well. See *Developing Cultural Competence: Cultural Responses to Perinatal Loss*.

Developing Cultural Competence Cultural Responses to Perinatal Loss

There is much information a nurse can learn about a particular culture's response to perinatal loss and grieving. While knowledge of specific beliefs and rituals is helpful when caring for a family from an unfamiliar culture, it is *most* important that the nurse simply remains open, curious, nonjudgmental, and unassuming. There are underlying threads that weave together the relevant factors affecting grief response, yet no two people will grieve alike, and even knowledge of a person's cultural and religious background does not offer the nurse a guaranteed blueprint to follow. This is particularly true where culture is concerned. Not only are there many country of origin and regional differences, but the extent of assimilation into American culture will factor in as well. Therefore, to say that all Hispanic Americans will respond to the death of a baby alike because they are Hispanic American would be akin to saying that all Protestants will worship alike because they are Protestant. One only has to consider the vast number of Protestant denominations with varying and often conflicting viewpoints to realize that such a generalization is useless to the nurse assisting grieving parents and families. Perinatal loss is unique in cultural awareness because one can never be sure to what extent culture, religious beliefs, or other factors will dominate the response to such an unexpected and unnatural event as the death of a baby (Allahdadian & Iraipour, 2015).

TABLE 36–4 Common Cultural Practices: Grief, Bereavement, and Perinatal Loss

CULTURE	FAMILY HIERARCHY AND REACTION TO MEDICAL COMMUNITY	COMMON BELIEFS AND EXPRESSIONS OF GRIEF	CARE AND HANDLING OF THE BODY: RELIGIOUS AND CULTURAL RITUALS
		Before and After Death	**Before and After Death**
African American	Matriarchal; family decision making. Family, religion, and community play a large role in grief recovery; considered collectivists. May distrust majority healthcare system; common to rely on internal resources. Healthcare providers should work to build trust and respect family dynamics.	Vary widely because of diversity in religious beliefs, countries of origin, and geographical regions. Some will cry or wail, while others will appear stoic, especially if mistrustful of healthcare providers. Many hold strong religious beliefs; will turn to clergy for assistance. Prayer for healing or comfort around the bedside is a common occurrence for Christians. May be averse to withdrawal of life support.	Will generally want pictures and mementos; naming of the baby is important for family heritage. Death is often called "home going" or "passing on," especially by Christians. May desire pre- or postdeath baptism. Common to wait for extended family to arrive for funeral services. Most likely to prefer burial to cremation. May have elaborate caskets and/or services as a way of showing respect and giving the baby a final tribute. Tend to view life as a continuous circle and therefore many have a steadfast belief of being reunited with their baby.
Old Order Amish	Patriarchal; strong family and community ties. Decisions dictated by religious beliefs; made by both parents, but father will usually relay. Will accept life-supporting medical technology. Most have eighth-grade education, so information should be provided appropriately. Will consent to legal dictates.	Children are a gift from God. Many losses occur due to advanced maternal age and consanguinity. The loss is profound, but viewed as God's will. Very private in grief; will keep to themselves for comfort. Rare for them to share with outsiders, known as the "English."	Do not believe in baby baptism. Family and friends will usually want to wash the body for burial in a white gown. Photos are not permitted (for the living or dead). May not accept mementos as community prepares casket and burial clothes, but offer should be made as less conservative families may accept. Bracelet may be accepted as legal identification. May want to transport body home, and burial will be at a designated funeral home or on the family farm as laws permit.
Asian American	Generally patriarchal, but strong community influence. In the more traditional families, older members are highly respected and should be included. Generally avoid confrontation and more traditional may avoid eye contact. Touching is impolite. Saying "no" directly may be considered rude, so healthcare provider should ask open-ended questions.	Community oriented. May believe that bad *karma* causes illness and death. May believe the number "4" is associated with death. Death of a baby is intensely mourned. Initial grief is acceptable and there may be crying and/or wailing at times. Death is not a usual topic for discussion and overt expressions of prolonged grief may be viewed as mental illness and therefore may alternately be expressed as somatic complaints (safer to be body related than mind related).	Usually a blend of Western and Eastern grieving and death ritual practices. The body should be handled with much care and always with respect. Family members may wear white clothing or headbands to mark mourning. Common to have an elaborate funeral ritual for the soul's passing.
European American	Family hierarchy is dependent upon faith values; Christian families tend toward patriarchy, while secular families tend toward companion marriage with equal decision making. Comfortable with technology and generally utilize to fullest extent possible. More likely to question authority and expect answers from healthcare providers.	Expressions of grief span the spectrum of responses; most often dictated by religious beliefs, geographical regions within the United States, and country of origin. Crying is acceptable; intense grief reactions are dependent upon previous factors noted. Usually no set mourning period and most likely to mourn longer than support is offered.	May or may not wish to bathe baby personally. May or may not wish to view and/or hold the baby. May or may not desire pictures. The nurse should inquire about all, but not place pressure for any. Naming of the baby and use of the name by healthcare providers are important. Burial or cremation preference may be determined by faith practices, financial status, or personal preference. May desire funeral services; baby areas in cemeteries are acceptable, especially to Catholics, who view babies as sinless. Baptism may or may not be desired and should not be done unless the parents request such. Pictures and mementos are usually appreciated.

TABLE 36–4 Common Cultural Practices: Grief, Bereavement, and Perinatal Loss *(continued)*

CULTURE	FAMILY HIERARCHY AND REACTION TO MEDICAL COMMUNITY	COMMON BELIEFS AND EXPRESSIONS OF GRIEF	CARE AND HANDLING OF THE BODY: RELIGIOUS AND CULTURAL RITUALS
Hindu (addressed separately, although Indian Americans are included in the Asian American minority group)	Patriarchal, though family oriented; needs of all over individual emphasized. Husband or eldest male will usually communicate decisions.	Combination of culture, philosophy, and religion. Believe in *karma* and reincarnation; seek to transcend birth and death by good deeds (karma), which ultimately frees the soul.	The body should be bathed, oils applied, and dressed in new clothes. Cremation should take place before the next sunrise in order to release the soul from the body. Eldest male member begins the cremation by physically pushing the button or flipping the switch (or, in older traditions, lighting the funeral pyre).
Hispanic and Latino American	Patriarchal; family decision making. Male to female, older to younger concept of *respeto* (respect) in social order. Applies to healthcare providers, and mutual respect is expected. More trusting of individual practitioners than system; expect warmth, caring, and attention. More traditional will expect handshake and formal use of last name upon introduction (*Senor* or *Senora*). Generally view human touch as respect from healthcare professionals.	View loss as God's will. Tend to rely on faith and prayer as tools for coping. Outward expression is encouraged, especially crying among women. Men tend toward stoicism for the family. Both may experience depressive symptoms. Support comes from family and friends. Extended family will usually travel for services. Support is found in family, friends, church, and community. Tend not to look toward medical community for support.	Baptism and naming are usually desired. Generally prefer burial to cremation. Pictures and other mementos are important, as they tend to utilize them for honoring the baby in the home. Country of origin will determine particular rituals involved in grief and death. Catholicism predominates. Prefer open-casket ceremonies. May wear traditional dark funeral clothing for an undefined mourning period. Continuing bonds with the deceased are important (hence, the "Day of the Dead" in Mexico). Belief of a fine line between the living and dead. Rituals include the lighting of candles, prayers for the dead, and shrines for honoring them.
Jewish	Traditionally patriarchal; modern Jewish families tend toward companion marriage with equal decision making.	For observant Jewish families, having children is commanded by God and considered a great blessing. Loss of a baby is profound and support may be sought from the family's rabbi. Some will tend toward stoicism, while others will openly grieve. Believe the soul begins the journey from the body immediately; this is why it is important to bury the body as soon as possible. The parents may not want to view the body, as they tend to want to remember the deceased as alive rather than dead.	Perinatal loss is a somewhat controversial topic in Judaism today. Traditionally, neonates (babies under 30 days of age) were not named or provided traditional bereavement practices such as sitting shiva. In recent times, the customs have changed, and many will observe full mourning and burial rituals for a perinatal loss. Adherence to traditional Jewish rites will entail body washing by a special group of people who ritually wash and dress the body in linen shrouds. Naming the baby will depend on whether the family adheres to the old traditions, as will sitting shiva. The baby may be named at the burial and given a name associated with comfort. Pictures of the dead are not permitted and autopsy not acceptable unless there is benefit to the living. Burial should take place within 24 hours and cremation is forbidden. Bodies should be whole, if possible. Burial is sometimes in a special section for babies, but always in a Jewish cemetery and usually in a wooden coffin with no metal to delay decomposition. Prefer monetary donations to charities in lieu of flowers, as the withering and dying of the flowers is considered a painful reminder of the loss.

(continued)

TABLE 36–4 Common Cultural Practices: Grief, Bereavement, and Perinatal Loss *(continued)*

CULTURE	FAMILY HIERARCHY AND REACTION TO MEDICAL COMMUNITY	COMMON BELIEFS AND EXPRESSIONS OF GRIEF	CARE AND HANDLING OF THE BODY: RELIGIOUS AND CULTURAL RITUALS
Muslim	Patriarchal, but decision making is shared. Information should be provided to both parents, even though the father may relay all decisions. Autopsy is usually forbidden unless for major concerns or demanded by law.	Death is considered a part of life. Children are a gift from Allah and are returned to Allah if they die, as they are considered sinless. The death of a fetus or baby is not minimized, but regarded as just as significant as that of an adult. Crying and solemn expressions of grief are permitted as long as control is maintained. Excessive grieving is considered not accepting of the will of Allah. The funeral is followed by 3 days of formal mourning (and 40 days of unofficial mourning), but for babies less than 4 months' gestation, the fetus may only be wrapped and buried.	If the child is born alive but death is imminent, the father may whisper the phrase "There is no God but Allah" in the baby's ear, securing the baby's call to worship. Naming is essential, as the mother and baby will be bound together in paradise. Parents may desire to perform a ritual washing of the body, usually by the same-sex parent. Conversely, they may not wish to see or hold the baby, as the viewing of bodies unnecessarily is discouraged. The legs should be straightened and sometimes the parents may request that the body face the right and face Mecca. Pictures are not usually desired, but should be offered. Locks of hair should not be removed; the body should be left intact and wrapped in a plain white shroud. Cremation is forbidden.
Native American	Patriarchal, though parents will make decisions together.	Navajo, the second largest Native American population, have traditional customs followed upon death. Tend to be stoic and grieve privately. Death is viewed as a transitional step on the journey to the next world, and the mourners must follow strict burial and bereavement rituals to ensure a successful journey.	Rituals must be completed within 4 days of death. The body is washed and painted for the journey. They do not speak of the dead after the fourth day because it is believed that it will impair the journey of the deceased. After a time, any discussion of the deceased is believed to bring ill health to the surviving family, and therefore support following the loss can be a challenge.

Note: It is unwise to attribute specific attitudes or beliefs to all members of a cultural group. The information in this table offers possible insights into caring for women from different cultural groups.

SOURCES: Data from Callister, 2006; Chichester, 2005, 2007; Clements et al., 2003; Hebert, 1998; Lobar, Youngblut, & Brooten, 2006; Schott & Henley, 2007; Whitaker & Kima, 2010.

A basic rule of thumb for cultural issues is to remember that curiosity is okay; avoidance is not. If you are not sure what the family needs, simply ask them how you can help to accommodate their wishes. Families appreciate an honest and caring attitude. See *Professionalism in Practice: Instituting Culturally Competent Care.*

Specific Circumstances

INFERTILITY

Infertility is not an episode, but an ongoing struggle for those who are caught in its grasp. The focus of treatment for infertility is a correct diagnosis, appropriate treatment, and successful live birth, yet infertility brings with it grief and loss issues that affect all realms of the couple's life. Not only are the medical and physical components extremely challenging, but the loss of infertility goes largely unrecognized by the usual support systems, placing it within the disenfranchised grief category. In the early phase, the patients are trying to assimilate the diagnosis of infertility and what the diagnosis actually means for them. Then they are faced with a gamut of decisions and difficulties such as:

- Treatment available (method that is best for them; when to begin; repercussion of choices; risk involved)
- Waiting (menstrual cycles; pregnancy; failed pregnancy; surgery; hormone treatments; in vitro fertilization)
- Psychologic roller coaster (spiritual impact; the strain on finances and primary, secondary, familial, and workplace relationships)
- When to discontinue treatment.

In supporting the patient dealing with infertility, the nurse should assess where the woman is in the process and respond accordingly. The nurse should be compassionate, give accurate and honest information, validate the many losses incurred, and support whatever decisions the couple makes regarding the continuation of treatment or decision to stop treatment. The nurse should not avoid the couple, offer pat answers or reasons for the infertility or the outcome, or relay unsolicited stories of others' successes or failures. For couples finally experiencing a pregnancy following infertility treatment, there may be heightened anxiety, for which additional reassurances will need to be offered. See Chapter 6 for a detailed discussion of infertility.

EARLY PREGNANCY LOSS

Early pregnancy loss, whether by ectopic or molar pregnancy, blighted ovum, or spontaneous abortion, is devastating for many couples. As attachment is based on the level of emotional bonding, it is necessary for the nurse to assess the situation in order to respond to actual patient needs and validate the loss for those who view the event as the death of their baby. Compounding early pregnancy loss is the extraordinary guilt the couple typically harbors, especially the mother. Mothers will often blame themselves, whether by

Professionalism in Practice Instituting Culturally Competent Care

There are ways that a nurse can provide culturally competent care in the challenging situation when a baby dies. A good place to start is with a formal or informal cultural awareness questionnaire similar to ones used for general nursing care. Questions pertaining to death, dying, and perinatal loss should provide answers for the following:

- What the family's beliefs are about what happens after death
- How the family views the death of a baby, in particular
- How the dying baby should be cared for as he or she approaches death, including who should be present and any ceremonies that should be performed at the moments before and after death
- How the body should be handled after death, including how the body should be cleansed and dressed, who should handle the body, and whether the body should be buried or cremated
- Whether grief should be expressed quietly and privately, or loudly and publicly, such as with public crying, keening, or wailing
- Whether there are different expectations on how a man should grieve versus a woman, or for children versus adults; what the family considers the role for each member in coping with the death
- What ceremonies and rituals should be performed and who should participate, such as children, community members, and friends.

SOURCE: Data from Cancer.net, 2018.

commission or omission, particularly in cultures where a woman's status is dominated by themes of motherhood and childrearing. The nurse should reassure the couple that they did not do anything to precipitate the loss and provide support materials specific to the type of loss incurred and what to expect in the immediate aftermath.

Assessment of future pregnancies will need to be dealt with gently, as some couples have no desire to try again. Healthcare professionals sometimes find it easier and more comfortable to refocus on something other than the loss; however, that tends to minimize the loss event and isolate the griever. Even if the parents are expressing an interest in trying again, it is important not to focus exclusively on the future pregnancy, but to provide opportunities to address the current loss. The nurse should prepare the couple for the fact that family members and friends will often underestimate the impact of the loss and may offer well-meaning, though often harmful, remarks or platitudes in an attempt to ease emotional pain. This is a common reaction in early pregnancy loss, as they may have not known about the pregnancy or feel as if the couple "didn't know the baby." The nurse should reassure the parents that they have a right to their feelings, thoughts, emotions, and reactions to the loss. An early pregnancy remembrance box (a remembrance journal, sachet pillow, and a baby ring) provides a sensitive and caring way to give parents something to take with them that contains memories of their baby (Figure 36–1). See *Case Study: Benita Cartier*.

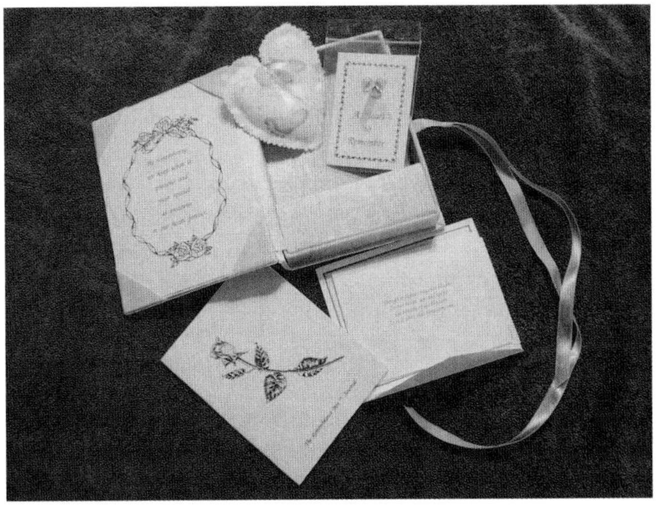

Figure 36–1 Early pregnancy remembrance box.

SOURCE: Share Pregnancy & Infant Loss Support, Inc.

MULTIFETAL PREGNANCY LOSS

In 2016 the U.S. live twin birth rate was 33.4 per 1000 births, and the high-order multiple-birth rate was 101.64 per 100,000 births, a decline since the 2015 statistics (Martin, Hamilton, Osterman, et al., 2018). Twin pregnancies demonstrated a mortality rate 2.5 times higher than singleton pregnancies, and triplets or higher multiples were five times the singleton mortality rate (MacDorman & Gregory, 2015). Multifetal pregnancy loss (MPL) may occur by spontaneous abortion, elective termination for unwanted pregnancy, selective reduction for fetal malformation, or selective reduction in high-risk multiple pregnancy to provide a greater chance of survival for remaining embryos. The loss of a baby in a multiple pregnancy may also occur by intrauterine demise, twin-to-twin transfusion syndrome, complications of monoamniotic twinning, placental problems, adverse intrapartum events, delayed interval delivery, postoperative complications, and the effects of prematurity. Parents whose multiples die have an increased risk of prolonged or delayed grief (Richards et al., 2015).

CASE STUDY: Benita Cartier

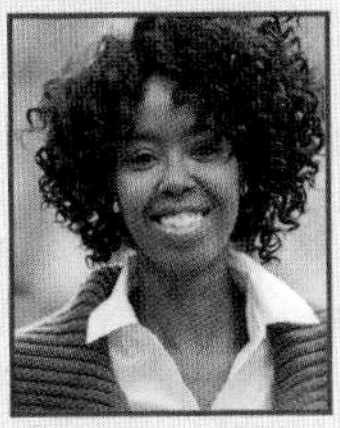

SOURCE: blvdone/Shutterstock

At her postpartum appointment, Benita expresses sadness to the nurse about her sister's situation. Her sister, Marcella, has had repeated pregnancy losses. She is now pregnant again, but is experiencing vaginal bleeding and has been diagnosed with a threatened abortion. Marcella and her family are devastated and worry that she will never be able to have a child.

Question to Ponder

What can nurses do to facilitate the grieving process for families like Marcella's that are experiencing loss?

Many aspects of multifetal pregnancy loss have historically been overlooked by healthcare professionals (Bhat & Byatt, 2016). Some of the predominant issues affecting parents are:

- Traumatic impact of diagnoses of malformation or birth defects
- Options and impact of difficult decisions
- Sudden death of a baby; fear and anxiety for surviving babies
- Prospect of infertility because of previous abortions
- Last attempt at in vitro fertilization (IVF) or other fertility intervention
- Guilt
- Cohabitation of mourning and joy, and resurgence of the body's remembering on special days and holidays.

In supporting bereaved parents caring for the surviving baby or babies in the loss of a multiple, the nurse should resist the urge to suggest the parents refocus on the positive aspect of having surviving siblings. Statements inferring that the death was meant to be, the death allowed the other baby(ies) to live, or the child who died would have had a compromised quality of life should never be made. The nurse needs to understand that the couple might have difficulty mourning their loss as they attempt to balance emotions of joy and sadness while caring for the surviving baby(ies). Parents will often imagine what the deceased baby might have looked like, what kind of personality the baby might have developed, and what the relationship with siblings might have been. They may harbor feelings of guilt if they feel relief for not having to care for numerous babies. The nurse should support parents by addressing these distinctive concerns and prepare them for the unique issues related to multifetal loss before they leave the hospital.

When creating visual memories for bereaved parents, an effort should be made to take pictures of the multiples together. The nurse should ask parents how they prefer to address surviving babies, for example, twins, triplets, quadruplets, and so forth. Additionally, the nurse should ask the couple whether they wish to delay funeral services until the mother is able to attend the ceremony. If the couple desires a delay, the nurse should contact appropriate disciplines to arrange for the delay in disposition of fetal remains (Adzich et al., 2016). The nurse should prepare the mother for the likelihood of her body missing and remembering the baby immediately after delivery, while caring for surviving baby(ies), and surrounding special days, milestones, and holidays. Finally, the nurse should be aware of the risk for complicated bereavement and refer the couple for appropriate support via resource materials (Adzich et al., 2016).

MATERNAL DEATH

Maternal death is defined by the World Health Organization (WHO, 2018) as "the death of a woman while pregnant or within 42 days of termination of pregnancy, irrespective of the duration and the site of the pregnancy, from any cause related to or aggravated by the pregnancy or its management, but not from accidental or incidental causes." The most common causes of maternal death are hemorrhage, hypertensive disorders, amniotic fluid embolism, infection, and preexisting chronic conditions, such as diabetes and cardiovascular disease. Obesity is also becoming a significant factor in maternal deaths because of the medical conditions that result. While they have been excluded from the definition of maternal death, some researchers have noted that maternal deaths related to homicide (and intimate partner or family violence) and suicide represent a small but significant number of deaths that occur during the pregnancy and postpartum period (Neimeyer, 2016).

The maternal mortality ratio in developing countries in 2015 was 239 per 100,000 live births versus 12 per 100,000 live births in developed countries (WHO, 2018). The California Department of Public Health (CDPH) launched a pregnancy-associated mortality review program with the aim of decreasing maternal mortality. As a result of the findings, CDPH reported in 2018 that in California maternal mortality decreased from a high in 2006 of 16.9 deaths per 100,000 live births to 7.3 deaths per 100,000 live births in 2013. In the rest of the United States, maternal mortality rates are triple the rates in California (CDPH, 2018).

For the spouse or partner, or the father of the child, the death of the mother is shocking (even if she had previous medical problems) and traumatic. There is an even deeper shock presenting here, in that the death is surrounding an expectedly joyous event, a birth. The initial shock experienced by the father or partner is traumatic and powerful. The grieving process is complicated by a number of factors (such as caring for the newborn while grieving the partner) and too comprehensive a topic for this text. What is important for nurses caring for the father, spouse, partner, and/or other family members is to recognize that initial grief reactions may be extremely intense. As long as no one is violating the fundamental principles of grief reaction (not hurting themselves, others, or personal property), the father/partner and family should be fully supported through this initial time with all support available to them and the facility in which the nurse is practicing. Interactions should be brief and direct, such as offering tissues and straightforward condolences (e.g., "I'm so sorry this is happening to you"). As with all losses, it is important to resist offering explanations or platitudes, which may prove harmful.

Across all settings, nurses are generally the only professionals whose care extends beyond the time of death. For the staff, a maternal death on the perinatal unit can be traumatic as well. When a death occurs on any unit, there are individual as well as group reactions to the event. The individual nurses involved may experience feelings of shock, sadness, anger, guilt, and other grief-associated reactions. The unit as a whole may experience feelings of inadequacy, anger, guilt, confusion, and depression. For the nurses directly involved, the father and family must still be cared for, and for everyone on the unit, nursing care continues.

It is important for obstetric nurses in situations of loss to be provided with adequate support within the work environment (Rondinelli, Long, Seelinger, et al., 2015). Staff members need the opportunity to express their feelings in a safe environment. Interventions for staff may include professional debriefing, professional counseling when needed, and the use of peer support. A model of peer training, in which nurses comfortable with caring for bereaved families act as peer mentors for less experienced nurses or for nurses who are uncomfortable caring for families with a perinatal loss, can provide a foundation for staff growth. Nurses need to take care of their own grief reactions and allow time for personal healing. Focusing on the positive aspects of the situation where they exist (such as personal kindness shown to the mother before the death or to the family in the aftermath) is an important step in the healing process as well as reflecting objectively on those things out of one's personal control (the mother's underlying medical issues or unforeseen complications). The idea, as with the loss of a baby, is to eventually memorialize the event with a balanced perspective, recognizing where personal effectiveness as well as limitations exist and learning to live with them, both personally and professionally. See *Professionalism in Practice: Bereavement Certification.*

Professionalism in Practice **Bereavement Certification**

Several organizations offer bereavement certification that focuses on perinatal loss and the needs of families during this difficult event. Ideally, each hospital should have a certified on-call specialist who can be brought in to meet the needs of families during the grief process.

●○● NURSING MANAGEMENT

For a Family Experiencing Perinatal Death

Nursing Assessment and Diagnosis

Cessation of fetal movement reported by the mother to the nurse is frequently the first indication of fetal death. It is followed by a gradual decrease in the signs and symptoms of pregnancy. Fetal heart tones are absent, and fetal movement is no longer palpable. In the clinical setting, once fetal demise is established, you will need to assess the family members' ability to adapt to their loss. Open communication among the mother, her partner, and the healthcare team members contributes to a realistic understanding of the medical condition and its associated treatments. You may discuss prior experiences the family has had with loss and what they feel were their perceived coping abilities at that time. Identifying the family's social supports and resources is also important.

Perinatal loss may also occur in the intrapartum period as a result of an intrapartum complication, such as an unresolved shoulder dystocia, prolapsed umbilical cord, abruptio placentae, or other complication. In such emergent situations, healthcare team members often focus on the physical needs of the mother and an attempt to save the life of the fetus. Commonly, it is not until the baby is delivered that the family is advised a perinatal death has occurred. Thus, the parents are faced with the sudden and completely unanticipated death of their baby. The most common response is protest or disbelief.

Although the physician/CNM informs the family of the death, you will continue one-on-one care with the family, providing both physical and emotional support throughout this crucial period. Assist the family in the mourning process and explore their immediate wishes for viewing and holding their deceased baby.

Nursing diagnoses that may apply include:

- *Grieving* related to the imminent loss of a child
- *Powerlessness* related to lack of control in current situational crisis
- *Family Processes, Dysfunctional*, related to death of a child/unresolved feelings regarding perinatal loss
- *Hopelessness* related to sudden, unexpected fetal loss
- *Spiritual Distress, Risk for*, related to intense suffering secondary to unexpected fetal loss

(NANDA-I © 2017)

Nursing Plan and Implementation

Most facilities have an established protocol to follow in the event of perinatal death. It typically provides a holistic focus for family-centered nursing care. It is important that the entire healthcare team be notified so interprofessional care can be initiated. When fetal death has been confirmed before admission, the entire staff on the unit is informed so they can avoid making inappropriate remarks. Many facilities have a symbol, such as a card with a leaf or a cluster of flowers, which is placed on the mother's door so that all of the staff is aware of the loss (Figure 36–2). This is something that should be discussed with the family before placement, as some may view the symbol as an identification of them as "damaged." As is stated throughout the chapter, it is important to allow the family to dictate their own experience.

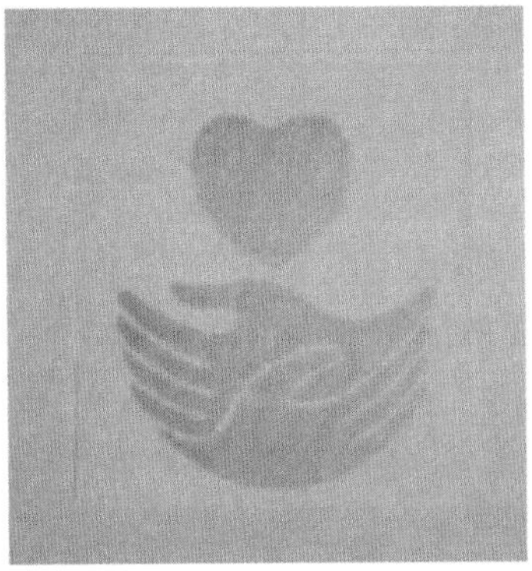

Figure 36–2 Door card.

SOURCE: Share Pregnancy & Infant Loss Support, Inc.

Clinical Tip

No matter how much nursing experience you have, when an expectant family is in pain because of their loss, and you feel you do not know the right thing to say, saying "I'm so sorry, I don't know what to say" is a start.

Avoiding the Use of Clichés

Inappropriate remarks are a hallmark of uninformed interactions, even though the intent behind them is honorable. Become familiar with statements that are helpful in facilitating the family's mourning process. Although grieving people often say that it is easier to forgive less-than-helpful remarks than to forgive those who do not reach out to them at all, the use of clichés can be harmful. Facilitate a healthy mourning process for the family by using active listening techniques and avoiding the use of clichés and platitudes. Sitting in silence with a family is often the most helpful form of intervention available. For a list of helpful versus unhelpful statements with rationales, see Table 36–5.

Facilitating the Family's Mourning Process

As mentioned at the opening of this chapter, there has been a paradigm shift in the field of grief and bereavement with regard to what constitutes a "normal" mourning process, as well as when and where early intervention is warranted. The standard of care has been centered on the notion that early and intense grief responses should be encouraged and even elicited for healing to begin. The relevant research, however, determined that many people are naturally resilient and will recover in their own time, without the benefit of assistance (Jaanista, Coombs, Donnelly, et al., 2017). For instance, stoic responses, when exhibited because of familial or cultural traits, are not always counterproductive and may not need intervention in order for the person to begin the path to recovery. Furthermore, not only is early intervention not always necessary, it can even be harmful in some instances. Although the research confirms that traumatic grief is usually best assisted by early intervention, perinatal

TABLE 36–5 Unhelpful versus Helpful Interactions with Grieving Families

UNHELPFUL	HELPFUL	RATIONALE
You're young; you can try again. At least you have your other children.	I am sure you'll miss [Sara] and no one will ever take her place in your heart.	Saying that they can try again diminishes their current pain. Saying that no one can ever take the deceased baby's place validates the loss as real and the baby as unique.
At least you didn't know him or her yet.	I'm sure you had many hopes and dreams for the future.	Never start a sentence with the words "at least." It diminishes whatever follows. Speaking of future plans validates the loss of the hoped-for child and the dreams that will never be.
It's a blessing in disguise.	I don't know why this terrible thing has happened to you. I just want you to know that I care and want to help you through it.	Statements like "It's a blessing in disguise" are often said when there are deformities involved. There is no adequate explanation for the family as to why this tragedy has befallen them and none should be offered. Instead, reassurance that they will not be alone should be given.
God needed another angel in heaven.	I'm so sorry this is happening to you. You are a good person and this is a terrible thing to have to go through. I'm here to listen if you would like to talk about it.	The family may make this statement as an indication of their belief system, and that is perfectly acceptable. It is not acceptable, however, for the nurse to impose her or his own belief system upon the family. It is much more effective to address the issue at hand (they are in pain) and reassure them of your caring presence.

loss does not *always* fall into this category, which leads to the current quandary: When is early intervention warranted and effective? The debate continues, but for the nurse caring for a family experiencing perinatal loss, avoiding the trap of "cookie-cutter" responses is not difficult if simple, caring guidelines are followed rather than rigid rules. Keep two goals in mind when assisting grieving parents and families. The first is to help the family navigate the medical/hospital system and the second is to facilitate the family's mourning process by allowing them to dictate their own experience.

Clinical Tip

Allowing families to meet their own needs in grief offers them the best path to learning to live with their loss; trying to force them into doing things the way that you think is best for them serves your own needs, not theirs, and can prove harmful.

The Caring Theory

The classic caring model developed by Swanson (1991) has sustained the test of time; it is as relevant today as when it was originally developed. Perhaps because of its lack of rigidity and concentration wholly on the overall *attitude* of the caregiver, it can best serve as a solid foundation for good nursing practice related to bereavement care. The **caring theory** consists of five attributes of the caregiver: (1) knowing, (2) being with, (3) doing for, (4) enabling, and (5) maintaining belief (Hutti et al., 2016; Kalfoss & Owe, 2015).

Knowing is defined as attempting to understand the event as it has meaning in the life of the parents. A thorough nursing assessment will facilitate the nurses' understanding of the significance of the loss to the parents. Nurses who operate from a level of knowing are perceived as sensitive, knowledgeable, and appropriate. Nurses who do not are often perceived as distant, cold, and uncaring. *Being with*, or being emotionally present, is the nurse's ability to reach beyond professionalism and give of herself or himself as a human being. *Doing for* is a restating of the golden rule. It means that the nurse does for the parents as she or he would have things done for her or him in the same situation. This does not mean detail by detail, as every family is unique in their needs; rather, this is an overall, treat-them-as-you-would-your-own-family type of behavior. *Enabling* means facilitation of the parents' passage through life transitions and unfamiliar events. Enabling encompasses all of the interventions listed throughout the text regarding perinatal loss and places the caregiver in the role of facilitator. Finally, *maintaining belief* is defined as believing in the parents' capacity to get through the event and face a future with meaning. If you ascribe to this model of care, you will well serve the needs of bereaved parents by compassionately helping them in the midst of their pain and imprinting positive memories to sustain them. It is important to recognize that nurses can become overwhelmed with providing the care that patients need and deserve. Coping strategies that are helpful for nurses come from sources such as their faith, their relationships with fellow nurses, and their own families (Hutti et al., 2016).

The Art of Responding

Employing the caring theory of behavior, you can then look to the responding model as a set of guidelines for successful interactions with grieving families. Keeping in mind the uniqueness of each situation, the **responding model** is offered to give you an overall set of guidelines for effectively interacting with families experiencing perinatal loss (see Table 36–6). The specific elements of the model are addressed throughout the rest of the chapter and within the nursing care plan that follows.

Preparing the Family for the Birth and Death

Upon arrival to the facility, the couple with a known or suspected fetal demise should immediately be placed in a private room. When possible, the woman should be in a room that is farthest away from other laboring women. Care should be taken not to leave the couple in the waiting room with other expectant parents or visitors waiting for news from other women in labor. Sit down for a moment with the woman and her spouse/partner, offer an introduction, and acknowledge the loss in the event of a known demise or impending death. A simple statement will go a long way toward establishing a relationship of trust between the nurse and the parents; for example, "My name is Brenda, and I'll be your nurse today. I'm so sorry; this must be very hard for you. I'd like to help you through it."

The couple should be allowed to remain together as much as they wish. Provide privacy as needed and maintain a supportive environment. Give the couple complete information about what to expect and what will happen. Encourage and answer questions clearly and straightforwardly; a review list for the parents to use may be helpful (Figure 36–3). Stay with the couple

TABLE 36–6 The Essential Elements of Responding Effectively to the Needs of Grieving Families

- **R**ecognition and validation of the loss
- **E**motional availability
- **S**piritual and cultural accommodation
- **P**hysical presence
- **O**pen communication
- **N**ormalization of grief reactions
- **D**ecision-making assistance
- **I**nterprofessional involvement
- **N**onjudgmental attitude
- **G**enuine caring

SOURCE: Shields, K. (2005). Preparing the family for the birth and death. *Healing Through Hope.* Used with permission.

PERINATAL COMFORT CARE PROGRAM
PLANNING FOR OUR BABY'S BIRTH A PARENT'S REVIEW LIST

♥ Let your doctor and Labor/Delivery staff know the name of your baby.

♥ Your baby's condition may be different at time of birth than expected right now. Your doctor may need to make immediate medical decisions at the time of your baby's birth in order to give your baby the best chance for a quality life. Some of your plans may not be possible in this situation. Please talk about this with your doctor before your baby's birth.

Mother's Name ____________ Father's Name ____________ Baby's Name ____________

Obstetrician ____________ Pediatrician ____________ EDC ____________ Diagnosis ____________

Completed by: ______________________ Name/Title ______________ Date

Section A

♥ **These are our wishes for the *personal care* of our baby at time of birth.**

	These are our wishes for the personal care of our baby at time of birth.	Comments/Date	Revisions/Date
	1. Hold our baby as soon as possible and as much as possible		
	2. Establish a plan for family and friends to celebrate our baby's birth/ visitation on the floor. Designate ____________ to give updates to family and friends.		
	3. Designate ____________ as adult chaperone for siblings.		
	4. After delivery and when I am stable to celebrate, stay in the same room for labor, delivery, and recovery if possible		
	5. Have a family member cut the umbilical cord		
	6. After delivery, give my baby to me after being quickly wiped, suctioned and wrapped.		
	7. Perform religious ceremonies		
	8. Videotape our baby		
	9. Take pictures of our baby		
	10. Make footprints & handprints of our baby		
	11. Take family photos and handprints		
	12. Have private time with our baby with minimal interruptions		
	13. Bathe our baby		
	14. Hold our baby while dying and after death		
	15. Obtain keepsakes such as : lock of hair, ID band, tape measure, crib card, hat, blanket and clothes		

St. Joseph Hospital
ST. JOSEPH HEALTH SYSTEM

PATIENT ID

PERINATAL COMFORT CARE PROGRAM
PLANNING FOR OUR BABY'S BIRTH
A PARENT'S REVIEW LIST

7401-0053 (6/22/07)

Page 1 of 2

Figure 36–3 St. Joseph perinatal comfort care program: Planning for our baby's birth, a parent's review list.

SOURCE: © St. Joseph Hospital, St. Joseph Health Systems, Orange, CA. https://www.sjo.org.

(continued)

	16. Allow teaching services (Medical residents and/or nursing students) present ☐ YES ☐ NO		
	17. Organ Donation Wishes		
	18. Autopsy -		
	19.		

Section B

	♥ These are our wishes for the *comfort care* of our baby at time of birth	Comments/Date	Revisions/Date
	1. Let me know if our baby has a heartbeat		
	2. Perform oral/nasal suctioning and blow by oxygen for comfort only		
	3. Do not perform advanced life support without explaining why it is necessary		
	4. Delay taking vital signs, weighing our baby, giving medications and obtaining lab work if not medically necessary		
	5. Allow our baby to feed: ___ breastfeed or ___ drops of expressed milk or formula		
	6. Provide our baby with medications if needed for comfort care		
	7.		

Section C

	♥ Discuss your *medical options* with your doctor prior to birth:	Comments/Date	Revisions/Date
	1. Medications to be used during labor		
	2. Management of milk suppression		
	3. Physical comfort measure after birth		
	4. Review your wishes for extended stay		
	5. Discuss plans for taking your baby home if this is an option		
	6.		

Plan of Care reviewed by: ____________________ ____________
(Signed by Hospital Staff) ____________________ ____________
____________________ ____________

The following changes have been made by the parent(s) upon admission to the hospital
____
____
____
____

St. Joseph Hospital
ST. JOSEPH HEALTH SYSTEM

PERINATAL COMFORT CARE PROGRAM
PLANNING FOR OUR BABY'S BIRTH
A PARENT'S REVIEW LIST

PATIENT ID

7401-0053 (6/22/07)

Page 2 of 2

Figure 36–3 *(Continued)* **St. Joseph perinatal comfort care program: Planning for our baby's birth, a parent's review list.**

SOURCE: © St. Joseph Hospital, St. Joseph Health Systems, Orange, CA. https://www.sjo.org.

so they do not feel alone and isolated; however, cues that the couple wants to be alone should be assessed continuously. Some couples may want outside support, such as family members or friends, to be present during the labor. You need to facilitate the couple's wishes.

When possible, the same nurse should provide care for the couple so that a therapeutic relationship can be established. As the relationship develops, provide solace by listening to the couple without offering explanations. Also provide ongoing opportunities for the couple to ask questions. It is not uncommon for the family to ask the same questions repeatedly. This is part of the initial process. Arrange for other members of the interprofessional team to interact with the family. The team should take great care to avoid inflicting further trauma on the couple by displaying conflicting words and behavior, such as using a falsely cheerful tone of voice while their body language clearly indicates sorrow. Offer to contact the hospital chaplain or another cleric for the couple, and a social worker should be involved. Typically, the nurse coordinates members of the collaborative care team so that a comprehensive plan of care can be initiated.

Women with Special Needs Intellectual Disability

For the woman with an intellectual disability, understanding of the cause and process of neonatal death may be difficult owing to cognitive abilities and grief responses. A grief counselor should be on hand and one-on-one support is warranted. Self-blame may be more common in these women, and reassurance, education, and support are imperative.

Explain details of the plan of care (Figure 36–4) and allow the family to ask questions and make decisions for their labor and birth preferences. The availability of anesthesia and analgesia

A THERAPEUTICALLY EQUIVALENT PRODUCT MAY BE DISPENSED AND ADMINISTERED UNLESS CHECKED IN THE LEFT COLUMN.

✓	DATE	TIME	⬅ DATE AND TIME MUST BE ENTERED	NEONATAL COMFORT CARE ORDERS	ROOM NO.

ALLERGIES: **Weight:** ____________ **kg**

Check (✓) all that apply and fill in the blank if applicable

1. **Medical Diagnosis:** ______________________________
2. **Code Status:** ☐ **Full Code** ☐ **See DNAR Form**
3. **Vital Signs:** every 4 hours and Prn
4. **Diet:** Breast milk or Formula ____________ as tolerated by breast, bottle, gavage, or syringe
   ☐ If needed place a Corpak for home care size ______ unweighted
5. **Offer Non-pharmacologic Comfort Measures Prn:** Swaddling, Holding, and Pacifier
6. **Offer Oral Sucrose per policy for mild to moderate pain Neonatal Infant Pain Scale (NIPS) less than 4**
7. **Pain Control:**
   A. **Short-acting or Breakthrough Pain Medications**
   Opioids need not be held for respiratory depression in actively dying patients.
   ☐ Morphine ____mg (0.2 – 0.5 mg/kg/dose) Po q ____ HRS Prn severe pain NIPS score greater than 4
   ☐ Acetaminophen ____mg (10 –15 mg/kg/dose) Po or PR q ____HRS Prn mild pain
   Note: Max dose = 90 mg/kg/day if greater than 36 weeks; 60 mg/kg/day if 32 – 36 weeks
   B. **Long-acting Pain Medications**
   Opioids need not be held for respiratory depression in actively dying patients.
   ☐ Methadone ____mg (0.05 – 0.1 mg/kg/dose) Po q ____HRS
   C. **Gastric Pain**
   ☐ Famotidine suspension (8 mg/mL) ______mg (0.5 mg/kg/dose) Po q 12 hours, **or**
   ☐ Other: ______________________________
8. **Dyspnea: Order opioids here if patient not already receiving opioids for pain.**
   ☐ Morphine _____mg (0.2 – 0.5 mg /kg/dose) Po q ___HRS Prn dyspnea
   or
   ☐ Lorazepam _____mg (0.1 mg /kg/dose) Po q ___HRS Prn dyspnea
   ☐ _____ % Oxygen _____ liters/min. by nasal cannula (indicated for hypoxemia; may be helpful in other cases)
9. **Anxiety/Agitation**
   ☐ Lorazepam ____mg (0.1 mg /kg/dose) Po q ____HRS Prn agitation.
   or
   ☐ Diphenhydramine ____mg (1 mg /kg/dose) Po q ____HRS Prn agitation
10. **Secretions**
   Control with medications is preferred as suctioning can be uncomfortable for the patient.
   Note: Minimizing fluids will help decrease symptoms
   ☐ Reposition q 2-4 HRS as tolerated
   ☐ Glycopyrrolate ____mCg (40 – 100 mCg /kg/dose) Po q ___HRS Prn secretions
11. **Fever**
   May consider additional non-pharmacologic measures such as bathing.
   ☐ Acetaminophen ____mg (10 –15 mg /kg/dose) Po or PR q ____HRS Prn Temp greater than ____°C
   Note: Max dose = 90 mg/kg/day if greater than 36 weeks; 60 mg/kg/day if 32 – 36 weeks
12. **Diarrhea**
   ☐ Loperamide ____ mg (0.08 – 0.24 mg /kg/DAY in divided doses) Po q ___ HRS Prn diarrhea (Do not exceed 2 mg/dose), **or**
   ☐ Other: ______________________________

12-hour Chart Check______________________ **RN** **DATE:** ____ / ____ / ____ **TIME:**__________

T.O. ______________________ Taken by: ______________________ Title: __________

TRANSCRIBED BY: __________ ___/___/___, TIME:________ NOTED BY:__________ ___/___/___, TIME:________

PHYSICIAN SIGNATURE: ______________________ DATE:__________ TIME: ________

PRINTED NAME/ID:. (FOR MEDICATION/BIOLOGICALS T.O. ORDERS ONLY, COUNTER-SIGN ABOVE WITHIN 48 HOURS, AND INCLUDE THE DATE/TIME AUTHENTICATED)

St. Joseph Hospital
ST. JOSEPH HEALTH SYSTEM

NEONATAL COMFORT CARE ORDERS

PATIENT ID

6381-2065 (5/07/07)

PHYSICIAN'S ORDERS

Figure 36–4 St. Joseph Hospital neonatal comfort care orders.

SOURCE: © St. Joseph Hospital, St. Joseph Health Systems, Orange, CA. www.sjo.org.

should be reviewed. The woman can typically have pain medication whenever she desires. Facilitate the participation of the woman and her partner in the labor and birth process.

It is important to remember that, in contrast to a typical birth experience, the birth of a terminal or stillborn baby marks both the beginning and the end. For this reason, it is imperative that the couple and family have all wishes and preferences respected. The family may be overwhelmed and may have difficulty making decisions in this period. You can strengthen the couples' ability to cope by providing a warm atmosphere of acceptance. Assist the couple in exploring their feelings and help them to make decisions about who will be present and what rituals will occur during and following the birth. Examples of birth preferences include:

- Use of music, dim lighting, or other environmental preferences
- Laboring or birthing in a specific position
- Having the baby placed on the mother's chest immediately after birth
- Allowing the father to cut the umbilical cord
- Including other family members or friends present at the birth.

Sometimes couples worry that others may view their preferences as "strange" or "wrong." Reassure the family that it is their experience and that there are no right or wrong feelings or wishes. Cultural diversity will play a vital role in how the couple responds or reacts during the birthing process.

The couple may have waves of overwhelming grief, disbelief, or sadness. Encourage them to experience the grief that they feel, but do not force the issue. It is not uncommon for one partner to attempt to put on a brave front, feeling that, by showing grief, he or she will make the other partner feel worse. It is also not uncommon for partners to have intense feelings that they are unable to share. Encourage partners to express their emotions freely to the extent they are able. Help them understand that they may each experience different feelings.

"At last, we are holding our beautiful baby. Swaddled in his hospital blanket decorated with pastel teddy bears and hot-air balloons, he is crying with some effort, his eyes squeezed tightly closed. He has the plump newborn cheeks his sisters had and a hint of downy dark hair. He is a little pale, and his fingernails are faintly blue. He is beautiful. We are overwhelmed with pride and love—and concern—for the newest member of our family."

—Amy Kuebelbeck*

Supporting the Family in Decision Making

It is important to remember that the family will need guidance throughout the process. The couple should be offered simple choices all along the way to help them retain as much control over their situation as possible. If the baby is born alive, but suffering from a complication that is incompatible with life, make every effort to allow the parents as much time as possible with the baby. In addition, the extended family should be allowed as much access as is comfortable for the parents.

Advocates of seeing the stillborn baby believe that viewing assists in dispelling denial and enables the couple to progress to the next step in the mourning process. This has become a topic of controversy in the field of death and dying. A study by Turton showed that there may be an increase in posttraumatic stress disorder among women who held their dead babies. Ironically, though the women wanted to hold and see their babies, the trauma appears to be related to the vivid imagery that is implanted during holding and seeing the dead baby (Adzich et al., 2016). One potential explanation for this aberrant finding is the possibility that if nurses who are uncomfortable with death and dying are rigidly following standard bereavement checklists rather than recognizing the uniqueness of each situation, the mother and father may be forced into uncomfortable situations they are not properly prepared for. Another proposed explanation is that when the parents view and hold the baby, further bonding occurs, which leads to a more intense grief reaction. It should be noted, however, that numerous other studies did not find an increase in anxiety and instead found that most women who held their babies did not regret it, while many who did not had subsequent feelings of regret (Adzich et al., 2016). Until more conclusive studies are reported, you should offer the couple the opportunity to see and hold the baby, assess possible motivations behind negative responses (such as a fear of the unknown), and reassure the couple that any decision they make for themselves is the right one. Careful listening on your part should allow the parent(s) to make clear their wishes. Additionally, you should not allow pressure from others to be put upon the couple either to see and hold or to not see and hold their stillborn baby. If they choose to see their stillborn baby, prepare the couple for what they will see by saying "She is going to feel cold," "He is going to be blue," or other appropriate statements. If the parents have shared with you the name they had chosen for their baby, use that name in discussing the baby; for example, "Jessie's face is bruised." If the couple is hesitant to view the baby out of a fear of what the baby will look like, offering a picture will sometimes help to allay their fears. With the development of digital bereavement photography, it is becoming easier for nurses to offer the family quality photos of their baby. Most facilities have a digital camera and printer for such use. There are also websites where parents can obtain digital photography or have photographs enhanced, edited, or have effects added, such as selective coloring (Adzich et al., 2016).

Clinical Tip

A picture that appears distressing in color may be comforting in black and white. A close-up of the baby's hand or foot lying in the parent's hand may provide a loving memory. Use your creativity in taking bereavement pictures.

Postmortem Care

Properly preparing the baby for viewing and holding is an essential step in the process. Stillborn babies are often misshapen, and the skin can be discolored or in a state of maceration. **Maceration** is the process of tissue breakdown, which begins from the moment an undelivered fetus dies. It is characterized by sloughing of the skin, which can help determine the interval between death and delivery of the baby; that is, the more sloughing, the greater length of time between the demise and delivery. When bathing the baby for viewing, care should be taken to cause as little additional disruption to the skin as possible. A gloved hand is preferable to a washcloth for these babies. After bathing, the baby should be placed in a suitable-sized gown and then wrapped in a blanket. A hat can be applied to cover birth defects. This allows the parents an opportunity to view the baby before seeing the birth defect. Many parents will eventually remove the covering to inspect the baby; however, applying a covering allows them time to adjust to the appearance at their own pace. In cases of extreme maceration, the parents should be fully informed of the condition of the skin, so that they can decide for themselves if they want to see, hold, and/or fully uncover the baby. Couples will often look to the assisting medical and nursing personnel for the "correct" attitude toward their stillborn baby. Carefully monitor your personal reactions and display acceptance of the choices the parents make. For step-by-step postmortem care instructions, see Table 36–7.

In a compromised or dying baby, bathing should be done quickly, so that the baby can be returned to the parents as soon as possible. Some parents may wish to participate in the bath process or complete it themselves. Some parents will hold their baby for a short time before returning him or her to the nurse, whereas others will wish to spend a great deal of time with their baby. Allow the baby to remain with the parents for as long as they desire.

Supporting Siblings and Extended Family Members

Some couples may want other family members, friends, or their other children to be with them in their experience and possibly view and hold the baby. Act as an advocate to ensure that the family's wishes are respected. Siblings will respond according to their age and maturity level. Children younger than 7 years of age may not recognize that the death is permanent, whereas older children may respond with concern for the parents' well-being. It is normal for them to regress slightly in social and cognitive behaviors when under stress. Children should be included as much as desired by the parents and told the truth in a simple, honest, and age-appropriate manner, avoiding the use of euphemisms when describing death and the aftermath. A **euphemism** is a substituted word or expression with a more pleasant association than the one that, although more direct, is considered to be harsher. Children will need reassurance of two things: That they are still going to be taken care of and that nothing they did caused the event to happen. In facilities in which child life specialists are present, their help can be elicited to assist the family

*Excerpt from *Waiting with Gabriel: A Story of Cherishing a Baby's Brief Life* by Amy Kuebelbeck (Loyola Press, 2003). Reprinted with permission of Loyola Press. To order copies call 1-800-621-1008 or go to www.loyolapress.com.

TABLE 36–7 Postmortem Care

Document time of death per physician.

Gather supplies per hospital protocol.

Appropriate forms.

Bathing—two basins, absorbent pads, diapers, clothing, washcloths, hat

Memory kit—memory card with foot or handprint area, memory box

Morgue kit—identification tags, pads for wrapping, paperwork

Remove tubes and wires when applicable.

Cap and leave all indwelling tubes and catheters if autopsy is to be performed.

Plug endotracheal tube (ETT) with cotton ball and tape over opening to hold in place and prevent seepage.

Bathe and dress fetus/baby.

Offer parents opportunity to assist with bathing and dressing baby as appropriate (if baby is stillborn, skin maceration may be traumatic for parents).

With gloved hands, place baby in lukewarm basin of water.

Rinse if skin breakdown is present; if skin integrity is intact, rub gently with washcloth. Soap is optional; based also on integrity of skin.

Place fetus/baby in second basin of lukewarm water to rinse.

Gently pat dry. Do not use scented (especially baby products) lotions or powders.

If seepage present from nasal cavity, place petroleum jelly in nostrils.

Diaper and dress fetus/baby in outfit provided either by parents, hospital, or volunteer organization. Consider the use of a hat, particularly where deformity is present.

Take pictures.

Cover imperfections and deformities when applicable.

Use mementos in pictures when available.

Use soft, yet vibrant, colors in background or consider black-and-white photos.

Place fetus/baby in a flattering and comforting position (different for every baby).

Offer parents opportunity to participate in picture taking, but do not force the issue.

If desired by parents, wrap in warm blanket and present baby for holding.

Prepare parents before holding fetus/baby by telling them what they will see, feel, and smell.

Offer a picture before holding.

Model normal nurturing behavior for parents.

Offer time alone with baby and check back frequently within previously specified time frame.

After holding, remove clothing for weight and measurements, footprints, handprints, memory card, and lock of hair (when applicable).

Prepare fetus/baby for pathology/morgue/family transport according to hospital protocol.

For morgue care:

Complete all hospital paperwork.

Place baby in supine position on top of folded diapers and pad to maintain body position and prevent disfigurement.

Use neck and body rolls to help with alignment.

Wrap baby according to hospital protocol.

Take memory box and bereavement information to parents.

Memory box should include pictures, ID bracelet, memory card, other personal items, and bereavement clothes.

Bereavement information should include pamphlets on grief and loss as well as local and national resources for support and information.

Document the events leading up to and following the death, including:

Time and pronouncement of death with physician's name.

Placement of tubes and catheters.

Postmortem care.

Comfort measures and bereavement care provided to family.

Preparation and transport to morgue.

in preparing the children for the death and provide an outlet for the children during the event (Bhat & Byatt, 2016).

Extended family members, especially grandparents, are doubly grieving, as they suffer through the pain their children are experiencing and the loss of their grandchild. They will have varied reactions, from the extreme of attempting to completely control the process for their child to a display of total passivity. Most reactions fall somewhere in the middle of the continuum. In addition, grandparents may have health issues related to the loss (O'Leary, Parker, & Wimmer, 2017). Help to validate the grandparents' grief by acknowledging the difficulty of their position and extending your support to them as well as to the parents. Even grandparents who are blaming, questioning, or demanding can be made a part of the team when approached in a nondefensive, nonjudgmental, and aid-enlisting manner.

Family support has been shown to be a major comfort to couples in families in which there is open communication and honest interaction. Less intense grief over time has been reported in families who are able to express their emotions with one another as compared with more stoic families. Provide every opportunity for family cohesion throughout the process, encouraging as much participation and interaction as desired by the couple.

Actualizing the Loss: Providing Memories

In a fetal demise, remember that mementos are some of the few memories the parents have to provide them comfort after the death of their baby. Every effort should be made to offer as many quality mementos as possible, such as pictures and hand- or footprint molds and cards (Figure 36–5). Most facilities prepare a remembrance box or package for the family to take home (Figure 36–6). This typically consists of a photograph taken of the baby or the family, a card with the baby's footprints, a crib card, identification band, a lock of hair, and, possibly, a blanket or clothing worn by the baby. In the event that the couple declines the package, it is common for the hospital to retain these items for a specific period of time in case they change their minds.

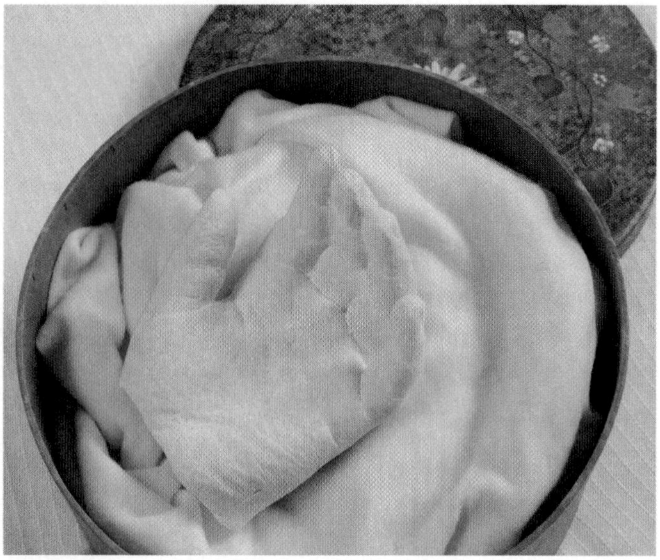

Figure 36–5 Foot- and handprint molds.

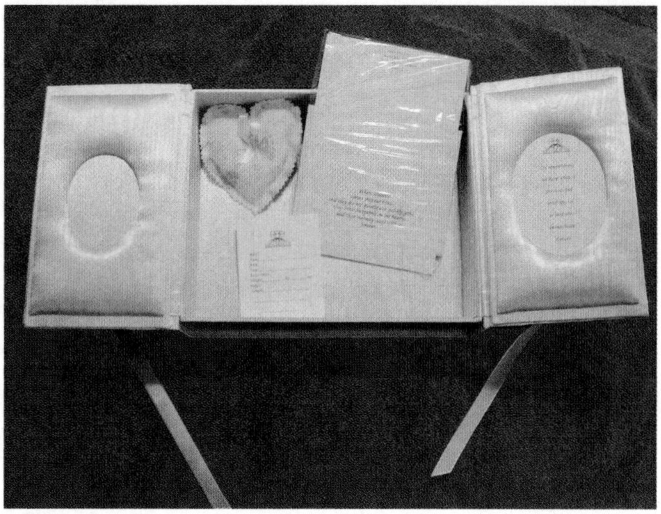

Figure 36–6 Personal memory box.

SOURCE: Share Pregnancy & Infant Loss Support, Inc.

> "Our night nurse, Cindy, encouraged us to take Gabriel's footprints before we went to sleep. She tenderly made several prints of his feet and his hands, and she helped us mix the plaster of Paris that we had brought along for a permanent imprint of his feet. While Mark held him, she carefully snipped a tiny lock of almost-black hair from the back of Gabriel's head.
>
> . . . So in the dim fluorescent light, I rearranged the pillows on my bed to make a place for him . . . My arm draped over his chest, my cheek touching his cool forehead, I fell asleep with my son for one last time."
>
> —Amy Kuebelbeck*

Providing Discharge Care

The family usually has three options open to them for disposition of the fetus or baby's body. The first is a traditional burial. Many funeral homes offer reduced fees for neonatal burial services. The family should contact the funeral home directly to make arrangements. Some families may wish to bury their baby on private land. This is state, county, and locally dictated, and it is up to the family to ascertain any restrictive ordinances as to transportation and burial. Hospitals with comprehensive bereavement programs in place usually have access to this information. The second option is cremation at a funeral home. Families will need to decide what to do with the cremains. The third option, and not one generally recommended, is hospital disposition. **Hospital disposition** at most facilities is incineration at regular intervals, usually with other body parts, and the family does not have the option to obtain the ashes. Some institutions, especially private and/or religiously affiliated facilities, offer mass burial options for hospital disposition, but not many. In the last decade or so, a few programs have been initiated that offer more individualized burial options for babies designated for hospital disposition. These programs are usually a coordinated effort between facilities within a specific area and one of the local funeral homes and cemeteries that serve their community. The program is usually offered at little or no charge to the family. Whatever option the family decides upon, support their decision and assist them in any way possible to achieve their goal for disposition and/or funeral services.

After the birth, the couple can be given the option of an early discharge (as early as 6 to 8 hours after the birth). Discharge focuses on the physical considerations and adaptation of the mother and emotional considerations of the couple. Provide postpartum directions for follow-up care. Written materials should be provided, and a phone number for questions can be given. Give the woman

*Excerpt from Waiting with Gabriel: A Story of Cherishing a Baby's Brief Life by Amy Kuebelbeck (Loyola Press, 2003). Reprinted with permission of Loyola Press. To order copies call 1-800-621-1008 or go to https://www.loyolapress.com.

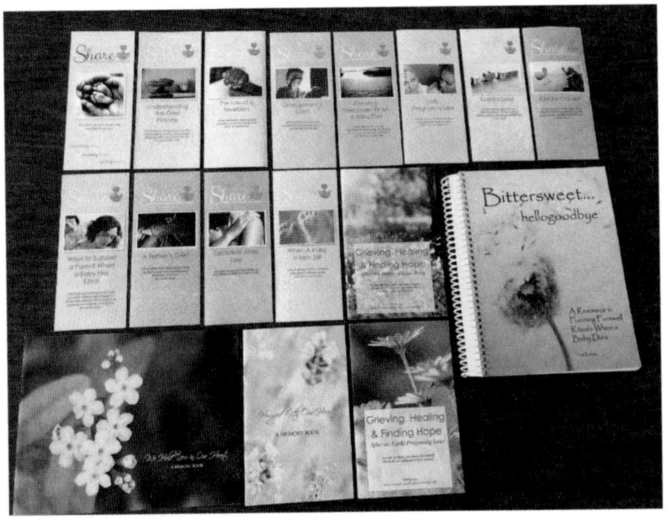

Figure 36–7 Bereavement literature.

SOURCE: Share Pregnancy & Infant Loss Support, Inc.

information about her milk coming in and interventions to follow to decrease the discomfort associated with engorgement.

Additional information should be given on the mourning process (Figure 36–7). Prepare the couple to return home by stressing that others may not know what to say, and that even loved ones may make inappropriate comments because they do not know how to respond to grief and loss. This can prepare the couple for the reactions of others. If there are siblings, each will usually progress through age-appropriate grieving. Provide the parents with information about normal grief reactions, both psychologic and physiologic.

The couple should be given information regarding depression as a normal part of grieving. Couples may feel empty and lost and may experience physical symptoms such as sleep disturbances, weight loss or gain, listlessness, fatigue, hyperactivity, inability to concentrate, and a lack of motivation. The onset of the symptoms of depression often coincides with the time when other people have moved on and withdrawn support for the couple, making it harder for them to cope. The couple should be informed that depression following perinatal loss is normal and unless debilitating or prolonged need not be medicated or treated and will subside in time. If depression is prolonged, outside help should be sought. Additionally, as the mourning process ensues, families should be encouraged to implement cultural, religious, or social customs that will assist them in their grief. Advise the family that certain upcoming milestones, such as holidays, future birthdays, Mother's Day, and Father's Day, and other social events such as baby showers, may trigger their grief. The family can better cope with these events if they are adequately prepared. Finally, the couple should be advised not to make any major life change decisions in the first year following the death, whenever possible. Making major life changes compounds grief reactions by adding other losses (such as moving away from the familiar) on top of the loss of the baby, often resulting in complicated mourning.

When caring for a family suffering from a perinatal loss, it is important to remember that you may experience many of the same grief reactions as the parents of a stillborn baby. It is important to have colleagues and family members available for counseling and support.

Following discharge, some families may need closure of the intrapartum event to continue their mourning process. A consultation can be scheduled with the practitioner who cared for them during the pregnancy and birth. Families may also wish to read the results of tests performed during the intrapartum period and the autopsy report. The couple should be provided with a copy of the medical record and encouraged to ask questions, express their feelings, and ask for clarification.

Families are routinely referred for counseling services after a perinatal loss has occurred. A counselor who specializes in perinatal issues can provide expertise and assist the couple in their grieving. Partners should be allowed to verbalize fears and concerns about future pregnancies. When appropriate, referrals to genetic counselors, religious support persons, and social service agencies should also be provided.

In addition to referral information, the parents should receive scheduled follow-up phone calls to assess the family's functioning and their progress with grief work, if they indicated the desire for follow-up contact. During these follow-up phone calls, pertinent information can be given and additional resources can be identified.

Referring the Family to Community Services

Most facilities have an established protocol for families experiencing perinatal loss. Programs that are more comprehensive are being established in communities to provide a systematic intervention program to assist these families. Community support groups that focus on perinatal loss can provide an important support network and resources. Specialized groups—such as those focused on early pregnancy loss, stillbirth, and perinatal loss associated with specific congenital anomalies—allow families the opportunity to interact with peers who have lost babies under similar circumstances. Provide the group name, contact person (if possible), and phone number. Offer bereavement resources that provide a list of relevant articles and books on death, dying, and grieving the loss of a baby. Provide information on supportive organizations such as Share Pregnancy & Infant Loss Support, Resolve Through Sharing (RTS) Bereavement Services, Centering Corporation, and The Compassionate Friends.

Internet technology has allowed large numbers of individuals to share resources and information and participate in online support groups. Internet resources can be effective for all families and may be the only resources available for families in rural underserved areas. Online perinatal loss support groups through social sharing can become "cultures," in that they have distinct beliefs, behaviors, norms, and attitudes that set a pattern of behavior for members of the online community. They can be very helpful in allowing mothers to interact with other mothers in similar circumstances.

Perinatal Hospice

Specialized hospice programs are another community resource that assists grieving families. **Perinatal hospice** offers a compassionate, structured program providing a context in which parents can find meaning in the intimate experience of the life and death of their child. In perinatal hospice programs, parents whose fetus has a known lethal congenital anomaly are given the opportunity to explore options, such as elective termination or waiting for the onset of spontaneous labor or a medically indicated induced labor. For families wishing to continue their pregnancies, the program typically assigns an interprofessional team that provides compassionate care, ongoing counseling, referral to support groups, and spiritual guidance (Wool, 2015). Perinatal hospice programs have been created in numerous international and U.S. hospitals, hospices, and clinics and are listed on the Perinatal Hospice website (Perinatal Hospice and Palliative Care, 2017). These programs offer parents much-needed support and guidance through the entire process of the pregnancy, birth, discharge, and/or death of the fetus or baby.

According to Suzanne Engelder, of the St. Joseph Perinatal Comfort Care program in Orange, California:

> "Regarding the future of perinatal hospice .... There has been tremendous growth over the past 4 years. More and more hospitals are looking at providing this special care. I think what is unique about our program (and a few others across the country) is that we are a collaborative program between hospice (outpatient) and hospital (inpatient). Most perinatal hospice care is being provided in the NICU setting and it really is more palliative care in the NICU versus hospice care, which focuses on care and support before the birth/death to prepare and educate parents/families. What I would like to see is more hospitals collaborating with hospices to provide care before and after. Another issue is reimbursement. Currently this is a non-reimbursable service. When adult hospice first came to the United States in the 1970s, it was run by volunteers and there was no reimbursement for it. In 1983, Medicare made it a benefit. My hope is that perinatal hospice will follow the same path—that insurance companies will see the benefit for the patient and family and be willing to pay for the care. The care provided on the front end saves resources at the time of birth/death and the back end (bereavement)."

The strength and success of these programs are a testament to the progress that has been made in bereavement care in the last decade. The challenge ahead is to move these programs into more awareness and ensure that healthcare providers are offered education to assist them in recognition of the need for these services.

Care of the Couple Who Has Experienced Loss in a Previous Pregnancy

A couple who has had a previous perinatal loss typically enters a subsequent pregnancy with conflicting feelings and may experience ambivalence, fear, and anxiety (Alghamdi & Jarrett, 2016; Meaney, Everard, Gallagher, et al., 2017). Many times, their experience is relived when another pregnancy occurs. Some couples conceive soon after a loss, whereas others wait years. Some couples enter a subsequent pregnancy with grief work largely completed, whereas others are still experiencing unresolved grief.

The nurse caring for a couple that has had a previous loss needs to be kind, compassionate, and patient. Couples need specific information and clear explanations of all prenatal information (Alghamdi & Jarrett, 2016; Meaney et al., 2017; Wool, 2015). Referrals to a genetic counselor should be made when appropriate. Some couples may wish to have a consultation with a perinatologist. If unresolved grief issues are present or the family experiences extreme anxiety, counseling may be beneficial.

Interventions to decrease anxiety can help the couple tremendously. At the first visit, an early ultrasound can be performed to verify the presence of the fetal heartbeat. In early pregnancy, women may be fearful when first-trimester pregnancy symptoms begin to resolve. Women with a previous loss typically receive additional antepartum testing throughout the pregnancy. Ultrasounds can be used to provide reassurance and assess fetal growth and development, placental functioning, and cord variations. Nonstress testing and biophysical profiles can be performed weekly after 32 weeks to ensure fetal well-being. Fetal kick counts should be initiated at 28 weeks and continue until the birth occurs. Women with a previous loss should undergo an induction at 39 weeks' gestation or once lung maturity has been established via amniocentesis because placental functioning can decline in postdate pregnancies. Great anxiety and stress are common in these mothers even after the birth of a healthy baby, and postpartum and nursery nurses should provide ongoing assessment and support to these mothers and families. See *Case Study: Melissa Bond-James*.

Evaluation

Caring for a family experiencing perinatal loss is a challenging, yet rewarding, opportunity for the nurse who offers her or his humanity, concern, and acceptance. There is nothing quite like helping a family through one of the most difficult events of their lives. The reward is often greater for the giver than for those who are receiving because the important life lessons learned and the sense of accomplishment achieved when reaching out to others in need is rarely rivaled. Nurses should remember to process their own grief reactions so that they remain healthy responders for the next family in need.

Expected outcomes of nursing care for the family experiencing perinatal loss include:

- Family members feel free to express their feelings about the death of their baby if they desire to do so.
- Family members participate in decision making regarding preferences for the labor, birth, and the immediate postpartum period.
- Family members participate in the decision of whether to see their baby and other decisions about the baby.
- The family has resources available for continued support.
- Family members know the community resources available and have names and phone numbers to use if they choose.

For more information, see *Nursing Care Plan: For a Family Experiencing Perinatal Loss*.

CASE STUDY: Melissa Bond-James

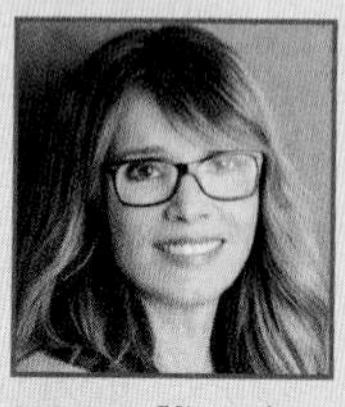

SOURCE: Kinga/Shutterstock.

Melissa presents for her 6-week checkup and is somewhat tearful. She tells the nurse her niece recently had a stillbirth at 37 weeks. Melissa is anxious that this could run in the family and is worried it will have implications for both her niece and herself in the future. She asks the nurse what factors could cause a stillborn.

Questions to Ponder

How would you explain to Melissa the possible causes of fetal demise? How would you encourage Melissa's niece to approach the grieving process? What interventions can be done by staff to support a family that has lost a baby?

Nursing Care Plan: For a Family Experiencing Perinatal Loss

Nursing Diagnosis: ***Coping: Family, Compromised*, related to perinatal loss as evidenced by crying/sadness, irritability/anger, guilt responses, and/or fear (NANDA-I © 2017)**

Goal: The woman will verbalize thoughts and feelings associated with the loss and understand the factual events surrounding the loss. She will begin to form a trust relationship with the nurse and freely ask for and accept support provided by nursing staff.

INTERVENTION	RATIONALE
• Normalize the experience by assuring parents that there is no right or wrong way to express grief.	• Grief reactions encompass a broad spectrum of thoughts and emotions. Providing a nonjudgmental, supportive environment validates the grief response, thereby establishing a trust relationship, which helps to facilitate a healthy mourning process.
• Crying. Offer tissues while allowing free expression of emotion.	• Crying is a normal reaction to the loss event and offering tissues is a tangible form of acceptance.
• Anger. Avoiding defensiveness, state the obvious and enlist the parents' assistance in exploring possible sources of, and solutions to, their anger.	• Anger as a part of the grief response usually stems from frustration at the circumstances and should not be taken personally. Allowing for the free expression of anger, as well as remaining neutral in responses, will help to defuse the situation. Utilizing a team approach will assist the woman in viewing hospital personnel as partners in care, rather than adversaries.
• Guilt responses. Reframe the event in a reality-based forum, reassuring the parents that they did nothing to precipitate the loss.	• Guilt is a predominant feature of grief following loss, especially in parents experiencing the death of a baby. Reality testing, which involves referencing factual information versus the parents' perceptions of culpability, assists them in coming to the conclusion that they did the best they could in the circumstance.
• Fear. Provide honest, simple explanations of what to expect before, during, and after the loss event.	• Families can cope with extreme situations when they are properly informed in an honest and forthright manner. Maintaining a close presence while providing factual information will help alleviate feelings of fear and isolation. Offering simple choices allows patients to maintain a semblance of control over their circumstances.

EXPECTED OUTCOMES: The woman and family acknowledge the loss as evidenced by verbalizing an understanding of the factual events surrounding the loss and openly expressing thoughts and feelings regarding the loss in a safe and constructive manner. The woman and family begin to form a trust relationship as evidenced by freely asking for and accepting support provided by nursing staff and relating to the nurse in an environment of acceptance.

Focus Your Study

- Perinatal loss poses a major nursing challenge to provide support and care for the parents.
- Perinatal loss is a tragic and often traumatic event in the life of most families experiencing it.
- Bereavement is the *event* of the loss, grief is the *reaction* to that loss, and mourning is the *process* by which we incorporate the loss into our lives with individual, cultural, religious, and social norms.
- Attachment theory with regard to perinatal loss is based on the premise that human beings are biologically predisposed to bond with emotionally significant persons in their lives and the grief response is a state of separation anxiety brought on by the disruption in the attachment bond.
- For mothers, there are nine events that are important to the formation of attachment to her baby. They are (1) planning the pregnancy, (2) confirming the pregnancy, (3) accepting the pregnancy, (4) feeling fetal movement, (5) accepting the fetus as an individual, (6) giving birth, (7) seeing the baby, (8) touching the baby, and (9) giving care to the baby.
- Meaning reconstruction focuses on redefining ourselves and how we interact with the world after a significant loss. The goal of recovery, as related to meaning reconstruction, is a positive change in self-identity by assigning the loss a meaning, thereby allowing the individual to assimilate the loss into her or his world.

- There are many normal physical, cognitive, emotional, behavioral, and spiritual early responses to loss. The recognition of normal responses helps to identify the presence of abnormal or exaggerated responses.
- Many factors will influence a couple's response to perinatal loss, including individual and family personality traits, as well as social, cultural, and religious customs.
- Cessation of fetal movement reported by the mother to the nurse is frequently the first indication of fetal death. The nurse continues one-on-one care with the family, providing both physical and emotional support throughout this crucial period.
- The nurse can facilitate a healthy mourning process for the family by using active listening techniques and avoiding the use of clichés. Sitting in silence with a family is often the most helpful form of intervention available.
- Traditionally, it was believed that early and intense grieving was necessary for healing, but studies show that many people are naturally resilient and will not necessarily grieve initially or intensely.
- The caring theory places the emphasis of care on the attitude adopted by the nurse toward the grieving family as paramount to successful intervention and includes knowing, doing for, enabling, and maintaining belief.
- The responding model describes 10 behaviors and actions necessary for effective interaction with the grieving family and includes recognition of the loss, emotional availability, spiritual and cultural accommodation, physical presence, open communication, normalization of grief reactions, decision-making assistance, interprofessional involvement, nonjudgmental attitude, and genuine caring.
- Upon arrival to the facility, the nurse should make introductions, acknowledge the loss, and establish the beginnings of a trust relationship with the family.
- The nurse functions as advocate for the family in organizing interprofessional involvement, maintaining continuity of care, offering the opportunity for open communication, and ensuring that the family's wishes regarding their loss experience are honored.
- Couples experiencing perinatal loss should be offered the opportunity to participate in postmortem care and to view, hold, and name their baby. In the event a couple declines the opportunity, the nurse should assess for fear of the unknown as a motivating factor and take steps to alleviate that fear. The couple should never be coerced into viewing and holding their baby if they choose not to do so, and the nurse should display a nonjudgmental, accepting attitude regardless of the decision made by the couple.
- Siblings and extended family members should be included in the plan of care to whatever extent the couple wishes. Children should be given information in an honest and age-appropriate manner, and grandparents should be recognized for the double grief they are experiencing through the pain of their child and death of their grandchild.
- Mementos are important links for the family to the deceased baby. A memory box should be offered with as many personal items of the baby as possible. Hand- and/or footprint cards are especially desired items.
- Follow-up care should include bereavement materials and community support information as well as a telephone call to assess the family's well-being and provide any further desired information.
- Couples experiencing pregnancy following a loss can be expected to have higher levels of fear and anxiety and will need to be treated with care and concern. Information may need to be repeated and details of time lines provided to raise the comfort level of the couple.

In order to make safe and effective judgments using NANDA-I © 2017 nursing diagnoses, it is essential that nurses refer to the definitions and defining characteristics of the diagnoses used in this text, which can be found in Appendix C.

References

Adzich, K., Davis, D., Hochberg, T., Kavanaugh, K., Kobler, K., Lammert, C. A., . . . & Press, J. N. (2016). *Pregnancy loss and infant death alliance (PLIDA) position statement on bereavement parents' right to self-determination regarding their baby* (Rev. ed.). Retrieved from http://www.hindshospice.org/uploads/1/5/2/5/15252368/plida_statement_holding_baby.pdf

Alghamdi, R., & Jarrett, P. (2016). Experiences of student midwives in the care of women with perinatal loss: A qualitative descriptive study. *British Journal of Midwifery, 24*(10), 715–722.

Allahdadian, M., & Iraipour, A. (2015).The role of religious beliefs in pregnancy loss. *Journal of Education and Health Promotion, 4*, 99. DOI: 10.4103/2277-9531.171813

American College of Obstetricians & Gynecologists (ACOG). (2009, reaffirmed 2016). *Management of stillbirth* (ACOG Practice Bulletin No. 102). Washington, DC: Author.

American College of Obstetricians & Gynecologists (ACOG). (2015, reaffirmed 2017). *Early pregnancy loss* (ACOG Practice Bulletin No. 150). Washington, DC: Author.

Ananth, C. V., Goldenberg, R. L., Friedman, A. M., Vintzileos, A. M. (2018). Association of temporal changes in gestational age with perinatal mortality in the United States, 2007–2015. *JAMA Pediatrics, 172*(7), 627–634. DOI: 10.1001/jamapediatrics.2018.0249

Beckett, C., & Dykeman, C. (2015). Preservice counselors' initial perceptions of client grief style: An analogue study. *OMEGA Journal of Death and Dying, 71*(3), 219–232.

Bennett, S. M., Litz, B. T., Lee, B. S., & Maguen, S. (2005). The scope and impact of perinatal loss: Current status and future directions. *Professional Psychology: Research and Practice, 36*(2), 180–187. DOI: 10.1037/0735-7028.36.2.180

Bhat, A., & Byatt, N. (2016). Infertility and perinatal loss: When the bough breaks. *Current Psychiatry Reports, 18*(3), 31. DOI: 10.1007/s11920-016-0663-8

Bowlby, J. (1969). *Attachment and loss: Vol. 1. Attachment.* New York, NY: Basic Books.

Brier, N. (2009). Grief following miscarriage: A comprehensive review of the literature. *Journal of Women's Health, 17*(3), 451–454. DOI: 10.1089/jwh.2007.0505

California Department of Public Health (CDPH). (2018). *Pregnancy-associated mortality review.* Retrieved from https://www.cdph.ca.gov/Programs/OPA/Pages/NR18-025.aspx

Callister, L. C. (2006). Perinatal loss: A family perspective. *Journal of Perinatal and Neonatal Nursing, 20*(3), 227–234.

Cancer.net. (2018). *Understanding grief within a cultural context.* Retrieved from https://www.cancer.net/coping-with-cancer/managing-emotions/grief-and-loss/understanding-grief-within-cultural-context

Chichester, M. (2005). Multicultural issues in perinatal loss. *AWHONN Lifelines, 9*(4), 312–320.

Chichester, M. (2007). Requesting perinatal autopsy: Multicultural considerations. *MCN, The American Journal of Maternal Child Nursing, 32*(2), 81–86.

Clements, P. T., Vigil, G. J., Manno, M. S., Henry, G. C., Wilks, J., Das, S., . . . Foster, W. (2003). Cultural perspectives of death, grief, and bereavement. *Journal of Psychosocial Nursing, 41*(7), 18–26.

DeSpelder, L. A., & Strickland, A. L. (2005). *The last dance: Encountering death and dying* (7th ed.). New York, NY: McGraw-Hill.

Doka, K. J. (Ed.). (2016). *Grief is a journey: Finding your path through loss.* New York, NY: Atria Books.

Doka, K. J., & Martin, T. L. (2010). *Grieving beyond gender: Understanding the ways men and women mourn.* New York, NY: Routledge.

Eutsey, D. E., & Di Lima, S. N. (Eds.). (2001). *Palliative care: Patient and family counseling manual.* Gaithersburg, MD: Aspen.

Gold, K. J., Leon, I., Boggs, M. E., & Sen, A. (2016). Depression and posttraumatic stress symptoms after perinatal loss in a population-based sample. *Journal of Women's Health (Larchmont), 25*(3), 263–269.

Gold, K. J., Mozurkewich, E. L., Puder, K. S., & Teadwell, M. C. (2016). Maternal complications associated with stillbirth delivery: A cross-sectional analysis. *Journal of Obstetrics and Gynaecology, 36*(2), 208–212. DOI: 10.3109/01443615.2015.1050646

Hebert, M. P. (1998). Perinatal bereavement in its cultural context. *Death Studies, 22*(1), 61–78.

Hutti, M., Myers, J., Hall, L., Polivka, B., White, S., Hill, J., . . . McGrew, M. (2017). Predicting grief intensity after recent perinatal loss. *Journal of Psychosomatic Research, 101*, 128–134.

Hutti, M., Polivka, B., White, S., Hill, J., Clark, P., Cooke, C., . . . & Abell, H. (2016). Experiences of nurses who care for women after fetal loss. *Journal of Obstetric, Gynecologic, & Neonatal Nursing, 45*(1), 17–27. Retrieved from https://www.jognn.org/article/S0884-2175(15)00011-8/fulltext

Jaanista, T., Coombs, S., Donnelly, T. J., Kelk, N., & Beston, D. (2017). Risk and resilience factors related to parental bereavement following the death with a life-limiting condition. *Children (Basel), 4*(11), 96. DOI: 10.3390/Children4110096

Kalfoss, M., & Owe, J. (2015) Empirical verification of Swanson's caring processes found in nursing actions: Systematic review. *Open Journal of Nursing, 5*(11), 976–986. DOI: 10.4236/ojn.2015.511104

Kingdon, C., O'Donnell, E., Givens, J., & Turner, M. (2015). The role of healthcare professionals in encouraging parents to see and hold their stillborn baby: A meta-synthesis of qualitative studies. *PloS One, 10*(7), e0130059. DOI: 10.1371/journal.pone.0130059

Klaus, M. H., & Kennell, J. H. (1976). *Maternal-infant bonding.* St. Louis, MO: Mosby.

Kuebelbeck, A. (2003). *Waiting with Gabriel: A story of cherishing a baby's brief life.* Chicago, IL: Loyola Press.

Lobar, S. L., Youngblut, J. M., & Brooten, D. (2006). Cross-cultural beliefs, ceremonies, and rituals surrounding death of a loved one. *Pediatric Nursing, 32*(1), 44–50.

MacDorman, M. F., & Gregory, C. W. (2015). Fetal and perinatal mortality, United States 2013. *National Vital Statistics Report, 6*(8), 1–24.

Martin, J. A., Hamilton, B. E., Osterman, M. J. K., Driscoll, A. K., & Drake, P. (2018). Births: Final data for 2016. *National Vital Statistics Report, 67*(1), 1–62.

Martin, T. L., & Doka, K. J. (2011). The influence of gender and socialization on grieving styles. In R. A. Neimeyer, D. L. Harris, H. R. Winokuer, & G. F. Thornton (Eds.), *Grief and bereavement in contemporary society: Bridging research and practice* (pp. 69–77). New York, NY: Routledge.

Mattingly, P. J. (2016). *Evaluation of fetal death.* Retrieved from https://emedicine.medscape.com/article/259165-overview

Neimeyer, R. A. (Eds.). (2016). *Techniques of grief therapy: Assessment and intervention.* New York, NY: Routledge.

O'Leary, J. M., Parker, L., & Wimmer, L. J. (2017). Bereaved grandparent—We didn't know our part. *Journal of Community Medicine and Public Health Care, 4*(2), 1–06. DOI: 10.24966/CMPH-1978/100029

Parkes, C. M., & Weiss, R. S. (1983). *Recovery from bereavement.* New York, NY: Basic Books.

Perinatal Hospice and Palliative Care. (2017). *Perinatal hospice/palliative care programs and support.* Retrieved from https://www.perinatalhospice.org/list-of-programs

Meaney, S., Everard, C. M., Gallagher, S., & O'Donoghue, K. (2017). Parents' concerns about future pregnancy after stillbirth: A qualitative study. *Health Expect, 20*(4), 555–562.

Romero, S. T., & Lockwood, C. J. (2016). Recurrent pregnancy loss. *Contemporary OB/GYN.* Retrieved from http://www.contemporaryobgyn.net/obstetrics-gynecology-womens-health/recurrent-pregnancy-loss

Richards, J., Graham, R., Embleton, N. D., Campbell, C., & Rankin, J. (2015). Mothers' perspectives on the perinatal loss of a co-twin: A qualitative study. *BMC Pregnancy and Childbirth, 15*(143), 1–12. DOI: 10.1186/s12884-015-0

Rondinelli, J., Long, K., Seelinger, C., Crawford, C. L., & Valdez, R. (2015). Factors related to nurse comfort when caring for families experiencing perinatal loss: Evidence for bereavement program enhancement. *Journal for Nurses in Professional Development, 31*(3), 158–163. DOI: 10.1097/NND.0000000000000163

Sagiv, R., Mizrachi, Y., Glickman, H., Kerner, R., Keidar, R., Bar, J., & Golan, A. (2015). Laminaria vs. vaginal misoprostol for cervical preparation before second-trimester surgical abortion: A randomized clinical trial. *Contraception, 91*(5), 406–411. DOI: 10.1016/j.contraception.2015.01.018

Schneider, J. M. (1994). *Finding my way.* Colfax, WI: Seasons Press.

Schott, J., & Henley, A. (2007). Pregnancy loss and death of a baby: The new Sands guidelines 2007. *British Journal of Midwifery, 15*(4), 195–198.

Steen, S. E. (2015). Perinatal death: Bereavement interventions used by US and Spanish nurses and midwives. *International Journal of Palliative Nursing 21*(2), 79–86.

Swanson, K. M. (1991). Empirical development of a middle range theory of caring. *Nursing Research, 40*(3), 161–166.

Wheeler, S. R. (1997). Adolescent pregnancy loss. In J. R. Woods & J. L. Esposito (Eds.), *Loss during pregnancy or in the newborn period: Principles of care with clinical cases and analyses* (pp. 387–410). Pittman, NJ: Jannetti.

Wheeler, S. R., & Sefton, M. G. S. (2016). Early pregnancy loss during adolescence. In B. P. Black, P. M. Wright, & R. Limbo (Eds.), *Perinatal and pediatric bereavement in nursing and other health professions* (pp. 132–157). New York, NY: Springer.

Whitaker, C., & Kima, C. (2010) Perinatal grief in Latino parents. *MCN: The American Journal of Maternal/Child Nursing, 35*(6), 341–345. DOI: 10.1097/NMC.0b013e3181f2a111

Wool, C. (2015). Clinician perspectives of barriers in perinatal palliative care. *MCN: The American Journal of Maternal/Child Nursing, 40*(1), 44–53.

Worden, J. W., & Winokuer, H. R. (2011). A task-based approach for counseling the bereaved. In R. A. Neimeyer, D. L. Harris, H. R. Winokuer, & G. F. Thornton (Eds.), *Grief and bereavement in contemporary society: Bridging research and practice* (pp. 57–67). New York, NY: Routledge.

World Health Organization. (2018). *Maternal mortality.* Retrieved from http://www.who.int/news-room/fact-sheets/detail/maternal-mortality

Appendix A:
Common Abbreviations in Maternal-Newborn and Women's Health Nursing

AC	Abdominal circumference
accel	Acceleration of fetal heart rate
AFAFP	Amniotic fluid alpha-fetoprotein
AFI	Amniotic fluid index
AFP	Alpha-fetoprotein
AFV	Amniotic fluid volume
AGA	Average for gestational age
AHT	Abusive head trauma
AI	Amnioinfusion *or* Adequate intake
AIDS	Acquired immune deficiency syndrome
AOP	Apnea of prematurity *or* Anemia of prematurity
AROM	Artificial rupture of membranes
ART	Assisted reproductive technology
AUB	Abnormal uterine bleeding
BAM	Becoming a mother
BAT	Brown adipose tissue (brown fat)
BBT	Basal body temperature
β-hCG	Beta-human chorionic gonadotropin
BL FHR	Baseline fetal heart rate
BL VAR	Baseline variability
BOW	Bag of waters
BPD	Biparietal diameter *or* Bronchopulmonary dysplasia
BPP	Biophysical profile
BRB	Bright red bleeding *or* Breakthrough bleeding
BRCA	Breast cancer
BSA	Breast self-awareness
BSE	Breast self-examination
BV	Bacterial vaginosis
cal	Calorie
CAM	Complementary and alternative medicine
CC	Chest circumference *or* Cord compression
CD	Cycle day
CEI	Continuous epidural infusion
cfDNA	Cell-free DNA
CLD	Chronic lung disease
CMV	Cytomegalovirus
CNM	Certified nurse-midwife
CNS	Clinical nurse specialist
COCs	Combined oral contraceptives
CPAP	Continuous positive airway pressure
CPD	Cephalopelvic disproportion *or* Citrate–phosphate–dextrose
CRL	Crown–rump length
CRNP	Certified registered nurse practitioner
C/S	Cesarean section (or C-section)
CST	Contraction stress test
CVS	Chorionic villus sampling
D&C	Dilatation and curettage
D&E	Dilatation and evacuation
decels	Deceleration of fetal heart rate
DFMR	Daily fetal movement response
DI	Donor insemination
dil	Dilatation
DNP	Doctor of Nursing Practice
DPNB	Dorsal penile nerve block
DRI	Dietary reference intake
DTR	Deep tendon reflexes
DUB	Dysfunctional uterine bleeding
DVT	Deep vein thrombosis
EAB	Elective abortion
EC	Emergency contraception
ECV	External cephalic version
EDB	Estimated date of birth
EDD	Estimated date of delivery
EFM	Electronic fetal monitoring
EFW	Estimated fetal weight
EIA	Enzyme immunoassay
ELBW	Extremely low birth weight
ELISA	Enzyme-linked immunosorbent assay
EMB	Endometrial biopsy
EOS	Early-onset sepsis
EP	Ectopic pregnancy
epis	Episiotomy
ERCS	Elective repeat cesarean section
FAB	Fertility awareness–based methods
FAD	Fetal activity diary
FAS	Fetal alcohol syndrome
FASD	Fetal alcohol spectrum disorder
FBM	Fetal breathing movements
FBS	Fetal blood sample *or* Fasting blood sugar test
FCC	Family-centered care
FECG	Fetal electrocardiogram
fFN	Fetal fibronectin
FGM	Female genital mutilation

FHR	Fetal heart rate
FHT	Fetal heart tones
Fhx	Family history
FISH	Fluorescence *in situ* hybridization
FL	Femur length
FMC	Fetal movement count
FMH	Fetal-maternal hemorrhage
FMR	Fetal movement record
FO	Foramen ovale
FPG	Fasting plasma glucose test
FRC	Female reproductive cycle *or* Functional residual capacity
FSE	Fetal scalp electrode
FSH	Follicle-stimulating hormone
FSHRH	Follicle-stimulating hormone–releasing hormone
$FSPO_2$	Fetal arterial oxygen saturation
G or grav	Gravida
GDM	Gestational diabetes mellitus
GIFT	Gamete intrafallopian transfer
GnRF	Gonadotropin-releasing factor
GnRH	Gonadotropin-releasing hormone
GTD	Gestational trophoblastic disease
GTPAL	Gravida, term, preterm, abortion, living children; a system of recording maternity history
HA	Head–abdominal ratio *or* headache
HC	Head compression
hCG	Human chorionic gonadotropin
HIV	Human immunodeficiency virus
hMG	Human menopausal gonadotropin
hPL	Human placental lactogen
HPT	Home pregnancy test
HPV	Human papillomavirus
HSG	Hysterosalpingography
HSV	Herpes simplex virus
HT	Hormone therapy
IAP	Intrapartum antimicrobial prophylaxis
IBCLC	International board-certified lactation consultant
IDM	Infant of a diabetic mother
IEM	Inborn errors of metabolism
IPV	Intimate partner violence
ISAM	Infant of a substance-abusing mother
IUC	Intrauterine contraception
IUD	Intrauterine device
IUFD	Intrauterine fetal death
IUGR	Intrauterine growth restriction
IUI	Intrauterine insemination
IUPC	Intrauterine pressure catheter
IUS	Intrauterine system
IVF	In vitro fertilization
kcal	Kilocalorie
LADA	Left-acromion-dorsal-anterior
LADP	Left-acromion-dorsal-posterior
LBC	Lamellar body count
LBW	Low birth weight
LDRP	Labor, delivery, recovery, and postpartum
LGA	Large for gestational age
LH	Luteinizing hormone
LHRH	Luteinizing hormone–releasing hormone
LLLI	La Leche League International
LMA	Left-mentum-anterior
LML	Left mediolateral (episiotomy)
LMP	Last menstrual period *or* Left-mentum-posterior
LMT	Left-mentum-transverse
LOA	Left-occiput-anterior
LOF	Low outlet forceps
LOP	Left-occiput-posterior
LOS	Length of stay
LOT	Left-occiput-transverse
L/S	Lecithin/sphingomyelin ratio
LSA	Left-sacrum-anterior
LSP	Left-sacrum-posterior
LST	Left-sacrum-transverse
MAS	Meconium aspiration syndrome
mec	Meconium
MEN	Minimal enteral nutrition
MHT	Menopausal hormone therapy
MLE	Midline episiotomy
MRA	Maternal role attainment
MSAF	Meconium-stained amniotic fluid
MSAFP	Maternal serum alpha-fetoprotein
multip	Multipara
NAS	Neonatal abstinence syndrome
NBS	New Ballard score
NEC	Necrotizing enterocolitis
NFP	Natural family planning
NICU	Neonatal intensive care unit
NNS	Nonnutritive sucking
NP	Nurse practitioner
NST	Nonstress test *or* Nonshivering thermogenesis
NSVD	Normal sterile vaginal delivery
NT	Nuchal translucency
NTD	Neural tube defects
NTE	Neutral thermal environment
NVP	Nausea and vomiting of pregnancy
OA	Occiput anterior
OCT	Oxytocin challenge test
OF	Occipitofrontal diameter of fetal head
OFC	Occipitofrontal circumference
OGTT	Oral glucose tolerance test

OM Occipitomental (diameter)
OP Occiput posterior
p Para
PABC Pregnancy-associated breast cancer
Pap smear Papanicolaou smear
PAPP-A Pregnancy-associated plasma protein A
PCA Patient-controlled analgesia
PCEA Patient-controlled epidural analgesia
PCOS Polycystic ovarian syndrome
PDA Patent ductus arteriosus
PG Phosphatidylglycerol *or* Prostaglandin
PGD Preimplantation genetic diagnosis
PGS Preimplantation genetic screening
PID Pelvic inflammatory disease
Pit Pitocin
PKU Phenylketonuria
PMDD Premenstrual dysphoric disorder
PMR Perinatal mortality rate
PMS Premenstrual syndrome
PNV Prenatal vitamins
PPHN Persistent pulmonary hypertension of the newborn
PPD Postpartum depression
PPH Postpartum hemorrhage
PPROM Preterm premature rupture of membranes
primip Primipara
PROM Premature rupture of membranes
PSI Prostaglandin synthesis inhibitor
PTB Preterm birth
PTL Preterm labor
PTSD Posttraumatic stress disorder
PUBS Percutaneous umbilical blood sampling
PUL Pregnancy of unknown location
RADA Right-acromion-dorsal-anterior
RADP Right-acromion-dorsal-posterior
RDA Recommended dietary allowance
RDS Respiratory distress syndrome
RhIg Rh immune globulin
RIA Radioimmunoassay
RMA Right-mentum-anterior
RMP Right-mentum-posterior
RMT Right-mentum-transverse
RNC Certified registered nurse
ROA Right-occiput-anterior
ROM Rupture of membranes
ROP Right-occiput-posterior *or* Retinopathy of prematurity
ROT Right-occiput-transverse
RPL Recurrent pregnancy loss
RRA Radioreceptor assay
RSA Right-sacrum-anterior
RSP Right-sacrum-posterior
RST Right-sacrum-transverse
SAB Spontaneous abortion
SBS Shaken baby syndrome
SET Surrogate embryo transfer
SGA Small for gestational age
SIDS Sudden infant death syndrome
SMB Submentobregmatic diameter
SMM Severe maternal morbidity
SOB Suboccipitobregmatic diameter *or* Shortness of breath
SPA Sperm penetration assay
SRBOW Spontaneous rupture of bag of waters
SROM Spontaneous rupture of membranes
SSC Skin-to-skin contact
STI Sexually transmitted infection
STS Serologic test for syphilis
SUID Sudden unexpected infant death
SVE Sterile vaginal exam
TAB Therapeutic abortion
TcB Transcutaneous bilirubin
TET Tubal embryo transfer
TOL Trial of labor
TOLAC Trial of labor after cesarean
TORCH Toxoplasmosis, rubella, cytomegalovirus, herpesvirus hominis type 2
TSS Toxic shock syndrome
TTN Transient tachypnea of the newborn
ū Umbilicus
UA Uterine activity
UAC Umbilical artery catheter
UC Uterine contraction
UNHS Universal newborn hearing screening
UPI Uteroplacental insufficiency
US Ultrasound
UTI Urinary tract infection
VBAC Vaginal birth after cesarean
VDRL Venereal Disease Research Laboratories
VIP Voluntary interruption of pregnancy
VLBW Very low birth weight
VTE Venous thromboembolism
VVC Vulvovaginal candidiasis
WIC Special supplemental nutrition program for women, infants, and children
ZIFT Zygote intrafallopian transfer

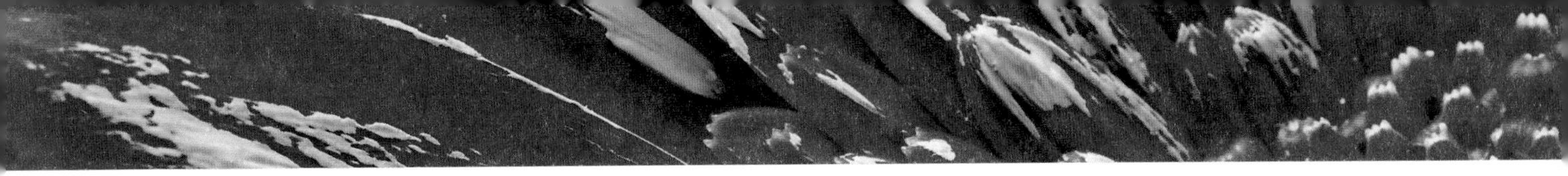

Appendix B:
Conversions and Equivalents

Temperature Conversion

(Fahrenheit temperature − 32) × 5/9 = Centigrade temperature
(Centigrade temperature × 9/5) + 32 = Fahrenheit temperature

Selected Conversion to Metric Measures

Known Value	Multiply by	To Find
inches	2.54	centimeters
ounces	28	grams
pounds	454	grams
pounds	0.45	kilogram

Selected Conversion from Metric Measures

Known Value	Multiply by	To Find
centimeters	0.4	inches
grams	0.035	ounces
grams	0.0022	pounds
kilograms	2.2	pounds

Conversion of Pounds and Ounces to Grams

	Ounces															
Pounds	0	1	2	3	4	5	6	7	8	9	10	11	12	13	14	15
0	—	28	57	85	113	142	170	198	227	255	283	312	340	369	397	425
1	454	482	510	539	567	595	624	652	680	709	737	765	794	822	850	879
2	907	936	964	992	1021	1049	1077	1106	1134	1162	1191	1219	1247	1276	1304	1332
3	1361	1389	1417	1446	1474	1503	1531	1559	1588	1616	1644	1673	1701	1729	1758	1786
4	1814	1843	1871	1899	1928	1956	1984	2013	2041	2070	2098	2126	2155	2183	2211	2240
5	2268	2296	2325	2353	2381	2410	2438	2466	2495	2523	2551	2580	2608	2637	2665	2693
6	2722	2750	2778	2807	2835	2863	2892	2920	2948	2977	3005	3033	3062	3090	3118	3147
7	3175	3203	3232	3260	3289	3317	3345	3374	3402	3430	3459	3487	3515	3544	3572	3600
8	3629	3657	3685	3714	3742	3770	3799	3827	3856	3884	3912	3941	3969	3997	4026	4054
9	4082	4111	4139	4167	4196	4224	4252	4281	4309	4337	4366	4394	4423	4451	4479	4508
10	4536	4564	4593	4621	4649	4678	4706	4734	4763	4791	4819	4848	4876	4904	4933	4961
11	4990	5018	5046	5075	5103	5131	5160	5188	5216	5245	5273	5301	5330	5358	5386	5415
12	5443	5471	5500	5528	5557	5585	5613	5642	5670	5698	5727	5755	5783	5812	5840	5868
13	5897	5925	5953	5982	6010	6038	6067	6095	6123	6152	6180	6209	6237	6265	6294	6322
14	6350	6379	6407	6435	6464	6492	6520	6549	6577	6605	6634	6662	6690	6719	6747	6776
15	6804	6832	6860	6889	6917	6945	6973	7002	7030	7059	7087	7115	7144	7172	7201	7228
16	7257	7286	7313	7342	7371	7399	7427	7456	7484	7512	7541	7569	7597	7626	7654	7682
17	7711	7739	7768	7796	7824	7853	7881	7909	7938	7966	7994	8023	8051	8079	8108	8136
18	8165	8192	8221	8249	8278	8306	8335	8363	8391	8420	8448	8476	8504	8533	8561	8590
19	8618	8646	8675	8703	8731	8760	8788	8816	8845	8873	8902	8930	8958	8987	9015	9043
20	9072	9100	9128	9157	9185	9213	9242	9270	9298	9327	9355	9383	9412	9440	9469	9497
21	9525	9554	9582	9610	9639	9667	9695	9724	9752	9780	9809	9837	9865	9894	9922	9950
22	9979	10,007	10,036	10,064	10,092	10,120	10,149	10,177	10,206	10,234	10,262	10,291	10,319	10,347	10,376	10,404

Appendix C:

NANDA-I © 2017 DIAGNOSES: Definitions and Defining Characteristics Used in This Text

AIRWAY CLEARANCE, INEFFECTIVE

Inability to clear secretions or obstructions from the respiratory tract to maintain a clear airway

Defining Characteristics

Subjective

Dyspnea

Objective

Adventitious breath sounds (e.g., rales, crackles, rhonchi, wheezes)
Changes in respiratory rate and rhythm
Cyanosis
Difficulty vocalizing
Diminished breath sounds
Excessive sputum
Ineffective or absent cough
Orthopnea
Restlessness
Wide-eyed

ANXIETY

Vague, uneasy feeling of discomfort or dread accompanied by an autonomic response (the source often nonspecific or unknown to the individual); a feeling of apprehension caused by anticipated danger. It is an alerting signal that warns of impending danger and enables the individual to take measures to deal with the threat

Defining Characteristics

Behavioral

Decreased productivity
Expressed concerns due to change in life events
Extraneous movement (e.g., foot shuffling, hand/arm movements)
Fidgeting, restlessness
Glancing about
Poor eye contact
Scanning and vigilance

Affective

Anguish
Apprehension
Distressed
Fearful
Feelings of inadequacy
Focus on self
Increased wariness
Irritability
Jittery
Overexcited
Helplessness
Rattled
Regretful
Scared
Uncertainty
Worried

Physiological

Facial tension
Increased perspiration
Increased tension
Shakiness
Trembling or hand tremors
Voice quavering

Parasympathetic

Abdominal pain
Decreased blood pressure
Decreased pulse
Diarrhea
Faintness
Fatigue
Nausea
Sleep disturbance
Tingling in extremities
Urinary frequency
Urinary hesitancy
Urinary urgency

Sympathetic

Anorexia
Cardiovascular excitation
Diarrhea
Dry mouth
Facial flushing
Heart pounding
Increased blood pressure
Increased pulse
Increased reflexes
Increased respiration
Pupil dilation
Respiratory difficulties
Superficial vasoconstriction
Twitching
Weakness

Cognitive

Awareness of physiologic symptoms
Blocking of thought
Confusion
Decreased perceptual field
Difficulty concentrating
Diminished ability to problem solve
Diminished learning ability
Fear of unspecific consequences
Forgetfulness
Impaired attention
Preoccupation
Rumination
Tendency to blame others

ATTACHMENT, RISK FOR IMPAIRED

Vulnerable to disruption of the interactive process between parent or significant other and child that fosters the development of a protective and nurturing reciprocal relationship

BLEEDING, RISK FOR

At risk for a decrease in blood volume that may compromise health

BODY TEMPERATURE: IMBALANCED, RISK FOR

Vulnerable to failure to maintain body temperature within normal parameters, which may compromise health

BREASTFEEDING, INEFFECTIVE

Difficulty providing milk to an infant or young child directly from the breasts, which may compromise nutritional status of the infant/child

Defining Characteristics

Subjective

Perceived inadequate milk supply

Objective

Inadequate infant stooling
Infant arching and crying at the breast
Infant crying or exhibiting fussiness within the first hour after breastfeeding
Infant inability to latch on to maternal breast correctly
Infant resisting latching on to breast
Infant unresponsiveness to other comfort measures
Insufficient emptying of each breast per feeding
Insufficient infant weight gain, or sustained infant weight loss
Insufficient signs of oxytocin release
Persistence of sore nipples beyond first week of breastfeeding
Unsustained suckling at the breast

BREASTFEEDING, READINESS FOR ENHANCED

A pattern of providing milk to an infant or young child directly from the breasts, which may be strengthened

Defining Characteristics

Subjective

Mother expresses desire to enhance ability to exclusively breastfeed
Mother expresses desire to enhance ability to provide breast milk for a child's nutritional needs

Objective

Adequate infant elimination patterns for age
Appropriate infant weight pattern for age
Eagerness of infant to nurse
Effective mother–infant communication patterns (e.g., infant cues, maternal interpretation or response)
Infant content after feeding
Mother able to position infant at breast to promote a successful latch-on response
Regular and sustained suckling and swallowing at breast
Signs and symptoms of oxytocin release (let-down or milk ejection reflex)

BREATHING PATTERN, INEFFECTIVE

Inspiration and/or expiration that does not provide adequate ventilation

Defining Characteristics

Subjective

Dyspnea

Objective

Abnormal breathing pattern (e.g., rate, rhythm, depth)
Altered chest excursion
Assumption of three-point position
Bradypnea
Decreased inspiratory–expiratory diameter
Nasal flaring
Orthopnea
Prolonged expiration phases
Pursed-lip breathing
Tachypnea
Use of accessory muscles to breathe

CARDIAC OUTPUT, DECREASED

Inadequate blood pumped by the heart to meet metabolic demands of the body

Defining Characteristics

Altered Heart Rate and Rhythm

Bradycardia
EKG exchange (e.g., arrhythmia, conduction abnormality, ischemia)
Palpitations
Tachycardia

Altered Preload

Edema
Fatigue
Heart murmur
Increased or decreased central venous pressure (CVP)
Increased or decreased pulmonary artery wedge pressure (PAWP)
Jugular vein distention
Weight gain

Altered Afterload

Abnormal skin color (e.g., pale, dusky, cyanotic)
Clammy skin
Decreased peripheral pulses
Dyspnea
Increased or decreased pulmonary vascular resistance (PVR)
Increased or decreased systemic vascular resistance (SVR)
Oliguria
Prolonged capillary refill
Variations in blood pressure

Altered Contractility

Adventitious breath sounds
Cough
Decreased cardiac index
Decreased ejection fraction, stroke volume index (SVI), and left-ventricular stroke work index (LVSWI)
Orthopnea or paroxysmal nocturnal dyspnea
S_3 or S_4 sounds

Behavioral/Emotional

Anxiety
Restlessness

CHILDBEARING PROCESS, INEFFECTIVE

Pregnancy and childbirth process and care of the newborn that does not match the environmental context, norm, and expectations

Defining Characteristics

During Pregnancy Subjective

Does not report appropriate prenatal lifestyle (e.g., nutrition, elimination, sleep, exercise, personal hygiene)

Does not satisfactorily manage unpleasant symptoms in pregnancy

Objective

Does not access support systems sufficiently

Failure to prepare necessary newborn care items

Inadequate prenatal visits

Inadequate preparation of the home environment

Insufficient respect for unborn baby

Unrealistic birth plan

During Labor and Delivery Subjective

Inadequate lifestyle (e.g., diet, elimination, sleep, bodily movement, personal hygiene) for the stage of labor

Objective

Decreased proactivity during labor and delivery

Does not demonstrate adequate attachment behavior to the newborn baby

Does not respond appropriately to onset of labor

Insufficient access to support systems

After Birth Objective

Does not demonstrate appropriate baby feeding techniques

Does not demonstrate appropriate breast care

Does not demonstrate basic baby care techniques

Does not demonstrate sufficient attachment to the baby

Does not provide safe environment for the baby

Inadequate postpartum lifestyle (e.g., elimination, exercise, nutrition, personal hygiene, sleep)

CONSTIPATION

Decrease in normal frequency of defecation accompanied by difficult or incomplete passage of stool and/or passage of excessively hard, dry stool

Defining Characteristics

Subjective

Abdominal pain

Abdominal tenderness with or without palpable muscle resistance

Anorexia

Feeling of rectal fullness or pressure

Generalized fatigue

Headache

Increased intra-abdominal pressure

Indigestion

Pain with defecation

Objective

Abdominal distention

Atypical presentations in older adults (e.g., change in mental status, urinary incontinence, unexplained falls, elevated body temperature)

Bright red blood with stool

Borborygmi (abdominal growling)

Change in bowel pattern

Decreased stool frequency

Decreased volume of stool

Hard, formed stools

Hypo- or hyperactive bowel sounds

Inability to defecate

Liquid stool

Palpable abdominal mass

Palpable rectal mass

Percussed abdominal dullness

Presence of soft paste-like stool in rectum

Severe flatus

Straining with defecation

Vomiting

CONSTIPATION, RISK FOR

Vulnerable to a decrease in normal frequency of defecation accompanied by difficult or incomplete passage of stool, which may compromise health

COPING: FAMILY, COMPROMISED

A usually supportive primary person (family member, significant other, or close friend) provides insufficient, ineffective, or compromised support, comfort, assistance, or encouragement that may be needed by the client to manage or master adaptive tasks related to his health challenge

Defining Characteristics

Subjective

Client concern or complaint about a significant person's response to his health problem

Support person describes preoccupation with personal reaction (e.g., fear, anticipatory grief, guilt, anxiety)

Support person reports an inadequate knowledge base or inadequate understanding that interferes with effective supportive behaviors

Objective

Communication limitation between support person and client

Support person's assistive or supportive behaviors produce unsatisfactory results

Support person displays protective behavior disproportionate (too little or too much) to the client's abilities or need for autonomy

Support person withdraws from client

COPING, INEFFECTIVE

Inability to form a valid appraisal of the stressors, inadequate choices of practiced responses, and inability to use available resources

Defining Characteristics

Subjective

Change in usual communication patterns

Fatigue

Inability to ask for help

Objective

Destructive behavior toward self and others

Difficulty organizing information

Difficulty sleeping

Frequent illness

Inability to attend to information

Inability to deal with a situation [cope]

Inability to meet basic needs

Inability to meet role expectations

Inadequate problem-solving skills

Insufficient access of social support

Lack of goal-directed behavior

Lack of resolution of problems

Poor concentration

Risk taking

Substance abuse

COPING: READINESS FOR ENHANCED

A pattern of cognitive and behavioral efforts to manage demands related to well-being, which can be strengthened

Defining Characteristics

Subjective

Aware of possible environmental changes

Objective

Expresses desire to enhance knowledge of stress management strategies

Expresses desire to enhance management of stressors

Seeks or expresses desire to enhance social support

Uses, or expresses desire to enhance use of, problem- and emotion-oriented strategies

Uses, or expresses desire to enhance use of, spiritual resources

DECISIONAL CONFLICT

Uncertainty about course of action to be taken when choice among competing actions involves risk, loss, or challenge to personal life values

Defining Characteristics

Subjective

Questioning moral rules, principles, and/or values while attempting a decision

Questioning personal values and/or beliefs while attempting a decision

Self-focusing

Verbalizes feelings of distress while attempting a decision

Verbalizes recognition of undesired consequences of actions being considered

Objective

Delayed decision making

Physical signs of distress or tension (e.g., increased heart rate, increased muscle tension, restlessness)

Uncertainty about choices

Vacillation among choices

DEVELOPMENT: DELAYED, RISK FOR

Vulnerable to delay of 25% or more in one or more of the areas of social or self-regulatory behavior or in cognitive, language, or gross- or fine-motor skills, which may compromise health

DYSREFLEXIA, AUTONOMIC

Life-threatening, uninhibited sympathetic response of the nervous system to a noxious stimulus after a spinal cord injury at T7 or above

Defining Characteristics

Subjective

Blurred vision

Chest pain

Headache (a diffuse pain in different portions of the head and not confined to any nerve distribution area)

Metallic taste in mouth

Paresthesia

Objective

Bradycardia (pulse rate of < 60 beats/minute)

Chills

Conjunctival congestion

Diaphoresis above injury

Horner syndrome [contraction of pupil, partial ptosis of eyelid, enophthalmos, and sometimes loss of sweating over affected side of face]

Nasal congestion

Pallor below injury

Paroxysmal hypertension

Pilomotor reflex

Red blotches on skin (above the injury)

Tachycardia (pulse rate > 100 beats/minute)

FAMILY PROCESSES, DYSFUNCTIONAL

Psychosocial, spiritual, and physiologic functions of the family unit are chronically disorganized, which leads to conflict, denial of problems, resistance to change, ineffective problem solving, and a series of self-perpetuating crises

Defining Characteristics

Behaviors

Agitation

Blaming

Broken promises

Chaos

Complicated grieving

Conflict avoidance

Contradictory communication

Controlling communication and power struggles

Criticizing

Decrease in physical contact

Denial of problems

Dependency

Difficulty having fun

Difficulty with intimate relationships

Diminished physical contact

Disturbances in academic performance in children

Disturbances in concentration

Enabling maintenance of substance use patterns (e.g., alcohol)

Escalating conflict

Failure to accomplish current or past developmental tasks and difficulty with life-cycle transitions

Harsh self-judgment

Immaturity

Inability to accept or receive help

Inability to adapt to change

Inability to deal with traumatic experiences constructively

Inability to express or accept a wide range of feelings

Inability to meet emotional needs of its members

Inability to meet security needs of its members

Inability to meet spiritual needs of its members

Inadequate understanding or knowledge of substance abuse

Inappropriate expression of anger

Ineffective communication skills

Lying

Manipulation

Nicotine addiction

Orientation toward tension relief rather than achievement of goals

Paradoxical communication pattern

Rationalization

Refusal to accept or get help

Seeking approval and affirmation

Self-blaming

Social isolation

Special occasions are substance-use centered

Stress-related physical illnesses

Substance abuse
Unreliable behavior
Verbal abuse of children, spouse, or parent

Feelings

Abandonment
Anger
Anxiety, tension, distress
Confuses love and pity
Confusion
Decreased self-esteem
Depression
Dissatisfaction
Embarrassment
Emotional isolation and loneliness
Emotionally controlled by others
Failure
Fear
Feeling different from other people
Feeling misunderstood
Feeling unloved
Frustration
Guilt
Hopelessness
Hostility
Hurt
Insecurity
Lingering resentment
Loneliness
Loss
Mistrust
Moodiness
Powerlessness
Rejection
Repressed emotions
Shame
Taking responsibility for substance abuser's behavior
Unhappiness
Vulnerability
Worthlessness

Roles and Relationships

Altered role function and disruption of family roles
Chronic family problems
Closed communication system
Conflict between partners
Deterioration in family relationships and disturbed family dynamics
Disrupted family rituals
Economic problems
Family denial
Family does not demonstrate respect for individuality and autonomy of its members
Inconsistent parenting and low perception of parental support
Ineffective spouse communication or marital problems
Intimacy dysfunction
Insufficient cohesiveness
Lack of skills necessary for relationships
Neglected obligations
Pattern of recognition
Reduced ability of family members to relate to each other for mutual growth and maturation
Triangulation of family relationships

FAMILY PROCESSES, INTERRUPTED

Change in family relationships or functioning

Defining Characteristics

Subjective

Changes in family satisfaction

Objective

Changes in:
Assigned tasks
Availability for affective responsiveness and intimacy
Availability of emotional support
Communication patterns
Effectiveness of task completion
Expressions of conflict with or isolation from community resources
Family conflict resolution
Intimacy
Mutual support (decreased)
Participation in decision making
Participation in problem solving
Power alliances
Relationship pattern
Rituals
Somatic complaints
Stress-reduction behaviors

FAMILY PROCESSES, READINESS FOR ENHANCED

A pattern of family functioning to support the well-being of family members, which can be strengthened

Defining Characteristics

Objective

Expresses desire to enhance:
Balance between autonomy and cohesiveness
Communication
Energy level of family to support ADLs
Family dynamics
Family adaptation to change
Family resilience
Growth of family members
Interdependence with the community
Maintenance of boundaries between family members
Positive family relationships
Respect for family members
Safety of family members

FEAR

Response to perceived threat that is consciously recognized as a danger

Defining Characteristics

Subjective

Report of:
Alarm
Apprehensiveness
Decreased self-assurance
Excitedness
Feeling dread
Feeling fear
Feeling scared
Increased tension
Jitteriness
Muscle tension/tightness

Nausea
Panic
Terror

Cognitive

Diminished productivity, learning ability, problem-solving ability
Identifies object of fear
Stimulus believed to be a threat

Objective

Pallor
Pupil dilation
Vomiting

Behaviors

Avoidance or attack behaviors
Impulsiveness
Increased alertness
Narrowed focus on the source of fear

Physiological

Anorexia
Diarrhea
Dry mouth
Changes in oxygen saturation and end-tidal CO_2
Fatigue
Increased perspiration
Increased pulse rate
Increased respiratory rate and shortness of breath
Increased systolic blood pressure

FLUID VOLUME, DEFICIENT

Decreased intravascular, interstitial, or intracellular fluid; this refers to dehydration—water loss alone without change in sodium

Defining Characteristics

Subjective

Thirst

Objective

Change in mental status
Decreased blood pressure, decreased pulse volume and pressure
Decreased skin and tongue turgor
Decreased urine output
Decreased venous filling
Dry skin and mucous membrane
Elevated hematocrit
Increased body temperature
Increased pulse rate
Increased urine concentration
Sudden weight loss (except in third-spacing)
Weakness

FLUID VOLUME: RISK FOR DEFICIENT

Vulnerable to experiencing decreased intravascular, interstitial, and/or intracellular fluid volumes, which may compromise health

FLUID VOLUME: RISK FOR IMBALANCED

Vulnerable to a decrease, increase, or rapid shift from one to the other of intravascular, interstitial, or intracellular fluid, which may compromise health; refers to body fluid loss, gain, or both

GAS EXCHANGE, IMPAIRED

Excess or deficit in oxygenation and/or carbon dioxide elimination at the alveolar-capillary membrane

Defining Characteristics

Subjective

Dyspnea
Headache on awakening
Visual disturbance

Objective

Abnormal arterial blood gases
Abnormal arterial pH
Abnormal rate, rhythm, depth of breathing
Abnormal skin color (e.g., pale, dusky)
Confusion
Cyanosis (in neonates only)
Decreased carbon dioxide level
Diaphoresis
Hypercapnia
Hypoxemia
Hypoxia
Irritability
Nasal flaring
Restlessness
Somnolence
Tachycardia

GRIEVING

A normal complex process that includes emotional, physical, spiritual, social, and intellectual responses and behaviors by which individuals, families, and communities incorporate an actual, anticipated, or perceived loss into their daily lives

Defining Characteristics

Subjective

Anger
Blaming
Despair
Detachment
Experiencing guilt about feeling relief
Pain
Personal growth
Psychological distress
Suffering

Objective

Alterations in activity level
Alterations in dream patterns
Alterations in immune function
Alterations in neuroendocrine function
Alterations in sleep patterns
Disorganization
Maintaining the connection to the deceased
Making meaning of the loss
Panic behavior

GRIEVING, COMPLICATED

A disorder that occurs after the death of a significant other, in which the experience of distress accompanying bereavement fails to follow normative expectations and manifests in functional impairment

Defining Characteristics

Subjective

Rumination
Verbalizes the following:
Anxiety

Decreased sense of well-being
Depression
Disbelief
Distress about the deceased
Feelings of anger
Excessive stress
Fatigue
Feeling dazed
Feeling detached from others
Feeling stunned
Feelings of emptiness
Insufficient sense of well-being
Longing for the deceased
Low level of intimacy
Mistrust
Persistent painful memories
Preoccupation with thought of the deceased
Self-blame
Shock
Yearning for the deceased

Objective

Decreased functioning in life roles
Experiencing somatic symptoms of the deceased
Grief avoidance
Lack of acceptance of the death
Searching for the deceased person
Self-blame
Separation distress
Traumatic distress

HEALTH MAINTENANCE, INEFFECTIVE

Inability to identify, manage, or seek out help to maintain health

Defining Characteristics

Subjective

Absence of expressed interest in improving health behaviors

Objective

Demonstrated lack of adaptive behaviors to environmental changes
Insufficient knowledge about basic health practices
History of lack of health-seeking behavior
Inability to take responsibility for meeting basic health practices
Inadequate social support system

HEALTH MANAGEMENT, INEFFECTIVE

Pattern of regulating and integrating into daily living a therapeutic regimen for the treatment of illness and its sequelae that is unsatisfactory for meeting specific health goals

Defining Characteristics

Subjective

Expresses or demonstrates difficulty with prescribed regimen

Objective

Failure to include treatment regimens in daily living
Failure to take action to reduce risk factors
Ineffective choices in daily living for meeting health goals

HEALTH MANAGEMENT, READINESS FOR ENHANCED

A pattern of regulating and integrating into daily living a therapeutic program for the treatment of illness and its sequelae, which can be strengthened

Defining Characteristics

Expresses desire to enhance:

Choices of daily living appropriate for meeting goals (e.g., treatment, prevention)
Immunization/vaccination status
Management of the illness (e.g., treatment, prevention of sequelae)
Management of prescribed regimens
Management of risk factors and symptoms

HOPELESSNESS

Subjective state in which an individual sees limited or no alternatives or personal choices available and is unable to mobilize energy on own behalf

Defining Characteristics

Subjective

Verbal cues (e.g., despondent content, "I can't," sighing)

Objective

Avoiding eye contact
Closing eyes
Decreased affect
Decreased appetite
Decreased response to stimuli
Decreased verbalization
Lack of initiative
Lack of involvement in care
Passivity
Shrugging in response to speaker
Sleep-pattern disturbance
Turning away from speaker

HYPOTHERMIA

Core body temperature below the normal diurnal range due to failure of thermoregulation

Defining Characteristics

Objective

Acrocyanosis
Bradycardia
Cyanotic nail beds
Decrease in blood glucose level
Decrease in ventilation
Hypertension
Hypoglycemia
Hypoxia
Increase in oxygen consumption
Increased metabolic rate
Peripheral vasoconstriction
Shivering
Skin cool to touch
Slow capillary refill
Tachycardia

INFANT BEHAVIOR: DISORGANIZED

Disintegrated physiological and neurobehavioral responses of infant to the environment

Defining Characteristics

Attention-Interaction System

Abnormal response to sensory stimuli (e.g., difficult to soothe, inability to sustain alert status)

Motor System

Altered primitive reflexes
Exaggerated startle response

Finger splay, fisting, or hands to face
Hyperextension of arms and legs
Increased, decreased, or limp motor tone
Jitteriness
Tremors, startles, twitches
Uncoordinated movement

Physiological

Bradycardia, tachycardia, or arrhythmias
Desaturation (oximetry reading)
Feeding intolerances (e.g., aspiration or emesis)
Skin color change (e.g., pale, cyanotic, mottled, or flushed color)
"Time-out" signals (e.g., gaze, grasp, hiccough, cough, sneeze, sigh, slack jaw, open mouth, tongue thrust)

Regulatory Problems

Inability to inhibit startle reflex
Irritability

State-Organization System

Active–awake (fussy, worried gaze)
Diffuse alpha EEG activity with eyes closed
Irritable crying
Quiet–awake (staring, gaze aversion)
State oscillation

INFECTION, RISK FOR

Vulnerable to invasion and multiplication of pathogenic organisms, which may compromise health

INJURY, RISK FOR

Vulnerable to physical damage due to environmental conditions interacting with the individual's adaptive and defensive resources, which may compromise health

KNOWLEDGE, DEFICIENT

Absence or deficiency of cognitive information related to specific topic

Defining Characteristics

Objective

Inaccurate follow-through of instruction
Inaccurate performance on tests
Inappropriate or exaggerated behaviors (e.g., hysteria, hostility, agitation, or apathy)
Insufficient knowledge

KNOWLEDGE, READINESS FOR ENHANCED

A pattern of cognitive information related to a specific topic, or its acquisition, that is sufficient for meeting health-related goals and can be strengthened

Defining Characteristics

Subjective

Expresses desire to enhance learning

MATERNAL/FETAL DYAD, RISK FOR DISTURBED

Vulnerable to disruption of the symbiotic maternal/fetal dyad as a result of comorbid or pregnancy-related conditions, which may compromise health

MOBILITY: PHYSICAL, IMPAIRED

Limitation in independent, purposeful physical movement of the body or of one or more of the extremities [specify level, using a standardized functional scale]:

Level 0: Is completely independent
Level 1: Requires use of equipment or device
Level 2: Requires help from another person for assistance, supervision, or teaching
Level 3: Requires help from another person and equipment or device
Level 4: Is dependent; does not participate in activity

Defining Characteristics

Objective

Decrease in reaction time
Decreased ability to perform fine-motor skills
Decreased ability to perform gross-motor skills
Decreased range of motion
Difficulty turning
Discomfort
Engages in substitutions for movement (e.g., increased attention to other's activity, controlling behavior, focuses on pre-illness or disability activity)
Exertional dyspnea
Gait changes (e.g., decreased walk speed, difficulty initiating gait, small steps, shuffles feet, exaggerated lateral postural sway)
Movement-induced tremor
Postural instability (e.g., during performance of routine ADLs)
Slowed movement
Uncoordinated or jerky movements

NAUSEA

A subjective phenomenon of an unpleasant feeling in the back of the throat and stomach that may or may not result in vomiting

Defining Characteristics

Subjective

Aversion toward food
Gagging sensation
Increased salivation
Increased swallowing
Report of nausea
Sour taste in mouth

NEUROVASCULAR DYSFUNCTION: PERIPHERAL, RISK FOR

Vulnerable to disruption in circulation, sensation, or motion of an extremity, which may compromise health

NUTRITION, IMBALANCED, LESS THAN BODY REQUIREMENTS

Intake of nutrients insufficient to meet metabolic needs

Defining Characteristics

Subjective

Abdominal cramping
Abdominal pain
Altered taste sensation
Aversion to food
Perceived inability to ingest food
Satiety immediately after ingesting food
Sore buccal cavity

Objective

Body weight 20% or more below ideal weight range
Capillary fragility
Diarrhea or steatorrhea
Excessive loss of hair
Food intake less than recommended daily allowance (RDA)
Hyperactive bowel sounds
Lack of information, misinformation

Lack of interest in food
Misinformation and/or misperceptions
Pale
Poor muscle tone
Weakness of muscles required for swallowing or mastication

OVERWEIGHT, RISK FOR

Vulnerable to abnormal or excessive fat accumulation for age and gender, which may compromise health

PAIN, ACUTE

An unpleasant sensory and emotional experience associated with actual or potential tissue damage, or described in terms of such damage (International Association for the Study of Pain); sudden or slow onset of any intensity from mild to severe with an anticipated or predictable end

Defining Characteristics

Subjective

Appetite change
Evidence of pain for those unable to communicate verbally, using standardized pain behavior checklist
Self-report of characteristics of pain using standardized instrument
Self-report of intensity
Verbalizes pain

Objective

Autonomic responses
Distraction behavior
Expressive behavior
Facial expression of pain
Guarding and/or protective behavior
Hopelessness
Narrowed focus
Positioning to avoid pain
Report of pain behavior/activity changes from family member, caregiver, etc.

PARENTING, IMPAIRED

Inability of the primary caretaker to create, maintain, or regain an environment that promotes the optimum growth and development of the child

Defining Characteristics

Infant or Child

Objective

Behavioral disorders
Delayed cognitive development
Diminished separation anxiety
Failure to thrive
Frequent accidents
Frequent illness
History of physical, psychological, or sexual trauma or abuse
Poor academic performance
Runaway

Parental

Subjective

Decreased ability to manage child
Reports frustration with child
Reports inability to control child
Perceived inability to meet child's needs
Perceived role inadequacy

Objective

Abandonment
History of childhood abuse
Inadequate child health maintenance
Inappropriate caretaking skills
Inappropriate child-care arrangements
Inappropriate visual, tactile, or auditory stimulation
Inconsistent behavior management
Inconsistent care
Inflexibility in meeting needs of child
Little cuddling
Negative statements about child
Neglect of child's needs
Parent–child interaction deficit
Punitive
Rejection of or hostility to child
Unsafe home environment

PARENTING, IMPAIRED, RISK FOR

Vulnerable to inability of the primary caretaker to create, maintain, or regain an environment that promotes the optimum growth and development of the child, which may compromise the well-being of the child

PARENTING, READINESS FOR ENHANCED

A pattern of providing an environment for children or other dependent person(s) to nurture growth and development, which can be strengthened

Defining Characteristics

Subjective

Children or other dependent person(s) express satisfaction with home environment
Expresses willingness to enhance parenting
Parent expresses desire to enhance emotional support

POWERLESSNESS

The lived experience of lack of control over a situation, including a perception that one's actions do not significantly affect an outcome

Defining Characteristics

Subjective

Reports alienation
Reports doubt regarding role performance
Reports frustration over inability to perform previous activities
Reports lack of a sense of control
Reports shame

Objective

Dependence on others
Depression
Inadequate participation in care

POWERLESSNESS, RISK FOR

Vulnerable to the lived experience or lack of control over a situation, including a perception that one's actions do not significantly affect an outcome, which may compromise health

SELF-ESTEEM, SITUATIONAL LOW, RISK FOR

Vulnerable to developing negative perception of self-worth in response to a current situation, which may compromise health

SEXUALITY PATTERN, INEFFECTIVE

Expressions of concern regarding own sexuality

Defining Characteristics

Subjective

Alterations in perceived sex role

Alterations in relationship with significant other
Values conflict

Objective

Reports changes in sexual activities or behaviors
Reports difficulties with sexual activities or behaviors

SKIN INTEGRITY, IMPAIRED

Altered epidermis and/or dermis

Defining Characteristics

Objective

Foreign matter piercing skin

SKIN INTEGRITY: IMPAIRED, RISK FOR

Vulnerable to alteration in epidermis and/or dermis, which may compromise health

SPIRITUAL DISTRESS, RISK FOR

Vulnerable to an impaired ability to experience and integrate meaning and purpose in life through connectedness with self, others, art, music, literature, nature, or a power greater than oneself

THERMOREGULATION, INEFFECTIVE

Temperature fluctuation between hypothermia and hyperthermia

Defining Characteristics

Objective

Cyanotic nail beds
Fluctuations in body temperature above or below normal range
Flushed skin
Hypertension
Increased body temperature, above normal range
Increased respiratory rate
Pallor (moderate)
Piloerection
Reduction in body temperature below normal range
Seizures
Shivering (mild)
Skin cold to the touch
Skin warm to the touch
Slow capillary refill
Tachycardia

TISSUE INTEGRITY, IMPAIRED

Damage to the mucous membrane, cornea, integumentary system, muscular fascia, muscle, tendon, bone, cartilage, joint capsule, and/or ligament

Defining Characteristics

Objective

Damaged or destroyed tissue (e.g., corneal, mucous membrane, integumentary, or subcutaneous)

TISSUE PERFUSION: CARDIAC, RISK FOR DECREASED

Vulnerable to a decrease in cardiac (coronary) circulation, which may compromise health

TISSUE PERFUSION: PERIPHERAL, INEFFECTIVE

Decrease in blood circulation to the periphery that may compromise health

Defining Characteristics

Absent peripheral pulses
Altered motor function
Altered skin characteristics (color, elasticity, hair, moisture, nails, sensation, temperature)
Ankle-brachial index < 0.90
Blood pressure decrease in extremities
Capillary refill time > 3 s
Color does not return to lowered leg after 1-min leg elevation
Delayed peripheral wound healing
Diminished peripheral pulses
Distances achieved in the 6-min walk test below normal range (400 m to 700 m in adults)
Edema
Extremity pain
Femoral bruit
Intermittent claudication
Shorter pain-free distance achieved in the 6-min walk test
Paresthesia
Skin color pale on elevated limb

TISSUE PERFUSION: PERIPHERAL, RISK FOR INEFFECTIVE

Vulnerable to a decrease in blood circulation to the periphery, which may compromise health

TRAUMA, RISK FOR

Vulnerable to accidental tissue injury (e.g., wound, burn, fracture), which may compromise health

URINARY ELIMINATION, IMPAIRED

Dysfunction in urine elimination

Defining Characteristics

Subjective

Dysuria
Urgency

Objective

Frequency
Hesitancy
Incontinence
Nocturia
Retention

URINARY RETENTION

Incomplete emptying of the bladder

Defining Characteristics

Subjective

Dysuria
Sensation of bladder fullness

Objective

Absence of urine output
Bladder distention
Dribbling of urine
Overflow incontinence
Residual urine
Small voiding

VIOLENCE: SELF-DIRECTED, RISK FOR

Vulnerable to behaviors in which an individual demonstrates that she can be physically, emotionally, or sexually harmful to self

Glossary

Abnormal uterine bleeding (AUB) Uterine bleeding in the absence of pregnancy that is abnormal in volume, frequency, regularity, or duration.

Abortion Loss of pregnancy before the fetus is viable outside the uterus (before 20 weeks' gestation or fetus-newborn who weighs less than 500 g); may occur spontaneously (miscarriage) or be induced by medical or surgical means.

Abruptio placentae Partial or total premature separation of a normally implanted placenta.

Abstinence Refraining voluntarily, especially from indulgence in food, alcoholic beverages, or sexual intercourse.

Abusive head trauma (AHT) Nonaccidental traumatic brain injury that results from violent shaking, with or without contact between the baby's head and an exterior surface; previously called *shaken baby syndrome*.

Acceleration Periodic increase in the baseline fetal heart rate.

Acculturation Process by which people adapt to a new cultural norm.

Acme Peak or highest point; time of greatest intensity (of a uterine contraction).

Acquaintance rape Rape in which the assailant is someone with whom the victim has had previous nonviolent interaction.

Acrocyanosis Cyanosis of the extremities.

Acrosomal reaction Breakdown of the hyaluronic acid in the corona radiata by enzymes from the heads of sperm; allows one spermatozoon to penetrate the ovum zona pellucida.

Active acquired immunity Formation of antibodies by the pregnant woman in response to illness or immunization.

Active alert state Alert state marked by an increase in facial and body movement, with periods of fussiness occurring. The newborn in this state has increased sensitivity to disturbing stimuli. Also called *active awake*.

Adequate intake (AI) Value cited for a nutrient when there are not sufficient data to calculate an estimated average requirement.

Adjustment reaction with depressed mood Maternal adjustment reaction occurring in the first few postpartum days, characterized by mild depression, tearfulness, anxiety, headache, and irritability. Also called *postpartum blues*.

Afterpains Cramplike pains due to contractions of the uterus that occur after childbirth. They are more common in multiparas, tend to be most severe during breastfeeding, and last 2 to 3 days.

AIDS (acquired immunodeficiency syndrome) Immunologic disorder caused by infection with the human immunodeficiency virus (HIV) and characterized by increasing susceptibility to opportunistic infections and rare cancers.

Alpha-fetoprotein (AFP) Fetal protein produced in the yolk sac for the first 6 weeks of gestation and then by the fetal liver.

Alternative therapy Any procedure or approach that is used in place of conventional medicine.

Amenorrhea Suppression or absence of menstruation.

Amniocentesis Removal of amniotic fluid by insertion of a needle into the amniotic sac; amniotic fluid is used to assess fetal health or maturity and for genetic diagnosis.

Amnioinfusion (AI) Procedure used to infuse a sterile fluid (such as normal saline) through an intrauterine catheter into the uterus in an attempt to increase the fluid around the umbilical cord to decrease or prevent cord compression during labor contractions; also used to dilute thick meconium-stained amniotic fluid.

Amnion Inner of the two membranes that form the sac containing the fetus and the amniotic fluid.

Amniotic fluid Liquid surrounding the fetus in utero. It absorbs shocks, permits fetal movement, and prevents heat loss.

Amniotic fluid index (AFI) Method of reporting fluid volume. The AFI is calculated by dividing the maternal abdomen into four quadrants with the umbilicus as the reference point. Then the deepest vertical pocket in each quadrant is measured. These measurements are summed to calculate the AFI.

Amniotomy Artificial rupturing of the amniotic membrane.

Ampulla Outer two-thirds of the fallopian tube; fertilization of the ovum by a spermatozoon usually occurs here.

Anaphylactoid syndrome of pregnancy Obstetrical emergency that occurs when a bolus of amniotic fluid, fetal cells, hair, or other debris enters the maternal circulation and then the maternal lungs. Also called *amniotic fluid embolism*.

Antepartum Time between conception and the onset of labor; usually used to describe the period during which a woman is pregnant.

Anterior fontanelle Diamond-shaped area between the two frontal and two parietal bones just above the newborn's forehead.

Apgar score Scoring system used to evaluate newborns at 1 minute and 5 minutes after birth. The total score is achieved by assessing five signs: Heart rate, respiratory effort, muscle tone, reflex irritability, and color. Each of the signs is assigned a score of 0, 1, or 2. The highest possible score is 10.

Apnea Condition that occurs when respirations cease for more than 20 seconds, with generalized cyanosis.

Areola Pigmented ring surrounding the nipple of the breast.

Assimilation Situation in which a person completely changes his or her cultural identity to become part of the majority culture.

Assisted reproductive technology (ART) Term used to describe the highly technologic approaches used to produce pregnancy.

Attachment Enduring bonds or relationship of affection between persons.

Attachment theory Framework for understanding perinatal loss that begins with the basic premise that human beings are biologically predisposed to bond with emotionally significant persons in their lives.

Babinski reflex Reflex found normally in babies under 6 months of age in which the great toe dorsiflexes when the sole of the foot is stimulated.

Bacterial vaginosis (BV) Bacterial infection of the vagina, formerly called *Gardnerella vaginalis* or *Hemophilus vaginalis*, characterized by a foul-smelling, grayish vaginal discharge that exhibits a characteristic fishy odor when 10% potassium hydroxide (KOH) is added. Microscopic examination of a vaginal wet prep reveals the presence of "clue cells" (vaginal epithelial cells coated with Gram-negative organisms).

Bag of waters (BOW) Membrane containing the amniotic fluid and the fetus.

Ballottement Technique of palpation to detect or examine a floating object in the body. In obstetrics, the fetus, when pushed, floats away and then returns to touch the examiner's fingers.

Barlow maneuver Test designed to detect subluxation or dislocation of the hip. A dysplastic joint will be felt to be dislocated as the femur leaves the acetabulum.

Basal body temperature (BBT) Lowest waking temperature.

Baseline fetal heart rate (BL FHR) Average fetal heart rate observed during a 10-minute period of monitoring.

Baseline variability (BL VAR) Changes in the fetal heart rate that result from the interplay between the sympathetic and the parasympathetic nervous systems.

Battledore placenta Placenta in which the umbilical cord is inserted on the periphery rather than centrally.

Becoming a mother (BAM) Transition process of becoming a mother that changes throughout the maternal–child relationship. Also called *maternal role attainment*.

Bed-sharing Newborn or infant sleeping in close social and/or physical contact with a committed caregiver (usually the mother). Also called *co-sleeping*.

Bereavement To have suffered the event of loss.

Beta human chorionic gonadotropin (beta hCG) Product of the trophoblast or placenta that is detected through serum testing and is a very accurate marker of the presence of pregnancy and placental health.

Biophysical profile (BPP) Assessment of five variables in the fetus that help to evaluate fetal risk: Breathing movement, body movement, tone, amniotic fluid volume, and fetal heart rate reactivity.

Birth center Setting for labor and birth that emphasizes a family-centered approach rather than obstetric technology and treatment.

Birth defects Structural abnormalities in the neonate present at birth.

Birth plan Written document prepared by the expectant parents that is used to identify available options in the birth setting and aspects of the childbearing experience that are most important to them.

Birth rate Number of live births per 1000 population.

Birthing room Room for labor and birth with a relaxed atmosphere.

Bishop score A prelabor scoring system to assist in predicting whether an induction of labor may be successful. The total score is achieved by assessing five components: Cervical dilatation, cervical effacement, cervical consistency, cervical position, and fetal station. Each of the components is assigned a score of 0 to 2 or 0 to 3, and the highest possible score is 13.

Blastocyst Inner solid mass of cells within the morula.

Bloody show Pink-tinged mucus secretions resulting from rupture of small capillaries as the cervix effaces and dilates.

Bogginess Softening of the uterus due to inadequate contraction of the muscle tissue.

Boggy uterus (uterine atony) Term used to describe the uterine fundus when it is not firmly contracted after the birth of the baby and in the early postpartum period; excessive bleeding occurs from the placental site, and maternal hemorrhage may occur.

Bonding Process of parent–newborn attachment occurring at or soon after birth.

Brachial plexus injury Injury due to improper or excessive traction applied to the fetal head during birth that results in damage to the network of nerves that send signals from the spine to the shoulder, arm, and hand.

Braxton Hicks contractions Intermittent painless contractions of the uterus that may occur every 10 to 20 minutes. They occur more frequently toward the end of pregnancy and are sometimes mistaken for true labor signs.

Brazelton Neonatal Behavioral Assessment Scale Assessment tool that identifies the newborn's repertoire of behavioral responses to the environment and also documents the newborn's neurologic adequacy and capabilities.

Breast self-awareness (BSA) Need for a woman to be aware of how her breasts normally look and feel; advocated as a good method for detecting breast masses early.

Breast self-examination (BSE) Manual examination conducted monthly by a woman to evaluate her own breasts for signs of masses, changes, nipple discharge, or evidence of abnormalities.

Breasts Mammary glands.

Breech presentation Birth in which the buttocks and/or feet are presented instead of the head.

Bronchopulmonary dysplasia (BPD) Chronic pulmonary disease of multifactorial etiology characterized initially by alveolar and bronchial necrosis, which results in bronchial metaplasia and interstitial fibrosis. Appears in x-ray films as generalized small, radiolucent cysts within the lungs; also called *chronic lung disease (CLD) of prematurity*.

Brown adipose tissue (BAT) Fat deposits in newborns that provide greater heat-generating activity than ordinary fat. Found around the kidneys, adrenals, and neck; between the scapulae; and behind the sternum. Also called *brown fat*.

Calorie (cal) Amount of heat required to raise the temperature of 1 kg of water 1°C.

Capacitation Removal of the plasma membrane overlying the spermatozoa's acrosomal area with the loss of seminal plasma proteins and the glycoprotein coat. If the glycoprotein coat is not removed, the sperm will not be able to penetrate the ovum.

Caput succedaneum Swelling or edema occurring in or under the fetal scalp during labor.

Cardinal movements Positional changes of the fetus as it moves through the birth canal during labor and birth. The positional changes are descent, flexion, internal rotation, extension, restitution, and external rotation. Also called *mechanisms of labor*.

Caring theory Consists of five attributes of the caregiver: (1) knowing, (2) being with, (3) doing for, (4) enabling, and (5) maintaining belief.

Carrier screening Genetic testing to see if a person is a carrier for specific autosomal recessive diseases.

Cell-free DNA (cfDNA) When performed prenatally, a test that screens for specific fetal chromosome abnormalities by measuring circulating cell-free DNA (DNA that circulates in a person's blood or plasma) in the maternal blood.

Centering Group prenatal care.

Cephalic presentation Birth in which the fetal head is presenting against the cervix.

Cephalohematoma Subcutaneous swelling containing blood found on the head of a newborn several days after birth; it usually disappears within a few weeks to 2 months.

Cephalopelvic disproportion (CPD) Condition in which the fetal head is of such a shape or size, or in such a position, that it cannot pass through the maternal pelvis.

Cerclage Surgical procedure in which a stitch is placed in the cervix to prevent a spontaneous abortion or premature birth.

Certified nurse-midwife (CNM) Registered nurse that has received special training and education in the care of the family during childbearing and the prenatal, labor and birth, and postpartum periods. After a period of formal education, the nurse-midwife takes a certification test to become a CNM.

Certified registered nurse (RNC) A registered nurse who has shown expertise in a specific field by passing a national certification examination.

Cervical dilatation Process in which the cervical os and the cervical canal widen from less than 1 cm to approximately 10 cm, allowing birth of the fetus.

Cervical insufficiency Painless dilatation of the cervix without contractions because of a structural or functional defect of the cervix.

Cervical ripening Softening of the cervix; occurs normally as a physiologic process before labor or is stimulated to occur through the process of induction of labor.

Cervix "Neck" between the external os and the body of the uterus. The lower end of the cervix extends into the vagina.

Cesarean birth Birth of fetus accomplished by performing a surgical incision through the maternal abdomen and uterus.

Chadwick sign Violet-bluish color of the vaginal mucous membrane caused by increased vascularity; visible from about the fourth week of pregnancy.

Chemical conjunctivitis Irritation of the mucous membrane lining of the eyelid; may be due to instillation of silver nitrate ophthalmic drops.

Chlamydial infection Caused by *Chlamydia trachomatis*, this infection is the most common bacterial sexually transmitted infection in the United States.

Chloasma Brownish pigmentation over the bridge of the nose and the cheeks during pregnancy and in some women who are taking oral contraceptives. Also called *melasma gravidarum* or *mask of pregnancy*.

Chorioamnionitis Inflammation of the amniotic membranes stimulated by organisms in the amniotic fluid, which then becomes infiltrated with polymorphonuclear leukocytes.

Chorion Fetal membrane closest to the intrauterine wall that gives rise to the placenta and continues as the outer membrane surrounding the amnion.

Chorionic villus sampling (CVS) Procedure in which a specimen of the chorionic villi is obtained from the edge of the developing placenta at about 9 completed weeks' gestation (usually between 10 and 12 weeks). The sample can be used for chromosomal, enzyme, and DNA tests.

Chromosomes Threadlike structures within the nucleus of a cell that carry the genes.

Circumcision Surgical removal of the prepuce (foreskin) of the penis.

Circumvallate placenta Placenta with a thick, white fibrous ring around the edge.

Cleavage Rapid mitotic division of the zygote; cells produced are called *blastomeres*.

Climacteric Period of time that marks the cessation of a woman's reproductive function; the "change of life," or menopause.

Clinical nurse specialist (CNS) Nurse possessing a master's degree and specialized knowledge and competence in a specific clinical area.

Clinical practice guidelines Comprehensive interdisciplinary care plans for a specific condition that describe the sequence and timing of interventions that should result in expected patient outcomes.

Coitus interruptus Method of contraception in which the male withdraws his penis from the vagina before ejaculation.

Cold stress Excessive heat loss resulting in compensatory mechanisms (increased respirations and nonshivering thermogenesis) to maintain core body temperature.

Colostrum Secretion from the breast before the onset of true lactation; contains mainly serum and white blood corpuscles. It has a high protein content, provides some immune properties, and cleanses the newborn's intestinal tract of mucus and meconium.

Colposcopy Use of an instrument inserted into the vagina to examine the cervical and vaginal tissues by means of a magnifying lens.

Combined oral contraceptives (COCs) Commonly called birth control pills or "the pill," a form of contraception that uses a combination of a synthetic estrogen and a progestin.

Complementary and alternative medicine (CAM) Group of diverse medical and healthcare systems, practices, and products that are not generally considered part of conventional medicine.

Complementary therapy Any procedure or product that is used together with conventional medical treatment.

Conception Union of male sperm and female ovum; fertilization.

Condom Latex, silicone, polyurethane, or lambskin sheath worn on a man's penis during sexual intercourse to prevent conception or disease.

Conduction Loss of heat to a cooler surface by direct skin contact.

Condylomata acuminata Known also as genital or venereal warts, this is a common sexually transmitted infection caused by the human papillomavirus (HPV).

Condylomata lata Wartlike growth of skin, usually seen on the external genitals or anus. There are two types, a pointed variety and a broad, flat form usually found with syphilis.

Congenital dermal melanocytosis Macular areas of bluish-black or gray-blue pigmentation found on the dorsal area and the buttocks of newborns; also called *Mongolian blue spots*.

Congenital hypothyroidism Thyroid deficiency in the newborn; early symptoms include prolonged newborn jaundice, poor feeding, constipation, low-pitched cry, poor weight gain, inactivity, and delayed motor development; an inborn enzymatic defect, lack of maternal dietary iodine, or maternal ingestion of drugs that depress or destroy thyroid tissue can be the cause.

Conjugate Important diameter of the pelvis, measured from the center of the promontory of the sacrum to the back of the symphysis pubis. The diagonal conjugate is measured and the true conjugate is estimated.

Contingent screening Additional screening in the second trimester based on the first-trimester screening results.

Contraception Prevention of conception or impregnation.

Contraction Tightening and shortening of the uterine muscles during labor, causing effacement and dilatation of the cervix; contributes to the downward and outward descent of the fetus.

Contraction stress test (CST) Method of assessing the reaction of the fetus to the stress of uterine contractions. This test may be utilized when contractions are occurring spontaneously or when contractions are artificially induced by the oxytocin challenge test (OCT) or breast self-stimulation test (BSST).

Convection Loss of heat from the warm body surface to cooler air currents.

Cornua Elongated portions of the uterus where the fallopian tubes open.

Corpus Upper two-thirds of the uterus.

Corpus luteum Small yellow body that develops within a ruptured ovarian follicle; it secretes progesterone in the second half of the menstrual cycle and atrophies about 3 days before the beginning of menstrual flow. If pregnancy occurs, the corpus luteum continues to produce progesterone until the placenta takes over this function.

Co-sleeping Newborn or infant sleeping in close social and/or physical contact with a committed caregiver (usually the mother).

Cotyledons Rounded portions into which the placenta's uterine surface is divided, each consisting of a mass of villi, fetal vessels, and an intervillous space.

Couplet care Family-centered approach for maternal–child nursing where both the mother and her baby are cared for by the same nurse, with the baby remaining at the mother's bedside. Also called *mother–baby care*.

Couvade In some cultures, the male's observance of certain rituals and taboos to signify the transition to fatherhood.

Crowning Appearance of the presenting fetal part at the vaginal introitus during labor.

Crying state State in the newborn sleep–wake cycle in which the baby exhibits increased motor activity, grimaces, tightly closed or open eyes, and extreme responsiveness to stimuli.

Cultural competence To be in possession of the skills and knowledge necessary to appreciate, understand, and work with individuals from different cultures.

Culture Beliefs, values, attitudes, and practices that are accepted by a population, community, or individual.

Cycle of violence Theory that postulates that battering takes place in a cyclic fashion through three phases: The tension-building phase, the acute battering incident, and the tranquil phase (honeymoon period).

Cystocele Downward displacement of the bladder, which appears as a bulge in the anterior vaginal wall.

Date rape Form of acquaintance rape that occurs between a dating couple; the male has usually planned to have sex and will do what he feels is necessary if denied.

Decelerations Periodic decreases in the baseline fetal heart rate.

Decidua Endometrium or mucous membrane lining of the uterus in pregnancy that is shed after childbirth.

Decidua basalis Part of the decidua that unites with the chorion to form the placenta. It is shed in lochial discharge after childbirth.

Decidua capsularis Part of the decidua surrounding the chorionic sac.

Decidua vera (parietalis) Nonplacental decidua lining the uterus.

Deep sleep State of sleep in which the newborn will be nearly still except for occasional startles, twitches, and sucking.

Diagonal conjugate Extends from the subpubic angle to the middle of the sacral promontory; may be obtained by manual measurement.

Diaphragm Flexible disk that covers the cervix to prevent pregnancy.

Diastasis recti abdominis Separation of the recti abdominis muscles along the median line. In women, it is seen with repeated childbirths or multiple gestations. In the newborn, it is usually caused by incomplete development.

Dietary reference intakes (DRIs) Set of reference values used to plan and assess nutrient intakes of healthy people, which include specific allowances for pregnant and lactating women. DRIs are subdivided into the recommended dietary allowance (RDA) and adequate intake (AI).

Dilatation of the cervix Expansion of the external os from an opening a few millimeters in size to an opening large enough to allow the passage of the neonate.

Dilation and curettage (D&C) Stretching of the cervical canal to permit passage of a curette, which is used to scrape the endometrium to empty the uterine contents or to obtain tissue for examination.

Diploid number of chromosomes Containing a set of maternal and a set of paternal chromosomes; in humans, the diploid number of chromosomes is 46.

Disability Impairment in one or more of five function categories: Cognition, communication, motor abilities, social abilities, or patterns of interactions.

Disenfranchised grief Grief that is not supported by the usual societal customs.

Donor insemination (DI) Procedure to produce a pregnancy in which sperm obtained from a donor is deposited in the woman's vagina.

Doula Supportive companion who assists a laboring woman and provides emotional, physical, and informational support and acts as an advocate for the woman and her family.

Down syndrome Abnormality resulting from the presence of an extra chromosome number 21 (trisomy 21); characteristics include intellectual disability and altered physical appearance.

Drowsy state State in the newborn sleep–wake cycle that occurs between light sleep and the quiet alert state. It is marked by babies opening and closing their eyes, but the eyes appear glazed and the face is often still. They may return to sleep or awaken further in response to stimuli.

Dual process model View of grief encompassing two competing facets: Loss and restoration. The loss orientation is concerned with the individual's need to confront the reality of the loss, and the restoration orientation seeks to regain balance and temper the pain of grief.

Ductus arteriosus Communication channel between the main pulmonary artery and the aorta of the fetus. It is obliterated after birth by rising PO_2 and changes in intravascular pressure in the presence of normal pulmonary functioning. It normally becomes a ligament after birth but sometimes remains patent (patent ductus arteriosus, a treatable condition).

Ductus venosus Fetal blood vessel that carries oxygenated blood between the umbilical vein and the inferior vena cava, bypassing the liver; it becomes a ligament after birth.

Duncan mechanism Occurs when the maternal surface of the placenta rather than the shiny fetal surface presents upon birth.

Duration Time length of each contraction, measured from the beginning of the increment to the completion of the decrement.

Dysfunctional uterine bleeding (DUB) Condition characterized by anovulatory cycles with abnormal uterine bleeding that does not have a demonstrable organic cause.

Dysmenorrhea Painful menstruation.

Dyspareunia Painful intercourse.

Dystocia Difficult labor due to mechanical factors produced by the fetus or the maternal pelvis or due to inadequate uterine or other muscular activity.

Early adolescence Term referring to adolescents who are age 14 and under.

Early decelerations Periodic change in fetal heart rate pattern caused by head compression; deceleration has a uniform appearance and early onset in relation to maternal contraction.

Early term Pregnancy extending from 37 0/7 through 38 6/7 weeks' gestation.

Eclampsia Major complication of pregnancy. Its cause is unknown; it occurs more often in the primigravida and is accompanied by elevated blood pressure, albuminuria, oliguria, tonic-clonic convulsions, and coma. It may occur during pregnancy (usually after the 20th week of gestation) or within 48 hours after childbirth.

Ectoderm Outer layer of cells in the developing embryo that gives rise to the skin, nails, and hair.

Ectopic pregnancy Implantation of the fertilized ovum outside the uterine cavity; common sites are the abdomen, fallopian tubes, and ovaries.

Effacement Thinning and shortening of the cervix that occurs late in pregnancy or during labor.

Elder abuse Any deliberate action or lack of action that causes harm to an elderly person.

Electronic fetal monitoring (EFM) Method of placing a fetal monitor on the fetus in order to obtain a continuous tracing of the fetal heart rate, which allows its many characteristics to be observed and evaluated.

Emancipated minors Minors who are legally considered to have assumed the rights of an adult. An adolescent may be considered emancipated if he or she is self-supporting and living away from home, married, pregnant, a parent, or in the military.

Embryo Early stage of development of the young of any organism. In humans the embryonic period is from about 2 to 8 weeks' gestation and is characterized by cellular differentiation and predominantly hyperplastic growth.

Embryonic membranes Amnion and chorion.

Emergency contraception (EC) Form of combined hormonal contraception that is used when a woman is worried about pregnancy because of unprotected intercourse, rape, or possible contraceptive failure (e.g., broken condom, slipped diaphragm, missed oral contraceptives, or too long a time between Depo-Provera injections).

Endoderm Inner layer of cells in the developing embryo that give rise to internal organs such as the intestines.

Endometrial biopsy (EMB) Procedure providing information about the effects of progesterone produced by the corpus luteum after ovulation and endometrial receptivity.

Endometriosis Ectopic endometrium located outside the uterus in the pelvic cavity. Symptoms may include pelvic pain or pressure, dysmenorrhea, dispareunia, abnormal bleeding from the uterus or rectum, and sterility.

Endometritis (metritis) Infection of the endometrium.

Endometrium Mucous membrane that lines the inner surface of the uterus.

En face Assumed position in which one person looks at another and maintains his or her face in the same vertical plane as that of the other.

Engagement Entrance of the fetal presenting part into the superior pelvic strait and the beginning of the descent through the pelvic canal.

Engorgement Vascular congestion or distention. In obstetrics, the swelling of breast tissue brought about by an increase in blood and lymph supply to the breast, preceding true lactation.

Engrossment Characteristic sense of absorption, preoccupation, and interest in the newborn demonstrated by fathers during early contact with their babies.

Environmental toxins Chemical compounds found in air, food, and water, whose bioaccumulation can lead to adverse health effects.

Epidural block Regional anesthesia effective through the first and second stages of labor; involves injection of a local anesthetic agent into the epidural space.

Episiotomy Incision of the perineum to facilitate birth and to avoid laceration of the perineum.

Epstein pearls Small, white blebs found along the gum margins and at the junction of the hard and soft palates; commonly seen in the newborn as a normal manifestation.

Erb-Duchenne paralysis (Erb palsy) Paralysis of the arm and chest wall as a result of a birth injury to the brachial plexus or a subsequent injury to the fifth and sixth cervical nerves.

Erythema toxicum Innocuous pink papular rash of unknown cause with superimposed vesicles; it appears within 24 to 48 hours after birth and resolves spontaneously within a few days.

Erythroblastosis fetalis Hemolytic disease of the newborn characterized by anemia, jaundice, enlargement of the liver and spleen, and generalized edema. Caused by isoimmunization due to Rh incompatibility or ABO incompatibility. Also called *alloimmune hemolytic disease*.

Estimated date of birth (EDB) During a pregnancy, the approximate date when childbirth will occur; the "due date."

Estrogens Hormones estradiol and estrone, produced by the ovary.

Ethnicity Social identity that is associated with shared beliefs, behaviors, and patterns.

Ethnocentrism Individual's belief that the values and practices of his or her own culture are the best ones.

Euphemism Substituted word or expression with a more pleasant association than the one that, although more direct, is considered to be harsher.

Evaporation Loss of heat incurred when water on the skin surface is converted to a vapor.

Evidence-based practice Approach to problem solving and decision making based on the consideration of data from research, statistical analysis, quality measures, risk management measurements, and other sources of reliable information.

Exchange transfusion Replacement of 70 to 80% of circulating blood by withdrawing the recipient's blood and injecting a donor's blood in equal amounts, for the purpose of preventing the accumulation of bilirubin or other by-products of hemolysis in the blood.

External cephalic version (ECV) Procedure involving external manipulation of the maternal abdomen to change the presentation of the fetus from breech to cephalic.

Extremely preterm births Births that occur prior to 28 gestational weeks.

Fallopian tubes Tubes that extend from the lateral angle of the uterus and terminate near the ovary; they serve as a passageway for the ovum from the ovary to the uterus and for the spermatozoa from the uterus toward the ovary. Also called *oviducts* and *uterine tubes*.

False labor Contractions of the uterus, regular or irregular, that may be strong enough to be interpreted as true labor but that do not dilate the cervix.

False pelvis Portion of the pelvis above the linea terminalis; its primary function is to support the weight of the enlarged pregnant uterus.

Family Two or more persons who are joined together by bonds of sharing and emotional closeness and who identify themselves as being part of a family.

Family assessment Process by which a nurse collects data regarding a family's current level of functioning, support systems, sociocultural influences, home and work environment, type of family, family structure, and needs.

Family-centered care Approach to health care based on the concept that a hospital can provide professional services to mothers, fathers, and babies in a homelike environment that would enhance the integrity of the family unit.

Family planning Actions an individual or a couple take to avoid a pregnancy, to space future pregnancies for a specific reason, or to gain control over the number of children conceived.

Female genital mutilation (FGM) Also known as *female genital cutting*, *female circumcision*, and *genital circumcision*, the practice of removing all or parts of a girl's or woman's genitalia for cultural reasons.

Female reproductive cycle (FRC) Monthly rhythmic changes in sexually mature women.

Feminization of later life Worldwide trend for women to comprise a majority of the older population.

Feminization of poverty Term used to describe the fact that, in the United States, women comprise a majority of the adult poor.

Ferning capacity Formation of a palm-leaf pattern by the crystallization of cervical mucus as it dries at mid-menstrual cycle. The formation can be helpful in determining time of ovulation. Observed via microscopic examination of a thin layer of cervical mucus on a glass slide. This pattern is also observed when amniotic fluid is allowed to air-dry on a slide and is a useful and quick test to determine whether amniotic membranes have ruptured.

Fertility awareness-based (FAB) methods Also known as *natural family planning*, methods founded on an understanding of the changes that occur throughout a woman's ovulatory cycle. All these methods require periods of abstinence and recording of certain events throughout the cycle; cooperation of the partner is important.

Fertilization Impregnation of an ovum by a spermatozoon; conception.

Fetal alcohol spectrum disorders (FASDs) Umbrella term that includes all categories of prenatal alcohol exposure, including fetal alcohol syndrome (FAS); it is not meant to be used as a clinical diagnosis.

Fetal alcohol syndrome (FAS) Syndrome caused by maternal alcohol ingestion and characterized in the child by microcephaly, intrauterine growth restriction, short palpebral fissures, and maxillary hypoplasia.

Fetal attitude Relationship of the fetal parts to one another; describes the posture the fetus assumes as it conforms to the shape of the uterine cavity. Normal fetal attitude is one of moderate flexion of the arms onto the chest and flexion of the legs onto the abdomen.

Fetal bradycardia Fetal heart rate less than 110 beats per minute during a 10-minute period of continuous monitoring.

Fetal demise Death of the developing fetus after 20 weeks' gestation. Also called *stillbirth*.

Fetal heart rate (FHR) Number of times the fetal heart beats per minute; normal range is 120 to 160.

Fetal lie Relationship of the cephalocaudal axis (spinal column) of the fetus to the cephalocaudal axis of the woman. The fetus may be in a longitudinal or transverse lie.

Fetal movement count (FMC) Method for tracking fetal activity taught to pregnant women. Also called *fetal movement record (FMR)*.

Fetal position Relationship of the landmark on the presenting fetal part to the front, sides, or back of the maternal pelvis.

Fetal presentation Fetal body part that enters the maternal pelvis first and leads through the birth canal during labor. The three possible presentations are cephalic, shoulder, and breech.

Fetal tachycardia Fetal heart rate greater than 160 beats per minute during a 10-minute period of continuous monitoring.

Fetus Child in utero from about the seventh to ninth week of gestation until birth.

Fibrocystic breast changes Benign breast changes characterized by bilateral, cyclic breast pain and breast nodularities that may be unilateral or bilateral and are often in the upper outer quadrants of the breasts. Also called *benign breast disorder (BBD)*.

Fimbria Any structure resembling a fringe; the fringelike extremity of the fallopian tubes.

First-trimester single screening tests Performed between 10 weeks and 0 days and 13 weeks and 6 days to determine if a fetus is at risk for a chromosomal disorder, these tests include nuchal translucency measurement, serum free β-hCG, or total human chorionic gonadotropin (hCG) along with pregnancy-associated plasma protein A analyte levels (PAPP-A).

Folic acid Important vitamin directly related to the outcome of pregnancy and to maternal and fetal health.

Follicle-stimulating hormone (FSH) Hormone produced by the anterior pituitary during the first half of the menstrual cycle, stimulating development of the graafian follicle.

Fontanelle In the fetus, an unossified space, or soft spot, consisting of a strong band of connective tissue lying between the cranial bones of the skull.

Foramen ovale Special opening between the atria of the fetal heart. Normally, the opening closes shortly after birth; if it remains open, it can be repaired surgically.

Forceps Obstetric instrument occasionally used to aid in childbirth.

Forceps-assisted birth Birth in which a set of instruments, known as *forceps*, is applied to the presenting part of the fetus to provide traction or to enable the fetal head to be rotated to an occiput-anterior position. Also known as *instrumental delivery*, *operative delivery*, or *operative vaginal delivery*.

Forceps marks Reddened areas over the cheeks and jaws caused by the application of forceps. The red areas usually disappear within 1 to 2 days.

Foremilk Breast milk obtained at the beginning of the breastfeeding episode.

Frequency Time between the beginning of one contraction and the beginning of the next contraction.

Full term Pregnancy extending from 39 0/7 through 40 6/7 weeks' gestation.

Functional residual capacity (FRC) Amount of air remaining in the lungs at the end of a normal expiration.

Fundus Upper portion of the uterus between the fallopian tubes.

Galactorrhea Nipple discharge not associated with lactation.

Gamete intrafallopian transfer (GIFT) Retrieval of oocytes by laparoscopy; immediately combining oocytes with washed, motile sperm in a catheter; and placement of the gametes into the fimbriated end of the fallopian tube.

Gametes Female or male germ cell; contains a haploid number of chromosomes.

Gametogenesis Process by which germ cells are produced.

General anesthesia State of induced unconsciousness that may be achieved through intravenous injection, inhalation of anesthetic agents, or a combination of both methods.

Genotype Total genetic composition of an individual.

Gestation Period of intrauterine development from conception through birth; pregnancy.

Gestational age Number of complete weeks of fetal development, calculated from the first day of the last normal menstrual cycle.

Gestational age assessment tools Systems used to evaluate the newborn's external physical characteristics and neurologic and/or neuromuscular development to accurately determine gestational age. These replace or supplement the traditional calculation from the woman's last menstrual period.

Gestational diabetes mellitus (GDM) Form of diabetes of variable severity with onset or first recognition during pregnancy.

Gestational trophoblastic disease (GTD) Collection of disorders characterized by pathologic proliferation of trophoblastic cells; classified into two types: Benign (hydatidiform mole) and malignant. Also called *molar pregnancy*.

Gonadotropin-releasing hormone (GnRH) Hormone secreted by the hypothalamus that stimulates the anterior pituitary to secrete FSH and LH.

Gonadotropins Hormones that stimulate the gonads (ovaries in women or testes in men).

Gonorrhea Sexually transmitted infection caused by the bacterium *Neisseria gonorrhoeae*.

Goodell sign Softening of the cervix that occurs during the second month of pregnancy.

Graafian follicle Ovarian cyst containing the ripe ovum; it secretes estrogen.

Grasping reflex Normal newborn reflex elicited by stimulating the palm with a finger or object, resulting in newborn firmly holding on to the finger or object.

Gravida Pregnant woman; any pregnancy, regardless of duration, including present pregnancy.

Grief Individual's reaction to loss, including physical symptoms, thoughts, feelings, functional limitations, and spiritual responses.

Gynecoid pelvis Typical female pelvis in which the inlet is round instead of oval.

Habituation Newborn's ability to diminish innate responses to specific repeated stimuli.

Haploid number of chromosomes Half the diploid number of chromosomes. In humans there are 23 chromosomes, the haploid number, in each germ cell.

Harlequin sign Rare color change that occurs between the longitudinal halves of the newborn's body, such that the dependent half is noticeably pinker than the superior half when the baby is placed on one side; it is of no pathologic significance.

Hegar sign Softening of the lower uterine segment found upon palpation in the second or third month of pregnancy.

HELLP syndrome Cluster of changes including ***h***emolysis, ***e***levated ***l***iver enzymes, and ***l***ow ***p***latelet count; sometimes associated with severe preeclampsia.

Hemolytic disease of the newborn Hyperbilirubinemia secondary to Rh incompatibility.

Herpes genitalis Lifelong, recurrent sexually transmitted infection caused by the herpes simplex virus (HSV).

Hindmilk Breast milk released after initial let-down reflex; high in fat content.

HIV (human immunodeficiency virus) Virus that causes a progressive disease that ultimately results in the development of acquired immunodeficiency syndrome (AIDS).

Hospital disposition Incineration at regular intervals of a dead fetus or neonate's body, usually with other body parts.

Human chorionic gonadotropin (hCG) Hormone produced by the chorionic villi and found in the urine of pregnant women. Also called *prolan*.

Human placental lactogen (hPL) Hormone synthesized by the syncytiotrophoblast that functions as an insulin antagonist and promotes lipolysis to increase the amounts of circulating free fatty acids available for maternal metabolic use.

Hydatidiform mole Condition in which a proliferation of trophoblastic cells results in the formation of an abnormal placenta characterized by hydropic (fluid-filled) grapelike clusters.

Hydramnios Excess (over 2000 mL) of amniotic fluid, leading to overdistention of the uterus. Frequently seen in diabetic pregnant women, even if there is no coexisting fetal anomaly. Also called *polyhydramnios*.

Hydrops fetalis Marked fetal edema caused by erythroblastosis fetalis, a severe hemolytic disease of the fetus and newborn (HDFN).

Hyperbilirubinemia Excessive amount of bilirubin in the blood; indicative of hemolytic processes due to blood incompatibility, intrauterine infection, septicemia, neonatal renal infection, and other disorders.

Hyperemesis gravidarum Excessive vomiting during pregnancy, leading to dehydration and altered nutritional status.

Hyperventilation Rapid breathing that occurs over a prolonged period of time, resulting in an imbalance of oxygen and carbon dioxide that can cause tingling or numbness in the tip of nose, lips, fingers, or toes; dizziness; spots before the eyes; or spasms of the hands or feet (carpal-pedal spasms).

Hypoglycemia Abnormally low level of sugar in the blood.

Hysterectomy Surgical removal of the uterus.

Hysterosalpingography (HSG) Testing by instillation of a radiopaque substance into the uterine cavity to visualize the uterus and fallopian tubes.

Hysteroscopy Use of a special endoscope to examine the uterus.

In vitro fertilization (IVF) Procedure during which oocytes are removed from the ovary, mixed with spermatozoa, fertilized, and incubated in a glass petri dish; then up to four viable embryos are placed in the woman's uterus.

Inborn errors of metabolism Group of hereditary disorders transmitted by mutant genes that cause enzyme defects.

Induction of labor Process of causing or initiating labor by use of medication or surgical rupture of membranes.

Infant Child between 29 days and 1 year of age.

Infant mortality rate Number of deaths of babies under 1 year of age per 1000 live births in a given population per year.

Infant of diabetic mother (IDM) At-risk baby born to a woman previously diagnosed as diabetic or who develops symptoms of diabetes during pregnancy.

Infant of substance-abusing mother (ISAM) A baby born to a mother who abuses or is addicted to drugs or alcohol.

Infertility Diminished ability to conceive.

Informed consent A legal concept that protects a person's rights to autonomy and self-determination by specifying that no action may be taken without that person's prior understanding and freely given consent.

Instrumental styles of coping Styles of coping by which persons generally use more cognitive skills to navigate loss, and to value care that includes an emphasis on problem solving.

Integrated test Includes the first trimester combined test, the nuchal translucency testing, PAPP-A, and second trimester maternal serum testing, also known as the quadruple screen (quad screen) which measures AFP, uE3, beta hCG, and inhibin A, to calculate the risk of having an affected fetus.

Integrative health approaches Practices that involve the use of complementary and conventional medical techniques together in a coordinated manner to relieve pain, address side effects of drug therapies and pain in cancer patients, and foster programs to promote healthy behaviors, among other practices.

Intellectual disability Most common type of developmental disability; formerly called *mental retardation*.

Intensity Strength of a uterine contraction during acme.

Intimate partner violence (IPV) Defined as the collective methods used to exert power and control by one individual over another in an adult intimate relationship. Forms of abuse typically fall into three categories: Psychologic abuse, physical abuse, and sexual abuse. Also called *domestic violence*.

Intrapartum Time from the onset of true labor until the birth of the baby and expulsion of the placenta.

Intrauterine contraception (IUC) Use of an intrauterine device (IUD) that is designed to be inserted into the uterus by a qualified healthcare provider and left in place for an extended period, providing continuous contraceptive protection for 3 to 10 years.

Intrauterine fetal surgery Surgery performed on a fetus to correct anatomic lesions that are not compatible with life if left untreated.

Intrauterine growth restriction (IUGR) Fetal inadequate growth due to any etiology, such as intrauterine infection, deficient nutrient supply, or congenital malformation; a term used to describe fetuses falling below the 10th percentile in ultrasonic estimation of weight at a given gestational age.

Intrauterine insemination (IUI) Procedure to produce a pregnancy in which sperm obtained from a woman's husband or partner (or a donor) is deposited in the woman's vagina.

Intrauterine pressure catheter (IUPC) Catheter that can be placed through the cervix into the uterus to measure uterine pressure during labor. Some types of catheters may be inserted for the purpose of infusing warmed saline to add additional intrauterine fluid when oligohydramnios is present.

Intuitive styles of coping Styles of coping by which persons generally feel their way through loss and prefer care with an emphasis on emotional and psychosocial support.

Involution Rapid reduction in size of the uterus and its return to a condition similar to its nonpregnant state.

Ischial spines Prominences that arise near the junction of the ilium and ischium and jut into the pelvic cavity; used as a reference point during labor to evaluate the descent of the fetal head into the birth canal.

Isthmus Straight, narrow part of the fallopian tube with a thick muscular wall and an opening (lumen) 2 to 3 mm in diameter; the site of tubal ligation. Also, a constriction in the uterus that is located above the cervix and below the corpus.

Jaundice Yellow pigmentation of body tissues caused by the presence of bile pigments.

Karyotype Pictorial analysis of an individual's chromosomes.

Kegel exercises Perineal muscle tightening that strengthens the pubococcygeus muscle and increases its tone.

Kernicterus Encephalopathy caused by deposition of unconjugated bilirubin in brain cells; may result in impaired brain function or death.

Kilocalorie (kcal) Equivalent to 1000 calories, it is the unit used to express the energy value of food.

Labor Process by which the fetus is expelled from the maternal uterus. Also called *childbirth*, *confinement*, or *parturition*.

Labor augmentation Stimulation of uterine contractions when spontaneous contractions have failed to result in progressive cervical dilation or descent of the fetus.

Labor induction Stimulation of uterine contractions before the spontaneous onset of labor, with or without ruptured fetal membranes, for the purpose of accomplishing birth.

Labor support Emotional, physical, and informational support of the woman during childbirth.

Lactase deficiency Condition characterized by difficulty digesting milk and dairy products. Results from an inadequate amount of the enzyme lactase, which breaks down the milk sugar lactose into smaller digestible substances.

Lactation Process of producing and supplying breast milk.

Lactogenesis II After the birth of a baby, the period of time during which there is an increased volume of breast milk in the new mother, often termed the *milk coming in*.

Lactose intolerance Condition in which an individual has difficulty digesting milk and milk products.

Lacto-ovovegetarians Vegetarians who include milk, dairy products, and eggs in their diet.

Lactovegetarians Vegetarians who include dairy products but no eggs in their diets.

La Leche League International (LLLI) Organization that provides information on and assistance with breastfeeding.

Lamaze method Method of childbirth preparation.

Lamellar body counts (LBCs) Concentrated phospholipids that are produced by type II alveoli cells and are representative of stored surfactant.

Lanugo Fine, downy hair found on all body parts of the fetus, with the exception of the palms of the hands and the soles of the feet, after 20 weeks' gestation.

Laparoscopy Procedure that enables direct visualization of pelvic organs.

Large-for-gestational-age (LGA) newborns Excessive growth of a fetus in relation to the gestational time period, resulting in newborns who plot above the 90th percentile curve on intrauterine growth curves.

Last menstrual period (LMP) Last normal menstrual period experienced by the woman before pregnancy; sometimes used to calculate the fetus's gestational age.

Late adolescence Term referring to adolescents who are ages 18 to 19 years.

Late decelerations Symmetrical decrease in fetal heart rate beginning at or after the peak of the contraction and returning to baseline only after the contraction has ended, indicating possible uteroplacental insufficiency and potential that the fetus is not receiving adequate oxygenation.

Late maternal mortality Maternal death that occurs more than 42 days but less than 1 year after termination of pregnancy.

Late preterm newborns Babies born between 34 and 36 6/7 weeks' gestation.

Late term Pregnancy extending from 41 0/7 through 41 6/7 weeks' gestation.

Lecithin/sphingomyelin (L/S) ratio Lecithin and sphingomyelin are phospholipid components of surfactant; their ratio changes during gestation. When the L/S ratio reaches 2:1, the fetal lungs are thought to be mature and the fetus will have a low risk of respiratory distress syndrome (RDS) if born at that time.

Leopold maneuvers Series of four maneuvers designed to provide a systematic approach whereby the examiner may determine fetal presentation and position.

Let-down reflex Pattern of stimulation, hormone release, and resulting muscle contraction that forces milk into the lactiferous ducts, making it available to the baby. Also called *milk ejection reflex*.

Leukorrhea Mucous discharge from the vagina or cervical canal that may be normal or pathologic, as in the presence of infection.

Light sleep State that makes up the highest proportion of newborn sleep and precedes awakening; characterized by some body movements, rapid eye movements (REM), and brief fussing or crying.

Lightening Moving of the fetus and uterus downward into the pelvic cavity.

Linea nigra Line of darker pigmentation extending from the umbilicus to the pubis noted in some women during the later months of pregnancy.

Local anesthesia Injection of an anesthetic agent into the subcutaneous tissue in a fanlike pattern.

Lochia Maternal discharge of blood, mucus, and tissue from the uterus; may last for several weeks after birth.

Lochia alba White vaginal discharge that follows lochia serosa and that lasts from about the 10th to the 21st day after birth.

Lochia rubra Red, blood-tinged vaginal discharge that occurs following birth and lasts 2 to 4 days.

Lochia serosa Pink, serous, and blood-tinged vaginal discharge that follows lochia rubra and lasts until the 7th to 10th day after birth.

Lung compliance Ease with which the lung is able to fill with air.

Luteinizing hormone (LH) Anterior pituitary hormone responsible for stimulating ovulation and for development of the corpus luteum.

Maceration Process of tissue breakdown that begins from the moment of death.

Macrosomia Condition seen in newborns of large body size and high birth weight (more than 4000 g [8 lb, 13 oz]), such as those born of mothers who have prediabetes or diabetes.

Malposition Abnormal position of the fetus in the birth canal.

Malpresentations Presentations of the fetus into the birth canal that are not "normal"—that is, shoulder or breech presentation.

Mammogram Soft-tissue radiograph of the breast without the injection of a contrast medium.

Mastitis Inflammation of the breast, with or without bacterial infection, that occurs primarily in lactating women.

Maternal mortality rate Number of maternal deaths from any cause during the pregnancy cycle per 100,000 live births.

Maternal role attainment (MRA) Process by which a woman learns mothering behaviors and becomes comfortable with her identity as a mother. Also called *becoming a mother*.

Maternal serum alpha-fetoprotein (MSAFP) Screening test performed between 16 and 22 gestational weeks that utilizes the multiple markers (the "triple screen") of alpha-fetoprotein (AFP), human chorionic growth hormone (hCG), and urine estriol (uE3) to screen pregnancies for neural tube defect, Down syndrome, and trisomy 18.

Mature milk Breast milk that contains 10% solids for energy and growth.

McDonald sign Probable sign of pregnancy characterized by an ease in flexing the body of the uterus against the cervix.

Meaning reconstruction Framework for understanding perinatal loss that focuses on redefining ourselves and how we interact with the world after a significant loss. The goal of recovery, as related to meaning reconstruction, is a positive change in self-identity by assigning the loss a meaning, thereby allowing the individual to assimilate the loss into her or his world.

Meconium Dark green or black material present in the large intestine of a full-term newborn; the first stools passed by the newborn.

Meconium aspiration syndrome (MAS) Respiratory disease of term, postterm, and small-for-gestational-age newborns caused by inhalation of meconium or meconium-stained amniotic fluid into the lungs; characterized by mild to severe respiratory distress, hyperexpansion of the chest, hyperinflated alveoli, and secondary atelectasis.

Meiosis Process of cell division that occurs in the maturation of sperm and ova that decreases their number of chromosomes by one half.

Menarche Beginning of menstrual and reproductive function in the female.

Mendelian (single-gene) inheritance Major category of inheritance whereby a trait is determined by a pair of genes on homologous chromosomes. Also called *single-gene inheritance*.

Menopausal hormone therapy (MHT) Administration of specific hormones to alleviate symptoms associated with the changes of menopause; formerly called *hormone replacement therapy*.

Menopause Permanent cessation of menses.

Menorrhagia Excessive or profuse menstrual flow.

Menstrual cycle Cyclic buildup of the uterine lining, ovulation, and sloughing of the lining occurring approximately every 28 days in nonpregnant females.

Menstruation Cyclic uterine bleeding in a woman in response to cyclic hormonal changes.

Mesoderm Intermediate layer of germ cells in the embryo that gives rise to connective tissue, bone marrow, muscles, blood, lymphoid tissue, and epithelial tissue.

Middle adolescence Term referring to adolescents who are ages 15 to 17 years.

Milia Tiny white papules appearing on the face of a newborn as a result of unopened sebaceous glands; disappear spontaneously within a few weeks.

Miscarriage Lay term for abortion that occurs naturally or spontaneously.

Mitosis Process of cell division whereby both daughter cells have the same number and pattern of chromosomes as the original cell.

Molding Shaping of the fetal head by overlapping of the cranial bones to facilitate movement through the birth canal during labor.

Monosomies Genetic conditions that occur when a normal gamete unites with a gamete that is missing a chromosome.

Morning sickness Term that refers to the nausea and vomiting that a woman may experience in early pregnancy. This lay term is sometimes used because these symptoms frequently occur in the early part of the day and disappear within a few hours.

Moro reflex Flexion of the newborn's thighs and knees accompanied by fingers that fan, then clench, as the arms are simultaneously thrown out and then brought together, as though embracing something. This reflex can be elicited by startling the newborn with a sudden noise or movement. Also called the *startle reflex*.

Morula Developmental stage of the fertilized ovum in which there is a solid mass of cells.

Mosaicism Condition of an individual who has at least two cell lines with differing karyotypes.

Mother–baby care Also called *couplet care*, a family-centered care approach in which the newborn remains at the mother's bedside and both are cared for by the same nurse.

Mottling Discoloration of the skin in irregular areas; may be seen with chilling, poor perfusion, or hypoxia.

Mourning Process by which individuals incorporate the loss experience into their lives, it is influenced by many factors including personality, gender, family dynamics, and social, religious, and cultural norms.

Mucous plug Collection of thick mucus that blocks the cervical canal during pregnancy.

Multigravida Woman who has been pregnant more than once.

Multipara Woman who has had two or more births at more than 20 weeks' gestation.

Multiple gestation More than one fetus in the uterus at the same time.

Myelination Begins in the second trimester of pregnancy and continues into adult life; involves myelin (a fatty covering that insulates the brain circuitry) deposition around axons, which enhances intracellular communication.

Myometrium Uterine muscular structure.

Nägele's rule Method of determining the estimated date of birth (EDB): After obtaining the first day of the last menstrual period, subtract 3 months and add 7 days.

Neonatal asphyxia Deprivation of oxygen to the fetus's brain and organs during the birth process; also called *perinatal asphyxia* or *birth asphyxia*.

Neonatal morbidity Number of potential cases per year of a disease, illness, or complication occurring in the neonatal period.

Neonatal mortality risk Chance of death within the newborn period.

Neonatal therapeutic hypothermia Therapy involving the cooling of a newborn's body; used in the care of the newborn with asphyxia to decrease injury to the brain during reperfusion, preventing cell death (or apoptosis) and improving long-term neurodevelopmental outcomes; also called *therapeutic cooling (TC)*.

Neonatal transition First few hours of life, in which the newborn stabilizes respiratory and circulatory functions.

Neonatology Specialty that focuses on the management of at-risk conditions of the newborn.

Neuronal organization Provides the basis for brain function and its complex circuitry by achieving stabilization of cell connections.

Neutral thermal environment (NTE) Environment that provides for minimal heat loss or expenditure.

Nevus flammeus Nonelevated, sharply demarcated, red to purple area of dense capillaries directly below the epidermis; a capillary angioma; also called *port-wine stain*.

Nevus vasculosus Raised, clearly delineated, dark-red, rough-surfaced birthmark commonly found in the head region; also called *strawberry mark*.

New Ballard score (NBS) Postnatal gestational age assessment tool, it is a refinement of a previous Ballard score tool with added criteria for more accurate assessment of the gestational age of newborns between 20 and 28 weeks' gestation and less than 1500 g.

Newborn Baby from birth through the first 28 days of life.

Newborn screening tests Tests that detect inborn errors of metabolism that, if left untreated, cause intellectual disability and physical handicaps.

Newborns' and Mothers' Health Protection Act (NMHPA) Legislation stating that women who have given birth vaginally cannot be forcibly discharged from the hospital within 48 hours of the time of birth for insurance reasons. Cesarean birth mothers are covered by their insurance for 96 hours following the time of birth.

Nidation Implantation of a fertilized ovum in the endometrium.

Nipple Protrusion about 0.5 to 1.3 cm in diameter in the center of each mature breast.

Non-Mendelian (multifactorial) inheritance Occurrence of congenital disorders that result from an interaction of multiple genetic and environmental factors.

Nonstress test (NST) Assessment method by which the reaction (or response) of the fetal heart rate (FHR) to fetal movement is evaluated; involves using an external electronic fetal monitor to obtain a tracing of the FHR and observation of acceleration of the FHR with fetal movement.

Nuchal cord Term used to describe the umbilical cord when it is wrapped around the neck of the fetus.

Nuchal fold Accumulation of fluid between the posterior cervical spine and the overlying skin in the fetal neck identified during an ultrasound examination.

Nulligravida Woman who has never been pregnant.

Nullipara Woman who has not given birth at more than 20 weeks' gestation.

Nurse practitioner Professional nurse who has received specialized education in either a master's degree program or a continuing education program and thus can function in an expanded role.

Nurse researcher Professional nurse who has an advanced doctoral degree, typically a Doctor of Philosophy (PhD), and assumes a leadership role in generating new research.

Nursing advocacy Approach to patient care in which the nurse educates and supports the patient and protects his or her rights.

Obstetric conjugate Extends from the middle of the sacral promontory to the upper inner point on the symphysis.

Oligohydramnios Decreased amount of amniotic fluid, which may indicate a fetal urinary tract defect.

Oocyte Early primitive ovum before it has completely developed.

Oogenesis Process during fetal life whereby the ovary produces oogonia, cells that become primitive ovarian eggs.

Ophthalmia neonatorum Purulent infection of the eyes or conjunctiva of the newborn, usually caused by gonococci.

Orientation Newborn's ability to respond to auditory and visual stimuli in the environment.

Ortolani maneuver Manual procedure performed to rule out the possibility of developmental dysplastic hip.

Osteoporosis Condition most common in postmenopausal women that is characterized by decreased bone strength related to diminished bone density and bone quality. It is thought to be associated with lowered estrogen and androgen levels. Osteoporosis puts an individual at increased risk for fractures of the hip, forearm, and vertebrae.

Ovaries Female sex glands in which the ova are formed and in which estrogen and progesterone are produced. Normally there are two ovaries, located in the lower abdomen on each side of the uterus.

Ovulation Normal process of discharging a mature ovum from an ovary approximately 14 days before the onset of menses.

Oxytocin Hormone normally produced by the posterior pituitary, responsible for stimulation of uterine contractions and the release of milk into the lactiferous ducts.

Palmar grasping reflex Reflex that is elicited by stimulating the newborn's palm with a finger or object; the newborn grasps and holds the object or finger firmly enough to be lifted momentarily from the crib.

Palpation Technique of assessing a uterine contraction by touch.

Pap smear Procedure to detect the presence of cancer of the uterus by microscopic examination of cells gently scraped from the cervix.

Para Woman who has given birth after 20 weeks' gestation, regardless of whether the baby is born alive or dead.

Parametritis Inflammation of the parametrial layer of the uterus.

Parent–newborn attachment Close affectional ties that develop between parent and child.

Passive acquired immunity Transfer of antibodies (IgG) from the mother to the fetus in utero.

Patient-controlled analgesia (PCA) Method of pain control where anesthesia, usually morphine or meperidine, is initially administered by the anesthesiologist, and subsequent doses are self-administered by pushing a button controlled by a special IV pump system.

Pedigree Graphic representation of a family tree.

Pelvic cavity Bony portion of the birth passages; a curved canal with a longer posterior than anterior wall.

Pelvic cellulitis (parametritis) Infection involving the connective tissue of the broad ligament or, in severe cases, the connective tissue of all the pelvic structures.

Pelvic floor Muscles and tissue that act as a buttress to the pelvic outlet.

Pelvic inflammatory disease (PID) Infection of the fallopian tubes that may or may not be accompanied by a pelvic abscess; may cause infertility secondary to tubal damage.

Pelvic inlet Upper border of the true pelvis.

Pelvic outlet Lower border of the true pelvis.

Pelvic tilt Exercise designed to reduce back strain and strengthen abdominal muscle tone. Also called *pelvic rocking*.

Penis Male organ of copulation and reproduction.

Perimenopause Term referring to the period of time before menopause during which the woman moves from normal ovulatory cycles to cessation of menses.

Perimetrium Outermost layer of the corpus of the uterus. Also known as the *serosal layer*.

Perinatal hospice Compassionate, structured program that provides a context in which parents can find meaning in the intimate experience of the life and death of their child.

Perinatal loss Death of a fetus or neonate from the time of conception through the end of the neonatal period 28 days after birth.

Perineal prep Aseptic cleansing of the woman's vulvar and perineal area before she gives birth.

Perineum Area of tissue between the anus and scrotum in a man or between the anus and vagina in a woman.

Periodic breathing Sporadic episodes of apnea, not associated with cyanosis, that last for about 10 seconds and commonly occur in preterm newborns.

Periods of reactivity Predictable patterns of newborn behavior during the first several hours after birth.

Peripartum major mood episodes Clinical postpartum depression, categorized by the fifth edition of the *Diagnostic and Statistical Manual of Mental Disorders (DSM-5)* as Major Depressive Disorder with Peripartum Onset.

Peritonitis Infection involving the peritoneal cavity.

Periviable birth Birth that occurs between 20 0/7 and 25 6/7 weeks of gestation.

Persistent occiput posterior (OP) position Malposition of the fetus in which the fetal occiput is posterior in the maternal pelvis.

Persistent pulmonary hypertension of the newborn (PPHN) Respiratory disease resulting from right-to-left shunting of blood away from the lungs and through the ductus arteriosus and patent foramen ovale.

Phenotype Observable physical or biochemical characteristics of an individual, as determined by both genetic makeup and environmental influences

Phenylketonuria (PKU) Common metabolic disease caused by an inborn error in the metabolism of the amino acid phenylalanine.

Phosphatidylglycerol (PG) Phospholipid present in fetal surfactant after about 35 weeks' gestation.

Phototherapy Treatment of jaundice by exposure to light.

Physiologic anemia of infancy Harmless condition in which the hemoglobin level drops in the first 6 to 12 weeks after birth and then reverts to normal levels.

Physiologic anemia of pregnancy Apparent anemia that results during pregnancy when the plasma volume increases more than the erythrocytes increase. Also called *pseudoanemia*.

Physiologic anemia of the newborn Condition in which the hemoglobin level drops in the first 6 to 12 weeks after birth and then reverts to normal levels.

Physiologic jaundice Harmless condition caused by the normal reduction of red blood cells, occurring 48 or more hours after birth, peaking at the 5th to 7th days, and disappearing between the 7th and 10th days.

Pica Eating of substances not ordinarily considered edible or to have nutritive value.

Placenta Specialized disk-shaped organ that connects the fetus to the uterine wall for gas and nutrient exchange. Also called *afterbirth*.

Placenta accreta Partial or complete absence of the decidua basalis and abnormal adherence of the placenta to the uterine wall.

Placenta increta High-risk condition that occurs when the placenta attaches to the uterine wall and invades or attaches itself within the myometrium.

Placenta percreta High-risk condition that occurs when the placenta penetrates the myometrium, sometimes attaching to peritoneal structures within the abdominal cavity, where the removal of the uterus (hysterectomy) is sometimes necessary.

Placenta previa Abnormal implantation of the placenta in the lower uterine segment.

Podalic version Procedure used for the vaginal birth of a second twin. The obstetrician inserts a hand into the uterus, grasps the feet of the fetus, and changes the fetus from a transverse to a breech presentation. Also *internal version*.

Polycystic ovarian syndrome (PCOS) Most common endocrine disorder affecting women of reproductive age, marked by menstrual dysfunction, androgen excess, obesity, hyperinsulinemia, and infertility.

Polycythemia Abnormal increase in the number of total red blood cells in the body's circulation.

Polypharmacy Act of taking multiple drugs to treat symptoms, when the etiology of the symptoms is actually a side effect from one or more prescribed medications.

Polyploidies Heritable conditions that occur when there are extra sets of chromosomes; generally not considered compatible with live birth.

Positive signs of pregnancy Indications that confirm the presence of pregnancy.

Postconception age periods Period of time in embryonic/fetal development calculated from the time of fertilization of the ovum (about 266 days [38 weeks] or 9½ calendar months).

Postmaturity Term that applies only to the newborn who is born after 42 completed weeks of gestation and also demonstrates characteristics of *postmaturity syndrome.*

Postpartum After childbirth; time from birth until the woman's body returns to an essentially prepregnant condition, typically about 6 weeks.

Postpartum blues Transient period of depression that occurs during the first few days of the puerperium. Also called *adjustment reaction with depressed mood*.

Postpartum depression Severe depression that occurs within the first year after giving birth with increased incidence at about the fourth week postpartum, just before resumption of menses, and upon weaning.

Postpartum endometritis (metritis) Reproductive tract infection limited to the uterus and associated with childbirth that occurs at any time up to 6 weeks postpartum.

Postpartum hemorrhage (PPH) ACOG 2017 definition: Blood loss greater than or equal to 1,000 mL or blood loss accompanied by signs or symptoms of hypovolemia within 24 hours after the birth process (includes intrapartum blood loss) regardless of route of delivery. Traditional definition: A loss of blood of greater than 500 mL following a vaginal delivery and 1000 mL following a cesarean delivery. The hemorrhage is classified as early (primary) if it occurs within the first 24 hours and late (secondary) if it occurs after the first 24 hours.

Postpartum home care Home visits for postpartum families occurring in the home setting. This provides opportunities for expanding information and reinforcing self- and newborn care techniques initially presented in the birth setting.

Postpartum mood episodes with psychotic features Most serious of postpartum psychiatric disorders with delusions and/or visual, auditory, or tactile hallucinations. Also called *postpartum psychosis*.

Postpartum psychosis Most serious of postpartum psychiatric disorders with delusions and/or visual, auditory, or tactile hallucinations.

Postterm labor Labor that occurs after 42 weeks' gestation.

Postterm newborn Any baby born after 42 weeks' gestation.

Postterm pregnancy Pregnancy extending 42 0/7 weeks or longer.

Posttraumatic stress disorder (PTSD) Intense psychologic distress resulting from a traumatic event and evidenced by recurrent, intrusive thoughts; flashbacks; persistent avoidance of stimuli associated with the trauma; a generalized feeling of "numbness"; and persistent signs of arousal.

Precipitous birth (1) Unduly rapid progression (3 hours or less) of labor and birth; (2) A birth in which no physician is in attendance.

Precipitous labor Labor lasting 3 hours or less.

Preeclampsia Toxemia of pregnancy, characterized by hypertension, albuminuria, and edema. See also *Eclampsia*.

Pregnancy of unknown location (PUL) Situation in which a woman has had a positive pregnancy test but before there is sonographic evidence of an intrauterine or extrauterine (ectopic) pregnancy.

Pregnancy-related death Death of a woman while pregnant or within 1 year of the termination of pregnancy (regardless of the length of the pregnancy or the site of implantation) from any cause aggravated by pregnancy or related to it.

Preimplantation genetic diagnosis (PGD) Term used when a pregnancy is at risk for a detectable single-gene disorder or chromosome abnormality and testing is performed to determine whether that mutation or unbalanced chromosomal complement has been passed to the embryo.

Premature rupture of membranes (PROM) Premature breaking-open of the amniotic membranes, releasing amniotic fluid.

Premenstrual dysphoric disorder (PMDD) Disorder associated with the luteal phase of the menstrual cycle (2 weeks before onset of menses) in which a woman experiences five or more affective (emotional) or somatic (physical) symptoms, which are relieved with menstruation and have occurred during most cycles during the previous year.

Premenstrual syndrome (PMS) Cluster of symptoms experienced by some women, typically occurring from a few days up to 2 weeks before the onset of menses.

Prenatal diagnosis Diagnosis based on detecting anatomic and physiologic problems in the fetus before birth.

Prenatal education Programs offered to expectant families, adolescents, women, or partners to provide education regarding the pregnancy, labor, and birth experience.

Presentation Fetal body part that enters the maternal pelvis first. The three possible presentations are cephalic, shoulder, and breech.

Presenting part Fetal part present in or on the cervical os; the portion of the fetus that is felt through the cervix on vaginal examination.

Presumptive signs of pregnancy Symptoms that suggest but do not confirm pregnancy, such as cessation of menses, quickening, Chadwick sign, and morning sickness.

Preterm labor Labor occurring after 20 and before 37 completed weeks of pregnancy. Also called *premature labor*.

Preterm newborn Any baby born before 37 weeks' gestation.

Preterm PROM (PPROM) Preterm premature rupture of membranes (before 37 weeks of gestation).

Primigravida Woman who is pregnant for the first time.

Primipara Woman who has had one birth at more than 20 weeks' gestation, regardless of whether the baby is born alive or dead.

Probable signs of pregnancy Manifestations that strongly suggest the likelihood of pregnancy, such as a positive pregnancy test, enlarging abdomen, and positive Goodell, Hegar, and Braxton Hicks signs.

Professional nurse Person who has graduated from an accredited basic program in nursing, has successfully completed the nursing licensure examination (NCLEX), and is currently licensed as a registered nurse (RN).

Progesterone Hormone produced by the corpus luteum, adrenal cortex, and placenta whose function is to stimulate proliferation of the endometrium to facilitate growth of the embryo.

Prolactin Hormone secreted by the anterior pituitary that stimulates and sustains lactation in mammals.

Prolapsed umbilical cord Umbilical cord that becomes trapped in the vagina before the fetus is born.

Prolonged decelerations Decelerations in which the fetal heart rate decreases from the baseline for 2 to 10 minutes.

Prolonged labor Labor lasting more than 24 hours.

Prolonged rupture of the membranes Rupture of the membranes more than 24 hours before birth.

Prostaglandins (PGs) Complex lipid compounds synthesized by many cells in the body.

Pseudomenstruation Blood-tinged mucus from the vagina in the female newborn; caused by withdrawal of maternal hormones that were present during pregnancy.

Psychologic disorders Abnormal mental or emotional conditions characterized by alterations in thinking, mood, or behavior.

Ptyalism Excessive salivation.

Puberty Developmental period between childhood and the attainment of adult sexual characteristics and functioning.

Pudendal block Injection of an anesthetizing agent at the pudendal nerve to produce numbness of the external genitals and the lower one-third of the vagina to facilitate childbirth and permit episiotomy, if necessary.

Puerperal infection Infection of the reproductive tract associated with childbirth and occurring any time up to 6 weeks postpartum.

Puerperal morbidity Maternal temperature of 38°C (100.4°F) or higher on any 2 of the first 10 postpartal days, excluding the first 24 hours. The temperature is to be taken by mouth at least four times per day.

Puerperium Period after completion of the third stage of labor until involution of the uterus is complete, usually 6 weeks.

Quadruple screen (Quad screen) Second-trimester maternal serum testing that measures AFP, uE3, beta hCG, and inhibin A.

Quickening First fetal movements felt by the pregnant woman, usually between 16 and 20 weeks' gestation.

Quiet alert state Alert state characterized by a brightening of the eyes and face. Newborns are most attentive to their environment in this state and provide positive feedback to caregivers. Also called *wide awake state*.

Race Concept that categorizes groups of people who share biologic similarities such as skin color, bone structure, and genetic traits.

Radiation Heat loss incurred when heat transfers to cooler surfaces and objects not in direct contact with the body.

Rape Sexual activity, often intercourse, against the will of the victim.

Rape trauma syndrome Term that refers to a variety of symptoms, clustered in phases, that a rape survivor experiences following an assault.

Reciprocity Interactional cycle that occurs simultaneously between mother and newborn. It involves mutual cueing behaviors, expectancy, rhythmicity, and synchrony.

Recommended dietary allowance (RDA) Daily dietary intake that is considered sufficient to meet the nutritional requirements of nearly all individuals in a specific life stage and gender group.

Recurrent pregnancy loss (RPL) Three or more consecutive pregnancy losses before 24 weeks' gestation.

Regional analgesia Temporary and reversible loss of sensation produced by injecting an anesthetic agent (called a *local anesthetic*) into an area that will bring the agent into direct contact with nervous tissue.

Regional anesthesia Injection of local anesthetic agents so that they come into direct contact with nervous tissue.

Relaxin Water-soluble protein secreted by the corpus luteum that causes relaxation of the symphysis and cervical dilatation.

Religion Institutionalized system that shares a common set of beliefs and practices.

Relinquishing mother Mother who chooses to give her baby up for adoption.

Respiratory distress syndrome (RDS) Respiratory disease of the newborn characterized by interference with ventilation at the alveolar level, thought to be caused by the presence of fibrinoid deposits lining the alveolar ducts; formerly called *hyaline membrane disease*.

Responding model Set of guidelines for successful interactions with grieving families.

Retained placenta Retention of the placenta beyond 30 minutes after birth.

Retinopathy of prematurity (ROP) Formation of fibrotic tissue behind the lens; associated with retinal detachment and arrested eye growth, seen with hypoxemia in preterm newborns.

Rh factor Antigens present on the surface of blood cells that make the blood cell incompatible with blood cells that do not have the antigen.

Rh immune globulin (RhIg) Anti-Rh *(D)* gamma globulin given after birth to an Rh-negative mother of an Rh-positive fetus or child. Prevents the development of permanent active immunity to the Rh antigen.

Risk factors Any findings that suggest the pregnancy may have a negative outcome, for either the woman or her unborn child.

Roles Patterns of behavior normatively defined and expected of an occupant of a given social position.

Room-sharing Arrangement in which the baby sleeps in the same room in close proximity to the parents, but in his or her own bed.

Rooting reflex Newborn's tendency to turn the head and open the lips to suck when one side of the mouth or cheek is touched.

Round ligaments Ligaments that arise from the side of the uterus near the fallopian tube insertion to help the broad ligament keep the uterus in place.

Rugae Transverse ridges of mucous membranes lining the vagina that allow the vagina to stretch during the descent of the fetal head.

Rupture of membranes (ROM) Breaking-open of the amniotic membranes, releasing amniotic fluid. Rupture may be PROM (premature), SROM (spontaneous), or AROM (artificial).

Sacral promontory Projection into the pelvic cavity on the anterior upper portion of the sacrum; serves as an obstetric guide in determining pelvic measurements.

Salpingitis Infection of the fallopian tubes.

Scarf sign Position of the elbow when the hand of a supine newborn is drawn across to the other shoulder until it meets resistance.

Schultze mechanism Expulsion of the placenta with the shiny, or fetal, surface presenting first.

Secondary infertility Condition in which couples are unable to conceive after one or more successful pregnancies.

Self-quieting ability Baby's ability to use personal resources to quiet and console him- or herself.

Semen Thick whitish fluid ejaculated by the male during orgasm and containing the spermatozoa and their nutrients.

Sepsis neonatorum Infection experienced by a newborn during the first month of life.

Sequential screening Screening approach in which women identified at highest risk after first-trimester screening are offered diagnostic testing or cell-free DNA testing.

Severe maternal morbidity (SMM) State of being unhealthful due to physical and psychologic conditions that result from or are aggravated by pregnancy and have an adverse effect on a woman's health.

Sex chromosomes X and Y chromosomes, which are responsible for sex determination.

Sexual assault Broad term that refers to a variety of types of unwanted sexual touching or penetration without consent, from unwanted sexual contact or touching of an intimate part of another person to forced anal, oral, or genital penetration.

Sexually transmitted infection (STI) Refers to infection ordinarily transmitted by direct sexual contact with an infected individual. Also called *sexually transmitted disease*.

Skin-to-skin contact (SSC) Physical contact between the mother and baby whereby the naked baby is placed prone on the mother's chest during the first 24 hours.

Skin turgor Elasticity of skin; provides information on hydration status.

Small-for-gestational-age (SGA) newborns Neonates who plot below the 10th percentile growth curve; inadequate weight or growth for gestational age.

Spermatogenesis Process by which mature spermatozoa are formed, during which the number of chromosomes is halved.

Spermatozoa Mature sperm cells of the male animal, produced by the testes.

Spermicide Available as a cream, foam, jelly, or suppository that, when inserted into the vagina before intercourse, destroys sperm or neutralizes any vaginal secretions and thereby immobilizes sperm.

Spinal block Injection of a local anesthetic agent directly into the spinal fluid in the spinal canal to provide anesthesia for vaginal and cesarean births.

Spirituality Belief in a transcendent power pertaining to the spirit or soul.

Spontaneous rupture of membranes (SROM) Breaking of the "water" or membranes marked by the expulsion of amniotic fluid from the vagina.

Station Relationship of the presenting fetal part to an imaginary line drawn between the pelvic ischial spines during labor.

Stepping reflex Reflex that is elicited when a newborn is held upright with one foot touching a flat surface and the newborn puts one foot in front of the other and "walks."

Stepwise screening Screening approach in which women identified at highest risk after first-trimester screening are offered diagnostic testing or cfDNA testing.

Sterility Term applied when there is an absolute factor preventing reproduction.

Sterilization Inclusive term that refers to surgical procedures that permanently prevent pregnancy. In the male, sterilization is achieved through a procedure called a *vasectomy*. In the female, sterilization is done by *tubal ligation*.

Stillbirth Baby born dead after 20 weeks' gestation.

Striae Stretch marks; shiny purplish lines that appear on the abdomen, breasts, thighs, and buttocks of pregnant women as a result of stretching the skin.

Subconjunctival hemorrhages Hemorrhages on the sclera of a newborn's eye, usually caused by changes in vascular tension during birth.

Subfertility Couple that has difficulty conceiving because both partners have reduced fertility.

Subinvolution Failure of a part to return to its normal size after functional enlargement, such as failure of the uterus to return to normal size after pregnancy.

Sucking reflex Normal newborn reflex elicited by inserting a finger or nipple in the newborn's mouth, resulting in forceful, rhythmic sucking.

Sudden infant death syndrome (SIDS) Sudden death of an infant not explained by autopsy, site investigation, and clinical history; the primary cause of infant death beyond the neonatal period in the United States.

Sudden unexpected infant death (SUID) Sudden death of an infant that includes SIDS as well as deaths that are explained by a thorough investigation.

Supine hypotensive syndrome Condition that can develop during pregnancy when the enlarging uterus puts pressure on the vena cava when the woman is supine. This pressure interferes with returning blood flow and produces a marked decrease in blood pressure with accompanying dizziness, pallor, and clamminess, which can be corrected by having the woman lie on her left side. Also called *vena cava syndrome* and *aortocaval compression*.

Surfactant Substance composed of phospholipid, which stabilizes and lowers the surface tension of the alveoli during extrauterine respiratory exhalation, allowing a certain amount of air to remain in the alveoli during expiration.

Sutures Membranous joints that unite the cranial bones in the fetal skull.

Symphysis pubis Fibrocartilaginous joint between the pelvic bones in the midline.

Syndactyly Malformation of the fingers or toes in which there may be webbing or complete fusion of two or more digits.

Syphilis Chronic, sexually transmitted infection caused by the spirochete *Treponema pallidum*.

Systemic analgesia Pain medication given intravenously that does not result in complete loss of sensation or a reduction of motor functioning.

Taboo Behavior or object that is avoided by individuals or groups.

Telangiectatic nevi Small clusters of pink-red spots appearing on the nape of the neck and around the eyes of newborns; localized areas of capillary dilatation; also called *stork bites*.

Teratogens Substances that adversely affect the normal growth and development of the fetus.

Term Normal duration of pregnancy; ACOG recommends that the label *term* be replaced by *early term*, *full term*, *late term*, and *postterm*.

Testes Male gonads, in which sperm and testosterone are produced.

Testosterone Male hormone; responsible for the development of secondary male characteristics.

Therapeutic abortion Medically induced termination of pregnancy when a malformed fetus is suspected or when the woman's health is in jeopardy.

Thermogenesis Newborn's physiologic mechanisms that increase heat production.

Thrombophlebitis Inflammation of a vein wall, resulting in thrombus.

Thrush Fungal infection of the oral mucous membranes caused by *Candida albicans*. Most often seen in newborns and infants; characterized by white plaques in the mouth.

Tocolysis Use of medications to arrest preterm labor.

Tonic neck reflex Postural reflex seen in the newborn. When the supine baby's head is turned to one side, the arm and leg on that side extend while the extremities on the opposite side flex. Also called the *fencing position*.

TORCH Acronym used to describe a group of infections that represent potentially severe problems during pregnancy. *TO*, toxoplasmosis; *R*, rubella; *C*, cytomegalovirus; *H*, herpesvirus.

Total bilirubin Sum of conjugated (direct) and unconjugated (indirect) bilirubin.

Transition First 6 hours of life, in which the newborn stabilizes respiratory and circulatory functions.

Transitional milk Breast milk produced from the end of colostrum production until about 2 weeks postpartum.

Transvaginal ultrasound Follicular monitoring test that is used in women undergoing induction cycles, for timing ovulation for insemination and intercourse, for retrieving oocytes for in vitro fertilization, and for monitoring early pregnancy.

Transverse diameter Largest diameter of the pelvic inlet; helps determine the shape of the inlet.

Transverse lie Lie in which the fetus is positioned crosswise in the uterus.

Transversus abdominis plane (TAP) block Guided by ultrasound, local anesthetic is injected bilaterally into the space between the transverse abdominus and the internal oblique muscles, filling the connective tissue and providing pain relief to the abdominal area; used for postoperative pain management after cesarean birth.

Trial of labor after cesarean (TOLAC) Planned attempt to labor by a woman who has previously undergone a cesarean delivery and desires a subsequent vaginal delivery.

Trichomoniasis Sexually transmitted infection caused by *Trichomonas vaginalis*, a microscopic motile protozoan that thrives in an alkaline environment.

Trimester Three months, or one-third of the gestational time for pregnancy.

Trisomies Abnormalities that occur as the result of the union of a normal gamete (egg or sperm) with a gamete that contains an extra chromosome; the presence of three homologous chromosomes rather than the normal two.

Trophoblast Outer layer of the blastoderm that will eventually establish the nutrient relationship with the uterine endometrium.

True conjugate One of three anteroposterior diameters of the pelvic inlet; extends from the middle of the sacral promontory to the middle of the pubic crest; also called *conjugate vera*.

True pelvis Portion of the pelvis that lies below the linea terminalis (pelvic brim), made up of the inlet, cavity, and outlet.

Tubal embryo transfer (TET) Procedure in which eggs are retrieved and incubated with the man's sperm and then transferred back into the woman's body at the embryo stage.

Tubal ligation Sterilization of a woman accomplished by transecting or occluding the fallopian tubes.

Ultrasound (US) High-frequency sound waves that may be directed, through the use of a transducer, into the maternal abdomen. The ultrasonic sound waves reflected by the underlying structures of varying densities allow identification of various maternal and fetal tissues, bones, and fluids.

Umbilical cord Structure connecting the placenta to the umbilicus of the fetus and through which nutrients from the woman are exchanged for wastes from the fetus.

Urinary tract infection (UTI) Significant bacteriuria in the presence of symptoms.

Uterine atony Relaxation of uterine muscle tone following birth.

Uterine inversion Prolapse of the uterine fundus through the cervix into the vagina; may occur just before or during expulsion of the placenta; associated with massive hemorrhage, requiring emergency treatment.

Uterine rupture Nonsurgical disruption of the uterine cavity.

Uterus Hollow muscular organ in which the fertilized ovum is implanted and in which the developing fetus is nourished until birth.

Vacuum extraction Obstetric procedure used to assist in the birth of a fetus by applying suction to the fetal head with a soft suction cup attached to a suction bottle (pump) by tubing and placing the device against the occiput of the fetal head.

Vagina Musculomembranous tube or passageway located between the external genitals and the uterus of a woman.

Vaginal birth after cesarean (VBAC) Practice of permitting a trial of labor and possible vaginal birth for women following a previous cesarean birth for nonrecurring causes such as fetal distress or placenta previa.

Variability Baseline fluctuations of two cycles per minute or greater in the fetal heart rate and classified by the visually quantified amplitude of peak-to-trough in beats per minute.

Variable decelerations Periodic changes in fetal heart rate caused by umbilical cord compression; decelerations vary in onset, occurrence, and waveform.

Vasa previa Condition occurring when the fetal vessels cross through membranes and are present at the cervical os. Although this is a rare cause of antepartum bleeding, it has a high rate of fetal death.

Vasectomy Surgical removal of a portion of the vas deferens (ductus deferens) to produce infertility.

Vegan "Pure" vegetarian; one who consumes no food from animal sources.

Vena cava syndrome Symptoms of dizziness, pallor, and clamminess that result from lowered blood pressure when a pregnant woman lies supine and the enlarged uterus presses on the vena cava. Also known as *supine hypotensive syndrome* and *aortocaval compression*.

Venous thromboembolism Term that includes deep vein thrombosis and pulmonary embolism and refers to formation of a blood clot (thrombus formation) at an area of impeded blood flow in a superficial or deep vein.

Vernix caseosa Protective, cheeselike, whitish substance made up of sebum and desquamated epithelial cells that is present on the fetal skin.

Version Turning of the fetus in utero.

Vertex Top or crown of the head.

Viability Potential for a pregnancy to result in a live birth.

Vulva External structure of the female genitals, lying below the mons veneris.

Vulvovaginal candidiasis (VVC) Genital infection most often caused by *Candida albicans*. Also called *moniliasis* or *yeast infection*.

Weaning Process of discontinuing breastfeeding and accustoming a baby to another feeding method.

Wharton jelly Yellow-white gelatinous material surrounding the vessels of the umbilical cord.

Zygote Fertilized egg.

Zygote intrafallopian transfer (ZIFT) Retrieval of oocytes under ultrasound guidance, followed by in vitro fertilization and laparoscopic replacement of fertilized eggs into the fimbriated end of the fallopian tube.

Index

Page numbers followed by f *indicate figures, and those followed by* t *indicate tables. The titles of special features (e.g., Evidence-Based Practice, Developing Cultural Competence, Safety Alert!, Clinical Tip, Ethics in Action!) are capitalized.*

A

B

C

I

O

P

T

U

Special Features

DRUG GUIDE

EVIDENCE-BASED PRACTICE

GENETIC FACTS

HEALTH PROMOTION

KEY FACTS TO REMEMBER